Significant websites

General websites

http://www.who.ch/
World Health Organization

http://www.ncbi.nlm.nih.gov/PubMed
PubMed – Medline on the Web

http://www.nih.gov/health
UK National Institute of Health website
(biomedical research, free)

http://chid.nih.gov
US combined Health Information Database of the
NIH: clearing house database, healthcare
information and a good search engine.

http://www.mayoclinic.com/index.cfm
US Mayo Clinic

http://www.nice.org.uk
UK National Institute for Clinical Excellence

http://www.nhsdirect.nhs.uk
UK NHS Direct online

http://www.doh.gov.uk/chi/index/htm
UK Commission for Health Improvement

Healthcare journal and magazines

http://www.jr2.ox.ac.uk/bandolier/
Bandolier (free abstracts and good links)

http://www.bmj.com/index.shtml
British Medical Journal

http://www.open.gov.uk/doh/cmo/cmoh.htm
CMO's letters

http://www.doh.gov.uk/cmo/publications.htm
CMO's publications

http://www.thelancet.com/index1.html
The Lancet

http://www.nejm.org/content/index.asp
New England Journal of Medicine

Medical societies and organizations

http://www.gmc-uk.org/
UK General Medical Council

http://www.mrc.ac.uk
UK Medical Research Council

http://www.rcplondon.ac.uk
Royal College of Physicians – England, Wales
and Northern Ireland

http://www.rcpe.ac.uk
Royal College of Physicians of Edinburgh

1 Ethics and communication

http://www.wma.net/e/policy.html
World Medical Association policy

http://www.bma.org.uk/ethics
British Medical Association ethics site

http://www.nih.gov/sigs/bioethics/
UK National Institute of Health website:
bioethics pages

http://www.clinical-skills-net.org.uk
UK Clinical Skills Network

http://www.nivel.nl/each
European Association for Communication in
Healthcare

2 Infectious diseases, tropical medicine and sexually transmitted diseases

http://www.idlinks.com
General starting point for infectious disease links

http://www.cdc.gov
US Centers for Disease Control

http://www.phls.co.uk/facts/index.htm
UK Public Health Laboratory Service – figures and
statistics on communicable diseases

http://www.medscape.com/Home/Topics/ID
/Infectious Diseases.html
Free registration – good source of latest information

http://www.who.int/emc/
World Health Organization Communicable Disease
Surveillance and Response

http://www.bt.cdc.gov/
US Centers for Disease Control (Atlanta)

http://www.phls.co.uk/
UK regional information on infections

3 Cell and molecular biology, and genetic disorders

http://www.genetichealth.com
US company

4 Clinical immunology

http://www-micro.msb.le.ac.uk/MCQs/
MCQ.html

http://www-micro.msb.le.ac.uk/MBChB/
ImmGloss.html
MCQs and immunology glossary
(University of Leicester)

http://www.antibodyresource.com/
Source of antibody resources for educators and
researchers

5 Nutrition

http://www.who.int/nutgrowthdb/
World Health Organization site, provides information
on world-wide nutritional issues, resources and
research

http://www.fao.org/
Food and Agriculture Organization (FAO) –
autonomous body within the United Nations, aims
to improve health through nutrition and agricultural
productivity, especially in rural populations

http://www.ific.org/
International Food Information Council (IFIC) –
non-profit organization providing access to health
and nutrition resources to improve communication
of health and nutrition information to consumers

http://www.ag.uiuc.edu/~food-lab/nat/
Free analysis of the nutrient content of food
available to anyone (at University of Illinois, USA)

Selected nutrition journals (for more extensive
website addresses see Journal of Nutrition 1997;
127:1527–1532):

http://www.faseb.org/ajcn
American Journal of Clinical Nutrition

http://www.nutrition.org/
The Journal of Nutrition

http://www.naturesj.com/ijo
International Journal of Obesity

http://www.[...]/[...]NALS/
BJN/In[...]
The British [...] of Nutrition

http://www.ilsi.org/publications/reviews.html
Nutrition Reviews

http://clinnutr.org/
Journal of Parenteral and Enteral Nutrition

http://www.naturesj.com/ejcn/
European Journal of Clinical Nutrition

6 Gastrointestinal disease

http://www.graylab.ac.uk/cancernet/10002
5.html
Gastric cancer

http://www.jr2.ox.ac.uk/bandolier/
band27/b27-7.html

band38/b38-4.html
Gastric ulcer and GORD

http://www.nacc.org.uk
UK National Association for Colitis and Crohn's
Disease

http://www.digestivedisorders.org.uk/leaflets
/ibs.html
Irritable bowel syndrome

http://www.coeliac.co.uk
Coeliac disease

7 Liver, biliary tract and pancreatic disease

http://www.gastrohep.com
Resources for gastroenterology, hepatology and
endoscopy

http://www-micro.msb.le.ac.uk/335/
Hepatitis.html
Viral hepatitis

http://www.emedicine.com/emerg/
topic98.htm
Cholecystitis, cholelithiafis

8 Haematological disease

http://www.bloodline.net
General website on haematology

http://www.transfusion.org
Journal of the American Association of Blood Banks

http://www.shot.demon.co.uk
Serious Hazards of Transfusion (SHOT) scheme,
covering UK and Ireland NHS and private hospitals,
affiliated to the Royal College of Pathologists
(based Manchester Blood Transfusion Centre)

http://www.blood.co.uk
UK National Blood Service

http://www.doh.gov.uk/bbt2
UK CMO's Better Blood Transfusion Conference

http://www.bcshguidelines.com
British Society for Haematology guidelines

http://www.wfh.org
World Federation of Hemophilia

http://www.hemophilia.org
US National Hemophilia Foundation

http://www.med.unc.edu/isth/
International Society on Thrombosis and
Haemostasis (ISTH)

9 Medical oncology including haematological malignancy

http://www.cancerbacup.org.uk
UK patient organization

http://www.cancerresearchuk.org/
UK charity (formed from merged Imperial Cancer Research Fund and Cancer Research Campaign).

http://www.cancer.org
US cancer organization

http://www.palliativemedjournal.com
Journal of Palliative Medicine

10 Rheumatology and bone disease

http://www.rheumatology.org
American College of Rheumatology

http://www.arc.org.uk
UK Arthritis Research Campaign

http://www.rheumatology.org.uk/
British Society of Rheumatology – useful, patient-oriented information

http://www.nos.org.uk/
UK National Osteoporosis Society – useful information and reviews of ongoing research

http://www.osteo.org/
US National Institute of Health's bone-diseases page, with useful links from there for osteoporosis, Paget's and osteomalacia

http://www.cbcu.cam.ac.uk/calreviews
Cambridge University site – links to quizzes, pathology images, etc.

11 Renal disease &
12 Water, electrolytes and acid–base balance

http://www.tinkershop.net/nephro.htm
Nephrology calculator

http://www.nephronline.org
For healthcare professionals involved in the management of patients with kidney disease

http://www.renalnet.org
Kidney information clearing house database

http://www.kidney.org.uk/
UK charity run by and for patients

http://www.nkrf.org.uk/
UK charity

13 Cardiovascular disease

http://www.doh.gov.uk/nsf/coronarych4.htm
UK National Service Framework for Coronary Heart Disease (2000)

http://www.americanheart.org/
American Heart Association

http://www.erc.edu/
European Resuscitation Council

http://www.resus.org.uk
UK Resuscitation Council

http://homepages.enterprise.net/djenkins/ecghome.html
ECG tracings library

14 Respiratory disease

http://www.brit-thoracic.org.uk
British Thoracic Society

http://www.thoracic.org
American Thoracic Society

http://www.asthma.org.uk
UK National Asthma Campaign

http://www.quitsmokinguk.com
Good site for those wanting to quit or to help patients to quit

15 Intensive care medicine

http://www.ics.ac.uk
UK Intensive Care Society

http://www.esicm.org
European Society of Intensive Care Medicine

16 Drug therapy and poisoning

http://www.nice.org.uk
UK National Institute for Clinical Excellence

http://cebm.jr2.ox.ac.uk/
UK Centre for Evidence-Based Medicine

http://www.spib.axl.co.uk
Toxbase poisons information

17 Environmental medicine

http://www.who.int/m/topicgroups/environment/en/index.html
WHO guidelines and information on various environmental topics

http://www.hypothermia.org/
Hypothermia

http://www.nlm.nih.gov/medlineplus/hypothermia.html
Hypothermia

http://www.high-altitude-medicine.com/
Altitude sickness

18 Endocrine disease

http://www.endocrinology.org
UK Society for Endocrinology

http://www.endo-society.org
Endocrine Society

http://www.niddk.nih.gov/health/endo/endo.htm
US National Institutes of Health, National Institute of Diabetes & Digestive & Kidney Diseases

http://www.endocrineweb.com
Endocrine web resource

http://www.pituitary.org.uk
The Pituitary Foundation (UK charity)

http://www.tss.org.uk
UK Turner Syndrome Support Society

http://www.medicalert.org.uk
Emergency identification system for people with hidden medical conditions

19 Diabetes mellitus and other disorders of metabolism

http://www.doh.gov.uk/nsf
UK Government's forthcoming National Service Framework draft information

http://www.sign.ac.uk/guidelines/published/index.html
Scottish Intercollegiate Guidelines Network – guidelines on a range of subjects including diabetes

http://www.dtu.ox.ac.uk
Diabetes Trials Unit (University of Oxford) – research information, particularly the UK Prospective Diabetes Study results

http://medweb.bham.ac.uk/easdec/
Diabetic retinopathy

http://www.diabetes.org.uk
Diabetes UK charity – information for patients, researchers and health professionals

http://www.diabetes.org
American Diabetes Association – heavyweight and authoritative, with an American flavour

http://www.diabetes.ca
Canadian Diabetes Association site – well designed practical site with many links to other diabetes-related sites; a good jumping off point

20 Neurological disease

http://www.theabn.org
Association of British Neurologists information service

http://jnnp.bmjjournals.com/
Journal of Neurosurgery and Psychiatry

http://www.epilepsynse.org.uk
UK National Society for Epilepsy

21 Psychological medicine

http://www.rcpsych.ac.uk
UK Royal College of Psychiatrists

http://www.Connects.org.uk
A free linking website for mental health in general

http://www.cebmh.com/
Centre for Evidence-Based Mental Health

http://www.mentalhealth.org.uk
Mental Health Foundation, a charity that funds research and services for people with mental health problems and learning difficulties

22 Skin disease

http://www.bad.org.uk
British Association of Dermatologists

http://www.aad.org/MedWebGuide.html
American Academy of Dermatology web guide

http://tray.dermatology.uiowa.edu/Dermlmag.htm
Dermatologic image database (adult)

http://www.usc.edu/hsc/nml/e-resources/info/dermis.html
Dermatologic image database (paediatric)

http://www.eczema.org
UK National Eczema Society (atopic eczema)

http://www.paalliance.org
Psoriatic Arthropathy Alliance (psoriasis)

Kumar & Clark

Clinical

Fifth Edition

MEDICINE

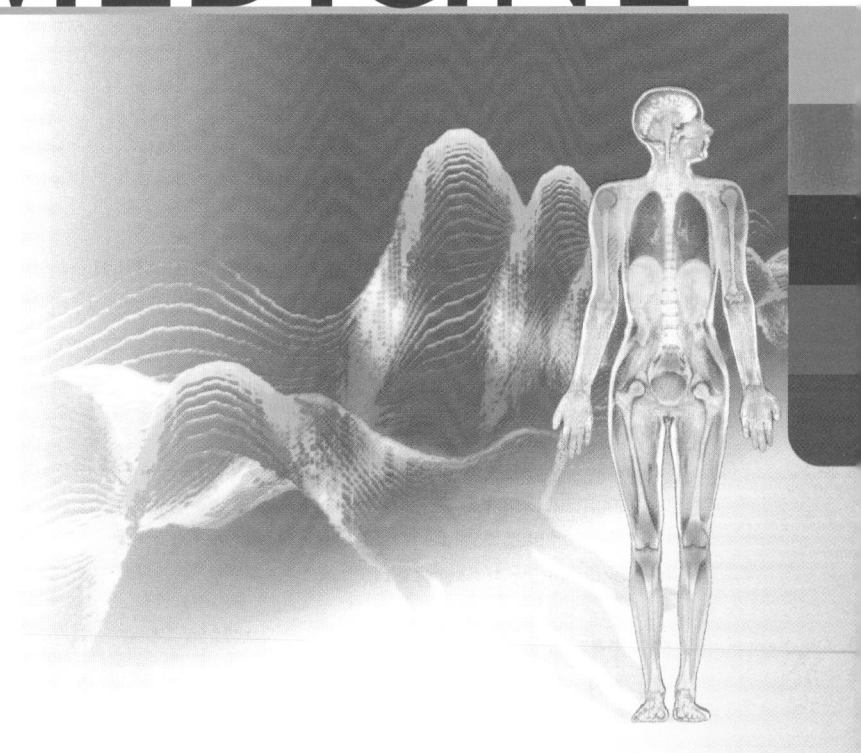

Edited by

Professor Parveen Kumar

CBE BSc MD FRCP FRCP (Edin)

Professor of Clinical Medical Education, Barts and The London,
Queen Mary's School of Medicine and Dentistry, University of London,
and Honorary Consultant Physician and Gastroenterologist, Barts and
The London NHS Trust and Homerton Hospital NHS Trust, London, UK.

Professor Kumar is also Chairman of the Medicines Commission UK,
and has held the appointments of Director of Continuing Professional
Development, Royal College of Physicians, London, and Non-Executive
Director, National Institute for Clinical Excellence (NICE). She was recently
awarded the CBE for services to medicine.

Dr Michael Clark

MD FRCP

Honorary Senior Lecturer, Barts and The London, Queen Mary's School of
Medicine and Dentistry, University of London, UK.

W.B. SAUNDERS

Edinburgh • London • New York • Philadelphia • St Louis • Sydney • Toronto 2002

Kumar & Clark
Clinical
Fifth Edition
MEDICINE

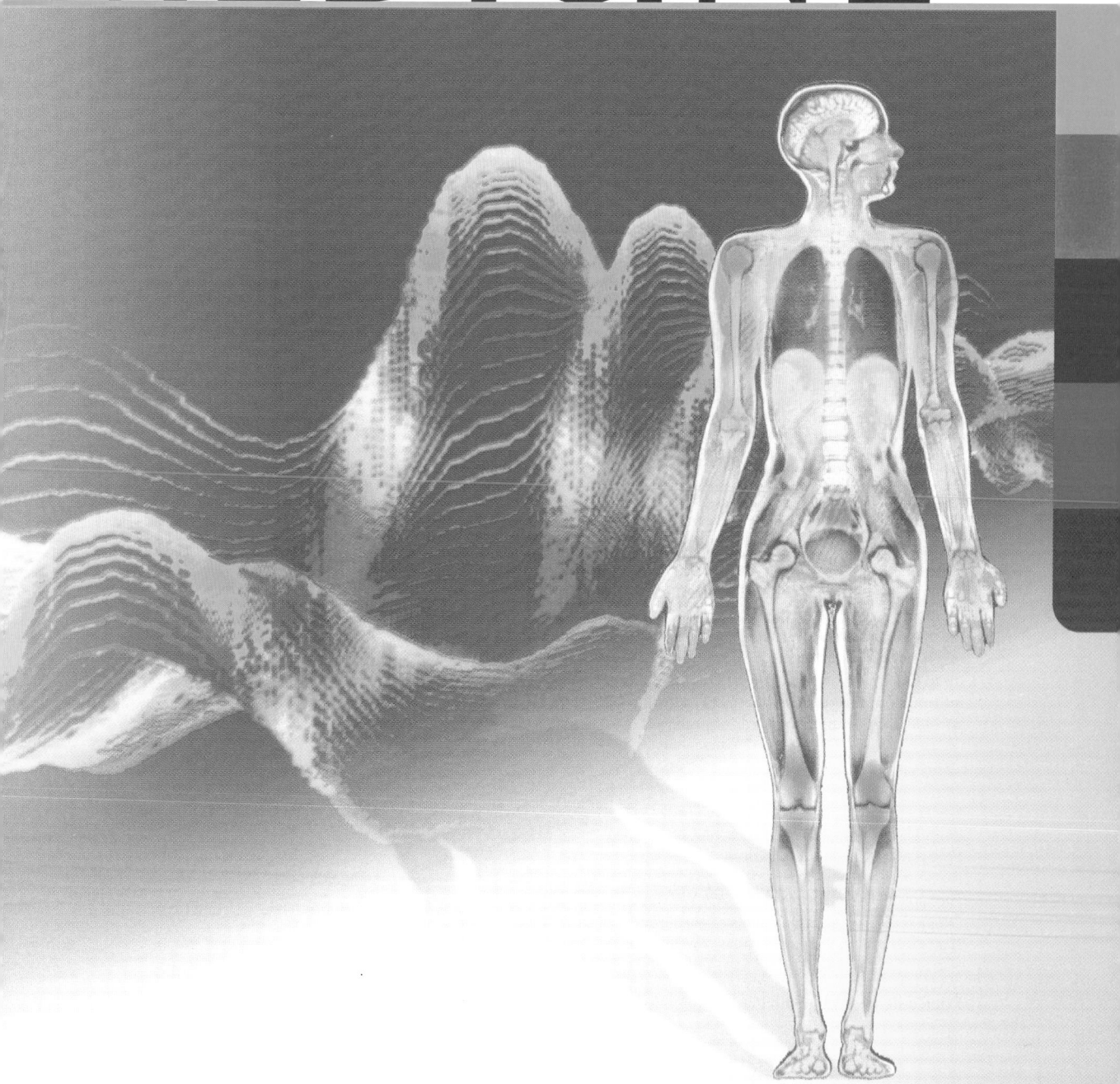

WB SAUNDERS
An imprint of Elsevier Science Limited

First edition 1987
Second edition 1990
Third edition 1994
Fourth edition 1998
Fifth edition 2002

ISBN 0 702 02579 8
International Student Edition ISBN 0 702 02606 9

British Library Cataloguing in Publication Data
A catalogue record for this book is available from the British Library

Library of Congress Cataloging in Publication Data
A catalog record for this book is available from the Library of Congress

Note
Medical knowledge is constantly changing. As new information
becomes available, changes in treatment, procedures, equipment and
the use of drugs become necessary. The editors and the publishers have
taken care to ensure that the information given in this text is accurate and
up to date. However, readers are strongly advised to confirm that the
information, especially with regard to drug usage, complies with the
latest legislation and standards of practice.

Commissioning Editor: Ellen Green
Project Development Manager: Fiona Conn
Project Manager: Frances Affleck
Designer: Sarah Russell
Page layout: Alan Palfreyman, Kate Walshaw
Original illustrations: Hardlines
New illustrations: Richard Morris

The
publisher's
policy is to use
**paper manufactured
from sustainable forests**

Printed in the UK by Bath Press Limited

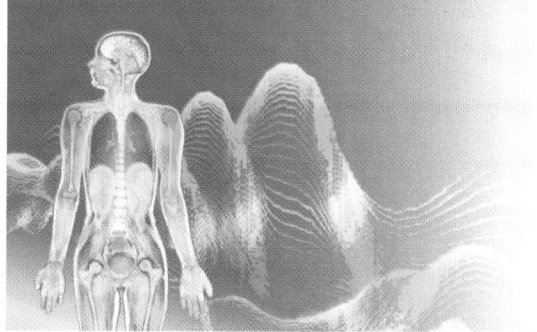

Contents

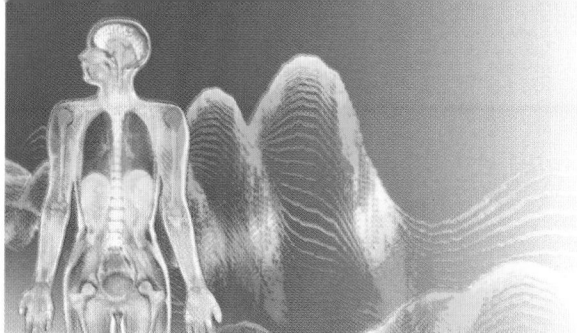

Contributors

Jane Anderson PhD MB BS FRCP
Senior Lecturer in HIV Medicine,
Honorary Consultant Physician
Barts and The London, Queen Mary's School of
Medicine and Dentistry, University of London, UK
Sexually transmitted diseases

John V Anderson MA MD MB BS FRCP
Senior Lecturer, Honorary Consultant Physician
in Diabetes and Metabolism
Barts and The London, Queen Mary's School of
Medicine and Dentistry, University of London and
Homerton Hospital NHS Trust, London, UK
Diabetes mellitus and lipids

Laurence R I Baker MA MD FRCP FRCP (Edin)
Emeritus Consultant Physician and Nephrologist
Barts and The London NHS Trust, London, UK
Renal disease

Nigel Benjamin DM FRCP (Edin) FMedSci
Professor of Clinical Pharmacology
Barts and The London, Queen Mary's School of
Medicine and Dentistry, University of London, UK
Drug therapy

Carol M Black CBE BA MD PRCP FRCP FACP FMedSci
Professor of Rheumatology and
Director of Centre for Rheumatology
University College London Hospitals NHS Trust,
London, UK
Connective tissue disorders, vasculitis

Andrew K Burroughs MB ChB (Hons) FRCP
Consultant Physician and Hepatologist
Royal Free Hampstead NHS Trust, London, UK
Liver disease

A John Camm MD FRCP
Professor of Clinical Cardiology
St George's Hospital Medical School,
University of London, UK
Cardiovascular disease

Anthony W Clare MD FRCPI FRCP FRCPsych MPhil
Professor of Clinical Psychiatry
Trinity College, Dublin;
Medical Director
St Patrick's Hospital, Dublin, Ireland
Psychological medicine

Michael L Clark MD FRCP
Honorary Senior Lecturer
Barts and The London, Queen Mary's School of
Medicine and Dentistry, University of London, UK
Gastrointestinal disease; Environmental medicine

Charles R A Clarke MA MB BCh FRCP
Consultant Neurologist
The National Hospital for Neurology and
Neurosurgery, University College London NHS Trust,
London, UK
Neurological disease; Environmental medicine

Brian T Colvin MB BChir FCRP FRCPath
Senior Lecturer in Haematology,
Director of the Haemophilia Centre
Barts and The London, Queen Mary's School of
Medicine and Dentistry, University of London, UK
Bleeding disorders, thrombosis

Juliet Compston MD FRCP FRCPath FMedSci
Reader, Honorary Consultant Physician
Department of Medicine, Addenbrooke's NHS Trust,
University of Cambridge School of Clinical Medicine, UK
Bone diseases

Len Doyal BA MSc
Professor of Medical Ethics, Honorary Consultant
Barts and The London, Queen Mary's School of
Medicine and Dentistry, University of London, UK
Ethics

Paul L Drury MA MB FRCP FRACP
Medical Director
Auckland Diabetes Centre, Auckland, New Zealand
Endocrine disease

Clinical Medicine

Marinos Elia BSc (Hons) MB ChB MD FRCP
Professor of Clinical Nutrition and Metabolism
University of Southampton, UK
Nutrition

Roger G Finch MB BS FRCP FRCPath FRCP (Edin) FFPM
Professor of Infectious Diseases
Nottingham City Hospital NHS Trust and the
University of Nottingham, UK
Infectious diseases and tropical medicine

Anthony J Frew MA MD FRCP
Professor of Allergy and Respiratory Medicine
University of Southampton, UK
Respiratory disease

Edwin A M Gale MB FRCP
Professor of Diabetic Medicine
University of Bristol, UK
Diabetes mellitus and other disorders of metabolism

Christopher J Gallagher MB ChB FRCP
Consultant Medical Oncologist
Barts and The London NHS Trust, London, UK
Medical oncology including haematological malignancy

Charles J Hinds FRCP FRCA
Consultant and Senior Lecturer in
Anaesthesia and Intensive Care
Barts and The London NHS Trust, London, UK
Intensive care medicine

Stephen T Holgate BSc MD DSc FRCP FRCPath
FMedSci
Medical Research Council Clinical Professor of
Immunopharmacology
University of Southampton, UK
Respiratory disease

Trevor A Howlett MD FRCP
Consultant Physician and Endocrinologist
University Hospitals of Leicester NHS Trust,
Leicester, UK
Endocrine disease

Ray K Iles BSc MSc PhD CBiol MBiol
Senior Lecturer (non-clinical) in Obstetrics and
Gynaecology, Director of the Williamson Laboratory
Barts and The London, Queen Mary's School of
Medicine and Dentistry, University of London;
Professor of Biomedical Science
University of North London, UK
Cell and molecular biology, and genetic disorders

Donald J Jeffries BSc MB BS FRCP FRCPath
FRCP (Edin) FFPM
Professor of Virology, Head of Medical Microbiology
Barts and The London, Queen Mary's School of
Medicine and Dentistry, University of London, UK
Virology

Stephen M Kelsey MB ChB MRCPath
Senior Lecturer, Honorary Consultant in Haematology
Barts and The London, Queen Mary's School of
Medicine and Dentistry, University of London, UK
Medical oncology including haematological malignancy

Christopher Mallinson FRCP
Consultant Physician and Gastroenterologist,
Director of Communications Research Group
Lewisham Hospital NHS Trust, London;
President of Forum for Communication in Health Care,
Royal Society of Medicine, London, UK
Communication

Peter J Moss MD MRCP DTMH
Consultant in Infectious Diseases
Hull and East Yorkshire Hospitals NHS Trust, UK
Infectious diseases and tropical medicine

Michael F Murphy MD FRCP FRCPath
Consultant Haematologist
National Blood Service and Department of Haematology,
Oxford Radcliffe Hospitals NHS Trust, Oxford;
Honorary Senior Clinical Lecturer in Blood Transfusion
University of Oxford, UK
Haematological disease

Donncha O'Gradaigh MB MRCP
Clinical Research Fellow
University of Cambridge School of Clinical Medicine, UK
Bone diseases

David G Paige MB BS MA FRCP
Consultant in Dermatology
Barts and The London NHS Trust, London;
Honorary Senior Lecturer
Centre for Cutaneous Research
Barts and The London, Queen Mary's School of
Medicine and Dentistry, University of London, UK
Skin disease

Jacqueline M Parkin PhD FRCP
Senior Lecturer, Honorary Consultant
in Clinical Immunology
Barts and The London, Queen Mary's School of
Medicine and Dentistry, University of London, UK
Clinical immunology

Anthony J Pinching BM BCh MA DPhil FRCP
Louis Freedman Professor of Immunology
Barts and The London, Queen Mary's School of
Medicine and Dentistry, University of London, UK
Clinical immunology

Sir Michael Rawlins MD FRCP FRCP (Edin) FFPM
FMedSci FRCA (Hon)
Professor of Clinical Pharmacology and Therapeutics
University of Newcastle;
Chairman, National Institute for Clinical Excellence, UK
Clinical trials and statistics

Michael Shipley MA MD FRCP
Consultant Rheumatologist
University College London Hospitals, London, UK
Rheumatology

David B Silk MD FRCP
Consultant Physician in Gastroenterology and Nutrition
North West London Hospitals NHS Trust, London, UK
Gastrointestinal disease

Teresa Tate FRCP FRCR
Consultant in Palliative Medicine
Barts and The London NHS Trust, London;
Medical Adviser, Marie Curie Cancer Care
London, UK
Palliative care

Allister Vale MD FCRP FRCPE FRCPG FFOM FAACT
Director, NPIS (Birmingham Centre) and
West Midlands Poisons Unit
City Hospital, Birmingham, UK
Poisoning

James Wainscoat FRCP FRCPath
Consultant Haematologist
Oxford Radcliffe Hospitals NHS Trust, Oxford, UK
Haematological disease

J David Watson MB BS FRCA
Consultant in Intensive Care
Barts and The London NHS Trust and Homerton
Hospital NHS Trust, London, UK
Intensive care medicine

David Westaby MA FRCP
Consultant Physician and Gastroenterologist
Chelsea and Westminster Healthcare NHS Trust,
London, UK
Biliary and pancreatic disease

Peter D White MD FRCP FRCPsych
Senior Lecturer in Psychological Medicine,
Honorary Consultant in Liaison Psychiatry
Barts and The London, Queen Mary's School of
Medicine and Dentistry, University of London, UK
Psychological medicine

Muhammad M Yaqoob MD FRCP
Consultant Nephrologist
Barts and The London NHS Trust, London, UK
Water, electrolytes and acid–base balance

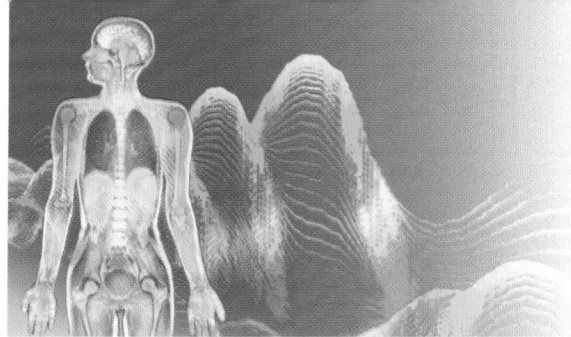

Preface to the Fifth Edition

This edition of *Clinical Medicine* takes us into a new century and a new millennium. Medicine continues to become more complex but nevertheless more interesting. We now know the outline of the human genome and increasingly more diseases can be explained by some genetic abnormality. As always, we have tried to keep up with these advances so that *Clinical Medicine* continues to remain at the cutting edge of medical science.

From the beginning we have had two aims in writing this book: firstly, to strike a balance between developments in medical research and the facts that students must absorb, and secondly, to link scientific advances with clinical practice so that the management of disease can be based on sound physiological concepts. We have remained constant to these aims throughout all editions, so inevitably the book has grown in size. The book's reputation as an easy-to-understand text has made us resist making widespread reductions in its content. For this edition, we have removed the appendices, but this has been counterbalanced by a new chapter on ethics and communications – an essential part of being a good clinician. Cell and molecular biology and genetics, and immunology have become separate chapters. Each chapter has been reviewed and revised and new authors have brought in fresh ideas to make the book better illustrated and easier to read.

The book continues to be 'the book' that everybody involved in clinical medicine must have. It is very widely read by undergraduate and postgraduate students, practising physicians, nurses and professionals allied to medicine. We are always grateful for their views and criticisms, which we have tried to incorporate: the uniformity of the 'boxes' in this edition is mainly due to readers' requests for simplification, as is the placement of the normal values on the inside back cover. We hope readers will also find the websites listed at the front of the book, and the kumarandclark.com website useful additions.

For an easier-to-carry version, *Clinical Medicine* is supplemented by the *Pocket Essentials of Clinical Medicine* by A. Ballinger and S. Patchett. This allows everyone to have a pocket version of the book as a constant companion.

Once again, we would like to thank the families of our authors as well as our own. As always, they have hugely supported us; inevitably this book has been written during evenings, weekends and of course whilst on holiday.

PJK
MLC

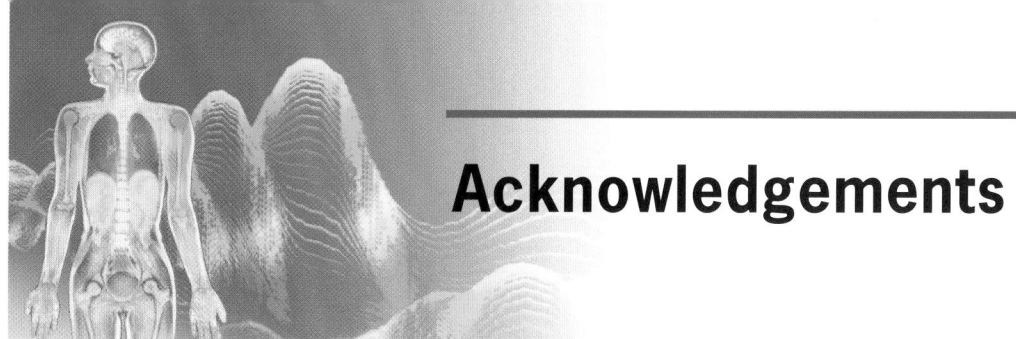

Acknowledgements

We would like to thank many of our colleagues who have helped in the preparation of this edition. Many have given us useful advice, helped us to collect photographs and indeed read the manuscripts to make sure that the contents are up-to-date. These include Alison McLean, David Leaver, Peter Fairclough, Paul Kelly, Paolo Domizio, Judy Webb, Rodney Reznek, Nick Wright, Beng Goh, Mona Bajaj-Elliott and Vince McDonald.

Some of our authors have left after many years of commitment and loyalty to the book. We would like to thank Professor Michael Farthing, Dr Richard Pearson and Professor Robert Davies who have been with us from that first edition and Dr Maurice Slevin, Professor Ama Rohatiner, Dr John Morrow and Professor Irene Leigh who have written for more recent editions. We welcome our new authors who have contributed much to this edition.

Our ward rounds and outpatient reviews are a continuing source of evidence-based education and we are grateful to our specialist registrars, senior house officers, house officers and our own medical students who continue to stimulate us by asking penetrating questions.

We are extremely grateful for the skill and support of our publishers. Ellen Green has now taken us through the last two editions. Fiona Conn has meticulously co-ordinated the whole project with unfailing good humour and patience. The production team, Frances Affleck, Kate Walshaw and Alan Palfreyman, and the designer, Sarah Russell, have produced a high quality edition of the book.

We are also grateful to the many people behind the scenes without whose help this book would not have been possible, in particular Nici Kingston who kept us in order!

We are particularly grateful to Ms Jillian Linton who did most of the preparation and co-ordination of the numerous chapters.

Special acknowledgements

Chapter 1 Ethics and communication
Professor Len Doyal would like to thank Sharon Burton of the General Medical Council.

Chapter 6 Gastrointestinal disease
Dr David Silk would like to thank Dr Iain Beveridge for his contribution to the colon polyps and cancer section of the chapter.

Chapter 9 Medical oncology including haematological malignancy
Dr Christopher J Gallagher would like to thank Prof A Rohatiner (St Bartholomew's Hospital Dept of Medical Oncology)

Chapter 10 Rheumatology and bone disease
Professor Carol M Black would like to thank Dr Christopher Denton (Senior Lecturer in Rheumatology, Royal Free Hospital) who assisted with manuscript preparations and proof corrections.

Chapter 13 Cardiovascular disease
Professor A J Camm would like to thank

Dr Aodhan Breathnach and Dr Derek Macallan (Dept of Infectious Diseases, PHLS Collaborating Centre & Dept of Medical Microbiology, St George's Hospital) for their work on the infective endocarditis section of the chapter.

Dr Naab Al-Saady (Senior Registrar, Cardiological Sciences, St George's Hospital Medical School) for general assistance with the chapter.

Crown copyright material is reproduced with the permission of the Controller of Her Majesty's Stationery Office.

Important note

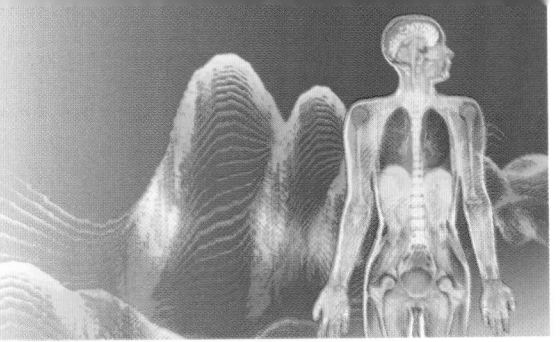

Every effort has been made to check the drug dosages given in this book. However, as it is possible that dosage schedules have been revised, the reader is strongly urged to consult the drug companies' literature before administering any of the drugs listed. Drugs mentioned in this book are given their generic Recommended International Non-Proprietary Names in accordance with Directive, 97/27/EEC. In some cases the UK name (BAN) is also given in brackets as recommended in the BNF. Please see the latest BNF for further details of the name changes.

The internet is now a growing source of medical information, so we have included a selection of websites at the front of the book. Although the websites were reviewed and chosen with care, the reader should recognize that such information changes constantly and should therefore be used with discretion.

Ethics and communication

Ethics

Why study ethics and law applied to medicine?

Professional concern about ethics and law

Many clinical choices created by advances in medical technology are essentially ethical rather than scientific. Doctors may be expert in understanding and applying clinical science, yet this expertise does not in itself answer many ethical questions about the circumstances in which such science should and should not be applied. For example, they may know a great deal technically about advanced life-support systems or the termination of pregnancy. Their knowledge, however, will not tell them whether or not it is ethical to withdraw ventilatory support from a severely brain-damaged patient who will not otherwise die or to perform a termination on a 13-year-old girl who does not want her parents to know that she is pregnant. Answers to these questions derive from moral beliefs and arguments.

Patients are increasingly aware of what they believe to be their human rights and expect doctors to respect them.

- Rights are claims for specific types of goods or services that individuals are believed to be entitled to make on others (e.g. free speech, access to primary and secondary education, access to an acceptable standard of medical care).
- In the UK, if patients believe their rights have been ignored by doctors, they may formally complain to the General Medical Council (GMC) or seek legal redress.
- As it pertains to medicine, the law establishes boundaries for what government and the courts – through statute and common law – have deemed to be acceptable professional practice. The GMC – the UK regulatory body – sets boundaries for acceptable standards of conduct and care through its guidance documents and decisions in cases heard by its Professional Conduct and Performance Committees.
- Whether or not legal actions or formal complaints against doctors are successful, they contribute toward bringing the medical profession into disrepute.

Ethics and communication

The three duties of clinical care

The rights of patients may be summarized by three corresponding duties of care which apply to all patients for whom doctors have clinical responsibility.

1. **Protect life and health.** Clinicians should practise medicine to a high standard, taking care not to cause unnecessary harm or suffering. Patients should only be given treatments which they need. Treatments should not be prescribed, for example, just because patients request them.
2. **Respect autonomy.** Humans have autonomy – the ability to reason, plan and make choices about the future. Respect for these attributes goes hand in hand with respect for human dignity. Doctors should respect the autonomy, and thus the dignity, of their patients. This respect for the autonomy of patients leads to two further rights – informed consent and confidentiality. Competent adult patients should be able to choose to accept proposed treatments and to control personal information which they divulge concerning such treatments. Denying patients such choice and control robs them of their human dignity.
3. **Protect life and health and respect autonomy with fairness and justice.** In the conduct of public and professional life, it is generally thought that people have the right to expect to be treated equally. Medicine is no exception and doctors have a duty to practise accordingly. The access to, and quality of, clinical care should be based only on the dictates of need rather than arbitrary prejudice or favouritism.

Why should doctors take the duties of care seriously?

Professional regulation

Within the UK, the practice of medicine is regulated by the General Medical Council (GMC). It is responsible for the registration of doctors, setting and monitoring the quality of their education and disciplining for unprofessional conduct. Doctors have no professional choice but to conform to the standards laid down by the GMC, which are based on the three duties of care (Box 1.1). These same duties are confirmed by other professional bodies like the Royal College of Physicians, the Royal College of Surgeons, the British Medical Association and the Medical Research Council.

The law

The three duties of care are also enshrined in statute and common law, which also regulate medical practice. Doctors may be sued in civil law for financial compensation for any harm that they may cause while failing in their professional duties. If it can be shown that this failure is intentional, or reckless in the extreme harm or death that results, doctors may face prosecution in the criminal courts and, if found guilty, imprisonment.

> ### Box 1.1
>
> **General Medical Council, Good Medical Practice: 2–4**
>
> The importance of protecting life and health:
>
> - 'an adequate assessment of the patient's condition …(and)… if necessary, an appropriate examination'
> - 'providing or arranging investigations or treatments where necessary'
> - 'competence when making diagnoses and when giving or arranging treatment'
>
> The importance of respect for autonomy:
>
> - 'listen to patients and respect their views and beliefs'
> - 'giving patients the information they ask for or need about their condition, its treatment and prognosis'
> - 'respecting patients' privacy and dignity'
>
> The importance of fairness and justice:
>
> - '…(not allowing)… views about a patient's lifestyle, culture, beliefs, race, colour, gender, sexuality, disability age or social or economic status, to prejudice … treatments'
> - '…(not refusing or delaying) treatment because you believe that patients' actions have contributed to their condition, or because you may be putting yourself at risk'
>
> Similar statements are made by a variety of professional bodies in many countries.

UK law now includes the Human Rights Act 1998. This law incorporates the European Convention on Human Rights making it legally binding in the UK (Box 1.2). The provisions of the Act impose duties on doctors to ensure that their clinical practice is not in violation of these rights – the same duties that all other doctors in Europe must observe. The Act also thus helps to ensure that what constitutes legal practice in the UK is judged by broader, trans-national moral standards.

> ### Box 1.2
>
> **European Convention on Human Rights**
>
> **Substantive rights which apply to evaluating good medical practice**
> Right to life (Article 2)
> Prohibition of torture, inhuman or degrading treatment or punishment (Article 3)
> Prohibition of slavery and forced labour (Article 4)
> Right to liberty and security (Artcle 5)
> Right to a fair trial (Article 6)
> No punishment without law (Article 7)
> Right to respect for private and family life (Article 8)
> Freedom of thought, conscience and religion (Article 9)
> Freedom of expression (Article 10)
> Right to marry (Article 12)
> Prohibition of discrimination (Article 14)

Rational self-interest

The most rational way for doctors to ensure that their own medical treatment meets high standards of care is to support the right of all patients to it through the professional and legal enforcement of these duties.

The clinical importance of trust

Patients will not trust doctors whom they suspect may ignore their human rights. Without trust, patients will not cooperate in their diagnosis and treatment, undermining the prospect for clinical success. Lack of trust also engenders a defensive and impersonal approach to medicine by both clinicians and patients, potentially spoiling the quality of patient care and professional life.

The doctor/patient relationship

Doctors are expected to treat patients, and their carers where appropriate, as active partners in the healing process.

FURTHER READING

British Medical Association (2000) *The Impact of the Human Rights Act 1998 on Medical Decision Making.* London: BMA.
General Medical Council (2001) *Good Medical Practice.* London: GMC.
Royal College of Surgeons (1997) *The Surgeon's Duty of Care.* London: RCS.

The nature of medical mistakes

Doctors have a duty to protect the life and health of patients to an acceptable professional standard. What does this mean in practice and what are the penalties for not doing so?

Clinical negligence

If clinicians are suspected not to have provided an acceptable standard of clinical care, they may be sued for negligence – a breach of their professional duty. To win a legal action and financial damages for negligence, patients/claimants must provide convincing evidence to a judge that:

- they were harmed
- the harm was caused by the accused doctor
- the action which caused the harm was a breach of professional duty.

However, in practice, such a demonstration may be more difficult. For example, the alleged harm may have occurred against the background of a complex medical condition or course of treatment, making it difficult to establish the actual cause.

When has a breach of professional duty occurred?

In the UK, whether or not a doctor has acted inconsistently with the duty to protect life and health to an acceptable standard, is ordinarily decided in civil cases by a judge on the basis of testimony from expert witnesses.

- Such experts are selected to represent a responsible body of professional opinion. The testimony of these experienced clinicians will be used to help the court determine a professional standard which doctors working in their specializations should meet in clinical practice of the kind under dispute. Both the patient/claimant and defendant/doctor will try to produce experts to support their case.
- There will be clinical conduct so unreasonable that its negligence speaks for itself (e.g. a dramatic mistake about drug overdose).
- If expert witnesses are found for the doctor/defendant who will state that under similar circumstances, they would have clinically responded in the same way as the doctor then the patient/claimant will probably lose. Provided that their testimony is logically consistent and compatible with other widely accepted professional beliefs about good clinical practice, it is likely that the doctor's actions will be found to be reasonable. This will be so irrespective of how representative the clinical opinions given in court are of other doctors practising in the same field. Experts can differ about what is and is not clinically acceptable.
- Because only a minority opinion is required for doctors to defend claims of negligence against them, the professional standard employed in deciding such claims can make it difficult for patients/claimants to win damages.

Inexperience is irrelevant

Lack of experience is not taken into account in legal determinations of negligence or the GMC's formal hearings. All doctors are expected to work to a professional standard of expertise based on similar clinical work of experienced clinicians. This does not mean that doctors have to be experts in everything. In the face of doubts about their ability or training to provide treatment to a reasonable standard, doctors should seek appropriate supervision and refuse to proceed otherwise.

Mistakes are not necessarily to be feared

Poor professional practice – for example, clinical care which is overly defensive – can result from unfounded fears of patients' readiness to make formal complaints or take legal action.

- All doctors make clinical mistakes in their professional careers. Yet it should be clear that a clinical error is not necessarily a negligent error. Responsible and experienced clinicians may testify that the erroneous action was and is unavoidable in that type of clinical practice. Under similar circumstances, they too sometimes make – or might make – the same error.

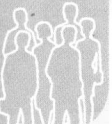

- Just because doctors can make professionally defensible mistakes does not mean that they should in any way relax their professional standards.
- Professional bodies within medicine, and the defence associations which insure doctors against negligence, recommend that doctors should be honest and apologetic about their mistakes, remembering that to do so is not necessarily an admission of negligence. As a result of such honesty and humility, there is mounting evidence that patients will feel that they have been respected and are less likely to take legal action or to make formal complaints.

For all of these reasons, there is less to fear legally from patients than doctors sometimes believe. The law offers wide protection for clinicians provided that they do their best to act reasonably and responsibly in protecting the lives and health of their patients.

Respect for autonomy

Legally valid consent

Obtaining the consent of patients to treatment is just as fundamentally a part of good medical care as is proper clinical diagnosis and good therapeutic management. Doctors seeking consent for a particular procedure must be competent in the knowledge of how the procedure is performed and its problems.

For agreement to treatment to be legally acceptable it must meet three conditions:

- Consent must be informed to an adequate standard.
- Patients must be competent to consent to treatment.
- Patients must not be coerced into accepting treatment against their wishes.

Patients need to weigh up the pros and cons of proposed treatments with other objective interests in their personal lives. They cannot do so without the basic ability to reason about information concerning what is wrong with them, what their doctors propose to do about it and with what potential benefits and risks. If patients are coerced into making choices about treatment, the ethical and legal right to exercise control over their personal life is ignored. In these circumstances, such choices become more those of clinicians who unduly pressure patients rather than of patients themselves.

Battery

It is an unlawful battery intentionally to touch a competent person without their consent.

- For competent adult patients to be touched lawfully, they must be given information in broad terms about the proposed treatment – what it is and why it is being suggested. Thus a clinician will commit a battery if such a patient is given an injection without permission, irrespective of the need for it.
- Treatment can be given legally to adult patients without consent if they are temporarily or permanently incompetent to provide it and the treatment is *necessary* to save their life, or to prevent them from incurring serious and permanent injury. Otherwise, consent must be obtained, however inconvenient this may be for the patient or clinician.

Negligence: information about risks

Clinicians may also be in breach of their professional duty to obtain adequate consent through not providing a reasonable amount of information about the *risks* of proposed treatment. Here the legal claim of a patient/claimant would be for negligence.

The reasonable doctor standard of disclosure.

- Success will depend on the court being convinced that the patient/claimant had been harmed by the treatment and would not have agreed to it if they had been given more information about its risks.
- The patient/claimant must also show the amount of information provided about risks was unreasonable. If the clinician/defendant can find expert witnesses deemed to constitute a reasonable body of medical opinion who will say that they too (at that point in time) would have provided no more information about risks, the patient/plaintiff will probably lose, just as we saw in the case of litigation for clinical negligence.
- This 'professional standard' of disclosure of information about risks is open to dispute.

The reasonable patient standard of disclosure.

Patients may disagree with clinicians about how much information they require to protect their personal interests. Indeed, in deciding what information to disclose to patients about risks, clinicians may know little about how they perceive their interests. Since it is the health and lives of patients that are potentially at risk, the moral focus of such disclosure should be on what is acceptable to them rather than the medical profession.

- It is increasingly argued that clinicians obtaining consent to treatment should ask what sort of information about risks a 'reasonable person' in the position of the patient would want before agreeing to treatment. To do otherwise constitutes an unacceptable threat to the moral rights and dignity of patients and entails a potential loss of trust in the medical profession.
- Practically, clinicians should interpret this standard of disclosure of the reasonable person as meaning that they should ask the patient what sort of information about risks they would want bearing in mind their particular experiences and needs. When in doubt, clinicians should also ask what sort of

information they would want for themselves, their families and friends. They should also remember that the graver the risk, the more important to disclose information about it, even when the chance of it occurring is small.

Express vs implied consent
Consent to treatment may be obtained in two ways:

- Express consent may be verbal or written, usually through the patient signing a consent form. Here consent is given explicitly in relation to specific information about the proposed treatment.
- Consent may also be implied by the fact that the patient accepts treatment without question, protest or any other physical sign that might be associated with rejection. Implied consent is ordinarily given against the background of an express consent to a specific treatment which has already been obtained. For example, patients have not given their implied consent to a specific treatment simply because they have presented themselves for care in a hospital. They must be given appropriate information about the proposed care and provide express consent to it.

Medical students or their supervisors should always obtain the explicit consent of patients to provide case histories or to be examined for purely educational purposes. Students should always make it clear to patients that they are not qualified doctors.

Confidentiality
If clinicians violate the confidentiality of their patients, they risk causing harm rather than protecting patients from it. Through violating the right of patients to control information which they divulge as part of their medical care, such clinicians disrespect autonomy, undermine trust and call the medical profession into disrepute. These rights are protected by common and statute law. Doctors who breach the confidentiality of patients face severe professional and legal sanctions.

Respecting confidentiality in practice
Patients should be informed of the ways in which information about them will need to be shared with other clinicians and health care workers involved in their treatment. Patients' express consent to such occurrences should be sought, or they might give implied consent as part of their general consent to undergo a specific treatment. Where they object to particular information being shared, generally this should be respected. Health professionals and others not involved in the care of a patient have no right of access to related information without the patient's consent, simply because such information is considered useful for other purposes. In almost all clinical circumstances, therefore, the confidentiality of patients must be respected.

When confidentiality must or may be breached
The principle of confidentiality in medicine is not absolute. Sometimes, the law dictates that clinicians must reveal private information about patients to others in contexts that they may or do object to. At other times, they have the discretion to do so, in accordance with good professional practice. Both circumstances highlight the difficult ethical tension which can be posed between the rights of individual patients and the interests of the public. The right to privacy does not entail the right to harm others in exercising it.

Therefore, clinicians must breach confidentiality when (among others):

- patients have infectious diseases which must be notified, through informing the relevant local authority officer
- police request information about patients who have been involved in a traffic accident
- patients are suspected of engaging in terrorist activity in the UK
- they are presented with a court order by a judge or asked to do so by a judge in judicial proceedings.

Clinicians have the discretion to breach confidentiality when they become aware of, for example:

- past or potential criminal and violent behaviour that has resulted, or is likely to result, in serious harm to the patient or others, such as child abuse.
- refusal of patients to comply with their own legal obligations to provide information about their medical condition to the relevant authority (e.g. to the Driver and Vehicle Licensing Agency)
- infectious patients who pose a threat to specific individuals through undisclosed risks.
- infectious patients who pose a potential threat to unknown members of the public through undisclosed risks.

In all these circumstances, patients should be informed of any intent to breach their confidentiality, unless doing so may place the clinician or others at risk of serious harm. Clinicians should always remember that they are professionally accountable for discretionary breaches and may be asked to justify their decision either in court or by the GMC.

Respect for autonomy in the treatment of vulnerable patients
We have seen that for consent to treatment to be valid, patients must be competent to give it.

What is competence?
Competence should be understood as task-oriented. People may be competent to do some things but incompetent to do others. This means that they should not be

judged to be either competent or incompetent in absolute terms. Legally, if patients are competent they must be able to:

- understand information about their condition and treatment
- remember this information
- deliberate about the therapeutic choices posed by the information
- believe that the information applies to them and is not, for example, being made up for other reasons.

Competence to consent to treatment may be compromised by many things – age, mental illness, congenital disease, accident and injury (among others).

Children

In the UK, the legal age of presumed competence to consent to treatment is 16. Below this age, those with parental responsibility are the legal proxies of their children and usually consent to treatment on their behalf. Yet:

- The age of 16 is somewhat arbitrary and many children below this age will also possess the abilities associated with competence. For example, they may be mature enough to understand and reason about information given to them about their condition and treatment.
- Clinicians should ordinarily respect the dignity of such children through asking them if they agree to the proposed treatment, even when the consent of parents is also obtained.
- If such children wish to have clinical consultations and clinically indicated care without the knowledge of their parents then this – along with their confidentiality – should be respected.
- Young children may be incompetent to make important decisions about their medical care, although they may have developed some degree of autonomy in this regard. They should be consulted about their care and due consideration given to their wishes.
- In England, unlike Scotland, young people do not acquire the right to refuse medical treatment thought to be in their best interest until the age of 18. In practice, the legal ability to force treatment on mature children against their wishes should only be contemplated in circumstances where life is at risk or there is a risk of serious and permanent injury. Doing otherwise is not in the best interests of young people because of the potentially dangerous alienation that it may create toward doctors and medicine.

Those with parental responsibility have no legal authority to direct clinicians to administer or withdraw treatments from children deemed necessary to protect them from death or serious harm. The court should be consulted about such disagreements, unless an emergency dictates otherwise.

Psychiatric illness

The vast majority of patients being treated for psychiatric illness are competent to consent and to refuse treatment. There is no difference between their rights and those of other competent patients. Because of the danger of stigma associated with mental illness, great care should be taken to protect their confidentiality. If patients with severe psychiatric illness are incompetent to understand the nature and consequences of their illness, they will be unable to provide valid consent to treatment. Here, the ethical duty of care shifts from respect for autonomy of such patients to protecting them.

The 1983 Mental Health Act. Mental illness may so compromise the autonomy of patients that they become a danger to themselves and/or to others. Provided that their illness is treatable, such patients may be detained under the 1983 Mental Health Act for further examination and treatment. Because of the terrible risks and ethical significance of denying someone their ordinary civil liberties, the conditions of detainment under the Act are highly specific: the longer the period of detainment, the more safeguards there are to ensure the clinical need for it (see Table 21.29, p. 1270).

Psychiatric treatment without consent. Under certain circumstances, detained patients may be given psychiatric treatment without their consent. However, attempts should be made to obtain consent, if possible. Unless their mental illness has made them incompetent to do so, such patients must still give their consent to proposed treatments for physical disorders. Again, incompetence in one respect does not entail incompetence in all respects. However, if patients are unable competently to consent because of the severity of their psychiatric condition – and treatment is required to save their life or to prevent serious and permanent disability – they can be given necessary care without it. If treatment can wait, without seriously compromising their interests, then patients should be asked to consent to it when they become competent to do so.

Other forms of incompetence to provide consent to treatment

Patients may also be incompetent because of congenital, developmental or accidental brain damage. Where they are children, those with parental responsibility consent to treatment on their behalf. With adults, there is no provision in English law for adults to act as legal proxies for other adults, although this is not so in other legal jurisdictions (e.g. Scotland). Ethically, since some people might not be motivated by protecting the best interests of their family members, relatives should not be asked to consent to proposed treatments. However, relatives should be asked their views about the wishes or concerns of the patient and consulted about medically relevant information which might be used to optimize the success of the patient's care. They should not be given the impression as a result of such consultation that it is they who are determining treatment decisions. Within the jurisdiction of English law, doctors and no-one else must decide what is and is not in the best clinical interests of patients. All forms of treatment can be administered to permanently incompetent adults on this basis.

FURTHER READING

British Medical Association (1999) *Confidentiality and the Disclosure of Health Information*. London: BMA.

British Medical Association (2001) *Consent, Rights, and Choices in Healthcare for Children and Young People*. London: BMJ Press.

Doyal L, Tobias J (eds) (2001) *Informed Consent in Medical Research*. London: BMJ Books.

General Medical Council (1998) *Seeking Patient's Consent: The Ethical Considerations*. London: GMC.

General Medical Council (2001) *Confidentiality: Protecting and Providing Information*. London: GMC.

Ethical and legal boundaries of the duty to protect life and health

Generally speaking, clinicians are professionally obligated to intervene to save the lives of patients for whom they have clinical responsibility. However, there are a range of circumstances where the duty of care to provide life-sustaining treatment is superseded by other ethical and legal responsibilities.

Competent refusal

The right of competent refusal supersedes the ordinary duty clinicians have to try to save the lives of such patients, along with any preferences others might have that they should be forced to accept treatment (Box 1.3). Patients may refuse life-sustaining treatment explicitly when it is offered or they may formulate an 'advance directive' which stipulates the circumstances under which they refuse it, should they become incompetent to do so in the future. Decisions not to provide life-sustaining treatment for competent patients (e.g. do not resuscitate (DNR) codes) should *not* be taken without their informed consent on the basis of clear information about the consequences of their refusal. Such patients may have arrangements which they need to make that their clinicians will know nothing about and it would be ethically wrong to pre-empt this.

The best interests of the incompetent

There will be some situations where the provision of life-sustaining treatment will not be regarded as being in the best interests of permanently incompetent patients, even though not providing it will lead to their death occurring before it otherwise would. This is when prolongation of patients' lives will be of no benefit to

---

> **Box 1.3**
>
> ### Competent refusal
>
> Prima facie every adult has the right and capacity to decide whether or not he will accept medical treatment, even if a refusal may risk permanent injury to his health or even lead to premature death. Furthermore, it matters not whether the reasons for the refusal were rational or irrational, unknown or even non-existent. This is so notwithstanding the very strong public interest in preserving the life and health of all citizens.
>
> *Re T* (adult: refusal of medical treatment) [1992]

---

them, against the background of their dire clinical circumstances. For example, it is acceptable not to use medical means to prolong the lives of patients when:

- it is believed on good evidence that further treatment will not save life
- patients are already imminently and irreversibly close to death
- patients are so permanently or irreversibly brain damaged that they are incapable of any future self-directed activity.

One ethical justification for the latter two provisions is that such patients have no further need for medical treatment because they have no further objective interest in continuing to live. Because of their clinical condition, they can no longer do or achieve anything in life. However, because of potential differences in moral and religious belief, decisions not to provide or continue life-sustaining treatment should always be made with as much consensus as possible among the clinical team responsible for the patient's care and people close to the patient who are consulted about their care.

Clinicians may decide not to prolong the lives of imminently dying and/or extremely brain-damaged patients for the legally acceptable reason that they are acting in the best interests of their patients to attempt to minimise their suffering rather than intending to kill them. To do the latter would be murder. Clearly, when contemplating not providing or withdrawing life-sustaining treatments, doctors should do their best to act within the law. However, it should also not be forgotten that much debate continues about whether or not there is a much closer ethical link between clinical decisions not to save life and decisions actively to end it. The law concerning such matters may change at some point in the future.

The duty as a doctor to be fair and just

The principle of equality of persons should dominate the way in which the duties of care are discharged in clinical practice. Clinicians may show technical mastery of treatment options and great ability and sensitivity in obtaining informed consent to treatment and maintaining confidentiality. However, if in the process of doing so, they actively discriminate against individual or groups of patients, they are still acting unprofessionally

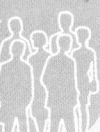

Box 1.4

The duty as a doctor to be fair and just

Injustice can occur in medicine through treating patients unequally according to (among others):

- race
- age
- fitness
- social worth
- class
- intelligence
- physical attractiveness
- profession
- parenthood.

---

and should be penalized accordingly. For example, discrimination on the basis of race, age, social worth, class, intelligence or occupation should not be tolerated (Box 1.4).

Scarce resources

As a matter of right, the National Health Service provides *equal* access to appropriate medical care on the basis of need alone. This right is mitigated by scarce resources and the courts have made it clear that they will not force Health Authorities or Trusts to provide treatments which are beyond their means. However, the courts also demand that decisions about such means must be made on reasonable grounds and that patients have a clear right to expect this. Thus on both ethical and legal grounds, prejudice or favouritism is not acceptable in the allocation of scarce resources. Where practically possible, resources should be allocated to patients on the basis of the similarity and extremity of their need (e.g. triage) and the time at which they presented themselves for treatment (e.g. the randomness imposed by the 'lottery of nature'). To the degree that this procedure of allocation is followed, all patients will be said to have had an equal opportunity to be treated on the basis of equal need. In the UK, the National Institute for Clinical Excellence (NICE) is a body set up to evaluate treatments on a clinical and cost effective basis, and to ensure equal access to care across the country. On both ethical and legal grounds, prejudice or favouritism is not acceptable in the allocation of scarce resources.

Lifestyle

Patients should not be denied potentially beneficial treatments on the grounds that their lifestyles have been more unhealthy than others with whom they compete for the same treatments. Patients are not equal in their abilities to lead healthy lives and to make correct healthcare choices for themselves. Some are better educated and informed, more emotionally confident and more supported by their social environment. To ignore this, to regard all patients as equal competitors and to reward the already better off is unjust and unfair.

FURTHER READING

British Medical Association (2001) *Withholding and Withdrawing Life-prolonging Medical Treatment*. London: BMJ Press.

Butler J (1999) *The Ethics of Health Care Rationing*. London: Cassell.

Harris J (1984) *The Value of Life*. London: Routledge.

GENERAL READING

Beauchamp T, Childress J (2001) *Principles of Biomedical Ethics*. New York: Oxford University Press.

Mason JK, McCall Smith RA (1999) *Law and Medical Ethics*. London: Butterworths.

Montgomery J (1997) *Health Care Law*. Oxford: Oxford University Press.

Parker M, Dickenson D (2001) *Medical Ethics Workbook*. Cambridge: Cambridge University Press.

Communication

Communication in healthcare

Communication is the way in which clinicians integrate clinical science with patient-centred, evidence-based, shared healthcare. It is the process of exchanging information and ideas and also making a trusting relationship upon which the collaborative partnership between patients and clinicians depends. In this chapter the word 'patient' is shorthand for the patient, the patient's family, work colleagues and whole social and environmental milieu while the term 'clinician' implies every sort of healthcare professional/multidisciplinary team.

Good communication is an absolute requirement for achieving best practice and outcome, giving patients the best experience of their illness. It is a major contributory factor to the personal and professional development and satisfaction of healthcare professionals themselves.

Failed communication adversely affects health and social outcomes, and the satisfaction of patients and clinicians. Unfortunately, poor communication is widespread in most healthcare systems and it is now recognized as a major healthcare issue.

Health outcomes

Effect of communication on biomedical care and its outcome

The best biomedical outcome obviously depends upon accurate diagnosis and appropriate treatment. Communication styles that are 'patient centred' provide a more complete clinical picture upon which diagnosis and treatment can be based and lead to improvement

Box 1.5

Communication improves health outcomes

Outcome improved with better communication
Symptom resolution
Psychological distress reduced
Health and functional status improved
Blood pressure control improved
Pain control improved
Patient anxiety reduced

From Stewart M (1995). Effective physician–patient communication and health outcomes: a review. *Canadian Medical Association Journal* **152**: 1423–1433.

Box 1.6

Failures of communication

Patients reported the following problems in interviews:

- 54% of their complaints were not elicited
- 45% of their concerns were not elicited
- 50% of psychological problems were not elicited
- In 50% of visits, patients and doctors disagreed on main presenting problem
- In 50% of cases, their history was blocked by interruption within 24 seconds.

Simpson M et al. (1991). The Toronto Consensus Statement. *British Medical Journal* **303**: 1385–1387.

Box 1.7

Problems identified as causing failure of adherence to clinical advice

In a random sample of 8303 patients from 66 hospitals in England and Wales:

- 22% reported that no named doctor was in charge of their care
- 64% reported that no named nurse was in charge of their care
- 20% reported that they were in pain all or most of the time
- 62% were not told on discharge when to resume their normal activities.

Bruster et al. (1994). National survey of patients. *British Medical Journal* **309**: 1542–1549.

Box 1.8

Factors in communication which improve patients' adherence to clinical advice

- Clinician understands the patient
- Clinician's tone of voice
- Clinician elicits all the patient's health concerns
- Patient is comfortable asking questions
- Patient perceives that sufficient time is spent with the clinician

Stewart M et al. (1999). Evidence on patient communication. *Cancer Prevention and Control* **3(i)**: 25–30.

in health outcomes (Box 1.5). Patients describe several consistent failures of communication (Box 1.6) which lead to an incomplete history and a poor professional relationship.

Adherence to treatment

Health outcomes also depend on the extent to which patients adhere to their clinical advice. Patients do not do so for many reasons (shown in Box 1.7). The correctable factors are all matters of communication: letting patients know why their treatment is being given and what benefits they stand to gain, what the pros and cons may be, what options exist, and doing so in a way which builds trust and collaboration. The annual economic cost of non-adherence to advice runs into many millions of pounds in the UK.

Social outcomes

Patient satisfaction is the result of their:

- knowing that they are getting the best appropriate biomedical healthcare
- knowing that they are being treated as individuals and not items on a conveyor belt
- being treated with humanity.

These are all strongly related to good communication (Box 1.8).

Satisfaction also affects psychological well-being and adherence to treatment, both of which have a knock-on effect on physical health outcomes.

Discord between patients and clinicians

Modern healthcare is carried out in a climate of consumerism and critical participation. With this has come an increasing number of complaints and lawsuits from what is nevertheless a small proportion of patients. The majority of complaints are not based on failures of biomedical practice but on poor communication (Box 1.9). In contrast, Box 1.10 shows the qualities that patients describe in interviews with primary care physicians who have never been sued.

Complaints and lawsuits, however, represent the tip of an iceberg. There is the widespread failure of even the most basic communication in hospital and general practice, at least in the UK in the middle 1990s. Box 1.9 shows the results of a very large study of what patients experience rather than their opinion of it. A very large proportion of patients were not provided with even basic civility let alone simple information about their future care.

The monetary costs of these failures of communication is enormous.

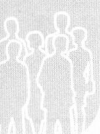

Clinician satisfaction

While staffing shortages and inadequate resources and facilities for biomedical care are commonly cited as causes of discontent amongst clinicians of all kinds, it is the quality of their relationships with their patients and colleagues which is the most reliable global indicator of clinician satisfaction and happiness. Healthcare professionals have a very high incidence of occupational morbidity, a major source of which is seen to be due to difficulties with personal relationships including the problem of clinician–patient relationships. The health of clinicians as well as their patients is closely connected with the development of skill, knowledge and above all attitude to communication.

The cost of loss of work, early retirement, healthcare for clinicians and poor performance is a further heavy burden on any health service.

In summary, the evidence for communication being central to healthcare is clear and the need for improved communication also. Communication is the individual responsibility of every healthcare practitioner; it cannot be delegated but fortunately it can be taught and learnt.

Poor communication between doctors and patients

Difficulties clinicians have in communicating with patients

Lack of knowledge

Clinicians usually concentrate on the biomedical model of clinical medicine rather than the psychosocial model, as they are often ignorant of the qualitative research on the latter. This can lead to major diagnostic and therapeutic errors, for example:

- numerous illnesses have physical symptoms without an organic basis
- physical illnesses are prolonged by psychological factors (p. 1232)
- 20% of medical patients have psychiatric disease (p. 1232).

Many clinicians 'know' that patients never remember what they are told so it is a waste of time giving them more than reassurance. The evidence is that patients' memory for even complicated matters is good if they are informed skilfully, as outlined on page 13.

Attitude

Clinicians who take an authoritarian role and have a negative attitude to shared care and multiprofessional teamwork tend to reveal themselves in their questioning styles and are unlikely to be self-critical of their communication skills even when they are shown the evidence of their poor performance.

Lack of skill

- *Time.* It takes coaching and practice to acquire the skill to integrate good communication into every interview and to make patients feel that they have had enough time devoted to them. Clinicians often see communication as desirable but too time-consuming. However, time skimped at a critical moment deprives the patient and involves someone else in more time later.
- *Uncomfortable topics and patients.* Lack of skill also leaves clinicians uneasy in certain difficult interviews, and Box 1.11 shows the different strategies patients notice clinicians use to avoid uncomfortable topics or 'difficult patients'. These strategies are largely the result of clinicians' fears and inadequate training. It is necessary for clinicians to find their own ways of managing patients who are widely found to be difficult.

Failure of empathy

One of the things which distinguishes the healthcare professions from others is that patients expect humanity from their doctors as well as competence. Clinicians provide this by demonstrating empathy (p. 13). This may require an effort to project from doctors who have never been ill themselves. It takes commitment as well

Box 1.11

Strategies which patients find their doctors use to distance themselves from their patients

Strategy	Example
Selective attention to cues	Chooses biomedical topics, avoids others
Normalizing	'Everyone feels that. Forget it.'
Premature reassurance	'I am sure everything will be OK.'
False reassurance	'Everything is OK.'
Switching the topic	'A headache? Tell me about your feet.'
Passing the buck	'Nurse will tell you all about that.'
Jollying along	'Worse things happen at sea.'
Physical avoidance	Waving but not stopping

Maguire P (2000). *Communication Skills for Doctors*. London: Arnold.

as skill to demonstrate empathy to a large number of similar patients in a morning.

Personal failures

Like anyone else, clinicians can be unhappy, short-tempered, rushed and interrupted, ignorant on some subjects, or charmless. But this is not the patients' problem and it is a professional obligation not to allow doctors' problems to affect a patient's experience or care.

Difficulties for patients in communicating with doctors

Inferiority

Patients commonly feel themselves to be in the weaker position in a medical interview. This may be exacerbated by their own problems or by their clinicians.

Anxiety and its consequences

Most patients are anxious to some extent and often try to hide it. Anxiety can make patients seem to regress in behaviour, mental power and memory. Free-floating anxiety may cause ideas which are worse than reality and contribute to complex misconceptions.

Misconceptions

Anxiety and medical ignorance can create misconceptions in patients' minds about their illnesses which in turn profoundly affect their symptoms and the ability to recover. Such misconceptions need detecting and uprooting, without which correct information will not register. Simple reassurance will not supplant a misconception.

Conflicting information

Apart from friends, family and the media, patients get varied information from many different healthcare professionals. These pieces of conflicting information are seldom recorded and in themselves help to contribute to misconceptions.

Forgetfulness

Patients, like most of us who are provided with numerous new and alarming facts, tend to forget all but a few, unless care is taken to aid their memory. This is compounded if they are told information in words they do not understand. However, if information is given carefully, 70–80% of the facts will be remembered by a patient after 6 weeks, or even indefinitely.

Disinclination to disclose their concerns

Patients may not disclose all their concerns if they feel nothing can be done, or they are wasting the doctors' time or fear being thought neurotic with non-physical problems. They are less likely to be forthcoming if their first questions are blocked or answered incomprehensibly, if they fear their effective treatment may be withdrawn, if they are distracted or distressed, or if they do not like or trust their doctor.

Impaired faculties of communication

Patients with impaired hearing or speech or vision or mental function or whose clinician does not speak their language all experience substandard healthcare as a direct result of their inability to communicate.

One in five medical patients have psychiatric illnesses, diagnosed or otherwise, which may affect their ability or inclination to communicate.

FURTHER READING

Lewin B (1995) The place of psychological therapies in coronary artery disease. In: *Psychiatric Aspects of Physical Disorder*. London: Royal College of Physicians/Royal College of Psychiatrists.

Maguire P (2000) *Communication Skills for Doctors*. London: Arnold.

Simpson M et al. (1991) The Toronto Consensus Statement. *British Medical Journal* **303**: 1385–1387.

Stewart M et al. (2000) The impact of patient-centred care on outcomes. *Journal of Family Practice* **49**: 796–804.

The medical interview

Clinicians conduct about 200 000 interviews during their careers. Such interviews often provide more critical information than do clinical tests and they also form the basis of the relationship which leads to collaborative partnership with their patients.

There is no single prescription for a medical interview because each patient is different, but well-researched guiding principles and well-coached skills will allow clinicians to use their time to the greatest benefit of their patients.

Box 1.12

The three phases of an interview

Opening
Exploring and focusing } During which the clinician will { Engage
Closing } { Empathize
{ Educate
{ Enlist

Table 1.1
Components of a medical interview

The nature of the key problems
Clarification of these problems
Date and time of onset
Development over time
Precipitating factors
Help given to-date
Impact of the problem on patient's life
Availability of support
Patient's ideas and fears
Patient's attitude to similar problems in others
Screening question

The overriding principle is to find out not only the medical facts in detail, but what patients have experienced and what impact this experience has had upon them. This information is essential to expand the diagnosis and recommend appropriate action and also to gain the confidence, the trust and the compliance of the patient.

The example below is in the context of a first medical interview in a consulting room. Obviously this is different from a follow-up interview, or an emergency.

It is helpful to regard the interview in three phases (Box 1.12).

Opening

The start of the interview will be helped by well-organized arrangements for appointments, reception and punctuality. If possible, the clinician should come out of the room to greet each patient. Otherwise it is polite to rise, look at the patient, establish eye contact and shake hands if appropriate. Greet them and find out the way the patient prefers to be addressed. The patient sits beside the clinician, not on the far side of a desk. The clinician sits in a posture which conveys attention and friendliness. Clinicians should introduce themselves indicating a name badge and their status and responsibility to the patient. On no account should the patient be undressed before the first meeting.

First impressions are critical. The patients' non-verbal cues indicate their emotional state, and the main influences on the emotional tone of the interview are the clinicians' own non-verbal messages, facial expression, body language and unspoken attitudes.

Start by discovering what the patient expects from the interview and indicate how long it will last.

Exploring and focusing

Taking a full history

The components of a complete history are shown in Table 1.1. A clear factual account of the biomedical details is, of course, essential, but is in itself not enough. The order of taking a history is not prescribed, for example many experienced clinicians begin with the social history: 'To start with, can you tell me something about yourself?'.

Listening skills and questioning styles

Questioning style determines whether the clinician or the patient talks more. The clinician will obtain more information by starting with open questions, letting the patients speak more than they do, then guiding the history by using closed questions for further detail, than if they occupy most of the time in asking closed questions of their own (Box 1.13). The aim is to obtain all the patients' concerns, remembering that they usually have at least three (range 1–12). Only then can the topics be prioritized, balancing the patients' concerns with the clinician's main points of interest.

It is a failure of opening and engaging the patient if an important point is raised only as the patient has a hand on the door knob, preparing to leave.

Facilitating the patient

If the clinician sits in complete silence, the patient will flounder and lose confidence. The patient will be helped by some eye contact or a smile to show that the clinician is listening attentively. Reflecting questions (see Box 1.13) guide the history, allowing the clinician to take up unexpected points as they arise or expand topics, without interrupting the patient. As the history unfolds, detail can be brought into focus by using screening and closed questions.

Leading questions may be helpful but they should not end in the rhetorical 'isn't it?', 'wouldn't it?' challenge

---

Box 1.13

Questioning style

Question	Example
Open question	'What has brought you to see me today?'
Open screening question	'Is there anything else you want to tell me?'
Open directive question	'How did the treatment for your headache go?'
Reflecting question	'Could you tell me a bit more about that?'
Closed question	'What date exactly did the headache start?'
Rhetorical leading question	'The headache has got better on my treatment hasn't it?'

which makes the question difficult to discuss even when it is completely wrong. They are a major cause of misunderstanding and are difficult for the patient to contradict even when they are completely wrong.

Ideas and fears and their validation

While the clinician may be mainly interested in the biomedical facts, patients usually seek help because of their own interpretation of their condition. Patients need to know that these ideas have been heard and acknowledged and are henceforth incorporated in their clinician's interpretation of their complaints. Otherwise the patient may tend to believe that the clinician has not got things right, which increases the risk of the patient not adhering to the recommendations that follow. So hearing these ideas and then acknowledging them, i.e. *validating* them, is an essential step in engaging a patient's trust, and beginning to 'treat the whole patient'.

Empathy

Empathy has been described as 'imagination for others'. An empathic response is one which demonstrates a genuine interest in patients' experiences. This is a key skill in building the patient–clinician relationship and is highly therapeutic. Like other communication skills, it can be taught and learnt and it cannot be counterfeited by a repertoire of routine mannerisms.

Techniques which demonstrate empathy are:

- seeing, hearing and accepting patients as they are – illustrated in Box 1.14
- acknowledging facial and bodily expressions, mode of dress and notable physical characteristics
- avoiding physical barriers; sitting or standing at the same level without objects between
- reflecting what the patient is feeling as they talk and what the patient sees as important and what the patient may be thinking
- using the patient's own words and ideas
- letting the patient correct any misunderstanding that arises
- using appropriate self-disclosure without capping the patient's story
- evaluating behaviour, not judging the person.

Giving information – educating the patient

When information is given skilfully, patients are able to understand what is said, to remember it and to find it helpful. Patients are more likely to adhere to clinical advice if they get comprehensible information, if it makes sense of their problems and if they can get easy access to more if they need it. The whole point of giving information is to allow patients to understand their problem and use their information to help themselves. This aspect of patient partnership is a keystone of modern medical practice.

One study of junior doctors showed that they gave information poorly because they lacked both clear objectives and a systematic technique of giving information.

There is a large amount of research to show that:

- Information must be related not only to the biomedical facts, but to the patients' ideas about their condition.
- While most patients are voracious for information, this is not invariably the case, particularly when the information is sensitive or threatening. The pacing of information is discussed further in 'Breaking bad news' on page 14.
- Most patients will understand and recall 70–80% of even the most unfamiliar, complex or alarming information if it is provided along the following guidelines:
  (a) Use a logical sequence to explain the cause and effect of the condition in the context of the patient's symptoms. (Be proactive about explaining causes; patients always want to know.)
  (b) Talk about one thing at a time and check that the patient understands before you move on to the next.
  (c) Use simple language; translate any unavoidable medical terms and write them down.
  (d) Make your information and instructions direct, detailed and concrete.
  (e) At the outset show patients that you will write down the key words, use a simple diagram, and can offer them other aids to memory as shown in Box 1.15. Otherwise, patients may be alarmed

---

Box 1.14

Demonstrating empathy by showing the patient that their experiences are recognized and accepted

Demonstration	Questioning style
The patient experiences being seen	'That last point made you look worried. Is there something more serious about that point you would like to tell me?'
The patient experiences being heard	'I notice that you have talked about the death of your mother but could I ask you to tell me something about how your brother died?'
The patient experiences being accepted	'I can tell you that most people in your circumstances get angry at some point, even with the people who have helped them.'
The clinician shows self-disclosure	'I'm a bit like you. Whenever I get heartburn I think it's a heart attack.'

Box 1.15

Possible aids to giving information

Method	Example
Write it down ⎫	As you go – make a copy for
Use a diagram ⎬	your records
Send the patient a	With a patient's paragraph
copy of your report	as a routine
Make an audio tape	Desk-top recorder £20; tapes
	50p each
Use prepared information	Leaflets, audio or video
Provide address of support	BACUP for cancer patients
organization	NHS Direct for help of all
	kinds. Tel: 0845 4647
Provide a website reference	Patient UK: www.patient.co.uk

---

to find that they are forgetting half of what you say, perhaps distracted by some of the earlier information. Write out the risks of operations for patients, which tend to be rapidly forgotten after operations, however well understood before.

(f) For the numerous patients who need more information than you can provide in the time, give them prepared information, or a source of it.

(g) Do not be exasperated when patients refer to the Internet; have a useful web-site reference ready and written out.

Negotiating the next steps – enlisting the patient's collaboration

To achieve optimum adherence, the clinician's suggestions about diagnosis or treatment must be negotiated with the patient. This requires an explanation of the benefits and disadvantages and the risks of these suggestions and any alternatives, all with the aim of enlisting patients to take an active part in their own care.

Patients adhere to suggestions about investigation and treatment when they are thus enlisted as partners as a result of:

- a frank exchange of information
- a negotiation of options
- involving the patient in decisions.

Summarizing

Any possible misunderstanding will be greatly reduced if a brief summary is made first of the patient's agenda and then of that of the clinician. This may include matters which have had to be postponed to a further interview, and certainly should include the arrangements for any such interview or the commitment to informing other healthcare professionals involved with the patient. It is good practice to make a note at this point of what the patient has been told and what has been understood.

Closing

Any human contact ends with an appropriate farewell, not forgetting some words of encouragement.

FURTHER READING

Bedell SE et al. (2001) The doctor's letter of condolence. *New England Journal of Medicine* **344**: 1162–1163.

Keller V (1994) A new model for physician–patient communication. *Patient Education and Counselling* **23**: 131–140.

Silverman J et al. (1998) *Skills for Communicating with Patients*. London: Radcliffe Press.

Interviews in which difficulties in communication can be expected

Some interviews are bound to be difficult for patients or doctors or both. Usually this is because they have a high emotional content – frightening, painful or embarrassing – and there is no straightforward medical solution. So clinicians have to rely on their personal qualities to an extent which their training may not have prepared them for.

The four commonest subjects requested on communication courses for doctors reflect problems commonly reported by patients:

- Breaking bad news
- Complaints and lawsuits
- Cultural differences
- Patients with impaired faculties for communication.

These are discussed below.

Other popular topics are: hostility and anger, difficult patients and colleagues, taking a sexual history, and eliciting a psychiatric history, which is discussed in detail on page 1226.

The techniques of explaining risk and informed consent are seldom requested even though they are the commonest examination subjects.

These are all interviews in which, patients find, many clinicians exhibit the distancing strategies listed in Box 1.11. Every clinician has a professional responsibility to recognize which interviews they find difficult and to overcome their shortcomings. Otherwise they will make difficult matters even worse for their patients than they need be.

The basic principles of the medical interview described above hold good for all of the above examples but certain details may need to be emphasized.

Breaking bad news

Bad news is any information which is likely to alter drastically a patient's view of the future. It is one of the most potent causes of distress and of complaints and lawsuits.

This may be difficult because:

- bad news usually means that biomedical measures cannot help, so the clinician's familiar basis of experience and authority is irrelevant
- the clinician is upset as well
- the patient can be expected to be upset, behave unpredictably and require emotional support which may be beyond what the clinician can give
- the patient may blame the clinician, and indeed there may be an element of medical mishap to complicate matters
- the clinician may have had little experience (being ushered out during training) or have had bad previous experiences and no help subsequently.

Breaking bad news is a professional skill which is acquired by practice under supervision. It should give a clinician confidence and satisfaction rather than alarm, although it can never be painless.

The way that bad news is broken has a major psychological and physical effect upon patients. For example, the main predictive factor for patients developing full-blown psychiatric disorders on learning of the diagnosis of cancer depends upon the way their bad news is broken. Likewise the memories and well-being of the relatives now and later depends on the way that the subject is introduced. The rehabilitation of patients after acute coronary events depends, damage for damage, on the way in which the news is broken and patients' ideas about it are educated.

The patient's relatives may ask that bad news is withheld from the patient. The information, however, does not belong to the relatives and the evidence is clear that patients:

- usually know more than anyone has guessed
- may imagine things to be worse than they are
- welcome clear information even about the worst news
- welcome the liberty to speak as they wish about their illness and their future rather than join in a charade of deception decided by others
- differ in how much they can take at a time.

The interview

The basic clinical interview described above is adjusted by particular attention to certain points:

Opening

- The patient is seen as soon as possible once the current information has been gathered.
- If possible, the patient should have someone with them.
- The interview should take place with everyone introduced, sitting in a quiet place.

- Clinicians must indicate their status and the extent of their responsibility toward the patient and the amount of time available.

Exploring and focusing

- The clinician should find out if anything new has happened since the last encounter.
- What does the patient know and how does the patient react to it? In detail.
- The clinician should then give the patient a warning that the news is bad: 'I'm afraid it looks more serious than we hoped.'
- At this point the clinician should pause and allow the patient to think this over and only continue when the patient gives some lead to follow. This pause may be a long one while thoughts go round in the patient's head and is often accompanied by shutdown which makes patients unable to hear anything further until these thoughts settle down and allow them to re-emerge.

The clinician should then:

- Discover how much the patient is likely to be able to take in at this point – methods for finding this out are shown in Table 1.2.
- Give the information without fudging, in small chunks and make sure that the patient understands each one before moving on.
- Be prepared for the patient to have disorderly emotional responses of some kind and acknowledge them early on as being what you expect and understand and wait for them to settle before continuing. The clinician must learn to judge which patients wish to be touched and which do not.
- Watch out for shutdown; when it occurs, just wait. When the patient emerges it is best to deal with what they then say, and only after that take up the clinical agenda again.
- Keep pausing to allow the patient to think.
- Stop the interview if necessary and arrange to resume later.

Focusing on planning and support

- The clinician can emphasize that some things are fixable and others are not. A broad time frame can be given for the fixable aspects of care.
- No time frame is ever accurate for the unfixable, but the clinician must be prepared for the question: 'How long have I got?' and avoid the trap of providing a figure which is bound to be inaccurate. Rather stress the importance of ensuring that the quality of life is made as good as possible from day to day.
- The patient must be provided with some positive information and hope tempered with realism.

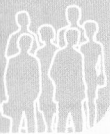
Table 1.2
Two ways to find out how much a patient in an oncology clinic wants to know

Buckman (Canada)	An open screening question: 'If this condition turns out to be something serious are you the type of person who likes to know exactly what is going on?'
Sanson–Fisher (Australia)	Explicit categorization by direct questions in succession: 'If you would like to know, I will tell you … 1. What the diagnosis is' 2. What the treatment will be' 3. What sort of symptoms you will have' 4. What examinations and tests will be necessary' 5. What can be done for any physical discomfort or pain you may have' 6. What the outcome might be.'

Buckman R (1994) *How to Break Bad News*. London, Papermac
Reynolds PM, Sansom-Fisher RW et al (1981) Cancer and Communication. *British Medical Journal* 282: 1449–1451.

Closing
The clinician must be sure that:

- the patient has understood what has been discussed so far
- the patient knows how to contact the appropriate team member and thus has a safety net in place
- the next interview date – preferably soon – has been agreed and for what purpose
- other members of the family have been invited to meet the clinicians as the patient wishes
- written material and further sources of information are readily available
- everyone is bid goodbye, starting with the patient.

After the bad news is broken
Patients who are facing the loss of life, limb or liberty can be expected to have many questions that are difficult to answer and to exhibit their own pattern of the disorderly emotions summarized in Table 1.3. The way questions are answered and emotions are empathically treated has a major long-term effect on patients and clinicians alike.

Patients want to know if they are going to die and if so when? Will they be able to stay at home? Will they be in pain? Patients facing the end of life have different priorities from the clinicians, and need clear information about their pain and symptom control, the extent to

Table 1.3
Emotional responses to the fact or threat of loss: some or all of these can be expected but in no particular pattern

Despair
Denial
Anger
Bargaining
Depression
Acceptance

Kubler Ross E 1970 *On Death and Dying*. New York: Macmillan

which they can influence this and how long active treatment will continue. Settling family matters and completing unfinished business come high on their agenda, and must be reconciled with attempts at palliation or treatment, particularly if these are of uncertain benefit. It is the clinician's responsibility to mediate between the patient, other medical staff and the patients' relatives.

Even if there is no medical solution, the clinician has a valuable role at this stage as an empathic experienced professional who can help the patient in many ways.

Dealing with adversity

Complaints and lawsuits
Unfortunately adversity is as unavoidable in healthcare as it is in life. However, hardworking clinicians doing their best do not always respond appropriately to adverse criticism of any kind. They tend not to deal effectively with grumbles and complaints at the appropriate time, which is as soon as they are made, but use avoiding strategies as for other forms of difficulty (Box 1.11).

In a recent national survey of patients' complaints, the two main recommendations were that all healthcare professionals should have training in communication and should be aware of their responsibility for dealing promptly with complaints made by patients in their care and not to involve managers or complaints officers immediately; even more so when patients have suffered the results of a mistake or a mishap.

Complaints
The majority of complaints come from the exasperation of patients who:

- have not been able to get clear information
- feel that they are owed an apology
- are concerned that other patients will go through what they have.

Many complaints are resolved satisfactorily once these points are satisfied. Clinicians should not take criticism as a personal affront but respond professionally by providing the information that patients need, not just by a defence or a medical account but in answer to the specific questions. A personal apology is, as medical defence organizations emphasize, not an expression of guilt; it is a common courtesy. Nor should it be wrapped up so cautiously as to become a worthless token.

Clinicians should work in a professional culture which regards complaints as a valuable source of feedback which deserve to be noted, collected systematically and acted upon if need be. The constructive use of complaints is built into the concept of patient involvement in achieving quality in healthcare.

When clinicians learn of a complaint they should:

- be objective, not resentful or defensive – remember that there is a duty of care to the patient in this as every way
- allow all the facts to speak through a clear account, verbal or written
- explain the reasons and circumstances behind the facts
- express regret
- explain how the things will improve
- remember that the patient is still a patient
- leave the medical records strictly unaltered.

Lawsuits

Lawsuits, an extreme form of complaint, are commonly rooted in poor communication arising from:

- misinformation which comes from unclear language and medical jargon
- different words being used by the large number of different healthcare professionals that many patients see
- no clear explanation being given to patients as situations change or when they are discharged
- misunderstanding of the medical records
- failure to provide adequate information during consent procedures.

The difficulty of unravelling these issues is usually complicated by the absence of any record of what the patient was told.

The communication styles which distinguish clinicians who have never been sued (shown in Box 1.10) can help to prevent these frustrations.

A lawsuit is the ultimately wasteful and damaging way of resolving these serious failures of communication. As in complaints procedures, many patients abandon a lawsuit when they get a clear exposition of the facts which they can see explains their circumstances; something which could usually have been provided long before and should not have arisen in the first place.

Certain points should be borne in mind when writing in response to a complaint or a court.

It is for the use of the tribunal (the judge in effect) and not just for representatives of one side. Therefore, the report should be the same regardless of whether the clinician is instructed by the plaintive or the defence.

Writing a legal report is complex and the clinician who takes on the work of expert witness would be well advised to seek training in the preparation of reports, court procedure and cross-examination. Training is best provided by the firms of solicitors which specialize in this work. Without preparation, the clinician risks failing the court and having a bruising experience.

Patients with impaired faculties for communication

All healthcare professionals need to exert particular patience and ingenuity, and acquire some special knowledge, when communicating with certain patients with impaired faculties for communication.

Patients with limited understanding or speech. With certain patients, for example with organic brain disease or severe mental disease, clinicians require energy and imagination to make the best of the limited lines of communication. Open questions are often impossible for them; open directive questions have to be adjusted to the ability of each patient together with every non-verbal gesture, mime or murmur that can help. Just as much ingenuity may be called upon to confirm the meaning of the responses. Third parties involved in the care of the patient can help. Much can be learnt by watching a specialized speech therapist at work.

Patients with impaired hearing. Patients with severely impaired hearing may be accompanied by a signer in one of the two sign languages. Deaf patients who do not use signing are helped by several factors shown in Table 1.4, many of which would not occur to the uninformed.

It is a help for deaf patients to have access to a Minicom – a telephone adapted for the deaf.

Table 1.4

Dos and don'ts of communicating with people who are deaf or hard of hearing (from RAD – Royal Association in Aid of Deaf People)

Smile and use eye contact

If you are stuck write it down

Speak normally, don't mouth slowly

Put your face in a good light

Stay still and don't put things in your mouth

Trim moustaches and beards, avoid sunglasses, big earrings or background activity

Never say 'forget it'

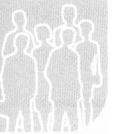

Patients whose doctors do not share their cultural background. Patients who do not have the language of their host country or their doctor suffer poor healthcare relative to their socio-economic status. When such patients depend upon a third party in the form of an interpreter, clinicians must remember to talk to the patient, and not to the interpreter or other third parties to avoid marginalizing the patient and missing what non-verbal communication occurs. Clinicians should also be aware of certain taboos concerning shaking hands, eye contact or topics that cannot be discussed, for example with unmarried women. It is difficult to produce prepared written material for every ethnic group, particularly when these change rapidly. However, members of the patient's community may be able to find appropriate material on the Internet or acquire it otherwise. Another source of help would be a fellow healthcare professional from the same cultural background.

The role of third parties. It has been suggested that all patients are in need of a third party advocate to help them through the foreign language and culture of healthcare. 'I speak perfect English, but I don't speak Biology.'

Patients in all three of the above groups often depend on third parties either for their care or as interpreters, as do very many other patients, particularly at the extremes of life.

With the best of intentions third parties may take over the patients in their care, reading their minds and taking responsibility for them. Whether the patient is with a carer, a relative, another doctor or an interpreter, the clinician should if possible speak to the patient and not to the third party and make a distinction between what is a straight translation and what is the contribution of the third party. However, third parties also deserve respect; paediatricians have often been found to communicate more considerately with children than with the parents, and the army of carers who look after the disabled are often disregarded by the professionals and family members who may know their charges much less well.

FURTHER READING

Littlewood R, Lipsedge M (1997) *Aliens and Alienists*, 3rd edn. London: Routledge.
Silverman J et al. (1998) *Skills for Communicating with Patients*. London: Radcliffe Press.

Improving communication

In the UK, improving communication is a stated objective in the policy statement of every national, governmental, professional and academic body concerned with healthcare, particularly in respect of increasing the extent to which patients take part in their own healthcare and its management and reducing the wastage of resources from complaints and nonadherence to treatment.

Most UK institutions which offer undergraduate and postgraduate diplomas to healthcare professionals now teach and examine the communication skills of the candidates. Such efforts, however, do not bear fruit in every graduate and those who graduated over 10 years ago did not have communication on the syllabus and do not necessarily regard patient-centred communication as an obligation or even a serious subject.

The challenge to the professional bodies and to healthcare management equally is:

- to provide facilities, time, resources and trained personnel to develop and support good communication practice in every healthcare professional
- at the same time to motivate healthcare professionals in communication
- to provide patients with accurate accessible information
- to organize systematic regular feedback from patients and the community and respond to the evidence therefrom.

This requires consistent and persistent strategic initiative, an effective programme for change management, and the capacity to provide the individual coaching that is needed to change the performance of individuals. In this sort of strategy it is the peer pressure of senior and influential professionals which has the greatest influence.

Improving communication in individuals

However individuals may be motivated to take these matters up, there are certain basic factors which contribute to improving communication skills:

- Having clear objectives about the work, the nature of communication and medical interviews and how the basic interview can be adapted to all others.
- Teaching in small groups of learners who get to know each other, all of whom go through the same process. This allows each member to reveal difficulties and weaknesses and to discuss and improve them comfortably.
- Experiential methods are needed; learning by doing it, not by reading the manual.
- Role-play is one cornerstone of learning communication skill – role-play with experienced simulated patients rather than amateur role-players selected from the group.
- Discussion of each simulated consultation is carried out along pre-decided rules of feedback, designed to explore what has happened; working from the strengths of the learner towards weaknesses; among

friendly, discreet and equally vulnerable colleagues. Learning from feedback can be enhanced by using a video-recording of the process.

- A few hours' work can only raise awareness. A new skill needs to be practised at least three times and often more before it will stick. Improvement in performance requires coaching until the skill is established, and like any other human activity communication skills need to be exercised regularly.

Teaching the teachers

Widespread improvement in communication will require a lot more teachers and well-motivated learners.

The best way of motivating and supporting such teachers has yet to be determined, and the resources for replacing their time will need to be found. At the moment the majority of substantive communication teachers are fully occupied, and many of the volunteer clinical faculty teach in spare time. Nevertheless, peer pressure from clinician teachers is essential to get the subject into everyday discussion as a matter of course, treated with the same respect that the details of biomedical care have long enjoyed.

Research

One reason that many clinicians do not know the results of research on communication is that the qualitative and meta-analytic methods used are unfamiliar and are dispersed in non-clinical literature.

Qualitative research seeks to ask broad questions concerning social phenomena in a natural rather than an experimental setting; questions about the meaning, the experience, the views and values of healthcare issues to all participants.

The methods used – observation, in-depth interviews, focus groups and detailed case studies – are complementary rather than antithetical to quantitative research. They are designed to answer the questions that quantitative research cannot reach. For example, while quantitative research demonstrates the dangers of smoking, qualitative research examines what makes people stop or continue smoking.

Many questions on communication issues remain to be answered:

- What are the most effective methods of practice and teaching?
- How can clinicians become more self-aware and why do they resist learning communication skills?
- How can clinicians get fast personal feedback?
- To what extent does improved communication influence outcome?
- How can cost–benefit calculations be made in communication practice and how can these best be explained to hard-pressed managers?

When all is said, at least it should be possible to show that investment in good communication will pay for itself.

FURTHER READING

Pope C et al. (1995) Reaching the parts other methods cannot reach: an introduction to qualitative methods in health and health services research. *British Medical Journal* **31**: 42–51.

GENERAL READING

Audit Commission of the UK (1993) *What seems to be the matter? Communication Between Hospital and Patients.* London: HMSO.

Di Blasiz Z et al. (2001) Influence of context effects on health outcomes: a systematic review. *Lancet* **357**: 757–762.

Royal College of Physicians of London (1997) *Improving Communications Between Doctors and Patients.* Royal College of Physicians of London.

The NHS Plan: A Plan for Investment. A Plan for Reform. (July 2000) London: The Stationery Office.

Infectious diseases, tropical medicine and sexually transmitted diseases

Infection and infectious disease

The world is full of microorganisms, the vast majority of which are harmless to man, and many of which are essential to life. Some of these organisms live on or within human hosts: most of these form part of our normal flora and are benign passengers or symbiotes. A minority, however, are pathogenic, causing illness or even death to their host. It is these viruses, bacteria, protozoa, and worms which are responsible for the infectious diseases.

Infection remains the main cause of morbidity and mortality in man, particularly in underdeveloped areas where it is associated with poverty and overcrowding. In the developed world increasing prosperity, universal immunization and antibiotics have reduced the prevalence of infectious disease. However, antibiotic-resistant strains of bacteria as well as viruses and 'new' diseases such as human immunodeficiency virus (HIV) infection and variant Creutzfeldt–Jakob disease (vCJD) have emerged. Increased global mobility has aided the spread of infectious disease and allowed previously localized pathogens to establish themselves world-wide. Deteriorating social conditions in the inner city areas of our major conurbations have facilitated the resurgence of tuberculosis and other infections. Changes in farming and food-processing methods have contributed to an increase in the incidence of food- and water-borne diseases.

In the developing world successes such as the eradication of smallpox have been balanced or outweighed by the new plagues. Infectious diseases cause nearly 25% of all human deaths (Table 2.1). Two billion people – one-third of the world's population – are infected with

Table 2.1
World-wide mortality from infectious diseases

Disease	Estimated deaths (in 1998)
Acute lower respiratory infection	3.5 million
HIV/AIDS	2.25 million
Diarrhoeal disease	2.25 million
Tuberculosis	1.5 million
Malaria	1.1 million
Measles	888 000
Tetanus	410 000
Whooping cough	350 000
Meningitis	143 000
Leishmaniasis	42 000

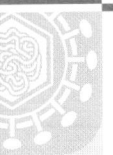

tuberculosis, 250–300 million people catch malaria every year, and 200 million are infected with schistosomiasis. Infections are often multiple, and there is synergy both between different infections, and between infection and other factors such as malnutrition. Many of the infectious diseases affecting developing countries are preventable or treatable, but continue to thrive owing to lack of money and political will.

Infectious agents

The causative agents of infectious diseases can be divided into four groups.

Prions are the most recently-recognized and the simplest infectious agents, consisting of a single protein molecule. They contain no nucleic acid and therefore no genetic information: their ability to propagate within a host relies on inducing the conversion of endogenous protein into prion protein.

Viruses contain both protein and nucleic acid, and so carry the genetic information for their own reproduction. However, they lack the apparatus to replicate autonomously, relying instead on 'hijacking' the cellular machinery of the host. They are small (usually less than 200 nanometres in diameter) and each virus possesses only one species of nucleic acid (either RNA or DNA).

Bacteria are usually, though not always, larger than viruses. Unlike the latter they have both DNA and RNA, with the genome encoded by DNA. They are enclosed by a cell membrane, and even bacteria which have adopted an intracellular existence remain enclosed within their own cell wall. Bacteria are capable of fully autonomous reproduction, and the majority are not dependent on host cells.

Eukaryotes are the most sophisticated infectious organisms, displaying sub-cellular compartmentalization. Different cellular functions are restricted to specific organelles, e.g. photosynthesis takes place in the chloroplasts, DNA transcription in the nucleus and respiration in the mitochondria. Eukaryotic pathogens include unicellular protozoa, fungi (which can be unicellular or filamentous), and multicellular parasitic worms.

Other higher classes, notably the insects and the arachnids, also contain species which can parasitize man and cause disease: these are discussed in more detail on page 120.

Host/organism interactions

Each of us is colonized with huge numbers of microorganisms (10^{14} bacteria, plus viruses, fungi, protozoa, and worms) with which we coexist. The relationship with some of these organisms is symbiotic, in which both partners benefit, while others are commensals, living on the host without causing harm. Infection and illness may be due to these normally harmless commensals and symbiotes evading the body's defences and penetrating into abnormal sites. Alternatively, disease may be caused by exposure to exogenous pathogenic organisms which are not part of our normal flora.

The symptoms and signs of infection are a result of the interaction between host and pathogen. In some cases, such as the early stages of influenza, symptoms are almost entirely due to killing of host cells by the invading organism. Usually, however, the harmful effects of infection are due to a combination of direct microbial pathogenicity, and the body's response to infection. In meningococcal septicaemia, for example, much of the tissue damage is caused by cytokines released in an attempt to fight the bacteria. In a few instances, such as chronic South American trypanosomiasis (Chagas' disease), morbidity is almost entirely immunological, with the parasite itself having little effect once the inflammatory process has been triggered. The molecular mechanisms underlying host–pathogen interactions are discussed in more detail on page 192.

Sources of infection

The endogenous skin and bowel commensals can cause disease in the host, either because they have been transferred to an inappropriate site (e.g. bowel coliforms causing urinary tract infection), or because host immunity has been attenuated (e.g. candidiasis in an immunocompromised host). Many infections are acquired from other people, who may be symptomatic themselves or be asymptomatic carriers. Some bacteria, like the meningococcus, are common transient commensals, but cause invasive disease in a small minority of those colonized. Infection with other organisms, such as the hepatitis B virus, can be followed in some cases by an asymptomatic but potentially infectious carrier state.

Zoonoses are infections that can be transmitted from wild or domestic animals to man. Infection can be acquired in a number of ways: direct contact with the animal, ingestion of meat or animal products, contact with animal urine or faeces, aerosol inhalation, via an arthropod vector, or by inoculation of saliva in a bite wound. Many zoonoses can also be transmitted from person to person. Some zoonoses are listed in Table 2.2.

Most microorganisms do not have a vertebrate or arthropod host but are free-living in the environment. The vast majority of these environmental organisms are non-pathogenic, but a few can cause human disease (Table 2.3). Person-to-person transmission of these infections is rare. Some parasites may have a stage of their life cycle which is environmental (for example the free-living larval stage of *Strongyloides stercoralis* and the hookworms) even though the adult worm requires a vertebrate host. Other pathogens can survive for periods in water or soil and may be transmitted from host to host via this route (see below): these should not be confused with true environmental organisms.

Table 2.2
Zoonotic infections

Disease	Pathogen	Animal reservoir	Mode of transmission
Prions			
vCJD	Prion protein	Cattle	Ingestion (CNS tissue)
Viral			
Lassa fever	Arenavirus	Multimammate rat	Direct contact
Japanese encephalitis	Flavivirus	Pigs	Mosquito bite
Rabies	Rhabdovirus	Dog and other mammals	Saliva, faeces (bats)
Yellow fever	Flavivirus	Primates	Mosquito bite
Bacterial			
	Escherichia coli 0157	Cattle, chickens	Ingestion (meat)
	Salmonella enteritidis and others	Chickens, cattle	Ingestion (meat, eggs)
Gastroenteritis	*Campylobacter jejuni*	Various	Ingestion (meat, milk, water)
Leptospirosis	*Leptospira icterohaemorrhagiae* and others	Rodents	Ingestion (urine)
Brucellosis	*Brucella abortus*	Cattle	Contact; ingestion of
	Brucella melitensis	Sheep, goats	milk/cheese
Anthrax	*Bacillus anthracis*	Cattle, sheep	Contact; ingestion
Lyme disease	*Borrelia burgdorferi*	Deer	Tick bite
Cat scratch fever	*Bartonella henselae*	Cats	Flea bite
Plague	*Yersinia pestis*	Rodents	Flea bite
Typhus	Various *Rickettsia* spp.	Various	Arthropod bite
Psittacosis (ornithosis)	*Chlamydia psittaci*	Psittacine and other birds	Aerosol
Others			
Toxoplasmosis	*Toxoplasma gondii*	Cats and other mammals	Ingestion (meat, faeces)
Cryptosporidiosis	*Cryptosporidium parvum*	Cattle	Ingestion (faeces)
Hydatid disease	*Echinococcus granulosus*	Dogs	Ingestion (faeces)
Cutaneous larva migrans	*Ancylostoma caninum*	Dogs	Penetration of skin by larvae

vCJD, variant Creutzfeldt–Jakob disease

Table 2.3
Environmental organisms which can cause human infection

Organism	Disease (most common presentations)
Bacteria	
Burkholderia pseudomallei	Melioidosis
Burkholderia cepacia	Lung infection in cystic fibrosis
Pseudomonas spp.	Various
Legionella pneumophila	Legionnaires' disease (pneumonia)
Bacillus cereus	Gastroenteritis
Listeria monocytogenes	Various
Clostridium tetani	Tetanus
Clostridium perfringens	Gangrene, septicaemia
Mycobacteria other than tuberculosis (MOTT)	Pulmonary infections
Fungi	
Candida sp.	Local and disseminated infection
Cryptococcus neoformans	Meningitis, pulmonary infection
Histoplasma capsulatum	Pulmonary infection
Coccidioides immitis	Pulmonary infection
Mucor spp.	Mucormycosis (rhinocerebral, cutaneous)
Sporothrix schenkii	Lymphocutaneous sporotrichosis
Blastomyces dermatitidis	Pulmonary infection
Aspergillus fumigatus	Pulmonary infection

Routes of transmission

Endogenous infection

The body's own endogenous flora can cause infection if the organism gains access to an inappropriate area of the body. This can happen by simple mechanical transfer, for example colonic bacteria entering the female urinary tract. The non-specific host defences may be breached, for example by cutting or scratching the skin and allowing surface commensals to gain access to deeper tissues; this is frequently the aetiology of cellulitis. There may be more serious defects in host immunity owing to disease or chemotherapy, allowing normally harmless skin and bowel flora to produce invasive disease.

Airborne spread

Many respiratory tract pathogens are spread from person to person by aerosol or droplet transmission. Secretions containing the infectious agent are coughed, sneezed, or breathed out, and are then inhaled by a new victim. Some enteric viral infections may also be spread by aerosols of faeces or vomit. Environmental pathogens such as *Legionella pneumophila*, and zoonoses such as psittacosis, are also acquired by aerosol inhalation, while rabies virus may be inhaled in the dust from bat droppings.

Faeco-oral spread

Transmission of organisms by the faeco-oral route can occur by direct transfer (usually in small children), by contamination of clothing or household items (usually in institutions or conditions of poor hygiene), or most commonly via contaminated food or water. Human and animal faecal pathogens can get into the food supply at any stage. Raw sewage is used as fertilizer in many parts of the world, contaminating growing vegetables and fruit. Poor personal hygiene can result in contamination during production, packaging, preparation or serving of foodstuffs. In the western world, the centralization of food supply and increased processing of food has allowed the potential for relatively minor episodes of contamination to cause widely disseminated outbreaks of food-borne infection.

Water-borne faeco-oral spread is usually the result of inadequate access to clean water and safe sewage disposal, and is common throughout the developing world. In wealthier countries it usually occurs in isolated outbreaks with a specific source.

Vector-borne disease

Many tropical infections, most importantly malaria, are spread from person to person or from animal to person by an arthropod vector. Vector-borne diseases are also found in temperate climates, but are relatively uncommon. In most cases part of the parasite life cycle takes place within the body of the arthropod, and each parasite species requires a specific vector. Simple mechanical transfer of infective organisms from one host to another can occur, but is rare. Some vector-borne diseases are shown in Table 2.4

Direct person-to-person spread

Organisms can be passed on directly in a number of ways. Sexually-transmitted infections are dealt with on page 120. Skin infections such as ringworm, and ectoparasites such as scabies and head lice, can be spread by simple skin-to-skin contact. Other organisms are passed on by blood- (or occasionally other body fluid) to-blood transmission. In some cases such as HIV and hepatitis B virus this is the only route: in others such as malaria and Chagas' disease it is an unusual alternative to the normal arthropod vector. Blood-to-blood transmission can occur during sexual contact, from mother to infant peripartum, between intravenous drug users sharing any part of their injecting equipment, when infected medical equipment is reused, if contaminated blood or blood products are transfused, or in any sporting or accidental contact when blood is spilled.

Table 2.4
Infections transmitted by arthropod vectors

Disease	Infective organism	Vector
Dengue	Flavivirus	Mosquito
Yellow fever	Flavivirus	Mosquito
Scrub typhus	*Rickettsia tsutsugamushi*	Mite
Rickettsial spotted fevers	*Rickettsia* sp.	Hard tick
Tick-borne relapsing fever	*Borrelia duttoni*	Soft tick
Louse-borne relapsing fever	*Borrelia recurrentis*	Body louse
Lyme disease	*Borrelia burgdorferi*	Hard tick
Plague	*Yersinia pestis*	Flea
Malaria	*Plasmodium* sp.	Mosquito
Lymphatic filariasis	*Wuchereria bancrofti*	Mosquito
	Brugia malayi	Mosquito
Onchocerciasis	*Onchocerca volvulus*	Blackfly
Leishmaniasis	*Leishmania* sp.	Sandfly
African trypanosomiasis	*Trypanosoma brucei*	Tsetse fly
South American trypanosomiasis	*Trypanosoma cruzi*	Reduviid bug

Direct inoculation

Infection can occur when pathogenic organisms breach the normal mechanical defences by direct inoculation. Some of the circumstances in which this can occur are covered under endogenous infection and blood-to-blood transmission above. Some environmental organisms may be inoculated by accident: this is a common mode of transmission of tetanus and certain fungal infections. Rabies virus may be inoculated by the bite of an infected animal.

Consumption of infected material

Although many food-related zoonotic infections are due to contamination of food with animal faeces (and are thus, strictly speaking, faeco-oral), several important diseases are transmitted directly in animal products. These include some strains of salmonella (eggs, chicken meat), brucellosis (unpasteurized milk), and the prion diseases kuru and vCJD (neural tissue).

Prevention and control

Methods of preventing infection depend upon the source and route of transmission, as described above.

- *Eradication of reservoir.* In a few diseases, for which man is the only natural reservoir of infection, it may be possible to eliminate disease by an intensive programme of case finding, treatment and immunization. This has been achieved in the case of smallpox. If there is an animal or environmental reservoir complete eradication is unlikely, but local control methods may decrease the risk of human infection (for example killing of rodents to control plague, leptospirosis, and other diseases).
- *For arthropod-vector-borne infections:*
  - destroying vector species (which may be practical in certain circumstances)
  - taking measures to avoid being bitten (e.g. insect repellent sprays, bed nets).
- *For food borne infections.* Improvement in food handling and preparation result in less contamination during processing, transport or preparation. Organisms intrinsically present in food can be killed by appropriate preparation and cooking. Improved surveillance and regulation of the food industry, as well as better health education for the public is necessary.
- *For faeco-oral infections.* Improvement in water supply. Thirty percent of the world's population do not have access to adequate safe drinking water, and over half do not have adequate sanitation.
- *For blood-borne infections.* Prevention of blood transfer, e.g. in blood transfusions and contaminated medical equipment. Donated blood is routinely tested for infection in most developed countries.

Table 2.5

Notifiable diseases in England & Wales under the Public Health (Infectious Diseases) Regulations 1988

Acute encephalitis
Acute poliomyelitis
Anthrax
Cholera
Diphtheria
Dysentery (amoebic or bacillary)
Food poisoning
Leprosy
Leptospirosis
Malaria
Measles
Meningitis
Meningococcal septicaemia (without meningitis)
Mumps
Ophthalmia neonatorum
Paratyphoid fever
Plague
Rabies
Relapsing fever
Rubella
Scarlet fever
Smallpox
Tetanus
Tuberculosis
Typhoid fever
Typhus
Viral haemorrhagic fever
Viral hepatitis
Whooping cough
Yellow fever

- *For infections spread by airborne and direct contact.* In theory some airborne-transmitted respiratory infections, and some infections spread by direct contact, could be controlled by isolating patients. This is usually impractical but isolation is useful in patients with severe immunodeficiency to protect them from infection.

Cases of some infectious diseases should be notified to the public health authorities so that they are aware of cases and outbreaks. Diseases that are notifiable in England and Wales are listed in Table 2.5.
   Immunization (p. 44).

FURTHER READING

Gorbach SL (2001) Antimicrobial use in animal feed – time to stop. *New England Journal of Medicine* **345**: 1202–1203.
Hart CA, Trees AJ, Duerden BI (1997) Zoonoses. *Journal of Medical Microbiology* **46**: 4–33.
PHLS website: www.phls.co.uk
WHO website: www.who.int/whosis/

Principles and basic mechanisms

Pathogenesis

Figure 2.1 summarizes some of the steps that occur during the pathogenesis of infection.

Specificity

Some infectious agents are strictly species-selective. Amoebiasis, for example, only naturally affects humans. Even within a species, relative resistance is apparent, such as the decreased susceptibility of Duffy blood group-negative individuals to *Plasmodium vivax* malaria (p. 100).

Microorganisms are also highly specific with respect to the organ or tissue they infect. For example, a number of viruses are hepatotropic, such as those responsible for hepatitis A, B, C and E and yellow fever. This predilection for specific sites in the body relates partly to the immediate environment in which the organism finds itself; for example, anaerobic organisms colonize the anaerobic colon, whereas aerobic organisms are generally found in the mouth, pharynx and proximal intestinal tract. Other organisms that show selectivity include:

- *Streptococcus pneumoniae* (respiratory tract)
- *Escherichia coli* (urinary and alimentary tract).

Even within a species of bacterium such as *E. coli*, there are clear differences between strains with regard to their ability to cause gastrointestinal disease (p. 72), which in turn differ from uropathogenic *E. coli* responsible for urinary tract infection.

Within an organ a pathogen may show selectivity for a particular cell type. In the intestine, for example, rotavirus predominantly invades and destroys intestinal epithelial cells on the upper portion of the villus, whereas reovirus selectively enters the body through the specialized epithelial cells, known as M cells, that cover the Peyer's patches (see p. 287).

Epithelial attachment

Many bacteria attach to the epithelial substratum by specific organelles called pili (or fimbriae) that contain a surface lectin(s) – a protein or glycoprotein that recognizes specific sugar residues on the host cell. This family of molecules is known as adhesins (see p. 192). Following attachment some bacteria, such as coagulase-negative staphylococci (*Staphylococcus epidermidis*), produce an extracellular slime layer and recruit additional bacteria, which cluster together to form a biofilm. These biofilms can be difficult to eradicate, and are a frequent cause of medical device-associated infections which affect prosthetic joints and heart valves as well as indwelling catheters. Some viruses (e.g. HIV) and protozoa (e.g. *Plasmodium* spp., *Entamoeba histolytica*) attach to specific target-cell receptors. Other parasites such as hookworm have specific attachment organs (buccal plates) that firmly grip the intestinal epithelium.

Colonization

Following epithelial attachment, pathogens may either remain on the surface epithelium or within the lumen of the organ they have colonized. Tissue invasion may follow.

Invasion may result in:
- an intracellular location for the pathogen (e.g. viruses, *Toxoplasma gondii*, *Leishmania* spp., *Plasmodium* spp.)
- an extracellular location for the pathogen (e.g. pneumococci, staphylococci and *Entamoeba histolytica*)

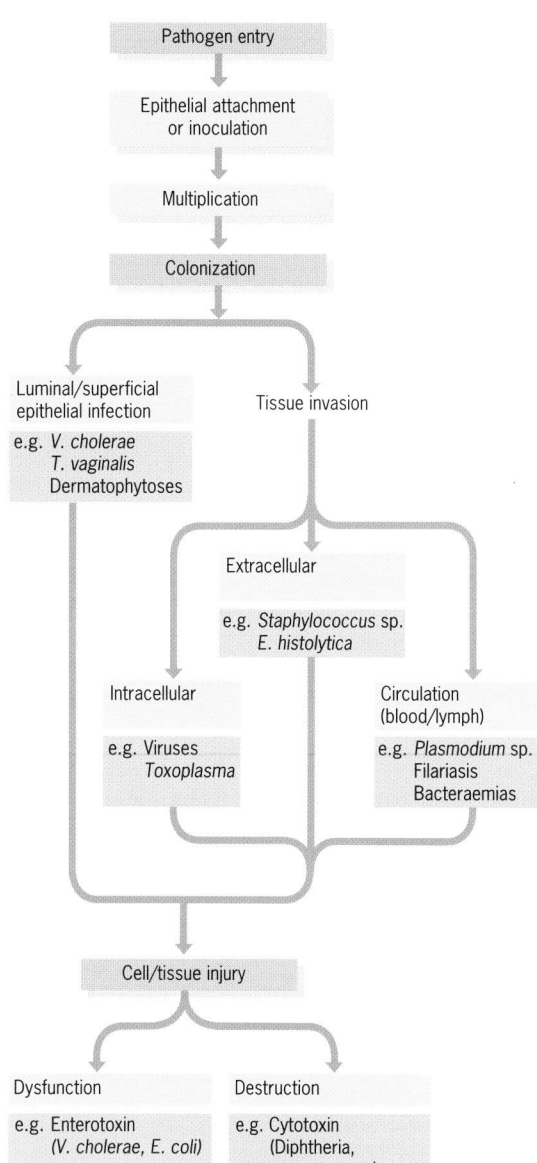

Fig. 2.1 **The pathogenesis of infection.**

- invasion directly into the blood or lymph circulation (e.g. schistosome schistosomula and trypanosomes).

Once the pathogen is firmly established in its target tissue, a series of events follows that usually culminates in damage to the host.

Tissue dysfunction or damage

Microorganisms produce disease by a number of well-defined mechanisms:

Exotoxins and endotoxins

- *Exotoxins* have many diverse activities including inhibition of protein synthesis (diphtheria toxin), neurotoxicity (*Clostridium tetani* and *C. botulinum*) and enterotoxicity, which results in intestinal secretion of water and electrolytes (*E. coli*, *Vibrio cholerae*).
- *Endotoxin* is a lipopolysaccharide (LPS) in the cell wall of Gram-negative bacteria. It is responsible for many of the features of septic shock (see p. 931), namely hypotension, fever, intravascular coagulation and, at high doses, death. The effects of endotoxin are mediated predominantly by release of tumour necrosis factor.

Tumour necrosis factor (TNF)

TNF-alpha is released from a variety of phagocytic cells (macrophages/monocytes) and TNF-beta from non-phagocytic cells (lymphocytes, natural killer cells) in response to infections and inflammatory stimuli (Fig. 2.2). TNF itself then stimulates the release of a cascade of other mediators involved in inflammation and tissue remodelling, such as interleukin (IL-1 and IL-6), prostaglandins, leukotrienes and corticotropin. TNF is therefore responsible for many of the effects of an infection.

Tissue invasion

Staphylococcus aureus has tissue-invasive qualities allowing abscess formation and bacteraemia, as well as producing toxins which can cause diarrhoea and widespread erythema (staphylococcal scalded skin syndrome). Table 2.6 summarizes the variety of infections produced by *S. aureus*, while some of the host factors that increase susceptibility to staphylococcal infections are shown in Table 2.7. Similarly, some pathogenic *E. coli* can produce tissue invasion without production of a specific toxin.

Table 2.6
Clinical conditions produced by *Staphylococcus aureus*

Due to invasion	Bones and joints
Skin	Osteomyelitis, arthritis
Furuncles	
Cellulitis	**Miscellaneous**
Impetigo	Parotitis
Carbuncles	Pyomyositis
	Septicaemia
Lungs	Enterocolitis
Pneumonia	
Lung abscesses	**Due to toxin**
	Staphylococcal food poisoning
Heart	Scalded skin syndrome
Endocarditis	Bullous impetigo
Pericarditis	Staphylococcal scarlet fever
	Toxic shock syndrome
Central nervous system	
Meningitis	
Brain abscesses	

Table 2.7
Examples of host factors that increase susceptibility to staphylococcal infections (predominantly *S. aureus*)

Injury to skin or mucous membranes	Abnormal leucocyte function
Abrasions	Job's syndrome
Trauma (accidental or surgical)	Chediak-Higashi syndrome
Burns	Steroid therapy
Insect bites	Drug-induced leucopenia
Metabolic abnormalities	**Postviral infections**
Diabetes mellitus	Influenza
Uraemia	
	Miscellaneous conditions
Foreign bodies*	Excess alcohol consumption
Intravenous and other indwelling catheters	Malnutrition
Cardiac and orthopaedic prostheses	Malignancies
Tracheostomies	Old age

* Often *Staphylococcus epidermidis*

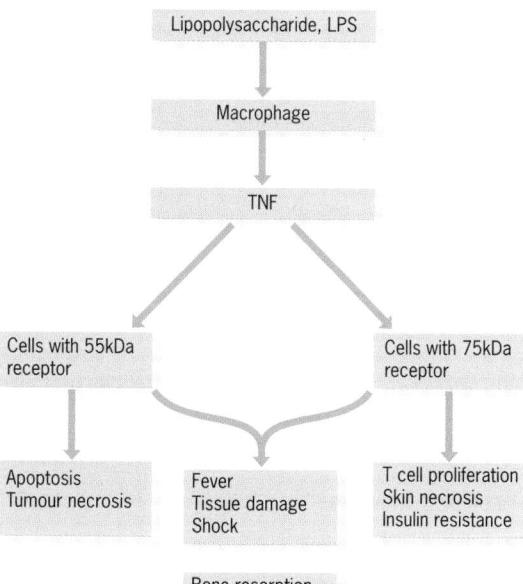

Fig. 2.2 Biology of tumour necrosis factor in infection. LPS acts on macrophages to stimulate TNF. TNF acts on its two receptors (55 kDa and 75 kDa), producing the effects shown. Both receptors mediate the general effects of fever, tissue damage, shock and bone resorption.

Secondary immunological phenomena

All organisms can initiate secondary immunological mechanisms, such as complement activation, immune complex formation and antibody-mediated cytolysis of cells. The immunological response to infection is described in Chapter 4.

Many infections are self-limiting, and immune and non-immune host defence mechanisms will eventually clear the pathogens. This is generally followed by tissue repair, which may result in complete resolution or leave residual damage.

Metabolic and immunological consequences of infection

Fever

Body temperature is controlled by the thermoregulatory centre in the anterior hypothalamus in the floor of the third ventricle. IL-1, IL-6 and TNF-α are released from a variety of cells involved in host defence, primarily blood monocytes and phagocytes, under the influence of microbial exogenous pyrogens such as lipopolysaccharide (LPS). These cytokines act on the thermoregulatory centre by increasing prostaglandin (PGE$_2$) synthesis. The antipyretic effect of salicylates is brought about, at least in part, through its inhibitory effects on prostaglandin synthetase.

Fever production has a positive effect on the course of infection. However, for every 1°C rise in temperature, there is a 13% increase in resting metabolic rate and oxygen consumption. Fever therefore leads to increased energy requirements at a time when anorexia leads to decreased food intake. The normal compensatory mechanisms in starvation (e.g. mobilization of fat stores) are inhibited in acute infections. This leads to an increase in skeletal muscle breakdown, releasing amino acids, which, via gluconeogenesis, are used to provide energy.

In chronic infection there is time for adaptation. The body is able to utilize fat stores more effectively, and thus weight loss is much slower.

Protein metabolism

During acute infection, three major changes occur in protein metabolism:

- There is a diversion of synthesis away from somatic and circulating proteins such as albumin towards acute-phase proteins (see Table 4.4, p. 194).
- Protein synthesis is also directed towards immunoglobulin production and there is increased production of lymphocytes, neutrophils and other phagocytic cells.
- There is a marked increase in nitrogen losses due to tissue breakdown (see p. 228), which may reach 10–15 g per day.

Nutrition and host defence

Undernutrition impairs host defence. Natural resistance to infection is lowered by alterations in the integrity of

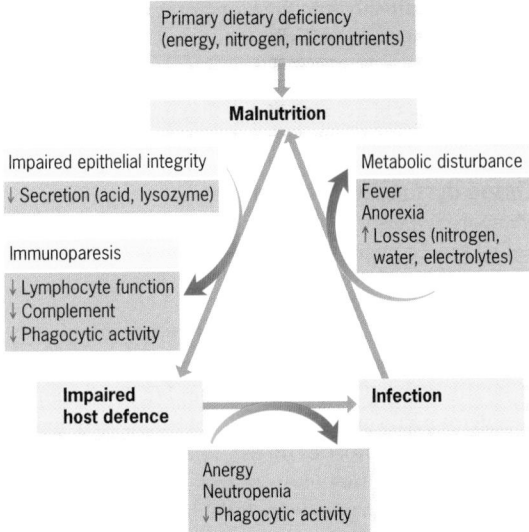

Fig. 2.3 **The malnutrition-impaired host defence and infection cycle is fairly well established.** The shaded boxes suggest likely mechanisms.

body surfaces, the reduced ability to repair epithelia, and the reduction in gastric acid production. In addition, with malnutrition, immunological abnormalities are found (Fig. 2.3).

Mineral metabolism and acid–base balance

Mineral metabolism and acid–base balance are disturbed during acute infection. In general, sodium and water are retained, principally owing to the effects of increased levels of aldosterone and inappropriate secretion of antidiuretic hormone. During the convalescent period after acute infection, a diuresis may occur. Acid–base balance disturbance is common. Causes include respiratory alkalosis following tachypnoea related to fever, respiratory acidosis and hypoxaemia associated with pneumonia, and metabolic acidosis associated with septicaemia.

In acute infection these changes are mild and resolve promptly without specific intervention. However, in situations where infections are prolonged and resolution is slow, supportive care may be necessary, particularly with respect to managing nutritional deficits and electrolyte and acid–base disturbances.

FURTHER READING

Dinarell CA (1999) Cytokines as endogenous pyrogens. *Journal of Infectious Diseases* **179** (Suppl 2): S294–S304.
Finlay BB, Falkow S (1997) Common themes in microbial pathogenicity revisited. *Microbiology and Molecular Biology Revues* **61**: 136–169.
Guiney DG (1997) Regulation of bacterial virulence gene expression by the host environment. *Journal of Clinical Investigation* **99**: 565–569.

Mackowiak PA, Barlett JG, Borden EC et al. (1997) Concepts of fever: recent advances and lingering dogma. *Clinical Infectious Diseases* **25**: 119–138.

Strauss EJ, Falkow S (1997) Microbial pathogenesis: genomics and beyond. *Science* **276**: 707–712.

Vallance BA, Finlay BB (2000) Exploitation of host cells by enteropathogenic *Escherichia coli*. *Proceedings of the National Academy of Sciences of the United States of America* **97**(16): 8799–8806.

Approach to the patient with a suspected infection

Infectious diseases can affect any organ or system, and can cause a wide variety of symptoms and signs. Fever is often regarded as the cardinal feature of infection, but not all febrile illnesses are infections, and not all infectious diseases present with a fever. History-taking and examination should aim to identify the site(s) of infection, and also the likely causative organism(s).

History

A detailed history is taken with specific questions about epidemiological risk factors for infection. These are based on the sources of infection and routes of transmission discussed above.

- Travel history: some diseases are more prevalent in certain geographical locations, and many infections common in the tropics are seen rarely if at all in the UK.
- Food and water history: systemic as well as gastroenteric infections can be caught via this route.
- Occupational history.
- Animal contact: domestic, farm and wild animals can all be responsible for zoonotic infection.
- Sexual activity: as well as the traditional sexually transmitted diseases, HIV, hepatitis B and very occasionally hepatitis C can all be transmitted sexually. Some enteric infections are more common among male homosexuals.
- Intravenous drug use: as well as blood-borne viruses, drug injectors are susceptible to a variety of bacterial and fungal infections due to inoculation. Tattooing, body piercing and receipt of blood products (especially outside the UK) are also risk factors for blood-borne viruses.
- Leisure activities: certain pastimes may predispose to water-borne infections or zoonoses.

Clinical examination

A thorough examination covering all systems is required. Skin rashes and lymphadenopathy are common features of infectious diseases, and the ears, eyes, mouth and throat should also be inspected. Infections commonly associated with a rash are listed in Box 2.1. Rectal, vaginal and penile examination is required in sexually transmitted infections.

The fever pattern may occasionally be helpful; many infectious diseases have a characteristic fever, e.g. the tertian fever of falciparum malaria, or the stepped fever of typhoid. However, these patterns tend to be found only in untreated disease, and are rarely seen in developed countries. In general, although the presence of fever is suggestive of infection, too much weight should not be placed on the pattern or degree.

Box 2.1

Infections commonly associated with a rash

Macular/maculopapular
Measles
Rubella
Enteroviruses
Human herpesvirus 6
Epstein–Barr virus
Cytomegalovirus
Parvovirus
Human immunodeficiency virus (HIV)
Dengue
Typhoid
Secondary syphilis

Vesicular
Chickenpox (herpes zoster virus)
Shingles (herpes zoster virus)
Herpes simplex virus
Hand, foot and mouth disease (Coxsackie virus)
Herpangina (Coxsackie virus)

Petechial/haemorrhagic
Meningococcal septicaemia
Any septicaemia with disseminated intravascular coagulation (DIC)
Tick typhus
Viruses (Table 2.22)

Erythematous
Scarlet fever
Lyme disease (erythema chronicum migrans)
Toxic shock syndrome

Urticarial
Toxocariasis
Strongyloidiasis
Schistosomiasis
Cutaneous larva migrans

Others
Tick typhus (eschar)
Primary syphilis (chancre)
Anthrax (ulcerating papule)

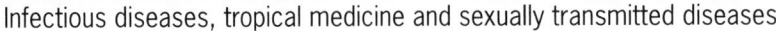

Investigations

In some infections such as chickenpox the clinical presentation is so distinctive that no investigations are normally necessary to confirm the diagnosis. Other cases require investigation.

General investigations (to assess health and identify organ(s) involved)

These will vary depending on circumstances:

- **Blood tests.** Routine blood count, ESR and C-reactive protein, biochemical profile, urea and electrolytes are performed in all cases (Box 2.2).
- **Imaging.** X-ray, ultrasound, echocardiography, CT and MR scanning are used to identify and localize infections. Biopsy or aspiration of tissue for microbiological examination may also be facilitated by ultrasound or CT guidance.
- **Radionuclide scanning** after injection of indium- or technetium-labelled white cells (previously harvested from the patient) may occasionally help to localize infection. It is most effective when the peripheral white cell count is raised, and is of particular value in localizing occult abscesses.

Microbiological investigations (to identify causative organism)

Diagnostic services range from simple microscopy to molecular probes. It is often helpful to discuss the clinical problem with a microbiologist to ensure that appropriate tests are performed, and that specimens are collected and transported correctly.

Microscopy and culture

Specimens to be sent for microscopy and culture (Box 2.3).

- *Blood and urine* should routinely be sent for bacterial culture regardless of whether fever is present at the time.
- *Cerebrospinal fluid, sputum, and biopsy* specimens are sent if clinically indicated.
- *Special culture techniques* are required for fungi, mycobacteria, and some other bacteria such as *Brucella* spp., and the laboratory must be informed if these are suspected.
- *Faeces* should not routinely be sent for viral investigations: viral gastroenteritis is rare except in infants and the institutionalized elderly, and is self-limiting. Protozoa should be considered as a cause of diarrhoea in returning travellers, immunocompromised patients, toddlers, homosexual men, farm workers, and in any cases of prolonged unexplained diarrhoea. Detection of a specific clostridial toxin is a more reliable test for diarrhoea caused by *Clostridium difficile* than culture of the organism itself. Stool culture is a costly routine test and is often requested indiscriminately.

Immunodiagnostic tests

These can be divided into two types:

- tests that detect viral or bacterial antigen, using a polyvalent antiserum or a monoclonal antibody
- tests that detect serological response to infection.

Box 2.2

General investigations for a patient with suspected infection

Investigation (results)	Possible cause
Full blood count	
Neutrophilia	Bacterial infection
Neutropenia	Viral infection
	Brucellosis
	Typhoid
	Typhus
	Overwhelming sepsis
Lymphocytosis	Viral infection
Lymphopenia	HIV infection (not specific)
Atypical lymphocytes	Infectious mononucleosis
Eosinophilia	Invasive parasitic infection
Thrombocytopenia	Overwhelming sepsis
	Malaria
Raised ESR or C-reactive protein	All
Urea and electrolytes	Potentially deranged in severe illness from any cause
Liver enzymes	
Minor elevation of transferases	Non-specific feature of many infections
	Mild viral hepatitis
Grossly deranged transferases, elevated bilirubin	Viral hepatitis (usually A,B or E)
Coagulation	May be deranged in hepatitis, and in overwhelming infection of any type

Box 2.3

Specimens and indications for microscopy and culture

Specimen	Investigation	Indication
Blood	Giemsa stain for malaria	Any symptomatic traveller returning from a malarious area
	Stains for other parasites	Specific tropical infections
	Culture	All suspected bacterial infections
Urine	Microscopy and culture	All suspected bacterial infections
	Tuberculosis (TB) culture	Suspected TB
		Unexplained leucocytes in urine
Faeces	Microscopy ± iodine stain	Suspected protozoal diarrhoea
	Culture	All unexplained diarrhoea
	Electron microscopy/viral culture	Suspected viral diarrhoea in children
	(not usually necessary to do both)	Viral meningitis
	Clostridium difficile toxin	Diarrhoea following hospital stay or antibiotic treatment
Throat swabs	Culture	Suspected bacterial tonsillitis and pharyngitis
	Viral culture	Viral meningitis
		Viral respiratory infections where urgent diagnosis is considered necessary
Sputum	Microscopy and culture	Unusual chest infections; pneumonia
	Auramine stain/TB culture	Suspected TB
	Other special stains/cultures	Immunocompromised patients
		Suspected fungal infections
Cerebrospinal fluid	Microscopy and culture	Suspected meningitis
	Auramine stain/TB culture	Suspected TB, meningitis
	Other special stains/cultures	Immunocompromised patients
		Suspected fungal infections
	Polymerase chain reaction	Suspected encephalitis or viral or bacterial meningitis
Rash aspirate:		
Petechial	Microscopy and culture	Meningococcal disease
Vesicular	Viral culture	Herpes simplex/zoster

These investigations are valuable in the identification of organisms that are difficult to culture, especially viruses and fungi, and can also be helpful when antibiotics have been administered before samples were obtained. However, care is needed in the interpretation of serological tests. Elevated antibody titres on a single occasion (especially of IgG) are rarely diagnostic, and in some infections it may be difficult to distinguish between old and acute infection. Paired serological tests a few weeks apart, or specific assays for IgM (indicating an acute infection) are more helpful.

Nucleic acid detection

Specific genes from many pathogenic microorganisms have been cloned and sequenced. Nucleic acid probes can be designed to detect these sequences, identifying pathogen-specific nucleic acid in body fluids or tissue. The utility of this approach has been greatly enhanced by the development of amplification techniques such as the polymerase chain reaction (PCR), which increases the amount of target DNA/RNA in the sample to be tested. However PCR assays for many organisms are still in the process of development.

Treatment

The mainstay of treatment for most infectious diseases is antimicrobial chemotherapy. The choice of antibiotic should be governed by:

- the clinical state of the patient
- the likely cause of their infection.

Many infections, particularly those caused by viruses, are self-limiting and require no treatment. More serious infections may require supportive therapy in addition to antibiotics. It is always preferable to have a definite microbial diagnosis before starting treatment, so that an antibiotic with the most appropriate spectrum of activity and site of action can be used. However, some patients are too unwell to wait for results (which in the case of culture may take days). In diseases such as meningitis or septicaemia delay in treatment may be fatal and therapy must be started on an empirical basis. Appropriate samples for culture should be taken before the first dose of antibiotic, and an antibiotic regimen chosen on the basis of the most likely causative organisms. Usually patients are less unwell, and specific therapy can be deferred pending results. Antibiotic therapy is discussed in more detail on page 34.

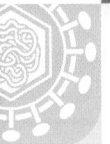

Special circumstances

Overseas travellers. A detailed travel itinerary, including any flight stopovers should be taken from anyone who is unwell after arriving in this country from abroad. Previous travel should also be covered as some infections may be chronic or recurrent. It is necessary to find out not just which countries were visited but also the type of environment: a stay in a remote jungle village carries different health risks from a holiday in an air-conditioned coastal holiday resort. Food and water consumption, bathing and swimming habits, animal and insect contact, and contact with human illness all need to be recorded. Enquiry should be made about sexual contacts, drug use and medical treatment (especially parenteral) while abroad. In some parts of the world over 90% of professional sex workers are HIV positive, and hepatitis B and C are very common in parts of Africa and Asia. In addition to the investigations described in the previous section, special tests may be needed depending on the epidemiological risks and clinical signs, and malaria films are mandatory in anyone who is unwell after being in a malarious area. Some of the more common causes of a febrile illness in returning travellers are listed in Table 2.8.

Immunocompromised patients. Advances in medical treatment over the past three decades have led to a huge increase in the number of patients living with immunodeficiency states. Cancer chemotherapy, the use of immunosuppressive drugs and the world-wide AIDS epidemic have all contributed to this. The presentation may be very atypical in the immunocompromised patient with few, if any, localizing signs or symptoms. Infection can be due to organisms which are not usually pathogenic, including environmental bacteria and fungi. The normal physiological responses to infection (e.g. fever, neutrophilia) may be diminished or absent. The onset of symptoms may be sudden, and the course of the illness fulminant. A high index of suspicion for infections in people who are known to be immunosuppressed is

required. These patients should usually be given early and aggressive antibiotic therapy without waiting for the results of investigations. Samples for culture should be sent before starting treatment, but therapy should not be delayed if this proves difficult. The choice of antibiotics should be guided by the likely causative organisms: these are shown in Box 2.4.

Pyrexia of unknown origin

History, clinical examination and simple investigation will reveal the cause of a fever in most patients. In a small number, however, no diagnosis is apparent despite continuing symptoms. The term pyrexia (or fever) of unknown origin (PUO) is sometimes used to describe this problem. Various definitions have been suggested for PUO: a useful one is 'a fever persisting for > 2 weeks, with no clear diagnosis despite intelligent and intensive investigation'. Patients who are known to have HIV or other immunosuppressing conditions are normally excluded from the definition of PUO, as the investigation and management of these patients is different.

Successful diagnosis of the cause of PUO depends on a knowledge of the likely and possible aetiologies. These have been documented in a number of studies, and are summarized in Box 2.5

A detailed history and examination is essential, taking into account the possible causes, and the examination should be repeated on a regular basis in case new signs appear. Investigation findings to date should be reviewed, obvious omissions amended and abnormalities followed up. Confirm that the patient does have objective evidence of a raised temperature: this may require admission to hospital if they are not already under observation. Some people have an exaggerated circadian temperature variation (usually peaking in the evening), which is not pathological.

The range of tests available is discussed above. Obviously investigation is guided by particular abnormalities on examination or initial test results, but in some cases 'blind' investigation is necessary. Some investigations, especially cultures, should be repeated regularly, and serial monitoring of inflammatory markers such as C-reactive protein allows assessment of progress.

Improvements in imaging techniques have diminished the need for invasive investigations in PUO, and scanning has now superseded the blind diagnostic laparotomy. Ultrasound, echocardiography, CT, MRI, and labelled white cell scanning can all help in establishing a diagnosis if used appropriately: the temptation to scan all patients with PUO from head to toe as a first measure should be avoided. Biopsy of liver and bone marrow may be useful even in the absence of obvious abnormalities, and temporal artery biopsy should be considered in the elderly (p. 566). Bronchoscopy can be used to obtain samples for microbiological and histological examination if sputum specimens are not adequate.

Table 2.8
Causes of febrile illness in travellers arriving in the UK

Tropical countries	Specific geographical areas (see text)
Malaria	Histoplasmosis
Schistosomiasis	Brucellosis
Dengue	
Tick typhus	**World-wide**
	Pneumonia
Economically less-developed countries	URTI
	UTI
Typhoid	Traveller's diarrhoea
Tuberculosis	Viral infection
Dysentery	
Hepatitis A	
Amoebiasis	

URTI, upper respiratory tract infection; UTI, urinary tract infection

---

Box 2.4

Common causes of infection in immunocompromised patients

Deficiency	Causes	Organisms
Neutropenia	Chemotherapy	*Escherichia coli*
	Bone marrow transplant	*Klebsiella pneumoniae*
	Immunosuppressant drugs	*Staphylococcus aureus*
		Staphylococcus epidermidis
		Aspergillus spp.
		Candida spp.
Cellular immune defects	HIV infection	Respiratory syncytial virus
	Lymphoma	Cytomegalovirus
	Bone marrow transplant	Epstein–Barr virus
	Congenital syndromes	Herpes simplex and zoster
		Salmonella spp.
		Mycobacterium spp. (esp. *M. avium-intracellulare*)
		Cryptococcus neoformans
		Candida spp.
		Cryptosporidium parvum
		Pneumocystis carinii
		Toxoplasma gondii
Humoral immune deficiencies	Congenital syndromes	*Haemophilus influenzae*
	Chronic lymphocytic leukaemia	*Streptococcus pneumoniae*
	Corticosteroids	Enteroviruses
Terminal complement deficiencies (C5–C9)	Congenital syndromes	*Neisseria meningitidis*
		N. gonorrhoeae
Splenectomy	Surgery	*Strep. pneumoniae*
	Trauma	*N. meningitidis*
		H. influenzae
		Malaria

Box 2.5

Causes of pyrexia of unknown origin

Infection (20–40%)
Pyogenic abscess
Tuberculosis
Infective endocarditis
Toxoplasmosis
Epstein Barr virus (EBV) infection
Cytomegalovirus (CMV) infection
Primary HIV infection
Brucellosis
Lyme disease

Malignant disease (10–30%)
Lymphoma
Leukaemia
Renal cell carcinoma
Hepatocellular carcinoma

Collagen vascular disease (15–20%)
Adult Still's disease
Rheumatoid arthritis
Systemic lupus erythematosus
Wegener's granulomatosis
Giant cell arteritis

Miscellaneous (10–25%)
Drug fevers
Thyrotoxicosis
Inflammatory bowel disease
Sarcoidosis
Granulomatous hepatitis
Factitious fever
Familial Mediterranean fever

Undiagnosed (5–25%)

Serological tests have greatly improved the diagnosis of infectious causes of PUO, but should be used with caution. The more tests that are done, the greater is the danger of a false positive or misleading result, and serological tests should only be ordered and interpreted in the context of the clinical findings and epidemiology.

Treatment of a patient with a persistent fever is aimed at the underlying cause, and if possible only symptomatic treatment should be used until a diagnosis is made. Blind antibiotic therapy may make diagnosis of an occult infection more difficult, and empirical steroid therapy may mask an inflammatory response without

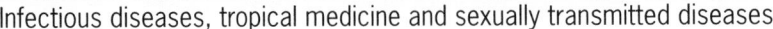

treating the underlying cause. In a few patients no cause for the fever is found despite many months of investigation and follow-up. In most the symptoms do eventually settle spontaneously, and if no definite cause has been identified after 2 years the long-term prognosis is good.

FURTHER READING

Humar A, Keystone J (1996) Evaluating fever in travellers returning from tropical countries. *British Medical Journal* **312**: 953–956.

Petersdorff R (1992) Fever of unknown origin: an old friend revisited. *Archives of Internal Medicine* **152**: 21.

Walter E, Bowden R (1995) Infections in the bone marrow transplant patient. *Infectious Disease Clinics of North America* **9**: 823–847.

Antimicrobial chemotherapy

Principles of use

Antibiotics are among the safest of drugs, especially those used to treat community infections. They have had a major impact on the life-threatening infections and reduce the morbidity associated with many common infectious diseases. This in turn is, in part, responsible for the overprescribing of these agents which has led to concerns with regard to the increasing incidence of antibiotic resistance.

Most antibiotic prescribing, especially in the community, is empirical. Even in hospital practice, microbiological documentation of the nature of an infection and the susceptibility of the pathogen is generally not available for a day or two. Initial choice of therapy relies on a clinical diagnosis and, in turn, a presumptive microbiological diagnosis. Such 'blind therapy' is directed at the most likely pathogen(s) responsible for a particular syndrome such as meningitis, urinary tract infection or pneumonia. Initial therapy in the severely ill patient is often broad spectrum in order to cover the range of possible pathogens but should be narrowed down once microbiological information becomes available.

Bactericidal versus bacteriostatic

In the majority of infections there is no firm evidence that bactericidal drugs (penicillins, cephalosporins, aminoglycosides) are more effective than bacteriostatic drugs, but it is generally considered necessary to use the former in the treatment of bacterial endocarditis and in patients in whom host defence mechanisms are compromised, particularly in those with neutropenia.

Combinations of drugs are occasionally required for reasons other than providing broad-spectrum cover. Tuberculosis is initially treated with three or four agents to avoid resistance emerging. Synergistic inhibition is achieved by using penicillin and gentamicin in enterococcal endocarditis or gentamicin and ceftazidime in life-threatening pseudomonas infection.

Pharmacokinetic factors

To be successful, sufficient antibiotic must penetrate to the site of the infection. Knowledge of the standard pharmacokinetic considerations of absorption, distribution, metabolism and excretion for the various drugs is required. Difficult sites include the brain, eye and prostate, while loculated abscesses are inaccessible to most agents.

Many mild-to-moderate infections can be treated effectively with oral antibiotics provided that the patient is compliant. Parenteral administration is indicated in the severely ill patient to ensure rapid high blood and tissue concentrations of drug. Some antibiotics can only be administered parenterally such as the aminoglycosides and extended spectrum cephalosporins. Parenteral therapy is also required in those unable to swallow or where gastrointestinal absorption is unreliable.

Dose and duration of therapy

This will vary according to the nature, severity and response to therapy.

Prolonged treatment (up to 6 weeks) is necessary for some varieties of infective endocarditis, while pulmonary tuberculosis is treated for at least 6 months. In treating many common infections, improvement occurs within 2–3 days; once the patient is afebrile or the leucocytosis has settled, oral administration should be considered for those commenced on parenteral therapy. Five to seven days' treatment is adequate for most infections. Shorter-course therapy (3 days or less) is appropriate for those with symptomatic uncomplicated bacteriuria (cystitis). Minimizing the duration of therapy lowers the risks of adverse reactions and superinfection with *Candida* spp. or *Clostridium difficile*, as well as the cost of therapy.

Drugs which are concentrated intracellularly, such as erythromycin, quinolones and tetracyclines are used in treating mycoplasma, brucella and legionella infections.

Renal and hepatic insufficiency

Many drugs require dose reduction in renal failure to avoid toxic accumulation. This applies to the β-lactams and especially the aminoglycosides. Nalidixic acid and the tetracyclines, other than doxycycline, should be avoided. In those with hepatic insufficiency, caution or dose reduction is required for agents such as isoniazid, ketoconazole, interferon and rifampicin.

Therapeutic drug monitoring

To ensure therapeutic yet non-toxic drug concentrations, serum concentrations of drugs such as the aminoglycosides and vancomycin are monitored, especially in those with impaired or changing renal function. Peak (1 hour post-dose) and trough (pre-dose) serum samples are assayed. However, with the increasing use of once-daily aminoglycoside dosage regimens, random but timed serum assays are being adopted.

Antibiotic chemoprophylaxis

There are a number of indications for the prophylactic use of antibiotics (Table 2.9). These include conditions where the risk of infection is high (colon surgery) or the consequences of infection are serious (endocarditis, post-splenectomy sepsis). The choice of agent(s) is determined by the likely infectious risk and the established efficacy and safety of the regimen.

Mechanisms of action and resistance to antimicrobial agents

Antibiotics act at different sites of the bacterium. Penicillins, cephalosporins and vancomycin act on the cell wall; erythromycin and aminoglycosides affect protein synthesis, rifampicin affects RNA synthesis; and the quinolones and metronidazole affect DNA synthesis. Sulphonamides and trimethoprim are folic acid antagonists and amphotericin B inhibits fungal sterol synthesis.

Resistance to an antibiotic can be the result of:

- failure to reach the target site, for example because impaired permeability causes a failure to penetrate the outer bacterial membrane (e.g. penicillins in Gram-negative bacteria)
- enzyme inactivation (e.g. β-lactamase enzymes – see p. 37)
- alteration of the target site (e.g. single point mutations in *E. coli* or a penicillin-binding protein in *Strep. pneumoniae* leading to acquired resistance – see below).

The development or acquisition of resistance to an antibiotic by bacteria invariably involves either a mutation at a single point in a gene or transfer of genetic material from another organism (Fig. 2.4).

Larger fragments of DNA may be introduced into a bacterium either by transfer of 'naked' DNA or via a bacteriophage (a virus) DNA vector. Both the former

Table 2.9

Antibiotic chemoprophylaxis (see *British National Formulary*)

Clinical problem	Aim	Drug regimen
Rheumatic fever	To prevent recurrence and further cardiac damage	Phenoxymethylpenicillin 250 mg twice-daily, or sulfadiazine 1 g when penicillin-allergic
Infective endocarditis	To prevent infection on abnormal, prosthetic or homograft heart valves, patent ductus or septal defect (see 'special'-risk patients)	*Dental/upper respiratory tract procedures* (LA) Oral amoxicillin 3 g 1 hour before procedure For penicillin-allergic individuals, clindamycin 600 mg 1 hour before procedure Chlorhexidine mouthwash may also be used *Dental under GA* At induction: i.v. amoxicillin. 1 g Six hours later: oral amoxicillin 500 mg **'Special'-risk patients only** (prosthetic valves and/or previous endocarditis): *Gastrointestinal, obstetric or gynaecological, dental (GA) and genitourinary procedures:* At induction i.v. amoxicillin 1 g i.v. gentamicin 120 mg Six hours after procedure, amoxicillin 500 mg (vancomycin for penicillin-allergic patient)
Splenectomy/spleen malfunction	To prevent serious pneumococcal sepsis	Phenoxymethylpenicillin 500 mg 12-hourly
Meningitis: Due to meningococci	To prevent infection in close contacts	Adults: rifampicin 600 mg twice-daily for 2 days Children < 1 month: 5 mg/kg Children > 1 month: 10 mg/kg
Due to *H. influenzae* type b	To reduce nasopharyngeal carriage and prevent infection in close contacts	Adults: rifampicin 100 mg daily for 4 days Children: 20 mg/kg
Tuberculosis	To prevent infection in exposed (close contacts) tuberculin-negative individuals, infants of infected mothers and immunosuppressed patients	Oral isoniazid 5 mg/kg daily for 6–12 months

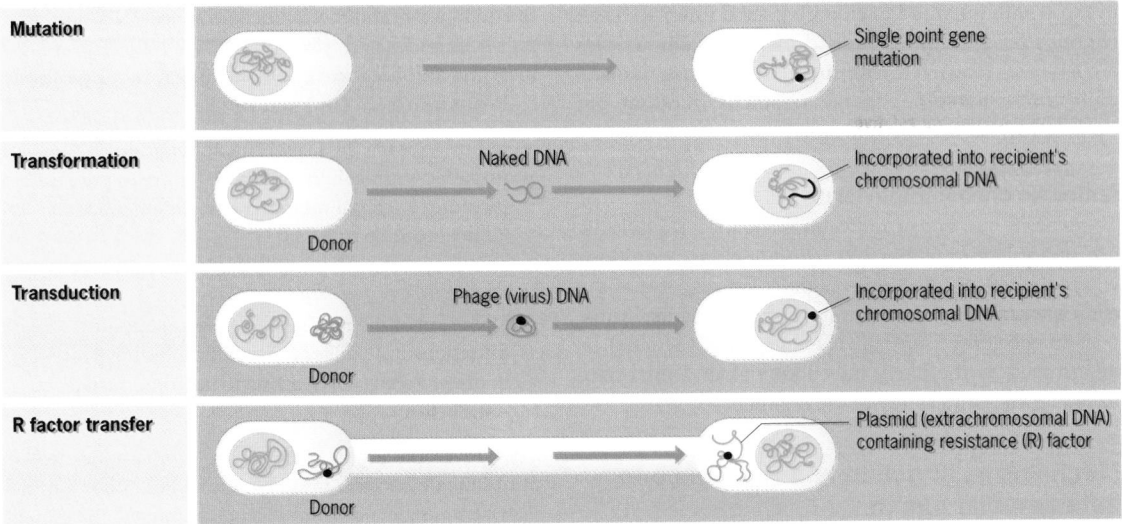

Fig. 2.4 Some mechanisms for the development of resistance to antimicrobial drugs. These involve either a single point mutation or transfer of genetic material from another organism (transformation, transduction or R factor transfer).

Table 2.10
Some bacteria that have developed resistance to common antibiotics

Pathogen	Previously fully sensitive to
Streptococcus pneumoniae	Penicillin, erythromycin, cefotaxime
Streptococcus pyogenes	Erythromycin, tetracycline
Staphylococcus aureus	Penicillin, methicillin, ciprofloxacin
Neisseria gonorrhoeae	Penicillin, ciprofloxacin
Haemophilus influenzae	Amoxicillin, chloramphenicol
Enterobacteria	Amoxicillin, trimethoprim, ciprofloxacin, gentamicin
Salmonella spp.	Amoxicillin, sulphonamides, ciprofloxacin
Shigella spp.	Amoxicillin, trimethoprim, tetracycline
Pseudomonas aeruginosa	Gentamicin

multiple antibiotic resistance in a single bacterium. Increasing resistance to many antibiotics has developed (Table 2.10).

FURTHER READING

Finch RG (1998) Antibiotic resistance. *Journal of Antimicrobial Chemotherapy* **42**: 125–128.
Finch RG, Williams RJ (eds) (1999) *Antibiotic resistance. Baillière's Clinical Infectious Diseases*. London: Baillière Tindall.
Murray BE (2000) Vancomycin-resistant enterococcal infections. *New England Journal of Medicine* **342**: 710–721.

(transformation) and the latter (transduction) are dependent on integration of this new DNA into the recipient chromosomal DNA. This requires a high degree of homology between the donor and recipient chromosomal DNA.

Finally, antibiotic resistance can be transferred from one bacterium to another by conjugation, when extrachromosomal DNA (a plasmid) containing the resistance factor (R factor) is passed from one cell into another during direct contact. Transfer of such R factor plasmids can occur between unrelated bacterial strains and involve large amounts of DNA and often codes for multiple antibiotic resistance.

Transformation is probably the least clinically relevant mechanism, whereas transduction and R factor transfer are usually responsible for the sudden emergence of

Antibacterial drugs

β-Lactams (penicillins, cephalosporins and monobactams)

Penicillins (Table 2.11)

Structure. The β-lactams share a common ring structure (Fig. 2.5). Changes to the side-chain of benzylpenicillin (penicillin G) render the phenoxymethyl derivative (penicillin V) acid resistant and allow it to be orally absorbed. The presence of an amino group in the phenyl radical of benzylpenicillin increases its antimicrobial spectrum to include many Gram-negative and Gram-positive organisms. More extensive modification of the side-chain (e.g. as in flucloxacillin) renders the drug insensitive to bacterial penicillinase. This is useful in treating infections caused by penicillinase (β-lactamase)-producing staphylococci.

Table 2.11
Classification of penicillins

Benzylpenicillin and its long-acting parenteral relatives
Benzylpenicillin
Benethamine penicillin*
Benzathine penicillin*
Clemizole penicillin*
Procaine benzylpenicillin
(procaine penicillin)

Oral alternatives to benzylpenicillin
Azidocillin*
Phenoxymethylpenicillin
(penicillin V)

β-lactamase-stable penicillins
Flucloxacillin
Oxacillin*
Methicillin*
Nafcillin*

Extended-spectrum penicillins
Ampicillin, pivampicillin,*
talampicillin*
Amoxicillin
Co-amoxiclav, pivmecillinam

Pencillins active against Pseudomonas
Azlocillin, mezlocillin,*
piperacillin, ticarcillin

* Not available in the UK

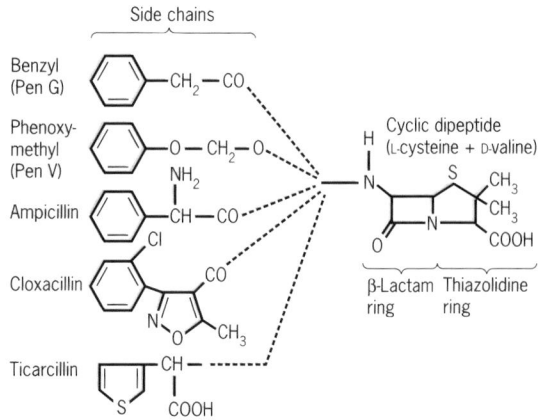

Fig. 2.5 The structure of penicillins.

Mechanisms of action. β-lactams block bacterial cell wall mucopeptide formation by binding to and inactivating specific penicillin-binding proteins (PBPs), which are peptidases involved in the final stages of cell wall assembly and division. Methicillin-resistant *Staph. aureus* (MRSA) (see p. 66) produce a low-affinity PBP which retains its peptidase activity even in the presence of high concentrations of methicillin.

Indications for use. Benzylpenicillin can only be given parenterally and is often the drug of choice for serious infections, notably infective endocarditis, meningococcal, streptococcal and gonococcal infections, clostridial infections (tetanus, gas gangrene), actinomycosis, anthrax, and spirochaetal infections (syphilis, yaws).

Phenoxymethylpenicillin (penicillin V) is an oral preparation that is used chiefly to treat streptococcal pharyngitis and as prophylaxis against rheumatic fever.

Flucloxacillin is used in infections caused by penicillinase-producing staphylococci.

Ampicillin is susceptible to penicillinase, but its antimicrobial activity includes streptococci, pneumococci and enterococci as well as Gram-negative organisms such as *Salmonella* spp., *Shigella* spp., *E. coli*, *H. influenzae* and *Proteus* spp. More recently, drug resistance has eroded its efficacy against these Gram-negatives. It is widely used in the treatment of respiratory tract infections. Amoxicillin has similar activity to ampicillin, but is better absorbed when given by mouth.

The extended-spectrum penicillin, ticarcillin is active against pseudomonas infections, as is the acylureidopenicillin piperacillin in combination with sulbactam.

Clavulanic acid is a powerful inhibitor of many bacterial β-lactamases and when given in combination with an otherwise effective agent such as amoxicillin (co-amoxiclav) or ticarcillin can broaden the spectrum of activity of the drug. Sulbactam acts similarly and is available combined with ampicillin, while tazobactam in combination with piperacillin is effective in appendicitis, peritonitis, pelvic inflammatory disease, and complicated skin infections. The penicillin β-lactamase combinations are also active against β-lactamase-producing staphylococci.

Pivmecillinam has significant activity against Gram-negative bacteria including *E. coli*, *Klebsiella*, *Enterobacter* and salmonellae but no activity against pseudomonas.

Interactions. Penicillins inactivate aminoglycosides when mixed in the same solution.

Toxicity. Generally, the penicillins are very safe. Hypersensitivity (skin rash (common), urticaria, anaphylaxis), encephalopathy and tubulointerstitial nephritis can occur. Ampicillin also produces a hypersensitivity rash in approximately 90% of patients with infectious mononucleosis who receive this drug. Co-amoxiclav causes a cholestatic jaundice six times more frequently than amoxicillin.

Cephalosporins (Fig. 2.6)
The cephalosporins have an advantage over the penicillins in that they are resistant to staphylococcal penicillinases (but are still inactive against methicillin-resistant staphylococci) and have a broader range of activity that includes both Gram-negative and Gram-positive organisms, but excludes enterococci and anaerobic bacteria. Ceftazidime and cefpirome are active against *Pseudomonas aeruginosa*.

Indications for use (Table 2.12). These potent broad-spectrum antibiotics are useful for the treatment of serious systemic infections, particularly when the precise nature of the infection is unknown. They are commonly used for serious sepsis in postoperative and immunocompromised patients, particularly during cytotoxic chemotherapy of leukaemia and other malignancies.

Cephalosporin

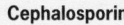

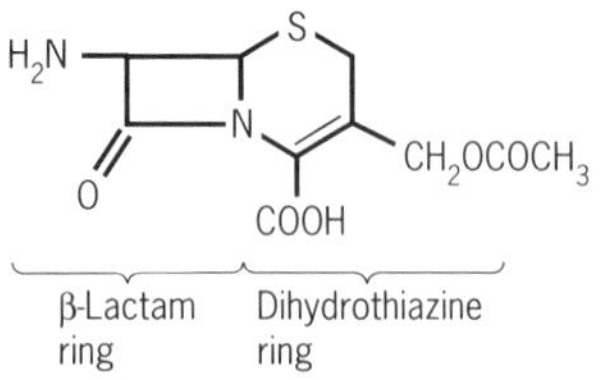

Fig. 2.6 **The structure of a cephalosporin.**

Interactions. There are relatively few interactions.

Toxicity. The toxicity is similar to the penicillins but is less common. Some 10% of patients are allergic to both groups of drugs. The early cephalosporins caused proximal tubule damage, although the newer derivatives have fewer nephrotoxic effects.

Monobactams

Aztreonam is currently the only member of this class available. It is a synthetic β-lactam and, unlike the penicillins and cephalosporins, has no ring other than the β-lactam, hence its description as a monobactam. Its mechanism of action is by inhibition of bacterial cell wall synthesis. It is resistant to most β-lactamases and does not induce β-lactamase production.

Indications for use. Aztreonam's spectrum of activity is limited to aerobic Gram-negative bacilli. With the exception of urinary tract infections, aztreonam should be used in combination with metronidazole (for anaerobes) and an agent active against Gram-positive cocci (a penicillin or erythromycin). It is a useful alternative to aminoglycosides in combination therapy, largely for the treatment of intra-abdominal sepsis.

Toxicity. As for the β-lactam antibiotics.

Carbapenems

The carbapenems are semisynthetic β-lactams and include imipenem, biapenem and meropenem. They are currently the most broad spectrum of antibiotics being active against the majority of Gram-positive and Gram-negative as well as anaerobic bacterial pathogens. Imipenem is partially inactivated in the kidney by enzymatic inactivation and is therefore administered in combination with cilastatin.

Indications for use. They are used for serious nosocomial infections when multiple-resistant Gram-negative bacilli or mixed aerobe and anaerobe infections are suspected.

Toxicity. This is similar to that of β-lactam antibiotics. Nausea, vomiting and diarrhoea occur in less than 5% of cases. Imipenem may cause seizures and should not be used to treat meningitis; meropenem is safe for this indication.

Aminoglycosides

Structure. These antibiotics are polycationic compounds of amino sugars (Fig. 2.7).

Table 2.12
Some examples of cephalosporins

	Activity	Use
First generation Cefalexin (oral) Cefaclor (oral) Cefradine (oral) Cefadroxil (oral)	Gram-positive cocci and Gram-negative organisms	Urinary tract infections Penicillin allergy
Second generation Cefuroxime Cefamandole Cefoxitin Cefuroxime (oral)	Extended spectrum More effective than first generation against *E. coli*, *Klebsiella* spp. and *Proteus mirabilis*, but less effective against Gram-positive organisms	Prophylaxis and treatment of Gram-negative infections and mixed aerobic–anaerobic infections
Third generation Cefotaxime Ceftazidime Cefpirome Cefodizime Ceftriaxone Cefpodoxime (oral) Cefixime (oral) Ceftibutin (oral)	Broad-spectrum More potent against aerobic Gram-negative bacteria than first or second generation	Especially severe infection with Enterobacteriaceae, *Pseudomonas aeruginosa* (ceftazidime, cefpirome) and *Neisseria gonorrhoeae*, Lyme disease (ceftriaxone)

Aminoglycoside

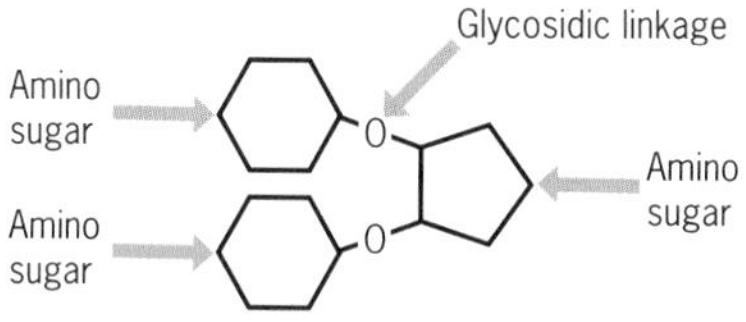

Fig. 2.7 **The structure of an aminoglycoside.**

Tetracycline

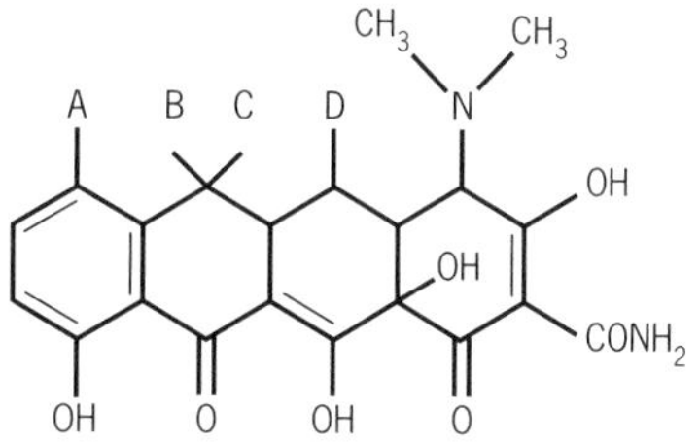

Fig. 2.8 **The structure of a tetracycline.** Substitution of CH_3, OH or H at positions A to D produces variants of tetracycline.

Mechanism of action. Aminoglycosides interrupt bacterial protein synthesis by inhibiting ribosomal function (messenger and transfer RNA).

Indications for use. Streptomycin is bactericidal and is rarely used except for the treatment of tuberculosis. Occasional indications include endocarditis (with penicillin/ampicillin). Neomycin is used only for the topical treatment of eye and skin infections and in the management of portosystemic encephalopathy. Even though it is poorly absorbed, prolonged oral administration can produce ototoxicity.

Gentamicin and tobramycin are given parenterally. They are highly effective against many Gram-negative organisms including *Pseudomonas* spp. They are synergistic with a penicillin against *Enterococcus* spp. Netilmicin and amikacin have a similar spectrum but are more resistant to the aminoglycoside-inactivating enzymes (phosphorylating, adenylating or acetylating) produced by some bacteria. Their use should be restricted to gentamicin-resistant organisms.

Interactions. Enhanced nephrotoxicity occurs with other nephrotoxic drugs, ototoxicity with some diuretics, and neuromuscular blockade with curariform drugs.

Toxicity. This is dose-related. Aminoglycosides are nephrotoxic and ototoxic (vestibular and auditory), particularly in the elderly. Therapeutic drug monitoring is important in ensuring therapeutic and non-toxic drug concentrations.

Tetracyclines
Structure. These are bacteriostatic drugs possessing a four-ring hydronaphthacene nucleus (Fig. 2.8). Included among the tetracyclines are tetracycline, oxytetracycline, demeclocycline, lymecycline, doxycycline and minocycline.

Mechanism of action. Tetracyclines inhibit bacterial protein synthesis by interrupting ribosomal function (transfer RNA).

Indications for use. Tetracyclines are active against Gram-positive and Gram-negative bacteria but their use is now limited, partly owing to increasing bacterial resistance. A tetracycline is used for the treatment of acne and rosacea. Tetracyclines are also active against *V. cholerae*, *Rickettsia* spp., *Mycoplasma* spp., *Coxiella burnetii*, *Chlamydia* spp. and *Brucella* spp. They were formerly used widely in lower respiratory tract infection, but resistance is now common among *Strep. pneumoniae*.

Interactions. The efficacy of tetracyclines is reduced by antacids and oral iron-replacement therapy.

Toxicity. Tetracyclines are generally safe drugs, but they may enhance established or incipient renal failure, although doxycycline is safer than others in this group. They cause brown discoloration of growing teeth, and thus these drugs are not given to children or pregnant women. Photosensitivity can occur.

Macrolides
Erythromycin
Structure. Erythromycin consists of a lactone ring with unusual sugar side-chains.

Mechanism of action. Erythromycin inhibits protein synthesis by interrupting ribosomal function.

Indications for use. Erythromycin has a similar (but not identical) antibacterial spectrum to penicillin and is useful in individuals with penicillin allergy. It can be given orally or parenterally. It is the preferred agent in the treatment of pneumonias caused by *Legionella* spp. and *Mycoplasma* spp. It is also effective in the treatment of infections due to *Bordetella pertussis* (whooping cough), *Campylobacter* spp., *Chlamydia* spp. and *Coxiella* spp.

Other macrolides
These include clarithromycin, roxithromycin and azithromycin. They have a broad spectrum of activity that includes Gram-negative organisms, mycobacteria and *Toxoplasma gondii*. Compared with erythromycin, they have superior pharmacokinetic properties with enhanced tissue and intracellular penetration and longer half-life that allows once or twice daily dosage. Clarithromycin is widely recommended as a component of triple therapy regimens (usually with a proton pump inhibitor and metronidazole) for the eradication of *Helicobacter pylori*. Azithromycin is now used for trachoma (see p. 86).

Interactions. Erythromycin and other macrolides interact with theophyllines, carbamazepine, digoxin and ciclosporin, occasionally necessitating dose adjustment of these agents.

Toxicity. Diarrhoea, vomiting and abdominal pain are the main side-effects of erythromycin (less with

Infectious diseases, tropical medicine and sexually transmitted diseases

clarithromycin and azithromycin) and are, in part, a consequence of the intestinal prokinetic properties of the macrolides. Macrolides may also rarely produce cholestatic jaundice after prolonged treatment. QT_c prolongation is a recognized cardiac effect of the macrolides. This may have serious consequences if the syndrome of 'torsades de pointes' is induced.

Chloramphenicol

Structure. Chloramphenicol is the only naturally occurring antibiotic containing nitrobenzene (Fig. 2.9). This structure probably accounts for its toxicity in humans and for its activity against bacteria.

Mechanism of action. Chloramphenicol competes with messenger RNA for ribosomal binding. It also inhibits peptidyl transferase.

Indications for use. Chloramphenicol is rarely used in developed countries. In developing countries it has been invaluable in the treatment of severe infections caused by *Salmonella typhi* and *S. paratyphi* (enteric fevers) and *H. influenzae* (meningitis and acute epiglottitis) which are still prevalent in countries where Hib vaccination has not been introduced. It is also active against *Yersinia pestis* (plague) and is used topically for the treatment of purulent conjunctivitis. Drug resistance is currently eroding the efficacy of chloramphenicol.

Interactions. Chloramphenicol enhances the activity of anticoagulants, phenytoin and oral hypoglycaemic agents.

Toxicity. Severe irreversible bone marrow suppression is rare but nevertheless now restricts the usage of this drug to only the severely ill patient. Chloramphenicol should not be given to premature infants or neonates because of their inability to conjugate and excrete this drug; high blood levels lead to circulatory collapse and the often fatal 'grey baby syndrome'.

Fusidic acid

Structure. Fusidic acid has a structure resembling that of bile salts (see p. 339).

Mechanism of action. It is a potent inhibitor of bacterial protein synthesis. Its entry into cells is facilitated by the detergent properties inherent in its structure.

Indications for use. Fusidic acid is mainly used for penicillinase-producing *Staph. aureus* infections such as osteomyelitis (it is well concentrated in bone) or endocarditis, and for other staphylococcal infections accompanied by septicaemia. The drug is well absorbed orally but is relatively expensive.

Resistance. Resistance may occur rapidly and is the reason why fusidic acid is given in combination with another antibiotic.

Toxicity. Fusidic acid may occasionally be hepatotoxic but is generally a safe drug and if necessary can be given during pregnancy.

Sulphonamides and trimethoprim

Structure. The sulphonamides are all derivatives of the prototype sulphanilamide. Trimethoprim is a 2,4-,diaminopyrimidine.

Mechanism of action. Sulphonamides block thymidine and purine synthesis by inhibiting microbial folic acid synthesis. Trimethoprim prevents the reduction of dihydrofolate to tetrahydrofolate (see Fig. 8.10).

Indications for use. Sulfamethoxazole is mainly used in combination with trimethoprim (as co-trimoxazole). Its use is now largely restricted to the treatment and prevention of *Pneumocystis carinii* infection and listeriosis in developed countries, although it is still in widespread use in developing countries. It may also be used for toxoplasmosis and nocardiosis and as a second-line agent in acute exacerbations of chronic bronchitis and in urinary tract infections. Trimethoprim alone is often used for urinary tract infections and acute-on-chronic bronchitis, as the side-effects of co-trimoxazole are most commonly due to the sulphonamide component. Sulfapyridine in combination with 5-aminosalicylic acid (i.e. sulfasalazine) is used in inflammatory bowel disease.

Resistance. Resistance to sulphonamides is often plasmid-mediated and results from the production of sulphonamide-resistant dihydropteroate synthetase from altered bacterial cell permeability to these agents.

Interactions. Sulphonamides potentiate oral anticoagulants and hypoglycaemic agents.

Toxicity. Sulphonamides cause a variety of skin eruptions, including toxic epidermal necrolysis, the Stevens–Johnson syndrome, thrombocytopenia, folate deficiency and megaloblastic anaemia with prolonged usage. It can provoke haemolysis in individuals with glucose-6-phosphate dehydrogenase deficiency and therefore should not be used in such people. Co-trimoxazole should also be avoided in the elderly if possible, as deaths have been recorded, probably owing to the sulphonamide component.

Quinolones

The quinolone antibiotics, such as ciprofloxacin, norfloxacin, ofloxacin and levofloxacin, are useful oral broad-spectrum antibiotics, related structurally to

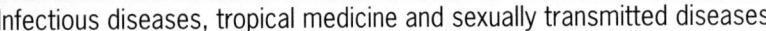

Chloramphenicol

Fig. 2.9 **The structure of chloramphenicol.**

Quinolone

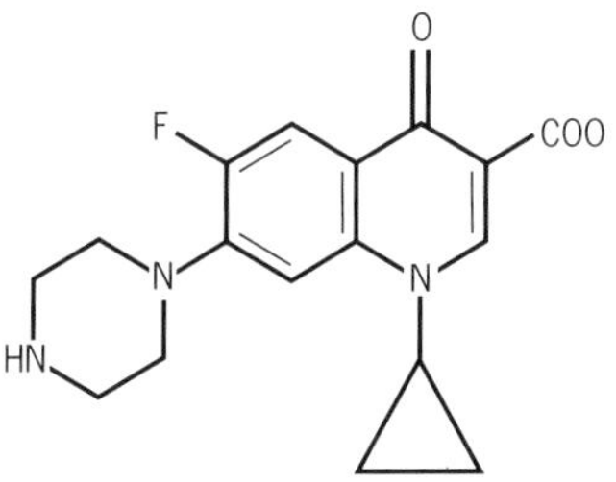

Fig. 2.10 The structure of a quinolone (ciprofloxacin).

Linezolid

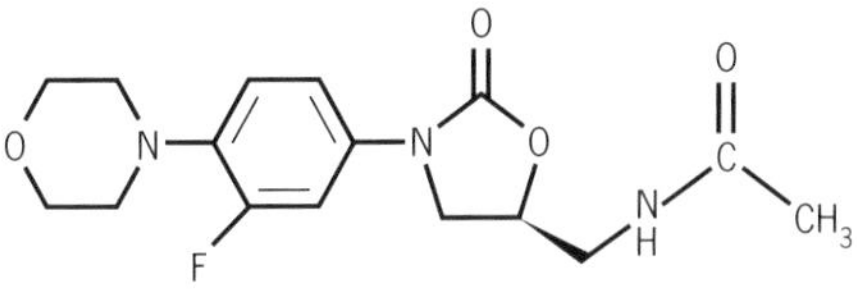

Fig. 2.11 The structure of linezolid, an oxazolidinone.

nalidixic acid. The latter achieves only low serum concentrations after oral administration and its use is limited to the urinary tract where it is concentrated. Newer quinolones, including moxifloxacin and gemifloxacin, have greater activity against Gram-positive pathogens. The structure is shown in Figure 2.10.

Mechanism of action. The quinolone group of bactericidal drugs inhibit bacterial DNA synthesis by inhibiting topoisomerase IV and DNA gyrase, the enzyme responsible for maintaining the superhelical twists in DNA.

Indications for use. The 4-fluoroquinolones should be reserved for infections caused by organisms resistant to standard drugs. The extended-spectrum quinolones such as ciprofloxacin have activity against Gram-negative, including *Pseudomonas aeruginosa*, and some Gram-positive bacteria. They are useful in Gram-negative septicaemia, skin and bone infections, urinary and respiratory tract infections, meningococcal carriage, in some sexually transmitted diseases such as gonorrhoea and non-specific urethritis due to *Chlamydia trachomatis*, and in severe cases of traveller's diarrhoea (see p. 72). The newer oral quinolones provide an alternative to β-lactams in the treatment of community-acquired lower respiratory tract infections.

Interactions. Ciprofloxacin can induce toxic concentrations of theophylline.

Toxicity. Gastrointestinal disturbances, photosensitive rashes and occasional neurotoxicity can occur. Avoid in pregnancy.

Oxazolidinones

Structure. The oxazolidinones are a novel class of antibacterial agents of which linezolid (Fig. 2.11) is the first to become available.

Mechanism of action. The oxazolidinones inhibit protein synthesis by binding to the bacterial 23S ribosomal RNA of the 59S sub-unit, thereby preventing the formation of a functional 70S complex essential to bacterial translation.

Indications for use. Linezolid is active against a variety of Gram-positive pathogens including vancomycin-resistant *Enterococcus faecium* (unfortunately resistant

organisms have already been reported), methicillin-resistant *Staphylococcus aureus* and penicillin-resistant *Streptococcus pneumoniae*. It is also active against group A and group B streptococci. To date, clinical experience has demonstrated efficacy in a variety of hospitalized patients with severe to life-threatening infections, such as bacteraemia, hospital-acquired pneumonia and skin and soft tissue infections. It can be given both intravenously and by mouth.

Interactions. Linezolid interacts reversibly as a non-selective inhibitor of monoamine oxidase, and has the potential for interacting with serotoninergic and adrenergic agents.

Toxicity. Side-effects include gastrointestinal disturbances, headache, rash, hypertension and reversible thrombocytopenia. Safety has not yet been shown in pregnancy.

Nitroimidazoles

Structure. These agents are active against anaerobic bacteria and some pathogenic protozoa. The most widely used drug is metronidazole (Fig. 2.12). Others include tinidazole and nimorazole.

Mechanism of action. After reduction of their nitro group to a nitrosohydroxyl amino group by microbial enzymes, nitroimidazoles cause strand breaks in microbial DNA.

Indications for use. Metronidazole is of major importance in the treatment of anaerobic bacterial infections, particularly those due to *Bacteroides* spp. It is also used prophylactically in colonic surgery. It may be given orally, by suppository (well absorbed and cheap) or intravenously (very expensive). It is also the treatment of choice for amoebiasis, giardiasis and infection with *Trichomonas vaginalis*.

Metronidazole

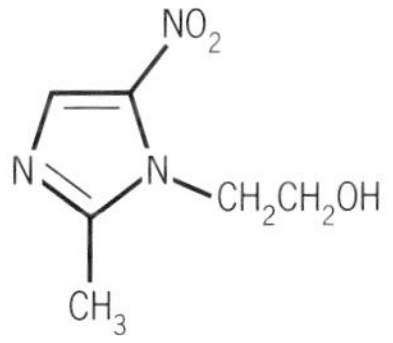

Fig. 2.12 The structure of metronidazole, a nitroimidazole.

Interactions. Nitroimidazoles can produce a disulfiram-like reaction with ethanol and enhance the anticoagulent effect of warfarin.

Toxicity. Nitroimidazoles are tumorigenic in animals and mutagenic for bacteria, although carcinogenicity has not been described in humans. They cause a metallic taste, and polyneuropathy with prolonged use. They should be avoided in pregnancy.

Glycopeptides

The glycopeptides are antibiotics active against Gram-positive bacteria and act by inhibiting cell wall synthesis.

Vancomycin

Vancomycin is given intravenously for methicillin-resistant *S. aureus* and other multiresistant Gram-positive organisms. It is also used for treatment and prophylaxis against Gram-positive infections in penicillin-allergic patients. It has recently been recommended for *S. pneumoniae* meningitis when caused by penicillin-resistant strains. By mouth it is an alternative to metronidazole for *Clostridium difficile*-associated colitis. Vancomycin-resistant enterococci (VRE) are increasingly being recognized.

Toxicity. Vancomycin can cause ototoxicity and nephrotoxicity and thus serum levels should be monitored. Care must be taken to avoid extravasation at the injection site as this causes necrosis and thrombophlebitis. Too rapid infusion can produce symptomatic release of histamine.

Teicoplanin

This glycopeptide antibiotic is less nephrotoxic than vancomycin. It has more favourable pharmacokinetic properties, allowing once-daily dosage.

Other antibiotics

Clindamycin is not widely used because of its toxic side effect, antibiotic associated colitis (pseudomembranous colitis). It is active against Gram-positive cocci including some penicillin-resistant staphylococci. It is also active against anaerobes, especially bacteroides. It is well concentrated in bone and used for osteomyelitis.

Quinupristin and dalfopristin. A combination of these streptogramin antibiotics is used for Gram-postive bacteria which have failed to respond to other antibacterials.

Antituberculosis drugs

These are described on page 895. Rifampicin is also used in other infections apart from tuberculosis.

Antifungal drugs (Table 2.13)

Polyenes

Polyenes react with the sterols in fungal membranes, increasing permeability and thus damaging the organism. The most potent is amphotericin B, which is used intravenously in severe systemic fungal infections. Nephrotoxicity is a major problem and dosage levels must take background renal function into account. Liposomal amphotericin B is less toxic but very expensive. Nystatin is not absorbed through mucous membranes and is therefore useful for the treatment of oral and enteric candidiasis and for vaginal infection. It can only be given orally or as pessaries.

Azoles

Imidazoles such as ketoconazole, miconazole and clotrimazole are broad-spectrum antifungal drugs. They act by inhibiting fungal sterol synthesis resulting in damage to the cell wall.

Clotrimazole is used topically for the treatment of ringworm and cutaneous and genital candidiasis. Econazole and tioconazole are used for the topical treatment of cutaneous and vaginal candidiasis and dermatophyte infections. Ketoconazole is active orally but can produce liver damage. It is effective in candidiasis and deep mycoses including histoplasmosis and blastomycosis but not in aspergillosis and cryptococcosis.

Triazoles. These include fluconazole and itraconazole. Fluconazole is noted for its ability to enter CSF and is used for candidiasis and for the treatment of central nervous system (CNS) infection with *Cryptococcus neoformans*. Itraconazole fails to penetrate CSF. It is the agent of choice for non-life-threatening blastomycosis and histoplasmosis. It is also moderately effective in invasive aspergillosis. Toxicity is mild. The problem associated with poor absorption of the capsules in the absence of food has been overcome with the liquid formulation. Voriconazole is a new agent.

Allylamines

Terbinafine has antifungal and anti-inflammatory activity orally and is useful for the treatment of superficial

---

Table 2.13
Antifungal agents

Polyenes	Allylamines
Amphotericin B, nystatin	Terbinafine
Azoles	**Other antifungals**
Miconazole, ketoconazole, fluconazole, itraconazole	Amorolfine (topical only)
Topical clotrimazole, sulconazole, econazole, tioconazole	Fluorinated pyrimidizine
	5-Flucytosine
	Griseofulvin

mycoses such as dermatophyte infections, onychomycosis and cutaneous candidiasis. A topical formulation is also available to treat fungal skin infections.

Other antifungals

Flucytosine. The fluorinated pyridine derivative, flucytosine, is used in combination with amphotericin B for systemic fungal infection. Side-effects are uncommon, although it may cause bone marrow suppression. It is active when given orally or parenterally.

Griseofulvin. Griseofulvin, a naturally occurring antifungal, is widely used for the treatment of more extensive superficial mycoses and onychomycosis.

Amorolfine. Amorolfine is available for the topical treatment of fungal skin and nail infections.

Antiviral drugs

Drugs for HIV infection are discussed on page 147.

Aciclovir

Aciclovir (Fig. 2.13) is an acyclic nucleoside analogue which acts as a chain terminator of herpesvirus DNA synthesis. This drug is converted to aciclovir monophosphate by a virus-encoded thymidine kinase produced by alpha herpesviruses, herpes simplex types 1 and 2 and varicella zoster virus (Table 2.14). Conversion to the triphosphate is then achieved by cellular enzymes. Aciclovir triphosphate competes with deoxyguanine triphosphate and the drug is incorporated into the growing chains of herpesvirus DNA. This highly specific mode of activity, targeted only to virus-infected cells, means that aciclovir has very low toxicity. Intravenous, oral and topical preparations are available for the treatment of herpes simplex types and varicella-zoster virus infections (Table 2.14).

A pro-drug of aciclovir, valaciclovir, has been developed. Coupling of the amino acid valine to the acyclic side-chain of aciclovir allows better intestinal absorption. The valine is removed by enzymic action and aciclovir is released into the circulation. A similar pro-drug of a related nucleoside analogue (penciclovir) is the antiherpes drug, famciclovir. The mode of action and efficacy of famciclovir are similar to those of aciclovir.

Ganciclovir

This guanine analogue is structurally similar to aciclovir, with extension of the acyclic side-chain by a carboxymethyl group. It is active against herpes simplex viruses and varicella zoster virus by the same mechanism as aciclovir. In addition, phosphorylation by a protein kinase encoded by the UL97 region of cytomegalovirus renders it potently active against this virus. Thus ganciclovir is currently the first-line treatment for cytomegalovirus disease. Intravenous and oral preparations are available. Unlike aciclovir, ganciclovir has a significant toxicity profile including neutropenia, thrombocytopenia and the likelihood of sterilization by inhibiting spermatogenesis. For this reason, it is reserved for the treatment or prevention of life-or sight-threatening cytomegalovirus infection.

Foscarnet

Foscarnet (sodium phosphonoformate) is a simple pyrophosphate analogue which inhibits viral DNA polymerases. It is active against herpesviruses and its main roles are as a second-line treatment for severe cytomegalovirus disease and for the treatment of aciclovir-resistant herpes simplex infection. It is given intravenously and the potential for severe side-effects, particularly renal damage, limits its use.

Table 2.14
Antiviral agents (for drugs against HIV see Table 2.53)

Drug	Use
Nucleoside analogues	
Aciclovir	Topical – HSV infection
	Oral and intravenous – VZV and HSV
Famciclovir	Oral – VZV and HSV
Valaciclovir	Oral – VZV and HSV
Ganciclovir	Intravenous and oral – CMV
Idoxuridine	HSV (topical eye treatment)
Trifluorothymidine	HSV (topical eye treatment)
Vidarabine	Topical – HSV (eye)
	Intravenous – severe VZV and HSV
Cidofovir	CMV
Pyrophosphate analogues	
Foscarnet	Intravenous – CMV
Adamantanes	
Amantadine	Oral – influenza A
Neuraminidase inhibitors	
Zanamivir	Topical (inhalation) – influenza A and B
Oseltamivir	Oral – influenza A and B
Ribavirin	Topical (inhalation) – RSV
	Intravenous – Lassa fever, hepatitis C
Interferon-α	HBV, HCV, some malignancies
	(e.g. renal cell carcinoma)
(Peg interferon-α)	(Given once weekly)

Acyclovir

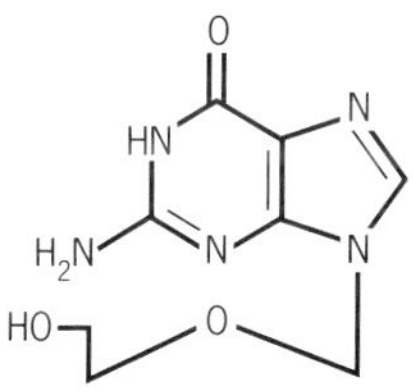

Fig. 2.13 **The structure of aciclovir.**

Cidofovir

This is a phosphonate derivative of an acyclic nucleoside which is a DNA polymerase chain inhibitor. It is administered intravenously for the treatment of severe cytomegalovirus (CMV) infections in patients with AIDS. It is given with probenecid, and as it is nephrotoxic, particular attention should be given to hydration and to monitoring renal function.

Idoxuridine

This is a nucleoside analogue with activity against herpesviruses (mainly HSV-1). Its use is confined mainly to the topical treatment of ophthalmic herpes simplex infection.

Amantadine

Amantadine is a synthetic symmetrical amine which is active prophylactically and therapeutically against influenza A virus (it is inactive against influenza B virus). Its prophylactic efficacy is similar to that of influenza vaccine and it is occasionally used to prevent the spread of influenza A in institutions such as nursing homes. Although CNS side-effects such as insomnia, dizziness and headache may occur (it is also used as a treatment for Parkinson's disease), these are not usually produced by the lower doses currently recommended.

Neuraminidase inhibitors

Two drugs that inhibit the action of the neuraminidase of influenza A and B have been introduced. Zanamavir is administered by inhalation and oseltamivir is an oral preparation. Both have been shown to be effective in reducing the duration of illness in influenza.

Ribavirin

This synthetic purine nucleoside derivative which interfaces with 5'-capping of messenger RNA, is active against several RNA viruses. It is administered by a small-particle aerosol generator (SPAG) to infants with acute respiratory syncytial virus (RSV) infection. In a clinical trial in Sierra Leone it was shown to reduce the mortality of Lassa fever virus infection. Individuals with hepatitis C virus infection, treated with interferon alpha-ribavirin combinations, have lower relapse rates than those receiving interferon alone.

Interferons (see also p. 197)

These are naturally occurring proteins produced by virus-infected cells, macrophages and lymphocytes. Interferons are stimulated by a number of factors, including viral nucleic acid, and render uninfected cells resistant to infection with the same – or in some circumstances different – viruses. They have been synthesized commercially by either culture of lymphoblastoid cells or by recombinant DNA technology and are licensed for therapeutic use. Currently, infection with hepatitis viruses B and C (and certain malignancies) are treated with regular injections of α-interferon.

The potency of α-interferon has been enhanced by coupling the protein with polyethylene glycol. The resulting peg interferon given once weekly has been shown to improve the response to treatment of hepatitis C.

FURTHER READING

Anyes SGB, Gemmell CG (1997) Antibiotic resistance. *Journal of Medical Microbiology* **33**: 436–470.

Blair E, Darby G, Gough G, Littler E, Rowlands D, Tisdale M (1998) *Antiviral Therapy*. Oxford: Bios.

Finch RG (1998) Antibiotic resistance. *Journal of Antimicrobial Chemotherapy* **42**: 125–128.

O'Grady FW, Lambert HP, Finch RG, Greenwood D (1997) *Antibiotic and Chemotherapy*, 7th edn. Edinburgh: Churchill Livingstone.

Patel R (1998) Antifungal agents. Part I. Amphotericin B preparations and flucytosine. *Mayo Clinic Proceedings* **73(12)**: 1205–1225.

Terrell CL (1999) Antifungal agents. Part II. The azoles. *Mayo Clinic Proceedings* **74**: 78–100.

Immunization against infectious diseases

Although effective antimicrobial chemotherapy is available for many diseases, the ultimate aim of any infectious disease control programme is to prevent infection occurring. This may be achieved either by:

- eliminating the source or mode of transmission of an infection (p. 25)
- reducing host susceptibility to environmental pathogens.

Immunization, immunoprophylaxis and immunotherapy

Immunization has changed the course and natural history of many infectious diseases. Passive immunization by administering preformed antibody, either in the form of immune serum or purified normal immunoglobulin, provides short-term immunity and has been effective in both the prevention (immunoprophylaxis) and treatment (immunotherapy) of a number of bacterial and viral diseases (Table 2.15). The active immunization schedule currently recommended is summarized in Box 2.6. Long-lasting immunity is achieved only by active immunization with a live attenuated or an inactivated organism (Table 2.16). Active immunization may also be performed with microbial toxin (either native or modified) – that is, a toxoid. Immunization should be kept up to date with booster doses throughout life. Travellers to developing countries, especially if visiting rural areas, should in addition enquire about further specific immunizations.

Table 2.15
Examples of passive immunization available

Infection	Antibody	Indication	Efficacy
Bacterial			
Tetanus	Human tetanus immune globulin	Prevention and treatment	+
Diphtheria	Horse serum	Prevention and treatment	±
Botulism	Horse serum	Treatment	+
Viral			
Hepatitis A Measles }	Human normal immune globulin	Prevention	+
Hepatitis B	Human hepatitis B immune globulin	Prevention	+
Varicella zoster	Human varicella zoster immune globulin	Prevention	+
Rabies	Human rabies immune globulin	Prevention	+

Table 2.16
Preparations available for active immunization

Live attenuated vaccines
Oral polio (Sabin)
Measles
Mumps
Rubella
Yellow fever
BCG
Typhoid (Ty 21a)

Inactivated conjugate vaccines
Hepatitis A
Pertussis
Typhoid – whole cell and Vi antigen
Polio (Salk)
Influenza
Cholera
Meningococci (groups A and C)
Meningococcus group C (conjugate)
Rabies
Pneumococcal
Haemophilus influenza type b

Toxoids
Diphtheria
Tetanus

Recombinant vaccines
Hepatitis B

BCG, bacille Calmette-Guérin

Box 2.6

Recommended immunization schedules: (i) in the UK; (ii) WHO model schedule for developing countries

Time of immunization	Vaccine
(i) UK	
2 months	DPT, Hib, OPV, MenC, BCG*
3 months	DPT, Hib, OPV, MenC
4 months	DPT, Hib, OPV, MenC
12–15 months	MMR
3–5 years	DT, OPV, MMR
10–14 years	BCG[†]
13–18 years	DT, OPV
(ii) Developing countries[‡]	
Birth (or first contact)	OPV, BCG
6 weeks	DPT, OPV, HBV
10 weeks	DPT, OPV, HBV
14 weeks	DPT, OPV, HBV
9 months	Measles, YF[§]

DPT, diphtheria, pertussis, tetanus triple vaccine; Hib, *Haemophilus influenzae* b vaccine; OPV, oral polio vaccine; MenC, meningococcus group C vaccine; BCG, bacille Calmette–Guérin (tuberculosis vaccine); MMR, measles, mumps, rubella triple vaccine; HBV, hepatitis B vaccine; YF, yellow fever vaccine

* Children at high risk of contact with tuberculosis
[†] Tuberculin-negative children at low risk of contact with tuberculosis
[‡] Model scheme, adapted locally depending on need and availability of vaccines
[§] In endemic areas

In 1974 the World Health Organization introduced the Expanded Programme on Immunization (EPI). Twenty years later more than 80% of the world's children had been immunized against tuberculosis, diphtheria, tetanus, pertussis, polio and measles. It is hoped that poliomyelitis will shortly be eradicated world-wide, which will match the past success of global smallpox eradication. Introduction of conjugate vaccines against *Haemophilus influenzae* type b (Hib) has proved highly effective in controlling invasive *H. influenzae* infection, notably meningitis (see p. 860).

FURTHER READING

Ada G (2001) Vaccines and vaccination. *New England Journal of Medicine* **345**: 1042–1053.

John TJ (2000) The final stages of the global eradication of polio. *New England Journal of Medicine* **343**: 806–807.

Salisbury DM, Begg NT (eds) (1996) *Immunization Against Infectious Diseases*. London: HMSO.

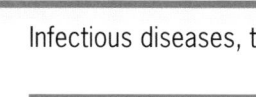

Viral infections: an introduction

Viruses are much smaller than other infectious agents (Tables 2.17 and 2.19) and contain either DNA or RNA, not both as in bacteria and other microorganisms. Since they are metabolically inert, they must live intracellularly, using the host cell for synthesis of viral proteins and nucleic acid. Viruses have a central nucleic acid core surrounded by a protein coat that is antigenically unique for a particular virus. The protein coat (capsid) imparts a helical or icosahedral structure to the virus. Some viruses also possess an envelope consisting of lipid and protein.

Hepatitis viruses are discussed on page 351.

DNA viruses

Details of the structure, size and classification of human DNA viruses are shown in Table 2.17.

Adenoviruses

Adenovirus infection commonly presents as an acute pharyngitis, and extension of infection to the larynx and trachea in infants may lead to croup. By school age the majority of children show serological evidence of previous infection. Certain subtypes produce an acute conjunctivitis associated with pharyngitis. In adults, adenovirus causes acute follicular conjunctivitis and rarely pneumonia that is clinically similar to that produced by *Mycoplasma pneumoniae* (see p. 887). Adenoviruses have also been implicated as a cause of gastroenteritis (see p. 54) without respiratory disease and may be responsible for acute mesenteric lymphadenitis in children and young adults. Mesenteric adenitis that is due to adenoviruses may lead to intussusception in infants.

Herpesviruses

Members of the herpesviruses are important causes of a wide range of human diseases. Details are summarized in Table 2.18. The hallmark of all herpesvirus infections is the ability of the viruses to establish latent (or silent) infections that then persist for the life of the individual.

Herpes simplex virus (HSV) infection
(Fig. 2.14)

Two types of HSV have been identified: HSV-1 is the major cause of herpetic stomatitis, herpes labialis ('cold sore'), keratoconjunctivitis and encephalitis, whereas HSV-2 causes genital herpes and may also be responsible for systemic infection in the immunocompromised host. These divisions, however, are not rigid, for HSV-1 can give rise to genital herpes and HSV-2 can cause pharyngitis.

The portal of entry of HSV-1 infection is usually via the mouth or occasionally the skin. The primary infection may go unnoticed or may produce a severe inflammatory reaction with vesicle formation leading to painful

Table 2.17
Human DNA viruses

Structure		Approximate size	Family	Viruses
Symmetry	Envelope			
Icosahedral	–	80 nm	Adenovirus	Adenoviruses
Icosahedral	+	100 nm (160 nm with envelope)	Herpesvirus	Herpes simplex virus (HSV) types 1 and 2 Varicella zoster virus Cytomegalovirus Epstein–Barr virus (EBV) Human herpesvirus type 6 (HHV-6) Human herpesvirus type 7 (HHV-7) Human herpesvirus type 8 (HHV-8)
Icosahedral	+	42 nm	Hepadnavirus	Hepatitis B virus (HBV)
Icosahedral	–	50 nm	Papovavirus	Human papillomavirus Polyomavirus
Icosahedral	–	23 nm	Parvovirus	Parvovirus B19
Complex	+	300 nm × 200 nm	Poxvirus	Variola virus Vaccinia virus Monkeypox Cowpox Orf Molluscum contagiosum

Table 2.18
Major diseases caused by human herpesviruses

Subfamily	Virus	Children	Adults	Immunocompromised
α-Herpesvirus	Herpes simplex type 1	Stomatitis*	Cold sores Keratitis Erythema multiforme	Dissemination
	Herpes simplex type 2		Primary genital herpes* Recurrent genital herpes	Dissemination
	Varicella zoster virus	Chickenpox*	Shingles	Dissemination
β-Herpesvirus	Cytomegalovirus	Congenital*		Pneumonitis Retinitis Gastrointestinal
	Human herpesvirus type 6	Roseola infantum*		Pneumonitis
	Human herpesvirus type 7	Roseola infantum*		
γ-Herpesvirus	Epstein-Barr virus		Infectious mononucleosis* Burkitt's lymphoma Nasopharyngeal carcinoma	Lymphoma
	Human herpesvirus type 8		Kaposi's sarcoma	Kaposi's sarcoma

* Signifies primary infections

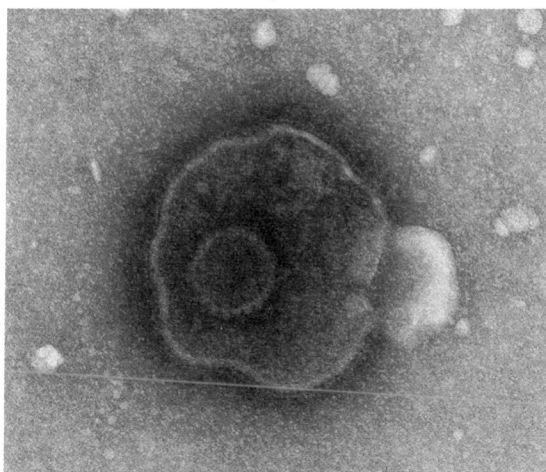

Fig. 2.14 **Electronmicrograph of herpes simplex virus.**

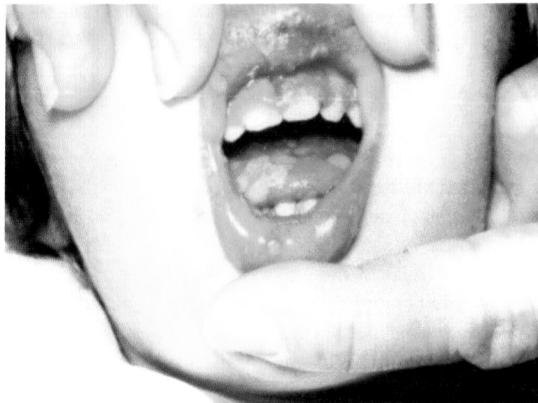

Fig. 2.15 **Primary herpes simplex type 1 (gingivostomatitis).**

ulcers (gingivostomatitis; see Fig. 2.15). The virus then remains latent, most commonly in the trigeminal ganglia, but may be reactivated by stress, trauma, febrile illnesses and ultraviolet radiation, producing the recurrent form of the disease known as herpes labialis ('cold sore'). Approximately 70% of the population are infected with HSV-1 and recurrent infections occur in one-third of individuals. Reactivation often produces localized paraesthesiae in the lip before the appearance of a cold sore.

Complications of HSV-1 infection include transfer to the eye (dendritic ulceration, keratitis), acute encephalitis (p. 1195), skin infections such as herpetic whitlow, and erythema multiforme (see p. 1297).

In genital herpes the primary infection is usually more severe and recurrences are common. The virus remains latent in the sacral ganglia and during recurrence can produce a radiculomyelopathy, with pain in the groin, buttocks and upper thighs. Primary anorectal herpes infection is common in male homosexuals (see p. 128).

Immunocompromised patients such as those receiving intensive cancer chemotherapy or those with the acquired immunodeficiency syndrome (AIDS) may develop disseminated HSV infection involving many of the viscera. In severe cases death may result from hepatitis and encephalitis.

Neonates may develop primary HSV infection following vaginal delivery in the presence of active genital HSV infection in the mother. The disease in the baby varies from localized skin lesions to widespread visceral disease often with encephalitis. Caesarean section should therefore be considered if active genital HSV infection is present during labour.

Humoral antibody develops following primary infection, but mononuclear cell responses are probably more important in preventing dissemination of disease.

The clinical picture, diagnosis and treatment are described on page 1276.

Varicella zoster virus (VZV) infection

VZV produces two distinct diseases, varicella (chickenpox) and herpes zoster (shingles). The primary infection is chickenpox. It usually occurs in childhood, the virus entering through the mucosa of the upper respiratory tract. It should be noted that in some countries (e.g. the Indian subcontinent) a different epidemiological pattern exists with most infections occurring in adulthood. Chickenpox rarely occurs twice in the same individual. Infectious virus is spread from fresh skin lesions by direct contact or airborne transmission and the period of infectivity in chickenpox extends from 2 days before the appearance of the rash until the skin lesions are all at the crusting stage. Following recovery from chickenpox the virus then remains latent in dorsal root and cranial nerve ganglia.

Clinical features of chickenpox

Fourteen to twenty-one days after exposure to VZV, a brief prodromal illness of fever, headache and malaise heralds the eruption of chickenpox, characterized by the rapid progression of macules to papules to vesicles to pustules in a matter of hours (Fig. 2.16). In young children the prodromal illness may be very mild or absent. The illness tends to be more severe in older children and can be debilitating in adults. The lesions occur on the face, scalp and trunk, and to a lesser extent on the extremities. It is characteristic to see skin lesions at all stages of development on the same area of skin. Fever subsides as soon as new lesions cease to appear. Eventually the pustules crust and heal without scarring.

Important complications of chickenpox include pneumonia, which generally begins 1–6 days after the skin eruption, and bacterial superinfection of skin lesions. Pneumonia is more common in adults than children and cigarette smokers are at particular risk. Pulmonary symptoms are usually more striking than the physical findings, although a chest radiograph usually shows diffuse changes throughout both lung fields. CNS involvement occurs in about 1 per 1000 cases and most commonly presents as an acute truncal cerebellar ataxia. The immunocompromised are susceptible to disseminated infection with multiorgan involvement.

Clinical features of shingles

Shingles (see p. 1277) occurs at all ages but is most common in the elderly, producing similar skin lesions to chickenpox, although classically they are unilateral and restricted to a sensory nerve (dermatomal) distribution (Fig. 2.17). Shingles never occurs as a primary infection but results from reactivation of latent VZV from dorsal root and/or cranial nerve ganglia. The onset of the rash of shingles is usually preceded by severe dermatomal pain, indicating the involvement of sensory nerves in its pathogenesis. Virus is disseminated from freshly formed vesicles and may cause chickenpox in susceptible contacts.

Diagnosis

The diseases are usually recognized clinically but can be confirmed by electronmicroscopy, immunofluorescence or culture of vesicular fluid and by serology.

Prophylaxis and treatment

Chickenpox usually requires no treatment in healthy children and infection results in lifelong immunity. However, the disease may be fatal in the immunocompromised, who can be offered protection, after exposure to the virus, with zoster immune immunoglobulin (ZIG).

Anyone with chickenpox who is over the age of 16 years should be considered for antiviral therapy with aciclovir, or a similar drug, if they present within 72 hours of onset. Women in pregnancy are prone to severe chickenpox and, in addition, there is a risk of intrauterine infection with structural damage to the fetus (mainly in the mid trimester – risk rate 2%). For these reasons ZIG is recommended for prophylaxis of women in pregnancy exposed to varicella zoster virus and, if chickenpox develops, aciclovir treatment should be considered. (NB: aciclovir has not been licensed for use in

Fig. 2.16 Chickenpox in an adult. Generalized VZV.

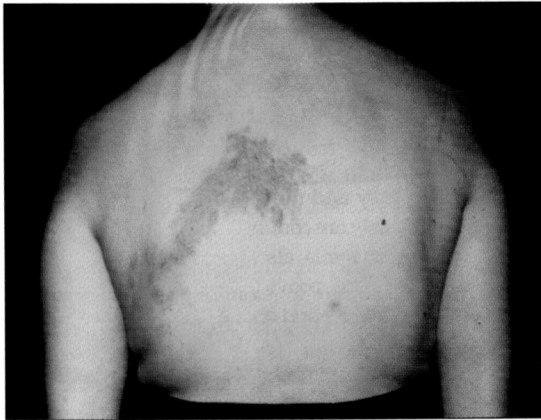

Fig. 2.17 Shingles – VZV affecting a dermatome.
Reproduced with kind permission of Imperial College School of Medicine.

pregnant women.) If a woman has chickenpox at term, her baby should be protected by ZIG if delivery occurs within 5 days of the onset of the mother's illness. An effective varicella vaccine is used in many parts of the USA; it is available on a named-patient basis in the UK.

Shingles is also treated with aciclovir and the duration of lesion formation and time to healing can be reduced by early treatment. Aciclovir, valaciclovir and famciclovir have all been shown to reduce the burden of zoster-associated pain when treatment is given at the acute phase. Shingles involving the ophthalmic division of the trigeminal nerve has an associated incidence of acute and chronic ophthalmic complications of 50%. Early treatment with aciclovir reduces this to 20% or less. As for chickenpox, all immunocompromised individuals should be given aciclovir at the onset of shingles.

Cytomegalovirus (CMV) infection

Infection with CMV is found world-wide and has its most profound effects as an opportunistic infection in the immunocompromised, particularly in recipients of bone-marrow and solid organ transplants and in patients with AIDS. Over 50% of the adult population have serological evidence of latent infection with the virus, although infection is generally symptomless. As with all herpesviruses, the virus persists for life, usually as a latent infection in which the naked DNA is situated extrachromosomally in the nuclei of the cells in the endothelium of the arterial wall and in T lymphocytes.

Clinical features

In healthy adults CMV infection is usually asymptomatic but may cause an illness similar to infectious mononucleosis, with fever, occasionally lymphocytosis with atypical lymphocytes, and hepatitis with or without jaundice. The Paul–Bunnell test for heterophile antibody is negative. Infection may be spread by kissing, sexual intercourse or blood transfusion, and transplacentally to the fetus. Disseminated fatal infection with widespread visceral involvement occurs in the immunocompromised (see p. 141) and may cause encephalitis, retinitis, pneumonitis and diffuse involvement of the gastrointestinal tract.

Intrauterine infection usually occurs in primary infection acquired during pregnancy and may have serious consequences in the fetus; CNS involvement may cause microcephaly and motor disorders. Jaundice and hepatosplenomegaly are common and thrombocytopenia and haemolytic anaemia also occur. Evidence of CNS involvement may be provided by demonstration of periventricular calcification on X-ray.

Diagnosis

Serological tests can identify latent (IgG) or primary (IgM) infection. The virus can also be identified in tissues by the presence of characteristic intranuclear 'owl's eye'

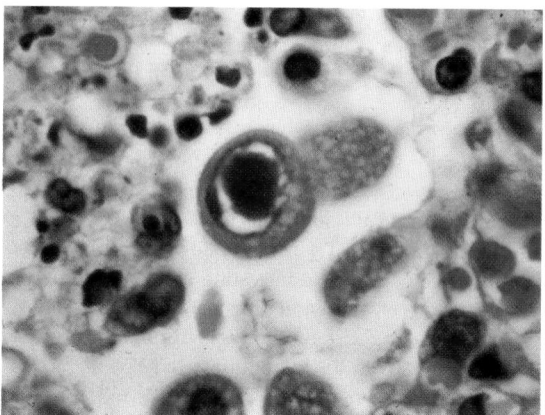

Fig. 2.18 Typical 'owl-eye' inclusion-bearing cell infected with cytomegalovirus.

inclusions (Fig. 2.18) on histological staining and by direct immunofluorescence. Culture in human embryo fibroblasts is usually slow but diagnosis can be accelerated by immunofluorescent detection of antigen in the cultures. The polymerase chain reaction, which can be quantitative, provides a sensitive way of detecting CMV in blood and other body fluids.

Treatment

In the immunocompetent, infection is usually self-limiting and no specific treatment is required. In the immunosuppressed, ganciclovir (5 mg/kg daily for 14–21 days) reduces retinitis and gastrointestinal damage and can eliminate CMV from blood, urine and respiratory secretions. It is less effective against pneumonitis. In patients who are continually immunocompromised, particularly those with AIDS, maintenance therapy may be necessary. Drug resistance has been reported in AIDS patients and transplant recipients. Bone marrow toxicity is common. No antiviral drugs are currently available for routine treatment of CMV in neonates and the toxicity of ganciclovir prohibits its use in most cases. Two other drugs, foscarnet and cidofovir, are currently in use for the treatment of CMV infection. Both are nephrotoxic and, as with ganciclovir, their use should be restricted to those with severe disease.

Epstein–Barr virus (EBV) infection

This virus causes an acute febrile illness known as infectious mononucleosis (glandular fever), which occurs world-wide in adolescents and young adults. EBV is probably transmitted in saliva and by aerosol.

Clinical features

The predominant symptoms are fever, headache, malaise and sore throat. Palatal petechiae and a transient macular rash are common, the latter occurring in 90% of patients who have received ampicillin (inappropriately) for the sore throat. Cervical lymphadenopathy, particularly of the posterior cervical nodes, and splenomegaly are characteristic. Mild hepatitis is common, but other complications such as myocarditis, meningitis, encephalitis, mesenteric adenitis and splenic rupture are rare.

Although some young adults remain debilitated and depressed for some months after infection, the evidence for reactivation of latent virus in healthy individuals is controversial, although this is thought to occur in immunocompromised patients. Following primary infection, EBV remains latent in resting memory B lymphocytes. It has been shown in vitro that of nearly 100 viral genes expressed during replication, approximately only 10 are expressed in the latently infected B cells. Severe, often fatal infectious mononucleosis may result from a rare X-linked immunoproliferative syndrome affecting young boys. Those who survive have an increased risk of hypogammaglobulinaemia and/or lymphoma.

EBV is the cause of oral hairy leucoplakia in AIDS patients and is the major aetiological agent responsible for Burkitt's lymphoma, nasopharyngeal carcinoma, post-transplant lymphoma and the immunoblastic lymphoma of AIDS patients. Different levels of expression of EBV latency genes occur in the various clinical conditions caused by the virus.

Diagnosis

EBV infection should be strongly suspected if atypical mononuclear cells (glandular fever cells) are found in the peripheral blood. It can be confirmed during the second week of infection by a positive Paul–Bunnell reaction, which detects heterophile antibodies (IgM) that agglutinate sheep erythrocytes. False-positives can occur in other conditions such as viral hepatitis, Hodgkin's disease and acute leukaemia. The Monospot test is a sensitive and easily performed screening test for heterophile antibodies. Specific EBV IgM antibodies indicate recent infection by the virus. Clinically similar illnesses are produced by CMV and toxoplasmosis but these can be distinguished serologically.

Treatment

The majority of cases require no specific treatment and recovery is rapid. Corticosteroid therapy is advised when there is neurological involvement (e.g. encephalitis, meningitis, Guillain–Barré syndrome) or when there is marked thrombocytopenia or haemolysis.

Human herpesvirus type 6 (HHV-6)

This human herpesvirus infects CD4+ T lymphocytes, occurs world-wide, and exists as a latent infection in over 85% of the adult population. The virus causes roseola infantum (exanthem subitum) which presents as a high fever followed by generalized macular rash in infants. HHV-6 is a common cause of febrile convulsions, and aseptic meningitis or encephalitis may occur as rare complications. Reactivation in the immunocompromised may lead to severe pneumonia.

Treatment

Supportive management only is recommended for the common infantile disease. Ganciclovir can be used in the immunocompromised.

Human herpesvirus type 7 (HHV-7)

This virus is similar to HHV-6 in being a T lymphotropic herpesvirus. It is also present as a latent infection in over 85% of the adult population and it is known to infect CD4+ helper T cells by using the CD4 antigen (the main receptor employed by HIV). The full spectrum of disease due to HHV-7 has not yet been fully characterized, but, like HHV-6, it is known to cause roseola infantum in infants.

Human herpesvirus type 8 (Kaposi's sarcoma-associated herpesvirus)

This human herpesvirus, first described in 1994, is strongly associated with the aetiology of classical and AIDS-related Kaposi's syndrome. Antibody prevalence is high in those with tumours but relatively low in the general population of most industrialized countries. High rates of infection (> 50% population) have been described in central and southern Africa and this matches the geographic distribution of Kaposi's sarcoma before the era of AIDS. HHV-8 can be sexually transmitted among homosexual men, through heterosexual sex and through exposure to blood from needle sharing. It is thought that salivary transmission may be the predominant route in Africa. HHV-8 RNA transcripts have been detected in Kaposi's sarcoma cells and in circulating mononuclear cells from patients with the tumour.

Papovaviruses

These viruses tend to produce chronic infections, often with evidence of latency. They are capable of inducing neoplasia in some animal species and were among the first viruses to be implicated in tumorigenesis. Human papillomaviruses, of which there are at least 70 types, are responsible for the common wart and have been implicated in the aetiology of carcinoma of the cervix (mainly types 16 and 18) and oral cancer (type 16). The human BK virus, a polyomavirus, is generally found in immunocompromised individuals and may be detected in the urine of 15–40% of renal transplant patients, in patients receiving cytotoxic chemotherapy, and in those with immunodeficiency states. A related virus, JC, is the cause of progressive multifocal leuco-encephalopathy (PML) which presents as dementia in the immunocompromised and is due to progressive cerebral destruction resulting from accumulation of the virus in brain tissue.

For genital warts see page 129.

Human parvovirus B19

Human parvovirus B19 produces erythema infectiosum (fifth disease), a common infection in schoolchildren. The rash is typically on the face (the 'slapped-cheek' appearance). The patient is well and the rash can recur over weeks or months. Asymptomatic infection occurs in 20% of children. Moderately severe self-limiting arthropathy (see p. 556) is common if infection occurs in adulthood. Aplastic crisis may occur in patients with chronic haemolysis (e.g. sickle cell disease). Chronic infection with anaemia may occur in immunocompromised subjects. Hydrops fetalis (3% risk) and spontaneous abortion (9% risk) may result from infection during the first and second trimesters of pregnancy.

Poxviruses

Smallpox (variola)

This disease was eradicated in 1977 following an aggressive vaccination policy and careful detection of new cases coordinated by the World Health Organization.

Monkeypox

This is a rare zoonosis that occurs in small villages in the tropical rainforests in several countries of western and central Africa. Its clinical effects, including a generalized vesicular rash, are indistinguishable from smallpox, but person-to-person transmission is unusual. Serological surveys indicate that several species of squirrel are likely to represent the animal reservoir.

Cowpox

Cowpox produces large vesicles which are classically on the hands in those in contact with infected cows. The lesions are associated with regional lymphadenitis and fever. Cowpox virus has been found in a range of species including domestic and wild cats, and the reservoir is thought to exist in a range of rodents.

Vaccinia virus

This is a laboratory virus and does not occur in nature in either humans or animals. Its origins are uncertain but it has been invaluable in its use as the vaccine to prevent smallpox. Vaccination is now not recommended except for laboratory personnel handling certain poxviruses for experimental purposes. It is being assessed experimentally as a possible carrier for new vaccines.

Orf

This poxvirus causes contagious pustular dermatitis in sheep and hand lesions in humans (see p. 1278).

Molluscum contagiosum

This is discussed on page 1278.

RNA viruses (Table 2.19)

Picornaviruses

Poliovirus infection (poliomyelitis)

Poliomyelitis occurs when a susceptible individual is infected with poliovirus type 1, 2 or 3. These viruses have a propensity for the nervous system, especially the anterior horn cells of the spinal cord and cranial nerve motor neurones. Poliomyelitis is found world-wide but its incidence has decreased dramatically following improvements in sanitation, hygiene and the widespread use of polio vaccines. Spread is usually via the faecal–oral route, as the virus is excreted in the faeces.

Clinical features

The incubation period is 7–14 days. Although polio is essentially a disease of childhood, no age is exempt. The clinical manifestations vary considerably.

Inapparent infection

Inapparent infection is common and occurs in 95% of infected individuals.

Abortive poliomyelitis

Abortive poliomyelitis occurs in approximately 4–5% of cases and is characterized by the presence of fever, sore throat and myalgia. The illness is self-limiting and of short duration.

Non-paralytic poliomyelitis

Non-paralytic poliomyelitis has features of abortive poliomyelitis as well as signs of meningeal irritation, but recovery is complete.

Paralytic poliomyelitis

Paralytic poliomyelitis occurs in approximately 0.1% of infected children (1.3% of adults). Several factors predispose to the development of paralysis:

- male sex
- exercise early in the illness
- trauma, surgery or intramuscular injection, which localize the paralysis
- recent tonsillectomy (bulbar poliomyelitis).

This form of the disease is characterized initially by features simulating abortive poliomyelitis. Symptoms subside for 4–5 days, only to recur in greater severity with signs of meningeal irritation and muscle pain, which is most prominent in the neck and lumbar region. These symptoms persist for a few days and are followed by the onset of asymmetric paralysis without sensory involvement. The paralysis is usually confined to the lower limbs in children under 5 years of age and the upper limbs in older children, whereas in adults it manifests as paraplegia or quadriplegia.

Table 2.19
Human RNA viruses

Structure		Approximate size	Family	Viruses
Symmetry	Envelope			
Icosahedral	–	30 nm	Picornavirus	Poliovirus Coxsackievirus Echovirus Enterovirus 68–72 Rhinovirus
Icosahedral	–	80 nm	Reovirus	Reovirus Rotavirus
Icosahedral	+	50–80 nm	Togavirus	Rubella virus Alphaviruses Flaviviruses
Spherical	+	80–100 nm	Bunyavirus	Congo-Crimean haemorrhagic fever Hantavirus
Spherical	–	35–40 nm	Calicivirus	Norwalk agent Hepatitis E
Spherical	–	28–30 nm	Astrovirus	Astrovirus
Helical	+	80–120 nm	Orthomyxovirus	Influenza viruses A, B and C
Helical	+	100–300 nm	Paramyxovirus	Measles virus Mumps virus Respiratory syncytial virus Nipah virus Hendra virus
Helical	+	60–175 nm	Rhabdovirus	Rabies virus
Helical	+	100 nm	Retrovirus	Human immunodeficiency viruses (HIV 1 and 2) Human T cell lymphotropic virus (HTLV 1 and 2)
Helical	+	100–300 nm	Arenavirus	Lassa virus Lymphocytic choriomeningitis virus
Pleomorphic	+	Filaments or circular forms; 100 × 130–2600 nm	Filovirus	Marburg virus Ebola virus

Bulbar poliomyelitis

Bulbar poliomyelitis is characterized by the presence of cranial nerve involvement and respiratory muscle paralysis. Soft palate, pharyngeal and laryngeal muscle palsies are common.

Aspiration pneumonia, myocarditis, paralytic ileus and urinary calculi are late complications of poliomyelitis.

Diagnosis

The diagnosis is a clinical one. Distinction from Guillain–Barré syndrome is easily made by the absence of sensory involvement and the asymmetrical nature of the paralysis in poliomyelitis. Laboratory confirmation and distinction between the wild virus and vaccine strains is achieved by virus culture, neutralization and temperature marker tests.

Treatment

Treatment is supportive. Bed rest is essential during the early course of the illness. Respiratory support with intermittent positive-pressure respiration is required if the muscles of respiration are involved. Once the acute phase of the illness has subsided, occupational therapy, physiotherapy and occasionally surgery have important roles in patient rehabilitation.

Prevention and control

Immunization has dramatically decreased the prevalence of this disease world-wide and global eradication of the virus, coordinated by the World Health Organization, is expected within the next 1–2 years. Trivalent oral poliovaccine (OPV) (active virus) is currently used (see Box 2.6); occasionally, inactivated poliovirus vaccine (IPV) is used intramuscularly for the immunocompromised and their family contacts and for women in pregnancy. Recent studies using inactivated poliovirus vaccine have revealed greater potency than the original Salk IPV. The greater reliability of IPV in hot climates and the scientific and ethical problems of continuing to use OPV in countries free from poliomyelitis, mean that IPV is likely to be recommended for immunization schedules in the future.

Coxsackievirus, echovirus and other enterovirus infections

These viruses are spread by the faecal–oral route. They each have a number of different types and are responsible for a broad spectrum of disease involving the skin and mucous membranes, muscles, nerves, the heart (Table 2.20) and, rarely, other organs, such as the liver and pancreas. They are frequently associated with pyrexial illnesses and are the most common cause of aseptic meningitis.

Herpangina

This disease is mainly caused by Coxsackie A viruses and presents with a vesicular eruption on the fauces, palate and uvula. The lesions evolve into ulcers. The illness is usually associated with fever and headache but is short-lived, recovery occurring within a few days.

Hand, foot and mouth disease

This disease is mainly caused by Coxsackievirus A16 or A10. Oral lesions are similar to those seen in herpangina but may be more extensive in the oropharynx. Vesicles and a maculopapular eruption also appear, typically on the palms of the hands and the soles of the feet, but also on other parts of the body. This infection commonly affects children. Recovery occurs within a week.

Neurological disease

Other enteroviruses in addition to poliovirus can cause a broad range of neurological disease, including meningitis, encephalitis, and a paralytic disease characteristic of poliomyelitis.

Heart and muscle disease

Enteroviruses are an important cause of acute myocarditis and pericarditis, from which, in general, there is complete recovery. However, these viruses can also cause chronic congestive cardiomyopathy and, rarely, constrictive pericarditis.

Skeletal muscle involvement, particularly of the intercostal muscles, is an important feature of *Bornholm disease*, a febrile illness usually due to Coxsackievirus B. The pain may be of such an intensity as to mimic pleurisy or an acute abdomen. The infection affects both children and adults and may be complicated by meningitis or cardiac involvement.

Rhinovirus infection

Rhinoviruses are responsible for the common cold (see p. 856). Chimpanzees and humans are the only species to develop the common cold. ICAM-1 is the cellular receptor (p. 192) for rhinovirus and it is only in these two species that the specific binding domain is present. Peak incidence rates occur in the colder months, especially spring and autumn. There are multiple rhinovirus immunotypes (> 100), which makes vaccine control impracticable. In contrast to enteroviruses, which replicate at 37°C, rhinoviruses grow at 33°C (the temperature of the upper respiratory tract), which explains the localized disease characteristic of common colds.

Reoviruses

Reovirus infection

Reovirus infection occurs mainly in children, causing mild respiratory symptoms and diarrhoea. A few deaths have been reported following disseminated infection of brain, liver, heart and lungs.

Rotavirus infection

Rotavirus (Latin *rota* = wheel) is so named because of its electronmicroscopic appearance with a characteristic

Table 2.20
Picornavirus infections (excluding poliovirus and rhinovirus)

Disease	Coxsackievirus		Echovirus (types 1–9, 11–27, 29–33)	Enterovirus (types 68–71)
	A (types A_1-A_{22}, A_{24})	B (types B_1-B_6)		
Cutaneous and oropharyngeal				
Herpangina	+++	+	+	
Hand, foot and mouth	+++	+		+
Erythematous rashes	+	+	+++	
Neurological				
Paralytic	+		±	+
Meningitis	++	++	+++	+
Encephalitis	++	++	±	+
Cardiac				
Myocarditis and pericarditis	+	+++	+	
Muscle				
Myositis (Bornholm disease)	+	+++	+	

+++, often causes: ++, sometimes causes; +, rarely causes; ±, possibly causes

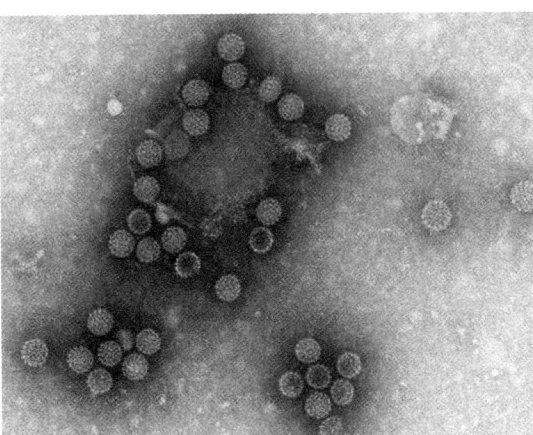

Fig. 2.19 Electronmicrograph of human rotavirus.

circular outline with radiating spokes (Fig. 2.19). It is responsible world-wide for both sporadic cases and epidemics of diarrhoea, and is currently one of the most important causes of childhood diarrhoea. More than 870 000 children under the age of 5 years are estimated to die annually in resource-deprived countries, compared with 75–150 in the USA. The prevalence is higher during the winter months in non-tropical areas. Asymptomatic infections are common, and bottle-fed babies are more likely to be symptomatic than breast-fed.

Adults may become infected with rotavirus but symptoms are usually mild or absent. The virus may, however, cause outbreaks of diarrhoea in patients on geriatric wards.

Clinical features

The illness is characterized by vomiting, fever, diarrhoea, and the metabolic consequences of water and electrolyte loss.

Diagnosis and treatment

The diagnosis can be established by ELISA for the detection of rotavirus antigen in faeces and by electron-microscopy of faeces. Histology of the jejunal mucosa in children shows shortening of the villi, with crypt hyperplasia and mononuclear cell infiltration of the lamina propria.

Treatment is directed at overcoming the effects of water and electrolyte imbalance with adequate oral rehydration therapy and, when indicated, intravenous fluids (see Box 2.10). Antibiotics should not be prescribed.

Rhesus–human reassortant vaccines have been developed whereby a human rotavirus VP7 is expressed on the surface of a rhesus rotavirus. The tetravalent vaccine contains three reassortants for human rotavirus G-types 1, 2 and 4 plus the rhesus rotavirus (G-type 3). This vaccine (IRRV-TV; rhesus (human) rotavirus – tetravalent vaccine) has been shown to give high levels

Table 2.21
Viruses associated with gastroenteritis

Rotavirus (groups A, B, C, D and E)
Enteric adenovirus (types 40 and 41)
Small round structured viruses (SRSV):
Calicivirus (Norwalk and related viruses)
Astrovirus

of protection in children in resource-deprived countries. Although initially licensed by the FDA in the USA, it has recently been withdrawn owing to an increased incidence of intussusception in the vaccinees.

Other viruses associated with gastroenteritis are shown in Table 2.21. These include members of two major families which can be recognized by their electron-microscopic appearance. Caliciviruses, which include the Norwalk agents, and astroviruses are collectively known as small round structured viruses (SRSVs) and are responsible for winter vomiting. Although gastroenteritis viruses are normally spread by the faecal–oral route, the high level of transmission of SRSVs within closed spaces indicates aerosol spread.

Togaviruses

This family comprises two genera: the rubiviruses, which include rubella virus; and the alphaviruses, which include some of the arthropod-borne viruses.

Rubella

Rubella ('German measles') is caused by a spherical, enveloped RNA virus which is easily killed by heat and ultraviolet light. While the disease can occur sporadically, epidemics are not uncommon. It has a world-wide distribution. Spread of the virus is via droplets; maximum infectivity occurs before and during the time the rash is present.

Clinical features

The incubation period is 14–21 days, averaging 18 days. The clinical features are largely determined by age, with symptoms being mild or absent in children under 5 years

During the prodrome the patient may develop malaise and fever. Mild conjunctivitis and lymphadenopathy may be present. The distribution of the lymphadenopathy is characteristic and involves particularly the sub-occipital, postauricular and posterior cervical groups of lymph nodes. Small petechial lesions on the soft palate (Forchheimer spots) are suggestive but not diagnostic. Splenomegaly may be present.

The eruptive or exanthematous phase usually occurs within the first 7 days of the initial symptoms. The rash first appears on the forehead and then spreads to involve the trunk and the limbs. It is pinkish red, macular and discrete, although some of these lesions may coalesce

Fig. 2.20 Rubella rash.

(Fig. 2.20). It usually fades by the second day and rarely persists beyond the third day after its appearance.

Complications

Complications are rare. They include superadded pulmonary bacterial infection, arthralgia, haemorrhagic manifestations due to thrombocytopenia, encephalitis and the congenital rubella syndrome. Rubella affects the fetuses of up to 80% of all women who contract the infection during the first trimester of pregnancy. The incidence of congenital abnormalities diminishes in the second trimester and no ill-effects result from infection in the third trimester.

Congenital rubella syndrome is characterized by the presence of fetal cardiac malformations, especially patent ductus arteriosus and ventricular septal defect, eye lesions (especially cataracts), microcephaly, mental retardation and deafness.

The expanded rubella syndrome consists of the manifestations of the congenital rubella syndrome plus other effects including hepatosplenomegaly, myocarditis, interstitial pneumonia and metaphyseal bone lesions.

Diagnosis and treatment

The diagnosis may be suspected clinically, but laboratory diagnosis is essential to distinguish the illness from other virus infections (e.g. echovirus) and drug rashes. This is achieved by demonstrating a rising antibody titre (measured using the sensitive haemagglutination-inhibiting antibody (HAI) test or ELISA) in two successive blood samples taken 14 days apart or by the detection of rubella-specific IgM. The virus can be cultured from throat swabs, urine and, in the case of intrauterine infection, the products of conception.

Treatment is supportive.

Prevention

Prevention of rubella is important. Human immunoglobulin can decrease the symptoms of this already mild illness, but does not prevent the teratogenic effects.

Several live attenuated rubella vaccines have been used with great success in preventing this illness and these have been successfully combined with the measles and mumps (MMR) vaccine. The side-effects of vaccination have been dramatically decreased by using vaccines prepared in human embryonic fibroblast cultures (RA 27/3 vaccine). Use of the vaccine is contraindicated during pregnancy or if there is a likelihood of pregnancy within 3 months of immunization. Inadvertent use of the vaccine during pregnancy has not, however, revealed a risk of teratogenicity.

Arbovirus (arthropod-borne) infection

Arboviruses are zoonotic viruses, with the possible exception of the O'nyong-nyong fever virus of which humans are the only known vertebrate hosts. They are transmitted through the bites of insects, especially mosquitoes, and ticks. Over 385 viruses are classified as arboviruses. *Culex*, *Aedes* and *Anopheles* mosquitoes account for the transmission of the majority of these viruses.

Although most arbovirus diseases are generally mild, epidemics are frequent and when these occur the mortality is high. In general, the incubation period is less than 10 days. The illness tends to be biphasic and, as in other viral fevers, pyrexia, conjunctival suffusion, a rash, retro-orbital pain, myalgia and arthralgia are common. Lymphadenopathy is seen in dengue. Lifelong immunity to a particular virus is usual. In some of these viral fevers, haemorrhage is a feature (Table 2.22). Increased vascular permeability, capillary fragility and

Table 2.22

Viral infections associated with haemorrhagic manifestations*

Togavirus
Flavivirus
Yellow fever (urban and sylvan)
Dengue haemorrhagic fever
Kyasanur Forest disease
Omsk haemorrhagic fever
Rift Valley fever
Alphavirus
Chikungunya

Bunyavirus
Congo-Crimean haemorrhagic fever
Hantavirus infections

Arenavirus
Argentinian haemorrhagic fever
Bolivian haemorrhagic fever
Lassa fever
Epidemic haemorrhagic fever

Filovirus
Marburg
Ebola

---

* Most of these are arboviruses. Some (e.g. hantavirus, Lassa fever) have a rodent vector. The source and transmission route of filoviruses is not known

consumptive coagulopathy have been implicated as causes of the haemorrhage. Encephalitis resulting from cerebral invasion may be prominent in some fevers.

Alphaviruses

The 24 viruses of this group are all transmitted by mosquitoes; eight result in human disease. These viruses are globally distributed and tend to acquire their names from the location where they were first isolated (such as Ross River, Eastern Venezuelan, and Western encephalitis viruses) or by the local expression for a major symptom caused by the virus (such as chikungunya, meaning 'doubled up'). Infection is characterized by fever, skin rash, arthralgia, myalgia and sometimes encephalitis.

Flaviviruses

There are 60 viruses in this group, some of which are transmitted by ticks and others by mosquitoes.

Yellow fever

Yellow fever, caused by a flavivirus, results in an illness of widely varying severity so that the disease is underreported. It is a disease confined to Africa (90% of cases) and South America between latitudes 15°N and 15°S. For poorly understood reasons, yellow fever has not been reported from Asia, despite the fact that climatic conditions are suitable and the vector, *Aedes aegypti*, is common. The infection is transmitted in the wild by *A. africanus* in Africa and the *Haemagogus* species in South and Central America. Extension of infection to humans (via the mosquito or from monkeys) leads to the occurrence of 'jungle' yellow fever. *A. aegypti*, a domestic mosquito which lives in close relationship to humans, is responsible for human-to-human transmission in urban areas (urban yellow fever). Once infected, a mosquito remains so for its whole life.

Clinical features

The incubation period is 3–6 days. When the infection is mild, the disease is indistinguishable from other viral fevers such as influenza or dengue.

Three phases in the severe (classical) illness are recognized. Initially the patient presents with a high fever of acute onset, usually 39–40°C, which then returns to normal in 4–5 days. During this time, headache is prominent. Retrobulbar pain, myalgia, arthralgia, a flushed face and suffused conjunctivae are common. Epigastric discomfort and vomiting are present when the illness is severe. Relative bradycardia (Faget's sign) is present from the second day of illness. The patient then makes an apparent recovery and feels well for several days. Following this 'phase of calm' the patient again develops increasing fever, deepening jaundice and hepatomegaly. Ecchymosis, bleeding from the gums, haematemesis and melaena may occur. Coma, which is usually a result of uraemia or haemorrhagic shock, occurs for a few hours preceding death. The mortality rate is up to 40% in severe cases. The pathology of the liver shows mid-zone necrosis, and eosinophilic degeneration of hepatocytes (Councilman bodies) (see p. 350).

Diagnosis and treatment

The diagnosis is established by a careful history of travel and vaccination status, and by isolation of the virus (when possible) from blood during the first 3 days of illness. Serodiagnosis is possible, but in endemic areas cross-reactivity with other flaviviruses is a problem.

Treatment is supportive. Bed rest (under mosquito nets), analgesics, and maintenance of fluid and electrolyte balance are important.

Prevention and control

Yellow fever is an internationally notifiable disease. It is easily prevented using the attenuated 17d chick embryo vaccine. Vaccination is not recommended for children under 9 months and immunosuppressed patients unless there are compelling reasons. For the purposes of international certification, immunization is valid for 10 years, but protection lasts much longer than this and probably for life. The WHO Expanded Programme of Immunization includes yellow fever vaccination in endemic areas.

Dengue

This is the commonest arthropod-borne viral infection in humans: 50–100 million cases occur every year in the tropics, with over 10 000 deaths from dengue haemorrhagic fever. Dengue is caused by a flavivirus and is found mainly in Asia, South America and Africa, although it has been reported from the USA. Four different antigenic varieties of dengue virus are recognized and all are transmitted by the daytime-biting *A. aegypti*. Humans are infective during the first 3 days of the illness (the viraemic stage). Mosquitoes become infective about 2 weeks after feeding on an infected individual, and remain so for the rest of their lives. The disease is usually endemic. Immunity after the illness is partial.

Clinical features

The incubation period is 5–6 days following the mosquito bite. Asymptomatic or mild infections are common. Two clinical forms are recognized.

Classic dengue fever

Classic dengue fever is characterized by the abrupt onset of fever, malaise, headache, facial flushing, retrobulbar pain which worsens on eye movements, conjunctival suffusion and severe backache, which is a prominent symptom. Lymphadenopathy, petechiae on the soft palate and skin rashes may also occur. The rash is transient and morbilliform. It appears on the limbs and then spreads to involve the trunk. Desquamation occurs subsequently. Cough is uncommon. The fever subsides after 3–4 days, the temperature returns to normal for a couple of days, and then the fever returns, together with the features already mentioned, but milder. This biphasic or saddleback pattern is considered characteristic. Severe fatigue, a feeling of being unwell and depression are common for several weeks after the fever has subsided.

Dengue haemorrhagic fever

Dengue haemorrhagic fever is a severe form of dengue fever and is believed to be the result of two or more sequential infections with different dengue serotypes. It is a disease of children and has been described almost exclusively in South East Asia. The disease has a mild start, often with symptoms of an upper respiratory tract infection. This is then followed by the abrupt onset of shock and haemorrhage into the skin and ear, epistaxis, haematemesis and melaena known as the dengue shock syndrome. Serum complement levels are depressed and there is laboratory evidence of a consumptive coagulopathy.

Diagnosis and treatment

Isolation of dengue virus by tissue culture in sera obtained during the first few days of illness is diagnostic. Demonstration of rising antibody titres by neutralization (most specific), haemagglutination inhibition (ELISA) or complement-fixing antibodies in sequential serum samples is evidence of dengue virus infection.

Treatment is supportive.

Prevention

Travellers should be advised to sleep under impregnated nets and to use topical insect repellents. Adult mosquitoes should be destroyed by sprays, and breeding sites should be eradicated.

Rift Valley fever

Rift Valley fever, caused by a flavivirus, is primarily an acute febrile illness of livestock – sheep, goats and camels. It is found in southern and eastern Africa. The vector in East Africa is *Culex pipiens* and in southern Africa, *Aedes caballus*. Following an incubation period of 3–6 days, the patient has an acute febrile illness that is difficult to distinguish clinically from other viral fevers. The temperature pattern is usually biphasic. The initial febrile illness lasts 2–4 days and is followed by a remission and a second febrile episode. Complications are indicative of severe infection and include retinopathy, meningoencephalitis, haemorrhagic manifestations and hepatic necrosis. Mortality approaches 50% in severe forms of the illness. Treatment is supportive.

Japanese encephalitis

Japanese encephalitis is a mosquito-borne encephalitis caused by a flavivirus. It has been reported most frequently from the rice-growing countries of South East Asia and the Far East. *Culex tritaeniorhynchus* is the most important vector and this feeds mainly on pigs as well as birds such as herons and sparrows. Humans are accidental hosts.

As with other viral infections, the clinical manifestations are variable. The onset is heralded by severe rigors. Fever, headache and malaise last 1–6 days. Weight loss is prominent. In the acute encephalitic stage the fever is high (38–41°C), neck rigidity occurs and neurological signs such as altered consciousness, hemiparesis and convulsions develop. Mental deterioration occurs over a period of 3–4 days and culminates in coma. Mortality varies from 7 to 40% and is higher in children. Residual neurological defects such as deafness, emotional lability and hemiparesis occur in about 70% of patients who have had CNS involvement. Convalescence is prolonged. Antibody detection in serum and CSF by IgM capture ELISA is a useful rapid diagnostic test. An inactivated mouse brain vaccine is effective and available. Treatment is supportive.

In 1999, the *West Nile virus* was first recognised in the Western hemisphere, in New York, USA. The outbreak produced thousands of symptomatic and symptomless infections with 1% resulting in encephalitis.

Bunyaviruses

Bunyaviruses belong to a large family of more than 200 viruses, most of which are arthropod-borne.

Congo–Crimean haemorrhagic fever

This is found mainly in Asia and Africa. The primary hosts are cattle and hares and the vectors are the *Hyalomma* ticks. Following an incubation period of 3–6 days there is an influenza-like illness with fever and haemorrhagic manifestations. The mortality is 10–50%.

Hantaviruses

Hantaviruses are enzootic viruses of wild rodents which are spread by aerosolized excreta and not by insect vectors. The most severe form of this infection is Korean haemorrhagic fever (or haemorrhagic fever with renal syndrome – HFRS). This condition has a mortality of 5–10% and is characterized by fever, shock and haemorrhage followed by an oliguric phase. Milder forms of the disease are associated with related viruses (e.g. Puumala virus) and may present as nephropathia epidemica, an acute fever with renal involvement. It is seen in Scandinavia and in other European countries in people who have been in contact with bank voles. In the USA, a new hantavirus (transmitted by the deer mouse) termed Sin Nombre was identified as the cause of outbreaks of acute respiratory disease in adults, referred to as hantavirus pulmonary syndrome (HPS). Since then, newly discovered hantavirus types and other rodent vector systems have been associated with this syndrome.

Diagnosis of hantavirus infection is made by an ELISA technique for specific antibodies.

Orthomyxoviruses

Influenza

Three types of influenza virus are recognized: A, B and C. The influenza virus is a spherical or filamentous enveloped virus. Haemagglutinin, a surface glycopeptide, aids attachment of the virus to the wall of susceptible host cells at specific receptor sites. Cell penetration, probably by pinocytosis, and release of replicated viruses from the cell surface is effected by budding through the cell membrane facilitated by the action of the enzyme neuraminidase which is also present on the viral envelope.

- Influenza A is generally responsible for pandemics and epidemics.
- Influenza B often causes smaller or localized and milder outbreaks, such as in camps or schools.
- Influenza C rarely produces disease in humans.

Antigenic shift (major antigenic change within an influenza A subtype) usually heralds the onset of a pandemic. This results from genetic recombination of the RNA of the virus, which is arranged in eight segments, with that of an animal orthomyxovirus.

Antigenic drift (minor changes in influenza A and B viruses) results from point mutations leading to amino acid changes in the two surface glycoproteins, haemagglutinin and neuraminidase, which are important in inducing humoral immunity.

Thus, changes due to antigenic shift or drift render the individual's immune response less able to combat the new variant. Purified haemagglutinin and neuraminidase from recently circulating strains of influenza A and B viruses are incorporated in current vaccines.

Sporadic cases of influenza and outbreaks among groups of people living in a confined environment are frequent. The incidence increases during the winter months. Spread is mainly by droplet infection but fomites and direct contact have also been implicated.

The clinical features, diagnosis, treatment and prophylaxis of influenza are discussed on page 860.

Paramyxoviruses

These are a heterogeneous group of enveloped viruses of varying size that are responsible for parainfluenza, mumps, measles and other respiratory infections (Fig. 2.21).

Parainfluenza

Parainfluenza is caused by the parainfluenza viruses types I–IV; these have a world-wide distribution and cause acute respiratory disease. Type IV appears to be less virulent than the other types and has been linked only to mild upper respiratory diseases in children and adults.

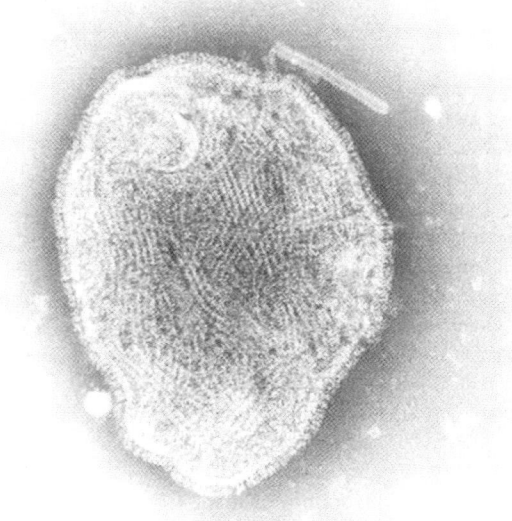

Fig. 2.21 Electronmicrograph of a paramyxovirus (mumps).

Parainfluenza is essentially a disease of children and presents with features similar to the common cold. When severe, a brassy cough with inspiratory stridor and features of laryngotracheobronchitis (croup) are present. Fever is usually present for 2–3 days and may be more prolonged if pneumonia develops. The development of croup is due to submucosal oedema and consequent airway obstruction in the subglottic region. This may lead to cyanosis, subcostal and intercostal recession and progressive airway obstruction. Infection in the immunocompromised is usually prolonged and may be severe. Treatment is supportive with oxygen, humidification and sedation when required. The role of steroids is controversial.

Measles (rubeola)

Measles is a highly communicable disease that occurs world-wide. With the introduction of aggressive immunization policies, the incidence of measles has fallen dramatically in the West, but it still remains one of the most common childhood infections in resource-deprived countries, where it is associated with a high morbidity and mortality. It is spread by droplet infection and the period of infectivity is from 4 days before until 2 days after the onset of the rash.

Clinical features
The incubation period is 8–14 days. Two distinct phases of the disease can be recognized.

Typical measles
- *The pre-eruptive and catarrhal stage*. This is the stage of viraemia and viral dissemination. Malaise, fever, rhinorrhoea, cough, conjunctival suffusion and the pathognomonic Koplik's spots are present during

this stage. Koplik's spots are small, greyish, irregular lesions surrounded by an erythematous base and are found in greatest numbers on the buccal mucous membrane opposite the second molar tooth. They occur a day or two before the onset of the rash.

- *The eruptive or exanthematous stage.* This is characterized by the presence of a maculopapular rash that initially occurs on the face, chiefly the forehead, and then spreads rapidly to involve the rest of the body (Fig. 2.22). At first the rash is discrete but later it may become confluent and patchy, especially on the face and neck. It fades in about 1 week and leaves behind a brownish discoloration.

Although measles is a relatively mild disease in the healthy child, it carries a high mortality in the malnourished and in those who have other diseases. Complications are common in such individuals and include bacterial pneumonia, bronchitis, otitis media and gastroenteritis. Less commonly, myocarditis, hepatitis and encephalomyelitis may occur. In those who are malnourished or those with defective cell-mediated immunity, the classical maculopapular rash may not develop and widespread desquamation may occur. The virus also causes the rare condition, subacute sclerosing panencephalitis, which may follow measles infection occurring early in life (< 18 months of age). Persistence of the virus with reactivation pre-puberty results in accumulation of virus in the brain, progressive mental deterioration and a fatal outcome (see p. 1197).

Maternal measles, unlike rubella, does not cause fetal abnormalities. It is, however, associated with spontaneous abortions and premature delivery.

Atypical measles

In the past, a severe illness called atypical measles occurred in individuals given an inactivated vaccine (now withdrawn). This vaccine conferred incomplete protection and on exposure to the wild measles virus they developed high fever, myalgia, abdominal pain and a variety of skin rashes which could be mistaken for scarlet fever, meningococcal disease or varicella. Pneumonia was invariably present and pulmonary infiltrates persisted for years in some cases.

Diagnosis and treatment

Most cases of measles are diagnosed clinically but, if necessary, immunofluorescence, virus culture and serological tests (complement fixation test (CFT), haemagglutination inhibition tests) are used to confirm the diagnosis.

Treatment is supportive. Antibiotics are indicated only if secondary bacterial infection occurs.

Prevention

A previous attack of measles confers a high degree of immunity and second attacks are uncommon. Normal human immunoglobulin given within 5 days of exposure effectively aborts an attack of measles. It is indicated for previously unimmunized children below 3 years of age, during pregnancy, and in those with debilitating disease.

Active immunization. Children are immunized with the combined mumps–measles–rubella (MMR) vaccine (Box 2.6).

Mumps

Mumps is the result of infection with a paramyxovirus. It is spread by droplet infection, by direct contact or through fomites. Humans are the only known natural hosts. The peak period of infectivity is 2–3 days before the onset of the parotitis and for 3 days afterwards.

Clinical features

The incubation period averages 18 days. Although no age is exempt, it is primarily a disease of school-aged children and young adults; it is uncommon before the age of 2 years. The prodromal symptoms are non-specific and include fever, malaise, headache and anorexia. This is usually followed by severe pain over the parotid glands, with either unilateral or bilateral parotid swelling. The enlarged parotid glands obscure the angle of the mandible and may elevate the ear lobe, which does not occur in cervical lymph node enlargement. Trismus due to pain is common at this stage. Submandibular gland involvement occurs less frequently.

Complications

CNS involvement is the most common extrasalivary-gland manifestation of mumps. Clinical meningitis occurs in 5% of all infected patients, and 30% of patients with CNS involvement have no evidence of parotid gland involvement.

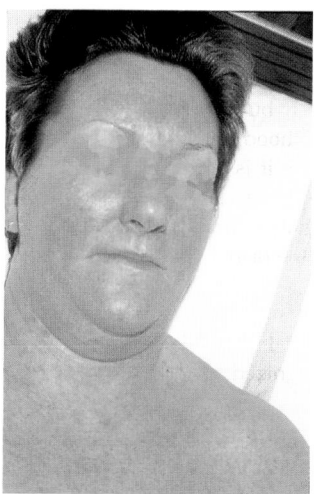

Fig. 2.22 **Measles.** Courtesy of Dr MW McKendrick, Royal Hallamshire Hospital, Sheffield.

Epididymo-orchitis develops in about one-third of patients who develop mumps after puberty. Bilateral testicular involvement results in sterility in only a small percentage of these patients.

Pancreatitis, oophoritis, myocarditis, mastitis, hepatitis and polyarthritis may also occur.

Diagnosis and treatment

The diagnosis of mumps is on the basis of the clinical features. In doubtful cases, serological demonstration of a fourfold rise in antibodies detected by complement fixation or indirect haemagglutination or neutralization tests on acute and convalescent sera is diagnostic. Virus can be isolated in cell culture from saliva, throat swab, urine and CSF and identified by immunofluorescence or haemadsorption.

Treatment is supportive. Attention should be given to adequate nutrition and mouth care. Analgesics should be used to relieve pain.

Prevention

Active immunization. Children are immunized with the MMR vaccine (Box 2.6). Vaccination is contraindicated in immunosuppressed individuals, during pregnancy, or in those with severe febrile illnesses.

Respiratory syncytial virus infection

Respiratory syncytial virus is a paramyxovirus that causes many respiratory infections in epidemics each winter. It is a common cause of bronchiolitis in infants, which is complicated by pneumonia in approximately 10% of cases. The infection normally starts with upper respiratory symptoms. After an interval of 1–3 days a cough and low-grade fever may develop. The onset of bronchiolitis is characterized by dyspnoea and hyperexpansion of the chest with subcostal and intercostal recession. The disease may be severe and potentially fatal in babies with underlying cardiac or respiratory disease. RSV infection has been associated with the occurrence of sudden infant death syndrome (SIDS). Immunity is short-lived and consequently reinfection can occur throughout life. RSV is occasionally the cause of outbreaks of pneumonia in the elderly and in the immunocompromised.

Transfer of infection between children in hospital commonly occurs unless infected patients are isolated or cohorted. Meticulous attention to handwashing and other infection control measures reduces the risk of transmission by staff members.

Diagnosis and treatment

Immunofluorescence on nasopharyngeal aspirates, virus culture and serology are the usual ways of confirming the diagnosis.

Treatment is generally supportive, but aerosolized ribavirin can be given to severe cases, particularly those with underlying cardiac or respiratory disease.

Prevention

No vaccine is available for RSV but high-risk children (including those with bronchopulmonary dysplasia and congenital heart disease) can be protected against severe disease by monthly administration of either a hyperimmune globulin against RSV, or a humanized monoclonal antibody, during the winter months.

Hendra and Nipah viruses

Hendra virus (formerly called equine morbillivirus) and Nipah virus are newly recognized zoonotic viruses that have caused disease in humans who have been in contact with infected animals (horses and pigs respectively). The viruses are named after the locations where they were first isolated, Hendra in Australia and Nipah in Malaysia, and both are classified as paramyxoviruses. Hendra virus has caused severe respiratory distress in horses and humans and Nipah virus caused a major outbreak of viral encephalitis (265 cases and 105 deaths) in Malaysia between September 1998 and April 1999. Treatment of these conditions is largely supportive, although there is some evidence that early treatment with ribavirin may reduce the severity of the diseases.

Rhabdoviruses

Rabies

Rabies is a major problem in some countries, and established infection is invariably fatal. The rabies virus is bullet-shaped and has spike-like structures arising from its surface containing glycoproteins that cause the host to produce neutralizing, haemagglutination-inhibiting antibodies. The virus has a marked affinity for nervous tissue and the salivary glands. It exists in two major epidemiological settings:

- *Urban rabies* is most frequently transmitted to humans through rabid dogs and, less frequently, cats.
- *Sylvan (wild) rabies* is maintained in the wild by a host of animal reservoirs such as foxes, skunks, jackals, mongooses and bats.

With the exception of Australia, New Zealand and the Antarctic, human rabies has been reported from all continents. Transmission is usually through the bite of an infected animal. However, the percentage of rabid bites leading to clinical disease ranges from 10% (on the legs) to 80% (on the head). Rabies has been transferred by corneal grafting, but anecdotal reports of human-to-human spread by kissing, biting and sexual intercourse have not been confirmed. Rabid animals can also transmit the disease by licking abraded skin or mucosa. Rarely, airborne droplet infection occurs from exposure to infected bats in caves, or in laboratory workers handling concentrated virus.

Having entered the human body, the virus replicates in the muscle cells near the entry wound. It penetrates the nerve endings and travels in the axoplasm to the spinal cord and brain. In the CNS the virus again proliferates before spreading to the salivary glands, lungs, kidneys and other organs via the autonomic nerves.

There have been only two recorded cases of survival from clinical rabies.

Clinical features

The incubation period is variable and may range from a few weeks to several years; on average it is 1–3 months. In general, bites on the head, face and neck have a shorter incubation period than those elsewhere. In humans, two distinct clinical varieties of rabies are recognized:

- furious rabies – the classic variety
- dumb rabies – the paralytic variety.

Furious rabies

The only characteristic feature in the prodromal period is the presence of pain and tingling at the site of the initial wound. Fever, malaise and headache are also present. About 10 days later, marked anxiety and agitation or depressive features develop. Hallucinations, bizarre behaviour and paralysis may also occur. Hyperexcitability, the hallmark of this form of rabies, is precipitated by auditory or visual stimuli. Hydrophobia (fear of water) is present in 50% of patients and is due to severe pharyngeal spasms on attempting to eat or drink. Aerophobia (fear of air) is considered pathognomonic of rabies. Examination reveals hyperreflexia, spasticity, and evidence of sympathetic overactivity indicated by pupillary dilatation and diaphoresis.

The patient goes on to develop convulsions, respiratory paralysis and cardiac arrhythmias. Death usually occurs in 10–14 days.

Dumb rabies

Dumb rabies, or paralytic rabies, presents with a symmetrical ascending paralysis resembling the Guillain–Barré syndrome. This variety of rabies commonly occurs after bites from rabid bats.

Diagnosis

The diagnosis of rabies is generally made clinically. Fluorescent antibody has been used to detect rabies antigen in corneal impressions or in salivary secretions; this is a useful test. The classic Negri bodies are detected at post-mortem in 90% of all patients with rabies; these are eosinophilic, cytoplasmic, ovoid bodies, 2–10 nm in diameter, seen in greatest numbers in the neurones of the hippocampus and the cerebellum. The diagnosis should be made pathologically on the biting animal.

Treatment

Once the disease is established, therapy is symptomatic as death is virtually inevitable. The patient should be nursed in a quiet, darkened room. Nutritional, respiratory and cardiovascular support may be necessary.

Drugs such as morphine, diazepam and chlorpromazine should be used liberally in patients who are excitable.

Prevention

The vaccine is the human diploid cell vaccine (HDCV).

Postexposure prophylaxis. Five 1.0 mL doses of HDCV should be given intramuscularly: the first dose is given on day 0 and is followed by injections on days 3, 7, 14 and 28. Reaction to the vaccine is uncommon. The wound should be cleaned carefully with soap and water, adequately debrided and left open. Human rabies immunoglobulin should be given immediately (20 IU/kg); half should be injected around the area of the wound and the other half should be given intramuscularly.

Pre-exposure prophylaxis. This is given to individuals with a high risk of contracting rabies, such as laboratory workers, animal handlers and veterinarians. Two doses of HDCV 1.0 mL deep subcutaneously or intramuscularly given 4 weeks apart should provide effective immunity. A reinforcing dose is given after 12 months and additional reinforcing doses are given every 1–3 years depending on the risk of exposure. Vaccines of nervous-tissue origin are still used in some parts of the world. These, however, are associated with significant side-effects and are best avoided if HDCV is available.

Control of rabies

Domestic animals should be vaccinated if there is any risk of rabies in the country. In the UK, control has been by quarantine of imported animals and no indigenous case of rabies has been reported for many years. The quarantine laws are under revision at the present time. The Pet Travel Scheme (PETS) introduced as a pilot scheme in 2000 enables certain pet animals to enter or re-enter Great Britain without quarantine if they come from qualifying countries via designated routes, are carried by authorized transport companies, and meet the conditions of the scheme. Wild animals in 'at risk' countries must be handled with great care.

Retroviruses

Retroviruses (Table 2.23) are distinguished from other RNA viruses by their ability to replicate through a DNA intermediate using an enzyme, reverse transcriptase.

Table 2.23
Human lymphotropic retroviruses

Subfamily	Virus	Disease
Lentivirus	HIV-1	AIDS
	HIV-2	AIDS
Oncovirus	HTLV-1*	Adult T cell leukaemia/lymphoma
		Tropical spastic paraparesis
	HTLV-2	Myelopathy

* HTLV, human T cell lymphotropic virus

HIV-1 and the related virus, HIV-2, are further classified as lentiviruses ('slow' viruses) because of their slowly progressive clinical effects.

HIV-1 and HIV-2 are discussed on page 132.

HTLV-1 causes adult T cell leukaemia/lymphoma and tropical spastic paraparesis (see p. 1145).

Arenaviruses

Arenaviruses are pleomorphic, round or oval viruses with diameters ranging from 50 to 300 nm. The virion surface has club-shaped projections, and the virus itself contains a variable number of characteristic electron-dense granules that represent residual, non-functional host ribosomes. The prototype virus of this group is lymphocytic choriomeningitis virus, which is a natural infection of mice. Arenaviruses are also responsible for Argentinian and Bolivian haemorrhagic fevers and Lassa fever.

Lassa fever

This illness was first documented in the town of Lassa, Nigeria, in 1969 and is confined to sub-Saharan West Africa (Nigeria, Liberia and Sierra Leone). The multimammate rat, *Mastomys natalensis*, is known to be the reservoir. Humans are infected by ingesting foods contaminated by rat urine or saliva containing the virus. Person-to-person spread by body fluids also occurs. Only 10–30% of infections are symptomatic.

Clinical features

The incubation period is 7–18 days. The disease is insidious in onset and is characterized by fever, myalgia, severe backache, malaise and headache. A transient maculopapular rash may be present. A sore throat, pharyngitis and lymphadenopathy occur in over 50% of patients. In severe cases epistaxis and gastrointestinal bleeding may occur – hence the classification of Lassa fever as a viral haemorrhagic fever. The fever usually lasts 1–3 weeks and recovery within a month of the onset of illness is usual. However, death occurs in 15–20% of hospitalized patients, usually from irreversible hypovolaemic shock.

Diagnosis

The diagnosis is established by serial serological tests (including the Lassa virus-specific IgM titre) or by culturing the virus from the throat, serum or urine. Molecular diagnosis by means of the reverse transcriptase polymerase chain reaction has recently become available and this provides a sensitive and reasonably rapid diagnostic test.

Treatment

Treatment is supportive. In addition, clinical benefit and reduction in mortality can be achieved with ribavirin therapy, if given in the first week.

In non-endemic countries, strict isolation procedures should be used, the patient ideally being nursed in a flexible-film isolator. Specialized units for the management of Lassa fever and other haemorrhagic fevers have been established in the UK. As Lassa fever virus and other causes of haemorrhagic fever (Marburg/Ebola and Congo–Crimean haemorrhagic fever viruses) have transmitted from patients to staff in health care situations, great care should be taken in handling specimens and clinical material from these patients.

Lymphocytic choriomeningitis (LCM)

This infection is a zoonosis, the natural reservoir of LCM virus being the house mouse. Infection is characterized by:

- non-nervous-system illness, with fever, malaise, myalgia, headache, arthralgia and vomiting
- aseptic meningitis in addition to the above symptoms.

Occasionally, a more severe form occurs, with encephalitis leading to disturbance of consciousness.

This illness is generally self-limiting and requires no specific treatment.

Marburg virus disease and Ebola virus disease

These severe, haemorrhagic, febrile illnesses are discussed together because their clinical manifestations are similar. The diseases are named after Marburg in Germany and the Ebola river region in the Sudan and Zaire where these viruses first appeared. The natural reservoir for these viruses has not been identified and the precise mode of spread from one individual to another has not been elucidated.

Epidemics have occurred periodically in recent years, mainly in sub-Saharan Africa. The mortality from Marburg and Ebola has ranged from 25% to 90% and recovery is slow in those who survive.

The illness is characterized by the acute onset of severe headache, severe myalgia and high fever, followed by prostration. On about the fifth day of illness a non-pruritic maculopapular rash develops on the face and then spreads to the rest of the body. Diarrhoea is profuse and is associated with abdominal cramps and vomiting. Haematemesis, melaena or haemoptysis may occur between the seventh and sixteenth day. Hepato-splenomegaly and facial oedema are usually present. In Ebola virus disease, chest pain and a dry cough are prominent symptoms.

Treatment is symptomatic. Convalescent human serum appears to decrease the severity of the attack.

Postviral/chronic fatigue syndrome (see also p. 1234)

Viral illnesses have been implicated aetiologically, including those due to EBV, Coxsackie B viruses, echoviruses, CMV and hepatitis A virus. Non-viral causes such as allergy to *Candida* spp. have also been proposed.

The proportion of patients with 'organic' diagnoses remains uncertain. Studies have suggested that two-thirds of patients with a symptom duration of more than 6 months may have an underlying psychiatric disorder.

Prion disease

A number of diseases of humans and animals have been loosely termed 'slow virus' diseases. These are now known as transmissible spongiform encephalopathies and are caused by the accumulation in the nervous system of a protein, termed a prion, which is an abnormal isoform of a normal, host protein.

Although familial forms of prion disease are known to exist, these conditions can be transmissible, particularly if brain tissue enters another host. There is no convincing evidence for the presence of nucleic acid in association with prions; thus these agents cannot be considered orthodox viruses and the current view is that the abnormal prion protein itself is infectious and can trigger a conversion of the normal protein into the atypical isoform. After infection a long incubation period is followed by CNS degeneration associated with dementia or ataxia which invariably leads to death. Histology of the brain reveals spongiform change with an accumulation of the abnormal prion protein in the form of amyloid plaques.

The human prion diseases are Creutzfeldt–Jakob disease, including the sporadic, familial, iatrogenic and variant forms of the disease, Gerstmann–Straussler–Scheinker syndrome, fatal familial insomnia, and kuru.

- *Creutzfeldt–Jakob disease (CJD)* usually occurs sporadically at an annual rate of one per million of the population. Although, in most cases, the epidemiology remains obscure, transmission to others has occurred as a result of administration of human cadaveric growth hormone or gonadotrophin, from dura mater and corneal grafting, and in neurosurgery from reuse of contaminated electrodes (iatrogenic CJD). In the UK, knowledge that large numbers of cattle with the prion disease, bovine spongiform encephalopathy (BSE) had gone into the human food chain, led to enhanced surveillance for emergence of the disease in humans. The evidence is now convincing, based on transmission studies in mice and on glycosylation patterns of prion proteins, that this has occurred and, to date, there have been over 100 confirmed and suspected cases of variant CJD (human BSE) in the UK. In contrast to sporadic CJD, which presents with dementia at a mean age of onset of 60 years, variant CJD presents with psychiatric and cerebellar signs at a mean age of onset of 29 years.
- *Gerstmann–Straussler–Scheinker syndrome* and fatal familial insomnia are rare prion diseases usually occurring in families with a positive history. The pattern of inheritance is as an autosomal dominant with some degree of variable penetrance.
- *Kuru* was described and characterized in the Fore highlanders in NE New Guinea. Transmission was associated with ritualistic cannibalism of deceased relatives. With the cessation of cannibalism by 1960, the disease has gradually diminished and recent cases had all been exposed to the agent before 1960.

The infectious agents of prion disease have remarkable characteristics. In the infected host there is no evidence of inflammatory, cytokine or immune reactions. The agent is highly resistant to decontamination, and infectivity is not reliably destroyed by autoclaving or by treatment with formaldehyde and most other gas or liquid disinfectants. It is very resistant to γ irradiation. Autoclaving at a high temperature (134–137°C for 18 minutes) is used for decontamination of instruments, and hypochlorite (20 000 p.p.m. available chlorine) or 1 molar sodium hydroxide are used for liquid disinfection. Uncertainty about the reliability of any methods for safe decontamination of surgical instruments has necessitated the introduction of guidelines for patient management (listed in the recommendations for further reading).

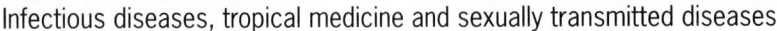

FURTHER READING

Advisory Committee on Dangerous Pathogens/Spongiform Encephalopathy Advisory Committee (1998) *Transmissible Spongiform Encephalopathy Agents; Safe Working and the Prevention of Infection*. London: The Stationery Office.

Centers for Disease Control and Prevention (1995) Update: management of patients with suspected haemorrhagic fever. *United States Morbidity and Mortality Weekly Report* **44**: 475–479.

Cohen JI (2000) Epstein–Barr virus infection. *New England Journal of Medicine* **242**: 481–492.

Couch R B (2000) Prevention and treatment of influenza. *New England Journal of Medicine* **343**: 1778–1787.

Department of Health (2000) *Memorandum on Rabies. Prevention and Control*. London: DoH.

Hall CB, Thompson WW, Cox N (2001) Respiratory syncytial virus and parainfluenza virus. *New England Journal of Medicine* **344**: 1917–1928.

Robertson SE, Hull BP, Tomori O et al. (1995) Yellow fever. A decade of resurgence. *Journal of the American Medical Association* **276**: 1157–1162.

Whirley B, Roizman B (2001) Herpes simplex virus infections. *Lancet* **357**: 1513–1518.

Bacterial infections

Classification of bacteria

Bacteria are unicellular organisms (prokaryotes). A small fraction are of medical importance. Unusual infections may result from exposure under circumstances of altered host defences, notably in the severely immunocompromised patient.

Bacteria have traditionally been classified according to the Gram stain which distinguishes Gram-positive from Gram-negative organisms. Using light microscopy, these can then largely be divided into cocci and bacilli (rods). Some have a spiral appearance (spirochaetes) while others, such as *Clostridium* spp., may contain spores (Table 2.24). The cell wall arrangement of Gram-positive cocci contains a phospholipid bilayer surrounded by peptidoglycan made up of repeating units of *N*-acetylglucosamine and *N*-acetylmuramic acid. In contrast, Gram-negative bacilli possess a second outer lipid bilayer containing protein and lipopolysaccharide (endotoxin). Some pathogens are encapsulated, which is an antiphagocytic virulence factor.

Table 2.24
Classification of bacteria affecting humans

Aerobic bacteria	Cocci	Bacilli
Gram-positive	*Staphylococcus aureus* *Staphylococcus epidermidis* *Streptococcus pneumoniae* *Streptococcus pyogenes* (group A) *Strep. agalactiae* (group B) Enterococci Viridans streptococci	*Listeria monocytogenes* *Corynebacterium diphtheriae* *Bacillus anthracis* *B. cereus*
Gram-negative	*Neisseria gonorrhoeae* *N. meningitidis* *Moraxella catarrhalis* *Bordetella pertussis*	*Escherichia coli* *Klebsiella* spp. *Proteus* spp. *Haemophilus influenzae* *Legionella* spp. *Salmonella* spp. *Shigella* spp. *Campylobacter jejuni* *Helicobacter pylori* *Pseudomonas* spp. *Brucella* spp. *Acinetobacter* spp. *Burkholderia* spp. *Vibrio cholerae*
Anaerobic bacteria	Peptococci Peptostreptococci	*Actinomyces* spp. *Clostridium perfringens* *C. difficile* *Bacteroides fragilis* group *Fusobacterium* spp.
Spirochaetes	*Treponema pallidum* *Leptospira* spp. *Borrelia* spp.	
Others	*Mycobacterium* spp. *Mycoplasma pneumoniae* *Ureaplasma* spp. *Chlamydia* spp.	

Bacteria can often be cultured in broth or on solid agar. Those growing in the absence of oxygen are strict anaerobes (e.g. *Bacteroides* spp.), whilst oxygen-dependent bacteria are known as aerobes (e.g. *Pseudomonas* spp.). Many pathogens can tolerate reduced concentrations of oxygen (e.g. *E. coli*). Some organisms are more demanding in their growth requirements and require special laboratory media (e.g. *Mycoplasma* spp. and *Mycobacterium* spp.); others require more prolonged incubation (e.g. *Brucella* spp.).

Genetic classification is now defining bacteria in terms of DNA sequence information and has led to the reclassification of several bacteria. DNA fingerprinting is also being increasingly applied to distinguishing similar isolates, which has applications in defining the epidemiology of infection.

Diagnosis and management of bacterial infections

The history and examination usually localizes the infection to a specific organ or body site. A systemic response may accompany such localized disease or, in the case of bloodstream infections, be the primary mode of presentation. The microbiological diagnosis is difficult to establish in most community-managed infections, and even in hospital where there is ready access to diagnostic laboratories only a minority of infections are documented. For these reasons, a clinical approach to bacterial diseases has been adopted.

Skin and soft tissue infection

Superficial infections

Infections of the skin and the soft tissues beneath are common. These are usually fungal (see p. 1278) or bacterial. Although a wide range of bacteria have been recovered from skin and soft tissue infections (Table 2.25),

the majority are caused by the Gram-positive cocci *Staphylococcus aureus* and *Streptococcus pyogenes*. Staphylococci are part of the normal microflora of the human skin and nasopharynx; up to 25% of people are carriers of *S. aureus*, which is the species responsible for the majority of staphylococcal infections. Although soft tissue infections are the most common manifestation of *S. aureus* disease, numerous other sites can be affected (Table 2.6).

The classification of soft tissue infections is complex, as imprecise and overlapping terms are in use. The commonly encountered infections (Table 2.26) are described in more detail on page 1274.

The majority of skin and superficial soft tissue infections are due to bacteria on the skin surface penetrating the dermis or the subcutaneous tissues. Infection can take place via hair follicles, insect bites, cuts and abrasions, or skin damaged by superficial fungal infection. Sometimes infection is introduced by an animal bite or a penetrating foreign body: in these cases more unusual organisms may be found. A number of factors predispose to cellulitis and other soft tissue infections (Table 2.27).

Table 2.25
Bacterial causes of superficial skin and soft tissue infection

Specific risk factors	Likely organisms
None	*Staphylococcus aureus*
	Streptococcus pyogenes
Diabetes, peripheral vascular disease	Group B streptococci
Animal bite	*Pasteurella multocida,*
	Capnocytophaga canimorsus
Fresh water exposure	*Aeromonas hydrophila*
Sea water exposure	*Vibrio vulnificans*
Lymphoedema, stasis dermatitis	Groups A, C and G streptococci
Hot tub exposure	*Pseudomonas aeruginosa*
Malignant otitis externa	*Pseudomonas aeruginosa*
Human bite	*Fusobacterium* spp.

Table 2.26
Classification of bacterial skin and superficial soft tissue infections

Infection	Subgroup	Site	Common cause
Pyoderma	Impetigo	Skin	*Streptococcus pyogenes*
			Staphylococcus aureus
	Bullous impetigo	Skin	*Staph. aureus*
	Folliculitis	Skin, hair follicles	*Staph. aureus*
Abscesses	Furuncle (boil)	Subcutaneous tissue	*Staph. aureus*
	Hydradenitis suppurativa	Multiple sweat gland furuncles (axillae, groins)	*Staph. aureus*, anaerobes
	Carbuncle	Dense group of furuncles: back of neck, shoulders	*Staph. aureus*
Cellulitis		Skin and subcutaneous tissue	*Staph. aureus*
			Strep. pyogenes
			Group C and G streptococci
Erysipelas		Skin	*Strep. pyogenes*
Ecthyma		Skin and subcutaneous tissue	*Strep. pyogenes*
			Staph. aureus

Table 2.27
Predisposing factors for skin and soft tissue infection

Diabetes mellitus
Chronic lymphoedema
Peripheral vascular disease
Steroid treatment
Malnutrition
Some immunodeficiency states (e.g. Job's syndrome)
Nasal carriage of *Staphylococcus aureus*

Pasteurellosis

Pasteurella multocida is found in the oropharynx of up to 90% of cats and 70% of dogs. It can cause soft tissue infections following animal bites. Although the infection initially resembles other forms of cellulitis, there is a much higher incidence of spread to deeper tissues, resulting in osteomyelitis, tenosynovitis or septic arthritis. The organism is sensitive to penicillin, however as infections following animal bites are often polymicrobial, co-amoxiclav is used.

Methicillin-resistant *Staphylococcus aureus* (MRSA)

S. aureus are commonly resistant to penicillin, and isolated resistance to other β-lactam antibiotics such as methicillin and flucloxacillin has been recognized since the development of the first semisynthetic penicillins in the early 1960s. However, in the last 25 years, strains of MRSA with resistance to a much wider range of antibiotics have emerged. In some cases only the glycopeptide antibiotics vancomycin and teicoplanin are effective, and a few organisms have been isolated with decreased sensitivity even to these (vancomycin-insensitive *Staphylococcus aureus*, VISA). Two new classes of antibiotics, the streptogramins (e.g. quinupristin with dalfopristin) and the oxazolidinones (e.g. linezolid) are effective against Gram-positive bacteria, including MRSA. They should usually be reserved for multi-resistant organisms.

MRSA is usually seen as a harmless skin commensal, especially in hospitalized patients or nursing home residents. However, it can cause a variety of infections in soft tissues and elsewhere. It is particularly associated with surgical wound infections. Eradication of the organism is difficult, and people who are known to be colonized should be isolated. Topical treatment with antibiotics is often used, but is of limited efficacy.

Cat scratch disease

Cat scratch disease is a zoonosis caused by *Bartonella henselae*. Asymptomatic bacteraemia is relatively common in domestic and especially feral cats, and human infection is probably due to cat flea bites. Regional lymphadenopathy appears 1–2 weeks after infection; the nodes become tender and may suppurate. Histology of the nodes shows granuloma formation, and the illness may be mistaken for mycobacterial infection or lymphoma.

There are usually few systemic symptoms in immunocompetent patients, although more severe disease may be seen in the immunocompromised. In these patients tender cutaneous or subcutaneous nodules are seen (bacillary angiomatosis) which may ulcerate. The lymphadenopathy resolves spontaneously over weeks or months, although surgical drainage of very large suppurating nodes may be necessary. *B. henselae* is sensitive to doxycycline, but the clinical benefit of treatment is unproven.

Toxin-mediated skin disease

A number of skin conditions, although caused by bacteria, are mediated by exotoxins rather than direct local tissue damage.

Staphylococcal scalded skin syndrome

The scalded skin syndrome is caused by a toxin-secreting strain of *Staph. aureus*. It principally affects children under the age of 5. The toxin, exfoliatin, causes intra-epidermal cleavage at the level of the stratum corneum leading to the formation of large flaccid blisters that shear readily. It is a relatively benign condition, and responds to treatment with flucloxacillin.

Toxic shock syndrome (TSS)

TSS is usually due to toxin-secreting staphylococci, although streptococci have also been implicated. Although historically associated with vaginal colonization and tampon use in women this is not always the case. The exotoxin (normally toxic shock syndrome toxin 1, TSST-1) causes abrupt onset of fever and shock, with a diffuse macular rash and desquamation of the palms and soles. Many patients are severely ill and mortality is about 10%. Treatment is mainly supportive, although the organism should be eradicated.

Scarlet fever (see p. 67)

Deep soft tissue infections

Infections of the deeper soft tissues are much less common than superficial infections, and tend to be more serious. Usually they are related to penetrating injuries or to surgery, and the causative organisms relate to the nature of the wound.

Necrotizing fasciitis

Necrotizing fasciitis is a fulminant, rapidly spreading infection associated with widespread tissue destruction and a high mortality. There are two forms. Type 1, caused by a mixture of aerobic and anaerobic bacteria, is usually seen following abdominal surgery or in diabetics. Type 2, caused by group A streptococci, arises spontaneously in previously healthy people. Both types are characterized by severe pain at the site of initial infection, rapidly followed by tissue necrosis. Infection tracks rapidly along the tissue planes, causing spreading erythema, pain and sometimes crepitus. The only chance of survival is with urgent surgical debridement and aggressive antibiotic therapy. Type 2 necrotizing fasciitis is treated with high doses of benzylpenicillin and clindamycin; type 1 with a broad-spectrum combination.

Gas gangrene

Gas gangrene is caused by deep tissue infection with *Clostridium* spp., especially *C. perfringens*, and follows contaminated penetrating injuries. It is particularly associated with battlefield wounds, but is also seen in intravenous drug users, and following surgery. The initial infection develops in an area of necrotic tissue caused by the original injury; toxins secreted by the bacteria kill surrounding tissue and enable the anaerobic organism to spread rapidly. Toxins are also responsible for the severe systemic features of gas gangrene. Treatment consists of urgent surgical removal of necrotic tissue, and treatment with benzylpenicillin and clindamycin

FURTHER READING

Gottlieb T, Mitchell D (1998) The independent evolution of resistance to ciprofloxacin, rifampicin and fusidic acid in methicillin-resistant *Staphylococcus aureus* in Australian teaching hospitals (1990–1995). *Journal of Antimicrobial Chemotherapy* **42**(1): 67–73.
Urschel JD (1999) Necrotising soft tissue infections. *Postgraduate Medical Journal* **75**: 645–649.

Respiratory tract infections

Infections of the respiratory tract are divided into infections of the upper and lower respiratory tract, which are separated by the carina. In health, the lower respiratory tract is normally sterile owing to a highly efficient defence system (p. 841). Infections of the upper respiratory tract are particularly common in childhood when they are usually the result of virus infection. The paranasal sinuses and middle ear are contiguous structures and can be involved secondary to viral infections of the nasopharynx. The lower respiratory tract is frequently compromised by smoking, air pollution, aspiration of upper respiratory tract secretions and chronic lung disease, notably chronic bronchitis and chronic obstructive pulmonary disease. Infections of the respiratory tract are defined clinically, sometimes radiologically, as in the case of pneumonia, and by appropriate microbiological sampling.

Upper respiratory tract infections
- The common cold (acute coryza) (p. 856)
- Sinusitis (p. 857)
- Rhinitis (p. 857)
- Pharyngitis (p. 860).

Scarlet fever

Scarlet fever occurs when the infectious organism (usually a group A streptococcus) produces erythrogenic toxin in an individual who does not possess neutralizing antitoxin antibodies.

Clinical features

The incubation period of this relatively mild disease, which mainly affects children, is 2–4 days following a streptococcal infection, usually in the pharynx. Regional lymphadenopathy, fever, rigors, headache and vomiting are present. The rash, which blanches on pressure, usually appears on the second day of illness; it initially occurs on the neck but rapidly becomes punctate, erythematous and generalized. It is typically absent from the face, palms and soles, and is prominent in the flexures. The rash usually lasts about 5 days and is followed by extensive desquamation of the skin (Fig. 2.23). The face is flushed with characteristic circumoral pallor. Early in the disease the tongue has a white coating through which prominent bright red papillae can be seen ('strawberry tongue'). Later the white coating disappears, leaving a raw-looking, bright red colour ('raspberry tongue'). The patient is infective for 10–21 days after the onset of the rash unless treated with penicillin.

Scarlet fever may be complicated by peritonsillar or retropharyngeal abscesses and otitis media.

Diagnosis

The diagnosis is established by the typical clinical features and culture of a throat swab. Elevated antistreptolysin O and anti-DNAse B levels in convalescent serum are indicative of streptococcal infection.

Treatment

Penicillin is the drug of choice and is given orally as phenoxymethylpenicillin 500 mg four times daily for 10 days. Individuals allergic to penicillin can be treated effectively with erythromycin 250 mg four times daily

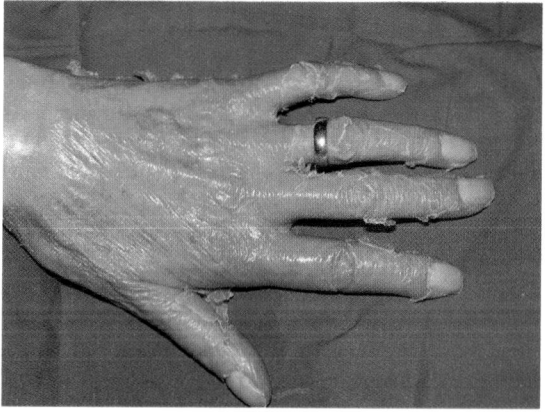

Fig. 2.23 Scarlet fever rash, showing desquamation.

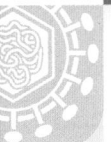

for 10 days. Treatment is usually effective in preventing rheumatic fever (p. 79) and acute glomerulonephritis (p. 607) which are non-suppurative complications of streptococcal pharyngitis. Unlike acute rheumatic fever, streptococcal nephritis may also complicate streptococcal skin infection.

Prevention

Chemoprophylaxis with penicillin or erythromycin should be given in epidemics.

Diphtheria

Diphtheria caused by *Corynebacterium diphtheriae* occurs world-wide. Its incidence in the West has fallen dramatically following widespread active immunization, but it is epidemic in Russia and Eastern Europe. Transmission is mainly through airborne droplet infection and rarely through fomites.

C. diphtheriae is a Gram-positive bacillus. Only strains which carry the tox+ gene, are capable of toxin production. The toxin has two subunits, A and B. Subunit A is responsible for clinical toxicity. Subunit B serves only to transport the toxin component to specific receptors, present chiefly on the myocardium and in the peripheral nervous system. Humans are the only natural hosts.

Clinical features

Diphtheria was formerly a disease of childhood but is increasingly affecting adults in countries where childhood immunization has been interrupted as in Russia and Eastern Europe. The incubation period is 2–7 days. The manifestations may be regarded as local (due to the membrane) or systemic (due to exotoxin). The presence of a membrane, however, is not essential to the diagnosis. The illness is insidious in onset and is associated with tachycardia but only low-grade fever. If complicated by infection with other bacteria such as *S. pyogenes*, fever is high and spiking.

Nasal diphtheria is characterized by the presence of a unilateral, serosanguineous nasal discharge that crusts around the external nares.

Pharyngeal diphtheria is associated with the greatest toxicity and is characterized by marked tonsillar and pharyngeal inflammation and the presence of a membrane. This tough greyish yellow membrane is formed by fibrin, bacteria, epithelial cells, mononuclear cells and polymorphs, and is firmly adherent to the underlying tissue. Regional lymphadenopathy, often tender, is prominent and produces the so-called 'bull-neck'.

Laryngeal diphtheria is usually a result of extension of the membrane from the pharynx. A husky voice, a brassy cough, and later dyspnoea and cyanosis due to respiratory obstruction are common features.

Clinically evident myocarditis occurs, often weeks later, in patients with pharyngeal or laryngeal diphtheria. Acute circulatory failure due to myocarditis may occur in convalescent individuals around the tenth day of illness and is usually fatal. Neurological manifestations occur either early in the disease (palatal and pharyngeal wall paralysis) or several weeks after its onset (cranial nerve palsies, paraesthesiae, polyneuropathy or, rarely, encephalitis).

Cutaneous diphtheria is increasingly being seen in association with burns and in individuals with poor personal hygiene. Typically the ulcer is punched-out with undermined edges and is covered with a greyish white to brownish adherent membrane. Constitutional symptoms are uncommon.

Diagnosis

This must be made on clinical grounds since therapy is usually urgent and bacteriological results of culture studies and toxin production cannot be awaited.

Treatment

The patient should be isolated and bed rest advised. Antitoxin therapy is the only specific treatment. It must be given promptly to prevent further fixation of toxin to tissue receptors, since fixed toxin is not neutralized by antitoxin. Depending on the severity, 20 000–100 000 units of horse-serum antitoxin should be administered intramuscularly after an initial test dose to exclude any allergic reaction. Intravenous therapy may be required in a very severe case. There is a risk of acute anaphylaxis after antitoxin administration and of serum sickness 2–3 weeks later (Box 2.7). However, the risk of death outweighs the problems of anaphylaxis. Antibiotics should be administered concurrently to eliminate the organisms and thereby remove the source of toxin production. Benzylpenicillin 1.2 g four times daily is given for 1 week.

The cardiac and neurological complications need intensive therapy.

Prevention

Diphtheria is prevented by active immunization in childhood (see p. 45). Booster doses should be given to those travelling to endemic areas if more than 10 years has elapsed following their primary course of

---

Box 2.7

Antitoxin administration

- Many antitoxins are heterologous and therefore dangerous
- Hypersensitivity reactions are common

Prior to treatment:
Question patient about:
(a) allergic conditions (e.g. asthma, hay fever)
(b) previous antitoxin administration.

Read instructions on antitoxin package carefully.
Always give a subcutaneous test dose.

immunization. All contacts of the patient should have throat swabs sent for culture; those with a positive result should be treated with penicillin or erythromycin and active immunization or a booster dose of toxoid given.

Pertussis (whooping cough)

Pertussis occurs world-wide. Humans are both the natural hosts and reservoirs of infection. The disease is caused by *Bordetella pertussis* which is a Gram-negative coccobacillus. *B. parapertussis* and *B. bronchiseptica* produce milder infections. Pertussis is highly contagious and is spread by droplet infection. In its early stages it is indistinguishable from other types of upper respiratory tract infection. Epidemic disease occurred in the UK when the safety of the whooping cough vaccine was questioned. Currently, uptake exceeds 95% and the disease is uncommon.

Clinical features

The incubation period is 7–10 days. It is a disease of childhood, with 90% of cases occurring below 5 years of age. However, no age is exempt.

During the catarrhal stage the patient is highly infectious, and cultures from respiratory secretions are positive in over 90% of patients. Malaise, anorexia, mucoid rhinorrhoea and conjunctivitis are present. The paroxysmal stage, so called because of the characteristic paroxysms of coughing, begins about a week later. Paroxysms with the classic inspiratory whoop are seen only in younger individuals in whom the lumen of the respiratory tract is compromised by mucus secretion and mucosal oedema. The whoop results from air being forcefully drawn through the narrowed tract. These paroxysms usually terminate in vomiting. Conjunctival suffusion and petechiae and ulceration of the frenulum of the tongue are usual. Lymphocytosis due to the elaboration of a lymphocyte-promoting factor by *B. pertussis* is characteristic; lymphocytes may account for over 90% of the total white blood cell count. This stage lasts approximately 2 weeks and may be associated with several complications, including pneumonia, atelectasis, rectal prolapse and inguinal hernia. Cerebral anoxia may occur, especially in younger children, resulting in convulsions. Bronchiectasis is a rare sequel.

Diagnosis

The diagnosis is suggested clinically by the characteristic whoop and a history of contact with an infected individual. It is confirmed by isolation of the organism. Cultures of swabs of nasopharyngeal secretions result in a higher positive yield than cultures of 'cough plates'.

Treatment

If the disease is recognized in the catarrhal stage, erythromycin will abort or decrease the severity of the infection. In the paroxysmal stage antibiotics have little role to play in altering the course of the illness.

Prevention and control

Affected individuals should be isolated to prevent contact with others, e.g. in hostels and boarding schools. Pertussis is an easily preventable disease and effective active immunization is available (Box 2.6). Convulsions and encephalopathy have been reported as rare complications of vaccination but they are probably less frequent than after whooping cough itself. Any exposed susceptible infant should receive prophylactic erythromycin.

Acute epiglottitis (p. 860)

This has been virtually eliminated among children in those countries which have introduced *Haemophilus influenzae* vaccine, as in the UK. Occasionally, infections are being recognized in adults. The clinical features are described on page 860.

Acute laryngotracheobronchitis (p. 860)

Influenza (pp. 58 and 860)

Lower respiratory tract infections

Pneumonia: community-acquired (p. 887); hospital-acquired (p. 891); in immunocompromised persons (p. 889).

Psittacosis (ornithosis)

Although originally thought to be limited to the psittacine birds (parrots, parakeets and macaws), it is known that the disease is widely spread amongst many species of birds, including pigeons, turkeys, ducks and chickens (hence the broader term 'ornithosis'). Human infection is related to exposure to infected birds and is therefore a true zoonosis. The causative organism, *Chlamydia psittaci*, is excreted in avian secretions; it can be isolated for prolonged periods from birds who have apparently recovered from infection. The organism gains entry to the human host by inhalation.

Clinical features and treatment

These are discussed on page 886.

Other respiratory infections (see also p. 887)

Chlamydia pneumoniae causes relatively mild pneumonias in young adults, clinically resembling infection caused by *Mycoplasma pneumoniae*. Diagnosis can be confirmed by specific IgM serology. Treatment is with erythromycin or tetracycline.

Other chlamydial infections include trachoma (p. 86), lymphogranuloma venereum (p. 125) and other genital infections.

Legionnaires' disease. This is caused by *Legionella pneumophila* and other *Legionella* spp. It is described on page 888.

Lung abscess (p. 891).
Tuberculosis (pp. 89 and 892).

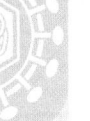

Gastrointestinal infections

Gastroenteritis

The most common form of acute gastrointestinal infection is gastroenteritis, causing diarrhoea with or without vomiting. Children in the developing world can expect, on average, three to six bouts of severe diarrhoea every year. Although oral rehydration programmes have cut the death toll significantly at least 2.25 million people die every year as a direct result of diarrhoeal disease. In the western world diarrhoea is both less common and less likely to cause death. However it remains a major cause of morbidity, especially in the elderly. Other groups who are at increased risk of infectious diarrhoea include travellers to developing countries, homosexual men, and infants in day care facilities. Viral gastroenteritis (p. 54) is a common cause of diarrhoea and vomiting in young children but is rarely seen in adults. Protozoal and helminthic gut infections (p. 109) are rare in the West but relatively common in developing countries. The most common cause of significant adult gastroenteritis world-wide is bacterial infection.

Mechanisms

Bacteria can cause diarrhoea in three different ways (Table 2.28). Some species may employ more than one of these methods.

Mucosal adherence

Most bacteria causing diarrhoea must first adhere to specific receptors on the mucosa. A number of different molecular adhesion mechanisms have been elaborated, for example, adhesions at the tip of the pili or fimbriae which protrude from the bacterial surface aid adhesion.

For some pathogens this is merely the prelude to invasion or toxin production but others such as enteropathogenic *Escherichia coli* (EPEC) damage the mucosa and produce a secretory diarrhoea directly as a result of adherence.

Mucosal invasion

Invasive pathogens such as *Shigella* spp. and *Campylobacter* spp. penetrate into the intestinal mucosa. They destroy the epithelial cells and produce the symptoms of dysentery: low-volume bloody diarrhoea, with abdominal pain. Other secretory systems are used by Gram-negative bacteria to actually transport molecules, e.g. toxins, from their cytoplasm to the outside. These systems vary from simple protein complexes on bacterial surfaces to highly complex mechanisms where a protruding hollow needle is formed to inject toxins into the host cell (e.g. *Yersinia*, *Salmonella*). The injected proteins have been shown to have a homology with the host cell kinases and phosphorylases and thus can modulate the host signalling mechanisms, for example, a tyrosine phosphate (called YopH) which causes cytoskeletal rearrangements and reduces the rate of phagocytosis in infected macrophages allowing continued multiplication.

Toxin production

Gastroenteritis can be caused by three different types of bacterial toxins:

- *Enterotoxins* induce excessive fluid secretion into the bowel lumen, leading to watery diarrhoea, without physically damaging the mucosa.
- *Neurotoxins* affect the autonomic nervous system, causing diarrhoea and vomiting.

Table 2.28

Pathogenic mechanisms of bacterial gastroenteritis

Pathogenesis	Mode of action	Clinical presentation	Examples
Mucosal adherence	Effacement of intestinal mucosa	Moderate watery diarrhoea	Enteropathogenic *E. coli* (EPEC)
Mucosal invasion	Penetration and destruction of mucosa	Dysentery	*Shigella* spp. *Campylobacter* spp. Enteroinvasive *E. coli* (EIEC)
Toxin production Enterotoxin	Fluid secretion without mucosal damage	Profuse watery diarrhoea	*Vibrio cholerae* *Salmonella* spp. *Campylobacter* spp. Enterotoxigenic *E. coli* (ETEC)
Neurotoxin	Paralysis of autonomic nervous system	Variable diarrhoea and vomiting	*Bacillus cereus* *Staphylococcus aureus* producing enterotoxin B
Cytotoxin	Damage to mucosa	Bloody diarrhoea	*Salmonella* spp. *Campylobacter* spp. Enterohaemorrhagic *E. coli* (EHEC)

- *Cytotoxins* damage the intestinal mucosa and, in some cases, vascular endothelium as well.

Usually these toxins are produced by bacteria adhering to the intestinal epithelium, but neurotoxins (often stable to heat and gastric acid) may be elaborated exogenously by pathogens in poorly prepared food. A typical example of this is 'fried rice poisoning', in which *Bacillus cereus* toxin is present in cooked rice left standing overnight at room temperature.

Clinical syndromes

Bacterial gastroenteritis can be divided on clinical grounds into two broad syndromes: *watery diarrhoea* (usually due to neuro- or enterotoxins, or adherence), and *dysentery* (usually due to mucosal invasion) (Box 2.8). With some pathogens such as *Campylobacter jejuni* there may be overlap between the two syndromes.

Salmonella

Gastroenteritis can be caused by many of the numerous serotypes of salmonella (all of which are members of a single species, *S. choleraesuis*), but the most commonly implicated are *S. enteritidis* and *S. typhimurium*. These organisms, which are found all over the world, are commensals in the bowels of livestock (especially poultry) and in the oviducts of chicken. They are usually transmitted to man in contaminated foodstuffs.

Salmonellae can affect both the large and small bowel, and induce diarrhoea both by production of enterotoxins and by epithelial invasion. The typical symptoms commence abruptly 12–48 hours after infection and consist of nausea, cramping abdominal pain, diarrhoea, and sometimes fever. The diarrhoea can vary from profuse and watery to a bloody dysentery

---

<table>
<tr><td colspan="2">Box 2.8</td></tr>
<tr><td colspan="2">Causes of watery diarrhoea and dysentery</td></tr>
</table>

Watery diarrhoea
Bacillus cereus ⎫
Staphylococcus aureus ⎬ plus profuse vomiting
Vibrio cholerae
Enterotoxigenic *Escherichia coli* (ETEC)
Enteropathogenic *Escherichia coli* (EPEC)
Salmonella spp.
Campylobacter jejuni
Clostridium perfringens
Clostridium difficile

Dysentery
Shigella spp.
Salmonella spp.
Campylobacter spp.
Enteroinvasive *Escherichia coli* (EIEC)
Enterohaemorrhagic *Escherichia coli* (EHEC)
Yersinia enterocolitica
Vibrio parahaemolyticus
Clostridium difficile

---

syndrome. Spontaneous resolution usually occurs in 3–6 days, although the organism may persist in the faeces for several weeks. Bacteraemia occurs in 1–4% of cases and is more common in the elderly and the immunosuppressed. Occasionally bacteraemia is complicated by metastatic infection, especially of atheroma on vascular endothelium, with potentially devastating consequences. In healthy adults salmonella gastroenteritis is usually a relatively minor illness, but young children and the elderly are at risk of significant dehydration.

Specific diagnosis is made by culturing the organism from blood or faeces, but management is usually empirical. Antibiotic therapy (ciprofloxacin 500 mg twice daily) may decrease the duration and severity of symptoms, but is rarely warranted (see Box 2.10).

Campylobacter jejuni

C. jejuni is also a zoonotic infection, existing as a bowel commensal in many species of livestock. It is found world-wide, and is a common cause of childhood gastroenteritis in developing countries. Adults in these countries may be tolerant of the organism, excreting it asymptomatically. In the West it is a common cause of sporadic food-borne outbreaks of diarrhoea, especially in the summer when barbecued beefburgers are a frequent vehicle.

Like salmonella, campylobacter can affect large and small bowel and can cause a wide variety of symptoms. The incubation period is usually 2–4 days, after which there is an abrupt onset of nausea, diarrhoea and abdominal cramps. The diarrhoea is usually profuse and watery, but an invasive haemorrhagic colitis is sometimes seen. Bacteraemia is very rare, and infection is usually self-limiting in 3–5 days. Diagnosis is made from stool cultures. If symptoms are severe, ciprofloxacin 500 mg twice daily is the drug of choice (see Box 2.10).

Shigella

Shigellae are enteroinvasive bacteria which cause classical bacillary dysentery. The principal species causing gastroenteritis are *S. dysenteriae*, *S. flexneri* and *S. sonnei*, which are found with varying prevalence in different parts of the world. All cause a similar syndrome, causing damage to the intestinal mucosa. Some strains of *S. dysenteriae* also secrete a cytotoxin affecting vascular endothelium. Although shigellae are found world-wide, transmission is strongly associated with poor hygiene. The organism is spread from person to person, and only small numbers need to be ingested to cause illness (< 200, compared to 10^4 for campylobacter and $>10^5$ for salmonella). Bacillary dysentery is far more prevalent in the developing world, where the main burden falls on children.

Symptoms start 24–48 hours after ingestion and typically consist of frequent small-volume stools containing blood and mucus. Dehydration is not as significant as in

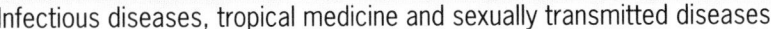

the secretory diarrhoeas, but systemic symptoms and intestinal complications are worse. The illness is usually self-limiting in 7–10 days, but in children in developing countries the mortality may be as high as 20%. Antibiotic treatment decreases the severity and duration of diarrhoea, and possibly reduces the risk of further transmission (see Box 2.11). Resistance to antibiotics is widespread: in some areas amoxicillin or co-trimoxazole may still be effective, but in many places nalidixic acid or ciprofloxacin is needed.

Enteroinvasive *Escherichia coli* (EIEC)
This causes an illness indistinguishable from shigellosis. Definitive diagnosis is made by stool culture.

Enterohaemorrhagic *Escherichia coli* (EHEC)
EHEC (usually serotype O157:H7, and also known as verotoxin-producing *E. coli*, or VTEC) is a recently recognized cause of gastroenteritis in man. It is a zoonosis usually associated with cattle, and there have been a number of major outbreaks (notably in Scotland and Japan) associated with contaminated food. EHEC secrete a toxin (Shiga-like toxin 1) which affects vascular endothelial cells in the gut and in the kidney. After an incubation period of 12–48 hours it causes diarrhoea (frequently bloody), associated with abdominal pain and nausea. Some days after the onset of symptoms the patient may develop thrombotic thrombocytopenic purpura (p. 459) or haemolytic uraemic syndrome (HUS, p. 611). This is more common in children, and may lead to permanent renal damage or death. Treatment is mainly supportive: it has been suggested that antibiotic therapy might precipitate HUS by causing increased toxin release.

Cholera
Cholera is the prototypic pure enterotoxigenic diarrhoea: it is described on page 87.

Enterotoxigenic *Escherichia coli* (ETEC)
ETEC produce both heat-labile and heat-stable enterotoxins which stimulate secretion of fluid into the intestinal lumen. The result is watery diarrhoea of varying intensity, which usually resolves within a few days. Transmission is normally from person to person via contaminated food. The organism is common in developing countries, and is a major cause of traveller's diarrhoea (see below).

Yersiniosis
Yersinia enterocolitica infection is a zoonosis of a variety of domestic and wild mammals. Human disease can arise either via contaminated food products or from direct animal contact. *Y. enterocolitica* can cause a range of gastroenteric symptoms including watery diarrhoea, dysentery, and mesenteric adenitis. The illness is usually self-limiting, but ciprofloxacin may shorten the duration.

Yersinia pseudotuberculosis is a much less common human pathogen: it causes mesenteric adenitis and terminal ileitis.

Staphylococcus aureus
Some strains of *S. aureus* can produce a heat-stable toxin (enterotoxin B) which causes massive secretion of fluid into the intestinal lumen, principally because of its effect on the autonomic nervous system. It is a common cause of food-borne gastroenteritis in Europe and the USA, outbreaks usually occurring as a result of poor food hygiene. Because the toxin is preformed in the contaminated food, onset of symptoms is rapid, often within 2–4 hours of consumption. There is violent vomiting, followed within hours by profuse watery diarrhoea. Symptoms have usually subsided within 24 hours. A very similar syndrome is caused by *Bacillus cereus*.

Clostridium difficile
C. difficile is found as part of the normal bowel flora in 3–5% of the population and even more commonly in hospitalized people. *C. difficile* produces two toxins: toxin A is an enterotoxin and toxin B is cytotoxic and causes bloody diarrhoea. It usually causes illness after other bowel commensals have been eliminated by antibiotic therapy. Almost all antibiotics have been linked with *C. difficile* diarrhoea, which can begin anything from 2 days to a month after taking antibiotics. Elderly hospitalized patients are most frequently affected. Symptoms can range from mild diarrhoea to haemorrhagic colitis: sometimes the ulcerated colonic mucosa may be covered by a membrane-like material (pseudomembranous colitis). The diarrhoea is caused by toxins released by the organism, and diagnosis is made by detecting A or B toxins in the stools by ELISA techniques. Treatment is with metronidazole 400 mg three times daily or vancomycin 125 mg four times daily; causative antibiotics should be discontinued if possible. The disease is usually more severe in the elderly, and can cause intractable diarrhoea leading to death.

Travellers' diarrhoea
Travellers' diarrhoea is defined as the passage of three or more unformed stools per day in a resident of an industrialized country travelling in a developing nation. Infection is usually food- or water-borne, and younger travellers are most often affected (probably reflecting behaviour patterns). Reported attack rates vary from country to country, but approach 50% for a 2-week stay in many tropical countries. The disease is usually benign and self-limiting: treatment with quinolone antibiotics may hasten recovery but is not normally necessary. Prophylactic antibiotic therapy may also be effective for short stays, but should not be used routinely. The common causative organisms are listed in Table 2.29.

Table 2.29

Common causes of travellers' diarrhoea (TD)

Organism	Frequency of recovery in TD (varies from country to country)
ETEC	30–70%
Shigella spp.	0–15%
Salmonella spp.	0–10%
Campylobacter spp.	0–15%
Viral pathogens	0–10%
Giardia intestinalis	0–3%

ETEC, enterotoxigenic *Escherichia coli*

Management of acute gastroenteritis

In children untreated diarrhoea has a high mortality due to dehydration, especially in hot climates. Death and serious morbidity are less common in adults but still occur, particularly in developing countries and in the elderly. The mainstay of treatment for all types of gastroenteritis is rehydration: antibiotics have a subsidiary role in some cases (Fig. 2.24; Boxes 2.9 and 2.10). It should also be remembered that other diseases, notably urinary tract infections and chest infections in the elderly, and malaria at any age, can present with acute diarrhoea.

Box 2.9

Rehydration fluids in moderate and severe diarrhoea

	Salts (mmol per litre)				Substance added (per litre of water)	
	Na	K	Cl	Glucose		
Intravenous						
Ringer's lactate	131	4	109	0	Pre-prepared	
Dacca solution	134	13	99	0	NaCl	5 g
					NaHCO$_3$	4 g
					KCl	1 g
Oral						
WHO/UNICEF	90	20	80	111	NaCl	3.5 g
					Na citrate	2.9 g
					KCl	1.5 g
					Glucose	20 g
Cereal-based	85	–	80	–	80 g cooked rice	
					5 g salt (NaCl)	
Household	85	–	80	111	20 g glucose	
					5 g salt (NaCl)	
UK/Europe	35–60	20	37	90–200	Pre-prepared	

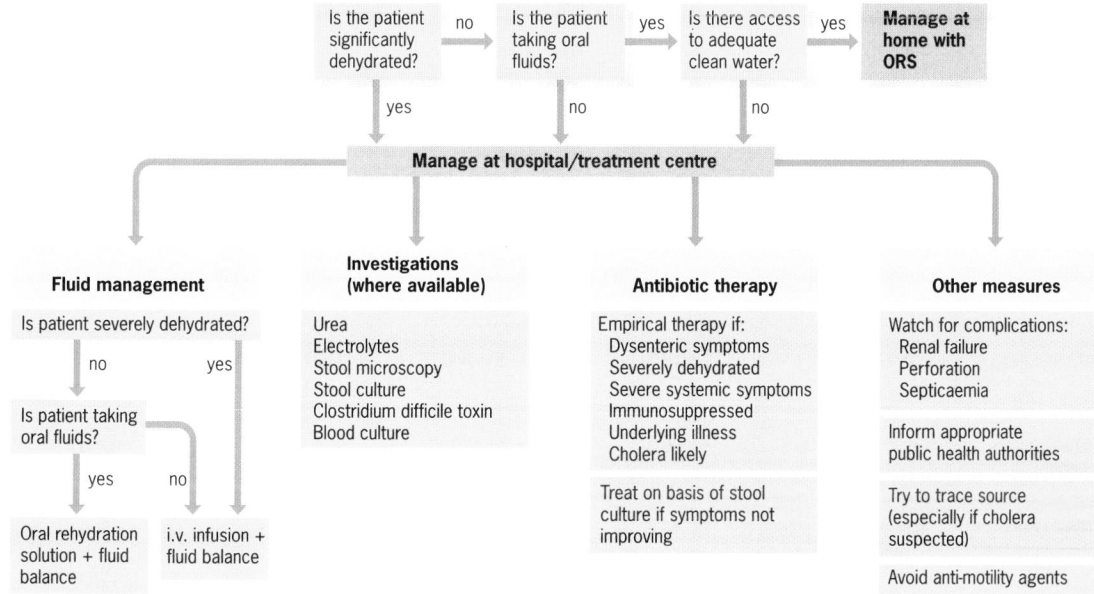

Fig. 2.24 Gastroenteritis – management plan. ORS, oral rehydration solution.

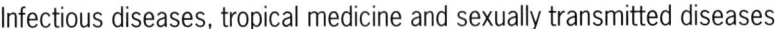

Box 2.10

Antibiotics in adult acute bacterial gastroenteritis

Condition	Indications	Drug of choice	Alternatives	Benefits
Dysentery	Most patients	Ciprofloxacin 500 mg twice daily	Nalidixic acid 1 g four times daily Ampicillin 500 mg four times daily Co-trimoxazole 960 mg twice daily	Relieve symptoms Shorten illness Decrease transmission
Cholera	All patients	Ciprofloxacin	Tetracycline 250 mg four times daily Nalidixic acid Co-trimoxazole	Relieve symptoms Shorten illness Decrease transmission
Empirical therapy of watery diarrhoea	Severe symptoms Prolonged illness Elderly patients Immunosuppressed	Ciprofloxacin	Erythromycin 500 mg four times daily Co-trimoxazole	Relieve symptoms Shorten illness May decrease complications
Travellers' diarrhoea	Rarely used	Ciprofloxacin	Co-trimoxazole	Relieve symptoms Shorten illness
Treatment of confirmed *Salmonella, Campylobacter, Shigella*	Symptoms not improving (rarely needed)	Ciprofloxacin	Erythromycin Co-trimoxazole	May shorten illness
Clostridium difficile	Most cases (unless symptoms resolved)	Metronidazole 400 mg three times daily	Vancomycin 125 mg four times daily	Relieve symptoms Shorten illness

Table 2.30
Bacterial causes of food poisoning

Organism	Source/vehicles	Incubation period	Symptoms	Diagnosis	Recovery
Staphylococcus aureus	Man – contaminated food and water	2–4 h	Diarrhoea, vomiting and dehydration	Culture organism in vomitus or remaining food	< 24 h
E coli O157:H7	Cattle – meat, milk	12–48 h	Watery diarrhoea ± haemorrhagic colitis, HUS	Stool culture	10–12 days
Bacillus cereus	Environment – contaminated food	1–6 h	Diarrhoea, vomiting and dehydration	Culture organism in faeces and food	Rapid
Clostridium perfringens	Environment – contaminated food	8–22 h	Watery diarrhoea and cramping pain	Culture organism in faeces and food	2–3 days
Clostridium botulinum	Environment – bottled or canned food	18–24 h	Brief diarrhoea and paralysis due to neuromuscular blockade	Demonstrate toxin in food or faeces	10–14 days
Salmonella spp.	Cattle and poultry – eggs, meat	12–48 h	Abrupt diarrhoea, fever and vomiting	Stool culture	Usually 3–6 days, but may be up to 2 weeks
Campylobacter jejuni	Cattle and poultry – meat, milk	48–96 h	Diarrhoea ± blood, fever, malaise and abdominal pain	Stool culture	3–5 days
Shigella spp.	Man – contaminated food and water	24–48 h	Acute watery, bloody diarrhoea	Stool culture	7–10 days

HUS, haemolytic uraemic syndrome

Table 2.31
Organic toxins causing food poisoning (see p. 988)

Toxin	Source	Illness
Scombotoxin	Tuna, mackerel	Histamine fish poisoning
Ciguatoxin	Barracuda, snapper	Ciguatera (diarrhoea and paraesthesia)
Dinoflagellate plankton toxin	Shellfish	Neurotoxic shellfish poisoning
Haemagglutinins	Inadequately-prepared dried kidney beans	Diarrhoea and vomiting
Unknown	Buffalo fish	Haff disease (toxic rhabdomyolysis)
Phallotoxins, amatoxins	Mushrooms	Various

Food poisoning

Food poisoning is a legally notifiable disease in England and Wales, and is defined as 'any disease of an infective or toxic nature caused by or thought to be caused by the consumption of food and water'. Not all cases of gastroenteritis are food poisoning, as the pathogens are not always food- or water-borne. Common bacterial causes of food poisoning are listed in Table 2.30. Food poisoning may also be caused by a number of non-infectious organic and inorganic toxins (Table 2.31). Illnesses such as botulism (p. 76) are also classified as food poisoning, even though they do not primarily cause gastroenteritis.

The recent increase in reported food poisoning in developed countries is at least in part due to changes in the production and distribution of food. Livestock raised and slaughtered under modern intensive farming conditions is frequently contaminated with salmonella or campylobacter. However, the main problem is not at this stage. Only 0.02–0.1% of the eggs from a flock of chickens infected with *S. enteritidis* will be affected, and then only at a level of less than 20 cells per egg – harmless to most healthy individuals. It is flaws in the processing, storage and distribution of food products which allow massive amplification of the infection, resulting in extensive contamination. The internationalization of food supply encourages widespread and distant transmission of the resulting infections.

Enteric fever (p. 88)

Other gastrointestinal infections

Gastric infection with *Helicobacter pylori* is discussed on page 271, Whipple's disease on page 295, and bacterial peritonitis on page 330.

FURTHER READING

Bartlett JG (2002) Antibiotic associated diarrhoea. *New England Journal of Medicine* **346**: 334–339.
Donnenberg MS (2000) Pathogenic strategies of enteric bacteria. *Nature* **406**: 768–774.
Moss PJ, McKendrick MW (1997) Bacterial gastroenteritis. *Current Opinion in Infectious Diseases* **10**: 402–407.
www.phls.co.uk/publications/cdrindex/99index.pdf

Infections of the cardiovascular system

- Infective endocarditis (p. 793).

Infections of the nervous system

The central and peripheral nervous systems can be affected by a variety of microorganisms either directly or via toxins, e.g. viral (p. 1192), protozoal (p. 100) and prion diseases (p. 1197).

Bacterial meningitis (see p. 1192)

The most common bacterial disease affecting the central nervous system is acute meningitis, which causes about 150 000 deaths per year, predominantly in the developing world. Epidemic meningitis due to *Neisseria meningitidis* (usually group A) is common in a broad belt across sub-Saharan Africa and is also seen in parts of Asia. In Europe and North America bacterial meningitis is usually sporadic, with B and C strains predominating. A new conjugate vaccine for serogroup C meningococcus may cause a fall in the number of cases.

Streptococcus pneumoniae is the other major cause throughout the world, while tuberculous meningitis (p. 1194) is common in sub-Saharan Africa and parts of Asia.

Haemophilus influenzae b (Hib). As an effective vaccine is available, serious *H. influenzae* infections are now rare in western countries (Fig. 14.21). Many developing countries have also instituted immunization programmes, but invasive *H. influenzae* infection remains common in some parts of the world.

Other less common causes of meningitis in adults include group B streptococci, *Listeria monocytogenes* (see p. 81), *Staphylococcus aureus*, and Gram-negative bacilli. These organisms are usually associated with an underlying illness or immunocompromising condition, or with a cerebrospinal fluid leak.

Cerebral abscess

This is covered on page 1198.

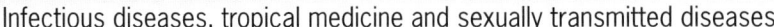
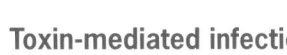

Toxin-mediated infections

Botulism

Clostridium botulinum is a common environmental organism, and produces spores which can survive heating to 100°C. It causes botulism, an illness caused by contamination of canned or bottled foodstuff, in which the anaerobic organism can multiply and elaborate a neurotoxin. After ingestion the toxin causes profound neuromuscular blockade, leading to autonomic and motor paralysis. The first symptoms, occurring 18–24 hours after ingestion, are nausea and diarrhoea. These are followed by cranial nerve weakness and then progressive symmetrical paralysis, leading to respiratory failure.

The diagnosis is usually clinical, and is confirmed by detection of toxin in faeces or in the contaminated food. Treatment is mainly supportive, with mechanical ventilation if necessary. Antitoxin is available in some countries (including the UK); the risk of anaphylaxis is relatively high, and it should only be used in severe cases. A subcutaneous test dose should be given before intravenous or intramuscular injection. Antibiotics have no proven role. The overall mortality from botulism is high, but patients who survive the acute paralysis can make a full recovery.

Botulism may also follow the contamination of wounds with *C. botulinum*, and in infants may be related to bowel colonization by the organism.

Tetanus

Tetanus is also due to a toxin-secreting clostridium: *C. tetani*. The organism is found in soil, and illness usually results from a contaminated wound. The injury itself may be trivial and disregarded by the individual. In developing countries neonatal tetanus follows contamination of the umbilical stump, often after dressing the area with dung.

The organism is not invasive, and clinical manifestations of the disease are due to the potent neurotoxin, tetanospasmin. Tetanospasmin acts on both the α and δ motor systems at synapses, resulting in disinhibition. It also produces neuromuscular blockade and skeletal muscle spasm, and acts on the sympathetic nervous system. The end result is marked flexor muscle spasm and autonomic dysfunction.

Clinical features

The incubation period varies from a few days to several weeks. The most common form of the disease is generalized tetanus. General malaise is rapidly followed by trismus (lockjaw) due to masseter muscle spasm. Spasm of the facial muscles produces the characteristic grinning expression known as risus sardonicus. If the disease is severe, painful reflex spasms develop, usually within 24–72 hours of the initial symptoms. The interval between the first symptom and the first spasm is referred to as the 'onset time'. The spasms may occur spontaneously but are easily precipitated by noise, handling of the patient, or by light. Respiration may be impaired because of laryngeal spasm; oesophageal and urethral spasm lead to dysphagia and urinary retention, respectively, and there is arching of the neck and back muscles (opisthotonus). Autonomic dysfunction produces tachycardia, a labile blood pressure, sweating and cardiac arrhythmias. Patients with tetanus are mentally alert.

Death results from aspiration, hypoxia, respiratory failure, cardiac arrest or exhaustion. Mild cases with rigidity usually recover. Poor prognostic indicators include short incubation period, short onset time, and extremes of age.

Localized tetanus is a milder form of the disease. Pain and stiffness are confined to the site of the wound, with increased tone in the surrounding muscles. Recovery usually occurs.

Cephalic tetanus is uncommon but invariably fatal. It usually occurs when the portal of entry of *C. tetani* is the middle ear. Cranial nerve abnormalities, particularly of the seventh nerve, are usual. Generalized tetanus may or may not develop.

Neonatal tetanus is usually due to infection of the umbilical stump. Failure to thrive, poor sucking, grimacing and irritability are followed by the rapid development of intense rigidity and spasms. Mortality approaches 100%. One aim of the WHO Expanded Programme on Immunization (EPI) is to eliminate this condition by immunizing all women of childbearing age, providing clean delivery facilities and strengthening surveillance in high-risk areas.

Diagnosis

Few diseases resemble tetanus in its fully developed form, and the diagnosis is therefore usually clinical. Rarely, *C. tetani* is isolated from wounds. Phenothiazine overdosage, strychnine poisoning, meningitis and tetany can occasionally mimic tetanus.

Management

When tetanus is suspected any wound must be cleaned and debrided if necessary, to remove the source of toxin. Human tetanus immunoglobin 250 units should be given along with an intramuscular injection of tetanus toxoid. If the patient is already protected a single booster dose of the toxoid is given; otherwise the full three-dose course of adsorbed vaccine is given (see below).

Management of established tetanus is supportive medical and nursing care. Improvement in this area has contributed more than any other single measure to the decrease in the mortality rate from 60% to nearer 20%. Patients are nursed in a quiet, isolated, well-ventilated, darkened room. Benzodiazepines are used to control spasm and sedate the patient; if the airway is compromised intubation and mechanical ventilation may be necessary.

Antibiotics and antitoxin should be administered, even in the absence of an obvious wound. Intravenous metronidazole is the drug of choice, although penicillin is also effective. Human tetanus immunoglobulin (HTIG) 250 IU should be given by intramuscular injection to neutralize any circulating toxin. If HTIG is not available immune equine tetanus immunoglobulin 10 000 IU should be given intramuscularly: this is probably as effective as HTIG, but there is a high incidence of severe allergic reactions. If the patient recovers, active immunization should be instituted, as immunity following tetanus is incomplete.

Prevention

Tetanus is an eminently preventable disease and all persons should be immunized regardless of age. Those who work in a contaminated environment, such as farmers, are particularly at risk and should have regular booster injections. Active immunization with the alum-adsorbed toxoid should be given. Initially two doses of 0.5 mL of the toxoid are given intramuscularly at 8-week intervals. The third dose is given 6–12 months later as a booster. Subsequent boosters are required at 5-year intervals. Infant immunization schedules in all countries include tetanus (Box 2.6). Protection by passive immunization with either the equine or human antitetanus immunoglobulin is short-lived, lasting only about 2 weeks.

FURTHER READING

Begg N, Cartwright KA, Cohen J, Kaczmarski EB, Innes JA, Leen CL, Nathwani D, Singer M, Southgate L, Todd WT, Welsby PD, Wood MJ (1999) Consensus statement on diagnosis, investigation, treatment and prevention of acute bacterial meningitis in immunocompetent adults. British Infections Society Working Party. *Journal of Infection* **39**(1): 1–15.

Bone and joint infections

- Infective arthritis (p. 554)
- Osteomyelitis (p. 557).

Urinary tract infections

- Complicated versus uncomplicated infections (p. 616)
- Acute pyelonephritis (p. 616)
- Reflux nephropathy (p. 616)
- Perinephric abscess (renal carbuncle) (p. 620)
- Bacterial prostatitis (p. 620)
- Tuberculosis of the urinary tract (p. 620)
- Peritonitis complicating continuous ambulatory peritoneal dialysis (p. 654).

Systemic/multisystem infections

Many infections are confined to a particular body organ or system, owing to the metabolic requirements of the organism, the route of infection, or the response of host defences. Other infections can potentially affect several systems or the entire body. Under unusual circumstances such as altered host immunity, infections which are normally circumscribed may become systemic. This section describes those infections which commonly cause multisystem disease in an immunocompetent host.

Bacteraemia and septicaemia

Bacteraemia, the transient presence of organisms in the blood, can occur in healthy people without causing symptoms. It can follow surgery, dental treatment, and even tooth-brushing. Bacteraemia can also occur from the bowel or bladder, especially in the presence of local inflammation. Unless a site of metastatic infection is established (such as the heart valves), most organisms are rapidly cleared from the blood.

Septicaemia. Some invading bacteria such as *Staphylococcus aureus* or *Escherichia coli* are less likely to be dealt with by the immune system and more likely to cause disease. Illness arising from such blood-borne infection is called septicaemia, and may occur in isolation or secondary to a focal infection. Septicaemia usually causes severe systemic symptoms including high fever, rigors, hypotension, myalgia and headache. It can also lead to the establishment of metastatic foci of infection and, in its most severe form, to septic shock.

Patients presenting with symptoms and signs suggesting septicaemia should be examined carefully for evidence of a source: common sites of infection and organisms leading to septicaemia are listed in Tables 2.32 and 2.33. Because of the potential severity of septicaemia, treatment with antibiotics should usually be started empirically as soon as appropriate cultures have been taken. The choice of agent is governed by the likely pathogen: if there are no clues a broad-spectrum regimen

---

Table 2.32
Causes of septicaemia in a previously healthy adult

Site of origin	Usual pathogen(s)
Skin	*Staphylococcus aureus* and other Gram-positive cocci
Urinary tract	*Escherichia coli* and other aerobic Gram-negative rods
Respiratory tract	*Streptococcus pneumoniae*
Gall bladder or bowel	*Enterococcus faecalis, Escherichia coli* and other Gram-negative rods *Bacteroides fragilis*
Pelvic organs	*Neisseria gonorrhoeae*, anaerobes

Table 2.33
Causes of septicaemia in hospitalized patients

Clinical problem	Usual pathogen(s)
Urinary catheter	*Escherichia coli*, *Klebsiella* spp., *Proteus* spp., *Serratia* spp., *Pseudomonas* spp.
Intravenous catheter	*Staphylococcus aureus* and *Staphylococcus epidermidis*, *Klebsiella* spp., *Pseudomonas* spp., *Candida albicans*
Peritoneal catheter	*Staphylococcus epidermidis*
Post-surgery:	
Wound infection	*Staphylococcus aureus*, *Escherichia coli*, anaerobes (depending on site)
Deep infection	Depends on anatomical location
Burns	Gram-positive cocci, *Pseudomonas* spp., *Candida albicans*
Immunocompromised patients	Any of the above

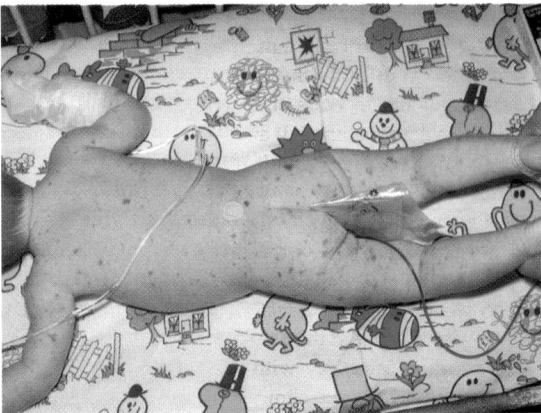

Fig. 2.25 **Meningococcal infections, showing a purpuric rash.**

should be used (e.g. piperacillin plus gentamicin, or cefotaxime, with or without metronidazole). Antibiotic therapy should be reviewed daily as the illness progresses and the results of investigations become available. The general management of septic shock is covered on page 937.

Meningococcal septicaemia

Neisseria meningitidis is found world-wide, in five major serogroups. In sub-Saharan Africa and parts of Asia where group A meningococcus is prevalent it usually causes epidemic disease. Groups Y and W can also cause epidemic infection, while groups B and C (which are the predominant strains in Europe and North America) tend to be sporadic. In England and Wales approximately 2000 cases of meningococcal disease are reported annually.

Man is the only known reservoir for the organism, which is carried asymptomatically in the nasopharynx of 5–20% of the general population. Meningococcal disease occurs when the bacteria invade the nasal mucosa and enter the bloodstream: this only happens in a small percentage of those colonized. Invasion depends on both host and bacterial factors. It is more likely to take place soon after colonization has taken place, and following viral upper respiratory infections.

Clinical features

Invasive meningococcal infection may cause meningitis, septicaemia, or both. Meningitic disease (see p. 1192) usually presents with the classical triad of headache, fever, and neck stiffness. Vomiting, diminished consciousness, and focal neurological signs occur although some patients, especially in the early stages, only have mild symptoms. Meningococcal septicaemia causes the typical features of septic shock such as fever, myalgia,

and hypotension (p. 931), and may be accompanied by a petechial or haemorrhagic rash (Fig. 2.25). In some cases the patient can deteriorate rapidly, with shock, disseminated intravascular coagulation, and multiorgan failure.

Diagnosis

The presence of menigitis and septicaemia with a typical rash is strongly suggestive of meningococcal disease. Antibiotics (benzyl penicillin 2.4 g i.v. slowly) should be given immediately. Gram-negative diplococci may be seen on Gram stain of CSF or of aspirate from petechiae, and meningococci can also be cultured from CSF or blood, or detected by PCR. A rising titre of antibody to meningococcal outer membrane protein (OMP) can also be used in diagnosis.

Management

N. meningitidis is sensitive to benzylpenicillin, chloramphenicol, and third-generation cephalosporins: antibiotic treatment for meningococcal meningitis should be continued parenterally for 7 days. Meningococcal septicaemia should be managed in the same way as any other septicaemic illness (p. 31). The mortality from meningococcal septicaemia in developed countries is currently approximately 10%, while that from meningococcal meningitis alone is less than 5% (see below). Mild neurological sequelae (especially vestibular nerve damage) are common, but serious brain damage is relatively unusual.

A conjugate *vaccine* against meningococcal serogroup C polysaccharide is now available. This may lead to an overall reduction of meningococcal disease in the UK but unfortunately an increase in infection of other serotypes may occur. A B vaccine is not available.

For close contacts of a case of meningococcal disease, household and 'kissing' contacts should be given prophylaxis with oral rifampicin or ciprofloxacin (the latter should not be given to children) to eradicate the bacteria from the nasopharynx. In the case of group C disease, contacts should be offered immunization.

Rheumatic fever

Rheumatic fever is an inflammatory disease that occurs in children and young adults (the first attack usually occurs at between 5 and 15 years of age) as a result of infection with group A streptococci. It affects the heart, skin, joints and central nervous system. It is common in the Middle and Far East, eastern Europe and South America. It is rare in the UK, western Europe and North America. This decline in the incidence of rheumatic fever (from 10% of children in the 1920s to 0.01% today) parallels the reduction in all streptococcal infections and is largely due to improved hygiene and the use of antibiotics.

Pharyngeal infection with group A streptococcus may be followed by the clinical syndrome of rheumatic fever. This is thought to develop because of an autoimmune reaction triggered by molecular mimicry between M proteins of the infecting *Streptococcus pyogenes* and cardiac myosin and laminin. The condition is not due to direct infection of the heart or to the production of a toxin. Chronic and progressive valvular heart disease follows in more than half those affected.

Pathology

All three layers of the heart may be affected. The characteristic lesion of rheumatic carditis is the Aschoff nodule, which is a granulomatous lesion with a central necrotic area occurring in the myocardium, particularly in the subendocardium of the left ventricle. Small, warty vegetations may develop on the endocardium, particularly on the heart valves. This leads to some degree of valvular regurgitation. A serofibrinous effusion characterizes the acute pericarditis that occurs.

The synovial membranes are acutely inflamed during rheumatic fever, and subcutaneous nodules (which are also granulomatous lesions) are seen in the acute stage of the disease.

Clinical features

The disease presents suddenly, with fever, joint pains, malaise and loss of appetite. The clinical features depend on the organs that are involved. Diagnosis relies on the presence of two or more major clinical manifestations or one major manifestation plus two or more minor features. These are known as the Duckett Jones criteria (Table 2.34).

Carditis manifests as:

- new or changed heart murmurs
- development of cardiac enlargement or cardiac failure
- appearance of a pericardial effusion and ECG changes of pericarditis (raised ST segments) or myocarditis (inverted or flattened T waves), first-degree or greater AV block or other cardiac arrhythmias
- transient diastolic mitral (Carey–Coombs) murmur due to mitral valvulitis.

Table 2.34
Revised Duckett Jones criteria for the diagnosis of rheumatic fever. The diagnosis is made on the basis of two or more major criteria or one major plus two or more minor criteria

Major criteria
Carditis
Polyarthritis
Chorea
Erythema marginatum
Subcutaneous nodules

Minor criteria
Fever
Arthralgia
Previous rheumatic fever
Raised ESR/C-reactive protein
Leucocytosis
Prolonged PR interval on ECG

Plus evidence of antecedent streptococcal infection, e.g. positive throat cultures for group A streptococci, elevated antistreptolysin O titre (> 250 U) or other streptococcal antibodies, or a history of recent scarlet fever

ESR, erythrocyte sedimentation rate

Non-cardiac features include the following:

- There is usually a fever with an apparently excessive tachycardia.
- The arthritis associated with rheumatic fever is classically a fleeting migratory polyarthritis affecting large joints such as the knees, elbows, ankles and wrists. The joints are swollen, red and tender. As the inflammation in one joint recedes, another becomes affected. Once the acute inflammation disappears, the rheumatic process leaves the joints normal.
- Sydenham's chorea (or St Vitus' dance, see p. 1187) is involvement of the central nervous system that develops late after a streptococcal infection. Sufferers are noticeably 'fidgety' and display spasmodic, unintentional choreiform movements. Speech is often affected.
- Skin manifestations include erythema marginatum, a transient pink rash with slightly raised edges, which occurs in 20% of cases. The erythematous areas found mostly on the trunk and limbs coalesce into crescent- or ring-shaped patches. Subcutaneous nodules, which are painless, pea-sized, hard nodules beneath the skin, may also occur, particularly over tendons, joints and bony prominences.

Investigations

- **Throat swabs** are cultured for the group A streptococcus.
- **Serological changes** may indicate a recent streptococcal infection. The antistreptolysin O titre, and sometimes others such as the antistreptokinase titre, are performed.

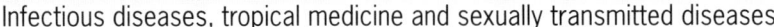

- **Non-specific indicators of inflammation** such as the ESR and the C-reactive protein levels are usually elevated.

Treatment

Patients with fever, active arthritis or active carditis should be completely rested in bed. When the clinical syndrome has subsided (e.g. no pyrexia, normal pulse rate, normal ESR, normal white cell count) the patient may be mobilized.

Residual streptococcal infections should be eradicated with a single intramuscular injection of 916 mg of benzathine penicillin or oral phenoxymethylpenicillin 500 mg four times daily for 1 week. This therapy should be administered even if nasal or pharyngeal swabs do not culture the streptococci.

High-dose salicylate (preferably acetylsalicylate, i.e. aspirin) therapy is given to the limit of tolerance determined by the development of tinnitus. If carditis is present, systemic corticosteroids may be given. Prednisolone 60–120 mg in four divided doses each day is administered until the clinical syndrome is improved and the ESR has fallen to normal. Steroids are then tapered off over 2–4 weeks. However, the efficacy of steroids is in doubt.

Recurrences are most common when persistent cardiac damage is present, and are prevented by the continued administration of oral phenoxymethylpenicillin 250 mg daily or by monthly injections of 916 mg of benzathine penicillin until the age of 20 years or for 5 years after the latest attack (see p. 35). A sulphonamide (e.g. sulfadiazine) may be used if the patient is allergic to penicillin. Any streptococcal infection that does develop should be treated very promptly.

Prognosis

More than 50% of those who suffer acute rheumatic fever with carditis will later (after 10–20 years) develop chronic rheumatic valvular disease, predominantly affecting the mitral and aortic valves (Table 13.35).

Leptospirosis

Leptospirosis is a zoonosis caused by the spirochaete *Leptospira interrogans*. There are over 200 serotypes: the main types affecting humans are *L. i. icterohaemorrhagiae* (rodents), *L. i. canicola* (dogs and pigs), *L. i. hardjo* (cattle), and *L. i. pomona* (pigs and cattle). Leptospires are excreted in the animal urine, and enter the host through a skin abrasion or through intact mucous membranes. Leptospirosis can also be caught by ingestion of contaminated water. The organism can survive for many days in warm fresh water, and for up to 24 hours in sea water.

In England and Wales only 20–30 cases of leptospirosis are diagnosed every year (although many mild infections probably go undiagnosed), and it remains largely an occupational disease of farmers, vets, and others who work with animals. In some parts of the world (e.g. Hawaii, where the annual incidence is about 130/100 000) it is associated with a variety of recreational activities which bring people into closer contact with rodents. Outbreaks of leptospirosis have also been associated with flooding.

Clinical features

Weil, in 1886, described a severe illness consisting of jaundice, haemorrhage, and renal impairment caused by *L. i. icterohaemorrhagiae*, but fortunately 90–95% of infections are subclinical or cause only a mild fever. The incubation period of leptospirosis is usually 7–14 days, and the illness typically has two phases. A leptospiraemic phase, which lasts for up to a week, is followed after a couple of days' interval by an immunological phase. The first phase is characterized by severe headache, malaise, fever, anorexia and myalgia. Most patients have conjunctival suffusion. Hepatosplenomegaly, lymphadenopathy and various skin rashes are sometimes seen. The second phase is usually mild. Fifty percent of patients have meningism, about a third of whom have a CSF lymphocytosis. The majority of patients recover uneventfully at this stage.

In severe disease there may not be a clear distinction between phases. Following the initial symptoms patients progressively develop hepatic and renal failure, haemolytic anaemia, and circulatory collapse. Cardiac failure and pulmonary haemorrhage may also occur. Even with full supportive care the mortality is around 10%, rising to 15–20% in the elderly.

Diagnosis

The diagnosis is usually a clinical one. Leptospires can be cultured from blood or CSF during the first week of illness, but culture requires special media and may take several weeks. A minority of patients may also excrete the organism in their urine from the second week onwards. Specific IgM antibodies start to appear from the end of the first week. There is typically a leucocytosis; other laboratory investigations may be abnormal but are non-specific.

Management

Early antibiotic therapy will limit the progress of the disease, but treatment should still be initiated whatever the stage of the infection. Oral doxycycline may be used in mild cases: intravenous penicillin or erythromycin are given in more severe disease. Intensive supportive care is needed for those patients who develop hepatorenal failure.

Brucellosis

Brucellosis (Malta fever, undulant fever) is a zoonosis and has a world-wide distribution, although it has been virtually eliminated from cattle in the UK. The highest incidence is in the Mediterranean countries, the Middle East and the tropics; there are about 500 000 new cases diagnosed per year (Table 2.35).

Table 2.35
Main geographical distribution and natural hosts of the _Brucella_ species

Organism	Geographical distribution	Natural host
B. abortus	World-wide, except northern Europe, Japan	Cattle
B. melitensis	Mediterranean region especially Malta	Goats, sheep and camels
B. suis	Far East, USA	Pigs
B. canis*		Beagles

* Rarely causes disease in humans

The organisms usually gain entry into the human body via the mouth; less frequently they may enter via the respiratory tract, genital tract or abraded skin. The bacilli travel in the lymphatics and infect lymph nodes. This is followed by haematogenous spread with ultimate localization in the reticuloendothelial system. Spread is usually by the ingestion of raw milk from infected cattle or goats, although occupational exposure is also common. Person-to-person transmission is rare.

Clinical features
The incubation period of acute brucellosis is 1–3 weeks. The onset is insidious, with malaise, headache, weakness, generalized myalgia and night sweats. The fever pattern is classically undulant, although continuous and intermittent patterns are also seen. Lymphadenopathy, hepatosplenomegaly and spinal tenderness may be present; arthritis, osteomyelitis, orchitis, epididymitis, meningoencephalitis and endocarditis have all been described.

Untreated brucellosis can give rise to chronic infection, lasting a year or more. This is characterized by easy fatiguability, myalgia, and occasional bouts of fever and depression. Splenomegaly is usually present. Occasionally infection can lead to localized brucellosis. Bones and joints, spleen, endocardium, lungs, urinary tract and nervous system may be involved. Systemic symptoms occur in less than one-third.

Diagnosis
Blood (or bone marrow) cultures are positive during the acute phase of illness in 50% of patients, but prolonged culture is needed. This is less helpful in chronic disease where serological tests are of greater value. The brucella agglutination test, which demonstrates a fourfold or greater rise in titre over a 4-week period, is highly suggestive of brucellosis. A single titre greater than 1 in 160 is also suggestive of brucellosis in the appropriate clinical setting. An elevated serum IgG level is evidence of current or recent infection; a negative test excludes chronic brucellosis. In localized brucellosis antibody titres are low, and diagnosis is usually established by culturing the organisms from the involved site.

Management and prevention
Brucellosis is treated with a combination of doxycycline 200 mg daily and rifampicin 600–900 mg daily for 6 weeks, but relapses occur. Alternatively, tetracycline can be combined with streptomycin, which is usually given for only the first 2 weeks of treatment. Prevention and control involve careful attention to hygiene when handling infected animals, eradication of infection in animals, and pasteurization of milk. No vaccine is available for use in humans.

Listeriosis
Listeria monocytogenes is an environmental organism which is widely disseminated in soil and decayed matter. It affects both animals and man: the most common route of human infection is in contaminated foodstuffs. The organism can grow at temperatures as low as 4°C, and the most commonly implicated foods are unpasteurized soft cheeses, raw vegetables and chicken pâtés. Listeriosis is a rare but serious infection affecting mainly neonates, pregnant women, the elderly, and the immunocompromised. _L. monocytogenes_ has also recently been recognized as a cause of self-limiting food-borne gastroenteritis in healthy adults, but the incidence of this is unknown.

In pregnant women listeria causes a flu-like illness, but infection of the fetus can lead to septic abortion, premature labour, and stillbirth. Early treatment of listeria in pregnancy may prevent this, but the overall fetal loss rate is about 50%. Listeria in the elderly and the immunocompromised usually causes meningoencephalitis, although septicaemia and a variety of other focal infections have been described.

The diagnosis is established by culture of blood, CSF, or other body fluids. The treatment of choice for adult listeriosis is ampicillin plus gentamicin. Co-trimoxazole is also effective, but the organism is resistant to cephalosporins.

Lyme disease
Lyme disease, caused by the spirochaete _Borrelia burgdorferi_, is a zoonosis of deer and other wild mammals. The syndrome was first recognized and named following an 'outbreak' of arthritis in the town of Lyme, Connecticut, in the mid-1970s. Since then the disease has increased in both incidence and detection: it is now known to be widespread in the USA and Europe. About 300 cases are reported in the UK annually (of which 15% are acquired abroad), although this probably underestimates the actual incidence. Infection is transmitted from animal to man by ixodid ticks, and is most likely to occur in rural wooded areas in spring and early summer.

Clinical features
The first stage of the illness, which follows 7–10 days after infection, is characterized by the skin lesion erythema chronicum migrans. This is often accompanied by headache, fever, malaise, myalgia, arthralgia and

lymphadenopathy. The second stage follows weeks or months later, when some patients develop neurological symptoms (meningoencephalitis, cranial or polyneuropathies), radiculopathies, cardiac problems (conduction disorders, myocarditis) or arthritis. These manifestations, which are often fluctuant and changing, usually resolve spontaneously over months or years. Some patients, however, develop chronic and persistent neurological disease (e.g. paraparesis) or rheumatological disease ('late Lyme disease').

Diagnosis

The clinical features and epidemiological considerations are usually strongly suggestive. The diagnosis can only rarely be confirmed by isolation of the organisms from blood, skin lesions or CSF. IgM antibodies are detectable in the first month, and IgG antibodies are invariably present late in the disease. However, false positive serological results do occur, and even a genuine positive IgG may be a marker of previous exposure rather than of ongoing infection.

Management

Amoxicillin or doxycycline given early in the course of the disease shortens the duration of the illness in approximately 50% of patients. Late disease should be treated with 2–4 weeks of intravenous benzylpenicillin or ceftriaxone. However, treatment is unsatisfactory, and preventative measures are necessary. In tick-infested areas, repellents and protective clothing should be worn. Prompt removal of any tick is essential as infection is unlikely to take place until the tick has been attached for more than 48 hours. Ticks should be grasped with forceps near to the point of attachment to the skin and then withdrawn by gentle traction. Antibiotic prophylaxis following a tick bite is not justified, even in areas where Lyme disease is common. A vaccine is available and may be offered to those at high risk of infection.

Tularaemia

Tularaemia is due to infection by *Francisella tularensis*, a Gram-negative organism. It is primarily a zoonosis, acquired mainly from rodents. Infection is normally transmitted by arthropod vectors, including ticks and blood-sucking flies. Humans may be infected by this route or by handling infected animals, when the microorganisms enter through minor abrasions or mucous membranes. Occasionally infection occurs from contaminated water or from eating uncooked meat. The disease is widely distributed in North America, Northern Europe and Asia. It is relatively rare, occurring mainly in hunters, trappers, and others in close contact with animals.

The incubation period of 2–7 days is followed by a generalized illness. The most common presentation is ulceroglandular tularaemia. A papule occurs at the site of inoculation. This ulcerates and is followed by tender,

suppurative lymphadenopathy. Rarely this can be followed by bacteraemia, leading to septicaemia, pneumonia, or meningitis. These forms of the disease carry a high mortality if untreated.

Diagnosis is by culture of the organism or by a rising titre seen on a bacterial agglutination test.

Tularaemia should be treated with streptomycin or gentamicin.

FURTHER READING

Astiz ME, Rachow EC (1998) Septic shock. *Lancet* **351**: 1501–1505.

Galvin JE, Hemric ME, Ward K, Cunningham MW (2000) Cytotoxic Mab from rheumatic carditis recognizes heart valves and laminin. *Journal of Clinical Investigation* **106**: 217–224.

Levett PN (1999) Leptospirosis: re-emerging or rediscovered disease? *Journal of Medical Microbiology* **48**: 417–418.

Rosenstein NE et al. (2001) Meningococcal disease. *New England Journal of Medicine* **344**: 1378–1389.

Steere AC (2001) Lyme disease. *New England Journal of Medicine* **345 (2)**: 115–125.

Stollerman GH (1997) Rheumatic fever. *Lancet* **349**: 935–942.

Bacterial infections seen in developing and tropical countries

Skin, soft tissue and eye disease

Leprosy

Leprosy (Hansen's disease) is caused by the acid-fast bacillus *Mycobacterium leprae*. Unlike other mycobacteria, it does not grow in artificial media or even in tissue culture. Apart from the nine-banded armadillo, man is the only natural host of *M. leprae*, although it can be grown in the footpads of mice.

Leprosy occurs in all tropical and warm temperate regions, particularly in Asia and Africa. Endemic foci are still present in Southern Europe and parts of the USA. The prevalence of the disease has fallen dramatically in the last 20 years, largely as a result of the use of supervised multidrug treatment regimens. There are currently estimated to be about 2.5 million people with leprosy world-wide, about half of whom are in South East Asia.

The precise mode of transmission of leprosy is still uncertain but it is likely that nasal secretions play a role. Infection is related to poverty and overcrowding. Once an individual has been infected, subsequent progression to clinical disease appears to be dependent on several factors. Males appear to be more susceptible than females, and there is evidence from twin studies of a genetic susceptibility. The main factor, however, is the response of the host's cell-mediated immune system.

Two *polar types* of leprosy are recognized:

- tuberculoid leprosy, a localized disease that occurs in individuals with a high degree of cell-mediated immunity (CMI)
- lepromatous leprosy, a generalized disease that occurs in individuals with impaired CMI (Fig. 2.26).

In practice many patients will fall between these two extremes and some may move along the spectrum as the disease progresses or is treated.

Clinical features

The incubation period varies from 2–6 years, although it may be as short as a few months or as long as 20 years. The onset of leprosy is generally insidious. Acute onset is known to occur, and patients may present with a transient rash, with features of an acute febrile illness, with evidence of nerve involvement, or with any combination of these. The major signs of leprosy are:

- Skin lesions, usually anaesthetic (generally tuberculoid).
- Thickened peripheral nerves, nerves of predelection which are superficial or lie in fibro-osseous tunnels – ulnar (elbow), median (wrist), radial cutaneous (wrist), common peroneal (knee), posterior tibial and sural (ankle), facial (crossing zygomatic arch) and greater auricular (posterior triangle of the neck).

The spectrum of disease can be divided into five clinical groups.

Tuberculoid leprosy (TT)

In tuberculoid leprosy the infection is localized because the patient has unimpaired cell-mediated immunity.

The characteristic, usually single, skin lesion is a hypopigmented, anaesthetic patch with thickened, clearly demarcated edges, central healing, and atrophy. The face, gluteal region and extremities are most commonly affected. The nerve leading to the hypopigmented patch, and the regional nerve trunk, are often thickened and tender. Unlike other parts of the body, a tuberculoid patch on the face is not anaesthetic. Nerve involvement leads to marked muscle atrophy. Tuberculoid lesions are known to heal spontaneously. The prognosis is good.

Borderline tuberculoid (BT) leprosy

This resembles TT but skin lesions are usually more numerous, smaller, and may be present as small 'satellite' lesions around larger ones. Peripheral but not cutaneous nerves are thickened, leading to deformity of hands and feet.

Borderline (BB) leprosy

Skin lesions are numerous, varying in size and form (macules, papules, plaques). The annular, rimmed lesion with punched-out, hypopigmented anaesthetic centre is characteristic (Fig. 2.27). There is widespread nerve involvement and limb deformity (Fig. 2.28).

Borderline lepromatous (BL) leprosy

There are a large number of florid asymmetrical skin lesions of variable form, which are strongly positive for

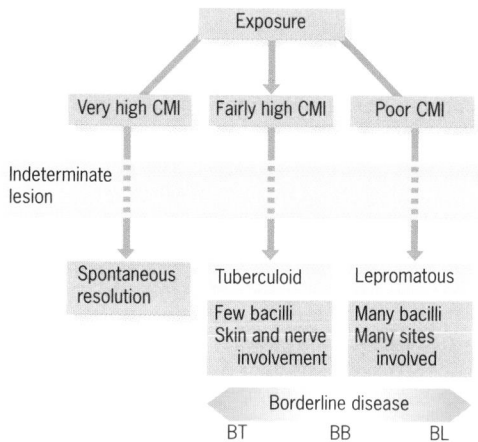

Fig. 2.26 **Clinical spectrum of leprosy.** BT, borderline tuberculoid; BB, borderline; BL, borderline lepromatous; CMI, cell mediated immunity.

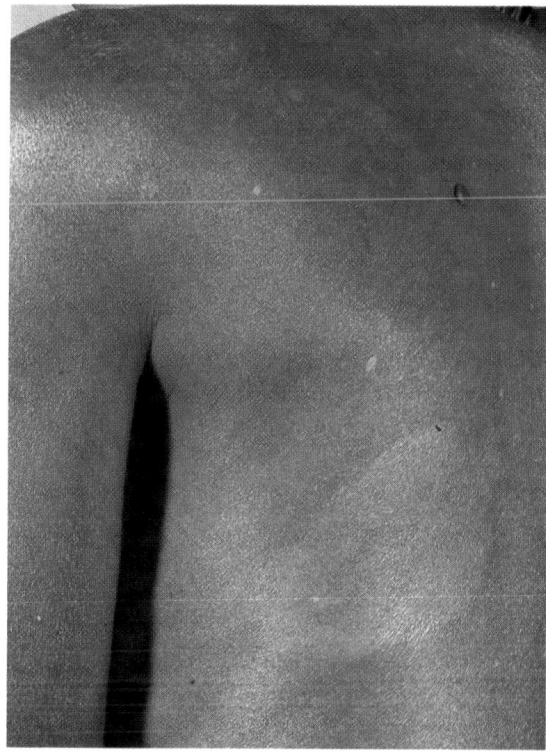

Fig. 2.27 **Multiple asymmetrical hypopigmented anaesthetic patches.** Courtesy of Dr P Matondo, Zambia.

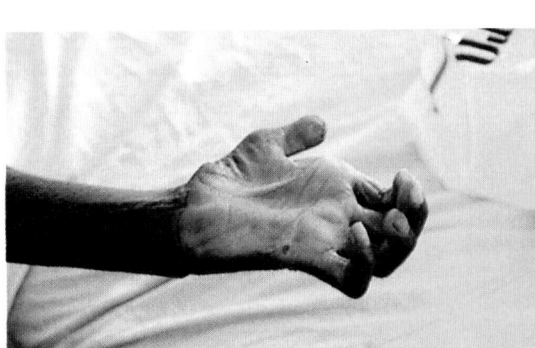

Fig. 2.28 Leprosy – claw hand due to median and ulnar nerve damage.

acid-fast bacilli. Skin between the lesions is normal and often negative for bacilli.

Lepromatous leprosy (LL)

Although practically every organ can be involved, the changes in the skin are the earliest and most obvious manifestation. Peripheral oedema and rhinitis are the earliest symptoms. The skin lesions predominantly occur on the face, the gluteal region and the upper and lower limbs. They may be macules, papules, nodules or plaques: of these, the macule is the first to appear. Infiltration is most noticeable in the ear lobes. Thinning of the lateral margins of the eyebrows is characteristic. The mucous membranes are frequently involved, resulting in nasal stuffiness, laryngitis and hoarseness of the voice. Nasal septal perforation with collapse of the nasal cartilages produces a saddle-nose deformity. With progression of the disease the typical leonine facies due to infiltration of the skin becomes apparent. Glove and stocking anaesthesia, gynaecomastia, testicular atrophy, ichthyosis and nerve palsies (facial, ulnar, median and radial) develop late in the disease. Neurotrophic atrophy affecting the phalanges leads to the gradual disappearance of fingers. Nerve involvement is less pronounced than in TT.

The lepromin test

This test, in which a suspension of dead bacilli is injected intradermally, is a measure of host resistance to leprosy and not a test for detecting leprosy. Two types of reaction are observed. *The early (Fernandez) reaction* becomes positive in 48 hours and reflects the sensitivity of the tissue to the leprosy bacilli protein. *The late (Mitsuda) reaction* develops in 4–5 weeks and reflects the resistance of the host to the bacteria: this reaction is strongly positive in TT and is negative in LL.

Lepra reactions

These are immunologically mediated acute reactions that occur in patients with the borderline or lepromatous spectrum of disease, usually during treatment. Two forms are recognized.

Non-lepromatous lepra reaction (type I lepra reaction). This is seen following treatment of patients with borderline disease; it is a type IV delayed hypersensitivity reaction. Both upgrading (or reversal) reactions (i.e. a clinical change towards a more tuberculoid form) and downgrading reactions (i.e. a change towards the lepromatous form) can occur. Neurological deficits such as an ulnar nerve palsy may occur abruptly.

Erythema nodosum leprosum (ENL; type II lepra reaction). This is a humoral antibody response to an antigen–antibody complex (i.e. a type III hypersensitivity reaction). It is seen in 50% of patients with treated LL. ENL is characterized by fever, arthralgia, iridocyclitis, crops of painful, subcutaneous erythematous nodules, and other systemic manifestations. It may last from a few days to several weeks.

Diagnosis

The diagnosis of leprosy is essentially clinical. Patients should be examined carefully for skin lesions in adequate natural light. Acid-fast bacilli may be seen in smears from the skin or nasal mucosa. Occasionally nerve biopsies are helpful. The definitive diagnosis is established by cultivating the organisms in the footpads of mice. Detection of *M. leprae* DNA is possible in all forms of leprosy using the polymerase chain reaction, and can be used to assess the efficacy of treatment.

Management

Multidrug therapy is now essential because of developing drug resistance (up to 40% of bacilli in some areas are resistant to dapsone). Dapsone, a folate synthetase inhibitor, is bacteriostatic. It is cheap and well tolerated; side-effects (which include haemolytic anaemia and sulphaemoglobinaemia) are rare. The other commonly used drugs are clofazimine (a phenazine dye, whose principal side-effect is persistent skin pigmentation) and rifampicin (p. 895). Recommended treatment regimens for leprosy are shown in Box 2.11. Three new drugs have

---

Box 2.11

Recommended treatment regimens for leprosy in adults

Multibacillary leprosy (LL, BL, BB)
Rifampicin 600 mg once-monthly, supervised
Clofazimine 300 mg once-monthly, supervised
Clofazimine 50 mg daily, self-administered
Dapsone 100 mg daily, self-administered

Treatment continued for 2 years

Paucibacillary leprosy (BT, TT)
Rifampicin 600 mg once-monthly, supervised
Dapsone 100 mg daily, self-administered

Treatment continued for 6 months

LL, lepromatous; BL, borderline lepromatous; BB, borderline; BT, borderline tuberculoid; TT, tuberculoid

been found to be active against *M. lepra* and are currently under evaluation in human infection: ofloxacin, minocycline, and clarithromycin. It is possible that use of these drugs will substantially reduce the duration of treatment in the future.

Leprosy should be treated in specialist centres with adequate physiotherapy and occupational therapy support. Surgery and physiotherapy also play a role in the management of trophic ulcers and deformities of the hands, feet and face.

Treatment of lepra reactions. This is urgent, as irreversible eye and nerve damage can occur. Antileprosy therapy must be continued. Type II lepra reactions (ENL) can be treated with analgesics, chloroquine, clofazimine and antipyretics. Thalidomide, a drug known for its potent teratogenic effects, is by far the most effective in the ENL reaction, but must be used with caution. Prednisolone 30–40 mg daily for a few weeks is effective in type I reactions.

Prevention

The prevention and control of leprosy depends on rapid treatment of infected patients, particularly those with LL and BL, to decrease the bacterial reservoir. *M. leprae* is spread by close contact, but only a small proportion of contacts – approximately 1% – develop the disease. Antileprosy vaccines are under clinical trial; the efficacy of the BCG vaccine against leprosy is debatable. Mass chemoprophylaxis is impracticable and its efficacy in household contacts has not been established.

Anthrax

Anthrax is caused by *Bacillus anthracis*. The spores of these Gram-positive bacilli are extremely hardy and withstand extremes of temperature and humidity. The organism is capable of toxin production and this property correlates most closely with its virulence. The disease occurs world-wide. Epidemics have been reported in The Gambia, in both North and South America and in southern Europe. Transmission is through direct contact with an infected animal; infection is most frequently seen in farmers, butchers, and dealers in wool and animal hides. Spores can also be ingested or inhaled.

Clinical features

The incubation period is 1–10 days. By far the most common form is cutaneous anthrax. The small, erythematous, maculopapular lesion is initially painless. It may subsequently vesiculate and ulcerate, with formation of a central black eschar. The illness is self-limiting in the majority of patients, but occasionally perivesicular oedema and regional lymphadenopathy may be marked, and toxaemia can occur.

Respiratory involvement (woolsorter's disease) follows inhalation of spores. A febrile illness is accompanied by non-productive cough and retrosternal discomfort;

pleural effusions are common. Untreated, the mortality is about 90%.

Gastrointestinal anthrax is due to consumption of contaminated meat. It presents as severe gastroenteritis; haematemesis and bloody diarrhoea can occur. Toxaemia, shock and death may follow.

Diagnosis

The diagnosis is established by demonstrating the organism in smears from cutaneous lesions or by culture of blood and other body fluids. Serological confirmation can be made using ELISAs detecting antibodies to both the organism and a toxin.

Management

Penicillin or ciprofloxacin are the best treatments. In mild cutaneous infections, oral therapy for 2 weeks is adequate. In more severe infections high doses of intravenous antibiotics are needed, along with appropriate supportive care.

Control

Any infected animal that dies should be burned and the area in which it was housed disinfected. Where animal husbandry is poor, mass vaccination of animals may prevent widespread contamination, but needs to be repeated annually. A human vaccine is available for those at high risk.

Mycobacterial ulcer (Buruli ulcer)

Buruli ulcer is seen in rural areas in the tropics. *Mycobacterium ulcerans*, the causative organism, is found in pools and rivers, and infection is usually due to bathing, swimming or collecting water. A small subcutaneous nodule at the site of infection gradually ulcerates, involving subcutaneous tissue, muscle and fascial planes. The ulcers are usually large with undermined edges and markedly necrotic bases. Smears taken from necrotic tissue generally reveal numerous acid-fast bacilli. The only effective treatment is wide surgical excision with skin grafts, but this is often unavailable in areas where the disease is prevalent. Antituberculous therapy is ineffective.

Endemic treponematoses (bejel, yaws and pinta)

These diseases are found in various parts of the tropics and subtropics, mainly in impoverished rural areas (Fig. 2.29). The WHO treated over 50 million cases in the 1950s and 1960s, reducing the prevalence of these diseases, but subsequently there has been a resurgence of infection. The latest estimate of global prevalence is 2.5 million cases. Improvements in sanitation and an increase in living standards will be required to eradicate the diseases completely as organisms are transmitted by bodily contact, usually in children.

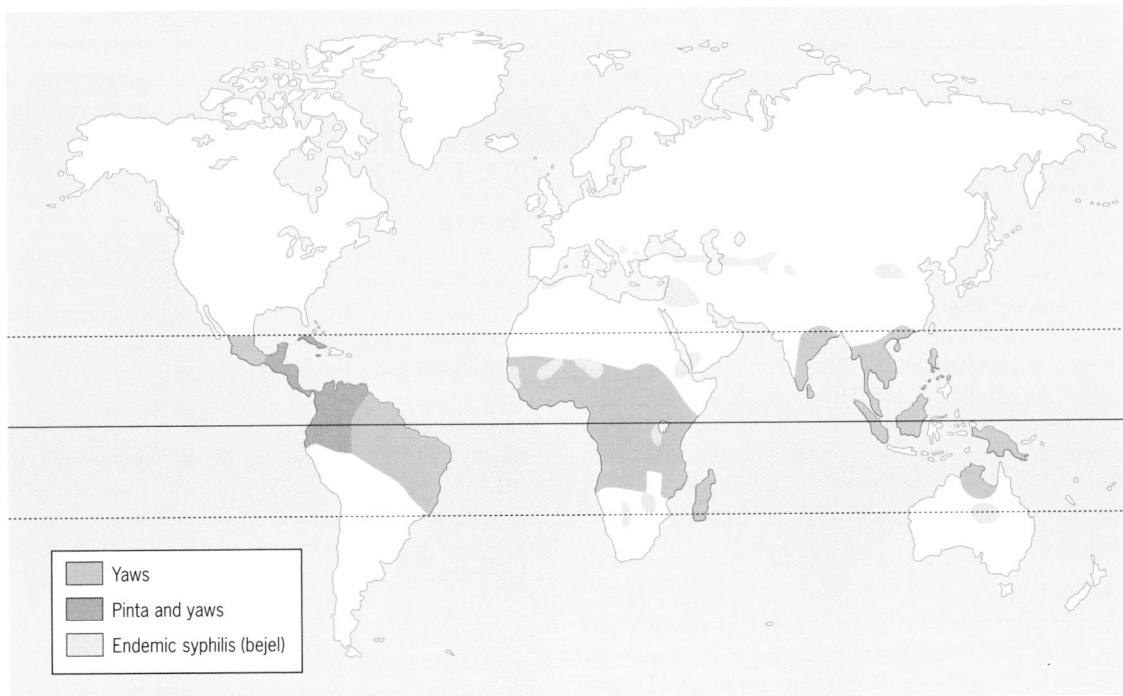

Fig. 2.29 Bejel, yaws and pinta – geographical distribution.

Clinical features

Yaws

Yaws (caused by *Treponema pertenue*) is the most wide-spread and common of the endemic treponemal diseases. It is spread by direct contact, the organism entering through damaged skin. After an incubation period of weeks or months a primary inflammatory reaction occurs at the inoculation site, from which organisms can be isolated. Dissemination of the organism leads to multiple papular lesions containing treponemes; these skin lesions usually involve the palms and soles. There may also be bone involvement, particularly affecting the long bones and those of the hand.

Approximately 10% of those infected go on to develop late yaws. Bony gummatous lesions may progress to cause gross destruction and disfigurement, particularly of the skull and facial bones, the interphalangeal joints and the long bones. Plantar hyperkeratosis is characteristic. Like syphilis, there may be a latent period between the early and late phases of the disease, but visceral, neurological and cardiovascular problems do not occur

Bejel (endemic syphilis)

Bejel is seen in Africa and the Middle East. The causative organism (*Treponema endemicum*) enters through abrasions in the skin or from contaminated drinking vessels. It differs from venereal syphilis in that a primary lesion is not commonly seen. The late stages resemble syphilis, but cardiological and neurological manifestations are rare.

Pinta

Pinta, caused by *Treponema carateum*, is restricted mainly to Central and South America. It is milder than the other trepanomatoses and is confined to the skin. The primary lesion is a pruritic red papule, usually on the hand or foot. It may become scaly but never ulcerates and is generally associated with regional lymphadenopathy. In the later stages similar lesions can continue to occur for up to 1 year, associated with generalized lymphadenopathy. Eventually the lesions heal leaving hyperpigmented or depigmented patches.

Diagnosis and management

In endemic areas the diagnosis is usually clinical. The causative organism can be identified from the exudative lesions under dark-ground microscopy. Serological tests for syphilis are positive but do not differentiate between the conditions.

The treatment is with long-acting penicillin (e.g. intramuscular benzathine penicillin, 1.2 million units) given as a single dose. Alternatives include erythromycin and tetracycline.

Trachoma

Trachoma, caused by the intracellular bacterium *Chlamydia trachomatis*, is the most common cause of blindness in the world. It is estimated that there are 500 million current infections, and 6 million people who have been blinded by trachoma. It is a disease of poverty which is found mainly in the tropics and the

Middle East: it is entirely preventable. Trachoma commonly occurs in children, and is spread by direct transmission or by flies. Isolated infection is probably self-limiting, and it is repeated infection which leads to chronic eye disease.

Clinical features

Infection is bilateral and begins in the conjunctiva, with marked follicular inflammation and subsequent scarring. Scarring of the upper eyelid causes entropion, leaving the cornea exposed to further damage with the eyelashes rubbing against it (trichiasis). The corneal scarring that eventually occurs leads to blindness.

Trachoma may also occur as an acute ophthalmic infection in the neonate.

Diagnosis and management

The diagnosis is generally established by the typical clinical picture. It can be confirmed by cell culture techniques or species-specific fluorescent monoclonal antibodies, but these are rarely available in endemic areas.

Tetracycline ointment applied locally each day for 6–8 weeks is effective, as is systemic therapy with a single dose of azithromycin. In endemic areas repeated courses of therapy are necessary. Once infection has been controlled, surgery may be required for eyelid reconstruction and for treatment of corneal opacities.

Prevention

Community health education, improvements in water supply and sanitation, and earlier case reporting could make a substantial impact on disease prevalence. This is reflected in the WHO 'SAFE' approach to trachoma prevention: surgery, antibiotics, facial cleanliness, environmental improvement.

Gastrointestinal infections

Cholera

Cholera is caused by the curved, flagellated Gram-negative bacillus, *Vibrio cholerae*. The organism is killed by temperatures of 100°C in a few seconds but can survive in ice for up to 6 weeks. The major pathogenic strain possesses a somatic antigen (O1) with two biotypes: classical and El Tor. The El Tor biotype has replaced the classical biotype as the major cause of cholera: this is because the El Tor *V. cholerae* is a hardier organism. Infection with the El Tor biotype generally causes milder symptoms, but can still cause severe and life-threatening disease.

The fertile, humid Gangetic plains of West Bengal have traditionally been regarded as the home of cholera. However, a series of pandemics have spread the disease across the world, usually following trade routes. The seventh pandemic, caused by the El Tor biotype, has affected large areas of Asia, North Africa, Kenya and southern Europe. It has spread to South and Central America in recent years, claiming thousands of lives. A newly recognized strain of *V. cholerae* (O139) is responsible for an increasing number of cases in India and South East Asia. It has a characteristic pattern of antibiotic resistance (sulfamethoxazole, trimethoprim and streptomycin), and may prove to be the cause of the next pandemic.

Transmission is by the faecal–oral route. Contaminated water plays a major role in the dissemination of cholera, although contaminated foodstuffs and contact carriers may contribute in epidemics. Achlorhydria or hypochlorhydria facilitates passage of the cholera bacilli into the small intestine. Here they proliferate, elaborating an exotoxin which produces massive secretion of isotonic fluid into the intestinal lumen (see p. 321). Cholera toxin also releases serotonin (5-HT) from enterochromaffin cells in the gut, which activates a neural secretory reflex in the enteric nervous system. This may account for at least 50% of cholera toxin's secretory activity. *V. cholerae* also produces other toxins (zona occludens toxin, ZOT, and accessory cholera toxin, ACT) which may contribute to its pathogenic effect.

Clinical features

The incubation period varies from a few hours to 6 days. The majority of patients with cholera have a mild illness that cannot be distinguished clinically from diarrhoea owing to other infective causes. Classically, however, three phases are recognized in the untreated disease.

The *evacuation phase* is characterized by the abrupt onset of painless, profuse, watery diarrhoea, associated with vomiting in the severe forms. 'Rice water' stools, so called because of mucus flecks floating in the watery stools, are typical of this stage.

If appropriate supportive treatment is not given, the patient passes on to the *collapse phase*. This is characterized by features of circulatory shock (cold clammy skin, tachycardia, hypotension and peripheral cyanosis) and dehydration (sunken eyes, hollow cheeks and a diminished urine output). The patient, though apathetic, is usually lucid. Muscle cramps may be severe. Children may present with convulsions owing to hypoglycaemia. At this stage renal failure and aspiration of vomitus present major problems.

If the patient survives the collapse stage the *recovery phase* starts, with a gradual return to normal clinical and biochemical parameters in 1–3 days.

Diagnosis

This is largely clinical. Examination of freshly passed stools may demonstrate rapidly motile organisms. This is not diagnostic, as *Campylobacter jejuni* may also give a similar appearance. However, demonstration of the rapidly motile vibrios by dark-field illumination and subsequent inhibition of their movement with type-specific antisera is diagnostic. Stool and rectal swabs should be taken for culture.

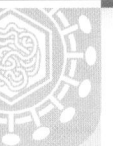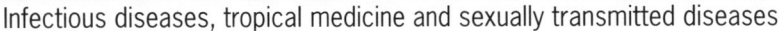
Management

The mainstay of treatment is rehydration, and with appropriate and effective rehydration therapy mortality has decreased to less than 1%. Oral rehydration is usually adequate, but intravenous therapy is occasionally required.

Oral rehydration solutions (ORS) are based on the observation that glucose (and other carbohydrates) enhances sodium absorption in the small intestine, even in the presence of secretory loss due to toxins. Additions such as amylase-resistant starch to glucose-based ORS have been shown to increase the absorption of fluid. Cereal-based electrolyte solutions have been found to be as effective as sugar/salt ORS, and actually reduce stool volume as well as rehydrating. Suitable solutions for rehydration are listed in Box 2.9.

Mildly dehydrated individuals are given ORS 50 mL/kg in the first 4 hours, followed by a maintenance dose of 100 mL/kg daily until the diarrhoea stops. For moderate dehydration, ORS 100 mL/kg is given within the first 4 hours followed by 10–15 mL/kg/hour.

Intravenous rehydration is required only for severely dehydrated individuals with features of collapse. Several litres of intravenous fluid are usually required to overcome the features of shock. Maintenance of hydration is effectively carried out by oral rehydration solutions.

Antibiotics such as tetracycline 500 mg four times daily for 3 days help to eradicate the infection, decrease stool output, and shorten the duration of the illness. Drug resistance is becoming an increasing problem, and ciprofloxacin is now used more frequently.

Immunization with currently available parenteral vaccines results in poor immunity and is no longer recommended. Newer killed whole-cell vaccines, and attenuated live vaccines are under intensive evaluation. Chemoprophylaxis with tetracycline 500 mg twice-daily for 3 days for adults, or 125 mg daily for children, is effective. The most important preventative measures, however, are good hygiene and improved sanitation.

Enteric fever

Enteric fever is an acute systemic illness characterized by fever, headache, and abdominal discomfort. *Typhoid*, the typical form of enteric fever, is caused by *Salmonella typhi*. A similar but generally less severe illness known as paratyphoid is due to infection with *S. paratyphi* A, B, or C. Man is the only natural host for *S. typhi*, which is transmitted in contaminated food or water.

Clinical features

After ingestion the bacteria invade the small bowel wall via Peyer's patches, from where they spread to the regional lymph nodes and then to the blood. The onset of illness is insidious and non-specific, with intermittent fever, headache, and abdominal pain. Physical findings in the early stages include abdominal tenderness, hepatosplenomegaly, lymphadenopathy, and a scanty maculopapular rash ('rose spots'). Without treatment (and occasionally even after treatment) serious complications can arise, usually in the third week of illness. These include meningitis, lobar pneumonia, osteomyelitis, intestinal perforation and intestinal haemorrhage. The fourth week of the illness is characterized by gradual improvement, but in developing countries up to 30% of those infected will die, and 10% of untreated survivors will relapse. This compares with a mortality rate of 1–2% in the USA.

After clinical recovery 5–10% of patients will continue to excrete *S. typhi* for several months: these are termed convalescent carriers. Between 1 and 4% will continue to carry the organism for more than a year: this is chronic carriage. The usual site of carriage is the gall bladder, and chronic carriage is associated with the presence of gallstones. However, in parts of the Middle East and Africa where urinary schistosomiasis is prevalent, chronic carriage of *S. typhi* in the urinary bladder is also common.

Diagnosis

The definitive diagnosis of enteric fever requires the culture of *S. typhi* or *S. paratyphi* from the patient. Organisms may be cultured from the blood, bone marrow, intestinal secretions, faeces, and urine, although in the last three cases care must be taken to distinguish acute infection from chronic carriage. Bone marrow culture is more sensitive than blood culture, but is rarely required except in patients who have already received antibiotics. Leucopenia is common but non-specific. Serological tests such as the Widal antigen test are of little practical value and are easily misinterpreted.

Management

Increasing antibiotic resistance is seen in isolates of *S. typhi*, especially in the Indian subcontinent. Chloramphenicol, co-trimoxazole and amoxicillin may all still be effective in some cases, but quinolones (e.g. ciprofloxacin 500 mg twice daily) are now the treatment of choice. Some resistance is emerging even to these agents. The patient's temperature may remain elevated for several days after starting antibiotics, and this alone is not a sign of treatment failure. Prolonged antibiotic therapy may eliminate the carrier state, but in the presence of gall bladder disease it is rarely effective. Cholecystectomy is not usually justified on clinical or public health grounds.

Systemic infections

Tuberculosis

Tuberculosis is caused by *Mycobacterium tuberculosis*, and occasionally *M. bovis* or *M. africanum*. These are slow-growing bacteria, and unlike other mycobacteria, are facultative intracellular organisms. Tuberculosis is found world-wide, but is particularly common in Africa and Asia. In all nearly 2 billion people, a third of the world's population, are infected. The prevalence of tuberculosis increases with poor social conditions, inadequate nutrition, and overcrowding. In developing countries it is most commonly acquired in childhood.

The impact of tuberculosis in the developing world has been magnified in the past 20 years by the emergence of the HIV pandemic (p. 131).

Widespread misuse of antibiotics, combined with the breakdown of healthcare systems in parts of Africa, Russia and East Europe, has led to the emergence of drug-resistant tuberculosis. The most serious form, known as multidrug resistant tuberculosis (MDRTB), is caused by bacteria that are resistant to both rifampicin and isoniazid, two drugs which form the mainstay of treatment. MDRTB is very difficult to treat, and has a significant mortality even with the best medical care.

In most people, the initial primary tuberculosis is asymptomatic or causes only a mild illness.

Occasionally the primary infection progresses locally to a more widespread lesion. Haematogenous spread at this stage may give rise to miliary tuberculosis.

Tuberculosis in the adult may be the result of reactivation of old disease (post-primary tuberculosis), primary infection, or more rarely reinfection.

Pulmonary tuberculosis is the most common form; this is described on page 892, along with the chemotherapeutic regimens. Tuberculosis also affects other parts of the body:

- The gastrointestinal tract, mainly the ileocaecal area, but occasionally the peritoneum producing ascites (see p. 296).
- The genitourinary system. The kidneys are most commonly involved, but tuberculosis can also cause painless, craggy swellings in the epididymis, and salpingitis, tubal abscesses, and infertility in females.

- The central nervous system, causing tuberculous meningitis and tuberculomas (p. 1198).
- The skeletal system, leading to septic arthritis and osteomyelitis.
- The skin, giving rise to lupus vulgaris.
- The eyes, where it can cause choroiditis or iridocyclitis.
- The pericardium, producing constrictive pericarditis (p. 818).
- The adrenal glands, causing destruction and producing Addison's disease.
- Lymph nodes. This is a common mode of presentation, especially in young adults and children. Any group of lymph nodes may be involved, but hilar and paratracheal lymph nodes are the most common. Initially the nodes are firm and discrete but later they become matted and can suppurate with sinus formation. Scrofula is the term used to describe massive cervical lymph node enlargement with discharging sinuses. Mycobacterial lymph node disease may also be caused by non-tuberculous mycobacteria.

Non-tuberculous mycobacterial infections

The majority of mycobacterial species are environmental organisms, and are rarely pathogenic. Some have been found to cause disease in man, particularly in immunocompromised patients or those with pre-existing chronic lung disease (Table 2.36).

Plague

Plague is caused by *Yersinia pestis*, a Gram-negative bacillus. Sporadic cases of plague (as well as occasional epidemics) occur world-wide: from 1980 to 1994 approximately 19 000 cases were reported to the WHO, with a 10% mortality. The vast majority of cases are seen in sub-Saharan Africa and South East Asia, although the disease is occasionally seen in developed countries in

Table 2.36
Non-tuberculous mycobacteria causing disease in man

Clinical	Common cause	Rare cause
Chronic lung disease	*Mycobacterium avium-intracellulare* *M. kansasii*	*M. malmoense* *M. xenopi*
Local lymphadenitis	*M. avium-intracellulare* *M. scrofulaceum*	*M. malmoense* *M. fortuitum*

Skin and soft tissue infection
  Fish tank granuloma
  Abscesses, ulcers, sinuses
	M. marinum
	M. fortuitum
	M. chelonae
		M. haemophilum

Bone and joint infection	*M. kansasii* *M. avium-intracellulare*	*M. scrofulaceum*
Disseminated infection (in HIV)	*M. avium-intracellulare*	

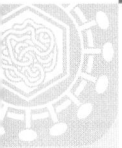

people undertaking outdoor pursuits. The main reservoirs are woodland rodents, which transmit infection to domestic rats (*Rattus rattus*). The usual vector is the rat flea, *Xenopsylla cheopis*. These fleas bite humans when there is a sudden decline in the rat population. Occasionally spread of the organisms may be through infected faeces being rubbed into skin wounds, or through inhalation of droplets.

Clinical features

Four clinical forms are recognized: bubonic, pneumonic, septicaemic and cutaneous.

Bubonic plague

This is the most common form and occurs in about 90% of infected individuals. The incubation period is about 1 week. The onset of illness is acute, with high fever, chills, headache, myalgia, nausea, vomiting and, when severe, prostration. This is rapidly followed by the development of lymphadenopathy (buboes), most commonly involving the inguinal region. Characteristically these are matted and tender, and suppurate in 1–2 weeks. Petechiae, ecchymoses and bleeding from the gastrointestinal tract, the respiratory tract and the genitourinary tract may occur. Mental confusion follows the development of toxaemia.

Pneumonic plague

This is characterized by the abrupt onset of features of a fulminant pneumonia with bloody sputum, marked respiratory distress, cyanosis and death in almost all affected patients.

Septicaemic plague

This presents as an acute fulminant infection with evidence of shock and disseminated intravascular coagulation (DIC). If left untreated, death usually occurs in 2–5 days. Lymphadenopathy is unusual.

Cutaneous plague

This presents either as a pustule, eschar or papule or an extensive purpura, which can become necrotic and gangrenous.

Diagnosis

The diagnosis is established by demonstrating the organism in lymph node aspirates, in blood cultures or on examination of sputum.

Management

Treatment is urgent and should be instituted before the results of culture studies are available. The treatment of choice is intramuscular streptomycin 1 g twice daily for 10 days, or for less severe cases, oral tetracycline 500 mg four times daily; chloramphenicol and gentamicin are also effective.

Prevention

Prevention of plague is largely dependent on the control of the flea population. Outhouses, or huts, should be sprayed with insecticides that are effective against the local flea. During epidemics rodents should not be killed until the fleas are under control, as the fleas will leave dead rodents to bite humans. Tetracycline 500 mg four times daily or sulphonamides 2–4 g daily for 7 days are effective chemoprophylactic agents. A partially effective formalin-killed vaccine is available for use by travellers to plague-endemic areas.

Relapsing fevers

These conditions are so named because, after apparent recovery from the initial infection, one or more recurrences may occur after a week or more without fever. They are caused by spirochaetes of the genus *Borrelia*.

Clinical features

Louse-borne relapsing fever

Louse-borne relapsing fever (caused by *B. recurrentis*) is spread by body lice, and only humans are affected. Classically it is an epidemic disease of armies and refugees, although it is also endemic in the highlands of Ethiopia, Yemen and Bolivia. Lice are spread from person to person when humans live in close contact in impoverished conditions. Infected lice are crushed by scratching, allowing the spirochaete to penetrate through the skin. Symptoms begin 3–10 days after infection and consist of a high fever of abrupt onset with rigors, generalized myalgia and headache. A petechial or ecchymotic rash may be seen. The general condition then deteriorates, with delirium, hepatosplenomegaly, jaundice, haemorrhagic problems and circulatory collapse. Although complete recovery may occur at this time, the majority experience one or more relapses of diminishing intensity over the weeks following the initial illness. The severity of the illness varies enormously, and some cases have only mild symptoms. However, in some epidemics mortality has exceeded 50%.

Tick-borne relapsing fever

Tick-borne relapsing fever is caused by *B. duttoni* and other *Borrelia* species, spread by soft (argasid) ticks. Rodents are also infected, and humans are incidental hosts, acquiring the spirochaete from the saliva of the infected tick. This disease is mainly found in countries where traditional mud huts are the form of shelter, but is occasionally associated with old houses and camp sites in the USA. The illness is generally similar to the louse-borne disease, although neurological involvement is more common.

Diagnosis and management

Spirochaetes can be demonstrated microscopically in the blood during febrile episodes: organisms are more numerous in louse-borne relapsing fever. Treatment is usually with tetracycline or doxycycline (see p. 39). A severe Jarisch–Herxheimer reaction (p. 127) occurs in many patients, often requiring intensive nursing care and intravenous fluids.

Prevention

Control of infection relies on elimination of the vector. Ticks live for years and remain infected, passing the infection to their progeny. These reservoirs of infection should be controlled by spraying houses with insecticides and by reducing the number of rodents. Patients infested with lice should be deloused by washing with a suitable insecticide. All clothes must be thoroughly disinfected.

Bartonellosis and ehrlichiosis

Bartonella spp. and *Ehrlichia* spp. are intracellular bacteria closely related to the rickettsiae. A number of human diseases can be caused by these organisms; like rickettsial disease, infection is usually spread from animals via an arthropod vector (Table 2.37).

Carrión's disease

This disease is restricted mainly to the habitat of its main vector, the sandfly, in the river valleys of the Andes mountains at an altitude of 500–3000 m. Two clinical presentations are seen, which may occur alone or consecutively. *Oroya fever* is an acute febrile illness causing myalgia, arthralgia, severe headache, and confusion, followed by a haemolytic anaemia. *Verruga peruana* consists of eruptions of reddish-purple haemangiomatous nodules, resembling bacillary angiomatosis. It may follow 4–6 weeks after Oroya fever, or be the presenting feature of infection. Spontaneous resolution may occur over a period of months or years. Carrión's disease is frequently complicated by superinfection, especially with *Salmonella* spp.

The diagnosis is made by culturing bacilli from blood or peripheral lesions. Serological tests have been developed but are not widely available.

Treatment with chloramphenicol or tetracycline is very effective in acute disease, but less so in verruga peruana.

Cat-scratch disease and bacillary angiomatosis

These are described on page 66.

Trench fever

Trench fever is caused by *Bartonella quintana*, and transmitted by human body lice. It is mainly seen in refugees and the homeless. It is characterized by cyclical fever (typically every 5 days), chills, and headaches, accompanied by myalgia and pretibial pain. The disease is usually self-limiting but it can be treated with erythromycin or doxycycline if symptoms are severe.

Melioidosis

The term melioidosis refers to infections caused by the Gram-negative bacteria *Burkholderia pseudomallei*. This environmental organism, which is found in soil and surface water, is distributed widely in the tropics and subtropics. The majority of clinical cases of melioidosis occur in South East Asia. Infection follows inhalation or direct inoculation. More than half of all patients with melioidosis have predisposing underlying disease: it is particularly common in diabetics.

B. pseudomallei causes a wide spectrum of disease, and the majority of infections are probably subclinical. Illness may be acute or chronic, localized or disseminated, but one form of the disease may progress to another and individual patients may be difficult to categorize. The most serious form is septicaemic melioidosis, which is often complicated by multiple metastatic abscesses: this is frequently fatal. Serological tests are available, but definitive diagnosis depends on isolating the organism from blood or appropriate tissue. *B. pseudomallei* has extensive intrinsic antibiotic resistance. The most effective agent is ceftazidime, which is given intravenously for 2–4 weeks; this should be followed by several months of co-amoxiclav to prevent relapses.

Actinomycosis

Actinomyces spp. are Gram-positive, branching higher bacteria which are normal mouth and intestine commensals; they are particularly associated with poor mouth hygiene. Actinomyces have a world-wide distribution but are a rare cause of disease in the West.

Table 2.37
Human infections caused by *Bartonella* spp. and *Ehrlichia* spp.

Disease	Organism	Reservoir	Vector
Bartonella			
Carrión's disease	*Bartonella bacilliformis*	Unknown	Sandfly
Cat scratch disease	*B. henselae*	Cat	Cat flea
Bacillary angiomatosis	*B. henselae*	Cat	Cat flea
Trench fever	*B. quintana*	Human	Body louse
Ehrlichia			
Human ehrlichiosis	*Ehrlichia chafeensis*	Deer	Hard ticks
	'Human granulocytic ehrlichia' (HGE)	Various mammals	Hard ticks

Clinical features

- *Cervicofacial actinomycosis*, the most common form, usually occurs following dental infection or extraction. It is often indolent and slowly progressive, associated with little pain, and results in induration and localized swelling of the lower part of the mandible. Lymphadenopathy is uncommon. Occasionally acute inflammation occurs. Sinuses and tracts develop with discharge of 'sulphur' granules.
- *Thoracic actinomycosis* follows inhalation of organisms, usually into a previously damaged lung. The clinical picture is not distinctive and is often mistaken for malignancy or tuberculosis. Symptoms such as fever, malaise, chest pain and haemoptysis are present. Empyema occurs in 25% of patients and local extension produces chest-wall sinuses with discharge of 'sulphur' granules.
- *Abdominal actinomycosis* most frequently affects the caecum. Characteristically, a hard indurated mass is felt in the right iliac fossa. Later, sinuses develop. The differential diagnosis includes malignancy, tuberculosis, Crohn's disease and amoeboma. The incidence of pelvic actinomycosis appears to be increasing with wider use of intrauterine contraceptive devices.

Occasionally actinomycosis becomes disseminated to involve any site.

Diagnosis and management

Diagnosis is by microscopy and culture of the organism. Treatment often involves surgery as well as antibiotics: penicillin is the drug of choice. Intravenous penicillin 2.4 g 4-hourly is given for 4–6 weeks, followed by oral penicillin for some weeks after clinical resolution. Tetracyclines are also effective.

Nocardia infections

Nocardia spp. are Gram-positive branching bacteria, which are found in soil and decomposing organic matter. *N. asteroides*, and less often *N. brasiliensis*, are the main human pathogens.

Clinical features

Mycetoma is the most common illness. This is a result of local invasion by *Nocardia* spp. and presents as a painless swelling, usually on the sole of the foot (Madura foot). The swelling of the affected part of the body continues inexorably. Nodules gradually appear which eventually rupture and discharge characteristic 'grains', which are colonies of organisms. Systemic symptoms and regional lymphadenopathy are rare. Sinuses may occur several years after the onset of the first symptom. A similar syndrome may be produced by other branching bacteria, and also by species of eumycete fungi such as *Madurella mycetomi* (p. 98).

Pulmonary disease, which follows inhalation of the organism, presents with cough, fever, and haemoptysis: it is usually seen in the immunocompromised. Pleural involvement and empyema occur. In severely immunosuppressed patients initial pulmonary infection may be followed by disseminated disease.

Diagnosis and management

The diagnosis is often difficult to establish, as *Nocardia* is not easily detected in sputum cultures or on histological section. Severe pulmonary or disseminated infection may require parenteral treatment: effective agents include ceftriaxone and amikacin. Local infection is usually treated with prolonged courses of oral sulphonamides, combined with surgical drainage of pus if necessary.

FURTHER READING

Jacobson RR, Krahenbuhl JL (1999) Leprosy. *Lancet* **353**: 655–660.

Rowe B, Ward LR, Threlfall EJ (1997) Multidrug-resistant *Salmonella typhi*: a worldwide epidemic. *Clinical Infectious Diseases* **24** (Suppl 1): S106–S109.

Sanchez JL, Taylor DN (1997) Cholera. *Lancet* **349**: 1825–1830.

Schachter J et al. (1999) Azithromycin in control of trachoma. *Lancet* **354**: 630–635.

Rickettsiae and similar organisms

Rickettsiae are Gram-negative, rod-shaped, spherical or pleomorphic organisms smaller than bacteria. They are spread to humans by arthropod vectors (body lice, fleas, ticks and larval mites). Rickettsiae inhabit the alimentary tract of these arthropods and the disease is spread to the human host by inoculation of their faeces through broken human skin, generally produced by scratching. Rickettsiae multiply intracellularly and can enter most mammalian cells, although the main lesion produced is a vasculitis due to invasion of endothelial cells of small blood vessels. Multisystem involvement is usual.

Typhus

Typhus is the collective name given to a group of diseases caused by *Rickettsia* species. Some rickettsial diseases are shown in Table 2.38.

Clinical features
Typhus fever group
Epidemic typhus

The vector of epidemic typhus is the human body louse, and like louse-borne relapsing fever, epidemics are associated with war and refugees. Outbreaks have occurred in Africa, Central and South America, and Asia.

Table 2.38
Infections caused by rickettsiae

Disease	Organism	Reservoir	Vector
Typhus fever group			
Epidemic typhus	*Rickettsia prowazekii*	Man	Human body louse
Endemic (murine) typhus	*R. typhi*	Rodents	Rat flea
Scrub typhus	*R. tsutsugamushi*	Trombiculid mite	Trombiculid mite
Spotted fever group			
African tick typhus	*R. conorii, R. africae*	Various mammals	Hard tick
Fièvre boutonneuse	*R. conorii*	Rodents, dog	Hard tick
Rocky Mountain spotted fever	*R. rickettsii*	Rodents	Hard tick
Rickettsial pox	*R. acari*	Rodents	Mite

The incubation period of 1–3 weeks is followed by an abrupt febrile illness associated with profound malaise and generalized myalgia. Headache is severe and there may be conjunctivitis with orbital pain. A measles-like eruption appears around the fifth day, the macules increasing in size and eventually becoming purpuric in character. At the end of the first week signs of meningo-encephalitis appear and CNS involvement may progress to stupor or coma, sometimes with extrapyramidal involvement. At the height of the illness splenomegaly, pneumonia, myocarditis, and gangrene at the peripheries may be evident. Oliguric renal failure occurs in fulminating disease, which is usually fatal. Recovery begins in the third week but is generally slow. The disease may recur many years after the initial attack owing to rickettsiae that lie dormant in lymph nodes. The recrudescence is known as Brill–Zinsser disease. The factors that precipitate recurrence are not clearly defined, although other infections may play a role.

Endemic (murine) typhus

This is an infection of rodents that is inadvertently spread to humans by rat fleas. The disease closely resembles epidemic typhus but is much milder and rarely fatal.

Scrub typhus

Found throughout Asia and the Western Pacific, this disease is spread by larval trombiculid mites (chiggers). An eschar (a black, crusted, necrotic papule) can often be found at the site of the bite. The clinical illness is very variable, ranging from a mild illness to fulminant and potentially fatal disease. The more severe cases resemble epidemic typhus. Unlike other types of typhus the organism is passed on to subsequent generations of mites, which consequently act as both reservoir and vector.

Spotted fever group

A variety of *Rickettsia* species, collectively known as the spotted fever group rickettsiae, cause the illnesses known as spotted fevers. In all except for rickettsial pox (which is transmitted by a rodent mite) the vector is a hard tick. Although the causative organism and the name of the illness vary from place to place the clinical course is common to all. After an incubation period of 4–10 days an eschar may develop at the site of the bite in association with regional lymphadenopathy. There is abrupt onset of fever, myalgia and headache, accompanied by a maculopapular rash which may become petechial. Neurological, haematological and cardio-vascular complications occur as in epidemic typhus, although these are uncommon.

Diagnosis

The diagnosis is generally made on the basis of the history and clinical course of the illness. It can be confirmed serologically by the indirect fluorescent antibody test (the most sensitive and specific), or the latex agglutination test. The Weil–Felix agglutination test, although previously widely used, is not specific or sensitive.

Treatment and prevention

Doxycycline or tetracycline given for 5–7 days is the treatment of choice. Ciprofloxacin is also effective. Doxycycline 200 mg weekly protects against scrub typhus; it is reserved for highly endemic areas. Rifampicin is also used.

Control of typhus is achieved by eradication of the arthropod vectors. Lice and fleas can be eradicated from clothing by insecticides (0.5% malathion or DDT). Control of rodents is necessary in endemic typhus and some of the spotted fevers. Areas of vegetation infested with trombiculid mites can be cleared by chemical spraying from the air. Bites from ticks and mites should be avoided by wearing protective clothing on exposed areas of the body. The likelihood of infection from ticks is related to the duration of feeding, and in high-risk areas the body should be inspected twice a day and any ticks removed (p. 82).

Q fever

Q fever is a zoonosis caused by the rickettsia-like organism *Coxiella burnetii*. Infection is widespread in domestic and farm animals: it is usually spread between animals by ticks which are a reservoir of infection. Modes of transmission to humans are by dust, aerosol, and unpasteurized milk from infected cows. *C. burnetii* can survive

in extreme environmental conditions for long periods, and the infective dose is very small, so that minimal animal contact is required. One reported outbreak occurred among inhabitants of a village through which infected sheep had passed.

Clinical features
Symptoms begin insidiously 2–4 weeks after infection. Fever is accompanied by flu-like symptoms with myalgia and headache. The acute illness usually resolves spontaneously, but in a few cases pneumonia or hepatitis may develop. Occasionally infection can become chronic, with endocarditis, myocarditis, uveitis, osteomyelitis or other focal infections.

C. burnetii is an obligate intracellular organism, and does not grow on standard culture media. Diagnosis is made serologically using complement fixation tests. Antibody tests for two different bacterial antigens allow distinction between acute and chronic infection.

Management
Treatment with doxycycline 200 mg daily reduces the duration of the acute illness, but it is not known whether this correlates with eradication of the organism. For chronic Q fever, including endocarditis, doxycycline is often combined with rifampicin or clindamycin. Even prolonged courses of treatment may not clear the infection.

FURTHER READING

Azad AF, Beard CB (1998) Rickettsial pathogens and their arthropod vectors. *Emerging Infectious Diseases* **4**: 179–186.

Fungal infections

Morphologically, fungi can be grouped into three major categories:

- yeasts and yeast-like fungi, which reproduce by budding
- moulds, which grow by branching and longitudinal extension of hyphae
- dimorphic fungi, which behave as yeasts in the host but as moulds in vitro (e.g. *Histoplasma capsulatum* and *Sporothrix schenckii*).

Despite the fact that fungi are ubiquitous, systemic fungal infections are uncommon. Fungal infections are transmitted by inhalation of spores or by contact with the skin. Opportunistic mycoses can cause disease in immunocompromised patients. Fungi do not produce endotoxin, but exotoxin (e.g. aflatoxin) production has been documented in vitro. Fungi may also produce allergic pulmonary disease. Some fungi such as *Candida*

Table 2.39	
Common fungal infections	
Systemic	**Subcutaneous**
Histoplasmosis	Sporotrichosis
Cryptococcosis	Subcutaneous zygomycosis
Coccidioidomycosis	Chromomycosis
Blastomycosis	Mycetoma
Zygomycosis (mucormycosis)	
Candidiasis	**Superficial**
Aspergillosis	Dermatophytosis
Pneumocystic carinii	Superficial candidiasis
(previously classed as a	*Malassezia* infections
protozoan)	

albicans are human commensals. Diseases are usually divided into systemic, subcutaneous or superficial (Table 2.39).

Systemic fungal infections

Candidiasis
Candidiasis is the most common fungal infection in humans and is caused by *Candida albicans*. Candida are small asexual fungi. Most species that are pathogenic to humans are normal oropharyngeal and gastrointestinal commensals. Candidiasis is found world-wide.

Clinical features
Any organ in the body can be invaded by candida, but vaginal infection and oral thrush are the most common forms. This latter is seen in the very young, in the elderly, following antibiotic therapy and in those who are immunosuppressed. Candidal oesophagitis presents with painful dysphagia. Cutaneous candidiasis typically occurs in intertriginous areas. It is also a cause of paronychia. Balanitis and vaginal infection are also common (see p. 130).

Chronic mucocutaneous candidiasis is a rare manifestation, usually occurring in children, and is associated with a T cell defect. It presents with hyperkeratotic plaque-like lesions on the skin, especially the face, and on the fingernails. It is associated with several endocrinopathies, including hypothyroidism and hypoparathyroidism. Dissemination of candidiasis may lead to haematogenous spread, with meningitis, pulmonary involvement, endocarditis or osteomyelitis.

Diagnosis and treatment
The fungi can be demonstrated in scrapings from infected lesions, tissue secretions or in invasive disease, from blood cultures.

Treatment varies depending on the site and severity of infection. Oral lesions respond to nystatin, oral amphotericin B or miconazole. For more severe systemic infections, parenteral therapy with fluconazole, itraconazole or amphotericin B may be necessary. Polysymptomatic patients often complaining of widespread candidiasis can have a psychiatric disorder (see p. 1236).

Histoplasmosis

Histoplasmosis is caused by *Histoplasma capsulatum*, a non-encapsulated, dimorphic fungus. Spores can survive in moist soil for several years, particularly when it is enriched by bird and bat droppings. Histoplasmosis occurs world-wide and is commonly seen in Ohio and the Mississippi river valley regions where over 80% of the population have been subclinically exposed. Transmission is mainly by inhalation of the spores.

Clinical features

Figure 2.30 summarizes the pathogenesis, main clinical forms and sequelae of histoplasma infection. Primary pulmonary histoplasmosis is usually asymptomatic. The only evidence of infection is conversion of a histoplasmin skin test from negative to positive, and radiological features similar to those seen with the Ghon primary complex of tuberculosis (see p. 892). Calcification in the lungs, spleen and liver occurs in patients from areas of high endemicity. When symptomatic, primary pulmonary histoplasmosis generally presents as a mild influenza-like illness, with fever, chills, myalgia and cough. The systemic symptoms are pronounced in severe disease.

Complications such as atelectasis, secondary bacterial pneumonia, pleural effusions, erythema nodosum and erythema multiforme may also occur.

Chronic pulmonary histoplasmosis is clinically indistinguishable from pulmonary tuberculosis (see p. 894). It is usually seen in white males over the age of 50 years. Radiologically, pulmonary cavities, infiltrates and characteristic fibrous streaking from the periphery towards the hilum are seen.

Disseminated histoplasmosis resembles disseminated tuberculosis clinically. Fever, lymphadenopathy, hepatosplenomegaly, weight loss, leucopenia and thrombocytopenia are common. Rarely, features of meningitis, hepatitis, Addison's disease, endocarditis and peritonitis may dominate the clinical picture.

Diagnosis

Definitive diagnosis is possible only by culturing the fungi or by demonstrating them on histological sections. The histoplasmin skin test is of limited diagnostic value and can be negative in acute disseminated disease. Antibodies usually develop within 3 weeks of the onset of illness and are best detected by the complement-fixation, immunodiffusion or the counter-immuno-electrophoretic tests.

Management

Only symptomatic acute pulmonary histoplasmosis, chronic histoplasmosis and acute disseminated histoplasmosis require therapy. Ketoconazole or itraconazole

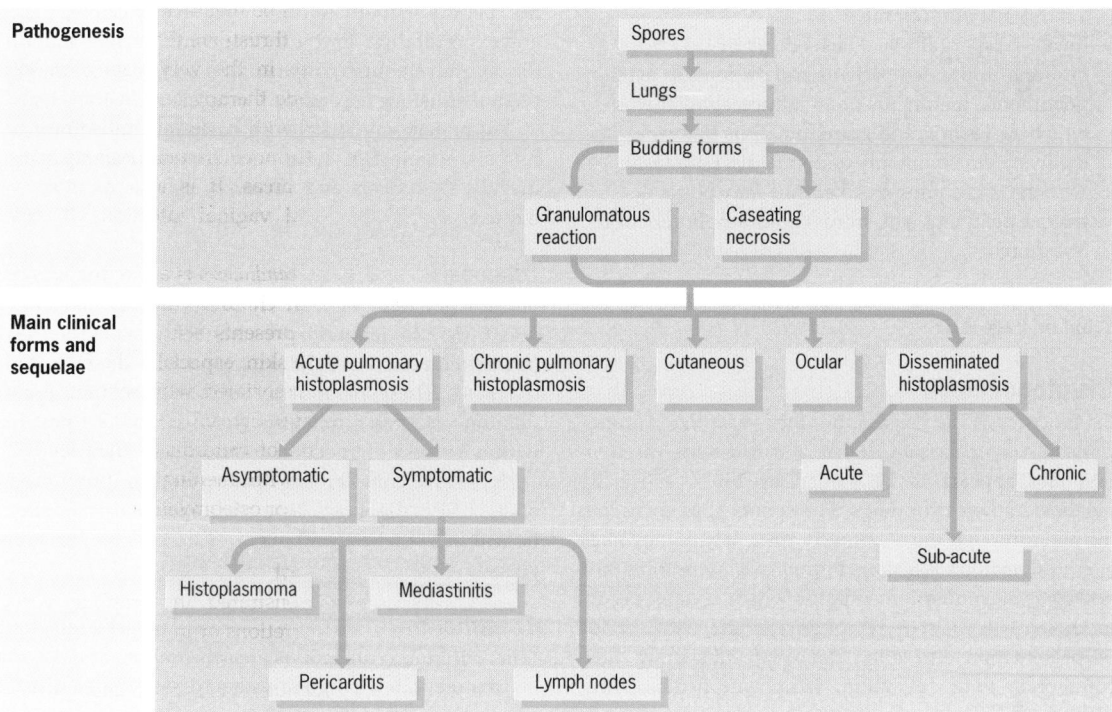

Fig. 2.30 **Histoplasma infection.** Summary of pathogenesis, main clinical forms and sequelae.

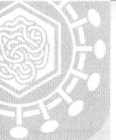

are indicated for moderate disease. Severe infection is treated with intravenous amphotericin B to a total dose of 1.5 g. Patients with AIDS usually require treatment with parenteral amphotericin B. Surgical excision of histoplasmomas (pulmonary granuloma due to *H. capsulatum*) or chronic cavitatory lung lesions and release of adhesions following mediastinitis is often required.

African histoplasmosis

This is caused by *Histoplasma duboisii*, the spores of which are larger than those of *H. capsulatum*. Skin lesions (e.g. abscesses, nodules, lymph node involvement and lytic bone lesions) are prominent. Pulmonary lesions do not occur. Treatment is similar to that for *H. capsulatum* infection.

Aspergillosis

Aspergillosis is caused by one of several species of dimorphic fungi of the genus *Aspergillus*. Of these, *A. fumigatus* is the most common, although *A. flavus* and *A. niger* are also recognized. These fungi are ubiquitous in the environment and are commonly found on decaying leaves and trees. Humans are infected by inhalation of the spores. Disease manifestation depends on the dose of the spores inhaled as well as the immune response of the host. Three major forms of the disease are recognized:

- Bronchopulmonary allergic aspergillosis (see p. 902) shows symptoms suggestive of bronchial asthma.
- Aspergilloma (see p. 903) is sometimes referred to as a pulmonary mycetoma.
- Invasive aspergillosis, which occurs in immunosuppressed patients and presents as acute pneumonia, meningitis or an intracerebral abscess, lytic bone lesions, and granulomatous lesions in the liver; less commonly endocarditis, paranasal *Aspergillus* granuloma or keratitis may occur. Urgent treatment with intravenous amphotericin B is required.

The diagnosis and treatment are described in more detail on page 902.

Cryptococcosis

Cryptococcosis is caused by the yeast-like fungus, *Cryptococcus neoformans*. It has a world-wide distribution and appears to be spread by birds, especially pigeons, in their droppings. The spores gain entry into the body through the respiratory tract, where they elicit a granulomatous reaction. Pulmonary symptoms are, however, uncommon; meningitis which usually occurs in those with HIV or lymphoma is the usual mode of presentation and often develops subacutely. Less commonly, lung cavitation, hilar lymphadenopathy, pleural effusions and occasionally pulmonary fibrosis occur. Skin and bone involvement is rare.

Diagnosis and treatment

This is established by demonstrating the organisms in appropriately stained tissue sections. A positive latex cryptococcal agglutinin test performed on the CSF is diagnostic of cryptococcosis.

Amphotericin B (0.3–0.5 mg/kg daily i.v.) alone or in combination with flucytosine (100–200 mg/kg daily) has reduced the mortality of this once universally fatal condition. Therapy should be continued for 3 months if meningitis is present. Fluconazole has greater CSF penetration and is used when toxicity is encountered with amphotericin B and flucytosine and as maintenance therapy in immunocompromised patients, especially those with HIV.

Coccidioidomycosis

Coccidioidomycosis is caused by the non-budding spherical form (spherule) of *Coccidioides immitis*. This is a soil saprophyte and is found in the southern USA, Central America and parts of South America. Humans are infected by inhalation of the thick-walled barrel-shaped spores called arthrospores. Occasionally epidemics of coccidioidomycosis have been documented following dust storms.

Clinical features

The majority of patients are asymptomatic and the infection is only detected by the conversion of a skin test using coccidioidin (extract from a culture of mycelial growth of *C. immitis*) from negative to positive. Acute pulmonary coccidioidomycosis presents, after an incubation period of about 10 days, with fever, malaise, cough and expectoration. Erythema nodosum, erythema multiforme, phlyctenular conjunctivitis and, less commonly, pleural effusions may occur. Complete recovery is usual.

Pulmonary cavitation with haemoptysis, pulmonary fibrosis, meningitis, lytic bone lesions, hepatosplenomegaly, skin ulcers and abscesses may occur in severe disease.

Diagnosis

Because of the high infectivity of this fungus, and consequent risk to laboratory personnel, serological tests (rather than culture of the organism) are widely used for diagnosis. These include the highly specific latex agglutination and precipitin tests (IgM) which are positive within 2 weeks of infection and decline thereafter.

A positive complement-fixation test (IgG) performed on the CSF is diagnostic of coccidioidomycosis meningitis within 4–6 weeks and may remain positive for many years.

Treatment

Mild pulmonary infections are self-limiting and require no treatment, but progressive and disseminated disease requires urgent therapy. Ketoconazole or itraconazole daily for 6 months is the treatment of choice for primary pulmonary disease with more prolonged courses for cavitating or fibronodular disease. Fluconazole in high dose (600–1000 mg daily) is given for meningitis. Amphotericin B is indicated for life-threatening infection. Surgical excision of cavitatory pulmonary lesions or localized bone lesions may be necessary. When occurring in those with HIV, amphotericin B, followed by maintenance itraconazole or fluconazole is indicated.

Blastomycosis

Blastomycosis is a systemic infection caused by the biphasic fungus *Blastomyces dermatitidis*. Although initially believed to be confined to certain parts of North America, it has been reported in Canada, Africa, Israel, Eastern Europe and Saudi Arabia.

Clinical features

Blastomycosis primarily involves the skin, where it presents as non-itchy papular lesions that later develop into ulcers with red verrucous margins. The ulcers are initially confined to the exposed parts of the body but later involve the unexposed parts as well. Atrophy and scarring may occur. Pulmonary involvement presents as a solitary lesion resembling a malignancy or gives rise to radiological features similar to the primary complex of tuberculosis. Systemic symptoms such as fever, malaise, cough and weight loss are usually present. Bone lesions are common and present as painful swellings.

Diagnosis and treatment

The diagnosis is confirmed by demonstrating the organism in histological sections or by culture, although results can be negative in 30–50% of cases. Serology is not useful because of the marked cross-reactivity of antibodies to blastomyces with histoplasma.

Itraconazole is preferred for treating mild to moderate disease in the immunocompetent for periods up to 6 months. Ketoconazole or fluconazole are useful alternatives. In severe or unresponsive disease and in the immunocompromised, amphotericin B is indicated.

Invasive zygomycosis

Invasive zygomycosis (mucormycosis) is rare and is caused by several fungi, including *Mucor* spp., *Rhizopus* spp. and *Absidia* spp. It occurs in severely ill patients. The hallmark of the disease is vascular invasion with marked haemorrhagic necrosis.

Rhinocerebral mucormycosis is the most common form. Nasal stuffiness, facial pain and oedema, and necrotic, black nasal turbinates are characteristic. It is rare and is mainly seen in diabetics with ketoacidosis. Other forms include pulmonary and disseminated infection (immunosuppressed), gastrointestinal infection (in malnutrition), and cutaneous involvement (in burns).

Treatment is with amphotericin B and sometimes judicious debridement. This condition is invariably fatal if left untreated.

Subcutaneous infections

Sporotrichosis

Sporotrichosis is due to the saprophytic fungus *Sporothrix schenckii*, which is found world-wide. Infection usually follows cutaneous inoculation, at the site of which a reddish, non-tender, maculopapular lesion develops – referred to as 'plaque sporotrichosis'. Pulmonary involvement and disseminated disease rarely occur.

Treatment with saturated potassium iodide (10–12 mL daily orally for adults) is curative in the cutaneous form. Itraconazole is a useful alternative.

Subcutaneous zygomycosis

Subcutaneous zygomycosis, a disease seen in children in Africa and Indonesia, is caused by several filamentous fungi of the *Basidiobolus* genus. The disease usually remains confined to the subcutaneous tissues and muscle fascia. It presents as a brawny, woody infiltration involving the limbs, neck and trunk. Less commonly, the pharyngeal and orbital regions may be affected.

Treatment is with saturated potassium iodide solution given orally.

Chromomycosis

Chromomycosis (chromoblastomycosis) is caused by fungi of the genera *Phialophora*, *Cladosporium* and *Fonsecaea*. These are found mainly in tropical and subtropical countries. It presents initially as a small papule, usually at the site of a previous injury. This persists for several months before ulcerating. The lesion later becomes warty and encrusted and gradually spreads. Satellite lesions may be present. Itching is frequent. The drug of choice is flucytosine, sometimes in combination with ketoconazole or amphotericin B. Itraconazole may also prove effective. Cryosurgery is used to remove local lesions.

Mycetoma (Madura foot)

Mycetoma may be due to subcutaneous infection with fungi (*Eumycetes* spp.) or bacteria (see p. 192). Infection results in local swelling which may discharge through sinuses. Bone involvement may follow.

Treatment is with ketoconazole or antibacterials according to the aetiological agent.

Pneumocystis carinii infection

Genetic analysis has shown this organism to be homologous with fungi. It exists as a trophozoite which is probably motile and reproduces by binary fission. After invasion the trophozoite wall thickens and forms a cyst. On maturation further division takes place to yield eight merozoites which after cell wall rupture develop into trophozoites. Infection probably occurs in infancy but in otherwise healthy infants it remains undetected. It is usually cleared from the lungs. *P. carinii* disease in

adults is associated with immunodeficiency states, particularly AIDS, and is discussed on page 131.

Superficial infections

Dermatophytosis

Dermatophytoses are chronic fungal infections of keratinous structures such as the skin, hair or nails. *Trichophyton* spp., *Microsporum* spp., *Epidermophyton* spp. and *Candida* spp. can also infect keratinous structures.

Malassezia infection

Malassezia spp. are found on the scalp and greasy skin and are responsible for seborrhoeic dermatitis, pityriasis versicolor (hypo- or hyperpigmented rash on trunk) and *Malassezia* folliculitis (itchy rash on back).

Treatment is with topical antifungals (e.g. terbinafine) or with oral agents if infection is extensive.

Protozoal infections

Protozoa are unicellular eukaryotic organisms. They are more complex than bacteria, and belong to the animal kingdom. Although many protozoa are free-living in the environment some have become parasites of vertebrates, including man, often developing complex life cycles involving more than one host species. In order to be transmitted to a new host, some protozoa transform into hardy cyst forms which can survive harsh external conditions. Others are transmitted by an arthropod vector, in which a further replication cycle takes place before infection of a new vertebrate host. Major protozoan parasites of man are listed in Table 2.40.

Blood and tissue protozoa

Malaria

Human malaria can be caused by four species of the genus *Plasmodium*: *P. falciparum*, *P. vivax*, *P. ovale* and *P. malariae*. It probably originated from animal malarias in central Africa, but was spread around the globe by human migration. Public health measures and changes in land use have eradicated malaria in most developed countries, although the potential for malaria transmission

Table 2.40
Major protozoal diseases of man

Blood	Tissues	Gastrointestinal tract
Malaria	Leishmaniasis	Giardiasis
Trypanosomiasis	Toxoplasmosis	Amoebiasis
		Cryptosporidiosis

still exists in many areas. Three hundred million people are infected every year, and over one million die.

Epidemiology

Malaria is transmitted by the bite of female anopheline mosquitoes. The parasite undergoes a temperature-dependent cycle of development in the gut of the insect, and its geographical range therefore depends on the presence of the appropriate mosquito species and on adequate temperature. The disease occurs in endemic or epidemic form throughout the tropics and subtropics (Fig. 2.31) except for areas above 2000 m: Australia, the USA, and most of the Mediterranean littoral are also malaria-free. In hyperendemic areas, where transmission of infection occurs year round, the bulk of the mortality is seen in infants. Those who survive to adulthood acquire significant immunity; low-grade parasitaemia is still present, but causes few symptoms. In mesoendemic areas there is regular seasonal transmission of malaria. Mortality is still mainly seen in infants, but older children and adults may develop chronic ill-health due to repeated infections. In holoendemic areas, where infection occurs in occasional epidemics, little immunity is acquired and the whole population is susceptible to severe and fatal disease.

Malaria can also be transmitted in contaminated blood transfusions. It has occasionally been seen in injecting drug users sharing needles and as a hospital-acquired infection related to contaminated equipment. Rare cases are acquired outside the tropics when mosquitoes are transported from endemic areas ('airport malaria'), or when the local mosquito population becomes infected by a returning traveller.

Parasitology

The female mosquito becomes infected after taking a blood meal containing gametocytes, the sexual form of the malarial parasite (Fig. 2.32). The developmental cycle in the mosquito usually takes 7–20 days (depending on temperature), culminating in infective sporozoites migrating to the insect's salivary glands. The sporozoites are inoculated into a new human host, and those which are not destroyed by the immune response are rapidly taken up by the liver. Here they multiply inside hepatocytes as merozoites: this is pre-erythrocytic (or hepatic) sporogeny. After a few days the infected hepatocytes rupture, releasing merozoites into the blood from where they are rapidly taken up by erythrocytes. In the case of *P. vivax* and *P. ovale*, a few parasites remain dormant in the liver as hypnozoites. These may reactivate at any time subsequently, causing relapsing infection.

Inside the red cells the parasites again multiply, changing from merozoite, to trophozoite, to schizont, and finally appearing as 8–24 new merozoites. The erythrocyte ruptures, releasing the merozoites to infect further cells. Each cycle of this process, which is called erythrocytic schizogeny, takes about 48 hours in

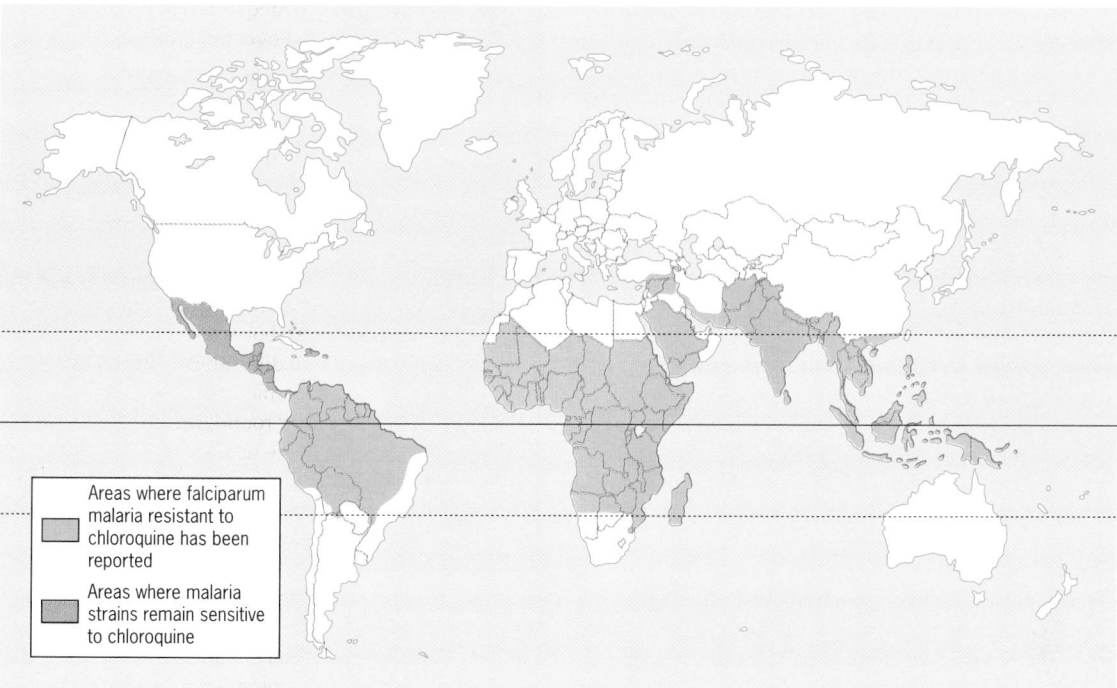

Fig. 2.31 **Malaria – geographical distribution.**

Legend:
Areas where falciparum malaria resistant to chloroquine has been reported

Areas where malaria strains remain sensitive to chloroquine

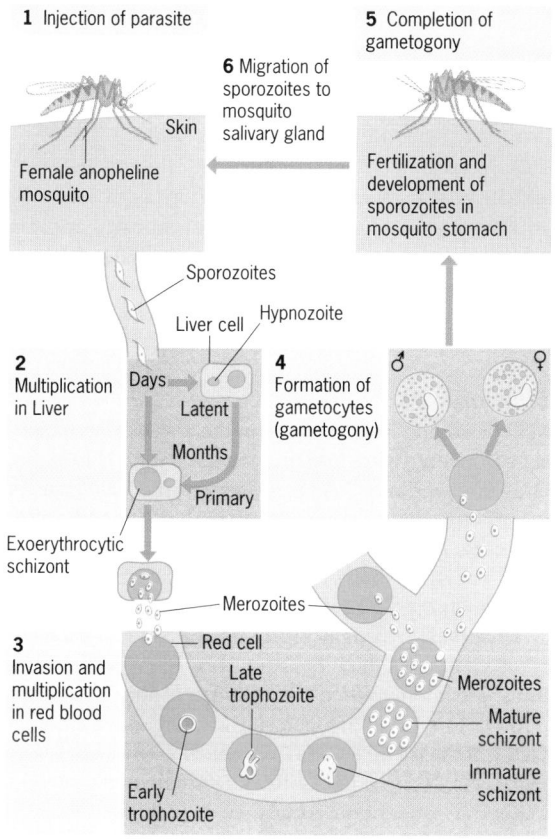

1 Injection of parasite

Female anopheline mosquito

Skin

6 Migration of sporozoites to mosquito salivary gland

5 Completion of gametogony

Fertilization and development of sporozoites in mosquito stomach

Sporozoites

Liver cell — Hypnozoite

2 Multiplication in Liver

Days

Latent

Months

Primary

4 Formation of gametocytes (gametogony)

♂   ♀

Exoerythrocytic schizont

Merozoites

3 Invasion and multiplication in red blood cells

Red cell

Late trophozoite

Merozoites

Mature schizont

Immature schizont

Early trophozoite

Fig. 2.32 **A schematic life cycle of *Plasmodium vivax*.**

P. falciparum, *P. vivax* and *P. ovale*, and about 72 hours in *P. malariae*. *P. vivax* and *P. ovale* mainly attack reticulocytes and young erythrocytes, while *P. malariae* tends to attack older cells; *P. falciparum* will parasitize any stage of erythrocyte.

A few merozoites develop not into trophozoites but into gametocytes. These are not released from the red cells until taken up by a feeding mosquito to complete the life cycle.

Pathogenesis

The pathology of malaria is related to anaemia, cytokine release, and in the case of *P. falciparum*, widespread organ damage due to impaired microcirculation. The anaemia seen in malaria is multifactorial (Table 2.41). In *P. falciparum* malaria, red cells containing schizonts adhere to the lining of capillaries in the brain, kidneys, gut, liver and other organs. As well as causing mechanical obstruction these schizonts rupture, releasing toxins and stimulating further cytokine release.

Table 2.41
Causes of anaemia in malaria infection

Haemolysis of infected red cells
Haemolysis of non-infected red cells (blackwater fever)
Dyserythropoiesis
Splenomegaly and sequestration
Folate depletion

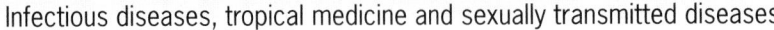

After repeated infections partial immunity develops, allowing the host to tolerate parasitaemia with minimal ill effects. This immunity is lost if there is no further infection for a couple of years. Certain genetic traits also confer some immunity to malaria. People who lack the Duffy antigen on the red cell membrane (a common finding in West Africa) are not susceptible to infection with *P. vivax*. Certain haemoglobinopathies (including sickle cell trait) also give some protection against the severe effects of malaria: this may account for the persistence of these otherwise harmful mutations in tropical countries. Iron deficiency may also have some protective effect. The spleen appears to be particularly important in controlling infection, and splenectomized people are at risk of overwhelming malaria. Some individuals appear to have a genetic predisposition for developing cerebral malaria following infection with *P. falciparum*. Pregnant women are especially susceptible to severe disease.

Clinical features

Typical malaria is seen in non-immune individuals. This includes children in any area, adults in hypoendemic areas, and any visitors from a non-malarious region.

The normal incubation period is 10–21 days, but can be longer. The most common symptom is fever, although malaria may present initially with general malaise, headache, vomiting, or diarrhoea. At first the fever may be continual or erratic: the classical tertian or quartan fever only appears after some days. The temperature often reaches 41°C, and is accompanied by rigors and drenching sweats.

P. vivax or P. ovale infection

The illness is relatively mild. Anaemia develops slowly, and there may be tender hepatosplenomegaly. Spontaneous recover usually occurs within 2–6 weeks, but hypnozoites in the liver can cause relapses for many years after infection. Repeated infections often cause chronic ill health due to anaemia and hyperreactive splenomegaly.

P. malariae infection

This also causes a relatively mild illness, but tends to run a more chronic course. Parasitaemia may persist for years, with or without symptoms. In children, *P. malariae* infection is associated with glomerulonephritis and nephrotic syndrome.

P. falciparum infection

This causes, in many cases, a self-limiting illness similar to the other types of malaria, although the paroxysms of fever are usually less marked. However it may also cause serious complications (Box 2.12), and the vast majority of malaria deaths are due to *P. falciparum*. Patients can deteriorate rapidly, and children in particular progress from reasonable health to coma and death within hours. A high parasitaemia (> 1% of red cells

---

> **Box 2.12**
>
> ### Some features of severe falciparum malaria
>
> **CNS**
> Cerebral malaria
> (coma, convulsion)
>
> **Renal**
> Haemoglobinuria
> (blackwater fever)
> Oliguria
> Uraemia (acute tubular necrosis)
>
> **Blood**
> Severe anaemia
> (haemolysis and
> dyserythropoiesis)
> Disseminated intravascular
> coagulation
> (DIC – haemorrhage)
>
> **Respiratory**
> Acute respiratory
> distress syndrome
>
> **Metabolic**
> Hypoglycaemia
> (particularly in children)
> Metabolic acidosis
>
> **Gastrointestinal/liver**
> Diarrhoea
> Jaundice
> Splenic rupture
>
> **Other**
> Shock – hypotensive
> Hyperpyrexia

---

infected) is an indicator of severe disease, although patients with apparently low parasite levels may also develop complications. *Cerebral malaria* is marked by diminished consciousness, confusion, and convulsions, often progressing to coma and death. Untreated it is universally fatal. *Blackwater fever* is due to widespread intravascular haemolysis, affecting both parasitized and unparasitized red cells, giving rise to dark urine.

Hyperreactive malarial splenomegaly (tropical splenomegaly syndrome, TSS)

This is seen in older children and adults in areas where malaria is hyperendemic. It is associated with an exaggerated immune response to repeated malaria infections, and is characterized by anaemia, massive splenomegaly, and elevated IgM levels. Malaria parasites are scanty or absent. TSS usually responds to prolonged treatment with prophylactic antimalarial drugs.

Diagnosis

Malaria should be considered in the differential diagnosis of anyone who presents with a febrile illness in, or having recently left, a malarious area. Falciparum malaria is unlikely to present more than 3 months after exposure, even if the patient has been taking prophylaxis, but vivax malaria may cause symptoms for the first time up to a year after leaving a malarious area.

Diagnosis is usually made by identifying parasites on a Giemsa-stained thick or thin blood film (thick films are more difficult to interpret, and it may be difficult to speciate the parasite, but they have a higher yield). At least three films should be examined before malaria is declared unlikely. An alternative microscopic method is quantitative buffy coat analysis (QBC), in which the centrifuged buffy coat is stained with a fluorochrome which 'lights up' malarial parasites. A number of antigen-detection methods for identifying malarial proteins and enzymes have been developed. Some of these are available in card or dipstick form, and are potentially suitable for use in resource-poor settings. Serological tests are of no diagnostic value.

Parasitaemia is common in endemic areas, and the presence of parasites does not necessarily mean that malaria is the cause of the patient's symptoms. Further investigation, including a lumbar puncture, may be needed to exclude bacterial infection.

Management

The drug of choice for susceptible parasites is chloroquine (Box 2.13). *P. vivax*, *P. ovale* and *P. malariae* are almost always sensitive to this drug, the only exception being some strains of *P. vivax* from Oceania.

There is now widespread chloroquine resistance among *P. falciparum*. Chloroquine acts by binding to ferriprotoporphyrin IX, which is released during digestion of haemoglobin in the lysosome of the parasite leading to its accumulation, which causes membrane damage. In chloroquine resistance there are mutations in at least two membrane proteins in the lysosome membrane which increase acidity and increases export of the drug from the lysosome. There are now few parts of the world where all infections will be susceptible. Despite this, cost and availability mean that it is still the most commonly used antimalarial.

Treatment should ideally be based on a knowledge of local sensitivity, but this is often not known. In developed countries *P. falciparum* is commonly treated with quinine, usually as quinine sulphate. In mild cases this can be given orally, but in more severe illness it is given by intravenous infusion. Tinnitus and nausea are predictable side-effects of quinine, and do not require dose reduction unless severe. Some resistance to quinine is emerging, and another antimalarial (either Fansidar (pyramethamine/sulfadoxine) or tetracycline) should be given at the end of the course of quinine.

Other available antimalarial drugs include mefloquine, artemesinin derivatives, and malarone (atovaquone/proguanil). The way in which these drugs should be distributed and used, particularly in the poorer developing countries, is still a matter for debate. It is possible that multidrug combinations will be more widely used in future, both to extend the usefulness of existing drugs and to limit the development of resistance to new agents.

Severe malaria, indicated by the presence of any of the complications discussed above, or a parasite count above 1% in a non-immune patient, is a medical emergency. Quinine should be given intravenously as shown in Emergency box 2.1: the loading dose should be omitted if the patient has already received quinine or mefloquine. Intensive care facilities may be needed, including mechanical ventilation and dialysis. Severe anaemia may require transfusion. Careful monitoring of fluid balance is essential: both pulmonary oedema and prerenal failure are common. Hypoglycaemia can be induced both by the infection itself and by quinine treatment. Superadded bacterial infection is common. In very heavy infections (parasitaemia > 10%), there may be a role for exchange transfusion, if the facilities are available.

Following successful treatment of *P. vivax* or *P. ovale* malaria, it is necessary to give a 2- to 3-week course of primaquine (15 mg daily) to eradicate the hepatic hypnozoites and prevent relapse. This drug can precipitate haemolysis in patients with G6PD deficiency (p. 433).

Prevention and control

As with many vector-borne diseases, control of malaria relies on a combination of case treatment, vector

---

Box 2.13

Drug treatment of uncomplicated malaria in adults

Type of malaria	Drug treatment
Plasmodium vivax, P. ovale, P. malariae, CQ-sensitive *P. falciparum*	Chloroquine: 600 mg 300 mg 6 hours later 300 mg 24 hours later 300 mg 24 hours later
CQ-resistant, SP-sensitive *P. falciparum*	Fansidar (SP): 3 tablets as single dose
CQ- and SP-resistant *P. falciparum*	Quinine: 600 mg 3 times daily for 7 days *plus* Tetracycline: 500 mg 4 times daily for 7 days or Fansidar (SP): 3 tablets as single dose at the end of 7 days Alternative therapy Mefloquine: 20 mg/kg in 2 doses 8 hours apart Alternative therapy Malarone: 4 tablets daily for 3 days

CQ, chloroquine; SP, Fansidar = pyramethamine/sulfadoxine; Malarone = atovaquone/proguanil
Chloroquine doses quoted are for base drug
Quinine dose applies to sulphate, hydrochloride or dehydrochloride

---

! Emergency box 2.1

Drug treatment of severe *Plasmodium falciparum* malaria in adults

	Full hospital facilities	**No infusion available**	**No injection available**

CQ-sensitive
P. falciparum
	Chloroquine: 10 mg/kg
	  infused over 8 hours,
	  followed by 15 mg/kg
	  over 24 hours
		Chloroquine: 2.5 mg/kg
		  every 4 hours by
		  intramuscular injection
		  (to total of 25 mg/kg)
			Chloroquine: by nasogastric tube
			  (as in oral regimen)
			or
			Artemisinin: rectally, 10 mg/kg at
			  0 and 4 hours, followed by
			  7 mg/kg at 24, 36, 48 and 60 hours

CQ-resistant
P. falciparum
	Quinine salt: 20 mg/kg
	  infused over 4 hours,
	  followed by 10 mg/kg
	  over 4 hours every 8 hours
	or
	Artesunate 2 mg/kg by
	  intravenous injection,
	  then 1 mg/kg at 12 hours,
	  then 1 mg/kg daily
		Quinine dihydrochloride given
		  by divided intramuscular
		  injection (regimen as for i.v.)
			Artemisinin: rectally as above

Chloroquine doses quoted are for base drug. Quinine doses apply to sulphate, hydrochloride and dihydrochloride.

---

eradication, and personal protection from vector bites. Mosquito eradication is usually achieved either by the use of insecticides, or by manipulation of the habitat (e.g. marsh drainage). After some initial successes, a WHO campaign to eliminate malaria foundered in the mid-1960s. Since then the emergence of both parasite resistance to drugs and mosquito resistance to insecticides has rendered the task more difficult. However, malaria is once again a priority for the WHO, which announced a new 'Roll Back Malaria' campaign in 1998.

Non-immune travellers to malarious areas should take measures to avoid insect bites, such as using insect repellent and sleeping under mosquito nets. Antimalarial prophylaxis should also be taken in most cases, although this is never 100% effective (Box 2.14). The precise choice of prophylactic regimen depends both on the individual traveller and on the specific itinerary; further details can be found in the British National Formulary or from travel advice centres. Despite considerable efforts, there is still no effective vaccine available for malaria.

Trypanosomiasis

African trypanosomiasis (sleeping sickness)

Sleeping sickness is caused by trypanosomes transmitted to humans by the bite of the tsetse fly (genus *Glossina*). It is endemic in a belt across sub-Saharan Africa, extending to about 14°N and 20°S: this marks the natural range of the tsetse fly. Two subspecies of trypanosome cause human sleeping sickness: *Trypanosoma brucei gambiense* ('Gambian sleeping sickness'), and *T. b. rhodesiense* ('Rhodesian sleeping sickness').

Epidemiology

Gambian sleeping sickness is found from Uganda in Central Africa, west to Senegal and south as far as Angola. Man is the major reservoir, and infection is transmitted by riverine *Glossina* species (e.g. *G. palpalis*). Sleeping sickness due to *T. b. rhodesiense* occurs in East and Central Africa from Ethiopia to Botswana. It is a zoonosis of both wild and domestic animals. In endemic

---

Box 2.14

Malaria prophylaxis for adult travellers

Area visited	Prophylactic regimen	Alternatives
No chloroquine resistance	Chloroquine 300 mg weekly	Proguanil 200 mg daily
Limited chloroquine resistance	Chloroquine 300 mg weekly *plus* Proguanil 200 mg daily	Doxycycline 100 mg daily *or* Mefloquine 250 mg weekly
Significant chloroquine resistance	Mefloquine 250 mg weekly	Doxycycline 100 mg daily *or* Malarone 1 tablet daily

Malarone = proguanil/atovaquone

---

situations it is maintained in game animals and transmitted by savanna flies such as *G. morsitans*. Epidemics are usually related to cattle, and the vectors are riverine flies. Recent political upheavals and wars have both disrupted established treatment and control programmes, and led to large population movements. This has resulted in major epidemics of *T. b. gambiense* disease in Angola and the Democratic Republic of Congo, and *T. b. rhodesiense* in Uganda. Although the majority of cases are unreported the incidence probably exceeds 300 000 per year.

Parasitology

Tsetse flies bite during the day, and unlike most arthropod vectors both males and females take blood meals. An infected insect may deposit metacyclic trypomastigotes (the infective form of the parasite) into the subcutaneous tissue. These cause local inflammation ('trypanosomal chancre') and regional lymphadenopathy. Within 2–3 weeks the organisms invade the bloodstream, subsequently spreading to all parts of the body including the brain.

Clinical features

T. b. gambiense causes a chronic, slowly progressive illness. Episodes of fever and lymphadenopathy occur over months or years, and hepatosplenomegaly may develop. Eventually infection reaches the central nervous system, causing headache, behavioural changes, confusion, and daytime somnolence. As the disease progresses patients may develop tremors, ataxia, convulsions and hemiplegias; eventually coma and death supervene. Histologically there is a lymphocytic meningoencephalitis, with scattered trypanosomes visible in the brain substance.

T. b. rhodesiense sleeping sickness is a much more acute disease. Early systemic features may include myocarditis, hepatitis and serous effusions, and patients can die before the onset of CNS disease. If they survive, cerebral involvement occurs within weeks of infection, and is rapidly progressive.

Diagnosis

Trypanosomes may be seen on Giemsa-stained smears of thick or thin blood films, or of lymph node aspirate. Blood films are usually positive in *T. b. rhodesiense*, but may be negative in *T. b. gambiense*: concentration techniques may increase the yield. The quantitative buffy coat test (QBC, see p. 100) developed for diagnosing malaria is also used to identify trypanosomes. Serological tests are useful for screening for infection: the card agglutination test for trypanosomiasis (CATT) is a robust and easy-to-use field assay. Examination of cerebrospinal fluid is essential in patients with evidence of trypanosomal infection. CNS involvement causes lymphocytosis and elevated protein in the CSF, and parasites may be seen in concentrated specimens.

Management

The treatment of sleeping sickness has remained largely unchanged for more than 40 years, although there have been recent developments in the management of *T. b. gambiense* infection. In both forms, treatment is usually effective if given before the onset of CNS involvement, but much less so in neurological disease. The drug of choice in early trypanosomiasis is suramin, given intravenously at a dose of 20 mg/kg at 5- to 7-day intervals up to a total dose of 5 g. Severe reactions are relatively common, and a test dose of 100 mg is usually given prior to this regimen. Intramuscular pentamidine is effective against *T. b. gambiense* only: a number of different regimens are in use. A single dose of suramin should be given to patients with parasitaemia prior to lumbar puncture, to avoid inoculation into the CSF.

Until very recently, the only effective drugs which penetrated the CSF in trypanocidal concentrations were the arsenicals, of which the most widely used is melarsoprol. These are given intravenously; a variety of dosing schedules are in use. Melarsoprol is extremely toxic: 2–10% of patients develop an acute encephalopathy, with a 50–75% mortality, and peripheral neuropathy and hepatorenal toxicity are also common. Prednisolone 1 mg/kg/day decreases the treatment-related mortality by 50% in *T. b. gambiense* infection; it has not been fully assessed in *T. b. rhodesiense* disease. Between 3 and 6% of patients relapse following melarsoprol treatment. In *T. b. gambiense* sleeping sickness a new drug, eflornithine, may be effective: it has no effect on *T. b. rhodesiense* infection. Eflornithine is much less toxic than the arsenical drugs, but cost prevents it from being used as a first-line treatment in most cases.

Control

The morbidity and mortality of sleeping sickness could be considerably reduced by early detection and treatment of cases. Control programmes have been effective in some areas, but many have been discontinued because of lack of funding, or political upheaval. As in many vector-borne diseases, prevention depends largely on elimination, control or avoidance of the vector. Again this requires considerable coordination and money, and has only been implemented in a few places.

South American trypanosomiasis (Chagas' disease)

Chagas' disease is widely distributed in rural areas of South and Central America. It is caused by *Trypanosoma cruzi*, which is transmitted to humans in the faeces of blood-sucking reduviid bugs (also called cone-nose, or assassin bugs). The bugs, which live in mud or thatch buildings, feed on a variety of vertebrate hosts at night, defecating as they do so. Faeces infected with *T. cruzi* trypomastigotes are rubbed in through skin abrasions, mucosa or conjunctiva. The parasites spread in the bloodstream, before entering host cells and multiplying.

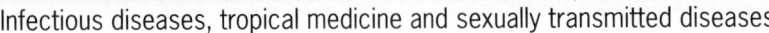
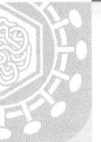

Cell rupture releases them back into the circulation, where they can be taken up by a feeding bug. Further multiplication takes place in the insect gut, completing the trypanosome life cycle. Human infection can also occur via contaminated blood transfusion, or occasionally by transplacental spread.

Clinical features

Acute infection, which usually occurs in children, often passes unnoticed. A firm reddish papule is sometimes seen at the site of entry, associated with regional lymphadenopathy. In the case of conjunctival infection there is swelling of the eyelid, which may close the eye (Romaña's sign). There may be fever, lymphadenopathy, hepatosplenomegaly, and rarely meningoencephalitis. Acute Chagas' disease is occasionally fatal in infants, but normally there is full recovery within a few weeks.

After a latent period of many years, some people go on to develop chronic Chagas' disease. The pathogenesis of this is unclear: it is probably due to an autoimmune response triggered by the initial infection rather than directly to the continued presence of parasites. The heart is commonly affected, with conduction abnormalities, arrhythmias, aneurysm formation and cardiac dilatation. Gastrointestinal involvement leads to progressive dilatation of parts of the gastrointestinal tract: this commonly results in megaoesophagus (causing dysphagia and aspiration pneumonia) and megacolon (causing severe constipation).

Diagnosis

Trypanosomes may be seen on a stained blood film during the acute illness. In chronic disease, parasites may be detected by xenodiagnosis: infection-free reduviid bugs are allowed to feed on the patient, and the insect gut subsequently examined for parasites. Serological tests can detect both acute and chronic Chagas' disease.

Management and control

Until recently, nifurtimox was the drug of choice for treating Chagas' disease, but it is no longer readily available. It has been replaced by benznidazole (5–10 mg/kg/day for 60 days), which has a cure rate of about 80% in acute infection. The drug treatment of chronic infection is controversial, as most of the tissue damage is thought to be immune-mediated and there is little clinical evidence that parasite elimination influences the outcome. Antiarrhythmic drugs and pacemakers may be needed in cardiac disease, and surgical treatment is sometimes needed for gastrointestinal complications. In the long term, prevention of Chagas' disease relies on improved housing and living conditions. In the interim, local vector control programmes may be effective and the countries of the 'Southern Cone' of South America have announced a joint programme to control the disease by spraying houses with insecticide.

Leishmaniasis

This group of diseases is caused by protozoa of the genus *Leishmania*, which are transmitted by the bite of the female phlebotomine sandfly (Table 2.42). Leishmaniasis is seen in localized areas of Africa, Asia, Europe, and South and Central America. Certain parasite species are specific to each geographical area. The clinical picture is dependent on the species of parasite, and on the host's cell-mediated immune response. Asymptomatic infection, in which the parasite is eradicated by a strong immune response, is common in endemic areas, as demonstrated by a high incidence of positive leishmanin skin tests. Symptomatic infection may be confined to the skin (sometimes with spread to the mucous membranes), or widely disseminated throughout the body (visceral leishmaniasis). Relapse of previously asymptomatic infection may be seen in patients who become immunocompromised, especially those with HIV infection.

In some areas leishmania is primarily zoonotic, whereas in others man is the main reservoir of infection. In the vertebrate host the parasites are found as oval amastigotes (Leishman–Donovan bodies). These multiply inside the macrophages and cells of the reticuloendothelial system, and are then released into the circulation as the cells rupture. Parasites are taken into the gut of a feeding sandfly (genus *Phlebotomus* in the Old World, genus *Lutzomyia* in the New World), where they develop into the flagellate promastigote form. These migrate to the salivary glands of the insect, where they can be inoculated into a new host.

Visceral leishmaniasis
Clinical features

Visceral leishmaniasis (kala azar) is caused by *L. donovani*, *L. infantum* or *L. chagasi*, and is prevalent in localized

Table 2.42
Leishmania species causing visceral and cutaneous disease in man

	Species complex	Species
Visceral leishmania	L. donovani	L. donovani
		L. infantum
		L. chagasi
Cutaneous leishmania	L. tropica	L. tropica
	L. major	L. major
	L. aethiopica	L. aethiopica
	L. mexicana	L. mexicana
		L. amazonensis
		L. garnhami
		L. pifanoi
		L. venezuelensis
	L. braziliensis	L. braziliensis
		L. guyanensis
		L. panamanensis
		L. peruviana
Mucocutaneous leishmania		L. braziliensis

areas of Asia, Africa, the Mediterranean littoral and South America. In India, where man is the main host, the disease occurs in epidemics. In most other areas it is endemic, and it is mainly children and visitors to the area who are at risk. The main animal reservoirs in Europe and Asia are dogs and foxes, while in Africa it is carried by various rodents.

The incubation period is usually 1–2 months, but may be several years. The onset of symptoms is insidious, and the patient may feel quite well despite markedly abnormal physical findings. Fever is common, and although usually low-grade, it may be high and intermittent. The liver, and especially the spleen, become enlarged, lymphadenopathy is common in African kala azar. The skin becomes rough and pigmented. If the disease is not treated profound pancytopenia develops, and the patient becomes wasted and immunosuppressed. Death usually occurs within a year, and is normally due to bacterial infection or uncontrolled bleeding.

Diagnosis
Specific diagnosis is made by demonstrating the parasite in stained smears of aspirates of bone marrow, lymph node, spleen or liver. The organism can also be cultured from these specimens. Specific serological tests are positive in 95% of cases. Pancytopenia, hypoalbuminaemia and hypergammaglobulinaemia are common. The leishmanin skin test is negative, indicating a poor cell-mediated immune response.

Management
The most widely used drugs for visceral leishmaniasis are the pentavalent antimony salts (e.g. sodium stibogluconate, which contains 100 mg of antimony per mL), given intravenously or intramuscularly at a dose of 20 mg of antimony per kg for 21 days. Resistance to antimony salts is increasing, and relapses may occur following treatment. The drug of choice where resources permit is intravenous amphotericin B (preferably given in the liposomal form). However, this drug is expensive and not widely available in many areas where the disease is prevalent. Intravenous pentamidine is also effective, and a new oral drug, miltefosine, has shown promising results. Intercurrent bacterial infections are common and should be treated with antibiotics. Blood transfusion may occasionally be required.

Successful treatment may be followed in a small proportion of patients by a nodular or hypopigmented skin eruption. This is called *post-kala azar dermal leishmaniasis* (PKDL).

Cutaneous leishmaniasis
Cutaneous leishmaniasis is caused by a number of geographically localized species, which may be zoonotic or anthroponotic. Following a sandfly bite, leishmania amastigotes multiply in dermal macrophages. The local response depends on the species of leishmania, the size of the inoculum, and the host immune response. Single or multiple painless nodules occur on exposed areas within 1 week to 3 months following the bite. These enlarge and ulcerate with a characteristic erythematous raised border. An overlying crust may develop. The lesions heal slowly over months or years, sometimes leaving a disfiguring scar.

L. major and *L. tropica* are found in Russia and Eastern Europe, the Middle East, Central Asia, the Mediterranean littoral, and sub-Saharan Africa. The reservoir for *L. major* is desert rodents, while *L. tropica* has a mainly urban distribution with dogs and humans as reservoirs. *L. aethiopica* is found in the highlands of Ethiopia and Kenya, where the animal reservoir is the hyrax. The skin lesions usually heal spontaneously with scarring: this may take a year or more in the case of *L. tropica*. Leishmaniasis recidivans is a rare chronic relapsing form caused by *L. tropica*.

L. mexicana is found predominantly in Mexico, Guatemala, Brazil, Venezuela and Panama: infection usually runs a benign course with spontaneous healing within 6 months. *L. braziliensis* infections (which are seen throughout tropical South America) also usually heal spontaneously, but may take longer.

L. mexicana amazonensis and *L. aethiopica* may occasionally cause diffuse cutaneous leishmaniasis. This is rare, and is characterized by diffuse infiltration of the skin by Leishman–Donovan bodies. Visceral lesions are absent.

Diagnosis and treatment
The diagnosis can often be made clinically in a patient who has been in an endemic area. Giemsa stain on a split skin smear will demonstrate leishmania parasites in 80% of cases; the same material can also be cultured. The leishmanin skin test is positive in over 90% of cases, but does not distinguish between active and resolved infection. Serology is unhelpful.

Small lesions usually require no treatment. Large lesions or those in cosmetically important sites can sometimes be treated locally, by curettage, cryotherapy or topical antiparasitic agents. In other cases systemic treatment (as for visceral leishmaniasis) is required, although treatment is less successful as antimonials are poorly concentrated in the skin; *L. aethiopica* is not sensitive to antimonials.

Mucocutaneous leishmaniasis
Mucocutaneous leishmaniasis occurs in 3–10% of infections with *L. b. braziliensis*, and is commonest in Bolivia and Peru. The cutaneous sores are followed months or years later by indurated or ulcerating lesions affecting mucosa or cartilage, typically on the lips or nose ('espundia'). The condition can remain static, or there may be progression over months or years affecting the nasopharynx, uvula, palate and upper airways.

Diagnosis and treatment

Biopsies usually show only very scanty organisms, although culture is often positive; serological tests are frequently positive.

Amphotericin B is the treatment of choice if available, although systemic antimonial compounds are widely used. Relapses are common following treatment. Patients may die because of secondary bacterial infection, or occasionally laryngeal obstruction.

Prevention

Prevention of leishmaniasis relies on control of vectors and/or reservoirs of infection. Insecticide spraying, control of host animals, and treating infected humans may all be helpful. Personal protection against sandfly bites is also necessary, especially in travellers visiting endemic areas.

Toxoplasmosis

Toxoplasmosis is caused by the intracellular protozoan parasite *Toxoplasma gondii*. The sexual form of the parasite lives in the gut of the definitive host, the cat, where it produces oocysts. After a period of maturing in the environment these oocysts become the source of infection for secondary hosts which may ingest them. In the secondary hosts (which include man, cattle, sheep, pigs, rodents, and birds) there is disseminated infection. Following a successful immune response the infection is controlled, but dormant parasites remain encysted in host tissue for many years. The life cycle is completed when carnivorous felines eat infected animal tissue. Humans are infected either from contaminated cat faeces, or by eating undercooked infected meat; transplacental infection may also occur.

Clinical features

Toxoplasmosis is common: seroprevalence in adults in the UK is about 25%, rising to 80% in some parts of Europe. Most infections are asymptomatic or trivial. Symptomatic patients usually present with lymphadenopathy, mainly in the head and neck. There may be fever, myalgia, and general malaise; occasionally there are more severe manifestations including hepatitis, pneumonia, myocarditis, and choroidoretinitis. Lymphadenopathy and fatigue can sometimes persist for months after the initial infection.

Congenital toxoplasmosis may also be asymptomatic, but can produce serious disease. Clinical manifestations include microcephaly, hydrocephalus, encephalitis, convulsions and mental retardation. Choroidoretinitis is common; occasionally this may be the only feature.

Immunocompromised patients, especially those with HIV infection, are at risk of serious infections with *T. gondii*. In acquired immunodeficiency states this is usually due to reactivation of latent disease (p. 140).

Diagnosis

Diagnosis is usually made serologically. IgG antibodies detectable by the Sabin–Feldman dye test remain positive for years; acute infection can be confirmed by demonstrating a rising titre of specific IgM.

Management

Acquired toxoplasmosis in an immunocompetent host rarely requires treatment. In those with severe disease (especially eye involvement) sulfadiazine 2–4 g daily and pyrimethamine 25 mg daily are given for 4 weeks, along with folinic acid. The management of pregnant women with toxoplasmosis aims to decrease the risk of fetal complications. Treatment of early infection (before the parasite has crossed the placenta) with spiramycin cuts the rate of fetal infection significantly. If the fetus has already been infected treatment with sulfadiazine and spiramycin (± pyrimethamine, which is itself teratogenic) appears to decrease the severity of complications. Infected infants should be treated from birth. The treatment of toxoplasmosis in HIV-positive patients is covered on page 140.

Babesiosis

Babesiosis is a tick-borne parasitic disease, diagnosed most commonly in North America and Europe. It is a zoonosis of rodents and cattle, and is occasionally transmitted to humans: infection is more common and more severe in those who are immunocompromised following splenectomy. The causative organisms are the plasmodium-like *Babesia microti* (rodents) and *B. divergens* (cattle).

The incubation period averages 10 days. In patients with normal splenic function, the symptoms are mild and usually comprise fever, nausea, myalgia, chills, vomiting and abdominal pain. Hepatosplenomegaly and haemolytic anaemia may also be present. In splenectomized individuals, systemic symptoms are more pronounced and haemolysis is associated with haemoglobinuria, jaundice and renal failure. Examination of a peripheral blood smear may reveal the characteristic plasmodium-like organisms.

The standard treatment was a combination of quinine 650 mg and clindamycin 600 mg orally three times daily for 7 days but a regimen of atovaquone and azithromycin is as effective, with fewer adverse reactions.

Gastrointestinal protozoa

The major gastrointestinal parasites of man are shown in Table 2.43.

Amoebiasis

The most important human disease due to amoebae is amoebiasis, which is caused by *Entamoeba histolytica*. The organism formerly known as *E. histolytica* is now known to consist of two distinct species: *E. histolytica*, which is pathogenic, and *E. dispar*, which is non-pathogenic. Cysts of the two species are identical, but can be distinguished by molecular techniques after culture of

Table 2.43
Pathogenic human intestinal protozoa

Amoebae
Entamoeba histolytica

Flagellates
Giardia intestinalis

Ciliates
Balantidium coli

Coccidia
Cryptosporidium parvum
Isospora belli
Sarcocystis spp.
Cyclospora cayetanensis

Microspora
Enterocytozoon bieneusi
Encephalitozoon spp.

the trophozoite. *E. histolytica* can be distinguished from all amoebae except *E. dispar*, and from other intestinal protozoa, by microscopic appearance. Amoebiasis occurs world-wide, although much higher incidence rates are found in the tropics and subtropics.

The organism exists both as a motile trophozoite and as a cyst that can survive outside the body. Cysts are transmitted by ingestion of contaminated food or water, or spread directly by person-to-person contact. Trophozoites emerge from the cyst in the small intestine and then pass on to the colon, where they multiply.

Clinical features

It is believed that many individuals can carry the pathogen without obvious evidence of clinical disease (asymptomatic cyst passers). However, this may be due in some cases to the misidentification of non-pathogenic *E. dispar* as *E. histolytica*, and it is not clear how often true *E. histolytica* infection is symptomless. In affected people *E. histolytica* trophozoites invade the colonic epithelium, probably with the aid of their own cytotoxins and proteolytic enzymes. The parasites continue to multiply and finally frank ulceration of the mucosa occurs. If penetration continues, trophozoites may enter the portal vein, via which they reach the liver and cause intrahepatic abscesses. This invasive form of the disease is serious and may even be fatal.

The incubation period of intestinal amoebiasis is highly variable and may be as short as a few days or as long as several months. The usual course is chronic, with mild intermittent diarrhoea and abdominal discomfort. This may progress to bloody diarrhoea with mucus, and is sometimes accompanied by systemic symptoms such as headache, nausea and anorexia. Less commonly, infection may present as acute amoebic dysentery, resembling bacillary dysentery or acute ulcerative colitis.

Complications are unusual, but include toxic dilatation of the colon, chronic infection with stricture formation, severe haemorrhage, amoeboma, and amoebic liver abscess. Amoebomas, which develop most commonly in the caecum or rectosigmoid region, are sometimes mistaken for carcinoma. They may bleed, cause obstruction or intussuscept. Amoebic liver abscesses often develop in the absence of a recent episode of colitis. Tender hepatomegaly, a high swinging fever and profound malaise are characteristic, although early in the course of the disease both symptoms and signs may be minimal. The clinical features are described in more detail on page 381.

Diagnosis

Microscopic examination of fresh stool or colonic exudate obtained at sigmoidoscopy is the simplest way of diagnosing colonic amoebic infection. To confirm the diagnosis motile trophozoites containing red blood cells must be identified: the presence of amoebic cysts alone does not imply disease. Sigmoidoscopy and barium enema examination may show colonic ulceration but are rarely diagnostic.

The amoebic fluorescent antibody test is positive in at least 90% of patients with liver abscess and in 60–70% with active colitis. Seropositivity is low in asymptomatic cyst passers.

Management

Metronidazole 800 mg three times daily for 5 days is given in amoebic colitis and a more prolonged course (10–14 days) in liver abscess or other extraintestinal spread. Dehydroemetine and chloroquine are alternative drugs, but are rarely used. After treatment of the invasive disease, the bowel should be cleared of parasites with a luminal amoebicide such as diloxanide furoate.

Prevention

Amoebiasis is difficult to eradicate because of the substantial human reservoir of infection. The only progress will be through improved standards of hygiene and better access to clean water. Cysts are destroyed by boiling, but chlorine and iodine sterilizing tablets are not always effective.

Giardiasis

Giardia intestinalis is a flagellate (Fig. 2.33) that is found world-wide. It causes small intestinal disease, with diarrhoea and malabsorption. Prevalence is high throughout the tropics, and it is the most common parasitic infection in travellers returning to the UK. In certain parts of Europe, and in some rural areas of North America, large water-borne epidemics have been reported. Person-to-person spread may occur in day nurseries and residential institutions. Like *E. histolytica*, the organism exists

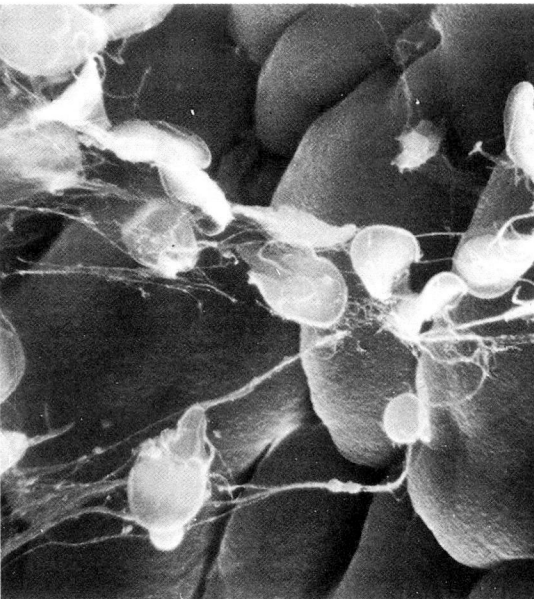

Fig. 2.33 *Giardia intestinalis* **on small intestinal mucosa.**
Courtesy of Dr A Phillips, Department of Electron Microscopy,
Royal Free Hospital, London.

both as a trophozoite and a cyst, the latter being the form in which the parasite is transmitted.

The organism sometimes colonizes the small intestine and may remain there without causing detriment to the host. In other cases, severe malabsorption may occur which is thought to be related to morphological damage to the small intestine. The changes in villous architecture are usually mild partial villous atrophy; subtotal villous atrophy is rare. The mechanism by which the parasite causes alteration in mucosal architecture and produces diarrhoea and intestinal malabsorption is unknown: there is evidence that the morphological damage may be immune-mediated. Bacterial overgrowth has also been found in association with giardiasis and may contribute to fat malabsorption.

Clinical features

Many individuals excreting giardia cysts have no symptoms. Others become ill within 1–3 weeks after ingesting cysts: symptoms include diarrhoea, often watery in the early stage of the illness, nausea, anorexia, and abdominal discomfort and bloating. In most people affected, these resolve after a few days, but in some the symptoms persist. Stools may then become paler, with the characteristic features of steatorrhoea. If the illness is prolonged, weight loss ensues, which can be marked. *Chronic giardiasis* frequently seen in developing countries can result in growth retardation in children.

Diagnosis

Both cysts and trophozoites can be found in the stool, but negative stool examination does not exclude the diagnosis since the parasite may be excreted at irregular intervals. The parasite can also be seen in duodenal aspirates (obtained either at endoscopy or with an Enterotest capsule), and in histological sections of jejunal mucosa.

Management

Metronidazole 2 g as a single dose on 3 successive days will cure the majority of infections, although sometimes a second or third course is necessary. Alternative drugs include tinidazole, mepacrine and albendazole. Preventative measures are similar to those outlined above for *E. histolytica*.

Cryptosporidiosis

This organism is found world-wide, cattle being the major natural reservoir. It has also been demonstrated in supplies of drinking water in the UK. The parasite is able to reproduce both sexually and asexually; it is transmitted by oocysts excreted in the faeces.

In healthy individuals cryptosporidiosis is a self-limiting illness. Acute watery diarrhoea is associated with fever and general malaise lasting for 7–10 days. In immunocompromised patients, especially those with HIV, diarrhoea is severe and intractable (see p. 140).

Diagnosis is usually made by faecal microscopy, although the parasite can also be detected in intestinal biopsies. As yet there is no effective antimicrobial treatment for this infection.

Balantidiasis

Balantidium coli is the only ciliate that produces clinically significant infection in humans. It is found throughout the tropics, particularly in Central and South America, Iran, Papua New Guinea and the Philippines. It is usually carried by pigs, and infection is most common in those communities that live in close association with swine. Its life cycle is identical to that of *E. histolytica*. *B. coli* causes diarrhoea, and sometimes a dysenteric illness with invasion of the distal ileal and colonic mucosa. Trophozoites rather than cysts are found in the stool. Treatment is with tetracycline or metronidazole.

Blastocystis hominis infection

B. hominis is a strictly anaerobic protozoan pathogen that inhabits the colon. For decades its pathogenicity for humans was questioned, but there is increasing evidence that it may cause diarrhoea. It is sensitive to metronidazole.

Cyclospora cayetanensis infection

Cyclospora cayetanensis, a coccidian protozoal parasite, was originally recognized as a cause of diarrhoea in travellers to Nepal. It has now been detected in stool specimens from immunocompetent and immuno-deficient people world-wide. Infection is usually self-limiting, but can be treated with co-trimoxazole.

Microsporidiosis

These protozoa are known to be a cause of diarrhoea in patients with HIV/AIDS (see p. 141).

FURTHER READING

Herwaldt BL (1999) Miltefosine – the long-awaited therapy for visceral leishmaniasis? *New England Journal of Medicine* **341**: 1840–1842.

Petri WA Jr, Singh U (1999) Diagnosis and management of amebiasis. *Clinical Infectious Diseases* **29**: 1117–1125.

Smith DH, Pepin J, Stich AHR (1998) Human African trypanosomiasis: an emerging public health crisis. *British Medical Bulletin* **54**: 341–343.

Warhurst DC (2001) Molecular marker for chloroquine-resistant falciparum malaria. *New England Journal of Medicine* **344**: 209–302.

White NJ (1996) Malaria. In: Cook GC (ed) *Manson's Tropical Diseases.* London: WB Saunders, 1087–1164.

Helminthic infections

Worm infections are very common in developing countries, causing much disease in both humans and domestic animals. They are frequently imported into industrialized countries. The most common human helminth infections are listed in Table 2.44.

Helminths are the largest internal human parasite. They reproduce sexually, generating millions of eggs or larvae. *Nematodes* and *trematodes* have a mouth and intestinal tract, while *cestodes* absorb nutrients directly through the outer tegument. All worms are motile, although once the adults are established in their definitive site they rarely migrate further. Adult helminths may be very long-lived: up to 30 years in the case of the schistosomes.

Many helminths have developed complex life cycles, involving more than one host. Both primary and intermediate hosts are often highly specific to a particular

Table 2.44
Helminths commonly infecting man

	Helminth	Common name
Nematodes (roundworms)		
Tissue-dwelling worms	*Wuchereria bancrofti*	Filariasis
	Brugia malayi/timori	Filariasis
	Loa loa	Loiasis
	Onchocerca volvulus	River blindness
	Dracunculus medinensis	Dracunculiasis
	Mansonella perstans	Mansonellosis
Intestinal human nematodes	*Enterobius vermicularis*	Threadworm
	Ascaris lumbricoides	Roundworm
	Trichuris trichiura	Whipworm
	Necator americanus	Hookworm
	Ancylostoma duodenale	Hookworm
	Strongyloides stercoralis	Strongyloidosis
Zoonotic nematodes	*Toxocara canis*	Toxocariasis
	Trichinella spiralis	Trichinellosis
Trematodes (flukes)		
Blood flukes	*Schistosoma* species	Schistosomiasis
Lung flukes	*Paragonimus* species	Paragonimiasis
Intestinal/hepatic flukes	*Fasciolopsis buski*	
	Fasciola hepatica	
	Clonorchis sinensis	
	Opisthorchis felineus	
Cestodes (tapeworms)		
Intestinal adult worms	*Taenia saginata*	Beef tapeworm
	Taenia solium	Pork tapeworm
	Diphyllobothrium latum	Fish tapeworm
	Hymenolepis nana	Dwarf tapeworm
Larval tissue cysts	*Taenia solium*	Cysticercosis
	Echinococcus granulosus	Hydatid disease
	Echinococcus multilocularis	Hydatid disease
	Spirometra mansoni	Sparganosis

species of worm. In some cases of human infection man is the primary host, while in others, humans are a non-specific intermediary or coincidentally infected.

Nematodes

Human infections can be divided into:

- *Tissue-dwelling worms* including the filarial worms, and the Guinea worm *Dracunculus medinensis.*
- *Human intestinal worms*, including the human hookworms, the common roundworm (*Ascaris lumbricoides*) and *Strongyloides stercoralis*, are the most common helminthic parasites of man. The adult worms live in the human gut, and do not usually invade tissues, but many species have a complex life cycle involving a migratory larval stage.
- *Zoonotic nematodes* which accidentally infect man are not able to complete their normal life cycle. They often become 'trapped' in the tissues, causing a potentially severe local inflammatory response.

Tissue-dwelling worms
Filariasis
Several nematodes belonging to the superfamily Filarioidea can infect humans. The adult worms are long and threadlike, ranging from 2–50 cm in length; females are generally much larger than males. Larval stages are inoculated by various species of biting flies, each specific to a particular parasite. The adult worms which develop from these larvae mate, producing millions of offspring (microfilariae), which migrate in the blood or skin. These are taken up by feeding flies, in which the remainder of the life cycle takes place. Disease, which may be caused by either the adult worms or by microfilariae, is caused by host immune response to the parasite and is

characterized by massive eosinophilia. Adult worms are long-lived (10–15 years), and reinfection is common, so that disease tends to be chronic and progressive.

Lymphatic filariasis
Lymphatic filariasis, which may be caused by different species of filarial worm, has a scattered distribution in the tropics and subtropics (Table 2.45). *Wuchereria bancrofti* is transmitted to man by a number of mosquito species, the most important of which is *Culex fatigans*. Adult female worms (which are 5–10 cm long) live in the lymphatics, releasing large numbers of microfilariae into the blood. Generally this occurs at night, coinciding with the nocturnal feeding pattern of *C. fatigans*. Non-periodic forms of *W. bancrofti*, transmitted by day-biting species of mosquito, are found in the South Pacific. *Brugia malayi* (and the closely related *B. timori*) are very similar to *W. bancrofti*, exhibiting the same nocturnal periodicity. The usual vectors are mosquitoes of the genus *Mansonia*, although other mosquitoes have been implicated.

Clinical features
Following the bite of an infected mosquito the larvae enter the lymphatics and are carried to regional lymph nodes. Here they grow and mature for 6–18 months.

Adult worms produce allergic lymphangitis. The clinical picture depends on the individual immune response, which in turn may depend on factors such as age at first exposure. In endemic areas many people have asymptomatic infection. Sometimes early infection is marked by bouts of fever accompanied by pain, tenderness and erythema along the course of affected lymphatics. Involvement of the spermatic cord and epididymis are common in Bancroftian filariasis. These acute attacks subside spontaneously in a few days, but usually recur. Recurrent episodes cause intermittent lymphatic obstruction, which in time can become

Table 2.45
Diseases caused by the filarial worms

Organism	Adult Worm	Microfilariae	Major vector	Clinical signs	Distribution
Wuchereria bancrofti	Lymphatics	Blood	*Culex species*	Fever Lymphangitis Elephantiasis	Tropics
Brugia timori/malayi	Lymphatics	Blood	*Mansonia* species	Fever Lymphangitis Elephantiasis	East and South East Asia, South India, Sri Lanka
Loa loa	Subcutaneous	Blood	*Chrysops* species	'Calabar' swellings Urticaria	West and Central Africa
Onchocerca	Subcutaneous	Skin, eye	*Simulium* species	Subcutaneous nodules Eye disease	Africa, South America
Mansonella perstans	Retroperitoneal	Blood	*Culicoides* species	Allergic eosinophilia	Sub-Saharan Africa, South America

fibrotic and irreversible. Obstructed lymphatics may rupture, causing cellulitis and further fibrosis; there may also be chylous pleural effusions and ascites. Over time there is progressive enlargement, coarsening, and fissuring of the skin, leading to the classical appearances of elephantiasis. The limbs or scrotum may become hugely swollen. Eventually the adult worms will die, but the lymphatic obstruction remains and tissue damage continues. Elephantiasis takes many years to develop, and is only seen in association with recurrent infection in endemic areas.

Occasionally the predominant features of filarial infection are pulmonary. Microfilariae become trapped in the pulmonary capillaries, generating intense local allergic response. The resulting pneumonitis causes cough, fever, weight loss, and shifting radiological changes, associated with a high peripheral eosinophil count. This is known as *tropical pulmonary eosinophilia* (see p. 903).

Diagnosis

The diagnosis of filariasis is usually made on clinical grounds, supported by a high eosinophil count. Serological tests are sensitive, especially in the earlier stages, but can cross-react with other nematodes: they become negative 1–2 years after effective treatment. Microfilaria start to appear in the peripheral blood about a year after infection, and may be detected on a stained nocturnal blood film. Parasitological diagnosis is difficult in elephantiasis. Filarial worms are responsible in the majority of cases, but similar lymphatic damage may occasionally be caused by silicates absorbed through the feet from volcanic soil.

Treatment

Diethylcarbamazine (DEC) kills both adult worms and microfilariae. Serious allergic responses may occur as the parasites are killed, and the dose must be increased slowly from 50 mg/day up to the full dose of 6–8 mg/kg/day (given in divided doses for 14 days). Associated bacterial infections should be treated promptly, and reconstructive surgery may be needed to remove excess tissue. Mass chemotherapy with DEC or ivermectin can decrease the prevalence and severity of infection in endemic areas. Early diagnosis and treatment prevents the development of elephantiasis. These approaches must be combined with vector control to achieve permanent results, while individual protection depends on avoidance of mosquito bites.

Loiasis

Loiasis, seen in humid forest areas of West and Central Africa, is caused by infection with *Loa loa*. This is a small (3–7 cm) filarial worm which is found in the subcutaneous tissues. The microfilariae circulate in the blood during the day, but cause no direct symptoms. The vectors are day-biting flies of the genus *Chrysops*.

Adult worms migrate around the body in subcutaneous tissue planes, frequently without causing symptoms. From time to time localized, tender, hot, soft tissue swellings (Calabar swellings) appear, often near to a joint. These are produced in response to the passage of a worm and usually subside over a few days or weeks. There may also be more generalized urticaria and pruritus. Occasionally a worm may be seen crossing the eye under the conjunctiva; they may also enter retro-orbital tissue, causing severe pain.

Microfilariae may be seen on stained blood films, although these are often negative. Serological tests are relatively insensitive, and cross-react with other microfilariae. There is usually massive eosinophilia.

DEC may cause severe allergic reactions (including fever, urticaria, myalgia, and occasionally encephalitis) associated with parasite killing: these symptoms require treatment with steroids. To minimize the risk of such reactions, the dose should be gradually increased over several days to the therapeutic dose of 5–10 mg/kg/day: this is then continued for 21 days. Ivermectin in single doses of 200–400 µg/kg is effective: it may occasionally cause severe reactions. Drug reactions are more likely if there is a high microfilarial load, or if there is co-infection with *Onchocerca volvulus*. Mass treatment with either DEC or ivermectin can decrease the transmission of infection, but the mainstay of prevention is vector avoidance and control.

Onchocerciasis

Onchocerciasis (river blindness) is found in well-defined areas of West and East Africa, Yemen, and parts of Central and South America. It is the result of infection with *Onchocerca volvulus*. Infection is transmitted by day-biting flies of the genus *Simulium*: principally *S. damnosum* in West Africa, *S. neavei* in East Africa, and *S. metallicum* in America. Onchocerciasis is a major cause of morbidity in parts of West Africa, where the whole adult population may be affected and blindness rates exceed 10%.

Pathogenesis

Infection occurs when larvae are inoculated by the bite of an infected fly. The worms mature in 2–4 months, and can live for more than 15 years. Adult worms, which can reach lengths of 50 cm (although less than 0.5 mm in diameter), live in the subcutaneous tissues. They may form fibrotic nodules, especially over bony prominences and sites of trauma. Huge numbers of microfilaria are distributed in the skin, and may invade the eyes. Live microfilariae cause relatively little harm, but dead parasites may cause severe allergic reactions, with hyaline necrosis and loss of tissue collagen and elastin. In the eye a similar process causes conjunctivitis, sclerosing keratitis, uveitis, and secondary glaucoma. Choroidoretinitis is also occasionally seen.

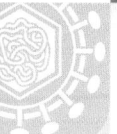

Clinical features

Symptoms usually start about a year after infection. Initially there is generalized pruritus, with urticaria and fleeting oedema. Subcutaneous nodules start to appear, and in dark-skinned individuals, hypo- and hyperpigmentation from excoriation and inflammatory changes. Over time more chronic inflammatory changes appear, with roughened, inelastic skin. Superficial lymph nodes become enlarged, and in the groin may hang down in loose folds of skin ('hanging groin'). Eye disease, which is associated with chronic heavy infection, usually first manifests as itching and conjunctival irritation. This gradually progresses to more extensive eye disease and eventually to blindness.

Diagnosis

In endemic areas the diagnosis can often be made clinically, especially if supported by finding eosinophilia on a blood film. In order to identify parasites, skin snips taken from the iliac crest or shoulder are placed in saline under a cover slip. After 4 hours, microscopy will show microfilariae wriggling free on the slide. If this is negative a 50 mg dose of DEC can be given: this will provoke an allergic rash in the majority of patients (the Mazzotti reaction). Serological tests are frequently positive in endemic areas, but may be negative in expatriates with a low worm load.

Management and prevention

Ivermectin, in a single dose of 150 µg/kg, kills microfilariae and prevents their return for 6–12 months. There is little effect on adult worms, so annual retreatment is needed. In patients co-infected with *Loa loa* ivermectin may occasionally induce severe allergic reactions.

Since 1974 the WHO Onchocerciasis Control Programme has had a considerable impact on onchocerciasis in West Africa. A combination of vector control measures and, more recently, mass treatment with ivermectin, has led to a decrease in both infection rates and progression to serious disease.

Mansonellosis

Mansonella perstans is a filarial worm transmitted by biting midges of the genus *Culicoides*. Small numbers of microfilaria are found in the blood, and although they do not cause serious disease there may be minor allergic reactions and an eosinophilia.

Dracunculiasis

Infection with the Guinea worm, *Dracunculus medinensis*, occurs when water fleas containing the parasite larvae are swallowed in contaminated drinking water. Ingested larvae mature, penetrate the intestinal wall, and mate, after which the male usually dies. The female worm, which can reach over a metre in length, migrates through connective and subcutaneous tissue for 9–18 months before surfacing, usually on the skin of the leg.

An allergic blister forms, and then bursts, exposing the anterior end of the worm. The uterus of the worm ruptures, releasing larvae: the worm is attracted to the surface by cooling, and so the larvae are likely to be deposited in water. They are ingested by the small crustacean water fleas, and the cycle is completed. The disease is found in sub-Saharan Africa, Egypt, the Arabian peninsula, and parts of Central Asia (India is now Guinea worm free). It is usually acquired by people collecting water at water holes.

A persistent skin ulcer may develop at the site of rupture: bacterial infection is common, and tetanus can occur. If the worm is broken there may be a systemic allergic reaction.

The diagnosis is usually clinical.

The traditional treatment, extracting the worm over several days by winding it round a stick, is probably still the most effective. It is important not to damage the worm, and antibiotics may be needed to control secondary infection. Anthelminthic drugs are of little value.

Water fleas (and thus infective larvae) can be removed from drinking water by chemical treatment or by simple filtration. Man is the only host of *D. medinensis*, and it should therefore be possible to completely eradicate this parasite.

Human intestinal nematodes

Adult intestinal nematodes (also sometimes referred to as soil-transmitted helminths, or geohelminths) live in the human gut. There are two main types of life cycle, both including a soil-based stage. In some cases infection is spread by ingestion of eggs (which often require a period of maturation in the environment), while in others the eggs hatch in the soil and larvae penetrate directly through the skin of a new host (Fig. 2.34). *Ascaris lumbricoides* deviates from the simplified life cycle shown in that the larvae invade the duodenum and enter the venous system, via which they reach the lungs. They are eventually expectorated and swallowed, entering the intestine where they complete their maturation. Strongyloides is also unusual, in that it is the only nematode that is able to complete its life cycle in humans. Larvae may hatch before leaving the colon, and so are able to reinfect the host by penetrating the intestinal wall and entering the venous system.

Ascariasis (roundworm infection)

A. lumbricoides is a pale yellow worm, 20–35 cm in length (Fig. 2.35). It is found world-wide but is particularly common in poor rural communities, where there is heavy faecal contamination of the immediate environment. Larvae migrate through the tissues to the lungs before being expectorated and swallowed; adult worms are found in the small intestine. Ova are deposited in faeces, and require a 2- to 4-month maturation in the soil before they are infective.

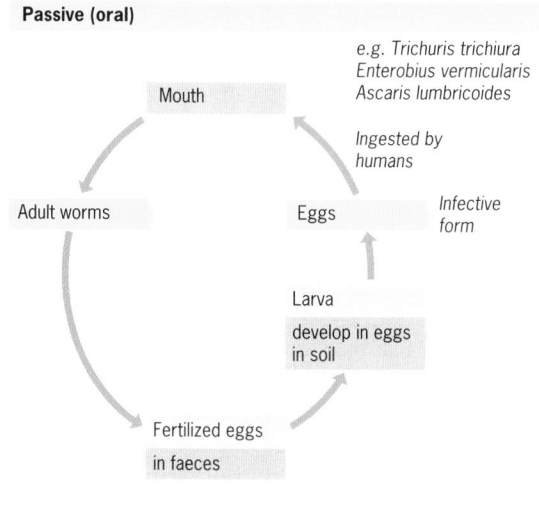

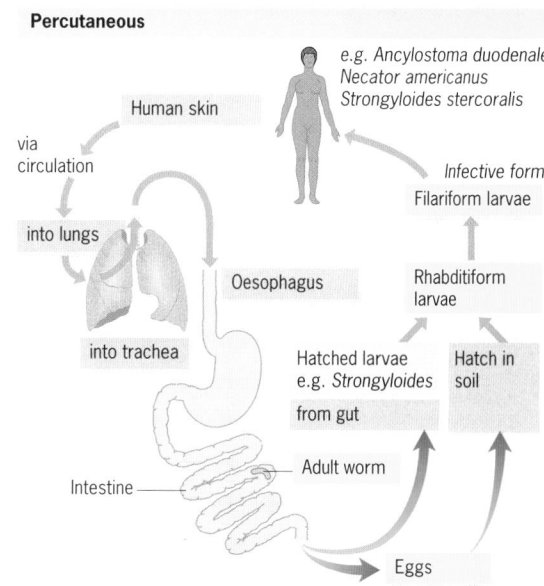

Fig. 2.34 A schematic life cycle of intestinal nematodes.

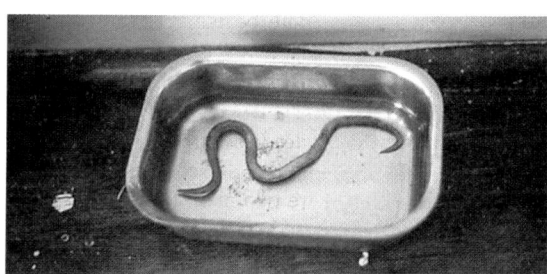

Fig. 2.35 *Ascaris lumbricoides*, approximately 20 cm long.

Infection is usually asymptomatic, although heavy infections are associated with nausea, vomiting, abdominal discomfort and anorexia. Worms can sometimes obstruct the small intestine, the most common site being at the ileocaecal valve. They may also occasionally invade the appendix, causing acute appendicitis, or the bile duct, resulting in biliary obstruction and suppurative cholangitis. Larvae in the lung may produce pulmonary eosinophilia. Heavy infection in children, especially those who are already malnourished, may have significant effects on nutrition and development. Serious morbidity and mortality are rare in ascariasis, but the huge number of people infected means that on a global basis roundworm infection causes a significant burden of disease, especially in children.

Ascaris eggs can be identified in the stool, and occasionally adult worms emerge from the mouth or the anus. They may also be seen on barium enema studies. Appropriate drug treatments are shown in Box 2.15. Very rarely surgical or endoscopic intervention may be required for intestinal or biliary obstruction.

Threadworm (*Enterobius vermicularis*)

E. vermicularis is a small (2–12 mm) worm, which is common throughout the world. Larval development takes place mainly in the small intestine, and adult worms are normally found in the colon. The gravid female deposits eggs around the anus causing intense itching, especially at night. Unlike *A. lumbricoides*, the eggs do not require a maturation period in soil, and infection is often directly transmitted from anus to mouth via the hands. Eggs may also be deposited on clothing and bedlinen, and are subsequently either ingested or inhaled. Apart from discomfort and local excoriation, infection is usually harmless.

Ova can be collected either using a moistened perianal swab, or by applying adhesive cellophane tape to the perianal skin. They can then be identified by microscopy.

The most commonly used drugs in the UK are mebendazole and piperazine (Box 2.15). However, isolated treatment of an affected person is often ineffective. Other family members (especially small children) may also need to be treated, and the whole family should be given advice about personal hygiene. Two courses of treatment 2 weeks apart may break the cycle of autoinfection.

Whipworm (*Trichuris trichiura*)

Infections with whipworm are common world-wide, especially in poor communities with inadequate sanitation. Adult worms, which are 3–5 cm long, inhabit the terminal ileum and caecum, although in heavy infection they are found throughout the large bowel. The head of the worm is embedded in the intestinal mucosa. Ova are deposited in the faeces, and require a period of 3–4 weeks maturation in the soil before becoming infective.

Box 2.15

Drugs used for treating human intestinal nematodes (single dose unless otherwise stated)

		Ascaris	Hookworm	Enterobius	Trichuris	Strongyloides
Piperazine	75 mg/kg	++	+	++	–	–
Pyrantal pamoate	10 mg/kg	++	++	++	–	–
Oxantel pamoate	10 mg/kg	–	–	–	++	–
Albendazole	400 mg[†]	++	++	++	+	+
Mebendazole	500 mg[*]	++	++	++	+	+
Tiabendazole	25 mg/kg[†]	n/a	n/a	n/a	n/a	++
Levamisole	5 mg/kg	++	+	n/a	n/a	–
Ivermectin	200 µg/kg	n/a	n/a	n/a	n/a	++

++, drug of choice; ++,highly effective; +, moderately effective; –, ineffective; n/a, drug not used for this indication

[*] WHO recommended dose for developing countries; in UK commonly given as 100 mg single dose for threadworm, or 100 mg twice daily for 3 days for whipworm
[†] Twice daily for 3 days in strongyloidiasis

Infection is usually asymptomatic, but mucosal damage can occasionally be so severe that there is colonic ulceration, dysentery, or rectal prolapse.

Diagnosis is made by finding ova on stool microscopy, or occasionally by seeing adult worms on sigmoidoscopy. Drug treatment is shown in Box 2.15.

Hookworm infection

Hookworm infections, caused by the human hookworms *Ancylostoma duodenale* and *Necator americanus*, are found world-wide. They are relatively rare in developed countries, but very common in areas with poor sanitation and hygiene: overall about 25% of the world's population are affected. Hookworm infection is a major contributing factor to anaemia in the tropics. *A. duodenale* is found mainly in East Asia, North Africa and the Mediterranean, while *N. americanus* is the predominant species in South and Central America, South East Asia and sub-Saharan Africa.

Adult worms (which are about 1 cm long) live in the duodenum and upper jejunum, where they are often found in large numbers. They attach firmly to the mucosa using the buccal plate, feeding on blood. Eggs passed in the faeces develop in warm moist soil, producing infective filariform larvae. These penetrate directly through the skin of a new host, and are carried in the bloodstream to the lungs. Having crossed into the alveoli the parasites are expectorated and then swallowed, thus arriving at their definitive home.

Clinical features

Local irritation as the larvae penetrate the skin ('ground itch') may be followed by transient pulmonary signs and symptoms, often accompanied by eosinophilia. Light infections, especially in a well-nourished person, are often asymptomatic. Heavier worm loads may be associated with epigastric pain and nausea, resembling peptic ulcer disease. Chronic heavy infection, particularly on a background of malnourishment, may cause iron deficiency anaemia. Blood loss has been estimated at about 0.15 mL/worm/day for *A. duodenale*, and 0.03 mL/worm/day for *N. americanus*; other factors may also be involved in the development of anaemia, which may be accompanied by hypoproteinaemia. Heavy infection in children is associated with delays in physical and mental development.

Diagnosis and treatment

The diagnosis is made by finding eggs on faecal microscopy. In infections heavy enough to cause anaemia these will be present in large numbers. The aim of treatment in endemic areas is reduction of worm burden rather than complete eradication: albendazole or mebendazole, which can both be given as a single dose, are the best drugs (Box 2.15). The WHO is promoting mass treatment programmes for schoolchildren in many parts of the world.

Strongyloidiasis

Strongyloides stercoralis is a small (2 mm long) worm which lives in the small intestine. It is found in many parts of the tropics and subtropics, and is especially common in Asia. Eggs hatch in the bowel, and larvae are found in the stool. Usually these are non-infective rhabditiform larvae, which require a further period of maturation in the soil before they can infect a new host, but sometimes this maturation can occur in the large bowel. Infective filariform larvae can therefore penetrate directly through the perianal skin, reinfecting the host. In this way autoinfection may continue for years or even decades. Some war veterans who were imprisoned in the Far East during the Second World War have been found to have active strongyloidiasis over 50 years later. After skin penetration the life cycle is similar to that of the hookworm, except that the adult worms may burrow into the intestinal mucosa, causing a local inflammatory response.

Clinical features

Skin penetration by *S. stercoralis* causes a similar local dermatitis to hookworm. In autoinfection this manifests as a migratory linear weal around the buttocks and lower abdomen (cutaneous larva currens). In heavy infections damage to the small intestinal mucosa can cause malabsorption, diarrhoea and even perforation. There is usually a persistent eosinophilia. In patients who are immunosuppressed (e.g. by corticosteroid therapy or intercurrent illness) filariform larvae may penetrate directly through the bowel wall in huge numbers, causing an overwhelming and usually fatal generalized infection (the strongyloidiasis hyperinfestation syndrome). This condition is often complicated by septicaemia due to bowel organisms.

Diagnosis and treatment

Motile larvae may be seen on stool microscopy, especially after a period of incubation. Serological tests are also useful. The best drug for treating strongyloidiasis is ivermectin (200 µg/kg daily for 2 days); albendazole and tiabendazole are also used.

Zoonotic nematodes

A number of nematodes which are principally parasites of animals may also affect man. The most common are described below.

Trichinosis

The normal hosts of *Trichinella spiralis*, the cause of trichinosis, include pigs, bears and warthogs. Man is infected by eating undercooked meat from these animals. Ingested larvae mature in the small intestine, where adults release new larvae which penetrate the bowel wall and migrate through the tissues. Eventually these larvae encyst in striated muscle.

Light infections are usually asymptomatic. Heavier loads of worms produce gastrointestinal symptoms as the adults establish themselves in the small intestine, followed by systemic symptoms as the larvae invade. The latter include fever, oedema, and myalgia. Massive infection may occasionally be fatal, but usually the symptoms subside once the larvae encyst.

The diagnosis can usually be made from the clinical picture, associated eosinophilia, and serological tests. If necessary it can be confirmed by muscle biopsy a few weeks after infection. Albendazole (20 mg/kg for 7 days) given early in the course of the illness will kill the adult worms and decrease the load of larvae reaching the tissues. Analgesia and steroids may be needed for symptomatic relief.

Toxocariasis (visceral larva migrans)

Eggs of the dog roundworm, *Toxocara canis*, are occasionally ingested by humans, especially children. The eggs hatch and the larvae penetrate the small intestinal wall and enter the mesenteric circulation, but are then unable to complete their life cycle in a 'foreign' host. Many are held up in the capillaries of the liver, where they generate a granulomatous response, but some may migrate into other tissues including lungs, striated muscle, heart, brain, and eye. In most cases infection is asymptomatic, and the larvae die without causing serious problems. In heavy infections there may be generalized symptoms (fever and urticaria) and eosinophilia, as well as focal signs related to the migration of the parasites. Pulmonary involvement may cause bronchospasm and chest X-ray changes. Ocular infection may produce a granulomatous swelling mimicking a retinoblastoma, while cardiac or neurological involvement may occasionally be fatal. Rarely, larvae survive in the tissues for many years, causing symptoms long after infection.

Isolation of the larvae is difficult, and the diagnosis is usually made serologically. Albendazole 400 mg daily for a week is the most effective treatment.

Cutaneous larva migrans (CLM)

CLM is caused by the larvae of the non-human hookworms *Ancylostoma braziliense* and *A. caninum*. Like human hookworms, these hatch in warm moist soil, and then penetrate the skin. In man they are unable to complete a normal life cycle, and instead migrate under the skin for days or weeks until they eventually die. The wandering of the larva is accompanied by a clearly-defined, serpiginous, itchy rash ('creeping eruption'), which progresses at the rate of about 1 cm per day. There are usually no systemic symptoms. The diagnosis is purely clinical. Single larvae may be treated with a 10% solution of topical tiabendazole; multiple lesions may require systemic therapy with tiabendazole or albendazole or ivermectin.

FURTHER READING

Bundy DAP, de Silva NR (1998) Can we deworm this wormy world? *British Medical Bulletin* **54**: 421–432.
Burnham S (1998) Onchocerciasis. *Lancet* **351**: 1341–1346.

Trematodes

Trematodes (flukes) are flat leaf-shaped worms. They have complex life cycles, often involving fresh water snails and intermediate mammalian hosts. Disease is caused by the inflammatory response to eggs or to the adult worms.

Water-borne flukes
Schistosomiasis

Schistosomiasis (bilharzia) affects over 200 million people in the tropics and subtropics. Chronic infection causes significant morbidity, and after malaria it is the most important parasitic disease in terms of socio-economic impact.

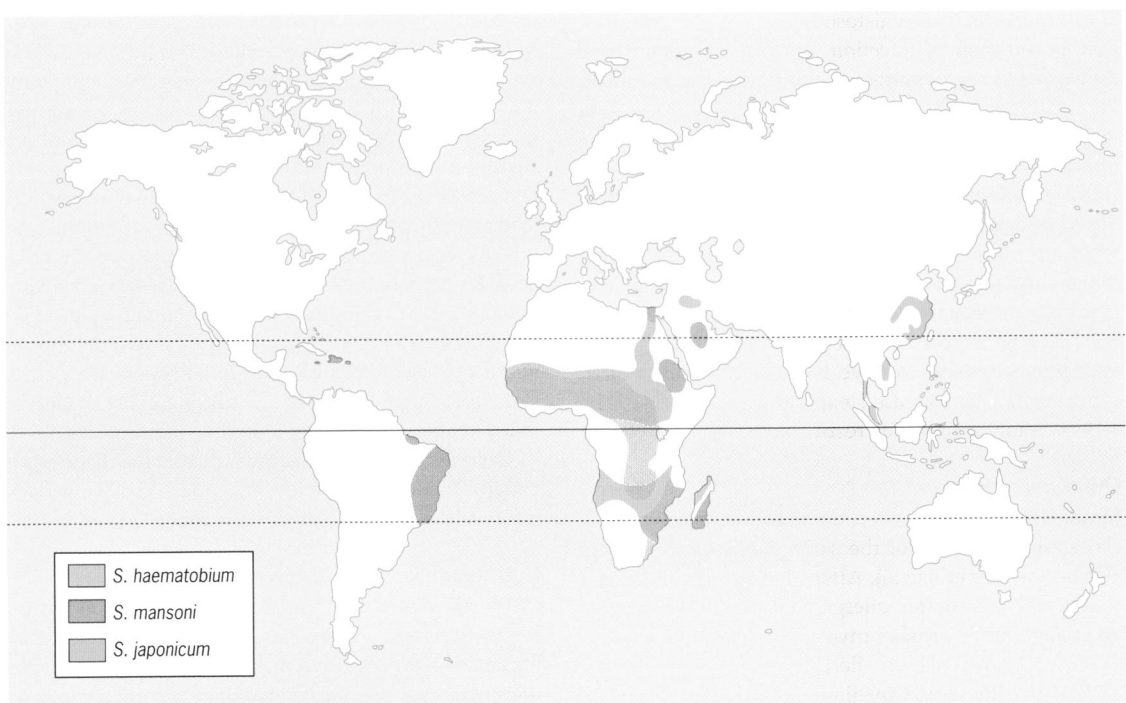

Fig. 2.36 Schistosomiasis – geographical distribution.

Schistosomiasis is largely a disease of the rural poor, but has also been associated with major development projects such as dams and irrigation schemes.

Parasitology and pathogenesis

There are three species of schistosome which commonly cause disease in man: *Schistosoma mansoni*, *S. haematobium*, and *S. japonicum*. The geographical distribution is shown in Figure 2.36. Eggs are passed in the urine or faeces of an infected person, and hatch in fresh water to release the miracidia (Fig. 2.37). These ciliated organisms penetrate the tissue of the intermediate host, a species of water snail specific to each species of schistosome. After multiplying in the snail, large numbers of fork-tailed cercariae are released back into the water, where they can survive for 2–3 days. During this time the cercariae can penetrate the skin or mucous membranes of the definitive host, man. Transforming into schistosomulae, they pass through the lungs before reaching the portal vein, where they mature into adult worms (the male is about 20 mm long, and the female a little larger). Worms pair in the portal vein before migrating to their final destination: mesenteric veins in the case of *S. mansoni* and *S. japonicum*, and the vesicular plexus for *S. haematobium*. Here they may remain for many years, producing vast numbers of eggs. The majority of these are released in urine or faeces, but a small number become embedded in the bladder or bowel wall, and a few are carried in the circulation to the liver or other distant sites.

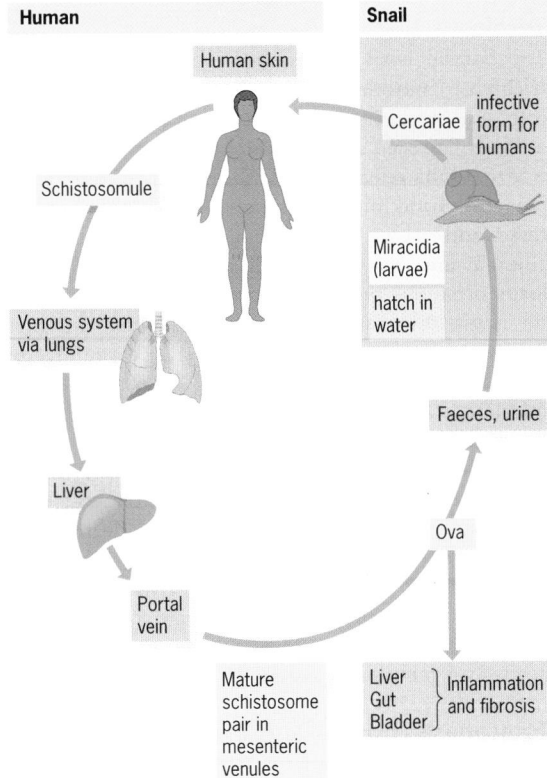

Fig. 2.37 A schematic life cycle of *Schistosoma*.

The pathology of schistosome infection varies with species and stage of infection. In the early stages there may be local and systemic allergic reactions to the migrating parasites. As eggs start to be deposited there may be a local inflammatory response in the bowel or bladder, while ectopic eggs may produce granulomatous lesions anywhere in the body. Chronic heavy infection, in which large numbers of eggs accumulate in the tissues, leads to fibrosis, calcification, and in some cases, dysplasia and malignant change. Morbidity and mortality are related to duration of infection and worm load, as well as to the species of parasite. Children in endemic areas tend to have the heaviest worm load, because of both increased exposure to infection, and differences in the immune response between adults and children.

Clinical features

Cercarial penetration of the skin may cause local dermatitis ('swimmer's itch'). After a symptom-free period of 3–4 weeks systemic allergic features may develop, including fever, rash, myalgia, and pneumonitis (Katayama fever). These allergic phenomena are common in non-immune travellers, but are rarely seen in local populations, who are usually exposed to infection from early childhood onwards. If infection is sufficiently heavy, symptoms from egg deposition may start to appear 2–3 months after infection

S. haematobium infection (bilharzia). The earliest symptom is usually painless terminal haematuria. As bladder inflammation progresses there is increased urinary frequency and groin pain. Obstructive uropathy develops, leading to hydronephrosis, renal failure, and recurrent urinary infection. There is a strong association between chronic urinary schistosomiasis and squamous cell bladder carcinoma. The genitalia may also be affected, and ectopic eggs may cause pulmonary or neurological disease.

S. mansoni usually affects the large bowel. Early disease produces superficial mucosal changes, accompanied by blood-stained diarrhoea. Later the mucosal damage becomes more marked, with the formation of rectal polyps, deeper ulceration, and eventually fibrosis and stricture formation. Ectopic eggs are carried to the liver, where they cause an intense granulomatous response. Hepatitis is followed by progressive periportal fibrosis, leading to portal hypertension, oesophageal varices and splenomegaly (p. 368). Hepatocellular function is usually well preserved.

S. japonicum, unlike the other species, infects numerous other mammals apart from man. It is similar to *S. mansoni,* but infects both large and small bowel, and produces a greater number of eggs. Disease therefore tends to be more severe, and rapidly progressive. Hepatic involvement is more common, and neurological involvement is seen in about 5% of cases.

Diagnosis

Schistosomiasis is suggested by relevant symptoms following fresh water exposure in an endemic area. In the early allergic stages the diagnosis can only be made clinically. When egg deposition has started, the characteristic eggs (with a terminal spine in the case of *S. haematobium,* and a lateral spine in the other species) can be detected on microscopy. In *S. haematobium* infection, the best specimen for examination is a filtered mid-day urine sample. Parasites may also be found in semen, and in rectal snip preparations. *S. mansoni* and *S. japonicum* eggs can usually be found in faeces or in a rectal snip. Serological tests are available, and may be useful in the diagnosis of travellers returning from endemic areas, but a parasitological diagnosis should always be made if possible. X-rays, ultrasound examinations, and endoscopy may show abnormalities of the bowel or urinary tract in chronic disease, although these are non-specific. Liver biopsy may show the characteristic periportal fibrosis.

Management

The aim of treatment in endemic areas is to decrease the worm load and therefore minimize the chronic effects of egg deposition. It may not always be possible (or even desirable) to eradicate adult worms completely, and reinfection is common. However, a 90% reduction in egg output has been achieved in mass treatment programmes, and in light infections where there is no risk of re-exposure the drugs are usually curative. The most widely used is praziquantel (40 mg/kg as a single dose), which is effective against all species of schistosome, well-tolerated, and reasonably cheap.

Prevention

Prevention of schistosomiasis is difficult, and relies on a combination of approaches. Mass treatment of the population (especially children) will decrease the egg load in the community. Health education programmes, the provision of latrines, and access to a safe water supply should decrease the contact with infected water. Attempts to eradicate the snail host have generally been unsuccessful, although man-made bodies of water can often be made less 'snail-friendly'. Travellers should be advised to avoid potentially infected water. Oral artemether is safe and shows a prophylactic effect against *S. mansoni.*

FURTHER READING

Davis A (1996) Schistosomiasis. In: Cook GC (ed) *Manson's Tropical Diseases.* London: WB Saunders, 1413–1456.

Food-borne flukes

Many flukes infect man via ingestion of an intermediate host, often fresh water fish.

Paragonimiasis

Over 20 million people are infected with lung flukes of the genus *Paragonimus*. The adult worms (of which the major species is *P. westermani*) live in the lungs, producing eggs which are expectorated or swallowed and passed in the faeces. Miracidia emerging from the eggs penetrate the first intermediate host, a fresh water snail. Larvae released from the snail seek out the second intermediate host, fresh water crustacea, in which they encyst as metacercariae. Humans and other mammalian hosts become infected after consuming uncooked shellfish. Cercariae penetrate the small intestinal wall, and migrate directly from the peritoneum to the lungs across the diaphragm. Having established themselves in the lung, the adult worms may survive for 20 years.

The common clinical features are fever, cough and mild haemoptysis. In heavy infections the disease may progress, sometimes mimicking pneumonia or pulmonary tuberculosis. Ectopic worms may cause signs in the abdomen or the brain.

The diagnosis is made by detection of ova on sputum or stool microscopy. Serological tests are also available. Radiological appearances are variable and non-specific. Treatment is with praziquantel 25 mg/kg three times daily for 3 days. Prevention involves avoidance of inadequately cooked shellfish.

Liver flukes

The human liver flukes, *Clonorchis sinensis*, *Opisthorchis felineus*, and *O. viverrini*, are almost entirely confined to East and South East Asia, where they infect more than 20 million people. Adults live in the bile ducts, releasing eggs into the faeces. The parasite requires two intermediate hosts, a fresh water snail and a fish, and humans are infected by consumption of raw fish. The cycle is completed when excysted worms migrate from the small intestine into the bile ducts.

Infection is often asymptomatic, but may be associated with cholangitis and biliary carcinoma. The diagnosis is made by identifying eggs on stool microscopy. Treatment is with a single dose of praziquantel (40 mg/kg), and infection can be avoided by cooking fish adequately.

Other fluke infections

Man can also be infected with a variety of animal flukes, notably the liver fluke *Fasciola hepatica*, and the intestinal fluke *Fasciolopsis buski*. Both require a water snail as an intermediate host; cercaria encyst on aquatic vegetation, and then are consumed by animals or man. After ingestion, *F. hepatica* penetrates the intestinal wall before migrating to the liver: during this stage it causes systemic allergic symptoms. After reaching the bile ducts it causes similar problems to the other liver flukes. *F. buski* does not migrate after it excysts, and causes mainly bowel symptoms.

Treatment is with tiabendazole 10 mg/kg as a single dose which may need repeating.

Cestodes

Cestodes (tapeworms) are ribbon-shaped worms which vary from a few millimetres to several metres in length. Adult worms live in the human intestine, where they attach to the epithelium using suckers on the anterior portion (scolex). From the scolex arises a series of progressively developing segments, called proglottids. The mature distal segments contain eggs, which may either be released directly into the faeces, or are carried out with an intact detached proglottid. The eggs are consumed by intermediate hosts, after which they hatch into larvae (oncospheres). These penetrate the intestinal wall and encyst in the tissues. Man ingests the cysts in undercooked meat or fish, and the cycle is completed when the parasites excyst in the stomach and develop into adult worms in the small intestine. Infections are usually solitary, but several adult tapeworms may coexist. The one exception to this life cycle is the dwarf tapeworm, *Hymenolepis nana*, which has no intermediate host and is transmitted from person to person by the faeco-oral route.

Taenia saginata

T. saginata, the beef tapeworm, may reach a length of several metres. It is common in all countries where beef is eaten. The adult worm causes few if any symptoms. Infection is usually discovered when proglottids are found in faeces or on underclothing, often causing considerable anxiety. Ova may also be seen on stool microscopy. Infection can be cleared with a single dose of praziquantel (10 mg/kg). It can be prevented by careful meat inspection, or by thorough cooking of beef.

Taenia solium and cysticercosis

T. solium, the pork tapeworm, is generally smaller than *T. saginata*, although it can still reach 6 metres in length. It is particularly common in South America, South Africa, China, and parts of South East Asia. As with *T. saginata* infection is usually asymptomatic. The ova of the two species are identical, but the proglottids can be distinguished on inspection. Treatment is with a similar dose of praziquantel: there is no evidence that this should be accompanied by a purgative, as was previously believed. Niclosamide 1 g repeated after 2 hours is the most widely used drug.

Man can act as both primary and intermediate host for *T. solium* (Fig. 2.38). The latter situation arises when eggs are ingested, or possibly when they are regurgitated from the small intestine to the stomach. Larvae are liberated, penetrate the intestinal wall, and are carried to various parts of the body where they develop into cysticerci. These are cysts, 0.5–1 cm diameter, containing the scolex of a new adult worm. Common sites for cysticerci include subcutaneous tissue, skeletal muscle and brain.

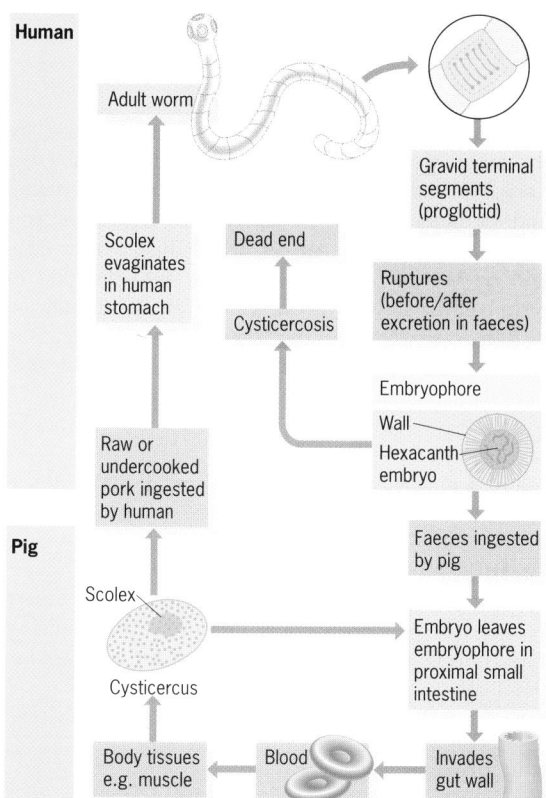

Fig. 2.38 A schematic life cycle of *Taenia solium*.

Diphyllobothrium latum

Infection with the fish tapeworm, *D. latum*, is common in northern Europe and Japan, owing to the consumption of raw fish. The adult worm reaches a length of several metres, but like the other tapeworms usually causes no symptoms. A megaloblastic anaemia (due to competitive utilization of B_{12} by the parasite) may occur. Diagnosis and treatment are the same as for *Taenia* species.

Hydatid disease

Hydatid disease occurs when humans become an intermediate host of the dog tapeworm, *Echinococcus granulosus* (Fig. 2.39). The adult worm lives in the gut of domestic and wild canines, and the larval stages are usually found in sheep, cattle and camels. Man may become infected either from direct contact with dogs, or from food or water contaminated with dog faeces. After ingestion the parasites excyst, penetrate the small intestine wall, and are carried to the liver and other organs in the bloodstream. A slow-growing, thick-walled cyst is formed, inside which further larval stages of the parasite develop. The life cycle cannot be completed unless the cyst is eaten by a dog. Hydatid disease is prevalent in areas where dogs are used in the control of livestock, especially sheep. It is common in Australia, Argentina, the Middle East, and parts of East Africa;

Superficial cysts may be felt under the skin, but usually cause no significant symptoms. Cysts in the brain can cause a variety of problems including epilepsy, personality change, hydrocephalus and focal neurological signs. These may only appear many years after infection.

Muscle cysts tend to calcify, and are often visible on X-rays. Cutaneous cysts can be excised and examined. Brain cysts are less prone to calcification, and are often only seen on CT or MRI scan. Serological tests may support the diagnosis.

Treatment of cerebral cysticercosis

Albendazole 15 mg/kg daily for 8 days is the drug of choice; the alternative is praziquantel 50 mg/kg daily (in divided doses) for 10 days. Successful treatment is accompanied by increased local inflammation, and corticosteroids should be given during and after the course of anthelminthic. Anticonvulsants should be given for epilepsy, and surgery may be indicated if there is hydrocephalus. Prevention of cysticercosis depends on good hygiene, as well as on the eradication of human *T. solium* infection.

The prognosis of cerebral cysticercosis is generally improved by anthelminthic chemotherapy, although the benefit in patients with old, calcified lesions is limited.

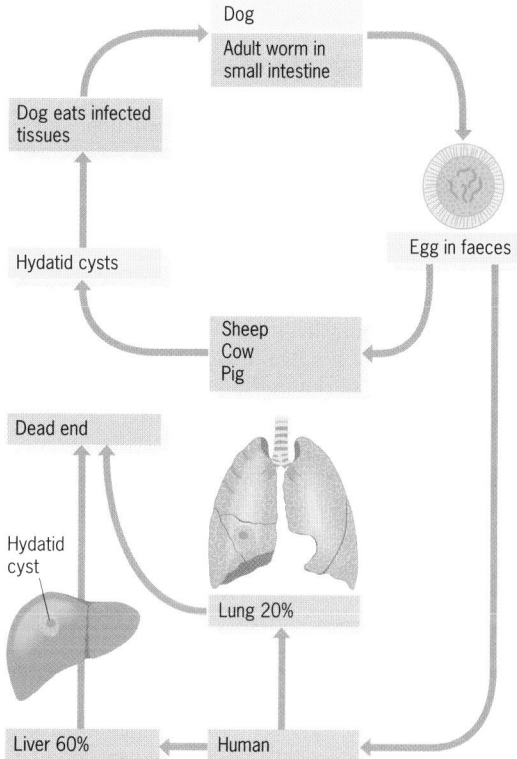

Fig. 2.39 A schematic life cycle of *Echinococcus granulosus*.

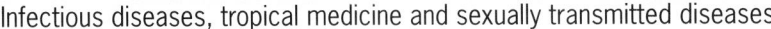

small foci of infection are still found in North Wales and rural Scotland.

Symptoms depend mainly on the site of the cyst. The liver is the most common organ affected (60%), followed by the lung (20%), kidneys (3%), brain (1%) and bone (1%). The symptoms are those of a slowly growing benign tumour. Pressure on the bile ducts may cause jaundice. Rupture into the abdominal cavity, pleural cavity or biliary tree may occur. In the latter situation, intermittent jaundice, abdominal pain and fever associated with eosinophilia result. A cyst rupturing into a bronchus may result in its expectoration and spontaneous cure, but if secondary infection supervenes a chronic pulmonary abscess will form. Focal seizures can occur if cysts are present in the brain. Renal involvement produces lumbar pain and haematuria. Calcification of the cyst occurs in about 40% of cases.

A related parasite of foxes, *E. multilocularis*, causes a similar but more severe infection, alveolar hydatid disease. These cysts are invasive and metastases may occur.

The diagnosis and treatment of hydatid liver disease are described on page 382.

Arthropod ectoparasites

Arthropods, which include the arachnid ticks and mites as well as insects, may be responsible for human disease in several ways.

Local hypersensitivity reactions

Local lesions may be caused by hypersensitivity to allergens in arthropod saliva. This common reaction, known as papular urticaria, is non-specific and is seen in the majority of people in response to the bite of a variety of blood-sucking arthropods including mosquitoes, bugs, ticks, lice, and mites. Occasionally tick bites may cause a more severe systemic allergic response, especially in previously sensitized individuals.

Most of these parasites alight on man only to feed, but some species of lice live in very close proximity to the skin: body lice in clothing, and head and pubic lice on human hairs (p. 1281).

Resident ectoparasite infections

Other ectoparasites are actually resident within the skin, causing more specific local lesions.

Scabies (p. 1281)

Jiggers

Jiggers is due to infection with the jigger flea, *Tunga penetrans*, and is common throughout South America and Africa. The pregnant female flea burrows into the sole of the foot, often between the toes. The egg sac grows to about 0.5 cm in size, before the eggs are discharged onto the ground. The main danger is bacterial infection or tetanus. The flea should be removed with a needle or scalpel, and the area kept clean until it heals.

Myiasis

Myiasis is caused by invasion of human tissue by the larva of certain flies, principally the Tumbu fly, *Cordylobia anthropophaga* (found in sub-Saharan Africa), and the human botfly, *Dermatobia hominis* (Central and South America). The larvae, which hatch from eggs laid on laundry and linen, burrow into the skin to form boil-like lesions: a central breathing orifice may be visible. Again the main risk is secondary infection. It is not always easy to extract the larva: covering it with petroleum jelly may bring it up in search of air.

Systemic envenomation

Many arthropods can cause local or systemic illness through envenomation (p. 989).

Arthropod vectors

The main role of arthropods in causing human disease is as vectors of parasitic and viral infections. Some of these infections are shown in Table 2.4, and discussed in detail elsewhere.

FURTHER READING

Moss PJ, Beeching NJ (1999) In: Armstrong D, Cohen J (eds) *Ectoparasites in Infectious Diseases*. London: Mosby.

Sexually transmitted infections

Sexually transmitted infections (STIs) are among the most common causes of illness in the world and remain epidemic in all societies. The public health, social and economic consequences are extensive, both of the acute infections and their longer-term sequelae. There has been a marked increase in the incidence of STIs in the UK (as in the rest of the world) over the past decade. New presentations at genitourinary medicine (GUM) clinics in the UK rose from 624 000 in 1990 to 1 170 000 in 1999.

Since 1995 there has been an increase in both gonorrhoea (55%) and syphilis (54%) infections. There has been a steady rise in the incidence of *Chlamydia trachomatis* with a 76% increase between 1995 and 1999. Viral conditions, particularly herpes simplex virus (HSV) and human papillomavirus, have also increased substantially. The recognition of acquired immune deficiency syndrome (AIDS) and human immunodefiency virus (HIV) has heightened awareness of STIs. Many people attend GUM clinics to seek information, advice and checks of their sexual health, but have no active STI.

People aged from 15 to 30 years are the most likely to acquire STIs. Changes in incidence reflect earlier sexual maturity and age at first intercourse. Widespread use of oral contraceptives has reduced the use of barrier methods of contraception. Increased travelling both within and between countries, recreational drug use, alcohol and more frequent partner change are also implicated. Multiple infections frequently coexist, some of which may be asymptomatic and facilitate spread.

Approach to the patient

Patients presenting with possible STIs are frequently anxious, embarrassed and concerned about confidentiality. Staff must be alert to these issues and respond sensitively. The clinical setting must ensure privacy and reinforce confidentiality.

History

The history of the presenting complaint frequently focuses on genital symptoms, the three most common being vaginal discharge (Table 2.46), urethral discharge (Table 2.47), and genital ulceration (Table 2.48). Details should be obtained of any associated fever, pain, itch, malodour, genital swelling, skin rash, joint pains and eye symptoms. All patients should be asked about dysuria, haematuria and loin pain. A full general medical, family and drug history, particularly of any recent antibacterial or antiviral treatment, allergies and use of oral contraceptives, must be obtained. In women, menstrual, contraception and obstetric history should be obtained. Any past or current history of drug misuse should be explored.

A detailed sexual history should be taken and include the number and types of sexual contacts (genital/genital, oral/genital, anal/genital, oral/anal) with dates, partner's sex, whether regular or casual partner, use of condoms and other forms of contraception, previous history of STIs including dates and treatment received, HIV testing and results and hepatitis B vaccination status.

Enquires should be made concerning travel abroad to areas where antibiotic resistance is known or where particular pathogens are endemic.

Examination

General examination must include the mouth, throat, skin and lymph nodes in all patients. Signs of HIV infection are covered on page 146. The inguinal, genital and perianal areas should be examined with a good light source. The groins should be palpated for lymphadenopathy and hernias. The pubic hair must be examined for nits and lice. The external genitalia must be examined for signs of erythema, fissures, ulcers, chancres, pigmented or hypopigmented areas and warts. Signs of trauma may be seen.

In men, the penile skin should be examined and the foreskin retracted to look for balanitis, ulceration, warts or tumours. The urethral meatus is located and the presence of discharge noted. Scrotal contents are palpated

Table 2.46
Causes of vaginal discharge

Infective	Non-infective
Candida albicans	Cervical polyps
Trichomonas vaginalis	Neoplasms
Bacterial vaginosis	Retained products
Neisseria gonorrhoeae	(e.g. tampons)
Chlamydia trachomatis	Chemical irritation
Herpes simplex	

Table 2.47
Causes of urethral discharge

Infective	Non-infective
Neisseria gonorrhoeae	Physical or chemical trauma
Chlamydia trachomatis	Urethral stricture
Mycoplasma genitilium	Non-specific (aetiology
Ureaplasma urealyticum	unknown)
Trichomonas vaginalis	
Herpes simplex virus	
Human papillomavirus (meatal warts)	
Urinary tract infection (rare)	
Treponema pallidum (meatal chancre)	

Table 2.48
Causes of genital ulceration

Infective	Non-infective
Syphilis	Behçet's syndrome
Primary chancre	Toxic epidermal necrolysis
Secondary mucous patches	Stevens-Johnson syndrome
Tertiary gumma	Carcinoma
Chancroid	Trauma
Lymphogranuloma	
venereum	
Donovanosis	
Herpes simplex	
Primary	
Recurrent	
Herpes zoster	

and the consistency of the testes and epididymis noted. A rectal examination/proctoscopy should be performed in patients with rectal symptoms, those who practise anoreceptive intercourse and patients with prostatic symptoms. A search for rectal warts is indicated in patients with perianal lesions.

In women, Bartholin's glands must be identified and examined. The cervix should be inspected for ulceration, discharge, bleeding and ectopy and the walls of the vagina for warts. A bimanual pelvic examination is performed to elicit adnexal tenderness or masses, cervical tenderness, and to assess the position, size and mobility of the uterus. Rectal examination and proctoscopy are performed if the patient has symptoms or practises anoreceptive intercourse.

Investigations

Although the history and examination will guide investigation, it must be remembered that multiple infections may coexist, some being asymptomatic. Full screening is indicated in any patient who may have been in contact with an STI.

In men

- Urethral smears for Gram staining
- Urethral swabs for gonococcal culture and *Chlamydia* testing
- Two-glass urine test and urinalysis
- Rectal swabs for Gram staining and culture for *N. gonorrhoeae* and *C. trachomatis*
- Throat swab for culture for *N. gonorrhoeae* and *C. trachomatis*
- Blood for syphilis and HIV serology (with full counselling).

In women

- Smears from the lateral vaginal wall for Gram staining
- Vaginal swab for culture of *Candida* and *Trichomonas*
- A wet preparation is made from the posterior fornix for *Trichomonas* and for the potassium hydroxide test for bacterial vaginosis
- The pH of vaginal secretions using narrow-range indicator paper
- Endocervical smears and swabs for Gram staining, gonococcal culture and *Chlamydia* tests
- Urethral smears and swabs for Gram staining and gonococcal culture
- Rectal and throat swabs for *N. gonorrhoeae* and *C. trachomatis*, if indicated
- Urinalysis
- Cervical cytology
- Blood for syphilis and HIV serology (with full counselling).

Additional investigations when appropriate

- Blood for hepatitis B and C serology
- Swabs for HSV and *Haemophilus ducreyi* from clinically suspicious lesions into special media
- Smears and swabs from the subpreputial area in men with balanoposthitis (inflammation of glans penis and prepuce) for candidiasis
- Scrapings from lesions suspicious of early syphilis for immediate dark-ground microscopy
- Pregnancy testing
- Cervical cytology
- Stools for *Giardia*, *Shigella* or *Salmonella* from those practising oral/anal sex.

Treatment, prevention and control

The treatment of specific conditions is considered in the appropriate section. Many GUM clinics keep basic stocks of medication and dispense directly to the patient.

Tracing the sexual partners of patients is crucial in controlling spread of STIs. The aims are to prevent the spread of infection within the community and to ensure that people with asymptomatic infection are properly treated. Appropriate antibiotic therapy may be offered to those who have had recent intercourse with someone known to have an active infection (epidemiological treatment). Interviewing people about their sexual partners requires considerable tact and sensitivity and specialist health advisors are available in GUM clinics.

Prevention starts with education and information. People begin sexual activity at ever-younger ages and education programmes need to include school pupils as well as young adults. Education of health professionals is also crucial. Appropriate and accessible services must be well advertised. Avoiding multiple partners, correct and consistent use of condoms and avoiding sex with people who have symptoms of infection may reduce the risks of acquiring an STI. For those who change their sexual partners frequently regular check-ups (approximately 3-monthly) are advisable. Once people develop symptoms they should be encouraged to seek medical advice as soon as possible to reduce complications and spread to others.

Clinical syndromes

HIV and AIDS

These are discussed in the section starting on page 131.

Gonorrhoea (GC)

Neisseria gonorrhoeae is a Gram-negative intracellular diplococcus (Fig. 2.40), which infects epithelium particularly of the urogenital tract, rectum, pharynx and conjunctivae. Humans are the only host and the organism is spread by intimate physical contact. It is very intolerant to drying and although occasional reports of spread by fomites exist, this route of infection is extremely rare.

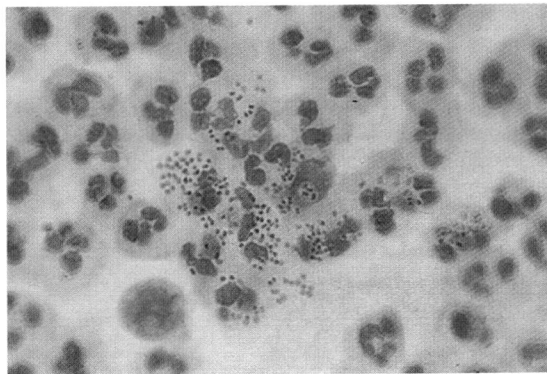

Fig. 2.40 *Neisseria gonorrhoeae* – **Gram-negative intracellular diplococci**. Courtesy of Dr B Goh.

Clinical features

Up to 50% of women and 10% of men are asymptomatic. The incubation period is 2–14 days with most symptoms occurring between days 2 and 5. In men the most common syndrome is one of anterior urethritis causing dysuria and/or urethral discharge (Fig. 2.42). Complications include ascending infection involving the epididymis or prostate leading to acute or chronic infection. In homosexual men rectal infection may produce proctitis with pain, discharge and itch.

In women the primary site of infection is usually the endocervical canal. Symptoms include an increased or altered vaginal discharge, pelvic pain due to ascending infection, dysuria, and intermenstrual bleeding. Complications include Bartholin's abscesses and in rare cases a perihepatitis (Fitzhugh–Curtis syndrome) can develop. On a global basis GC is one of the most common causes of female infertility. Rectal infection, due to local spread, occurs in women and is usually asymptomatic, as is pharyngeal infection. Conjunctival infection is seen in neonates born to infected mothers and is one cause of ophthalmia neonatorum.

Disseminated GC leads to arthritis (usually monoarticular or pauci-articular) (see p. 555) and characteristic papular or pustular rash with an erythematous base in association with fever and malaise. It is more common in women.

Diagnosis

N. gonorrhoeae can be identified from infected areas by culture on selective media with a sensitivity of at least 95%. Microscopy of Gram-stained secretions may demonstrate intracellular, Gram-negative diplococci, allowing rapid diagnosis. The sensitivity ranges from 90% in urethral specimens from symptomatic men to

50% in endocervical specimens. Microscopy should not be used for pharyngeal specimens. Blood culture and synovial fluid investigations should be performed in cases of disseminated GC. Coexisting pathogens such as *Chlamydia*, *Trichomonas* and syphilis must be sought.

Treatment

Treatment is indicated in those patients who have a positive culture for GC, or positive microscopy. Epidemiological treatment is given to patients who have had recent sexual intercourse with someone with confirmed GC infection. Although sensitive to a wide range of antimicrobial agents an increase in antibiotic resistant strains has been seen over the past two decades. This is especially marked in South East Asia. In the UK some form of antibiotic resistance is seen in 10% of the strains. Immediate therapy based on Gram-stained slides is usually initiated in the clinic, prior to culture and sensitivity results. Antibiotic choice is influenced by travel history or details known from contacts.

Single-dose oral therapy with either ciprofloxacin (500 mg) or ofloxacin (400 mg) successfully treats uncomplicated anogenital infection. Single-dose amoxicillin 3 g with probenecid 1 g are used in areas with low prevalence of penicillin resistance or in patients with quinolone sensitivity. Ceftriaxone 250 mg i.m. or spectinomycin 2 g i.m. (not generally available in the UK) are also used where penicillin resistance is high.

Longer courses of antibiotics are required for complicated infections. There should be at least one follow-up assessment, and culture tests should be repeated at least 72 hours after treatment is complete. All sexual contacts should be examined and treated as necessary.

Chlamydia trachomatis (CT)

Genital infection with CT is common, with up to 5% of sexually active women in the UK infected. It is regularly found in association with other pathogens: 20% of men and 40% of women with gonorrhoea have been found to have coexisting chlamydial infections. In men 40% of non-gonococcal and post-gonococcal urethritis is due to *Chlamydia*. As CT is often asymptomatic much infection goes unrecognized and untreated, which sustains the infectious pool in the population. The long-term complications associated with *Chlamydia* infection, especially infertility, impose significant morbidity in the UK. The organism has a world-wide distribution.

Clinical features

In men CT gives rise to an anterior urethritis with dysuria and discharge; infection is asymptomatic in up to 50% and detected by contact tracing. Ascending infection leads to epididymitis. Rectal infection leading to proctitis occurs in men practising anoreceptive intercourse. *In women* the most common site of infection is the endocervix where it may go unnoticed; up to 80% of infection in women is asymptomatic. Symptoms include

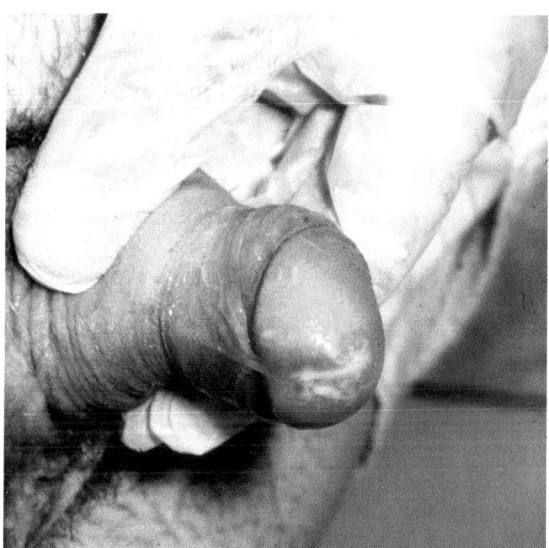

Fig. 2.41 *Neisseria gonorrhoeae* – **purulent urethral discharge.** Courtesy of Dr B Goh.

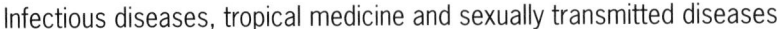

vaginal discharge, post-coital or intermenstrual bleeding and lower abdominal pain. Ascending infection causes acute salpingitis. Reiter's disease (see p. 551) has been related to infection with *C. trachomatis*. Neonatal infection, acquired from the birth canal, can result in mucopurulent conjunctivitis and pneumonia.

Diagnosis

CT is an obligate intracellular bacterium, which complicates diagnosis. Cell culture techniques provide the 'gold standard' but are expensive and require considerable expertise. Indirect diagnostic tests include direct fluorescent antibody (DIF) tests, enzyme immunoassays (EIA) and nucleic acid amplification techniques (NAAT) such as PCR or LCR: none are diagnostic.

In men first-voided urine samples are tested, or urethral swabs obtained. In women endocervical swabs are the best specimens and up to 20% additional positives will be detected if urethral swabs are also taken. Urine specimens are much less reliable than endocervical swabs in women and are not recommended. Specimen quality is critical and it must contain cellular material.

Treatment

Tetracyclines or macrolide antibiotics are most commonly used to treat *Chlamydia*. Doxycycline 100 mg 12-hourly for 7 days or azithromycin 1 g as a single dose are both effective for uncomplicated infection. Tetracyclines are contraindicated in pregnancy. Other effective regimens include erythromycin 500 mg four times daily. Routine test of cure is not necessary after treatment with doxycycline or azithromycin, although if symptoms persist or reinfection is suspected then further tests should be taken. Sexual contacts must be traced and treated, particularly as so many infections are clinically silent.

Urethritis

Urethritis is usually characterized in men by a discharge from the urethra, dysuria and varying degrees of discomfort within the penis. In 10–15% of cases there are no symptoms. A wide array of aetiologies can give rise to the clinical picture which are divided into two broad bands: gonococcal or non-gonococcal urethritis (NGU). NGU occurring shortly after infection with gonorrhoea is known as postgonococcal urethritis (PGU). Gonococcal urethritis and chlamydial urethritis (a major cause of NGU) are discussed above.

Trichomonas vaginalis, *Mycoplasma genitilium*, *Ureaplasma urealyticum* and *Bacterioides* spp. are responsible for a proportion of cases. HSV can cause urethritis in about 30% of cases of primary infection, considerably fewer in recurrent episodes. Other causes include syphilitic chancres and warts within the urethra. Non-sexually transmitted NGU may be due to urinary tract infections, prostatic infection, foreign bodies and strictures.

Clinical features

The urethral discharge is often mucoid and worse in the mornings. Crusting at the meatus or stains on underwear occur. Dysuria is common but not universal. Discomfort or itch within the penis may be present. The incubation period is 1–5 weeks with a mean of 2–3 weeks. Asymptomatic urethritis is a major reservoir of infection. Reiter's disease causing conjunctivitis and/or arthritis occurs, particularly in HLA B27-positive individuals.

Diagnosis

Smears should be taken from the urethra when the patient has not voided urine for at least 4 hours and should be Gram stained and examined under a high-power (×1000) oil-immersion lens. The presence of five or more polymorphonucleoleucocytes per high-power field is diagnostic. Men who are symptomatic but have no objective evidence of urethritis should be re-examined and tested after holding urine overnight. Cultures for gonorrhoea must be taken together with swabs for *Chlamydia* testing.

Treatment

Therapy for NGU is with tetracycline initially, using either doxycycline 100 mg 12-hourly or oxytetracycline 500 mg 6-hourly for 7 days. Sexual intercourse should be avoided. The vast majority of patients will show partial or total response. Sexual partners must be traced and treated; *C. trachomatis* can be isolated from the cervix in 50–60% of the female partners of men with PGU or NGU, many of whom are asymptomatic. This causes long-term morbidity in such women, acts as a reservoir of infection for the community, and may lead to reinfection in the index case if not treated.

Recurrent/persistent NGU

This is a common and difficult clinical problem. The usual time for patients to re-present is 2–3 weeks following treatment. Tests for organisms, e.g. *Mycoplasma*, *Chlamydia* and *Ureaplasma* are usually negative. It is necessary to document objective evidence of urethritis, check adherence to treatment and establish any possible contact with untreated sexual partners. Investigations should include wet preparation and culture of urethral material for *Trichomonas vaginalis*. Cultures should be taken for HSV. A mid-stream urine sample should be examined and cultured. A further 1 week's treatment with erythromycin and metronidazole 400 mg three times daily may be given and any specific additional infection treated appropriately. If symptoms are mild and all partners have been treated, patients should be reassured and further antibiotic therapy avoided. In cases of frequent recurrence and/or florid unresponsive urethritis, the prostate should be investigated and urethroscopy or cystoscopy performed to investigate possible strictures, periurethral fistulae or foreign bodies.

Lymphogranuloma venereum (LGV)

Chlamydia trachomatis types LGV 1, 2 and 3 are responsible for this sexually transmitted infection. It is endemic in the tropics, with the highest incidences in Africa, India and South East Asia.

Clinical features

The primary lesion is a painless ulcerating papule on the genitalia occurring 7–21 days following exposure. It frequently is unnoticed. A few days after this heals, regional lymphadenopathy develops. The lymph nodes are painful and fixed and the overlying skin develops a dusky erythematous appearance. Finally, nodes may become fluctuant (buboes) and can rupture. Acute LGV also presents as proctitis with perirectal abscesses, the appearances sometimes resembling anorectal Crohn's disease. The destruction of local lymph nodes can lead to lymphoedema of the genitalia.

Diagnosis

The diagnosis is often made on the basis of the characteristic clinical picture after other causes of genital ulceration or inguinal lymphadenopathy have been excluded. Syphilis and genital herpes must be excluded.

- Isolation of *C. trachomatis* in tissue culture. The sensitivity is 75–85%.
- Antigen-detection methods with material from bubo aspirates or ulcer scrapes:
  - direct immunofluorescence using monoclonal antibodies
  - enzyme immunoassay (EIA).
  Sensitivity 70–80%.
- Positive *C. trachomatis* serology (complement fixation tests, L-type immunofluorescence or micro-immunofluorescence test, IF). A fourfold rise in antibody titre in the course of the illness is diagnostic. *NB:* Micro-IF is the only serological means of distinguishing different serotypes of CT.

Treatment

Early treatment is critical to prevent the chronic phase. Doxycycline (100 mg twice daily for 21 days) or erythromycin (500 mg four times daily for 21 days) are efficacious. Follow-up should continue until signs and symptoms have resolved, usually 3–6 weeks. Chronic infection may result in extensive scarring and abscess and sinus formation. Surgical drainage or reconstructive surgery is sometimes required. Sexual partners in the 30 days prior to onset should be examined and treated if necessary.

Syphilis

Syphilis is a chronic systemic disease, which is acquired or congenital. In its early stages diagnosis and treatment are straightforward but untreated it can cause complex sequelae in many organs and eventually lead to death.

The causative organism, *Treponema pallidum* (TP) is a motile spirochaete that is acquired either by close sexual contact or can be transmitted transplacentally. The organism enters the new host through breaches in squamous or columnar epithelium. Primary infection of non-genital sites may occasionally occur but is rare.

Both acquired and congenital syphilis have early and late stages, each of which has classic clinical features (Table 2.49).

Primary

Between 10 and 90 days (mean 21 days) after exposure to the pathogen a papule develops at the site of inoculation. This ulcerates to become a painless, firm chancre. There is usually painless regional lymphadenopathy in association. The primary lesion may go unnoticed especially if it is on the cervix or within the rectum. Healing occurs spontaneously within 2–3 weeks.

Secondary

Between 4 and 10 weeks after the appearance of the primary lesion constitutional symptoms with fever, sore throat, malaise and arthralgia appear. Any organ may be affected – leading, for example, to hepatitis, nephritis, arthritis and meningitis. In a minority of cases the primary chancre may still be present and should be sought.

Signs include:

- generalized lymphadenopathy (50%)
- generalized skin rashes involving the whole body including the palms and soles but excluding the

Table 2.49
Classification and clinical features of syphilis

	Clinical features
Acquired	
Early stages	
Primary	Hard chancre
	Painless, regional lymphadenopathy
Secondary	*General*: Fever, malaise, arthralgia, sore throat and generalized lymphadenopathy
	Skin: Red/brown maculopapular non-itchy, sometimes scaly rash; condylomata lata
	Mucous membranes: Mucous patches, 'snail-track' ulcers in oropharynx and on genitalia
Late stages	
Tertiary	*Late benign*: Gummas (bone and viscera)
	Cardiovascular: Aortitis and aortic regurgitation
	Neurosyphilis: Meningovascular involvement, general paralysis of the insane (GPI) and tabes dorsalis
Congenital	Stillbirth or failure to thrive
Early stages	'Snuffles' (nasal infection with discharge)
	Skin and mucous membrane lesions as in secondary syphilis
Late stages	'Stigmata': Hutchinson's teeth, 'sabre' tibia and abnormalities of long bones
	Keratitis, uveitis, facial gummas and CNS disease

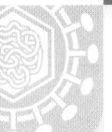

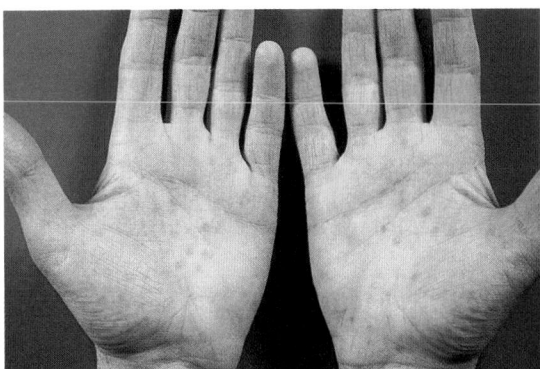

Fig. 2.42 **Rash of secondary syphilis on the palms.** Courtesy of Dr B Goh.

face (75%) – the rash, which rarely itches, may take many different forms, ranging from pink macules, through coppery papules, to frank pustules (Fig. 2.42)

- condylomata lata – warty, plaque-like lesions found in the perianal area and other moist body sites
- superficial confluent ulceration of mucosal surfaces – found in the mouth and on the genitalia, described as 'snail track ulcers'
- acute neurological signs in less than 10% of cases (e.g. aseptic meningitis).

Untreated early syphilis in pregnant women leads to fetal infection in at least 70% of cases and may result in stillbirth in up to 30%.

Latent
Without treatment, symptoms and signs abate over 3–12 weeks, but in up to 20% of individuals may recur during a period known as early latency, a 2-year period in the UK (1 year in USA). Late latency is based on reactive syphilis serology with no clinical manifestations for at least 2 years. This can continue for many years before the late stages of syphilis become apparent.

Tertiary
Late benign syphilis, so called because of its response to therapy rather than its clinical manifestations, generally involves the skin and the bones. The characteristic lesion, the gumma (granulomatous, sometimes ulcerating, lesions), can occur anywhere in the skin, frequently at sites of trauma. Gummas are commonly found in the skull, tibia, fibula and clavicle, although any bone may be involved. Visceral gummas occur mainly in the liver (hepar lobatum) and the testes.

Cardiovascular and neurosyphilis are discussed on pages 831 and 1196.

Congenital syphilis
Congenital syphilis usually becomes apparent between the second and sixth week after birth, early signs being nasal discharge, skin and mucous membrane lesions, and failure to thrive. Signs of late syphilis generally do not appear until after 2 years of age and take the form of 'stigmata' relating to early damage to developing structures, particularly teeth and long bones. Other late manifestations parallel those of adult tertiary syphilis.

Investigations for diagnosis
Treponema pallidum is not amenable to in vitro culture – the most sensitive and specific method is identification by dark-ground microscopy. Organisms may be found in variable numbers, from primary chancres and the mucous patches of secondary lesions. Individuals with either primary or secondary disease are highly infectious.

Serological tests used in diagnosis are either treponemal-specific or non-specific (cardiolipin test) (Table 2.50):

- **Treponemal specific.** The *T. pallidum* enzyme immunoassay (EIA). *T. pallidum* haemagglutination or particle agglutination assay (TPHA/TPPA) and fluorescent treponemal antibodies absorbed (FTA-abs) test are both highly specific for treponemal disease but will not differentiate between syphilis and other treponemal infection such as yaws. These tests usually remain positive for life, even after treatment.

Table 2.50
Syphilis serology

Stage of infection	Results			
	EIA	FTA-abs	TPHA/TPPA	VDRL/RPR
Very early primary	–	–	–	–
Early primary	+ (IgM)	+	–	–
Primary	+ (IgM)	+	±	+
Secondary or latent	+	+	+	+
Late latent	+	+	+	±
Treated	+	+	+	±
Biological false-positive	–	–	–	+

EIA, enzyme immunoassay; FTA-abs, fluorescent *Treponema* antibodies absorbed; TPHA/TPPA, *Treponema pallidum* haemagglutination/particle agglutination assay; VDRL, Venereal Disease Research Laboratory; RPR, rapid plasma reagin

- **Treponemal non-specific.** The Venereal Disease Research Laboratory (VDRL) or rapid plasma reagin (RPR) tests are non-specific, becoming positive within 3–4 weeks of the primary infection. They are quantifiable tests which can be used to monitor treatment efficacy and are helpful in assessing disease activity. They generally become negative by 6 months after treatment in early syphilis. The VDRL may also become negative in untreated patients (50% of patients with late-stage syphilis) or remain positive after treatment in late stage. False-positive results may occur in other conditions – particularly: infectious mononucleosis, hepatitis, *Mycoplasma* infections, some protozoal infections, cirrhosis, malignancy, autoimmune disease and chronic infections.

The EIA is the screening test of choice and can detect both IgM and IgG antibodies. A positive test is then confirmed with the TPHA/TPPA and VDRL/RPR tests. All serological investigations may be negative in early primary syphilis; the EIA IgM and the FTA-abs being the earliest tests to be positive. The diagnosis will then hinge on positive dark-ground microscopy and treatment should not be delayed if serological tests are negative in such situations.

In certain cases, examination of the CSF for evidence of neurosyphilis and a chest X-ray to determine the extent of cardiovascular disease will be indicated.

Treatment

Treponemocidal levels of antibiotic must be maintained in serum for at least 7 days in early syphilis to cover the slow division time of the organism (30 hours). In late syphilis treponemes may divide even more slowly requiring longer therapy.

Early syphilis (primary or secondary) should be treated with long-acting penicillin such as procaine benzylpenicillin (procaine penicillin) (e.g. Jenacillin A which also contains benzylpenicillin) 600 mg intramuscularly daily for 10 days. For late-stage syphilis, particularly when there is cardiovascular or neurological involvement, the treatment course should be extended for a further week. For patients sensitive to penicillin, either doxycycline 200 mg daily or erythromycin 500 mg four times daily is given orally for 2–4 weeks depending on the stage of the infection. Non-compliant patients can be treated with a single dose of benzathine penicillin G 2.4 g intramuscularly. These long-acting penicillins are not generally available in the UK but are imported directly by GUM clinics.

The Jarisch–Herxheimer reaction, which is due to release of TNF-α, IL-6 and IL-8 is seen in 50% of patients with primary syphilis and up to 90% of patients with secondary syphilis. It occurs about 8 hours after the first injection and usually consists of mild fever, malaise and headache lasting several hours. In cardiovascular or neurosyphilis the reaction, although rare, may be severe and exacerbate the clinical manifestations. Prednisolone given for 24 hours prior to therapy may ameliorate the reaction but there is little evidence to support its use. Penicillin should not be withheld because of the Jarisch–Herxheimer reaction; since it is not a dose-related phenomenon, there is no value in giving a smaller dose.

The prognosis depends on the stage at which the infection is treated. Early and early latent syphilis have an excellent outlook but once extensive tissue damage has occurred in the later stages the damage will not be reversed although the process may be halted. Symptoms in cardiovascular and neurosyphilis may therefore persist.

All patients treated for early syphilis must be followed up at regular intervals for the first year following treatment. Serological markers should be followed and a fall in titre of the VDRL/RPR of at least four-fold is consistent with adequate treatment for early syphilis. The sexual partners of all patients with syphilis and the parents and siblings of patients with congenital syphilis must be contacted and screened. Babies born to mothers who have been treated for syphilis in pregnancy may be retreated at birth.

Chancroid

Chancroid or soft chancre is an acute STI caused by *Haemophilus ducreyi*. It is probably the commonest cause of genital ulceration world-wide, and is prevalent in parts of Africa and Asia. Epidemiological studies in Africa have shown an association between genital ulcer disease, frequently chancroid, and the acquisition of HIV infection. A new urgency to control chancroid has resulted from these observations.

Clinical features

The incubation period is 3–10 days. At the site of inoculation an erythematous papular lesion forms which then breaks down into an ulcer. The ulcer frequently has a necrotic base, a ragged edge, bleeds easily and is painful. Several ulcers may merge to form giant serpiginous lesions. Ulcers appear most commonly on the prepuce and frenulum in men and can erode through tissues. In women the most commonly affected site is the vaginal entrance and the perineum. The lesions in women sometimes go unnoticed.

At the same time, inguinal lymphadenopathy develops (usually unilateral) and can progress to form large buboes which suppurate.

Diagnosis and treatment

Chancroid must be differentiated from other genital ulcer diseases (see Table 2.48). Co-infection with syphilis and herpes simplex is common. Isolation of *H. ducreyi* in specialized culture media is definitive but difficult. Swabs should be taken from the ulcer and material aspirated from the local lymph nodes for culture.

Polymerase chain reaction (PCR) techniques are now available. Gram stains of clinical material may show characteristic coccobacilli.

Single-dose regimens include azithromycin 1 g orally or ceftriaxone 250 mg i.m. Other regimens include ciprofloxacin 500 mg twice daily for 3 days, erythromycin 500 mg four times daily for 7 days. Clinically significant plasmid-mediated antibiotic resistance in *H. ducreyi* is developing.

Patients should be followed up at 3–7 days, when if treatment is successful ulcers will be responding.

Sexual partners should be examined and treated epidemiologically, as asymptomatic carriage has been reported.

HIV-infected patients should be closely monitored as healing may be slower. Multiple-dose regimens are needed in HIV patients since treatment failures have been reported with single-dose therapy.

Donovanosis

Donovanosis is the least common of all STIs in North America and Europe, but is endemic in the tropics and subtropics, particularly the Caribbean, South East Asia and South India. Infection is caused by *Klebsiella granulomatis*, a short, encapsulated Gram-negative bacillus. The infection was also known as granuloma inguinale. Although sexual contact appears to be the most usual mode of transmission, the infection rates are low, even between sexual partners of many years' standing.

Clinical features

In the vast majority of patients, the characteristic, heaped-up ulcerating lesion with prolific red granulation tissue appears on the external genitalia, perianal skin or the inguinal region within 1–4 weeks of exposure. It is rarely painful. Almost any cutaneous or mucous membrane site can be involved, including the mouth and anorectal regions. Extension of the primary infection from the external genitalia to the inguinal regions produces the characteristic lesion, the 'pseudo-bubo'.

Diagnosis and treatment

The clinical appearance usually strongly suggests the diagnosis but *K. granulomatis* (Donovan bodies) can be identified intracellularly in scrapings or biopsies of an ulcer. Successful culture has only recently been reported and PCR techniques and serological methods of diagnosis are being developed, but none are routinely available.

Antibiotic treatment should be given until the lesions have healed. A minimum of 3 weeks' treatment is recommended. Regimens include doxycycline 100 mg twice daily, co-trimoxazole 960 mg twice daily, azithromycin 500 mg daily, or ceftriaxone 1 g daily.

Sexual partners should be examined and treated if necessary.

Herpes simplex (p. 46)

Genital herpes is one of the most common STIs worldwide. In 1999 in the UK over 17 000 new cases and 14 000 recurrent infections were seen in GUM clinics. The peak incidence is in 16- to 24-year-olds of both sexes. Transmission occurs during close contact with a person who is shedding virus. Most genital herpes is due to type 2. Genital contact with oral lesions caused by HSV-1 can also produce genital infection.

Susceptible mucous membranes include the genital tract, rectum, mouth and oropharynx. The virus has the ability to establish latency in the dorsal root ganglia by ascending peripheral sensory nerves from the area of inoculation. It is this ability which allows for recurrent attacks.

Clinical features

Asymptomatic infection has been reported but is rare. Primary genital herpes is usually accompanied by systemic symptoms of varying severity including fever, myalgia and headache. Multiple painful shallow ulcers develop which may coalesce (Fig. 2.43). Atypical lesions are common. Tender inguinal lymphadenopathy is usual. Over a period of 10–14 days the lesions develop crusts and dry. In women with vulval lesions the cervix is almost always involved. Rectal infection may lead to a florid proctitis. Neurological complications can include aseptic encephalitis and/or involvement of the sacral autonomic plexus leading to retention of urine.

Recurrent attacks occur in a significant proportion of people following the initial episode. Precipitating factors vary as does the frequency of recurrence. A symptom prodrome is present in some people prior to the appearance of lesions. Systemic symptoms are rare in recurrent attacks.

The clinical manifestations in immunosuppressed patients (including those with HIV) may be more severe, and recurrences occur with greater frequency. Systemic spread has been documented (see p. 142).

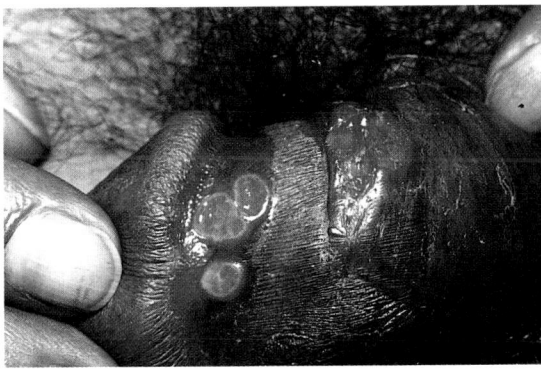

Fig. 2.43 **Herpes simplex rash on the penis.** Courtesy of Dr B Goh.

Diagnosis

Although the history and examination can be highly suggestive of HSV infection, a firm diagnosis can be made only on the basis of isolation of virus from lesions. Swabs should be taken and placed in viral transport medium. Virus is most easily isolated from new lesions.

Management

Primary

Saltwater bathing or sitting in a warm bath is soothing and may allow the patient to pass urine with some degree of comfort. Aciclovir, famciclovir and valaciclovir are useful if patients are seen whilst lesions are still moist. If lesions are already crusting, antiviral therapy will do little to change the clinical course. Secondary bacterial infection occasionally occurs and should be treated. Rest, analgesia and antipyretics should be advised. In rare instances patients may need to be admitted to hospital and aciclovir given intravenously, particularly if HSV encephalitis is suspected.

Recurrence

Recurrent attacks tend to be less severe and can be managed with simple measures such as saltwater bathing. Psychological morbidity is associated with recurrent genital herpes and frequent recurrences impose strains on relationships; patients need considerable support. Long-term suppressive aciclovir therapy is given in patients with frequent recurrences. An initial course of 400 mg twice daily or valaciclovir 500 mg daily for 6–12 months usually reduces the frequency of attacks, although there may still be some breakthrough.

HSV in pregnancy

The potential risk of infection to the neonate needs to be considered in addition to the health of the mother. Infection occurs either transplacentally or via the birth canal. If HSV is acquired for the first time during pregnancy, transplacental infection of the fetus may, rarely, occur. Management of primary HSV in the first or second trimester will depend on the woman's clinical condition and aciclovir can be prescribed in standard doses. Aciclovir therapy during the last 4 weeks of pregnancy may prevent recurrence at term.

Primary acquisition in the third trimester or at term with high levels of viral shedding usually leads to delivery by caesarean section.

For women with previous infection, concern focuses on the baby acquiring HSV from the birth canal. The risk is very low in recurrent attacks. For women with recurrent episodes only those with genital lesions at the onset of labour are delivered by caesarean section. Sequential cultures during the last weeks of pregnancy to predict viral shedding at term are no longer indicated.

Prevention and control

Patients must be advised that they are infectious when lesions are present; sexual intercourse should be avoided during this time or during prodromal stages. Condoms may not be effective as lesions may occur outside the areas covered. Sexual partners should be examined and may need information on avoiding infection.

Warts

Anogenital warts are amongst the most common sexually acquired infections. The causative agent is human papillomavirus (HPV) especially types 6 and 11 (p. 50). HPV is acquired by direct sexual contact with a person with either clinical or subclinical infection. Neonates may acquire HPV from an infected birth canal, which may result either in anogenital warts or in laryngeal papillomas. The incubation period ranges from 2 weeks to 8 months or even longer.

Clinical features

Warts develop around the external genitalia in women, usually starting at the fourchette, and involve the perianal region. The vagina may be infected. Flat warts may develop on the cervix and are not easily visible on routine examination. Such lesions are associated with cervical intraepithelial neoplasia. In men the penile shaft and subpreputial space are the most common sites although warts involve the urethra and meatus. Perianal lesions are more common in men who practise anoreceptive intercourse but can be found in any patient. The rectum may become involved. Warts become more florid during pregnancy or in immunosuppressed patients.

Diagnosis

The diagnosis is essentially clinical. It is critical to differentiate condylomata lata of secondary syphilis. Unusual lesions should be biopsied if the diagnosis is in doubt. Up to 30% of patients have coexisting infections with other STIs and a full screen must be performed.

Treatment

Local agents include podophyllin extract 10–25%, podophyllotoxin, imiquimod and trichloroacetic acid. In extensive or recalcitrant infection, cryotherapy, electrocautery or laser ablation is indicated. Podophyllin and podophyllotoxins are contraindicated in pregnancy.

Sexual contacts should be examined and treated if necessary. In view of the difficulties of diagnosing subclinical HPV, condoms should be used for up to 8 months after treatment. Because of the association of HPV with cervical intraepithelial neoplasia, women with warts and female partners of men with warts are advised to have regular cervical screening, i.e. every 3 years. Colposcopy may be useful in women with vaginal and cervical warts.

Hepatitis B

This is discussed in Chapter 7. Sexual contacts should be screened and given vaccine if they are not immune (see p. 355).

Trichomoniasis

Trichomonas vaginalis (TV) is a flagellated protozoon which is predominantly sexually transmitted. It is able to attach to squamous epithelium and can infect the vagina and urethra. *Trichomonas* may be acquired perinatally in babies born to infected mothers.

Infected women may, unusually, be asymptomatic. Commonly the major complaints are of vaginal discharge which is offensive and of local irritation. Men usually present as the asymptomatic sexual partners of infected women although they may complain of urethral discharge, irritation or urinary frequency.

Examination often reveals a frothy yellowish vaginal discharge and erythematous vaginal walls. The cervix may have multiple small haemorrhagic areas which lead to the description 'strawberry cervix'.

Diagnosis and treatment

Phase-contrast, dark-ground microscopy of a drop of vaginal discharge shows TV swimming with a characteristic motion. Many polymorphonuclear leucocytes are also seen. Culture techniques are good and confirm the diagnosis. *Trichomonas* is sometimes observed on cervical cytology with a 60–80% accuracy in diagnosis.

Metronidazole is the treatment of choice, either 2 g orally as a single dose or 400 mg twice-daily for 7 days. There is some evidence of metronidazole resistance and nimorazole is effective in these cases. Topical therapy with clotrimazole is effective, but if extravaginal infection exists this may not be eradicated and vaginal infection reoccurs. Male partners should be treated, especially as they are likely to be asymptomatic and more difficult to detect.

Candidiasis

Vulvovaginal infection with *Candida albicans* is extremely common. The organism is also responsible for balanitis in men. *Candida* can be isolated from the vagina in a high proportion of women of childbearing age, many of whom will have no symptoms.

The role of *Candida* as pathogen or commensal is difficult to disentangle and it may be changes in host environment which allow the organism to produce pathological effects. Predisposing factors include pregnancy, diabetes, and the use of broad-spectrum antibiotics and corticosteroids. Immunosuppression can result in more florid infection.

Clinical features

In women, pruritus vulvae is the dominant symptom. Vaginal discharge is present in varying degree. Many women have only one or occasional isolated episodes. Recurrent candidiasis (four or more symptomatic episodes annually) occurs in up to 5% of healthy women of reproductive age. Examination reveals erythema and swelling of the vulva with broken skin in severe cases. The vagina may contain adherent curdy discharge.

Men may have a florid balanoposthitis. More commonly, self-limiting burning penile irritation immediately after sexual intercourse with an infected partner is described. Diabetes must be excluded in men with balanoposthitis.

Diagnosis

Microscopic examination of a smear from the vaginal wall reveals the presence of spores and mycelia. Culture of swabs should be undertaken but may be positive in women with no symptoms. *Trichomonas* and bacterial vaginosis must be considered in women with itch and discharge.

Treatment

Topical. Pessaries or creams containing one of the imidazole antifungals such as clotrimazole 500 mg single dose used intravaginally are usually effective. Nystatin is also useful.

Oral. The triazole drugs such as fluconazole 150 mg as a single dose or itraconazole 200 mg twice in 1 day are used systemically where topical therapy has failed or is inappropriate. Recurrent candidiasis may be treated with fluconazole 100 mg weekly for 6 months, or clotrimazole pessary 500 mg weekly for 6 months.

The evidence for sexual transmission of *Candida* is slight and there is no evidence that treatment of male partners reduces recurrences in women.

Bacterial vaginosis

Bacterial vaginosis (BV) is a disorder characterized by an offensive vaginal discharge. The aetiology and pathogenesis are unclear but a mixed flora of *Gardnerella vaginalis*, anaerobes including *Bacteroides*, *Mobiluncus* spp. and *Mycoplasma hominis*, replaces the normal lactobacilli of the vagina. Amines and their breakdown products from the abnormal vaginal flora are thought to be responsible for the characteristic odour associated with the condition. As vaginal inflammation is not part of the syndrome the term vaginosis is used rather than vaginitis. It is not clear to what extent BV is a sexually transmitted condition.

Clinical features

Vaginal discharge and odour are the most common complaints although a proportion of women are asymptomatic. A homogeneous, greyish white, adherent discharge is present in the vagina, the pH of which is raised (greater than 5). Associated complications are ill-defined but may include chorioamnionitis and an increased incidence of premature labour in pregnant women. Whether BV disposes non-pregnant women to upper genital tract infection is unclear.

Diagnosis

Different authors have differing criteria for making the diagnosis of BV. In general it is accepted that three of the following should be present for the diagnosis to be made:

- characteristic vaginal discharge
- the amine test: raised vaginal pH using narrow range indicator paper (> 4.7)
- a fishy odour on mixing a drop of discharge with 10% potassium hydroxide
- the presence of clue cells on microscopic examination of the vaginal fluid.

Clue cells are squamous epithelial cells from the vagina which have bacteria adherent to their surface giving a granular appearance to the cell. A Gram stain gives a typical reaction of partial stain uptake.

Treatment

Metronidazole given orally in doses of 400 mg twice daily for 5–7 days is usually recommended. A single dose of 2 g metronidazole is less effective. Topical 2% clindamycin cream 5 g intravaginally is effective.

Recurrence is high, with some studies giving a rate of 80% within 9 months of completing metronidazole therapy. There is debate over the treatment of asymptomatic women who fulfil the diagnostic criteria for BV. The diagnosis should be fully discussed and treatment offered if the woman wishes. Until the relevance of BV to other pelvic infections is elucidated the treatment of asymptomatic women with BV is not to be recommended. There is no convincing evidence that simultaneous treatment of the male partner influences the rate of recurrence of BV and routine treatment of male partners is not indicated.

Infestations (see also p. 1281)

Pediculosis pubis

The pubic louse (*Phthirus pubis*) is a blood-sucking insect which attaches tightly to the pubic hair. They may also attach to eyelashes and eyebrows. It is relatively host-specific and is transferred only by close bodily contact. Eggs (nits) are laid at hair bases and usually hatch within a week. Although infestation may be asymptomatic the most common complaint is of itch.

Diagnosis

Lice may be seen on the skin at the base of pubic and other body hairs. They resemble small scabs or freckles but if they are picked up with forceps and placed on a microscope slide will move and walk away. Blue macules may be seen at the feeding sites. Nits are usually closely adherent to hairs. Both are highly characteristic under the low-power microscope.

As with all sexually transmitted infections, the patient must be screened for coexisting pathogens.

Treatment

Both lice and eggs must be killed with 0.5% malathion, permethrin or 0.5% carbaryl. The preparation should be applied to all areas of the body from the neck down and washed off after 12 hours. In a few cases a further application after 1 week may be necessary. For severe infestations, antipruritics may be indicated for the first 48 hours. All sexual partners should be seen and screened.

Scabies

This is discussed on page 1281.

FURTHER READING

Adler M (1998) *The ABC of Sexually Transmitted Diseases*, 4th edn. London: BMA Books.

PHLS (Dec 2000) *Trends in STI*. Public Health Laboratory Service.

Radcliffe K, Ahmedjushuf I, Cowan F, Fitzgerald M, Wilson J (1999) UK national guidelines on sexually transmitted infections and closely related conditions. *Sexually Transmitted Infections* **75** (Suppl 1).

Sobel JD (1997) Vaginitis. *New England Journal of Medicine* **337**: 1896–1903.

Human immune deficiency virus (HIV) and AIDS

Epidemiology

HIV, the cause of the acquired immune deficiency syndrome (AIDS) continues to spread and AIDS is now the fourth commonest cause of death world-wide, causing over 2.5 million deaths in 1999. In the year 2000, 34.5 million people were infected with HIV world-wide of whom 24.5 million are in sub-Saharan Africa. Approximately 16 000 new infections occur daily, the majority in young adults.

The human and economic costs are huge – 33% of 15-year-olds in high-prevalence countries in Africa will die of HIV, life expectancy in some African countries is set to fall by 16 years by 2010 with an inevitable impact on economic growth and stability. Although in the UK and other wealthy countries deaths from HIV have fallen, new HIV diagnoses continue (2500/year in the UK) with the result that prevalence is rising. Demographics have varied greatly within different regions, influenced by social, behavioural, cultural and political factors. Despite the fact that HIV can be isolated from a wide range of body fluids and tissues, the majority of infections are transmitted via semen, cervical secretions and blood. The character of the epidemic in different regions of the world has been influenced by the relative frequency of each of the routes of transmission.

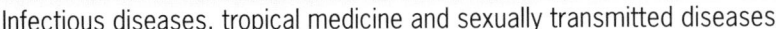

Sexual intercourse (vaginal and anal)

Globally, heterosexual intercourse accounts for the vast majority of infections, and coexistent STIs, especially those causing genital ulceration, enhance transmission. Passage of HIV appears to be more efficient from men to women, and to the passive partner in anal intercourse, than vice versa.

In the UK sex between men still accounts for over half the infections reported, but there is now an increasing rate of heterosexual transmission. At the end of 1999 an estimated 32% of prevalent infections were a result of heterosexual exposure. Of these infections 22% were in women compared to 5% in the late 1980s. In central and sub-Saharan Africa the epidemic has always been heterosexual and more than half the infected adults in these regions are women. South East Asia and the Indian subcontinent are still in the early phases of a possible explosive epidemic, driven by heterosexual intercourse and a high incidence of other sexually transmitted diseases.

Mother to child (parentally, perinatally, breast-feeding)

Vertical transmission is the most common route of HIV infection in children. UN estimates are of 600 000 children being infected globally in 1999. European studies suggest that, without intervention, 15% of babies born to HIV-infected mothers are likely to be infected although rates of up to 40% have been reported from Africa and the USA. Increased vertical transmission is associated with advanced disease in the mother, high maternal viral load, prolonged and premature rupture of membranes, and chorioamnionitis. Transmission can occur in utero although the majority of infections take place perinatally. Breast-feeding has been shown to increase the risk of vertical transmission by up to 20%. In the developed world interventions to reduce vertical transmission, including the use of antiretroviral agents, delivery by caesarean section and the avoidance of breast-feeding have led to a dramatic fall in the numbers of infected children. Access to these interventions in resource-poor countries in which 90% of infections occur is a major issue.

Contaminated blood, blood products and organ donations

In some developing countries where blood is not screened or treated, and in areas where the rate of new HIV infections is very high, transfusion-associated transmission remains significant.

Contaminated needles (intravenous drug misuse, injections, needle-stick injuries)

The practice of sharing needles and syringes for intravenous drug use continues to be a major route of transmission of HIV in both developed countries and parts of South East Asia, Latin America and parts of Eastern Europe. In some areas successful education and needle exchange schemes have reduced the rate of transmission by this route. Iatrogenic transmission from needles and syringes used in developing countries is reported. Healthcare workers have a risk of approximately 0.3% following a single needle-stick injury with known HIV-infected blood.

There is no evidence that HIV is spread by social or household contact nor by blood-sucking insects such as mosquitoes and bed bugs.

The virus

HIV belongs to the lentivirus group of the retrovirus family. There are at least two types, HIV-1 and HIV-2. HIV-2 is almost entirely confined to West Africa although there is evidence of some spread to the Indian subcontinent. HIV-2 is associated with an AIDS-type illness although it may be more indolent in nature. The structure of the virus is shown in Figure 2.44.

Retroviruses are characterized by the possession of the enzyme reverse transcriptase, which allows viral RNA to be transcribed into DNA, and thence incorporated into the host cell genome. Reverse transcription is an error-prone process with a significant rate of misincorporation of bases. This combined with a high rate of viral turnover, leads to considerable genetic variation and a diversity of viral subtypes or clades. On the basis of DNA sequencing, HIV-1 is divided into two subtypes:

- *Group M (major) subtypes.* There are at least 10, which are denoted A–J. There is a predominance of subtype B in Europe, North America and Australia, but areas of central and sub-Saharan Africa have multiple M subtypes.

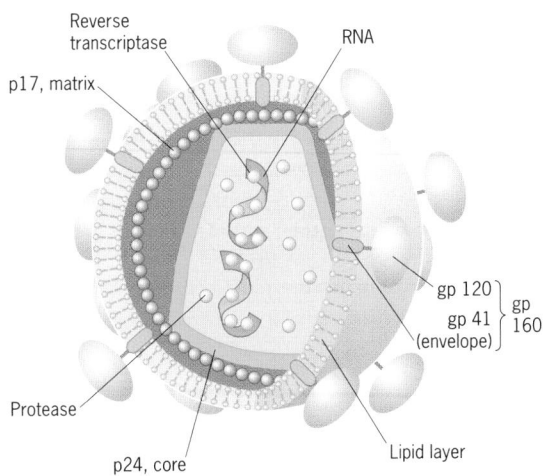

Fig. 2.44 **Structure of HIV.** Two molecules of single-stranded RNA are shown within the nucleus. The reverse transcriptase polymerase converts viral RNA into DNA (a characteristic of retroviruses). The protease includes integrase (p32 and p10). The p24 (core protein) levels can be used to monitor HIV disease. p17 is the matrix protein. gp120 is the outer envelope glycoprotein which binds to cell surface CD4 molecules. gp41, a transmembrane protein, influences infectivity and cell fusion capacity.

- *Group O (outlier) subtypes.* This is highly divergent from group M and is confined to small numbers centred on the Cameroons.

Recombination of viral material generates an array of circulating recombinant forms (CRFs) which increases the genetic diversity that may be encountered.

Connections between genetic diversity and biological effects, in particular pathogenicity, rates of transmission and response to therapy, are being sought.

Pathogenesis

The interrelationship between HIV and the host immune system is the basis of the pathogenesis of HIV disease. The host cellular receptor that is recognized by HIV surface glycoprotein is the CD4 molecule, which defines the cell populations that are susceptible to infection (Fig. 2.45). The interaction between CD4 and HIV surface glycoprotein together with chemokine co-receptors CCR5 and CXCR4 is responsible for HIV entry into cells. Mutations in the gene expressing the receptor for chemokine CCR5 may impair entry of HIV into cells and therefore confer some resistance to this infection. Auxiliary viral proteins such as those coded by the *Nef*

gene have a role in influencing host cell membrane proteins and signal transduction pathways. CD4 receptors and HIV surface glycoprotein interactions mediate the process of syncytium formation, which is a cytopathic effect of HIV infection.

Studies of viral turnover in HIV-infected individuals have demonstrated a virus half-life in the circulation of about 6 hours. To maintain observed levels of plasma viraemia, 10^8–10^9 virus particles need to be released and cleared daily. Virus production by infected cells lasts for about 2 days and is probably limited by the death of the cell owing to direct HIV effects, linking HIV replication to the process of CD4 destruction and depletion. Studies suggest that immunopathogenesis is a result of defective T cell homeostasis in HIV infection. The progressive and severe depletion of CD4 helper lymphocytes has profound repercussions for the functioning of the immune system (see p. 211). Cell-mediated immunodeficiency, which is the major consequence, leaves the host open to infections with intracellular pathogens, whilst the coexisting antibody abnormalities predispose to infections with capsulated bacteria. HIV also has a direct effect on certain tissues, notably the nervous system.

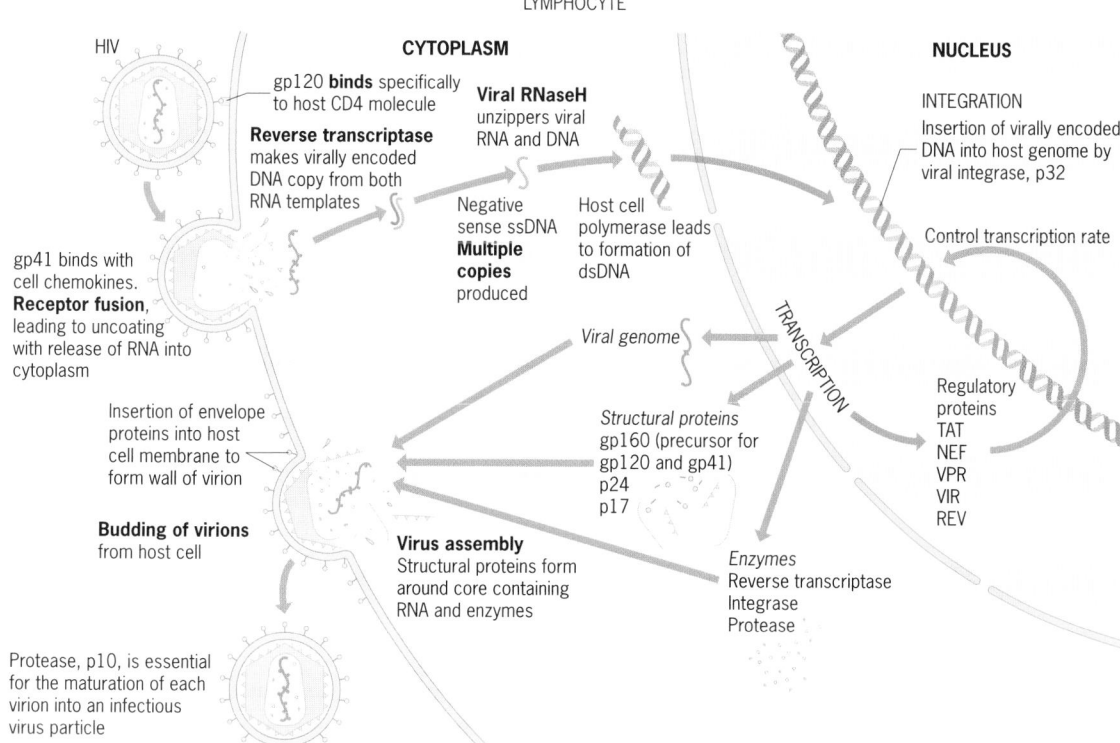

Fig. 2.45 HIV entry and replication in CD4 T lymphocytes. The human immune deficiency virus binds to the host CD4 inoculate via the envelope glycoprotein gp120. Gp41 binds to the cell chemokine causing receptor fusion and uncoating of RNA. DNA copies are made from both RNA templates (reverse transcriptase). The enzyme polymerase from the host cell leads to formation of dsDNA. In the nucleus the virally encoded DNA is inserted into the host genome (integration). Regulatory proteins control transcription (a process in which an RNA molecule is synthesized from a DNA template). The virus is re-assembled in the cytoplasm and budded out from the host cell. Adapted from original figure, courtesy of Bryony Cohen, Barts and The London NHS Trust.

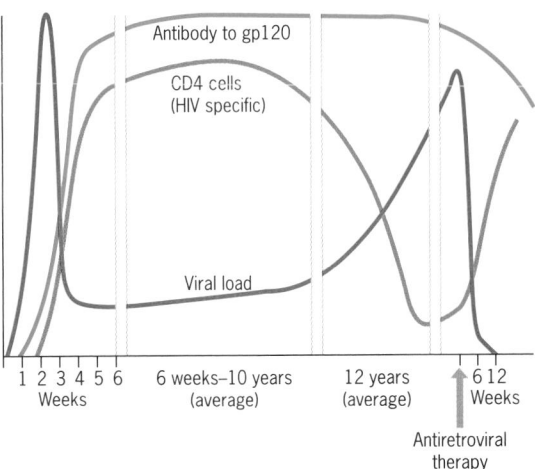

Fig. 2.46 The immune response to HIV (seroconversion).

Diagnosis and natural history (Fig. 2.46)

HIV infection is diagnosed either by the detection of virus-specific antibodies (anti-HIV) or by direct identification of viral material.

Detection of IgG antibody to envelope components (gp120 and its subunits). This is the most commonly used marker of infection. The routine tests used for screening are based on ELISA techniques, which may be confirmed with Western blot assays. Up to 3 months may elapse from initial infection to antibody detection (serological latency, or window period). These antibodies to HIV have no protective function and persist for life. As with all IgG antibodies, anti-HIV will cross the placenta. All babies born to HIV-infected women will thus have the antibody at birth. In this situation, anti-HIV antibody is not a reliable marker of active infection and in uninfected babies will be gradually lost over the first 18 months of life.

Other than in exceptional circumstances, HIV antibody testing should be carried out only after full discussion of the implications with the patient and with the patient's express consent.

IgG antibody to p24 (anti-p24). This can be detected from the earliest weeks of infection and through the asymptomatic phase. It is frequently lost as disease progresses.

Antigen assays. Nucleic acid-based assays are available which amplify and test for components of the HIV genome. All are based on HIV-1 subtype B material, and there are potential inaccuracies with other subtypes, especially group O variants. These assays are used to aid diagnosis of HIV in the babies of HIV-infected mothers or in situations where serological tests may be inadequate such as subtyping HIV variants for medicolegal reasons. (See the discussion of viral load monitoring, p. 145.)

Viral p24 antigen (p24ag). This is detectable shortly after infection but has usually disappeared by 8–10 weeks after exposure. It can be a useful marker in individuals who have been infected recently but have not had time to mount an antibody response. It may reappear at low levels intermittently during the period of clinical latency and in some people as infection progresses. Its use as a surrogate marker of viral activity has been superseded by HIV RNA assays in many areas (see p. 145).

Isolation of virus in culture. This is a specialized technique available in some laboratories to aid diagnosis and as a research tool.

Clinical features of HIV infection

The spectrum of illnesses associated with HIV infection is broad and is the result of both direct HIV effects and the associated immune dysfunction. Several classification systems exist, the most widely used being the 1993 Centers for Disease Control (CDC) classification (Box 2.16). This classification depends to a large extent on definitive diagnoses of infection, which makes it more difficult to use in those areas of the world without sophisticated laboratory support. As immunosuppression progresses the patient is susceptible to an increasing range of opportunistic infections and tumours, certain of which meet the criteria for the diagnosis of AIDS (Box 2.17).

Box 2.16

Summary of CDC classification of HIV infection

Absolute CD4 count (/mm³)	A: Asymptomatic OR persistent generalized lymphadenopathy OR acute seroconversion illness	B: HIV-related conditions,* not A or C	C: Clinical conditions listed in AIDS surveillance case definition (see Box 2.17)
>500	A1	B1	C1
200–499	A2	B2	C2
<200	A3	B3	C3

*Examples of category B conditions include: bacillary angiomatosis, candidiasis (oropharyngeal), constitutional symptoms, oral hairy leucoplakia, herpes zoster involving more than one dermatome, idiopathic thrombocytopenic purpura, listeriosis, pelvic inflammatory disease especially if complicated by tubo-ovarian abscess, peripheral neuropathy.

Since 1993 the definition of AIDS has differed between the USA and Europe. The USA definition includes individuals with CD4 counts below 200 in addition to the clinical classification based on the presence of specific indicator diagnoses shown in Box 2.17. In Europe the definition remains based on the diagnosis of specific clinical conditions with no inclusion of CD4 lymphocyte counts.

Incubation

The 2–4 weeks immediately following infection are usually silent both clinically and serologically.

Seroconversion/primary illness

The majority of HIV seroconversions are also clinically silent. In a proportion, a self-limiting non-specific illness occurs 6–8 weeks after exposure. Symptoms include fever, arthralgia, myalgia, lethargy, lymphadenopathy, sore throat, mucosal ulcers and occasionally a transient faint pink maculopapular rash. Neurological symptoms are common, including headache, photophobia, myelopathy, neuropathy and in rare cases encephalopathy. The illness lasts up to 3 weeks and recovery is usually complete.

Box 2.17

AIDS-defining conditions

- Candidiasis of bronchi, trachea or lungs
- Candidiasis, oesophageal
- Cervical carcinoma, invasive
- Coccidioidomycocis, disseminated or extrapulmonary
- Cryptococcosis, extrapulmonary
- Cryptosporidiosis, chronic intestinal (1-month duration)
- Cytomegalovirus (CMV) disease (other than liver, spleen or nodes)
- CMV retinitis (with loss of vision)
- Encephalopathy, HIV-related
- Herpes simplex, chronic ulcers (1-month duration); or bronchitis, pneumonitis or oesophagitis
- Histoplasmosis, disseminated or extrapulmonary
- Isosporiasis; chronic intestinal (1-month duration)
- Kaposi's sarcoma
- Lymphoma, Burkitt's
- Lymphoma, immunoblastic (or equivalent term)
- Lymphoma (primary) of brain
- *Mycobacterium avium* complex or *M. kansasii*, disseminated or extrapulmonary
- *Mycobacterium tuberculosis*, any site
- *Mycobacterium*, other species or unidentified species, disseminated or extrapulmonary
- *Pneumocystis carinii* pneumonia
- Pneumonia, recurrent
- Progressive multifocal leucoencephalopathy
- *Salmonella* septicaemia, recurrent
- Toxoplasmosis of brain
- Wasting syndrome, due to HIV

Laboratory abnormalities include lymphopenia with atypical reactive lymphocytes noted on blood film, thrombocytopenia and raised liver enzymes. CD4 lymphocytes may be markedly depleted and the CD4 : CD8 ratio reversed. Antibodies to HIV may be absent during this early stage of infection although the level of circulating viral RNA is high and p24 core protein may be detectable. Patients experiencing a seroconversion illness may have a more rapidly progressive course of infection.

Clinical latency

The majority of people with HIV infection are asymptomatic for a substantial but variable length of time. However, the virus continues to replicate and the person is infectious. Studies suggest a median time of 10 years from infection to development of AIDS, although some patients progress much more rapidly and others have remained symptom-free for up to 15 years. Older age is associated with more rapid progression, and the influence of putative protective genetic factors is under scrutiny. Gender and pregnancy per se do not appear to influence the rate of progression, although women may fare less well for a variety of reasons. A subgroup of patients with asymptomatic infection have persistent generalized lymphadenopathy (PGL), defined as lymphadenopathy (> 1 cm) at two or more extrainguinal sites for more than 3 months in the absence of causes other than HIV infection. The nodes are usually symmetrical, firm, mobile and non-tender. There may be associated splenomegaly. The architecture of the nodes shows hyperplasia of the follicles and proliferation of the capillary endothelium. Biopsy is rarely indicated. Similar disease progression has been noted in asymptomatic patients with or without PGL. Nodes may disappear with disease progression.

Symptomatic HIV infection

As HIV infection progresses the viral load rises, the CD4 count falls, and the patient develops an array of symptoms and signs. The clinical picture is the result of direct HIV effects and of the associated immunosuppression.

In an individual patient the clinical consequences of HIV-related immune dysfunction will depend on at least three factors:

- *The microbial exposure of the patient throughout life.* Many clinical episodes represent reactivation of previously acquired infection, which has been latent. Geographical factors determine the microbial repertoire of an individual patient. Those organisms requiring intact cell-mediated immunity for their control are most likely to cause clinical problems.
- *The pathogenicity of organisms encountered.* High-grade pathogens such as *Mycobacterium tuberculosis*, *Candida* and the herpesviruses are clinically relevant even when immunosuppression is mild, and will

thus occur earlier in the course of the disease. Less virulent organisms occur at later stages of immunodeficiency.

- *The degree of immunosuppression of the host.* When patients are severely immunocompromised (CD4 count < 100/mm³) disseminated infections with organisms of very low virulence such as *M. avium-intracellulare* (MAI) and *Cryptosporidium* are able to establish themselves. These infections are very resistant to treatment, mainly because there is no functioning immune response to clear organisms. This hierarchy of infection allows for appropriate intervention with prophylactic drugs.

Effects of HIV infection

Neurological disease

Infection of the nervous tissue occurs at an early stage but clinical neurological involvement increases as HIV advances. This includes AIDS dementia complex (ADC), sensory polyneuropathy and aseptic meningitis (see p. 1196). These conditions are much less common since the introduction of HAART (highly active anti-retroviral therapy). The pathogenesis is thought to be due both to the release of neurotoxic products by HIV itself and to cytokine abnormalities secondary to immune dysregulation.

ADC has varying degrees of severity, ranging from mild memory impairment and poor concentration through to severe cognitive deficit, personality change and psychomotor slowing. Changes in affect are common and depressive or psychotic features may be present. The spinal cord may show vacuolar myelopathy histologically. In severe cases brain CT scan shows atrophic change of varying degrees. MRI changes consist of white matter lesions of increased density on T2-weighted sections. EEG may show non-specific changes consistent with encephalopathy. The CSF is usually normal, although the protein concentration may be raised. Patients with mild neurological dysfunction may be unduly sensitive to the effects of other insults such as fever, metabolic disturbance or psychotropic medication, any of which may lead to a marked deterioration in cognitive functioning.

Sensory polyneuropathy is seen frequently in HIV infection, most commonly in the legs and feet although hands may be affected in advanced disease. In its most severe form it causes intense pain, usually in the feet, which may disrupt sleep, impair mobility and generally reduce the quality of life.

Autonomic neuropathy may also occur with postural hypotension and diarrhoea. Autonomic nerve damage is found in the small bowel.

Zidovudine has a beneficial effect on HIV neurological disease, with startling improvement in cognitive function in many patients with ADC. It may also have a neuroprotective role. Zalcitabine, didanosine and stavudine produce a similar neuropathy as a major toxic side-effect and must be used with caution in patients with HIV neuropathy.

Eye disease

Eye pathology is a regular finding in HIV infection, usually in the later stages. The most serious is cytomegalovirus retinitis (see p. 141) which is sight-threatening. Retinal cotton wool spots due to HIV per se are rarely troublesome but they may be confused with CMV retinitis. Anterior uveitis can present as acute red eye associated with rifabutin therapy for mycobacterial infections in HIV. Steroids used topically are usually effective but modification of the dose of rifabutin is required to prevent relapse. Pneumocystis, toxoplasmosis, syphilis and lymphoma can all affect the retina and the eye may be the site of first presentation.

Mucocutaneous manifestations (see Table 2.52)

The skin is a common site for HIV-related pathology as the function of dendritic and Langerhans' cells, both target cells for HIV, is disrupted. Delayed-type hypersensitivity (p. 214), a good indicator of cell-mediated immunity, is frequently reduced or absent even before clinical signs of immunosuppression appear. Pruritus is a common complaint at all stages of HIV. Generalized dry, itchy, flaky skin is typical and the hair may become thin and dry. An intensely pruritic papular eruption favouring the extremities may be found, particularly in patients from sub-Saharan Africa. Eosinophilic folliculitis presents with urticarial lesions particularly on the face, arms and legs.

Drug reactions with cutaneous manifestations are extremely frequent, with rashes developing notably to sulphur-containing drugs amongst others (see Fig. 22.38, p. 1314). Recurrent aphthous ulceration, which is severe and slow to heal is common and can impair the patient's ability to eat. Biopsy may be indicated to exclude other causes of ulceration. Topical steroids are useful and resistant cases may respond to thalidomide.

In addition to the above the skin is a common site of opportunistic infections (see below).

Haematological complications

Anaemia, neutropenia and thrombocytopenia are all common in advanced HIV infection.

- *Lymphopenia* – this progresses as the CD4 count falls
- *Anaemia of chronic HIV infection* is usually mild, normochromic and normocytic.
- *Neutropenia* is common and usually mild.
- *Isolated thrombocytopenia* may occur early in infection and be the only manifestation of HIV for some time. Platelet counts are often moderately reduced but can fall dramatically to $10–20 \times 10^9$/L producing easy bleeding and bruising. Circulating antiplatelet antibodies lead to peripheral destruction.

Megakaryocytes are increased in the bone marrow but their function is impaired. Effective anti-retroviral therapy usually produces a rise in platelet count. Thrombocytopenic patients undergoing dental, medical or surgical procedures may need therapy with human immunoglobulin, which gives a transient rise in platelet count, or be given platelet transfusion. Steroids are best avoided.

- *Pancytopenia* occurs because of underlying opportunistic infection or malignancies, in particular *Mycobacterium avium-intracellulare*, disseminated cytomegalovirus and lymphoma.
- *Other complications.* Myelotoxic drugs include zidovudine (megaloblastic anaemia, red cell aplasia, neutropenia), lamivudine (anaemia, neutropenia), ganciclovir (neutropenia), systemic chemotherapy (pancytopenia) and co-trimoxazole (agranulocytosis).

Gastrointestinal effects (see p. 324)

Weight loss and diarrhoea are extremely common in HIV-infected patients. Wasting is a common feature of advanced HIV infection, which although originally attributed to direct HIV effects on metabolism, is usually a consequence of anorexia. There is a small increase in resting energy expenditure in all stages of HIV, but weight and lean body mass usually remain normal during periods of clinical latency when the patient is eating normally.

HIV enteropathy is a term that has been used to describe a syndrome of diarrhoea, malabsorption and weight loss for which no other pathology has been found. HIV infection of the lymphocytes (in the lamina propria) which are distributed throughout both the large and small bowel, with disturbance of cytokine production, may be responsible. Villous atrophy is a common histological finding in the small bowel.

Hypochlorhydria is reported in patients with advanced HIV disease and may have consequences for drug absorption and bacterial overgrowth in the gut.

Rectal lymphoid tissue cells are the targets for HIV infection during penetrative anal sex and may be a reservoir for infection to spread through the body.

Renal complications

HIV-associated nephropathy (HIVAN) (see p. 607), although rare, can cause significant renal impairment particularly in more advanced disease. It is most frequently seen in black African male patients and appears to be exacerbated by heroin use.

Nephrotic syndrome subsequent to *focal glomerulosclerosis* is the usual pathology, which may be a consequence of HIV cytopathic effects on renal tubular epithelium. The course is usually relentlessly progressive and dialysis may be required.

Many nephrotoxic drugs are used in the management of HIV-associated pathology, particularly foscarnet, amphotericin B, pentamidine, sulfadiazine and indinavir.

Respiratory complications

The upper airway and lungs serve as a physical barrier to airborne pathogens and any damage will decrease the efficiency of protection, leading to an increase in upper and lower respiratory tract infections. The sinus mucosa may also function abnormally in HIV infection and is frequently the site of chronic inflammation. Response to antibacterial therapy and topical steroids is usual but some patients require surgical intervention. A similar process is seen in the middle ear, which can lead to chronic otitis media.

Lymphoid interstitial pneumonitis (LIP) is well described in paediatric HIV infection but is uncommon in adults. There is an infiltration of lymphocytes, plasma cells and lymphoblasts in alveolar tissue. Epstein–Barr virus may be present. The patient presents with dyspnoea, and a dry cough, which may be confused with pneumocystis infection (see p. 889). Reticular nodular shadowing is seen on chest X-ray. Therapy with steroids may produce clinical and histological benefit in some patients.

Endocrine complications

Various endocrine abnormalities have been reported, including reduced levels of testosterone and abnormal adrenal function. The latter may assume clinical significance in more advanced disease when intercurrent infection superimposed upon borderline adrenal function may precipitate clear adrenal insufficiency requiring replacement doses of gluco- and mineralocorticoid. CMV is also implicated in adrenal-deficient states.

Cardiac complications

Cardiomyopathy associated with HIV may lead to congestive cardiac failure. Lymphocytic and necrotic myocarditis have been described. Ventricular biopsy should be performed to ensure other treatable causes of myocarditis are excluded. Antiretrovirals, particularly zidovudine, may be helpful.

Conditions due to immunodeficiency

Immunodeficiency allows the development of opportunistic infections (OI) (Table 2.51). These are diseases caused by organisms that are not usually considered pathogenic, unusual presentations of known pathogens, and the occurrence of tumours that may have an oncogenic viral aetiology. Susceptibility increases as the patient becomes more immunosuppressed. CD4 T lymphocyte numbers are used as markers to predict the risk of infection. Patients with CD4 counts above 200 are at low risk for the majority of AIDS-defining OIs. A hierarchy of thresholds for specific infectious risks can be constructed. Mechanisms include defective T cell function against protozoa, fungi and viruses, impaired

Table 2.51
Major HIV-associated pathogens

Protozoa	Bacteria
Toxoplasma gondii	*Salmonella* spp.
Cryptosporidium parvum	*Mycobacterium tuberculosis*
Microsporidia spp.	*Mycobacterium avium-intracellulare*
Leishmania donovani	*Streptococcus pneumoniae*
Isospora belli	*Staphylococcus aureus*
	Haemophilus influenzae
Viruses	*Moraxella catarrhalis*
Cytomegalovirus	*Rhodococcus equii*
Herpes simplex	*Bartonella quintana*
Varicella zoster	*Nocardia*
Human papillomavirus	
Papovavirus	

Fungi and yeasts
Pneumocystis carinii
Cryptococcus neoformans
Candida spp.
Dermatophytes (*Trichophyton*)
Aspergillus fumigatus
Histoplasma capsulatum
Coccidioides immitis

macrophage function against intracellular bacteria such as mycobacteria and salmonella and defective B cell immunity against capsulated bacteria such as *Strep. pneumoniae* and *Haemophilus*. Many of the organisms causing clinical disease are ubiquitous in the environment or are already carried by the patient.

Diagnosis in an immunosuppressed patient may be complicated by a lack of typical signs, as the inflammatory response is impaired. Examples are lack of neck stiffness in cryptococcal meningitis or minimal clinical findings in early *Pneumocystis carinii* pneumonia (PCP). Multiple pathogens may coexist. Indirect serological tests are frequently unreliable. Specimens must be obtained from the appropriate site for examination and culture in order to make a diagnosis.

Opportunistic infections in the highly active antiviral treatment (HAART) era

In many developed countries of the world the mortality and morbidity associated with HIV infection have declined dramatically since the introduction of potent antiretroviral therapy. In the USA the age-adjusted death rate from AIDS fell 48% between 1996 and 1997 and death rates across Europe fell fivefold between 1995 and 1998. Recent European data show a fall in AIDS-defining illnesses (ADI) from 30.7 per 100 patient years of observation to 2.5 per 100 patient years between 1994 and 1998, with patients on HAART having a lower rate of ADIs than patients not on HAART. However, the decline has been steeper for some OIs than others suggesting that the immune reconstitution due to

HAART may not be functionally equal against all HIV-associated complications. Not all patients have adequate responses to these medications, even if they are available and tolerable. Immune reconstitution with HAART may produce unusual responses to opportunistic pathogens and confuse the clinical picture. Thus prevention and treatment of OIs still remains part of the management of HIV infection.

Prevention of opportunistic infection in HIV-infected patients

Avoid infection
Exposure to certain organisms can be avoided in those known to be HIV infected. Attention to food hygiene will reduce exposure to salmonella, toxoplasmosis, *Cryptosporidium* and protected sexual intercourse will reduce exposure to herpes simplex virus (HSV), hepatitis B and papilloma viruses. Cytomegalovirus (CMV)-negative patients should be given CMV-negative blood products.

Immunization strategies
Immunization may not be as effective in HIV-infected individuals. Live virus vaccines should not be used (e.g. yellow fever, live polio).

Hepatitis A and B vaccines should be given for those without natural immunity who are at risk, particularly if there is coexisting liver pathology, e.g. hepatitis C.

Chemoprophylaxis
In the absence of a normal immune response many OIs are hard to eradicate using antimicrobials, and the recurrence rate is high. Primary and secondary chemoprophylaxis has reduced the incidence of many OIs. Advantages must be balanced against the potential for toxicity, drug interactions and cost with each medication added to what are often complex drug regimens.

Primary prophylaxis has been shown to be effective in reducing the risk of *Pneumocystis carinii*, toxoplasmosis and *Mycobacterium avium-intracellulare*.

Primary prophylaxis is not normally recommended against cytomegalovirus, herpesviruses or fungi.

With the introduction of HAART and immune reconstitution, ongoing chemoprophylaxis for previously life-threatening conditions (e.g. *Pneumocystis carinii*, cytomegalovirus retinitis, cryptococcus, toxoplasmosis, MAI) can be discontinued in those patients with CD4 counts that remain consistently above 200 and who have a low viral load. American guidelines for stopping and restarting prophylaxis have been published. It is necessary to review such decisions as clinical and laboratory parameters change. In developing countries unable to obtain HAART, long-term secondary prophylaxis is advocated. Other less severe but recurrent infections may also warrant prophylaxis (e.g. herpes simplex, candidiasis).

Specific conditions encountered in HIV infection

Fungal infections

Pneumocystis carinii (see p. 889)

This organism most commonly causes pneumonia (PCP) but can cause disseminated infection. It is not usually seen until patients are severely immunocompromised with a CD4 count below 200. The infection remains common although the use of primary prophylaxis in patients with CD4 < 200 has reduced the incidence. The organism damages alveolar epithelium, which impedes gas exchange and reduces lung compliance.

The onset is often insidious over a period of weeks, with a prolonged period of increasing shortness of breath (usually on exertion), non-productive cough, fever and malaise. Clinical examination reveals tachypnoea, tachycardia, cyanosis and signs of hypoxia. Fine crackles are heard on auscultation, although in mild cases there may be no auscultatory abnormality. In early infection the chest X-ray is normal but the typical appearances are of bilateral perihilar interstitial infiltrates, which can progress to confluent alveolar shadows throughout the lungs. High-resolution CT scans of the chest demonstrate a characteristic ground-glass appearance even when there is little to see on the chest X-ray. The patient is usually hypoxic and desaturates on exercise. Definitive diagnosis rests on demonstrating the organisms in the lungs via bronchoalveolar lavage. As the organism cannot be cultured in vitro it must be directly observed either with silver staining or immunofluorescent techniques.

Treatment should be instituted as early as possible. First-line therapy is with intravenous co-trimoxazole (100 mg/kg per day sulfamethoxazole and 20 mg/kg per day trimethoprim in divided doses) for 21 days. Up to 40% of patients receiving this regimen will develop some adverse drug reaction, including typical allergic rash. Mutations in the gene for dihydropteroate synthetase in *P. carinii*, which may theoretically lead to co-trimoxazole resistance, have been reported. There is, however, no evidence that co-trimoxazole is becoming less efficacious clinically. If the patient is sensitive to co-trimoxazole, intravenous pentamidine (4 mg/kg per day) or dapsone and trimethoprim are given for the same duration. Atovaquone or a combination of clindamycin and primaquine is also used. In severe cases (P_aO_2 less than 9.5 kPa), systemic corticosteroids have been shown to reduce mortality and should be added. Continuous positive airways pressure (CPAP) or mechanical ventilation (see p. 949) may be required if the patient remains severely hypoxic or becomes too tired. Pneumothorax not uncommonly complicates the clinical course in an already severely hypoxic patient.

Long-term secondary prophylaxis is required in developing countries *without* HAART in patients whose CD4 count remains below 200, and to prevent relapse, the usual regimen being co-trimoxazole 960 mg three times a week. Patients sensitive to sulphonamide are given either dapsone or pyrimethamine or nebulized pentamidine. The latter only protects the lungs and does not penetrate the upper lobes particularly efficiently; hence if relapses occur on this regimen they may be either atypical or extrapulmonary.

Cryptococcus (see p. 96)

The most common presentation of cryptococcus in the context of HIV is meningitis, although pulmonary and disseminated infections can also occur. The organism, *C. neoformans*, is widely distributed – often in bird droppings – and is usually acquired by inhalation. The onset may be insidious with non-specific fever, nausea and headache. As the infection progresses the conscious level is impaired and changes in affect may be noted. Fits or focal neurological presentations are uncommon. Neck stiffness and photophobia may be absent as these signs depend on the inflammatory response of the host, which in this setting is abnormal.

The diagnosis is made on examination of the CSF (a CT scan must be carried out before lumbar puncture to exclude space-occupying pathology). Indian ink staining shows the organisms directly and CSF cryptococcal antigen is positive at variable titre. It is unusual for the cryptococcal antigen to become negative after treatment, although the levels should fall substantially. Cryptococci can also be cultured from CSF and/or blood.

Factors associated with a poor prognosis include a high organism count in the CSF, a low white cell count in the CSF, and an impaired consciousness level at presentation.

Treatment. Initial treatment is usually with intravenous amphotericin B (0.7 mg/kg per day), although intravenous fluconazole (400 mg daily) is useful if renal function is impaired or if amphotericin side-effects are troublesome. Oral fluconazole can be substituted if the organism is shown to be fully sensitive and the patient is responding.

The mortality from a first episode of cryptococcal meningitis is up to 20%. Relapse is very common, possibly from a prostatic reservoir in men. Lifelong secondary prophylaxis is required in the absence of HAART.

Candida (see p. 94)

Mucosal infection with *Candida* is very common in HIV-infected patients. Oral *Candida* is one of the most common conditions. *C. albicans* is the usual organism, although *C. krusei* and *C. glabrata* occur. Pseudomembranous candidiasis consisting of creamy plaques in the mouth and pharynx is the best recognized. *Erythematous Candida* is more subtle and appears as reddened areas on the hard palate or as atypical areas on the tongue. Angular cheilitis can occur in association with either form or more rarely alone. Vulvovaginal *Candida* is often problematic.

Oesophageal Candida infection produces dysphagia with retrosternal discomfort (see p. 268). Barium swallow or endoscopy shows multiple areas of ulceration throughout the length of the oesophagus. Fluconazole or itraconazole are the agents of choice. With prolonged exposure to these agents in HIV-infected patients, azole-resistant *C. albicans* is becoming an increasing problem. Switching azoles may produce a response. Symptom relief may require intravenous amphotericin. *Disseminated Candida* is uncommon in the context of HIV infection. *C. krusei* may colonize patients who have been treated with fluconazole, as it is fluconazole-resistant. Amphotericin is useful in the treatment of this infection and an attempt to type *Candida* from clinically azole-resistant patients should be made.

Aspergillus (see p. 96)

Infection with *Aspergillus fumigatus* occurs in advanced HIV disease. *Aspergillus* is controlled by functioning neutrophils, and patients with long-standing neutropenia (often due to chemotherapy) and those on ganciclovir therapy for CMV and myelotoxic antiretrovirals, are prone to this infection. Spores are airborne and ubiquitous. Following inhalation, lung infection proceeds to haematogenous spread to other organs. Sinus infection occurs.

The prognosis is very poor, with amphotericin B being the mainstay of therapy. Itraconazole is also effective. It is almost impossible to deal effectively with *Aspergillus* unless the neutrophil count can be sustained, and neutropenic patients should be supported with granulocyte colony-stimulating factors.

Histoplasmosis (see p. 95)

This infection is a well-recognized complication of HIV in the USA where it is endemic in soil. The most common manifestation is with pneumonia, which may be confused with *Pneumocystis carinii* in its presentation (see above).

Superficial dermatophyte infections

These are common. Nail infection with *Tricophyton rubrum* causes onychomycosis (see p. 1279 and Table 2.52).

Protozoal infections

Toxoplasmosis (see p. 106)

Toxoplasma gondii most commonly causes encephalitis and cerebral abscess in the context of AIDS, usually as a result of reactivation of previously acquired infection. The incidence depends on the rate of seropositivity to toxoplasmosis in the particular population. High levels are found in France where up to 90% of the adult population is seropositive. About 50% of the adult UK population is toxoplasmosis seropositive. AIDS patients who have these antibodies may develop cerebral toxoplasmosis.

The clinical presentation is of a focal neurological lesion with convulsions, fever, headache and possible confusion. Examination reveals focal neurological signs in more than 50% of cases. Eye involvement with chorioretinitis may also be present. In most but not all cases toxoplasmosis serology is positive. Typically CT scan of the brain shows multiple ring-enhancing lesions. A single lesion on CT may be found to be one of several on MRI. A solitary lesion on MRI, however, makes a diagnosis of toxoplasmosis unlikely.

The definitive method of diagnosis is brain biopsy, but in most cases an empirical trial of anti-toxoplasmosis therapy is instituted and if this leads to radiological improvement within 3 weeks this is considered diagnostic. The differential diagnosis includes cerebral lymphoma, tuberculoma or focal cryptococcal infection.

Treatment is with pyrimethamine for at least 6 weeks (loading dose 200 mg, then 50 mg daily) combined with sulfadiazine and folinic acid. Clindamycin and pyrimethamine may be used in patients allergic to sulphonamide. Anticonvulsants should be given. Lifelong maintenance is required to prevent relapse unless the CD4 count can be restored by HAART. There is some evidence to suggest that co-trimoxazole as PCP prophylaxis has some ability to reduce the incidence of toxoplasmosis.

Cryptosporidiosis (see p. 108)

Cryptosporidium parvum can cause a self-limiting acute diarrhoea in an immunocompetent individual. In HIV

Table 2.52

Some mucocutaneous manifestations of HIV infection (see also Ch. 22)

Skin	Mucous membranes
Dry skin and scalp	Candidiasis
Onychomycosis	oral
Seborrhoeic dermatitis	vulvovaginal
Tinea	Hairy oral leucoplakia
cruris	Aphthous ulcers
pedis	Herpes simplex
Pityriasis	genital
versicolor	oral
rosea	labial
Folliculitis	Periodontal disease
Acne	Warts
Molluscum contagiosum	oral
Warts	genital
Herpes zoster	
multidermatomal	
disseminated	
Papular pruritic eruption	
Scabies	
Ichthyosis	
Kaposi's sarcoma	

infection it can cause severe and progressive watery diarrhoea which may be associated with anorexia, abdominal pain, nausea and vomiting. Cysts attach to the epithelium of the small bowel wall causing secretion of fluid into the gut lumen and failure of fluid absorption. It is associated with sclerosing cholangitis (see p. 393). The cysts are seen on stool specimen microscopy using Kinyoun acid-fast stain. The organism is readily identified in small bowel biopsy specimens.

Treatment is largely supportive, as there are no effective antimicrobial agents available other than a non-absorbable aminogylycoside, paromamycin, which may have a limited effect on diarrhoea.

Microsporidiosis (see p. 109)

Enterocytozoon bieneusi and *Septata intestinalis* are associated with diarrhoeal illness in HIV infection. Spores can be detected in stools using a trichrome or fluorescent stain that attaches to the chitin of the spore surface. Albendazole eradicates the infection with amelioration of symptoms.

Leishmaniasis (see p. 104)

This is a cause of illness in immunosuppressed HIV-infected individuals who have been in endemic areas, which include South America, tropical Africa and much of the Mediterranean. Symptoms are frequently non-specific with fever, malaise, diarrhoea and weight loss. Splenomegaly, anaemia and thrombocytopenia are significant findings. Amastigotes may be seen on bone marrow biopsy or from splenic aspirates. Serological tests exist for *Leishmania* but they are not reliable in this setting.

Treatment is based on sodium stibogluconate (pentavalent antimony) but in HIV infection the response may be better to liposomal amphotericin. Relapse is common unless long-term secondary prophylaxis is given.

Viral infections

Cytomegalovirus (see p. 49)

CMV can be a cause of considerable morbidity in HIV-infected individuals, especially in the later stages of disease. The major problems encountered are retinitis, colitis, oesophageal ulceration, encephalitis and pneumonitis. CMV infection is associated with an arteritis, which may be the major pathogenic mechanism. CMV also causes polyradiculopathy and adrenalitis.

CMV retinitis

This tends to occur once the CD4 count is below 100 and is found in up to 30% of AIDS cases. It is the most common cause of eye disease and blindness. Although usually unilateral to begin with, the infection frequently progresses to involve both eyes. Presenting features depend on the area of retina involved (loss of vision being most common with macular involvement) and include floaters, loss of visual acuity, field loss and scotomata, orbital pain and headache.

Examination of the fundus (Fig. 2.47) reveals haemorrhages and exudates, which follow the vasculature of the retina (so called 'pizza pie' appearances). The features are highly characteristic and the diagnosis is made clinically. Retinal detachment and papillitis may occasionally occur. If untreated, retinitis spreads within the eye, destroying the retina within its path. Routine fundoscopy should be carried out on all HIV-infected patients to look for evidence of early infection. Any patient with symptoms of visual disturbance should have a thorough examination with pupils dilated, and if no evident pathology is seen a specialist ophthalmologic opinion should be sought.

Treatment for CMV should be started as soon as possible with either ganciclovir (10 mg/kg daily) or foscarnet (60 mg/kg 8-hourly) given intravenously for at least 3 weeks, or until retinitis is quiescent. Reactivation is common, leading to blindness. The major side-effect of ganciclovir is myelosuppression and foscarnet is nephrotoxic. Maintenance therapy requires long-term vascular access through either a Hickman line or subcutaneous reservoir device. An oral form of ganciclovir is available which has some long-term benefit when used as maintenance therapy, but has a lower efficacy than intravenous ganciclovir. Ganciclovir can be given directly into the vitreous cavity but regular injections are required. A sustained-release implant of ganciclovir can be surgically inserted into the affected eye. Cidofovir is available for use when the above drugs are contraindicated. It has renal toxicity.

CMV colitis

The usual presenting features include abdominal pain, often generalized or left iliac, diarrhoea which may be bloody, generalized abdominal tenderness with rebound in some cases, and a low-grade fever. Loops of dilated large bowel may be seen on abdominal X-ray.

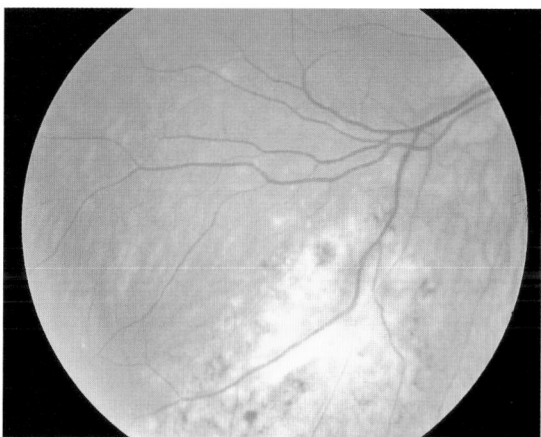

Fig. 2.47 Untreated CMV retinitis.

Sigmoidoscopy shows a friable or ulcerated mucosa, which should be biopsied. The diagnosis is made on the histological appearances with characteristic 'owls eye' cytoplasmic inclusion bodies (see Fig. 2.18).

Treatment with either intravenous ganciclovir or foscarnet for 3 weeks improves symptoms and the histological changes are reversed. However, relapse is common once therapy is stopped, unless HAART is available. The issue of long-term maintenance therapy in this situation is controversial since, unlike CMV retinitis, repeated attacks of colitis do not necessarily have significant long-term sequelae of the sort associated with retinitis. Given the complications associated with maintenance anti-CMV therapy there may be no overall benefit.

Other sites along the gastrointestinal tract also are prone to CMV infection. Solitary ulceration of the oesophagus, usually in the lower third, causes painful dysphagia. CMV can also cause hepatitis.

CMV neurological conditions

CMV polyradiculopathy usually affects the lumbosacral roots, leading to paraparesis and sphincter disturbance. The CSF has an increase in white cells, which surprisingly are almost all neutrophils. Although progression may be arrested by anti-CMV medication, functional recovery may not occur. The encephalopathy of CMV has clinical similarities to that caused by HIV itself. It tends to respond poorly to therapy.

Herpesviruses (see pp. 46 and 128)

Herpes simplex infection occurs with greater frequency and severity, presenting in an ulcerative rather than vesicle form in profoundly immunosuppressed individuals. Genital, oral and occasionally disseminated infection is seen. Viral shedding may be prolonged in comparison with immunocompetent patients.

Varicella zoster can occur at any stage of HIV but tends to be more aggressive and longer-lasting in the more immunosuppressed patient. Multidermatomal zoster may occur.

Herpesvirus 8 (HHV-8) is associated with Kaposi's sarcoma (see p. 50).

Therapy with aciclovir is usually effective. Frequent recurrences need suppressive therapy. Aciclovir-resistant strains (usually due to thymidine kinase deficient mutants) in HIV-infected patients have become more common. Such strains may respond to foscarnet.

Epstein–Barr virus (see p. 49)

Patients with HIV have been shown to have high levels of EBV colonization. There are increased EBV titres in oropharyngeal secretions and high levels of EBV-infected B cells. The normal T cell response to EBV is depressed in HIV. EBV is strongly associated with primary cerebral lymphoma and non-Hodgkin's lymphoma (see below). Hairy oral leucoplakia caused by EBV is a sign of immunosuppression first noted in HIV but now also recognized in other conditions. It appears intermittently on the lateral borders of the tongue or the buccal mucosa as a pale ridged lesion. Although usually asymptomatic, patients may find it unsightly and occasionally painful. The virus can be identified histologically and on electronmicroscopy. There is a variable response to aciclovir.

Human papillomavirus (see p. 50)

HPV produces genital, plantar and occasionally oral warts, which may be slow to respond to therapy and recur repeatedly. HPV is associated with the more rapid development of cervical and anal intraepithelial neoplasia, which in time may progress to squamous cell carcinoma of the cervix or rectum in HIV-infected individuals.

Papovavirus (see p. 50)

JC virus, a member of the papovavirus family, which infects oligodendrocytes, causes progressive multifocal leucoencephalopathy (PML). This leads to demyelination particularly within the white matter of the brain. The features are of progressive neurological and/or intellectual impairment, often including hemiparesis or aphasia. The course is usually inexorably progressive but a stuttering course may be seen. Radiologically the lesions are usually multiple and confined to the white matter. They do not enhance with contrast and do not produce a mass effect. MRI (Fig. 2.48) is more sensitive than CT and reveals enhanced signal on T2-weighted images of the lesions. Definitive diagnosis is made on histological and viral examination of brain tissue obtained at biopsy. There is no specific therapy. HAART which enhances the immune response has, however, produced both clinical and radiological remission in a number of cases. Addition of cidofovir to HAART may improve outcome in some patients.

Bacterial infections

Bacterial infection in HIV is common and frequently disseminated. Cell-mediated immune responses normally control infection against intracellular bacteria,

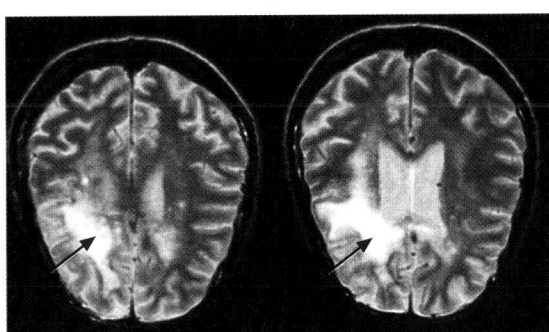

Fig. 2.48 MRI scans showing progressive multifocal leucoencephalopathy.

e.g. *Mycobacterium*. The abnormalities of B cell function associated with HIV lead to infections with encapsulated bacteria, as reduced production of IgG_2 cannot protect against the polysaccharide coat of such organisms. These functional abnormalities may be present well before there is a significant decline in CD4 numbers and so bacterial sepsis may be seen at early stages of HIV infection. *Streptococcus pneumonia, Haemophilus influenzae* and *Moraxella catarrhalis* infections are examples. Bacterial infection is often disseminated and, although usually amenable to standard antibiotic therapy, may reoccur. Long-term prophylaxis is required if recurrent infection is frequent.

Skin conditions such as folliculitis, abscesses and cellulitis are common and are usually caused by *Staphylococcus aureus*. Periodontal disease, which may be necrotizing, causes pain and damage to the gums. It is more common in smokers, but no specific causative agent has been identified. Therapy is with local debridement and systemic antibiotics.

Salmonella (non-typhoidal) (see p. 71) is a frequent pathogen in HIV infection. Salmonellas are able to survive within macrophages, this being a major factor in their pathogenicity. Organisms are usually acquired orally and frequently result in disseminated infection. Gastrointestinal disturbance may be disproportionate to the degree of dissemination, and once the pathogen is in the bloodstream any organ may be infected. Salmonella osteomyelitis and cystitis have been reported. Diagnosis is from blood and stool cultures.

Response to standard antibiotic therapy, depending on laboratory sensitivities, is usually good. Recurrent infection is, however, common and long-term prophylaxis may be required.

Education on food hygiene should be provided.

Mycobacteria

Mycobacterium tuberculosis (see p. 894)

The interaction between HIV and TB has several particular characteristics. Many parts of the world with a high prevalence of TB also have high rates of HIV infection. The respiratory transmission of TB means both HIV-positive and -negative people are being infected. Although more common in immunosuppressed patients, TB can cause disease when there is only minimal immunosuppression and thus often appears early in the course of HIV infection. In many countries where HIV is spreading and TB is endemic there has been a substantial increase in the incidence of tuberculosis. HIV-related TB frequently represents reactivation of latent TB, but there is also clear evidence of newly acquired infection and nosocomial spread in HIV-infected populations.

The pattern of disease differs with immunosuppression. Patients with relatively well preserved CD4 counts have a clinical picture similar to that seen in HIV-negative patients with pulmonary infection.

In more advanced HIV disease atypical pulmonary presentations without cavitation and prominent hilar lymphadenopathy, or extrapulmonary TB affecting lymph nodes, bone marrow or liver occur. Bacteraemia may be present.

The diagnosis depends on demonstrating the organisms in appropriate tissue specimens. The response to tuberculin testing is blunted in HIV-positive individuals and is unreliable. Sputum microscopy may be negative even in pulmonary infection and culture techniques are the best diagnostic tool.

M. tuberculosis infection usually responds well to standard treatment regimens, although the duration of therapy may be extended, especially in extrapulmonary infection. Multidrug resistance is becoming a problem, particularly in the USA where it is becoming a nosocomial danger. Cases from HIV units in the UK have been reported. Compliance with antituberculous therapy needs to be emphasized. Treatment of TB in the HIV-infected individual is not curative and long-term isoniazid prophylaxis may be given. In patients from TB endemic areas, primary prophylaxis may prevent emergence of infection. Immune reconstitution phenomenon as a result of HAART occurs (p. 150).

Mycobacterium avium-intracellulare

Atypical mycobacteria, particularly *M. avium-intracellulare* (MAI), generally appear only in the later stages of HIV infection when patients are profoundly immunosuppressed. It is a saprophytic organism of low pathogenicity that is ubiquitous in soil and water. Entry may be via the gastrointestinal tract or lungs with dissemination via infected macrophages.

The major clinical features are fevers, malaise, weight loss, anorexia and sweats. Dissemination to the bone marrow causes anaemia. Gastrointestinal symptoms may be prominent with diarrhoea and malabsorption. At this stage of disease patients frequently have other concurrent infections, so differentiating MAI is difficult on clinical grounds. Direct examination and culture of blood, lymph node, bone marrow or liver give the diagnosis most reliably.

MAI is typically resistant to standard antituberculous therapies, although ethambutol may be useful. Drugs such as rifabutin in combination with clarithromycin or azithromycin reduce the burden of organisms and in some ameliorate symptoms. A common combination is ethambutol, rifabutin and clarithromycin. Addition of amikacin to a drug regimen may produce a good symptomatic response. Primary prophylaxis with rifabutin or azithromycin may delay the appearance of MAI, but no corresponding increase in survival has been shown.

Infections due to other organisms

Strongyloides (see p. 114), a nematode found in tropical areas, may produce a hyperinfection syndrome in HIV-infected patients. Larvae are produced which invade through the bowel wall and migrate to the lung and occasionally to the brain. Albendazole or ivermectin may be used to control infection. Gram-negative septicaemia can develop (see p. 931).

Scabies (see p. 1281) may be much more severe in HIV infection. It may be widely disseminated over the body and appear as atypical, crusted papular lesions known as 'Norwegian scabies' from which mites are readily demonstrated. Superadded staphylococcal infection may occur. Treatment with conventional agents such as lindane may fail, and ivermectin has been used to good effect in some patients.

Neoplasms

The mortality and morbidity associated with neoplasia in HIV is substantial, with Kaposi's sarcoma and non-Hodgkin's lymphoma being the most significant tumours.

Kaposi's sarcoma (see p. 1308)

Kaposi's sarcoma (KS) in association with HIV (epidemic KS) behaves more aggressively than that associated with HIV-negative populations (endemic KS). The incidence has fallen significantly since the introduction of HAART. The tumour is most common in homosexual men and others who have acquired HIV sexually, particularly from a partner who has KS, implicating a sexually transmitted cofactor in the pathogenesis. Human herpesvirus 8 (HHV-8) is involved in pathogenesis. KS skin lesions are characteristically pigmented well circumscribed and occur in multiple sites. It is a multicentric tumour consisting of spindle cells and vascular endothelial cells, which together form slit-like spaces in which red blood cells become trapped. This process is responsible for the characteristic purple hue of the tumour. In addition to the skin lesions, KS affects lymphatics and lymph nodes, the lung and gastrointestinal tract, giving rise to a wide range of symptoms and signs. Most patients with visceral involvement also have skin or mucous membrane lesions. Visceral KS carries a worse prognosis than that confined to the skin. Kaposi's sarcoma is seen around the eye (Fig. 2.49), particularly in the conjunctivae, which can lead to periorbital oedema.

Treatment with local radiotherapy gives good results in skin lesions and is helpful in lymph node disease. Initiation of HAART may cause regression of lesions and prevent new ones emerging. For patients with aggressive disease, systemic chemotherapy is indicated using combinations of vincristine and bleomycin or the newer liposomal preparations of doxorubicin. Response is often very good although of uncertain duration. Interferon-α is also effective.

Lymphoma

A significant proportion of patients with HIV will at some stage develop lymphoma, mostly of the non-Hodgkin's, large B cell type. These are frequently extranodal, often

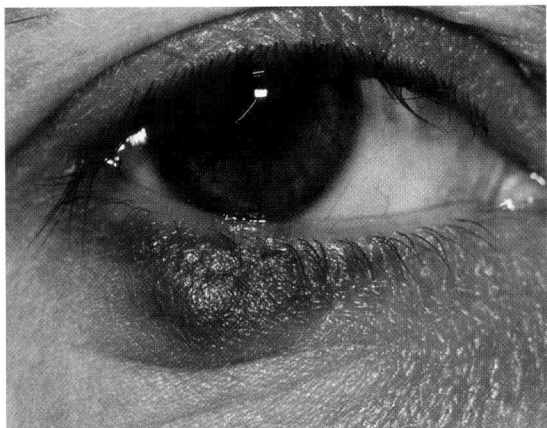

Fig. 2.49 **Kaposi's sarcoma of the eyelid.**

affecting the brain, lung and gastrointestinal tract. Many of these tumours are strongly associated with Epstein–Barr virus (EBV), with evidence of expression of latent gene nuclear antigens such as EBNA 1–6, some of which are involved in the immortalization of B cells and drive a neoplastic pathway.

HIV-associated lymphomas are frequently very aggressive. Patients often present with systemic 'B' syndromes and progress rapidly despite chemotherapy. Primary cerebral lymphoma is variably responsive to radiotherapy but overall carries a poor prognosis. Lymphomas occurring early in the course of HIV infection tend to respond better to therapy and carry a better prognosis, occasionally going into complete remission.

Squamous cell carcinoma

Squamous cell carcinoma, especially of the cervix and anus, is associated with HIV. Human papillomavirus may have a role in the pathogenesis of these malignancies. Women with HIV infection should have yearly cervical cytology for detection of premalignant change.

Investigations and monitoring

Initial assessment

A full history should be taken, followed by examination. Baseline investigations will depend on the clinical setting, but those for an asymptomatic person in the UK are shown in Box 2.18.

Monitoring

Patients are regularly monitored to assess the progression of the infection. Clinical examination will identify signs of immunosuppression (such as oral hairy leucoplakia) and detect early evidence of major opportunistic events. Decisions about appropriate intervention can be made.

Box 2.18

Baseline investigations in a newly diagnosed asymptomatic patient with HIV infection

Haematology
Full blood count, differential count and film
Erythrocyte sedimentation rate

Biochemistry
Serum, liver and renal function
Serum lipid profile
Blood glucose

Immunology
Lymphocyte subsets

Virology
HIV antibody (confirmatory)
HIV viral load
Hepatitis serology (A, B, and C)
Cytomegalovirus antibody

Microbiology
Toxoplasmosis serology
Syphilis serology
Screen for other sexually transmitted infections

Other
Cervical cytology

Immunological monitoring

CD4 lymphocytes. The absolute CD4 count and the percentage of total lymphocytes that this represents falls as HIV progresses. These figures bear a relationship to the risk of the occurrence of HIV-related pathology, with patients with counts below 200 cells at greatest risk. Rapidly falling CD4 counts and those below 350 are an indication to consider HAART. Routine assays measure numbers of circulating CD4 lymphocytes but are unable to assess cellular function, which may be abnormal, even when numbers are relatively well preserved. Factors other than HIV (e.g. smoking, exercise, intercurrent infections and diurnal variation) also affect CD4 numbers. CD4 counts are performed at approximately 3-monthly intervals unless values are approaching critical levels for intervention, in which case they are performed more frequently.

Virological monitoring

Viral load (HIV RNA)

The replication of HIV continues at a high rate throughout the course of infection, with many billion new virus particles being produced daily. The rate of viral clearance is relatively constant in any individual and thus the level of viraemia is a reflection of the rate of virus replication. This has both prognostic and therapeutic value.

The commonly used term 'viral load' has been coined to encompass viraemia and HIV RNA levels. Three HIV RNA assays for viral load are in current use:

- branched-chain DNA (bDNA)
- reverse transcription polymerase chain reaction (RT-PCR)
- nucleic acid sequence-based amplification (NASBA).

Results are given in copies of viral RNA per millilitre of plasma, or converted to a logarithmic scale and there is good correlation between tests. The most sensitive test is able to detect as few as 20 copies of viral RNA per

millilitre. Transient increases in viral load are seen following immunizations (e.g. for influenza and *Pneumococcus*) or during episodes of acute intercurrent infection (e.g. tuberculosis); and viral load measurements should not be carried out within a month of these events.

By about 6 months after seroconversion to HIV, the viral set-point for an individual is established and there is a correlation between HIV RNA levels and long-term prognosis, independent of the CD4 count. Those patients with a viral load consistently greater than 10 000 copies per millilitre have a 10 times higher risk of progression to AIDS over the ensuing 5 years than those consistently below 10 000 copies/mL. Although a correlation exists between viral load and CD4 cell numbers, the viral load appears to be the best predictor of the long-term prognosis, whilst the CD4 count will give warning of the risks of immediate or shorter-term problems.

HIV RNA is a useful marker of treatment efficacy, with levels falling in response to the introduction of effective antiretroviral medication (see below). Both duration and magnitude of virus suppression are pointers to clinical outcome. None of the currently available therapies is able to suppress viral replication indefinitely, and a rising viral load indicates drug failure.

Various guidelines exist for viral load monitoring in clinical practice. Baseline measurements are followed by repeat estimations at intervals of 3–4 months, ideally in conjunction with CD4 counts to allow both pieces of evidence to be used together in decision-making. Following initiation of antiretroviral therapy or changes in therapy, effects on viral load should be seen by 4 weeks, reaching a maximum at 10–12 weeks, when repeat viral load testing should be carried out (see Fig. 2.46).

Phenotype determination

Two phenotypes of HIV, syncytium-inducing (SI) and non-syncytium-inducing (NSI), exist and appear to correlate with disease progression. This is a specialized technique that is currently available only as a research tool.

Genotype determination

Clear genotype variations exist within HIV and there are increasing numbers of well-identified point mutations associated with antiretroviral drugs. Viral genotype is now entering routine practice to guide therapy, particularly in treatment-experienced patients and women who are pregnant.

Management of the HIV-infected patient (Box 2.19)

Despite the introduction of new antiretroviral agents there is still no cure for HIV and AIDS, and patients must live with a chronic, progressive, infectious and unpredictable condition. The aims of management in HIV infection are to maintain physical and mental health, to avoid transmission of the virus, and to maximise quality of life. The complexity of HIV infection means that it is best managed via a multidisciplinary team approach. Confidentiality must be strictly observed and care taken over establishing who is aware of the patient's diagnosis and who is excluded from that knowledge. Psychological support is needed not only for the patient but also for family, friends and carers. Dietary assessment and advice and support for adherence to medication should be freely accessible.

Clear advice on reducing the risk of HIV transmission and on childbearing must be provided.

Antiretroviral drugs (ARVs)

Highly active antiretroviral therapy (HAART), with at least three drugs used in combination, has led to a marked decline in the mortality and morbidity associated with HIV infection in the industrialized world. The aim of antiretroviral drug therapy is to suppress viral replication for as long as possible.

None of the current drug combinations eradicates HIV. Plasma RNA levels rise when therapy is stopped. Studies suggest that even in patients in whom viral replication is suppressed below the limits of detection for prolonged periods viral replication is ongoing.

Reasons include the existence of reservoirs of long-lived infected cells and reduced drug penetration into sanctuary sites.

The current drugs available for the treatment of HIV infection are shown in Table 2.53. Various events in the HIV life cycle have been identified as potential targets for antiretroviral therapy. Inhibitors of HIV reverse transcriptase and of HIV protease are so far the most developed (Table 2.53). Newer agents of these classes with improved pharmacokinetic and resistance profiles are coming into production.

Novel approaches in development are compounds that inhibit fusion of HIV to the host cell surface. These

---

Box 2.19

An approach to sick HIV-positive patients

Potential problems include
Acute opportunistic infections
Presentation or complication of malignancy
Adverse drug reactions
Immune reconstitution phenomenon
Infection in an immunocompromised host
Organic or functional brain disorders
Non-HIV-related pathology must not be forgotten

Full medical history
Remember:

● Antiretroviral drugs, prophylaxis, travel, previous HIV-related pathology, potential source of infectious agents (food hygiene, pets, contacts with acute infections, contact with TB, sexually transmitted infections)
● Secure confidentiality. Check with patient who is aware of HIV diagnosis.

Full physical examination
Remember:

● Signs of disseminated sepsis
● Clinical evidence of immunosuppression, e.g. oral candida, oral hairy leucoplakia
● Signs of adverse drug reactions, e.g. skin rashes, oral ulceration
● Focal neurological signs and/or meningism
● Evidence of altered mental state – organic or functional
● Examine:
  – the genitalia, e.g. herpes simplex, syphilis, gonorrhoea
  – the fundi, e.g. CMV retinitis
  – the mouth
● Lymphadenopathy.

Immediate investigations
Full blood count and differential count
Liver and renal function tests
Blood glucose
Blood gases including acid–base balance
Blood cultures, including specimens for mycobacterial culture
Microscopy and culture of available/appropriate specimens: stool, sputum, urine, CSF
Malaria screen in recently returned travellers
Serological tests for cryptococcal antigen, toxoplasmosis: save serum for viral studies
Chest X-ray
CT scan brain if focal neurological signs, and ALWAYS before lumbar puncture

NB: Lymphocyte subsets and HIV viral load assays may yield misleading results during intercurrent illness.

---

include peptides such as T-20 and T1249 and an anti-CCR5 monoclonal antibody PRO 140. HIV integrase is another target but development of inhibitors has been slow and complicated by the intricate workings of the enzyme. Drugs are unlikely to be available for clinical use for some years.

Table 2.53
Antiretroviral drugs

Drug	Daily dose and pill burden	Metabolism/food	Side-effects
Nucleoside reverse transcriptase inhibitors (nucleoside analogues, NA)			
Abacavir	300 mg × 2 daily 2 tablets/day	No food restrictions.	Hypersensitivity reaction, fever, rash, vomiting. Association with mitochondrial dysfunction and lactic acidosis.
Didanosine (DDI)	400 mg daily 1 capsule/day	30–60 minutes before food.	Nausea, diarrhoea, peripheral neuropathy, pancreatitis. Association with mitochondrial dysfunction and lactic acidosis.
Lamivudine (3TC)	150 mg × 2 daily 2 tablets/day	No food effects, well absorbed with high bioavailability.	Nausea, headache, rash, peripheral neuropathy, myelosuppression. Association with mitochondrial dysfunction and lactic acidosis.
Stavudine (D4T)	40 mg × 2 daily 2 capsules/day Reduce to 30 mg × 2 daily for persons less than 60 kg	High bioavailability. Competes with zidovudine for phosphorylation so do not use together.	Polyneuropathy. May be able to tolerate reduced dosage. Megaloblastic changes. Association with mitochondrial dysfunction and lactic acidosis.
Zalcitabine (DDC)	0.75 mg × 3 daily 3 tablets/day	No food effects.	Polyneuropathy, aphthous ulceration. Association with mitochondrial dysfunction and lactic acidosis.
Zidovudine (AZT)	250–300 mg × 2 daily 2 capsules/day	Well absorbed with good bioavailability. No food effects.	Nausea, headache, insomnia, skin and nail pigmentation, myelosuppression, megaloblastic changes. Myelopathy with extended use. Association with mitochondrial dysfunction and lactic acidosis.
Non-nucleoside reverse transcriptase inhibitors (NNRTI)			
Efavirenz	600 mg daily 3 capsules at night	Metabolised by cytochrome p450 (3A, mixed inducer and inhibitor). Do not take with high fat foods.	Rash, Stevens–Johnson syndrome, central nervous system effects (vivid dreams, agitation, hallucinations, and depression amongst others). Contraindicated in pregnancy.
Nevirapine	200 mg od for first 14 days then 200 mg × 2 daily 2 tablets/day	High bioavailability, long half-life, wide tissue distribution. Induces its own metabolism hence dose escalation. No food effects.	Rash, Stevens–Johnson syndrome, hepatic toxicity.
Protease inhibitors (Single drugs)			
Amprenavir (not licensed for ARV naive patients)	1200 mg × 2 daily 16 capsules/day	Cytochrome p450 inhibitor. High-fat meals lead to reduction in plasma drug levels.	Diarrhoea, nausea, rash, oral paraesthesia, abnormal liver function, body fat redistribution and abnormal plasma lipids.
Indinavir	800 mg × 3 daily 6 capsules/day	Food reduces plasma levels. Take one hour before or two hours after food. Drink additional 1.5 L water/day.	Nephrolithiasis and crystalluria, dry skin, nail dystrophy, alopecia, hyperbilirubinaemia, fat redistribution, raised plasma lipids, hyperglycaemia.
Nelfinavir	1250 mg × 2 daily 10 tablets/day	Take with food. Cytochrome p450 3A inhibitor.	Diarrhoea, fat redistribution, raised plasma lipids, hyperglycaemia.
Ritonavir	600 mg × 2 daily 12 capsules/day	Take with meals. Potent cytochrome p450 3A4 inhibitor.	Nausea/vomiting, diarrhoea, taste distortion, perioral paraesthesia, fat redistribution, hepatotoxicity, hyperglycaemia.
Saquinavir (soft gel)	1200 mg × 3 daily or 1800 mg × 2 daily 18 capsules/day	Take with food.	Nausea, diarrhoea, abdominal pain, fat redistribution, abnormal plasma lipids, hyperglycaemia.
Protease inhibitors boosted with ritonavir			
Lopinavir R	3 capsules × 2 daily 6 capsules/day	Take with food.	Diarrhoea, nausea, fat redistribution, abnormal plasma lipids.
Ritonavir/indinavir	100 mg/800 mg × 2 daily 6 capsules/day	With a light meal/snack.	As ritonavir and indinavir.
Ritonavir/saquinavir	400 mg/400 mg × 2 daily 12 capsules/day	With a light meal.	As ritonavir and saquinavir.

Reverse transcriptase inhibitors

These are of three classes, nucleoside analogues (NA), non-nucleoside analogues (NNRTI) and nucleotide analogues (NT).

- *Nucleoside analogues (NAs)* inhibit reverse transcription by binding to viral DNA and also act as DNA chain terminators. These were the first group of agents to be used against HIV, initially as monotherapy and later as dual drug combinations. Usually two drugs of this class are combined to provide the 'backbone' of a HAART regimen. Standard combinations are shown in Table 2.54. Zidovudine and lamivudine have been combined into a single tablet (Combivir), as also have zidovudine, lamivudine and abacavir (Trizavir), which helps reduce the pill burden. All NAs have been associated with lactic acidosis and mitochondrial toxicity.
- *Non-nucleoside reverse transcriptase inhibitors (NNRTIs)* interfere with reverse transcriptase by direct binding to the enzyme. They are generally small molecules that are widely disseminated throughout the body and have a long half-life. NNRTIs have clinically significant effects on cytochrome p450. They are ineffective against HIV-2. The level of cross-resistance across the class is very high. All have been associated with rashes and elevation of liver enzymes.
- *Nucleotide analogues (NT)* are competitive reverse transcriptase inhibitors and DNA chain terminators. There is no effect on cytochrome p450 and excretion is mainly via the kidney. Tenofovir has been approved in the USA (October 2001) and is available on a named patient basis in Europe.

Protease inhibitors (PIs)

These act competitively on the HIV aspartyl protease enzyme, which is involved in the production of functional viral proteins and enzymes. In consequence, viral maturation is impaired and immature dysfunctional viral particles are produced. Most of the protease inhibitors are active at very low concentrations and in vitro are found to have synergy with reverse-transcriptase inhibitors. However, there are marked differences in toxicity, pharmacokinetics and resistance patterns which influence prescribing. Cross-resistance is common across the PI group, which makes it difficult to use the drugs sequentially. There appears to be no activity against human aspartyl proteases (e.g. renin), although there are clinically significant interactions with the cytochrome p450 system. All PIs have been linked with abnormalities of fat metabolism and control of blood sugar, and some have been associated with deterioration in clotting function in people with haemophilia.

Drug resistance

Resistance to ARVs is a result of point mutations in the protease and reverse transcriptase genes of the virus. HIV has a rapid turnover with 10^7 replications occurring per day resulting in a high error rate with drug-resistant mutants. When drugs only partially inhibit virus replication there will be a selection pressure for the emergence of drug-resistant strains. The rate at which resistance develops depends on the frequency of pre-existing variants and the number of mutations required. Resistance to zidovudine occurs with an accumulation of mutations, whilst a single point mutation will confer high-level resistance to both NNRTIs.

Assays that measure the genetic structure of the reverse transcriptase and protease genes of HIV are

Table 2.54
Summary of combinations of antiretroviral drug combinations that may be used to initiate HIV therapy.
(Modified from BHIVA Guidelines 2001)

Nucleoside analogue backbone	Combined with one of	Drug class (listed alphabetically)	Dose	Potency	Adherence	Long term toxicity
Combination of two NAs e.g. (listed alphabetically)	Abacavir	NA	300 mg × 2	++	+++	+
	Efavirenz	NNRTI	600 mg daily	+++	+++	+
	Nevirapine	NNRTI	200 mg × 2	++	+++	+
	Indinavir	PI	800 mg × 3	++	+	+++
Stavudine + didanosine	Nelfinavir	PI	1250 mg × 2	++	++	++
Stavudine + lamivudine	Ritonavir	PI	600 mg × 2	++	++	++
Zidovudine + didanosine	Saquinavir soft gel	PI	1800 mg × 2	++	+	++
Zodovudine + lamivudine Zidovudine + zalcitabine	Lopinavir/ritonavir	Ritonavir boosted PI	400 mg/ 100 mg × 2	+++	++	++
Abacavir is usually included as a third drug but may be used to construct backbone	Ritonavir/indinavir	Ritonavir boosted PI	100 mg/ 800 mg × 2	++	++	+++
	Ritonavir/saquinavir	Ritonavir boosted PI	400 mg/ 400 mg × 2	++	++	++

+ low   ++ medium   +++ high

available. Such 'resistance tests' give an indication of drug susceptibility in only the predominant viral variants that are circulating and may miss changes in minor strains. Wild type virus reappears rapidly once drugs are stopped. For patients who are changing therapy resistance tests should be taken on treatment. Reliability is improved if the circulating level of virus is at least 1000 copies per mL. Studies of genotyping in patients in whom therapy is failing have shown a clear virological benefit in testing over not testing when selecting new drug combinations.

There is clear evidence for the transmission of HIV that is resistant to all or some classes of drugs. This is a matter for considerable concern and the testing of treatment-naive patients may be indicated. Resistance testing in pregnancy is recommended in the UK to guide therapy to prevent vertical transmission to the fetus.

Starting therapy

Although clear clinical benefit has been demonstrated with the use of antiretroviral drugs in advanced HIV disease, the evidence for the introduction of medication at earlier stages of infection is less clear-cut. None of the current therapeutic regimens is likely to be able to eradicate the virus from an individual, and there is a lack of data on the long-term effectiveness and toxicity of antiretrovirals. Strategic planning in antiretroviral use is becoming increasingly necessary.

Various national guidelines and treatment frameworks exist (e.g. British HIV Association (BHIVA) Guidelines, NHS Guidelines, and International AIDS Society (IAS) Recommendations). A combination of clinical assessment and laboratory marker data, including viral load and CD4 counts, guide therapeutic decision-making. Current UK guidance (BHIVA 2001) on starting antiretroviral drugs in adults is as follows:

- Patients should start therapy before the CD4 count falls below 200 cells/microlitre
- Treatment is not indicated in patients with a CD4 count greater than 350 cells/microlitre
- Patients with a CD4 count between 200 and 350 who have a high viral load or rapidly falling CD4 count may consider earlier intervention.

Special situations (seroconversion, pregnancy, post-exposure prophylaxis) in which antiretrovirals may be used are described on page 151.

Choice of drugs

The drug regimen used for starting therapy must be individualised to suit particular patient needs. Treatment is initiated with at least three drugs, two NAs in combination with either a NNRTI, a protease inhibitor, or with abacavir as a third NA (see Table 2.54). The choice of which drugs to include in initial therapy will be governed by potency, adherence issues, toxicity and side-effect profiles, potential drug–drug interactions,

resistance and cross-resistance patterns of the drugs and viral sensitivity. Virological success is a fall in viral load to less than 50 copies per mL within 6–9 months of staring treatment. Given that long-term patient adherence is essential to gain the most enduring viral suppression and to impede the emergence of drug resistance it is crucial that patients be fully involved in therapeutic decision making. Drug regimens that can be incorporated into normal, day to day life are more likely to produce overall benefits.

Adherence

Adherence to treatment is pivotal to success. Adherence levels less than 90–95% compromise virological and immunological responses. Many of the drugs used have a short half-life and require frequent dosing. Poor absorption and low bioavailability mean that for some compounds trough levels are barely adequate to suppress viral replication. For some regimens missing even a single dose will result in plasma drug levels falling dangerously low. Patchy adherence facilitates the emergence of drug-resistant variants, which in time will lead to virological failure. Cross-resistance within drug classes will further limit future options.

Monitoring therapy (Box 2.20)

Once ARV has been initiated the viral load should be measured at 4–8 weeks to assess efficacy. A drop of at least 0.5–1.0 log is a minimum if treatment is to be considered adequate. The durability of the virological response is linked both to the rate of viral load fall and the absolute nadir attained. The goal should be to achieve a viral load below the limits of detection. This is usually feasible for those starting therapy for the first time but may not be a realistic objective for heavily pretreated patients. Viral load and CD4 count should be measured at 12 weeks and then at 3-monthly intervals. Patients should be monitored.

Treatment failure

Failure of antiretroviral treatment, i.e. persistent viral replication causing immunological deterioration and

---

Box 2.20

Monitoring patients on highly active antiretroviral therapy (HAART)

- Clinical history and examination
- Weight
- HIV viral load
- Lymphocyte subsets
- Full blood count
- Liver and renal function
- Fasting lipid profile
- Blood glucose

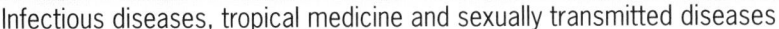

eventual clinical evidence of disease progression, is caused by a variety of factors. Even HAART drug regimens have limited potency. Food or other medication may compromise drug absorption. Drug interactions may interfere with metabolism and elimination of medication. There may be limited penetration of drug into sanctuary sites such as the CNS, permitting viral replication. Side-effects and other patient-related elements might contribute to poor adherence.

Changing therapy

A rise in viral load, a falling CD4 count or new clinical events that imply progression of HIV disease, are all reasons to review therapy. Reasons for treatment failure include the emergence of resistant viral strains, poor patient adherence, drug intolerance or adverse drug reactions.

If the patient has a viral load below the limit of detection and a change needs to be made because of intolerance then one or more drugs are altered.

If the patient is deteriorating clinically, virologically or immunologically then at least two or more drug changes should be made. A resistance test (see p. 149) is recommended. Salvage therapy, i.e. treatment following exposure to all classes of antiretroviral agents, is complex and may involve the use of at least five agents (mega HAART). Toxicity and benefit are often finely balanced in such circumstances.

Stopping therapy

Stopping antiretroviral drugs may be the proper course of action in a number of circumstances. Examples are cumulative toxicity, or potential drug interactions with medications needed to deal with another more pressing problem. Poor quality of life and the view of the patient on the matter must be considered.

Structured treatment interruptions (STIs) are being examined in those with well-controlled viral loads to look for potential HIV-specific immune responses. The adverse effects of viral rebound on the immune system are, however, a cause for concern. 'Drug holidays' in those who are virologically failing therapy and have multidrug-resistant viral strains may be considered. There is a suggestion that wild-type virus may re-emerge in such patients.

Complications of antiretroviral therapy

With increasing 'real life' use of these drugs a variety of complications of therapy are emerging. A syndrome of lipodystrophy comprising loss of subcutaneous fat in the arms, legs and face (lipoatrophy), deposition of intra-abdominal fat ('protease paunch'), increase in the dorsocervical fat pad (Buffalo hump) and breast enlargement is now well recognized although the exact aetiology is still unclear. Associated abnormalities in serum lipids, cholesterol and glucose are frequently seen. Many classes of ARVs are also implicated.

Mitochondrial toxicity, mostly involving the NA class, leads to raised lactate and lactic acidosis, which has in some cases been fatal. Symptoms are often vague and insidious and may include anorexia, nausea, abdominal pain and general malaise. Osteopenia, osteoporosis and avascular necrosis of bone occur with protease inhibitor-associated use.

Immune reconstitution can produce symptoms. This occurs usually in people who have been profoundly immunosuppressed who begin therapy. As their immune system recovers they are able to mount an inflammatory response to a range of pathogens. Examples include unusual mass lesions or lymphadenopathy associated with mycobacteria, inflammatory retinal lesions in association with cytomegalovirus, deterioration in liver function in chronic hepatitis B carriers and vigorous vesicular eruptions with herpes zoster.

Therapeutic drug monitoring. Poor bioavailability, variation in drug metabolism, drug–drug interactions and patient adherence can all lead to variations in circulating drug levels. Low plasma drug levels, in particular of protease inhibitors, have been shown to correlate with virological failure. Assays are mostly used to inform individual clinical situations rather than for routine use.

Specific therapeutic situations

Acute seroconversion

Antiretroviral therapy in patients presenting with an acute seroconversion illness is controversial. Preliminary evidence shows that the viral load can be reduced substantially by aggressive therapy at this stage, although it rises when treatment is withdrawn. The longer-term clinical sequelae are not yet known. If treatment is contemplated in this situation entry into a clinical trial may be considered. If patients are treated outside a clinical trial then a standard regimen is likely to be most appropriate, although the risk of limiting future options must be assessed.

Pregnancy

HIV-positive women should be advised against breast-feeding, which doubles the risk of vertical transmission. Delivery by caesarean section reduces the risk of transmission. The specific antiviral therapy drug choices are based on both maternal and fetal considerations. Risk of vertical transmission increases with viral load. Although the fetus will be exposed to more drugs the chances of reducing the viral load and hence preventing infection are greatest with a potent triple therapy regimen in the mother. Based on existing evidence the regimen should contain zidovudine, as this is the only agent shown to have an effect on vertical transmission. Treatment may start from 12–14 weeks of pregnancy and continue during delivery. The baby should receive zidovudine for 6 weeks postpartum. The woman should remain on treatment with appropriate monitoring and support. Women who do not need treatment for themselves may consider short-course triple therapy or zidovudine monotherapy to reduce vertical transmission. Treatment of the mother with zidovudine monotherapy is at variance with the data on combination therapy for adults as described on page 149. This may have longer-term implications for the course of the mother's HIV infection, particularly with regard to the possible emergence of zidovudine-resistant virus.

Post-exposure prophylaxis

Healthcare workers following occupational exposure to HIV must consider antiretroviral therapy. The British recommendation is zidovudine, lamivudine and indinavir for 4 weeks. Post-sexual-exposure prophylaxis may be appropriate in some situations. Drug regimens are guided by knowledge of the drug experience of the source patient.

Prevention and control

Antiretroviral drugs are not a cure and are accessible only to a privileged minority of the world's population. Vaccine development has been hampered by the genetic variability of the virus and the complex immune response that is required from the host. Prevention of new infection is fundamental to the control of the epidemic. Strategies that have been shown to be effective include treatment of sexually transmitted infections, consistent use of condoms, use of clean needles and syringes for drug users and antiretroviral drugs to reduce mother-to-child transmission. Topical microbicides for intravaginal use are in development.

Screening of blood products has reduced iatrogenic infection in developed countries but is expensive and not globally available.

Partner notification schemes are developing but are sensitive and controversial. Availability and accessibility of confidential HIV testing provides an opportunity for individual health education and risk reduction to be discussed.

Understanding and changing behaviour is crucial but notoriously difficult, especially in areas that carry as many taboos as sex, HIV and AIDS. Poverty, social unrest and war all contribute to the spread of HIV. Political will, not always readily available, is required if progress in these areas is to occur.

FURTHER READING

AIDS 2000 a year in review (2000) *AIDS* **14** (Suppl 3).
Antman K, Chang Y (2000) Kaposi's sarcoma. *New England Journal of Medicine* **342**: 1027–1038.
British HIV Association (BHIVA) (2001) Guidelines for the treatment of HIV-infected adults with antiretroviral therapy. BHIVA Writing Committee on behalf of the BHIVA Executive Committee. *HIV Medicine* **2**: 276–313.
Carpenter CC et al. (2000) Antiretroviral therapy in adults. Updated recommendations of the International AIDS Society. USA panel. *Journal of the American Medical Association* **283**: 381–391.
Centers for Disease Control and Prevention (April 2001) *Guidelines for the Use of Antiretroviral Agents in HIV – Infected Adults and Adolescents (the Living Document).* HIV/AIDS Treatment Information Service (ATIS) Atlanta GA. http://www.hivatis.org
The EuroGuidelines Group for HIV Resistance (2001) Clinical and laboratory guidelines for the use of HIV-1 drug resistance testing as part of treatment management: recommendations for the European setting. *AIDS* **15**: 309–320.
Kovacs, JA, Masur H (2000) Prophylaxis against opportunistic infections in patients with human immunodeficiency virus infection. *New England Journal of Medicine* **342(19)**: 1416–1429.
London Department of Health (1997). *Guidelines on Post-exposure Prophylaxis for Health Care Workers Occupationally Exposed to HIV.* Expert Advisory Group on AIDS.
Lyall EGH, Blott M, de Ruiter A et al. (2001) Guidelines for the management of HIV in pregnant women and the prevention of mother to child transmission. British HIV Association. *HIV Medicine* **2**: 314–334.
Mocroft, A, Katlama C, Johnson MA et al. (2000) AIDS across Europe 1994-1998: The EUROSIDA Study. *Lancet* **356**: 291–296.
Piscitelli SC, Gallicano KD (2001) Interaction among drugs for HIV and opportunistic infections. *New England Journal of Medicine* **344**: 984–996.
World AIDS Series (2000) Supplement to *Lancet* **356**: WA1–WA40.

Cell and molecular biology, and genetic disorders

3

The cell and cell biology

The cell (Fig. 3.1) is a highly organized structure and consists of various common organelles held by an adaptive internal scaffolding (the cytoskeleton), which radiates from the nuclear membrane to the cell plasma membrane. The number and finer detail of these common organelles varies according to the specialized function a cell might perform. For example, the muscle cell contains mitochondria with many infolded cristae, as it produces large amounts of ATP from the electron transport chain that sits on the inner membrane. However, the mitochondria of liver cells are smaller and rounded as they produce low levels of ATP, but many products from the inner matrix feed other metabolic pathways. Each cell is a component unit but can 'talk' to an adjacent cell via specific channels and receptors. Within a cell there is a constant flow of traffic between the organelles.

The cell membrane

The plasma cell membrane interfaces between the cell's internal mechanisms and the extracellular environment. It is a bilayer of amphipathic phospholipids that consist of a polar hydrophilic head (e.g. phosphatidyl choline) and an insoluble non-polar lipid hydrophobic tail (commonly two long-chain fatty acids). The phospholipids spontaneously form bilayers that, as complete circular structures, form an effective barrier that is impermeable to most water-soluble molecules. This barrier defines the interior environment of the cell and the exchanges across the plasma membrane are regulated by various proteins that are embedded in the lipid bilayer (Fig. 3.2). The lipids' hydrophobic structure means that relatively weak bonds hold the plasma membrane together. However, this strongly opposes the transverse movement of hydrophilic molecules but allows considerable freedom for lateral 'fluid' movement by molecules such as membrane proteins that are embedded in it. The plasma membrane is thus a very dynamic structure. Cell-to-cell communication is the key to many diseases and chemotherapeutic interventions.

The membrane proteins embedded in the lipid bilayer either traverse the whole membrane or are associated only with the outer or inner leaflet of the bilayer (Fig. 3.2). These proteins are responsible for the cell's

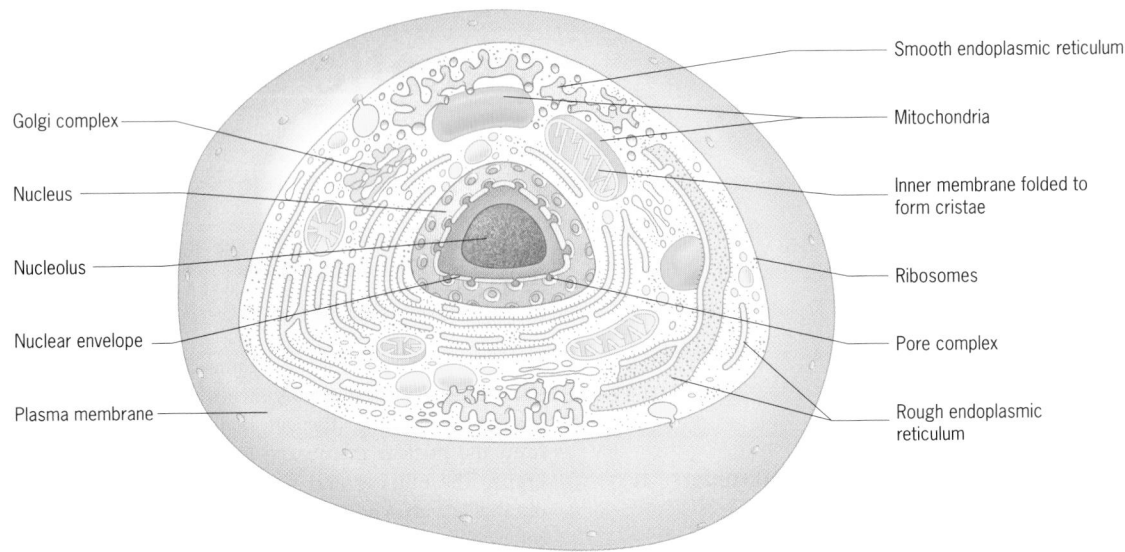

Fig. 3.1 Diagrammatic representation of the cell, illustrating the major organelles.

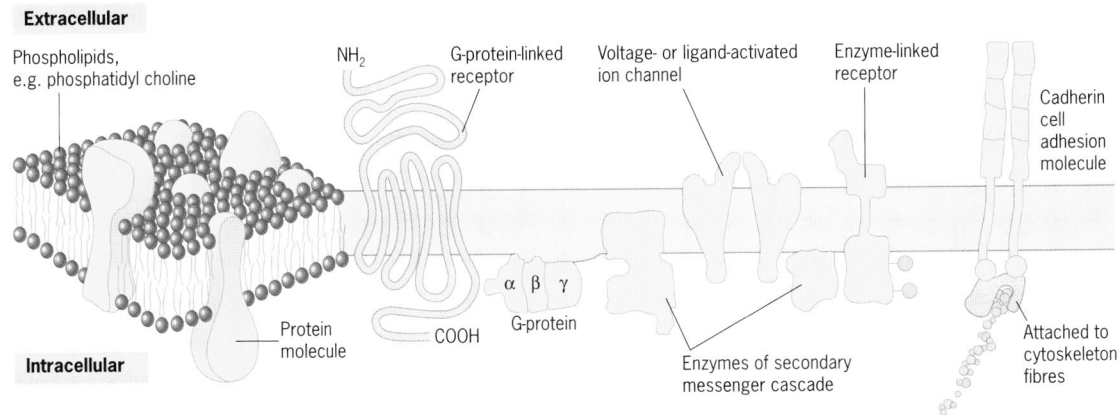

Fig. 3.2 Cell membrane showing lipid structures and main types of integral proteins such as receptors, G-proteins, channels, secondary messenger enzyme complexes and cell adhesion molecules.

interaction with its external environment. The molecules involved are either *channels*, *receptors* or *cell adhesion molecules* (see below).

Cell dynamics

Like all systems, the component proteins – and even organelles – of the cell are continually being formed and degraded. Most of the degradation steps involve ATP-dependent multienzyme complexes. Old cellular proteins are mopped up by a small cofactor molecule called '*ubiquitin*', which interacts with these worn proteins via their exposed lysine residues. The ubiquitin acts as a signal for destruction, and a complex containing more than five ubiquitin molecules is rapidly degraded by a large proteolytic multienzyme array termed '26S proteasome'. The failure to remove worn proteins

can result in the development of chronic debilitating disorders. Alzheimer and fronto-temporal dementias are associated with the accumulation of ubiquinated proteins (prion-like proteins), which are resistant to ubiquitin-mediated proteolysis. Similar proteolytic-resistant ubiquinated proteins give rise to inclusion bodies found in myositis and myopathies. This resistance can be due to point mutation in the target protein itself (e.g. mutant *p53* in cancer; see p. 184) or as a result of an external factor altering the conformation of the normal protein to create a proteolytic-resistant shape, as in variant Creutzfeldt–Jakob disease (vCJD).

Phagocytosis, pinocytosis and exocytosis

Specialized cells such as macrophages and neutrophils can engulf about 20% of their surface area in the pursuit of large particles such as bacteria. Lysosomes rapidly fuse with phagosomes, giving equally rapid digestion of the contents, and recycling as much of the internalized membrane as possible. *Phagocytosis* is only triggered when specific cell surface receptors – such as the macrophage Fc receptor – are occupied by their ligand. *Pinocytosis* is a much smaller-scale model of phagocytosis and is continually occurring in all cells. In contrast to phagocytosis, receptors for smaller molecular complexes, such as low-density lipoprotein (LDL) (Fig. 3.3) result in surface clumping and the internal accumulation of a protein called *clathrin*. Clathrin-coated pits pinch inwards as clathrin-coated vesicles. Clathrin prevents fusion of lysosomes, and thus its removal will result in lysosomal fusion and degradation of the contents. Maintenance of a clathrin coat can result in transcellular transit of the contents and their *exocytosis* at another side of the plasma membrane, i.e. apical-to-basal surface transcytosis. Similarly, cell organelles bud off vesicles coated in clathrin to prevent lysosomal fusion and degradation. Some of these vesicles rapidly fuse with the plasma membrane and exocytose their contents. Other vesicles do not immediately fuse with the plasma membrane (or indeed any other organelle). The clathrin-coated vesicles have additional lipid bilayer-embedded proteins called v-SNAREs, which interact with target

organelle membrane proteins called t-SNAREs. Vesicle fusion is therefore specific, comprising fusion in the correct place (at a particular organelle or part of the plasma membrane) at the correct time (e.g. the fusion of neuronal transmitter vesicles and release of the transmitter at the synaptic membrane when stimulated).

Membrane transport and ion channels

The plasma membrane is freely permeable to gases such as O_2, CO_2 and N_2, and to small uncharged molecules such as H_2O (*not* H^+ and OH^-) and urea. Whilst larger hydrophobic lipid-soluble molecules – like steroids – also pass freely through the membrane, large uncharged molecules (glucose, amino acids and nucleotides) and small charged ions (K^+, Na^+, Ca^{2+}, Cl^-, Mg^{2+} and HCO_3^-) cannot pass unless via a specific transport protein embedded in the plasma membrane. Two structural types of transport molecules/complexes exist (Fig. 3.2):

- *Channel proteins* literally open a channel in the lipid membrane to allow a specific solute to pass through.
- *Carrier proteins* are slower in action, shuttling the solute across and either facilitating diffusion down a gradient across the membrane, or actively pumping solutes against the gradient using ATP as an energy source.

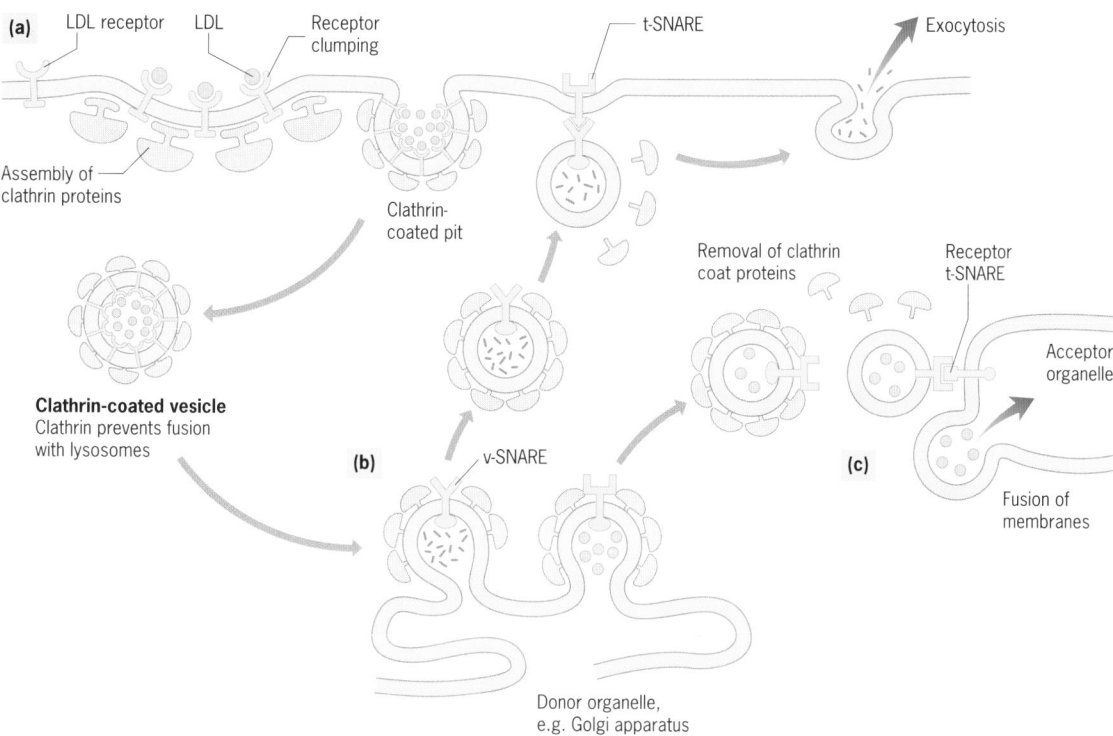

Fig. 3.3 **Intracellular transport. (a)** Receptor-mediated pinocytosis. **(b)** Trafficking of vesicles containing synthesized proteins to the cell surface (e.g. hormones). **(c)** Traffic between organelles is also mediated by v- and t-SNARE-containing organelles. v-SNARE, vesicle-specific SNARE; t-SNARE, target-specific SNARE.

Active carrier pumps and gated ion channels work together in neural transmission. These carrier proteins pump Na$^+$ and K$^+$ across the neuronal cell membrane to create a differential gradient, but ion channels open in response to stimuli to cause a rapid depolarization, allowing the ions to flow back. At synaptic junctions these ion channels open in response to chemical signals such as the release of glutamate, epinephrine (adrenaline) or acetylcholine.

ATP-dependent transport molecules (ATPases) belong to a superfamily called the '*ABC transporter superfamily*'. These include the multidrug-resistance protein (MDR), which pumps out hydrophobic drugs and is overexpressed by tumour cells, and the chloride ion pump coded by the cystic fibrosis gene (see Fig. 3.21). All share a common structure of six transmembrane domains interrupted by a cytoplasmic ATPase domain, followed by a further six transmembrane domains and another cytoplasmic ATPase. The cystic fibrosis chloride ion channel is unusual in that it requires the binding and hydrolysis of both ATP and cAMP for activation.

Receptors

Membrane surface receptors pass their extracellular signal across the plasma membrane to cytoplasmic secondary signalling molecules. Examples of these receptors include the non-lipid-soluble ligands such as growth hormone (GH), insulin, insulin-like growth factor (IGF) and luteinizing hormone (LH). These membrane-bound receptors can be subclassified according to the mechanism by which they activate signalling molecules:

- ion channel linked (see above)
- G-protein linked
- enzyme linked.

Structurally these plasma membrane receptors can be:

- serpentine (seven transmembrane domains, e.g. the LH receptor)
- transmembrane with large extra- and intracellular domains (e.g. the epidermal growth factor (EGF) receptor)
- transmembrane with a large extracellular domain only
- entirely linked onto the outer membrane leaflet by a lipid moiety known as a GPI (glycan phosphatidylinositol) anchor (e.g. T-cell receptor).

The function of these membrane receptors is to initiate a secondary message that ultimately results in activation of a DNA-binding protein. This translocates to the nucleus and initiates transcription of a specific set of genes.

G-protein-linked receptors

The G-protein-linked receptor, once activated by a ligand, binds a trimeric complex (α,β,γ) which is anchored to the inner surface of the plasma membrane. This complex is a GTP-binding protein, or G-protein. The G-protein binds GTP rather than GDP, and then interacts with enzyme complexes anchored into the inner leaflet of the membrane. These complexes in turn activate one or all three of the secondary messengers:

- cyclic AMP (cAMP)
- Ca^{2+} ions
- inositol 1,4,5-trisphosphate/diacylglycerol (IP$_3$/DAG).

Enzyme-linked surface receptors

These receptors usually have a single transmembrane-spanning region, and a cytoplasmic domain that has intrinsic enzyme activity or will bind and activate other membrane-bound or cytoplasmic enzyme complexes. Four classes of enzymes have been designated:

- *Guanylyl cyclase-linked receptors* (e.g. the atrial natriuretic peptide receptor), which produce cyclic GMP. This in turn activates a cGMP-dependent kinase (G-kinase), which binds to and phosphorylates serine and threonine residues of specific secondary messengers.
- *Tyrosine kinases receptors* (e.g. the platelet-derived growth factor (PDGF) receptor), which either specifically phosphorylate kinases on a small set of intracellular signalling proteins, or associate with proteins that have tyrosine kinase activity.
- *Tyrosine phosphatase receptors* (e.g. CD45), which remove phosphates from tyrosine residues of specific intracellular signalling proteins.
- *Serine/threonine kinase receptors* (e.g. the transforming growth factor-beta (TGF-β) receptor), which phosphorylate specific serine and threonine residues of intracellular signalling proteins.

There are many intracellular receptors that bind lipid-soluble ligands such as steroid hormones (e.g. progesterone, cortisol, T$_3$ and T$_4$). These cytoplasmic receptors often change shape in response to binding their ligands, form dimers, enter the nucleus and interact directly with specific DNA sequences (see DNA-binding proteins, p. 166).

Cytoplasm

This is the fluid component inside the cell membrane and contains many specialized organelles. It contains a scaffolding or cytoskeleton that regulates the passage and direction in which the interior solutes and storage granules flow. The cytoplasm contains:

- *Endoplasmic reticulum (ER).* This consists of interconnecting tubules or flattened sacs (cisternae) of lipid bilayer membrane. It may contain ribosomes on the surface (termed rough endoplasmic reticulum (RER) when present, or smooth endoplasmic reticulum (SER) when absent). The ER is involved in the processing of proteins: the ribosomes translate mRNA into a primary sequence of amino acids of a protein peptide chain (see Fig. 3.4). This chain is synthesized into the ER where it is first folded and modified into mature peptides. ER is the major site of drug metabolism.

- *Golgi apparatus*. This consists of flattened cisternae similar to the ER. It is characterized as a stack of cisternae from which vesicles bud off from the thickened ends. The primary processed peptides of the ER are exported to the Golgi apparatus for maturation into functional proteins (e.g. glycosylation of proteins which are to be excreted occurs here) before packaging into secretory granules and cellular vesicles that bud off the end.

- *Lysosomes*. These are dense cellular vesicles containing acidic digestive enzymes. They fuse with phagocytotic vesicles from the outer cell membrane, digesting the contents into small biomolecules that can cross the lysosomal lipid bilayer into the cell cytoplasm. Lysosomal enzymes can also be released outside the cell by fusion of the lysosome with the plasma membrane. Lysosomal action is crucial to the function of macrophages and polymorphs in killing and digesting infective agents, tissue remodelling during development and osteoclast remodelling of bone. Not surprisingly, many metabolic disorders result from impaired lysosomal function (p. 1116).

- *Peroxisomes*. These are dense cellular vesicles so named because they contain enzymes that catalyse the breakdown of hydrogen peroxide. They are involved in the metabolism of bile and fatty acids, and are primarily concerned with detoxification, for example D-amino acid oxidase and H_2O_2 catalase. The inability of the peroxisomes to function correctly can lead to rare metabolic disorders such as Zellweger's syndrome and rhizomelic dwarfism.

- *Mitochondria*. These organelles are the power house of the cell. Each mitochondrion comprises two lipid bilayer membranes and a central matrix. It also possesses several copies of its own DNA in a circular genome. The *outer membrane* contains many gated receptors responsible for the import of raw materials like pyruvate and ADP, and the export of products such as oxaloacetate (precursor of amino acids and sugars) and ATP. An interesting caveat to our symbiotic relationship is that proteins of the *Bcl2–bax* family are incorporated in this outer membrane and can release mitochondrial enzymes that trigger apoptosis (see pp. 162 and 184). The *inner membrane* is often highly infolded to form cristae to increase its effective surface area. It contains transmembrane enzyme complexes of the electron transport chain, which generate an H^+ ion gradient. This gradient then drives the adjacent transmembrane ATPase complex to form ATP from ADP and P_i. The *inner matrix* contains the enzymes of the Krebs cycle that generate the substrates of both the electron transport chain ($FADH_2$ and NADH) and central metabolism (e.g. succinyl CoA, α-oxoglutarate, oxaloacetate).

Secondary messengers

Secondary messengers are molecules that transduce a signal from a bound receptor to its site of action (e.g. the nucleus). There are essentially four mechanisms by which secondary messengers act but they cross talk and are rarely activated independently of each other (Fig. 3.4). These mechanisms are cyclic AMP, IP_3/DAG, Ca^{2+} ions and protein phosphorylation.

Cyclic AMP, IP_3/DAG and Ca^{2+} ions

The generation of cAMP by G-protein-linked receptors results in an increase in cellular cAMP (Fig. 3.4(a)), which binds and activates specific cAMP-binding proteins. These dimerize and enter the cell nucleus to interact with set DNA sequences (the cAMP response elements). In addition, cofactors in the cAMP-binding proteins are co-activated and interact with the phosphorylation pathway.

Other G-protein complexes activate inner membrane-bound phospholipase complexes. These in turn cleave membrane phospholipid-polyphosphoinositide (PIP_2) into two components (Fig. 3.4(b)). The first is the water-soluble molecule inositol trisphosphate, IP_3. This floats off into the cytoplasm and interacts with gated ion channels in the endoplasmic reticulum (or sarcoplasmic reticulum in muscle cells), causing a rapid release of Ca^{2+}. The lipid-soluble component diacylglycerol (DAG) (Fig. 3.4(c)) remains at the membrane, but activates a serine/threonine kinase, protein kinase C (see phosphorylation section below).

Although the cellular calcium-binding proteins and ion pumps rapidly remove Ca^{2+} from the cytoplasm back into a storage compartment (such as the endoplasmic reticulum), free Ca^{2+} interacts with target proteins in the cytoplasm, inducing a phosphorylation/dephosphorylation cascade, resulting in activated DNA-binding proteins entering the nucleus.

Protein phosphorylation

Although phosphorylation of the cytoplasmic secondary messengers is often a consequence of secondary activation of cAMP, Ca^{2+} and DAG, the principal route for the protein phosphorylation cascades is from the dimerization of surface protein kinase receptors, which have bound their ligands. The tyrosine kinase receptors phosphorylate each other when ligand binding brings the intracellular receptor components into close proximity (see Fig. 3.4(ii)). The inner membrane and cytoplasmic targets of these activated receptor complexes are

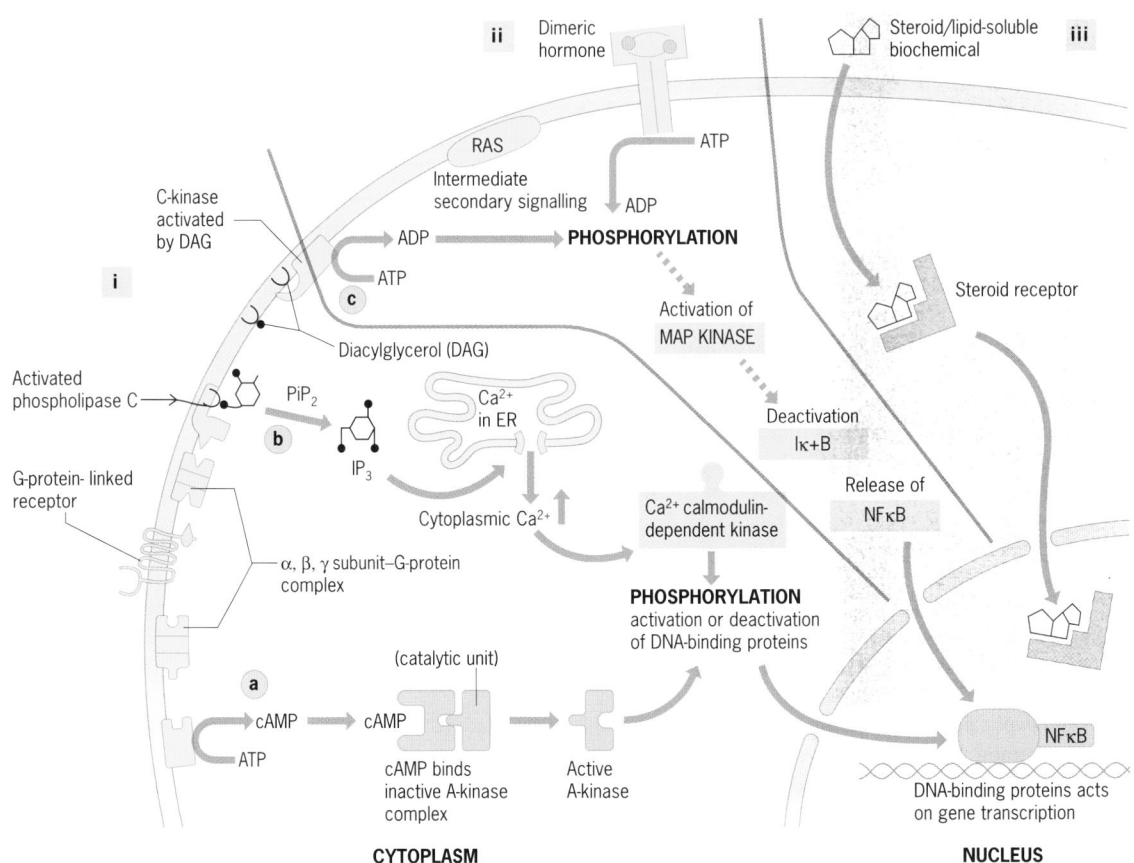

Fig. 3.4 Receptor and secondary messengers. (i) G-protein receptor binds ligand (e.g. hormone) and activates G-protein complex. The G-protein complex can activate three different secondary messengers: (a) cAMP generation; (b) inositol 1,4,5-trisphosphate (IP$_3$) and release of Ca^{2+}; (c) diacylglycerol (DAG) activation of C-kinase and subsequent protein phosphorylation. **(ii)** Dimeric hormone binds receptor subunits bringing them into close association. Intracellular domains cross-phosphorylate and link to the phosphorylation cascades via molecules such as RAS. **(iii)** Lipid-soluble molecules, e.g. steroids, pass through the cell membrane and bind to cytoplasmic receptors, which enter the nucleus and bind directly to DNA. ER, endoplasmic reticulum; IκB, inhibitory factor kappa B; NFκB, nuclear factor kappa B.

ras, protein kinase C and ultimately the MAP (microtubule associated protein) kinase, Janus-Stat pathways or phosphorylation of IκB causing it to release its DNA-binding protein, nuclear factor kappa B (NFκB). These intracellular signalling proteins usually contain conserved non-catalytic regions called SH2 and SH3 (serc homology regions 2 and 3). The SH2 region binds to phosphorylated tyrosine. The SH3 domain has been implicated in the recruitment of intermediates that activate *ras* proteins. Like G-proteins, *ras* (and its homologous family members *rho* and *rac*) switches between an inactive GDP-binding state and an active GTP-binding state. This starts a phosphorylation cascade of the MAP kinase, Janus-Stat protein pathways, which ultimately activate a DNA-binding protein. This undergoes a conformational change, enters the nucleus and initiates transcription of specific genes.

Lipid-soluble ligands (e.g. steroids) do not need secondary messengers; their cytoplasmic receptors, once activated, enter the nucleus as DNA-binding proteins and alter gene expression directly.

The cytoskeleton

This is a complex network of structural proteins which regulates not only the shape of the cell, but also its ability to traffic internal cell organelles and even move in response to external stimuli (see Fig. 3.2). The major components are microtubules, intermediate filaments and microfilaments.

• *Microtubules* (Fig. 3.5). These are made up of two protein subunits, α and β tubulin (50 kDa), and are continuously changing length. They form a 'highway', transporting organelles through the cytoplasm. There are two motor microtubule-associated proteins (MAP) – dynein and kinesin – allowing antegrade and retrograde movement. Dynein is also responsible for the beating of cilia. During interphase the microtubules are rearranged by the microtubule-organizing centre (MTOC), which consists of centrosomes containing tubulin and provides a structure on which the daughter

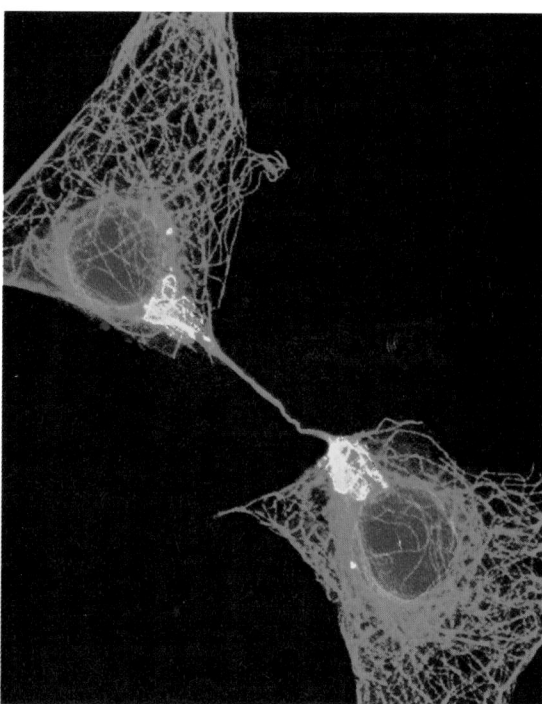

Fig. 3.5 **Immunofluorescent micrograph of dividing fibroblasts showing the cytoskeleton.** Microtubules are shown in green, Golgi apparatus in yellow and the nuclei in blue. Reproduced with permission of Dr Philip Huie, Stanford University, from *Biotechniques* July/August 1995.

chromosomes can separate. Another protein involved in the binding of organelles to microtubules is the cytoplasmic linker protein (CLIP). Drugs that disrupt the microtubule assembly (e.g. colchicine and vinblastine) affect the positioning and morphology of the organelles. The anticancer drug paclitaxel causes cell death by binding to microtubules and stabilizing them so much that organelles cannot move, and thus mitotic spindles cannot form.

- *Intermediate filaments.* These form a network around the nucleus and extend to the periphery of the cell. They make cell-to-cell contacts with the adjacent cells via desmosomes, and with basement matrix via hemidesmosomes (Fig. 3.6). Their function appears to be in structural integrity; they are prominent in cellular tissues under stress. The term cytoskeleton was first used to describe the crossing web of these intermediate (thickness) filaments (Fig. 3.6). The intermediate filament fibre proteins are specific to the embryonic lineage of the cell concerned, for example keratin intermediate fibres are only found in epithelial cells whilst vimentin is only found in mesothelial (fibroblastic) cells.
- *Microfilaments.* Muscle cells contain a highly ordered structure of actin (a globular protein, 42–44 kDa) and myosin filaments, which form the contractile system.

These filaments are also present throughout the non-muscle cells as truncated myosins (e.g. myosin 1), in the cytosol (forming a contractile actomyosin gel), and beneath the plasma membrane. Cell movement is mediated by the anchorage of actin filaments to the plasma membrane at adherent junctions between cells (Fig. 3.6). This allows a non-stressed coordination of contraction between adjacent cells of a tissue. Similarly vertical contraction of tissues is anchored across the cell membrane to the basement matrix at focal adhesion junctions where actin fibres converge (Fig. 3.6). Actin-binding proteins (e.g. fimbria) modulate the behaviour of microfilaments and their effects are often calcium-dependent. The actin-associated proteins can be tissue type specific, for example actin-binding troponin is a complex of three subunits and two of these have isomers which are only found in cardiac muscle. Cardiac troponin I and T are released into the blood circulation after the onset of a heart attack (p. 777).

Alterations in the cell's actin architecture are also controlled by the activation of small *ras*-like GTP-binding proteins *rho* and *rac*. These are important in rearrangement of the cell during division, and thus dysfunctions of these proteins are associated with malignancy.

Intercellular connections

The cytoskeleton and plasma membrane interconnect, and extracellular domains form junctions between cells to form tissues. There are three types of junction between cells: tight junctions, adherent junctions and gap junctions (Fig. 3.6).

Tight junctions

Tight junctions (zonula occludens) hold cells together. They are at the ends of margins adjacent to epithelial cells (e.g. intestinal and renal cells) and form a barrier to the movement of ions and solutes across the epithelium, although they can be variably 'leaky' to certain solutes. The proteins responsible for the intercellular tight junction closure are called *claudins*. They show selective expression within tissue and regulate what small ions may pass through the gaps between cells. For example, the kidney displays a differential expression of these claudin proteins. Mutations of claudin-16 (which is only expressed in the thick ascending limb of the loop of Henle, where magnesium is reabsorbed) are responsible for some forms of Gitelman's syndrome – a rare inherited hypomagnesaemia and hypokalaemia characterized by massive urinary magnesium and potassium loss, hypercalciuria and seizures at an early age (see p. 683). Since magnesium reabsorption is paracellular, tight junctions (which contain claudin-16) presumably prevent these divalent ions rapidly diffusing back between the cells into renal tubules.

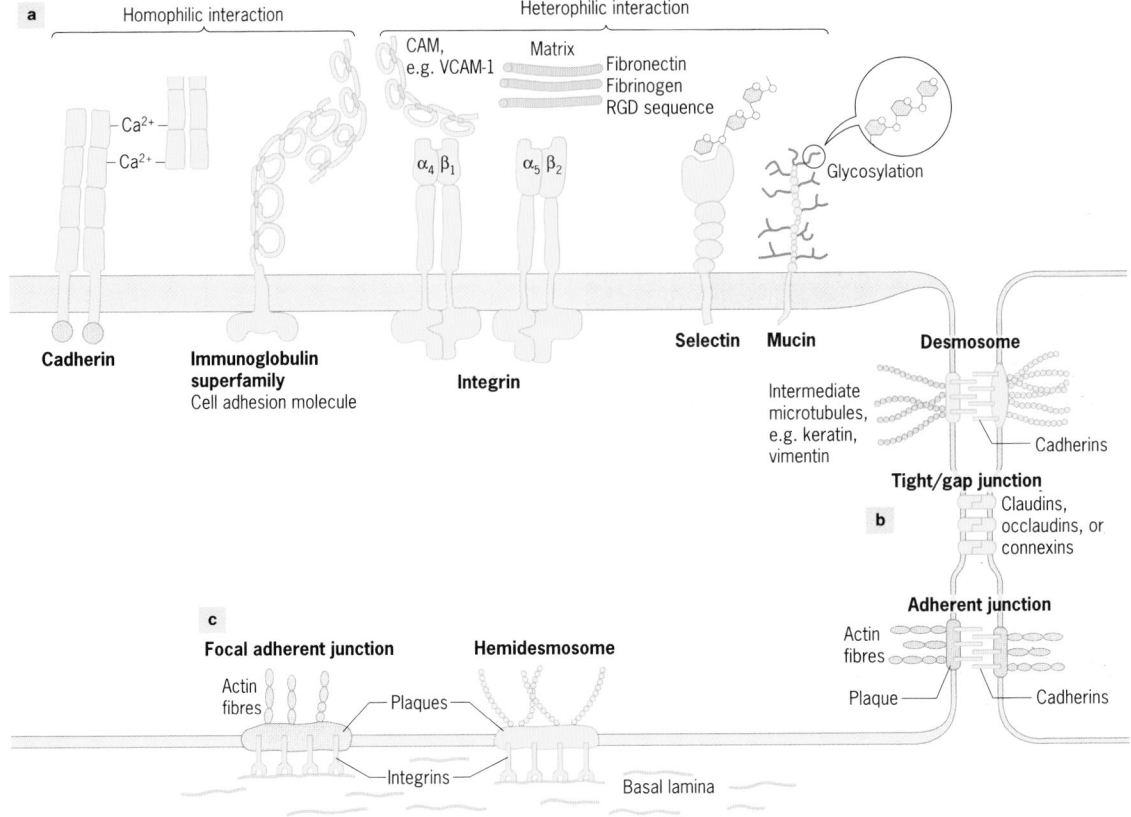

Fig. 3.6 Cell adhesion molecules and cellular junctions.

(a) Five main groups of adhesion molecules. The cadherins have a Ca^{2+}-dependent homodimer homophilic interaction and their intracellular domains link to the cytoskeleton. Immunoglobulin superfamily cell adhesion molecules (CAMs) have both homophilic and heterophilic (integrin) interactions. Binding is Ca^{2+} independent and the intracellular domains are cell signalling. Integrins have heterophilic interactions mostly with basement matrix components. They have an α–β chain structure and their intracellular domains are predominantly cell signalling but can directly interact with cytoskeletal complexes. Selectins have a weak binding affinity for specific sugar molecules found on mucins. Mucins are long random-repeat peptides which protrude from the cell membrane and are covered in glycosylation moieties.

(b) Adjacent cells form focal adhesion junctions. *Desmosomes* are where the membrane forms a proteinaceous plaque containing molecules like desmoglein, from which cadherins protrude and bind cadherins of the adjacent cell. Intracellularly the plaque binds loops of cytoskeleton intermediate filaments, e.g. keratin in epithelial cells and vimentin in fibroblasts. *Tight junctions* are mediated by integral membrane proteins, claudins and diclaudins, which associate to form subunits bridging the intercellular gap. *Gap junctions* consists of connexin subunits that form a regulated hollow tube. *Adherent junctions* are similar to desmosomes in that cell-to-cell adhesion is mediated by cadherins but the membrane proteinaceous plaque components are different and bind contractile cytoskeletal fibres like actin at the terminus.

(c) Basement membrane adhesion. This is similar to desmosomes and adherent junctions in that membrane plaques link intercellular intermediate filaments (e.g. keratin or vimentin) in *hemidesmosomes* and contractile cytoskeleton actin in *focal adherent junctions* to the basement matrix. However, integrins replace cadherins as the surface adhesion molecules.

Adherent junctions

Adherent junctions (zonula adherens) are continuous on the basal side of cells. They contain cadherins and are the major site of attachment of intracellular microfilaments. Intermediate filaments attach to *desmosomes*, which are apposed areas of thickened membranes of two adjacent cells. *Hemidesmosomes* attach cells to the basal lamina and are also connected to intermediate filaments. Transmembrane *integrins* link the extracellular matrix to microfilaments at focal areas where cells also attach to their basal laminae. In blistering dermatological disorders autoantibodies cause damage by attacking tight junction desmosomal proteins such as desmoglein-3 in *pemphigus vulgaris* and desmoglein-1 in *pemphigus foliaceus* (p. 1302).

Gap junctions

Gap junctions allow substances to pass directly between cells without entering the extracellular fluids. Protein channels (*connexons*) are lined up between two adjacent cells and allow the passage of solutes up to molecular weight 1000 kDa (e.g. amino acids and sugars), as well as ions, chemical messengers and other factors. The diameter of these channels is regulated by intracellular Ca^{2+}, pH and voltage. Connexons are made up of six subunits surrounding a channel and their isoforms in tissues are encoded by different genes. Mutant connexons can cause disorders, such as the X-linked form of Charcot–Marie–Tooth disease (p. 1216).

Cell adhesion molecules

(see also p. 193)

Adhesion molecules and adhesion receptors are essential for tissue structural organization. Differential expression of such molecules is implicit in the processes of cell growth and differentiation, such as wound repair and embryogenesis. There are four major families of cell adhesion molecules: cadherins, integrins, the immunoglobulin superfamily and selectins (Fig. 3.6).

Cadherins

The cadherins establish molecular links between adjacent cells. They form zipper-like structures at 'adherens junctions', areas of the plasma membrane where cells make contact with other cells. Through these junctions, bundles of actin filaments run from cell to cell. Related molecules such as desmogleins form the main constituents of desmosomes, the intercellular contacts found abundantly between epithelial cells. Desmosomes serve as anchoring sites for intermediate filaments of the cytoskeleton. When dissociated embryonic cells are grown in a dish, they tend to cluster according to their tissue of origin. The homophilic (like with like) interaction of cadherins is the basis of this separation, and has a key role in segregating embryonic tissues. The expression of specific adhesion molecules in the embryo is crucial for the migration of cells and the differentiation of tissues. For example, when neural crest cells stop producing N-CAM and N-cadherin and start to display integrin receptors they can separate, and begin to migrate on the extracellular matrix. Changes in cadherin expression are often associated with tumour metastatic potential.

Integrins

These are membrane glycoproteins with α and β subunits and exist in active and inactive forms. The integrins principally bind to extracellular matrix components such as fibrinogen, elastase and laminin. The amino acid sequence arginine–glycine–aspartic acid (RGD) is a potent recognition sequence for integrin binding, and integrins replace cadherins in the focal membrane anchorage of hemidesmosomes and focal adhesion junctions (Fig. 3.6). A feature of integrins is that the active form can come about as a result of a cytoplasmic signal that causes a conformational change in the extracellular domain, increasing affinity for its ligand. This 'inside-out' signalling occurs when leucocytes are stimulated by bacterial peptides, rapidly increasing leukocyte integrin affinity for immunoglobulin superfamilies structures such as the Fc portion of immunoglobulin. The 'outside-in' signalling follows the binding of the ligand to the integrin and stimulates secondary signals resulting in diverse events such as endocytosis, proliferation and apoptosis. Defective integrins are associated with many immunological and clotting disorders such as Bernard–Soulier syndrome and Glanzmann's thrombasthenia (p. 460).

Immunoglobulin superfamily cell adhesion molecules (CAMs)

These molecules contain domain sequences which are immunoglobulin-like structures. The neural-cell adhesion molecule (N-CAM) is found predominantly in the nervous system. It mediates a homophilic (like with like) adhesion. When bound to an identical molecule on another cell, N-CAM can also associate laterally with a fibroblast growth factor receptor and stimulate the tyrosine kinase activity of that receptor to induce the growth of neurites. Thus adhesion molecules can trigger cellular responses by indirect activation of other types of receptors. The placenta and gastrointestinal tract also express immunoglobulin superfamily members, but their function is not completely understood.

Selectins

Unlike most adhesion molecules (which bind to other proteins), the selectins interact with carbohydrate-ligands or *mucin* complexes on leucocytes and endothelial cells (vascular and haematological systems). Selectins were named after the tissues in which they were first identified. *L-selectin* is found on leucocytes and mediates the homing of lymphocytes to lymph nodes. *E-selectin* appears on endothelial cells after they have been activated by inflammatory cytokines; the small basal amount of E-selectin in many vascular beds appears to be necessary for the migration of leucocytes. *P-selectin* is stored in the alpha granules of platelets and the Weibel–Palade bodies of endothelial cells, but it moves rapidly to the plasma membrane upon stimulation of these cells. All three selectins play a part in leucocyte rolling (p. 192).

The nucleus and its responses

A nucleus is present in all eukaryotic cells that divide. It contains the human genome and is bound by two bilayer lipid membranes. The outer of the two is continuous with the endoplasmic reticulum. Nuclear pores are present in the membranes, allowing the passage of nuleotides and DNA interacting proteins in, and mRNA out (see Fig. 3.4). The genome consists of DNA and all the apparatus for replication and transcription into RNA (see p. 164). There are two types of cell division – meiosis and mitosis. In *meiosis*, which occurs only in germ cells, the chromosome complement is halved (haploid) and, at fertilization, the union of two cells restores the full complement of 46 chromosomes. *Mitosis* occurs in dividing cells after fertilization, and results in two identical daughter cells. It is only during cell division that chromosomes (see p. 175) become visible.

A nucleolus is a dense area within the nucleus. It is rich in proteins and RNA and is chiefly concerned with the synthesis of ribosomal RNA (rRNA) and ribosomes.

The cell cycle (Fig. 3.7)

Regulation of the cell cycle is complex. Cells in the quiescent G0 phase (G, gap) of the cycle are stimulated by the receptor-mediated actions of growth factors (e.g. EGF, epithelial growth factor; PDGF, platelet-derived growth factor; IGF, insulin-like growth factor) via intracellular second messengers. Stimuli are transmitted to the nucleus (see below) where they activate transcription factors and lead to the initiation of DNA synthesis, followed by mitosis and cell division. Cell cycling is modified by the cyclin family of proteins that activate or deactivate proteins involved in DNA replication by phosphorylation (via kinases and phosphatase domains). Thus from G0 the cell moves on to G1 (gap 1) when the chromosomes are prepared for replication. This is followed by the synthetic (S) phase, when the 46 chromosomes are duplicated into chromatids, followed by another gap phase (G2), which eventually leads to mitosis (M).

Apoptosis (programmed cell death)

(see also p. 184)

Necrotic cell death is where some external factor (e.g. hypoxia, chemical toxins) damages the cell's physiology and results in the disintegration of the cell. Characteristically there is an influx of water and ions, after which cellular organelles swell and rupture. Cell lysis induces acute inflammatory responses in vivo owing to the release of lysosomal enzymes into the extracellular environment. In apoptosis, physiological cell death occurs through the deliberate activation of constituent genes whose function is to cause their own demise. Apoptotic cell death has characteristic morphological features:

- chromatin aggregation, with nuclear and cytoplasmic condensation into distinct membrane-bound vesicles which are termed apoptotic bodies
- organelles remain intact
- cell 'blebs' (which are intact membrane vesicles)
- there is no inflammatory response
- cellular 'blebs' and remains are phagocytosed by adjacent cells and macrophages.

This process requires energy (ATP), and several Ca^{2+}- and Mg^{2+}-dependent nuclease systems are activated which specifically cleave nuclear DNA at the inter-histone residues.

An endonuclease destroys DNA following apoptosis. This involves the enzyme CASPASE (cysteine-containing aspartase-specific protease) which activates the CAD (caspase-activated DNase)/ICAD (inhibitor of CAD) system which can destroy DNA.

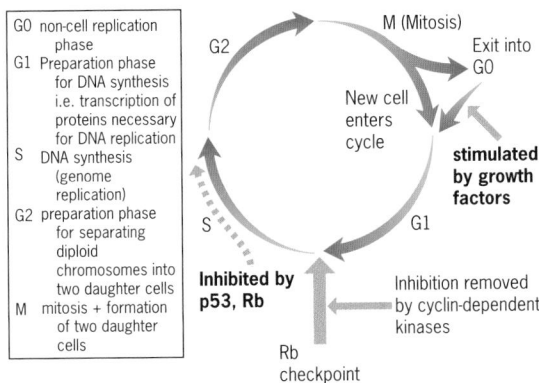

Fig. 3.7 **The cell cycle.** Cells are stimulated to leave non-cycle G0 to enter G1 phase by growth factors. During G1, transcription of the DNA synthesis molecules occurs. Rb is a 'checkpoint' (inhibition molecule) between G1 and S phases and must be removed for the cycle to continue. This is achieved by the action of the cyclin-dependent kinase produced during G1. During the S phase any DNA defects will be detected and *p53* will halt the cycle (see p. 184). Following DNA synthesis (S phase) cells enter G2, a preparation phase for cell division. Mitosis takes place in the M phase. The new daughter cells can now either enter G0 and differentiate into specialized cells, or re-enter the cell cycle.

It is now recognized that regulated apoptosis is essential for many life processes from tissue structure formation in embryogenesis and wound healing to normal metabolic processes such as autodestruction of the thickened endometrium to cause menstruation in a non-conception cycle. In oncology it has become clear that chemotherapy and radiotherapy regimes only work if they can trigger the tumour cells' own apoptotic pathways. Failure to do so in resistant tumours can result in the accumulation of further genetic damage to the surviving cells.

FURTHER READING

Ashcroft FM (2000) *Ion Channels and Disease.* San Diego: Academic Press

Blobe GC, Schiemann WP, Lodish HF (2000) Role of transforming growth factor-β in human disease. *New England Journal of Medicine* **342**: 1350–1358.

Cohen N (ed) (1991) *Cell Structure, Function and Metabolism.* London: Hodder and Stoughton.

Green KJ, Jones JCR (1996) Desmosomes and hemidesmosomes: structure and function of molecular components. *FASEB Journal* **10**: 871–881.

Mitic LL, Van Itallie CM, Anderson JM (2000) Molecular physiology and pathophysiology of tight junctions 1. Tight junction structure and function: lessons from mutant animals and proteins. *Gastrointestinal and Liver Physiology* **279**: 250–254.

Mitch WE, Goldberg AL (1996) The role of the ubiquitin–proteasome pathway. *New England Journal of Medicine* **335**: 1897–1905.

Molecular biology and genetic disorders

Over 200 genetic disorders have been identified, and the role of molecular biology in the diagnosis of monogenic disease is clear cut. The interaction of 'at risk' genes in multifactorial diseases has also increased the role of genetics in rheumatology, cancer, schizophrenia and many other more common human afflictions. The future promise of direct gene therapy makes the understanding of the principles and the basic tools of molecular genetics essential.

DNA structure and function

Genetic information is stored in the form of double-stranded deoxyribonucleic acid (DNA). Each strand of DNA is made up of a deoxyribose–phosphate backbone and a series of purine (adenine (A) and guanine (G)) and pyrimidine (thymine (T) and cytosine (C)) bases of the nucleic acid. For practical purposes the length of DNA is generally measured in numbers of base-pairs (bp).

The monomeric unit in DNA (and in RNA) is the nucleotide, which is a base joined to a sugar–phosphate unit (Fig. 3.8a). The two strands of DNA are held together by hydrogen bonds between the bases. There are only four possible pairs of nucleotides – TA, AT, GC

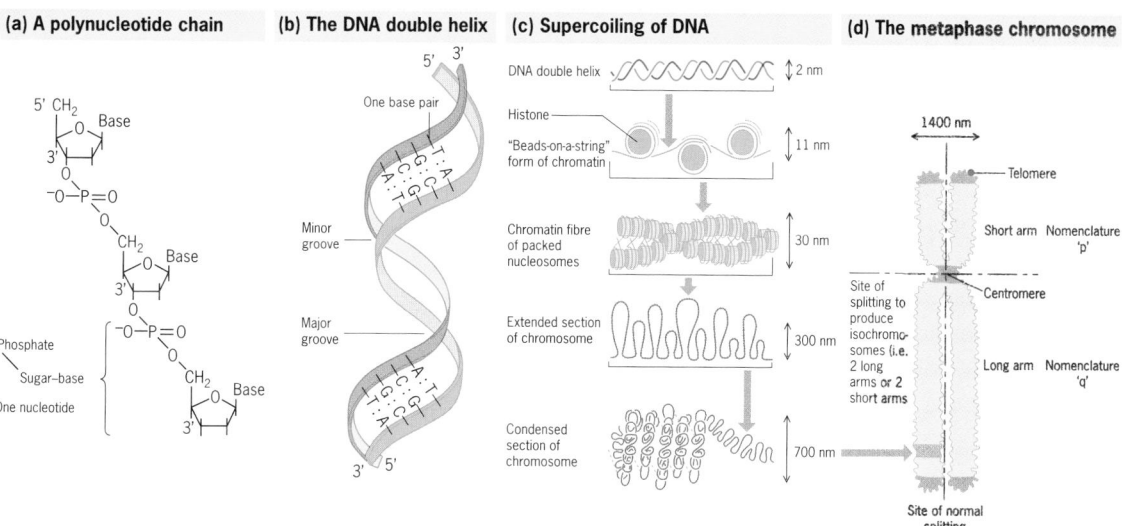

Fig. 3.8 DNA and its structural relationship to human chromosomes.

(a) A polynucleotide strand with the position of the nucleic bases indicated. Individual nucleotides form a polymer linked via the deoxyribose sugars. The 5′ carbon of the heterocyclic sugar structure links to the 3′ carbon of the next via a phosphate molecule forming the sugar–phosphate backbone of the nucleic acid. The 5′–3′ linkage gives an orientation to a sequence of DNA.

(b) Double-stranded DNA. The two strands of DNA are held together by hydrogen bonds between the bases. As T always pairs with A, and G with C, there are only four possible pairs of nucleotides – TA, AT, GC and CG. The orientation of the complementary single strands of DNA (ssDNA) is always opposite; i.e. one will be 5′–3′ whilst the partner will be 3′–5′. CG base-pairs form three hydrogen bonds whilst the AT bonds form only two. Thus, CG bonds are stronger than AT bonds, which affects the biophysical nature of different sequences of DNA. In a random sequence of DNA with equal proportions of CG and AT base-pairs, complementary strands form a helical 3D structure. This helix will have major and minor grooves and a complete turn of the helix will contain 12 base-pairs. These grooves are structurally important, as DNA-binding proteins predominantly interact with the major grooves. DNA sequences rich in repetitive CG base-pairs distort the helical shape whereby the minor grooves become more equal in size to the major grooves, giving a Z-like structure. These CG-rich regions are sites were DNA-binding proteins are likely to bind.

(c) Supercoiling of DNA. In humans, and other higher organisms, the large stretches of helical DNA are coiled to form nucleosomes and further condensed into the chromosomes that can be seen at metaphase. DNA is first packaged by winding around nuclear proteins – histones – every 180 bp. This can then be coiled and supercoiled to compact nucleosomes and eventually visible chromosomes.

(d) At the end of the metaphase DNA replication will result in a twin chromosome joined at the centromere. This picture shows the chromosome, its relationship to supercoiling, and the positions of structural regions: centromeres, telomeres and sites where the double chromosome can split.

Nomenclature of chromosomes. This is the assigned number or X or Y, plus short arm (p) or long arm (q). The region or subregion is defined by the transverse light and dark bands observed when staining with Giemsa (hence G-banding) or quinacrine and numbered from the centromere outwards. **Chromosome constitution** = chromosome number + sex chromosomes + abnormality; e.g.

    46XX = normal female
    47XX+21 = Down's syndrome (trisomy 21)
    46XYt (2;19) (p21;p12) = male with a normal number of chromosomes but a translocation between chromosome 2 and 19 with breakages at short-arm bands 21 and 12 of the respective chromosomes.

and CG (Fig. 3.8b). The two strands twist to form a double helix with major and minor grooves, and the large stretches of helical DNA are coiled around histone proteins to form nucleosomes and further condensed into the chromosomes that are seen at metaphase (Fig. 3.8c and d).

Genes

A gene is a portion of DNA that contains the codes for a polypeptide sequence. Three adjacent nucleotides (a codon) code for a particular amino acid, such as AGA for arginine, and TTC for phenylalanine. There are only 20 common amino acids, but 64 possible codon combinations that make up the genetic code. This means that some amino acids are encoded for by more than one triplet; other codons are used as signals for 'initiating' or 'terminating' polypeptide-chain synthesis, while others read as 'nonsense' and no amino acid is produced.

Genes consist of lengths of DNA that contain sufficient nucleotide triplets to code for the appropriate number of amino acids in the polypeptide chains of a particular protein. Genes vary greatly in size: most extend over 20–40 kbp, but a few (such as the gene for the muscle protein dystrophin) can extend over millions of base-pairs. In bacteria the coding sequences are continuous, but in higher organisms these coding sequences (exons) are interrupted by intervening sequences that are non-coding (introns) at various positions (see Fig. 3.9). Some genes code for RNA molecules which will not be further translated into proteins. These code for functional ribosomal RNA (rRNA) and transfer RNA (tRNA), which play vital roles in polypeptide synthesis.

Transcription and translation

(Fig. 3.9)

The conversion of genetic information to polypeptides and proteins relies on the transcription of sequences of bases in DNA to messenger RNA molecules; mRNAs are found mainly in the nucleolus and the cytoplasm, and are polymers of nucleotides containing a ribose–phosphate unit attached to a base. The bases are adenine, guanine, cytosine and uracil (U) (which replaces the thymine found in DNA). RNA is a single-stranded molecule but it can hybridize with a complementary sequence of single-stranded DNA (ssDNA). Genetic information is carried from the nucleus to the cytoplasm by mRNA, which in turn acts as a template for protein synthesis.

Each base in the mRNA molecule is lined up opposite to the corresponding base in the DNA: C to G, G to C, U to A and A to T. A gene is always read in the 5'–3' orientation and at 5' promoter sites which specifically bind

the enzyme RNA polymerase and so indicate where transcription is to commence. Eukaryotic genes have two AT-rich promoter sites. The first, the TATA box, is located about 25 bp upstream of (or before) the

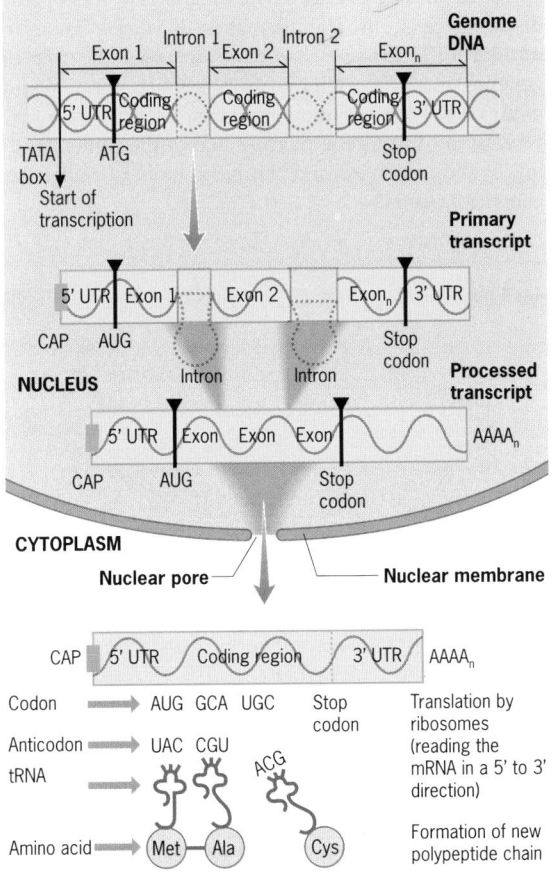

Fig. 3.9 **Transcription and translation (DNA to RNA to protein).** RNA polymerase creates an RNA copy of the gene sequence. This primary transcript is processed: capping of the 5' free end of the mRNA precursor involves the addition of an inverted guanine residue to the 5' terminal which is subsequently methylated, forming a 7-methylguanosine residue. (The corresponding position on the gene is thus called the CAP site.) The 3' end of an mRNA defined by the sequence AAUAAA acts as a cleavage signal for an endonuclease, which cleaves the growing transcript about 20 bp downstream from the signal. The 3' end is further processed by a Poly A polymerase which adds about 250 adenosine residues to the 3' end, forming a Poly A tail (polyadenylation). Without these additions the mRNA sequence will be rapidly degraded 5'–3' but the inverted cap nucleotide prevents nuclease attachment. The activity of specific 5' mRNA nucleases to remove the cap is further regulated by the Poly A tail which must first be removed by other degradation enzymes. Splicing out of the introns then produces the mature mRNA (prokaryote genes do not contain introns). This then moves out of the nucleus via nuclear pores and aligns on endoplasmic reticulum. Ribosomal subunits assemble on the mRNA moving along 5' to 3'. With the transport of amino acids to their active sites by specific tRNAs, the complex translates the code, producing the peptide sequence. Once formed the peptide is released into the cytoplasmic reticulum for post-translational modification into a mature protein.

transcription start site, while the second, the CAAT box, is 75 bp upstream of the start site. The initial or primary mRNA is a complete copy of one strand of DNA and therefore contains both introns and exons. While still in the nucleus, the mRNA undergoes post-transcriptional modification whereby the 5' and 3' ends are protected by the addition of an inverted guanidine nucleotide (CAP) and a chain of adenine nucleotides (Poly A) (see Fig. 3.9). In higher organisms, the primary transcript mRNA is further processed inside the nucleus whereby the introns are spliced out. Splicing is achieved by small nuclear RNA in association with specific proteins. Furthermore, alternative splicing is possible whereby an entire exon can be omitted. Thus more than one protein can be coded from the same gene. The processed mRNA then migrates out of the nucleus into the cytoplasm. Polysomes (groups of ribosomes) become attached to the mRNA; the ribosomes consist of subunits composed of small RNA molecules (rRNA) and proteins. The rRNA components are key to the binding and translation of the genetic code. Held by the ribosomes, triplets of adjacent bases on the mRNA called codons are exposed and recognized by complementary sequences, or anti-codons, in transfer RNA (tRNA) molecules. Each tRNA molecule carries an amino acid that is specific to the anti-codon. As the ribosome passes along the mRNA in the 5'–3' direction, amino acids are transferred from tRNA molecules and sequentially linked by the ribosome in the order dictated by the order of codons. The ribosome, in effect, moves along the mRNA like a 'zipper', linking the assembled amino acids to form a polypeptide chain. The first 20 or more nucleotides are recognition and regulatory sequences and are untranslated but necessary for translation and possibly earlier transcription. Translation begins when the triplet AUG (methionine) is encountered. All proteins start with methionine but this is often lost as the leading sequence of amino acids of the native peptides are removed during protein folding and post-translational modification into a mature protein. Similarly the Poly A tail is not translated (3' untranslated region) and is preceded by a stop codon, UAA, UAG or UGA.

The control of gene expression

Gene expression can be controlled at many points in the steps between the translation of DNA to proteins. Proteins and RNA molecules are in a constant state of turnover; as soon as they are produced, processes for their destruction are at work. For many genes transcriptional control is the most important point of regulation. Deleterious, even oncogenic, changes to a cell's biology may arise through no fault in the expression of a particular gene. Apparent over-expression may be due to non-breakdown of mRNA or protein product.

Transcriptional control

Gene transcription (DNA to mRNA) is not a spontaneous event and is possible only as a result of the interaction of a number of DNA-binding proteins with genomic DNA. Regulation of a gene's expression must first start with the opening up of the double helix of DNA in the correct region of the chromosome. In order to do this, a class of protein molecules that recognize the outside of the DNA helix have evolved. These DNA-binding proteins preferentially interact with the major groove of the DNA double helix (see Fig. 3.8). The base-pair composition of the DNA sequence can change the geometry of a DNA helix to facilitate the fit of a DNA-binding protein with its target region: CG-rich areas form the Z-structure DNA helix; sequences such as AAAANNN cause a slight bend, and if this is repeated every 10 nucleotides it produces pronounced curves. DNA-binding proteins that recognize these distorted helices result either in the opening up of the helix so that the gene may be transcribed, or in the prevention of the helix being opened.

Structural classes of DNA-binding proteins

There are four basic classes of DNA-binding protein, classified according to their structural motifs (see Fig. 3.10 and Table 3.1).

Control regions and proteins

DNA-binding proteins act as regulators of gene expression in three different ways. They are the promoters, the operators and the enhancers. The primary gene expression regulators are the *promoters*. The RNA polymerases bind to a promoter region, normally adjacent to the transcribed sequence of DNA. In prokaryotes these are single DNA-binding proteins, but in eukaryotes active transcription is possible only when a number of DNA-binding and associated proteins come together and interact. Known as 'general transcription factors', these proteins are thought to assemble at promoter sites used by the enzyme RNA polymerase II (Pol II) that are characterized by the TATA sequence.

Other DNA regulator proteins operate in close proximity to the site of promoter binding. These are called operator proteins/regions and act either as repressors by binding to DNA sequences within the promoter site (Fig. 3.11a), or as positive regulators facilitating RNA polymerase binding (Fig. 3.11b).

The third class of regulator proteins operate as enhancer sequences a considerable distance from the site of transcription initiation. Binding of regulator proteins to enhancer regions upregulates the expression of a gene up to several kilobases from the promoter site. This turns out to be a distance favourable for DNA to loop back on itself without straining the backbone bonds of the DNA double helix.

The GAL4 enhancer of yeast physically aids the binding of transcription factors to the TATA region of

(a) Helix–turn–helix

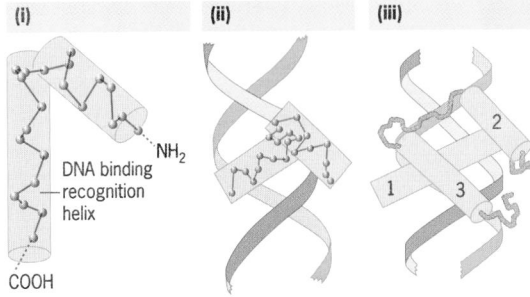

(b) Zinc finger

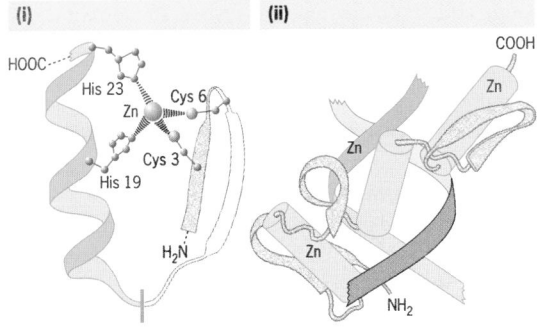

(c) Leucine zipper

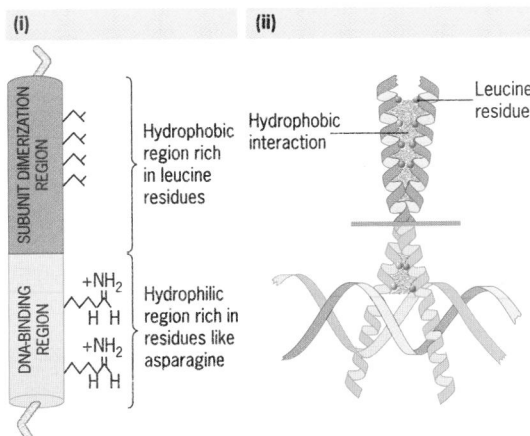

(d) Helix–loop–helix

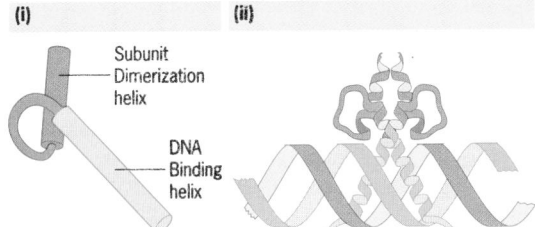

Fig. 3.10 **The four classes of DNA-binding proteins.**

(a) **Helix–turn–helix (HTH) motifs.** The simplest and most common, it consists of a helix connected by a fixed angle to a second helix. This represents the 'core' motif of HTH DNA-binding proteins but considerable modifications occur **(i)**. Like all DNA-binding proteins they interact as dimers, binding at exactly one turn of the double helix (3.4 nm or 12 bp) apart **(ii)**. The homeodomain HLH DNA-binding proteins are a special class of HTH proteins. Discovered in the 1980s during investigation of the gene controlling *Drosophila* development, they contain an almost identical stretch of 60 amino acids. They have a third helix which holds the DNA-binding region in a fixed orientation. Indeed, all homeodomain proteins appear to have specific conserved amino acid positions and residues which interact with DNA. Furthermore, random orientation extension chains at the N-terminal can interact with the minor groove **(iii)**.

(b) **Zinc finger motifs,** characterized by the incorporation of zinc, in some form, into the protein's quartenary structure. The term originated from the structural model of a *Xenopus laevis* protein which uses a zinc ion to hold a loop in a 'finger'-shape by cross-linking two histidine residues with two cysteine residues. The Cys–Cys–His–His family of zinc finger DNA regulator proteins typically consists of an anti-parallel sheet forming a tight tertiary association with its own helix by zinc interaction with Cys and His residues within each of the two secondary structures. Several clusters of zinc fingers are found together and form a repeating structure which can interact with repetitive sequences in DNA **(ii)**.

(c) **Leucine zipper motif,** consisting of a long α-helix which has many hydrophobic leucine residues at one end, responsible for dimer formation, whilst the opposite hydrophilic ends interact with DNA across the major groove of the double helix **(i)**. The quaternary structure of the leucine zippers need not be homodimeric, and indeed heterodimers are extremely common **(ii)**. Thus multiple sequences may be recognized by two or three DNA leucine zipper proteins depending on the type of dimer formed.

(d) **Helix–loop–helix (HLH) motifs.** These consist of a DNA-binding α-helix joined to a protein dimerization secondary α-helix via a loop **(i)**. These combine leucine zipper properties with those of helix motif DNA-binding proteins. A helix interacting with DNA is linked via a loop to a large second helix which non-covalently binds to a similar HLH protein. Homo- and heterodimers can form, but the loop gives flexibility in the orientation of the given DNA-binding α-helix domain **(ii)**.

Table 3.1

Examples of DNA-binding proteins

Class of DNA-binding protein	Examples
Helix-turn-helix	CREB (cAMP response element binding protein)
Zinc finger	Steroid and thyroid hormone receptors Retinoic acid and vitamin D receptors *bcl6* oncogene product (lymphoma) *WT1* oncogene product (Wilms' tumour) GATA-1 erythrocyte differentiation and Hb expression factor
Leucine zippers	*c-jun* cell replication oncogene *c-fos* cell replication oncogene
Helix-loop-helix	*myc* oncogene *mad* oncogene *max* oncogene

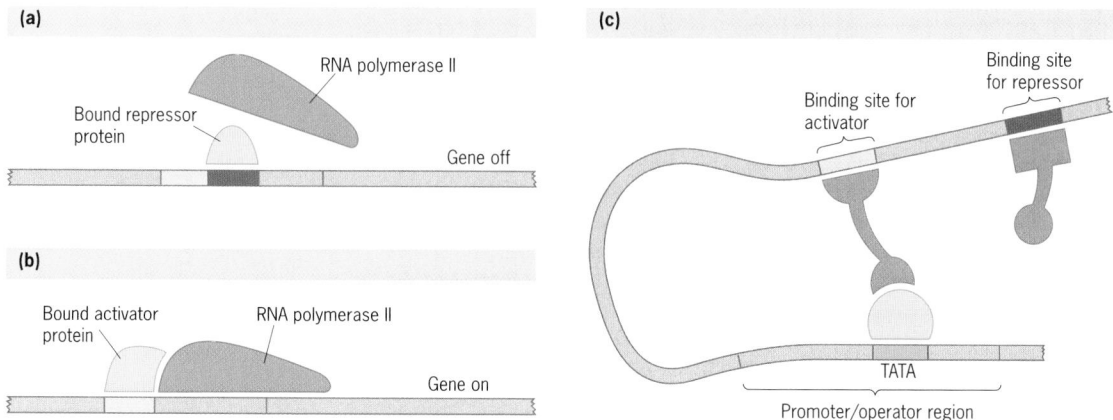

Fig. 3.11 The general transcription factors – operators and enhancers. DNA-binding proteins/regions can **(a)** bind to recognition sequences which lie within the binding region of the RNA polymerase and therefore prevent gene transcription, or **(b)** bind to regions adjacent to the RNA polymerase assembly point and facilitate its binding/assembly and promote gene transcription. **(c)** DNA-binding proteins/regions are usually at least 500 bp away from the promoter region of gene transcription. The DNA loops back on itself, and the DNA-binding protein is brought into close proximity to the target gene. This can either facilitate the assembly of factors such as the general factors of transcription and hence enhance gene expression, or hinder such assembly. © 1994 from *Molecular Biology of the Cell*, 3rd edn, by Alberts et al. Reproduced by permission of Routledge Inc., part of the Taylor and Francis Group.

the promoter, and thus acts like a catalyst for general transcription factor assembly, and consequently also the rate of RNA polymerase activity. In mammals, it is frequently a region termed the 'cyclic AMP response element' (CRE) that acts in this manner. Increasing intracellular cAMP levels cause activation and release of CRE-binding protein (CREB). This binds to the CRE sequence and enhances the transcription rate.

These relatively remote regulatory regions need not just enhance gene expression but may also repress transcription. Indeed, loops can be formed from regulatory regions downstream as well as upstream of the gene's coding sequence. Repressors can inhibit the transcription of a given gene by binding to the regulatory sequence and blocking positive regulators, binding and thus inactivating the positive regulator, or by interfering with the promoter protein assembly. Multiple regulatory regions and DNA-binding proteins can surround a given gene and precisely control its expression at a basal level and in response to a cellular stimulus (Table 3.1).

The reason for chromosomes and introns

Human genetics differs from that of bacteria in structural components of the genetic code and in the way DNA is packaged. The fact that humans have chromosomes and introns affects how much DNA we require to code for all our proteins in an unusual way. We have far more DNA than protein-coding genes, whereas simple bacteria appear to have a much more economic DNA to gene ratio. Simple organisms like bacteria that have

circular genomes which are not contained within a membrane-bound organelle (the nucleus) are termed 'prokaryotes'. Higher eukaryotic organisms have their linear genomic packages – chromosomes – separated from the general cytoplasm by the nuclear envelope. In eukaryotes, genomic DNA is associated with nuclear proteins called histones.

Coiling around histones requires regions of DNA devoted specifically to the purpose of packaging and not coding for a protein (see Fig. 3.8c). Most of human DNA is highly repetitive (or 'satellite' DNA) consisting of long arrays of tandem repeats. These regions tend to be supercoiled around histones in condensed regions termed *heterochromatin*, even when the cell is not undergoing division. In contrast, most other DNA regions – in particular, those coding for proteins – are relatively uncondensed during interphase and constitute the euchromatin. This remaining DNA is either moderately repetitive ($50–100 \times 10^3$), accounting for about 1% of the total, or codes for unique genes and gene families, some $50–100 \times 10^3$, occupying some 2% of the genome.

Thus the reason for chromosomes is that supercoiling around histones gives tighter control of specific gene expression. Introns enable the production of alternative proteins for one gene, e.g. parathyroid-like proteins for the parathyroid hormone (PTH) gene.

FURTHER READING

Aberts B, Bray D, Lewis J, Raff M, Roberts K, Watson JD (1994) *Molecular Biology of the Cell*, 3rd edn. New York: Garland Publishing.

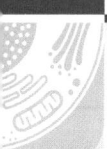

Tools for molecular biology

Preparation of genomic DNA

The first step in studying the DNA of an individual involves preparation of genomic DNA. This is a simple procedure in which any cellular tissue including blood (the nucleated cells are isolated from the erythrocytes) can be used. The cells are lysed in order to open their cell and nuclear membranes, releasing chromosomal DNA. Following digestion of all cellular protein by the addition of proteolytic enzymes, the genomic DNA is isolated by chemical extraction with phenol. DNA is stable and can be stored for years.

Restriction enzymes and gel electrophoresis

Genomic DNA can be cut into a number of fragments by enzymes called 'restriction enzymes', which are obtained from bacteria. Restriction enzymes recognize specific DNA sequences and cut double-stranded DNA at these sites. For example, the enzyme EcoRI will cut DNA wherever it reads the sequence GAATTC, and so human genomic DNA is cut into hundreds of thousands of fragments. Whenever the genomic DNA from an individual is cut with EcoRI, the same 'restriction fragments' are produced. As DNA is a negatively charged molecule, the genomic DNA that has been digested with a restriction enzyme can be separated according to its size and charge, by electrophoresing the DNA through a gel matrix. The DNA sample is loaded at one end of the gel, a voltage is applied across the gel, and the DNA migrates towards the positive anode. The small fragments move more quickly than the large fragments, and so the DNA fragments separate out. Fragment size can be determined by running fragments of known size on the same gel.

Pulsed-field gel electrophoresis (PFGE) can be used to separate very long pieces of DNA (hundreds of kilobases) which have been cut by restriction enzymes that cut at rare sites in the genome. In this technique, DNA molecules are subjected to two perpendicular electric fields that are switched on alternately. The DNA molecules are separated on the basis of molecular size, and this technique can be used for long-range mapping of the genome to detect major deletions and rearrangements.

Southern blotting and DNA probes

This technique allows the visualization of individual DNA fragments (Fig. 3.12). A DNA probe is used to indicate where the fragment of interest lies. DNA probes are useful because a fundamental property of DNA is that when two strands are separated, for example by heating, they will always reassociate and stick together again because of their complementary base sequences. Therefore the presence or position of a particular gene can be identified using a gene 'probe' consisting of DNA with a base sequence that is complementary to that of

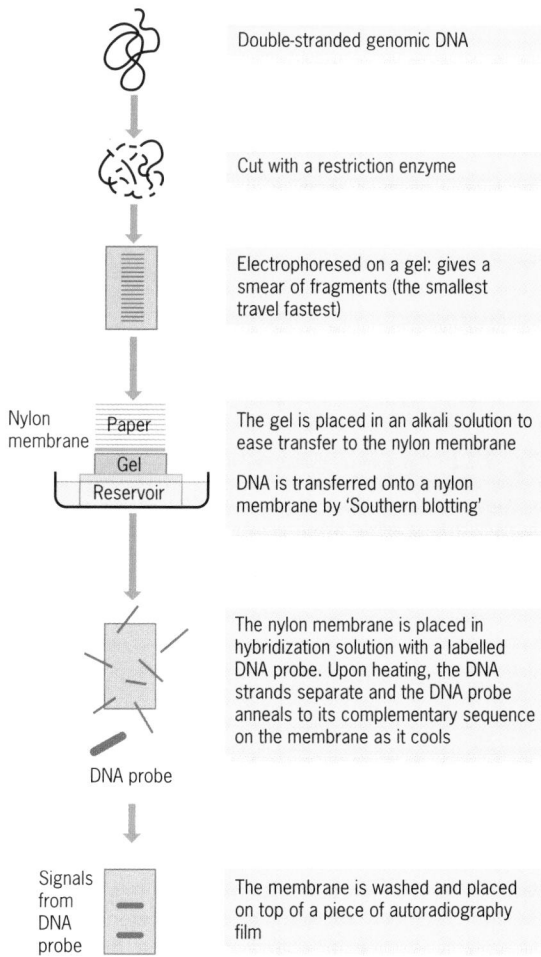

Fig. 3.12 Southern blotting and DNA probes.

the sequence of interest. A DNA probe is thus a piece of single-stranded DNA that can be labelled with a radioactive isotope (usually ^{32}P) or a fluorescent signal. The probe is added to a hybridization solution into which the membrane with the DNA is also placed. The single-stranded probe will locate and bind to its complementary sequence on the blot and can be identified by autoradiography or fluorescence.

A similar technique for blotting RNA fragments (which are not cut by restriction enzymes, but which are blotted as full-length mRNAs) on to membranes is called Northern blotting and one for blotting proteins is called Western blotting.

The polymerase chain-reaction (PCR)

Minute amounts of DNA can be amplified over a million times within a few hours using this in vitro technique (Fig. 3.13). The exact DNA sequence to be amplified needs to be known because the DNA is amplified between two short (generally 17–25 bp) single-stranded

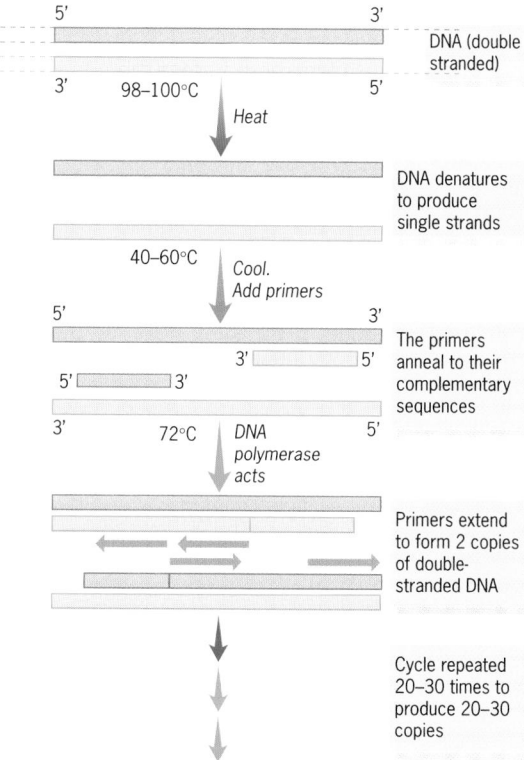

5'   3'

DNA (double
stranded)

3'   98–100°C   5'

Heat

DNA denatures
to produce
single strands

40–60°C   Cool.
Add primers

5'   3'

3'   5'

5'   3'

3'   72°C   DNA   5'
polymerase
acts

The primers
anneal to their
complementary
sequences

Primers extend
to form 2 copies
of double-
stranded DNA

Cycle repeated
20–30 times to
produce 20–30
copies

Fig. 3.13 **Polymerase chain reaction.**

DNA fragments ('oligonucleotide primers') which are complementary to the sequences at each end of the DNA of interest.

The technique has three steps. First, the double-stranded genomic DNA is denatured by heat into single-stranded DNA. The reaction is then cooled to favour DNA annealing, and the primers bind to their target DNA. Finally, a DNA polymerase is used to extend the primers in opposite directions using the target DNA as a template. After one cycle there are two copies of double-stranded DNA, after two cycles there are four copies, and this number rises exponentially with the number of cycles. Typically a polymerase chain-reaction is set for 25–30 cycles, allowing millions of amplifications, i.e. 2^n where n = number of cycles.

This technique has revolutionized genetic research because minute amounts of DNA not previously amenable to analysis can be amplified, such as from buccal cell scrapings, blood spots, or single embryonic cells.

DNA cloning

A particular DNA fragment of interest can be isolated and inserted into the genome of simple self-replicating organisms or organelles such as viruses and plasmids. When used for this purpose they are referred to as vectors. Replication by the million of the vector results in multiple copies or clones of the inserted sequence.

Thus, after removal from the host vector, cloned gene sequences can be prepared in large quantities independently of other sequences. Vectors include: bacteriophage viruses; plasmids, which are self-replicating episomal circular DNA molecules found in bacteria that carry antibody resistance genes; and 'yeast artificial chromosomes' (YACs), which are derived from centromeric and telomeric DNA sequences found in yeast. Each vector takes an optimum size of cloned DNA insert. Typically, viruses can accommodate only small sequences up to a maximum of a kilobase, larger fragments of 2–10 kilobases can be inserted into a plasmid, and sequences of several hundred kilobases can be inserted into a YAC. Each has its relative merits – viruses being very efficient, but the vectors which take large clones being considerably less so. A hybrid between a plasmid and a bacteriophage (called a cosmid) has been constructed artificially. This has the ability to clone reasonably large sequences as plasmids within a host bacteria. However, cosmids trick bacteriophages into packaging them into a viral body, and this viral body is then able to infect the target bacteria, giving efficient transfection rates.

The DNA fragment of interest is inserted into the vector DNA sequence using an enzyme called a ligase. This takes place in vitro. The next step, cloning, creates many copies of the 'recombinant DNA molecule' and takes place in vivo when the plasmid or other vector is placed back into the bacterial (or yeast) host. Bacteria that have successfully taken up the recombinant plasmid can be selected if the plasmid also carries an antibiotic resistance gene (so bacteria without the plasmid die in the presence of antibiotic) (Fig. 3.14).

The DNA fragment of interest to be cloned may be a restriction fragment. Alternatively it could be DNA (cDNA) which has been copied from an mRNA sequence. mRNA provides the template from which a viral enzyme called reverse transcriptase (RT) can synthesize a complementary single-stranded DNA copy (cDNA). A DNA polymerase may then be used to produce a double-stranded copy by PCR. A cDNA molecule contains all the sequences necessary for a functional gene, but unlike genomic DNA it lacks introns.

DNA libraries

These are pools of isolated and cloned DNA sequences that form a permanent resource for further experiments. Two types of library are used:

- Genomic libraries are prepared from genomic DNA that has been digested with restriction enzymes, ligated into a vector and each individual clone passed into a bacterial (plasmid, bacteriophage, cosmid) or yeast (YAC) host. A genomic library usually contains almost every sequence in the genome.
- cDNA libraries are prepared from the total mRNA of a tissue, which is copied into cDNA by reverse

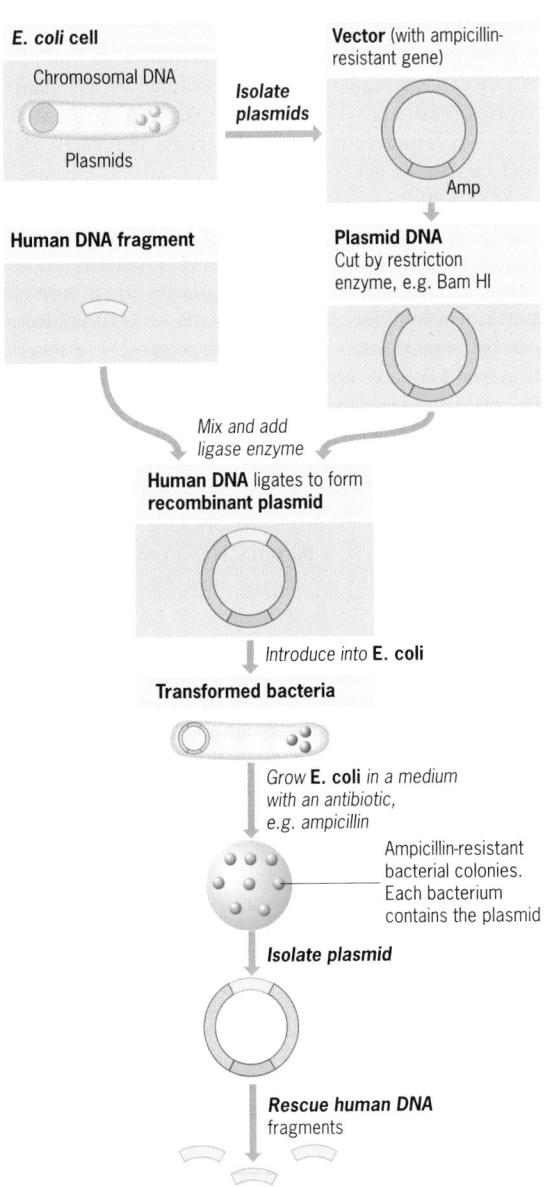

Fig. 3.14 **DNA cloning.** Recombinant DNA technique, showing incorporation of foreign DNA into a plasmid. The ampicillin-resistant genes can be used to distinguish transformed *Escherichia coli* cells.

transcriptase. The cDNA is ligated into a vector and passed into a host as above. A cDNA library should contain sequences derived from all the mRNAs expressed in that tissue type.

DNA sequencing

A chemical process known as dideoxy-sequencing allows the identification of the exact nucleotide sequence of a piece of DNA. The DNA of interest is single-stranded and an oligonucleotide primer is annealed adjacent to the region of interest. This primer acts as the starting point for a DNA polymerase to build a new DNA chain that is complementary to the sequence under investigation.

The reaction is carried out in four tubes to each of which a mixture of nucleotides is added, one of which is radioactive. To each tube one dideoxytriphosphate of either adenine, guanine, cytosine or thymine is also added at a low level. These are incorporated into the growing chain and stop enzymatic synthesis (because they lack the necessary 3'-hydroxyl group). As the dideoxynucleotides are present at a low concentration, not all the chains in a reaction tube will incorporate a dideoxynucleotide in the same place, so the tubes contain sequences of different lengths but which all terminate with a particular dideoxynucleotide. These fragments are electrophoresed in four columns and a sequence of DNA is deduced by autoradiography.

Sequencing machines work by using fluorescent labels on the four nucleotides. By laser scanning a gel these machines can rapidly sequence a stretch of DNA.

FURTHER READING

Brown TA (1990) *Gene Cloning: An Introduction*, 2nd edn. London: Chapman & Hall.

Maniatis T, Fritsch EF, Sambrook J (1989) *Molecular Cloning: A Laboratory Manual*, 2nd edn. New York: Cold Spring Harbour.

Papavassilioy AG (1995) Transcription factors. *New England Journal of Medicine* **332**: 45–47.

Smith CA, Wood EJ (1991) *Molecular Biology and Biotechnology*. London: Chapman & Hall.

The biology of chromosomes

Human chromosomes

The nucleus of each diploid cell contains 6×10^9 bp of DNA in long molecules called *chromosomes*. Chromosomes are massive structures containing one linear molecule of DNA that is wound around histone proteins into small units called nucleosomes, and these are further wound to make up the structure of the chromosome itself. Diploid human cells have 46 chromosomes, 23 inherited from each parent; thus there are 23 'homologous' pairs of chromosomes (22 pairs of 'autosomes' and two 'sex chromosomes'). The sex chromosomes, called X and Y, are not homologous but are different in size and shape. Males have an X and a Y chromosome; females have two X chromosomes. (Primary male sexual characteristics are determined by the *SRY* gene – sex determining region, Y chromosome.)

The chromosomes can be classified according to their size and shape, the largest being chromosome 1. The constriction in the chromosome is the centromere, which can be in the middle of the chromosome (metacentric) or at one extreme end (acrocentric). The centromere divides the chromosome into a short arm and a long arm, which are referred to as the p arm and the q arm respectively (see Fig. 3.8d). In addition, chromosomes can be stained when they are in the metaphase stage of the cell cycle and are very condensed. The stain gives a different pattern of light and dark bands that is diagnostic for each chromosome. Each band is given a number, and gene mapping techniques allow genes to be positioned within a band within an arm of a chromosome. For example, the *CFTR* gene (in which a defect gives rise to cystic fibrosis) maps to 7q21; that is, on chromosome 7 in the long arm in band 21.

During cell division (mitosis), each chromosome divides into two so that each daughter nucleus has the same number of chromosomes as its parent cell. During gametogenesis, however, the number of chromosomes is halved by meiosis, so that after conception the number of chromosomes remains the same and is not doubled. In the female, each ovum contains one or other X chromosome but, in the male, the sperm bears either an X or a Y chromosome.

Chromosomes can only be seen easily in actively dividing cells. Typically, lymphocytes from the peripheral blood are stimulated to divide and are processed to allow the chromosomes to be examined. Cells from other tissues can also be used – for example amniotic fluid, placental cells from chorionic villus sampling, bone marrow and skin (Box 3.1).

Box 3.1

Indications for chromosomal analysis

Chromosome studies may be indicated in the following circumstances.

Antenatal
- Pregnancies in women over 35 years
- Positive maternal serum screening test for trisomy 21
- Ultrasound markers of chromosomal abnormalities
- Severe fetal growth retardation
- Sexing of fetus in X-linked disorders

In the neonate
- Congenital malformations
- Suspicion of trisomy or monosomy
- Ambiguous genitalia

In the adolescent
- Primary amenorrhoea or failure of pubertal development
- Growth retardation

In the adult
- Screening parents of a child with a chromosomal abnormality for further genetic counselling
- Infertility or recurrent miscarriages
- Learning difficulties
- Certain malignant disorders (e.g. leukaemias)

The X chromosome and inactivation

Although female chromosomes are XX, females do not have two doses of X-linked genes (compared with just one dose for a male XY), because of the phenomenon of X inactivation or Lyonization (after its discoverer, Dr Mary Lyon). In this process, one of the two X chromosomes in the cells of females becomes transcriptionally inactive, so the cell has only one dose of the X-linked genes. Inactivation is random and can affect either X chromosome.

Telomeres and immortality

The ends of chromosomes, telomeres (see Fig. 3.8d) do not contain genes but many repeats of a hexameric sequence TTAGGG. Replication of linear chromosomes starts at coding sites (origins of replication) within the main body of chromosomes and not at the two extreme ends. The extreme ends are therefore susceptible to single-stranded DNA degradation back to double-stranded DNA. Thus cellular ageing can be measured as a genetic consequence of multiple rounds of replication with consequential telomere shortening. This leads to chromosome instability and cell death.

Stem cells have longer telomeres than their terminally differentiated daughters. However, germ cells replicate without shortening of their telomeres. This is because they express an enzyme called telomerase, which protects against telomere shortening by acting as a template primer at the extreme ends of the chromosomes. Most somatic cells (unlike germ and embryonic cells) switch off the activity of telomerase after birth and die as a result of apoptosis. Many cancer cells, however, reactivate telomerase, contributing to their immortality. Conversely, cells from patients with progeria (premature ageing syndrome) have extremely short telomeres.

The mitochondrial chromosome

In addition to the 23 pairs of chromosomes in the nucleus of every diploid cell, the mitochondria in the cytoplasm of the cell also have their own chromosomes. The mitochondrial chromosome is a circular DNA (mtDNA) molecule of approximately 16 500 bp, and every basepair makes up part of the coding sequence. These genes principally encode proteins or RNA molecules involved in mitochondrial function. These proteins are components of the mitochondrial respiratory chain involved in oxidative phosphorylation (OXPHOS) producing ATP. They also have a critical role in apoptotic cell death. Every cell contains several hundred mitochondria, and therefore several hundred mitochondrial chromosomes.

All mitochondria are inherited from the mother as sperm contain no (or very few) mitochondria. Disorders are described on p. 173.

FURTHER READING

Buys C (2000) Telomeres, telomerase and cancer. *New England Journal of Medicine* **342**: 1282–1283.

Human genetic disorders

The spectrum of inherited or congenital genetic disorders can be classified as the chromosomal disorders, including mitochondrial chromosome disorders, the Mendelian and sex-linked single-gene disorders, a variety of non-Mendelian disorders, and the multifactorial and polygenic disorders (Table 3.2 and Box 3.2). All are a result of a mutation in the genetic code. This may be a change of a single base-pair of a gene, resulting in functional change in the product protein (e.g. thalassaemia) or gross rearrangement of the gene within a genome (e.g. Down's syndrome). These mutations can be congenital (inherited at birth) or somatic (arising during a person's life). The latter are responsible for the collective disease known as cancer, and the principles underlying Mendelian inheritance act in a similar manner to dominant and recessive traits. Both gross chromosomal and point mutations occur in somatic genetic disease.

Chromosomal disorders

Chromosomal abnormalities are much more common than generally appreciated. Over half of spontaneous abortions have chromosomal abnormalities, compared with only 4–6 abnormalities per 1000 live births. Specific

Table 3.2
Prevalence of genetic disease

Type	Estimated prevalence per 1000 population
Single-gene disorders	
Autosomal dominant	2–10
Autosomal recessive	2
X-linked recessive	1–2
Chromosomal abnormalities	6–7
Common disorders with a genetic component	7–10
Congenital malformation	20
Total	38–51

From Kingston H (1989) Clinical genetic services. *British Medical Journal* **298**: 306–307

chromosomal abnormalities can lead to well-recognized and severe clinical syndromes, although autosomal aneuploidy (a differing from the normal diploid number) is usually more severe than the sex-chromosome aneuploidies. Abnormalities may occur in either the number or the structure of the chromosomes.

Abnormal chromosome numbers

If a chromosome or chromatids fail to separate ('non-disjunction') either in meiosis or mitosis, one daughter cell will receive two copies of that chromosome and one daughter cell will receive no copies of the chromosome. If this non-disjunction occurs during meiosis it can lead to an ovum or sperm having either (i) an extra chromosome, so resulting in a fetus that is 'trisomic' and has three instead of two copies of the chromosome; or (ii) no chromosome, so the fetus is 'monosomic' and has one instead of two copies of the chromosome. Non-disjunction can occur with autosomes or sex chromosomes. However, only individuals with trisomy 13, 18 and 21 survive to birth, and most children with trisomy 13 and trisomy 18 die in early childhood. Trisomy 21 (Down's syndrome) is observed with a frequency of 1 in 700 live births regardless of geography or ethnic background. This should be reduced with widespread screening (p. 186). Full autosomal monosomies are extremely rare and very deleterious. Sex-chromosome trisomies (e.g. Klinefelter's syndrome, XXY) are relatively common.

> ### Box 3.2
>
> ### Genetic disorders
>
> **Mendelian**
> - Inherited or new mutation
> - Mutant allele or pair of mutant alleles at single locus
> - Clear pattern of inheritance (autosomal or sex-linked) dominant or recessive
> - High risk to relatives
>
> **Chromosomal**
> - Loss, gain or abnormal rearrangement of one or more of 46 chromosomes in diploid cell
> - No clear pattern of inheritance
> - Low risk to relatives
>
> **Multifactorial**
> - Common
> - Interaction between genes and environmental factors
> - Low risk to relatives
>
> **Mitochondrial**
> - Due to mutations in mitochondrial genome
> - Transmitted through maternal line
> - Different pattern of inheritance from Mendelian disorders
>
> **Somatic cell**
> - Mutations in somatic cells
> - Somatic event is not inherited
> - Often give rise to tumours

The sex-chromosome monosomy in which the individual has an X chromosome only and no second X or Y chromosome is known as Turner's syndrome and is estimated to occur in 1 in 2500 live-born girls (Table 3.3).

Occasionally, non-disjunction can occur during mitosis shortly after two gametes have fused. It will then result in the formation of two cell lines, each with a different chromosome complement. This occurs more often with the sex chromosome, and results in a 'mosaic' individual.

Very rarely the entire chromosome set will be present in more than two copies, so the individual may be triploid rather than diploid and have a chromosome number of 69. Triploidy and tetraploidy (four sets) result in spontaneous abortion.

Abnormal chromosome structures

As well as abnormal numbers of chromosomes, chromosomes can have abnormal structures, and the disruption to the DNA and gene sequences may give rise to a genetic disease.

- *Deletions.* Deletions of a portion of a chromosome may give rise to a disease syndrome if two copies of the genes in the deleted region are necessary, and the individual will not be normal with just the one copy remaining on the non-deleted homologous chromosome. Many deletion syndromes have been well described. For example, Prader–Willi syndrome (p. 241) is the result of cytogenetic events resulting in deletion of part of the long arm of chromosome 15, Wilms tumour is characterized by deletion of part of the short arm of chromosome 11, and microdeletions in the long arm of chromosome 22 give rise to the DiGeorge syndrome.
- *Duplications.* Duplications occur when a portion of the chromosome is present on the chromosome in two copies, so the genes in that chromosome portion are present in an extra dose. A form of the neuropathy, Charcot–Marie–Tooth disease (p. 1216), is due to a small duplication of a region of chromosome 17.

- *Inversion.* Inversions involve an end-to-end reversal of a segment within a chromosome; e.g. abcdefgh becomes abcfedgh.
- *Translocations.* Translocations occur when two chromosome regions join together, when they would not normally. Chromosome translocations in somatic cells may be associated with tumourigenesis (see p. 489).

Translocations can be very complex, involving more than two chromosomes, but most are simple and fall into one of two categories. Reciprocal translocations occur when any two non-homologous chromosomes break simultaneously and rejoin, swapping ends. In this case the cell still has 46 chromosomes but two of them are rearranged. Someone with a balanced translocation is likely to be normal (unless a translocation breakpoint interrupts a gene); but at meiosis, when the chromosomes separate into different daughter cells, the translocated chromosomes will enter the gametes and any resulting fetus may inherit one abnormal chromosome and have an unbalanced translocation, with physical manifestations.

Robertsonian translocations occur when two acrocentric chromosomes join and the short arm is lost, leaving only 45 chromosomes. This translocation is balanced as no genetic material is lost and the individual is healthy. However, any offspring have a risk of inheriting an unbalanced arrangement. This risk depends on which acrocentric chromosome is involved. Clinically important is the 14/21 Robertsonian translocation. A woman with this karyotype has a 1 in 8 risk of delivering a baby with Down's syndrome (a male carrier has a 1 in 50 risk). However, they have a 50% risk of producing a carrier like themselves, hence the importance of genetic family studies. Relatives should be alerted about the increased risk of Down's syndrome in their offspring, and should have their chromosomes checked.

Table 3.4 shows some of the syndromes resulting from chromosomal abnormalities.

Mitochondrial chromosome disorders

The mitochondrial chromosome (p. 171) carries its genetic information in a very compact form; for example there are no introns in the genes. Therefore any mutation has a high chance of having an effect. However, as every cell contains hundreds of mitochondria, a single altered mitochondrial genome will not be noticed. As mitochondria divide there is a statistical likelihood that there will be more mutated mitochondria, and at some point this will give rise to a mitochondrial disease.

Most mitochondrial diseases are myopathies and neuropathies with a maternal pattern of inheritance. Other abnormalities include retinal degeneration, diabetes mellitus and hearing loss. Many syndromes have been described. Myopathies include chronic progressive external ophthalmoplegia (CPEO); encephalomyopathies include myoclonic epilepsy with ragged red fibres (MERRF) and mitochondrial encephalomyopathy, lactic

---

Table 3.3
Examples of chromosomal disorders in live births

Abnormal chromosome disorders

Autosomal disorders

Trisomy 21 (Down's syndrome)	1 in 650
Trisomy 18 (Edward's syndrome)	1 in 3000
Trisomy 13 (Patau's syndrome)	1 in 5000

Sex-chromosome disorders

47, XXY (Klinefelter's syndrome)	1 in 1000 males
47, XYY	1 in 800 males
47, XXX	1 in 1000 females
45, X (Turner's syndrome)	1 in 2500 females

Abnormal chromosome structures

Balanced translocations	1 in 500
Unbalanced translocations	1 in 2000

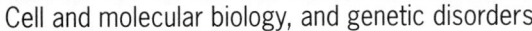

Table 3.4
Chromosomal abnormalities: examples of a few syndromes

Syndrome	Chromosome karyotype	Incidence and risks	Clinical features	Mortality
Autosomal abnormalities				
Trisomy 21 (Down's syndrome)	47, +21 (95%) Mosaicism Translocation 5%	1:650 (risk with 20- to 29-year-old mother 1:1000; >45-year-old mother 1:30)	Flat face, slanting eyes, epicanthic folds, small ears, simian crease, short stubby fingers, hypotonia, variable learning difficulties, congenital heart disease (up to 50%)	High in first year, but many now survive to adulthood
Trisomy 13 (Patau's syndrome)	47, +13	1:5000	Low-set ears, cleft lip and palate, polydactyly, micro-ophthalmia, learning difficulties	Rarely survive for more than a few weeks
Trisomy 18 (Edwards' syndrome)	47, +18	1:3000	Low-set ears, micrognathia, rocker-bottom feet, mental retardation	Rarely survive for more than a few weeks
Sex-chromosome abnormalities				
Fragile X syndrome	46, XX, fra (X) 46, XY, fra (X)	1:2000	Most common inherited cause of learning difficulties predominantly in males Macro-orchidism	
Female				
Turner's syndrome	45, XO	1:2500	Infantilism, primary amenorrhoea, short stature, webbed neck, cubitis valgus, normal IQ	
Triple X syndrome	47, XXX	1:1000	No distinctive somatic features, learning difficulties	
Others	48, XXXX 49,XXXXX	Rare	Amenorrhoea, infertility, learning difficulties	
Male				
Klinefelter's syndrome	47, XXY (or XXYY)	1:1000 (more in sons of older mothers)	Decreased crown–pubis:pubis–heel ratio, eunuchoid, testicular atrophy, infertility, gynaecomastia, learning difficulties (20%; related to number of X chromosomes)	
Double Y syndrome	47, XYY	1:800	Tall, fertile, minor mental and psychiatric illness, high incidence in tall criminals	
Others	48, XXXY 49, XXXXY		Learning difficulties, testicular atrophy	

acidosis and stroke-like episodes (MELAS) (see p. 1224). Kearus–Sayre syndrome includes ophthalmoplegia, heart block, cerebellar ataxia, deafness and mental deficiency due to long deletions and rearrangements. Leber's hereditary optic neuropathy (LHON) is the commonest cause of blindness in young men, with bilateral loss of central vision and cardiac arrhythmias, and is an example of a mitochondrial disease caused by a point mutation in one gene. Multisystem disorders include Pearson's syndrome (sideroblastic anaemia, pancytopenia, exocrine pancreatic failure, subtotal villous atrophy, diabetes mellitus and renal tubular dysfunction). In some families, hearing loss is the only symptom and one of the mitochondrial genes implicated may predispose parents to aminoglyceride ototoxicity.

Analysis of chromosome disorders

The analysis of gross chromosomal disorders has traditionally involved the culture of isolated cells in the presence of toxins such as colchicine. These toxins arrest the cell cycle at mitosis and, following staining, the chromosomes with their characteristic banding can be seen. A highly trained cytogeneticist can then identify each chromosome pair and any abnormalities (Fig. 3.15).

New molecular biology techniques have made things simpler: YAC-cloned probes are available and cover large genetic regions of individual chromosomes. These probes can be labelled with fluorescently tagged nucleotides and used in in situ hybridization of the nucleus of isolated tissue from patients. These tagged probes allow rapid and relatively unskilled

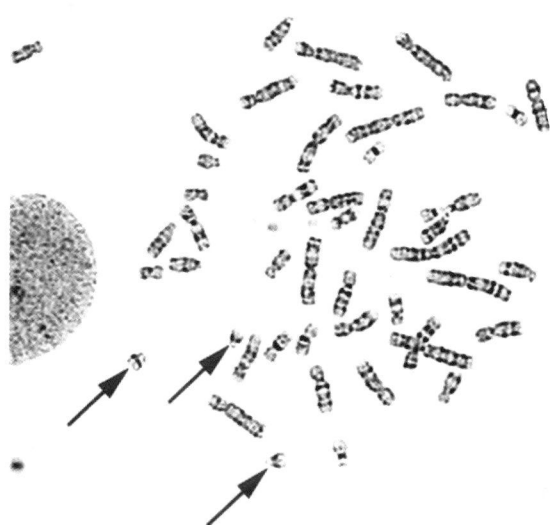

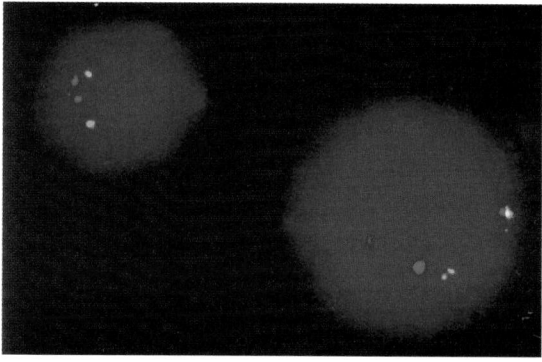

Fig. 3.16 Fluorescence in situ hybridization (FISH).
Two-coloured FISH using a red paint for the *ABL* gene on chromosome 9 and a green paint for the *BCR* gene on chromosome 22 in the anaphase cell nucleus. Where a translocation has occurred the two genes become juxtaposed on the Philadelphia chromosome and a hybrid yellow florescence can be seen only in the affected cell nucleus on the right. Courtesy of D Lillington, Medical Oncology Unit, St. Bartholomew's Hospital.

Fig. 3.15 Karyotyping. G-banded spread of metaphase chromosomes, showing trisomy 21 (arrowed) Down's syndrome. Courtesy of D Lillington, Medical Oncology Unit, St Bartholomew's Hospital.

identification of metaphase chromosomes, and allow the identification of chromosomes dispersed within the nucleus. Furthermore, tagging two chromosome regions with different fluorescent tags allows easy identification of chromosomal translocations (Fig. 3.16).

Gene defects

Mendelian and sex-linked single-gene disorders are the result of mutations in coding sequences and their control elements. These mutations can have various effects on the expression of the gene, as explained below, but all cause a dysfunction of the protein product.

Mutations

Although DNA replication is a very accurate process, occasionally mistakes occur to produce changes or mutations. These changes can also occur owing to other factors such as radiation, ultraviolet light or chemicals. Mutations in gene sequences or in the sequences which regulate gene expression (transcription and translation) may alter the amino acid sequence in the protein encoded by that gene. In some cases protein function will be maintained; in other cases it will change or cease, perhaps producing a clinical disorder. Many different types of mutation occur.

Point mutation

This is the simplest type of change and involves the substitution of one nucleotide for another, so changing the codon in a coding sequence. For example, the triplet AAA, which codes for lysine, may be mutated to AGA, which codes for arginine. Whether a substitution produces a clinical disorder depends on whether it changes a critical part of the protein molecule produced. Fortunately, many substitutions have no effect on the function or stability of the proteins produced as several codons code for the same amino acid. However, some mutations may have a severe effect; for example, in sickle cell disease a mutation within the globin gene changes one codon from GAG to GTG, so that instead of glutamic acid, valine is incorporated into the polypeptide chain, which radically alters its properties.

Insertion or deletion

Insertion or deletion of one or more bases is a more serious change, as it results in the alteration of the rest of the following sequence to give a frame-shift mutation. For example, if the original code was:

TAA GGA GAG TTT

and an extra nucleotide (A) is inserted, the sequence becomes:

TAA AGG AGA GTT T

Alternatively, if the third nucleotide (A) is deleted, the sequence becomes:

TAG GAG AGT TT

In both cases, different amino acids are incorporated into the polypeptide chain. This type of change is responsible for some forms of thalassaemia (p. 427). Insertions and deletions can involve many hundreds of base-pairs of DNA. For example, some large deletions in the dystrophin gene remove coding sequences and this results in Duchenne muscular dystrophy. Insertion/deletion (ID) polymorphism in the angiotensin-converting enzyme (ACE) gene has been shown to result in the genotypes II, ID and DD. The deletion is of a 287 bp repeat sequence and DD is associated with higher concentrations of circulating ACE and possibly cardiac disease (see p. 768).

Splicing mutations

If the DNA sequences which direct the splicing of introns from mRNA are mutated, then abnormal splicing may occur. In this case the processed mRNA which is translated into protein by the ribosomes may carry intron sequences, so altering which amino acids are incorporated into the polypeptide chain.

Termination mutations

Normal polypeptide chain termination occurs when the ribosomes processing the mRNA reach one of the chain termination or 'stop' codons (see above). Mutations involving these codons will result in either late or premature termination. For example, Haemoglobin Constant Spring is a haemoglobin variant where instead of the 'stop' sequence, a single base change allows the insertion of an extra amino acid (see p. 430).

Single-gene disease

Monogenetic disorders involving single genes can be inherited as dominant, recessive or sex-linked characteristics. Inheritance occurs according to simple Mendelian laws, making predictions of disease in offspring and therefore genetic counselling more straightforward.

Autosomal dominant disorders (Fig. 3.17 and Table 3.5)

Each diploid cell contains two copies of all the autosomes. An autosomal dominant disorder occurs when one of the two copies has a mutation and the protein produced by the normal form of the gene cannot compensate. In this case a heterozygous individual who has two different forms (or alleles) of the same gene will manifest the disease. The offspring of heterozygotes have a 50% chance of inheriting the chromosome carrying the disease allele, and therefore also of having the disease. However, estimation of risk to offspring for counselling families can be difficult because of three factors:

- These disorders have a great variability in their manifestation. 'Incomplete penetrance' may occur if patients have a dominant disorder but it does not manifest itself clinically in them. This gives the appearance of the gene having 'skipped' a generation.
- Dominant traits are extremely variable in severity (variable expression) and a mildly affected parent may have a severely affected child.
- New cases in a previously unaffected family may be the result of a new mutation. If it is a mutation, the risk of a further affected child is negligible. Most cases of achondroplasia are due to new mutations.

The overall incidence of autosomal dominant disorders is 7 per 1000 live births.

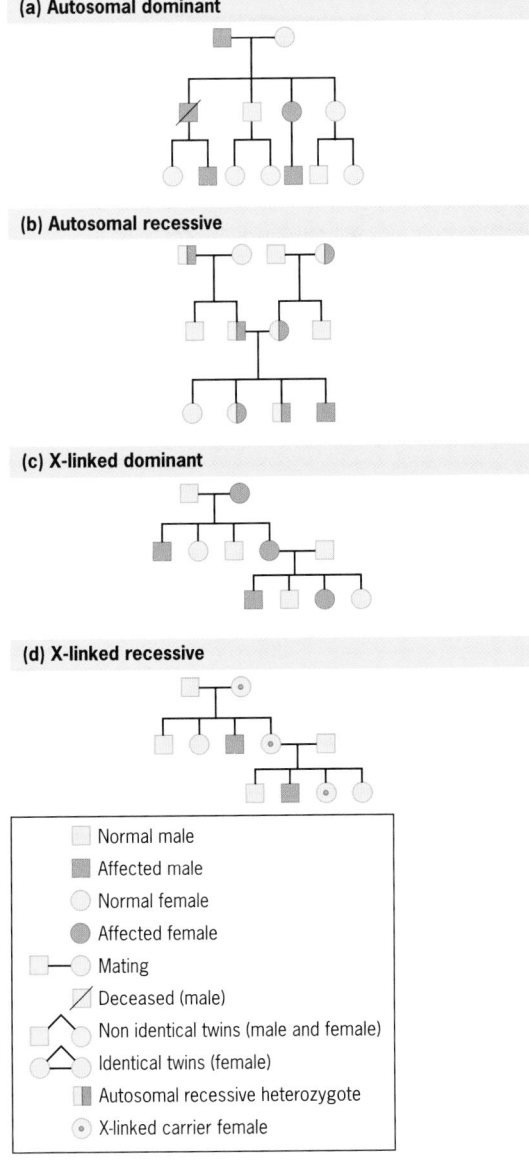

Fig. 3.17 Modes of inheritance of simple gene disorders, with a key to the standard pedigree symbols.

Autosomal recessive disorders (Fig. 3.17 and Table 3.6)

These disorders manifest themselves only when an individual is homozygous for the disease allele, i.e. both chromosomes carry the mutated gene. In this case the parents are generally unaffected, healthy carriers (heterozygous for the disease allele). There is usually no family history, although the defective gene is passed from generation to generation. The offspring of an affected person will be healthy heterozygotes unless the other parent is also a carrier. If carriers marry, the offspring have a 1 in 4 chance of being homozygous and affected, a

Table 3.5
Examples of autosomal disorders with chromosome and gene defect

Achondroplasia	4p	FGFR3
Alzheimer's disease (some)	1q	Presenelin II
	14q	Presenelin I
	21q	Amyloid precursor protein (APP)
		Mitochondrial DNA
α_1-antitrypsin deficiency	14q	α_1-protease inhibitor
Breast carcinoma (familial, early onset)	17q	BRCA1
	13q	BRCA2
C_1 esterase deficiency	6p	C1 1NH
Charcot–Marie–Tooth disease (HMSN)	1q	Myelin protein (HMSN 1B)
	17q	Myelin protein 22 (HMSN 1A)
Congenital spherocytosis	8p	Ankyrin
Crigler–Najjar syndrome type II		UDP glucuronyl transferase mutation
Cutis laxa	7q	Elastin
Distal renal tubular acidosis	17q	SLC4A1
Dystrophia myotonica	19q	DM kinase (CTG triple repeat expansion disorder)
Ehlers–Danlos syndrome	Many, e.g.	
	7q	COL1A1
	7q	COL1A2
	2q	COL3A1
	9q	COL5A1
Epidermolysis bullosa (some)	12q, 17q	Keratin 5, 14; Laminin 5 etc.
Facioscapulohumeral dystrophy type I		LGMD
Familial adenomatous polyposis	5q	APC
Familial hypercholesterolaemia	19p	LDL receptor
Familial Mediterranean fever	16p	Marenostrin
Hereditary elliptocytosis	1q	α-spectrin
	14q	β-spectrin
Hereditary haemorrhagic telangiectasia	9q	Endoglin (HHT1)
	12q	ALK1 (HHT2)
Hirschsprung's disease	Complex	
	10q	RET proto-oncogene mutation (recessive 13q endothelin 3B receptor)
Huntington's disease	4p	Huntingtin (CAG triple repeat expansion disorder)
Hypertrophic cardiomyopathy	1q	Troponin-T
	11q	Cardiac myosin-binding protein
	14q	Cardiac myosin-binding heavy chain
	15q	α-tropomyosin
Li–Fraumeni syndrome	17q	p53
Malignant hyperpyrexia	19q	
Marfan's syndrome	15q	Fibrillin 1
Motor neurone disease	21q	SOD-1
Multiple endocrine neoplasia (MEN)	10q	RET proto-oncogene (MEN 2A and 2B)
	11q	Menin (MEN1)
Neurofibromatosis	17q	Neurofibromin (NF1)
	22q	Merlin (NF2)
Osteogenesis imperfecta	Many, e.g.	
	7q	COL1A1
	7q	COL1A2
	2q	COL4A1
Peutz–Jegher's syndrome		STK 11 (LKB1)
Polycystic kidney disease (PKD)	16p	PKD1
Porphyria cutanea tarda	1q	Uropophyrinogen decarboxylase
Retinitis pigmentosa	>18 genes, e.g.	
	3q	Rhodopsin
	6p	Peripherin
Retinoblastoma	13q	RB
Tuberous sclerosis (TS)	9q	Hamartin (TS1)
	16q	Tuberin (TS2)
von Hippel–Lindau syndrome	3p	VHL
von Willebrand's disease	12p	vWF
Wilm's tumour	11p	WT1
	11p	WT2

Table 3.6
Examples of autosomal recessive disorders with chromosome and gene defects

Abetalipoproteinaemia	4q	Mic TG transfer protein
Adenosine deaminase deficiency (ADA)	20q	ADA
Albinism	11q (9p, 15q)	Tyrosinase
Alkaptonuria	3q	Homogen β1, 2 dioxide
Ataxia telangiectasia	11q	ATM
Crigler-Najjar syndrome		Hepatic UDP glucuronide transferase
Cystic fibrosis	7q	CFTR
Deafness	Many forms, e.g.	
	13q	GJB2 (connexin 26), Myosin genes
Dubin–Johnson syndrome		MRP2 gene
Epidermolysis bullosa (some)		Collagen VII
Friedreich's ataxia	9q	Frataxia (GAA triple repeat expansion disorder)
Galactosaemia		Galactose-1-phosphate uridyl transferase
Gaucher's disease	1q	Glucocerebrosidase
Glycogen storage disease	1p3p, 11, 12, 14, 17	See Table 19.17
Haemolytic uraemic syndrome	1q	Factor H
Hereditary haemochromatosis	6p	HFE
Homocystinuria type I	21q	Cystathionine β synthetase
Hurler's syndrome type I	4p	α-L-iduronidase
Phenylketonuria	12q	Phenylalanine hydroxylase
Refsum's disease	10q	Phytanoyl-CoA hydroxylase
Sickle cell disease	11p	β-globin
β-thalassaemia	11p	β-globin
α-thalassaemia	16 and 11	α-globin
Tay–Sach's disease	15q	Hexosaminidase A
Wilson's disease	13q	ATP7B (copper transporter)
Zellweger's syndrome	Multiple	Peroxins

1 in 2 chance of being a carrier, and a 1 in 4 chance of being genetically normal. Consanguinity increases the risk. The clinical features of autosomal recessive disorders are usually severe; patients often present in the first few years of life and have a high mortality.

Many inborn errors of metabolism are recessive diseases. The most common recessive disease in the UK is cystic fibrosis (see pp. 188 and 871). The overall incidence of autosomal recessive disorders is about 2.5 per 1000 live births in the UK. World-wide, diseases such as thalassaemia and sickle cell disease are very common; the frequency of these diseases may be as high as 20 per 1000 births in some populations. Prenatal diagnosis for recessive disorders may be possible by analysing the DNA of the fetus for mutations known in the parents.

Tables 3.6 and 3.7 list some autosomal dominant and autosomal recessive genetic diseases with their chromosomal localization. Some diseases show a racial or geographical prevalence. Thalassaemia (see p. 427) is seen mainly in Greeks, South East Asians and Italians, porphyria variegata occurs more frequently in the South African white population, and Tay–Sachs (p. 1117) disease particularly occurs in Ashkenazi Jews.

Sex-linked disorders (Fig. 3.17 and Table 3.7)
Genes carried on the X chromosome are said to be 'X-linked', and can be dominant or recessive in the same way as autosomal genes. As females have two

Table 3.7
Examples of X-linked disorders with chromosome and gene defects

Recessive

Alport's syndrome	Xq22	COL4A5
Becker's muscular dystrophy	Xp21	Dystrophin
Charcot–Marie–Tooth disease (HMSN)	Xq13	Connexin 32
Duchenne muscular dystrophy	Xp21	Dystrophin
Fabry's disease	Xq22	α-galactosidase
Fragile X syndrome	Xq27	FRAXQ27*RFA
Haemophilia A	Xq28	Factor VIII
Haemophilia B	Xq27	Factor IX
G6PD deficiency	Xq28	Glucose-6-phosphate dehydrogenase
Mucopolysaccharidosis type II (Hunter's sydnrome)	Xq28	Iduronate sulphatase
Nephrogenic diabetic insipidus	Xq28	Arginine vasopressin receptor
Turner's syndrome	Xq13	Ribosomal protein S4
X-linked severe combined immunodeficiency	Xq13	1L-2 receptor γ chain

Other recessive disorders include albinism (ocular), colour blindness, Lesch–Nyhan syndrome, Menkes syndrome, mental retardation (with or without fragile sites), and Wiskott–Aldrich syndrome.

Dominant

Vitamin D-resistant rickets	Xq22	PEX

X chromosomes they will be unaffected carriers of X-linked recessive diseases. However, since males have just one X chromosome, any deleterious mutation in an X-linked gene will manifest itself because no second copy of the gene is present.

X-linked dominant disorders

These are rare. Vitamin D-resistant rickets is the best-known example. Females who are heterozygous for the mutant gene and males who have one copy of the mutant gene on their single X chromosome will manifest the disease. Half the male or female offspring of an affected mother and all the female offspring of an affected man will have the disease. Affected males tend to have the disease more severely than the heterozygous female.

X-linked recessive disorders

These disorders present in males and present only in (usually rare) homozygous females. X-linked recessive diseases are transmitted by healthy female carriers or affected males if they survive to reproduce. An example of an X-linked recessive disorder is haemophilia A (see p. 460), which is caused by a mutation in the X-linked gene for factor VIII. It has recently been shown that in 50% of cases there is an intrachromosomal rearrangement (inversion) of the tip of the long arm of the X chromosome (one break point being within intron 22 of the factor VIII gene).

Of the offspring from a carrier female and a normal male:

- 50% of the girls will be carriers as they inherit a mutant allele from their mother and the normal allele from their father; the other 50% of the girls inherit two normal alleles and are themselves normal
- 50% of the boys will have haemophilia as they inherit the mutant allele from their mother (and the Y chromosome from their father); the other 50% of the boys will be normal as they inherit the normal allele from their mother (and the Y chromosome from their father).

The male offspring of a male with haemophilia and a normal female will not have the disease as they do not inherit his X chromosome. However, all the female offspring will be carriers as they all inherit his X chromosome.

Y-linked genes

Genes carried on the Y chromosome are said to be Y-linked and only males can be affected. However, there are no known examples of Y-linked single-gene disorders which are transmitted.

Sex-limited inheritance

Occasionally a gene can be carried on an autosome but manifests itself only in one sex. For example, frontal baldness is an autosomal dominant disorder in males but behaves as a recessive disorder in females.

Other single-gene disorders

These are disorders which may be due to mutations in single genes but which do not manifest as simple monogenic disorders. They can arise from a variety of mechanisms, including the following.

Triplet repeat mutations

In the gene responsible for myotonic dystrophy (p. 1224), the mutated allele was found to have an expanded 3'UTR region in which three nucleotides, GCT, were repeated up to about 35 times. In families with myotonic dystrophy, people with the late-onset form of the disease had 20–40 copies of the repeat, but their children and grandchildren who presented with the disease from birth had vast increases in the number of repeats, up to 2000 copies. It is thought that some mechanism during meiosis causes this 'triplet repeat expansion' so that the offspring inherit an increased number of triplets. The number of triplets affects mRNA and protein function. See also page 186 for the phenomenon of 'anticipation'.

Imprinting

It is known that normal humans need a diploid number of chromosomes, 46. However the maternal and paternal contributions are different and, in some way which is not yet clear, the fetus can distinguish between the chromosomes inherited from the mother and the chromosomes inherited from the father, although both give 23 chromosomes. In some way the chromosomes are 'imprinted' so that the maternal and paternal contributions are different. Imprinting is relevant to human genetic disease because different phenotypes may result depending on whether the mutant chromosome is maternally or paternally inherited. A deletion of part of the long arm of chromosome 15 (15q11–q13) will give rise to the Prader–Willi syndrome (PWS) if it is paternally inherited. A deletion of a similar region of the chromosome gives rise to Angelman's syndrome (AS) if it is maternally inherited. Recently the affected gene has been identified as ubiquitin (*UBE3A*). Significantly maternal chromosome 15 *UBE3A* is expressed in the brain and hypothalamus. Defective maternal ubiquitin in Angelman's syndrome is thus responsible for accumulation of undegraded protein, and hence neuronal damage.

Complex traits: multifactorial and polygenic inheritance

Characteristics resulting from a combination of genetic and environmental factors are said to be multifactorial; those involving multiple genes can also be said to be polygenic.

Measurements of most biological traits (e.g. height) show a variation between individuals in a population and a unimodal, symmetrical (Gaussian) frequency distribution curve can be drawn. This variability is due to variation in genetic factors and environmental factors. Environmental factors may play a part in determining some characteristics, such as weight, whilst other characteristics such as height may be largely genetically determined. This genetic component is thought to be due to the additive effects of a number of alleles at a number of loci, many of which can be individually identified using molecular biological techniques, for example studying identical twins in different environments.

A common genetic variation in the 3′ untranslated region of the prothrombin gene is associated with elevated prothrombin (up to fourfold), increased risk of venous thrombosis, and myocardial infarction. Presumably the 3′ mutation induces overexpression of the prothrombin gene by increasing mRNA stability. In some pedigree studies those homozygous for this mutation and heterozygous for factor V Leiden mutation have an even greater risk of thrombotic events (p. 466). Conversely, downregulation of α_1-antitrypsin gene (due to similar mutation in the 3′ and 5′ untranslated regions) is associated with emphysema and cirrhosis (p. 377). There are sex differences. Congenital pyloric stenosis is most common in boys, but if it occurs in girls the latter have a larger number of affected relatives. This difference suggests that a larger number of the relevant genes are required to produce the disease in girls than in boys. Most of the important human diseases, such as heart disease, diabetes and common mental disorders, are multifactorial traits (Table 3.8).

Table 3.8
Examples of disorders that may have a polygenic inheritance

Disorder	Frequency (%)	Heritability (%)*
Hypertension	5	62
Asthma	4	80
Schizophrenia	1	85
Congenital heart disease	0.5	35
Neural tube defects	0.5	60
Pyloric stenosis	0.3	75
Ankylosing spondylitis	0.2	70
Cleft palate	0.1	76

* Percentage of the total variation of a trait which can be attributed to genetic factor

FURTHER READING

Brock DJH (1993) *Molecular Genetics for the Clinician.* Cambridge: Cambridge University Press.
Connor JM, Ferguson-Smith MA (1997) *Essential Medical Genetics,* 5th edn. Oxford: Blackwell Scientific.
Gelehrter TD, Collins FS, Ginsburg D (1997) *The Principles of Medical Genetics,* 2nd edn. Baltimore: Williams and Wilkins.
Leonard JV, Shapira AHV (2000) Mitochondrial respiratory chain disorders I and II. *Lancet* **355**: 299–304, 389–394.
Saenger P (1996) Turner's syndrome. *New England Journal of Medicine* **335**: 1749–1754.

Analysis of mutations and genetic disease

Tracking a disease gene
Of the estimated 3400 inherited genetic disorders, only a very small number have been characterized in terms of their biochemistry and genetics. Their clinical phenotype may have been described extensively but the identity of the culpable gene is still unknown. However, it is not necessary to identify the gene because two genes that are situated close together on a chromosome are nearly always co-inherited. Only on rare occasions do they segregate during meiosis when the two chromosomes of a diploid pair cross over and exchange parts (recombination) – even then the crossover point must be between the two genes. The closer the genes, the less chance of a segregating crossover, such that two genes that are one million base-pairs apart will only have a 1% chance of being separated by recombination. This might be an enormous distance in molecular terms, but for clinical genetic analysis this is acceptable for diagnosis. If a known gene or non-coding repetitive DNA sequence is within this one million base-pairs of the disease gene, it will act as the tag or marker probe for the disease.

The large amount of non-coding DNA between genes, like all DNA, accumulates random base-pair changes throughout many generations. If these changes occur within genes, then they cause inherited disorders. The rate of mutation in some genes is quite low as there is a strong genetic selection against variants, but this is not true of non-coding DNA where a base-pair change has no deleterious effect. The frequency of change can approach 1 in 100 base-pairs. These changes occur randomly throughout the non-coding DNA, as do restriction enzyme sites. Sometimes a base-pair change will create or destroy a particular restriction site. Generally two members of a chromosome pair (homologues) will have broadly the same restriction patterns at any one point (Fig. 3.18a). However, owing to a random base-pair change, one chromosome will show a different restriction pattern for one enzyme (BamHI in Fig. 3.18a) compared with its homologue. These differences in restriction pattern are inherited, and are known as polymorphisms. Because they are observable as differences in length of particular restriction fragments, they are known as *restriction fragment length polymorphisms* (RFLPs).

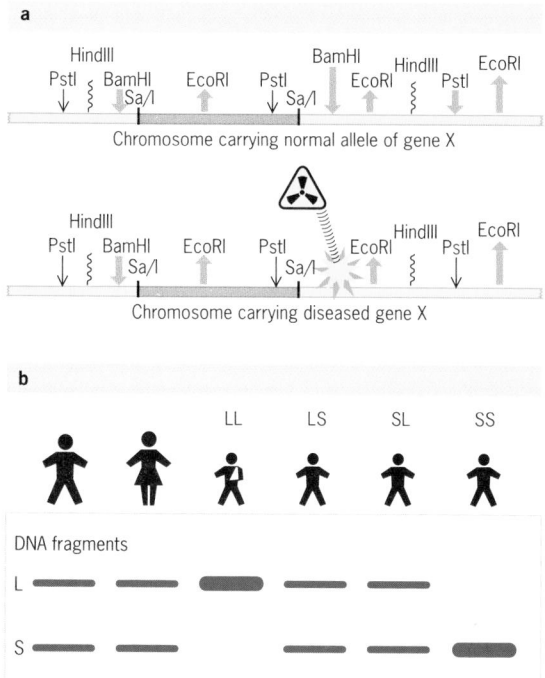

Fig. 3.18 **(a) Restriction fragment length polymorphism.**
Diagrammatic representation of two allelic sections of DNA from a
chromosome pair. The restriction site map of the two is identical
except for a BamHI sequence which has been mutated by
environmental radiation resulting in a restriction fragment length
polymorphism (RFLP). The blue area represents a cloned sequence
which acts as a marker probe or tag for the polymorphism. This
polymorphism is within one million base pairs of a disease gene and
co-segregates with the disease. **(b) RFLP and disease tracking.**
A family with four children whose parents are heterozygous for the
polymorphism shown in (a). The bands below show DNA fragments
(large, L, and small, S) on a Southern blot of DNA. If the RLFP which
gives the L fragment is on the chromosome carrying the defective
gene then only the fetus which is homozygous for the large fragment
(LL) will be affected. The fetus homozygous for the small fragment (SS)
will not be a sufferer. The heterozygous fetuses (LS and SL) will also be
unaffected but will be carriers.

The inheritance of RFLPs

The blue area in Figure 3.18a shows a cloned area of
DNA from two chromosomes. If this is used as a probe,
it will detect any restriction fragment that contains an
identical piece of DNA sequence, and thus it can be used
to detect the BamHI polymorphism shown. A person
with these two chromosomes will be heterozygous for
the BamHI polymorphism, as the two chromosomes are
different. The person will produce gametes that have
only one of these chromosomes: 50% of the cells will
have one type, 50% the other. If the mate of this person
is also heterozygous for the same polymorphism, he or
she will produce gametes that are 50% of one type and
50% the other. At fertilization there is a random chance
that any one gamete will fuse with any gamete from the
other parent, and thus four types of progeny will be produced. Two will be heterozygous for the polymorphism

(Fig. 3.18b), one will be homozygous for the large
BamHI fragment, the other will be homozygous for the
small BamHI fragment.

If the chromosome carrying the BamHI polymorphism has a closely linked gene that when defective
causes an inherited disorder, then by studying the family
pedigree, the inheritance of both the disorder and the
RFLP can be monitored. Generally, inherited disorders
are caused by recessive genes. Both parents can therefore
be carriers without being affected. If both parents come
from families that have affected relatives, or they themselves have produced affected children, then they may
wish to know if any subsequent children will also be
sufferers. Suppose that the large BamHI fragment of
the polymorphism is on the same chromosome as the
defective gene, the small fragment being on the same
chromosome as the normal allele. This can be checked by
showing that any sufferers of the condition must be
homozygous for the defective gene and thereby homozygous for the large BamHI fragment. To determine if
any subsequent children are likely sufferers, DNA from
a chorionic villus or amniocentesis sample can be
digested with BamHI and electrophoresed on an agarose
gel. It can then be probed with a cloned fragment using
a Southern blot.

DNA can be amplified from very small tissue samples using PCR. If a polymorphism is reasonably well
characterized, PCR across the RFLP will yield a suitable
fragment to test for its presence. Other markers used to
trace disease genes are simple sequence repeats. More
common and more polymorphic (i.e. having greater
variability) than RFLPs, these are short di-, tri-, tetra-
or pentanucleotide repeats (such as (CA)n) which are
present throughout the genome and have highly variable
lengths. By designing primers to the sequence either
side of one of these repeats, the repeat can be amplified
by PCR. The amplified product is electrophoresed on
a gel and different-sized products are produced from
different people. If the mutant gene is close by, then
a particular size repeat in that region will always
segregate with the disease allele.

The likelihood of recombination between the marker
under study and the disease allele must be taken into
account. This measure of likelihood is known as the 'lod
score' (the logarithm of the odds) and is a measure of the
statistical significance of the observed co-segregation of
the marker and the disease gene, compared with what
would be expected by chance alone. Positive lod scores
make linkage more likely; negative lod scores make it
less likely. By convention a lod score of +3 is taken to be
definite evidence of linkage because this indicates 1000
to 1 odds that the co-segregation of the DNA marker
and the disease did not occur by chance alone.

Linkage analysis has provided many breakthroughs
in mapping the positions of genes that cause genetic
diseases, such as the gene for cystic fibrosis which was
found to be tightly linked to a marker on chromosome 7,

or the gene for Friedreich's ataxia which is tightly linked to a marker on chromosome 9.

Gene hunting

Two approaches to the identification of a disease gene are possible – functional or positional cloning (Fig. 3.19).

Functional cloning

Functional cloning requires a working knowledge of the biochemistry of the disease such that the defective protein/enzyme has previously been characterized in some way. Extracted mRNA from tissue expressing the disease gene (from both normal and affected individuals) is cloned into a vector. The clones are engineered such that the gene product is expressed by the host organism (i.e. bacteria) which may then be screened by antibodies or functional (enzyme–substrate) assay for those clones producing the desired gene product. The selected clones are isolated, propagated and the insert sequenced. The isolated cDNA insert can then be used as a probe to identify the location of the gene on a chromosome by in situ hybridization and to identify the genomic sequence from genome libraries.

As already stated, the biochemistry of most genetic disease is unknown and positional cloning is required.

Positional cloning

Positional cloning is used to isolate genes whose protein products are not known, but whose existence can be inferred from a disease phenotype. The process involves narrowing the search to a chromosome, then to a region of the chromosome, and finally to a gene in which a mutation is always present in affected individuals and absent in normal individuals.

The first step in the analysis is to study the pattern of inheritance. This may provide valuable clues about whether a single gene is affected, and whether this gene is likely to be autosomal or on the sex chromosomes or the mitochondrial chromosome. Gross chromosome analysis can be useful and geneticists look for chromosomal aberrations (for example deletions), which are present at an unusually high frequency in individuals affected with the disease, compared with the normal population.

If there are no further clues, often the next stage in locating the gene that is mutated in the disease is to look for genetic markers as described earlier. Once polymorphic markers from across the genome have been tested, it should be possible by linkage analysis to see if any segregate with the disease allele in a family. If the position of the polymorphic marker is known, then the affected gene is likely to be close by and is therefore mapped to a region of the genome (i.e. a specific band on a chromosome arm).

Isolating the gene

Once linkage analysis has established which chromosome and which region of the chromosome contains the disease gene, the next step is to identify the gene. The region of DNA which contains the gene may span several million base-pairs, and a variety of techniques exist for cloning cDNAs and gene sequences from such regions. Genes which have been cloned and are very tightly linked to a genetic disease may be 'candidate genes' for that disease, and researchers have to show that a mutation in the gene is likely to give rise to the disease.

However, most are unknown and markers which span the disease gene's physical location on the chromosome are traced through the affected families' genetic samples. These markers define the target interval of genetic code – often several million base-pairs – within which the disease gene lies. Essentially the whole target interval is cloned and partially or entirely sequenced by 'chromosome walking' or searching cDNA libraries for uncharacterized sequences which hybridize to regions of the target interval. Sequencing approaches require searching for motif sequences, such as areas rich in repetitive cytosine and guanidine base-pairs, which are characteristic of a gene. A further criterion for candidacy is that the gene is expressed in the affected tissues. It is unlikely that a gene giving rise to a liver disease might give the instructions for making protein purely in neuronal tissue. Probably the most important criterion is to find a mutation in the gene in affected and not unaffected individuals.

When candidate genes have been identified, they are cloned and expressed in order to establish the function of the protein product.

The genetic basis of cancer

Cancers are genetic diseases and involve changes to the normal function of cellular genes. However, multiple genes interact during oncogenesis and an almost stepwise progression of defects leads from an overproliferation of a particular cell to the breakdown of control mechanisms such as apoptosis (programmed cell death). This would be triggered if a cell were to attempt to survive in an organ other than its tissue of origin. For

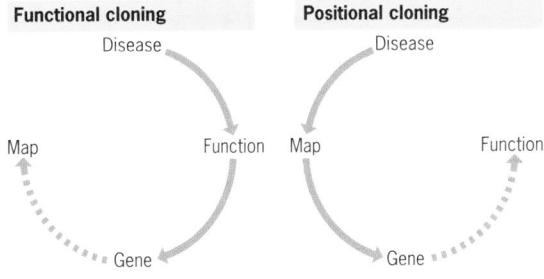

Fig. 3.19 Diagrammatic representation of the two approaches to gene cloning.

the vast majority of cancer cases (especially those in older people) we believe that the multiple genetic changes which occur are somatic. However, it is clear that susceptibility to the development of a particular form of cancer can be inherited. Indeed for some rare cancers a dominant single-gene defect can give rise to an almost Mendelian trend. In some other cancers (e.g. forms of breast cancer) the mode of inheritance is much more complex. In these cases close relatives may have an increased susceptibility to cancer (Table 9.3), and the genetics are clearly those of a multifactorial trait.

- Cancer tissues are clonal, and tumours arise from changes in only one cell which then proliferates in the body.
- The genes that are primarily damaged by the genetic changes which lead to cancer fall into two categories: oncogenes and tumour suppressor genes.
- Oncogenesis is a multistep process in that a number of mutations or alterations to key genes are required before a malignant phenotype is expressed.
- Once mutations have begun to cause unchecked clonal expansion of the primary tumour cells, further mutations occur within the subsequent generations of daughter cells that give rise to clones which are invasive and/or form metastases.

Oncogenes (see p. 477)

The genes coding for proteins which are either growth factors, growth factor receptors, secondary messengers or even DNA-binding proteins would act as promoters of abnormal cell growth if mutated. This concept was verified when viruses were found to carry genes which, when integrated into the host cell, promoted oncogenesis. These were originally termed viral or 'v-oncogenes', and later their normal cellular counterparts, c-oncogenes, were found. Thus, oncogenes encode proteins that are known to participate in the regulation of normal cellular proliferation e.g. *erb-A* on chromosome 17q11–q12 encodes for the thyroid hormone receptor. See also Table 9.4.

Activation of oncogenes

Non-activated oncogenes which are functioning normally have been referred to as 'proto-oncogenes'. Their transformation to oncogenes can occur by three routes.

Mutation

Carcinogens such as those found in cigarette smoke, ionizing radiation and ultraviolet light can cause point mutations in genomic DNA. By chance some of these point mutations will occur in regions of the oncogene which lead to activation of that gene. Not all bases in an oncogene cause cancer if mutated, but some (e.g. those in the coding region) do.

Chromosomal translocation

If during cell division an error occurs and two chromosomes translocate, so that a portion swaps over, the translocation breakpoint may occur in the middle of two genes. If this happens then the end of one gene is translocated on to the beginning of another gene, giving rise to a 'fusion gene'. Therefore sequences of one part of the fusion gene are inappropriately expressed because they are under the control of the other part of the gene.

An example of such a fusion gene occurs in chronic myeloid leukaemia (CML). In patients with CML a translocated chromosome (the Philadelphia chromosome; see p. 489) is seen in the leukaemic cells. This chromosome arises from a translocation between chromosomes 9 and 22 in which they exchange a portion of their long arms. Consequently the *ABL* gene on chromosome 9 becomes joined to the *BCR* gene on chromosome 22. The resulting fusion protein is thought to cause the changes which lead to CML. Similarly in Burkitt's lymphoma a translocation causes the regulatory segment of the *myc* oncogene to be replaced by a regulatory segment of an unrelated immunoglobulin.

Viral stimulation

When viral RNA is transcribed by reverse transcriptase into viral cDNA and in turn is spliced into the cellular DNA, the viral DNA may integrate within an oncogene and activate it. Alternatively the virus may pick up cellular oncogene DNA and incorporate it into its own viral genome. Subsequent infection of another host cell might result in expression of this viral oncogene. For example, the Rous sarcoma virus of chickens was found to induce cancer because it carried the *ras* oncogene.

After the initial activation event other changes occur within the DNA. A striking example of this is amplification of gene sequences, which can affect the *myc* gene for example. Instead of the normal two copies of a gene, multiple copies of the gene appear either within the chromosomes (these can be seen on stained chromosomes as homogeneously staining regions) or as extrachromosomal particles (double minutes). N-*myc* sequences are amplified in neuroblastomas as are N-*myc* or L-*myc* in some lung small-cell carcinomas.

Tumour suppressor genes

These genes restrict undue cell proliferation (in contrast to oncogenes), and induce the repair or self-destruction (apoptosis) of cells containing damaged DNA. Therefore mutations in these genes which disable their function lead to uncontrolled cell growth in cells with active oncogenes. An example is the germline mutations in genes found in non-polyposis colorectal cancer which are responsible for repairing DNA mismatches (p. 317).

The first tumour suppressor gene to be described was the *RB* gene. Mutations in *RB* lead to retinoblastoma which occurs in 1 in 20 000 young children and can be sporadic or familial. In the familial variety, the first mutation is inherited and by chance a second somatic mutation occurs with the formation of a tumour. In the sporadic variety, by chance both mutations occur in both the *RB* genes in a single cell. Since the finding of *RB*, other tumour suppressor genes have been described, including the gene *p53*. Mutations in *p53* have been found in almost all human tumours, including sporadic colorectal carcinomas, carcinomas of breast and lung, brain tumours, osteosarcomas and leukaemias. The protein, encoded by *p53*, is a cellular 53 kDa nuclear phosphoprotein that plays a role in DNA repair and synthesis, in the control of the cell cycle and cell differentiation and programmed cell death – apoptosis. *p53* is a DNA-binding protein which activates many gene expression pathways but it is normally only short-lived. In many tumours, mutations that disable *p53* function also prevent its cellular catabolism. Although in some cancers there is a loss of *p53* from both chromosomes, in most cancers (particularly colorectal carcinomas; see Fig. 6.38) such long-lived mutant *p53* alleles can disrupt the normal alleles' protein. As a DNA-binding protein, *p53* is likely to act as a dimer. Thus, a mutation in a single copy of the gene can promote tumour formation because a heterodimer of mutated and normal *p53* subunits would still be dysfunctional.

How tumour suppressor genes work

Tumour suppressor gene products are intimately involved in control of the cell cycle (see Fig. 3.7). Progression through the cell cycle is controlled by many molecular gateways, which are opened or blocked by the cyclin group of proteins that are specifically expressed at various stages of the cycle. The RB and p53 proteins control the cell cycle and interact specifically within many cyclin proteins. The latter are affected by INK 4α acting on p16 proteins. The general principle is that being held at one of these gateways will ultimately lead to programmed cell death. p53 is a DNA-binding protein which induces the expression of other genes and is a major player in the induction of cell death. Its own expression is induced by broken DNA. The induction of *p53* by damage initially causes the expression of DNA repair enzymes. If DNA repair is too slow or cannot be effected, then other proteins that are induced by *p53* will effect programmed cell death.

One gateway event that has been largely elucidated is that between the G1 and the S phase of the cell cycle. The transcription factor dimer E2F-DP1 causes progression from the G1 to the S phase. However, the RB protein binds to this transcription factor, preventing its induction of DNA synthesis. Other, cyclin D-related molecules inactivate the RB protein thus allowing DNA synthesis to proceed. This period of rapid DNA synthesis is susceptible to mutation events and will propagate a pre-existing DNA mistake. Damaged DNA-induced

p53 expression rapidly results in the expression of a variety of closely related (and possibly tissue-specific) proteins WAF-1/p21, p16, p27. These inhibit the inactivation of *RB* by cyclin D-related molecules. As a result *RB*, the normal gate which stops the cell cycle, binds to the E2F-DP1 transcription factor complex, halting S phase DNA synthesis. If the DNA damage is not repaired apoptosis ensues.

Viral inactivation of tumour suppressors

The suppression of normal tumour suppressor gene function can be achieved by disabling the normal protein once it has been transcribed, rather than by mutating the gene. Viruses have developed their own genes which produce proteins to do precisely this. The main targets of these proteins are *RB* and *p53* to which they bind and thus disable. The best understood are the adenovirus E1A and human papillomavirus (HPV) E7 gene products which bind *RB*, whilst the adenovirus E1B and HPV E6 gene products bind *p53*. The SV40 virus large T antigen binds both *RB* and *p53*.

Cancer aetiology: inheritance or environment?

It is clear that a mutation causing the dysfunction of a single oncogene or tumour supressor gene is not sufficient to induce unregulated clonal expansion. The Knudson multi-hit hypothesis elegantly unites the genetics of familial and sporadic tumour development: an inherited mutation in one gene allele may be insufficient to cause a tumour but will cause a significant susceptibility to the development of a particular cancer. Subsequent lifetime exposure to environmental carcinogens (viral, chemical, radiation), along with simple mistakes during cell division, may deregulate the normal allele. Other mutations which accumulate in a similar manner then lead to tumour development. Research has clearly shown that germline mutations in particular genes, such as *p53* and *RB*, have a much stronger influence on the chance of subsequent tumour development than others.

The genetics of apoptosis

Programmed cell death has been principally studied in the nematode *Caenorhabditis elegans*. The genes identified as responsible for the process are termed *ced* (cell death defective). Of particular interest are those termed *ced3*, *ced4* and *ced9* since the first two need to be active for apoptosis to occur and the last protects cells from undergoing apoptosis if triggered. In mammals, at least 10 homologues of *ced3* have been found. The first of these to be discovered is the protease interleukin caspase-1 (**c**ysteine-containing **asp**artase-specific prote**ase**). Subsequently several classes of homologous proteins have been discovered (e.g. caspase 2–10 proteases). The genes for these cysteine proteases are initially transcribed to produce inactive precursors, which are constitutively expressed in most cells. Thus they are always present, ready to be immediately activated. Several factors initiate apoptosis but in general there are two signalling pathways: the extrinsic apoptotic pathway triggered by death receptors on the cell surface and the intrinsic pathway initiated at the mitochondrial level. Death receptors are all members of the TNF receptor superfamily and include CD95 (APO-1/Fas), TRAIL (TNF-related apoptosis ligand)-R1, TRAIL-R2, TNF-R1, DR3 and DR6.

The mammalian homologue of *ced9* is the known oncogene *Bcl-2*. The expression of the *Bcl-2* protein and other inhibitors of apoptosis proteins (IAPs), is protective against apoptosis and heightens the threshold to which a cell will respond to a signal to undergo apoptosis (Fig. 3.20). Thus, over-expression of *Bcl-1* is a component of oncogenesis for some tumours and proliferative states (e.g. polycythaemia vera). There are several homologues of *Bcl-2* termed *Bax*, *Bclx* and *Mcl*. *Bcl-2* forms a dimer when acting as an inhibitor of apoptosis. However, its dimeric partner can be any of the proteins arising from the homologous genes. This disrupts *Bcl-2*'s function to varying degrees, and *Bax–Bax* homodimers are in fact enhancers of apoptosis. Thus the ratio of pro-apoptotic to anti-apoptotic proteins is necessary for the survival of a cell.

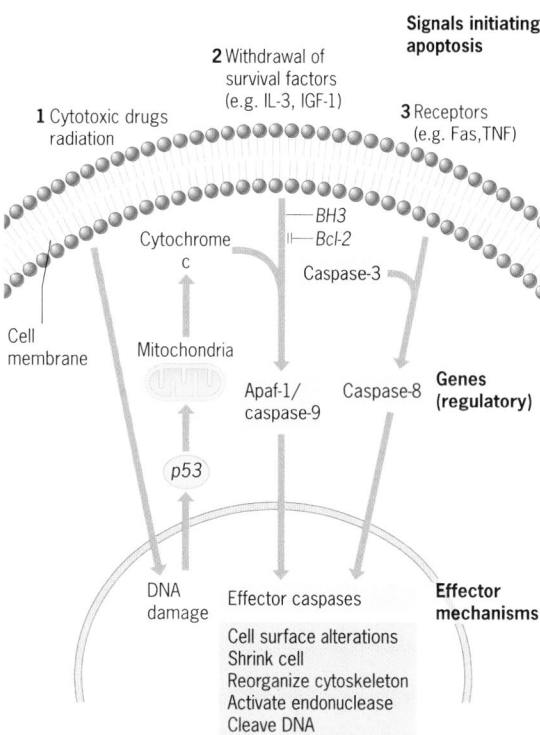

Fig. 3.20 **Mechanisms of apoptosis in a human cell.** Three initiating factors that signal apoptosis (1, 2 and 3) have an effect on gene regulation leading to effector mechanisms in the nucleus. These initiators include anticancer drugs, γ and UV irradiation, loss of survival factors, e.g. interleukin (IL), insulin-like growth factor (IGF) and cytokines that activate 'death' receptors, e.g. Fas and tumour necrosis factor (TNF). These stimuli cause a variety of regulatory genes to be expressed. An example shown in the figure is *Bcl-2* (an anti-apoptotic gene) whilst *BH3* is a pro-apoptotic gene of the *Bcl-2* family. The tumour suppressor gene *p53* is a well-known apoptotic agent. Apaf-1, apoptosis proteases activating factor; Caspase, cysteine-containing aspartase-specific protease. Modified from Renehan et al 2001 *BMJ* **322**: 1537.

FURTHER READING

Duke RC, Ojcius DM, Young JD-E (1996) Cell suicide in health and disease. *Scientific American* December: 48–56.

Eichhorst ST, Krammer PH (2001) Derangement of apoptosis in cancer. *Lancet* **358**: 345–346.

Krontiris TG (1995) Oncogenes. *New England Journal of Medicine* **333**: 303–306.

Macdonald F, Ford CHJ (1997) *Molecular Biology of Cancer.* Oxford: BIOS Science Publishers.

Wyllie AH (ed) (1997) Apoptosis: an overview. *British Medical Bulletin* **53**: 451–465.

Population genetics

The genetic constitution of a population depends on many factors. The Hardy–Weinberg equilibrium is a concept, based on a mathematical equation, that describes the outcome of random mating within populations. It states that 'in the absence of mutation, non-random mating, selection and genetic drift, the genetic constitution of the population remains the same from one generation to the next'.

This genetic principle has clinical significance in terms of the number of abnormal genes in the total gene pool of a population. The Hardy–Weinberg equation states that:

$$p^2 + 2pq + q^2 = 1$$

where p is the frequency of the normal gene in the population, q is the frequency of the abnormal gene, p^2 is the frequency of the normal homozygote, q^2 is the frequency of the affected abnormal homozygote, $2pq$ is the carrier frequency, and $p + q = 1$.

Example. The equation can be used, for example, to find the frequency of heterozygous carriers in cystic fibrosis. The incidence of cystic fibrosis is 1 in 2000 live births. Thus $q^2 = 1/2000$, and therefore $q = 1/44$. Since $q = 1 - q$, then $q = 43/44$. The carrier frequency is represented by $2pq$, which in this case is $1/22$. Thus 1 in 22 individuals in the whole population is a heterozygous carrier for cystic fibrosis.

Clinical genetics and genetic counselling

Genetic disorders pose considerable health and economic problems because often there is no effective therapy. In any pregnancy the risk of a serious developmental abnormality is approximately 1 in 30 pregnancies; approximately 15% of paediatric inpatients have a multifactorial disorder with a predominantly genetic element.

People with a history of a congenital abnormality in a member of their family often seek advice as to why it happened and about the risks of producing further abnormal offspring. Interviews must be conducted with great sensitivity and psychological insight, as parents may feel a sense of guilt and blame themselves for the abnormality in their child.

Genetic counselling should have the following aims:

- *Obtaining a full and careful history.* The pregnancy history, drug and alcohol ingestion during pregnancy and maternal illnesses (e.g. diabetes) should be detailed.
- *Establishing an accurate diagnosis.* Examination of the child may help in diagnosing a genetically abnormal child with characteristic features (e.g. trisomy 21) or whether a genetically normal fetus was damaged in utero.
- *Drawing a family tree is essential.* Questions should be asked about abortions, stillbirths, deaths, marriages, consanguinity and medical history of family members. Diagnoses may need verification from other hospital reports.
- *Estimating the risk of a future pregnancy being affected or carrying a disorder.* Estimation of risk should be based on the pattern of inheritance. Mendelian disorders (see earlier) carry a high risk; chromosomal abnormalities carry a low risk. Empirical risks may be obtained from population or family studies.
- *Information giving.* On prognosis and management.
- *Continued support and follow-up.* Explanation of the implications for other siblings and family members.
- *Genetic screening.* This includes prenatal diagnosis if requested, carrier detection and data storage in genetic registers.

Genetic counselling should be non-directive, with the couple making their own decisions on the basis of an accurate presentation of the facts and risks in a way they can understand.

Carrier detection

This is offered in autosomal recessive disorders for conditions that are relatively common such as thalassaemia (Asian and Mediterranean populations), cystic fibrosis (Caucasian populations), sickle cell disease (African origin) and Tay–Sachs disease (Ashkenazi Jews). Families with the severe form of haemophilia A can now have more accurate genetic counselling to detect the inversion of the X chromosome (flip-tip inversion) using Southern blotting.

Genetic anticipation

It has been noted that successive generations of patients with, for example, myotonic dystrophy and Huntington's chorea, present earlier and with progressively worse symptoms. This 'anticipation' is due to unstable mutations occurring within the disease gene. Trinucleotide repeats such as CTG (myotonic dystrophy) and CAG (Huntington's chorea) expand within the disease gene with each generation, and somatic expansion with cellular replication is also observed. This novel type of genetic mutation can occur within the translated region or untranslated (and presumably regulatory) regions of the target genes. This genetic distinction has been used to subclassify a number of genetic diseases which have now been shown to be caused by trinucleotide repeat expansion and display phenotypic 'anticipation' (Table 3.9).

Prenatal diagnosis

This is offered to all pregnant women in the UK. Practice varies in different maternity units, with some only offering screening to high risk mothers. Prediction factors for high risk include women who are older than 35 years and those with a history or family history of chromosomal abnormalities.

Investigations
First trimester
- Ultrasound (high resolution) for nuchal translucency to exclude major chromosomal abnormalities (e.g. trisomies and Turner's syndrome).

Table 3.9
The location of the trinucleotide repeat in 'anticipation' genetic diseases*

Trinucleotide repeat (untranslated)
Myotonic dystrophy (19q13)
Fragile X (Xq28)
Friedreich's ataxia (9q13–21)

Trinucleotide repeat (translated)
Huntington's chorea (4p16)
Spinobulbar muscular atrophy – SBMA (Xq21)
Spinocerebellar ataxia 1 and 2 – SCA1/2 (6p21)
Machado–Joseph ataxia – SCA-3 (14p32)
Dento-rubro-pallido-Luysian atrophy – DRPLA (12p12)

* The chromosomal locations of the genes are given in in parentheses

- Maternal serum for pregnancy-associated plasma protein-A (PAP-A from the syncytial trophoblast) for trisomy 21. This is more accurate than the triple test at 16 weeks.

Second trimester

- Ultrasound for structural abnormalities (e.g. neural tube defects, congenital heart defects). Serum screening has been superseded by high resolution ultrasound (above) in specialist centres.
- Triple test (used by some) for chromosomal abnormalities. This consists of a serum α-fetoprotein (low), unconjugated oestradiol (low) and human chorionic gonadotrophin (high).
- α-fetoprotein (high for neural tube defects).

All markers are corrected for gestational ages a multiple of the mean (MOM) value for the appropriate week of gestation. If abnormalities are detected, it is necessary to continue invetsigations with chorionic villus sampling (CVS) via transcervical or transabdominal route at 11–13 weeks for confirmation of abnormalities of nuchal translucence. Amniocentesis under ultrasound control can be performed at 15 weeks to sample amniotic fluid and fetal cells.

These tests may well be superseded by salvage of fetal cells from the maternal blood sample at 12 weeks.

The following points must be borne in mind when considering a prenatal screening test for aneuploidies:

- The most common congenital chromosomal aneuploidy in which the afflicted individual lives into old age is Down's syndrome – trisomy 21
- Most Down's individuals have an IQ of between 20 and 80; 61% will require surgery for congenital heart, gastrointestinal and ophthalmic defects; there is a strong association with the development of acute childhood leukaemia; and 60–70% will develop Alzheimer-like neuronal degeneration after the age of 40 years.
- The risk of having a Down's child increases with maternal age, such that at age 35 the risk is 1 in 380.
- Although women over 35 are at higher risk, they account for only 7% of pregnancies. In fact, 70–80% of all Down's children are born to women under this age.
- Karyotyping is the only definitive test, but cannot be offered to all as it is expensive and time-consuming and requires skilled technicians.
- Fetal tissue sampling is associated with a 1% risk of spontaneous termination.
- Screening aims to select a high-risk group, irrespective of maternal age, to be offered a diagnostic procedure; it does not provide a diagnosis itself.
- Of paramount importance is the ability of screening to give parents a more informed choice.

FURTHER READING

Harper PS (1996) New genes for old diseases: the molecular basis of myotonic dystrophy and Huntington's disease. *Journal of the Royal College of Physicians of London* **30**: 221–231.

Harper PS (1999) *Practical Genetic Counselling*, 5th edn. Oxford: Butterworth.

Stranc LC et al. (1997) CVS and amniocentesis in prenatal diagnosis. *Lancet* **349**: 711–714.

Applications of molecular genetics

The use of molecular biological techniques in genetics is having a massive impact on the investigation, diagnosis, treatment and control of genetic disorders.

The avoidance and control of genetic disease

Some genetic disorders, such as phenylketonuria or haemophilia, can be managed by diet or replacement therapy, but most have no effective treatment. By understanding what causes genetic damage, potential mutagens such as radiation, environmental chemicals, viruses or drugs (e.g. thalidomide) can be avoided.

Gene therapy

There are many technical problems to overcome in gene therapy, particularly in finding delivery systems to introduce DNA into a mammalian cell. Very careful control and supervision of gene manipulation will be necessary because of its potential hazards and the ethical issues.

Treatment of congenital genetic disease

Conventional therapy consists of controlling rather than curing the genetic defect. In some conditions, gene product replacement may ameliorate the symptoms; examples are the production of insulin (from recombinant DNA) for the treatment of diabetes, and factor VIII replacement in haemophilia A.

Gene therapy entails placing a normal copy of a gene into the cells of a patient who has a defective copy of the gene.

Experiments have concentrated on *recessive* disorders, such as cystic fibrosis where the disease is due to the absence of a normal gene product. In *dominant* disorders the pathogenic potential of the mutant allele is normally expressed in the presence of a normal allele. This requires gene correction, whereby the mutant sequence is replaced by an equivalent sequence from a normal allele, or the mutant allele is inactivated. Such procedures are more difficult.

Two major factors are involved in gene therapy:

- the introduction of the functional gene sequence into target cells
- the expression and permanent integration of the transfected gene into the host cell genome.

Suitable diseases for current gene therapy experiments include cystic fibrosis, adenosine deaminase deficiency, and familial hypercholesterolaemia.

Cystic fibrosis (see also p. 871)

The gene responsible for cystic fibrosis was first localized to chromosome 7 by linkage analysis. The cystic fibrosis transmembrane regulator gene (*CFTR*) was then isolated by chromosome-mediated gene transfer, chromosome walking and jumping. The *CFTR* gene spans about 250 kbp and contains 27 exons. The DNA sequence analysis predicts a polypeptide sequence of 1480 amino acids. The *CFTR* gene also encodes a simple chloride ion channel within the cystic fibrosis transmembrane regulator (Fig. 3.21). In most patients there is a single mutation with a 3 bp deletion in exon 10 resulting in the removal of a codon specifying phenylalanine. There are also over 100 different minor mutations of the *CFTR* gene with most mapping to the ATP-binding domains. This has led to the improved diagnosis of cystic fibrosis as well as new strategies for conventional drug-based therapies.

Gene therapy experiments are underway that take two different routes to putting a normal version of the *CFTR* gene into the lung epithelial cells of a patient who is homozygous for a defect in this gene. One route entails placing the *CFTR* gene in an adenovirus vector, and infecting the epithelial cells of the patient with the virus (Fig. 14.30). Infection causes the *CFTR* gene to be taken into the cell where it may start functioning normally. A second route entails placing the DNA for the *CFTR* gene into a liposome. Liposomes are then conveyed to the lung using an aerosol spray, and the fatty surface of the liposome fuses with the cell membrane to deliver the *CFTR* DNA into the cell, where again the gene should function normally. Ultimately this type of gene therapy should give cystic fibrosis patients a normal life without the need for drugs and intensive physiotherapy.

Adenosine deaminase (ADA) deficiency

Gene therapy for this rare immunodeficiency disease entails introducing a normal human *ADA* gene into the patient's lymphocytes to reconstitute the function of the cellular and humoral immune system in severe combined immunodeficiency (SCID). Lymphocytes have been tried for short-term therapy, but for longer-term treatment bone marrow transplantation would be the definitive approach (see p. 485).

Familial hypercholesterolaemia

This disorder is a result of a defective low-density lipoprotein (LDL) receptor gene. In therapy, a receptor gene is inserted into hepatocytes, removed by liver biopsy from the patient. Gene-corrected hepatocytes are then reinjected into the portal circulation of the patient. These cells migrate back to the liver where they are reincorporated and should start to produce LDL receptor protein, which would dramatically lower the patient's cholesterol level.

Muscle-cell-mediated gene therapy

Much of the problem associated with gene therapy of chronic genetic disease is how long the transfected cells will survive. Isolated myoblasts transfected with a retrovirus have been shown to function and live for the lifetime of mouse models (2 years). The myoblasts fuse with the patient's muscle fibres and express the transfected protein. The long life of the muscle fibres and their rich blood supply make them an ideal site for treatment of diseases in which functional serum-born factors are missing (e.g. human growth hormone, coagulation factors and erythropoietin).

Obviously, myoblast transfection would appear to be the best option for the treatment of Duchenne muscular dystrophy. However, the Duchenne gene is far too large to fit into any current viral vector, and reimplanted myoblasts do not colonize muscles fibres distant from the site of injection.

Treatment of somatic disease

Gene therapy which requires only a transient expression of the transfected genetic material circumvents the problems currently plaguing gene therapy of inherited disorders. This may also prove to be the front-line of gene therapy.

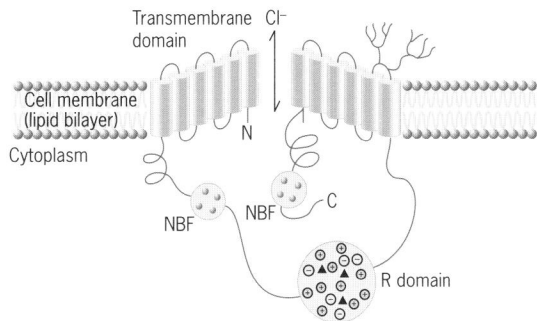

Fig. 3.21 Model of cystic fibrosis transmembrane regulator (CFTR). This is an integral membrane glycoprotein, consisting of two repeated elements. The cylindrical structures represent six membrane-spanning helices in each half of the molecule. The nucleotide-binding folds (NBFs) are in the cytoplasm, and the dots in these shaded areas represent the means of entry by the nucleotide. The regulatory (R) domain links the two halves and contains charged individual amino acids and protein kinase phosphorylation sites (black triangles). N and C are the N and C terminals. The branched structure on the right half represents potential glycosylation sites. The chloride channel is shown.

Vascular disease

The ideal therapy in heart disease would be neovascularization to increase blood flow and the repair of cardiac tissue after a myocardial infarction. In fact, any vascular disease might require regeneration or new blood vessel growth. Temporary expression of angiogenic factors at the site of a blockage would induce new blood vessels. Alternatively, local temporary expression of clot-disintegrating enzymes such as streptokinase and lipases may repair damaged and diseased arteries. It is quite possible to deliver liposomes loaded with DNA or, in fact, directly inject DNA plasmids into the tissue, and the protein will be expressed by the cells which take it up. Only 1–3% will do so, but this is sufficient for the local effect required and it is a transient expression. This gives a controllable gene therapy.

Neuronal disease

Neurotrophic factors can be transiently expressed as described above for vascular diseases. The local expression of neurotrophins is essential for nerve cell regeneration and maintenance. It is possible to extend the expression period of the neurotrophin by injecting transfected myocytes into the damaged area. They will fuse with any adjacent muscle tissue to give a prolonged expression of the factor gene.

Cancer

Cancer is a genetic disease and many genes are deregulated. *p53* is a tumour suppressor gene; the reintroduction and overexpression of a functional *p53* in tumours is being investigated with some success. Since *p53* will induce apoptosis in cells with damaged genetic material, the transient expression of high levels in a tumour cell with *p53* pathway defects should induce its own (apoptotic) demise. Since this is only likely to occur in rapidly dividing cells, this is a perfect target for cancer gene therapy. Transient expression induced by repeat exposure to vectors such as retroviruses, liposomes and naked DNA plasmids is all relatively straightforward. Trials using aerosols of these vectors in patients with lung cancer are being performed.

Tumour growth depends on the development of new blood vessels (angiogenesis), and inhibitors of this process are also being used in trials.

Creating and using animal models

There is a need for model systems in which to test gene therapies prior to use in patients. To some extent gene 'knock-out' experiments in mice are providing new animal models of disease. In these experiments the normal gene of interest in a mouse is targeted using recombinant DNA techniques so that gene function is impaired, in analogy to the situation in the particular gene of a human patient. However, mice and humans are different and it will not be possible to mimic some human genetic diseases in mice. Transgenic mice are created when exogenous DNA carrying a gene of interest is injected into a mouse egg. If this egg is fertilized then all the cells of the resulting animal will carry the extra gene sequences. Transgenic mice have also been used as animal models of human diseases in which new therapies may be tested.

Other animal models have paved the way for gene therapy techniques. For example, some of the first experiments in the transfer of globin genes (which will be useful for gene therapy for sickle cell disease and thalassaemia) have taken place in mice. These include transplanting normal donor cells with normal genes into lethally irradiated mice, which results in engraftment of the donor cells.

The human genome project (HGP)

An international effort to sequence the entire human genome, all 3×10^9 bp on the 24 different chromosomes, was officially launched in 1986. An initial aim was to construct genetic and physical maps of the chromosomes: 40 three-generation families were studied for microsatellite and restriction enzyme (RFLP) polymorphisms. Some 70 000 polymorphisms were characterized and physically assigned to chromosomal band locations. These landmarks in the genome are used as reference points in the subsequent genome mapping project. However, as already described, these polymorphisms are the first step in positional cloning of a disease gene and are used as genetic markers if they co-segregate with the disease. As of 2000, a first-draft map has been completed. Having the complete sequence of the genome will make it much easier to identify candidate genes in genetic disorders, and will be a great aid to genetic research.

As only 2% of the genome codes for actual proteins, it has been suggested that we should only sequence cDNA, which would be cheaper and much quicker. However, many genetic disorders are the result of deregulation of expression and it is the control elements surrounding the coding that are deregulated. Thus complete sequencing will eventually give rise to an understanding of how genes are packaged as euchromatin or heterochromatin.

The human proteome project

A more direct route to understanding genetic and somatic disease is by studying the protein expression characteristics of normal and diseased cells – the proteome. This relies on the separation of proteins expressed by a given tissue by molecular size and charge on a simple two-dimensional display and is achieved by using two-dimensional gel electrophoresis. The pattern of dots corresponds to the different proteins

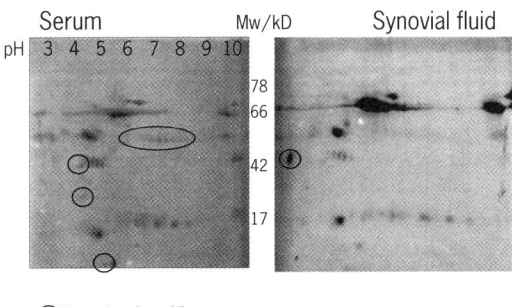

Serum   Mw/kD   Synovial fluid

○ Peaks lost from SF   ○ New peak in SF

Fig. 3.22 Two-dimensional gel electrophoresis comparing paired serum and synovial fluid in a patient with rheumatoid arthritis. Biofluids were first separated according to isoelectric point on a linear immobilized pH gradient followed by SDS-PAGE in a 10% gel. The circled proteins indicate major proteins which differ between the two biofluids. Although serum contained many proteins not found in synovial fluid, one major protein was found to be present in the synovial fluid electropherogram but not in the serum electropherogram. This indicates that synovial fluid is not a simple transudate of serum. Courtesy of Prof. D Perrett and Dr R Bevan, Department of Medicine, Barts and The London School of Medicine.

expressed. With the improvement in technology the patterns are reproducible and can be stored as electronic images. Non-, over- and underexpression of a given protein can be detected by a corresponding change on the proteome two-dimensional electrophoresis image. As can be seen in Figure 3.22, the protein profile of synovial fluid from a diseased joint shows a new protein arising with disease. Such proteins have been identified as inflammatory cytokines. Furthermore, post-translational modifications of the protein show up as a change in either size or charge on the proteome picture. This cannot be detected by genome analysis. Looking for such changes has already lead to the discovery of new protein markers for the diagnosis of Creutzfeldt–Jakob disease, multiple sclerosis, schizophrenia, Parkinson's disease (spinal fluid protein) and Alzheimer's disease (blood and brain proteins). The proteome approach may prove more useful to medical advances than the genome project.

Ethical considerations

Ethical considerations must be taken into account in any discussion of clinical genetics. For example, prenatal diagnosis with the option of termination may be unacceptable on moral or religious grounds. With diseases for which there is no cure and currently no treatment (e.g. Huntington's), genetic tests can predict accurately which family members will be affected; however, many people would rather not know this information. One very serious outcome of the new genetic information is that disease susceptibility may be predictable, for example in Alzheimer's disease, so the medical insurance companies can decline to give policies for individuals at high risk.

Society has not yet decided who should have access to an individual's genetic information and to what extent privacy should be preserved.

FURTHER READING

Blau HM, Springer ML (1995) Gene therapy: a novel form of drug delivery. *New England Journal of Medicine* **333**: 1204–1207.

Blau HM, Springer ML (1995) Muscle-mediated gene therapy. *New England Journal of Medicine* **333**: 1554–1556.

McDonnell WM, Askari FK (1996) DNA vaccines. *New England Journal of Medicine* **334**: 42–46.

Super M (2000) CFTR and disease: implications for drug development. *Lancet* **355**: 1840–1842.

Weatherall DJ (1996) *Basic Molecular and Cell Biology*, 3rd edn. London: BMJ Publishing.

CHAPTER BIBLIOGRAPHY

Brock DJH (1993) *Molecular Genetics for the Clinician*. Cambridge: Cambridge University Press.

Connor JM, Ferguson–Smith MA (1997) *Essential Medical Genetics*, 5th edn. Oxford: Blackwell Scientific.

McKusick VA (1998) *Mendelian Inheritance in Man*, 12th edn. London: Johns Hopkins Press.

Vogel F, Motulsky AG (1997) *Human Genetics*, 3rd edn. New York: Springer

Clinical immunology

4

The immune system protects against infections and tumours. It is made up of a network of lymphoid organs, cells, humoral factors and soluble messengers called cytokines. However, this system does not work in isolation. There are intimate interactions with the neurological and endocrine systems, giving new insight into regulation of immune responses. The functions of the immune system become most clear when it fails. Abnormalities are a common cause of disease, overactivity of the immune response leading to allergic and autoimmune disorders, or underactivity resulting in immunodeficiency. Manipulation of the immune response, for example by vaccination with organisms or their proteins to protect from infection, or immuno-suppression to enable organ and bone marrow trans-plantation is well established in clinical practice. The development of therapeutic monoclonal antibodies, genetic engineering of cytokines or their receptors, and DNA vaccine technology are changing the approach to the treatment of many diseases.

The immune system in health

Host defence

Throughout life we are exposed to millions of organisms which are inhaled, swallowed or contact our skin or mucous membranes. Whether these organisms invade and cause disease is determined by the balance of the pathogenicity of the organism (i.e. the virulence factors that it has at its disposal) and the integrity of the host defence mechanisms. Immunity is often divided into two types termed innate and specific (acquired or adap-tive), although in practice these overlap.

Innate immunity

Innate immunity consists of the immediately active but non-specific host defence mechanisms. A major part of this immunity does not involve the immune system but uses physical and chemical barriers. Disruption of these is a common cause of susceptibility to infection in clini-cal practice, even if the immune system itself is fully functioning (Table 4.1).

The elements of the immune system itself that mount an innate response are phagocytic cells (neutrophils,

191

Table 4.1
Non-immunological host defence mechanisms

Normal barriers	Examples of defects leading to infection
Physical barriers	
Skin and mucous membranes	Breach, e.g. trauma, burns, eczema, cannulae
Cough reflex	Suppression, e.g. by opiates, neurological disease
Mucociliary escalator	Ciliary paralysis (smoking, primary ciliary dyskinesis syndromes)
	Increased mucus production (asthma)
	Abnormally viscid secretions (cystic fibrosis)
Washing, tears, saliva, urine	Decreased fluid, e.g. sicca syndromes, drugs
	Urinary stasis, e.g. prostatic hypertrophy
Chemical barriers, e.g. gastric acid	Gastric acid secretion inhibitors
Colonization resistance provided by non-pathogenic commensal organisms of skin and gut	Use of broad-spectrum antibiotics

and monocytes in the blood, macrophages in tissues), eosinophils, mast cells and basophils, as well as humoral components (mainly complement). These are directly activated by infectious agents, tissue damage or tumours.

The immediate immune response to infection

The non-specific immune responses utilized in the first stages of a local infection are a good illustration of the normal mechanisms of cell production, recruitment and activation used by the immune system. The same mechanisms that lead to protective inflammation can also cause extensive damage if not regulated.

Initiation of the inflammatory response

The neutrophil (polymorphonuclear, or PMN cell) is a specialized microbicidal (microbe-killing) phagocyte. The human body contains over 10^{11} polymorpho-nuclear leucocytes/kg, most of which are in the bone marrow. A series of events leads to the recruitment and activation of these cells at the site of tissue damage.

Adhesion molecules (Table 4.2)

Neutrophils, like most of the cells involved in immune responses, are not static within a particular tissue but are mobile cells. Neutrophils travel within the blood, either flowing freely as part of the circulating pool or rolling along the vascular endothelium as the marginating pool (see below).

Recruitment of cells of the immune system (phagocytes and lymphocytes) to tissue sites involves cell surface adhesion molecules (CAM) (p. 160, Fig. 3.6). The main ones are the intercellular adhesion molecules (ICAM), integrins, selectins and cadherins (calcium-dependent adherins). Adhesion molecules associate with cytoskeletal components to cause cytoskeletal re-organization, migration and spreading, allowing the cells to move independently. The binding of adhesion molecules to their ligand also causes signal transduction with increased expression of other receptors, altered gene expression and effects on protein synthesis and cell survival and often leads to cell activation.

Cell recruitment

Cells move towards the site of inflammation in response to chemoattractants (chemicals which attract cells) at sites of infection or tissue damage. The main chemoattractants for neutrophils *in vivo* are N-formyl-methionyl-leucylphenylalanine (FMLP) from bacterial cell walls, which in turn causes the release of another chemoattractant, leukotriene B_4 (LTB_4) from tissue mast cells; the chemokine (chemoattractant cytokine) interleukin-8 (from macrophages); and C5a from the activation of complement. These substances cause migration of neutrophils by three mechanisms:

- *Upregulation of neutrophil adhesion molecules*, L-selectin and the integrin LFA-1 (leucocyte function antigen), which increases the stickiness of the cells.
- *Increase in vascular endothelial cell expression of the adhesion molecules* E-selectin and ICAM-1 which causes increased stickiness of the endothelium. The selectin expression causes the circulating neutrophil to be tethered and roll along the endothelium slowly (margination), whereas the reaction between the integrins LFA-1 and ICAM-1 is much stronger, causing the cells to stop moving.
- *Stimulation of neutrophil chemotaxis* (directed movement along the chemoattractant gradient towards the stimulus).

The cells pass between endothelial cells into the tissues by the formation of foot-like processes (pseudopodia) that push through the intercellular spaces, this is called diapedesis. The cells continue to move along the chemoattractant gradient to the site of infection (Fig. 4.1). When the cells reach the highest concentration of chemoattractant the receptor on the cell surface is downregulated, ensuring that the phagocytes remain at the site of inflammation.

The exodus of neutrophils leads to the inflammatory response and if it involves large numbers causes the formation of pus, the characteristic yellow colour being due to the cytochromes within the cells. Patients with congenital deficiencies of adhesion molecules or those

Table 4.2
Adhesion molecules

Adhesion molecule	Tissue distribution	Ligand
Immunoglobulin superfamily		
ICAM-1 (CD54)	Endothelial cells, monocytes, T and B cells, dendritic cells, keratinocytes, chondrocytes, epithelial cells	LFA-1
ICAM-2 (CD102)	Endothelial cells, monocytes, dendritic cells, subpopulations of lymphocytes	LFA-1
ICAM-3	Lymphocytes	LFA-1, Mac-1
VCAM-1 (CD106)	Endothelial cells, kidney epithelium, macrophages, dendritic cells, myoblasts, bone marrow fibroblasts	VLA-4
PECAM-1	Platelets, T cells, endothelial cells, monocytes, granulocytes	Unknown
MAdCAM-1	Endothelial venules in mucosal lymph nodes	$\alpha4\beta7$ integrin and L-selectin
Selectin family		
E-selectin (CD62E)/ELAM-1	Endothelial cells	Unknown
L-selectin (CD62L)	Lymphocytes, neutrophils, monocytes	CD34
P-selectin (CD62P)	Megakaryocytes, platelets and endothelial cells	Unknown
Integrin family		
VLA subfamily		
VLA-1 to VLA-4	Endothelial cells, resting T cells, monocytes, platelets and epithelial cells	Various molecules including laminin, fibronectin, collagen and VCAM-1
VLA-5 (fibronectin receptor)	Endothelial cells, monocytes and platelets	Laminin
VLA-6 (laminin receptor)	Endothelial cells, monocytes and platelets	Laminin
$\beta1\alpha7$	Endothelial cells, ? others	Laminin
$\beta1\alpha8$	Endothelial cells, ? others	Unknown
$\beta1\alpha$	Platelets and megakaryocytes	Fibronectin
$\beta2$	Widely distributed	Collagen, laminin, vitronectin
Leucam subfamily		
LFA-1	Leucocytes	ICAMs 1 to 3
Mac-1	Endothelial cells, ? others	ICAM-1, fibrinogen, C3bi
Cytoadhesin subfamily		
Vitronectin receptor	Platelets and megakaryocytes	Vitronectin, fibrinogen, laminin, fibronectin, von Willebrand factor, thrombospondin
$\beta4\alpha6$	Endothelial cells, thymocytes and platelets	Laminin
$\beta5\alpha$	Platelets and megakaryocytes, ? others	Vitronectin, fibronectin
$\beta6\alpha$	Platelets and megakaryocytes, ? others	Fibronectin
$\beta7\alpha4$/LPAM-1	Endothelial cells, thymocytes, monocytes	Fibronectin, VCAM-1
$\beta8\alpha$	Platelets and megakaryocytes, ?	Unknown

E-selectin or ELAM, endothelial leucocyte adhesion molecule; ICAM, intercellular adhesion molecule;
LPAM, lymphocyte Peyer's patch adhesion molecule; MAdCAM-1, mucosal addressin; PECAM, platelet/endothelial cell adhesion molecule;
VCAM vascular cell adhesion molecule; VLA, very late antigen; LFA, leucocyte function antigen

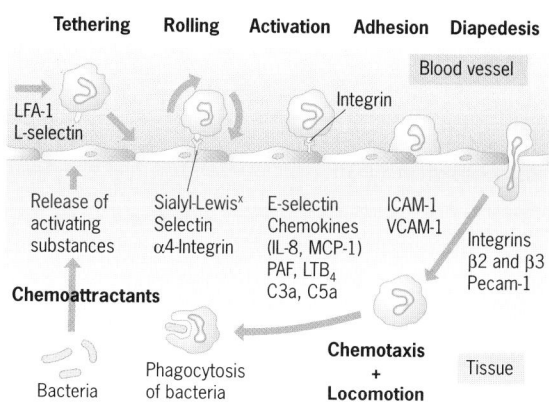

Fig. 4.1 Neutrophil migration. Neutrophils arrive at the site of the inflammation, attracted by chemoattractants. They roll along the blood-vessel wall and their progress is halted by L-selectin, on their surface, binding to a carbohydrate structure, e.g. sialyl-Lewis^x, an adhesion molecule. On activation, the L-selectin is replaced by another cell surface adhesion molecule, e.g. integrin which binds to E-selectin. Various other chemokines, e.g. interleukin-8 (IL-8), macrophage chemoattractant factor (MCP), TNF-α and other inflammatory mediators are involved. These inflammatory markers attract the activated neutrophil into the tissue where it phagocytoses and destroys C3b-coated bacteria. The inflammation releases activating substances attracting more neutrophils. LFA, leucocyte function antigen; PAF, platelet-activating factor, LTB$_4$, leukotriene B$_4$; ICAM, intracellular adhesion molecule; VCAM, vascular cell adhesion molecule; PECAM, platelet/endothelial cell adhesion molecule.

on systemic corticosteroids who have acquired adhesion molecule defects (steroids reduce ICAM-1 expression on endothelial cells) cannot target their neutrophils to sites of infection. As a result of this they suffer with recurrent infections. The peripheral blood characteristically shows a leucocytosis as the cells cannot leave the circulation.

Similar mechanisms of cell recruitment and trafficking by the use of adhesion molecules are described for other cells within the immune system, for example L-selectin facilitates 'homing' of lymphocytes to lymph nodes.

Phagocytosis and intracellular killing

Once the neutrophils have been recruited, phagocytosis (ingestion) and intracellular killing of microbes begins. Phagocytosis occurs by the formation of pseudopodia (projections of cytoplasmic membrane) around the organism or particle to be ingested (see Fig. 4.11a). Owing to the fluidity of the cell membrane, the tips eventually fuse to form a membrane-bound vesicle called a phagosome. This fuses with the neutrophil cytoplasmic granules (Table 4.3) to form a phagolysosome. Within this localized environment killing occurs, the cytoplasm being protected. There are two major mechanisms:

1. O_2-dependent response or 'respiratory burst', in which there is production of reactive oxygen metabolites, such as hydrogen peroxide, hydroxyl radicals and singlet oxygen, via the reduction of oxygen by a cytochrome-dependent NADPH oxidase.
2. O_2-independent response, due to the toxic action of preformed cationic proteins and enzymes contained within the cytoplasmic granules.

Ingestion and killing of organisms is much more effective if the particle is first coated or opsonized ('made ready to eat') with specific antibody and complement. This is because neutrophils have receptors for the Fc portion of antibody molecules (FcR), and complement (CR). Binding of cell-surface receptors to complement and antibody on the particle both increases the strength of adhesion and causes transduction of intracellular signals, which activate the cell to promote phagocytic and killing activity. The role of antibody in this situation demonstrates the interaction of the innate (neutrophil) and antigen-specific (antibody) immune responses.

Granulocyte and granulocyte–macrophage colony-stimulating factors (G-CSF and GM-CSF) are cytokines which are released by activated endothelial cells and macrophages at the site of infection and act on the bone marrow to stimulate stem cell division to release more neutrophils into the circulation. This causes the characteristic neutrophil leucocytosis observed in the peripheral blood in infectious or inflammatory disease. Interleukin-6 is also produced and induces the liver synthesis of large amounts of the acute-phase reactants, particularly complement components, C-reactive protein (CRP), mannan-binding lectin and fibrinogen (Table 4.4). Many of these are opsonins. CRP and fibrinogen (the main factor which affects the ESR reading) are measured diagnostically to monitor infection and inflammatory conditions.

Neutrophils can only ingest particles smaller than themselves and are therefore mainly active against extracellular infections, particularly bacteria and some fungi, protecting the blood and viscera from these types of organisms. Monocytes and macrophages act in the same way using similar types of receptors. Phagocytes also remove particles of foreign material and tissue debris.

Eosinophils in host defence

In developed countries eosinophilia is most commonly associated with allergic disease, but their physiological function is in parasite control. Eosinophils have receptors for IgE which is the major antiparasite antibody, particularly against nematodes. Eosinophils bind via the FcεR, and toxic metabolites are released from the eosinophil granules directly onto the parasite surface. Examples are major basic protein (MBP), which produces ballooning and detachment of the helminth tegumental membrane, and eosinophil cationic protein (ECP), which is present in smaller amounts but is eight to ten times more toxic than MBP, producing complete fragmentation and disruption of the parasites.

Table 4.3
Neutrophil granule proteins (there are two types distinguished by staining characteristics)

Primary granule (azurophilic)
Defensins
Lysozyme
Elastase
Bactericidal/permeability-increasing factor
Cathepsin G
Myeloperoxidase
Acid glycolases
Collagenase

Secondary granule (specific)
Lysozyme
Lactoferrin
Collagenase
Cytochrome B
Vitamin B_{12}-binding protein

Table 4.4
Acute-phase proteins

Pentraxins – C-reactive protein, serum amyloid P protein
Complement components
Fibrinogen
Haptoglobulin
Caeruloplasmin
α_1-Antitrypsin
Mannose-binding lectin
Ferritin

Basophils and mast cells

Mast cells consist of two populations, which are distinguished by their enzyme content. The T mast cells contain trypsin alone and are also termed mucosal mast cells owing to their location near mucosal surfaces. The TC mast cells contain both trypsin and chymotrypsin and are called connective tissue mast cells. Mast cell function appears to be in the initiation of inflammatory responses (increased vascular permeability, bronchoconstriction) by the release (following degranulation) of pro-inflammatory mediators such as histamine, leukotrienes and platelet-activating factor (PAF). Basophils are morphologically similar to mast cells but are found in very small numbers in the blood. These cells bear high-affinity IgE receptors FcεR1 (CD23) which rapidly absorb any local IgE and also participate in immediate-type hypersensitivity reactions (see p. 213).

Complement

The complement system comprises a series of at least 20 glycoproteins that are activated in a cascade sequence, similar to the coagulation pathway, with proenzymes that undergo sequential proteolytic cleavage to their active forms. It is a major part of the innate immune system.

Three main pathways of C′ activation exist, termed the classical, alternative and manose-binding lectin (MBL) pathways (Fig. 4.2). The *terminology* of the complement proteins is that components of the classical pathway are named by 'C' followed by a number (the numbering sequence is in order of their discovery not position in the sequence). Alternative pathway components are called factors followed by a specific letter. During activation some components are initially cleaved into fragments. The smaller fragment, designated 'a', is released; the larger 'b' fragment is usually deposited on the surface of the activating cell. Further fragmentation may occur to 'c', 'd' and 'g' fragments.

The complement pathways are triggered by different factors:

- **Classical pathway** by antigen–antibody immune complexes, apoptotic cells, C-reactive protein bound to ligand and certain viruses and bacteria.
- **Alternative pathway** by bacterial endotoxin, fungal cell walls, viruses and tumour cells.
    The pathways converge in the activation of C3 (by the formation of either classical or alternative C3 convertase). This leads into a final common pathway with the assembly of components C5–C9 to form the membrane attack complex (MAC) which assembles into a 'doughnut-like' transmembrane channel leading to cell lysis by osmotic shock.
- **Mannose-binding lectin (MBL) pathway** is activated by microbes with terminal mannose groups. MBL has a similar structure to C1q and activates through the classical pathway without the requirement for antibody.

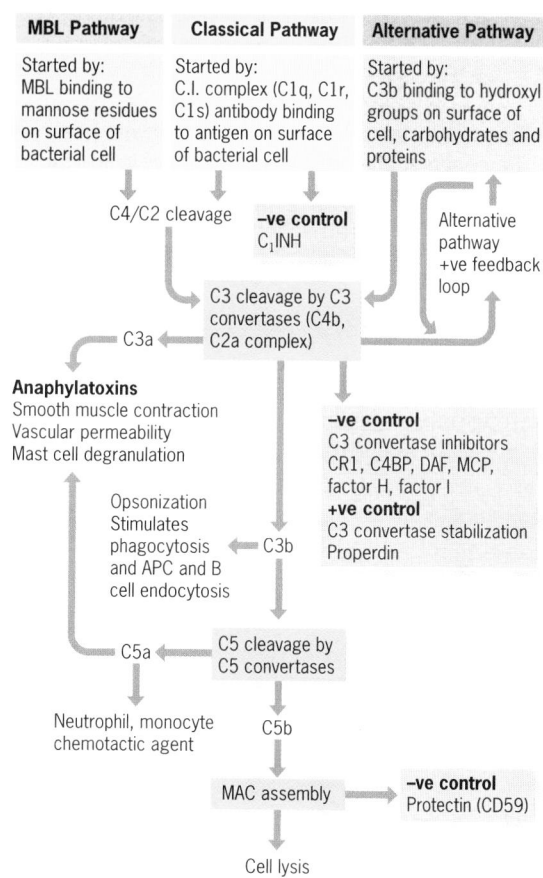

Fig. 4.2 Complement pathway. The three activation pathways (mannose-binding lectin (MBL), classical and alternative) converge at the central C3 component. This leads to a final common pathway with the assembly of C5 to C9 forming a transmembrane pore (membrane attack complex MAC) in the cell surface and death by osmotic lysis. C1INH, C1 esterase inhibitor; factors H and I, regulatory factors; DAF, decay-accelerating factor; MCP, macrophage chemoattractant protein; APC, antigen-presenting cell; CR1, complement receptor 1; C4BP, C4 binding protein.

Complement activation is focused at cell membranes. Host cells are protected from complement-mediated lysis by inhibitory surface molecules, for example decay accelerating factor (DAF). The importance of this factor is demonstrated in paroxysmal nocturnal haemoglobinuria where there are severe episodes of uncontrolled complement-mediated haemolyis. Most organisms lack any protective molecules and are therefore susceptible to lysis.

Functions of complement

- *Anti-infective function*:
    - oponization of C3b- and C4b-coated particles
    - chemotaxis – attraction of phagocytes by chemoattractant activation products

- activation of leucocytes by anaphylatoxins (C5a, C3a and C4a); there are anaphylatoxin receptors on leucocytes
- lysis of bacteria and cells (C5b–C9).
- *Interplay between innate and adaptive immune system.* Immunomodulation of B-cell responses to specific antigen through binding of complement receptors on B-cell surface, thus augmenting antibody responses and immunological memory.
- *Clearance of:*
  - immune complexes (C1q, C3 and C4)
  - apoptotic cells (C1q, C3 and C4).

Other cells or factors active in non-specific immunity
Natural killer (NK) cells
These non-phagocytic cells have the morphology of lymphocytes but do not bear the markers for T or B cells. They are distinguished by the presence of numerous cytoplasmic granules. They have non-specific antiviral and antitumour activity, causing lysis of cells with which they react.

NK cells recognize abnormal cells in two ways. Firstly, they bear immunoglobulin receptors (FcR) and bind antibody-coated targets leading to antibody-dependent cellular cytotoxicity (ADCC). Secondly, they have surface receptors for MHC class I. If these MHC receptors are not bound on interaction with a cell, the NK cell is programmed to lyse this target cell. It does this by making holes in its cell membrane by secreting 'perforins'; granzymes are injected through these pores and cause the induction of apoptosis. As normal host cells are MHC class I positive, the 'death pathway' is inhibited by the NK cell binding to this receptor. However, tumour cells and viruses often cause downregulation of class I and thus it leaves them open to NK cell attack.

Table 4.5
Origins and biological functions of cytokines (including chemokines)

Cytokine	Source	Mode of action
IL-1	Macrophages/monocytes	Immune activation: induces an inflammatory response
IL-2	Primarily Th1 cells	Activates T (and NK) cells and supports their growth
IL-3	T cells	Primarily promotes growth of haematopoietic cells
IL-4	Th2 cells	Lymphocyte growth factor; involved in IgE responses
IL-5	Th2 cells	Promotes growth of B cells and eosinophils
IL-6	Th2 cells and macrophages	Promotes B-cell growth and antibody production
IL-7	Stromal cells	Lymphocyte growth factor, important in the growth of immature cells
IL-10	CD4 cells, activated monocytes	Inhibits the production of IFN-γ, IL-1, IL-6, TNF-α and antigen presentation
IL-12	Monocytes/macrophages	Augments Th1 responses and induces IFN-γ
IL-13	Activated T cells	Stimulates B cells
IL-15	Many tissues, not T cells	Similar action to IL-2
G-CSF	Primarily monocytes	Promotes growth of myeloid cells
M-CSF	Primarily monocytes	Promotes growth of macrophages
GM-CSF	Primarily T cells	Promotes growth of mono-myelocytic cells
IFN-α	Leucocytes	Immune activation and modulation (following viral infection)
IFN-β	Fibroblasts	Immune activation and modulation (following viral infection)
IFN-γ	Th1 and NK cells	Immune activation and modulation (inhibits Th2 cells, activates macrophages)
TNF-α	Macrophages, NK, T, B and mast cells	Stimulates generalized immune activation as well as tumour necrosis; formerly known as *cachectin*
TNF-β	T and B cells, macrophages, mast cells	Stimulates immune activation and generalized vascular effects; also known as *lymphotoxin*
TGF-β	Platelets	Immunoinhibitory but stimulates tumourigenesis, angiogenesis and fibrosis
Chemokine (class defined in brackets)*		
MCP-1 (-CC-)	Monocytes, macrophages, fibroblasts, keratinocytes	Attracts monocytes and memory T cells to inflammatory sites
MIP-1α (-CC-)	Macrophages	Attracts monocytes and T cells
MIP-1β (-CC-)	Monocytes, macrophages, endothelial cells, T and B cells	Attracts monocytes and CD8+ T cells
Eotaxin (-CC-)	Macrophages, activated leucocytes, endothelial cells	Attracts eosinophils, basophils
RANTES (-CC-)	Platelets and T cells	Attracts monocytes, T cells, eosinophils
IL-8 (-CXC-)	Macrophages	Attracts neutrophils, naive T cells

* Refers to a double cysteine amino acid structure (**-CC-**) within the cytokine; in some cases this is interspersed with another amino acid (**-CXC-**)
G-CSF, granulocyte colony-stimulating factor; GM-CSF, granulocyte–macrophage colony-stimulating factor; IFN, interferon; IL, interleukin; M-CSF, monocyte colony-stimulating factor; TGF, transforming growth factor; TNF, tumour necrosis factor; MCP, macrophage chemoattractant protein; MIP, macrophage inflammatory protein; RANTES, regulated on activation, normal T-cell expressed and secreted

NK cells also bear chemokine receptors CCR2 and CCR5 which bond the chemokines, e.g. MCP, MIP and RANTES (see Table 4.5).

Cytokines

Cytokines are small soluble intercellular messengers that exert their effect by binding to specific receptors on target cells. They act as autocrine, paracrine or endocrine messengers. Cytokines produced by white blood cells and having major effects on other white cells are termed interleukins. Cytokines that have chemoattractant function are called chemokines Those that cause differentiation and proliferation of stem cells are called colony-stimulating factors. Cytokines are produced by any cell. Their biological effect varies according to the cytokine and the cell involved (Table 4.5), but typically these molecules will signal certain cell populations to activate, divide or home in on a particular site in the body.

Interferons (IFN) are a major class of cytokine. They are divided into type I (alpha and beta) and type II (gamma or 'immune' interferon). Type I interferons are antiviral agents produced mainly by fibroblasts and monocytes as a reaction to viral infection. Alpha and beta IFN bind the same cellular receptor and protect uninfected cells by inducing the intracellular production of molecules that inhibit viral RNA and DNA production. They also increase the expression of MHC class I molecules leading to enhanced lysis of virally infected cells by specific cytotoxic T lymphocytes. Type I interferons also have antiproliferative function. IFN-α is used in the treatment of chronic hepatitis B and C infections as well as in some forms of leukaemia. IFN-β reduces the relapse rate in multiple sclerosis.

Gamma-interferon has different functions, acting mainly on the immune response. It activates macrophage and neutrophil intracellular killing, stimulates natural killer cells and enhances T-cell responses by increasing MHC class II expression on antigen-presenting cells. IFN-γ is only produced by cells of the immune system and uses a separate receptor from the type I interferons. It is used therapeutically in the congenital neutrophil defect (chronic granulomatous disease), in patients with defects in IFN-γ production or receptor expression, and in the adjunct therapy of some infections (leishmaniasis, atypical mycobacterial disease).

Other cytokines are also involved in innate immunity. Tumour necrosis factor (TNF) alpha increases phagocyte function. Interleukin-6 mediates the acutephase reaction through hepatic induction. Interleukin-8 is a powerful chemoattractant. The release of granulocyte and macrophage–granulocyte colony-stimulating factors (G- and GM-CSF) will increase phagocyte numbers for recruitment to the site of infection and to replace the cells that will die during the inflammatory process.

Heat-shock proteins (HSP)

Heat-shock proteins are a family of highly conserved proteins which act as immunodominant antigens in many infections. They act as molecular chaperones, housekeeping proteins within cells, preserving the cell's protein structure. They are similar in configuration to antigens found on certain microorganisms and may induce autoimmunity through molecular mimicry.

Pattern recognition receptors (Fig. 4.3)

The innate immune response is essential for host survival as it is immediately active. It is not antigen specific but can discriminate foreign molecules from 'self'. Phagocytic cells (macrophages, dendritic and B cells – antigen-presenting cells) bear pattern-recognition receptors with lectin-like activity which recognize pathogen-associated molecular patterns present on microbes but not host cells. These include:

- Mannose-binding lectin, which initiates complement activity inducing opsonization (p. 195).

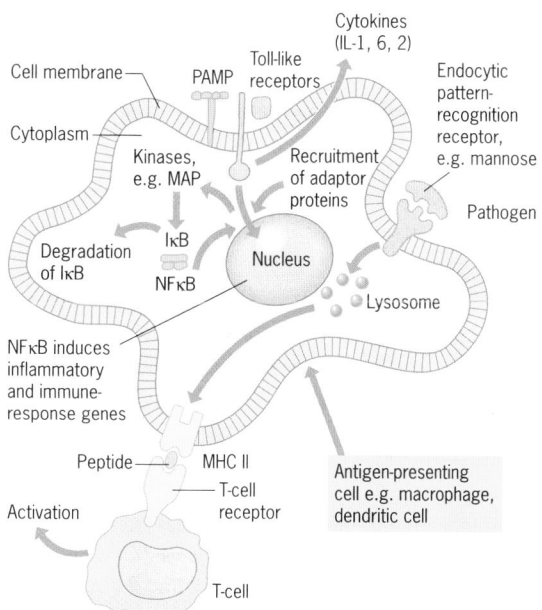

Fig. 4.3 Pattern recognition receptors in the innate and adaptive immune systems. The innate immune system has pattern-recognition receptors, e.g. toll-like receptors, which recognize microbial products by their pathogen-associated molecular pattern (PAMP). This leads to activation of kinases (e.g. mitogen-activated protein – MAP), which in turn leads to degradation of inhibitory κB (IκB) and release of NFκB. NFκB induces inflammatory and immune-response genes in the nucleus and is activated by the recognition of PAMP. An antigen-presenting cell, e.g. macrophage, dendritic cell, has endocytic pattern-recognition receptors (e.g. macrophage mannose receptor) through which it binds to and phagocytoses pathogens. These are processed by lysosomes to produce peptides which form a complex with the major histocompatibility complex (MHC) on the surface. These are recognized by T cell receptors leading to activation of this cell. NF, nuclear factor.

- Endocytic pattern recognition receptors, which act by enhancing antigen presentation on macrophages, by recognizing microorganisms with mannose-rich carbohydrates on their surface or by binding to bacterial cell walls and scavenging bacteria from the circulation. All lead to phagocytosis.
- Signalling receptors that initiate nuclear factor kappa B induction (e.g. toll-like receptor TLR-4) and immune response genes leading to cell activation.
- TREM-1 (triggering receptor expressed on myeloid cells), a member of aminoglobulin superfamily, is a cell surface receptor which, when bound to its ligand, associates with a signal transduction molecule called DAP-12 and triggers secretion of proinflammatory cytokines. It is upregulated by bacterial lipopolysaccharides (e.g. pseudomonas), but not in non-infective disorders. It is a mechanism that links bacteria on the outside of the cell membrane with gene transcription of cytokines in the cell nucleus (p. 197).

Nuclear factor kappa B (NFκB)

NFκB is a pivotal transcription factor in chronic inflammatory diseases. It is a heterodimer of two proteins (p. 158) and is found in the cytoplasm bound to an inhibitor (IκB), which prevents it from entering the nucleus. It is released from IκB on stimulation of the cell and passes into the nucleus where it binds to specific sequences in the promoter regions of target genes. It is stimulated by, for example, cytokines, protein C activators and viruses and itself regulates various proteins (e.g. pro-inflammatory cytokines, chemokines, adhesion molecules, inflammatory enzymes and receptors).

immune system to recognize a wider range of antigens. The response takes time to develop so that although specific immunity has the benefit of being very focused it cannot provide immediate protection on first meeting an antigen. However, another characteristic is the development of memory so that subsequent exposure leads to a more rapid response. The role of T and B lymphocytes in specific immunity is shown in Figure 4.4.

T and B cell immunity extends the ability to combat infection and tumours. Phagocytes only recognize extracellular organisms, mostly bacteria. In contrast, T cells are able to combat intracellular infections, such as viruses that can infect any cells, as well as the organisms that parasitize macrophages such as facultative bacteria (mycobacteria, legionella, listeria, brucella, salmonella), many fungi and protozoa. Such intracellular infections are controlled by two separate T-cell mechanisms.

- *Cytotoxic T cells* recognize tiny fragments of virus or tumour antigen that are expressed on the surface of affected cells and are able to destroy the cell and pathogen within it. These cells usually bear CD8.
- *Helper T cells* are unable to destroy pathogens or cells directly, but through cytokine production are able to activate macrophages to kill organisms within them and further activate cytotoxic T cells. These cells are usually CD4 positive.

Helper cells also activate the non-specific killing of virally infected and tumour cells by NK cell attack. Antibody enhances the innate response by opsonizing foreign particles, but also has potent neutralizing activity against viruses and toxins and plays a part in antigen presentation.

Specific (adaptive or acquired) immunity

Specific or 'adaptive' immunity is the hallmark of the immune system of higher animals. The characteristic of this response is the use of antigen-specific receptors on T lymphocytes (T-cell receptor, TCR) and B lymphocytes (surface and secreted antibody) to direct the response. Specificity is achieved by an unusual mechanism involving multiple rearrangements of original (germline) DNA in T and B lymphocytes. The altered DNA codes for proteins with hypervariable regions and creates the specific antigen-binding T-cell receptor and antibody sites. This diversity allows the production, for example, of over 10^8 different antibodies and 10^7 distinct TCRs, enough to cover the spectrum of pathogenic antigens encountered by man. T and B cells do not recognize exactly the same part of any antigen. T-cell receptors recognize peptide fragments, whereas antibody identifies the shape of epitopes. This increases the ability of the

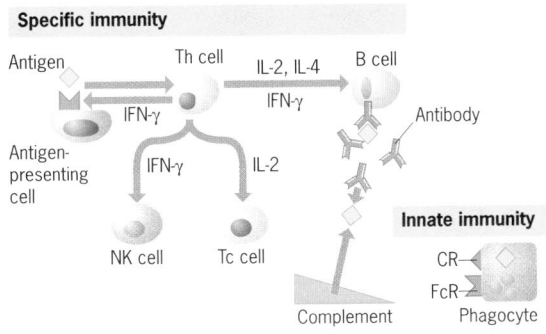

Fig. 4.4 Components of the immune response. Antigen is presented to T-helper cells (Th cells) by an antigen-presenting cell. Th cells secrete lymphokines, which activate cytotoxic T cells (Tc cells) that are involved in antiviral activity. The lymphokines also activate NK cells, which are involved in tumour surveillance. B cells are activated when the antigen binds to the surface immunoglobulins in the presence of lymphokines. This leads to secretion of antibodies. Antibody and complement coat the antigen (opsonize), leading to phagocytosis by phagocytes via binding to the complement receptor (CR) and Fc receptor (FcR). NK, natural killer cell.

Organization of the lymphoid system

Most lymphocyte maturation and activation occurs within several masses of lymphoid tissue/organs located throughout the body. Populations of lymphoid cells of different types originate from pluripotent stem cells in the bone marrow (Fig. 4.5). Immature B lymphocytes remain in the bone marrow to mature. Lymphoid precursors destined to be T cells move to the thymus where their maturation process occurs. These are termed the primary lymphoid tissues. Once cells have matured, they are released into the circulation and populate secondary lymphoid tissue such as lymph nodes, tonsils and spleen where they are ready to respond to foreign antigens.

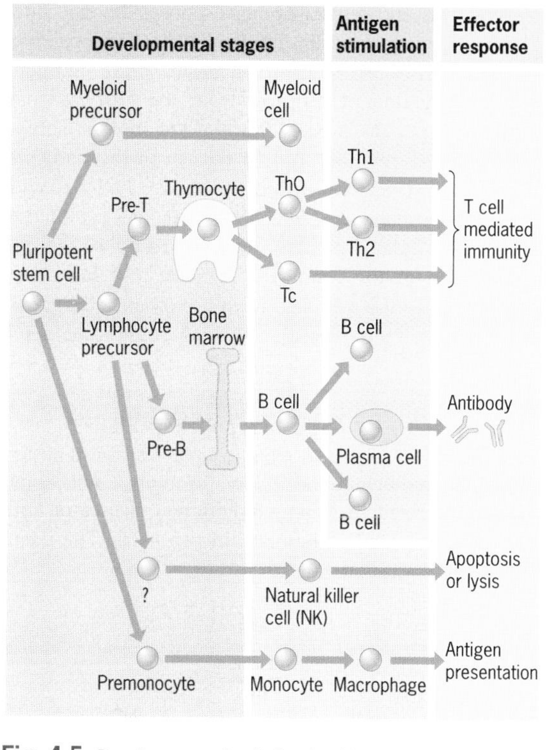

Mucosa-associated lymphoid tissue (MALT)

Lymphoid tissue is frequently found distributed in mucosal surfaces in non-encapsulated patches. This is termed mucosa-associated lymphoid tissue (MALT), consisting of gut-associated lymphoid tissue (GALT, mainly Peyer's patches), bronchus-associated lymphoid tissue (BALT, found in the lobes of the lungs along the main bronchi) and skin-associated lymphoid tissue (SALT).

B cells

These cells comprise approximately 25% of lymphocytes. In response to antigen binding to the B cell receptor (BCR) and usually with T-cell help, B cells divide and are activated to become plasma cells which secrete large amounts of antibody (Fig. 4.5).

Antibody molecules (immunoglobulins)

Antibodies are glycoproteins. They consist of (Fig. 4.6) two heavy chains and two light chains (either κ or λ

Fig. 4.5 Development of cells involved in immune responses. Cells destined to be lymphocytes or of the myeloid lineage are derived from a common pluripotent stem cell in the bone marrow. Immature T cells leave the bone marrow to enter the thymus as thymocytes. In this site, gene rearrangement takes place to form the antigen-specific T-cell receptor; positive and negative selection occur to ensure that only cells that are likely to be effective and non-autoreactive survive and further differentiation to CD4[+] or CD8[+] cells occurs. These antigen-naive T cells leave the thymus to populate peripheral lymphoid tissue. On encountering their specific antigen, proliferation and activation occur to armed effector cells, having either helper (CD4[+] cell) or cytotoxic (CD8[+] cell) function. B cells undergo development to maturity within the bone marrow, including gene rearrangement for production of antigen-specific antibody molecules (initially surface-bound and acting as antigen receptors). The mature cells are released and populate the follicles of lymph nodes, including the mucosa-associated lymphoid tissue (MALT). On interaction with their specific antigen, B cells proliferate and differentiate to antibody-secreting plasma cells. Cells of the myeloid lineage develop within the marrow under the influence of colony-stimulating factors. Tc, cytotoxic T cell.

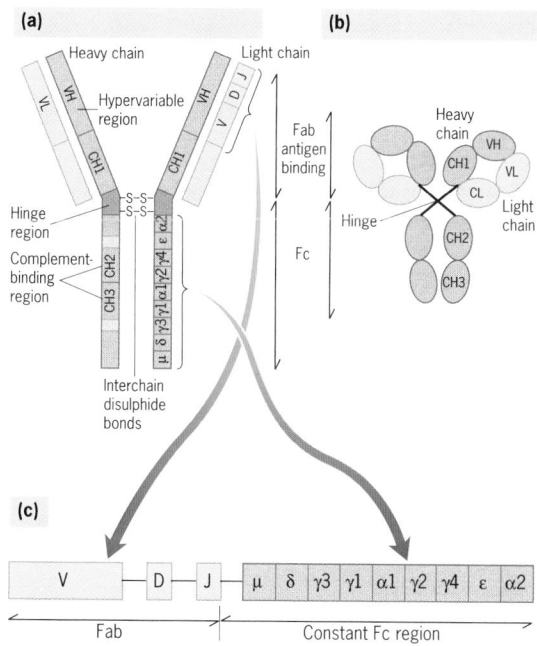

Fig. 4.6 Immunoglobulin structure. (a) Basic subunit consisting of two heavy and two light chains. **(b) Schematic diagram of the same molecule.** C and V, constant and variable domains; H and L, heavy and light chains; Fab, fragment antigen binding; Rc fragment crystalline. **(c) Genes on the Fab and Fc regions of an immunoglobulin.** The chain is made up of a V (variable) gene which is translocated to the J (joining) chain. The VJ segment is then spliced to the C (constant) gene. Heavy chains have an additional D (diversity) segment which forms the VDJ segment that bears the antigen-binding site determinants.

polypeptides). The heavy chain determines the antibody *isotype* or class, i.e. IgG, A, M, D or E. The major regions of immunoglobulin are as follows:

Variable 'V' domains, which have great variation in amino acid sequence between immunoglobulins, with short segments of hypervariable regions. Antigen binding occurs in the area where the loops bearing the hypervariable regions of the light and heavy chains come together, called the *Fab* (*fragment antigen binding*) region. The shape of the binding site determines the 'goodness of fit' or affinity/avidity of any particular antibody for an antigen.

Idiotypes are markers found in the hypervariable region and are associated with the antigen-binding site. The idiotype is antigenic and idiotypes and anti-idiotypes are thought to make a network regulating the production of antibody.

The Fc (fragment crystalline) region is formed from the constant domains in which the amino acid sequences are relatively conserved. This is the part that binds to cell-surface immunoglobulin receptors (FcR) or causes complement fixation; hence it controls the effects of the antibody molecule after it has bound its antigen.

Genetics of antibody production

Rearrangement of the germline DNA occurs within immature B cells in the bone marrow, leading to production of antibodies with many different antigen-binding sites or *clonal diversity* (Fig. 4.6). There are three main areas of the gene called the variable (V), diversity (D) and joining (J) regions which need to be spliced together to form the final sequence from which protein will be transcribed to form the antibody molecule. It is during this splicing that much of the variability occurs. Firstly, there is a multiplicity of all these regions within the DNA (V = 25–100 genes, D = 10 genes and J = 5–6 genes).

Any one of the multiple genes within a region can join any other (called *combinational freedom*) to form the final VDJ sequence. Secondly, splicing of the genes together is frequently inaccurate and 'frame-shift' in base-pairs leads to misreading and production of the 'wrong' amino acid (junctional diversity). Thirdly, somatic mutation in the genes may occur during cell division.

Once the VDJ region is spliced it combines successively to the IgM, IgD, IgG, IgA, and IgE constant genes to cause progressive switching in the isotype of the antibody. However, as the Fab gene is not further altered the same antigen-binding region is maintained. Thus, a mature but naive B cell that has rearranged its VDJ gene will initially make an IgM response on antigen stimulation, as this is the first to be translocated. The primary immune response is therefore always of the IgM isotype, IgG and other isotype responses develop later and usually require additional T-cell help (T-independent responses are restricted to polysaccharide antigens and usually do not progress from the IgM isotype). However, once the 'switch' from IgM to another isotype has occurred, memory B cells remain in the body for many years. These react rapidly to any re-challenge with the same antigen, and the characteristic IgG production of the secondary or late primary response occurs. Knowledge of the timing of primary and secondary antibody responses is used in the serological diagnosis of infections, the presence of IgM suggesting acute infection.

Immunoglobulin isotypes and their functions

The main biological features of the human antibodies are summarized in Table 4.6. Different classes of antibody tend to predominate at different sites. The major functions of antibody are:

Table 4.6
Characteristics of the immunoglobulins

	IgG Dominant class of antibody	IgM Produced first in immune response	IgA Found in mucous membrane secretions	IgE Responsible for symptoms of allergy; used in defence against nematode parasites	IgD Found almost solely on lymphocyte membrane
Heavy chain	γ	μ	α	ε	δ
Mean adult serum levels (mg/mL):	IgG (total) = 8–16 G_1 = 6.5 G_2 = 2.5 G_3 = 0.7 G_4 = 0.3	0.5–2	IgA (total) = 1.4–4 A_1 = 1.5 A_2 = 0.2	17–450 ng/ml	0–0.4
Half-life (days)	21	10	6	2	3

Complement fixation
    Classical
    Alternative
	++
	–
		+++
		–
			–
			+
				–
				–
					–
					–

Binding to mast cells	–	–	–	+	–
Crosses placenta	+	–	–	–	–

- elimination of infective organisms by:
  - binding to prevent adhesion and invasion of organisms (e.g. preventing the entry of poliovirus and other enteroviruses)
  - opsonization of particles for phagocytosis
  - lysis (in combination with complement)
- antitoxin activity (e.g. in prevention of tetanus)
- sensitization of cells for antibody-dependent cell cytotoxicity (ADCC)
- immune regulation, acting as the antigen receptor on B cells and presenting the antigen to helper T cells.

IgM

The antibody is confined mainly to the intravascular pool. It is a large pentameric molecule, the single IgM molecules being bound together by the joining 'J' chain. It is the major antibody of the primary immune response. It does not cross the placenta, and is not normally produced in the child until after birth. Therefore, if present in the newborn infant, antigen-specific IgM is a good marker for intrauterine infection.

IgG

This is the most abundant immunoglobulin in serum, present as a monomer. IgG is the antibody of secondary response, and has high antigen affinity. It is the only antibody to cross the placenta in significant quantities. There are four subclasses: IgG_1, IgG_2, IgG_3 and IgG_4. IgG_1 and IgG_3 are produced mainly in response to protein antigens, such as tetanus toxin and many viruses. These subclasses are good opsonins, binding *Fc* receptors on neutrophils and activating complement. IgG_2 and IgG_4 are produced in response to polysaccharide antigen (e.g. the capsule of bacteria such as pneumococcus and *Haemophilus influenzae*) and are the major opsonins for such organisms. IgG appears to be the most important antibody in resistance to infection, as patients who are lacking in IgG suffer with recurrent, even life-threatening bacterial infections. Those with isolated IgA or IgM deficiency have much less severe problems.

IgA

This is mainly the antibody of secretions, being present in the respiratory, gastrointestinal and urinary tracts. There are two subclasses, IgA_1 and IgA_2, but their functions appear to be similar. IgA is mainly monomeric in the serum, but dimeric in secretions, the two molecules being complexed by a joining (J) chain. The mechanism for transport from serum to mucosal surface is well established for the gut. IgA in serum binds to a poly Fc receptor for IgA and IgM on the basal surface of enterocytes and hepatocytes. Transcellular transport delivers the immunoglobulin to the luminal surface where it is secreted still bound to the receptor, which is termed the *secretory component* (SC). For IgA responses, localized antigen exposure gives rise to generalized mucosal immunity, which is of importance in vaccination. This is because after encountering antigen, IgA precursor B cells in the mucosal lymphoid follicles journey to regional lymph nodes. After clonal expansion the cells return to the systemic circulation via the thoracic duct and circulate to settle widely in the mucosa-associated lymphoid tissue (MALT; see p. 199), not just the area where antigen exposure occurred.

IgD

Serum levels are very low and its function at this site is uncertain. IgD is present on the surface of B lymphocytes, and may have an immunoregulatory role. Levels are high in conditions with B-cell activation such as systemic lupus erythematosus (SLE), AIDS and Hodgkin's disease.

IgE

IgE is a monomer that is normally present in very low levels in serum, as most is membrane-bound to the high-affinity receptors on mast cells and basophils. Its main physiological role is its antinematode activity, but its most common clinical relevance is in the pathogenesis of type 1 hypersensitivity (atopic or allergic) disease.

T lymphocytes

T cells are classified according to function into CD4 (mainly cytokine-secreting) helper cells, making up about 75% of peripheral blood T cells, and CD8, mainly cytotoxic killer cells, which account for the remainder. These functional cell types are indistinguishable morphologically, but can be separated by the presence of cell-surface molecules detected by monoclonal antibodies.

Helper/inducer cells

T-helper cells can be distinguished by the presence of the CD4 protein on their surface and the ability to recognize antigen only when expressed with MHC class II on antigen-presenting cells. T-helper cells are viewed as orchestrating the immune response. They cannot directly destroy their target, but recognize specific foreign antigen and proceed to activate other parts of the system which can eradicate it (Fig. 4.7).

T-helper cells have been categorized into two major functional subpopulations based on their pattern of cytokine production. A single clone of T cells can differentiate to either type, depending on antigen route and dose as well as the cytokine environment in which the response occurs and hereditary tendency. The T-helper 1 (Th1) class produces IL-2, IL-3 and gamma-interferon. These cytokines will promote immune responses that are primarily cell-mediated/inflammatory by activating cytotoxic T cells, NK cells and macrophages. Cells in the T-helper 2 (Th2) category produce cytokines that favour induction of antibody responses by B cells, i.e. IL-4, IL-5, IL-6, IL-10, and are thought to be involved in the development of allergic disease.

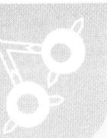

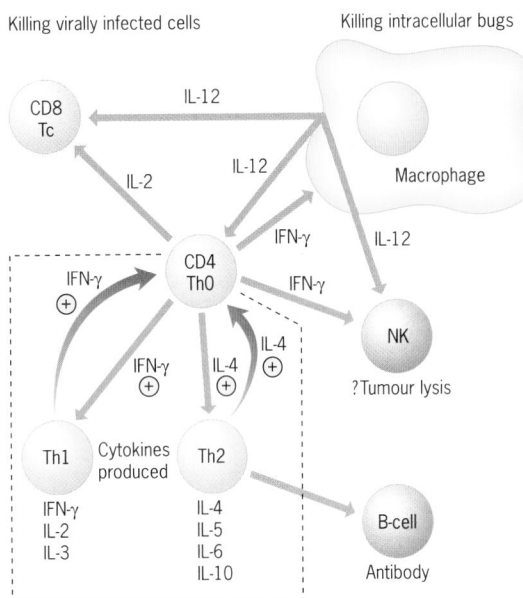

Killing virally infected cells   Killing intracellular bugs

Fig. 4.7 CD4⁺ orchestration of the immune response.
CD4 T helper cells differentiate into either Th1 or Th2 from Th0 cells.
The type of cell produced depends on the cytokine environment. The
presence of IGN-γ leads to production of Th1 cells; IL-4 leads to Th2
predominance. Stimulation of B cells leads to antibody production and
NK cells to tumour lysis.

Cytotoxic/suppressor cells

The cytotoxic/suppresser lymphocyte can be recognized by the presence of the CD8⁺ cell surface molecule and its ability to recognize antigen only when presented with MHC class I molecules. Cytotoxic T cells kill other cells, either by inserting perforins into target cell membranes, producing pores through which granzyme is inserted and causing the action of granule-associated osmotic lysis of the cell (similar to the membrane attack complex (MAC) of complement) or via activation of caspases to induce apoptosis (programmed cell death) in the target. This kind of response is used in controlling viral infections and possibly malignancies. The suppressor cell downregulates immune responses. It may function by releasing soluble factors which act on B lymphocytes to reduce their output of antibodies.

Cluster of differentiation (CD) classification

The CD nomenclature classifies monoclonal antibodies that identify numerous molecules both within and outside the immune system. Classification of cell surface molecules uses their monoclonal antibody-binding characteristics. As the surface molecule has many different epitopes (antibody-binding sites), several different antibodies may react (a cluster). As initially most of the surface molecules defined the stage of development of the cell, they were termed 'differentiation' molecules. The term CD therefore refers to a specific target molecule on a cell that is recognized by one or more antibodies

and defines a particular cell type or function. A list of CD molecules that are commonly mentioned is given in Table 4.7.

Antigen recognition – the T-cell receptor complex

Antigen recognition by T cells is accomplished by a mechanism similar to that employed by immunoglobulin. Essentially, a limited set of gene segments can recombine to encode a highly diverse set of receptor specificities; however, the receptor is not released, forming a permanent part of the cell surface. The T-cell receptor (TCR) is on the surface of all thymus-derived lymphocytes. It comprises two transmembrane glycoprotein chains, termed α and β (αβ cells) (although analogous structures named γ and δ (γδ cells) can be found on some immature T cells). The αβ cells play a role in adaptive immune responses, whereas the γδ cells are involved in epithelial defence (see p. 292). As with antibody, the polypetide chains have both a variable (V) and a constant region (C) of amino acid residues. In the β chain the variable region is encoded by V-, D- and J-like elements. The α chain is made up of V- and J-like elements (Fig. 4.6). The polypeptide chains of the receptor are linked by disulphide bridges. The molecule is arranged on the T-cell membrane as a complex with another structure known as CD3. This association is necessary for the antigen receptor to be expressed at the cell surface. The receptor also has a transmembrane tail. When an antigenic peptide is received by the receptor, a signal, manifesting as a series of enzyme phosphorylation reactions, is transmitted to the nucleus and the cell then responds accordingly by becoming activated, releasing cytokines and/or proliferating. Binding of the receptor with appropriate costimuli leads to anergy or death.

Antigen presentation

The term antigen means any structure that can be recognized by the specific immune response and is not restricted to microbial pathogens and toxins but includes foreign organs (i.e. following transplantation) and certain tumour-associated structures. It can be said that the immune system has the ability to discriminate between 'self' and 'non-self' antigens. This process is facilitated by a recognition system called the *major histocompatibility complex* (MHC) which dictates the way antigen is processed and recognized as foreign.

Human leucocyte antigens
(Fig. 4.8)

In humans the MHC is a cluster of genes located on the short arm of chromosome 6. It encodes a series of molecules known as the *human leucocyte antigens* (HLA). The

Table 4.7

Major CD antigens and their cellular distribution*

Cluster designation	Tissue distribution	Function
CD1	Cortical thymocytes	
CD2	All T cells and NK cells	Ligand for CD58; pair (e.g. between T cell and antigen-presenting cell)
CD3	Found on all mature T cells Intimately associated with the T cell receptor	Signal transduction following antigen presentation
CD4	T-helper/inducer lymphocytes Comprise 2/3 circulating T cells	Interacts with class II MHC molecules associated with processed antigen fragments
CD5	T cells; also B cells	Ligand for CD72
CD8	Cytotoxic/suppressor T cells	Interacts with class I MHC molecules associated with processed antigen fragments
CD11a	Lymphocytes (especially memory T cells), granulocytes, monocytes and macrophages	Part of adhesion molecule LFA-1
CD14	Macrophages	Receptor for bacterial lipopolysaccharide
CD15 (also known as Lewis X)	Granulocytes	Ligand for selectins
CD16	Natural killer cells and macrophages	CD16 is a low-affinity *Fc* receptor involved in signal transduction
CD18	Leucocytes	Common β-chain of LFA family (beta integrins)
CD19	All mature B cells	Signal transduction
CD20	All mature B cells	Involved in cell activation; may be a calcium channel
CD21	Mature B cells, follicular dendritic cells, pharyngeal and cervical epithelial cells	Complement C3d receptor
CD23	B cells, macrophages, eosinophils	Low-affinity receptor for IgE
CD25	T, B cells, macrophages	IL-2 receptor
CD28	Activated T cells and some B cells	Activation of naive T cells
CD34	Precursors of haemopoietic cells	Unknown
CD40	B cells	B cell activation, induced by T-cell interaction
CD45	All cells of a haematopoietic origin; also called leucocyte common antigen	Two isoforms, RO and RA. RO is associated with memory. Functions by cell signalling through the T-cell receptor; RA identifies naive cell
CD56	NK cell marker	Mediates cell adhesion
CD62	Endothelial cells, leucocytes and platelets (E-, L-, P-selectin)	Adhesion
CD72	All mature B cells	Ligand for CD5; involved in signalling
CD80/86	Antigen-presenting cells	Costimulatory ligands for CD28
CD95 (Fas Ag, APO-1)	Multiple cells	Induction of programmed cell death

* This list is far from exhaustive and has been confined to CD types most commonly encountered in a clinical immunology setting

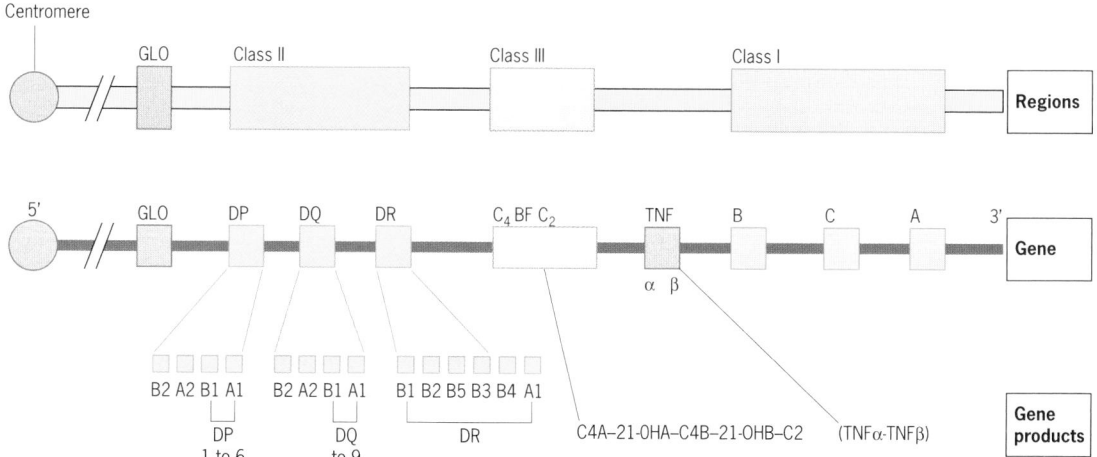

Fig. 4.8 **The major histocompatibility complex,** showing the regions, genes and gene products on the short arm of chromosome 6. GLO, glyoxalase; TNF, tumour necrosis factor.

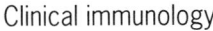

MHC is used in transplantation reactions, determining the acceptance of an organ or tissue graft between individuals. The system comprises six genetic loci – HLA-A, -B, -C, -D, -DR and -DQ. Each locus may be one of many polymorphic forms or alleles, which number over 40 in the case of HLA-B. The combination or segregation of the A, B, C, D, DR and DQ alleles in any one individual is called the haplotype. A list of the currently recognized HLA antigens is presented in Table 4.8. The HLA molecules are distributed throughout the body tissues and it is through differences in HLA that cells are classified as self or non-self. The possibility of two different individuals having the same combination of HLA molecules is very remote. It is this particular aspect of the immune system that presents problems for organ transplantation. Unless the HLA type of the donor and the recipient are virtually identical, the organ graft will be recognized as non-self and rejected by the immune system of the host. Thus donors and recipients have to be tissue typed to find the best-matched organ or bone marrow. This involves the identification of the set of HLA antigens in the tissues of a given individual.

Genetic linkage

The genes at a given locus are inherited as co-dominants, so that each individual expresses both alleles, one from the mother and the other from the father. Because of the close linkage between the loci, all the genes in the MHC tend to be inherited together. 'Crossing over' can occur within the HLA region. However, certain alleles occur more frequently in the same haplotype than expected by chance and this is known as 'linkage disequilibrium'; for example, the haplotype A1 B8 occurs more frequently than would be expected from the individual gene frequencies of A1 or B8. There is a wide inter-racial variation in HLA antigens.

Products of the HLA genes

The HLA genes code for cell-surface glycoproteins that extend from the plasma membrane to the cytoplasm and are known as class I and class II molecules. These glycoproteins consist of two chains of unequal size (α and β chains). The chains form a groove in which an antigenic peptide sits ready for presentation to T cells.

Class I molecules

Class I (HLA-A, -B and -C) antigens are expressed on all cell types except erythrocytes and trophoblasts. Striated muscle cells and liver parenchymal cells are normally negative but become strongly positive in inflammatory reactions. Class I molecules interact with CD8 T cells during antigen presentation and therefore are involved in driving mainly cytotoxic reactions.

Class II molecules

Class II antigens (HLA-D and -DR, D-related) are constitutively expressed only on professional antigen-presenting cells (B cells, monocytes/macrophages, Langerhans' cells, dendritic cells) and activated T cells. Other cells do not normally express this antigen but may be induced to do so in the presence of gamma-interferon at sites of inflammation and can then become antigen-presenting cells. Class II antigens link with CD4 molecules during antigen presentation and the reaction induced by cells bearing this molecule is therefore of the helper type.

Regulation of antigen-specific responses

Activation of antigen-specific cells is closely regulated. This is essential as the receptors on T cells are very

Table 4.8
Diseases associated with HLA

A1, B8, DR3	Polymyositis and dermatomyositis
A3, B14	Hereditary haemochromatosis
A28	Schizophrenia
B5	Behcet's syndrome Polycystic kidney disease Ulcerative colitis
B8	Tuberculoid leprosy (Asians)
B8, DR3	Autoimmune hepatitis Dermatitis herpetiformis Graves' disease Idiopathic membranous glomerulonephritis Myasthenia gravis (without thymoma) Addison's disease Sjögren's syndrome Systemic lupus erythematosus
B8, DR3, DR7, DQ2	Coeliac disease
B18	Hodgkin's disease
B27	Acute anterior uveitis Ankylosing spondylitis Psoriatic arthropathy Reiter's syndrome Juvenile arthritis
B47	Congenital adrenal hyperplasia
C6, B13, 17	Psoriasis
DR7, DR2	Goodpasture's syndrome (anti-GBM) Multiple sclerosis Narcolepsy (100% association)
DR4	Rheumatoid arthritis Vitiligo
DR4, DR6	Pemphigus vulgaris
DR4, DR3 (B8, 15 [62] 18)	Diabetes mellitus (insulin-dependent)
DR5	Hashimoto's thyroiditis Systemic sclerosis
DR5, DQ3	Associated with spontaneous clearance of hepatitis C virus
DR7	Minimal change disease (nephrotic)
MHC class III	C4A associated with SLE

GBM, glomerular basement membrane

sensitive and a cell can be activated by interaction with a very few molecules of the relevant antigen, leading to the potential for inappropriate and excessive responses. The antigen-presentation system ensures that only antigens that have invaded far enough to be within cells, or those which are recognized and engulfed by antigen-presenting cells, are presented to T lymphocytes.

Antigen presentation to T cells (Fig. 4.9)

For T-cell activation to occur, several interactions between the antigen and the T-cell receptor have to take place. Firstly, the antigen must be presented to the T cell as a peptide fragment within the groove of the MHC molecules on the antigen-presenting cell. This is necessary as the TCR only recognizes the combined shape of the foreign antigen together with self-MHC. Free antigen will have no effect. The combination of T-cell receptor, MHC molecule and antigen fragment is known as the trimolecular complex. The antigen gains access to the MHC molecule during intracellular processing in which the peptide enters the MHC cleft during the assembly of this molecule. The whole molecule is then expressed on the surface of the cell. $CD8^+$ cells recognize antigen with class I MHC. As this molecule is present on all nucleated cells, nearly all cells can present to cytotoxic cells. Antigen expressed with class I is endogenous, i.e. the molecules are produced from within the cell, such as viral proteins and tumour antigens. CD4 cells are more limited as they can only be stimulated by cells that bear MHC class II. Such cells are mainly cells of the immune system that have the specific function of antigen presentation, sometimes termed *accessory cells*. These cells take up exogenous antigen by endocytosis and degrade it intracellularly. The processed antigen is then re-expressed on the cell surface with class II.

As there are differences in the three-dimensional shape of the MHC molecules owing to genetic variation, some antigens may be more effective than others in inducing immune responses, because they present an optimum shape or conformation to the T cells. Immune responses that only occur with certain antigen–MHC combinations are called MHC restricted. The host MHC reacts with either CD4 (MHC class II) (Fig. 4.10) or CD8 accessory molecules (MHC class I) on the T cell. These interactions stabilize the TCR/MHC/antigen reaction and act as costimulatory molecules to further activate the T cell through intracellular signalling cascades. The interaction of another molecule, B7 on antigen-presenting cells with its ligand CD28 on T cells is also a major costimulating interaction. Cytokines produced during the reaction by the antigen-presenting cell (interleukins-1 and -12) and the early activation steps of the T cells (interleukin-2) enhance the reaction by decreasing the threshold for T-cell activation.

Antigen-presenting cells

The main antigen-presenting cells are macrophages (which are widely distributed throughout the tissues), Langerhans' cells (found in skin) and dendritic or veiled cells (found in lymph and blood). These cells are of the same lineage. Follicular dendritic cells are of a different lineage and are located in the germinal centres of lymph nodes (follicles). They are surrounded by B lymphocytes to which they present antigen, usually complexed with antibody, on the surface of their dendrites. Their surfaces are rich in Fc and C3b receptors to facilitate antigen trapping. B cells are also class II positive and trap antigen in immune complexes through their Fc receptors. They are able to present to T cells.

Antibody-dependent cytotoxic cells (ADCC)

These are populations of lymphocytes that are not characterized by their surface molecules, but by function. ADCC are non-T and non-B lymphocyte-like cells that bear Fc receptors on their surface, and recognize target cells coated with immunoglobulin. They may have a role in eradicating virus-infected and tumour cells.

Lymphokine-activated killer (LAK) cells

Incubation of lymphocytes with interleukin-2 (IL-2) causes them to become highly cytotoxic (hence

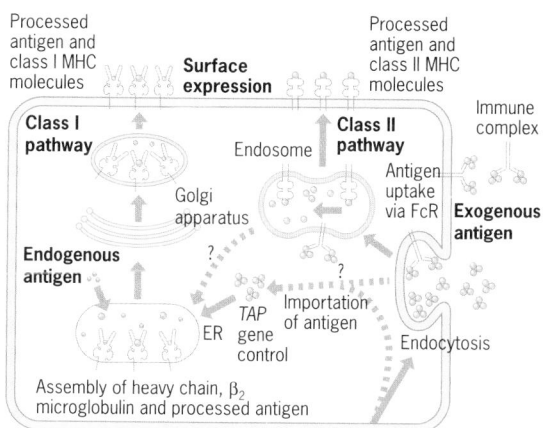

Fig. 4.9 Antigen presentation. Antigen processing is different for endogenous antigens (such as those produced by cellular viral infection and tumours) compared to exogenous antigens which have to be taken up by antigen-presenting cells prior to processing. *Endogenous antigen* peptide fragments are transported from the cytoplasm into the endoplasmic reticulum, where they are picked up in the peptide-binding groove of MHC class I molecules. The antigen-bearing MHC molecules are then expressed on the surface of the cell. Any nucleated cell is able to perform this process, as all such cells produce class I molecules. *Exogenous antigen* (usually as proteins) is internalized by specialized antigen-presenting cells. Acidification occurs within the endosome, causing breakdown of the protein and peptide fragments. Antigen-presenting cells manufacture MHC class II molecules within the endoplasmic reticulum The molecules are transported to the endosome via the Golgi apparatus. The peptides within the endosome then bind to the class II molecules, which are then expressed on the cell surface. The normal restriction of MHC class II molecule expression to antigen-presenting cells means that only a few can perform this process. ER, endoplasmic reticulum. Modified from a figure in *Immunology Today* **14**, Raychaudhuri S, Morrow WJW pp344–348. © 1993, with permission from Elsevier Science.

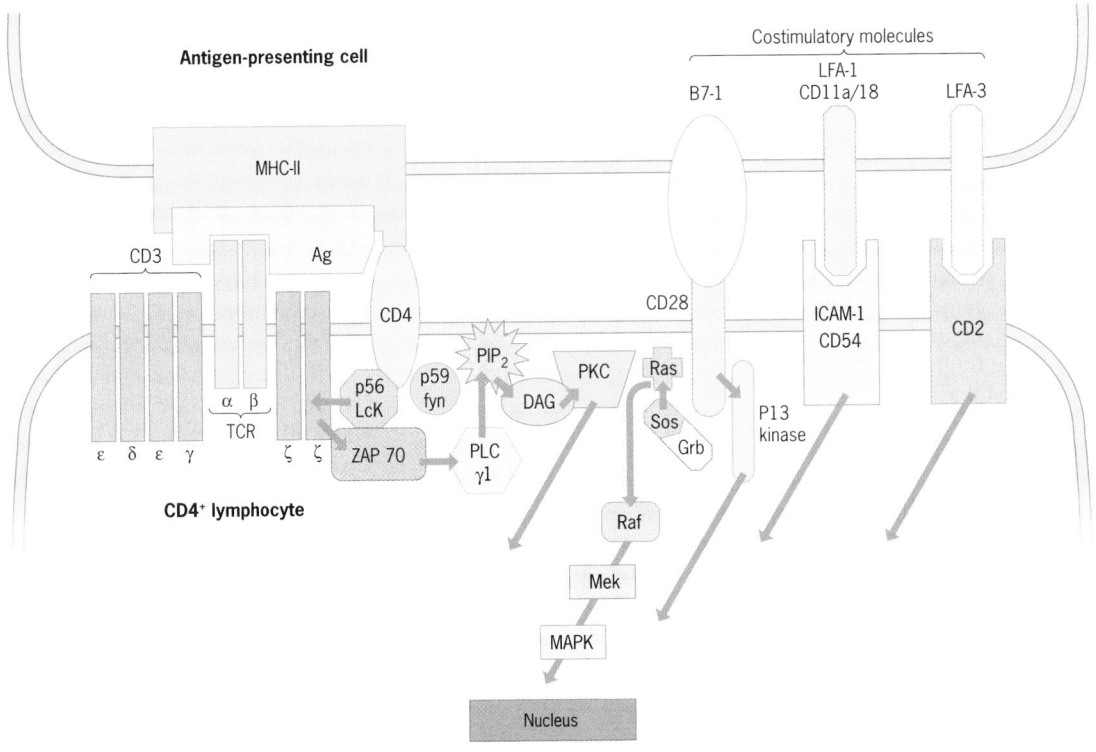

Fig. 4.10 Activation of T cells. This figure shows the complex interaction of the antigen-presenting cell with the CD4⁺ T lymphocyte. Cross-linking of the T-cell receptor causes aggregation with the CD3 complex containing ε, δ and γ chains together with the three dimers. This leads to activation of phosphorylation and differentiation. If the costimulatory molecules are not activated at the same time, a different sequence of signals is activated, leading to cell death and apoptosis. Lck, lymphocyte cytoplasmic kinase; ZAP, zeta-associated protein; DAG, diacyl glycerol; Ras, rous adenosarcoma; Sos, son of sevenless; Raf, raf-associated factor; Mek, mitogenic extracellular kinase; MAPK, mitogenic-associated proliferation kinase; PKC, protein kinase C; PLC, phospholipase C. From *Lancet* (2001) **357**: 1786. Courtesy of Dr Keith Nye, Barts and The London School of Medicine and Dentistry.

'lymphokine activated') particularly to tumour cells. These artificially stimulated cells have been used in the treatment of malignancies, where patients' blood lymphocytes have been harvested, cultured with IL-2 and then re-infused to target tumours.

The immune system in concert

The immune system is not fixed, but dynamic. Cells traffic to different sites within the body via blood and lymphatic vessels, using adhesion molecules and chemokines/chemoattractants. Following an antigenic stimulus, the components of the immune system co-operate to meet and eliminate the challenge. The cells return to lymphoid tissue, bringing antigen to these specialized processing and presenting sites. Activated lymphocytes proliferate and leave the lymphoid tissue as armed effector cells to return to the site of infection. The immune system communicates intimately with and is likely to be regulated by the neuroendocrine axis. Corticosteroids inhibit T-cell responses by reducing IL-2 and other pro-inflammatory cytokine production. Reduction in adhesion molecule expression also affects

neutrophil function. Neuropeptides such as prolactin, which antagonizes corticosteroids and activates T cells, B cells and macrophages, are produced by both the pituitary and peripheral blood mononuclear cells. Another cytokine, macrophage inhibitory factor (MIF), which was thought to be exclusively a product of the immune system, has also been found to be produced by the pituitary. Substance P, produced by sensory nerves on stimulation, binds to receptors on endothelial cells and lymphocytes and induces an inflammatory reaction.

Therefore, infection, tumour, autoimmune disease, pain or other stress, may induce immune reaction and a change in hypothalamic–pituitary–adrenal hormone production which prepares the body to repair tissues and regulates the inflammatory response.

Immunodeficiency – congenital and acquired

General principles
While many specific congenital immunodeficiencies are relatively rare, AIDS and the widespread use of corticosteroid and immunosuppressive therapies mean

that immunosuppression is a major aspect of clinical practice in many fields. Prompt recognition, appropriate management and referral of patients with suspected immunodeficiency are vital. Furthermore, the occurrence of infections in the context of specific immune defects can illuminate the physiological role of those parts of immune defence in the normal control of infection.

The main categories of immunodeficiency, by host mechanism, are:

- reduced neutrophil (and monocyte/macrophage) numbers and/or function
- deficiencies of individual complement components
- B cell defects, causing antibody deficiency
- T cell defects, impairing cell-mediated immunity
- combined T and B cell defects.

Congenital immunodeficiencies (Table 4.9)

These are usually due to specific genetic defects, leading to abnormalities in defined molecular and cellular mechanisms; most are rare. They usually present in childhood, but some types and less severe forms may not beome apparent until adult life. In some cases the abnormalities are restricted to the immune system, but in others the immune defects are part of a wider range of congenital defects.

Acquired immunodeficiencies (Table 4.9)

These are much more common, but often less-precisely defined in terms of immunological mechanisms. They can result from malnutrition, splenectomy, some infections and autoimmune disorders, tumours of the immune system, immunosuppressive therapy or drug side-effects (Table 4.9). The most common infective cause is HIV infection, which leads to the acquired immunodeficiency syndrome (AIDS); this is covered in some detail (see p. 131).

Opportunist infections

Infection is the result of microbial virulence on the one hand and host defence on the other. Pathogenic organisms have mechanisms of evading normal defence mechanisms. Organisms of low virulence can only cause disease if the host defence mechanisms that normally control them are defective. Organisms taking advantage of the opportunity of impaired host defence mechanisms are called *opportunists*. Different host defence defects cause increased susceptibility to different groups of organisms. Therefore, recognizing a pattern of infections can provide the best clinical clue to the type of underlying defence defect.

Patterns of opportunist infection

Examples of opportunist organisms in the setting of non-immunological innate defence defects include: staphylococci and *Pseudomonas* in burns patients; *Haemophilus influenzae* and pneumococci in smokers;

Table 4.9
Congenital and acquired immunodeficiencies

Congenital	Acquired
Phagocytes	
Congenital neutropenia	Neutropenia due to
Cyclical neutropenia	myelosuppression
Leucocyte adhesion defects	Hypersplenism
Hyper-IgE syndrome	Autoimmune
Shwachman's syndrome	neutropenia
Chronic granulomatous disease	Corticosteroid therapy
Other intrinsic killing defects	Diabetes mellitus
Storage diseases	Hypophosphataemia
Chediak–Higashi syndrome	Myeloid leukaemias
	Influenza
Complement deficiency	
C3, Clq, I, H deficiencies	
C5, 6, 7, 8, 9, deficiencies	
Mannan-binding lectin deficiency	
Complement-dependent opsonization defects	
Antibody deficiency (B-cell defects)	
X-linked hypogammaglobulinaemia	Myeloma, lymphoma
Common variable immunodeficiency	Splenectomy
IgA (±IgG$_2$) deficiency	Congenital rubella
Specific antibody deficiencies	
T-cell deficiencies	
DiGeorge anomaly	AIDS
IL-2 deficiency	Measles
Signal transduction defect	Corticosteroid therapy
	Ciclosporin, tacrolimus
Combined T and B cell immunodeficiencies	
Severe combined immunodeficiency:	
Adenosine deaminase deficiency	Protein–calorie
Purine nucleoside phosphorylase	malnutrition
deficiency	Immunodeficiency of
Non-expression of MHC class II	prematurity
Reticular dysgenesis	
Wiskott–Aldrich syndrome	
Ataxia telangiectasia	
EBV-associated immunodeficiency	

Pseudomonas in cystic fibrosis patients; Gram-negative infections where there is urinary obstruction; staphylococcal and candidal infections with indwelling venous catheters and other foreign bodies; *Candida* and pathogenic *Escherichia coli* following elimination of gut flora after antibiotic therapy.

Table 4.10 shows the main infecting organisms for the principal classes of immunodeficiency. In broad terms, the following principles apply:

- *Neutrophil defects*. Extracellular infections mainly consist of bacterial diseases (e.g. staphylococci, Gram-negative organisms) and systemic fungal infections. These organisms are able to survive and replicate in the extracellular environment. The main defence against such infections is through neutrophil phagocytosis and intracellular killing, which is enhanced 100-fold by coating (opsonization) of

Table 4.10
Immune defects and some opportunist organisms

Neutropenia and defective neutrophil function	Lytic complement pathway defects (C5–9)
Staphylococcus aureus	Meningococcus
Staphylococcus epidermidis	Gonococcus (disseminated)
Escherichia coli	
Klebsiella pneumoniae	**Cell-mediated**
Proteus mirabilis	**immunodeficiency**
Pseudomonas aeruginosa	*Listeria monocytogenes*
Serratia marcescens	*Legionella pneumophilia*
Bacteroides spp.	*Salmonella* spp. (non-typhi)
Aspergillus fumigatus	*Nocardia asteroides*
Candida spp. (systemic)	*Mycobacterium tuberculosis*
Mucor spp.	Atypical mycobacteria, especially *M. avium-intracellulare*
	Candida spp. (mucocutaneous)
Opsonin defects	*Cryptococcus neoformans*
(antibody/complement	*Histoplasma capsulatmn*
deficiency, splenectomy)	*Pneumocystis carinii*
Pneumococcus	*Toxoplasma gondii*
Haemophilus influenzae	Herpes simplex
Meningococcus	Herpes zoster
Streptococcus spp. (capsulated)	Cytomegalovirus
	Epstein–Barr virus
Antibody deficiency only	Measles virus
Campylobacter spp.	Papovaviruses
Mycoplasma spp.	
Ureaplasma spp.	
Echovirus	

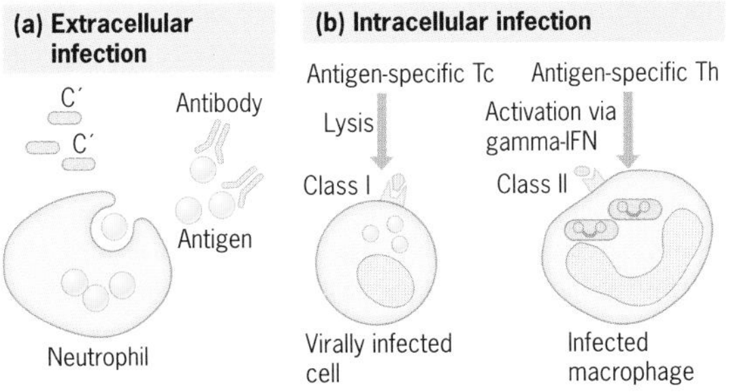

Fig. 4.11 **Control of infection.** **(a) Control of extracellular infection.** Neutrophils phagocytose and kill antibody- and complement- (C') coated antigens, e.g. bacteria. **(b) Control of intracellular infection** by two immune mechanisms. Intracellular viral proteins are complexed with MHC class I molecules and expressed on the surface of the virally infected cell. Antigen-specific CD8+ cytotoxic T cells (Tc) lyse the infected cells. Infected macrophages activate specific CD4+ helper T cells (Th) that produce gamma-interferon (IFN) which activates macrophages to kill the intracellular infection.

organisms by complement and antibody to specific receptors on the neutrophil surface (Fig. 4.11a). Failure of neutrophils to eradicate these extracellular organisms leads to infection.

- *Opsonic defects* due to antibody deficiencies or defects of the main complement pathways, and splenectomy lead to infection with capsulated organisms. These cannot be eliminated by neutrophils alone, as the capsule prevents phagocytosis unless opsonized by either antibody or complement.
- *Defects of the lytic pathway of complement* cause susceptibility to disseminated infections with Gram-negative cocci (mainly *Neisseria*, meningococcal meningitis).
- *Cell-mediated immune defects.* Neutrophils, antibody and complement react with the surface of the organism and therefore cannot detect intracellular infections. These are mainly due to viruses which require the intracellular environment for their replication, as well as fungi and protozoa which often parasitize macrophages. Some bacteria, especially mycobacteria, are facultative intracellular parasites that can also live within macrophages. The immune system has two mechanisms to eradicate such pathogens (Fig. 4.11b). Virally infected cells produced endogenous viral proteins that are complexed with MHC class I molecules and expressed on the cell surface. These are recognized by antigen-specific CD8+ cytotoxic T cells, which

lyse the infected cell. Organisms within macrophages are killed through a different mechanism. This involves activation of specific CD4+ helper T cells that produce gamma-interferon locally. This activates the macrophages to kill the intracellular infections. The different mechanisms of control explain why patients with neutrophil, complement or antibody deficiency tend to have bacterial infections, whereas those with T-cell defects have viral, fungal and protozoal disease.

Phagocyte defects

Neutropenia

Congenital neutropenias are rare and, if severe, are often fatal at an early age. Most, however, are relatively mild and benign and may even be incidental findings. They generally reflect defects of maturation and release of neutrophils from bone marrow. A particular and typically benign variant is cyclical neutropenia, with cycles of 3–5 weeks.

Acquired neutropenias are due to myelosuppression by disease, such as the leukaemias, or due to drug therapy. Myelosuppressive drugs used in the treatment of tumours, for prevention or treatment of transplant rejection, and in severe autoimmune disease are common causes. A number of other drugs, such as some antiviral drugs (e.g. zidovudine, ganciclovir) are myelosuppressive and can cause neutropenia; agranulocytosis can also be an idiosyncratic side-effect (e.g. chloramphenicol). Neutropenia due to an increased rate of destruction of neutrophils is seen in hypersplenism and in autoimmune neutropenia.

The risk of infection rises steeply once the neutrophil count falls below 0.5×10^9/litre, regardless of cause. The risk is less if the monocyte count is preserved, as these cells can serve as a back-up phagocyte population. (In cyclical neutropenia, monocytes usually have cycles of opposite phase, which is probably why serious infections are uncommon.) Infections are typically disseminated, with septicaemia, fungaemia and deep abscess formation. Colonization of the gut with pathogens can readily lead to septicaemia. Local infections often affect the mouth, perianal area and sites of skin damage, including indwelling vascular catheters, and these can readily lead to systemic infection. Pus, which largely comprises neutrophils, may be scanty and may appear serous.

If myelosuppressive agents are being used, the dose should be reduced, or the drug stopped. The duration of neutropenia can be reduced by the use of G-CSF or GM-CSF, which appear to reduce infective episodes. Antibiotic or antifungal prophylaxis may be valuable. Otherwise, prompt antimicrobial therapy for febrile episodes during neutropenia is essential, using agents with broad cover for the common organisms encountered (see p. 34).

Defects of neutrophil function

Defects of neutrophil function (some of which also affect monocyte/macrophage function) interfere with migration into the tissues through vascular endothelium, locomotion in tissues, phagocytosis or intracellular killing.

Clinical features

Mucocutaneous sepsis in the mouth and perianal areas is common and local infections often lead to chronic abscess formation in the tissues or draining lymph nodes. Granulomas may be seen, because of failure of neutrophils to degrade microbes effectively. Systemic spread is less common than with neutropenia. Congenital causes may first present with infection or delayed separation of the umbilical stump.

Congenital

Leucocyte adhesion defect

This is an autosomal recessive disorder caused by abnormal synthesis of the β-chain CD18 that is shared by the CD11a, b and c molecules to form leucocyte function antigen (LFA) LFA-1, the C3bi (inactivated C3b) receptor and the C3dg receptor (p150/95). There is impaired leucocyte tissue localization, locomotion and endocytosis. Bone marrow transplantation has been successful in a few cases.

Hyper-IgE syndrome

The syndrome is characterized by very high levels of IgE (much of it anti-staphylococcal), impaired neutrophil locomotion and severe eczema, with frequent staphylococcal secondary infections and abscesses. Other immune defects may be seen, causing a wider spectrum of pyogenic and fungal infections.

Shwachman's syndrome

This may resemble cystic fibrosis clinically, with exocrine pancreatic insufficiency and pyogenic infections, in which mild neutropenia is associated with a defect of neutrophil migration.

Chronic granulomatous disease (CGD)

This is the prototype congenital defect of neutrophil (and monocyte) killing.

Pathogenesis

In this disorder, the oxidative pathway of microbial killing is severely impaired, either owing to a defective cytochrome b558 (X-linked CGD) or components of the associated NADPH oxidase (autosomal recessive CGD). Production of superoxide is abnormal, this being the first of a cascade of microbicidal oxygen radicals, including hydrogen peroxide, hypohalites, hydroxyl radicals and singlet oxygen. Impaired production of oxygen radicals can also affect the efficiency of non-oxidative killing.

Clinical features

Patients have chronic suppurative granulomas or abscesses affecting skin, lymph nodes and sometimes lung and liver, as well as osteomyelitis. They may present during early or late childhood years, depending on the severity of the defect. Most of the typical infections associated with neutrophil defects can be seen, particularly those that produce catalase, which inactivates any endogenous microbial peroxide that can kill organisms inside the phagocytic vacuole. Because macrophages are also affected, cell-mediated opportunist infections may also be seen, such as atypical mycobacteria, *Nocardia* and salmonellae.

Diagnosis

Diagnosis is made with the nitroblue tetrazolium (NBT) test, which uses a coloured dye reaction to assay the oxidative pathway; it can also be used to screen carriers.

Treatment

Infections respond to appropriate antimicrobial therapy and surgical measures as needed; in some patients prophylaxis may be merited. Regular gamma interferon can reduce the frequency of infections, probably through enhanced monocyte/macrophage killing.

Chédiak–Higashi syndrome

This, an autosomal recessive disorder, is characterized by giant granules in myeloid cells and large granular lymphocytes. Abnormal microbial killing, and hence recurrent infections, are due to defective phagolysosome fusion; NK cell activity is similarly impaired. Similar fusion abnormalities in melanocytes cause partial oculocutaneous albinism.

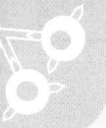

A wide variety of other rare disorders can impair microbial killing, including other inborn errors in microbicidal mechanisms, such as leucocyte G6PD deficiency (much less common than that affecting red cells) and myeloperoxidase deficiency. Storage diseases, such as Gaucher's and glycogen storage diseases, can impair phagocyte function.

Acquired

The most important and common of these is corticosteroid therapy, which also affects T cell–macrophage cooperation, causing cell-mediated immunodeficiency. The main effect of corticosteroids on neutrophils is to impair leucocyte–endothelial adhesion. This reduces the marginated pool of leucocytes and impairs their attachment to endothelium at the site of tissue injury or infection. Corticosteroids thus prevent neutrophils reaching the tissues. The corollary of reduced margination is a rise in the neutrophil count; this can be deceptive if its significance is not appreciated.

The effect of corticosteroid therapy on neutrophil function is reflected by increased focal and systemic infections with staphylococci and Gram-negative bacteria. The effect is usually apparent above doses of 15 or 20 mg prednisolone daily or equivalent, and can be substantially reduced (as can other side-effects) by alternate-day therapy.

An important infective cause of acquired neutrophil dysfunction is influenza, which causes a specific transient impairment of phagosome–lysosome fusion. This is the main reason for the high risk of staphylococcal pneumonia in influenza epidemics.

Myeloid leukaemias can cause defective neutrophil function, as well as causing neutropenia. Neutrophil and macrophage function can also be impaired in abnormal metabolic states, such as uncontrolled diabetes mellitus and hypophosphataemia. The latter may be seen during intravenous feeding of critically ill patients. Inhibitors of endogenous chemotactic factors for neutrophils may be seen in Hodgkin's disease and alcoholic cirrhosis, and may be responsible for their increased pyogenic infections.

Complement deficiencies

There are two major patterns of infection associated with complement deficiencies:

- *Deficiencies of C3, C1q or of factors H or I* cause increased susceptibility to capsulated bacteria. These patients may also develop immune complex disorders and SLE-like disorders, as do patients with deficiencies of other classical pathway components of complement.
- *Deficiencies of the lytic complement pathway, C5–9,* cause susceptibility to disseminated neisserial infections, meningococcaemia and gonococcaemia;

the latter has also been seen in association with disorders of complement function.

These complement deficiencies are rare, but functional defects of complement deposition on microbial surfaces are common. These are responsible for increased infections with *Haemophilus* and pneumococcal infections, especially in the early childhood years before a sufficiently wide specific antibody repertoire is acquired.

A common and well-defined opsonization defect is caused by *mannan-binding lectin* (*MBL*) deficiency. MBL is a member of the *collectin* family, which is in the serum in the form of multimers of the basic 32 kDa peptide. It activates the classical complement C1 complex in the absence of other activating factors. Mutations in codons 52, 54 or 57 prevent the formation of the multimers, leading to intracellular degradation or defective function. The defect is present in up to 5% of Caucasian populations, but appears to be associated with recurrent viral and pyogenic infections in children.

The C3 depletion caused by C3nef, an autoantibody that stabilizes the alternative pathway convertase and is seen in association with partial lipodystrophy, may also increase the risk of pyogenic infection.

C1 esterase inhibitor deficiency (see p. 1290) is not associated with infection but with hereditary angio-oedema, with episodes of localized oedema in skin of limbs or face, and the mucosa of the larynx or gut; the latter can cause life-threatening respiratory obstruction or severe episodes of abdominal pain.

Antibody deficiencies

Congenital
X-linked hypogammaglobulinaemia

There is a profound reduction in all immunoglobulin classes; B cells and plasma cells are reduced. The defect is in the differentiation of pre-B cells into B cells; T cells are normal. The specific gene defect has now been shown to be in the *btk* gene for a tyrosine kinase signal transducing molecule involved in the maturation of B cells; the gene is at a position Xq 21.2-22 on the long arm of the X chromosome. It typically presents with infections, e.g. meningitis, mycoplasmal infections, after the first 3–6 months of life, when the protection from passively transferred maternal antibody has largely been lost. Immunoglobulin replacement therapy is very successful and is now generally given intravenously. Many patients treat themselves at home.

Common variable immunodeficiency (CVI)

This is a late-onset antibody deficiency, which may present in childhood or adult life. IgG levels are especially low. B-cell numbers are usually normal; the defect appears to result from failure of their further differentiation. Some tests of T-cell function may be abnormal but few clinical manifestations of T-cell immunodeficiency are documented. CVI is probably a heterogeneous group of disorders in its cellular and molecular origins, reflecting defective interactions between T and B cells, with arrested maturation of B cells.

The patients have similar infections to those with the X-linked variety. However, a particular feature is follicular hyperplasia of lymph nodes, which in the gut takes the form of nodular lymphoid hyperplasia, and there may be splenomegaly. CVI patients may develop autoimmune disease and there is also an increased risk of lymphoreticular malignancy. The finding of reduced immunoglobulin levels and normal B-cell numbers indicates the diagnosis. Most of the manifestations are satisfactorily prevented by regular immunoglobulin replacement therapy.

IgA deficiency

This is an extremely common disorder (affecting 1 in 600 of the UK population) but is often symptomless. Only a small proportion have an increased risk of pyogenic infection and many of these have another defect, such as IgG_2 subclass deficiency. Some have allergic disorders or gluten hypersensitivity, and autoimmune disorders may also occur.

Isolated IgG_2 subclass deficiency

This is a rare cause of increased infection with capsulated organisms, for which it is the main immunoglobulin subclass; intravenous immunoglobulin replacement provides effective restoration.

A variety of other rare immunoglobulin deficiencies exist, including *hypogammaglobulinaemia with raised IgM*, in which there is a defect in isotype switching; the genetic basis has been shown to be due to the mutations in the gene for CD40 ligand, which is at Xq26 on the long arm of the X chromosome. Patients have recurrent bacterial infections and are susceptible to *Pneumocystis carinii* pneumonia. Other patients with increased bacterial infections have apparently normal levels of immunoglobulin but fail to produce specific antibodies to certain organisms, so-called *functional dysgammaglobulinaemia*.

Acquired

Hypogammaglobulinaemia is seen in the immune paresis of patients with myeloma and chronic lymphatic leukaemia or lymphoma. Infection with capsulated bacteria may be seen, especially with myeloma. Splenectomy causes impairment of defence against capsulated bacteria, especially pneumococcus, partly because T-independent antibody responses are largely made in the spleen and partly because of its role as part of the fixed reticuloendothelial system. Hyposplenism associated with severe sickle cell disease is responsible for the increased risk of infection in such patients. Pneumococcal, meningococcal and Hib vaccination (see p. 444) before elective splenectomy and the use of penicillin prophylaxis can largely eliminate risk of serious infection. Hypogammaglobulinaemia can be seen in congenital rubella.

T-cell immunodeficiencies

Congenital
DiGeorge anomaly

A defect of branchial arch development leads to abnormal thymic development. This is of varying severity and is associated with other branchial arch defects: dysmorphic facies, hypoparathyroidism and cardiac defects. Patients present with infections including mucocutaneous candidiasis and *Pneumocystis carinii* pneumonia, together with chronic diarrhoea, due to a variety of pathogens. The absent thymus can be documented radiologically. CD3 T cells are variably reduced in number, but the CD4 subset is usually reduced and T-cell proliferative responses are impaired. Immunoglobulin production is typically normal. Thymic transplants and thymic hormone have been reported to have reconstituted some patients with severe disease and bone marrow transplants have also had some success. The defect for this condition has been found on chromosome 22.

Other causes of cellular immunodeficiency

Various other rare congenital defects have been reported that predominantly affect T-cell responses, including:

- isolated CD4 lymphopenia
- IL-2/IL-2-receptor deficiency
- defects in signal transduction via the T-cell receptor (e.g. *Zap*-70 deficiency).

Acquired
Acquired immunodeficiency syndrome (AIDS)

By far the most common immunodeficiency worldwide is that due to infection with the human immunodeficiency virus (HIV), the cause of AIDS.

Pathogenesis

The primary cellular receptor for HIV is the CD4 molecule, which defines the cells that are susceptible and includes the following cells within the immune system:

1. CD4$^+$ T lymphocytes (which are most affected)
2. monocytes
3. macrophages and other antigen-presenting cells:
   - dendritic cells in the blood
   - Langerhans' cells of the skin
   - follicular dendritic cells of the lymph nodes (the site where much of the early replication of HIV takes place).

Binding of the HIV envelope glycoprotein gp120 to CD4 causes the virus to adhere to the cell. A second receptor is required for fusion with the cell membrane and

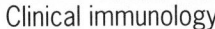
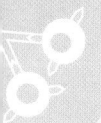

Table 4.11
Mechanisms of CD4 loss/dysfunction in HIV infection

Direct cytopathic effects of HIV

Lysis of infected cells by HIV-specific cytotoxic T cells

Tc-mediated lysis of uninfected CD4$^+$ T cells that have bound gp120 to the CD4 molecule

Immunosuppressive effects of soluble HIV proteins on uninfected cells, e.g. gp120 envelope protein leading to decreased proliferation

Molecular mimicry between gp120/160 and MHC class I inducing autoimmune destruction

Signal transduction defects and induction of programmed cell death (apoptosis) by unknown mechanisms

release of the virus into the cell. The second receptor is CXCR4 in lymphocytes and CCR5 in cells of the monocyte/macrophage lineage; these normally function as chemokine receptors.

A number of pathogenic mechanisms have been described to account for the profound cellular immunodeficiency of HIV infection (Table 4.11) leading to progressive clinical changes (see Fig. 2.46).

Immunological abnormalities

The central and most characteristic is the progressive and severe depletion of CD4$^+$ 'helper' lymphocytes. As described earlier, these cells orchestrate the immune response, responding to antigen presented to them via antigen-presenting cells in the context of class II MHC. They proliferate and release cytokines, in particular IL-2, which leads to proliferation of other reactive T-cell clones, including cytotoxic T cells, to eradicate viral infections, and gamma-interferon, which activates NK cells to cytotoxicity and macrophages to microbicidal activity against intracellular pathogens. Loss of this single cell type can therefore explain nearly all the immunological abnormalities of AIDS, as other cells' functions are so dependent on it. In addition other cells are also affected, if not infected, by HIV. Antigen-presenting cells are directly and productively infected; B cells are polyclonally activated by the soluble envelope proteins of HIV released into plasma.

The effects of highly affective antiretroviral therapy (HAART) on immune function in HIV infection

Antiretroviral therapy, using combinations of drugs against the reverse transcriptase and protease enzymes, has proved effective in controlling HIV replication. On these regimes, many patients show a marked improvement in CD4 cell numbers within a matter of 4–8 weeks, mainly due to redistribution of lymphocytes from the tissues. Functional improvement with regeneration of T cells showing the naive phenotype, and antigen-specific responses (immune reconstitution) takes about 6 months. Immune reconstitution disorders due to intensive lymphocyte reactions may occur. For the presentation and management of HIV infection and AIDS, see page 134.

Measles

Measles can cause a transient T-cell immunodeficiency, but it is rarely long-lasting enough for severe clinical problems to ensue.

Immunosuppressive therapy

Immunosuppressive therapy with cytotoxic agents such as cyclophosphamide and azathioprine tends to cause predominant T-cell immunosuppression. Ciclosporin and tacrolimus are potent immunosuppressive agents, which interfere with T-cell activation mechanisms at an intracellular level. Surprisingly, they are associated with only modest increases in infection, unless combined with corticosteroids or other agents. In such combinations, increased risk of Epstein–Barr virus (EBV)-associated lymphoma has been reported. Antilymphocyte immunoglobulin or monoclonal anti-CD3 antibody therapy also suppresses T-cell responses transiently.

Corticosteroid therapy

This interferes with cell-mediated immunity, in particular T cell–macrophage cooperation. This is due to effects on T-cell traffic and impairment of macrophage responses to cytokines, together with impaired antigen presentation. Mucocutaneous candidiasis, *Pneumocystis carinii* pneumonia, cytomegalovirus infection, mycobacterial infection, *Nocardia*, non-typhi *Salmonella* septicaemia and cryptococcosis are some of the very many infections seen with prolonged high-dose steroid therapy.

Combined T and B immunodeficiencies

The most severe immunodeficiencies are those that affect both B- and T-cell responses. These can stem from a variety of defective mechanisms in lymphocyte function, but tend to have rather similar clinical features, combining the opportunist infections of cell-mediated immunodeficiency with those of antibody deficiency.

Congenital

Severe combined immunodeficiency (SCID)

This typically presents in the first weeks of life. Failure to thrive, absent lymphoid tissue, lymphopenia and hypogammaglobulinaemia with multiple severe infections are characteristic.

There are primary X-linked and autosomal recessive variants of SCID. The X-linked defect has been mapped to Xq13 which leads to mutations in the gamma chain common to the IL-2, IL-4, IL-7, IL-11 and IL-15 receptors, leading to failure to respond to these growth factors in T and B cells. Other causes include adenosine deaminase (ADA) deficiency, in which a defective purine salvage enzyme that is expressed in all cells, has a particular effect on lymphocytes because of the accumulation of substrates and metabolites that interfere with lymphocyte function. An analogous disorder is seen in purine nucleoside phosphorylase deficiency. Non-expression of MHC class II, owing to a variety of defects in class II transactivating proteins, and reticular dysgenesis cause similar syndromes. Milder expressions of these defects exist, some presenting in later life, and are sometimes termed benign combined immunodeficiency or Nezelof's syndrome.

Even with supportive and antimicrobial therapy, most of these conditions have a very poor prognosis without reconstitutive therapy. Immunoglobulin therapy is effective for the antibody deficiency, but the cell-mediated opportunists are the main determinant of outcome. Bone marrow transplantation is the definitive approach and has had significant success, especially if undertaken before extensive infection has set in. Recent approaches have included attempts to restore the defective enzymes in ADA deficiency, and gene therapy has had some success.

Wiskott–Aldrich syndrome

This is an X-linked defect (at Xp11-23 on the short arm) with associated eczema and thrombocytopenia; a mainly cell-mediated defect with falling immunoglobulins is seen and autoimmune manifestations and lymphoreticular malignancy may develop.

Ataxia telangiectasia

These patients have defective DNA repair mechanisms and have cell-mediated defects with low IgA and IgG_2; lymphoid malignancy is again common.

EBV-associated immunodeficiency (Duncan's syndrome)

Apparently normal, but genetically predisposed (usually X-linked) individuals develop overwhelming EBV infection, polyclonal EBV-driven lymphoproliferation, combined immunodeficiency, aplastic anaemia and lymphoid malignancy. EBV appears to act as a trigger for the expression of a hitherto silent immunodeficiency.

Acquired

Protein–calorie malnutrition

This is a very common cause of acquired combined immunodeficiency, with predominantly cell-mediated defects. Mechanisms are not fully established. Measles is a major cause of morbidity and mortality among children and *Pneumocystis carinii* pneumonia is also a major pathogen; indeed, *Pneumocystis* was first recognized in this setting, in the Warsaw ghetto.

The immunodeficiency of prematurity

An immune response is not essential for normal fetal development and growth, but is necessary for survival after birth. Premature infants of 26 weeks' gestation and under are now surviving and have several immunological deficiencies and problems:

- *Antibody deficiency.* IgM synthesis does not occur before 30 weeks' gestation; IgG production does not occur until several weeks after birth. As active placental transfer of maternal antibody does not occur until the third trimester, babies born before 28 weeks have hypogammaglobulinaemia, and antibody levels continue to drop further after birth owing to loss of maternal IgG.
- *Neutropenia and impaired chemotaxis.*
- *Disruption of host defence barriers:*
  - insertion of foreign bodies, such as indwelling catheters and ventilator tubes
  - antibiotic therapy, which reduces resistance.

Hypersensitivity diseases

Allergy or hypersensitivity was initially defined by Von Pirquet in 1906 as: 'Specifically changed reactivity of an host to an agent on a second or subsequent occasion'. This definition would apply to all specific immune responses, and allergy is now taken to mean a damaging reaction. Hypersensitivity reactions underlie a number of autoimmune and allergic conditions. The immunological classification of these reactions is shown in Table 4.12. This scheme devised by Gel and Coombs is useful to group conditions with a similar underlying pathogenesis.

Allergic disease (type I reaction or immediate hypersensitivity reactions)

The type I reaction is an allergic response produced within 5–10 minutes of exposure to a specific allergen. Type I reactivity is mediated by IgE, although later in the reaction other mechanisms of inflammation including infiltration with eosinophils and lymphocytes may contribute. Allergens (antigens that evoke allergic responses), e.g. house-dust mite, pollens, animal danders or moulds, only elicit significant IgE reactions in genetically predisposed individuals, who are said to be *atopic*. Atopic diseases include, extrinsic asthma, some forms of eczema, allergic rhinitis/conjunctivitis, food allergies, anaphylaxis and angio-oedema. The diagnosis is made by a typical clinical history and examination in conjunction with either skin-prick testing (when a type I weal and flare reaction is elicited by pricking the skin through a solution of the test antigens) or by measuring specific IgE in the serum.

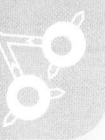
Table 4.12
Hypersensitivity reactions

	I (immediate)	II (cytotoxic)	III (immune complex)	IV (delayed)	V (stimulating/ blocking)*
Antigens	Pollens, moulds, mites, drugs, food and parasites	Cell surface or tissue bound	Exogenous (viruses, bacteria, fungi, parasites) Autoantigens	Cell/tissue bound	Cell surface receptors
Mediators	IgE and mast cells	IgG, IgM and complement	IgG, IgM, IgA and complement	TD, Tc, activated macrophages and lymphokines	IgG
Diagnostic tests	Skin-prick tests: weal and flare Specific IgE in serum	Coombs' test Indirect immunofluorescence (antibodies) Red cell agglutination Precipitating antibodies ELISA	Immune complexes	Skin test: erythema induration (e.g. tuberculin test)	Indirect immunofluorescence
Time taken for reaction to develop	5–10 min	6–36 hours	4–12 hours	48–72 hours	Variable
Immunopathology	Oedema, vasodilation, mast cell degranulation, eosinophils	Antibody-mediated damage to target cells	Acute inflammatory reaction, neutrophils, vasculitis	Perivascular inflammation, mononuclear cells, fibrin Granulomas Caseation and necrosis in TB	Hypertrophy or normal
Diseases and conditions produced	Asthma (extrinsic) Urticaria/oedema Allergic rhinitis Anaphylaxis	Autoimmune haemolytic anaemia Transfusion reactions Haemolytic disease of newborn Goodpasture's syndrome Addisonian pernicious anaemia Myasthenia gravis	Autoimmune (e.g. SLE, glomerulonephritis, rheumatoid arthritis) Low-grade persistent infections (e.g. viral hepatitis) Disease caused by environmental antigens (e.g. farmer's lung)	Pulmonary TB Contact dermatitis Graft-versus-host disease Insect bites Leprosy	Neonatal hyperthyroidism Graves' disease Myasthenia gravis
Treatment	Antigen avoidance Antihistamines Corticosteroids (usually topical) Sodium cromoglicate Epinephrine (adrenaline) for life-threatening conditions	Exchange transfusion Plasmapheresis Immunosuppressives/ cytotoxics	Corticosteroids Immunosuppressives Plasmapheresis	Immunosuppressives Corticosteroids Removal of antigen	Treatment of individual disease

* Type V hypersensitivity may also be classified with type II reactions
RAST, radioallergosorbent test; SLE, systemic lupus erythematosus; TB, tuberculosis; Tc, T cytotoxic; TD, T delayed hypersensitivity

Susceptibility to atopic disease

In all cases of true allergic disease the individual must have been previously sensitized to the allergen. There is an inherited component, because if one parent is atopic the child has a 25–40% of also being atopic; if both parents are affected the risk rises to 50–75%. This is compared to a background incidence in the developed world of approximately 15% (this figure is continually rising). There is also an association with HLA-A1, B8, Dw3 and HLA-A3, Dw2, although no specific 'allergy gene' has been identified. However, not all individuals who make IgE antibody to environmental allergens suffer with atopic disease; other factors play a part:

Age. Exposure in the first few years of life is more likely to induce atopic disease. In addition, childhood atopic disease tends to improve with age.

Intercurrent infections. Viral infections may induce atopic disease, potentially by damaging the respiratory mucosa and allowing greater allergen penetration and sensitization.

Non-specific irritants. Pollutants such as diesel emission particles (DEPs) and cigarette smoke increase bronchial reactivity and may also damage the mucosa.

Immunodeficiency. Patients with underlying immuno-deficiency are more susceptible to atopic disease. This may be due to greater allergen exposure after damage to the respiratory or gut mucosa by infection or due to decreased T cell regulation of IgE production.

Mechanisms of allergic disease

High-affinity FcεRI on mast cells tightly bind locally produced allergen-specific IgE. On subsequent allergen exposure, cross-linkage of the surface IgE molecules causes *degranulation* of the mast cell and release of preformed (granule-derived) and newly formed (mem-brane-derived) mediators. These initiate the allergic response through increasing vascular permeability (causing swelling of the tissue), inducing chemotaxis of neutrophils and eosinophils and later lymphocytes (inflammation) and increasing airways hyperactivity (bronchoconstriction) (Box 4.1).

Arachidonic acid metabolites

Arachidonic acid is generated in sensitized cells from membrane lipids following the binding of specific allergen. It is subsequently metabolized to produce prostaglandins (cyclo-oxygenase pathway), leukotrienes (lipoxygenase pathway) or platelet-activating factor (PAF acetylation), depending on which cell type is being activated. Leukotrienes and prostaglandins are together termed eicosanoids. The arachidonic acid metabolites involved in type 1 hypersensitivity reactions are PAF, leukotrienes (LT) B_4, C_4, D_4 and E_4 and prostaglandins (PG) D_2, E_2 and F_2. They have four main actions:

- *Inflammatory cell mucosal infiltration.* This is mediated by LTB_4 and PAF, which attract and activate neutrophils, eosinophils and monocytes/macrophages. LTB_4 is released by activated mast cells and macrophages, and PAF is released by mast cells, neutrophils and eosinophils.
- *Bronchoconstriction.* This is mediated by several metabolites including PAF, LTC_4, LTD_4, LTE_4, PGD_2 and PGF_2. LTC_4 and PGD_2 are the major arachidonic acid metabolites released by mast cells. The remaining eicosanoids are generated by human lung tissue and/or alveolar macrophages.
- *Bronchial mucosal oedema* is mediated by LTC_4, LTD_4 and PGE_2. PGE_2 is released from alveolar macrophages and human lung tissue.
- *Mucus hypersecretion* is mediated by LTC_4 and LTD_4.

This reaction is termed the *early-phase response*. The *late-phase reaction* comes 4–6 hours later and is characterized by inflammatory cell infiltrates with neutrophils, eosinophils and lymphocytes. It is likely that this reaction is important in asthma.

Regulation of IgE production

The regulation of IgE production appears to be con-trolled by functional subsets of helper T lymphocytes termed *Th1* and *Th2*, which develop after antigen stimu-lation from an undifferentiated population termed *Th0* (p. 202).

Th1 cells produce the cytokines gamma-interferon and interleukin-2 and suppress IgE production by B cells. Th2 cells produce mainly IL-4 and IL-5. IL-4 is the switch factor for B cells to produce IgE. IL-5 attracts eosinophils. Thus Th2 cells drive an atopic response and Th1 cells suppress it. There appears to be a dysregula-tion towards a Th2 response in atopic individuals.

Therapeutic interventions

Various therapeutic agents act at different stages of the pathways described above to control allergic disease. Sodium cromoglicate stabilizes mast cell membranes to reduce degranulation, antihistamine-receptor (H_1) blockers reduce the effect of histamine release, cortico-steroids reduce production of mediators and the inflam-matory response. A recent addition are leukotriene receptor blockers used in asthma. All these agents, in conjunction with β-adrenergic drugs, help to control allergic disease but do not alter the underlying sensi-tivity. *Hyposensitization* is a technique used to reduce IgE responses. This involves the injection of gradually increasing doses of the allergen, starting at very tiny amounts. This leads to a switch from an IgE to an IgG response. However, there is the risk of anaphylaxis

---

> ### Box 4.1
>
> **Mediators involved in the allergic response**
>
> **Preformed mediators**
> - Histamine and serotonin:
>   - Bronchoconstriction
>   - Increased vascular permeability
> - Neutrophil and eosinophil chemotactic factors (NCF and ECF):
>   - Induce inflammatory cell infiltration.
>
> **Newly formed mediators (membrane-derived)**
> - Leukotriene (LT) B4:
>   - Chemoattractant
> - LTC4, -D4, -E4 (slow-reacting substance of anaphylaxis, SRS-A):
>   - Sustained bronchoconstriction and oedema
> - Prostaglandins and thromboxanes:
>   - Platelet-activating factor (PAF)
>   - Prolonged airway hyperactivity.

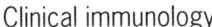

and its use is largely confined to the treatment of life-threatening allergy (e.g. that to bee or wasp venom) and only at specialist centres with on-site resuscitation facilities. Experimental approaches using anti-IL-4 agents are under investigation.

Autoimmunity (type II hypersensitivity)

An autoimmune disease occurs when the immune system fails to recognize the body's own tissues as 'self' and attacks itself. Autoimmune disorders comprise some common diseases, such as rheumatoid arthritis, multiple sclerosis, insulin-dependent diabetes and thyroiditis. Illnesses are often divided into those that are organ specific and organ non-specific or multisystemic (Table 4.13). The diseases are characterized by the presence of autoantibodies or autoreactive T cells. These autoreactive antibodies or cells may be directly pathogenic (for example the autoantibodies in autoimmune cytopenias and antiglomerular antibody in Goodpasture's disease). In other circumstances autoantibodies may not directly cause damage (such as antinuclear antibodies in various connective tissue diseases) but are a marker of an autoimmune state.

Table 4.13
Autoimmune diseases as classified by organ specificity

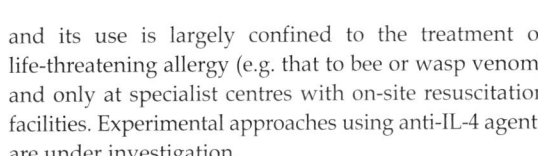

Disease	Organ specificity
Graves' disease	Single organ involvement
Hashimoto's thyroiditis	(organ-specific autoimmunity)
Pernicious anaemia	
Addison's disease	
Diabetes mellitus (insulin-dependent)	
Goodpasture's syndrome	
Myasthenia gravis	
Pemphigus vulgaris	
Pemphigoid	
Multiple sclerosis	
Haemolytic anaemia	
Thrombocytopenic purpura	
Autoimmune hepatitis	
Primary biliary cirrhosis	
Crohn's disease (?)	
Ulcerative colitis (?)	
Wegener's granulomatosis	
Psoriatic arthritis (?)	
Sjögren's syndrome	
Rheumatoid arthritis	
Polymyositis/dermatomyositis	
Scleroderma	Multiple organ involvement
Overlap syndrome	(non-organic-specific
Systemic lupus erythematosus	autoimmunity)

Mechanism of development of autoimmune disease

In the healthy individual the immune system is made tolerant to self-antigens at an early stage of immune development (tolerance is a state in which the immune system fails to respond to a given antigen). On occasions when tolerance fails or is incomplete, autoimmunity can result.

Several factors influence the balance between the development of either tolerance or immunity. Continuous antigenic stimulation over several days, e.g. by self antigens, usually transmits tolerogenic stimuli. A sudden increase in antigens, e.g. infection, usually transmits an immunologenic signal. Binding of antigens during immature lymphocyte formation in the bone marrow/thymus produces tolerance, whereas binding of mature lymphocytes produces immunity.

Tolerance
Positive and negative selection (central tolerance)
(see Fig. 4.5)

There are several mechanisms of T-cell tolerance. One occurs in the thymus by means of a complicated, multi-step selection mechanism. In the first stage of this process, immature T cells which do not bear either of the CD4 and CD8 molecules (double-negative cells) enter the subcapsular region of the thymus, divide and proliferate. T-cell receptors, CD4 and CD8 molecules, are then co-expressed simultaneously; these cells are termed 'double-positive'. Maturing cells migrate towards the cortex of the thymus where the selection process occurs. T cells that can engage with MHC class I or II molecules on the epithelium of the thymic cortex are said to be 'positively selected' and they undergo further processing. They will lose either the CD4 or CD8 co-receptor, depending on which particular MHC molecule they engage. Cells that do not interact with the MHC undergo programmed cell death (apoptosis). Thus after positive selection, only cells that can recognize MHC molecules (and thus antigenic peptides presented in association with these structures) remain.

However, another step is necessary to remove cells that can react with self-peptides, and this occurs through negative selection. This part of the selection process occurs in the corticomedullary junction, which is rich in dendritic cells and macrophages. If either CD4 or CD8 cells engage with cells bearing MHC class I or II molecules containing self-peptide (i.e. autoreactive T cells) they undergo apoptosis and are clonally deleted. The remaining cells pass through the thymus and become part of the mature T-cell pool. Negative selection is probably the most significant aspect of tolerance induction. The loss of thymocytes through the positive and negative selection process is high, with over 90% of cells undergoing apoptosis.

Peripheral tolerance

Self-reactive cells occasionally escape the elimination process in the thymus and become part of the circulating pool of T cells. While these lymphocytes may become auto-aggressive there are other forms of tolerance that occur outside the thymus. Although poorly understood, processes exist to eliminate (by specialized cytotoxic T cells) or inactivate (anergize) both self-reactive T and B lymphocytes. In the case of B cells, anti-idiotypic antibodies (which bind to the idiotype marker on the autoreactive B cell) may also play a part.

Mechanism of loss of tolerance

There are several mechanisms proposed to account for a change from tolerance to immunity.

Immune dysregulation

T cells regulate any autoreactive T and B cells that have survived clonal deletion. It is hypothesized that dysregulation of T-cell function could therefore lead to loss of control and the development of autoimmune disease. This is backed up by the observation that immunodeficiency diseases such as hypogammaglobulinaemia and HIV infection are commonly associated with autoimmune phenomena. However, most patients with autoimmune disease do not have obvious immune deficiency.

Tissue damage

There are some autoantigens to which the developing immune system is not usually exposed because these antigens are 'hidden' within the cells or tissues. Therefore clonal deletion of self-reactive cells does not occur. Normally these self-antigens remain hidden, so no autoimmune disease develops. If, however, the tissue is damaged by trauma, infection or tumour, the antigens may be released and evoke an autoimmune response. Examples of this in clinical practice are Dressler's syndrome in which patients with myocardial infarction develop acute pericarditis secondary to the production of antimyocardial antibodies, or the association of coxsackie virus infection with the development of insulin-dependent diabetes. The presence of inflammatory cytokines at the site of injury may enhance the expression of costimulatory molecules on local antigen-presenting cells and increase the likelihood of an autoreactive T-cell response still further. This hypothesis may be supported by the observation that patients given alpha-interferon (which upregulates class I expression) develop thyroid autoantibodies on therapy.

T-cell bypass

This is a mechanism by which T cells are tricked into providing help to autoreactive B cells rather than suppressing them. For this to occur the self-antigen needs to be attached to a foreign antigen that is recognized by the T cell. T-cell activation will occur with the production of cytokines such as IL-4. If an autoreactive B cell has also bound the self-antigen it will then receive the signals to proliferate and produce autoantibody. There are several examples of this in drug-induced autoimmune responses. Quinine binds to platelets, creating a foreign epitope for T cells and inducing autoreactive B cells to make antiplatelet antibodies with sometimes fatal thrombocytopenia developing. Methyldopa or infection with mycoplasma causes changes in red cell epitopes to induce a similar autoantibody response to red cells with haemagglutination or lysis.

Molecular mimicry

This occurs when an organism has a similar antigenic structure to self-molecules. The infection generates antigen-specific T cells and antibodies that cross-react with host tissues and cause autoimmune disease. Examples where there is known cross-reaction between an infective agent and host antigen are in the production of anticardiac antibodies (antimyosin) after streptococcal infection leading to rheumatic fever, between klebsiella and HLA-B27 in ankylosing spondylitis, and coxsackie and glutamic acid decarboxylase in insulin-dependent diabetes.

The development of autoimmune disease can be viewed as either a loss of tolerogenic signals to lymphocytes, or an increase in immunogenic signals. The underlying mechanism appears to be the activation of lymphocytes by different pathways.

HLA and autoimmunity

There is a strong association between certain HLA types and the development of (or sometimes protection from) autoimmune diseases (Table 4.8). These may represent linkage-disequilibrium with a true disease-susceptibility gene that has not yet been identified (this seems particularly likely in those conditions such as narcolepsy where there is a strong HLA association, but in a disease that is not immunologically mediated). The other possibilities are that HLA types determine the degree of immune response to antigens (the polymorphisms of HLA will determine how well a particular antigen fits within the cleft for presentation) and therefore the ease of autoimmune reactions.

Immunopathology of autoimmune disease
(Fig. 4.12)
Formation of autoantibodies may be a normal physiological process and help to remove tissue debris. Many autoantibodies are detectable at low levels in normal individuals or may rise temporarily in inflammatory conditions without any evidence of pathogenicity. However, excessive and persistent production of such antibodies can be harmful. Antibodies may directly react with a specific tissue, resulting in inflammation and tissue damage by complement activation, neutrophil, mast cell, or antibody-dependent cellular cytotoxic attack (Fig. 4.12a). Autoantibodies in some situations do

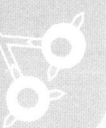

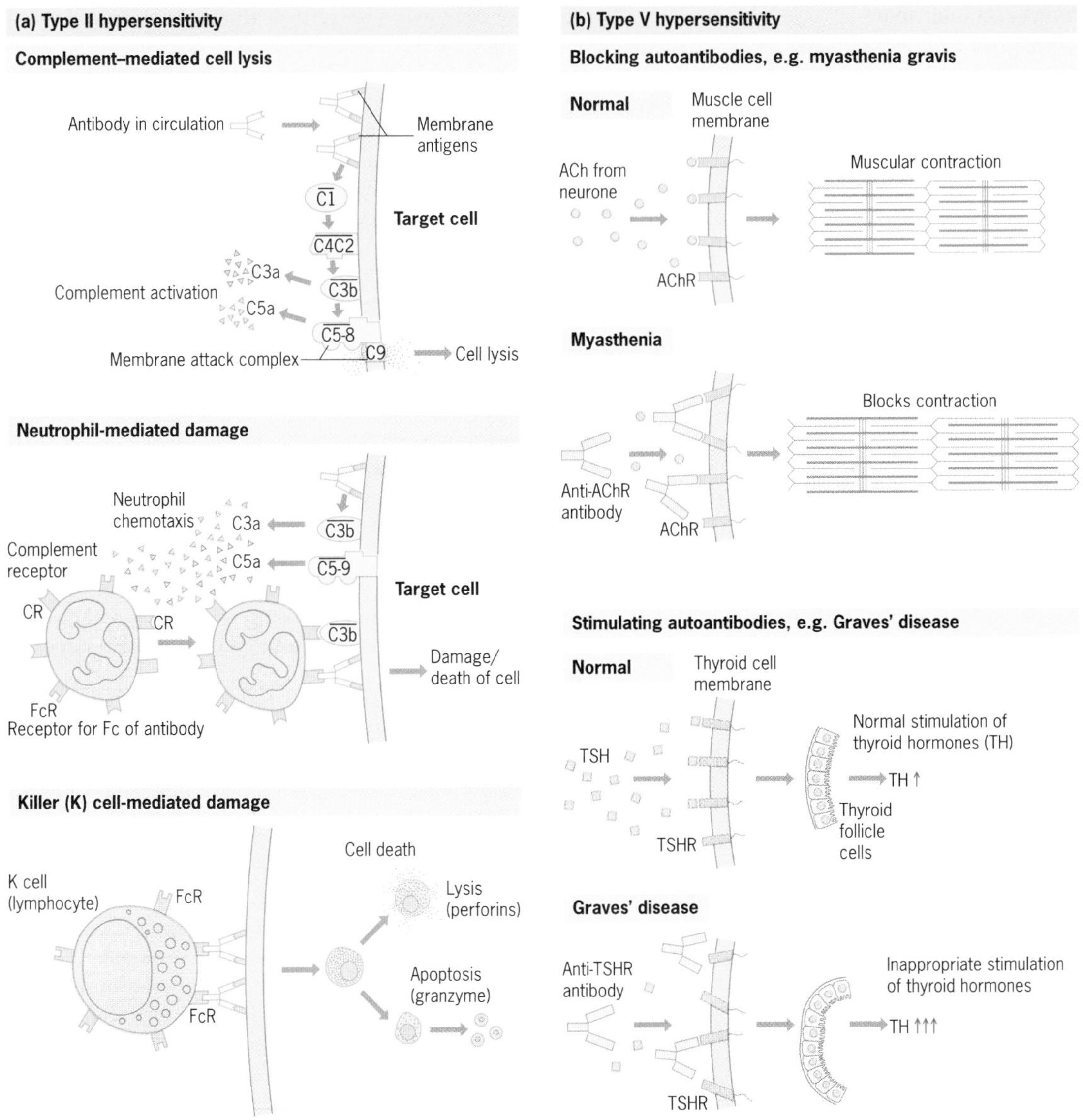

(a) Type II hypersensitivity

Complement–mediated cell lysis

Antibody in circulation → Membrane antigens

C1 → Target cell

C4C2

C3a ← C3b

Complement activation

C5a

C5-8

Membrane attack complex — C9 → Cell lysis

Neutrophil-mediated damage

Neutrophil chemotaxis ← C3a ← C3b

Complement receptor ← C5a ← C5-9

CR

CR → C3b → Target cell

Damage/death of cell

FcR
Receptor for Fc of antibody

Killer (K) cell-mediated damage

Cell death

K cell (lymphocyte) — FcR → Lysis (perforins)

Apoptosis (granzyme)

FcR

(b) Type V hypersensitivity

Blocking autoantibodies, e.g. myasthenia gravis

Normal — Muscle cell membrane

ACh from neurone → Muscular contraction

AChR

Myasthenia

Blocks contraction

Anti-AChR antibody — AChR

Stimulating autoantibodies, e.g. Graves' disease

Normal — Thyroid cell membrane

TSH → Normal stimulation of thyroid hormones (TH)

TH ↑

Thyroid follicle cells

TSHR

Graves' disease

Anti-TSHR antibody → Inappropriate stimulation of thyroid hormones

TH ↑↑↑

TSHR

Fig. 4.12 Mechanisms of autoimmunity (type II and V hypersensitivity). **Type II hypersensitivity** occurs when a cell-bound autoantigen is recognized by the immune system. Damage occurs in several different ways.

(a) Antibody binding to the autoantigen leads to local complement activation and lysis of the cells. Complement activation products recruit neutrophils, which bind to the IgG and release their granules directly onto the surface of the cell. Lymphocytes binding antigen-specific Ig (killer cells) can bind to the autoantigens on cells and induce their killing by apoptosis.

(b) Type V hypersensitivity. Some autoantibodies do not cause tissue destruction, but affect cellular regulation. In myasthenia gravis an anti-acetylcholine-receptor antibody binds to the receptors at the neuromuscular junction and blocks any further activation. In Graves' disease the autoantibody, thyroid-stimulating immunoglobulin (TSI), binds to TSH receptors on thyrocytes and causes prolonged excess thyroid hormone secretion. Modified from an original figure courtesy of Bryony Cohen, Barts and The London NHS Trust.

not damage the tissue but block or stimulate function, Type V hypersensitivity which in turn leads to disease (Fig. 4.12b). The activation of autoantigen-specific T cells causes infiltration of the tissues with lymphocytes and damage.

A third type of hypersensitivity reaction is caused by immune complex formation. The immune complexes may either be formed from antibody binding pathogen or autoantigen.

Immune complex disease (type III hypersensitivity)

Immune complexes are often found in healthy individuals; for example after eating, circulating complexes with food antigens are normal. However, if the complexes are persistent, disease may develop. Immune complexes are normally removed from the circulation attached to receptors on red blood cells and removed by the liver or spleen. Complexes with antibody or antigen excess are either easily removed or remain soluble but those at around equivalence are more difficult to remove, yet precipitate easily.

Immune complexes can be formed in tissues causing a local (Arthus) reaction, or in the circulation, causing systemic disease. Examples of the former are extrinsic allergic alveolitis (e.g. farmer's lung) where repeated inhaled exposure to an antigen such as mouldy hay leads to the production of high levels of specific antibody in the lung. Further exposure causes local immune complex production and inflammatory responses leading to chronic progressive lung fibrosis. Examples of diseases where systemic immune complexes play a major role are listed in Table 4.13, and include the major vasculitides such as systemic lupus erythematosus and other connective tissue diseases, as well as accounting for the vasculitic component of rheumatoid arthritis and other conditions. Serum sickness used to be common in patients receiving horse antisera for the treatment of tetanus and diphtheria (before effective vaccination programmes) as they made anti-horse

immunoglobulin antibodies which formed immune complexes with the antiserum. A similar reaction is once again being observed as an adverse effect of the newly developed mouse-derived monoclonal antibodies under investigation as immunosuppressants (owing to anti-mouse immunoglobulin antibodies) and in patients receiving streptokinase post-myocardial infarction (who may have unsuspected high circulating antistreptococcal antibody levels because of intercurrent streptococcal infections).

Immunopathogenesis of immune complex disease (Fig. 4.13)

Immune complexes activate the classical pathway of complement, releasing C3a and C5a, which cause increased adhesion molecule expression on the vascular endothelial cells and on circulating neutrophils. This causes the circulating neutrophils to adhere to the vascular endothelial cells. The neutrophils bind the immune complexes via their Fc and C' receptors and are activated, leading to the release of toxic oxygen metabolites through the respiratory burst, which results in tissue damage. The inflammatory mediators cause

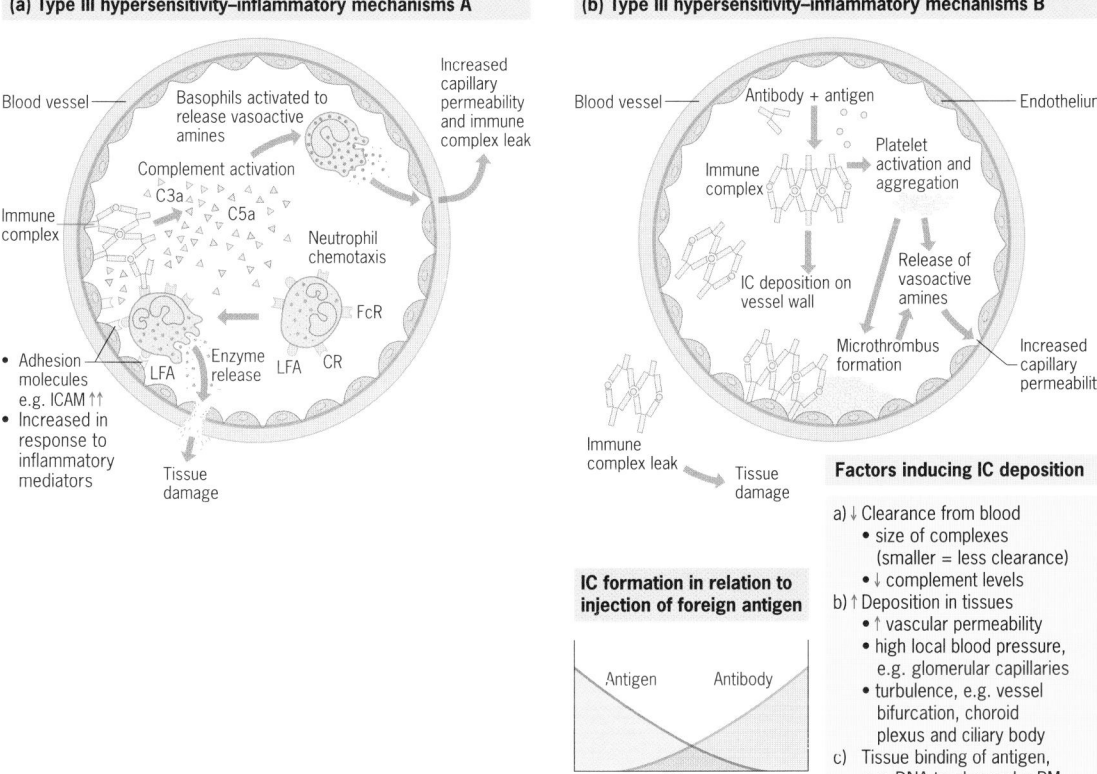

Fig. 4.13 Mechanisms of immune complex (IC) disease (type III hypersensitivity). LFA, leucocyte function antigen; ICM, intercellular adhesion molecule; FcR, receptor for Fc antibody; CR, complement receptor. Modified from an original figure courtesy of Bryony Cohen, Barts and The London NHS Trust.

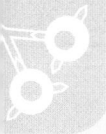

separation of the vascular endothelial cells and immune complexes and neutrophils pass into the tissues. Immune complexes also activate *platelets* with release of vasoactive amines and clumping, resulting in micro-thrombus formation and tissue infarction. Immune complexes tend to be deposited in the walls of vessels at sites of turbulence (such as bifurcations), at hydrostatic pressure gradients (such as in the glomerulus and synovium), or where the complex contains an antigen that binds to tissue (such as in the presence of DNA in immune complexes in SLE, which is attracted by charge differences to the glomerular basement membrane). Inflammation in larger vessels causes weakening of the blood vessel wall and microaneurysm formation (e.g. in polyarteritis nodosa, PAN). In smaller vessels the inflammation and thrombus formation leads to infarction and necrosis of tissue.

Principles of immunosuppressive therapy

Treatment to suppress the inflammation caused by autoimmune reactions includes systemic steroids to suppress neutrophil-driven inflammation and cytotoxics, such as methotrexate, azathiaprine and cyclophosphamide, to suppress lymphocyte numbers and function, including antibody production. More intense lymphocyte suppression is provided by ciclosporin A, tacrolimus, mycophenolate and monoclonal anti-lymphocyte immunoglobulin and anti-TNF. Opportunist infection and tumours are major side-effects of these therapies. Where the antibody is known to be directly damaging (e.g. Goodpasture's syndrome), plasmapheresis can be used to reduce the levels rapidly.

Immunological interventions

A number of products of the immune response can now be produced for therapeutic use by purification from blood (immunoglobulins and C1 esterase inhibitor), cell culture (e.g. monoclonal antibodies, fibroblast interferons) and molecular techniques (recombinant interferons, interleukin-2, colony-stimulating factors). Some are still in trials (Table 4.14).

Table 4.14
Immunological interventions

Intravenous immunoglobulin
Replacement (e.g. in hypogammaglobulinaemic states)
Fc-receptor blockade (e.g. in autoimmune cytopenias; idiopathic thrombocytopenic purpura)
Immunomodulation in autoimmune disease
Guillain–Barré syndrome
Chronic inflammatory demyelinating polyneuropathies
Lambert–Eaton myasthenic syndrome
Adult dermatomyositis

Interferons
Antiproliferative agents (e.g. hairy cell leukaemia; Kaposi's sarcoma)
Antiviral and immunomodulatory agents (e.g. chronic hepatitis B and C infection; multiple sclerosis)
Immunomodulation (e.g. gamma-interferon in chronic granulomatous disease)

Colony stimulating factors
e.g. Granulocyte and granulocyte–monocyte colony-stimulating factors (G-CSF and GM-CSF) in neutropenia

Monoclonal antibodies
Immunosuppressives (e.g. anti-T-cell antibody to prevent graft-versus-host disease; anti-CD4 in treatment of rheumatoid arthritis)
Anti-inflammatory agents (e.g. anti-TNF in rheumatoid arthritis, inflammatory bowel disease and Behçets disease; leukotriene antagonist, e.g. montelukast sodium, in asthma)

CHAPTER BIBLIOGRAPHY

Kamradt T, Mitchison NA (2001) Advances in immunology: tolerance and autoimmunity. *New England Journal of Medicine* **344**: 655–664.

Kay AB (2001) Advances in immunology: allergy and allergic diseases (Parts I and II). *New England Journal of Medicine* **344**: 30–37, 109–113.

Lancet (2001) Immunology series. *Lancet* **357**: June.

Medzhitov R, Janeway C (2000) Advances in immunology: innate immunity. *New England Journal of Medicine* **343**: 338–344.

von Andrian UH, Mackay CR (2000) Advances in immunology: T-cell function and migration – two sides of the same coin. *New England Journal of Medicine* **343**: 1020–1034.

Walport MJ (2001) Advances in immunology: complement (Parts I and II). *New England Journal of Medicine* **343**: 1058–1066, 1140–1144.

General aspects

In developing countries, lack of food and poor usage of the available food can result in protein–energy malnutrition (PEM); 50 million pre-school African children have PEM. In developed countries, excess food is available and the most common nutritional problem is obesity.

Diet and disease are interrelated in many ways. Excess energy intake, particularly when high in animal (saturated) fat content, is thought to contribute to a number of diseases, including ischaemic heart disease and diabetes. A relationship between food intake and cancer has been found in many epidemiological studies; an excess of energy-rich foods (i.e. fat and sugar containing), often with physical inactivity, plays a role in the development of certain cancers, while diets high in vegetables and fruits reduce the risk of most epithelial cancers. Numerous carcinogens, either intentionally added to food (e.g. nitrates for preserving foods) or accidental contaminants (e.g. moulds producing aflatoxin and fungi), may also be involved in the development of cancer.

The proportion of processed foods eaten may affect the development of disease. A number of processed convenience foods have a high sugar and fat content and therefore predispose to dental caries and obesity respectively. They also have a low fibre content, and dietary fibre is possibly important in the prevention of a number of diseases (see p. 226). Some epidemiological data suggest that there are long-term effects of undernutrition; low growth rates in utero being associated with high death rates from cardiovascular disease in adult life.

In 1991 the Department of Health published the dietary reference values for food and energy and nutrients for the UK. Values were based on all of the available information including data from the 1985 Food and Agriculture Organization (FAO–WHO), United Nations University (UNU) expert committee, so that there is broad agreement on the reference values given. In the United Kingdom recommended daily amounts (RDAs) are no longer used, but have been replaced by the reference nutrient intake (RNI) to provide more help in interpreting dietary surveys.

The RNI is roughly equivalent to the previous RDA, and is sufficient or more than sufficient to meet the nutritional needs of 97.5% of healthy people in a population. Most people's daily requirements are less than this, and so an estimated average requirement (EAR) is also given, which will certainly be adequate for most. A lower reference nutrient intake (LRNI) which fails to meet the requirement of 97.5% of the population is also given. The RNI figures quoted in this chapter are for the age group 19–50 years. These represent values for healthy subjects and are not always appropriate for patients with disease.

FURTHER READING

O'Brian PMS et al. (1999) *Fetal Programming Influences on Development and Disease in Later Life*. London: Royal College of Obstetricians and Gynaecologists Press.
Panel on Dietary Reference Values of the Committee on Medical Aspects of Food Policy (1991) *Dietary Reference for Food Energy and Nutrients for the United Kingdom* (Report 41DOH). London: HMSO.

Water and electrolyte balance

Water and electrolyte balance is dealt with fully in Chapter 12. About 1 L of water is required in the daily diet to balance insensible losses, but much more is usually drunk, the kidneys being able to excrete large quantities. The daily RNI for sodium is 70 mmol (1.6 g) but daily sodium intake varies in the range 90–440 mmol (2–10 g). These are needlessly high intakes of sodium which are thought by some to play a role in causing hypertension (see p. 819).

Dietary requirements

Energy

Food is necessary to provide the body with energy (Fig. 5.1). The SI unit of energy is the joule (J), and 1 kJ = 0.239 kcal. The conversion factor of 4.2 kJ, equivalent to 1 kcal, is used in clinical nutrition.

Energy balance

Energy balance is the difference between energy intake and energy expenditure. Weight gain or loss is a simple, but accurate, way of indicating differences in energy balance.

Energy requirements

There are two approaches to assessing energy requirements for subjects who are weight stable and close to energy balance:

- assessment of energy intake
- assessment of total energy expenditure.

Energy intake

This can be estimated from dietary surveys and in the past has been used to decide daily energy requirements.

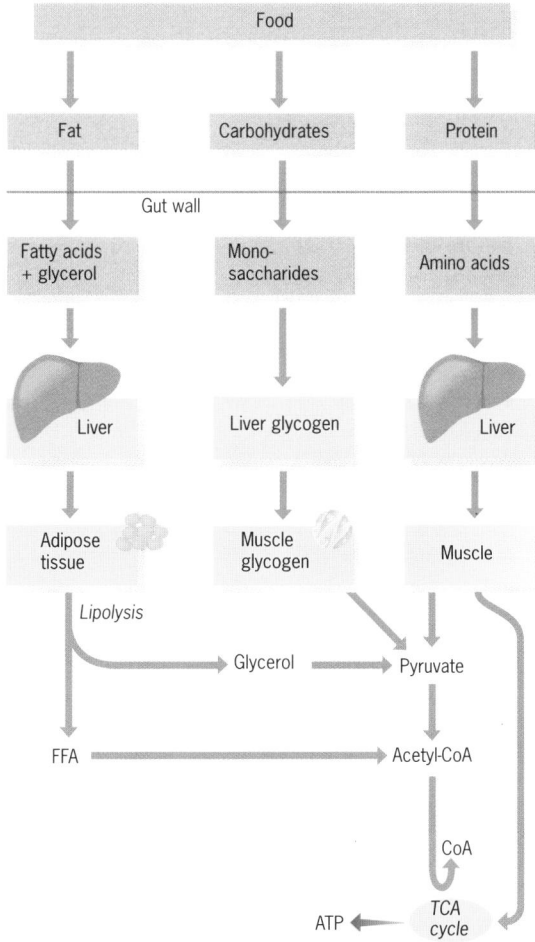

Fig. 5.1 The production of energy from the main constituents of food. Alcohol produces up to 5% of total calories, but the variation between individuals is wide. 1 mol of glucose produces 36 mol of ATP. FFA, free fatty acids; ATP, adenosine triphosphate.

However, measurement of energy expenditure gives a more accurate assessment of requirements.

Energy expenditure

Daily energy expenditure (Fig. 5.2) is the sum of:

- the basal metabolic rate (BMR)
- the thermic effect of food eaten
- occupational activities
- non-occupational activities.

Total energy expenditure can be measured using a double-labelled water technique. Water containing the stable isotopes ^2H and ^{18}O is given orally. As energy is expended carbon dioxide and water are produced. The difference between the rates of loss of the two isotopes is used to calculate the carbon dioxide production, which is then used to calculate energy expenditure. This can be done on urine samples over a 2- to 3-week period with the subject ambulatory. The technique is accurate, but it is expensive and requires the availability

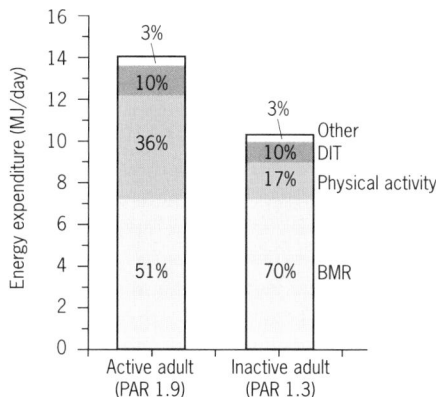

Fig. 5.2 **Daily energy expenditure in an active and a sedentary 70 kg adult.** BMR, basal metabolic rate; DIT, dietary induced thermogenesis; PAR, physical activity ratio.

Table 5.1

Equations for the prediction of basal metabolic rate (in MJ per day)

Age range (years)	Prediction equation (BMR =)	95% confidence limits
Men		
10–17	0.074 (wt)* + 2.754	± 0.88
18–29	0.063 (wt)* + 2.896	± 1.28
30–59	0.048 (wt)* + 3.653	± 1.40
60–74	0.0499 (wt)* + 2.930	N/A
75+	0.0350 (wt)* + 3.434	N/A
Women		
10–17	0.056 (wt)* + 2.898	± 0.94
18–29	0.062 (wt)* + 2.036	± 1.00
30–59	0.034 (wt)* + 3.538	± 0.94
60–74	0.0386 (wt)* + 2.875	N/A
75+	0.0410 (wt)* + 2.610	N/A

*Bodyweight (wt) in kilograms
Data reproduced with permission of Department of Health, 1991

Table 5.2

Physical activity ratio (PAR) for various activities (expressed as multiples of BMR)

	PAR
Occupational activity	
Professional/Housewife	1.7
Domestic helper/Sales person	2.7
Labourer	3.0
Non-occupational activity	
Reading/Eating	1.2
Household/Cooking	2.1
Gardening/Golf	3.7
Jogging/Swimming/Football	6.9

of a mass spectrometer. An alternative tracer technique for measuring total energy expenditure is to estimate CO_2 production by isotopic dilution. A subcutaneous infusion of labelled bicarbonate is administered continuously by minipump and urine is collected to measure isotopic dilution by urea, which is formed from CO_2. Other methods for estimating energy expenditure, such as heart rate monitors or activity monitors, are also available but are less accurate.

Basal metabolic rate. The BMR can be calculated by measuring oxygen consumption and CO_2 production, but it is more usually taken from standardized tables (Table 5.1) that require knowledge of the subject's age, weight and sex.

Physical activity. The physical activity ratio (PAR) is expressed as multiples of the BMR for both occupational and non-occupational activities of varying intensities (Table 5.2).

Total daily	BMR × [Time in bed +
energy =	(Time at work × PAR) +
expenditure	(Non-occupational time × PAR)].

Thus, for example, to determine the daily energy expenditure of a 55-year-old, 50 kg female doctor, with a BMR of 5240 kJ per day spending one-third of a day sleeping, working or engaged in non-occupational activities, the latter at a PAR of 2.1, the following calculation ensues:

(5240 kJ/day) × [0.3 + (0.3 × 1.7) + (0.3 × 2.10)]
= 7550 kJ or 1806 kcal/day.

In the UK the estimated 'average' daily requirement is:

- for a 55-year-old female – 8100 kJ (1940 kcal)
- for a 55-year-old male – 10 600 kJ (2550 kcal).

This is made up of 50% carbohydrate, 35% fat, 15% protein plus or minus 5% alcohol. In developing countries, however, carbohydrate may be more than 75% of the total energy input, and fat less than 15% of the total energy input.

Energy requirements increase during the growing period, with pregnancy and lactation, and sometimes following infection or trauma. In general, the increased BMR associated with inflammatory or traumatic conditions is counteracted or more than counteracted by a decrease in physical activity, so that total energy requirements are not increased.

In the basal state, energy demands for resting muscle are 20% of the total energy required, abdominal viscera 35–40%, brain 20% and heart 10%. There can be more than a 50-fold increase in muscle energy demands during exercise.

Energy stores

Although virtually all body fat and glycogen are available for oxidation , less than half the protein is available for oxidation. Figure 5.3 shows that fat accounts for the largest reserves of energy in both lean and obese subjects. The size of the stores determines survival during starvation.

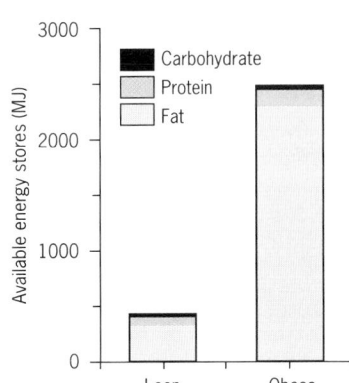

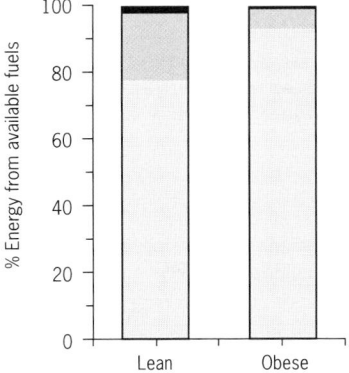

Fig. 5.3 Available energy reserves from different fuels expressed in MJ (upper) and as a percentage of total (lower) in a lean hypothetical 70 kg adult and an obese 140 kg adult.

Bodyweight

Bodyweight depends on energy balance. Intake depends not only on food availability but also on a number of complex interrelationships that include the stimulus of good food, the role of hunger, metabolic changes (e.g. hypoglycaemia), and the pleasure and habit of eating. Some people are able to keep their bodyweight constant within a few kilograms for many years, but most gradually increase their weight owing to a small but continuous increase of intake over expenditure. A gain or loss of energy of 25–29 MJ (6000–7000 kcal) would respectively increase or decrease bodyweight by approximately 1 kg.

Protein

In the UK the adult daily RNI for protein is 0.75 g/kg, with protein representing at least 10% of the total energy intake. Most affluent people eat more than this, consuming 80–100 g of protein per day. The total amount of nitrogen excreted in the urine represents the balance between protein breakdown and synthesis. In order to maintain nitrogen balance, at least 40–50 g of protein are needed. The amount of protein oxidized can be calculated from the amount of nitrogen excreted in the urine over 24 hours using the following equation:

Grams of protein required = Urinary nitrogen × 6.25 (most proteins contain about 16% of nitrogen).

In practice, urinary urea is more easily measured and forms 80–90% of the total urinary nitrogen (N). In healthy individuals urinary nitrogen excretion reflects protein intake. However, urine N excretion does not match intake either in catabolic conditions (negative N balance) or during growth or repletion following an illness (positive N balance).

Protein contains many amino acids, of which nine are indispensable (essential). These amino acids cannot be synthesized and must be provided in the diet. The dispensable (non-essential) amino acids can be synthesized in the body, but some may still be needed in the diet unless adequate amounts of their precursors are available. Animal proteins, such as in milk, meat and eggs, are of high nutritional value as they contain all indispensable amino acids. Conversely, many proteins from vegetables are deficient in at least one indispensable amino acid.

In developing countries, adequate protein intake is achieved mainly from vegetable proteins. By combining foodstuffs with different low concentrations of indispensable amino acids (e.g. maize with legumes), protein intake can be adequate provided enough vegetables are available.

Loss of protein from the body (negative N balance) occurs not only because of inadequate protein intake, but also owing to inadequate energy intake. When there is loss of energy from the body, more protein is directed towards oxidative pathways and eventually gluconeogenesis for energy. Of all the amino acids, glutamine is quantitatively the most important one in the circulation and in inter-organ exchange. Alanine is also an important amino acid released from muscle; it is deaminated and converted into pyruvic acid before entering the citric acid cycle. Homocysteine is a sulphur-containing amino acid which is derived from methionine in the diet. A raised plasma concentration is an independent risk factor for vascular disease (see p. 768).

Amino acids may be utilized to synthesize products other than protein or urea. For example:

- haem requires glycine
- melanin and thyroid hormones require tyrosine
- nucleic acid bases require glutamine, aspartate and glycine
- glutathione, which is part of the defence system against free radicals, requires glutamate, cysteine and glycine.

Fat

Dietary fat is chiefly in the form of triglycerides, which are esters of glycerol and free fatty acids. Fatty acids vary in chain length and in saturation (Table 5.3). Unsaturated fatty acids are monounsaturated or polyunsaturated. The hydrogen molecules related to

Table 5.3
The main fatty acids in foods

Saturated
Lauric C12:0
Myristic C14:0
Palmitic C16:0
Stearic C18:0

Monosaturated
Oleic C18:1 (n-9)
Elaidic C18:1 (n-9 *trans**)

Polyunsaturated
Linoleic C18:2 (n-6)
α-Linolenic C18:3 (n-3)
Arachidonic C20:4 (n-6)
Eicosapentaenoic C20:5 (n-3)
Docosahexaenoic C22:6 (n-3)

The number of carbon atoms is indicated before the colon; the number of double bonds after the colon. In parentheses the positions of the double bonds (designated either n as here or ω) are shown counted from the methyl end of the molecule. All double bonds are in the *cis* position except the*

Box 5.1

Dietary sources of fatty acids

Type of acid	Sources
Saturated fatty acids	Mainly animal fat
n-6 fatty acids	Vegetables oils and other plant foods
n-3 fatty acids	Vegetable foods, rapeseed oil, fish oils
trans fatty acids	Hydrogenated fat or oils, often in margarine

these double bonds can be in the *cis* or the *trans* position, most natural fatty acids in food being in the *cis* position (Box 5.1).

The essential fatty acids (EFAs) are linoleic and α-linolenic acid, both of which are precursors of prostaglandins (see Fig. 14.32). Eicosapentaenoic and docosahexaenoic are physiologically important, but can be made to a limited extent in the tissues from linoleic and linolenic and thus a dietary supply is not essential.

Synthesis of triglycerides, sterols and phospholipids is very efficient, and even with low-fat diets subcutaneous fat stores can be normal.

Dietary fat provides 37 kJ (9 kcal) of energy per gram. A high fat intake has been implicated in the causation of:

- cardiovascular disease
- cancer (e.g. breast, colon and prostate)
- obesity
- type 2 diabetes.

The data on causation are largely epidemiological and disputed by many. Nevertheless, it is often suggested that the consumption of saturated fatty acids should be reduced, accompanied by an increase in monounsaturated fatty acids (the 'Mediterranean diet') or polyunsaturated fatty acids. Any increase in polyunsaturated fats should not, however, exceed 10% of the total food energy, particularly as this requires a big dietary change.

Increased consumption of hydrogenated vegetable and fish oils in margarines has led to an increased *trans* fatty acid consumption and their intake should not, on present evidence, increase more than the current estimated average of 5 g per day or 2% of the dietary energy. The current recommendations for fat intake for the UK are as follows:

- Saturated fatty acids should provide approximately 10% of the dietary energy.
- *cis*-monounsaturated acids (mainly oleic acid) should continue to provide approximately 12% of the dietary energy.
- *cis*-polyunsaturated acids should provide 6% of dietary energy, and are derived from n-6 and n-3 polyunsaturated fatty acids.
- Total fat intake should be no more than 35% of the total dietary energy, and restriction to 30% is desirable.

Cholesterol is found in all animal products. Eggs are particularly rich in cholesterol, which is virtually absent from plants. The average daily intake in the UK is 300–500 mg. Cholesterol is also synthesized (see p. 337) and only very high or low dietary intakes will significantly affect blood levels.

Essential fatty acid deficiency

Essential fatty acid deficiency may accompany protein energy malnutrition (PEM), but it has been clearly defined as a clinical entity only in patients on long-term parenteral nutrition given glucose, protein and no fat. Alopecia, thrombocytopenia, anaemia and a dermatitis occur within weeks with an increased ratio of triene (n-9) to tetraene (n-6) in plasma fatty acids.

Carbohydrate

Carbohydrates are readily available in the diet, providing 17 kJ (4 kcal) per gram of energy (15.7 kJ (3.75 kcal) per gram monosaccharide equivalent).

Carbohydrate intake comprises the polysaccharide starch, the disaccharides (mainly sucrose) and monosaccharides (glucose and fructose). Carbohydrate is cheap compared with other foodstuffs; a great deal is therefore eaten, usually more than required.

Dietary fibre, which is largely *non-starch polysaccharide* (NSP) (entirely NSP according to some authorities), is often removed in the processing of food. This leaves highly refined carbohydrates such as sucrose which contribute to the development of dental caries and obesity.

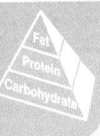

Lignin is included in dietary fibre in some classification systems, but it is not a polysaccharide. It is only a minor component of the human diet. The principal classes of NSP are:

- cellulose
- hemicelluloses
- pectins
- gums.

None of these is digested by gut enzymes. However, NSP is partly broken down in the gastrointestinal tract, mainly by colonic bacteria, producing gas and volatile fatty acids, e.g. butyrate.

All plant food, when unprocessed, contains NSP, so that all unprocessed food eaten will increase the NSP content of the diet. *Bran*, the fibre from wheat, provides an easy way of adding additional fibre to the diet: it increases faecal bulk and is helpful in the treatment of constipation.

The average daily intake of NSP in the diet is approximately 16 g. *NSP deficiency* is accepted as an entity by many authorities in the UK. It is suggested that the total NSP be increased to up to 30 g daily. This could be achieved by increased consumption of bread, potatoes, fruit and vegetables, with a reduction in sugar intake in order not to increase total calories. Each extra gram of fibre daily adds approximately 5 g to the daily stool weight. A high intake of fruits and vegetables probably reduces the risk of cancer. A high intake of dietary fibre reduces blood lipids (p. 1109).

Pectins and gums have been added to food to slow down monosaccharide absorption, particularly in type 2 diabetes.

Health promotion

Many chronic diseases – particularly obesity, diabetes mellitus and cardiovascular disease – cause premature mortality and morbidity and are potentially preventable by dietary change.

Box 5.2 suggests the composition of the 'ideal healthy diet'. The values given are based on the principle of:

- reducing total fat in the diet, particularly saturated fat
- increasing consumption of fish which contain n-3 (or ω-3) polyunsaturated fatty acids
- increasing intake of whole-grain cereals, green and orange vegetables and fruits, leading to an increase in fibre and antioxidants.

Reductions in dietary sodium and cholesterol have also been suggested. There would be no disadvantage in this, and most studies have suggested some benefit.

Fortification of foods with specific nutrients is common. In the UK *margarine* and *milk* are fortified with vitamins A and D, *flour* with calcium, iron, thiamin and niacin, and *breakfast cereals* with several vitamins and iron. Not all substances used in fortification have

---

Box 5.2

Recommended healthy diet

Intake	Approximate amounts (%)	Helpful hints
Energy % derived from:		
Carbohydrates	40	Increase fruit, vegetables,
Sugar	10	beans, as well as bread and pasta
Protein	12	Decrease red meat
Total fat	30	Decrease meat and cheese, and increase olive and other vegetable oils
Saturated fat	10	
Cholesterol (mg/day)	< 300	Decrease meat and eggs
NSP (g/day)	30	Increase bran and cereal
Salt (g/day)	6	Decrease prepared meats and do not add salt to food

NSP, non-starch polysaccharides

---

nutritive value. For example, *Olestra* is a polymer of sucrose and six or more triglycerides which has been introduced to combat obesity. It is not absorbed and is therefore used particularly in savoury snack foods (where it has FDA approval) as a 'fake fat'. Therefore, it results in a reduction in total calories. It has side-effects (mainly in the gut) and its use is being carefully monitored.

The interests of the individual are often different from those associated with government policy. A distinction needs to be made about nutrient goals and dietary guidelines. Nutrient goals refer to the national intakes of nutrients that are considered appropriate for optimal health in the population, whereas dietary guidelines refer to the dietary methods used to achieve these goals. Since dietary habits in different countries vary, dietary guidelines may also differ, even when the nutrient goals are the same. Nutrient goals are based on scientific information that links nutrient intake to disease. Although the information is incomplete, it includes evidence from a wide range of sources, including experimental animal studies, clinical studies and both short-term and long-term epidemiological studies.

FURTHER READING

Calder PC (1997) n-3 polyunsaturated fatty acids and cytokine production in health and disease. *Annals of Nutrition and Metabolism* **41**: 203–234.

Connor WE, Connor SJ (1997) Should a ω-fat high-carbohydrate diet be recommended for everyone? for and against. *New England Journal of Medicine* **337**: 562–567.

Willett WC, Sampson L (eds) (1997) Dietary assessment methods. *American Journal of Clinical Nutrition* **65** (Suppl 4).

Protein–energy malnutrition

In developed countries

Starvation uncomplicated by disease is relatively uncommon in developed countries, although some degree of undernourishment is seen in very poor areas. Most nutritional problems occurring in the population at large are due to eating wrong combinations of foodstuffs, such as an excess of refined carbohydrate or a diet low in fresh vegetables. Undernourishment associated with disease is common in hospitals and nursing homes and Table 5.4 gives a list of conditions in which malnutrition is often seen. Surgical complications, with sepsis, are a common cause. Many patients are admitted to hospital undernourished, and a variety of chronic conditions predispose to this state (Table 5.5).

The majority of the weight loss, leading to malnutrition, *is due to poor intake secondary to the anorexia associated with the underlying condition.* Disease may also contribute by causing malabsorption and increased catabolism,

which is mediated by complex changes in cytokines, hormones, side-effects of drugs, and immobility. The elderly are particularly at risk of malnutrition because they often suffer from diseases and psychosocial problems such as social isolation or bereavement (Table 5.5).

Pathophysiology of starvation (Fig. 5.4)

In the first 24 hours following low dietary intake, the body relies on the breakdown of hepatic glycogen to glucose for energy. Hepatic glycogen stores are small and therefore gluconeogenesis is soon necessary to maintain glucose levels. Gluconeogenesis takes place mainly from pyruvate, lactate, glycerol and amino acids, especially alanine and glutamine. The majority of protein breakdown takes place in muscle, with eventual loss of muscle bulk.

Lipolysis, the breakdown of the body's fat stores, also occurs. It is inhibited by insulin, but the level of this hormone falls off as starvation continues. The stored triglyceride is hydrolysed by lipase to glycerol, which is used for gluconeogenesis, and also to non-esterified fatty acids that can be used directly as a fuel or oxidized in the liver to ketone bodies.

As starvation continues, *adaptive processes* take place lest the body's available protein be completely utilized. There is a decrease in metabolic rate and total body energy expenditure. Central nervous metabolism changes from glucose as a substrate to ketone bodies, which now become the main source of energy for the brain. Gluconeogenesis in the liver decreases with a consequent reduction of protein breakdown in muscle, both of these processes being inhibited directly by ketone bodies, which are derived from fat. Most of the energy

Table 5.4

Common conditions associated with protein–energy malnutrition

Sepsis	Psychological: anorexia
Trauma	nervosa, depression
Surgery, particularly of GI	Dementia
tract with complications	Malignancy
GI disease, particularly	Metabolic disease: renal failure
involving the small bowel	Any very ill patient

Table 5.5

Nutritional consequences of disease and the underlying risk factors (physical/psychosocial problems)

Risk factors	Consequence
Underlying disease	
Almost any moderate/severe chronic disease	Anorexia, increased requirements for some nutrients, and *other effects*
Recovery from severe acute/subacute disease	*indicated below (depending on condition)*
Physical problems	
Muscle weakness (respiratory and peripheral muscles) and/or incoordination	Problems with shopping, cooking and eating
Severe arthritis in hands and arms	
Swallowing problem (neurological causes), painful or obstructive conditions of mouth and gastrointestinal tract (GIT)	Inadequate food intake, and/or risk of aspiration pneumonia
GIT symptoms (e.g. nausea, vomiting, diarrhoea, jaundice)	Food aversion, malabsorption (small bowel disease), anorexia
Sensory deficit (e.g. impaired sight, hearing and other deficits)	Difficulties in shopping, cooking and/or decreased intake of food
Psychosocial problems	
Loneliness, depression, bereavement, confusion, living alone, poverty, alcoholism, drug addiction	Self-neglect, inadequate intake of food or quality of food
Multiple drug use (polypharmacy)	Indicates severe disease or multiple physical and psychosocial problems; drugs may lead to confusion, sedation, depression and GIT side-effects (including malabsorption of nutrients)

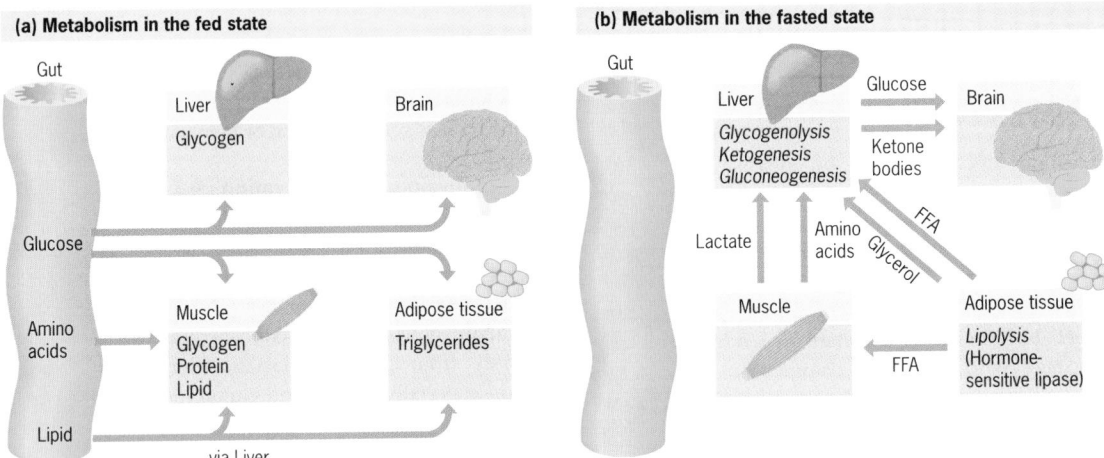

Fig. 5.4 **Metabolism in (a) the fed and (b) the fasted state.** FFA, free fatty acids.

at this stage comes from adipose tissue, with some gluconeogenesis from amino acids, particularly from alanine in the liver, and glutamine in the kidney.

The metabolic response to prolonged starvation differs between lean and obese individuals. One of the major differences concerns the proportion of energy derived from protein oxidation, which determines the proportion of weight loss due to lean tissues. This proportion may be up to three times smaller in obese subjects than lean subjects. It can be regarded as an adaptation which depends on the compensation of the initial reserves (Fig. 5.3). This means that deterioration in body function is more rapid in lean subjects. Furthermore, survival time is much less in lean subjects (~ 2 months), compared to the obese (can be at least several months).

Following trauma or shock, some of the adaptive changes do not take place. Glucocorticoid and cytokines (see below) stimulate the ubiquitin–proteasome pathway in muscle, which is responsible for accelerated proteolysis in muscle in many catabolic illnesses. In contrast to starvation, which is associated with a decrease in BMR, in inflammatory and traumatic disease it is often increased. These changes all result in continuing gluconeogenesis with massive muscle breakdown, and further reduction in survival time.

Regulation of metabolism

The unavailability of the various substrates in starvation produces dramatic changes in hormone levels, which are one of the main factors controlling intracellular metabolism.

- *In the fed state*, insulin/glucagon ratios are high. Insulin promotes synthesis of glycogen, protein and fat, and inhibits lipolysis and gluconeogenesis.
- *In the fasted state*, the insulin/glucagon ratios are low. Glucagon acts mainly on the liver and has no action on muscle. It increases glycogenolysis and

gluconeogenesis, as well as increasing ketone body production from fatty acids. It also stimulates lipolysis in adipose tissue. Catecholamines have a similar action to glucagon but also affect muscle metabolism. These agents both act via cyclic adenosine monophosphate (cAMP) to stimulate lipolysis, producing free fatty acids that can then act as a major source of energy.

Cytokines, such as interleukin-1, interleukin-6 and tumour necrosis factor (TNF), have also been shown to play a role in regulating metabolism. TNF, which inhibits lipoprotein lipase, has been identified as the cachexia factor in patients with cancer. It is unclear how these cytokines interact with central feeding pathways to cause anorexia. However, in both animal models of cancer and inflammatory bowel disease, many peripheral and central mediators of appetite are involved. For example, neuropeptide Y levels in the hypothalamus are often inappropriately low, so there is a reduced drive to feeding.

Clinical features

Patients are sometimes seen with loss of weight or malnutrition as the primary symptom (failure to thrive in children). Mostly, however, malnourishment is only seen as an accompaniment of some other disease process, such as malignancy. Severe malnutrition is seen mainly with advanced organic disease or after surgical procedures followed by complications. Three key features which help in the detection of chronic protein energy malnutrition (PEM) in adults are:

1. *The body mass index* (BMI):
   - Probable chronic PEM: < 18.5 kg/m²
   - Possible chronic PEM: 18.5–20 kg/m²
   - Little or no risk of chronic PEM: > 20 kg/m².
   In patients with oedema or dehydration the BMI may be somewhat misleading.

2. *Weight loss in previous 3–6 months:* > 10%, high risk; 5–10%, possible risk; < 5% low/no risk of developing PEM.

3. *Other factors:*
   - history of decreased food intake/loss of appetite
   - clothes becoming loosely fitting (weight loss) and general appearance, which may indicate obvious wasting
   - physical and psychosocial disturbances likely to have contributed to the weight loss.

These factors act as a link between detection and management. If the underlying physical or psychosocial problems are not adequately addressed, treatment may not be successful.

PEM leads to a depression of the immunological defence mechanism, resulting in a decreased resistance to infection (see p. 28). It also detrimentally affects muscle strength and fatigue, reproductive function (e.g. in anorexia nervosa, which is common in adolescent girls; p. 1266), wound healing, and psychological function (depression, anxiety, hypochondriasis, loss of libido).

Treatment (see also pp. 245 and 248)

When malnutrition is obvious and the underlying disease cannot be corrected at once, some form of nutritional support is necessary. Nutrition should be given enterally if the gastrointestinal tract is functioning adequately. This can most easily be done by encouraging the patient to eat more often and by giving a high-calorie supplement. If this is not possible, a liquefied diet may be given intragastrically via a fine-bore tube or by a percutaneous endoscopic gastrostomy (PEG). If both of these measures fail, parenteral nutrition is given.

In developing countries

In many areas of the world, people are on the verge of malnutrition. In addition, if events such as drought, war or changes in political climate occur, millions suffer from starvation. Although the basic condition of PEM is the same in all parts of the world from whatever cause, malnutrition resulting from long periods of near-total starvation produces unique clinical appearances in children virtually never seen in the West.

The term 'protein–energy malnutrition' covers the spectrum of clinical conditions seen in adults and children. The World Health Organization (WHO) classification of chronic undernutrition in children is based on standard deviation scores. Thus, children with a standard deviation score of less than –2 (2 standard deviation scores below the median – corresponding to 2.3 centile) can be regarded as being at high risk of undernutrition. The following terminology is used:

- low weight-for-age: underweight
- low height-for-age: shortness (stunting when pathological)

Table 5.6
Wellcome classification of protein–energy malnutrition

Weight (% of standard for age)	Oedema present	Oedema absent
80–60	Kwashiorkor	Undernourished
< 60	Marasmic kwashiorkor	Marasmus

- low weight for height: thinness (wasted when pathological).

This classification, which is widely used and employs the National Center for Health Statistics (USA)/WHO reference standards, does not take into account oedema. On the other hand the Wellcome classification, shown in Table 5.6, includes oedema in its clinical classification. The mildly-to-moderately undernourished child is the most common.

Marasmus is the childhood form of starvation, which is associated with obvious wasting.

Kwashiorkor occurs typically in a young child displaced from breast-feeding by a new baby and fed a diet with a very low protein content relative to energy, such as cassava. Underlying diseases are common, and a variety of acute diseases, such as measles, may precipitate kwashiorkor. This diet – which has sufficient energy but an inadequate amount of protein – results in a high plasma insulin and a low plasma cortisol. This hormonal pattern leads to an uptake of amino acids in the muscle (diverting these from the liver), leading to reduced albumin synthesis and, therefore, oedema (i.e. kwashiorkor). Conversely, when total energy is insufficient, there is an opposite hormonal pattern (i.e. low insulin and high cortisol). Amino acids are now released from the muscles, albumin is synthesized normally, and this results in marasmus rather than kwashiorkor. This classical hypothesis of protein deficiency with adequate carbohydrates as the aetiology of kwashiorkor is difficult to substantiate as most infants will have deficiency of total calorie intake as well as other unspecified nutrients. Alternatively, it has been suggested that kwashiorkor results from an imbalance of free radicals and their safe disposal, causing cell membrane damage and oedema. Disease, which frequently co-exists, probably has a role in the aetiology of kwashiorkor while infections such as measles, malaria and diarrhoea can affect the clinical picture and children with one form of PEM may change to another form.

Clinical features
Adults

Starvation in adults leads to extreme loss of weight depending upon the severity and duration. They crave for food, are apathetic and complain of cold and weakness with a loss of subcutaneous fat and muscle wasting.

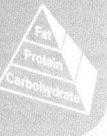

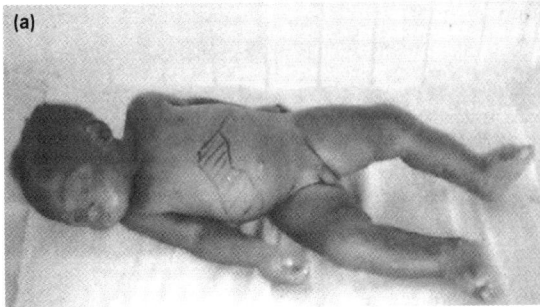

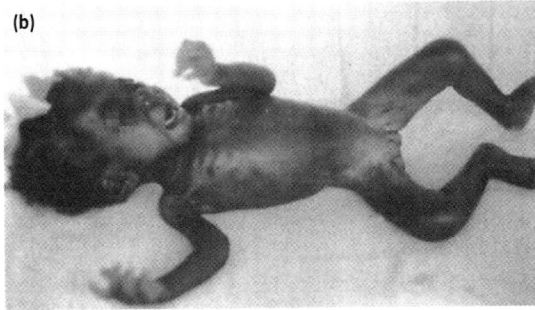

Fig. 5.5 Malnourished children: (a) kwashiorkor and (b) marasmus. Courtesy of Professor J Garrow.

Infections such as gastrointestinal or bronchopneumonia are common.

Children under the age of 5 years (Fig. 5.5)

- *Marasmus* is the type of *severe* PEM seen most commonly. A child looks emaciated, there is obvious muscle wasting and loss of body fat. There is no oedema. The hair is thin and dry. The child is not so apathetic or anorexic as with kwashiorkor. Diarrhoea is frequently present and signs of infection must be looked for carefully.
- *Kwashiorkor* shows the child to be apathetic and lethargic with severe anorexia. There is generalized oedema with skin pigmentation and thickening. The hair is dry, sparse and may become reddish or yellow in colour. The abdomen is distended owing to hepatomegaly and/or ascites. The serum albumin is always low.

The undernourished child

Many children in developing countries are underweight, and subclinical PEM is often present if looked for carefully using anthropometric criteria. Mild-to-moderate malnutrition can be detected in children by the mid upper-arm circumference (MUAC).

Nutritional dwarfism is a term used to describe a child who appears normal until it is realized that he or she is short for age. Reduced linear growth occurs in response to undernutrition; dental development is less retarded so that the facial appearance is inappropriate for the age.

As with an adult, the undernourished child is very susceptible to respiratory and gastrointestinal infections, leading to an increased mortality in this group.

Investigation

It must be realized that this is not always practicable.

- **Blood tests**
  - (a) Anaemia due to folate, iron and copper deficiency is often present, but the haematocrit may be high owing to dehydration.
  - (b) Eosinophilia suggests parasitic infestation.
  - (c) Electrolyte disturbances are common.
  - (d) Malarial parasites should be looked for.
  - (e) HIV tests.
- **Stools** should be examined for parasitic infestations.
- **Chest X-ray** – tuberculosis is common and is easily missed if a chest X-ray is not performed.

Treatment

Treatment must involve the provision of protein and energy supplements and the control of infection.

Resuscitation

The severely ill child will require correction of fluid and electrolyte abnormalities, but intravenous therapy should be avoided if possible because of the danger of fluid overload.

Glucose–electrolyte mixtures (such as the WHO formulation, p. 73) are sometimes necessary. Diarrhoea is often due to bacterial or protozoal overgrowth; metronidazole is very effective and is often given routinely. Parasites are also common and, as facilities for stool examination are usually not available, mebendazole 100 mg twice daily should be given for 3 days. In high-risk areas, antimalarial therapy is given.

Refeeding

This needs to be planned carefully. During the initial treatment of the acute situation, a balanced diet with sufficient protein and energy is given to maintain a steady state. Large increases in energy lead to heart failure, circulatory collapse and death. A child requires approximately 450 kJ/kg (100 kcal/kg) daily, which is provided by 0.6 g/kg of protein. This is often given as milk with additional water, flour, maize or whatever is available locally in a palatable mixture. Sugar mixed with dried skimmed milk and small amounts of cotton-seed oil (DISCO) is frequently used. Attempts should be made to give the feeds as slowly and as often as possible, although anorexia is often a problem and can be exacerbated by excessive feeding. If necessary, fluids and food should be given by nasogastric tube. The child is then gradually weaned to liquids and then solids by mouth.

Hypothermia and hypoglycaemia occur in severely ill children, often with an accompanying infection, and need to be treated urgently. Because of the cold temperatures at night, blankets and sometimes additional heat are necessary.

Supplements of vitamins (A, D, B and C) should always be given, together with folic acid and iron. Many children are deficient in minerals such as zinc, copper and selenium, and supplements should be given if deficiency is suspected.

Rehabilitation

Gradually, as the child improves, more energy can be given, and during rehabilitation maximum weight gain is achieved in the shortest time by extra calories ('catch-up weight gain'). Children who have been severely ill need constant attention right through the convalescent period, as often home conditions are poor and feeds are refused.

Adults do not usually suffer such severe malnutrition, but the same principles of treatment should be followed.

Prognosis

Children with extreme malnutrition have a mortality of over 50%. By careful management this can be reduced significantly to 1–2%, depending on the availability of facilities. Brain development takes place in the first years of life, a time when severe PEM frequently occurs. There is evidence that intellectual impairment and behavioural abnormalities occur in severely affected children. Physical growth is also impaired. Probably both of these effects can be alleviated if it is possible to maintain a high standard of living with a good diet and freedom from infection over a long period.

Prevention

Prevention of PEM depends not only on adequate nutrients being available but also on education of both governments and individuals in the importance of good nutrition and immunization (Box 5.3). Short-term programmes are useful for acute shortages of food, but long-term programmes involving improved agriculture are equally important. Bad feeding practices and infections are more prevalent than actual shortage of food in many areas of the world. However, good surveillance is necessary to avoid periods of famine.

Food supplements (and additional vitamins) should be given to 'at-risk' groups by adding high-energy food (e.g. milk powder, meat concentrates) to the diet. Pregnancy and lactation are times of high energy requirement and supplements have been shown to be beneficial.

FURTHER READING

Khanu MS, Ashworh A, Huttley SR (1994) Controlled trial of three approaches to the treatment of severe malnutrition. *Lancet* **334**: 1728–1732.

Schwarz MW, Seeley RT (1997) Neuro-endocrine responses to starvation and weight loss. *New England Journal of Medicine* **336**: 1802–1811.

Waterlow JC (1992) *Protein energy malnutrition*. London: Edward Arnold.

Vitamins

Deficiencies due to inadequate intake associated with PEM (Table 5.7) are commonly seen in the developing countries. This is not, however, invariable. For example, vitamin A deficiency is never seen in Jamaica, but is common in PEM in Hyderabad, India. In the West, deficiency of vitamins is rare except in the specific groups shown in Table 5.8. The widespread use of vitamins as 'tonics' is unnecessary and should be discouraged. Toxicity from excess fat-soluble vitamins is occasionally seen.

Fat-soluble vitamins

Vitamin A

Vitamin A (retinol) is part of the family of retinoids which is present in food and the body as esters combined with long-chain fatty acids. The richest food source is liver, but it is also found in milk, butter, cheese, egg yolks and fish oils. Retinol or carotene is added to margarine in the UK and other countries.

Beta-carotene is the main carotenoid found in green vegetables, carrots and other yellow and red fruits. Other carotenoids, lycopene and lutein, are probably of little quantitative importance as dietary precursors of vitamin A.

Beta-carotene is cleaved in the intestinal mucosa by carotene dioxygenase, yielding retinaldehyde which can be reduced to retinol. Between a quarter and a third of dietary vitamin A in the UK is derived from retinoids. Nutritionally, 6 μg of β-carotene is equivalent to 1 μg of preformed retinol; vitamin A activity in the diet is given as retinol equivalents.

Box 5.3

Prevention of protein–energy malnutrition – GOBIF (a WHO priority programme)

- **G**rowth monitoring: The WHO has a simple growth chart that the mother keeps
- **O**ral rehydration, particularly for diarrhoea
- **B**reast-feeding supplemented by food after 6 months
- **I**mmunization: against measles, tetanus, pertussis, diphtheria, polio and tuberculosis
- **F**amily planning

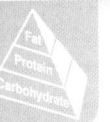

Table 5.7
Fat-soluble and water-soluble vitamins: reference nutrient intake (RNI) and lower reference nutrient intake (LRNI)

Vitamin	RNI/day (sufficient)	LRNI/day (insufficient)	Major clinical features of deficiency
Fat-soluble			
A (retinol)	700 µg	300 µg	Xerophthalmia, night blindness, keratomalacia, follicular hyperkeratosis
D (cholecalciferol)	No dietary intake required	10 µg (living indoors)	Rickets, osteomalacia
K	1 µg/kg bodyweight		Coagulation defects
			Neurological disorders, e.g. ataxia
E (α-tocopherol)	10°*		
Water-soluble			
B$_1$ (thiamin)	0.4 mg per 1000 kcal**	0.23 mg per 1000 kcal**	Beriberi, Wernicke–Korsakoff syndrome
B$_2$ (riboflavin)	1.3 mg	0.8 mg	Angular stomatitis
Niacin	6.6 mg per 1000 kcal	4.4 mg per 1000 kcal	Pellagra
B$_6$ (pyridoxine)	15 µg per g of dietary protein	11 µg per g of dietary protein	Polyneuropathy
B$_{12}$ (cobalamin)	1.5 µg	1.0 µg	Megaloblastic anaemia, neurological disorders
Folate	200 µg	100 µg	Megaloblastic anaemia
C (ascorbic acid)	40 mg	10 mg	Scurvy

*No official RNI because amount varies depending upon polyunsaturated fatty acid content of diet
**Thiamin requirements are related to energy metabolism

Table 5.8
Some causes of vitamin deficiency in developed countries

Decreased intake
Alcohol dependency: chiefly B vitamins (e.g. thiamin)
Small bowel disease: chiefly folate, occasionally fat-soluble vitamins
Vegans: vitamin D (if no exposure to sunlight), vitamin B$_{12}$
Elderly with poor diet: chiefly vitamin D (if no exposure to sunlight), folate
Anorexia from any cause: chiefly folate

Decreased absorption
Ileal disease/resection: only vitamin B$_{12}$
Liver and biliary tract disese: fat-soluble vitamins
Intestinal bacterial overgrowth: vitamin B$_{12}$
Oral antibiotics: vitamin K

Miscellaneous
Long-term enteral or parenteral nutrition: usually vitamin supplements are given
Renal disease: vitamin D
Drug antagonists (e.g. methotrexate interfering with folate metabolism)

Table 5.9
Classification of xerophthalmia by ocular signs

Night blindness (XN)
Conjunctival xerosis (XIA)
Bitot's spot (X2)
Corneal xerosis (X2)
Corneal ulceration/keratomalacia < ⅓ corneal surface (X3A)
Corneal ulceration/keratomalacia ≥ ⅓ corneal surface (X3B)
Corneal scar (XS)
Xerophthalmic fundus (XF)

Reproduced with permission from WHO/Unicef/IVACG 1988

Deficiency
Vitamin A deficiency and xerophthalmia (see below) is the major cause of blindness in young children despite intensive preventative programmes. The WHO estimates that between six and seven million new cases of xerophthalmia occur each year, with 20% of survivors being totally blind and 50–56% partially blind. South and East Asia, parts of Africa and Latin America as well as the Middle East are the most severely affected.

Xerophthalmia has been classified by the WHO (Table 5.9). Impaired adaptation followed by night blindness is the first effect. There is dryness and thickening of the conjunctiva and the cornea (xerophthalmia occurs as a result of keratinization). Bitot's spots – white plaques of keratinized epithelial cells – are found on the conjunctiva of young children with vitamin A deficiency. These spots can, however, be seen without vitamin A deficiency, possibly caused by exposure. Corneal softening, ulceration and dissolution (keratomalacia) eventually occur; superimposed infection is a frequent accompaniment and both lead to blindness.

Function
Retinol is stored in the liver and is transported in plasma bound to an α-globulin, retinol-binding protein (RBP). Vitamin A has several metabolic roles:

- Retinaldehyde in its *cis* form is found in the opsin proteins in the rods (rhodopsin) and cones (iodopsin) of the retina. Light causes retinaldehyde to change to its *trans* isomer, and this leads to changes in membrane potentials that are transmitted to the brain.
- Retinol and retinoic acid are involved in the control of cell proliferation and differentiation.
- Retinyl phosphate is a cofactor in the synthesis of most glycoproteins containing mannose.

In PEM, retinol-binding protein along with other proteins is reduced. This suggests vitamin A deficiency, although body stores are not necessarily reduced.

Vitamin A in malnourished children

Vitamin A supplementation appears to improve morbidity and mortality from measles. It has also been suggested that supplementation reduces morbidity and/or mortality from diarrhoeal diseases and respiratory infections and improves growth. However, despite the large number of studies in both developed and developing countries over the last two decades, the results remain controversial. Furthermore, although low circulating concentrations of vitamin A in HIV-infected individuals are associated with increased risk of vertical transmission of HIV, vitamin A supplementation during pregnancy and the interpartum period are unlikely to reduce vertical transmission to the child.

Diagnosis

In parts of the world where the deficiency is common, diagnosis is made on the basis of the clinical features, and deficiency should always be suspected if any degree of malnutrition is present. Blood levels of vitamin A will usually be low, but the best guide to the diagnosis is a response to replacement therapy.

Treatment

Urgent treatment with retinol palmitate 30 mg orally should be given on two successive days. In the presence of vomiting and diarrhoea, 30 mg of vitamin A is given intramuscularly. Associated malnutrition must be treated and superadded bacterial infection should be treated with antibiotics. Referral for specialist ophthalmic treatment is necessary in severe cases.

Prevention

Most Western diets contain enough dairy products and green vegetables, but vitamin A is added to foodstuffs (e.g. margarine) in some countries. Vitamin A is not destroyed by cooking.

In some developing countries vitamin A supplements are given at the time the child attends for measles vaccination. Food fortification programmes are another approach. Education of the population is necessary and people should be encouraged to grow their own vegetables. In particular, pregnant women and children should be encouraged to eat green vegetables.

Other effects of vitamin A
Possible beneficial effects
- *Protection against cancer.* In epidemiological studies, β-carotene (which acts as an antioxidant), and to a lesser extent vitamin A, have been shown to have a possible protective effect against certain cancers. Controlled trials using β-carotene supplements have, however, not confirmed this protective effect.

- *Reduction in cardiovascular events.* Epidemiological studies have shown an association between increased intake of antioxidant vitamins (β-carotene, vitamin E, vitamin C) and reduced morbidity and mortality from coronary artery disease. Randomized trials have so far shown no reduction with β-carotene supplementation.
- *Dermatological applications.* Retinoic acid and some synthetic retinoids are used in dermatology (p. 1293).

Possible adverse effects
- *High intakes of vitamin A.* Chronic ingestion of retinol can cause liver and bone damage, hair loss, double vision, vomiting, headaches and other abnormalities. Single doses of 300 mg in adults or 100 mg in children can be harmful.
- *Retinol is teratogenic.* The incidence of birth defects in infants is high with vitamin A intakes of more than 3 mg a day during pregnancy. In pregnancy, extra vitamin A or consumption of liver is not recommended in the UK. However, β-carotene is not toxic.

Vitamin D
See page 576.

Vitamin K

Vitamin K is found as phylloquinone (vitamin K_1) in green leafy vegetables, dairy products, rape seed and soya bean oils. Intestinal bacteria can synthesize the other major form of vitamin K, menaquinone (vitamin K_2), in the terminal ileum and colon. Vitamin K is absorbed in a similar manner to other fat-soluble substances in the upper small gut. Some menaquinones must also be absorbed as this is the major form found in the human liver.

Function

Vitamin K is a cofactor necessary for the production not only of blood clotting factors (p. 463), but also for proteins necessary in the formation of bone.

Vitamin K is a cofactor for the post-translational carboxylation of specific protein-bound glutamate residues in γ-carboxyglutamate (Gla). Gla residues bind calcium ions to phospholipid templates, and this action on factors II, VII, IX and X, and on proteins C and S, is necessary for coagulation to take place.

Bone osteoblasts contain three vitamin K dependent proteins, osteocalcin, matrix Gla protein and protein S, which have a role in bone matrix formation. Osteocalcin contains three Gla residues which bind tightly to the hydroxyapatite matrix depending on the degree of carboxylation; this leads to bone mineralization. There is, however, no convincing evidence that vitamin K deficiency or antagonism affects bone other than rapidly growing bone.

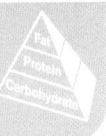

Vitamin K deficiency

Vitamin K deficiency results in inadequate synthesis of clotting factors (p. 463), which leads to an increase in the prothrombin time and haemorrhage. Deficiency occurs in the following circumstances:

The newborn

Deficiency occurs in the newborn owing to:

- poor placental transfer of vitamin K
- little vitamin K in breast milk
- no hepatic stores of menaquinone (no intestinal bacteria in the neonate).

Deficiency leads to a haemorrhagic disease of the newborn which can be prevented by prophylactic vitamin K. However, in the UK there is no agreement on whether prophylactic therapy is necessary.

Cholestatic jaundice

When bile flow into the intestine is interrupted, malabsorption of vitamin K occurs as no bile salts are available to facilitate absorption and the prothrombin time increases. This can be corrected by giving 10 mg of phytomenadione intramuscularly. (Note that an increased prothrombin time because of liver disease does not respond to vitamin K injection, there being no shortage of vitamin K, just bad liver function.) In patients with chronic cholestasis (e.g. primary biliary cirrhosis) oral therapy using a water-soluble preparation, menadiol sodium phosphate 10 mg daily, is used.

Concomitant vitamin K antagonists

Oral anticoagulants antagonize vitamin K (p. 469). Antibacterial drugs also interfere with the bacterial synthesis of vitamin K.

Vitamin E

Vitamin E includes eight naturally occurring compounds divided into tocopherols and tocotrienoles. The most active compound and the most widely available in food is the natural isomer d- (or RRR) α-tocopherol, which accounts for 90% of vitamin E in the human body. Vegetables and seed oils, including soya bean, saffron, sunflower, cereals and nuts, are the main sources. Animal products are poor sources of the vitamin.

Vitamin E is absorbed with fat, transported in the blood largely in low-density lipoproteins (LDL).

An individual's vitamin E requirement depends on the intake of polyunsaturated fatty acids (PUFAs). Since this varies widely, no daily requirement is given in the UK. The requirement stated in the USA is approximately 7–10 mg per day, but average diets contain much more than this. If PUFAs are taken in large amounts, more vitamin E is required.

Function

The biological activity of vitamin E results principally from its antioxidant properties. In biological membranes it contributes to membrane stability. It protects cellular structures against damage from a number of highly reactive oxygen species, including hydrogen peroxide, superoxide and other oxygen radicals. Vitamin E may also affect cell proliferation and growth.

Vitamin E deficiency

The first deficiency to be demonstrated was a haemolytic anaemia described in premature infants. Infant formulations now contain vitamin E.

Deficiency is seen only in children with abetalipoproteinaemia (p. 298) and in patients on long-term parenteral nutrition. The severe neurological deficit (gross ataxia) can be prevented by vitamin E injection.

Plasma or serum levels of α-tocopherol can be measured and should be corrected for the level of plasma lipids by expressing the value as milligrams per milligram of plasma lipid.

Epidemiological data

Animals fed an atherogenic diet supplemented with α-tocopherol develop many fewer new atheromatous lesions than do those fed an atherogenic diet alone, and there may be regression of existing lesions.

There is also evidence for vitamin E intake and blood α-tocopherol levels as an independent risk factor for the development of ischaemic heart disease (IHD) in healthy, well-nourished individuals eating a Western diet. This has been shown in comparisons of different communities in the WHO 'MONICA' observational study. It may account for the 'Mediterranean paradox' of communities in Southern Europe – who eat a high-fat diet with a high prevalence of cigarette smoking – having an incidence of premature IHD just 10% of that of communities in Northern Europe, such as the Clyde Valley or Finland.

Several trials have examined the effect of vitamin E supplementation in slowing down the development and progression of coronary heart disease. Most suggest benefit, although a recent study reports no significant benefit in secondary prevention of cardiovascular disease. Most trials have been undertaken with a dose of 100–800 IU/day which compares with up to about 30 IU/day provided by the normal diet. On the available evidence, many cardiologists recommend the use of vitamin E to prevent coronary heart disease in high-risk patients. One study has found that vitamin E and aspirin is more beneficial that aspirin alone. Other studies with positive results have combined a supplement of vitamin E with vitamin C, which makes it difficult to assess the independent effects of each antioxidant vitamin. Vitamin E may also be beneficial in preventing cerebrovascular disease and peripheral vascular disease, although these effects have been less studied than those on ischaemic heart disease.

Antioxidants may also have a role in the prevention of cancer, and vitamin E has also been shown to have some benefit in patients with Alzheimer's disease (p. 1264).

Water-soluble vitamins

Water-soluble vitamins are non-toxic and relatively cheap and can therefore be given in large amounts if a deficiency is possible. The daily requirements of water-soluble vitamins are given in Table 5.7.

Thiamin (vitamin B$_1$)

Thiamin consists of pyrimidine and thiazole rings. The alcohol side-chain is esterified with one, two or three phosphates (Fig. 5.6).

Function

Thiamin diphosphate, often called thiamin pyrophosphate (TPP), is an essential cofactor, particularly in carbohydrate metabolism.

TPP is involved in the oxidative decarboxylation of acetyl CoA in mitochondria. In the Krebs cycle, TPP is the key enzyme for the decarboxylation of a-ketoglutarate to succinyl CoA. TPP is also the cofactor for transketolase, a key enzyme in the hexose monophosphate shunt.

Thiamin is found in many foodstuffs, including cereals, grains, beans, nuts, as well as pork and duck. It is often added to food (e.g. in cereals) in developed countries. The dietary requirement (see Table 5.7) depends on energy intake, more being required if the diet is high in carbohydrates.

Following absorption, thiamin is found in all body tissues, the majority being in the liver. Body stores are small and signs of deficiency quickly develop with inadequate intake.

There is no evidence that a high oral intake is dangerous, but ataxia has been reported after high parenteral therapy.

Thiamin deficiency

Thiamin deficiency is seen:

- as beriberi, where the only food consumed is polished rice
- in chronic alcohol-dependent patients who are consuming virtually no food at all
- rarely in starved patients (e.g. with carcinoma of the stomach), and in severe prolonged hyperemesis gravidarum, especially when treated by intravenous fluids alone.

Beriberi

This is now confined to the poorest areas of South East Asia. It can be prevented by eating undermilled or parboiled rice, or by fortification of rice with thiamine. Probably the most important factor in the reduction of beriberi is the general increase in overall food consumption so that the staple diet is varied and contains legumes and pulses, which contain a large amount of thiamin. There are two main clinical types of beriberi, which, surprisingly, only rarely occur together.

Dry beriberi usually presents insidiously with a symmetrical polyneuropathy. The initial symptoms are heaviness and stiffness of the legs, followed by weakness, numbness, and pins and needles. The ankle jerk reflexes are lost and eventually all the signs of polyneuropathy that may involve the trunk and arms are found (p. 1215). Cerebral involvement occurs, producing the picture of the Wernicke–Korsakoff syndrome (p. 1216). In endemic areas, mild symptoms and signs may be present for years without unduly affecting the patient.

Wet beriberi causes oedema. Initially this is of the legs, but it can extend to involve the whole body, with ascites and pleural effusions. The peripheral oedema may mask the accompanying features of dry beriberi.

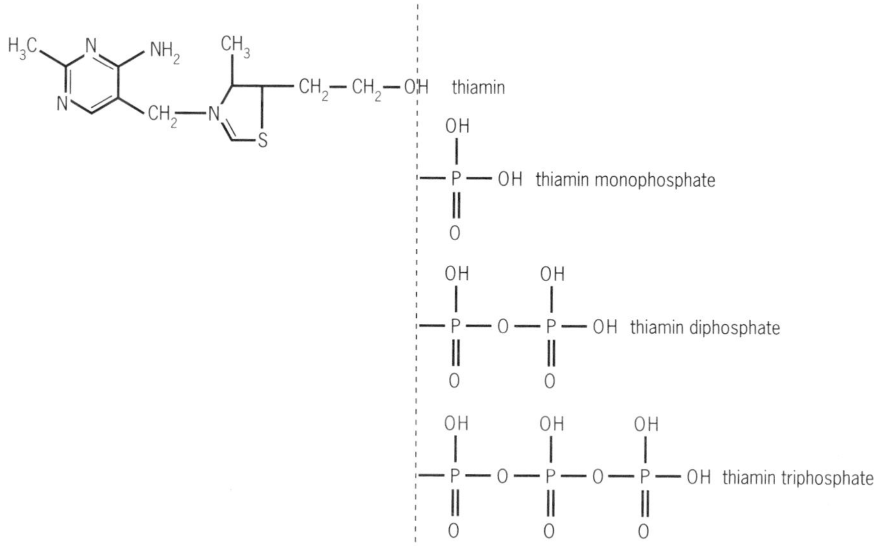

Fig. 5.6 Thiamin.

Thiamin deficiency impairs pyruvate dehydrogenase with accumulation of lactate and pyruvate, producing peripheral vasodilatation and eventually oedema. The heart muscle is also affected and heart failure occurs, causing a further increase in the oedema. Initially there are warm extremities, a full, fast, bounding pulse and a raised venous pressure ('high-output state'), but eventually heart failure advances and a poor cardiac output ensues. The electrocardiogram may show conduction defects.

Infantile beriberi occurs, usually acutely, in breast-fed babies at approximately 3 months of age. The mothers show no signs of thiamin deficiency but presumably their body stores must be virtually nil. The infant becomes anorexic, develops oedema and has some degree of aphonia. Tachycardia and tachypnoea develop and, unless treatment is instituted, death occurs quickly.

Diagnosis

In endemic areas the diagnosis of beriberi should always be suspected and if in doubt treatment with thiamine should be instituted. A rapid disappearance of oedema after thiamine (50 mg i.m.) is diagnostic. Other causes of oedema must be considered (e.g. renal or liver disease), and the polyneuropathy is indistinguishable from that due to other causes. The diagnosis is confirmed by measurement of transketolase activity in red cells using fresh heparinized blood. This enzyme is dependent on TPP. The assay is performed with and without added TPP; an increase in activity of 25% with TPP indicates deficiency.

Treatment

Thiamine 50 mg i.m. is given for 3 days, followed by 25 mg of thiamine daily by mouth. The response in wet beriberi occurs in hours, giving dramatic improvement, but in dry beriberi improvement is often slow to occur. In most cases all the B vitamins are given because of multiple deficiency. Infantile beriberi is treated by giving thiamine to the mother, which is then passed on to the infant via the breast milk.

Thiamin deficiency in patients with alcohol dependence

In the West such patients and those with severe acute illness receiving high carbohydrate infusions without vitamins are the only major groups to suffer from thiamin deficiency. Rarely they develop wet beriberi, which must be distinguished from alcoholic cardiomyopathy. More usually, however, thiamin deficiency presents with poly-neuropathy or with the Wernicke–Korsakoff syndrome.

This syndrome, which consists of dementia, ataxia, varying ophthalmoplegia and nystagmus (see p. 1216), presents acutely and should be suspected in all heavy drinkers. If treated promptly it is reversible; if left it becomes irreversible. It is a major cause of dementia in the USA.

Urgent treatment with thiamine 50–100 mg i.m. or i.v. is given for 3 days, often combined with other B-complex vitamins. Thiamine must always be given before any intravenous glucose infusion.

Riboflavin

Riboflavin is widely distributed throughout all plant and animal cells. Good sources are dairy products, offal and leafy vegetables. Riboflavin is not destroyed appreciably by cooking, but is destroyed by sunlight. Riboflavin is a flavoprotein that is a cofactor for many oxidative reactions in the cell.

There is no definite deficiency, although many communities have low dietary intakes. Studies in volunteers taking a low riboflavin diet have produced:

- angular stomatitis or cheilosis (fissuring at the corners of the mouth)
- a red, inflamed tongue
- seborrhoeic dermatitis, particularly involving the face (around the nose) and the scrotum or vulva.

Conjunctivitis with vascularization of the cornea and opacity of the lens has also been described. It is probable, however, that many of the above features are due to multiple deficiencies rather than the riboflavin itself.

Riboflavin 5 mg daily can be tried for the above conditions, usually given as the vitamin B complex.

Niacin

This is the generic name for the two chemical forms, nicotinic acid and nicotinamide, the latter being found in the two pyridine nucleotides, nicotinamide adenine dinucleotide (NAD) and nicotinamide adenine dinucleotide phosphate (NADP). Both act as hydrogen acceptors in many oxidative reactions, and in their reduced forms (NADH and NADPH) act as hydrogen donors in reductive reactions. Many oxidative steps in the production of energy require NAD, and NADP is equally necessary in the hexose monophosphate shunt (p. 433) for the generation of NADPH, which is necessary for fatty-acid synthesis.

Niacin is found in many foodstuffs, including plants, meat (particularly offal) and fish. Niacin is lost by removing bran from cereals but is added to processed cereals and white bread in many countries.

Niacin can be synthesized in humans from tryptophan, 60 mg of tryptophan being converted to 1 mg of niacin (Fig. 5.7). The amount of niacin in food is given as the 'niacin equivalent', which is equal to the amount of niacin plus one-sixtieth of the tryptophan content. Eggs and cheese contain tryptophan.

Kynureninase and kynurenine hydroxylase are both B_6 and riboflavin dependent and deficiency of these B vitamins can also produce pellagra.

Pellagra

This is rare and is found in people who eat virtually only maize, for example in parts of Africa. Maize contains

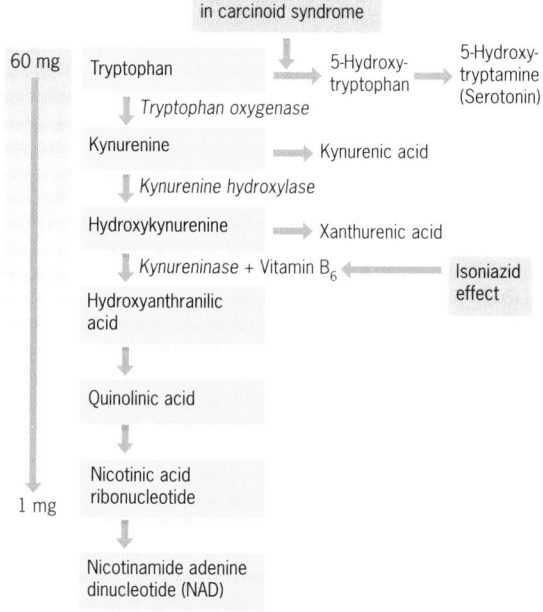

Fig. 5.7 The oxidative pathway of tryptophan metabolism.

niacin in the form of niacytin, which is biologically unavailable, and has a low content of tryptophan. In central America, pellagra has always been rare because maize (for the cooking of tortillas) is soaked overnight in calcium hydroxide which releases niacin. Many of the features of pellagra can be explained purely by niacin deficiency; but some are probably due to multiple deficiencies, including deficiencies of proteins and of other vitamins.

Clinical features

The classical features are of dermatitis, diarrhoea and dementia. Although this is an easily remembered triad, not all are always present and the mental changes are not a true dementia.

- *Dermatitis*. In the areas of skin exposed to sunlight, initially there is redness followed by cracks with occasional ulceration. Chronic thickening, dryness and pigmentation develop. The lesions are always symmetrical and often affect the dorsal surfaces of the hands. The perianal skin and vulva are frequently involved. Casal's necklace or collar is the term given to the skin lesion around the neck, which is confined to this area by the clothes worn.
- *Diarrhoea*. This is often a feature but constipation is occasionally seen. Other gastrointestinal manifestations include a painful, red, raw tongue, glossitis and angular stomatitis. Recurring mouth infections occur.
- *Dementia*. This occurs in chronic disease. In milder cases there are symptoms of depression, apathy and

sometimes thought disorders. Tremor and an encephalopathy frequently occur. Hallucinations and acute psychosis are seen with more severe cases.

Pellagra may also occur in the following circumstances:

- Isoniazid therapy can lead to a deficiency of vitamin B_6, which is needed for the synthesis of nicotinamide from tryptophan. Vitamin B_6 is now given concomitantly with isoniazid (Fig. 5.7).
- In Hartnup's disease, a rare inborn error, in which basic amino acids including tryptophan are not absorbed by the gut. There is also loss of this amino acid in the urine.
- In generalized malabsorption (rare).
- Alcohol-dependent patients who do not eat.
- Very low protein diets given for renal disease or taken as a food fad.
- In the carcinoid syndrome and phaeochromocytomas, tryptophan metabolism is diverted away from the formation of nicotinamide to form amines.

Diagnosis

In endemic areas this is based on the clinical features, remembering that other vitamin deficiencies can produce similar changes (e.g. angular stomatitis). Nicotinamide (approximately 300 mg daily by mouth) with a maintenance dose of 50 mg daily is given with dramatic improvement in the skin and diarrhoea. Mostly, however, vitamin B complex is given, as other deficiencies are often present.

An increase in the protein content of the diet and treatment of malnutrition and other vitamin deficiencies is essential.

Vitamin B_6

Vitamin B_6 exists as pyridoxine, pyridoxal and pyridoxamine, and is found widely in plant and animal foodstuffs. Pyridoxal phosphate is a cofactor in the metabolism of many amino acids. Dietary deficiency is extremely rare. Some drugs (e.g. isoniazid, hydralazine and penicillamine) interact with pyridoxal phosphate, producing B_6 deficiency. The polyneuropathy occurring after isoniazid usually responds to vitamin B_6. Sideroblastic anaemia occasionally responds to vitamin B_6 (see p. 416). A polyneuropathy has occurred after high doses (> 200 mg) given over many months. Vitamin B_6 is used for premenstrual tension: a daily dose of 10 mg should not be exceeded.

Biotin and pantothenic acid

Biotin is involved in a number of carboxylase reactions. It occurs in many foodstuffs and the dietary requirement is small. Deficiency is extremely rare and is confined to a few people who consume raw eggs, which contain an antagonist (avidin) to biotin. It has also been reported in patients receiving long-term parenteral

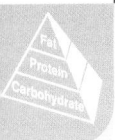

nutrition without adequate amounts of biotin. It causes a dermatitis that responds to biotin replacements.

Pantothenic acid is widely distributed in all foods and deficiency in humans has not been described.

Vitamin C

Ascorbic acid is a simple sugar and a powerful reducing agent, its main role being to control the redox potential within cells. It is involved in the hydroxylation of proline to hydroxyproline, which is necessary for the formation of collagen. The failure of this biochemical pathway in vitamin C deficiency accounts for virtually all of the clinical effects seen.

Humans, along with a few other animals (e.g. primates and the guinea-pig), are unusual in not being able to synthesize ascorbic acid from glucose.

Vitamin C is present in all fresh fruit and vegetables. Unfortunately, ascorbic acid is easily leached out of vegetables when they are placed in water and it is also oxidized to dehydro-ascorbic acid during cooking, exposure to copper or alkalis. Potatoes are a good source as many people eat a lot of them, but vitamin C is lost during storage.

It has been suggested that ascorbic acid in high dosage (1–2 g daily) will prevent the common cold. While there is some scientific support for this, clinical trials have shown no significant effect. Vitamin C supplements have also been advocated to prevent atherosclerosis and cancer, but again a clear benefit has not been demonstrated.

Vitamin C deficiency is seen mainly in infants fed boiled milk and in the elderly and single people who cannot be bothered to eat vegetables. In the UK it is also seen in Asians eating only rice and chapatis, and in food faddists.

Scurvy

In adults the early symptoms may be non-specific, with weakness and muscle pain. Other features are shown in Table 5.10. In infantile scurvy there is irritability, painful legs, anaemia and characteristic subperiosteal haemorrhages, particularly into the ends of long bones.

Diagnosis

The anaemia is usually hypochromic but occasionally a normochromic or megaloblastic anaemia is seen. The type of anaemia depends on whether iron deficiency

Table 5.10
Clinical features of vitamin C deficiency

Keratosis of hair follicles with 'corkscrew' hair
Perifollicular haemorrhages
Swollen, spongy gums with bleeding and superadded infection, loosening of teeth
Spontaneous bruising
Spontaneous haemorrhage
Anaemia
Failure of wound healing

(owing to decreased absorption or loss due to haemorrhage) or folate deficiency (folate being largely found in green vegetables) is present.

Plasma ascorbic acid is very low in obvious deficiency and a vitamin C level of less than 11 μmol/L (0.2 mg per 100 mL) indicates vitamin C deficiency. The leucocyte–platelet layer (buffy coat) of centrifuged blood corresponds to vitamin C concentrations in other tissues. The normal level of leucocyte ascorbate is 1.1–2.8 pmol per 10^6 cells.

Treatment

Initially the patient is given 250 mg of ascorbic acid daily and encouraged to eat fresh fruit and vegetables. Subsequently, 40 mg daily will maintain a normal exchangeable body pool of about 900 mg (5.1 mmol).

Prevention

Orange juice should be given to bottle-fed infants. The intake of breast-fed infants depends on the mother's diet. In the elderly, eating adequate fruit and vegetables is the best way to avoid scurvy. Careful surveillance of the elderly, particularly those who live alone, is necessary. Ascorbic acid supplements should only be necessary occasionally.

Vitamin B₁₂ and folate

These are dealt with on page 417 and daily requirements are shown in Table 5.7. In many developed countries, up to 15% of the population have a partial deficiency of 5,10-methylene-tetrahydrofolate reductase, a key folate-metabolizing enzyme. This is due to a point mutation and is associated with an increase in neural tube defects and hyperhomocysteinaemia, which may lead to cardiovascular damage. In the USA folic acid fortification of enriched cereals at 1.4 mg per kg grain is done and other countries may also increase their daily folate requirements.

FURTHER READING

Gerster H (1997) Vitamin A. Functions, dietary requirements and safety in humans. *International Journal of Vitamin and Nutrition Research* **67**: 71–90.
Kusti LH, Folsom AR, Prineas RJ et al. (1996) Dietary antioxidants, vitamins and death from coronary disease in postmenopausal women. *New England Journal of Medicine* **334**: 1156–1162.
Jones A (1995) [Series of review articles on vitamins A, D, E and K]. *Lancet* **345**.

Minerals

A number of minerals have been shown to be essential in animals and an increasing number of deficiency syndromes are becoming recognized in humans. Long-term total parenteral nutrition allowed trace element deficiency to be studied in controlled conditions; now trace elements are always added to long-term parenteral nutrition regimens. It is highly probable (but difficult to study because of multiple deficiencies) that trace-element deficiency is also a frequent accompaniment of all PEM states. Sodium (RNI 70 mmol/day), potassium (RNI 90 mmol/day), magnesium (RNI 12.3 mmol/day for men and 10.9 for women) and chloride are discussed in Chapter 12.

Iron (see also p. 412)

The daily RNI for men is 160 μmol (8.7 mg) and for women 260 μmol (14.8 mg). Iron deficiency is common world-wide, affecting both developing and developed countries. It is particularly prevalent in women of a reproductive age. Dietary iron overload is seen in the South African Bantu men who cook and brew in iron pots.

Copper

The daily RNI of copper is 1.2 mg (19 μmol). Shellfish, legumes, cereals and nuts are good dietary sources.

Deficiency

Menkes' kinky hair syndrome is a rare condition caused by malabsorption of copper. Infants with this sex-linked recessive abnormality develop growth failure, mental retardation, bone lesions and brittle hair. Anaemia and neutropenia also occur. This condition, which serves as a model for copper deficiency, supports the idea that some of the clinical features seen in PEM are due to copper deficiency. Breast and cows' milk are low in copper and supplementation is occasionally necessary when first treating PEM.

Copper toxicity

This occurs in Wilson's disease; see page 376.

Zinc

The daily RNI of zinc is 9.5 mg (145 μmol) for men, 7 mg (110 μmol) for women and it is widely available in food. Zinc is involved in many metabolic pathways, often acting as a coenzyme; it is essential for the synthesis of RNA and DNA.

Deficiency

Acrodermatitis enteropathica is an inherited disorder caused by malabsorption of zinc. Infants develop growth retardation, severe diarrhoea, hair loss and associated *Candida* and bacterial infections. This condition provides a model for zinc deficiency. Zinc supplementation results in a complete cure. Deficiency probably also plays a role in PEM.

Zinc levels have been shown to be low in some patients with malabsorption or skin disease, and in patients with AIDS, but the exact role of zinc in these situations is disputed. Zinc has low toxicity, but high zinc levels from water stored in galvanized containers interfere with iron and copper metabolism. Wound healing is impaired with moderate zinc deficiency and is improved by zinc supplements. Impaired taste and smell, hair loss and night blindness are also features of severe zinc deficiency.

Iodine

The daily RNI of iodine is 140 μg (1.1 μmol for men and women) and it is found in milk, meat and seafoods. It exists in foodstuffs as inorganic iodines which are efficiently absorbed. Iodine is a constituent of the thyroid hormones (p. 1035).

Deficiency

Many mountainous areas throughout the world lack iodine in the soil, and so iodine deficiency, which impairs brain development, is a WHO priority. Endemic goitre occurs in remote areas where the daily intake is below 70 μg, and in those parts 1–5% of babies are born with cretinism. In these areas, iodized oil should be given intramuscularly to all reproductive women every 3–5 years. In developed countries, salt is iodized and endemic goitre has disappeared.

Fluoride

In areas where the level of fluoride in drinking water is less than 1 p.p.m. (0.7–1.2 mg/L), dental caries is relatively more prevalent. Fluoridation of the water provides 1–2 mg daily, resulting in a reduction of about 50% of tooth decay in children. There is little fluoride in food except for seafish and tea, the latter providing 70% of the daily intake. Fluoride-containing toothpaste may add up to 2 mg a day.

Excessive fluoride intake in areas where the water fluoride level is above 3 mg/L can result in fluorosis, in which there is infiltration into the enamel of the teeth, producing pitting and discoloration.

Selenium

The daily RNI of selenium is 60 μg (0.8 μmol for men and women). Selenium is a component of several enzymes, including glutathione peroxidase and super-oxide dismutase. These enzymes prevent oxidative and free radical damage to cells. Selenium works in conjunction with vitamin E. Selenium is also involved in the conversion of thyroxine to triiodothyronine.

Clinical deficiency of selenium is rare except in areas of China where Keshan disease, a selenium-responsive cardiomyopathy, occurs. Selenium deficiency may also cause a myopathy. Toxicity has been described with very high intakes.

Calcium (see also p. 1059)

In the UK, the daily RNI of calcium is 700 mg (17.5 mmol), but substantially higher values are now recommended in the USA. It is found in many foodstuffs, with two-thirds

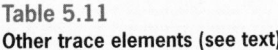

Table 5.11
Other trace elements (see text)

Element	Deficiency
Cadmium	?
Chromium	Glucose intolerance
Cobalt	Anaemia
Manganese	Growth retardation, skeletal abnormalities, glucose intolerance
Molybdenum	? Animals only
Nickel	? Animals only
Vanadium	? Nutritional oedema

of the intake coming from milk and milk products, only 5% from vegetables. In the UK most flour is fortified. Calcium absorption from the gastrointestinal tract is vitamin D-dependent. Ninety-nine per cent of body calcium is in the skeleton.

Increased calcium is required in pregnancy and lactation, when dietary intake must be increased. Calcium deficiency is usually due to vitamin D deficiency.

Phosphate (see also p. 688)

The daily RNI of phosphate is the same as that of calcium, i.e. 17.5 mmol. Phosphates are present in all natural foods and dietary deficiency has not been described. Patients taking large amounts of aluminium hydroxide can, however, develop phosphate deficiency owing to binding in the gut lumen. It can also be seen in total parenteral nutrition. Symptoms include anorexia, weakness and osteoporosis.

Other trace elements

The possible significance of cadmium, chromium, cobalt, manganese, molybdenum, nickel and vanadium is shown in Table 5.11.

FURTHER READING

Bender DA, Bender AE (1997) *Nutrition – a reference handbook.* Oxford: Oxford University Press.

Nutrition and ageing

Many animal studies have shown that life expectancy can be extended by restricting food intake. It is, however, not known whether the ageing process in humans can be altered by nutrition.

The ageing process

The process of ageing is not well understood. While wear and tear may play a role, it is an insufficient explanation for the causation of ageing. A number of theories have been postulated.

- *Programmed ageing theory* suggests a predetermined, presumably genetic, age-related alteration in cellular function that leads to susceptibility to disease and death.
- *Genomic instability theory* suggests errors in genetic transcription and translation, resulting in impaired protein synthesis and deterioration in cell function as age increases.
- *Free radical theory* suggests that these highly reactive molecules are no longer metabolized rapidly; accumulation occurs, leading to irreversible cell damage.
- *Random genetic errors* have also been implicated; an accumulation of errors over time is said to result in impaired protein synthesis and a decrease in cellular function.

Several other mechanisms have been suggested, but it is still unclear whether one universal or several independent mechanisms are involved.

Nutritional requirements in the elderly

These are qualitatively similar to the requirements of younger adults, but as energy expenditure is less, there is a lower energy requirement. However, maintaining physical activity is required for the overall health of the elderly.

The daily energy requirement of 'elderly people' (aged 60 and above, irrespective of age) has been set to be approximately 1.5 × BMR. The BMR is reduced, owing to a fall in the fat-free mass, from an average of 60 kg to 50 kg in men and from 40 kg to 35 kg in women. The diet should contain the same *proportions* of nutrients, and essential nutrients are still required.

Nutritional deficits in the elderly may be due to many factors, such as dental problems, lack of cooking skills (particularly in widowers), depression and lack of motivation. Significant malnourishment in developed countries is usually secondary to social problems or disease. In the elderly who are institutionalized, vitamin D supplements may be required because often these people do not go into the sunlight.

Owing to the high prevalence of osteoporosis in elderly people, daily calcium intake of 1–1.5 g/day is often recommended.

FURTHER READING

American Journal of Clinical Nutrition (1997) Special issue on aging and nutrition. **66** (4).
Finch S, Doyle W, Lowe C, Bates CJ, Prentice A, Smithers G et al. (1998) *National Diet and Nutrition Survey: People Aged 65 Years and Over.* London: The Stationery Office.
Schurch B, Scrimshaw NS (2000) Impact of human ageing on energy and protein metabolism and requirements. Proceeding of an IDECG workshop, Boston USA, May 3–6, 1999. *European Journal of Clinical Nutrition* **54** (Suppl 3): S1–S165.

Obesity

Obesity is almost invariable in developing countries and almost all people accumulate some fat as they get older. The World Health Organization now also acknowledges that obesity is a world-wide problem which also affects many developing countries. Obesity implies an excess storage of fat, and this can most easily be detected by looking at the undressed patient.

Most patients suffer from *simple obesity*, but in certain conditions obesity is an associated feature (Table 5.12). Even in the latter situation, the intake of calories must have exceeded energy expenditure over a prolonged period of time. Hormonal imbalance is often incriminated in women (e.g. postmenopause or when taking contraceptive pills), but most weight gain in such cases is usually small and due to water retention.

'Simple' obesity

Not all obese people eat more than the average person, but all obviously eat more than they need.

Suggested mechanisms

Genetic and environmental factors

These have always been difficult to separate when studying obesity. However, refeeding experiments in both monozygotic and dizygotic twins, reared together or apart, suggest that genetic influences account for 70% of the difference in body mass index (BMI) later in life, and that the childhood environment has little or no influence.

The refeeding experiments also showed that weight gain did not occur in all pairs of twins, suggesting that in some a facultative increase in thermogenesis occurred so that part of their extra dietary energy was expended inefficiently. Genetic factors have led to the discovery of a putative gene, firstly in the obese (*ob ob*) mouse and now in humans. The *ob* gene was shown to be expressed solely in both white and brown adipose tissue. The *ob* gene is found on chromosome 7 and produces a 16 kDa protein called leptin. In the *ob ob* mouse a mutation in the *ob* gene leads to production of a non-functioning protein. Administration of normal leptin to these obese mice reduces food intake and corrects the obesity. A similar situation has been described in a very rare genetic condition in humans, in which leptin is not expressed.

In massively obese subjects, leptin mRNA in subcutaneous adipose tissue is 80% higher than in controls. Plasma levels of leptin are also very high, correlating with the BMI. Weight loss due to food restriction decreases plasma levels of leptin. However, in contrast to the *ob ob* mouse, the leptin structure is normal and abnormalities in leptin are not the prime cause of human obesity.

Leptin secreted from fat cells could act as a feedback mechanism between the adipose tissue and the brain, acting as a 'lipostat' (adipostat), controlling fat stores by

Table 5.12
Conditions in which obesity is an associated feature

Genetic syndromes associated with hypogonadism
  (e.g. Prader–Willi syndrome, Laurence–Moon–Biedl syndrome)
Hypothyroidism
Cushing's syndrome
Stein–Leventhal syndrome
Drug-induced (e.g. corticosteroids)
Hypothalamic damage (e.g. due to trauma, tumour)

regulating hunger and satiety (see below). However, many other signals are involved and a unified theory of appetite regulation and its links to obesity is lacking. From an evolutionary perspective it seems that humans evolved to defend against energy deficit better than excess energy, which has been a relatively recent phenomenon in human history. Therefore, it is not surprising that obesity is largely restricted to humans, and animals that are domesticated or in zoos.

Food intake

Many factors related to the home environment, such as finance and the availability of sweets and snacks, will affect food intake. Some patients eat more during periods of heavy exercise or during pregnancy and are unable to get back to their former eating habits. The increase in obesity in social class 5 can usually be related to the type of food consumed (i.e. food containing sugar and fat). Psychological factors and how food is presented may override complex biochemical interactions.

It has been shown that obese patients eat more than they admit to eating, and over the years a very small daily excess can lead to a large accumulation of fat. For example, a 44 kJ (10.5 kcal) excess would lead to a 10 kg weight gain over 20 years.

Control of appetite

This is complex and depends partly on external stimuli, such as the company, the type of food, the surroundings and the person's habitual behaviour.

Appetite is the desire to eat and this usually initiates food intake. Following a meal, satiation occurs. This depends on gastric and duodenal distension and the release of many substances peripherally and centrally.

Following a meal, cholecystokinin (CCK), bombesin, glucagon-like peptide 1 (GLP1), enterostatin, and somatostatin are released from the small intestine, and glucagon and insulin from the pancreas. All of these hormones have been implicated in the control of satiety. Centrally, the hypothalamus – particularly ventromedial, dorsomedial, paraventricular and arcuate nuclei – plays an important role in integrating signals involved in appetite and bodyweight regulation (Fig. 5.8). Leptin receptors have been found in the above hypothalamic nuclei and their activation produces complex responses, which can be viewed functionally as: (a) inhibition of

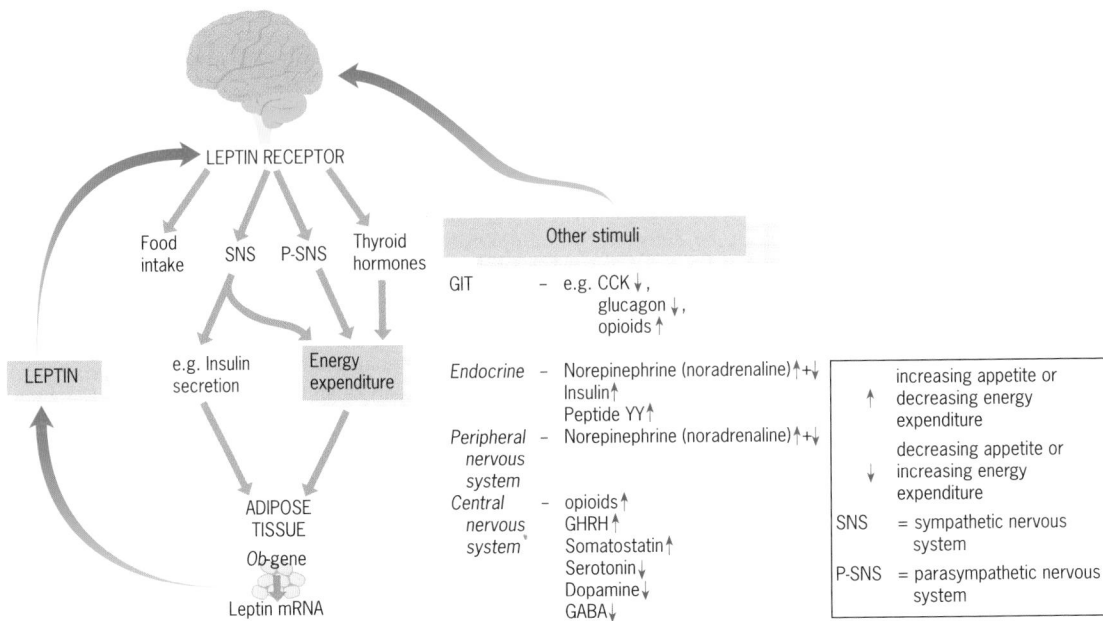

Fig. 5.8 **The proposed feedback loop between peripheral adipose tissue and central feeding pathways.** Peripheral and central factors (listed under 'other stimuli') influence food intake; some may interact with leptin.

signals that have a positive effect on appetite (orexigenic signals), such as melanin-concentrating hormone in the lateral hypothalamus and neuropeptide Y (NPY) in the arcuate nucleus; (b) stimulation of signals that have a negative effect on appetite (anorexigenic signals), such as alpha melanin-stimulating hormone (alpha MSH), which has effects on the melanocortin-4 (MC4) receptors in the paraventricular nucleus, preopiomelanocortin (POMC) precursor polypeptide and cocaine- and amphetamine-regulated transcript (CART) in the arcuate nucleus, and corticotrophin-releasing factor (CRF) in the paraventricular nucleus. This system potentially provides sensitive feedback regulation, whereby a reduction in leptin release, resulting from a reduction in adipose tissue mass, stimulates appetite and restores the energy deficit. In contrast, excess adipose tissue results in more leptin release, which is expected to reduce appetite.

The system is more complex than might first appear for at least three reasons. First, although obese individuals have excess adipose tissue and increased circulating leptin concentrations, appetite is not reduced. This has led to the notion of leptin resistance, which may be due to changes in leptin receptors or other downstream effects. Secondly, in some circumstances, leptin release from adipose tissue may occur independently of adipose tissue mass, e.g. during starvation, when the circulating concentration rapidly decreases far below that expected from loss of adipose tissue mass. Thirdly, new signals are being discovered in mammals and their role in appetite regulation still remains to be defined. Amongst these are central hypothalamic signals

such as orexins, and peripheral signals, such as Ghrelin, an endogenous growth hormone secretagogue which is surprisingly produced by the stomach (and kidney) and not the hypothalamus. Animal studies suggest that acute illness may increase circulating leptin concentrations, at least partly through cytokine action, but the effects disease has on leptin in humans are not so clear cut. Lastly, the effects of some appetite signals are not mediated by leptin. It is known that cytokines, such as TNF and IL-2, which are elevated in a wide range of inflammatory and traumatic conditions, also suppress appetite, although the exact pathways involved are not entirely clear.

Energy expenditure
Basal metabolic rate (BMR). BMR in obese subjects is higher than in lean subjects, which is not surprising since obesity is associated with an increase in lean body mass.

Physical activity. Obese patients tend to expend more energy during physical activity as they have a larger mass to move. On the other hand, many obese patients decrease their amount of physical activity. The energy expended on walking at 3 miles per hour is only 15.5 kJ/min (3.7 kcal/min) and therefore increasing exercise plays only a small part in losing weight. Nevertheless, because increased body fat develops insidiously over many years, any change in energy balance is helpful.

Thermogenesis
About 10% of ingested energy is dissipated as heat and is unconnected with physical activity. This dietary

induced thermogenesis has been reported to be lower in obese and post-obese subjects than lean subjects. This would tend to favour energy deposition in obesity and those predisposed to obesity. However, other workers have found no difference in dietary induced thermogenesis between lean and obese subjects.

Brown adipose tissue in animals, when stimulated by cold or food, dissipates in the form of heat the energy derived from ingested food. This can be a major component of overall energy balance in small mammals. However, the importance of brown adipose tissue thermogenesis in adult humans is likely to be very small, and of doubtful clinical significance. β_3-Adrenergic receptors are the principal receptors mediating catecholamine-stimulated lipolysis in brown adipose tissue and to a lesser extent at other sites. Drugs with β_3-adrenergic activities have been developed, but side-effects have limited their use.

Morbidity and mortality

Obese patients are at risk of early death, mainly from diabetes, coronary heart disease and cerebrovascular disease. The greater the obesity the higher the morbidity and mortality rates. For example, men who are 10% overweight have a 13% increased risk of death, while the increase in mortality for those 20% overweight is 25%. The rise is less in women, and in men over 65 obesity is not an independent risk factor. Weight reduction reduces this mortality and therefore should be strongly encouraged. The benefits are probably greater in more obese subjects (Table 5.13).

Clinical features

Most patients recognize their own problems, although often they are unaware of the main foods that cause obesity. Many symptoms are related to psychological problems or social pressures, such as the woman who cannot find fashionable clothes to wear.

The degree of obesity can be assessed by comparison with tables of ideal weight for height, from the BMI (Box 5.4), and by measuring skinfold thickness. The latter should be measured over the middle of the triceps muscle; normal values are 20 mm in a man and 30 mm in a woman. A central distribution of body fat (a waist/hip circumference ratio of > 1.0 in men and > 0.9 in women) is associated with a higher risk of morbidity and mortality than is a more peripheral distribution of body fat (waist/hip ratio < 0.85 in men and < 0.75 in women). This is because fat located centrally, especially inside the abdomen, is more sensitive to lipolytic stimuli, with the result that the abnormalities in circulating lipids are more severe.

Table 5.14 shows the conditions and complications that are associated with obesity. The relationship between cardiovascular disease (hypertension or ischaemic heart disease), hyperlipidaemia, smoking, physical exercise and obesity is complex. Difficulties arise in interpreting mortality figures because of the number of factors involved. Many studies of obesity do not, for instance, differentiate between smokers and non-smokers or between the types of physical exercise taken. Many do not take into account the cuff-size artefact in the measurement of blood pressure (an artefact will occur if a large cuff is not used in patients with a large arm). Nevertheless, obesity almost certainly plays a part in all of these diseases and should be treated. The only exception is that stopping smoking, even if accompanied by weight gain, is more important than any of the other factors.

Box 5.4

Ranges of body mass index (BMI) used to classify degrees of overweight and associated risk of co-morbidities

WHO classification	BMI (kg/m²)	Risk of co-morbidities
Overweight	25–30	Mildly increased
Obese	> 30	
Class I	30–35	Moderate
Class II	35–40	Severe
Class III	> 40	Very severe

Table 5.13
Potential benefits that may result from the loss of 10 kg in patients who are initially 100 kg and suffer from co-morbidities

Mortality	20–25% fall in total mortality 30–40% fall in diabetes-related deaths 40–50% fall in obesity-related cancer deaths
Blood pressure	Fall of about 10 mmHg (systolic and diastolic)
Diabetes	Reduces risk of developing diabetes by > 50% Fall of 30–50% in fasting blood glucose Fall of 15% in HbA1c
Serum lipids	Fall of 10% in total cholesterol Fall of 15% in LDL cholesterol Fall of 30% in triglycerides Increase of 8% in HDL cholesterol

---

Table 5.14
Conditions and complications associated with obesity

Psychological	Hypertension
Osteoarthritis of knees and hips	Breathlessness
Varicose veins	Ischaemic heart disease
Hiatus hernia	Stroke
Gallstones	Diabetes mellitus (NIDDM)
Postoperative problems	Hyperlipidaemia
Back strain	Menstrual abnormalities
Accident proneness	Increased morbidity and mortality

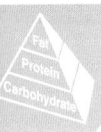

Treatment
Dietary control
This largely depends on a reduction in calorie intake.

The most common diets allow a daily intake of approximately 4200 kJ (1000 kcal), although this may need to be nearer 6300 kJ (1500 kcal) for someone engaged in physical work. Very low calorie diets are also advocated by some, usually over shorter periods of time, but unless they are accompanied by changes in lifestyle, weight regain is likely. Patients must realize that prolonged dieting is necessary for large amounts of fat to be lost. Furthermore, a permanent change in eating habits is required to maintain the new low weight. It is relatively easy for most people to lose the first few kilograms, but long-term success in moderate obesity is poor, with an overall success rate of no more than 10%.

Many dietary regimens aim to produce a weight loss of approximately 1 kg per week. Weight loss will be greater initially owing to accompanying protein and glycogen breakdown and consequent water loss. After 3–4 weeks, incremental weight loss may be very small because only adipose tissue is broken down and there is less accompanying water loss.

Patients must understand the principles of energy intake and expenditure, and the best results are obtained in educated, well-motivated patients. Constant supervision by a doctor, by close relatives or through membership of a slimming club helps to encourage compliance. It is essential to establish realistic aims. A 10% weight loss, which is regarded by some as a 'success' (see Table 5.13) is a realistic initial aim.

An increase in exercise will increase energy expenditure and should be encouraged – provided there is no contraindication – since weight control is usually not achieved without exercise. The effects of exercise are complex and not entirely understood. However, exercise alone will usually produce little long-term benefit. On the other hand there is evidence to suggest that in combination with dietary therapy, it can prevent weight being regained. In addition, regular exercise will improve general health.

The diet should contain adequate amounts of protein, vitamins and trace elements. A diet of 4200 kJ (1000 kcal) per day should be made up of more than 50 g protein, approximately 100 g of carbohydrate, and 40 g of fat. The carbohydrate should be in the form of complex carbohydrates such as vegetables and fruit rather than simple sugars. Alcohol contains 29 kJ/g (7 kcal/g) and should be discouraged. It can be substituted for other foods in the diet, but it often reduces the willpower. With a varied diet, vitamins and minerals will be adequate and supplements are not necessary. A balanced diet, attractively presented, is of much greater value and safer than any of the slimming regimens often advertised in magazines.

Most obese people oscillate in weight; they often regain the lost weight, but many manage to lose weight again. This 'cycling' in bodyweight may play a role in the development of coronary artery disease.

Behavioural modification
The aim of behavioural modification is to encourage the patient to take personal responsibility for changing lifestyle, which will determine dietary habits and physical activity. Family therapy may also be useful, especially when it involves obese children. It can be time-consuming and expensive. Cognitive behavioural therapy is even more time-consuming and expensive.

Drug therapy
Drugs can be used in the short term (up to 3 months) as an adjunct to the dietary regimen, but they do not substitute for strict dieting.

Centrally acting drugs.

- Drugs acting on the noradrenergic pathways do suppress appetite but all have been withdrawn in the UK due to cardiovascular side-effects.
- Drugs acting on both serotoninergic and noradrenergic pathways, e.g. sibutramine.

Peripherally acting drugs. Orlistat is an inhibitor of pancreatic and gastric lipases. It reduces dietary fat absorption and aids weight loss. Weight regain occurs after the drug is stopped. It has been used continuously in a large-scale trial for up to 2 years. The patients may complain of diarrhoea during treatment and to avoid this take a low fat diet resulting in weight loss.

Surgical treatment
Operations that involve bypassing parts of the small intestine have fallen out of favour because of their side-effects and cannot be recommended. Jejunoileal bypass was the most common operation and involved the anastomosis of approximately 18 cm of jejunum to the terminal 18 cm of the ileum. Complications are chiefly those of intestinal resection (p. 294). A fatty liver often occurs and in a few patients cirrhosis is seen.

Surgical procedures are still performed in cases of severe morbid obesity (BMI >40 kg/m^2) or BMI >35 with obesity-related medical co-morbidities:

- *Wiring the jaws* to prevent eating. This permits liquid feeds only. It can be used as a temporary measure but good dental hygiene is essential. Weight gain usually occurs after the wires have been removed, but in some individuals this can be controlled by the use of a tight waist cord. This procedure can be used to reduce postoperative complications after a major elective operation.
- *Gastroplasty.* A small gastric pouch is created by vertically stapling across the wall of the stomach. Good results have been claimed but slow weight regain occurs owing to change in eating patterns, e.g. ingestion of small frequent meals that do not cause discomfort.

- *Gastric banding.* An adjustable band is encircled around the proximal stomach to compartmentalize it into a small pouch and a large remnant. This can be performed laparoscopically. The results are variable.
- *Gastric bypass.* A Roux-en-Y gastrojejunostomy is performed. Loss of excess weight of 50–60% has been reported at 10 years but there are many long-term complications which need careful surveillance.
- *Liposuction.* The removal of large amounts of fat by suction does not deal with the underlying problem and weight regain frequently occurs.

Prevention

Preventing obesity must always be the goal because most obese people find it difficult to maintain any weight loss they have managed to achieve. All health professionals must be aware of the dangers of obesity and encourage children, young as well as older adults, from gaining too much weight. A small gain each year over a long period produces an obese individual for whom treatment is difficult.

FURTHER READING

Calle EE, Thun MJ, Petrelli JM, Rodriguez C, Heath CW (1999) Body-mass index and mortality in a prospective cohort of U.U. adults. *New England Journal of Medicine* **341**: 1097–1105.

Davidson MH, Hauptman J, Foreyt JP, Halsted CH, Heber D, Heimburger DC et al. (1999) Weight control and risk reduction in obese subjects treated for 2 years with orlistat. *Journal of the American Medical Association* **281**: 235–242.

Jung R (1997) Obesity as a disease. *British Medical Bulletin* **53**: 307–321.

Kopelman P (1999) *Appetite and obesity.* Royal College of Physicians of London.

Mun EC, Blackburn GL, Mathews JB (2001) Medical and surgical therapy for obesity. *Gastroenterology* **120**: 669–681.

Rosenbaum M, Leibel RL, Hirsch J (1997) Medical progress: obesity. *New England Journal of Medicine* **337**: 396–407.

Royal College of Physicians (1998) *Clinical management of overweight and obese patients, with particular reference to the use of drugs.* London: Royal College of Physicians.

Scott J (1996) New chapter for the fat controller. *Nature* **379**: 113–114.

WHO (1998) *Obesity: preventing and managing the global epidemic.* Geneva: WHO.

Nutritional support in the hospital patient

Nutritional support is recognized as being necessary in many hospitalized patients. The pathophysiology and hallmarks of malnutrition have been described earlier (p. 228); here the forms of nutritional support that are available are discussed, along with special nutritional requirements in some diseases.

Principles

Some form of nutritional supplementation is required in those patients who cannot eat, should not eat, will not eat or cannot eat enough. It is usually necessary to provide nutritional support for:

- all severely malnourished patients on admission to hospital
- moderately malnourished patients who, because of their physical illness, are not expected to eat for more than 3–5 days
- normally nourished patients not expected to eat for more than 5 days or eat less than half their intake for more than 8–10 days.

Enteral rather than parenteral nutrition should be used if the gastrointestinal tract is functioning normally.

Nutritional requirements for adults

- *Water.* Typical requirements are ~ 2–3 L/day. Increased requirements occur in patients with large-ouput fistulae, nasogastric aspirates and diarrhoea. Reduced requirements occur in patients with oedema, hepatic failure, renal failure (oliguric and not dialysed) and brain oedema.
- *Energy.* Typical requirements are ~ 7.5–10.0 MJ/day (1800–2400 kcal/day). Disease increases resting energy expenditure but decreases physical activity. Extra energy is given for repletion and reduced energy for obesity.
- *Protein.* Typically 10–15 g N/day (62–95 g protein/day) or 0.15–0.25 g N/kg/day (0.94–1.56 g protein/kg/day). Extra protein may be needed in severely catabolic conditions, such as extensive burns.
- *Major minerals.* Typical requirements for sodium and potassium are 70–100 mmol/day. Increased requirements occur in patients with gastrointestinal effluents. The excretion of these minerals in various effluents can provide an indication of the additional requirements (Table 12.9, p. 680). Low requirements may be necessary in those with fluid overload (or patients with hypernatraemia and hyperkalaemia. The requirements of calcium and magnesium are higher for enteral than for parenteral nutrition because only a proportion of these minerals is absorbed by the gut.
- *Trace elements.* For trace elements such as iodide, fluoride, and selenium that are well absorbed, the requirements for enteral and parenteral nutrition are similar. For other trace elements, such as iron, zinc, manganese and chromium, the requirements for parenteral nutrition are substantially lower than for enteral nutrition (Fig. 5.9).
- *Vitamins.* Many vitamins are given in greater quantities in patients receiving parenteral nutrition

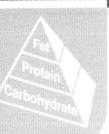

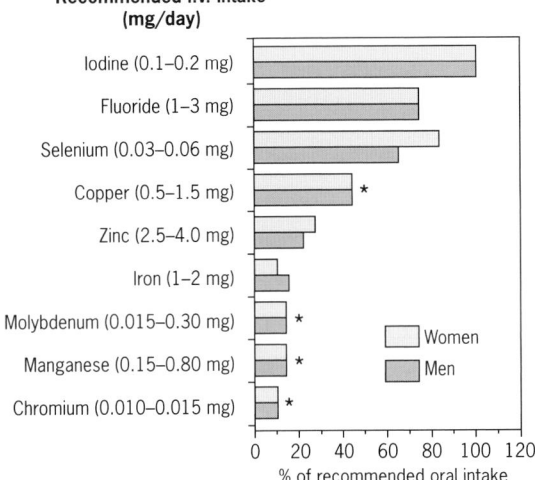

Fig. 5.9 **Recommended intravenous intake of trace elements in absolute values and as a percentage of recommended oral intake.** Trace elements marked with an asterisk are those for which there was too little information to establish recommended value for dietary oral intake: therefore the midpoint of estimated safe and adequate oral intake is used for comparison.

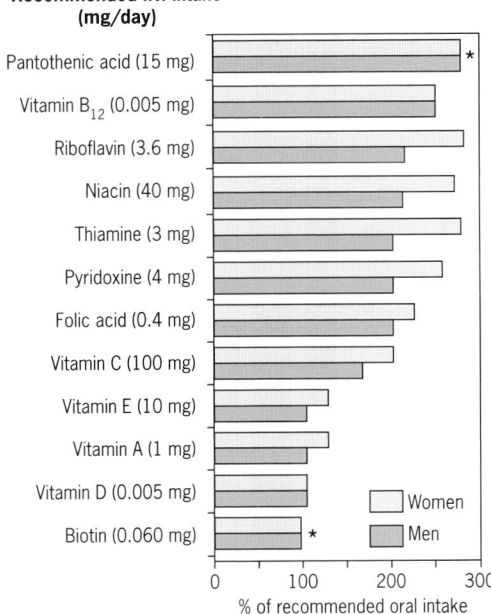

Fig. 5.10 **Recommended intravenous intake of vitamins** in absolute values and as a percentage of recommended oral intake. Vitamins marked with an asterisk are those for which there was too little information to establish recommended dietary oral intake: therefore the midpoint of estimated safe and adequate oral intake is used for comparison.

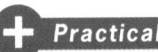

Practical box 5.1

Enteral feeding

Procedure
- Insert fine-bore tube intranasally with wire stylet.
- Confirm position of tube in stomach by aspiration of gastric contents and auscultation of the epigastrium.
- Check by X-ray if aspiration or auscultation is unsuccessful.

Problems
No satisfactory way of keeping nasogastric tubes in place (up to 60% come out).

Main complications
- Regurgitation and aspiration into bronchus.
- Blockage of the nasogastric tube.
- Gastrointestinal side-effects, the most common being diarrhoea.
- Metabolic complications including hyperglycaemia and hypokalaemia, as well as low levels of magnesium, calcium and phosphate, occur.

severe disease, partly because they may already have depleted pools of vitamins, and partly because some vitamins degrade during storage. Vitamin K is usually absent from parenteral nutrition regimens and therefore it may need to be administered separately.

Enteral nutrition (EN) (Practical box 5.1)
Feeds can be given by various routes:

- By mouth.
- By fine-bore nasogastric tube.
- Percutaneous endoscopic gastrostomy (PEG) is useful for patients who need enteral nutrition for a prolonged period (e.g. more than 30 days), such as those with swallowing problems following a head injury or in elderly people after a stroke. A catheter is placed percutaneously into the stomach under endoscopic control.
- With needle catheter jejunostomy, a fine catheter is inserted into the jejunum at laparotomy and brought out through the abdominal wall.

Diet formulation (see Table 5.15)
A polymeric diet with whole-protein and fat can be used, except in patients with severely impaired gastro-intestinal function who may require a predigested (i.e. elemental) diet. In these patients, the nitrogen source is purified low-molecular-weight peptides or amino acid mixtures, with sometimes the fat being given partly as medium-chain triglycerides.

Management
Daily amounts of diet vary between 2 and 2.5 L and the full amount can be started immediately.

than in those receiving enteral nutrition (Fig. 5.10). This is because patients on parenteral nutrition may have increased requirements, partly because of

Table 5.15
Standard enteric diet, providing 8.4 MJ per day (≈2000 kcal)

Energy
Carbohydrate as glucose polymers (49–53% of total energy)
Fat as triglycerides (30–35% of total energy)

Nitrogen
Whole protein (6–7 g of nitrogen/L)
Additional electrolytes, vitamins and trace elements

Features
Ratio of energy to nitrogen kJ:g = 620:1 (kcal:g = 150:1)
Osmolality = 285–300 mOsmol/kg

Hypercatabolic patients require a high supply of nitrogen (15 g daily) and often will not achieve positive nitrogen balance until the primary injury is resolved.

The success of enteral feeding depends on careful supervision of the patient with monitoring of weight, biochemistry and diet charts.

Total parenteral nutrition (TPN)
Peripheral parenteral nutrition
Specially formulated mixtures for peripheral use are available, with a low osmolality and containing lipid emulsions. Heparin and corticosteroids can be added to the infusion and local application of glyceryl trinitrate patches reduces the occurrence of thrombophlebitis and prolongs catheter life. Peripheral parenteral nutrition is often preferred initially (each catheter will last for about 5 days), allowing time to consider the necessity for having to insert a central venous catheter.

Parenteral nutrition via a central venous catheter
(see Practical box 5.2)
A silicone catheter is placed into a central vein, usually using the infraclavicular approach to the subclavian vein. The skin-entry site should be dressed carefully and not disturbed unless there is a suggestion of catheter-related sepsis.

Complications of catheter placement include central vein thrombosis, pneumothorax and embolism, but the major problem is catheter-related sepsis. Organisms, mainly staphylococci, enter along the side of the catheter, leading to septicaemia. Sepsis can be prevented by careful and sterile placement of the catheter, by not removing the dressing over the catheter entry site, and by not giving other substances (e.g. blood products, antibiotics) via the central vein catheter.

Sepsis should be suspected if the patient develops fever and leucocytosis. In two-thirds of cases, organisms can be grown from the catheter tip. Treatment involves removal of the catheter and appropriate systemic antibiotics.

Nutrients
With TPN it is possible to provide sufficient nitrogen for protein synthesis and calories to meet energy

Practical box 5.2

Central catheter placement for parenteral nutrition

This should be performed only by experienced clinicians under aseptic conditions in an operating theatre.

- The patient is placed supine with 5° of head-down tilt to avoid air embolism.
- The skin below the midpoint of the left clavicle is infiltrated with 1–2% lignocaine and a 1 cm skin incision is made.
- A 20-gauge needle on a syringe is inserted beneath the clavicle and first rib and angled towards the tip of a finger held in the suprasternal notch.
- When blood is aspirated freely, the needle is used as a guide to insert the cannula through the skin incision and into the subclavian vein.
- The catheter is advanced so that its tip lies in the distal part of the superior vena cava.
- A skin tunnel is created under local anaesthetic using an introducer inserted through a point about 10 cm below and medial to the incision and passed upwards to the incision.
- The proximal end of the catheter (with hub removed) is passed backwards through the introducer to emerge 10 cm below the clavicle, where it is sutured to the chest wall.
- The original infraclavicular entry incision is now sutured.

requirements. Electrolytes, vitamins and trace elements are also necessary. All of these substances are infused simultaneously.

Nitrogen source
Most patients receive at least 11–15 g N per day, in the form of synthetic L-amino acids.

Energy source
This is provided by glucose, with additional calories provided by a fat emulsion. Fat infusions provide a greater number of calories in a smaller volume than can be provided by carbohydrate. Fat infusions are not hypertonic and they also prevent essential fatty acid deficiency.

Essential fatty acid deficiency has been reported in long-term parenteral nutritional regimens without fat emulsions. It causes a scaly skin, hair loss and a delay in healing.

The calorie-to-nitrogen ratio (kcal:g N) is typically 150:1.

Electrolytes and trace elements (see Figs 5.9 and 5.10)
Initially, the electrolyte status should be monitored on a daily basis and electrolyte solutions given as appropriate. Water-soluble vitamins can be given daily but fat-soluble vitamins should be given weekly, as overdose can occur. A trace-metal solution is available for patients on long-term parenteral nutrition, but if the patient requires blood transfusions trace-metal supplements are not needed.

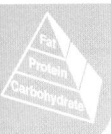

Nutrition

Administration and monitoring

Peripheral parenteral nutrition is administered via 3 L bags over 24 hours, with the constituents being premixed under sterile conditions by the pharmacy. Table 5.16 shows the composition which provides 9 g of nitrogen and 1750 calories in 24 hours.

For a central venous TPN regimen, most hospitals now use premixed 3 L bags. A standard parenteral nutrition regimen which provides 14 g of nitrogen and 2250 calories over 24 hours is given in Table 5.16.

Essential monitoring includes daily plasma electrolytes and weekly assessments of nutritional status (weight and skinfold thickness if appropriate callipers are available). Nitrogen balance could also be assessed but complete collections of urine are necessary.

Complications

- Catheter-related (see above)
- Metabolic (e.g. hyperglycaemia – insulin therapy is usually necessary)
- Fluid and electrolyte disturbances
- Hypercalcaemia
- Liver dysfunction.

Nutritional support in the home patient

In both high- and low-income countries there is considerably more undernutrition in the community than in hospital. However, the principles are very similar: detection of malnutrition and the underlying risk factors; treatment of underlying disease processes and disabilities; correction of specific nutrient deficiencies and provision of appropriate nutritional support. This typically begins with dietary advice, and may involve the provision of 'meals on wheels' by social services. A systematic review of the use of nutritional supplements in the community came to the following conclusions:

- Supplements are generally of more value in patients with a BMI < 20 kg/m² and children with growth failure (weight for height < 85% of ideal) than in those with better anthropometric indices. They are likely to be of little or no value in patients with little weight loss and a BMI > 20 kg/m². The supplemental energy intake in such subjects largely replaces oral food intake.
- Supplements may be of value in weight-losing patients (e.g. > 10% weight loss compared to pre-illness) with a BMI > 20 kg/m², and in children with deteriorating growth performance without chronic protein–energy undernutrition.
- The functional benefits varied according to the patient group. In patients with chronic obstructive airways disease the functional benefits were increased respiratory muscle strength, increase in

Table 5.16
Examples of total parenteral nutrition regimens

Central: all mixed in 3 L bags and infused over 24 hours

Nitrogen	L-Amino acids 14 g/L	1 L
Energy	Glucose 50%	0.5 L
	Glucose 20%	0.5 L
	plus	
	Lipid 10%	0.5 L
	as either Intralipid	Fractionated soya oil 100 g/L
	or Lipofundin	Soya oil 50 g, medium-chain triglycerides 50 g/L

+ Electrolytes, water-soluble vitamins, fat-soluble vitamins, trace elements, heparin and insulin may be added if required. Nitrogen 14 g non-protein calories 9305 kJ (2250 kcal)

Peripheral: all mixed in 3 L bags and infused over 24 hours

Nitrogen	L-Amino acids 9 g/L	1 L
Energy	Glucose 20%	1 L
	Lipid 20%	0.5 L

+ Trace elements, electrolytes, and water-soluble and fat-soluble vitamins. Heparin 1000 UL and hydrocortisone 100 mg insulin is added if required. Nitrogen 9 g non-protein calories 7206 kJ (1700 kcal)

handgrip strength, and an increase in walking distance/duration of exercise. In the elderly the benefits were reduced number of falls, or increase in activities of daily living, and reduced pressure sore surface area. In patients with HIV/AIDS there were changes in immunological function and improved cognition. Patients with liver disease experienced a lower incidence of severe infections and had a lower frequency of hospitalization.

- Acceptability and compliance are likely to be better when a choice of supplements (of type, flavour, consistency) and schedule are decided in conjunction with the patient and/or carer. Changes in these may be necessary when there is a change in patterns of daily activities, disease status, and 'taste fatigue' with prolonged use of the same supplement.
- Nutritional counselling and monitoring is recommended before and after the start of supplements (see also below).

Some patients receive enteral tube feeding and parenteral nutrition at home. At any one point in time in developed countries enteral tube feeding occurs more frequently at home than in hospital. In adults the commonest reason for starting home tube feeding is for swallowing difficulties. This involves patients with neurological disorder, such as motor neurone disease, multiple sclerosis and Parkinson's disease, but the commonest single diagnosis is cerebrovascular disease.

Table 5.17
Outcome of patients at 1 year after starting home enteral tube feeding (HETF)*

	All patients (n = 15 143) %	Cerebrovascular disease (n = 5660) %	Motor neurone disease (n = 874) %	Multiple sclerosis (n = 856) %
Continuing on HETF	50.2	53.0	35.8	81.0
Returned to oral feeding	14.2	12.9	1.1	3.7
Died	33.5	32.6	62.1	13.7
Other†	2.2	1.5	1.0	1.6

* Based on the British Artificial Nutrition Survey (1996–2000). Patients who returned to oral feeding or refused/withdrew from HETF may have died subsequently
† Withdrew or refused HETF, or in hospital

In 1998 it was estimated that almost 2% of patients who had a stroke in the UK received home enteral tube feeding (HETF). The outcome of this is indicated in Table 5.17. Fifteen per cent of patients were able to resume full oral nutrition after a year. It is therefore necessary to intermittently assess the swallowing capabilities of patients in order to avoid unnecessary tube feeding. The patients and/or carers should have adequate training, contacts with appropriate health professions, and a reliable delivery service for feeds and ancillary equipment. They should also be clear about how to manage simple problems associated with the feeding tube, which is usually a gastrostomy tube rather than a nasogastric tube.

Home parenteral nutrition is practised much less frequently, usually under the supervision of specialist centres. The potential value of intestinal transplantation in patients with long-term intestinal failure is still being assessed.

FURTHER READING

Payne-James JJ, Grimble G, Silk D (2000) *Artificial nutrition support in clinical practice*, 2nd edn. Greenwich Medical Media Ltd.

Sauba WW (1997) Nutritional support. *New England Journal of Medicine* **336**: 41–48.

Strutton R, Elia M (1999) A critical systematic analysis of the use of nutritional supplement in the community. *Clinical Nutrition* **18** (suppl 2): 29–84.

Food allergy and food intolerance

Many people ascribe their various symptoms to food allergy or food sensitivity, and there are a number of clinics in the UK where such sufferers are seen and started on exclusion diets. The scientific evidence that food does harm in most instances is incomplete, but certainly some evidence supports the following disease 'entities':

- *Acute hypersensitivity*. Some patients develop acute reactions to a particular food; an example is urticaria, vomiting or diarrhoea after eating nuts, strawberries or shellfish. These reactions are presumably immunological hypersensitivity reactions mediated by IgE. This is usually not a clinical problem as the patients have already learned to avoid the suspected food.
- *Eczema and asthma*. Particularly in young children, these have sometimes been treated successfully by removal of eggs from the diet, suggesting some form of food allergy.
- *Rhinitis and asthma*. These have been produced by foods such as milk and chocolate, mainly in atopic subjects, again suggesting a food allergy.
- *Chronic urticaria*. This has been treated successfully by an exclusion diet.
- *Migraine*. In some subjects this seems to follow the intake of foods such as chocolate, cheese and alcohol, suggesting a trigger mechanism, although probably not a true allergic phenomenon.
- *Irritable bowel syndrome*. In some patients this seems to be related to ingestion of certain food items, such as wheat, but the mechanisms are not clearly defined.

In addition, some people suffer a reaction due to:

- a constituent of food (e.g. the histamine in mackerel or canned food, or the tyramine in cheeses)
- chemical mediators released by food (e.g. histamine may be released by tomatoes or strawberries)
- toxic chemicals found in food (e.g. the food additive tartrazine)
- an enzyme deficiency (e.g. milk-induced diarrhoea in alactasia or fava-bean-induced haemolytic anaemia in glucose-6-phosphate dehydrogenase deficiency).

Many other additives and compounds with certain E numbers have been implicated as causing reactions, but here the evidence is less than complete.

There is little or no evidence to suggest that diseases such as arthritis, behaviour and affective disorders and Crohn's disease are due to ingestion of a particular food.

Multiple vague symptoms such as tiredness or malaise are also not due to food allergy. Most of the patients in this group are suffering from a psychiatric disorder.

Management

- **A careful history** may help to delineate the causative agent, particularly when the effects are immediate.
- **Skin-prick testing** with allergen and measurement in the serum of antigen or antibodies have not correlated with symptoms and are usually misleading. 'Fringe' techniques such as hair analysis, although widely advertised, are of limited value.
- **Diagnostic exclusion diets** are sometimes used, but they are time-consuming. They can occasionally be of value in identifying a particular food causing problems.
- **Dietary challenge** consists of the food and the test being given sublingually or by inhalation in an attempt to reproduce the symptoms. Again this may be helpful in a few cases.

Most people who have acute reactions to food realize it and stop the food, and do not require medical attention. In the remainder of patients, a small minority seem to be helped by modifying their diet, but there is no good scientific evidence to support these exclusion diets.

FURTHER READING

Guidelines for the Evaluation of Food Allergy (2001) *Gastroenterology* **120**: 1023–1025.

Review on the Evaluation of Food Allergy in GI Disorder, Official Recommendation of American Gastroenterology Association (2001) *Gastroenterology* **120**: 1026–1040.

Sampson HA (1997) Food allergies. In: *Sleisenger and Fordtran's Gastrointestinal and Liver Disease*. Philadelphia: WB Saunders.

Alcohol

Alcohol is a popular 'nutrient' consumed in large quantities all over the world. In many countries, alcohol consumption is becoming a major problem (see p. 1256).

Ethanol (ethyl alcohol) is oxidized, in the steps shown in Box 5.5, to acetaldehyde. Acetaldehyde is then converted to acetate, mainly in the liver mitochondria. Acetate is released into the blood and oxidized by peripheral tissues to carbon dioxide, fatty acids and water.

Alcohol dehydrogenases are found in many tissues and it has been suggested that enzymes present in the

---

> **Box 5.5**
>
> **The main pathways of ethanol oxidization**
>
> - Alcohol dehydrogenase:
>
> $$CH_3CH_2OH + NAD^+ \xrightarrow{ADH} CH_3CHO + NADH + H^+$$
> (ethanol) (acetaldehyde)
>
> - The liver microsomal enzyme oxidizing system (MEOS) including the specific p450 enzyme, p450 11E1, which is induced by ethanol;
>
> $$CH_3CH_2OH + NADPH + H^+ + O_2$$
> $$\xrightarrow{MEOS} CH_3CHO + NADP + 2H_2O$$

gastric mucosa may contribute substantially to ethanol metabolism.

Ethanol itself produces 29.3 kJ/g (7 kcal/g), but many alcoholic drinks also contain sugar, which increases their calorific value. For example, one pint of beer provides 1045 kJ (250 kcal), so the heavy drinker will be unable to lose weight if he or she continues to drink.

Effects of excess alcohol consumption

Excess consumption of alcohol leads to two major problems, both of which can be present in the same patient:

- alcohol dependence syndrome (p. 1256)
- physical damage to various tissues.

Each unit of alcohol (defined as one half pint of normal beer, one single spirit, or one small glass of wine) contains 8 g of ethanol (Fig. 5.11). All the long-term effects of excess alcohol consumption are due to excess ethanol, irrespective of the type of alcoholic beverage; i.e. beer and spirits are no different in their long-term effects. Short-term effects, such as hangovers, depend on additional substances, particularly other alcohols such as isoamyl alcohol, which are known as congeners. Brandy and bourbon contain the highest percentage of congeners.

The amount of alcohol that produces damage varies and not everyone who drinks heavily will suffer physical damage. For example, only 20% of people who drink heavily develop cirrhosis of the liver. The effect of alcohol on different organs of the body is not the same; in some patients the liver is affected, in others the brain or muscle. The differences may be genetically determined.

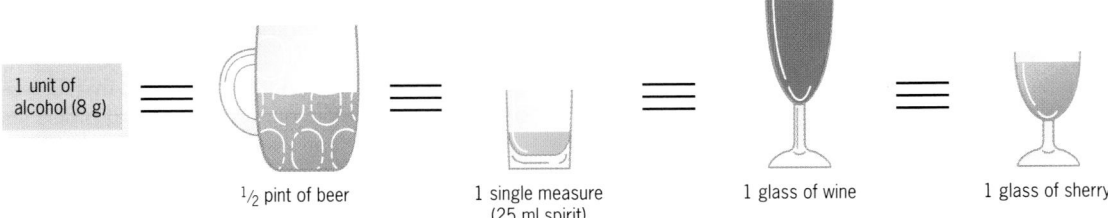

1 unit of alcohol (8 g) = ½ pint of beer = 1 single measure (25 ml spirit) = 1 glass of wine = 1 glass of sherry

Fig. 5.11 Measures of 1 unit of alcohol.

Guide to sensible drinking of alcohol

Daily maximum

3 units for men

2 units for women

To help achieve this

Use a standard measure.

Do not drink during the daytime.

Have alcohol-free days each week.

Remember

Health can be damaged without being 'drunk'.

Regular heavy intake is more harmful than occasional binges.

Do not drink to 'drown your problems'.

In the UK the drink-before-driving limit of alcohol in the blood is 800 mg/L (80 mg%).

One unit of alcohol is eliminated per hour, therefore spread drinking time.

Food decreases absorption and therefore results in a lower blood alcohol level.

4–5 units are sufficient to put the blood alcohol level over the legal driving limit in a 70 kg man (less in a lighter person).

Table 5.18
Physical effects of excess alcohol consumption

Central nervous system
Epilepsy
Wernicke–Korsakoff syndrome
Polyneuropathy

Muscles
Acute or chronic myopathy

Cardiovascular system
Cardiomyopathy
Beriberi heart disease
Cardiac arrhythmias
Hypertension

Metabolism
Hyperuricaemia (gout)
Hyperlipidaemia
Hypoglycaemia
Obesity

Endocrine system
Pseudo-Cushing's syndrome

Respiratory system
Chest infections

Gastrointestinal system
Acute gastritis
Carcinoma of the oesophagus or large bowel
Pancreatic disease
Liver disease

Haemopoiesis
Macrocytosis (due to direct toxic effect on bone marrow or folate deficiency)
Thrombocytopenia
Leucopenia

Bone
Osteoporosis
Osteomalacia

Thiamin deficiency contributes to both neurological (confusion, Wernicke–Korsakoff syndrome; see p. 1216) and some of the non-neurological manifestations (cardiomyopathy). Susceptibility to damage of different organs is variable and the figures in Box 5.6 are given only as a guide. Heavy persistent drinkers for many years are at greater risk than heavy sporadic drinkers.

Liver disease

In general the effects of a given intake of alcohol seem to be worse in women. The following figures are for men and should be reduced by 50% for women:

- 160 g ethanol per day (20 single drinks) carries a high risk
- 80 g ethanol per day (10 single drinks) carries a medium risk
- 40 g ethanol per day (five single drinks) carries little risk.

Alcohol consumption in pregnancy

Women are advised not to drink alcohol at all during pregnancy because even small amounts of alcohol consumed can lead to 'small babies'. The *fetal alcohol syndrome* is characterized by mental retardation, dysmorphic features and growth impairment; it occurs in fetuses of alcohol-dependent women.

Summary

A summary of the physical effects of alcohol is given in Table 5.18. Details of these diseases are discussed in the relevant chapters. The effects of alcohol withdrawal are discussed on page 1257.

FURTHER READING

Lieber CS (1995) Medical disorders of alcoholism. *New England Journal of Medicine* **333**: 1058–1063.

CHAPTER BIBLIOGRAPHY

Elia M (1995) Changing concepts of nutrient requirements in disease: implications for artificial nutritional support. *Lancet* **345**: 1279–1284.

Elia M, Stubbs RE, Henry CJK (1999) Differences in fat carbohydrate, and protein metabolism between lean and obese subjects undergoing total starvation. *Obesity Research* **7**: 597–604.

Green C (1999) Existence, causes and consequences of disease-related malnutrition in the hospital and community, and clinical and financial benefits of nutritional intervention. *Clinical Nutrition* **18** (Suppl 2): 3–28.

Lennard-Jones JE (1999) Ethical and legal aspects of clinical hydration and nutritional support. A report for the British Association for Parenteral and Enteral Nutrition (BAPEN). London: BAPEN.

Mohan IV, Stanby G (1999) Nutritional homocysteinaemia. *British Medical Journal* **318**: 1569–1571.

Nutrition Reviews (1997) Comparative nutrition policies in Europe: an international expert conference for the World Health Organization. *Nutrition Reviews* **55** (11 part II): S1–S75.

Stratton RJ, Elia M (1999) A critical systematic analysis of the use of oral nutritional supplements in the community. *Clinical Nutrition* **18** (Suppl 2): 29–84.

Gastrointestinal disease 6

In developed countries gastrointestinal problems are a common reason for attendance at the primary care clinic as well as the outpatient clinic of the hospital. The ever-increasing problem is that many of these consultations (approximately 75%) are for symptoms related to non-organic disease. The clinician's main task is to separate out the patients who require investigation, remembering that 20% of all cancers occur in the gastrointestinal tract (Fig. 6.1).

In developing countries, poor hygiene and malnutrition allow the spread of infective organisms. The clinician's main role here is to treat infections promptly and to help with prevention by encouraging improved sanitation and education.

In this chapter, the essential anatomy and principles of physiology are divided and discussed under the relevant sections.

Clinical approach to gastrointestinal symptoms and signs

Dyspepsia and indigestion

Dyspepsia is the term used by healthcare workers to describe upper abdominal symptoms, e.g. nausea, heartburn, acidity, pain or discomfort, wind, fullness or belching. Patients seldom use the term 'dyspepsia'; they are more likely to refer to indigestion to describe any symptom that is food related. Indigestion is common; 80% of the population will have had indigestion at some time.

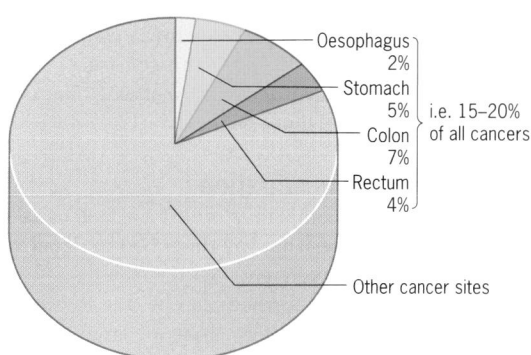

Fig. **6.1** Incidence (approximate) of cancers at various sites of the gastrointestinal tract.

There are no precise definitions and a careful history should be taken, particularly to elicit any 'alarm' features:

- dysphagia
- weight loss
- anorexia
- haematemesis or melaena.

Nausea and vomiting

There are three phases:

- nausea – a feeling of wanting to vomit, often associated with autonomic effects including hypersalivation, pallor and sweating
- retching – a strong involuntary effort to vomit
- vomiting – the expulsion of gastric contents through the mouth.

The vomiting centres are located in the lateral reticular formation of the medulla and are stimulated by the chemoreceptor trigger zones (CTZs) in the floor of the fourth ventricle, and also by vagal afferents from the gut. These zones are directly stimulated by drugs, motion sickness and metabolic causes.

Many gastrointestinal conditions are associated with vomiting (Table 6.1), but nausea and vomiting without pain are frequently non-gastrointestinal in origin.

Haematemesis is vomiting blood or 'coffee-grounds' from the stomach.

Large volumes of vomit suggest intestinal obstruction; *faeculent vomit* suggests low intestinal obstruction or the presence of a gastrocolic fistula, while *projectile vomiting* is due to gastric-outflow obstruction.

Chronic nausea and vomiting with no other abdominal symptoms is usually due to a psychological cause (p. 326).

Early-morning vomiting is seen in pregnancy, alcohol dependence and some metabolic disorders (e.g. uraemia).

Flatulence

This is the term used to describe excessive wind. It includes belching, abdominal distension, 'wind' or the passage of flatus per rectum. Swallowing air (aerophagia) is described on p. 326. Some of the swallowed air is passed into the intestine where most of it is absorbed. Intestinal bacterial breakdown of food also produces a small amount of gas. Flatus consists of nitrogen, carbon dioxide, hydrogen and methane. Flatus is normally passed 13–20 times per day.

Diarrhoea and constipation

These are common complaints which are not usually due to serious disease. They are described in detail on pages 320 and 309 respectively.

A single episode of diarrhoea can be due to dietary indiscretion or anxiety. Watery stools of large volume are always due to organic disease. Bloody diarrhoea usually implies colonic disease.

Table 6.1
Causes of vomiting

Any gastrointestinal disease*	Drugs, e.g.
Acute infections, e.g.	digoxin toxicity
influenza	opiates
pertussis	chemotherapy
Central nervous disease, e.g.	immunotherapy
raised intracranial pressure	Reflex, e.g.
meningitis	severe pain: myocardial
vestibular disturbances	infarction
migraine	Psychogenic
Metabolic causes, e.g.	Pregnancy
uraemia	Alcohol excess
diabetes: ketoacidosis or	
gastroparesis	
hypercalcaemia	

Acute diarrhoea lasting 2–5 days is often due to an infective cause and stool cultures are necessary.

Patients often consider themselves constipated if their bowels are not open on most days. The difficult passage of hard stool is also regarded as constipation, irrespective of stool frequency.

Abdominal pain

Pain is stimulated mainly by the stretching of smooth muscle or organ capsules. Severe acute abdominal pain can be due to a large number of gastrointestinal conditions, and normally presents as an emergency (p. 328). An 'acute abdomen' can occasionally be due to referred pain from the chest, as in pneumonia, or to metabolic causes, such as diabetic ketoacidosis.

In patients with abdominal pain the following should be ascertained:

- the site, intensity, character, duration and frequency of the pain
- the aggravating and relieving factors
- associated symptoms, including non-gastrointestinal symptoms.

Upper abdominal pain

Epigastric pain is very common; it is often a dull ache, but sometimes sharp and severe. Its relationship to food intake should be ascertained. It is a common feature of peptic ulcer disease, but also occurs in functional dyspepsia.

Right hypochondrial pain is usually from the gall bladder or biliary tract. Hepatic congestion (e.g. in hepatitis) and sometimes peptic ulcer can present with pain in the right hypochondrium. Chronic, often persistent, pain in the right hypochondrium is a frequent symptom in healthy females suffering from functional bowel disorders. This chronic pain is not due to gall bladder disease (p. 393).

Lower abdominal pain

Acute pain in the left iliac fossa is usually colonic in origin (e.g. acute diverticulitis). *Chronic pain* is most commonly associated with functional bowel disorders. In females, lower abdominal pain occurs in a number of gynaecological disorders and the differentiation from GI disease is often difficult.

Persistent pain in the right iliac fossa over a long period is not due to chronic appendicitis.

Proctalgia is a severe pain deep in the rectum that comes on suddenly but lasts only for a short time. It is not due to organic disease.

Abdominal wall pain

Recurrent localized abdominal pain with local tenderness can very rarely arise from the abdominal wall itself. Causes are thought to include nerve entrapment, external hernias and entrapment of internal viscera (commonly omentum) within traumatic ruptures of abdominal wall musculature.

Weight loss

This is due to anorexia (loss of appetite) and is a frequent accompaniment of all gastrointestinal disease. Anorexia is also common in systemic disease and may be seen in psychiatric disorders, particularly anorexia nervosa. Anorexia often accompanies carcinoma but it is a late symptom and not of diagnostic help. Weight loss with a normal or increased dietary intake occurs with hyperthyroidism. Malabsorption is never so severe as to cause weight loss without anorexia. Weight loss should be assessed objectively as patients often 'think' they have lost weight. Appetite is described on page 241.

Clinical examination

A general examination is performed, with particular emphasis on the examination of all lymph nodes and noting the presence of anaemia or jaundice. Detailed examination of the gastrointestinal tract starts with the mouth and tongue, before examining the abdomen.

Examination of the abdomen

Inspection

Abdominal distension, whether due to flatus, fat, fetus, fluid or faeces, must be looked for. Lordosis may give the appearance of a distended abdomen; it is a common feature of the 'abdominal distension' seen in functional bowel disorder.

Palpation

The abdominal organs may be felt in some normal subjects (Fig. 6.2) but this is not common and such organs are usually only just palpable. A Reidel's lobe is

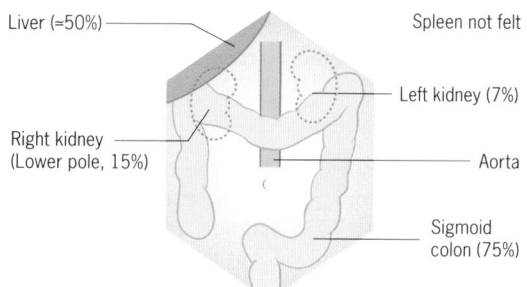

Fig. 6.2 The organs sometimes palpable in thin subjects.

an extension of the lateral portion of the right lobe of the liver and can occasionally be palpated. Figure 6.3 shows a normal CT scan at the T12 level.

Any palpable mass is carefully felt to decide which organ is involved and also to evaluate its size, shape and consistency and whether it moves with respiration.

The hernial orifices should be examined if intestinal obstruction is suspected.

A succussion splash suggests gastric outlet obstruction if the patient has not drunk for 2–3 hours; the splash of fluid in the stomach can be heard with a stethoscope laid on the abdomen when the patient is moved.

Percussion

This is performed in the usual way to detect the area of dullness caused by the liver and spleen, and possibly bladder enlargement. The presence of fluid in the peritoneal cavity (i.e. ascites) is detected by shifting dullness. The percussion note changes from resonance to dullness when the patient is moved from one side to the other. It is a good physical sign if performed carefully, but 1–2 L of fluid must be present to elicit it. A fluid

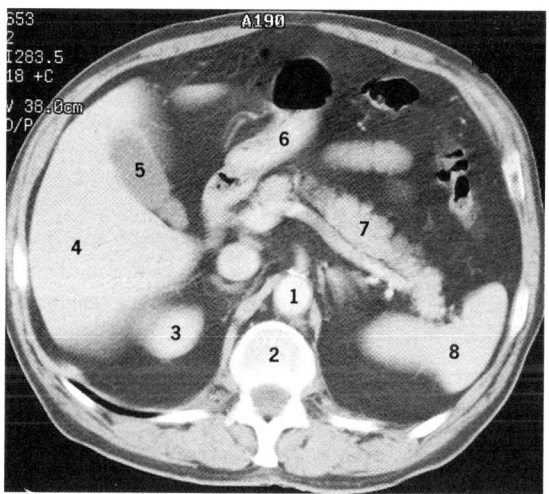

Fig. 6.3 CT scan of the normal abdomen at the level of T12.
1, aorta; 2, spine; 3, top of right kidney; 4, liver; 5, gall bladder; 6, stomach (containing air); 7, pancreas; 8, spleen.

'thrill' can be elicited, but is not always helpful. A large ovarian cyst can sometimes produce an enlarged abdomen, but the dullness is more centrally placed than in ascites.

Auscultation

Auscultation is not of great value in gastrointestinal disease, apart from in the evaluation of the acute abdomen (see p. 328). Abdominal bruits are often present in normal subjects, but these are not clinically significant. Intestinal sounds do not help in diagnosis.

Examination of the rectum and sigmoid colon

Digital examination of the rectum should be performed in all patients with a change in bowel habit and rectal bleeding.

Rigid sigmoidoscopy (Practical box 6.1) should, in hospital, be part of the routine examination in all cases of diarrhoea and in patients with lower abdominal symptoms such as a change in bowel habit or rectal bleeding.

Proctoscopy (Practical box 6.1) is performed in all patients with a history of bright red blood per rectum; the narrow sigmoidoscope does not distend the lumen and haemorrhoids can be missed.

Flexible sigmoidoscopy

The rigid sigmoidoscope allows inspection of only the lower 20–25 cm of the bowel. A 60 cm flexible sigmoidoscope can be readily used in the outpatient department after minimal bowel preparation (a disposable enema). Specialist nurse practitioners use this technique in many outpatient clinics. Seventy per cent of colonic neoplasms occur within the range of the flexible sigmoidoscope. It is used to biopsy lesions in the sigmoid area seen on barium enema and for the follow-up of patients with distal colitis. It is useful as an initial test for patients with left-sided colonic symptoms and rectal bleeding but a full colonoscopy will be needed if no pathology is found.

Stool examination

This can be useful occasionally to confirm the patient's symptoms (e.g. passing of blood or steatorrhoea). The shape and size may be helpful (e.g. rabbity stools in the irritable bowel syndrome). Stool charts for recording volume and frequency of defecation are useful in inpatients to follow the progress of diarrhoea.

Investigations

Radiology and endoscopy are the principal investigations. These are usually preceded by routine haematology and biochemistry. The investigation of small

 Practical box 6.1

Sigmoidoscopy and proctoscopy

Sigmoidoscopy
- The technique using a 25 cm rigid sigmoidoscope is easy to learn, provides valuable information and is safe in competent hands.
- No bowel preparation is required.
- The technique is relatively painless. In the irritable bowel syndrome, the patient's pain is often reproduced by air insufflation.

1 Rectal examination is initially performed.
2 The sigmoidoscope is passed into the anus, pointing towards the symphysis pubis. The obturator is removed, and the instrument passed under direct vision to the rectosigmoid junction and beyond if possible (using air insufflation).
3 The mucosa of the anus and rectum is inspected. The normal mucosa is shiny with superficial vessels and no contact bleeding.
4 Biopsies can be taken of any lesions that are seen or from apparently normal-looking mucosa which occasionally shows histological evidence of inflammation.

Proctoscopy
1 The proctoscope is passed into the anus directed towards the symphysis pubis and the obturator is removed.
2 The patient strains down as the proctoscope is removed.
3 Haemorrhoids are seen as purplish veins in the left lateral, right posterior or right anterior positions.
4 Fissures may also be seen, but pain often prevents the procedure from being performed.

bowel disease is discussed in more detail on page 289. Manometry is mainly used in oesophageal disease (p. 263) and rectal disorders (p. 312).

Barium contrast studies (Box 6.1)

These are performed after an overnight fast. The radiologist should be given correct clinical information and directed to the particular area under suspicion. X-rays should be reviewed with the radiologist, if possible.

- **Barium swallow.** The oesophagus is visualized as barium is swallowed in the upright and prone positions. Motility abnormalities as well as anatomical lesions can then be observed. Reflux of barium from the stomach into the oesophagus is demonstrated with the patient tipped head down. The severity of this reflux can be gauged by administering an effervescent tablet and asking the patient to drink water (water siphon test). Swallowing bread with the barium (to add bulk) is sometimes useful in a case of dysphagia.
- **Double-contrast barium meal.** This is performed to examine the stomach and duodenum. A small amount of barium is given together with effervescent granules or tablets to produce carbon

The use of barium contrast studies

Barium contrast study	Main use	Comments
Barium swallow	Dysphagia	Particularly useful in motility disorders
Barium meal	Epigastric pain Vomiting	Gastroscopy is replacing barium meal as biopsy and histology is possible for *Helicobacter pylori* and carcinoma
Small bowel follow-through	Diarrhoea Abdominal pain	Only practical way of studying gross small bowel anatomy
Barium enema	Altered bowel habit Abdominal pain	Colonoscopy has largely replaced this examination for rectal bleeding, inflammatory bowel disease and polyp follow-up

dioxide so that a double contrast between air and barium is obtained. This technique has a high accuracy rate when performed carefully but many prefer gastroscopy to examine the stomach.

- **Small bowel follow-through.** This is used to examine the small bowel and ideally should be performed separately from a barium meal as a different technique is employed. Barium is swallowed and allowed to pass into the small intestine through the jejunum and into the ileum. This technique is the only way of demonstrating the gross anatomy of the small intestine. Specific views of the terminal ileum are routinely obtained using compression to separate the loops.
- **Small bowel enema** (enteroclysis). A tube is passed through the duodenum and a large volume of dilute barium is introduced. In some centres this is the examination of choice for the assessment of small bowel disease. It is particularly useful where there is suspicion of obstruction, to evaluate the strictures.
- **Barium enema.** Patients are given a low-fibre diet for 3 days and the colon thoroughly cleansed with oral laxative preparations. Barium and air are insufflated via a rectal catheter and double-contrast views obtained of the entire colon. Rectal examination and sigmoidoscopy should precede this examination. Many patients find the procedure rather unpleasant and it can be difficult in the elderly and frail patient. An 'instant' barium enema involving no bowel preparation is used in colitis (p. 306).

Plain X-rays

Plain X-rays of the chest and abdomen are chiefly used in the investigation of an acute abdomen (see p. 330) including patients presenting with acute colitis (p. 306). Areas of calcification can be seen in chronic pancreatitis (see p. 397). Faecal loading is seen in constipation.

Ultrasound, computed tomography (CT) and magnetic resonance imaging (MRI)

These techniques are used to define the intra-abdominal organs (e.g. liver, spleen, pancreas) but also to detect thickened bowel, masses, abscesses or fistulae. Ultrasound is often performed first as it is cheap and easy to perform although very operator dependent.

- **Ultrasound.** This requires no radiation and is best for fluid-filled lesions. Mesenteric glands and thickened bowel can be visualized, but mucosal detail is not seen. In the acute abdomen it can be used to diagnose acute cholecystitis, aortic aneurysms or appendicitis. It has a complementary role to CT and is useful for follow-up and for draining collections.
- **Endoscopic ultrasound (EUS).** A gastroscope incorporating an ultrasound probe at the tip is used to assess oesophageal and gastric wall thickening for detailed staging of oesophageal/gastric cancer. This is currently the most sensitive technique for the detection of small pancreatic tumours.
- **Endo-anal ultrasonography** involves the passage of a transducer into the rectum. It is used to define the anatomy of the anal sphincters (p. 314) to detect perianal disease and to stage rectal carcinomas.
- **Computed tomography.** CT, particularly helical (spiral) CT, gives excellent anatomical definition. It can detect thickened bowel wall and gives good visualization of the mesentery, the retroperitoneal structures and the aorta. It can detect a perforated viscus, subdiaphragmatic abscesses, extraluminal abscesses in appendicitis and diverticulitis. It can assess the extent of Crohn's disease and is of value in the diagnosis of the presence and cause of high-grade bowel obstruction. Contrast extravasated from the gut lumen can be detected, as can free air. It is being used widely in the management of the acute abdomen (p. 330) CT-guided fine-needle biopsies can be taken from tumours and lymph nodes. Cancer can be staged prior to surgery. Air insufflation into the colon prior to spiral CT (spiral pneumocolon/CT colography) provides an alternative to a barium enema for evaluation of colonic mass lesions. Unprepared CT is particularly useful in the elderly or immobile patient and has a reasonably good sensitivity in the detection of significant tumours.

- **Magnetic resonance imaging.** MRI has the advantage of using no ionizing radiation. It is particularly useful in the evaluation of abscesses and fistulae in the perianal region. There is likely to be an increasing role in the evaluation of luminal gut disease (MR enteroclysis). MRI is currently used more in hepatobiliary and pancreatic disease (see p. 343).

Radioisotope imaging

Radionuclides are used to a varying degree depending on local enthusiasm and expertise. Indications are:

- to demonstrate oesophageal reflux using [^{99m}Tc] technetium–sulphur colloid
- to determine the rate of gastric emptying using [^{99m}Tc] technetium–sulphur colloid
- to demonstrate a Meckel's diverticulum using [^{99m}Tc] pertechnetate, which has an affinity for gastric mucosa
- to show the extent of inflammation and the presence of any inflammatory collections in inflammatory bowel disease using ^{99m}Tc HMPAO (hexamethylpropylene amine oxime) labelled white cells.

Isotopes can also be used for assessing:

- gastrointestinal loss of red cells by giving ^{51}Cr red cells and measuring radioactivity in the faeces, or by labelling red cells with ^{99m}Tc and scanning the abdomen, e.g. Meckel's diverticulum
- albumin loss in the stools in protein-losing enteropathy by giving ^{51}CrCl$_3$ intravenously (p. 291)

- bile salt malabsorption by whole-body scanning and counting the activity in the faeces following oral ^{75}Se-homochoyl taurine (SeHCAT)
- bacterial overgrowth by measuring ^{14}CO$_2$ in the breath following ^{14}C glycocholic acid orally
- neuroendocrine tumours using radiolabelled octreotide and whole-body scanning
- B$_{12}$ malabsorption using ^{57}Co-B$_{12}$ (see p. 419).

Endoscopy (Practical box 6.2)

Video endoscopes have largely replaced the old fibre-optic types. They have three chips (for blue, green and red light) mounted at the tip of the instrument. These chips relay colour images via an image processor to a television monitor. A permanent record of the procedure can be obtained.

The tip of the endoscope can be angulated in all directions. Channels are present in the endoscope for air insufflation, water injection, suction and for the passage of biopsy forceps or brushes for obtaining tissue. These latter channels can also be used for other therapeutic interventions (e.g. injection of varices).

- **Oesophagogastroduodenoscopy (OGD).** This is often used as the investigation of choice for upper GI disorders by gastroenterologists because of easy access, the possibility of interventional therapy and obtaining mucosal biopsies. Relative contraindications include severe chronic obstructive pulmonary disease, a recent myocardial infarction, or instability of the atlanto-axial joints. The mortality for diagnostic endoscopy is 0.001% with significant complications in 1:1000.

Practical box 6.2

Gastroscopy and colonoscopy

- Explain to the patient the nature of the procedure (pamphlets are available).
- Get written consent.
- Tell the patient that i.v. sedation may be given.

Gastroscopy

1 The patient is fasted for at least 4 hours.
2 The throat is sprayed with lidocaine (lignocaine).
3 Intravenous sedation is given for the very anxious patient or for additional procedures.
4 Oxygen saturation is monitored.
5 Oxygen via nasal prongs is given to elderly patients.
6 The instrument is passed into the pharynx under direct vision, then down the oesophagus into the stomach and duodenum.
7 The patient must be 'nil by mouth' for approximately $1^1/_2$ hours following the procedure and may complain of a sore throat and abdominal discomfort.
8 Complications include local perforation and aspiration pneumonia.

Colonoscopy

1 *Two days before* the procedure, start a low-residue diet.
2 *One day before* the procedure
- Light lunch followed by clear fluids only.
- In the morning take one sachet of sodium picosulfate with one pint of water.
- In the afternoon take second sachet of sodium picosulfate with water.
- In the evening take senna tablets with one pint of water.
3 *Day of procedure* take clear fluids only.
4 *Procedure*
- Intravenous sedation with a benzodiazepine and pethidine is required.
- Oxygen saturation is monitored.
- The instrument is passed under direct vision and manoeuvred around to the caecum and into the terminal ileum.
- Observation is required for approximately 2 hours following the procedure.
- Complications include perforation or haemorrhage following a biopsy or polypectomy.

- **Colonoscopy.** This allows good visualization of the whole colon and terminal ileum. Biopsies can be obtained and polyps removed. The success rate for reaching the terminal ileum is approximately 90%. Perforation occurs in 1:2500 examinations and in 1% after polypectomy. The mortality is 0.02% for diagnostic colonoscopy.
- **Enteroscopy.** The small bowel from the duodenum to the ileum can be visualized by enteroscopes. The indications for this technique are limited (mainly gastrointestinal blood loss), the instruments are expensive, and consequently they are used only in a few centres.

FURTHER READING

Mallery S, Van Dam J (2000) Endoscopic practice at the start of the new millennium. *Gastroenterology* **118**: 5129–5147.

The mouth

The oral cavity extends from the lips to the pharynx and contains the tongue, teeth and gums. Its primary functions are mastication, swallowing and speech.

Problems in the mouth are extremely common and although they may be trivial, they can produce severe symptoms. Poor dental hygiene is often a factor.

Stomatitis is inflammation in the mouth from any cause, such as ill-fitting dentures. Angular stomatitis is inflammation of the corners of the mouth.

The burning mouth syndrome consists of a burning sensation in the context of a clinically normal oral mucosa. It occurs more commonly in middle-aged and elderly females. It is probably psychogenic in nature. Halitosis is a common symptom; causes are shown in Box 6.2.

Oral ulceration

Recurrent ulceration

Recurrent aphthous ulceration of unknown aetiology is a common oral mucosa disorder affecting 20% of the population. It consists of recurrent bouts of one or more

---

Box 6.2

Causes of halitosis

- Poor oral hygiene
- Anxiety when halitosis is more imaginary than real
- Rare causes:
  - oesophageal stricture
  - pulmonary sepsis

---

rounded, shallow, painful ulcers recurring at intervals of days to a few months. There are three main clinical types:

- *Minor aphthous ulcers* are the most common. They are less than 10 mm diameter, have a grey/white centre with a thin erythematous halo and heal within 14 days without scarring.
- *Major aphthous ulcers* are less common. They are larger (more than 20 mm diameter), often persist for weeks or months and heal with scarring. They present after puberty.
- *Herpetiform aphthous ulcers* are characterized by multiple (10–100), 2–3 mm diameter lesions. The term 'herpetiform' is purely descriptive and does not imply an infective aetiology.

Most patients with recurrent ulcers are otherwise well. Various nutritional deficiencies of iron, folic acid or vitamin B_{12} (with or without gastrointestinal disorders) are occasionally found.

There are no specific, effective therapies. Corticosteroids may lessen the duration and severity of the attacks. Chlorhexidine gluconate mouthwash, dapsone, colchicine, systemic steroids and azathioprine have all been tried.

Ulceration associated with systemic disorders

Oral ulceration is seen in gastrointestinal disorders, such as Crohn's disease, ulcerative colitis and coeliac disease in approximately 10–20% of cases. Other diseases associated with oral ulceration include lupus erythematosus (systemic and discoid), Behçet's disease, neutropenia (p. 452) and immunodeficiency disorders. In Reiter's disease, ulceration occurs in approximately 25–30% of patients.

Ulceration associated with dermatological disorders

These include erythema multiforme major, toxic epidermal necrolysis, lichen planus, pemphigus vulgaris, mucous membrane pemphigoid, 'epidermolysis bullosa' and dermatitis herpetiformis.

Ulceration associated with viral infection

Herpes simplex virus. Primary herpes simplex (usually type I but rarely type II) presents with fever and widespread confluent painful ulcers. After resolution, the virus remains latent and recurs as herpes labialis ('cold sores', see p. 1276). Reactivation of persistent herpes simplex virus occurs secondary to a viral infection, fever, sunlight exposure or menstruation. There is a prodrome of lip burning or pricking sensation. Treatment with soluble tetracycline mouthwash three times daily gives pain relief. Oral systemic aciclovir shortens the course of the disease.

Coxsackie. Hand, foot and mouth disease due to Coxsackie A virus produces small ulcers. Herpangina, due to a different Coxsackie A, or rarely B, infection presents with an acute pharyngitis, cervical lymphadenopathy and pyrexia with multiple ulcers of the soft palate and pharyngeal mucosa.

Other viruses. Herpes zoster and cytomegalovirus are among many viruses that can produce mouth ulceration, usually during the acute infective phase.

Ulceration associated with bacterial infection

Syphilis and tuberculosis can rarely cause oral ulcerations and are seen mainly in developing countries.

Ulceration associated with drugs

Certain drugs can cause oral lichenoid eruptions. They include antimalarials, methyldopa, tolbutamide, penicillamine and gold salts.

Trauma

Traumatic ulcers may be due to ill-fitting dentures, toothbrushing or lacerations by sharp teeth.

Neoplastic lesions (squamous cell carcinoma)

Malignant tumours of the mouth account for 1% of all malignant tumours in the UK. The majority develop on the floor of the mouth or lateral borders of the tongue. Early tumours may be painless, but advanced tumours are easily recognizable as indurated aphthous ulcers with raised and rolled edges. Aetiological agents include tobacco, heavy alcohol consumption and the areca nut. Intra-oral lesions which undergo malignant transformation include leucoplakia, lichen planus, submucous fibrosis and erythroplakia (a red patch). The previous male predominance has declined. Treatment is by surgical excision and/or radiotherapy.

Oral white patches

White lesions may be transient or persistent. Transient white patches are either due to *Candida* infection or are very occasionally seen in systemic lupus erythematosus. Oral candidiasis in adults is seen in seriously ill or immunocompromised patients, or following therapy with broad-spectrum antibiotics or inhaled steroids.

Local causes include mechanical, irritative or chemical trauma from drugs (e.g. aspirin).

Leucoplakia describes white patches for which no local cause can be found. It is associated with alcohol and (particularly) smoking, and is regarded as a premalignant condition. A biopsy should always be undertaken; histology shows alteration in the keratinization and dysplasia of the epithelium. Treatment with isotretinoin reduces disease progression. Oral lichen planus presents as white striae.

Oral pigmented lesions
Non-neoplastic lesions

Racial pigmentation is scattered and symmetrically distributed. Amalgam tattoo is the most common form of localized oral pigmentation and consists of blue-black macules involving the gingivae and results from the dental amalgam sequestering into the tissues. Diseases causing pigmentation include Peutz–Jegher's syndrome, Addison's disease and lichen planus. Heavy metals, such as lead, bismuth and mercury, and drugs (e.g. phenothiazines and antimalarials) all cause gingival pigmentation.

Neoplastic lesions

These include melanotic naevi on the hard palate and buccal mucosa. These are rarer in the mouth than on the skin. Malignant melanomas are rare, more common in males, and occur mainly on the upper jaw. The 5-year survival is only 5%.

The tongue

The tongue may be involved in a generalized stomatitis with similar lesions to those described above. Glossitis is a red, smooth, sore tongue seen in anaemia due to B_{12}, folate or iron deficiency. It is also seen in infections due to *Candida* and in riboflavin and nicotinic acid deficiency.

A black hairy tongue is due to a proliferation of chromogenic microorganisms causing brown-staining of elongated filiform papillae. The causes are unknown, but heavy smoking and the use of antiseptic mouth washes have been implicated. A geographic tongue is an idiopathic condition occurring in 1–2% of the population and may be familial. There are erythematous areas surrounded by well-defined, slightly raised irregular margins. The lesions are usually painless and the patient should be reassured.

The gums

The gingivae consist of the mucus membranes covering the alveolar process of the mandible and the maxilla.

Chronic gingivitis is the most common cause of bleeding gums and is an inflammation following the accumulation of bacterial plaque. It resolves when the plaque is removed.

Acute (necrotizing) ulcerative gingivitis (Vincent's gingivitis) is characterized by the proliferation of spirochaete and fusiform bacteria. Young male smokers with poor oral hygiene are predominantly affected. It responds to oral metronidazole 200 mg three times daily for 3 days, used with chlorhexidine gluconate mouthwash.

Desquamatous gingivitis is a clinical description of smooth, red atrophic gingivae caused by lichen planus or mucus membrane pemphigoid. The diagnosis is confirmed by biopsy.

Gingival swelling is due to fibrous hyperplasia or as a result of inflammatory changes. Fibrous gingival hyperplasia is a result of hereditary gingival fibromatosis or associated with drugs (e.g. phenytoin, ciclosporin, nifedipine). Inflammatory swellings are seen in pregnancy, gingivitis and scurvy. Swelling due to infiltration is seen in acute leukaemia and Wegener's granulomatosis.

The teeth
Streptococcus mutans is the main bacterial cause of dental caries in man. These bacteria are cariogenic only in the presence of dietary sugar. Dental caries can progress to pulpitis and pulp necrosis, and spreading infection can cause dentoalveolar abscesses. If there is soft tissue swelling, antibiotics (e.g. amoxicillin or metronidazole) should be prescribed prior to dental intervention. Erosion of the teeth can also result from exposure to acid (e.g. in bulimia nervosa – p. 1267) or, very occasionally, in patients with gastro-oesophageal reflux disease.

Oral manifestations of HIV infection
In the UK, 60% of HIV-infected patients have characteristic oral lesions. Lesions strongly associated with HIV infection include candidiasis (with erythema and/or white exudates), erythematous candidiasis, oral hairy leucoplakia, Kaposi's sarcoma, non-Hodgkin's lymphoma, necrotizing ulcerative gingivitis, and necrotizing ulcerative periodontitis.

Oral hairy leucoplakia is almost pathognomonic of HIV infection and may be an early sign. It is more common in HIV-infected homosexual men than in any other high-risk group. It is characterized by white vertical corrugations on the lateral borders of the tongue and immunostaining shows Epstein–Barr virus. Treatment is rarely necessary.

Kaposi's sarcoma presents as a red, purple or blue macule or nodule, most commonly on the palate. It is diagnostic of AIDs. The lesion is associated with herpesvirus 8 (p. 50).

FURTHER READING

Lehner T (1996) The mouth and salivary glands. In: Weatherall DJ, Ledingham JG, Warrell DA (eds) *Oxford Textbook of Medicine*, 3rd edn. Oxford: Oxford University Press, 1846–1865.
Rees TD (2000) Orofacial granulomatosis and related conditions. *Periodontology* **21**: 145–157.

The salivary glands

Ptyalism (excessive salivation)
Ptyalism occurs prior to vomiting, but may be secondary to other intra-oral pathology. It can be psychogenic.

Xerostomia (dry mouth)
This can result from:

- Sjögren's syndrome
- drugs (e.g. anticholinergic, antiparkinsonian, antihistamines, lithium, monoamine oxidase inhibitors, tricyclic and related antidepressants, and clonidine)
- radiotherapy
- psychogenic causes
- dehydration, shock and renal failure.

The principles of management are to preserve what flow remains, stimulate flow and replace saliva (glycerine and lemon mouthwash and artificial saliva).

Sialadenitis
Acute sialadenitis is due to mumps (parotitis) or bacteria. Bacteria include *Staphylococcus aureus*, *Streptococcus pyogenes* and *Streptococcus pneumoniae*. There is an ascending infection, usually secondary to secretory failure. Pus can be expressed from the affected duct.

Salivary duct obstruction due to calculus
Obstruction to salivary flow is usually due to a calculus. There is a painful swelling of the submandibular gland after eating and stones can sometimes be felt in the floor of the mouth. Sialography and plain X-ray films will show the calculus. Removal of the obstruction gives complete relief.

Sarcoidosis (see also p. 897)
Sarcoidosis can involve the major salivary glands and forms part of Heerfordt's syndrome (parotitis, uveitis, low-grade fever). When combined with lacrimal gland enlargement it is known as the Mikulicz syndrome.

Neoplasms
Salivary gland neoplasms account for 3% of all tumours world-wide. The majority occur in the parotid gland. The pleomorphic adenoma is the most common and 15% of these undergo malignant transformation. Recurrence following surgical excision is common. Malignant tumours classically result in 7th cranial nerve lower motor neurone signs.

The pharynx and oesophagus

Structure and function
The oesophagus is a muscular tube, approximately 25 cm long, connecting the pharynx to the stomach. The muscle coat has two layers – an outer longitudinal layer and an inner circular layer of fibres. In the upper portion both muscle layers are striated. They gradually change to smooth muscle in the lower oesophagus, where they are continuous with the muscle layer of the stomach.

The oesophagus joins to the stomach, just below the diaphragm after a short intra-abdominal segment (the gastro-oesophageal junction).

The oesophagus is lined by stratified squamous epithelium; the squamo-columnar junction lies 2 cm above the gastro-oesophageal junction and is recognized endoscopically by an irregular white Z line.

The oesophagus is separated from the pharynx by the *upper oesophageal sphincter*, which is normally closed by the continuous contraction of the cricopharyngeus muscle. The *lower oesophageal sphincter* (LOS) consists of an area of the distal end of the oesophagus that has a high resting tone and is largely responsible for the prevention of gastric reflux. The reduction in tone and relaxation of the LOS that occurs with swallowing is under the control of cholinergic excitatory neurones and non-adrenergic non-cholinergic (NANC) neurones as well as hormonal mechanisms. The presynaptic neurotransmittter is acetylcholine. The postsynaptic neurotransmitter, which inhibits relaxation, is nitric oxide (NO), with vasoactive intestinal peptide (VIP) and other peptides playing a role.

During swallowing, the bolus of food is moved from the mouth to the pharynx voluntarily. Immediately, the upper sphincter relaxes and food enters the oesophagus. A primary peristaltic wave starts in the pharynx at the onset of swallowing and sweeps down the whole oesophagus (Fig. 6.4). Secondary peristalsis occurs locally in response to direct stimulation (e.g. distension by the bolus) and helps to clear food residue from the oesophagus. Non-peristaltic, non-propulsive tertiary waves are frequent in the elderly. The LOS relaxes when swallowing is initiated, before the arrival of the peristaltic wave.

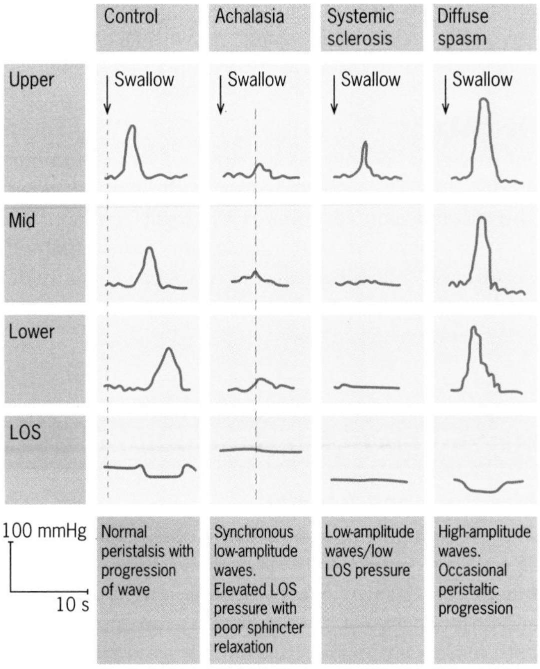

Symptoms of oesophageal disorders

Major oesophageal symptoms are:

- dysphagia
- substernal discomfort/heartburn
- acid regurgitation
- painful swallowing (odynophagia).

Dysphagia

This is difficulty in swallowing which is due to a local lesion or is part of a generalized disease. Patients will complain of something sticking in their throat or chest during swallowing or immediately afterwards. It is always a serious symptom and the cause must be found (Table 6.2); benign and malignant oesophageal strictures are the most common causes seen in hospital practice. *Globus* is described on page 325.

Substernal discomfort/heartburn

This is a common symptom of acid reflux. It is usually a retrosternal burning pain that can spread to the neck, across the chest, and can be difficult to distinguish from the pain of ischaemic heart disease. It can occur at night when the patient lies flat or after bending or stooping. Hot drinks and alcohol often precipitate the pain.

Acid regurgitation

Acid regurgitation is the effortless reflux of gastric contents into the mouth and pharynx. It occurs infrequently in normal subjects but frequently in patients with gastro-oesophageal reflux disease.

Painful swallowing

Painful swallowing without real difficulty is a symptom of candidiasis and herpes simplex infection. Both these

Fig. 6.4 Oesophageal manometric patterns in normals and diseased states. LOS, lower oesophageal sphincter.

Table 6.2
Causes of dysphagia

Disease of mouth and tongue (e.g. tonsillitis)	Extrinsic pressure:
Neuromuscular disorders:	Mediastinal glands
Pharyngeal disorders	Goitre
Bulbar palsy (e.g. motor	Enlarged left atrium
neurone disease)	Intrinsic lesion:
Myasthenia gravis	Foreign body
Oesophageal motility disorders:	Stricture
Achalasia	benign – peptic, corrosive
Scleroderma	malignant – carcinoma
Diffuse oesophageal spasm	Lower oesophageal rings
Presbyoesophagus	Oesophageal web
Diabetes mellitus	Pharyngeal pouch
Chagas' disease	

conditions are seen in AIDS patients. Ingestion of tablets such as bisphosphonates and potassium (slow release) will produce local ulceration if they lodge in the gullet when swallowed lying down and without water.

Signs of oesophageal disorders
There are very few signs associated with oesophageal disease, the main one being of weight loss as a consequence of dysphagia.

Investigation of oesophageal disorders
- **Barium swallow and meal.**
- **Oesophagoscopy.**
- **Manometry** (Fig. 6.4) is performed by passing a catheter through the nose into the oesophagus and measuring the pressures generated within the region of the lower oesophageal sphincter (LOS) and body of oesophagus either for a short fixed time period (static) or up to 24 hours (ambulatory).
- **pH monitoring** – 24-hour ambulatory monitoring using a pH-sensitive probe positioned in the lower oesophagus is used to identify reflux episodes (pH < 4) and when combined with manometry is a valuable means of correlating episodes of acid reflux and oesophageal dysmotility with patients' symptoms (see Fig. 6.6).
- **Radioisotope studies** with technetium–sulphur colloid incorporated into food can also be used to study reflux. It is not widely used in the UK.
- **The Bernstein test** (alternate dilute acid and alkali infused into the oesophagus to reproduce the pain) is hardly ever used. A positive test suggests oesophagitis, but there are many false negatives.

Hiatus hernia

This describes the 'herniation' of part of the stomach into the chest.

In a *sliding hiatus hernia*, the gastro-oesophageal junction 'slides' through the hiatus so that it lies above the diaphragm. This type of hernia occurs in approximately 30% of people of 50 years of age and by itself is of no diagnostic significance. It does not produce symptoms on its own; symptoms occur because of the presence of associated reflux (see below).

A *para-oesophageal or rolling hernia* is when a small part of the fundus of the stomach rolls up through the hernia alongside the oesophagus. The sphincter remains below the diaphragm and remains competent. Occasionally a rolling para-oesophageal hernia will produce severe pain and require surgical treatment for gastric volvulus or strangulation.

Gastro-oesophageal reflux disease (GORD)

Gastro-oesophageal reflux occurs as a normal event, and the clinical features of GORD occur only when the antireflux mechanisms fail sufficiently to allow gastric contents to make prolonged contact with the lower oesophageal mucosa. Definitions of terms used in oesophageal disease are showed in Box 6.3.

Antireflux mechanisms (Fig. 6.5)
The lower oesophageal sphincter (LOS) is formed by the distal 4 cm of oesophageal smooth muscle. It rapidly regains its normal tone (following relaxation to allow a bolus to enter the stomach) and thereby prevents reflux. It is capable of increasing tone in response to rises in intra-abdominal and intragastric pressures.

Other antireflux measures involve the intra-abdominal segment of the oesophagus, which acts as a flap valve, and the mucosal rosette formed by folds of the gastric mucosa also helps to occlude the gastro-oesophageal junctional lumen. In addition, contraction of the crural diaphragm exerts a 'pinchcock-like' action at the LOS.

The oesophagus is normally rapidly cleared of any reflux contents by secondary peristalsis.

Pathogenesis
The following mechanisms have been implicated:

- Transient LOS relaxations.
- Low resting LOS tone which fails to increase when the patient is lying flat, as occurs normally.
- The LOS tone fails to increase when intra-abdominal pressure is increased by tight clothing or pregnancy.
- There is increased oesophageal mucosal sensitivity to acid.

Box 6.3

Definitions in oesophageal disease

- **Hiatus hernia** – anatomical abnormality with part of the stomach in the chest, usually asymptomatic.
- **Gastro-oesophageal reflux** – reflux of gastric contents which can occur normally with no symptoms.
- **Gastro-oesophageal reflux disease (GORD)** – patient with reflux who has persistent symptoms.
- **Reflux oesophagitis** – inflammation of the lower oesophagus produced by persistent episodes of reflux. Patients may be asymptomatic.
- **Barrett's oesophagus** – presence of intestinal metaplastic columnar epithelium which has replaced squamous epithelium as a consequence of acid reflux.

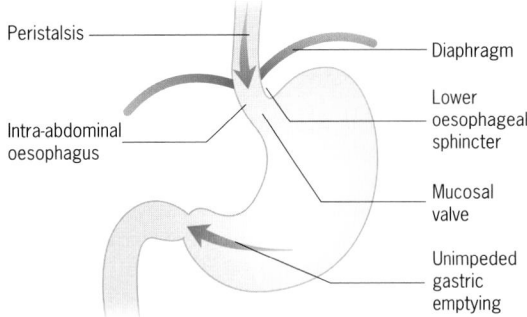

Peristalsis

Intra-abdominal oesophagus

Diaphragm

Lower oesophageal sphincter

Mucosal valve

Unimpeded gastric emptying

Fig. 6.5 The main antireflux mechanisms.

- There is reduced oesophageal clearance of acid because of poor oesophageal peristalsis. The reduced acid clearance is exacerbated with a hiatus hernia owing to trapping of acid within the hernial sac.
- A large hiatus hernia can impair the 'pinchcock' mechanism of the crural diaphragm.
- Delayed gastric emptying occurs, which may increase the chance of reflux.
- Prolonged episodes of gastro-oesophageal reflux which occur at night and postprandially.

Factors associated with increased gastro-oesophageal reflux are shown in Table 6.3. All or some of these features play a role in the individual patient and can occur whether or not a hiatus hernia is present. GORD can undoubtedly occur without a hiatus hernia.

Clinical features

Heartburn is the major feature of GORD. Pain is mainly due to direct stimulation of the hypersensitive oesophageal mucosa, but is also partly due to spasm of the distal oesophageal muscle. The burning is aggravated by bending, stooping or lying down and may be relieved by antacids. The patient may complain of pain on drinking hot liquids or alcohol. The correlation between heartburn and oesophagitis is poor. Some patients have mild oesophagitis, but severe heartburn; others have severe oesophagitis without symptoms, and present with a haematemesis or an iron deficiency anaemia from chronic blood loss.

Table 6.3
Factors associated with increased gastro-oesophageal reflux

Pregnancy or obesity
Fat, chocolate, coffee or alcohol ingestion
Large meals
Cigarette smoking
Drugs – anticholinergic, calcium-channel blockers, nitrates
Systemic sclerosis
After treatment for achalasia
Hiatus hernia

Regurgitation of food and 'acid' into the mouth occurs, particularly when the patient is bending or lying flat. Aspiration into the lungs, producing pneumonia, is unusual without an accompanying stricture, but cough and nocturnal asthma from regurgitation and aspiration can occur. The differential diagnosis of the retrosternal pain from angina can be difficult; 20% of cases admitted to a coronary care unit have GORD (Box 6.4).

Diagnosis and investigations

GORD is a clinical diagnosis and in many patients the diagnosis can be made without investigation. Under the age of 45 years, all patients should be treated initially without investigations, unless there are alarm symptoms (see p. 254).

Documenting reflux

- Barium swallow when combined with the water siphon test is a reliable way of assessing the potential severity of reflux. It will also show the presence of a hiatus hernia.
- 24-Hour intraluminal pH monitoring combined with manometry (see p. 263), which should always be performed to confirm GORD before considering surgery. There should be a good correlation between reflux (pH < 4.0) and symptoms (Fig. 6.6). It is also necessary to exclude oesophageal dysmotility as the cause of symptoms.
- Radiolabelled technetium (see p. 263) is used in some centres to demonstrate reflux.

Assessing oesophagitis (Fig. 6.7)

Fibreoptic oesophagoscopy is used to confirm the presence of oesophagitis, i.e. a red friable mucosa with ulceration in severe cases (erosive oesophagitis). The technique is also used to diagnose Barrett's oesophagus (p. 265).

Treatment

Many patients with reflux symptoms (approximately 50%) can be treated successfully with simple antacids,

---

Box 6.4

Features of gastro-oesophageal reflux and myocardial ischaemia

Gastro-oesophageal reflux
Burning pain produced by bending stooping or lying down
Pain seldom radiates to the arms
Pain precipitated by drinking hot liquids or alcohol
Relieved by antacids

Myocardial ischaemia
Gripping or crushing pain
Pain radiates into neck, shoulders and both arms
Pain produced by exercise
Accompanied by dyspnoea

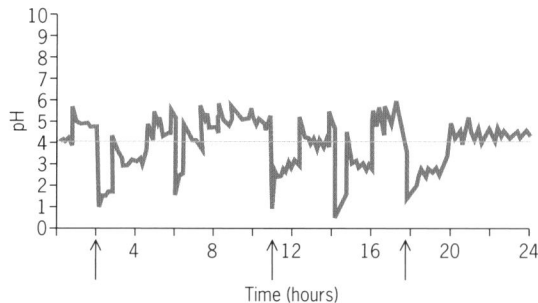

Fig. 6.6 **24-hour intraluminal pH monitoring.** Five reflux episodes (pH < 4) occurred, but only three gave symptoms (arrows).

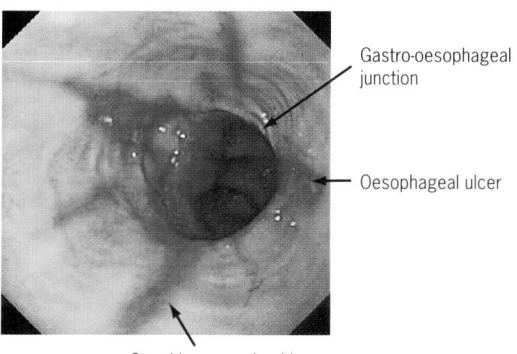

Gastro-oesophageal junction

Oesophageal ulcer

Streaking oesophagitis

Fig. 6.7 **Endoscopic picture, showing oesophagitis.**
Courtesy of Dr Geoff Smith, Barts and The London NHS Trust.

loss of weight, and raising the head of the bed at night. Precipitating factors should be avoided with a reduction in alcohol consumption and cessation of smoking. These measures are simple to say, difficult to carry out, but are useful in mild cases.

Drugs

Simple antacids magnesium trisilicate and aluminium hydroxide are readily available and are often used initially by patients. The former tends to cause diarrhoea whilst the latter causes constipation. Many antacids contain sodium which may exacerbate fluid retention; aluminium hydroxide has less sodium than magnesium trisilicate.

Alginate-containing antacids (10 mL three times daily) are the most frequently prescribed agents for GORD. They form a gel or 'foam raft' with gastric contents and thereby reduce reflux. They are available over the counter and are often used by the patient before consultation.

H_2-*receptor antagonists* (e.g. cimetidine, ranitidine, famotidine and nizatadine) are used for acid suppression if the above measures fail and now they can be obtained over the counter; they are frequently used.

Proton pump inhibitors (PPIs) (e.g. omeprazole, rabeprazole, lansoprazole, pantoprazole, esomeprazole) inhibit gastric hydrogen–potassium-ATPase (see Fig.

6.10). PPIs produce almost complete reduction of gastric acid secretion and are the drugs of choice for all but mild cases. Patients with severe symptoms need prolonged treatment, often for years. Sometimes a lower dose, e.g. omeprazole 10 mg, is sufficient for maintenance.

The prokinetic agents metoclopramide and domperidone are dopamine antagonists. They are occasionally helpful as they enhance peristalsis and speed gastric emptying. Cisapride increases the QT_c interval and has been withdrawn because of the risk of arrhythmias.

Helicobacter pylori eradication in GORD is controversial. Some believe that after eradication, acid secretion increases and worsens reflux symptoms. Others believe that prolonged acid suppression therapy without eradication of *H. pylori* results in migration of the organism into areas of Barrett's oesophagus where it acts as an oncogenic agent.

Surgery

Surgery should never be performed for a hiatus hernia alone. The properly selected case with severe reflux symptoms confirmed by pH monitoring and with oesophagitis on oesophagoscopy responds well to surgery. Repair of the hernia and some sort of additional antireflux surgery (e.g. a modified Nissen fundoplication) is performed laparoscopically. Results show an improvement in symptoms in up to 80% of cases. The indications for surgery are not always clear as medical therapy with PPIs is so effective; the young patient needing years of drug treatment is one common indication.

Patients with oesophageal dysmotility unrelated to acid reflux tend to do less well as do those with underlying functional bowel disease.

Management of reflux oesophagitis

There is a poor correlation between GORD symptoms and the presence of endoscopic oesophagitis. Using the treatments above, most patients can be kept symptom-free but symptoms usually return when treatment is stopped.

Many gastroenterologists also treat severe oesophagitis with long-term PPIs with regular surveillance oesophagoscopy in an attempt to reduce the risk of complications. Long term omeprazole use appears very safe.

Complications

Peptic stricture usually occurs in patients over the age of 60. The symptoms are those of intermittent dysphagia over a long period. Treatment is by dilatation of the stricture and management of the reflux usually medically with a proton-pump inhibitor to achieve anacidity. Occasionally surgery is required.

Barrett's oesophagus. This is thought to occur from long-standing reflux. It consists of columnar epithelium with intestinal metaplasia extending upwards into the lower oesophagus replacing normal squamous epithelium. It is seen in up to 20% of patients undergoing endoscopy for gastro-oesophageal reflux disease. Endoscopically Barrett's may be seen as a continual sheet, a finger like projection extending upwards from the squamo-columnar junction or as islands of columnar mucosa interspersed in areas or residual squamous mucosa. It is very common in middle-aged men. Barrett's oesophagus (even a short segment < 3 cm) is premalignant for adenocarcinoma. An indocarmine spray down the endoscope can detect intestinal metaplasia and possibly dysplasia. The dysplasia is patchy and biopsies from all four quadrants (every 2 cm) of the Barrett's segment must be performed. There is no evidence that treatment with PPIs or surgery leads to Barrett's regression. Surveillance – looking for severe dysplasia/cancer – is costly and subject to observer error. In the view of a number of gastroenterologists, endoscopy should be performed 6-monthly with intensive medical therapy in a patient with low-grade dysplasia, while high-grade dysplasia is treated by endoscopic mucosal ablation or surgery.

Adenocarcinoma. Patients with weekly reflux symptoms are nearly 8 times more likely to develop adenocarcinoma compared with those without symptoms. The greater the frequency, severity and the duration of reflux symptoms, the greater the risk.

Motility disorders

Achalasia

Achalasia is a disease characterized by aperistalsis in the body of the oesophagus and failure of relaxation of the lower oesophageal sphincter on initiation of swallowing. In the majority of cases the aetiology is unknown (idiopathic). A similar clinical picture is seen in Chagas' disease (American trypanosomiasis, p. 103) where there is damage to the neural plexus of the gut.

Pathogenesis

Degenerative lesions are found in the vagus as well as a decrease in ganglionic cells in the myenteric nerve plexus of the oesophageal wall. Nitric oxide-containing neurones are affected more than the cholinergic nerves, and thus the relaxation of the sphincter is impaired in its absence. Some patients have autoantibodies to a dopamine-carrying protein on the surface of the cells in the myenteric plexus.

Clinical features

The disease can present at any age but is rare in childhood. The incidence is about 1 per 100 000 per year. Patients usually have a long history of intermittent dysphagia for both liquids and solids. Regurgitation of food from the dilated oesophagus may be induced by the patient or may occur spontaneously, particularly at night, and aspiration pneumonia may result. Occasionally food gets stuck but patients often learn to overcome this by drinking large quantities, thereby increasing the head of pressure in the oesophagus and forcing the food through. Severe retrosternal chest pain occurs particularly in younger patients with vigorous non-peristaltic contraction of the oesophagus. The dysphagia in these patients can be mild and the pain misdiagnosed as cardiac in origin. Weight loss is usually not marked.

Investigations

- **Chest X-ray** may show a dilated oesophagus, sometimes with a fluid level seen behind the heart. The fundal gas shadow is not present.
- **Barium swallow** will show dilatation of the oesophagus, lack of peristalsis and often synchronous contractions. The lower end gradually narrows ('swan neck deformity'); this appearance is due to failure of the sphincter to relax (Fig. 6.8).
- **Oesophagoscopy** is necessary to exclude a carcinoma at the lower end of the oesophagus, as an intramucosal carcinoma can produce a similar X-ray appearance. When there is marked dilatation, extensive cleansing is necessary to remove food debris in order to obtain a clear view. In achalasia the oesophagoscope easily flops through the apparent narrowing without resistance.

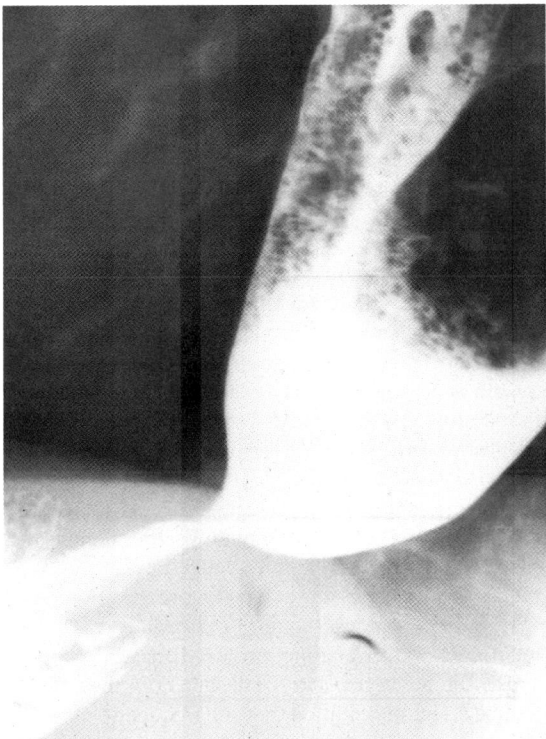

Fig. 6.8 **Barium swallow showing achalasia** with atonic body of the oesophagus and a narrowed distal end. Note food residue in dilated oesophagus.

- **CT scan.** This is helpful, particularly in detecting an intramucosal carcinoma.
- **Manometry** shows aperistalsis of the oesophagus as well as the failure of relaxation of the lower oesophageal sphincter (see Fig. 6.4).

Treatment

The treatment of choice is endoscopic dilatation of the LOS using a pneumatic bag (passed under X-ray control). This weakens the sphincter and is successful in 80% of cases. Endoscopic injection of botulinum toxin into the LOS has been used with variable success. If these measures fail, surgical division of the muscle at the lower end of the oesophagus (cardiomyotomy or Heller's operation) is performed laparoscopically. Reflux oesophagitis complicates all procedures and the aperistalsis of the oesophagus remains. In older patients, nifedipine (20 mg sublingually) or sildenafil can be tried initially.

Complications

There is a slight increase in the incidence of squamous carcinoma of the oesophagus in both treated and untreated cases (7% after 25 years).

Systemic sclerosis (see also p. 561)

There is oesophageal involvement in 90% or more of patients with this disease. Diminished peristalsis, detected manometrically (see Fig. 6.4) or by barium swallow, is due to replacement of the smooth muscle layers by fibrous tissue. The lower oesophageal sphincter pressure is also decreased, allowing reflux; mucosal damage occurs as a consequence. Strictures may develop. Initially there are no symptoms, but dysphagia and heartburn occur as the oesophagus becomes severely involved.

Similar motility abnormalities may be found in other connective-tissue disorders, particularly if Raynaud's phenomenon is present. Treatment is as for reflux (see p. 264) and stricture formation.

Diffuse oesophageal spasm

This is a severe form of abnormal oesophageal motility that can sometimes produce retrosternal chest pain and dysphagia. It can accompany GORD. Swallowing is accompanied by bizarre and marked contractions of the oesophagus without propagation of the waves (see Fig. 6.4). On barium swallow the appearance may be that of a 'corkscrew'. However, changes in oesophageal motility 'dysmotility' are not infrequent, particularly in patients over the age of 60 years (presbyoesophagus). Care must therefore be taken that the symptoms, the manometry and X-ray findings of oesophageal spasm are not falsely correlated; functional dyspepsia is commoner than oesophageal spasm.

A variant of diffuse oesophageal spasm is the 'nutcracker' oesophagus, which is characterized by finding very high-amplitude peristalsis (pressures > 200 mmHg) within the oesophagus. Chest pain and dysphagia occur.

Treatment

True oesophageal spasm producing severe symptoms is uncommon and treatment is often difficult. Antispasmodics, nitrates, or calcium-channel blockers – such as sublingual nifedipine 10 mg three times daily – may be tried. Occasionally, balloon dilatation or even myotomy is necessary. When the spasm is associated with GORD, acid suppression is given.

Miscellaneous motility disorders

Abnormalities of motility that are mostly asymptomatic but occasionally produce dysphagia are found in the elderly, in diabetes mellitus, myotonica dystrophica and myasthenia gravis, as well as neurological disorders involving the brainstem.

Other oesophageal disorders

Oesophageal diverticulum

This is a pouch lined with epithelium that can produce dysphagia and regurgitation. It is usually asymptomatic and often detected accidentally on a barium swallow performed for other reasons. Diverticula can occur:

- immediately above the upper oesophageal sphincter (pharyngeal pouch) – if large, it may cause dysphagia as well as spillage of contents into the trachea
- near the middle of the oesophagus (traction diverticulum produced by extrinsic inflammation)
- just above the lower oesophageal sphincter (epiphrenic diverticulum).

Only when symptoms are severe should surgery be undertaken.

Rings and webs

A number of rings and webs have been described throughout the oesophagus.

Upper oesophageal web

This is a constriction near the upper oesophageal sphincter in the post-cricoid region and appears radiologically as a web. The web may be asymptomatic or may produce dysphagia. In the Plummer–Vinson syndrome (Paterson–Brown–Kelly syndrome) this web is associated with iron deficiency anaemia, glossitis and angular stomatitis. This rare syndrome affects mainly women and its aetiology is not understood. At oesophagoscopy the web may be difficult to see. Dilatation of the web is rarely necessary. Iron is given for the iron deficiency.

Cricopharyngeal dysfunction

There is poor relaxation of the cricopharyngeal muscle during swallowing so that a prominent indentation or 'bar' is seen on a barium swallow. It occurs in the elderly. Dysphagia is treated with dilatation but surgical myotomy may be necessary.

Lower oesophageal or Schatzki ring

This is a narrowing of the lower end of the oesophagus due to a ridge of mucosa or a fibrous membrane. The ring may be asymptomatic, but it can very occasionally produce dysphagia after swallowing a large bolus of bread or meat. A barium swallow (with the oesophagus well distended with barium) often shows the narrowing; barium-coated bread will lodge at the narrowing. Treatment is with reassurance and dietary advice, but dilatation is occasionally necessary.

Benign oesophageal stricture

Peptic stricture secondary to reflux is the most common cause of benign strictures (for treatment, see p. 265). They also occur after the ingestion of corrosives, after radiotherapy, after sclerosis of varices, and following prolonged nasogastric intubation. All strictures give rise to dysphagia. They are usually treated by dilatation, but occasionally surgery is necessary.

Oesophageal infections

Infection is a cause of painful swallowing and is seen particularly in immunosuppressed debilitated patients and patients with AIDS. Infection can occur with:

- *Candida*
- herpes simplex
- cytomegalovirus.

It is occasionally difficult to distinguish between these either on barium swallow or oesophagoscopy, as only widespread ulceration is seen. In candidiasis the characteristic white plaques on top of friable mucosa are frequently found but oral candidiasis is not always present. The diagnosis of *Candida* infection can be confirmed by examining a direct smear taken at endoscopy, but often infections are mixed and cultures and biopsies must be performed.

Treatment

Most patients on large doses of immunosuppressive agents are treated prophylactically with nystatin or amphotericin. Other antifungal or antiviral treatment is given appropriately (see Ch. 1).

The Mallory–Weiss syndrome

This is described on page 282.

Oesophageal perforation or rupture

Oesophageal perforation usually occurs at the time of endoscopic dilatation or very occasionally following insertion of a nasogastric tube. Patients with a malignant, corrosive or post-radiotherapy stricture are more likely to perforate than one with a benign peptic stricture.

Management usually involves placement of an oesophageal stent (p. 270), which dilates the usually malignant stricture and seals the hole. A water-soluble contrast X-ray is performed after 2–3 days to check the perforation has sealed.

Oesophageal rupture occurs with violent vomiting, producing severe chest pain and collapse. It may follow alcohol ingestion. A chest X-ray shows a hydro-pneumothorax. The diagnosis is made radiologically using water-soluble contrast. Treatment is surgical; mortality is high.

Oesophageal tumours

Cancer of the oesophagus

This is the eighth most common cancer seen throughout the world. Approximately 40% occur in the middle third of the oesophagus and are squamous carcinomas. Adenocarcinomas (approx 45%) occur in the lower third of the oesophagus and at the cardia. Tumours of the upper third are rare (15%).

Epidemiology and aetiological factors
Squamous cell carcinoma (SCC)
The incidence of this carcinoma varies throughout the world, being high in China, parts of Africa and in the Caspian regions of Iran (where the incidence is the highest observed for any type of cancer anywhere in the world). In the UK it is 5–10 per 100 000 and represents 2.2% of all malignant disease. The variation in incidence throughout the world is greater than for any other carcinoma and is unusual in that sharp differences occur in regions very close to one another.

SCC of the oesophagus is more common in men; risk factors are shown in Table 6.4. Monotonous diets very high in cereals and *N*-nitroso compounds in preserved food, possibly increase the risk. Diets high in carotenoids and vitamin C (vegetables and fruit) possibly decrease the risk.

Table 6.4
Risk factors for cancer of the oesophagus

Squamous cell carcinoma	Adenocarcinoma
Tobacco smoking	Long-standing GORD
Heavy alcohol intake	Barrett's oesophagus
Plummer–Vinson syndrome	Tobacco smoking
Achalasia	
Coeliac disease	
Tylosis*	
Diet deficient in vitamins; high dietary carotenoids and vitamin C possibly decrease the risk	

* Tylosis is an autosomal dominant condition with hyperkeratosis of the palms and soles

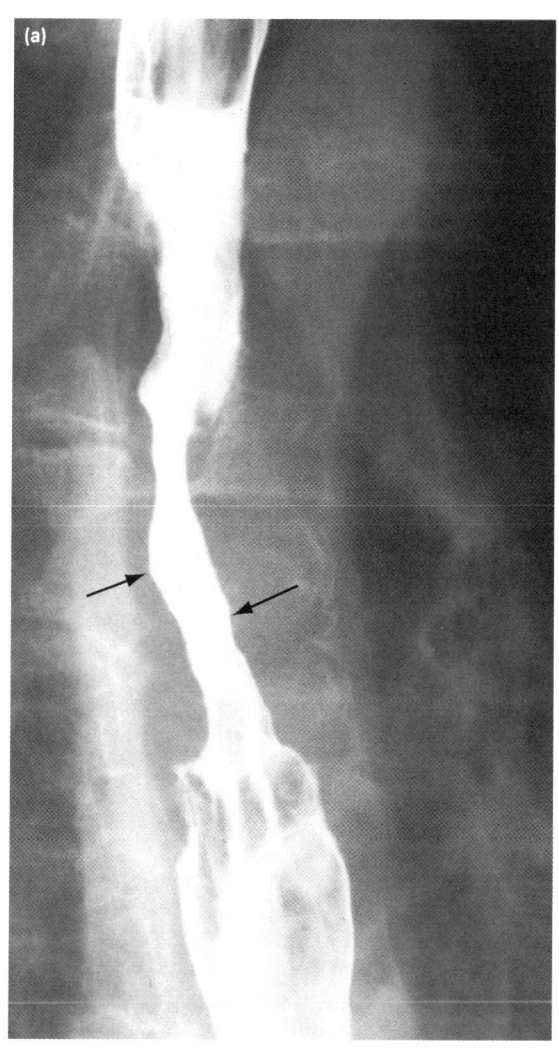

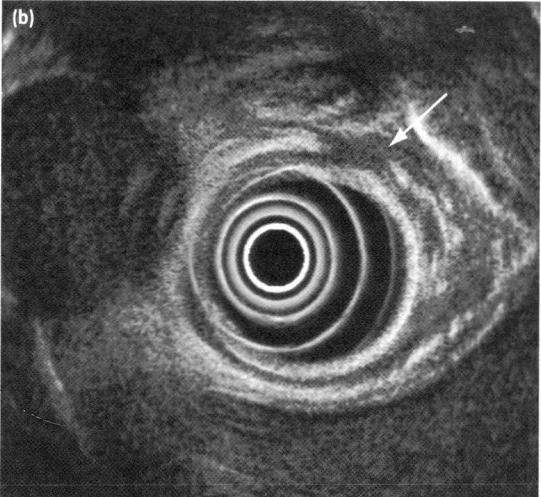

Fig. 6.9 **Carcinoma of the oesophagus. (a) Barium swallow,** showing an irregular narrowed area (arrows) at the lower end of the oesophagus. **(b) Endoscopic ultrasound.** The central concentric circles are the probe. The arrow points to a break in the muscle layer and the soft tissue mass of the carcinoma.

Adenocarcinoma

These tumours arise in the columnar-lined epithelium of the lower oesophagus (Barrett's oesophagus, p. 265). This columnarization results from long-standing reflux, although some patients will have no preceding symptoms. This premalignant lesion increases the chances of developing an adenocarcinoma 30–40-fold. Extension of an adenocarcinoma of the gastric cardia can cause oesophageal obstruction. The incidence rate of this tumour is increasing.

Clinical features

Carcinoma of the oesophagus occurs mainly in those aged 60–70 years, although it is now occurring in younger age groups. Dysphagia is the most common single symptom and is progressive and unrelenting. Initially there is difficulty in swallowing solids, but eventually dysphagia for liquids also occurs. Benign strictures, on the other hand, initially produce intermittent dysphagia. Impaction of food causes pain, but more persistent pain implies infiltration.

The lesion is usually ulcerative, extending around the wall of the oesophagus to produce a stricture. Direct invasion of the surrounding structures occurs rather than widespread metastases. Weight loss, due to the dysphagia as well as to anorexia, frequently occurs. The oesophageal obstruction eventually causes difficulty in swallowing saliva, and coughing and aspiration into the lungs is common.

Signs are often absent. Weight loss, anorexia and lymphadenopathy are occasionally found.

Investigation
Diagnostic
Endoscopy/barium swallow. Many gastroenterologists like to go directly to oesophagoscopy which provides histological or cytological proof of the carcinoma; 90% of oesophageal carcinomas can be confirmed with this technique. Barium swallow (Fig. 6.9a) is also a very sensitive technique and is useful in the younger patient with dysphagia where the differential diagnosis includes a motility disorder.

Staging for surgery
The TNM staging system is used (p. 478). Extent of tumour invasion (T), presence of tumour in lymph nodes (N) or metastases (M) are combined into stage categories.

- ***CT scan and MRI*** of the thorax and upper abdomen will show the volume of the tumour, local invasion and lymph node involvement.
- ***Endoscopic ultrasound*** (Fig. 6.9b) has an accuracy rate of nearly 90% for assessing depth of tumour and infiltration and 80% for staging lymph node involvement.

Treatment

This depends on the age and fitness of the patient and the stage of the disease. Five-year survival with stage 1 is 80% (T_1/T_2, N_0, M_0), stage 2 is 30%, stage 3 is 18% and stage 4 is 4%. Most patients present with stage 3 disease, so that overall survival is 27% at 1 year and only 9% at 5 years.

Surgery

Surgery provides the best chance of a cure and should be used only when screening (see above) has shown that the tumour has not infiltrated outside the oesophageal wall. Surgery in this group shows an 80% 5-year survival rate if the postoperative pathology confirms the staging.

Radiotherapy

This is used, with limited success, for squamous carcinoma of the upper and middle third of the oesophagus with a 20% 5-year survival for stage 3 disease. Oesophagitis and stricture formation occur. Adenocarcinoma is less radiosensitive.

Chemotherapy

5FU, cisplatinum and combined chemoradiation are being used (see p. 505) before surgical resection in some centres with some prolongation of survival.

Palliative therapy

This is often the only realistic possibility. Repeated dilatation or dilatation of the stricture with the insertion of an expanding metal stent to keep the oesophageal lumen open is performed via an endoscope. This allows liquids and soft foods to be eaten. Fizzy drinks are recommended to keep the tubes from blocking.

Tumours can be photocoagulated using a laser beam delivered through an endoscope, or necrosed using alcohol injections. This relieves the dysphagia, but repeated treatments are necessary. Photodynamic therapy is being tried to reduce the tumour bulk.

Nutritional support, as well as support for the patient and their family, is vital in this distressing condition.

Other oesophageal tumours

Most other tumours are rare. Leiomyomas are found usually by chance. They can cause dysphagia or bleeding. Surgical removal is performed for symptomatic lesions.

Kaposi's sarcoma is found in the oesophagus as well as the mouth (see p. 1308) and hypopharynx in patients with AIDS.

FURTHER READING

Armstrong D (2000) Long term safety and efficacy of omeprazole in GORD. *Lancet* **356**: 610–612.

Baron TH (2001) Expandable metal stents for the treatment of cancerous obstruction of the gastrointestinal tract. *New England Journal of Medicine* **344**: 1681–1687.

Jankowski J A et al. (2000) Barrett's metaplasia. *Lancet* **356**: 2079–2085.

Katzha DA, Rustgi AK (2000) Gastro-oesophageal reflux disease and Barrett's oesophagus. *Medical Clinics of North America* **84**: 1137–1161.

Lagergreen J et al. (1999). Symptomatic gastro-oesophageal reflux as a risk factor for oesophageal adenocarcinoma. *New England Journal of Medicine* **340**: 825–831.

Mittal RK, Balaban DH (1997) The esophago-gastric junction. *New England Journal of Medicine* **336**: 924–932.

Richter JE (2001) Oesophageal motility disorders. *Lancet* **358**: 823–828.

The stomach and duodenum

Structure

The stomach, which varies considerably in size, is divided into a small area immediately distal to the oesophagus (the cardia), the upper region (the fundus which lies under the left diaphragm), the mid-region or body, and the antrum, which extends into the pyloric region.

There are two sphincters, the gastro-oesophageal sphincter and the pyloric sphincter; the latter is largely made up of a thickening of the circular muscle layer. The muscle wall of the stomach has three layers – an outer longitudinal, an inner circular, and an innermost oblique layer of smooth muscle.

The duodenum has outer longitudinal and inner smooth muscle layers. It is C-shaped and the pancreas sits in the concavity. It terminates in the jejunum at the duodenojejunal flexure.

The mucosal lining of the stomach, particularly in the greater curvature, is thrown into thick folds or rugae. The upper two-thirds of the stomach contains parietal cells, which secrete hydrochloric acid, and chief cells, which secrete pepsinogen (which initiates proteolysis). The junction between the body and the antrum of the stomach can often be seen macroscopically, but can be confirmed by measuring surface pH. The antrum contains mucus-secreting and G cells, which secrete gastrin. There are two major forms of gastrin, G17 and G34, depending on the number of amino-acid residues. G17 is the major form found in the antrum. Mucus-secreting cells are present throughout the stomach and secrete mucus and bicarbonate which is trapped in the mucus gel. The mucus is made of glycoproteins called mucins. Somatostatin is also produced by specialized antral cells (D cells).

The mucosal barrier, made up of the surface membranes of mucosal cells and the mucus, protects the gastric epithelium from damage by, for example, alcohol, aspirin, NSAIDs, and bile salts. Prostaglandins stimulate mucus secretion and their synthesis is inhibited by aspirin and NSAIDs which inhibit cyclooxygenase (see Fig. 14.32).

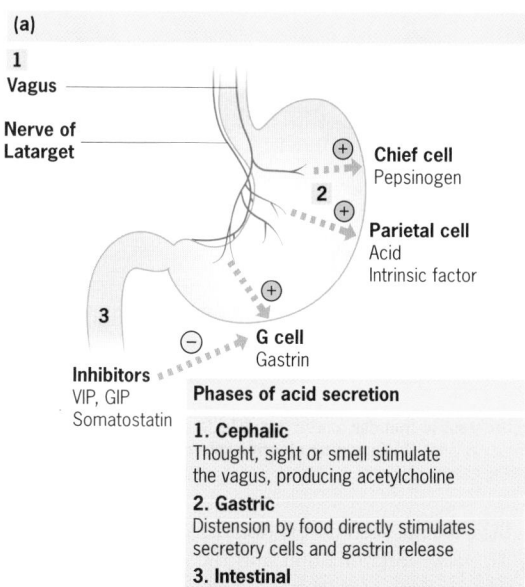

(a)

1 Vagus

Nerve of Latarget

Chief cell
Pepsinogen

2

Parietal cell
Acid
Intrinsic factor

3

G cell
Gastrin

Inhibitors
VIP, GIP
Somatostatin

Phases of acid secretion

1. Cephalic
Thought, sight or smell stimulate the vagus, producing acetylcholine

2. Gastric
Distension by food directly stimulates secretory cells and gastrin release

3. Intestinal
Passage of food into duodenum stimulates GI hormone release

(b)

H^+

Acid secretion

Apical surface

ATP-ase

K^+

Parietal cell

Protein kinases

ATP

Cyclic AMP

Ca^{2+} Ca^{2+}

G_s Ac G_i

Histamine   PGE$_2$ Acetylcholine   Gastrin

Fig. 6.10 **(a) Control of acid secretion. (b) Mechanisms involved in acid secretion.** Gastrin and acetylcholine also ct through enterochromaffin cells, stimulating histamine releas G_s, G_i, G-proteins – stimulatory and inhibitory; Ac, adenylate clase; PGE$_2$, prostaglandin E$_2$.

The duodenal mucosa contains Brunner's glands, which secrete alkaline mucus. This, along with the pancreatic and biliary secretions, helps to neutralize the acid secretion from the stomach when it reaches the duodenum.

Function

The factors controlling acid secretion are shown in Figure 6.10. Secretion is under neural and hormonal control. Both stimulate acid secretion through the direct release of histamine on the parietal cell. Acetylcholine and gastrin also release histamine via the enterochromaffin cells. Somatostatin inhibits both histamine and gastrin release and therefore acid secretion.

Other major gastric functions are:

- acting as a reservoir for food
- the emulsification of fat and mixing of gastric contents
- the secretion of intrinsic factor
- absorption (of only minimal importance).

Gastric emptying depends on many factors. There are osmoreceptors in the duodenal mucosa that control gastric emptying by local reflexes and the release of gut hormones. In particular, intraduodenal fat delays gastric emptying by negative feedback through duodenal receptors.

Helicobacter pylori infection

H. pylori is a spiral-shaped Gram-negative urease-producing bacterium (Fig. 6.11). Its complete genomic sequence is known. It is found in the gastric antrum and in areas of gastric metaplasia in the duodenum. *H. pylori* is found in greatest numbers under the mucus layers in gastric pits, where it adheres specifically to gastric epithelial cells.

Colonization in the acid environment of the gastric mucosa occurs because:

- Sheathed flagella allow the organisms to move quickly from the acidic lumen of the stomach through the mucus layer where the pH is higher. (Mutant strains that are non-motile do not colonize.)
- Acute infection produces transient hypochlorhydria.
- *H. pylori* produces urease (see Fig. 6.12). The ammonia produced neutralizes the acid.
- It possesses a proton pump.

Epidemiology

The exact mode of transmission is unclear, but intra-familial clustering suggests person-to-person spread, either oral–oral or faeco-oral mainly in childhood. The prevalence of *H. pylori* is high in developing countries (80–90% of the population) and its presence is associated with lower socio-economic status world-wide. Between one- and two-thirds of the western populations have this infection and the prevalence is high in the older population – presumably acquired in their childhood when hygiene was less good than today.

Pathogenesis

H. pylori infection produces a gastritis mainly in the antrum of the stomach. The mucosa appears reddened endoscopically and there is epithelial cell damage from local release of cytokines such as IL-6 and IL-8. This leads to recruitment and activation of an inflammatory

271

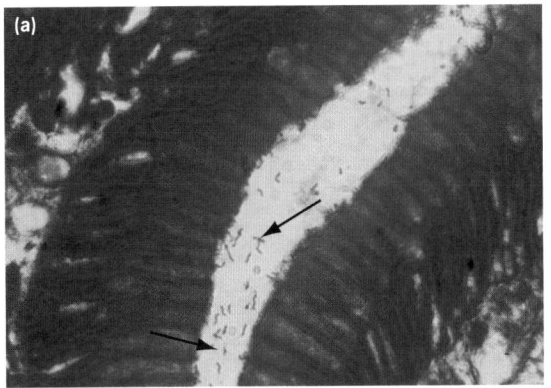
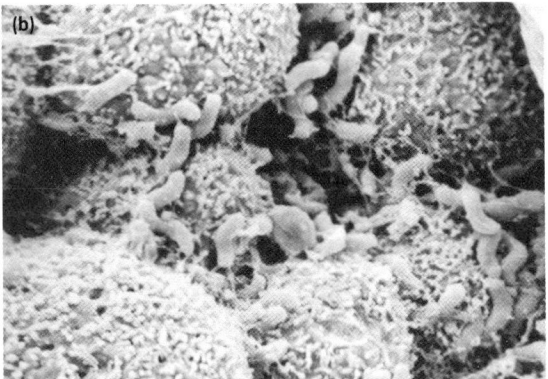

Fig. 6.11 *Helicobacter pylori.* **(a) Organisms (arrowed) are shown on the gastric mucosa** (cresyl fast violet (modified Giemsa) stain). Courtesy of Dr Alan Phillips, Department of Paediatric Gastroenterology, Royal Free Hospital. **(b) Scanning electron microscopy,** showing the spiral-shaped bacterium.

infiltrate in the lamina propria. This consists of polymorphonuclear leucocytes, eosinophils, lymphocytes, monocytes and plasma cells.

In some individuals this chronic superficial gastritis can involve the body of the stomach and this leads to atrophic gastritis. Intestinal metaplasia which is a premalignant pathological change, occurs in some of these (see Fig. 6.15).

Duodenal ulcer (DU) disease

H. pylori is causally associated with DU disease because in patients with DU:

- 95% are infected with *H. pylori*
- cure of the infection stops duodenal ulcer recurrence.

The precise mechanism of how duodenal ulceration occurs is unclear as only 15% of patients infected with *H. pylori* (approximately 50–60% of the adult population world-wide) develop duodenal ulcers. Factors that have been implicated include:

- Increased acid secretion because of:
  - increased parietal cell mass
  - increased gastrin secretion.
- Smoking impairing gastric mucosal healing.
- Virulence factors: *H. pylori* produces toxins, Vac A (vacuolating toxin) and Cag A (cytotoxic associated protein) as well as urease and adherence factors. There is controversy over their role in producing duodenal ulcer disease.
- Decreased inhibition of acid secretion, possibly by *H. pylori* damaging somatostatin-producing cells in the antrum.
- Genetic susceptibility may play a role. DUs are more common in patients who have blood group O and are non-secretors of blood group substances in saliva.

These factors lead to an increased acid load to the duodenum, which precipitates bile salts which would normally inhibit the growth of *H. pylori*.

Bicarbonate secretion is decreased in the duodenum by *H. pylori* inflammation and the damage and repair leads to gastric metaplasia which *H. pylori* colonizes, causing local release of cytokines and further damage.

Gastric ulcers (GU)

Gastric ulcers are associated with a gastritis affecting the body as well as the antrum of the stomach (pangastritis). Parietal cell damage occurs so that acid production is normal or low.

The ulcers occur because of local epithelial damage by cytokines released by *H. pylori* and also because of abnormal mucus production.

Clinical syndromes

H. pylori gastritis

This is usually asymptomatic; whether *H. pylori* gastritis itself produces epigastric discomfort, i.e. functional dyspepsia, is controversial.

Peptic ulcer disease

Epidemiology

DUs are very common and are two to three times more common than gastric ulcers (GUs). Approximately 10–15% of the population will suffer from a DU. Ulcer rates are declining rapidly for younger men and increasing for older individuals, particularly women. Both DUs and GUs are common in the elderly. There is a considerable geographical variation; for example, DUs are more common in northern England and Scotland than in other parts of the UK.

Pathology

Gastric ulcers are found in any part of the stomach, but are most commonly seen on the lesser curve. Most duodenal ulcers are found in the duodenal cap; the surrounding mucosa appears inflamed, haemorrhagic or friable (duodenitis). Erosions are superficial mucosal defects, while in a peptic ulcer there is a break in the superficial epithelial cells penetrating down to the muscularis mucosa at the site of the ulcer; there is a fibrous base and an increase in inflammatory cells. *H. pylori*-induced gastritis is present, confined to the antrum in DU disease but also involves the body in gastric ulcer disease.

Clinical features

The characteristic feature is epigastric pain. It has been shown that if a patient points to the epigastrium as the site of the pain this has a high discriminatory value for diagnosis. The relationship of the pain to food is variable and on the whole not helpful in the diagnosis. The pain of a DU classically occurs at night (as well as during the day) and is worse when the patient is hungry. Both gastric and duodenal ulcers are helped by antacids.

Nausea may accompany the pain; vomiting is infrequent but often relieves the pain. Heartburn occurs owing to acid regurgitation. Anorexia and weight loss may occur, particularly with gastric ulcers. If the patient complains of persistent and severe pain, complications such as penetration into other organs should be considered. Back pain suggests a penetrating posterior duodenal ulcer. Severe ulceration can occasionally be symptomless as 50% of patients who have died from the complications of peptic ulceration were unaware of the diagnosis prior to the final event. Patients can present for the first time with either a haematemesis or melaena or a perforation.

Untreated, the symptoms of a DU are periodic with spontaneous relapses and remissions. The natural history is for the disease to remit over many years with the onset of atrophic gastritis and a decrease in acid secretion.

Examination. This is usually unhelpful; epigastric tenderness is quite common in non-ulcer dyspepsia.

Diagnosis of *Helicobacter pylori* infection

Non-invasive methods

- ^{13}C Urea breath test (Fig. 6.12). This is a quick and easy way of detecting the presence of *H. pylori* and is used as a screening test. The measurement of $^{13}CO_2$ in the breath, after ingestion of ^{13}C urea, requires a mass spectrometer, which is expensive, but the test is very sensitive (98%) and specific (95%). The breath test is also used to demonstrate eradication of the organism following treatment.
- **Serological tests** detect IgG antibodies and are reasonably sensitive (80%) and specific. They are used in the diagnosis and in epidemiological studies. IgG titres may take up to 1 year to fall by 50% after eradication therapy and therefore are not useful for confirming eradication or the presence of a current infection. Antibodies can also be found in the saliva, but tests are currently not as sensitive or specific as serology.

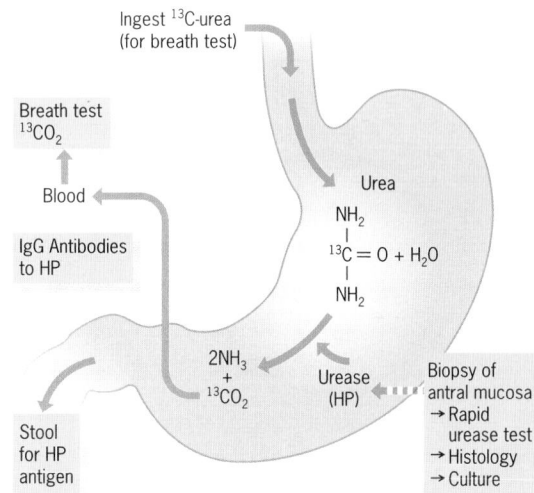

Fig. 6.12 Metabolism of urea by *Helicobacter pylori* (HP), showing the different tests that are available for the detection of *H. pylori*.

- **Stool test.** A specific immunoassay for the qualitative detection of *H. pylori* antigen is now widely available. The overall sensitivity is about 90% with a specificity of 95%. It is useful in the diagnosis of *H. pylori* infection and for monitoring efficacy of eradication therapy. (Patients should be off PPIs for 1 week but can continue with H_2 blockers.)

Invasive (endoscopy)

- **Rapid urease test.** Gastric biopsies are added to a urea solution containing phenol red. If *H. pylori* are present, the urease enzyme splits the urea to release ammonia which raises the pH of the solution and causes a rapid colour change.
- **Culture.** Biopsies obtained can be cultured on a special medium and sensitivities to antibiotics can be ascertained.
- **Histology.** *H. pylori* can be detected histologically on routine (Giemsa) stained sections of gastric mucosa obtained at endoscopy.

Investigation of suspected peptic ulcer disease

- *Patients under 45 years of age* with symptoms suggestive of peptic ulcer disease who are *H. pylori* positive often require no further investigation and can start eradication therapy.
- *In older patients*, confirmation of peptic ulcer is required. Endoscopy is the preferred investigation (Fig. 6.13) although barium studies are still often used depending on availability. All gastric ulcers (Fig. 6.14) must be biopsied.
- *In all patients* with 'alarm symptoms', (p. 254) endoscopy is required.

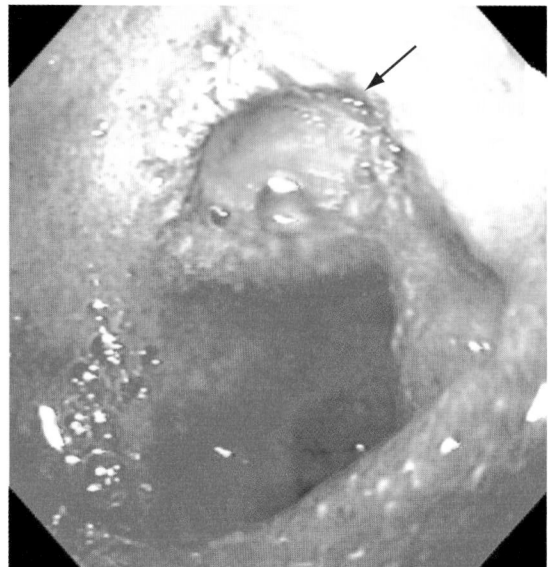

Fig. 6.13 Endoscopic picture of a benign gastric ulcer.

Eradication therapy

Current recommendations are that all patients with duodenal and gastric ulcers should have *H. pylori* eradication therapy.

Many patients, however, are now tested for *H. pylori* (see above) without the specific pathology in the stomach/duodenum being known. Some of these patients will have incidental *H. pylori* infection with no gastric/duodenal lesion and whether all such patients should have eradication therapy is controversial (see Functional dyspepsia, p. 325). There has been an increase in the prevalence of GORD and adenocarcinoma of the lower oesophagus in the last few years and some gastroenterologists thought this might be linked to eradication of *H. pylori*. This now seems unlikely and eradication of *H. pylori* is often advised in the hope that symptoms will be reduced and because of the link between *H. pylori* and gastric cancer.

All eradication therapies are successful in approximately 90% of patients.

Reinfection is very uncommon (1%) in developed countries. In developing countries, where compliance with treatment may be poor and metronidazole resistance is high (>50%) failure of eradication is common.

There are several regimens for eradication, but all regimens must take into account the following factors:

- the necessity of good compliance with the chosen treatment regimen
- the high incidence of antibiotic resistance to metronidazole (25%+)
- the side-effects of treatment with oral metronidazole
- bismuth chelate is unpleasant to take, even as tablets.

Currently favoured regimens are triple therapy with a PPI along with two antibiotics for 1 week. For example:

- omeprazole 20 mg + metronidazole 400 mg and clarithromycin 500 mg (all twice daily)
- omeprazole 20 mg + clarithromycin 500 mg and amoxicillin 1 g (all twice daily).

Resistance to amoxicillin has not yet been demonstrated.

Tripotassium dicitratobismuthate (bismuth chelate) binds to the ulcer crater and stimulates prostaglandin secretion. It is effective against *H. pylori* and is used in

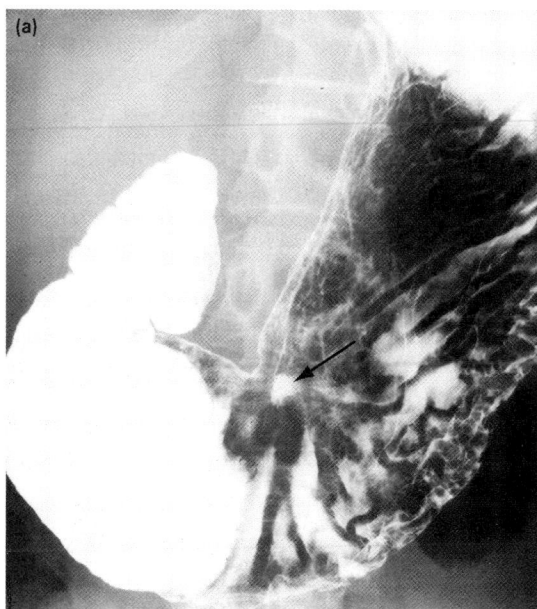

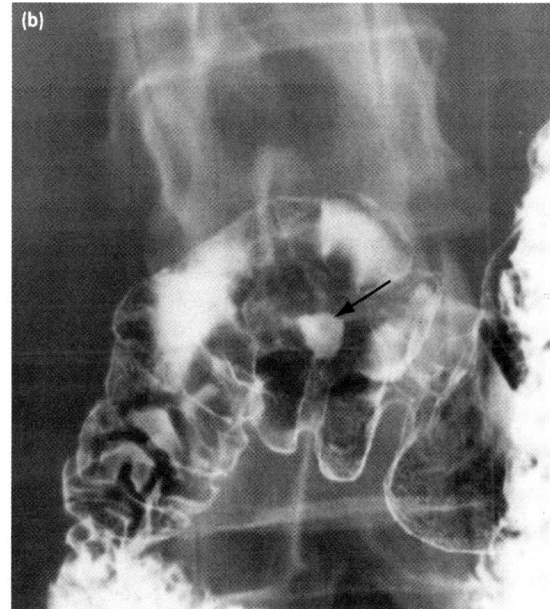

Fig. 6.14 **Barium meal,** showing **(a)** a large gastric ulcer (arrow) and **(b)** a chronic duodenal ulcer (arrow) on the posterior wall of the cap.

some eradication therapies with two antibiotics. It blackens the tongue and stools.

In some regimens, H_2-receptor antagonists, e.g. ranitidine or ranitidine bismuth citrate, are included instead of a PPI.

General measures
Stopping smoking should be strongly encouraged as smoking slows mucosal healing. Patients with peptic ulcers usually require 3–4 weeks' further treatment with a proton pump inhibitor after eradication therapy.

The effectiveness of treatment should be assessed symptomatically. If symptoms persist, a ^{13}C urea breath test or stool test for *H. pylori* should be performed to check eradication. Patients with complications, i.e. haemorrhage or perforation should always be tested to be sure eradication is successful.

A patient with a gastric ulcer should be re-endoscoped at 6 weeks to exclude a malignant tumour.

Complications of peptic ulcer
Haemorrhage
This is discussed on page 282.

Perforation (Box 6.5; see also p. 331)
The frequency of perforation of peptic ulceration is decreasing; this is partly attributable to better medical therapy. Duodenal ulcers perforate more commonly than gastric ulcers, usually into the peritoneal cavity; perforation into the lesser sac may occur.

Management of perforation
Detailed management is described on page 331. Surgery is performed to close the perforation and drain the abdomen. Conservative management using nasogastric suction, intravenous fluids and antibiotics is occasionally used in elderly and very sick patients.

Pyloric stenosis or obstruction
This is more accurately called gastric outflow obstruction, as the obstruction may be prepyloric or in the duodenum. The obstruction occurs either because of an active ulcer with surrounding oedema or because the healing of an ulcer has been followed by scarring. The obstruction can also be due to a gastric malignancy or external compression from a pancreatic carcinoma.

The main symptom of this condition is vomiting, usually without pain as the characteristic ulcer pain has abated owing to healing.

Vomiting is projectile and huge in volume, and the vomitus contains particles of yesterday's food. On examination of the abdomen the patient may have a succussion splash.

Severe or persistent vomiting causes loss of acid from the stomach and a metabolic alkalosis occurs (see p. 696).

Box 6.5

Management of a suspected perforated peptic ulcer

Look for:
- other acute gastrointestinal conditions (e.g. cholecystitis, pancreatitis – check serum amylase)
- non-GI conditions (e.g. myocardial infarction)
- silent perforations in the elderly or patients on steroids.

Remember:
- There is harm in leaving an undiagnosed perforation.
- Avoid laparotomy if pancreatitis is diagnosed.

The diagnosis is made by barium meal examination (less commonly by endoscopy) but can be suspected when large quantities of fluid are removed by gastric intubation in the fasting state. Fluid and electrolyte replacement is necessary, together with the regular removal of gastric contents via a nasogastric tube. In some patients with oedema rather than scarring, the symptoms will settle with this conservative management including acid suppression therapy. Most patients will require surgery although in some, endoscopic dilatation is successful.

Surgical treatment and its long-term consequences
Since the introduction of H_2-receptor antagonists in the 1970s and the eradication of *H. pylori*, surgery for peptic ulceration is used only for the complications:

- recurrent uncontrolled haemorrhage, when the bleeding vessel is ligated
- perforation, which is oversewn.

For both of these conditions no other procedure, such as a gastrectomy or vagotomy, is required.

Two types of operation were performed:

- *Partial gastrectomy*. The principle for this was to remove the antral area that secretes gastrin which stimulates acid production. In Billroth I partial gastrectomy, the lower part of the stomach was removed and the stomach remnant connected to the duodenum; in Billroth II (Polya gastrectomy), the stomach remnant was connected to the first loop of jejunum (a gastroenterostomy) and the duodenum closed. There was a very low recurrence of ulcer but a high complication rate (see below).
- *Vagotomy:*
  - (a) Truncal vagotomy plus gastroenterostomy/pyloroplasty.
  - (b) Selective vagotomy (preserving the hepatic and coeliac branch of the vagus) plus gastroenterostomy/pyloroplasty.

(c) Highly selective vagotomy or proximal gastric vagotomy, in which only the nerves supplying the parietal cells were transected, and therefore no drainage was required. With this type of operation there was less diarrhoea but the recurrence rate was still 5–10%.

Long-term complications of surgery are still seen occasionally.

A recurrent ulcer

This often occurred at the stoma. Epigastric pain is the main symptom although patients may present with haemorrhage. Endoscopy to visualize the ulcer and for the detection of *H. pylori* is performed. Treatment is with acid suppression and eradication of *H. pylori*, if present. Consideration should be given to the possibility of the Zollinger–Ellison syndrome (see p. 404).

Dumping

This is the term used to describe a number of upper abdominal symptoms (e.g. nausea and distension associated with sweating, faintness and palpitations) that occur in patients following gastrectomy or gastroenterostomy. It is due to 'dumping' of food into the jejunum, which is followed by rapid fluid dilution of the high osmotic load. A number of patients had mild symptoms of dumping but learned to cope with them. It was rare for it to be a clinical problem and, if it was, the symptoms had a functional element.

Diarrhoea

This was chiefly seen after vagotomy with occasional urgency and recurrent severe episodes (1%). Treatment is with antidiarrhoeals. The diarrhoea or steatorrhoea can be due to bacterial overgrowth in the blind loop of a Polya gastrectomy (see p. 275).

Nutritional complications

- Anaemia – mainly iron deficiency due to poor absorption.
- Occasionally folate deficiency due to poor intake.
- B$_{12}$ deficiency due to intrinsic factor deficiency.
- Patients often fail to gain weight owing to anorexia after gastric surgery.

Other *H. pylori*-associated diseases

Gastric adenocarcinoma

The incidence of gastric cancer parallels that of *H. pylori* infection in countries with a high incidence of gastric cancer. Serological studies show that people infected with *H. pylori* have a higher incidence of gastric carcinoma. For further discussion, see page 277.

Gastric B cell lymphoma

Over 70% of patients with gastric B cell lymphomas (mucosal-associated lymphoid tissue – MALT) have *H. pylori*. *H. pylori* gastritis has been shown to contain the clonal B cell that eventually gives rise to the MALT lymphoma. Some low-grade tumours regress with *H. pylori* eradication.

Gastropathy and gastritis

Gastropathy is the term used when there is epithelial/endothelial damage in the mucosa but there is little or no accompanying inflammation. Erosions and sub-epithelial haemorrhage are most commonly seen at endoscopy.

Gastritis is inflammation of the gastric mucosa.

The terms are often used loosely, particularly at endoscopy when any redness of the gastric mucosa may be described as 'gastritis'. Gastritis (as opposed to gastropathy) can only be readily diagnosed histologically.

The Sydney classification of gastritis was introduced in 1990 but has not been widely adopted because of the poor correlation between histological and endoscopic findings.

The commonest cause of *gastropathy* is mucosal damage associated with the use of aspirin and other NSAIDs and alcohol.

The commonest cause of *gastritis* is *H. pylori* infection (80%) and this is fully discussed on page 271. Auto-immune gastritis is seen in 5% while the remaining causes include viruses (e.g. CMV and herpes simplex), disorders of duodenogastric reflux and specific causes, e.g. Crohn's.

Erosive and haemorrhagic gastropathy

Aspirin and other NSAIDs deplete mucosal prostaglandins by inhibiting the cyclo-oxygenase (COX) pathway, which leads to mucosal damage. Cyclo-oxygenase occurs in two forms: COX-1, the constitutive enzyme, and COX-2, the inducible form which is produced by cytokine stimulation in areas of inflammation. NSAIDs more specific for COX-2 are now available (see p. 532) and these drugs have less effect on the COX-1 enzyme in the gastric mucosa. They still produce gastric mucosal damage but less than with COX-1 drugs.

Fifty per cent of patients on regular NSAIDs will develop gastric mucosal damage and approximately 30% will have ulcers on endoscopy. Only a small proportion of patients have symptoms (about 5%) and only 1–2% have a major problem, i.e. GI bleed. Because of the large number of patients on NSAIDs including low-dose aspirin for vascular prophylaxis, this is still a significant problem, particularly in the elderly.

H. pylori and NSAIDs are independent risk factors for the development of ulcers. There is little evidence to suggest that *H. pylori* infection increases the risk of ulceration in NSAID users.

Alcohol in high concentration damages the gastric mucosal barrier and is associated with acute gastric mucosal erosions and subepithelial haemorrhage which can lead to upper GI bleeding.

Acute erosive/haemorrhagic gastropathy can also be seen after severe stress (stress ulcers) and secondary to burns (Curling ulcers), trauma, shock, renal or liver (called portal gastropathy) disease. The underlying mechanism for these ulcers is unknown but may be related to an alteration in mucosal blood flow.

Management

In patients who develop problems, NSAIDs or alcohol should be stopped. For established ulcers, a PPI should be prescribed. There is a little evidence that *H. pylori* eradication is helpful.

In many patients with severe arthritis, stopping NSAIDs may not be possible. Use:

- an NSAID with low GI side-effects at lowest dose possible
- prophylactic therapy, e.g. PPI or misoprostol (see below) for all high-risk patients, i.e. over 65 years; those with a peptic ulcer history, particularly with complications, and patients on therapy with corticosteroids or anticoagulants
- COX-2 therapy (p. 532).

Other treatments

- Proton-pump inhibitors (PPIs) (p. 265). Recent evidence shows higher healing rates (80%) than with H_2-receptor antagonists and better patient compliance than with misoprostol.
- H_2-receptor antagonists can produce healing of ulcers, particularly duodenal.
- Misoprostol is a synthetic analogue of prostaglandin E_1 and inhibits gastric acid secretion. It is mainly used as a cytoprotective agent against NSAID-associated gastric ulcers, particularly in the elderly. Prophylaxis is 200 µg, two to four times per day. The main side-effects are diarrhoea and abdominal pain.

Autoimmune gastritis

This affects the fundus and body of the stomach (pangastritis), leading to atrophic gastritis with loss of parietal cells.

This leads to achlorhydria and intrinsic factor deficiency causing pernicious anaemia. Autoantibodies to gastric parietal cells and intrinsic factor are found in the serum (see p. 419).

Ménétrier's disease

This is a rare condition consisting of giant gastric folds, mainly in the fundus and the body of the stomach. Histologically there is hyperplasia of the gastric pits, atrophy of glands and an increase overall of mucosal thickness. Hypochlorhydria is usually present.

The patient may complain of epigastric pain and occasionally peripheral oedema may occur because of hypoalbuminaemia resulting from protein loss

through the gastric mucosa. It is possibly premalignant. Treatment is unclear as some patients improve spontaneously. Anti-secretory drugs are usually given. A few patients will require surgery.

Management of dyspepsia in the community

Dyspepsia (or indigestion) is very common in the general population. Over-the-counter antacids and H_2-receptor antagonists are available and are widely used.

Some patients' history is very suggestive of gastro-oesophageal reflux disease (GORD) and this subgroup of dyspepsia patients should be treated (see p. 265).

In young people (< 45 years) with dyspepsia, significant gastrointestinal pathology is very uncommon. Investigation with endoscopy is therefore not necessary. Their *H. pylori* status can be assessed serologically and, if positive, eradication therapy instituted. Further investigation should be reserved for those who remain symptomatic after successful eradication (p. 274). Patients who are *H. pylori*-negative on testing should be treated as functional dyspepsia (p. 326) which is much commoner than organic disease.

Older people (> 45 years) with new-onset dyspepsia and all patients with 'alarm symptoms' such as dysphagia, weight loss or gastrointestinal bleeding, must be investigated with endoscopy to exclude significant organic disease. Even in this age group, functional dyspepsia is very common and management of symptoms must reflect life event problems.

Therapies

Antacids are described on page 265.

H_2-receptor antagonists have molecular structures that fit the H_2-receptors on the parietal cells. They can produce up to 80% reduction in nocturnal acid production. They are useful in the management of dyspepsia and are part of some *H. pylori* eradication regimens. There is little difference between the several H_2-receptor antagonists available, but some have side-effects and cross-react with other medication, such as warfarin.

Proton pump inhibitors (p. 265) are also widely used. They are very effective for reflux symptoms and are also used in functional dyspepsia despite their cost as many find them helpful.

Gastric tumours

Adenocarcinoma

Carcinoma of the stomach (see Fig. 6.17) is one of the most common malignant tumours of the GI tract and is the sixth most common fatal cancer in the UK. The frequency varies throughout the world, being high in Japan and Chile and relatively low in the USA.

In the UK, 15 per 100 000 males are affected per year. Although the overall world-wide incidence of gastric carcinoma appears to be falling, even in Japan, proximal gastric cancers are increasing in the West. The incidence increases with age, being rare under the age of 30 years, and more men than women are affected.

Epidemiology and pathogenesis

There is a strong link between *H. pylori* infection and gastric cancer. *H. pylori* infection results in chronic gastritis which eventually leads to atrophic gastritis and intestinal metaplasia – a premalignant pathological change (Fig. 6.15). Much of the earlier epidemiological data (i.e. the increase of cancer in lower socio-economic groups) can be explained by the intrafamilial spread of *H. pylori*. *H. pylori* is recognized by WHO as a Class 1 gastric carcinogen.

Dietary factors may still be involved, as both initiators and promoters may have separate roles in carcinogenesis. Diets high in salt probably increase the risk. Dietary nitrates can be converted into nitrosamines by bacteria at neutral pH, and nitrosamines are known to be carcinogenic in animals. Nitrosamines are also present in the stomach of patients with achlorhydria, who have an increased cancer risk. Consumption of diets high in vegetables and fruits, and low in salt, protect against cancer. Smoking is also associated with an increased incidence of stomach cancer.

Genes underlying the inherited susceptibility to gastric cancer have not yet been identified, but certain patterns are emerging, as seen in colonic cancer. There is a higher incidence of gastric cancer in blood group A patients.

Benign gastric ulcers (see Fig. 6.14) have not been shown to develop into gastric cancer. It can, however, be difficult to differentiate a benign ulcer from a malignant ulcer, as even malignant ulcers can partially heal on medical treatment. For these reasons it was originally thought that gastric ulcers could become malignant.

Pernicious anaemia carries a small increased risk of developing gastric carcinoma. Atrophic gastritis present in the body and fundus of the stomach of these patients may be a precancerous lesion.

There is an increased risk of gastric cancer after a partial gastrectomy (postoperative stomach) whether performed for a gastric or a duodenal ulcer. This may be a reflection of *H. pylori* causing the original ulceration.

Screening

Gastric cancer has an appalling prognosis despite treatment, and earlier diagnosis has been advocated in an attempt to improve this. Unfortunately, earlier diagnosis does not necessarily mean longer survival. The patient is merely operated on at an earlier date and, although the survival may appear longer, death will still occur at the same time from the point of genesis of the cancer (called lead time bias) (Fig. 6.16).

With length time bias a greater number of slowly growing tumours are detected when screening asymptomatic individuals. In Japan, mass screening with mobile X-ray units has increased the proportion of early gastric cancers diagnosed. Early gastric cancer is defined as a carcinoma that is confined to the mucosa or submucosa. It is associated with 5-year survival rates of approximately 90%. In a large series of patients with gastric cancer from the UK, only 0.7% were identified as having early gastric cancer and therefore screening would not be warranted.

An effective screening procedure should:

- be cheap
- be acceptable to all social groups so that they attend for examination
- have a good discriminatory index from benign lesions
- result in an improvement in prognosis.

Unless all these criteria are fulfilled, screening is unwarranted except possibly in individuals with an increased

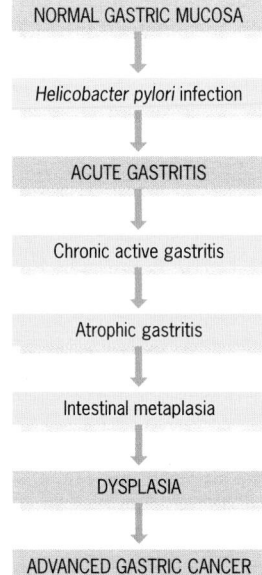

Fig. 6.15 Flow diagram showing the development of gastric cancer associated with *H. pylori* infection.

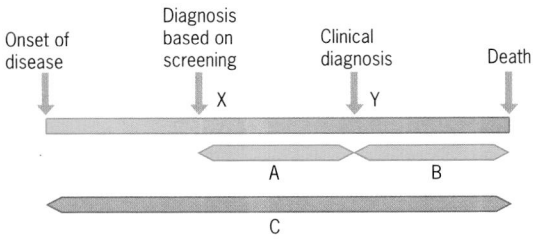

Fig. 6.16 **Lead time bias.** Earlier diagnosis, at X, made by screening tests before the clinical diagnosis, at Y, suggests an increased survival time of A + B compared with B. The actual survival time (C) remains unchanged.

risk for the disease (see above). Nevertheless, even in this high-risk group, screening asymptomatic subjects is not justified as the overall benefit is minimal.

An alternative approach to screening asymptomatic patients is to investigate symptomatic patients as quickly as possible in the UK. The mean interval between the onset of symptoms and attendance at hospital is approximately 6–9 months. However, dyspepsia is very common in the general population without any gastric lesions and it would obviously be impracticable for every dyspeptic member of the general population to consult a physician. Even if they did, most primary physicians would think it unjustified to arrange a complicated series of investigations on the first visit.

Thus, the detection of early gastric cancer in symptomatic patients is not a feasible proposition at present in the UK.

Pathology

Most gastric cancers occur in the antrum and are almost invariably adenocarcinomas. The common type is 'intestinal' and the tumours are polypoid or ulcerating lesions with heaped-up, rolled edges. Intestinal metaplasia is seen in the surrounding mucosa, often with *H. pylori*. The diffuse type is composed of scattered or small clusters of cells, often with extensive submucosal spread which may result in the picture of 'linitis plastica', where the stomach appears rigid on X-ray.

Clinical features

Symptoms

The most common symptom is epigastric pain, which is indistinguishable from the pain of peptic ulcer disease, both being relieved by food and antacids. The pain can vary in intensity, but may be constant and severe. Most patients with carcinoma of the stomach have advanced disease at the time of presentation, and also have nausea, anorexia and weight loss. Vomiting is frequent and can be severe if the tumour is near the pylorus. Dysphagia can occur with tumours involving the fundus. Gross haematemesis is unusual, but anaemia from occult blood loss is frequent.

Patients can present with metastases causing abdominal swelling due to ascites or jaundice due to liver involvement. Metastases also occur in bone, brain and lung, producing appropriate symptoms.

Signs

Nearly 50% of patients have a palpable epigastric mass with abdominal tenderness. Often weight loss is the only feature. A palpable lymph node is sometimes found in the supraclavicular fossa (Virchow's node) and signs of metastases are present in up to one-third of patients. Carcinoma of the stomach is the cancer most frequently associated with dermatomyositis (p. 563) and acanthosis nigricans.

Investigations

- **Routine full blood count and liver biochemistry.**
- **Gastroscopy** (Fig. 6.17). Gastroscopy is usually performed as the primary procedure and has the advantage that biopsies can be performed for histological assessment and to exclude lymphoma. Positive biopsies can be obtained in almost all cases of obvious carcinoma, but a negative biopsy does not necessarily rule out the diagnosis. For this reason, 8–10 biopsies should be taken from around the ulcer margin and its base. Superficial brushings for cytology will further improve the diagnostic rate.
- **Barium meal.** A good-quality double-contrast barium meal has a diagnostic accuracy of up to 90%. The carcinoma is usually seen as a filling defect or an irregular ulcer with rolled edges. With a diffuse (linitis plastica) infiltrating type, the X-ray may show a rigid stomach.

Staging

Imaging. CT can demonstrate gastric wall thickening, but has limited value in determining tumour invasion into adjacent tissues. Ultrasound can demonstrate masses and wall thickening. Liver secondaries can be detected. Endoscopic ultrasound can demonstrate the penetration of the cancer through the gastric wall and extension into lymph nodes. It complements CT and ultrasound.

The TNM classification is used (p. 478). The tumour (T) indicates depth of tumour invasion, N denotes the presence or absence of lymph nodes, M indicates presence or absence of metastases.

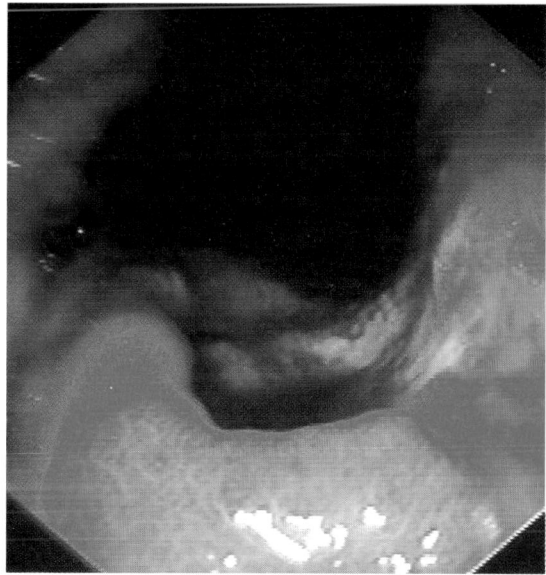

Fig. 6.17 Carcinoma of the stomach. Endoscopic picture showing a large irregular ulcer with rolled edges.

TNM classification is then combined with stage categories 0 to stage 4. At presentation, two thirds of patients are at stage 3 or 4, i.e. advanced disease.

Treatment

The 5-year survival rate of patients operated on for early gastric cancer (EGC) in Japan is 90%, but outside Japan EGC is rare. Surgery remains the best form of treatment if the patient is operable. Better preoperative staging has reduced the numbers undergoing surgery and has improved the overall surgical 5-year survival rates to around 30%. Five-year survival rates in 'curative' operations are as high as 50%. Despite these improved figures, the overall survival rate for a patient with gastric carcinoma has not dramatically improved, with a 10% 5-year survival.

Treatment with chemotherapy (see p. 505) is often given for unresectable lesions. Survival may be prolonged by a few months and better results are being obtained with a combination of cytotoxic agents. Adjuvant chemotherapy following apparently curative surgery has not been clinically successful but chemoradiotherapy may be effective.

Palliative care with relief of pain and counselling is essential, as described on page 507.

Stromal tumour

These tumours were known as leiomyomas or leiomyosarcomas. They are not of smooth muscle origin but are from the stroma and are thought to share a common ancestry with the interstitial cells of Cajal. They have a varying pattern of differentiation. There is a mutation in the cellular proto-oncogene *KIT* which leads to activation and cell-surface expression of the tyrosine kinas KIT (CD 117). They are usually asymptomatic and found by chance but they can occasionally ulcerate and produce a haematemesis.

Treatment is surgical. These tumours grow slowly and were thought to be benign, but histologically, tumours with more than 10 mitoses per 10 high-power fields are malignant and recurrences occur. Radiotherapy and chemotherapy have been advocated for these malignant tumours. A tyrosine kinase inhibitor is being used.

Primary lymphoma

Lymphoma of the stomach can account for 10% of all gastric malignancies in the developed world. It is a non-Hodgkin's lymphoma of the B-cell type. Gastric lymphomas in mucosal-associated lymphoid tissue (MALT) are caused by *H. pylori* (p. 271). The clinical presentation is the same as with gastric carcinoma. Some lymphomas due to *H. pylori* can be treated successfully by eradication therapy. Otherwise, treatment is surgical with postoperative radiotherapy and chemotherapy. Prognosis is good, with a 75% 5-year survival depending on the type of lymphoma.

Gastric polyps

These are uncommon and again are found usually by chance. They produce no symptoms. The most common are regenerative or hyperplastic polyps, which are often multiple and require no treatment. Rarely adenomatous polyps are found and endoscopic removal is recommended because of possible malignant potential. Most gastric cancers appear not to arise from pre-existing adenomas (in contrast to colonic carcinomas).

FURTHER READING

Blok N (1997) Carcinoma of the stomach. *Quarterly Journal of Medicine* **90**: 735.

Delaney et al. (2000) Cost effectiveness of initial endoscopy for dyspepsia in patients over 50 years of age. *Lancet* **356**: 1965–1969.

Fox JG, Wang TC (2001) Helicobacter pylori - not a good bug after all. *New England Journal of Medicine* **345**: 829–831.

Graham DY (2001) Therapy of H. pylori: current status and issues. *Gastroenterology* **118**: 52–58.

Hawkey CJ (2000) Non-steroidal anti-inflammatory drug gastropathy. *Gastroenterology* **119**: 521–535.

Laine L (2001) Approach to NSAID use in high risk patient. *Gastroenterology* **120**: 594–606.

Acute and chronic gastrointestinal bleeding

This section should be read in conjunction with the descriptions of the specific conditions mentioned.

Acute upper gastrointestinal bleeding

Haematemesis is the vomiting of blood from a lesion proximal to the distal duodenum. Melaena is the passage of black tarry stools; the black colour is due to altered blood – 50 mL or more is required to produce this. Melaena can occur with bleeding from any lesion from areas proximal to and including the caecum. Following a massive bleed from the upper GI tract, unaltered blood (owing to rapid transit) can appear per rectum, but this is rare. The colour of the blood appearing per rectum is dependent not only on the site of bleeding but also on the time of transit in the gut.

Aetiology

Chronic peptic ulceration still accounts for approximately half of all cases of upper GI haemorrhage. This and other causes are shown in Figure 6.18. The relative incidences of these causes vary depending on the patient population.

Drugs. Aspirin (even 75 mg a day) and other NSAIDs can produce gastric lesions. These agents are also responsible for GI haemorrhage from both duodenal and gastric ulcers, particularly in the elderly. Remember,

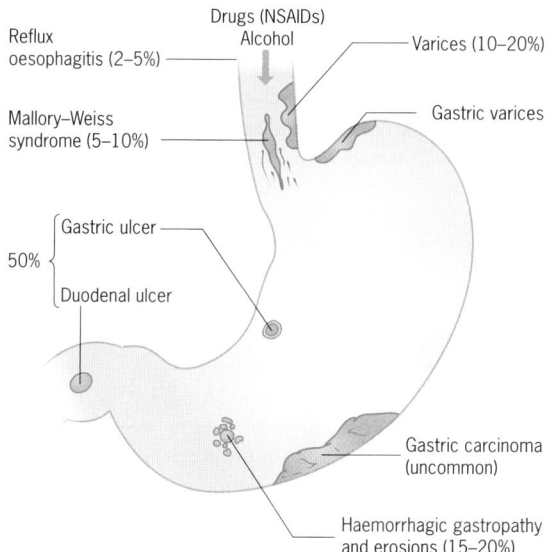

Reflux
oesophagitis (2–5%)

Drugs (NSAIDs)
Alcohol

Varices (10–20%)

Gastric varices

Mallory–Weiss
syndrome (5–10%)

Gastric ulcer

50%

Duodenal ulcer

Gastric carcinoma
(uncommon)

Haemorrhagic gastropathy
and erosions (15–20%)

Other uncommon causes
Hereditary telangiectasia (Osler–Weber–Rendu syndrome)
Pseudoxanthoma elasticum
Blood dyscrasias
Dieulafoy gastric vascular abnormality
Portal gastropathy
Aortic graft surgery with fistula

Fig. 6.18 **Causes of upper gastrointestinal haemorrhage.**
The approximate frequency is also given.

these drugs are available over the counter and careful questioning is necessary. Corticosteroids in the usual therapeutic doses probably have no influence on GI haemorrhage. Anticoagulants do not cause acute GI haemorrhage per se but bleeding from any cause is greater if the patient is anticoagulated.

Clinical approach to the patient

All cases with a recent (i.e. within 48 hours) significant gastrointestinal bleed should be sent to hospital. In many, no immediate treatment is required as often there has been only a small amount of blood loss and the patient's cardiovascular system can compensate for this. Approximately 85% of patients stop bleeding spontaneously within 48 hours. The cause of the haemorrhage may be obvious from the history, such as a long history of indigestion or, more significantly, previous haemorrhage from an ulcer. A history of aspirin or other NSAID ingestion suggests acute ulceration.

The following are additional factors that will affect the management:

- age (see below)
- the amount of blood lost, which may give some guide to the severity
- continuing visible blood loss
- signs of chronic liver disease on examination
- evidence of co-morbidity, e.g. cardiac failure, ischaemic heart disease, renal disease and malignant disease

---

> **!** **Emergency box 6.1**

Management of acute gastrointestinal bleeding

- History and examination.
- Monitor the pulse and blood pressure half-hourly.
- Take blood for haemoglobin, urea, electrolytes, grouping and cross-matching (2 units initially).
- Establish intravenous access – central line if brisk bleed.
- Give blood transfusion/colloid if necessary. *Indications for blood transfusion are:*
  (a) SHOCK (pallor, cold nose, systolic BP below 100 mmHg, pulse > 100 bpm)
  (b) haemoglobin < 10 g/dL in patients with recent or active bleeding.
- Oxygen therapy for shocked patients.
- Urgent endoscopy in shocked patients/liver disease.
- Continue to monitor pulse and BP.
- Re-endoscope for continued bleeding/hypovolaemia.
- Surgery if bleeding persists.

- presence of the classical clinical features of shock (pallor, cold nose, tachycardia and low blood pressure – see Emergency box 6.1).

With liver disease, the bleeding is often severe and recurrent if it is from varices. Splenomegaly suggests portal hypertension but its absence does not rule out oesophageal varices. Liver failure can develop.

With shock, remember that the peripheral arterial constriction that occurs may keep the blood pressure falsely high.

Immediate management

- Rapid history and examination.
- Note age of patient.
- Rapid assessment of haemodynamic state.
- Look for evidence of co-morbidity.
- Take blood for haemoglobin, urea, electrolytes, liver function, coagulation studies and for grouping and crossmatching.
- Stop drugs, e.g. NSAIDs, warfarin (see p. 470).

Urgent resuscitation is required in patients with large bleeds and the clinical signs of shock. Details of the management of shock are given in Figure 15.21. Many hospitals have multidisciplinary specialist teams with agreed protocols and these should be followed carefully. Such patients should be managed in high-dependency beds. Oxygen should be given by face mask.

Blood volume

The major principle is to rapidly restore the blood volume to normal. This can be best achieved by transfusion of whole blood via one or more large-bore intravenous cannulae. It may be necessary to give a blood substitute initially to a severely shocked patient or to a patient with blood compatibility problems.

The rate of blood transfusion must be monitored carefully to avoid overtransfusion and consequent heart failure. The pulse rate and venous pressure are the best guides to transfusion rates. All patients with organ failure and requiring blood transfusion as well as patients with severe hypotension should have a central venous pressure line.

Anaemia does not develop immediately as haemodilution has not taken place, and therefore the haemoglobin level is a poor indicator of the need to transfuse. If the level is low (less than 10 g/dL) and the patient has either bled recently or is actively bleeding, transfusion may be necessary. In most patients the bleeding stops, albeit temporarily, so that further assessment can be made.

Endoscopy

Endoscopy should be performed within 24 hours in most patients. Early endoscopy helps to make a diagnosis and to make decisions regarding discharge from hospital, particularly in patients with minor bleeds and under 60 years of age. Clinical risk scores are used in some centres to identify patients at low risk who do not require endoscopy.

Urgent endoscopy (i.e. after resuscitation) should be performed in patients with shock, suspected liver disease or with continued bleeding. Endoscopy can detect the cause of the haemorrhage in 80% or more of cases. In patients with a peptic ulcer, if the stigmata of a recent bleed are seen (i.e. a spurting artery, active oozing, fresh or organized blood clot or black spots) the patient is more likely to re-bleed.

At first endoscopy:

- varices should be injected – see page 368 for management of varices
- all bleeding ulcers should be either injected with epinephrine (adrenaline) and a sclerosant or the vessel coagulated either with a heater probe or with laser therapy.

These methods reduce the incidence of re-bleeding, although they do not significantly improve mortality as re-bleeding still occurs in 20% within 72 hours. In one study intravenous omeprazole substantially reduced the re-bleeding rate in this group and therefore should be given.

Drug therapy

There is little evidence that H_2-receptor antagonists or proton-pump inhibitors (PPIs) affect the mortality rate of GI haemorrhage, but PPIs are usually given to patients with ulcers because of their longer-term benefits. Somatostatin (which reduces the splanchnic blood flow as well as acid secretion) can be given as an infusion if the bleeding is difficult to stop, although a meta-analysis of clinical trials has shown no clear benefit.

Reassessment

- Age is clearly significant. Below the age of 60 years mortality from GI bleeding is small, <0.1%, but above the age of 80 the mortality is greater than 20%.
- Patients with recurrent haemorrhage have an increased mortality.
- Most re-bleeds (approximately 20% of all cases) occur within 48 hours.
- Co-morbidity invariably increases mortality.
- Melaena is usually less hazardous than haematemesis.

Uncontrolled or repeat bleeding

Endoscopy should be repeated to assess the bleeding site and to treat, if possible. Surgery is necessary only if bleeding is persistent and/or uncontrollable and should be limited to controlling the haemorrhage.

Discharge policy

The patient's age, diagnosis on endoscopy, co-morbidity and the presence or absence of shock should be taken into consideration. In general, all patients who are dynamically stable and have no stigmata of recent haemorrhage on endoscopy, can be discharged from hospital within 24 hours. All shocked patients need careful observation.

Specific conditions

Chronic peptic ulcer. Eradication of *H. pylori* is started as soon as possible (see p. 274). A proton-pump inhibitor is continued for 4 weeks to ensure ulcer healing. Eradication of *H. pylori* should always be checked in a patient who has bled. If necessary to control haemorrhage, surgery with ligation of the bleeding vessel is performed, but no other surgical procedure is undertaken.

Gastric carcinoma. Most patients do not have large bleeds with this condition but surgery is occasionally necessary for uncontrolled or repeat bleeding. Definitive surgery for the carcinoma should be delayed until the patient has been staged (p. 279).

Oesophageal varices. These are discussed on page 368.

Mallory–Weiss tear. This is a linear mucosal tear occurring at the oesophagogastric junction and produced by a sudden increase in intra-abdominal pressure. It often occurs after a bout of coughing or retching and is classically seen after an alcohol binge. There may, however, be no antecedent history of retching. The haemorrhage may be large but most patients stop spontaneously. Early endoscopy confirms diagnosis and allows early discharge from the hospital (within 24 hours). Rarely, surgery with oversewing of the tear will be required.

Prognosis

The mortality from gastrointestinal haemorrhage has not changed from 5–12% over the years, despite many changes in management, mainly because more patients are elderly. The lowest mortality rates are achieved in dedicated medical/surgical GI units. Early therapeutic endoscopy has not so far reduced the mortality, although bleeding episodes are reduced.

Acute lower gastrointestinal bleeding

Massive bleeding from the lower GI tract is rare. On the other hand, small bleeds from haemorrhoids occur very commonly. Massive bleeding is usually due to diverticular disease or ischaemic colitis. The causes of lower gastrointestinal bleeding are shown in Figure 6.19.

Management

Most acute lower GI bleeds start spontaneously. The few patients that continue bleeding and are haemodynamically unstable need resuscitation using the same principles as for upper GI bleeding (p. 281). Surgery is rarely required. Then a diagnosis is made using the history and the following investigations as appropriate:

- rectal examination (e.g. carcinoma)
- proctoscopy (e.g. anorectal disease particularly haemorrhoids)
- sigmoidoscopy (e.g. inflammatory bowel disease)
- barium enema – ischaemic colitis
- colonoscopy – for any mucosal lesion and removal of polyps
- angiography – vascular abnormality (e.g. angiodysplasia, which can be sometimes treated with argon plasma coagulation).

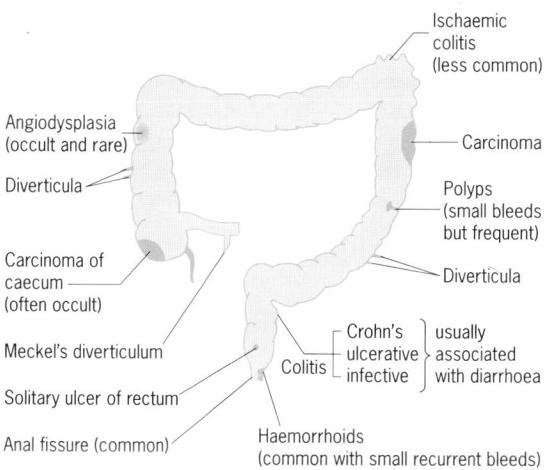

Angiodysplasia (occult and rare)

Diverticula

Carcinoma of caecum (often occult)

Meckel's diverticulum

Solitary ulcer of rectum

Anal fissure (common)

Ischaemic colitis (less common)

Carcinoma

Polyps (small bleeds but frequent)

Diverticula

Colitis — Crohn's / ulcerative / infective — usually associated with diarrhoea

Haemorrhoids (common with small recurrent bleeds)

Fig. 6.19 Causes of lower gastrointestinal bleeding. The sites shown are illustrative – many of the lesions can be seen in other parts of the colon.

Isolated episodes of rectal bleeding in the young (<45 years) only require rectal examination and sigmoidoscopy. Colorectal cancer is rare in this age group without a strong family history.

Individual lesions are treated as appropriate.

Chronic gastrointestinal bleeding

Patients with chronic bleeding usually present with iron-deficiency anaemia (see Ch. 8).

Chronic blood loss producing iron deficiency anaemia in all men and all women after the menopause is always due to bleeding from the gastrointestinal tract, often a right-sided colonic neoplasm which must be excluded. Occult blood tests are therefore not necessary (Box 6.6).

Diagnosis

Chronic blood loss can occur with any lesion of the gastrointestinal tract that produces acute bleeding (see Figs 6.18 and 6.19). It is, however, usual for oesophageal varices to bleed severely and rarely to present as chronic blood loss. It should be remembered that, world-wide, hookworm is the most common cause of chronic gastrointestinal blood loss.

Careful history and examination may indicate the most likely site of the bleeding, but if no clue is available it is usual to investigate both the upper and lower gastrointestinal tract endoscopically at the same session ('top and tail').

For practical reasons an upper gastrointestinal endoscopy is performed first as this takes only minutes, followed by colonoscopy when any lesion can be removed or biopsied. A barium enema is performed only if colonoscopy is unavailable.

A small bowel follow-through is the next investigation, but the diagnostic yield is very low.

Following negative investigations, a coeliac axis and mesenteric angiography may show the site of bleeding although the yield is low. Occasionally intravenous technetium-labelled colloid may be used to demonstrate

---

Box 6.6

Measurement of faecal occult blood

This is frequently performed *unnecessarily*. It is *only* of value in:

- premenopausal women – if a history of menorrhagia is uncertain and the cause of iron deficiency is unclear
- mass population screening for large bowel malignancy.

Advantages: cheap and easy to perform.

Disadvantages: high false-positive rate, leading to unnecessary investigations.

the bleeding site in a Meckel's diverticulum. Endoscopes to visualize the whole of the small bowel (enteroscopy) are available at specialist centres.

Treatment

The cause of the bleeding should be treated, if found. Oral iron is given to treat anaemia (see p. 465).

FURTHER READING

Jensen D M et al. (2000) Urgent colonoscopy for the diagnosis and treatment of severe diverticular haemorrhage. *Gastroenterology* **342**: 78–82.

Langman MJS, Weil J, Wainwright P et al. (1994) Risk of bleeding peptic ulcer associated with individual non-steroidal anti-inflammatory drugs. *Lancet* **343**: 1075–1078.

Lau JY et al. (2000) Effect of intravenous omeprazole on recurrent bleeding of peptic ulcers. *New England Journal of Medicine* **343**: 310–316.

Rockall TA et al. (1996) National audit for acute upper gastrointestinal haemorrhage. *Lancet* **347**: 1138–1140.

Rockall TA, Logan RFA, Devlin HB, Northfield TC (1995) Incidence of and mortality from upper gastrointestinal haemorrhage in the UK. *British Medical Journal* **311**: 222–226.

The small intestine

Structure

The small intestine extends from the duodenum to the ileocaecal valve. It is approximately 6 m in length, the upper 40% – the jejunum, the remainder – the ileum. Its surface area is enormously increased by mucosal folds. In addition, the mucosa has numerous finger-like projections called villi and the surface area is further increased by microvilli (Fig. 6.20). Each villus consists of a core containing blood vessels, lacteals (lymphatics) and cells (e.g. plasma cells and lymphocytes), and is covered by epithelial columnar cells that are absorptive. The crypts of Lieberkühn open into the lumen, between the villi.

The epithelial cells are formed at the bottom of these crypts and migrate to the tops of the villi, from where they are shed. This process takes 3–4 days. On its luminal side the epithelial cell has a brush border of microvilli that is covered by the glycocalyx. The lamina propria contains plasma cells, lymphocytes, macrophages, eosinophils and mast cells. Scattered throughout the gut are peptide-secreting cells.

Most of the blood supply to the small intestine is via branches of the superior mesenteric artery. The terminal branches are end arteries – there are no local anastomotic connections.

The *enteric nervous system* is linked to the central nervous system via the autonomic. The nerve plexuses in the mucosa, submucosa and muscularis propria are of three types:

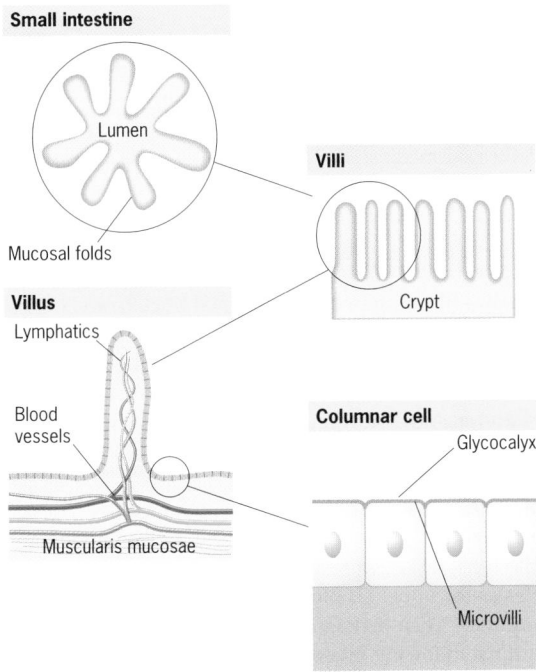

Fig. 6.20 Structure of the small intestine.

- cholinergic parasympathetic (with muscarinic or nicotinic receptors)
- adrenergic sympathetic (with both α and β receptors)
- non-cholinergic non-adrenergic (NANC).

For NANC the transmitters are thought to be either cyclic nucleotides and ATP (the purinergic system) or intestinal hormones (e.g. VIP – the peptidergic hypothesis) or nitric oxide.

Functions (Table 6.5)

The epithelial cells form a physical barrier permeable to ions, small molecules and macromolecules. The small intestine is concerned with the digestion and absorption of nutrients, salt and water. Digestive enzymes (e.g. proteases, disaccharidases) are produced by intestinal cells; some of these enzymes are membrane-bound whilst

---

Table 6.5
Functions of the small intestine

Digestion and absorption
Continuous cell renewal and cell death
Defence against antigen entry
    Structural
    Immunological – innate (see p. 191); e.g. antimicrobial peptides, trefoil peptides
    Immunological – acquired
Neuroendocrine peptide production
Motor function – transit of nutrients

others (e.g. lipases produced by the pancreas) are associated with the glycocalyx. Nutrients can be absorbed throughout the small intestine, but vitamin B$_{12}$ and bile salts have specific receptors in the terminal ileum.

General principles of absorption

Simple diffusion

This process requires no energy and takes place if there is a concentration gradient from the intestinal lumen (high concentration) to the bloodstream (low concentration).

Active transport

This requires energy and can work against a concentration gradient. A carrier protein is required and the process in the enterocyte is sodium-dependent. For example, glucose enters the enterocyte on the luminal side via a sodium-dependent carrier molecule (sodium/glucose cotransporter I, SGLTI) and leaves on the serosal side via a sodium-independent carrier (Glut-2) that is found in the basolateral membrane. A Na$^+$ gradient is maintained across the membrane by an energy-dependent sodium pump (Na$^+$–K$^+$-ATPase) that keeps the intracellular sodium concentration low (Fig. 6.21).

Facilitated diffusion

This is an energy-independent carrier-mediated transport system (Glut-5) that allows a faster absorption rate than simple diffusion (e.g. fructose absorption). Glut-5 has a very low affinity for glucose.

Absorption in the small intestine

Carbohydrate

Dietary carbohydrate consists mainly of starch with some sucrose and a small amount of lactose. Starch is a polysaccharide made up of numerous glucose units. Its hydrolysis begins in the mouth by salivary amylase. The majority of hydrolysis takes place in the upper intestinal lumen by pancreatic amylase. This hydrolysis is limited by the fact that amylases have no specificity for some glucose–glucose branching links.

The breakdown products of starch digestion, together with sucrose and lactose, are hydrolysed on the brush border membrane by their appropriate oligo- and disaccharidases to form the monosaccharides glucose, galactose and fructose. These monosaccharides are transported into the cells (Fig. 6.21).

Protein

Dietary protein is digested by pancreatic enzymes prior to absorption. These proteolytic enzymes are secreted by the pancreas as proenzymes and transformed to active enzymes in the lumen. The presence of protein in the lumen stimulates the release of enterokinase, which activates trypsinogen to trypsin, and this in turn activates the other proenzymes, chymotrypsin and elastase. These enzymes break down protein into oligopeptides.

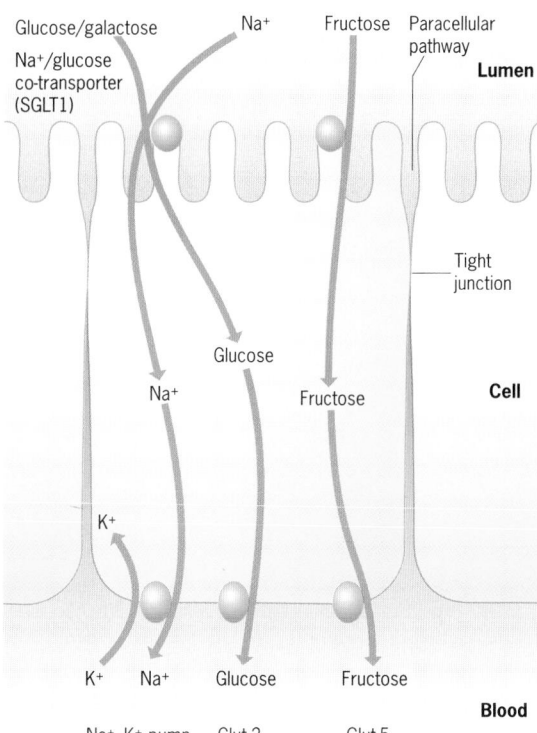

Fig. 6.21 **Solute (glucose, galactose, fructose) transport across the apical membrane,** showing glucose/galactose sodium-linked transport. Galactose is transported by the same mechanism as glucose. Fructose is transported across the apical and basolateral membranes down the concentration gradient. The sodium–potassium-ATPase pump is located in the basolateral membrane.

Some di- and tripeptides are absorbed intact by a carrier-mediated process, while the remainder are broken down into free amino acids by peptidases on the microvillus membranes of the cell, prior to absorption in a similar way to disaccharides. These amino acids are transported into the cell by a variety of carrier systems.

Fat (Fig. 6.22)

Dietary fat consists mainly of triglycerides with some cholesterol and fat-soluble vitamins. Emulsification of fat occurs in the stomach and is followed by hydrolysis of triglycerides in the duodenum by pancreatic lipase to yield fatty acids and monoglycerides.

Bile enters the duodenum following gall bladder contraction. Bile contains phospholipids and bile salts, both of which are partially water-soluble and act as detergents. They aggregate together to form micelles with their hydrophilic ends on the outside. Trapped in the hydrophobic centre of the micelles are the monoglycerides, fatty acids and cholesterol; these are then transported to the intestinal cell membrane. At the cell membrane the lipid contents of the micelles are absorbed, while the bile salts remain in the lumen. Inside the cell the monoglycerides and fatty acids are

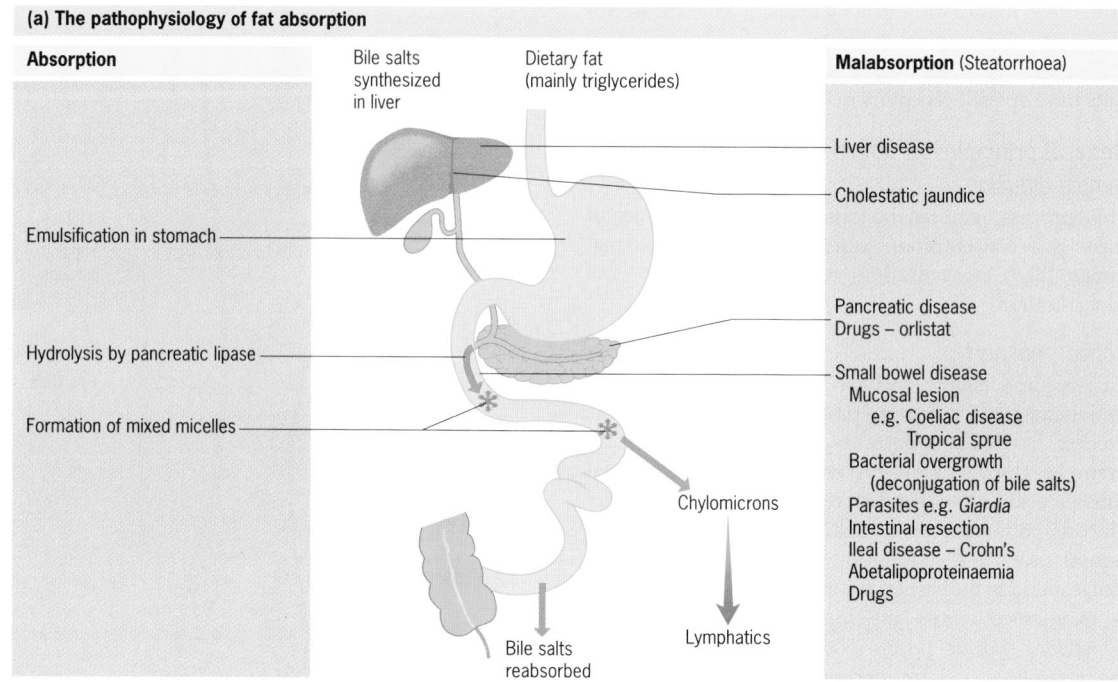

(a) The pathophysiology of fat absorption

| Absorption | Bile salts synthesized in liver | Dietary fat (mainly triglycerides) | Malabsorption (Steatorrhoea) |

Emulsification in stomach — Liver disease

Cholestatic jaundice

Hydrolysis by pancreatic lipase —

Pancreatic disease
Drugs – orlistat

Formation of mixed micelles —

Small bowel disease
    Mucosal lesion
        e.g. Coeliac disease
                Tropical sprue
    Bacterial overgrowth
        (deconjugation of bile salts)
    Parasites e.g. *Giardia*
    Intestinal resection
    Ileal disease – Crohn's
    Abetalipoproteinaemia
    Drugs

Chylomicrons

Bile salts reabsorbed

Lymphatics

(b) The formation of mixed micelles

Pancreatic lipase

Triglyceride   2-Monoglyceride   Bile salts micelle   Mixed micelle

Fig. 6.22 (a) **The pathophysiology of fat absorption.**
(b) **Diagram showing the formation of mixed micelles.**

re-esterified to triglycerides. The triglycerides and other fat-soluble molecules (e.g. cholesterol, phospholipids) are then incorporated into chylomicrons to be transported into the lymph.

Medium-chain triglycerides (which contain fatty acids of chain length 6–12) as well as a small amount of long-chain fatty acids are transported via the portal vein.

Bile salts are not absorbed in the jejunum, so that the intraluminal concentration in the upper gut is high. They pass down the intestine to be absorbed in the terminal ileum and are transported back to the liver. This enterohepatic circulation prevents excess loss of bile salts (see p. 339).

The pathophysiology of fat absorption is shown in Figure 6.22. Interference with absorption can occur at all stages, as indicated, giving rise to steatorrhoea.

Water and electrolytes

A large amount of water and electrolytes, partly dietary, but mainly from intestinal secretions, are absorbed coupled with monosaccharides, amino acids and bicarbonate in the upper jejunum. Some water and electrolytes are absorbed in the ileum and right side of the colon, where active sodium transport occurs but this is not coupled to solute absorption. Intestinal secretion also takes place and abnormalities of this mechanism cause secretory diarrhoea (see p. 320).

Water-soluble vitamins, essential metals and trace elements

These are all absorbed in the small intestine. Vitamin B_{12} (see p. 418) is the only substance other than bile salts that is specifically absorbed in the terminal ileum, and malabsorption of both these substances will always occur following ileal resection.

Calcium absorption

Calcium absorption is discussed on page 576.

Iron absorption

Iron absorption is discussed on page 412.

Defence against antigens (see also p. 191)

The small bowel excludes the entry of pathogens in several ways. Firstly, cells in the GI tract, including the surface epithelium, phagocytic and goblet cells, actively participate in the innate immune response. The mucus

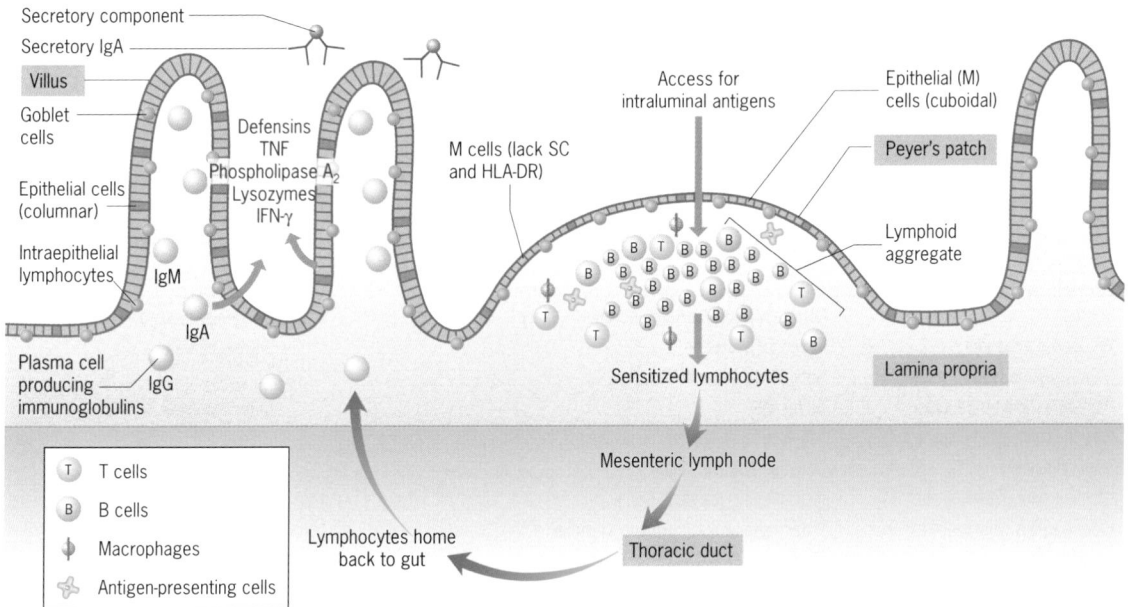

Fig. 6.23 Small intestinal mucosa with a Peyer's patch, showing the gut-associated lymphoid tissue (GALT). SC, secretory component; HLA-DR, human lymphocyte antigen-DR; TNF, tumour necrosis factor; IFN-γ, gamma-interferon.

layer overlaying the epithelium provides a physical barrier, and enzymes such as lysozyme, phospholipase A$_2$ and tumour necrosis factor secreted by the goblet cells ensure a sterile, infection-free environment in the gut, even in the presence of commensal bacteria. The epithelium and paneth cells also secrete various antimicrobial peptides (e.g. the defensin family) in response to infection and inflammation. These peptides have been shown to exhibit potent activity against various classes of pathogens including Gram-positive and -negative bacteria, fungi and viruses.

An additional source of long-term host defence is provided by the immune cells that participate in the adaptive immune response. Intestinal T cells occur principally in three major compartments: (a) organized gut-associated lymphoid tissue (GALT) such as the Peyer's patches; (b) the mucosal lamina propria, and (c) the surface epithelium where they are referred to as intraepithelial lymphocytes (IELs) (Fig. 6.23). GALT is the major site of antigen priming as it is dominated by a population of naive T and B cells.

Local mucosal immunity is provided by the secretory immunoglobulin (sIg) system. There are approximately 10^{10} Ig-producing immunocytes (plasma cells and plasmablasts) per metre of human small bowel, of which 70–90% are IgA immunocytes. Dimeric and polymeric IgA (pIgA) and IgM, containing a disulphide-linked polypeptide called 'J' (or 'joining') chain, are transported through the glandular epithelium via the transmembrane pIg receptor called 'secretory component' (SC) into the gut lumen. These antibodies are the first-line defence antigens in the lumen and may take part in the immunological homeostasis within the mucosa (e.g. dampening T-cell-mediated hypersensitivity responses against harmless absorbed luminal antigens). SC expression can be upregulated by lymphokines (e.g. IFNγ and TNFα) secreted by activated T cells and macrophages respectively, thus promoting the transport of IgA and IgM into the lumen.

A specialized epithelial cell above the Peyer's patches, called the 'M' or 'membrane' cell, lacks SC and HLA-DR expression; these cells allow non-selective inward transport of luminal antigens. Antigens may also be taken up by other epithelial cells (expressing HLA-DR) on a genetically restricted basis and may subsequently be presented directly by antigen-presenting cells (macrophages) to primed (memory) T lymphocytes.

In contrast to GALT, the lamina propria and the surface epithelium are effector compartments that receive primed T cells; while the CD4$^+$ subset is mainly retained in the former compartment, the CD8$^+$ subset predominates in the latter. At present, identification of the exact role of various T cell subsets in the pathogenesis of inflammatory gut diseases is being actively pursued in various laboratories.

Neuroendocrine peptide production

The hormone-producing cells of the gut are scattered diffusely throughout its length and also occur in the pancreas. The cells that synthesize these hormones are derived from neural ectoderm and are known as APUD (amine precursor uptake and decarboxylation) cells.

Table 6.6
Gut regulatory peptides

Hormone	Physiological action	Main gut localization
Gastrin family		
Cholecystokinin (CCK)	Stimulates gall bladder contraction and colonic motility	Duodenum and jejunum (I cells)
	Pancreatic secretion (minor role)	Enteric nerves
	Role in satiety	
Gastrin	Stimulates acid secretion	Gastric antrum, duodenum
	Stimulates growth of gut mucosa	
Secretin and related peptides (all possess structural homology with secretin)		
Secretin	Pancreatic bicarbonate secretion	Duodenum and jejunum (G cells)
Vasoactive intestinal polypeptide (VIP)	Intestinal secretion	Enteric nerves
	Splanchnic vasodilation	
Peptide-histidine methionine	As for VIP	Enteric nerves
Glucose-dependent insulinotropic peptide (GIP)	Facilitates insulin release by islets	Duodenum
	? Inhibits acid secretion	
Glucagon-like peptide-1 (GLP-1)	Increases insulin secretion	Ileum – pancreas
Glucagon-like peptide-2 (GLP-2)	Enterocyte-specific growth hormone	Ileum and colon (L cells)
Growth hormone-releasing factor (GHRF)	Unclear	Small gut
Other		
Pancreatic polypeptide	? Inhibitor of pancreatic and biliary secretion	Pancreas
Peptide YY	Inhibition of pancreatic exocrine secretion; slows gastric and small bowel transit ('ileal brake')	Ileum and colon (L cells)
Neuropeptide Y	Regulation of intestinal blood flow	Enteric nerves
Motilin	Increases gastric emptying and small bowel contraction	Whole gut
Ghrelin	Appetite stimulation, increases gastric emptying	Stomach
Bombesin	Stimulates pancreatic exocrine secretion and gastric acid secretion	Whole gut and pancreas
Somatostatin	Inhibits secretion and action of most hormones	Stomach and pancreas (D cells)
Galanin	Inhibits insulin secretion	Enteric nerves
Pancreastatin	Inhibits pancreatin exocrine and endocrine secretion	Pancreas
Substance P	? Unclear	Enteric nerves
Calcitonin gene-related peptide	? Unclear	Enteric nerves
Neurotensin	Affects gut motility. Increases jejunal and ileal fluid secretion	Ileum

Many of these hormones have very similar structures. Although they can be detected by radioimmunoassay in the circulation, their action is often local.

Table 6.6 shows some gut neuroendocrine peptides and their possible physiological actions. Many are also found in other tissues, particularly the brain. A number do not act as true hormones but act as neurotransmitters or have local effects on adjacent cells only (paracrine effects).

The exact physiological role of these peptides continues to be evaluated. Their importance clinically is that they may be secreted in excess, particularly in endocrine tumours of the pancreas (see p. 404).

Trefoil peptides

The trefoil factor family (TFF) of small proteins each consist of a three-loop structure. They help to protect the lining of the gastrointestinal tract by stabilizing the mucus in normal conditions and by upregulating and stimulating the repair process (e.g. epithelial restitution) in acute injury. TFF1 is produced predominantly by mucin-secreting cells of the stomach, small and large intestine. TFF2 is produced by mucus-producing cells of the stomach and by Brunner's glands and goblet cells in the small intestine, and is absent in the colon. TFF3 is absent from the stomach but secreted in the small intestine and colon. All three trefoil peptides can also be secreted ectopically in the cells around damaged areas (e.g. in inflammatory bowel disease and peptic ulceration).

Gut motility

The contractile patterns of the small intestinal muscular layers are primarily determined by integrated neural circuits within the gut wall – the enteric nervous system. The CNS and gut hormones also have a modulatory role on motility. The interstitial cells of Cajal lie within the smooth muscle. These mesenchymal cells appear to govern rhythmic contractions. During fasting, a distally migrating sequence of motor events termed the migrating motor complexes (MMC) occurs in a cyclical fashion. The MMC consists of a period of motor quiescence (phase I) followed by a period of irregular contractile activity (phase II), culminating in a short (5–10 minutes) burst of regular phasic contractions (phase III). Each MMC cycle lasts for approximately 90 minutes. In the duodenum, phase III is associated with increased gastric, pancreatic and biliary secretions. The role of the MMC is unclear, but the strong phase III contractions propel secretions, residual food and desquamated cells towards the colon, acting as an 'intestinal housekeeper'.

After a meal, the MMC pattern is disrupted and replaced by irregular contractions. This seemingly chaotic-fed pattern lasts typically for 2–5 hours, depending on the size and nutrient content of the meal. The irregular contractions of the fed pattern have a mixing function, moving intraluminal contents to and fro, aiding the digestive process.

Presenting features of small bowel disease

Regardless of the cause, the common presenting features of small-bowel disease are:

- *Diarrhoea.* This is a common feature of small bowel disease but approximately 10–20% of patients will have no diarrhoea or any other gastrointestinal symptoms. Steatorrhoea is occasionally present (Box 6.7).
- *Abdominal pain and discomfort.* Abdominal distension can cause discomfort and flatulence. The pain has no specific character or periodicity and is not usually severe.
- *Weight loss.* Weight loss is due to the anorexia that invariably accompanies small bowel disease. Although malabsorption occurs, the amount is small relative to intake.
- *Nutritional deficiencies.* Deficiencies of iron, B_{12}, folate or all of these, leading to anaemia, are the only common deficiencies. Occasionally malabsorption of other vitamins or minerals occurs, causing bruising (vitamin K deficiency), tetany (calcium deficiency), osteomalacia (vitamin D deficiency), or stomatitis, sore tongue and aphthous ulceration (multiple vitamin deficiencies). Ankle oedema may be seen and is partly nutritional and partly due to intestinal loss of albumin.

Physical signs of small bowel disease

These are few and non-specific. If present they are associated with anaemia and the nutritional deficiencies described above.

Abdominal examination is often normal, but sometimes distension and, rarely, hepatomegaly or an abdominal mass are found. In the severely ill patient, gross malnutrition with muscle wasting is seen. A neuropathy, not always due to B_{12} deficiency, can be present.

Box 6.7

Steatorrhoea

The stools:
- are pale, bulky, offensive and contain fat (> 17 mmol/day)
- float in the lavatory pan because of their increased air content
- are difficult to flush away.

Investigation of small bowel disease (Fig. 6.24)

Blood tests

- **Full blood count and film.** Anaemia can be microcytic (low mean corpuscular volume – MCV) or macrocytic (high MCV). The blood film may therefore be dimorphic and also show other abnormal cells (e.g. Howell–Jolly bodies which are seen in splenic atrophy associated with coeliac disease).
- *If the MCV is low,* serum ferritin and the serum soluble transferrin receptor are measured (p. 415).
- *If the MCV is high,* serum B_{12}, and serum and red cell folate are measured. However, with mixed deficiencies, the MCV may be normal. The red cell folate is a good indicator of the presence of small bowel disease. It is frequently low in both coeliac disease and Crohn's disease, which are the two most common causes of small bowel disease in developed countries.
- **Serum albumin** gives some indication of the nutritional status.
- **Low serum calcium and raised alkaline phosphatase.** These may indicate the presence of osteomalacia.
- **Autoantibodies.** Measurement in the serum of antibodies to endomysium, tissue transglutaminase, reticulin and gliadin are useful for the diagnosis of coeliac disease.

Small bowel anatomy

The macroscopic and microscopic appearances of the small bowel are studied unless the diagnosis has already been made (e.g. the presence of endomysial antibodies in coeliac disease).

- **Small bowel follow-through** (see p. 257). This detects gross anatomical defects such as diverticula, strictures and Crohn's disease. Dilatation of the bowel and a changed fold pattern may suggest malabsorption but, as these are not specific findings, the diagnosis should not be based on these alone. Gross dilatation is seen in myopathic pseudo-obstruction.
- **Jejunal biopsy.** This is used to assess the microanatomy of the small bowel. Biopsies are usually obtained via an endoscope passed into the

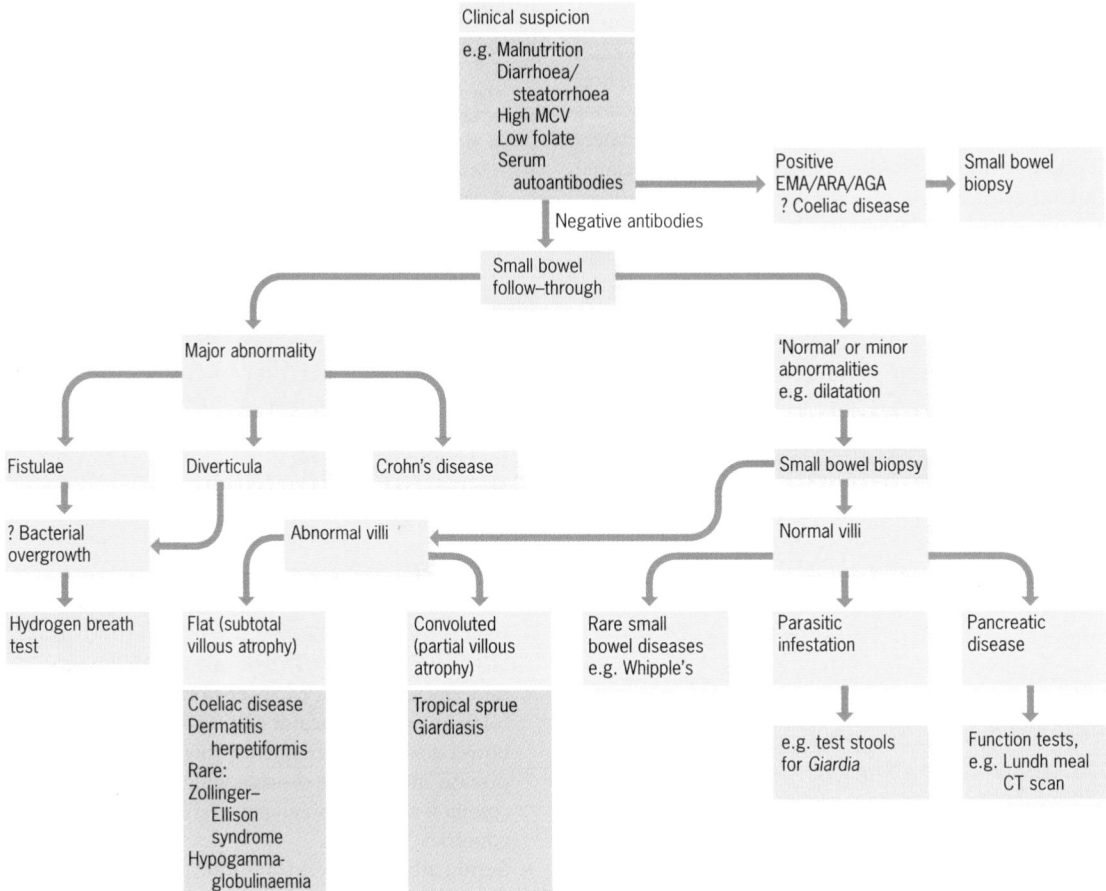

Fig. 6.24 **Flow diagram for investigation of patients with suspected small bowel disease.** EMA, endomysial antibody; ARA, anti-reticulin antibody; AGA, anti-gliadin antibody.

duodenum using large forceps. An adequate piece of tissue, well-orientated, is necessary for correct evaluation initially under a dissecting microscope. The histological appearances are described in the sections on individual diseases.

A smear of the jejunal juice or a mucosal impression can also be made and is helpful in the diagnosis of *Giardia intestinalis* (see p. 107).

Tests of absorption

These are required only in *complicated* cases.

- **Fat malabsorption.** The confirmation of the presence of steatorrhoea is only occasionally necessary. The fat content of stools is measured using a 3-day collection of faeces with the patient on a diet containing 100 g of fat daily. Normal faecal fat excretion is less than 17 mmol (6 g) per day. Spot samples of faeces can be used to avoid faecal collections but these are less sensitive. Fat absorption can also be measured using breath

analysis. Following oral administration of a radiolabelled fat load, the amount of $^{14}CO_2$ in the expired breath gives an indication of the amount of fat malabsorption. Comparison between a labelled triglyceride (^{14}C triolein) and a labelled fatty acid (tritiated oleic acid) is used to diagnose pancreatic disease, when fatty-acid absorption will be normal.

- **Lactose tolerance test.** This involves the oral ingestion of 50 g of lactose and the measurement of blood glucose. The test is of little use in adults as lactose intolerance is not a clinical problem since these patients avoid milk by choice. There is a high incidence of lactase deficiency in many parts of the world (e.g. the Mediterranean countries, and parts of Africa and Asia). It should be remembered that a glass of milk contains only approximately 11 g of lactose.

- **B_{12} absorption studies.** A Schilling test or whole-body counting technique is used (p. 419). In gastrointestinal disease, absorption studies are occasionally used in:

(a) pernicious anaemia (p. 418)
(b) ileal disease (when oral vitamin B$_{12}$ given with intrinsic factor will show malabsorption)
(c) bacterial overgrowth (measurement of vitamin B$_{12}$ plus intrinsic factor absorption is repeated after antibiotics).

Other tests

- **Hydrogen breath test.** This is frequently used as a screening test to detect bacterial overgrowth. Oral lactulose or glucose is metabolized by bacteria with the production of hydrogen. An early rise in the breath hydrogen will indicate bacterial breakdown in the small intestine. Rapid transit of the lactulose to the large intestine will also produce a rise in breath hydrogen. As bacteria are present in the oral cavity, the mouth should be rinsed out with an antiseptic mouthwash prior to the test being performed. This test is simple to perform and it does not involve radioisotopes. However, interpretation is often difficult with a low sensitivity and specificity.
- **^{14}C-glycocholic acid breath test.** This was performed to look for bacterial overgrowth. Bacteria deconjugate the bile salts, releasing [^{14}C]-glycine, which is metabolized and appears in the breath as ^{14}CO$_2$. It has largely been replaced by the hydrogen breath test.
- **Direct intubation.** Aspiration of intestinal juices is another method by which bacterial contamination can be detected, but is now seldom used. Bacterial counts are performed on aerobic and anaerobic cultures. Chromatography of bile salts can also be performed on the aspirate to detect evidence of deconjugation by bacteria.
- **Pancreatic tests** (see p. 396). These are used in the differential diagnosis of steatorrhoea.
- **Other blood tests.** Serum immunoglobulins are measured to exclude immune deficiencies. Hormones (e.g. vasoactive intestinal peptide – VIP) are measured in high-volume secretory diarrhoea.
- **Test for protein-losing enteropathy.** Intravenous radioactive chromium chloride (^{51}CrCl$_3$) is used to label circulating albumin. In excess gastrointestinal protein loss, the faeces will contain radioactivity. This test is rarely required unless a low serum albumin is a major clinical feature.
- **Bile salt loss.** This can be demonstrated by giving oral ^{75}Se-homochoyl taurine (SeHCAT – a synthetic taurine conjugate) and measuring the retention of the bile acid by whole-body counting at 7 days.

Malabsorption

In many small bowel diseases, malabsorption of specific substances occurs, but these deficiencies do not dominate the clinical picture. An example is Crohn's disease, in which malabsorption of vitamin B$_{12}$ can be demonstrated, but this is not usually a problem and diarrhoea and general ill-health are the major features.

Steatorrhoea – malabsorption of fat – is discussed on page 286.

The major disorders of the small intestine that cause malabsorption are shown in Table 6.7.

Coeliac disease (gluten-sensitive enteropathy)

Coeliac disease is a condition in which there is an inflammation of the jejunal mucosa that improves when the patient is treated with a gluten-free diet and relapses when gluten is reintroduced. Gluten is contained in the cereals wheat, rye and barley. Pure oats are not harmful.

It is closely related to dermatitis herpetiformis, a skin disorder that has an associated gluten-sensitive enteropathy (see below).

Incidence

Coeliac disease is common in Northern Europe, with an incidence in the UK of approximately 1 in 1000 although in Ireland it is 1 in 300. Population studies have shown a much higher prevalence of 1 in 200 as in many patients the disease is 'silent'. It occurs throughout the world, but is rare in the black African.

There is an increased incidence of coeliac disease within families but the exact mode of inheritance is unknown; 10–15% of first-degree relatives will have the condition, although it may be asymptomatic. The haplotype HLA-A1, B8, DR3, DR7, DQ2 (DQA °0501, DQB1 °0201) is seen in coeliac disease. Over 90% of patients will have DQ2, compared with 20–30% of the general population. However, the fact that not all patients have this haplotype, and that as many as 30% of identical twins are discordant for the condition, suggests an additional factor, e.g. environmental.

Aetiology

Gluten is a high-molecular-weight, heterogeneous compound that can be fractionated to produce α-, β-, γ- and ω-gliadin peptides. α-gliadin is the main damaging peptide to the small intestinal mucosa although the other peptides are also 'toxic'. There are many other immunological abnormalities that revert to normal on

---

Table 6.7

Disorders of the small intestine causing malabsorption

Coeliac disease
Dermatitis herpetiformis
Tropical sprue
Bacterial overgrowth
Intestinal resection
Whipple's disease
Radiation enteritis
Parasite infestation (e.g. *Giardia intestinalis*)

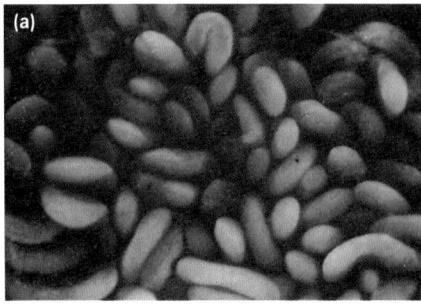

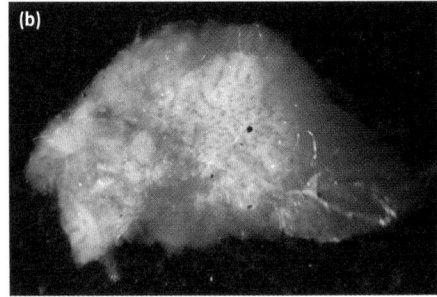

Fig. 6.25 Small bowel appearances on dissecting microscopy (DM) and histology. **(a) Normal mucosa DM. (b) Coeliac disease DM** – flattened mucosa. **(c) Normal mucosal histology. (d) Coeliac disease** – showing subtotal villous atrophy.

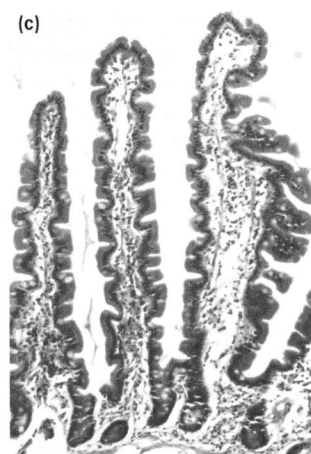

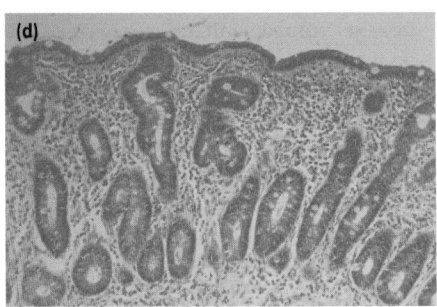

treatment. T cells play a central role in the aetopathogenesis and react with the enzyme tissue transglutaminase (the main antigen of the endomysial antibody). This enzyme is one of the targets of the autoimmune response; it modifies gliadin and enhances gliadin-specific T cell response in genetically predisposed individuals. An environmental factor, such as a viral infection, may play a role (e.g. adenovirus 12 which shows a sequence homology with gliadin). There are many other immunological abnormalities that revert to normal on treatment.

Pathology

The mucosa of the proximal small bowel is predominantly affected, the mucosal damage decreasing in severity towards the ileum as the gluten is digested into smaller non-toxic fragments.

Under the dissecting microscope there is an absence of villi, making the mucosal surface flat. Histological examination shows crypt hyperplasia with chronic inflammatory cells in the lamina propria (Fig. 6.25). The lesion is described as subtotal villus atrophy, although true atrophy of the mucosa is not present because the crypt hyperplasia compensates for villus atrophy and the total mucosal thickness is normal. A partial villus atrophy can also be found.

The surface cells become cuboidal. There is an increase in the number of intraepithelial lymphocytes (IELs) which show an increased expression of the γ/δ T-cell receptor, instead of the α/β receptor, and this is specific to coeliac disease and remains after treatment. In the lamina propria there is an increase in lymphocytes and plasma cells. A few patients just show an increase in IELs (latent coeliac disease) and others, e.g. relatives, a coeliac-like antibody pattern (potential coeliac disease).

Clinical features

Coeliac disease can present at any age. In infancy it appears after weaning on to gluten-containing foods. The peak incidence in adults is in the fifth decade, with a female preponderance. The symptoms are very variable and often non-specific with tiredness and malaise often associated with an anaemia. Common GI symptoms include diarrhoea or steatorrhoea, abdominal discomfort, bloating or pain and weight loss. Mouth ulcers and angular stomatitis are frequent and can be intermittent. Infertility and neuropsychiatric symptoms of anxiety and depression occur. Osteoporosis is common and occurs even in patients on long-term gluten-free diets. Rare complications include tetany, osteomalacia, or gross malnutrition with peripheral oedema. Neurological symptoms such as paraesthesia, muscle weakness or a polyneuropathy occur.

There is an increased incidence of atopy and autoimmune disease, including thyroid disease, insulin-dependent diabetes, primary biliary cirrhosis and Sjögren's syndrome. Other associated diseases include inflammatory bowel disease, chronic liver disease, fibrosing allergic alveolitis and epilepsy. IgA deficiency is more common than in the general population.

Physical signs are usually few and non-specific and are related to anaemia and malnutrition.

Investigations

- **Endomysial (EMA) and tissue transglutaminase (tTG) antibodies (IgA).** These antibodies have a high sensitivity and specificity for the diagnosis of untreated coeliac disease and can also be used as screening tests. They are now the investigation of first choice. An immunofluorescent test for endomysial antibodies can be performed on umbilical cord tissue or monkey oesophagus and the antigen is tissue transglutaminase. Anti-tissue transglutaminase antibodies are measured using an ELISA. In the presence of a typical clinical picture and the presence of these antibodies, a confirmatory small bowel biopsy may not always be required although most doctors prefer to have one.
- **Anti-reticulin antibodies (ARA)** are also very sensitive but not so specific, as they are seen in other gastrointestinal conditions (e.g. Crohn's disease). Anti-gliadin antibodies (AGA) are less sensitive.
- **Duodenal/jejunal biopsy.** The mucosal appearance (Fig. 6.25) of a small bowel biopsy specimen is diagnostic and regarded as the 'gold standard'. Other causes of a flat mucosa in adults are rare and are shown in Figure 6.24. At endoscopy, a dye can be injected on to the duodenal mucosa to accentuate the smoothness of the mucosa (positive dye test) before the biopsy is taken.
- **Haematology.** A mild or moderate anaemia is present in 50% of cases. Folate deficiency is almost invariably present in coeliac disease, giving rise in most instances to a high MCV. B_{12} deficiency is rare but iron deficiency due to malabsorption of iron and increased loss of desquamated cells is common. A blood film may therefore show microcytes and macrocytes as well as hypersegmented polymorphonuclear leucocytes and Howell–Jolly bodies due to splenic atrophy found in most patients.
- **Absorption tests** are often abnormal (see p. 290) but are seldom performed.
- **Radiology.** A small bowel follow-through may show dilatation of the small bowel with a change in fold pattern. Folds become thicker and in the severer forms total effacement is seen. Radiology is now mainly used when a complication, e.g. lymphoma, is suspected.
- **Bone densitometry** should be performed on all patients because of the increased risk of osteoporosis.
- **Biochemistry.** *In the severely ill patient*, biochemical abnormalities, e.g. hypoalbuminaemia, low calcium and high phosphate (osteomalacia) are seen.

Treatment and management

Treatment with a gluten-free diet usually produces a rapid clinical and morphological improvement. Replacement haematinics, e.g. iron, folic acid, calcium, are given initially to replace body stores. The usual cause for failure to respond to the diet is poor compliance. Dietary adherence can be monitored by serial tests for EMA, tTG. A repeat intestinal biopsy should be performed if clinical progress is suboptimal. A gluten challenge, i.e. reintroduction of gluten with evidence of jejunal morphological change, confirms the diagnosis, but is only performed if the diagnosis is equivocal. A transient gluten intolerance can occur in early childhood.

Despite advice, many patients do not keep to a strict diet but nevertheless maintain good health. The long-term effects of this low gluten intake are uncertain but osteoporosis is seen even in the treated case.

Patients should have pneumococcal vaccinations (because of splenic atrophy) once every five years.

Complications

A few patients do not improve on a strict diet (unresponsive 'coeliac disease'). Often no cause for this is found, but intestinal lymphoma, ulcerative jejunitis or carcinoma are sometimes responsible. The incidence of enteropathy-associated T-cell lymphoma (EATCL) (see p. 298) is increased in coeliac disease. Ulcerative jejunitis may present with fever, abdominal pain, perforation and bleeding. Diagnosis for these conditions is barium studies but laparotomy with full-thickness biopsies is often required. Steroids and immunosuppressive agents, e.g. azathioprine, are used. Carcinoma of the small bowel and oesophagus as well as extragastrointestinal cancers are also seen. Malignancy seems to be unrelated to the duration of the disease but the incidence may be reduced by a gluten-free diet.

Dermatitis herpetiformis (see also p. 1303)

This is an uncommon blistering subepidermal eruption of the skin associated with a gluten-sensitive enteropathy. Rarely there may be gross malabsorption, but usually the jejunal morphological abnormalities are not as severe as in coeliac disease. The inheritance and immunological abnormalities are the same as for coeliac disease. The skin condition responds to dapsone but both the gut and the skin will improve on a gluten-free diet.

Tropical sprue

This is a condition presenting with malabsorption that occurs in residents or visitors to a tropical area where the disease is endemic.

Malabsorption of a mild degree, sometimes following an enteric infection, is quite common and is usually asymptomatic. This is sometimes called tropical malabsorption. The term tropical sprue is reserved for severe malabsorption (of two or more substances) that is usually accompanied by diarrhoea and malnutrition. Tropical sprue is endemic in most of Asia, some Caribbean islands, Puerto Rico and parts of South America. Epidemics occur, lasting up to 2 years, and in some areas repeated epidemics occur at varying intervals of up to 10 years.

Aetiology

The aetiology is unknown, but is likely to be infective because the disease occurs in epidemics and patients improve on antibiotics.

A number of agents have been suggested but none has been shown to be unequivocally responsible. Different agents could be involved in different parts of the world.

Clinical features

These vary in intensity and consist of diarrhoea, anorexia, abdominal distension and weight loss. The onset is sometimes acute and occurs either a few days or many years after being in the tropics. Epidemics can break out in villages, affecting thousands of people at the same time. The onset can also be insidious, with chronic diarrhoea and evidence of nutritional deficiency.

The clinical features of tropical sprue vary in different parts of the world, particularly as different criteria are used for diagnosis.

Diagnosis

Acute infective causes of diarrhoea must be excluded (see p. 322), particularly *Giardia*, which can produce a syndrome very similar to tropical sprue.

Malabsorption should be demonstrated, particularly of fat and B_{12}.

The jejunal mucosa is abnormal, showing some villus atrophy (partial villus atrophy). In most cases the lesion is less severe than that found in coeliac disease, although it affects the whole small bowel. Mild changes can be seen in asymptomatic individuals in the tropics, so jejunal mucosal changes must be interpreted carefully.

Treatment and prognosis

Many patients improve when they leave the sprue area and take folic acid (5 mg daily). Most patients also require an antibiotic (usually tetracycline 1 g daily) to ensure a complete recovery; it may be necessary to give this for up to 6 months.

The severely ill patient requires resuscitation with fluids and electrolytes for dehydration; any nutritional deficiencies should be corrected. Vitamin B_{12} (1000 µg) is also given to all acute cases.

The prognosis is excellent. Mortality is usually associated with water and electrolyte depletion, particularly in epidemics.

Bacterial overgrowth

The upper part of the small intestine is almost sterile, containing only a few organisms derived from the mouth. Gastric acid kills most organisms and intestinal motility keeps the jejunum empty. The normal terminal ileum contains faecal-type organisms, mainly *Escherichia coli* and anaerobes. Bacterial overgrowth is normally only found associated with a structural abnormality of the small intestine, although it can occur occasionally in the elderly without.

Aspiration of the upper jejunum will reveal the presence of *E. coli* and/or *Bacteroides,* both in concentrations greater than 10^6/mL as part of a mixed flora. These bacteria are capable of deconjugating and dehydroxylating bile salts, so that unconjugated and dehydroxylated bile salts can be detected in aspirates by chromatography. Steatorrhoea (see p. 286) occurs as a result of conjugated bile salt deficiency.

The bacteria are able to metabolize B_{12} and interfere with its binding to intrinsic factor, thereby leading to B_{12} deficiency; this can be demonstrated with B_{12} absorption studies (p. 419). Conversely some bacteria produce folic acid giving a high serum folate.

Bacterial overgrowth has only minimal effects on other substances absorbed from the small intestine. The *clinical features* are chiefly diarrhoea and steatorrhoea. The vitamin B_{12} deficiency is not so severe as to produce a neurological deficit. Confirmation of bacterial overgrowth is with the hydrogen breath test (p. 291); aspiration studies are not routinely performed.

Although bacterial overgrowth may be responsible for the presenting symptoms, it must be remembered that many of the symptoms may be due to the underlying small bowel pathology.

Treatment

If possible, the underlying lesion should be corrected (e.g. a stricture should be resected). With multiple diverticula, grossly dilated bowel, or in Crohn's disease, this may not be possible and rotating courses of antibiotics are necessary, such as metronidazole, a tetracycline, or ciprofloxacin.

Intestinal resection (Fig. 6.26)

Intestinal resection is usually well tolerated, but massive resection is followed by the short-bowel syndrome. The effects of resection depend on the extent and the areas involved. Because the gut is long, a 30–50% resection can usually be tolerated without undue problems. Residual jejunum shows less capacity for structural and functional adaptation than residual ileum.

Ileal resection

The ileum has specific receptors for the absorption of bile salts and vitamin B_{12}, so that relatively small resections will lead to malabsorption of these substances.

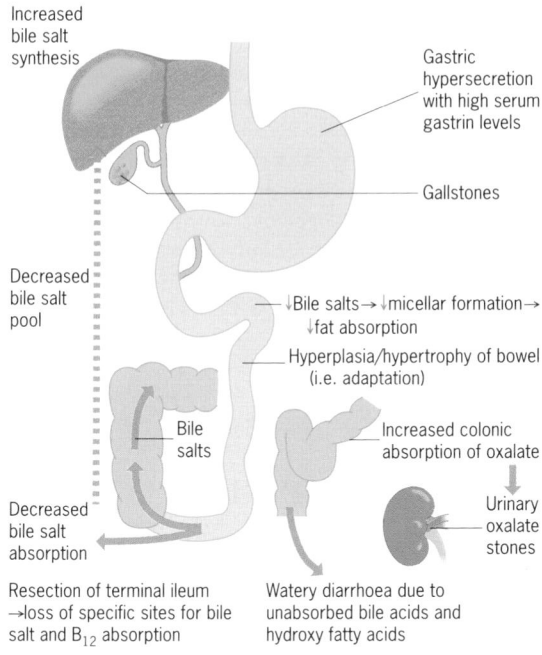

Increased bile salt synthesis

Gastric hypersecretion with high serum gastrin levels

Gallstones

Decreased bile salt pool

↓Bile salts→↓micellar formation→ ↓fat absorption

Hyperplasia/hypertrophy of bowel (i.e. adaptation)

Bile salts

Increased colonic absorption of oxalate

Urinary oxalate stones

Decreased bile salt absorption

Resection of terminal ileum →loss of specific sites for bile salt and B₁₂ absorption

Watery diarrhoea due to unabsorbed bile acids and hydroxy fatty acids

Fig. 6.26 **The effects of resection of distal small bowel.**

Removal of the ileocaecal valve increases the incidence of diarrhoea. The following occur in ileal resection:

- Bile salts and fatty acids enter the colon and cause malabsorption of water and electrolytes leading to diarrhoea (p. 322).
- Increased bile salt synthesis can compensate for loss of approximately one-third of the bile salts in the faeces. Greater loss than this results in decreased micellar formation and steatorrhoea, and lithogenic bile and gallstone formation.
- Increased oxalate absorption is caused by the presence of bile salts in the colon. This gives rise to renal oxalate stones.
- There is a low serum B₁₂ and macrocytosis.
- Glucagon-like peptide 2 (GLP-2) is low following ileal resection. GLP-2 is a specific growth hormone for the enterocyte and this deficiency may explain the lack of adaptation with an ileal resection.

Investigations include a small bowel follow-through, measurement of B₁₂, bile salts and occasionally fat absorption (see p. 291). A hydrogen breath test will show rapid transit (p. 291). Many patients require B₁₂ replacement and some need a low-fat diet if there is steatorrhoea. If diarrhoea is a problem, colestyramine, which binds bile salts, often helps.

Jejunal resection

The ileum can take over the jejunal absorptive function. Jejunal resection may lead to gastric hypersecretion with high gastrin levels; the exact mechanism of this is

unclear. Structural and functional intestinal adaptation take place over the course of a year, with an increase in the absorption per unit length of bowel.

Massive intestinal resection (short-bowel syndrome)

This most often occurs following resection for Crohn's disease, mesenteric vessel occlusion (p. 297), radiation enteritis (see p. 296) or trauma. There are two types of short-bowel syndrome:

Shortened small intestine ending at a terminal stoma
The major problem is of sodium and fluid depletion and the majority of patients with 100 cm or less of jejunum remaining will require parenteral supplements of fluid and electrolytes, often with nutrients. Sodium losses can by minimized by increasing salt intake, restricting clear fluids between meals and administering oral glucose–electrolyte mixture with a sodium concentration >90 mmol/L. Jejunal transit time can be increased and stomal effluent loss of fluids and electrolytes reduced by treatment with the somatostatin analogue octreotide, and to a much lesser extent, with loperamide, codeine phosphate or co-phenotrope. There is no benefit of a low-fat diet, but fat assimilation can be increased on treatment with colestyramine and synthetic bile acids.

Shortened small intestine in continuity with colon
Only a small proportion of these patients require parenteral supplementation of fluid, electrolytes and nutrients because of the absorptive capacity of the colon for fluid and electrolytes. Unabsorbed fat results in impairment of colonic fluid and electrolyte absorption so patients should be on a low-fat diet. A high carbohydrate intake is advised as unabsorbed carbohydrate is metabolized anaerobically to short-chain fatty acids (SCFAs). SCFAs are absorbed and act as an energy source (1.6 kcal/g) and stimulate fluid and electrolyte absorption in the colon. Patients are often treated with colestyramine, which binds dihydroxy bile acids which otherwise have a deleterious effect on colonic fluid and electrolyte absorption and increase colonic oxalate absorption to form renal stones.

Whipple's disease
This is a rare disease usually affecting males. It presents with steatorrhoea and abdominal pain along with systemic symptoms of fever and weight loss. Peripheral lymphadenopathy, arthritis and involvement of the heart, lung and brain may occur. Histologically, in the small bowel, the villi are stunted and contain diagnostic periodic acid–Schiff (PAS)-positive macrophages. On electron microscopy, bacilli can be seen 'within' the macrophages. The organism was identified by the polymerase chain reaction but can be cultured; it is similar to the actinomycetes and has been given the name *Tropheryma whippeii*. A dramatic improvement occurs

with antibiotic therapy, which should include an antibiotic that crosses the blood–brain barrier (e.g. co-trimoxazole) for 6 months.

Radiation enteritis

Radiation of more than 40 Gy will damage the intestine. The ileum and rectum are the areas most often involved, as pelvic irradiation is frequently used for gynaecological and urinary tract malignancies. There may be nausea, vomiting, diarrhoea and abdominal pain at the time of the irradiation. These symptoms usually improve within 6 weeks after completion of therapy. Chronic radiation enteritis is diagnosed if symptoms persist for 3 months or more. The prevalence is more than 15%. Many patients suffer from an increased bowel frequency.

Radiation produces muscle fibre atrophy, ulcerative changes due to ischaemia, and obstruction due to strictures produced by radiation-induced fibrosis. Abdominal pain is the main symptom due to the obstruction, which is usually partial but eventually may be complete. Malabsorption due to mucosal damage as well as bacterial overgrowth in dilated segments can occur. Treatment is symptomatic although often unsuccessful in chronic enteritis. Surgery should be avoided if at all possible, being reserved for life-threatening situations such as complete obstruction or occasionally perforation. Radiation damage to the rectum produces a radiation proctitis with diarrhoea, with or without blood and tenesmus. Local steroids sometimes help initially. The telangiectasia that form and cause persistent bleeding can be treated with argon plasma coagulation or by placing a formalin-soaked swab in the rectum (for 2 min), both of which heal the lesions.

Parasite infestation

Giardia intestinalis (see p. 107) not only produces diarrhoea but can produce malabsorption with steatorrhoea. Minor changes are seen in the jejunal mucosa and the organism can be found in the jejunal fluid or mucosa.

Cryptosporidiosis (see p. 96) can also produce malabsorption.

Patients with HIV infection are particularly prone to parasitic infestation (see Table 6.21).

Other causes of malabsorption

- Drugs that bind bile salts (e.g. colestyramine) and some antibiotics (e.g. neomycin) produce steatorrhoea.
- Orlistat (p. 244) inhibits gastric and pancreatic lipase, reducing fat absorption. It is used in obesity; its side-effect is diarrhoea and steatorrhoea.
- Diarrhoea, rarely with steatorrhoea, occurs in thyrotoxicosis owing to increased gastric emptying and increased motility. Steatorrhoea occurs in the Zollinger–Ellison syndrome (see p. 404).

- Intestinal lymphangiectasia produces diarrhoea and rarely steatorrhoea (see p. 289).
- Lymphoma that has infiltrated the small bowel mucosa causes malabsorption.
- In some patients with diabetes mellitus, diarrhoea, malabsorption and steatorrhoea occur, sometimes due to bacterial overgrowth from stasis.
- Hypogammaglobulinaemia, which is seen in a number of conditions including lymphoid nodular hyperplasia, causes steatorrhoea due either to an abnormal jejunal mucosa or to secondary infestation with *Giardia intestinalis.*

Miscellaneous intestinal diseases

Protein-losing enteropathy

Protein-losing enteropathy is seen in many gastrointestinal and systemic conditions. Increased protein loss across an abnormal mucosa causes hypoalbuminaemia. Causes include inflammatory or ulcerative lesions (e.g. Crohn's disease), tumours, Ménétrier's disease, coeliac disease and lymphatic disorders (e.g. lymphangiectasia). Usually protein-losing enteropathy forms a minor part of the generalized disorder, but occasionally hepatic synthesis of albumin cannot compensate for the hypoalbuminaemia, and the peripheral oedema produced may dominate the clinical picture. The investigations are described on page 291 and treatment is that of the underlying disorder.

Meckel's diverticulum

This is the most common congenital abnormality of the GI tract, affecting 2–3% of the population. The diverticulum projects from the wall of the ileum approximately 60 cm from the ileocaecal valve. It is usually symptomless, but 50% contain gastric mucosa that secretes hydrochloric acid. Peptic ulcers can occur and may bleed (see p. 283) or perforate.

Acute inflammation of the diverticulum also occurs and is indistinguishable clinically from acute appendicitis. Obstruction from an associated band rarely occurs. Treatment is surgical removal, often laparoscopically.

Tuberculosis

Tuberculosis (TB) can affect the intestine as well as the peritoneum (see p. 333).

Intestinal tuberculosis is due to reactivation of primary disease caused by *M. tuberculosis*. Bovine TB occurs in areas where milk is unpasteurized and is very rare in the UK. The ileocaecal area is most commonly affected, but the colon, and rarely other parts of the gastrointestinal tract, can be involved too.

Tuberculosis is being seen more frequently in patients with HIV infection.

Clinical features

These are chiefly diarrhoea and abdominal pain with generalized systemic manifestations, including fever, anorexia and weight loss. One-third of patients present acutely with intestinal obstruction or generalized peritonitis.

On examination, a mass may be palpable in the right iliac fossa and 50% have X-ray evidence of pulmonary tuberculosis.

Diagnosis

In the West, TB must be differentiated from Crohn's disease and should always be considered as a possible diagnosis in Asian immigrants. A caecal carcinoma can present with similar symptoms. A small bowel follow-through will show transverse ulceration, diffuse narrowing of the bowel with shortening of the caecal pole. An ultrasound or CT may show additional mesenteric thickening and lymph node enlargement. Histological verification and culture of tissue is highly desirable, but it is not always possible to obtain bacteriological confirmation and treatment should be started if there is a high degree of suspicion. Specimens can be obtained by colonoscopy but laparotomy is required in some cases.

Treatment

Drug treatment is similar to that for pulmonary TB – rifampicin, isoniazid and pyrazinamide (see p. 895) – but treatment should last 1 year.

Amyloid (see also p. 1118)

In systemic amyloidosis there is usually diffuse involvement that may affect any part of the GI tract. Occasionally amyloid deposits occur as polypoid lesions. The symptoms depend on the site of involvement; amyloidosis in the small intestine gives rise to diarrhoea.

Connective-tissue disorders

Systemic sclerosis (see p. 561) most commonly affects the oesophagus (p. 267), although the small bowel and colon are often found to be involved if the appropriate radiological studies are performed. Frequently there are no symptoms of this involvement, but diarrhoea and steatorrhoea can occur. This is usually due to bacterial overgrowth of the small bowel as a result of reduced motility, dilatation and the presence of diverticula.

In *rheumatoid arthritis* (p. 537) and systemic lupus erythematosus (p. 557), gastrointestinal symptoms may occur, but rarely predominate.

Intestinal ischaemia

Intestinal ischaemia results from occlusion of arterial inflow, occlusion of venous outflow or failure of perfusion; these factors may act singularly or in combination and usually occur in the elderly.

- *Arterial inflow occlusion:*
  - atheroma
  - thrombosis
  - embolus (cardiac arrhythmia) including cholesterol (p. 624)
  - aortic disease (occluding ostia of mesenteric vessels)
  - vasculitis (see p. 567), thromboangiitis and Takayasu's syndrome (p. 831)
  - neoplasia (occlusion of vessels-rare).
- *Venous outflow occlusion:* 5–15% of cases and usually occurs in sick patients with circulatory failure.
- *Infarction without occlusion.* Approximately one third of patients dying with acute ischaemic necrosis of the small intestine have no demonstrable occlusion of a major vessel. Reduced cardiac output, hypotension and shock are the main causes of reduced intestinal blood flow leading to non-occlusive infarction.

Acute small intestinal ischaemia

Patients present with sudden abdominal pain and vomiting. An embolus from the heart in a patient with atrial fibrillation is the commonest cause, usually occluding the superior mesenteric artery. The abdomen is usually distended, tender and bowel sounds are absent. The patient is hypotensive and ill. Treatment is surgical and gangrenous bowel is resected. Mortality is high (up to 90%) and is related to coexisting disease, the development of multiorgan failure (MOF) (p. 943) and massive fluid and electrolyte losses in the postoperative period. Survivors go on to develop nutritionally inadequate short-bowel syndrome (see p. 295).

Ischaemic colitis

See page 314.

Chronic small intestinal ischaemia

This is due to atheromatous occlusion or cholesterol emboli of the mesenteric vessels, particularly in the elderly. Such an occlusion does not always produce clinical effects because of the collateral circulation. The characteristic symptom is abdominal pain occurring after food. This may be followed by acute mesenteric vascular occlusion. Loud bruits may be heard but, as these are heard in normal subjects, they are of doubtful significance. The diagnosis is made using angiography.

The term 'coeliac axis compression syndrome' has been used in young patients with chronic abdominal pain, bruits and minor angiographic changes. Despite its plausible title, it is not an organic syndrome. Its suggested existence results from the false correlation of pain and bruits.

Eosinophilic gastroenteritis

In this condition of unknown aetiology there is eosinophilic infiltration and oedema of any part of the gastrointestinal mucosa. The gastric antrum and proximal small intestine are usually involved either as a localized lesion (eosinophilic granuloma) or diffusely with sheets of eosinophils seen in the serosal and submucosal layers. An association with asthma, eczema and urticaria has been described.

The condition occurs mainly in the third decade. The clinical presentation depends on the site of gut involvement. Abdominal pain, nausea and vomiting and upper GI bleeding occur. Eosinophilia occurs in only 20% of patients. Radiology or endoscopy will demonstrate the lesion. Steroids are used for the widespread infiltration, particularly if peripheral eosinophilia is present.

In some adults the condition appears to be allergic (allergic gastroenteritis) and is associated with peripheral eosinophilia and high levels of blood and tissue IgE.

Intestinal lymphangiectasia

Dilatation of the lymphatics may be primary or secondary to lymphatic obstruction, such as occurs in malignancy or constrictive pericarditis. In the rare primary form it may be detected incidentally as dilated lacteals on a jejunal biopsy or it can produce steatorrhoea of varying degrees. Hypoproteinaemia with ankle oedema is the other main feature. Serum immunoglobulin levels are reduced with low circulating lymphocytes. Treatment is with a low-fat diet.

Abetalipoproteinaemia

In this rare condition, there is failure of apo B-100 synthesis in the liver and apo B-48 in the intestinal cell, so that chylomicrons are not formed. This leads to fat accumulation in the intestinal cells, giving a characteristic histological appearance to the jejunal mucosa. Clinical features include acanthocytosis (spiky red cells owing to membrane abnormalities), a form of retinitis pigmentosa, and mental and neurological abnormalities. The latter can be prevented by vitamin E injections.

GI problems in patients with HIV infection
See Table 6.21.

Tumours of the small intestine

The small intestine is relatively resistant to the development of neoplasia and only 3–6% of all GI tumours and fewer than 1% of all malignant lesions occur here. The reasons for the rarity of tumours is unknown. Explanations include the fluidity and relative sterility of small bowel contents and the rapid transit time, reducing the time of exposure to potential carcinogens. It is also possible that the high population of lymphoid tissue and secretion of IgA in the small intestine protects against malignancy.

Adenocarcinoma of the small intestine is rare and found most frequently in the duodenum (in the periampullary region) and in the jejunum. It is the most common tumour of the small intestine, accounting for up to 50% of primary tumours.

Lymphomas are most frequently found in the ileum. These are of the non-Hodgkin's type and must be distinguished from peripheral or nodal lymphomas involving the gut secondarily.

In developed countries, the most common type of lymphoma is the B-cell type arising from MALT (see p. 199). These lymphomas tend to be annular or polypoid masses in the distal or terminal ileum, whereas most T-cell lymphomas are ulcerated plaques or strictures in the proximal small bowel.

A tumour similar to Burkitt's lymphoma also occurs and commonly affects the terminal ileum of the children in North Africa and the Middle East.

Predisposing factors for adenocarcinoma and lymphoma
Coeliac disease
There is an increased incidence of lymphoma of the T-cell type and adenocarcinoma of the small bowel in coeliac disease, as well as an unexplained increase in all malignancies both in the GI tract and elsewhere. The reason for the local development of malignancy is unknown. It is now accepted that coeliac disease is a premalignant condition, but there is no association with the length of the symptoms. Treatment of coeliac disease with a gluten-free diet reduces the risk of both lymphoma and carcinoma.

Crohn's disease
There is a small increase in the incidence of adenocarcinoma of the small bowel in Crohn's disease.

Immunoproliferative small intestinal disease (IPSID)
IPSID is a B cell disorder in which there is proliferation of plasma cells in the lamina propria of the upper small bowel. These cells produce truncated monoclonal heavy chains, but lack associated light chains. The α heavy chains are found in the gut mucosa on immunofluorescence and can also be detected in the serum. IPSID occurs usually in countries surrounding the Mediterranean, but it has also been found in other developing countries in South America and the Far East. IPSID predominantly affects people in lower socio-economic groups in areas with poor hygiene and·a high incidence of bacterial and parasitic infection of the gut. IPSID presents itself as a malabsorptive syndrome associated with diffuse lymphoid infiltration of the small bowel and neighbouring lymph nodes. This then progresses in some cases to a lymphoma. Recently the condition has been documented in the developed world.

Clinical features
Patients present with abdominal pain, diarrhoea, anorexia, weight loss and symptoms of anaemia.

There may be a palpable mass, and a small bowel follow-through will detect most lesions. Ultrasound and CT will show bowel wall thickening and the involvement of lymph nodes, which is common with lymphoma.

Treatment
Adenocarcinoma. Most patients are treated surgically with a segmental resection. The overall 5-year survival rate is 20–35%; this varies with the histological grade and the presence or absence of lymph node involvement. Radiotherapy and chemotherapy are used in addition.

IPSID. If there is no evidence of lymphoma, antibiotics, e.g. tetracycline, should be tried initially. In the presence of lymphoma, combination chemotherapy is used; in one series the 3- to 5-year survival was 58%.

Lymphoma. Most patients require surgery and radiotherapy with chemotherapy for more extensive disease. The prognosis varies with the type.

The 5-year survival rate for T cell lymphomas is 25%, but is better for B cell lymphomas, varying from 50% to 75%, depending on the grade of lymphoma.

Carcinoid tumours
These originate from the enterochromaffin cells (APUD cells) of the intestine. They make up 10% of all small bowel neoplasms, the most common sites being in the appendix, terminal ileum and the rectum. It is often difficult to be certain histologically whether a particular tumour is benign or malignant. Clinically most carcinoid tumours are asymptomatic until metastases are present. Ten per cent of carcinoid tumours in the appendix present as acute appendicitis, the inflammation being secondary to obstruction. Surgical resection of the tumour is usually performed.

Carcinoid syndrome occurs in only 5% of patients with carcinoid tumours and only when there are liver metastases. Patients complain of spontaneous or induced bluish-red flushing, predominantly on the face and neck. This can lead to permanent changes with telangiectasis. Gastrointestinal symptoms consist of abdominal pain and recurrent watery diarrhoea. Cardiac abnormalities are found in 50% of patients and consist of pulmonary stenosis or tricuspid incompetence. Examination of the abdomen reveals hepatomegaly.

The tumours secrete a variety of biologically active amines and peptides, including serotonin (5-hydroxytryptamine; 5-HT), bradykinin, histamine, tachykinins and prostaglandins.

The diarrhoea and cardiac complications are probably caused by 5-HT itself, but the cutaneous flushing is thought to be produced by one of the kinins, such as bradykinin, which is known to cause vasodilatation, bronchospasm and increased intestinal motility.

Diagnosis and treatment
Ultrasound examination confirms the presence of liver secondary deposits, and the major metabolite of 5-HT,

5-hydroxyindoleacetic acid (5-HIAA), is found in high concentration in the urine.

Octreotide and lanreotide are octapeptide somatostatin analogues that have been shown to inhibit the release of many gut hormones. They alleviate the flushing and diarrhoea and can control a carcinoid crisis. Octreotide is given subcutaneously in doses up to 200 μg three times daily, lanreotide 50 mg every 2 weeks.

Long-acting octreotide also sometimes inhibits tumour growth and, since its introduction, other therapy is usually unnecessary. Interferon and other chemotherapeutic regimens occasionally reduce tumour growth, but have not been shown to increase survival. Most patients survive for 5–10 years after diagnosis.

Peutz–Jeghers syndrome
This consists of mucocutaneous pigmentation (circumoral, hands and feet) and gastrointestinal polyps and has an autosomal dominant inheritance. The gene *LKB1* responsible for Peutz–Jeghers is a serine protein kinase and can be used for genetic analysis. The brown buccal pigment is characteristic of this condition. The polyps, which are hamartomas, can occur anywhere in the GI tract but are most frequent in the small bowel. They may bleed or cause small bowel obstruction or intussusception. The polyps can occasionally contain areas of epithelial dysplasia which can become malignant. Treatment is by individual polypectomy. Multiple polypectomies may have to be performed, but bowel resection should be avoided. Follow-up is every 2 years with X-ray and endoscopy.

Other tumours
Adenomas, lipomas and stromal tumours (p. 280) are rarely found and are usually asymptomatic and picked up incidentally. They occasionally present with iron deficiency anaemia. In familial adenomatous polyposis the upper gut, particularly the duodenum, is affected in one-third of patients.

FURTHER READING

Brands LT, Boley ST (2000) Intestinal ischaemia. *Gastroenterology* **118**: 954–968.
Farrell RJ, Kelly CP (2002) Celiac sprue. *New England Journal of Medicine* **346**: 180–188.
Fasano A, Catassi C (2001) Diagnosis and treatment of coeliac disease. *Gastroenterology* **120**: 636–651.
Johnson LR (1994) *Physiology of the Gastrointestinal Tract.* New York: Raven Press.
Lennard-Jones JE (1994) Practical management of the short bowel. *Alimentary Pharmacology and Therapeutics* **8**: 563–577.
Scott E M et al. (2000) Guidelines for osteoporosis in coeliac disease and inflammatory bowel disease. *Gut* **46** (Suppl I): i1–i8.

Inflammatory bowel disease (IBD)

Two major forms of *non-specific* inflammatory bowel disease are recognized: Crohn's disease (CD), which can affect any part of the GI tract, and ulcerative colitis (UC), which affects only the large bowel.

There is overlap between these two conditions in their clinical features, and histological and radiological abnormalities; in 10% of cases of colitis a definitive diagnosis of either colitis or Crohn's disease is not possible. Currently it is necessary to distinguish between these two conditions because of certain differences in their management. However, it is possible that these conditions represent two aspects of the same disease.

Three additional forms of non-specific inflammatory bowel disease are also recognized, namely microscopic ulcerative colitis, microscopic lymphocytic and collagenous colitis (see p. 308).

Epidemiology

The incidence of Crohn's disease is rising. It varies from country to country but is approximately 5–6 per 100 000 annually, with a prevalence of 27–106 per 100 000. The incidence of ulcerative colitis is stable at 6–15 per 100 000 annually, with a prevalence of 80–150 per 100 000.

Both conditions have a world-wide distribution but are more common in the West. The incidence is lower in the non-white races. Jews are more prone to inflammatory bowel disease than non-Jews, and the Ashkenazi Jews have a higher risk than the Sephardic Jews.

Crohn's disease is slightly commoner in females (M : F = 1 : 1.2) and occurs at a younger age (mean 26 years) than ulcerative colitis (M : F = 1.2:1; mean 34 years).

Aetiopathogenesis

The aetiology is unknown, but racial differences and geographical clusterings suggest both genetic and environmental causes.

- *Familial.* Both Crohn's disease (CD) and ulcerative colitis (UC) are more common amongst relatives of patients than in the general population. Thus 6–10% of patients affected with CD or UC have one or more relatives with the disease. The risk of CD in first-degree relatives of a CD patient is 10–14 times higher than in the general population, with the risk of UC being about 8 times higher. In CD, but not UC, affected patients are more likely to be siblings than first-degree relatives.
- *Genetic.* Based on studies of monozygotic twins, the coefficient of hereditability of CD is high (equivalent to that in type 1 diabetes mellitus). In UC it is much lower, which argues for a stronger environmental component in susceptibility. Current gene studies provide evidence for heterogeneity between and within CD and UC. To date it appears that the relative contribution of the HLA region to genetic susceptibility is stronger in UC than CD.
  - *In UC*, linkage analyses suggest that specific HLA alleles encode susceptibility in UC and may predict disease severity (DRB1*1502, DRB1*0103, DR*12). The allelic associations differ between ethnic groups, which is consistent with the concept of heterogeneity.
  - *In CD* the contribution of the HLA system to disease susceptibility and severity remains controversial. Currently there is considerable interest in the role of genes encoding the cytokines (interleukin-1, -10, -17 and tumour necrosis factor-α), as well as genes encoding proteins involved in mucosal integrity in relationship to determination of disease susceptibility and behaviour.
- *Diet.* To prove an aetiopathogenic role for specific nutrients in CD and UC it is necessary to demonstrate deficiencies or excesses in active disease with improvements following repletion or depletion. Examples currently under investigation are butyric acid, sulphides, L-arginine/inducible nitric oxide synthase, glutamine and omega-3 (n-3) fatty acids.
- *Smoking.* Patients with CD are more likely to be smokers, and smoking has been shown to exacerbate CD. In contrast there is an increased risk of UC in non- or ex-smokers and nicotine has been shown to be an effective treatment in UC .
- *Infective agent.* Considerable controversy surrounds the role of all infective agents implicated in the aetiopathogenesis of inflammatory bowel disease which include:
  - *Mycobacterium* – in cattle and sheep, Johne's disease, which is a chronic inflammatory disorder of the distal ileum, is caused by *M. paratuberculosis*. Isolation of mycobacteria from Crohn's disease has been inconsistent and current evidence is against this being an aetiological agent. Antituberculosis therapy has not been beneficial.
  - Measles virus – has been implicated following the demonstration of the virus within the vascular epithelium and the association of vascular injury and focal enteritis in the muscularis propria in affected intestine. However RT-PCR did not detect the virus in mucosal biopsies from patients. There may be antigen mimicry between the measles virus and an unidentified agent.
  - *Listeria monocytogenes.*
  - *Helicobacter hepaticus, H. cinaedi* and *H. fenelliae*.
  - Yeast (*Saccharomyces cerevisiae*).
- *Endogenous bacteria.* Experimental data do support a role for normal luminal bacteria or bacterial products in the initiation and perpetuation of chronic intestinal inflammation. Current interest is

focused on *Bacteroides* spp. and strains of *E. coli*. It is postulated that adhesins produced by some of the latter strains promote adhesion ability and synthesis of cytotoxins, allowing bacteria to colonize intestinal epithelium, damage intestinal cells and participate in the inflammatory response. The role of the natural bacterial flora (probiotics) is being investigated (Box 6.8).

- *Immunopathogenesis.* Many immunological abnormalities have been described. It is suggested that genetically susceptible patients with defective immunoregulation or barrier function/healing lack the ability to appropriately downregulate immune (antigen-specific) or antigen-non-specific inflammatory responses to endogenous luminal antigens. Specifically there is upregulation of macrophages and Th1 lymphocytes in Crohn's disease. This produces an excess of cytokines, interleukin-1β (IL-1β), IL-1 receptor antagonist (IL-IRA), IL-6, the chemokine IL-8 and TNFα. UC is a modified Th2 response with IL-5 and IL-10. Nuclear factor kappa B (NFκB) plays a central regulatory role by controlling the transcription of genes for these pro-inflammatory cytokines. There is also activation of other cells (eosinophils, mast cells, neutrophils and fibroblasts) which leads to excess production of chemokines (lymphokines, arachidonic acid metabolites, neuropeptides and free oxygen radicals), all of which can lead to tissue damage.

Pathology

- *Crohn's disease* is a chronic inflammatory condition that may affect any part of the gastrointestinal tract from the mouth to the anus but has a particular tendency to affect the terminal ileum and ascending colon (ileocolonic disease). The disease can involve one small area of the gut such as the terminal ileum, or multiple areas with relatively normal bowel in between (skip lesions). It may also involve the whole of the colon (total colitis) sometimes without small bowel involvement.

- *Ulcerative colitis* can affect the rectum alone (proctitis), can extend proximally to involve the sigmoid and descending colon (left-sided colitis), or may involve the whole colon (total colitis). In a few of these patients there is also inflammation of the distal terminal ileum (backwash ileitis).

Macroscopic changes

In *Crohn's disease* the involved small bowel is usually thickened and narrowed. There are deep ulcers and fissures in the mucosa, producing a cobblestone appearance. Fistulae and abscesses may be seen in the colon. An early feature is aphthoid ulceration, usually seen at colonoscopy (see Fig. 6.27); later, larger and deeper ulcers appear in a patchy distribution, again producing a cobblestone appearance.

In *ulcerative colitis* the mucosa looks reddened, inflamed and bleeds easily. In severe disease there is extensive ulceration with the adjacent mucosa appearing as inflammatory polyps.

In fulminant colonic disease of either type, most of the mucosa is lost, leaving a few islands of oedematous mucosa (mucosal islands), and toxic dilatation occurs. On healing, the mucosa can return to normal, although there is usually some residual glandular distortion.

Microscopic changes

In *Crohn's disease* the inflammation extends through all layers (transmural) of the bowel, whereas in ulcerative colitis a superficial inflammation is seen. In Crohn's disease there is an increase in chronic inflammatory cells and lymphoid hyperplasia, and in 50–60% of patients granulomas are present. These granulomas are non-caseating epithelioid cell aggregates with Langhans' giant cells.

In *ulcerative colitis* the mucosa shows a chronic inflammatory cell infiltrate in the lamina propria. Crypt abscesses and goblet cell depletion are also seen.

The differentiation between these two diseases can usually be made not only on the basis of clinical and radiological data but also on the histological differences seen in the rectal and colonic mucosa obtained by biopsy (Table 6.8).

It is occasionally not possible to distinguish between the two disorders, particularly if biopsies are obtained in the acute phase, and such patients are considered to have an indeterminate inflammatory colitis. Serological testing may be of value in differentiating the two conditions.

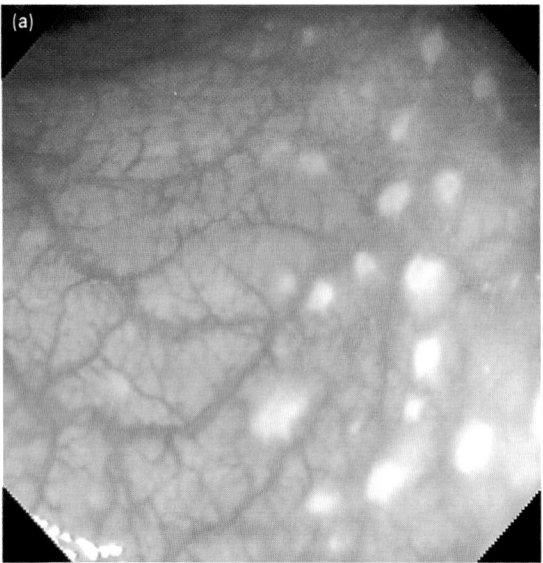 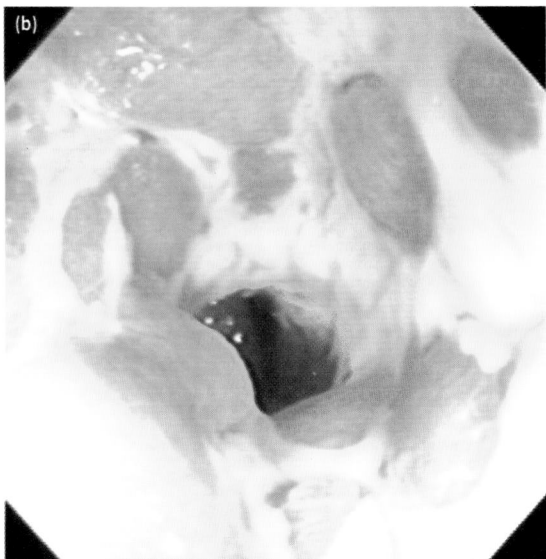

Fig. 6.27 Crohn's disease. Colonoscopic appearances of (a) aphthoid ulcers typical of Crohn's disease (b) cobblestone appearance.

Extragastrointestinal manifestations

These occur with both diseases. Joint complications are commonest, and the peripheral arthropathies are now classified as type 1 (pauci-articular) and type 2 (polyarticular). Type 1 attacks are acute, self-limiting (<10 weeks) and occur with IBD relapses; they are associated with other extraintestinal manifestations of IBD activity. Type 2 arthropathy lasts longer (months to years), is independent of IBD activity and usually associated with uveitis. The incidence of joint and other extragastrointestinal manifestations is shown in Table 6.9.

Differential diagnosis

All causes of diarrhoea should be excluded (Table 6.18) and stool cultures are always performed. Crohn's disease should be considered in all patients with evidence of malabsorption e.g. megaloblastic anaemia, or malnourishment, as well as in children with small stature. Ileo-colonic tuberculosis is common in developing countries, e.g. India, and makes a diagnosis of Crohn's disease difficult. Microscopy and culture for TB of any available tissue is essential in these countries. A therapeutic trial of antituberculosis therapy is often required.

Lymphomas can occasionally involve the ileum and caecum.

Crohn's disease

Clinical features

The major symptoms are diarrhoea, abdominal pain and weight loss. Constitutional symptoms of malaise, lethargy, anorexia, nausea, vomiting and low-grade fever may be present and in 15% of these patients there are no gastrointestinal symptoms. Despite the recurrent nature of this condition, many patients remain well and

Table 6.8
Histological differences between Crohn's disease and ulcerative colitis

	Crohn's disease	Ulcerative colitis
Inflammation	Deep (transmural)	Mucosal
	Patchy	Continuous
Granulomas	++	Rare
Goblet cells	Present	Depleted
Crypt abscesses	+	++

have an almost normal lifestyle. However, patients with extensive disease often have frequent recurrences, necessitating multiple hospital admissions.

The clinical features are very variable and depend partly on the region of the bowel that is affected. The disease may present insidiously or acutely. The abdominal pain can be colicky, suggesting obstruction but it usually has no special characteristics and sometimes in colonic disease only minimal discomfort is present. Diarrhoea is present in 80% of all cases and in colonic disease it usually contains blood, making it difficult to differentiate from ulcerative colitis. Steatorrhoea can be present in small bowel disease.

Crohn's disease may present as an emergency with acute right iliac fossa pain mimicking appendicitis. If laparotomy is undertaken, an oedematous reddened terminal ileum is found. There are other causes of an acute ileitis (e.g. infections such as *Yersinia*). Up to 30% of patients presenting with acute ileitis turn out eventually to have Crohn's disease. Crohn's disease can be complicated by anal and perianal disease and this is the presenting feature in 25% of cases, often preceding colonic and small intestinal symptoms by many years (Table 6.10).

Table 6.9
Extragastrointestinal manifestation of inflammatory bowel disease (percentage of cases)

	Ulcerative colitis	Crohn's disease
Eyes		
Uveitis	2	5
Episcleritis / Conjunctivitis	5–8	3–10
Joints		
Arthropathy (peripheral)	7	10
Arthralgia	5	14
Ankylosing spondylitis	1	1
Inflammatory back pain	4	9
Skin		
Erythema nodosum	1	4
Pyoderma gangrenosum	1	2
Liver and biliary tree		
Sclerosing cholangitis	2.5–7.5	1–2
Fatty liver	Common	Common
Chronic hepatitis	Uncommon	Uncommon
Cirrhosis	Uncommon	Uncommon
Nephrolithiasis	–	5–10 oxalate stones in patients with small bowel disease or after resection
Gallstones	As normal population	15–30
Venous thrombosis	5	1

Enteric fistulae, e.g. to bladder or vagina, occur in 20–40% of cases, equally divided between internal and external fistulae; the latter usually occurring after surgery.

Examination

Physical signs are few, apart from loss of weight and general ill-health. Aphthous ulceration of the mouth is often seen. Abdominal examination is often normal although tenderness and a right iliac fossa mass are occasionally found. The mass is due either to inflamed loops of bowel that are matted together or to an abscess. The anus should always be examined to look for oedematous anal tags, fissures or perianal abscesses.

Extragastrointestinal features of inflammatory bowel disease should be looked for (Table 6.9).

Sigmoidoscopy should always be performed in a patients with Crohn's disease. With small bowel involvement the rectum may appear normal, but a biopsy must be taken as non-specific histological changes can sometimes be found in the mucosa. Even with extensive colonic Crohn's disease the rectum may be spared and be relatively normal, but patchy involvement with an oedematous haemorrhagic mucosa can be present.

Table 6.10
Anal and perianal complications of Crohn's disease

Fissure in ano (multiple and indolent)
Haemorrhoids
Skin tags
Perianal abscess
Ischiorectal abscess
Fistula in ano (may be multiple)
Anorectal fistulae

Investigations
Blood tests

- Anaemia is common and is usually the normocytic, normochromic anaemia of chronic disease. Deficiency of iron and/or folate also occurs. Despite terminal ileal involvement in Crohn's disease, megaloblastic anaemia due to B_{12} deficiency is unusual, although serum B_{12} levels can be low.
- Raised ESR and CRP and a raised white cell count.
- Hypoalbuminaemia is present in severe disease.
- Liver biochemistry may be abnormal.
- Blood cultures are required if septicaemia is suspected.
- Serological tests. *Saccharamyces cerevisiae* antibody is usually present while p-ANCA antibody is negative. The reverse is true in UC but the clinical value of these tests is limited.

Stool cultures

These should always be performed on presentation if diarrhoea is present.

Radiology and imaging

A *barium follow-through* examination should always be performed in patients suspected of having Crohn's disease. The findings include an asymmetrical alteration in the mucosal pattern with deep ulceration, and areas of narrowing or stricturing. Although commonly confined to the terminal ileum (Fig. 6.28), other areas of the small bowel can be involved and skip lesions with normal bowel are seen between affected sites.

Imaging of the small bowel may also be performed by magnetic resonance enteroclysis. Colonoscopy is performed if colonic involvement is suspected except in patients presenting with severe acute disease. The findings vary from mild patchy superficial (aphthoid) ulceration to more widespread larger and deeper ulcers producing a cobblestone appearance (Fig. 6.27).

In patients presenting acutely with colonic symptoms an *instant barium enema* will show changes varying from patchy superficial ulceration to more widespread deep (rose thorn) ulceration, cobblestone appearance and narrowing due to fibrosis.

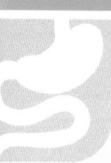
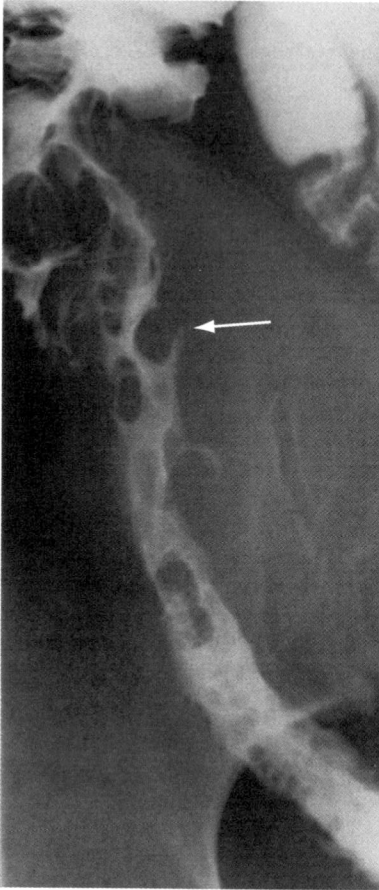

Fig. 6.28 **Terminal ileum on small bowel follow-through in Crohn's disease,** showing narrowing and ulceration of the terminal ileum (arrow). Note the presence of deep 'rose thorn' type ulcers and 'cobblestoning' in the terminal ileum.

High-resolution ultrasound and spiral CT scanning are both helpful techniques in defining thickness of the bowel wall and mesentery as well as intra-abdominal and para-intestinal abscesses.

Radionuclide scans with gallium-labelled polymorphs or indium- or technetium-labelled leucocytes are used in some centres to identify small intestinal and colonic disease and to localize extraintestinal abscesses.

Disease activity

This can be assessed using simple parameters such as Hb, white cell count, inflammatory markers (ESR CRP) and serum albumin. Formal clinical activity indices (e.g. Crohn's disease activity index) are used in research studies.

Medical management of Crohn's disease

(Box 6.9)

The aim of management is to induce and then maintain a remission. Patients with mild symptoms may require

---

Box 6.9

Options for medical treatment of Crohn's disease

Induction of remission
- Oral or i.v. glucocorticosteroids
- Enteral nutrition
- Oral glucocorticosteroids + azathioprine or mercaptopurine (6MP)

Maintenance of remission
- Aminosalicylates
- Azathioprine, 6MP, mycophenolate mofetil

Treatment of glucocorticosteroid/immunosuppressive therapy-resistant disease
- Methotrexate
- Intravenous ciclosporin
- Infliximab (TNFα antibody)

Perianal disease
- Ciprofloxacin and metronidazole

---

only symptomatic treatment. Cigarette smoking should be stopped. Diarrhoea can be controlled with loperamide, codeine phosphate or co-phenotope. Diarrhoea in long-standing inactive disease may be due to bile acid malabsorption (p. 322) and should be treated with cholecystyramine. Anaemia, if due to vitamin B_{12}, folic acid or iron deficiency, should be treated with the appropriate haematinics. Anaemia in more active disease is usually normochromic and normocytic (anaemia of chronic disease, p. 417) and will usually improve as the patient gets better. Patients with active (moderate/severe) attacks may have to be admitted to hospital. Patients with moderate to severe total *Crohn's colitis* are treated as for UC (p. 306).

Glucocorticosteroids are commonly used to induce remission in moderate and severe attacks of Crohn's disease. Steroids are usually administered as oral prednisolone (30–60 mg/day). In patients with ileocaecal, but not colonic Crohn's disease, slow-release formulations of budesonide are as equally efficacious as oral prednisolone. Budesonide has high topical potency and because of its extensive hepatic inactivation has low systemic availability which induces less suppression of endogenous cortisol and reduces frequency and intensity of steroidal side-effects. Overall remission/response rates vary from 60–90% depending on type, site and extent of disease.

Enteral nutrition is an underutilized means of inducing remission in moderate and severe attacks of Crohn's disease, and efficacy is independent of nutritional status. If enteral diets with a low fat (1.3% of total calories) and a low linoleic acid content are administered as the sole source of nutrition for 28 days, rates of induction of remission are similar to those obtained with steroids.

Relapse rates are high, however, particularly in those with colonic involvement.

Flare-ups commonly occur after steroid dosages are tapered and/or enteral nutrition stopped and alternative treatment strategies have to be introduced, e.g. steroid dosage may have to be temporarily increased, to re-induce and maintain remission. Aminosalicylates are particularly useful in Crohn's colitis. In contrast the immunosuppressive agents azathioprine (AZA) and its metabolite 6-mercaptourine (6MP) are both effective in inducing and maintaining remission and have steroid-sparing properties. Mycophenolate mofetil, which suppresses the proliferation of T and B lymphocytes, is also effective in maintaining remission.

Long-term treatment with AZA and 6MP is necessary as the rate of relapse on discontinuation of treatment is high (70%). Regular blood counts should be performed after commencing treatment as the key enzyme involved in AZA and 6MP metabolism (thiopurine methyltransferase, TPMT) has significant genetic variation in the population, with deficiencies resulting in high levels of active thioguanine nucleotides which result in immune and bone marrow suppression. In unresponsive patients, remission is sometimes induced and maintained by raising the dose of AZA to levels that make patients leucopenic.

In patients with corticosteroid/immunosuppressive therapy-resistant Crohn's disease, methotrexate or i.v. (but not oral) ciclosporin has been shown to be effective in inducing remission, but not in maintaining it. Biological treatments directed against specific inflammatory mediators, e.g. anti-TNFα antibody (infliximab), are being used. A single infusion of this has been shown to be effective in producing clinical improvement in up to 60% of patients with steroid-resistant disease, and in those responding to the initial infusion, a further four doses at 8-weekly intervals had maintained remission in 50% of patients by 8 weeks after the final infusion. Three doses of infliximab have also been shown to close fistulae (predominantly perianal) in half the patients treated.

Allergic reactions are seen in 5% of infusions. Low-titre human antichimeric antibodies occur in 13% of treated patients. Infliximab may also induce auto-antibodies such as ANA, ds DNA and TB. Isolated cases of lymphoma have been reported but may not be a primary association with treatment. A humanized antibody to TNFα has been developed and preliminary trials show this to be effective in inducing remission in moderately to severely active Crohn's disease.

Surgical management of Crohn's disease

Approximately 80% of patients will require an operation at some time during the course of their disease. Nevertheless, surgery should be avoided if possible and only minimal resections undertaken, as recurrence (15% per year) is almost inevitable. The indications for surgery are:

- failure of medical therapy, with acute or chronic symptoms producing ill-health
- complications (e.g. toxic dilatation, obstruction, perforation, abscesses, enterocutaneous fistula)
- failure to grow in children.

In patients with small bowel disease, some strictures can be widened (stricturoplasty), whereas others require resection and end-to-end anastomosis.

When colonic Crohn's disease involves the entire colon and the rectum is spared or minimally involved a subtotal colectomy and ileorectal anastomosis may be performed. An eventual recurrence rate of 60–70% in the ileum, rectum or both is to be expected. Two-thirds of these patients retain a functional rectum for 10 years. If the whole colon and rectum are involved a panproctocolectomy with an end ileostomy is the standard operation. In this operation the colon and rectum are removed and the ileum is brought out through an opening in the right iliac fossa and attached to the skin. The patient wears an ileostomy bag, which is stuck on to the skin over the ileostomy spout. The bag needs to be emptied once or twice daily, so this is compatible with a near-normal lifestyle. Stoma care therapists are readily available with help and advice.

Problems associated with ileostomies include:

- mechanical problems
- dehydration, particularly in hot climates
- psychosexual problems
- infertility in men
- recurrence of Crohn's disease.

Ulcerative colitis

Clinical features

The major symptom in ulcerative colitis is diarrhoea with blood and mucus, sometimes accompanied by lower abdominal discomfort. General features include malaise, lethargy and anorexia. Aphthous ulceration in the mouth is seen. The disease can be mild, moderate or severe, and in most patients runs a course of remissions and exacerbations. Ten per cent of patients have persistent chronic symptoms, while some patients may have only a single attack.

When the disease is confined to the rectum (proctitis), blood mixed with the stool, urgency and tenesmus are common. There are normally very few constitutional symptoms, but patients are nevertheless greatly inconvenienced by the frequency of defecation.

In an acute attack of UC, patients have bloody diarrhoea, passing up to 10–20 liquid stools per day. Diarrhoea also occurs at night, with urgency and incontinence that is severely disabling for the patient. Occasionally blood and mucus alone are passed.

The definition of a severe attack is given in Table 6.11. The patient is often very ill and needs urgent treatment in hospital.

Table 6.11
Definition of a severe attack of ulcerative colitis

Stool frequency	> 6 stools per day with blood
Fever	> 37.5°C
Tachycardia	> 90 per minute
ESR	> 30 mm per hour
Anaemia	Haemoglobin < 10 g/dL
Albumin	< 30 g/L

Examination

In general there are no specific signs in ulcerative colitis. The abdomen may be slightly distended or tender to palpation. The anus is usually normal. Rectal examination will show the presence of blood. Rigid sigmoidoscopy is usually abnormal showing an inflamed, bleeding, friable mucosa. Very occasionally rectal sparing occurs in which case sigmoidoscopy will be normal.

Investigations

Blood tests

- In moderate to severe attacks an iron deficiency anaemia is commonly present and the white cell and platelet counts are raised.
- The ESR and CRP are often raised; liver biochemistry may be abnormal, with hypoalbuminaemia occurring in severe disease.
- pANCA may be positive. This is contrary to Crohn's where pANCA is usually negative (p. 000).

Stool cultures

These should always be performed to exclude infective causes of colitis.

Imaging

A *plain abdominal X-ray* with an *abdominal ultrasound* are the key investigations in moderate to severe attacks. The extent of disease can be judged by the air distribution in the colon and the presence of colonic dilatation can be noted. Thickening of the colonic wall can be detected on ultrasound as can the presence of free fluid within the abdominal cavity. An instant *unprepared barium enema* is a good investigation to show extent of disease. Findings may include superficial ulceration and a shortened and narrowed colon in long-standing disease (see Fig. 6.29).

Colonoscopy

A *colonoscopy* should not be performed in severe attacks of disease for fear of perforation. In more long-standing and chronic disease it is useful in defining extent and activity of disease, and in patients with total ulcerative colitis of 10 years' duration or more, *colonoscopy* and multiple biopsies should be performed to exclude dysplasia and carcinoma.

Radionuclide scans

These can be used to assess colonic inflammation (p. 000).

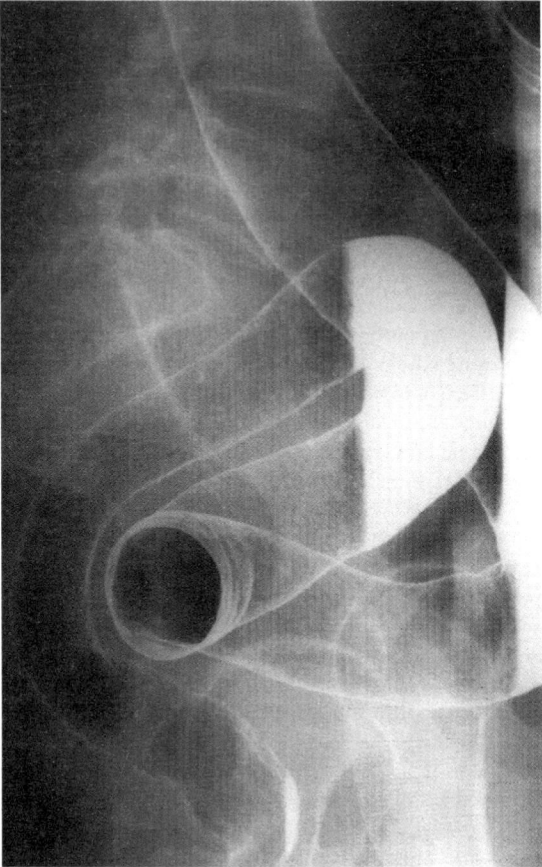

Fig. 6.29 **Unprepared barium enema in ulcerative colitis.** Showing a tubular featureless colon with fine ulceration.

Medical management of ulcerative colitis (UC)

Wherever possible patients with ulcerative colitis and Crohn's disease should be managed in patient-focused inflammatory bowel disease clinics. All patients with ulcerative colitis should be treated with an aminosalicylate. The active moiety of these is 5-aminosalicylic acid (5-ASA). 5-ASA is absorbed in the small intestine (and may be nephrotoxic) so the design of the various aminosalicylate preparations is based on the binding of 5-ASA by an azo bond to sulfapyridine (sulfasalazine), 4-aminobenzoyl-ß-alanine (balsalazide) or to 5-ASA itself (olsalazine), coating with a pH-sensitive polymer or packaging of 5-ASA in microspheres.

The azo bonds are broken down by colonic bacteria to release 5-ASA within the colon. The pH-dependent forms are designed to release 5-ASA in the terminal ileum. Luminal pH profiles in patients with inflammatory bowel disease are abnormal and in some patients the pH-dependent salicylate may pass through into the faeces intact. 5-ASA is released from microspheres throughout the small intestine and colon. The mode of action of 5-ASA in inflammatory bowel disease is unknown, but the aminosalicylates have been shown to be effective in inducing remission in mild to moderately active disease and maintaining remission in all forms of disease. Sulfasalazine is being used more infrequently because of its wider side effect profile.

Proctitis

Oral aminosalicylates plus a local rectal steroid preparation (10% hydrocortisone foam; prednisolone 20 mg enemas or foam) are the first-line treatment. Mesalazine enemas and budesonide enemas can be tried. Some cases of proctitis can be 'resistant' to treatment. In these, oral corticosteroids alone or in combination with azathioprine are used and in rare cases short-chain fatty acid enemas may help.

Left-sided proctocolitis

Oral aminosalicylates plus local rectal steroid preparations may be effective but in moderate to severe attacks oral prednisolone will be required. If patients do not respond within 2 weeks they should be admitted to hospital.

Total colitis (moderate to severe attacks) (Table 6.12)

Patients should be admitted to hospital and treated initially with hydrocortisone 100 mg i.v. 6-hourly with oral aminosalicylates. Full investigations (see above) should be performed initially and full supportive therapy administered (i.v. fluids, nutritional support via the enteral and not parenteral route if required).

Patients who have been previously admitted within 2–3 years with moderate to severe attacks of total colitis can be started on azathioprine if not already on this treatment as it takes time to work. The clinical status of patients should subsequently be monitored carefully (fever, tachycardia, abdominal signs) and daily FBC, ESR, CRP, electrolytes and urea, tests of liver function,

including serum albumin, straight abdominal X-ray, and stool weights should be performed. Success or failure of medical treatment of a severe attack of ulcerative colitis must be judged by an experienced gastroenterologist. A persistent fever, tachycardia, falling Hb, rising white cell count, falling potassium, falling albumin and persistently raised stool weights (> 500 g/day) with loose blood-stained stool are all signs that the patient is not responding to treatment and that surgery may be indicated.

Toxic dilatation of the colon in which the plain abdominal X-ray shows a dilated thin-walled colon with a diameter of more than 5 cm that is gas filled and contains mucosal islands (Fig. 6.30) is a particularly dangerous stage of advanced disease with impending perforation and high mortality (15–25%). Urgent surgery is required in all patients in whom toxic dilatation has not resolved within 48 hours.

In patients responding to i.v. hydrocortisone treatment, oral prednisolone therapy should be substituted and doses slowly tailed off (5–10 mg weekly). Maintenance of remission is with aminosalicylates. In patients in whom it is not possible to reduce the dose of prednisolone without flare-up, azathioprine is used.

Surgical management of ulcerative colitis

While the treatment of ulcerative colitis remains primarily medical, surgery continues to have a central role because it may be life-saving, is curative and eliminates the long-term risk of cancer. The main indication for surgery is for a severe attack which fails to respond to medical therapy. Other indications are listed in Box 6.10.

In acute disease, subtotal colectomy with end ileostomy and preservation of the rectum is the operation of choice. At a later date a number of surgical options are available. These include proctectomy with a permanent ileostomy. To avoid a permanent ileostomy, ileorectal anastomosis can be performed; annual biopsies of the rectal mucosa must be carried out to exclude dysplasia, a histological change that precedes the development of a rectal stump carcinoma. With an ileo-anal

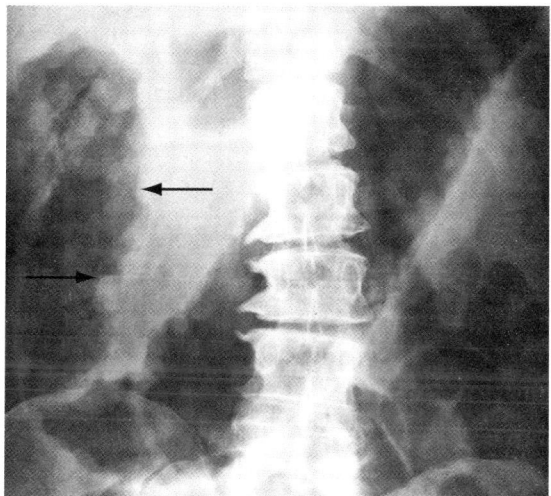

Fig. 6.30 **Plain abdominal X-ray, showing toxic dilatation in ulcerative colitis.** The arrows indicate mucosal islands.

Box 6.10

Indications for surgery in ulcerative colitis

Fulminant acute attack
- Failure of medical treatment
- Toxic dilatation
- Haemorrhage
- Perforation

Chronic disease
- Incomplete response to medical treatment
- Excessive steroid requirement
- Non-compliance with medication, Risk of cancer

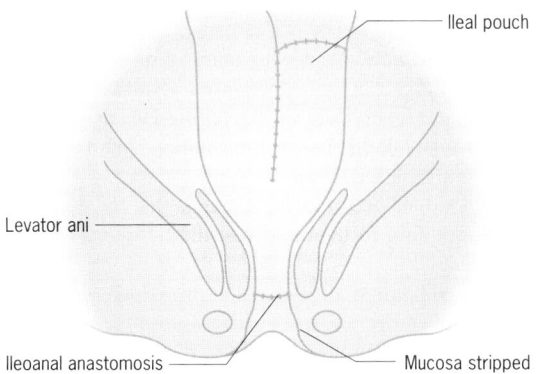

Ileal pouch

Levator ani

Ileoanal anastomosis

Mucosa stripped

Fig. 6.31 An ileo-anal pouch for ulcerative colitis.

anastomosis (Fig. 6.31), a pouch of ileum is formed that acts as a reservoir. The pouch is anastomosed to the anus at the dentate line following endoanal excision of the mucosa of the distal rectum and anal canal. Continence is usually achieved. A third of patients, however, will experience 'pouchitis' in which there is inflammation of the pouch mucosa with clinical symptoms of diarrhoea, bleeding, fever and at times exacerbation of extracolonic manifestations. Treatment is not always satisfactory and includes topical 5-ASA and corticosteroids, metronidazole, ciprofloxacin and probiotic therapy (see p. 301). The incidence of pouchitis is twice as high in patients with primary sclerosing cholangitis. In the hopes of improving night-time continence some surgeons advocate stapling the reservoir to the lower rectal or upper anal mucosa (ileal pouch–distal rectal anastomosis). The disadvantage of this technique is the cancer risk associated with the residual diseased mucosa.

Cancer in inflammatory bowel disease

Patients with extensive ulcerative colitis of more than 10 years' duration are at an increased risk of developing colorectal cancer. (Cumulative risk 5% after 20 years, 12% at 25 years). Although patients with Crohn's colitis are also at risk, this is lower than with ulcerative colitis. Many centres recommend that colonoscopy and multiple biopsies should be under taken at 1- to 2-year intervals in patients with extensive ulcerative colitis of more than 10 years' duration and those with evidence of high-grade dysplasia should undergo colectomy. There is, however, no supportive evidence for this strategy. There is insufficient evidence to support the use of a surveillance program in patients with Crohn's colitis.

Course and prognosis

A third of patients with distal inflammatory proctitis due to ulcerative colitis will develop more proximal disease, with 5–10% developing total colitis. A third of patients with ulcerative colitis will have a single attack and the others will have a relapsing course. A third of patients with ulcerative colitis will undergo colectomy within 20 years of diagnosis. About 60–70% will require a second operation.

Pregnancy and inflammatory bowel disease

Women with inactive IBD have normal fertility. Fertility, however, may be reduced in those with active disease, and patients with active disease are twice as likely to suffer spontaneous abortion than those with inactive disease.

Although the risk of an exacerbation of IBD is not increased in pregnancy, when exacerbations occur they do so most commonly in the first trimester and during the immediate postpartum period.

Aminosalicylates, steroids and azathioprine are safe at the time of conception and during pregnancy. The sulfapyridine moiety of sulfasalazine impairs spermatogenesis, so males trying to conceive should be treated with an alternative aminosalicylate.

Microscopic inflammatory colitis

Patients with this group of disorders present with chronic or fluctuating watery diarrhoea. Although the macroscopic features on colonoscopy are normal, the histopathological findings on biopsy are abnormal. There are three distinct forms of microscopic inflammatory colitis:

- microscopic ulcerative colitis
- microscopic lymphocytic colitis
- microscopic collagenous colitis.

In *microscopic ulcerative colitis*, there is a chronic inflammatory cell infiltrate in the lamina propria, with deformed crypt architecture, and goblet cell depletion with or without crypt abscesses. *Treatment* is as for ulcerative colitis although many patients respond to treatment with aminosalicylates alone.

In *microscopic lymphocytic colitis* there is surface epithelial injury, prominent lymphocytic infiltration in the surface epithelium and increased lamina propria mononuclear cells. It affects males and females equally and is associated with a high prevalence of antibiotic use.

In *microscopic collagenous colitis* there is a thickened subepithelial collagen layer ($> 10\,\mu m$) adjacent to the basal membrane with increased infiltration of the lamina propria with lymphocytes and plasma cells and surface epithelial cell damage. It is predominantly a disorder of middle-aged or elderly females, and is associated with a variety of autoimmune disorders (arthritis, thyroid disease, CREST syndrome and primary biliary cirrhosis). The prevalence of collagenous colitis has been shown to be $15.7/10^5$ population with an annual incidence of $1.8/10^5$ population. There are a number of reports linking drugs to the development of collagenous colitis (non-steroidal anti-inflammatory drugs, simvastatin, H_2-receptor antagonists).

There are no controlled clinical trials of treatment in microscopic lymphocytic or collagenous colitis. Treatment is usually with aminosalicylates, prednisolone and azathioprine in that order. In general patients with microscopic collagenous colitis are easier to treat than those with the lymphocytic form of the disease.

FURTHER READING

Farrell RJ, Peppercorn MA (2002) Ulcerative colitis. *Lancet* **359**: 331–340.

Gionchetti P, Rizzello F, Venturi A et al. (2000) Oral bacteriotherapy as maintenance treatment for patients with chronic pouchitis: a double-blind placebo-controlled trial. *Gastroenterology* **119**: 305–309.

Present DH, Rutgeerts P, Targan S (1999) Infliximab for the treatment of fistulas in patients with Crohn's disease. *New England Journal of Medicine* **240**: 1398–1405.

Rutgeerts P, Vermeire S (2000) Serological diagnosis of inflammatory bowel disease. *Lancet* **356**: 2117.

Rutgeerts P, Colombel J-F, Hanover SB, Scholmerich J, Tytgat GNJ, Van Gossum A (eds) (1995) *Advances in inflammatory bowel diseases.* London: Kluwer Academic Publishers.

Sands B E (2000) Therapy of inflammatory bowel disease. *Gastroenterology* **118**: 568–582.

Shanahan F (2002) Crohn's disease. *Lancet* **259**: 62–69.

Shanahan F (2001) Inflammatory bowel disease: immunodiagnostics, immunotherapeutics and ecotherapeutics. *Gastroenterology* **120**: 622–635.

Targan SR, Hanover SB, Van Deventer SJH et al. (1997) A short term study of the chimeric monoclonal antibody CA$_2$ to tumour necrosis factor α for Crohn's disease. *New England Journal of Medicine* **337**: 1029–1035.

The colon and rectum

Structure

The large intestine starts at the caecum, on the posterior medial wall of which is the appendix. The colon is made up of ascending, transverse, descending and sigmoid parts, which join the rectum at the rectosigmoid junction.

The muscle wall consists of an inner circular layer and an outer longitudinal layer. The outer layer is incomplete, coming together to form the taenia coli, which produce the haustral pattern seen in the normal colon.

The mucosa of the colon is lined with epithelial cells with crypts but no villi, so that the surface is flat. The mucosa is full of goblet cells. A variety of cells, mainly lymphocytes and macrophages, are found in the lamina propria.

The blood supply to the colon is from the superior and inferior mesenteric vessels. Generally there are good anastomotic channels, but the caecum and splenic flexure are areas where ischaemia can occur.

The rectum is about 12 cm long. Its interior is divided by three crescentic circular muscles producing shelf-like

Table 6.12

Input and output of water and electrolytes in the gastrointestinal tract over 24 hours

	Water (mL)	Sodium (mmol)	Potassium (mmol)
Input			
Diet	1500	150	80
GI secretions	7500	1000	40
Totals	9000	1150	120
Output			
Faeces	150	5	12
Ileostomy (adapted)	500–1000	60–120	4

folds. These are the rectal valves that can be seen at sigmoidoscopy. The anal canal has an internal and an external sphincter.

Physiology of the colon

The main roles of the colon are the absorption of water and electrolytes (Table 6.12) and the propulsion of contents from the caecum to the anorectal region. Approximately 1.5–2 L of fluid pass the ileocaecal valve each day. Absorption is stimulated by short-chain fatty acids which are produced predominantly in the right colon by the anaerobic metabolism of dietary fibre by bacterial polysaccharidase enzyme systems. Mixing of colonic contents (which aids this reaction) and absorption, is achieved as a consequence of non-propagative segmenting muscular contractions. Propulsion is achieved by the action of high-amplitude propagative colonic contractions. Normal colonic transit time is 24–48 h with normal stool weights of up to 250 g/day.

Physiology of defecation

The role of the rectum and anus in defecation is complex. The rectum is normally empty. Stool is propelled into the rectum by propagated colonic contractions. Sensation of fullness, a desire to defecate and urgency to defecate are experienced with increasing volumes of content (threshold 100 mL). The sensations are associated with rectal contraction and a relaxation of the internal anal sphincters, both of which serve to push the stool down into the proximal anal canal. This increases the defecatory urge, which can only be suppressed by vigorous contraction of the external sphincter and puborectalis. If conditions are appropriate for defecation the subject sits or squats, contracts the diaphragm and abdominal muscles and the levatores, while relaxing the external sphincter and possibly the puborectalis.

Constipation

'Constipation' is a symptom and thus a term that people use to express sensations or bodily functions that they perceive to be abnormal. The commonest

Table 6.13
Causes of constipation

General
Pregnancy
Inadequate fibre intake
Immobility

Metabolic/endocrine
Diabetes mellitus
Hypercalcaemia
Hypothyroidism
Porphyria

Functional
Irritable bowel syndrome
Idiopathic slow transit

Drugs
Opiates
Anticholinergics
Calcium-channel blockers,
   e.g. verapamil
Antidepressants
Iron

Neurological
Spinal cord lesions
Parkinson's disease

Psychological
Depression
Anorexia nervosa
Repressed urge to defecate

Gastrointestinal disease
Intestinal obstruction and
   pseudo-obstruction
Colonic disease, e.g. carcinoma,
   diverticular disease
Hirschprung's disease
Megarectum
Painful anal conditions,
   e.g. anal fissure

Obstructive constipation
Rectal prolapse, intussusception
   and solitary rectal ulcer
   syndrome
Large rectocoele
Pelvic floor dyssynergia

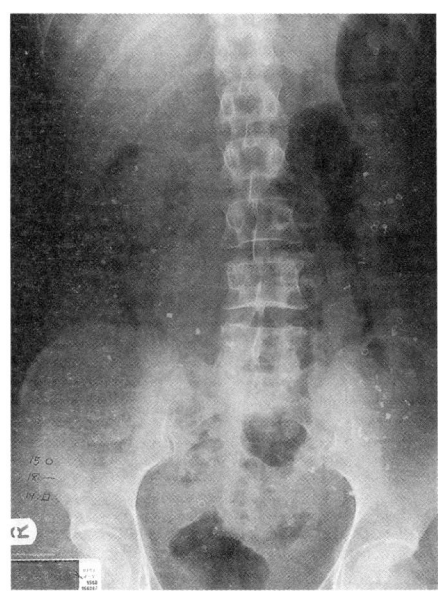

Fig. 6.32 Slow-transit constipation. Straight abdominal X-ray taken on day 5 after ingestion of capsules each containing 21 radio-opaque shapes, which were administered daily on days 1, 2 and 3. Fifty-two shapes are retained, confirming the diagnosis of severe slow-transit constipation.

definitions of constipation are infrequent passage of stools (< 2/week), straining > 25% of time, passage of hard stools and incomplete evacuation. According to these definitions 'constipation' affects more than 1 in 5 of the population.

Many symptoms are attributed by patients to constipation and include headaches, malaise, nausea and a bad taste in the mouth. Other symptoms include abdominal bloating and/or discomfort as well as local and perianal pain. The causes of constipation are shown in Table 6.13.

Assessment of constipation

This relies on a careful history. When there has been a recent change in bowel habit in association with other symptoms (e.g. rectal bleeding) a barium enema or colonoscopy will be indicated. A barium enema should always be preceded by a rectal examination and rigid sigmoidoscopy to exclude anorectal lesions that can otherwise be missed. By these means, colorectal cancer, narrowed segments due to diverticular disease and other rarer colonic causes of constipation (Table 6.13) can be excluded.

There are broadly two *clinical* types of constipation:

- *the slow transit form*, in which patients rarely experience a call to stool
- *an 'obstructive' form* in which patients experience a call to stool but because of coexisting organic and functional anorectal disease are not able to evacuate properly.

Slow-transit constipation

The causes of all types of constipation are shown in Table 6.13. The severity of slow-transit constipation can be assessed by undertaking a simple abdominal X-ray to show constipation and in more problematical cases by undertaking marker studies of colonic transit.

Capsules containing 21 radio-opaque shapes are swallowed on days 1, 2 and 3 and an abdominal X-ray obtained 120 hours after ingestion of the first capsule. Each capsule contains shapes of different configuration and the presence of more than 4 shapes from the first capsule, 6 from the second and 12 from the third denotes moderate to severe slow transit (Fig. 6.32).

'Obstructive' constipation

The common causes of 'obstructive' disorders of defecation includes the presence of an anterior rectocele whereby a weakness of the rectovaginal septum results in protuberances of the anterior wall of the rectum with trapping of stool if the diameter is > 3 cm. In some patients the mucosa of the anterior rectal wall prolapses downwards during straining impeding the passage of stool and in others there may be a higher mucosal intussusception. Finally, in other patients a 'paradoxical' contraction rather than the normal relaxation of the puborectalis and external anal sphincter and associated muscles during straining may prevent evacuation (pelvic floor dyssynergia, anismus). The obstructive disorders of defecation can often be characterized by performing evacuation proctography (Fig. 6.33).

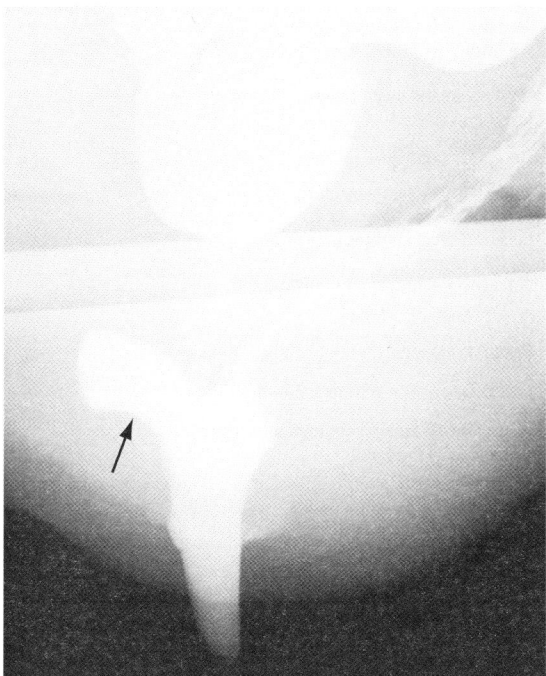

Fig. 6.33 **Evacuating proctogram** showing the presence of an anterior rectocoele (arrowed).

In the megarectum, a very large volume of constipated stool accumulates before evacuation is initiated, with severe symptoms of constipation resulting. In contrast, in some patients the rectum becomes unduly sensitive to the presence of small volumes of stool, resulting in the urge to pass frequent amounts of small-volume stool and the sensation of incomplete evacuation; these disorders can be characterized by anorectal manometry.

Treatment

Treatment of constipation is that of the underlying cause. In patients with slow-transit constipation the main focus should be directed to increasing the fibre content of the diet in conjunction with increasing fluid intake. Fibre intake should be increased by dietary means rather than by prescribing commercially available fibre sources in order to avoid substrate inducibility of colonic bacterial polysaccharidase enzyme systems. Patients with slow-transit constipation should be referred to a dietitian.

The use of laxatives should be restricted to severe cases. Types of laxatives available are listed in Box 6.11. Osmotic laxatives act by increasing colonic inflow of fluid and electrolytes; this acts not only to soften the stool but to stimulate colonic contractility. Magnesium sulphate 5–10 g dissolved in a glass of hot water should be taken before breakfast; it works in 2–4 hours. The polyethylene glycols (Macrogols) have the advantage over the synthetic disaccharide lactulose in that they are not fermented anaerobically in the colon to gas which

---

Box 6.11

Laxatives and enemas

Bulking agents
- Dietary fibre
- Wheat bran
- Methyl cellulose
- Mucilaginous gums – sterculia
- Mucilaginous seeds and seed coats, e.g. ispaghula husk

Stimulant laxatives (stimulate motility and intestinal secretion)
- Phenolphthalein
- Bisacodyl
- Anthraquinones – senna, cascara and dantron
- Dioctyl sodium sulphosuccinate

Osmotic laxatives
- Magnesium sulphate
- Lactulose
- Lactitol
- Macrogols

Suppositories
- Bisacodyl
- Glycerol

Enemas
- Olive oil
- Arachis oil
- Dioctyl sodium sulphosuccinate
- Hypertonic phosphate
- Sodium citrate

---

can distend the colon to cause pain. The osmotic laxatives are preferred to the stimulatory laxatives, which act by stimulating colonic contractility and by causing intestinal secretion. The use of irritant suppositories can be helpful in overcoming minor obstructive causes of constipation. The use of enemas should be restricted to the management of elderly, infirm and immobile patients and those with neurological disorders.

In patients with obstructive defecation due to an anatomical abnormality (e.g. anterior rectocoele, internal anal mucosal intussusception) surgery may be indicated. Anterior mucosal prolapse can be treated by injection and those with pelvic floor dyssynergia (anismus) can benefit from biofeedback therapy.

Megacolon

The term 'megacolon' is used to describe a number of congenital and acquired conditions in which the colon is dilated. In many instances it is secondary to chronic constipation and in some parts of the world Chagas' disease is a common cause.

All young patients with megacolon should have Hirschsprung's disease excluded. In this disease, which presents in the first years of life, an aganglionic segment of the rectum gives rise to constipation and subacute obstruction. Occasionally Hirschsprung's disease affecting only a short segment of the rectum and can be missed in childhood. A preliminary rectal biopsy is performed and stained with special stains for ganglion cells in the submucosal plexus. In doubtful cases full-thickness biopsy, under anaesthesia, should be obtained. A frozen section is stained for acetylcholinesterase, which is elevated in Hirschsprung's disease. Manometric studies show failure of relaxation of the internal sphincter, which is diagnostic of Hirschsprung's disease. This disease can be successfully treated surgically.

Treatment of megacolon is similar to slow transit constipation, but saline washouts and manual removal of faeces are sometimes required.

Faecal incontinence

Seven per cent of the healthy population over the age of 65 experience incontinence at least weekly. Incontinence occurs when the intrarectal pressure exceeds the intra-anal pressure and is classified as minor (inability to control flatus or liquid stool, causing soiling) or major (frequent and inadvertent evacuation of stool of normal consistency). The common causes of incontinence are shown in Table 6.14. Endoanal ultrasonography in women with enhancing per vaginal views is the investigation of choice in the assessment of anal sphincter damage. Neurophysiological investigation of pudendal nerve function, anal sensation and anal sphincter function may be required to elicit the cause of the problem.

Initial management of minor incontinence is bowel habit regulation. Loperamide is the most potent antidiarrhoeal agent which also increases internal sphincter tone.

Surgery may be required for anal sphincter trauma and should be carried out in specialist centres.

Diverticular disease

Diverticula are frequently found in the colon and occur in 50% of patients over the age of 50 years. They are most frequent in the sigmoid, but can be present over the whole colon.

The term *diverticulosis* indicates the presence of diverticula; *diverticulitis* implies that these diverticula are inflamed. It is perhaps better to use the more general term *diverticular disease*, as it is often difficult to be sure whether the diverticula are inflamed. The precise mechanism of diverticula formation is not known. There is thickening of the muscle layer and, because of high intraluminal pressures, pouches of mucosa extrude through the muscular wall through weakened areas near blood vessels to form diverticula. Diverticular disease seems to be related to the low-fibre diet eaten in developed countries.

Table 6.14
Aetiology of faecal incontinence

Anal sphincter dysfunction
Structural damage
  Surgery
  Obstetric injury
  Trauma
  Radiation
Pudendal nerve damage
  Childbirth
Perineal descent
  Prolonged straining at stool

Rectal prolapse

Faecal impaction with overflow diarrhoea

Neurological and psychological disorders
Spinal trauma (S_2–S_4)
Spina bifida
Multiple sclerosis
Dementia
Psychological illness
Diabetes mellitus (with autonomic involvement)

Diverticulitis occurs when faeces obstruct the neck of the diverticulum causing stagnation and allowing bacteria to multiply and produce inflammation. This can then lead to bowel perforation (peridiverticulitis), abscess formation, fistulae into adjacent organs, or even generalized peritonitis.

Clinical features and management

Diverticular disease is asymptomatic in 95% and is usually discovered incidentally on a barium enema examination. No treatment other than dietary advice is required in those patients. In symptomatic patients intermittent left iliac fossa pain or discomfort and an erratic bowel habit commonly occur. In severe disease luminal narrowing can occur in the sigmoid colon, giving rise to severer pain and constipation. In the absence of clinical signs of acute diverticulitis a barium enema is the investigation of choice (Fig. 6.34), combined with an abdominal ultrasound scan to assess bowel wall thickness and to exclude paracolic inflammatory disease. Technically it is sometimes difficult to obtain adequate views of the sigmoid region in diverticular disease and if this is the case a fibreoptic sigmoidoscopy may be required. Treatment of uncomplicated symptomatic disease is with a well-balanced (*soluble* and *insoluble*, see p. 225) fibre diet (20 g/day) with smooth muscle relaxants if required.

Acute diverticulitis

This most commonly affects diverticula in the sigmoid colon. It presents with severe pain in the left iliac fossa, often accompanied by fever and constipation. These symptoms and signs are similar to appendicitis but on the left side. On examination the patient is often febrile

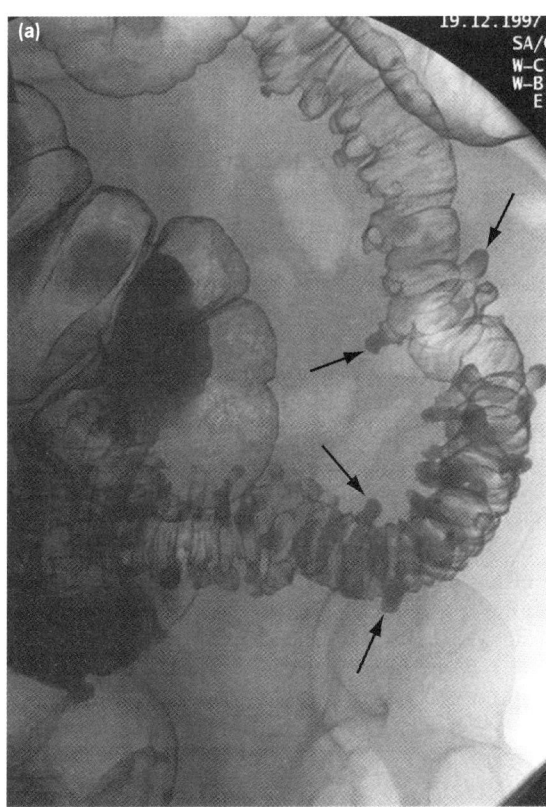

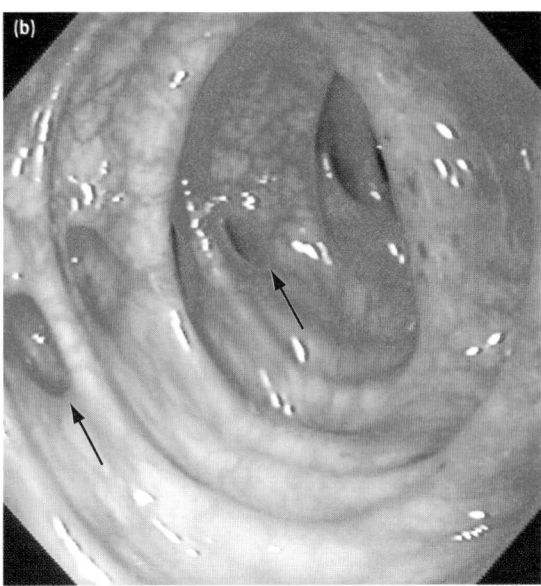

Fig. 6.34 **(a) Double-contrast enema, showing diverticular disease** (the diverticula are arrowed). The barium is black on these films. **(b) Diverticula seen on colonoscopy** (arrows).

with a tachycardia. Abdominal examination shows tenderness, guarding and rigidity on the left side of the abdomen. A palpable tender mass is sometimes felt in the left iliac fossa.

Investigations

- **Blood tests.** A polymorphonuclear leucocytosis is often present. The ESR is raised.
- **Spiral CT of the lower abdomen** (Fig. 6.35) will show colonic wall thickening, diverticula and often pericolic collections and abscesses. There is usually a streaky increased density extending into the immediate pericolic fat with thickening of the pelvic fascial planes. These findings are diagnostic of acute diverticular disease and differ from malignant disease.

Ultrasound examination is often more readily available and is cheaper. It can demonstrate thickened bowel and large pericolic collections, but is less sensitive than CT.

Treatment

Acute attacks can be treated on an outpatient basis using a cephalosporin and metronidazole. Patients who are more ill will require admission for bowel rest, intravenous fluids and antibiotic therapy (e.g. gentamicin, or a cephalosporin) and metronidazole.

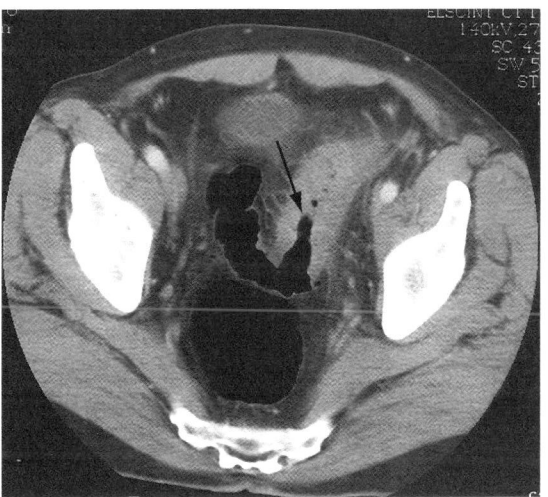

Fig. 6.35 **Spiral CT of lower abdomen, showing acute diverticulitis** (arrow). The bowel wall is thickened and there is loss of clarity of the pericolic fat. A narrow segment of bowel is seen to the left of the diseased segment.

Complications of diverticular disease

- Perforation, which usually, but not always, occurs in association with acute diverticulitis, can lead to formation of a paracolic or pelvic abscess or generalized peritonitis. Surgery is usually required.
- Fistula formation into the bladder, causing dysuria or pneumaturia, or into the vagina, causing discharge.
- Intestinal obstruction (see p. 331) usually after repeated episodes of acute diverticulitis.

- Bleeding, which is sometimes massive. In most cases the bleeding stops and the cause of the bleeding can be established by X-ray, colonoscopy and sometime angiography. Persistent bleeding can often be arrested by undertaking an 'instant' barium enema, which acts to plug the offending diverticulum. In rare cases emergency segmental colectomy is required.

Ischaemic disease of the colon (ischaemic colitis)

Occlusion of branches of the superior mesenteric (SMA) or inferior mesenteric arteries (IMA) often in the older age group commonly presents with sudden onset of abdominal pain and the passage of bright red blood per rectum, with or without diarrhoea. There may be signs of shock and evidence of underlying cardiovascular disease. The majority of cases affect the splenic flexure and left colon. This condition has also been described in women taking the contraceptive pill and in patients with thrombophilia (p. 567) and small- or medium-vessel vasculitis (p. 466).

On examination the abdomen is distended and tender. A straight abdominal X-ray often shows thumb printing (a characteristic sign of ischaemic disease) at the site of the splenic flexure.

The differential diagnosis is of other causes of acute colitis. A rigid sigmoidoscopy (normal mucosa appearances often with presence of blood) and a gentle instant enema is preferred to colonoscopy (to avoid perforation) in cases where the diagnosis is in doubt. A barium enema should be performed when the patient recovers to exclude the formation of a stricture at the site of disease. Patients without evidence of underlying cardiovascular disease should be screened for thrombophilia and vasculitis.

Treatment

Most patients settle on symptomatic treatment. A few develop gangrene and perforation and require urgent surgery.

Pneumatosis cystoides intestinalis

This is a rare condition in which multiple gas-filled cysts are found in the submucosa of the intestine, chiefly the colon. The cause is unknown but some cases are associated with chronic obstructive pulmonary disease. Patients are usually asymptomatic, but abdominal pain and diarrhoea do occur and occasionally the cysts rupture to produce a pneumoperitoneum. This condition is diagnosed on X-ray of the abdomen, barium enema or sigmoidoscopy when cysts are seen.

Treatment is often unnecessary but continuous oxygen therapy will help to disperse the largely nitrogen-containing cysts. Metronidazole may help.

Anorectal disorders

Pruritus ani

Pruritus ani, or an itchy bottom, is common. Perianal excoriation results from itching. Usually the condition results from seepage from haemorrhoids or overactivity of sweat glands. Treatment consists of salt baths, keeping the area dry with powder; the use of all creams should be avoided. Secondary causes include threadworm (*Enterobius vermicularis*) infestation, fungal infections (e.g. *Candidiasis*) and perianal eczema, which should be treated appropriately.

Haemorrhoids

Haemorrhoids (primary, internal, second degree, prolapsing, third degree prolapsed) usually cause rectal bleeding, discomfort and pruritus ani. Patients may notice red blood on their toilet paper and blood on the outside of their stools. They are the most common cause of rectal bleeding (see Fig. 6.19). *Diagnosis* is made by inspection, rectal examination and proctoscopy. If symptoms are minor no treatment is required; depending on severity of symptoms, treatment is with injection of sclerosant, rubber band ligation or surgery.

Anal fissures

An anal fissure is a tear in the sensitive skin-lined lower anal canal which produces pain on defecation. It can be an isolated primary problem in young to middle-aged adults or occur in association with Crohn's disease or ulcerative colitis, in which case perianal abscesses and anal fistulae can complicate the fissure. Diagnosis can usually be made on the history alone. Rectal examination is usually not possible because of pain and sphincter spasm. In severe cases proctoscopy and sigmoidoscopy should be performed under anaesthesia to exclude other anorectal disease. Initial treatment is with local anaesthetic gel. Use of 0.2% glyceryl trinitrate (which donates nitric oxide) ointment is of benefit. Lateral subcutaneous internal sphincterotomy may be required in severe cases.

Fistula in ano

Subcutaneous, low and high anal fistulae are the commonest types (Fig. 6.36). Anorectal fistulae are rarer forms. The fistulae usually present as abscesses and heal after the abscess is incised. In other cases a small discharging sinus may be noted by the patient. Endoanal ultrasonography and/or examination under anaesthetic is usually required to define the primary and any secondary tracks and detect any associated disease. Management is usually surgical with approximately 90% of fistulae being laid open or excised.

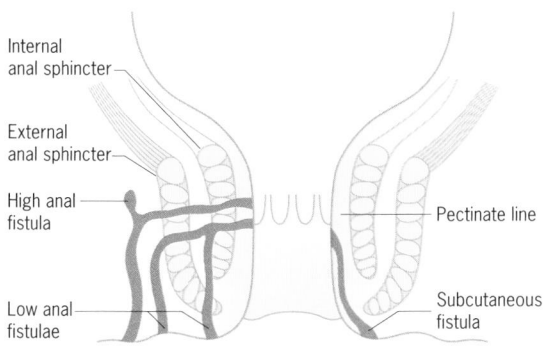

Fig. 6.36 Common sites of anal fistulae. Note subcutaneous fistulae do not traverse the sphincters whereas low and high fistulae do.

Anorectal abscesses

Anorectal abscesses are a common causes of admission to hospital. They are two to three times commoner in men, particularly in homosexual men who indulge in penetrative anal sex. They may be the first manifestation of Crohn's disease, ulcerative colitis and tuberculosis. Perianal and ischiorectal abscess, the commonest forms, present with painful, tender swellings and require surgical incision and drainage.

Rectal prolapse, intussusception and solitary rectal ulcer syndrome (SRUS)

All these conditions are thought to be related, with rectal prolapse being the unifying pathology. Some patients with SRUS do not have prolapse but strain excessively and ulcerate the anterior rectal wall which is forced into the anus during futile straining efforts.

Rectal prolapse starts as an intussusception of the upper rectum which passes into the lower part of the viscus and progression results in its protrusion through the anal canal to emerge as an external prolapse. Constipation and chronic straining are the likely causes. In addition the presence of an intussuscepting rectum will mimic presence of stool in the rectum and lead to straining efforts to evacuate the prolapse. In some patients repeated straining leads to traumatic ulceration of the mucosa and formation of SRUS, commonly on the anterior wall of the rectum within 13 cm of the anal verge. Sometimes difficult to distinguish from cancer and Crohn's disease, SRUS has typical histological features of non-specific inflammatory changes with bands of smooth muscle extending into the lamina propria.

Patients commonly present with slight bleeding and mucus on defecation, tenesmus and sensation of anal obstruction. Asymptomatic SRUS should not be treated. Symptomatic patients should be advised to stop straining and measures taken to soften the stool. If rectal prolapse can be demonstrated during defecation, this should be repaired; in severe cases surgical treatment by resection rectopexy may be indicated. Surgical treatment for complete rectal prolapse is also required.

Colonic tumours

Colon polyps and polyposis syndromes

A polyp is an elevation above the mucosal surface. The majority of colorectal polyps are adenomas with malignant potential. Polyps range in size from a few millimetres to several centimetres in diameter. They may be single or multiple and in the polyposis syndromes hundreds may be found.

Larger polyps in the rectum and 70–80% of all polyps in the colon are adenomas and 5% of these may contain invasive carcinoma at discovery. Most polyps are asymptomatic and found by chance when patients are investigated for pain, altered bowel habit, rectal bleeding or some other cause.

Classification of colorectal polyps (Table 6.15)

Non-neoplastic polyps

Hamartomatous polyps are commonly large and stalked.

Juvenile polyps (occurring in children and teenagers) are confined mainly to the colon and histologically show mucus retention cysts. Juvenile polyposis (more than 10 colonic polyps) is inherited in an autosomal dominant fashion and the relevant gene has recently been identified (Box 6.12). The polyps may be a cause of bleeding and intussusception in the first decade of life. There is also an increased risk of colonic cancer, and surveillance and removal of polyps must be undertaken.

Peutz–Jeghers syndrome (see p. 299).

Table 6.15
Classification of colorectal polyps

Type of polyp	Pathogenesis	Polyposis syndrome
Adenoma	Neoplastic	Familial adenomatous polyposis
Juvenile	Hamartoma	Juvenile polyposis
Peutz–Jeghers	Hamartoma	Peutz–Jeghers syndrome
Metaplastic	Unknown	Metaplastic polyposis
Lymphoid	Hyperplasia	Lymphoid polyposis
Inflammatory	Inflammation	Inflammatory polyposis

Box 6.12

Inherited syndromes of colon cancer and their responsible genes

Syndrome	Responsible gene
Adenomatous polyps	
FAP	*APC*
HNPCC	*MMR*
Hamartomatous polyps	
Peutz–Jeghers syndrome	*STK11 (LKB1)*
Juvenile polyposis	*SMAD4/DPC4*
Cowden syndrome	*PTEN*

Cowden syndrome is an autosomal dominant disease associated with skin stigmata and intestinal polyps regarded as harmartomas but with a mixture of cell types. These patients have an increased risk of various extraintestinal malignancies (thyroid, breast, uterine and ovarian).

Metaplastic polyps are frequently found in the rectum and sigmoid colon. These pale, sessile mucosal nodules usually measure <5 mm and are non-neoplastic lesions without significant malignant potential.

Neoplastic polyps

Port-mortem studies have shown the incidence of adenomas to be 30–40% in western populations, and most colorectal cancers develop from sporadic adenomatous polyps. Flat adenomas, which were first described in Japan, may be difficult to detect at endoscopy. They account for up to 10% of all polyps and may have a higher rate of malignant change.

Polyps rarely produce symptoms and most are diagnosed on X-ray or on colonoscopy performed for other reasons. Large polyps (Fig. 6.37) may bleed intermittently and cause anaemia. Large sessile villous adenomas of the rectum can present with profuse diarrhoea and hypokalaemia.

Several factors influence the risk of cancer developing in an adenoma (see Box 6.13).

Once a polyp has been found it is usually possible to remove it endoscopically. The National Polyp Study conducted in the USA showed that colonoscopic polypectomy with surveillance reduced colorectal cancer incidence by 76–90%. Current recommendations, based on this study, suggest that surveillance colonoscopy intervals of around 6 years after polypectomy are appropriate. If any doubt exists about the excision margins of any polyp then an earlier repeat examination is suggested.

Familial adenomatous polyposis (FAP) arises from germline mutations of the *APC* gene located on chromosome 5q and is inherited in an autosomal dominant fashion. The disease is characterized by the presence of hundreds to thousands of colorectal adenomas. The mean age of adenoma development is 16 years, whereas the average age for developing colorectal cancer is 39 years. Tracing and screening of relatives is essential (usually after 12 years of age) and affected individuals should be offered a prophylactic colectomy, often before the age of 20. Surgical options include colectomy and ileorectal anastomosis, which requires life-long surveillance of the rectal stump or a restorative proctocolectomy or pouch procedure.

Gastric fundic gland polyps and duodenal adenomas are frequently found in FAP, as well as other extraintestinal lesions such as osteomas, epidermoid cysts and desmoid tumours. Congenital hypertrophy of the retinal pigment epithelium (CHRPE) occurs in many families

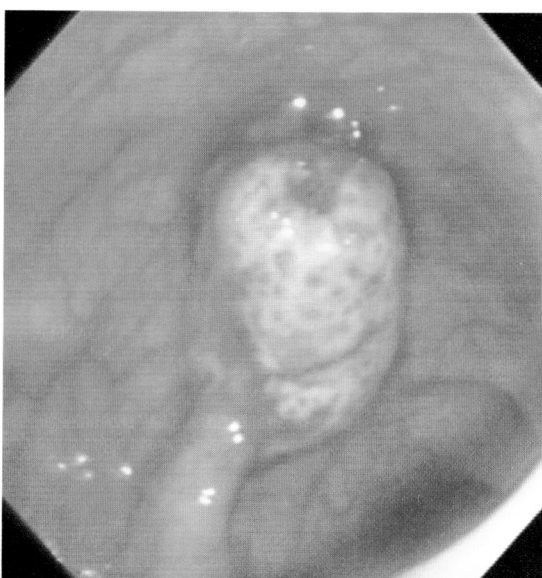

Fig. 6.37 Colonoscopic appearance of a large peduncular polyp.

Box 6.13

Factors affecting risk of malignant change in an adenoma

	Higher risk	**Lower risk**
Size	>1.5 cm	<1 cm
Type	Sessile or flat	Pedunculated
Histology	Severe dysplasia Villous architecture Squamous metaplasia	Mild dysplasia Tubular architecture
Number	Multiple polyps	Single polyp

---

with FAP. Other cancers that are observed in FAP include thyroid, pancreatic and hepatoblastomas.

APC gene mutations can be found on screening in about 80% of families with FAP. Once the disease-causing mutation has been identified in an index case known to have FAP, other family members can be tested for the mutation and screening can then be directed at mutation carriers. If a mutation cannot be found in a known FAP case, then all family members should undergo clinical screening with regular endoscopy.

Colorectal carcinoma

Colorectal cancer (CRC) is the second most common cause of cancer death in the UK. It was responsible for over 15 000 deaths in England and Wales in 1996 (68% colon, 32% rectal cancer). The prevalence rate per 100 000 (all ages) is 53.5 for men and 36.7 for women. The incidence increases with age, the average age at

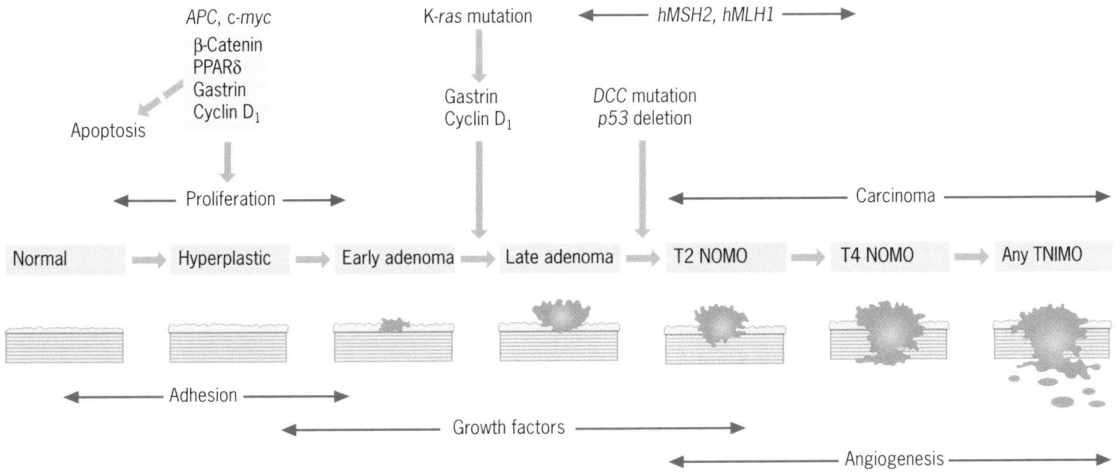

Fig. 6.38 **Genetic model for colorectal tumorigenesis, showing the progression from adenoma to carcinoma.** The stages are shown at which mutations occur in the genes. *APC* (adenomatous polyposis coli), *K-ras, DCC, p53, hMSH2,* and *hMLH1*.

diagnosis being 60–65 years. The disease is much more common in westernized countries than in Asia or Africa. Western diets are low in dietary fibre, which increases faecal bulk and reduces transit time and thus has been proposed as accounting for these differences. Fibre has many components and there may also be other properties in fruits and vegetables that contribute a protective effect. There is a positive correlation between the consumption of meat and intake of animal fat with CRC. There is also evidence that exercise reduces the risk of CRC and that the risk of developing both adenomas and cancers is reduced among those taking aspirin and other NSAIDs. There is also increasing evidence that there may be an association between hormone replacement therapy and a reduced risk of CRC.

Genetics

Most colorectal cancers develop as a result of a stepwise progression from normal mucosa to adenoma to invasive cancer. This progression is controlled by the accumulation of alterations or mutations in a number of critical growth-regulating genes. Germline mutations of the *APC* gene are responsible for FAP (see above), but inactivation of this tumour suppressor gene and β-catenin (a transcription activator) is also seen in up to 70% of sporadic colorectal cancers. A cytoplasmic complex consisting of the APC protein, β-catenin, conduction/axin and glycogen synthase kinase-3β (GSK-3β) ensures the tight control of β-catenin. GSK-3β is a serine–threonine kinase which destroys β-catenin. Other factors which regulate β-catenin include cyclin D_1, gastrin and perioxisome, proliferator-activated receptor β (PPARβ) which mediates transcription of prostaglandins and fatty acids. Inactivation of *APC* appears to occur at an early stage in the development of an adenoma, which has led to it being described as a 'gatekeeper' gene. The

sequence is usually followed by K-*ras* mutations which appear to facilitate the growth of adenomatous tissue and then by *DCC* (deleted in colon cancer) and *p53* gene mutations which occur around the adenoma–carcinoma transition (Fig. 6.38). The exact order of these mutations may vary but in around 15% of sporadic colorectal cancers there are insertions or deletions of nucleotides within repeated sequences of DNA – microsatellite instability (MSI) due to defective repair of mismatched nucleotides.

Cancer families

A family history of colon cancer confers an increased risk to relatives. Family history is, next to age, the most common risk factor for colon cancer. FAP (Fig. 6.39) is the best-recognized syndrome predisposing to colorectal cancer but represents less than 1% of all colorectal cancers. *Hereditary non-polyposis colorectal cancer* (HNPCC) arises from germline mutations in any one of five mismatch repair (MMR) genes. Mutations in two of these, *hMLH1* and *hMSH2*, account for >95% of HNPCC families. Mutations in these genes lead to microsatellite instability in the tumours of affected individuals. Other cancers frequently occur in HNPCC including endometrial, gastric, biliary tract, urinary tract, ovarian and small bowel malignancies. Diagnostic criteria, based on family history, were devised to help identify those affected and have subsequently (Modified Amsterdam Criteria) been modified to include non-colonic tumours (Box 6.14).

Patients with HNPCC tend to develop right-sided cancers at an early age and regular surveillance with colonoscopy is recommended.

In addition to the above syndromes CRC arises, at least in part, from an inherited predisposition, the so-called familial risk (Table 6.16). Estimates of their frequency range from 10–30% of all CRC but the genes

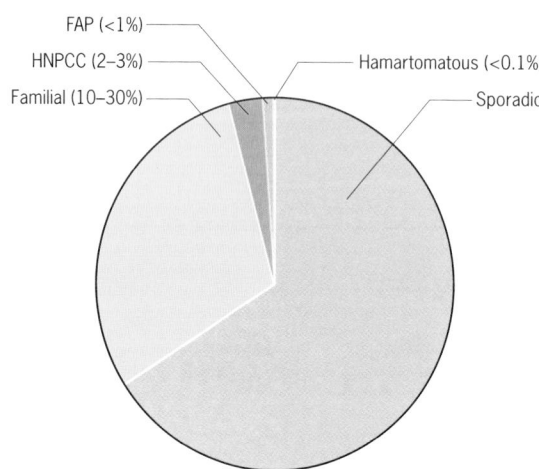

Fig. 6.39 **Percentages of colon cancer according to family risk.** HNPCC, hereditary non-polyposis colorectal cancer; FAP, familial adenomatous polyposis.

Box 6.14

Modified Amsterdam Criteria for hereditary non-polyposis colorectal cancer

- Three or more cases of colorectal cancer in a minimum of two generations.
- One affected individual must be a first-degree relative of the other two (or more) cases.
- One case must be diagnosed at age < 50.
- Colorectal cancer can be replaced by endometrial or small bowel cancer.
- Familial adenomatous polyposis (FAP) should be excluded.

---

involved have yet to be identified. The risk of CRC can be estimated from a careful family history matched with empirical risk tables so that appropriate advice regarding screening can be offered.

Most colorectal cancers are, however, sporadic and occur in individuals without a strong family history. More than half these cancers arise in the rectosigmoid area (Fig. 6.40).

Pathology

CRC, which is usually a polypoid mass with ulceration, spreads by direct infiltration through the bowel wall. It involves lymphatics and blood vessels with subsequent spread, most commonly to the liver. Synchronous tumours are present in 2% of cases. *Histology* is adenocarcinoma with moderately to well differentiated glandular epithelium with mucin production. 'Signet ring' cells in which mucin displaces the nucleus to the side of the cell is characteristic.

Clinical features

Alteration in bowel habit, with or without abdominal pain, is a common symptom of left-sided colonic

Table 6.16
Lifetime risk of colorectal cancer in first-degree relatives of a patient with colorectal cancer.

Population risk	1 in 50
One first-degree relative affected (any age)	1 in 17
One first-degree and one second-degree relative affected	1 in 12
One first-degree relative affected (age < 45)	1 in 10
Two first-degree relatives affected	1 in 6
Autosomal dominant pedigree	1 in 2

Houlston et al. 1990 *BMJ* 301: 366–368

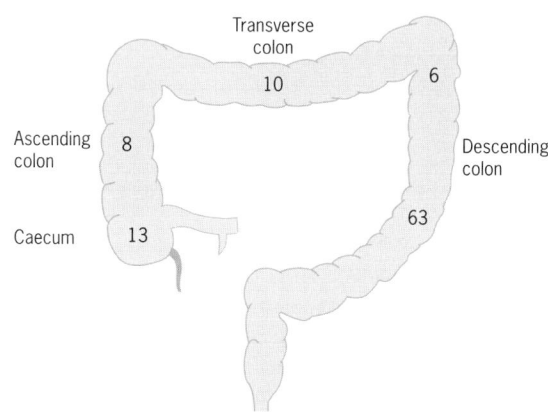

Fig. 6.40 **Distribution of sporadic colorectal cancer.**

lesions. Rectal and sigmoid cancers often bleed, blood being mixed in with the stool. Cancers arising in the caecum and right colon may often be asymptomatic and may present as an iron deficiency anaemia. The elderly often present with intestinal obstruction.

Patients aged greater than 35–40 presenting with new large bowel symptoms should be investigated. *The alarm symptoms*, suggestive of colorectal cancer include; change in bowel habit, rectal bleeding, anorexia and weight loss, faecal incontinence, tenesmus and passing mucus per rectum.

Examination is usually unhelpful but a mass may be palpable. Hepatomegaly may be found with liver metastases. Digital examination of the rectum is essential and rigid sigmoidoscopy should be performed in all cases.

Investigations

- **Blood count and routine biochemistry.**
- **Colonoscopy** (Fig. 6.41) is the gold standard for investigation and allows biopsies and polypectomies to obtain specimens for histological examination.
- **Double-contrast barium enema** can visualize the large bowel and may be superseded in the future by CT pneumocolon.
- **Ultrasound, CT and MRI** may help evaluate tumour size and local and secondary spread, including hepatic metastases.

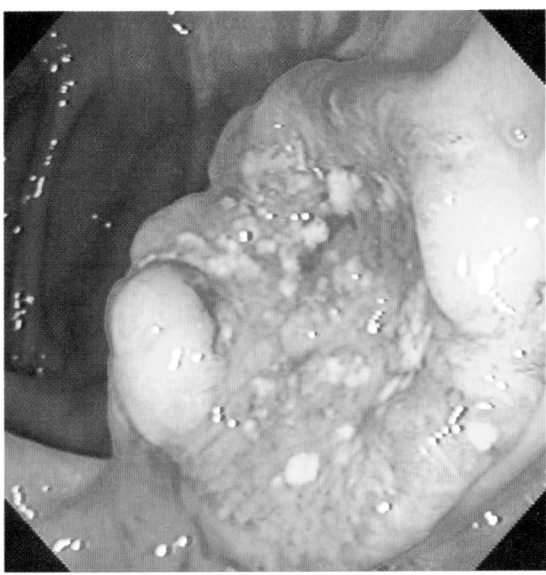

Fig. 6.41 Colonoscopic appearance of a carcinoma in the ascending colon – a large irregular ulcer.

Faecal occult blood tests have been used for mass screening but are no value in hospital practice.

Treatment

About 80% of patients with colorectal cancer undergo surgery though fewer than half survive more than 5 years. The operative procedure depends on the cancer site and long-term survival relates to the stage of the primary tumour and the presence of metastatic disease (see Table 6.17). There has been a gradual move from using Dukes' classification to using the TNM classification system.

Table 6.17
Staging and survival of colorectal cancers

TNM classification	Modified Dukes' classification	5-Year survival (%)
Stage 0 – carcinoma in situ		
Stage I – no nodal involvement no metastases: tumour invades submucosa (T1,N0,M0); tumour invades muscularis propria (T2,N0,M0)	A	90–100
Stage II – no nodal involvement, no metastases; tumour invades into subserosa (T3,N0,M0); tumour invades other organs (T4,N0,M0)	B	75–85
Stage III – regional lymph nodes involved (any T, N1,M0)	C	30–40
Stage IV – distant metastases (any T, any N)	D	< 5

Long-term survival is only likely when the cancer is completely removed. Total mesorectal excision (TME) is an approach to rectal surgery in which meticulous care is taken to remove all the tissue surrounding the cancer. There is some evidence from studies that TME may reduce recurrence rates in rectal cancer and improve survival. Preoperative radiotherapy offers patients with rectal cancer improved survival rates and radiotherapy can also be highly effective as palliation in locally advanced rectal cancer. Adjuvant postoperative chemotherapy will improve disease-free survival and overall survival in TNM stage III (Dukes' C) colon cancer. The most widely used agent is 5-fluorouracil with promising results with agents such as irinotecan. Cancers with high levels of microsatellite instability may have a more favourable outlook.

Prevention and screening

Healthcare agencies advocate a low-fat, high-fibre diet for the prevention of sporadic colorectal cancer, and endoscopic screening is a recommendation for high-risk patients with inherited syndromes (e.g. FAP, HNPCC) and those with an increased family risk. Faecal occult blood (FOB) tests have been used as a screening test for colorectal cancer. Several large randomized studies have demonstrated a reduction in cancer-related mortality of 15–33%. The disadvantage of screening with FOB is its relatively low sensitivity which means many unnecessary colonoscopies.

Colonoscopy is the gold-standard technique for the examination of the colon and rectum and is the investigation of choice for high-risk patients. Its expense, the need for full bowel preparation and sedation and the small risk of perforation obviate its use as a population screening tool at present, though trials are underway in the USA. In the future CT pneumocolon or 'virtual colonoscopy' and the refinement of genetic testing may contribute to screening programmes. Universal screening strategies have been recommended in the USA but not as yet in the UK.

FURTHER READING

Boland CR et al. (2000) Colorectal cancer: prevention and treatment. *Gastroenterology* **118**: 5115–5128.

Giardiello FM, Brensinger JD (2001) AGA technical review of hereditary colorectal cancer and genetic testing. *Gastroenterology* **121**: 198–213.

Lieberman DA et al. (2000) Use of colonoscopy to screen asymptomatic adults for colorectal cancer. *New England Journal of Medicine* **343**: 162–168.

Woolf SH (2001) The best screening test for colorectal cancer. *New England Journal of Medicine* **343**: 1641–1642.

Diarrhoea

Diarrhoea is a common clinical problem and there is no uniformly accepted definition of diarrhoea. Organic causes (stool weights > 250 g per day) have to be distinguished from 'functional causes' and is the first step in the assessment of the history. Sudden onset of bowel frequency associated with crampy abdominal pains, and a fever will point to an infective cause; bowel frequency with loose blood-stained stools to an inflammatory basis; and the passage of pale offensive stools that float, often accompanied by loss of appetite and weight loss, to steatorrhoea. Nocturnal bowel frequency and urgency usually points to an organic cause. Passage of frequent small-volume stools (often formed) points to a functional cause (see Functional gastrointestinal disorders, p. 328).

Mechanisms

Osmotic diarrhoea

The gut mucosa acts as a semipermeable membrane and fluid enters the bowel if there are large quantities of non-absorbed hypertonic substances in the lumen. This occurs because:

- the patient has ingested a non-absorbable substance (e.g. a purgative such as magnesium sulphate or magnesium-containing antacid)
- the patient has generalized malabsorption so that high concentrations of solute (e.g. glucose) remain in the lumen
- the patient has a specific absorptive defect (e.g. disaccharidase deficiency or glucose–galactose malabsorption).

The volume of diarrhoea produced by these mechanisms is reduced by the absorption of fluid by the ileum and colon. The diarrhoea stops when the patient stops eating or the malabsorptive substance is discontinued.

Secretory diarrhoea

In this disorder, there is both active intestinal secretion of fluid and electrolytes as well as decreased absorption. The mechanism of intestinal secretion is shown in Figure 6.42(a).

Common causes of secretory diarrhoea are:

- enterotoxins (e.g. cholera, E. coli – thermolabile or thermostable toxin)
- hormones (e.g. vasoactive intestinal peptide in the Verner–Morrison syndrome, p. 404)
- bile salts (in the colon) following ileal resection
- fatty acids (in the colon) following ileal resection
- some laxatives (e.g. dioctyl sodium sulphosuccinate).

Inflammatory diarrhoea (mucosal destruction)

Diarrhoea occurs because of damage to the intestinal mucosal cell so that there is a loss of fluid and blood (Fig. 6.42(b)). In addition, there is defective absorption of fluid and electrolytes. Common causes are infective conditions (e.g. dysentery due to *Shigella*), and inflammatory conditions (e.g. ulcerative colitis and Crohn's disease).

Abnormal motility

Diabetic, post-vagotomy and hyperthyroid diarrhoea are all due to abnormal motility of the upper gut. In many of these cases the volume and weight of the stool is not all that high, but frequency of defection occurs; this therefore is not true diarrhoea.

Causes of diarrhoea are shown in Table 6.18. It should be noted that the irritable bowel syndrome, colorectal cancer, diverticular disease and faecal impaction with overflow in the elderly do not cause 'true' organic diarrhoea (i.e. > 250 g/day), even though the patients may complain of diarrhoea. World-wide, infection and infestation are a major problem and these are discussed under the causative organisms in Chapter 2.

Table 6.18
Causes of diarrhoea

Infective causes	Diverticular disease
Bacterial	Ischaemic colitis
Campylobacter jejuni	Gastrointestinal lymphoma
Salmonella sp.	Carcinoma of the colon
Shigella	(change in bowel habit)
Escherichia coli (particularly	Malabsorption
enterohaemorrhagic	Gut resection
E. coli 0157:H7)	Bile acid malabsorption
Staphylococcus enterocolitis	Drugs, e.g.
Bacillus cereus	laxatives
Clostridium perfringens	biguanides
Clostridium botulinum	anticancer drugs
Gastrointestinal tuberculosis	Faecal impaction with overflow
Viral	Irritable bowel syndrome
Rotavirus	
Fungal	**Endocrine**
Histoplasmosis	Zollinger–Ellison syndrome
Parasitic	Vipoma
Amoebic dysentery	Somatostatinoma
(*Entamoeba histolytica*)	Glucagonoma
Schistosomiasis	Carcinoid syndrome
Giardia intestinalis	Thyrotoxicosis
	Medullary carcinoma of thyroid
Non-infective causes of	Diabetic autonomic neuropathy
diarrhoea	
Inflammatory bowel disease	**Factitious diarrhoea (4%)**
Pseudomembranous colitis	Purgative abuse
Radiation proctitis or colitis	Dilutional diarrhoea
Behçet's disease	

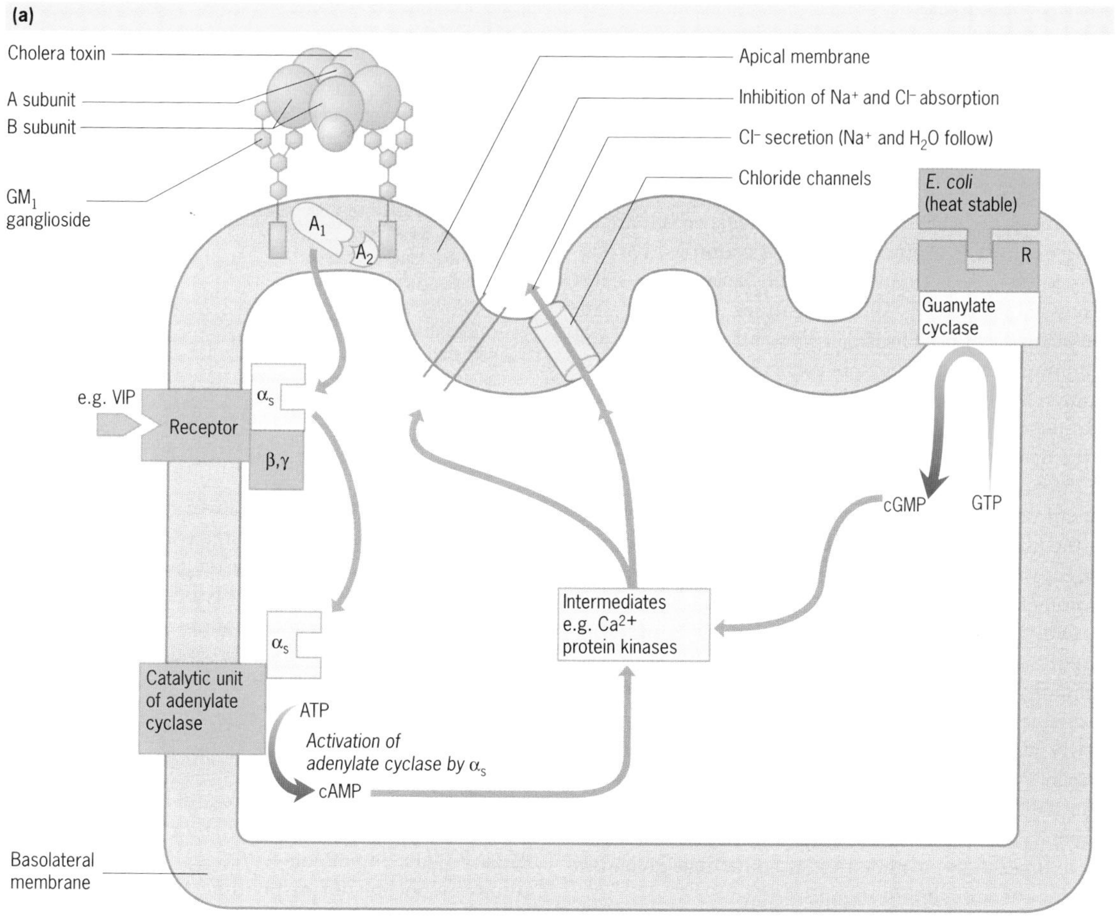

(a)

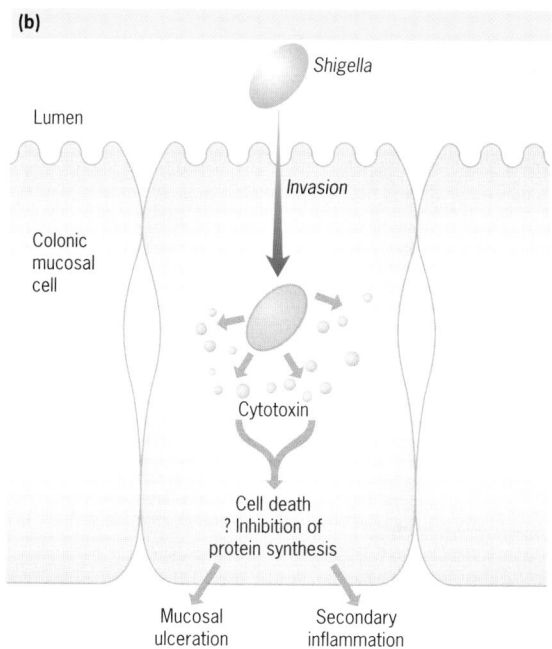

Cholera toxin

A subunit

B subunit

GM$_1$ ganglioside

Apical membrane

Inhibition of Na$^+$ and Cl$^-$ absorption

Cl$^-$ secretion (Na$^+$ and H$_2$O follow)

Chloride channels

E. coli (heat stable)

R

Guanylate cyclase

A$_1$

A$_2$

e.g. VIP

Receptor

α_s

β, γ

cGMP   GTP

Intermediates e.g. Ca^{2+} protein kinases

α_s

Catalytic unit of adenylate cyclase

ATP

Activation of adenylate cyclase by α_s

cAMP

Basolateral membrane

(b)

Lumen

Colonic mucosal cell

Shigella

Invasion

Cytotoxin

Cell death ? Inhibition of protein synthesis

Mucosal ulceration

Secondary inflammation

Fig. 6.42 **Mechanisms of diarrhoea.**

(a) Small intestinal cell. Cholera toxin binds to its receptor (monosialoganglioside GM$_1$) via its B subunit. The enzymatically active A$_1$ subunit activates G$_s$ protein, shown as its three subunits γ, β and α_s. α_s dissociates from G$_s$ protein and activates the catalytic unit of adenylate cyclase on the basolateral membrane. The resulting increase in cAMP activates intermediates (e.g. protein kinases and Ca^{2+}), which act on the apical microvillous membrane to cause Cl$^-$ secretion and inhibition of Na$^+$ and Cl$^-$ absorption. Heat-labile *E. coli* shares the same receptor as cholera toxin. Heat-stable *E. coli* (ST) binds to its receptor protein R and this complex activates guanylate cyclase, which produces the same effect. The ST receptor is specific for the intestine. In both mechanisms, stimulation occurs without invasion.

(b) Colonic mucosal cell. This demonstrates one of the mechanisms by which an invasive pathogen (e.g. *Shigella*) acts. Following penetration, the pathogens generate cytotoxins which lead to mucosal ulceration and cell death.

Acute diarrhoea

(excluding cholera, discussed on p. 87)

Diarrhoea of sudden onset is very common, often short-lived and requires no investigation or treatment. This type of diarrhoea is seen after dietary indiscretions, but diarrhoea due to viral agents also lasts 24–48 hours (see p. 54). The causes of other infective diarrhoeas are shown on page 71. Traveller's diarrhoea, which affects people travelling outside their own countries, particularly to developing countries, usually lasts 2–5 days; it is discussed on page 73. Clinical features associated with the acute diarrhoeas include fever, abdominal pain and vomiting. If the diarrhoea is particularly severe, dehydration can be a problem; the very young and very old are at special risk from this. Investigations are necessary if the diarrhoea has lasted more than 1 week. Stools (up to three) should be sent immediately to the laboratory for culture and examination for ova, cysts and parasites. If the diagnosis has still not been made, a sigmoidoscopy and rectal biopsy should be performed and radiological studies should be considered.

Oral fluid and electrolyte replacement is of prime importance in the treatment. Special oral rehydration solutions (e.g. sodium chloride and glucose powder) are available for use in severe episodes of diarrhoea, particularly in infants. Antidiarrhoeal drugs are thought to impair the clearance of any pathogen from the bowel but may be necessary for short-term relief (e.g. codeine phosphate 30 mg four times daily, or loperamide 2 mg three times daily). Antibiotics are sometimes given (see p. 74) depending on the organism.

Chronic diarrhoea

This always needs investigation. All patients should have a sigmoidoscopy and rectal biopsy. The flow diagram in Figure 6.43 is illustrative; whether the large or the small bowel is investigated first will depend on the clinical story of, for example, bloody diarrhoea or steatorrhoea. The investigations and treatment are described in detail under the individual diseases.

When difficulties exist in distinguishing between functional and organic causes of diarrhoea hospital admission for a formal 72-h assessment of stool weights is helpful and will also lead to the diagnosis of factitious causes of diarrhoea.

Antibiotic-associated diarrhoea (pseudomembranous colitis) (see p. 72)

Pseudomembranous colitis may develop following the use of any antibiotic. Diarrhoea occurs in the first few days after taking the antibiotic or even up to 6 weeks after stopping the drug. The causative agent is *Clostridium difficile* (p. 72).

Bile acid malabsorption

Bile acid malabsorption is an underdiagnosed cause of chronic diarrhoea and many patients with this disorder

---

Table 6.19
Causes of bile acid malabsorption

Ileal resection
Ileal disease, e.g. active or inactive Crohn's disease
Idiopathic or primary bile acid malabsorption (structurally normal ileum)
Postinfective gastroenteritis
Associated with:
    post-cholecystectomy diarrhoea
    diabetic diarrhoea
    post-vagotomy diarrhoea
    chronic pancreatitis
    cystic fibrosis
    coeliac disease
    microscopic inflammatory colitis
    drugs (e.g. colchicine, biguanides)

---

are assumed to have irritable bowel syndrome. Bile acid diarrhoea occurs when the terminal ileum fails to reabsorb bile acids. Bile acids (particularly the dihydroxy bile acids – deoxycholate and chenodeoxycholate) when present in increased concentrations in the colon lead to diarrhoea by reducing absorption of water and electrolytes and, at higher concentrations, inducing secretion as well as increasing colonic motility. A variety of causes of bile acid malabsorption are now recognized (Table 6.19).

Bile acid malabsorption should be considered not only in patients with chronic diarrhoea of unknown cause but also in patients with diarrhoea and associated disease who are not responding to standard therapy (e.g. patients with terminal ileal Crohn's disease, microscopic inflammatory colitis).

Diagnosis is made using the SeHCAT test in which a radiolabelled bile acid analogue is administered and percentage retention at 7 days calculated (<19% retention abnormal). Treatment is with colestyramine, a resin which binds and inactivates the action of bile acids in the colon. The best results of treatment are obtained in patients with a SeHCAT retention of <5%.

Factitious diarrhoea

Factitious diarrhoea accounts for up to 4% of new patients with diarrhoea attending gastroenterology clinics.

Purgative abuse

This is most commonly seen in females who surreptitiously take high-dose purgatives and are often extensively investigated for chronic diarrhoea. The diarrhoea is usually of high volume (>1 L daily) and patients may have a low serum potassium. Sigmoidoscopy may show pigmented mucosa, a condition known as melanosis coli. Histologically the rectal biopsy shows pigment-laden macrophages in patients taking an anthraquinone purgative (e.g. senna). Melanosis coli is also seen in people regularly taking purgatives in normal doses.

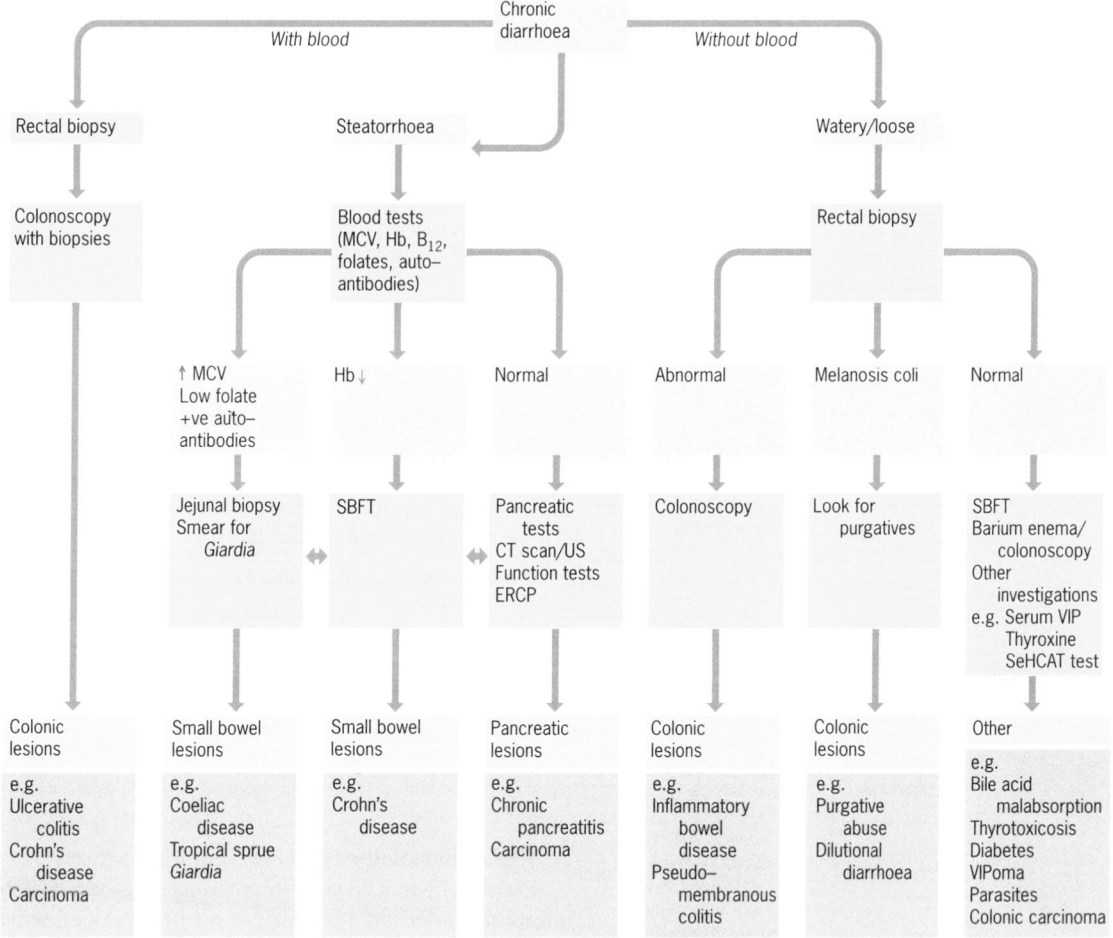

Fig. 6.43 Flow diagram for the investigation of chronic diarrhoea. NB: All patients should have had stool cultures. SBFT, small bowel follow-through; VIP, vasoactive intestinal polypeptide; ERCP, endoscopic retrograde cholangiopancreatography; SeHCAT, ^{75}Se-homochoyl taurine.

In advanced cases a barium enema may show a dilated colon and loss of haustral pattern.

Phenolphthalein laxatives can be detected by pouring an alkali (e.g. sodium hydroxide) on the stools, which then turn pink; a magnesium-containing purgative will give a high faecal magnesium content. Anthraquinones can also be measured in the urine. If the diagnosis is suspected a locker or bed search (while the patient is out of the ward) is occasionally necessary. Management is difficult as most patients deny purgative ingestion. Purgative abuse often occurs in association with eating disorders and all patients needs psychiatric help.

Dilutional diarrhoea

In this condition raised stool weights occur as a consequence of patients deliberately diluting their stool with urine or tap water. The diagnosis is made by measuring stool osmolality and electrolyte concentrations in order to calculate the faecal osmolar gap. Measurement of stool creatinine content is helpful in excluding dilution of stools with urine and early admission to hospital for formal assessment of stool weights may avoid unnecessary invasive investigations being carried out.

Diarrhoea in patients with HIV Infection

Chronic diarrhoea is a common symptom in HIV infection, but HIV's role in the pathogenesis of diarrhoea is unclear. *Cryptosporidium* (see p. 108) is the pathogen most commonly isolated. *Isospora belli* and microsporidia have also been found.

The cause of the diarrhoea is often not found and treatment is symptomatic. Table 6.20 shows the conditions affecting the gastrointestinal tract in patients with AIDS.

Table 6.20
Gastrointestinal problems in patients with AIDS

Site	Symptoms	Causes
Mouth/oesophagus	Dysphagia Retrosternal discomfort Oral ulceration	Candidiasis Herpes simplex virus (HSV) Cytomegalovirus (CMV)

Small bowel/colon	Chronic
	  diarrhoea
	Steatorrhoea
	Weight loss
		Parasites:
		  Entamoeba histolytica
		  Giardia intestinalis
		  Cryptosporidium
		  Blastocystis hominis
		  Isospora belli
		  Microsporidia
		  Cyclospora cayetanensis
		Viruses:
		  CMV/HSV, adenovirus
		Bacteria:
		  Salmonella
		  Campylobacter
		  Shigella
		  Mycobacterium
		    avium-intracellulare
		Non-infective enteropathy –
		  cause unknown

Rectum/colon	Bloody
	  diarrhoea
		Bacterial infection
		  (e.g. *Shigella*)

Any	Weight loss
	Diarrhoea
		Neoplasia:
		  Kaposi's sarcoma
		  Lymphoma
		  Squamous carcinoma
		Infection – disseminated,
		  e.g. *Mycobacterium*
		    avium-intracellulare
		Retroviral therapy

Functional gastrointestinal disorders

There is a large group of gastrointestinal disorders that are termed 'functional' because symptoms occur in the absence of any demonstrable abnormalities in the digestion and absorption of nutrients, fluid and electrolytes and no structural abnormality can be identified in the gastrointestinal tract.

Table 6.21 lists some of the symptoms that are suggestive of a functional gastrointestinal disorder; modern classification systems (e.g. Rome II 1999, p. 327) are based on the premise that for each disorder there is a symptom cluster that 'breeds true' across clinical and population groups. There is inevitably overlap with some symptoms being common to more than one disorder.

Table 6.22 lists the common functional gastrointestinal disorders. These conditions are extremely common world-wide, making up to 80% of patients seen in the gastroenterology clinic.

Table 6.21
Chronic gastrointestinal symptoms suggestive of a functional gastrointestinal disorder (FGID)

Nausea alone
Vomiting alone
Belching
Chest pain unrelated to exercise
Postprandial fullness
Abdominal bloating
Abdominal discomfort/pain (right or left iliac fossae)
Passage of mucus per rectum
Frequent bowel actions with urgency first thing in morning

Table 6.22
Common functional gastrointestinal disorders

Functional oesophageal disorders
Globus
Rumination syndrome
Chest pain of presumed oesophageal origin

Functional gastroduodenal disorders
Functional dyspepsia
Aerophagia
Vomiting

Functional bowel disorders
Irritable bowel syndrome
Pain/gas/bloat syndrome
Diarrhoea

Pathophysiology and brain–gut interactions

People with functional gastrointestinal disorders (FGID), are characterized by having a greater gastrointestinal motility response to life stress when compared to normal subjects. There is, however, a poor association between measured gastrointestinal motility changes and pain in many of the FGIDs. Patients with FGID have been shown to have abnormalities in visceral sensation and have a lower pain threshold when tested with balloon distension (visceral hyperalgesia). Visceral hypersensitivity possibly relates to:

- altered receptor sensitivity at the viscus itself
- increased excitability of the spinal cord dorsal horn neurones
- altered central modulation of sensations.

Symptoms are likely to be generated as a consequence of disturbed gastrointestinal motility that leads to distension with visceral hyperalgesia accentuating the pain. In one study, patients who developed the irritable bowel syndrome following an acute enteric infection, demonstrated micro-inflammatory changes in the enteric mucosa or neural plexus. These were thought to also contribute to symptom development.

The brain–gut axis describes a combination of intestinal motor, sensory and CNS activities (Fig. 6.44). Thus extrinsic (e.g. vision, smell) and intrinsic (e.g., emotion,

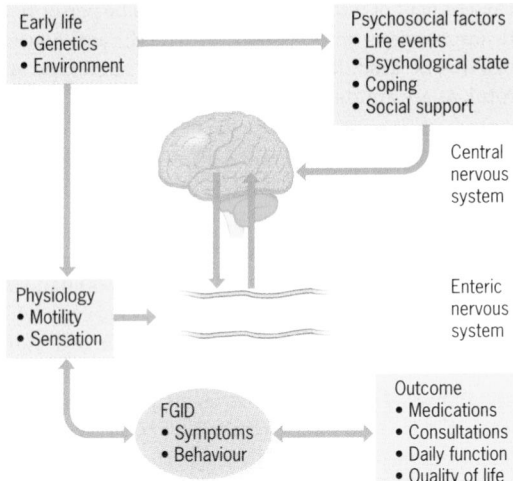

Fig. 6.44 **A biopsychosocial conceptualization of the pathogenesis and clinical expression of functional gastrointestinal disorders (FGID),** showing how genetic, environmental and psychological factors may interact to cause dysregulation of brain–gut function. Modified from *GUT* **45** (suppl) 1999.

thought) information can affect gastrointestinal sensation due to the neural connections from high centres. Conversely viscerotropic events can affect central pain perception, mood and behaviour.

Psychological stress can exacerbate gastrointestinal symptoms and psychological disturbances are more common in patients with FGIDs. They alter attitude to illness, promote healthcare seeking, often lead to a poor clinical outcome and have psychosocial consequences with poor quality of life at home and work. Early in life, genetics and environmental influences (e.g. family attitudes towards bowel training, verbal or sexual abuse, exposure to an infection) may affect one's psychosocial development (susceptibility to life stress, psychological state, coping skills, development of social support) or the development of gut dysfunction (abnormal motility or visceral hypersensitivity).

FGID should be regarded as a dysregulation of brain–gut function.

Functional oesophageal disorders

The criteria for diagnosis rest mainly on compatible symptoms. However *pathological gastro-oesophageal reflux and other causes may need full investigation,* particularly in the elderly with a short history.

Globus
Diagnostic criteria
- Persistent or intermittent sensation of a lump or foreign body in the throat.

- Occurrence of the sensation between meals.
- The absence of dysphagia and pain on swallowing (odynophagia).

Treatment
Reassurance and a trial of antireflux therapy are the mainstays of treatment.

Rumination syndrome
Diagnostic criteria
- Persistent or recurrent effortless regurgitation of recently ingested food into the mouth with subsequent re-mastication and re-swallowing.
- Absence of nausea and vomiting, abdominal discomfort, heartburn.
- Cessation of the process when the regurgitated material becomes acidic.

Central factors contribute significantly to the occurrence of rumination and the disorder is common in individuals with learning difficulties. A range of medical, behavioural and nutritional approaches have been attempted in these patients with varying success.

Functional chest pain, of presumed oesophageal origin
This is characterized by episodes of mainly midline chest pain, not burning in nature, that are potentially of oesophageal origin and which occur in the absence of a cardiological cause, gastro-oesophageal reflux and achalasia.

More than half of patients will respond to high-dose acid-suppression therapy in the first week; some will respond to nitrates and calcium-channel blockers. A history of psychiatric disorder is found in more than 60% of patients and low-dose antidepressant therapy has been shown to be effective.

Functional gastroduodenal disorders

Functional dyspepsia
This is the second most common functional gastrointestinal disorder (after irritable bowel syndrome). Patients can present with a spectrum of symptoms including upper abdominal pain/discomfort, fullness, early satiety, bloating and nausea.

These patients have no structural abnormality as an explanation for their symptoms.

Functional dyspepsia subgroups
Two subgroups based on the predominant (or most bothersome) single symptoms are suggested:

- *Ulcer-like dyspepsia* with pain centred in the upper abdomen as the predominant (most bothersome) symptom.

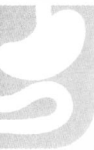
- *Dysmotility-like dyspepsia* with an unpleasant or troublesome non-painful sensation (discomfort) centred in the upper abdomen, being the predominant symptom. This sensation may be associated with upper abdominal fullness, early satiety, bloating and nausea.

The value of such subdivision is controversial.

Investigations

Many young patients (<45) require no investigation. Older patients or those with alarm symptoms require investigation (p. 254).

Treatment

The range of therapies prescribed for functional dyspepsia reflects the uncertain pathogenesis and the lack of satisfactory treatment options. Management is further confounded by high placebo response rates (20–60%). A proportion of patients will respond satisfactorily to reassurance, explanations and lifestyle changes, but anti-secretory or prokinetic agents are used for patients with ulcer-like and dysmotility-like dyspepsia respectively. Reducing intake of fat, coffee, alcohol and cigarette smoking may help.

H. pylori eradication therapy is often used in functional dyspepsia but there is little evidence to recommend its use. Most gastroenterologists usually try such therapy if only for its possible long-term benefit.

In one study omeprazole produced symptomatic relief in patients with *H. pylori* and did not help *H. pylori*-negative patients.

Aerophagia

Aerophagia refers to a repetitive pattern of swallowing or ingesting air and belching. It is usually an unconscious act unrelated to meals. Usually no investigation is required. Explanation that the symptoms are due to swallowed air and reassurance are necessary, as is treatment of associated psychiatric disease.

Functional vomiting

Functional vomiting is a rare condition in clinical practice but often extensive investigation is required before reaching a diagnosis. Clinically functional vomiting is characterized by

- frequent episodes of vomiting, occurring on at least three separate days in a week
- absence of criteria for an eating disorder, rumination, or major psychiatric disease
- absence of self-induced and medication-induced vomiting
- absence of abnormalities in the gut or central nervous system and metabolic disease to explain the recurrent vomiting.

An assessment of nutritional status should be performed and appropriate intervention provided; anti-nausea drugs maybe tried. Behavioural and psychotherapy are helpful, as are antidepressants.

Functional bowel disorders

Irritable bowel syndrome (IBS)

IBS is the commonest FGID. In western populations, up to 1 in 5 people report symptoms consistent with IBS. Only approximately 50% will consult their doctors and of these up to 30% will be referred by their GP to a hospital specialist. Up to 40% of all patients seen in specialist gastroenterology clinics will have IBS. Latest estimates in the UK put the annual cost of IBS to healthcare resources as £45.6 million; in the US the cost is higher at $8 billion. In the UK approximately a quarter of IBS patients lose time off work for periods ranging from 7–13 days each year.

The factors that determine whether an IBS sufferer in the community seeks medical advice include the demonstration that consulters have higher illness attitude scores and higher anxiety and depression scores than non-consulters. Consulters perceive that their symptoms are severer than non-consulters, and consulting behaviour may be determined by the number of presenting symptoms. Female consulters outnumber male consulters by a factor of 2–3. Reasons for this include the fact that anxiety and depression scores are higher in women than men and the gut may be more sensitive to various stimuli in women than in men. It is likely that women perceive internal events in the abdomen differently than men and that they may be more focused on these events. Food and eating are of more special psychological significance for women, as evidenced by a much higher incidence of eating disorders in women. The whole pelvic region carries a more specific significance for women, being associated not only with defecation, urination and sexuality but additionally with menstruation, pregnancy and childbirth. Finally, women in western society in general seem more willing than men to seek medical attention for a whole variety of disorders.

IBS – a multisystem disorder

IBS patients suffer from a number of non-intestinal symptoms (Table 6.23). The non-intestinal symptoms of IBS can be more intrusive than the classical features of IBS. IBS coexists with chronic fatigue syndrome (see p. 1234), fibromyalgia (see p. 531) and temporomandibular joint dysfunction.

The biopsychosocial conceptualization of the pathogenesis and clinical expression of FGIDs (Fig. 6.44) is particularly relevant to IBS and Box 6.15 lists some

Table 6.23
Non-gastrointestinal features of IBS

Gynaecological symptoms
Painful periods (dysmenorrhoea)
Pain following sexual intercourse (dyspareunia)
Premenstrual tension

Urinary symptoms
Frequency
Urgency
Passing urine at night (nocturia)
Incomplete emptying of bladder

Other symptoms
Back pain
Headaches
Bad breath, unpleasant taste in the mouth
Poor sleeping
Fatigue

Box 6.16

Approaches to management of irritable bowel syndrome

End-organ treatment
- Explore dietary triggers
- High-fibre diet ± fibre supplements for constipation
- Antidiarrhoeal drugs for bowel frequency
- Smooth muscle relaxants for pain

Central treatment
- Physiological explanation of symptoms
- Counselling
- Psychotherapy
- Hypnotherapy
- Cognitive behavioural therapy
- Antidepressants

Box 6.15

Some factors that can trigger onset of irritable bowel symptoms

- Gastrointestinal infection
- Antibiotic therapy
- Pelvic surgery
- Psychological stress
- Psychological trauma
- Sexual, physical, verbal abuse
- Mood disturbances
- Anxiety, depression
- Eating disorders
- Food intolerance

---

common factors that have been shown to trigger IBS symptoms. Infectious diarrhoea precedes the onset of IBS symptoms in 7–30% of patients. Whether this is a factor for all patients or just a small subgroup remains controversial. Risk factors in these patients have been shown to include female gender, severity and duration of diarrhoea, pre-existing life events and high hypochondriacal anxiety and neurotic scores at the time of the initial illness. Symptoms of anxiety and depression are more common in IBS patients and stress or life events often precede the onset of chronic bowel symptoms.

Diagnostic Criteria (Rome II 1999)
These criteria state that, in the preceding 12 months there should be at least 12 weeks (consecutive) of abdominal discomfort or pain that has two of three of the following features:

- relieved with defecation; and/or
- onset associated with a change in frequency of stool; and/or
- onset associated with a change in form (appearance) of stool.

The following symptoms cumulatively support the diagnosis of IBS:

- abnormal stool frequency ('abnormal' may be defined as >3/day and <3/week)
- abnormal stool form (lumpy/hard or loose/watery stool)
- abnormal stool passage (straining, urgency, or feeling of incomplete evacuation)
- passage of mucus
- bloating or feeling of abdominal distension.

These symptoms can be used to subclassify patients into diarrhoea- and constipation-predominant forms of IBS. In practice a third subgroup of alternating IBS exists, in which constipation and diarrhoea alternate. The three forms have equal frequency. Many patients with constipation (p. 310) have abdominal discomfort or pain with bloating or distension so there is considerable overlap with constipation-predominant IBS.

The decision as to whether to investigate and if so what choice of investigations is required should be based on clinical judgement. Pointers to the need for thorough investigation are the presence of the above symptoms in association with rectal bleeding, nocturnal pain, fever and weight loss.

Treatment
Current strategies for treatment of IBS are based on the biopsychosocial conceptualization of IBS (Fig. 6.44) with targeting of central and end-organ therapies (Box 6.16). End-organ and central approaches to treatment should not be mutually exclusive and can be used in sequence and in combinations. New end-organ therapies will shortly become available, including hydroxytryptamine (HT_3)-receptor antagonists for diarrhoea-predominant IBS, HT_4-receptor agonists for constipation-predominant IBS as well as kappa opioid agonists for use in patients in whom visceral hyperalgesia plays a predominant role in the pathogenesis of their symptoms.

Pain/gas/bloat syndrome

There exist a group of patients with functional bowel disease whose abdominal pain and other clinical features are likely to occur as a consequence of disordered motility and visceral sensation that predominantly affects the small intestine or midgut. The symptom-based diagnostic criteria are *abdominal pain*, not relieved by opening the bowels and not associated with the passage of more frequent or looser stools than normal and not associated with constipation. *Abdominal distension* that is not restricted to the upper abdomen occurs, as well as postprandial fullness, nausea and, on occasions, anorexia and weight loss.

Treatment of these patients is not easy; and pain can be chronic and severe, with attendant difficulties in achieving control. Narcotics should always be avoided. Central and end-organ targeted treatment approaches should be combined. Success can be achieved employing the central and end-organ properties of the selective serotonin re-uptake inhibitor paroxetine combined with a prokinetic agent or smooth muscle relaxant.

Functional diarrhoea

In this form of functional bowel disease, symptoms occur in the absence of abdominal pain and commonly are:

- The passage of several stools in rapid succession usually first thing in the morning. No further bowel action may occur that day or defecation only after meals.
- The first stool of the day is usually formed, the later ones mushy, looser or watery.
- Urgency of defecation.
- Anxiety, uncertainty about bowel function with restriction of movement (e.g. travelling).
- Exhaustion after the 'morning rush'.

Chronic diarrhoea without pain is caused by many diseases indistinguishable by history from functional diarrhoea (p. 322). Features atypical for a functional disorder (e.g. large-volume stools, rectal bleeding, nutritional deficiency, and weight loss) call for more extensive studies of intestinal structure and function. In cases where it proves difficult to distinguish between functional and organic causes of diarrhoea patients should be admitted to hospital for a formal 3-day analysis of stool weights and faecal fat levels, and a purgative screen together with stool osmolality and creatinine contents to exclude factitious causes of diarrhoea (see p. 322). Outpatient analysis of stool weights is unreliable as brain–gut dysrhythmia may result in increased stool weights in the normal home environment.

FURTHER READING

Camilleri M (2001) Management of the irritable bowel syndrome. *Gastroenterology* **120**: 652–668.

Rome II (1999) A multinational consensus document on functional gastrointestinal disorder. *Gut* **45** (Suppl II): II1–II81.

Spiller RG, Jenkins D, Thornley JP, Hebden JM, Wright T, Skinner M, Neal KR (2000) Increased rectal mucosal enteroendocrine cells, T lymphocytes and increased gut permeability following acute campylobacter enteritis and in post-dysenteric irritable bowel syndrome. *Gut* **47**: 804–811.

The acute abdomen

This section deals with the acute abdominal conditions that cause the patient to be hospitalized within a few hours of the onset of pain (Table 6.24). The diagnosis when made quickly reduces morbidity and mortality. Although a specific diagnosis should be attempted, the immediate problem in management is to decide whether an 'acute abdomen' exists and whether surgery is required.

History

This should include previous operations, any gynaecological problems and whether any concurrent medical condition is present.

Pain

The onset, site, type and subsequent course of the pain should be determined as accurately as possible. In general, the pain of an acute abdomen can either be constant (usually owing to inflammation) or colicky because of a blocked 'tube'. The inflammatory nature of a *constant pain* will be supported by a raised temperature, tachycardia and/or a raised white cell count. If these are normal, then other causes (e.g. musculoskeletal, aortic aneurysm) or rare causes (e.g. porphyria) should be considered. Colicky pain can be due to an obstruction of the gut, biliary system, urogenital system or the uterus. These will probably initially require conservative management along with analgesics. If a colicky pain becomes a constant pain, then inflammation of the organ may have supervened (e.g. strangulated hernia, ascending cholangitis or salpingitis).

A *sudden onset of pain* suggests:

- a perforation (e.g. of a duodenal ulcer)
- a rupture (e.g. of an aneurysm)
- torsion (e.g. of an ovarian cyst)
- acute pancreatitis

Back pain suggests:

- pancreatitis
- rupture of an aortic aneurysm
- renal tract disease.

Inflammatory conditions (e.g. appendicitis) produce a more gradual onset of pain. With peritonitis the pain is continuous and may be made worse by movement.

Table 6.24
Common causes of acute abdominal pain

Diagnosis	No. of patients
Non-specific abdominal pain	466
Acute appendicitis	449
Renal colic	61
Gynaecological disorders	44
Intestinal obstruction	32
Urinary tract infection	30
Gall bladder disease	12
Perforated ulcer/dyspepsia	10
Diverticular disease	6
Other diagnoses	58
No diagnosis established	39

Data drawn from a series of 1204 patients reported by Dixon et al. 1991

Table 6.25
Medical causes of acute abdomen

Referred pain
Pneumonia
Myocardial infarction

Functional gastrointestinal disorders

Renal causes
Pelviureteric colic
Acute pyelonephritis

Metabolic causes
Diabetes mellitus
Acute intermittent porphyria
Lead poisoning

Haematological causes
Haemophilia and other bleeding disorders
Henoch–Schönlein purpura
Sickle cell crisis
Polycythaemia vera

Vasculitis
Embolic

Vomiting

Vomiting may accompany any acute abdominal pain but, if persistent, it suggests an obstructive lesion of the gut. The character of the vomit should be asked – does it contain blood, bile or small bowel contents?

Other symptoms

Any change in bowel habit or of urinary frequency should be documented and, in females, a gynaecological history should be taken.

Physical examination

The general condition of the person should be noted. Does the patient look ill? Is he or she shocked? Large volumes of fluid may be lost from the vascular compartment into the peritoneal cavity or into the lumen of the bowel giving rise to hypovolaemia, i.e. a pale cold skin, a weak rapid pulse and hypotension.

The abdomen

- **Inspection.** Look for the presence of scars, distension or masses.
- **Palpation.** The abdomen should be examined gently for sites of tenderness and the presence or absence of guarding. Guarding is involuntary spasm of the abdominal wall and it indicates peritonitis. This can be localized to one area or it may be generalized, involving the whole abdomen.
- **Bowel sounds.** Increased high-pitch tinkling bowel sounds indicate fluid obstruction; this occurs because of fluid movement within the large dilated bowel lumen. Absent bowel sounds suggest peritoneal involvement. In an obstructed patient, absent bowel sound suggest strangulation or ischaemia or ileus. It is essential that the hernial orifices be examined if intestinal obstruction is suspected.

Pelvic and rectal examination

Pelvic examination can be very helpful, particularly in diagnosing gynaecological causes of an acute abdomen (e.g. a ruptured ectopic pregnancy). Rectal examination is less helpful as localized tenderness may be due to any cause; it may show blood on the finger stall.

Sigmoidoscopy

If diarrhoea is present, sigmoidoscopy is indicated to aid exclusion of infective, inflammatory and ischaemic causes of acute pain. A specimen of stool should be taken for stool culture for bacterial pathogens (e.g. campylobacter, salmonella, shigella) when diarrhoea is present – stool should also be tested for *Clostridium difficile* toxin if antibiotic therapy precedes onset of diarrhoea and acute abdominal pain (see p. 721).

Other observations

- **Mouth.** The tongue is furred in some cases and a fetor is present.
- **Temperature.** Fever is more common in acute inflammatory processes.
- **Urine.** Examine for:
  - blood – suggests urinary tract infection or renal colic
  - glucose and ketones – ketoacidosis can present with acute pain
  - protein and white cells – to exclude acute pyelonephritis.
- Think of medical causes (Table 6.25).

Investigations

- **Blood count.** A raised white cell count occurs in inflammatory conditions.

- **Serum amylase.** High levels (more than five times normal) indicate acute pancreatitis. Raised levels below this can occur in any acute abdomen and should not be considered diagnostic of pancreatitis.
- **Serum electrolytes.** These are not particularly helpful for diagnosis but useful for general evaluation of the patient.
- **Pregnancy.** A urine dipstick is used with women of child-bearing age.
- **X-rays.** A CXR is useful to detect air under the diaphragm owing to a perforation. Dilated loops of bowel or fluid levels are suggestive of obstruction (supine abdominal X-ray).
- **Ultrasound.** This is useful in the diagnosis of acute cholangitis, cholecystitis and aortic aneurysm and in expert hands is reliable in the diagnosis of acute appendicitis. Gynaecological and other pelvic causes of pain can be detected.
- **CT scan.** Spiral CT is the most accurate investigation in most acute emergencies.
- **Laparoscopy.** This has gained increasing importance as a diagnostic tool prior to proceeding with surgery, particularly in men and women over the age of 50 years. In addition, therapeutic manoeuvres, such as appendicectomy, can be performed.

Acute appendicitis

This is the most common surgical emergency. It affects all age groups. Appendicitis should always be considered in the differential diagnosis if the appendix has not been removed.

Acute appendicitis mostly occurs when the lumen of the appendix becomes obstructed with a faecolith; however, in some cases there is only generalized acute inflammation. If the appendix is not removed at this stage, gangrene occurs with perforation, leading to a localized abscess or to generalized peritonitis.

Clinical features and management

Most patients present with abdominal pain; in many it starts vaguely in the centre of the abdomen, becoming localized to the right iliac fossa in the first few hours. Nausea, vomiting and occasional diarrhoea can occur. Because of the motile position of the appendix, symptoms and signs are variable.

Examination of the abdomen reveals tenderness in the right iliac fossa, with guarding due to the localized peritonitis. There may be a tender mass in the right iliac fossa. Laboratory tests are unhelpful, except that the white cell count may be raised. An ultrasound is accurate for the detection of an inflamed appendix and will also indicate an appendix mass or other localized lesion. CT is now used more frequently. It is highly sensitive and specific, and reduces the incidence of removing the 'normal' appendix.

Differential diagnosis

- Non-specific mesenteric lymphadenitis – may mimic appendicitis.
- Acute terminal ileitis due to Crohn's disease or *Yersinia* infection.
- Acute salpingitis – should be considered in women; there is usually a vaginal discharge and on vaginal examination, adnexal tenderness is found.
- Inflamed Meckel's diverticulum.
- Functional bowel disease.

It should be noted that 45% of women aged 15–45 years who have an appendicectomy have a normal appendix removed.

Treatment

The appendix is removed by open surgery or laparoscopically. If an appendix mass is present, the patient is usually treated conservatively with intravenous fluids and antibiotics. The pain subsides over a few days and the mass usually disappears over a few weeks. Interval appendicectomy is recommended at a later date to prevent further acute episodes.

Gynaecological causes

Ruptured ectopic pregnancy. The fallopian tube is the commonest extrauterine site of implantation. Delayed diagnosis is the major cause of morbidity. Most patients will present with recurrent low abdominal pain associated with vaginal bleeding. Diagnosis is usually made with abdominal and transvaginal ultrasound. Most patients can be managed by laparoscopic salpingostomy or salpingectomy.

Ovarian:

- Rupture of 'functional' ovarian cysts in the middle of the cycle (Mittelschmerz).
- Torsion or rupture of ovarian cysts.

Acute salpingitis. Most cases are associated with sexually transmitted infection. Patients commonly present with bilateral low abdominal pain, a fever and vaginal discharge. In the Fitz-Hughes–Curtis syndrome the chlamydia infection tracks up the right paracolic gutter to cause a perihepatitis. Patients can present with acute right hypochondrial pain, fever and mildly abnormal liver biochemistry.

Acute peritonitis

Localized peritonitis

There is virtually always some degree of localized peritonitis with all acute inflammatory conditions of the gastrointestinal tract (e.g. acute appendicitis, acute cholecystitis). Pain and tenderness are largely features of this localized peritonitis. The treatment is for the underlying disease.

Generalized peritonitis

This is a serious condition resulting from irritation of the peritoneum owing to infection (e.g. perforated appendix), or from chemical irritation due to leakage of intestinal contents (e.g. perforated ulcer). In the latter case, superadded infection gradually occurs; *E. coli* and *Bacteroides* are most common organisms.

The peritoneal cavity becomes acutely inflamed with production of an inflammatory exudate that spreads throughout the peritoneum, leading to intestinal dilatation and paralytic ileus.

Clinical features and management

In perforation, the onset is sudden with acute severe abdominal pain, followed by general collapse and shock. The patient may improve temporarily, only to become worse later as generalized toxaemia occurs.

When the peritonitis is secondary to inflammatory disease, the onset is less rapid with the initial features being those of the underlying disease.

Investigations should always include an erect chest X-ray to detect free air under the diaphragm, and a serum amylase to diagnose acute pancreatitis, which is treated conservatively. Imaging with ultrasound and/or CT should also be performed for diagnosis.

Peritonitis is always treated surgically after adequate resuscitation with the re-establishment of a good urinary output. This includes insertion of a nasogastric tube, intravenous fluids and antibiotics. Surgery has a twofold objective:

- peritoneal lavage of the abdominal cavity
- specific treatment of the underlying condition.

Complications

Any delay in treatment of peritonitis produces more profound toxaemia and septicaemia. In addition, local abscess formation occurs and should be suspected if a patient continues to remain unwell postoperatively with a swinging fever, high white cell count and continuing pain. Abscesses are commonly pelvic or subphrenic and can be localized and drained using ultrasound and CT scanning techniques.

Intestinal obstruction

Most intestinal obstruction is due to a mechanical block. Sometimes the bowel does not function, leading to a paralytic ileus. This occurs temporarily after most abdominal operations and with peritonitis. Some causes of intestinal obstruction are shown in Table 6.26.

Obstruction of the bowel leads to bowel distension above the block, with increased secretion of fluid into the distended bowel. Bacterial contamination occurs in the distended stagnant bowel. In strangulation the blood supply is impeded, leading to gangrene, perforation and peritonitis unless urgent treatment of the condition is undertaken.

Table 6.26
Some causes of intestinal obstruction

Small intestinal obstruction
Adhesions (80% in adults)
Hernias
Crohn's disease
Intussusception
Obstruction due to extrinsic involvement by cancer

Colonic obstruction
Carcinoma of the colon
Sigmoid volvulus
Diverticular disease

Clinical features

The patient complains of abdominal colic, vomiting and constipation without passage of wind. In upper gut obstruction the vomiting is profuse but in lower gut obstruction it may be absent.

Examination of the abdomen reveals distension with increased bowel sounds. Marked tenderness suggests strangulation and urgent surgery is necessary. Examination of the hernial orifices and rectum must be performed. X-ray of the abdomen reveals distended loops of bowel proximal to the obstruction. Fluid levels are seen in small bowel obstruction on an erect film. In large bowel obstruction, the caecum and ascending colon are distended. An instant water-soluble barium enema without air insufflation may help to demonstrate the site of the obstruction.

Management

Initial management is by resuscitation with intravenous fluids (mainly isotonic saline with potassium) and decompression. Many cases will settle on conservative management, but an increasing temperature, raised pulse rate, increasing pain and a rising white cell count require exploratory laparotomy.

Laparotomy with removal of the obstruction is necessary in most cases of small bowel obstruction. If the bowel is gangrenous owing to strangulation, gut resection will be required. A few patients (e.g. those with Crohn's disease) may have recurrent episodes of incomplete intestinal obstruction that can be managed conservatively. In large bowel obstruction, if surgery is necessary, primary resection with or without primary anastomosis should be performed. In critically ill patients, a defunctioning colostomy may be the only alternative. Volvulus of the sigmoid colon can be managed by the passage of a flexible sigmoidoscope or a rectal tube to un-kink the bowel, but recurrent volvulus may require sigmoid resection.

Intestinal pseudo-obstruction

It is now recognized that a clinical picture mimicking mechanical obstruction may develop in patients who do

Box 6.17

Treatment of acute colonic pseudo-obstruction

- Neostigmine 2.0 mg i.v. over 3–5 minutes in presence of doctor with ECG monitor.
- 0.3–1 mg atropine if symptomatically bradycardic. Nurse the patient supine for 60 min.
- Monitor abdominal circumference and the diameter of the caecum, ascending, transverse and descending colon on straight abdominal X-ray.

Table 6.27
Disease of the peritoneum

Infective (bacterial) peritonitis	**Neoplasia**
Secondary to gut disease, e.g. appendicitis perforation of any organ	Secondary deposits (e.g. from ovary, stomach)
Chronic peritoneal dialysis	**Primary mesothelioma**
Spontaneous, usually in ascites with liver disease	**Vasculitis**
Tuberculosis	Connective tissue disease
	Polyserositis (e.g. familial Mediterranean fever)

not have a mechanical cause. Colonic pseudo-obstruction is the commonest form. In more than 80% of cases it complicates other clinical conditions, for example:

- intra-abdominal trauma, pelvic spinal and femoral fractures
- post operatively (abdominal, pelvic, cardiothoracic, orthopaedic, neurosurgical)
- intra-abdominal sepsis
- pneumonia
- metabolic (e.g. electrolyte disturbances, malnutrition, diabetes mellitus, Parkinson's disease)
- drugs – opiates (particularly after orthopaedic surgery) antidepressants, anti-Parkinsonian drugs.

Patients present with rapid and progressive abdominal distension and pain. X-ray shows a gas filled large bowel. Management is of the underlying problem (e.g. withdraw opiate analgesia) together with a trial of i.v. neostigmine therapy (Box 6.17). Patients should be monitored carefully and consideration should be given to surgery if the diameter of the caecum exceeds 14 cm.

Small intestinal pseudo-obstruction is a rare condition and is of the myopathic or neuropathic type. The former is usually due to degenerative disorders of the smooth muscle which may be familial. Patients present with functional small intestinal failure with bacterial overgrowth and steatorrhoea. The neurogenic form is commonly due to an autoimmune ganglionitis of the enteric nervous system and can occur in systemic lupus erythematosus (SLE). Patients commonly present with a long history of intractable postprandial small intestine pain.

FURTHER READING

Steinbrook RA (2001) An opioid antagonist for postoperative ileus. *New England Journal of Medicine* **345**: 988–989.

The peritoneum

The peritoneal cavity is a closed sac lined by mesothelial cells. The peritoneal mesothelial cells produce surfactant that acts as a lubricant within the peritoneal cavity.

The cavity contains less than 100 ml/L of serous fluid containing less than 30 g/L of protein.

The mesothelial cells lining the diaphragm have gaps that allow communication between the peritoneum and the diaphragmatic lymphatics. Approximately one-third of fluid drains through these lymphatics, the remainder through the parietal peritoneum. These mechanisms allow particulate matter to be removed rapidly from the peritoneal cavity.

Complement activation is an early defence mechanism followed rapidly by upregulation of the peritoneal mesothelial cells and migration of polymorphonuclear neutrophils and macrophages into the peritoneum.

Mast cells release potent mediators of inflammation and interact with T cells to generate an immune response.

The peritoneal-associated lymphoid tissue includes the omental milky spots, the lymphocytes within the peritoneal cavity and the draining lymph nodes. B cells with a unique CD5$^+$ are common. This defence system plays a major role in localizing peritoneal infection. Some conditions that can affect the peritoneum are shown in Table 6.27.

Peritonitis can be acute or chronic, as seen in tuberculosis. Most cases of infective peritonitis are secondary to gastrointestinal disease, but it occurs occasionally without intra-abdominal sepsis in ascites due to liver disease. Very rarely, fungal and parasitic infections can also cause primary peritonitis (e.g. amoebiasis, candidiasis). Peritonitis is discussed further on page 330.

The peritoneum can be involved by *secondary malignant deposits*, and the most common cause of ascites in a young to middle-aged woman is an ovarian carcinoma.

A *subphrenic abscess* is usually secondary to infection in the abdomen and is characterized by fever, malaise, pain in the right or left hypochondrium and shoulder-tip pain. An erect chest X-ray shows gas under the diaphragm, impaired movement of the diaphragm on screening and a pleural effusion. Ultrasound is usually diagnostic.

Ascites is associated with all diseases of the peritoneum. The fluid that collects is an exudate with a high protein content. It is also seen in liver disease. The mechanism, causes and investigation of ascites are discussed on page 370.

Retroperitoneal fibrosis (periaortitis)

This is a rare condition in which there is a marked fibrosis over the posterior abdominal wall and retroperitoneum. The aetiology is usually unknown but it has been associated with the drug methysergide and occasionally with the carcinoid syndrome. The disease usually presents in middle age with malaise, fever, and loss of weight. There is often anaemia and a raised ESR/CRP – a CT scan is diagnostic (see Fig. 11.35). The major complication is urinary tract obstruction from ureteric involvement, which may require surgery.

Tuberculous peritonitis

This is the second most common form of abdominal TB.

Three subgroups can be identified: wet, dry and fibrous.

- In patients with the wet type, ascitic fluid should be examined for protein concentration (> 20 g/L) and tubercle bacilli (rarely found).
- In the dry form, patients present with subacute intestinal obstruction which is due to tuberculous small bowel adhesions.
- In the fibrous form, patients present with abdominal pain, distension and ill-defined irregular tender abdominal masses.

The diagnosis of peritoneal TB can be supported by findings on ultrasound or CT screening (mesenteric thickening and lymph node enlargement). A histological diagnosis is not always required before instituting treatment. In some patients careful laparoscopy (to avoid perforation) may have to be performed and rarely laparotomy.

Treatment

Drug treatment is similar to that for pulmonary TB (see p. 895) and should be supervised by chest physicians who have experience in dealing with contacts.

FURTHER READING

Hall JC et al. (1998) The pathobiology of peritonitis. *Gastroenterology* **114**: 188–196.

CHAPTER BIBLIOGRAPHY

Feldman et al. (1997) *Sleisenger and Fordtran's Gastrointestinal and Liver Disease* 6th edn. Philadelphia: WB Saunders.

Liver, biliary tract and pancreatic disease

In the West, alcohol is the major cause of liver disease, whilst elsewhere the hepatitis B virus is still a significant factor. Hepatitis C virus is now the second most common cause of liver disease in many western countries and a major cause in countries surrounding the Mediterranean basin and in South America. Health education and the improvement of social conditions should help to stop the spread of viral infections, as should widespread vaccination against hepatitis A and B.

Imaging techniques including magnetic resonance imaging enable the liver and biliary tree to be visualized with precision, resulting in earlier diagnosis. Therapeutic endoscopy, and laparoscopic and minimally invasive surgery, avoid the necessity of major surgery, particularly for biliary tract disease. Finally, liver transplantation is established for the treatment of acute and chronic liver disease.

The liver

Structure of the liver and biliary system

The liver

The liver is the largest internal organ in the body and is situated in the right hypochondrium. Functionally, it is divided into right and left lobes by the middle hepatic vein. The right lobe is larger and contains the caudate and quadrate lobes. The liver is further subdivided into a total of eight segments (Fig. 7.1) by divisions of the right, middle and left hepatic veins. Each segment receives its own portal pedicle, permitting individual segment resection at surgery.

The blood supply to the liver constitutes 25% of the resting cardiac output and is via two main vessels:

- The *hepatic artery*, which is a branch of the coeliac axis, supplies 25% of the total blood flow. Autoregulation of blood flow by the hepatic artery ensures a constant total liver blood flow.
- The *portal vein* drains most of the gastrointestinal tract and the spleen. It supplies 75% of the blood flow. The normal portal pressure is 5–8 mmHg; flow increases after meals.

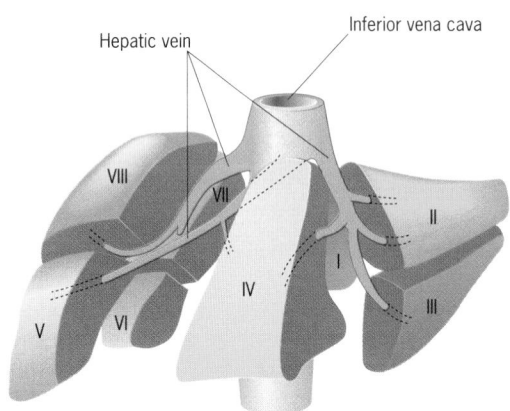

Fig. 7.1 **Segmental anatomy of the liver showing the eight hepatic segments.** I, caudate lobe; II–IV the left hemiliver; V–VIII the right hemiliver. Modified from Bismuth H (1982) *World Journal of Surgery* **6**: 38 (Springer–Verlag) with permission.

Both vessels enter the liver via the hilum (porta hepatis). The blood from these vessels is distributed to the segments and passes into the sinusoids via the portal tracts.

Blood leaves the sinusoids, entering branches of the hepatic vein which join into three main branches before entering the inferior vena cava.

The caudate lobe is an autonomous segment as it receives an independent blood supply from the portal vein and hepatic artery, and its hepatic vein drains directly into the inferior vena cava.

Lymph, formed mainly in the perisinusoidal space, is collected in lymphatics which are present in the portal tracts. These small lymphatics enter larger vessels which eventually drain into the hepatic ducts.

The functional unit of the liver is the acinus. This consists of parenchyma supplied by the smallest portal tracts containing portal vein radicles, hepatic arterioles and bile ductules (Fig. 7.2). The hepatocytes near this triad (zone 1) are well supplied with oxygenated blood and are more resistant to damage than the cells nearer the terminal hepatic (central) veins (zone 3).

The sinusoids lack a basement membrane and are loosely surrounded by specialist fenestrated endothelial cells and Kupffer cells (phagocytic cells). Sinusoids are separated by plates of liver cells (hepatocytes). The subendothelial space that lies between the sinusoids and hepatocytes is the space of Disse which contains a matrix of basement membrane constituents and stellate cells.

Stellate cells store retinoids in their resting state and contain the intermediate filament, desmin. When activated they are contractile and probably regulate sinusoidal blood flow. Endothelin and nitric oxide play a major role in modulating stellate cell contractility. Stellate cells, after activation, produce collagen types I, III and IV (see p. 364).

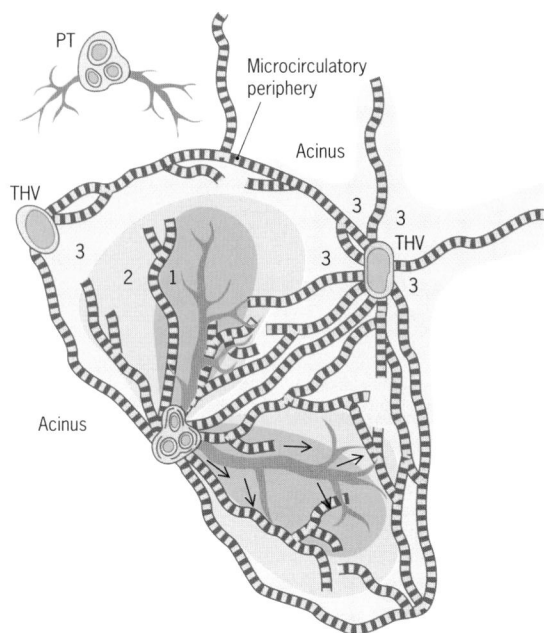

Fig. 7.2 **Diagram of an acinus.** Zones 1, 2 and 3 represent areas supplied by blood, with zone 1 being best oxygenated. Zone 3 is supplied by blood remote from afferent vessels and is in the microcirculatory periphery of the acinus. The perivascular area (star shaped) is formed by the most peripheral parts of zone 3 of several adjacent acini and is the least well oxygenated. THV, terminal hepatic venule; PT, portal triad.

The biliary system

Bile canaliculi form a network between the hepatocytes. These join to form thin bile ductules near the portal tract, which in turn enter the bile ducts in the portal tracts. These then combine to form the right and left hepatic ducts that leave each liver lobe. The hepatic ducts join at the porta hepatis to form the common hepatic duct. The cystic duct connects the gall bladder to the lower end of the common hepatic duct. The gall bladder lies under the right lobe of the liver and stores and concentrates hepatic bile; it has a capacity of approximately 50 mL. The common bile duct is formed by the combination of the cystic and hepatic ducts and is approximately 8 mm in diameter, narrowing at its distal end to pass into the duodenum. The common bile duct and pancreatic duct open into the second part of the duodenum through a common channel at the ampulla of Vater. The lower end of the common bile duct contains the muscular sphincter of Oddi, which contracts rhythmically and prevents bile from entering the duodenum in the fasting state.

FURTHER READING

Sherlock S, Dooley J (2001) *Anatomy and Function in Diseases of the Liver and Biliary System*, 11th edn. Oxford: Blackwell Science.

Functions of the liver

Protein metabolism (see also p. 227)
Synthesis
The liver is the principal site of synthesis of all circulating proteins apart from γ-globulins, which are produced in the reticuloendothelial system. The liver receives amino acids from the intestine and muscles and, by controlling the rate of gluconeogenesis and transamination, regulates levels in the plasma. Plasma contains 60–80 g/L of protein, mainly in the form of albumin, globulin and fibrinogen.

Albumin has a half-life of 16–24 days and 10–12 g are synthesized daily. Its main functions are first to maintain the intravascular oncotic (colloid osmotic) pressure, and second to transport water-insoluble substances such as bilirubin, hormones, fatty acids and drugs. Reduced synthesis of albumin over prolonged periods produces hypoalbuminaemia and is seen in chronic liver disease and malnutrition. Hypoalbuminaemia is also found in hypercatabolic states (e.g. trauma with sepsis) and in diseases where there is an excessive loss (e.g. nephrotic syndrome, protein-losing enteropathy).

Transport or carrier proteins such as transferrin and caeruloplasmin, acute-phase and other proteins (e.g. α_1-antitrypsin and α-fetoprotein) are also produced in the liver.

The liver also synthesizes all factors involved in coagulation (apart from factor VIII) – that is, fibrinogen, prothrombin, factors V, VII, IX, X and XIII, protein C and S and antithrombin (see Ch. 8) as well as components of the complement system.

Degradation (nitrogen excretion)
Amino acids are degraded by transamination and oxidative deamination to produce ammonia, which is then converted to urea and excreted by the kidneys. This is a major pathway for the elimination of nitrogenous waste. Failure of this process occurs in severe liver disease.

Carbohydrate metabolism
Glucose homeostasis and the maintenance of the blood sugar is a major function of the liver. It stores approximately 80 g of glycogen. In the immediate fasting state, blood glucose is maintained either by glucose released from the breakdown of glycogen (glycogenolysis) or by newly synthesized glucose (gluconeogenesis). Sources for gluconeogenesis are lactate, pyruvate, amino acids from muscles (mainly alanine and glutamine) and glycerol from lipolysis of fat stores. In prolonged starvation, ketone bodies and fatty acids are used as alternative sources of fuel and the body tissues adapt to a lower glucose requirement (see Ch. 5).

Lipid metabolism
Fats are insoluble in water and are transported in the plasma as protein–lipid complexes (lipoproteins). These are discussed in detail on page 1104.

The liver has a major role in the metabolism of lipoproteins. It synthesizes very-low-density lipoproteins (VLDLs) and high-density lipoproteins (HDLs). HDLs are the substrate for lecithin–cholesterol acyltransferase (LCAT), which catalyses the conversion of free cholesterol to cholesterol ester (see below). Hepatic lipase removes triglyceride from intermediate-density lipoproteins (IDLs) to produce low-density lipoproteins (LDLs) which are degraded by the liver after uptake by specific cell-surface receptors (see Fig. 19.19).

Triglycerides are mainly of dietary origin but are also formed in the liver from circulating free fatty acids (FFAs) and glycerol and incorporated into VLDLs. Oxidation or de novo synthesis of FFA occurs in the liver, depending on the availability of dietary fat.

Cholesterol may be of dietary origin but most is synthesized from acetyl-CoA mainly in the liver, intestine, adrenal cortex and skin. It occurs either as free cholesterol or is esterified with fatty acids; this reaction is catalysed by LCAT. This enzyme is reduced in severe liver disease, increasing the ratio of free cholesterol to ester, which alters membrane structures. One result of this is the red cell abnormalities (e.g. target cells) seen in chronic liver disease. Phospholipids (e.g. lecithin) are synthesized in the liver.

The complex interrelationships between protein, carbohydrate and fat metabolism are shown in Figure 7.3.

Formation of bile
Bile secretion
Bile consists of water, electrolytes, bile acids, cholesterol, phospholipids and conjugated bilirubin. Two processes are involved in bile secretion across the canalicular membrane of the hepatocyte – a *bile salt-dependent* and a *bile salt-independent* process – each contributing about 230 mL per day. The remainder of the bile (about 150 mL daily) is produced by the epithelial cells of the bile ductules.

Bile formation requires firstly the uptake of bile acids and other organic and inorganic ions across the basolateral (sinusoidal) membranes by multiple transport proteins. This process is driven by Na^+–K^+-ATPase in the basolateral membrane. Intracellular transport across the hepatocyte is partly through microtubules and partly by cytosol transport proteins. The canalicular membrane contains additional transporters, mainly ATPase-dependent, which carry molecules into the biliary canaliculi against a concentration gradient. The canalicular multispecific organic anion transporter (cMOAT) also known as multidrug-resistance protein 2 (MRP2) mediates transport of a broad range of compounds

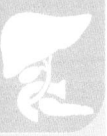

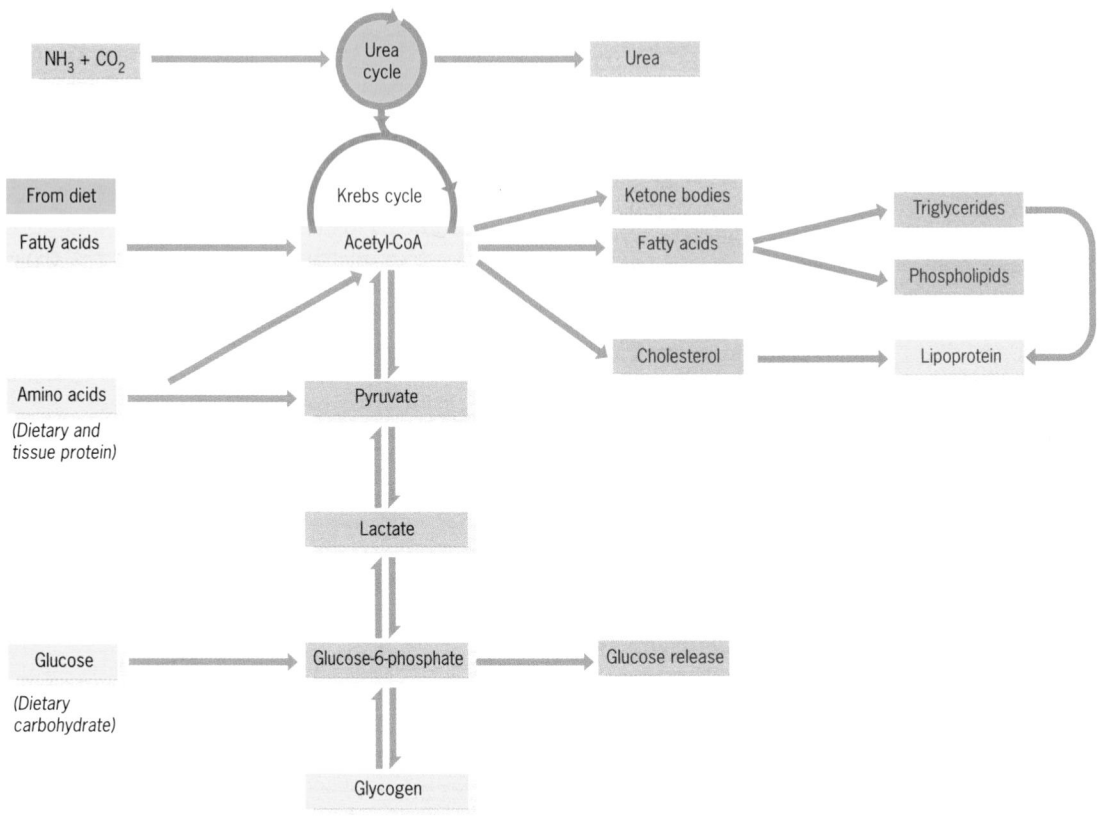

Fig. 7.3 Interrelationships of protein, carbohydrate and lipid metabolism in the liver.

including bilirubin diglucuronide, glucuronidated and sulphated bile acids and other organic anions. Na^+ and water follow the passage of bile salts into the biliary canaliculus by diffusion across the tight junction between hepatocytes (a bile salt-dependent process). In the bile salt-independent process water flow is due to other osmotically active solutes such as glutathione and bicarbonate.

Secretion of a bicarbonate-rich solution is stimulated mainly by secretin and is inhibited by somatostatin. In this process several membrane proteins are involved, including the Cl^-/HCO_3^- exchanger and the cystic fibrosis transmembrane conductance regulator which controls Cl^- secretion, as well as water channels (aquaporins) in cholangiocyte membranes.

The average total bile flow is approximately 600 mL per day. In the fasted state half of the bile flows directly into the duodenum and half is diverted into the gall bladder. The mucosa of the gall bladder absorbs 80–90% of the water and electrolytes, but is impermeable to bile acids and cholesterol. Following a meal, cholecystokinin is secreted by the duodenal mucosa and stimulates contraction of the gall bladder and relaxation of the sphincter of Oddi, so that bile enters the duodenum. An adequate bile flow is dependent on bile salts being returned to the liver by the enterohepatic circulation.

Bile acid metabolism

Bile acids are synthesized in hepatocytes from cholesterol. The rate-limiting step in their production is that catalysed by cholesterol-7α-hydroxylase. They are excreted into the bile and then pass into the duodenum. The two primary bile acids – cholic acid and chenodeoxycholic acid (Fig. 7.4) – are conjugated with glycine or taurine (in a ratio of 3:1 in humans) and this process increases their solubility. Intestinal bacteria convert these acids into secondary bile acids, deoxycholic and lithocholic acid. Figure 7.5 shows the enterohepatic circulation of bile acids.

Bile acids act as detergents; their main function is lipid solubilization. Bile acid molecules contain both a hydrophilic and a hydrophobic end. In aqueous solutions they aggregate to form micelles, with their hydrophobic (lipid-soluble) ends in the centre. Micelles are expanded by cholesterol and phospholipids (mainly lecithin), forming mixed micelles.

Bilirubin metabolism

Bilirubin is produced mainly from the breakdown of mature red cells in the Kupffer cells of the liver and in the reticuloendothelial system; 15% of bilirubin comes from the catabolism of other haem-containing proteins, such as myoglobin, cytochromes and catalases.

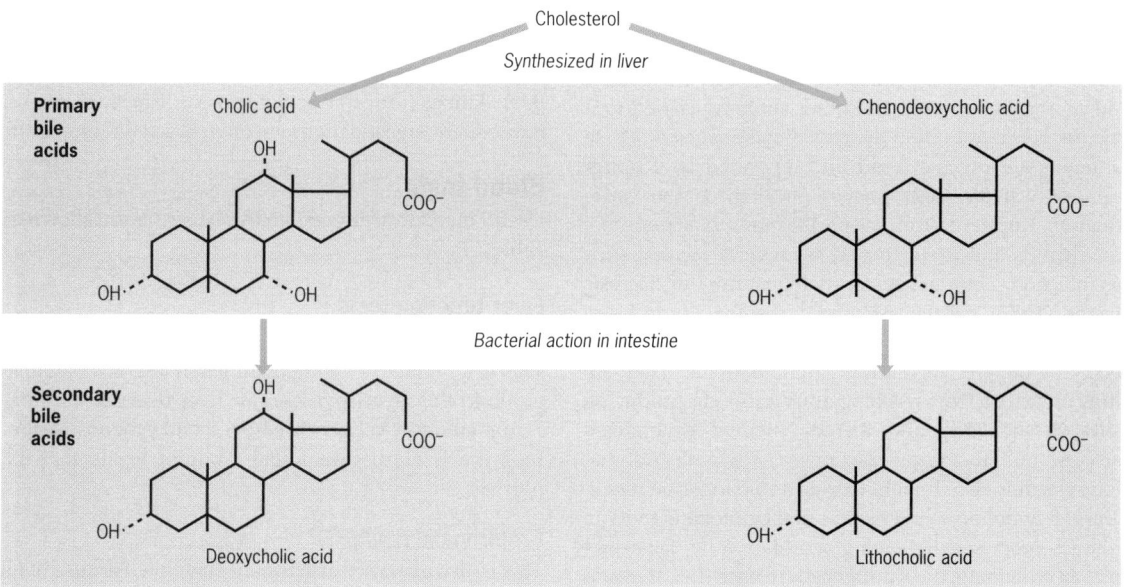

Fig. 7.4 **Primary and secondary bile acids.** All bile acids are normally conjugated with glycine or taurine.

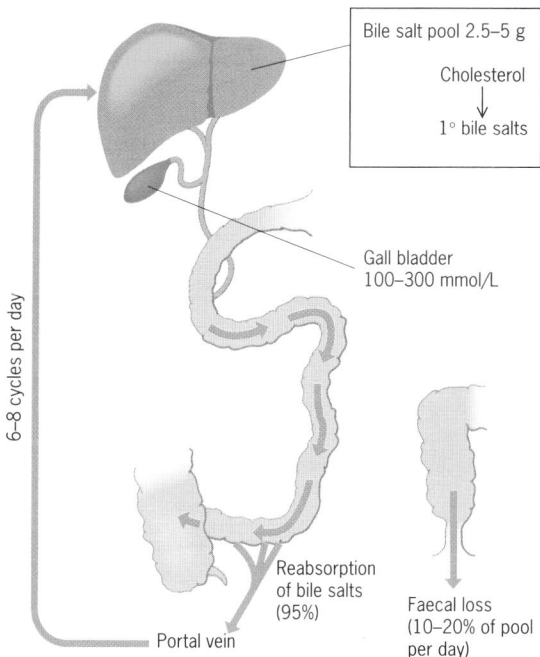

Fig. 7.5 **Recirculation of bile acids.** The bile salt pool is relatively small and the entire pool recycles 6–8 times via the enterohepatic circulation. Up to 40 g are excreted daily into the bile and the synthesis of new bile acids only compensates for faecal loss.

Normally, 250–300 mg of bilirubin are produced daily. The iron and globin are removed from the haem and are reused. Biliverdin is formed from the haem and this is reduced to form bilirubin. The bilirubin produced is unconjugated and water-insoluble, and is transported to the liver attached to albumin. Bilirubin dissociates from albumin and is taken up by the hepatic cell membrane and transported to the endoplasmic reticulum by cytoplasmic proteins, where it is conjugated with glucuronic acid and excreted into bile. The microsomal enzyme, uridine diphosphoglucurosyl transferase, catalyses the formation of bilirubin monoglucuronide and then diglucuronide. This conjugated bilirubin is water-soluble and is actively secreted into the bile canaliculi and excreted into the intestine within the bile (Fig. 8.5). It is not absorbed from the small intestine because of its large molecular size. In the terminal ileum, bacterial enzymes hydrolyse the molecule, releasing free bilirubin, which is then reduced to urobilinogen. Some of this is excreted in the stools as stercobilinogen. The remainder is absorbed by the terminal ileum, passes to the liver via the enterohepatic circulation, and is re-excreted into the bile. Urobilinogen bound to albumin enters the circulation and is excreted in the urine via the kidneys. When hepatic excretion of conjugated bilirubin is impaired, a small amount of conjugated bilirubin is found strongly bound to serum albumin. It is not excreted by the kidneys and accounts for the continuing hyperbilirubinaemia for a short time after cholestasis has resolved.

Hormone and drug inactivation

The liver catabolizes hormones such as insulin, glucagon, oestrogens, growth hormone, glucocorticoids and parathyroid hormone. It is also the prime target organ for many hormones (e.g. insulin). It is the major site for the metabolism of drugs (see p. 958) and alcohol (see p. 250). Fat-soluble drugs are converted to water-soluble substances that facilitate their excretion in the bile or urine.

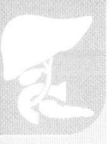

Immunological function

The reticuloendothelial system of the liver contains many immunologically active cells. The liver acts as a 'sieve' for the bacterial and other antigens carried to it via the portal tract from the gastrointestinal tract. These antigens are phagocytosed and degraded by Kupffer cells, which are macrophages attached to the endothelium. Kupffer cells have specific membrane receptors for ligands and are activated by several factors, such as infection. They secrete interleukins, tumour necrosis factor (TNF), collagenase and lysosomal hydrolases. Antigens are degraded without the production of antibody, as there is very little lymphoid tissue. They are thus prevented from reaching other antibody-producing sites in the body and thereby prevent generalized adverse immunological reactions. The reticuloendothelial system is also thought to play a role in tissue repair, T and B lymphocyte interaction, and cytotoxic activity in disease processes. Following stimulation by, for example, an endotoxin, the Kupffer cells release IL-6, IL-8 and TNF-α and play a key role in producing parenchymal damage. These cytokines stimulate the sinusoidal cells, stellate cells and natural killer cells to release pro-inflammatory cytokines. The stimulated hepatocytes themselves express adhesion molecules and release IL-8, which is a potent neutrophil chemoattractant. Homing of mucosal lymphocytes (enterohepatic circulation) has been proposed. These exogenous leucocytes again release more cytokines – all damaging the function of the hepatocyte, including hepatocellular bile formation which leads to cholestasis. Cytokines also stimulate hepatic apoptosis.

Investigations

Investigative tests can be divided into:

- **Blood tests**
  - (a) Liver 'function' tests:
    - (i) serum albumin
    - (ii) prothrombin time
  - (b) Liver biochemistry:
    - (i) serum aspartate and alanine aminotransferases – reflecting hepatocellular damage
    - (ii) serum alkaline phosphatase, γ-glutamyl transpeptidase – reflecting cholestasis
    - (iii) total protein
  - (c) Viral markers
  - (d) Additional blood investigations; haematological, biochemical and immunological.
- **Urine tests** – for bilirubin and urobilinogen.
- **Imaging techniques** – to define gross anatomy.
- **Liver biopsy** – for histology.

Most routine 'liver function tests' sent to the laboratory will be processed by an automated multichannel analyser to produce serum levels of bilirubin, aminotransferases, alkaline phosphatase, γ-glutamyl transpeptidase (γ-GT) and total proteins. These routine tests are markers of liver damage, but not actual tests of 'function' per se. Subsequent investigations are often based on these tests.

Blood tests

Useful blood tests for certain liver diseases are shown in Table 7.1.

Liver function tests

Serum albumin

This is a marker of synthetic function and is a valuable guide to the severity of chronic liver disease. A falling serum albumin in liver disease is a bad prognostic sign. In acute liver disease initial albumin levels may be normal.

Prothrombin time (PT)

This is also a marker of synthetic function. Because of its short half-life, it is a sensitive indicator of both acute and chronic liver disease. Vitamin K deficiency should be excluded as the cause of a prolonged PT by giving an intravenous bolus (10 mg) of vitamin K. Vitamin K deficiency commonly occurs in biliary obstruction, as the low intestinal concentration of bile salts results in poor absorption of vitamin K.

Prothrombin times vary in different laboratories depending upon the thromboplastin used in the assay. The International Normalized Ratio (INR) is therefore used in the UK (see p. 469).

Liver biochemistry

Bilirubin

In the serum, bilirubin is normally almost all unconjugated. In liver disease, increased serum bilirubin is usually accompanied by other abnormalities in liver

Table 7.1
Useful blood tests for certain liver diseases

Test	Disease
Antimitochondrial antibody	Primary biliary cirrhosis
Antinuclear, smooth muscle (actin), liver/kidney microsomal antibody	Autoimmune hepatitis
Raised serum immunoglobulins: IgG	Autoimmune hepatitis
IgM	Primary biliary cirrhosis
Viral markers	Hepatitis A, B, C, D and others
α-Fetoprotein	Hepatocellular carcinoma
Serum iron, transferrin saturation, serum ferritin	Hereditary haemochromatosis
Serum and urinary copper, serum caeruloplasmin	Wilson's disease
α$_1$-Antitrypsin	Cirrhosis (± emphysema)
Antinuclear cytoplasmic antibodies	Sclerosing cholangitis

biochemistry. Determination of whether the bilirubin is conjugated or unconjugated is only necessary in congenital disorders of bilirubin metabolism (see below) or to exclude haemolysis.

Aminotransferases

These enzymes (often referred to as transaminases) are present in hepatocytes and leak into the blood with liver cell damage. Two enzymes are measured:

- *Aspartate aminotransferase* (AST) is primarily a mitochondrial enzyme (80%; 20% in cytoplasm) and is also present in heart, muscle, kidney and brain. High levels are seen in hepatic necrosis, myocardial infarction, muscle injury and congestive cardiac failure.
- *Alanine aminotransferase* (ALT) is a cytosol enzyme, more specific to the liver so that a rise only occurs with liver disease.

Alkaline phosphatase (ALP)

This is present in the canalicular and sinusoidal membranes of the liver, but is also present in many other tissues, such as bone, intestine and placenta. If necessary, its origin can be determined by electrophoretic separation of isoenzymes or bone-specific monoclonal antibodies. Alternatively, if there is also an abnormality of, for example, the γ-GT, the ALP can be presumed to come from the liver.

Serum ALP is raised in cholestasis from any cause, whether intrahepatic or extrahepatic disease. The synthesis of ALP is increased and this is released into the blood. In cholestatic jaundice, levels may be four to six times the normal limit. Raised levels may also occur in conditions with infiltration of the liver (e.g. metastases) and in cirrhosis, frequently in the absence of jaundice. The highest serum levels due to liver disease (>1000 IU/L) are seen with hepatic metastases and primary biliary cirrhosis.

γ-Glutamyl transpeptidase

This is a microsomal enzyme that is present in many tissues as well as the liver. Its activity can be induced by such drugs as phenytoin and by alcohol. If the ALP is normal, a raised serum γ-GT is a good guide to alcohol intake and can be used as a screening test (see p. 1256). Mild elevation of the γ-GT is common even with a small alcohol consumption and does not necessarily indicate liver disease if the other liver biochemical tests are normal. In cholestasis the γ-GT rises in parallel with the ALP as it has a similar pathway of excretion. This is also true of the 5-nucleotidase, another microsomal enzyme that can be measured in blood.

Total proteins

This measurement, in itself, is of little value. Serum albumin is discussed above. The globulin fraction consists of many proteins that can be separated on electrophoresis.

A raised globulin fraction, seen in liver disease, is usually due to increased circulating immunoglobulins and is polyclonal (see below).

Viral markers

Viruses are a major cause of liver disease. Virological studies have a key role in diagnosis; markers are available for most common viruses that cause hepatitis.

Additional blood investigations
Haematological

A full blood count is always performed. Anaemia may be present. The red cells are often macrocytic and can have abnormal shapes – target cells and spur cells – owing to membrane abnormalities. Vitamin B_{12} levels are normal or high, while folate levels are often low owing to poor dietary intake. Other changes are caused by the following:

- Bleeding produces a hypochromic, microcytic picture.
- Alcohol causes macrocytosis, sometimes with leucopenia and thrombocytopenia.
- Hypersplenism results in pancytopenia.
- Cholestasis can often produce abnormal-shaped cells and also deficiency of vitamin K.
- Haemolysis accompanies acute liver failure and jaundice.
- Aplastic anaemia is present in up to 2% of patients with acute viral hepatitis.
- A raised serum ferritin with transferrin saturation (>60%) is seen in hereditary haemochromatosis.

Biochemical

- α_1-*Antitrypsin*. A deficiency of this enzyme can produce cirrhosis.
- *α-Fetoprotein*. This is normally produced by the fetal liver. Its reappearance in increasing and high concentrations in the adult indicates hepatocellular carcinoma. Increased concentrations in pregnancy in the blood and amniotic fluid suggest neural-tube defects of the fetus. Blood levels are also slightly raised with regenerative liver tissue in patients with hepatitis, chronic liver disease and also in teratomas.
- Serum and urinary copper and serum caeruloplasmin – for Wilson's disease (see p. 376).

Immunological tests

There are no specific antibodies to the liver itself that are measured routinely.

Serum immunoglobulins

Increased γ-globulins are thought to be due to reduced phagocytosis by sinusoidal and Kupffer cells of the antigens absorbed from the gut. These antigens then stimulate antibody production in the spleen, lymph nodes and lymphoid and plasma cell infiltrate in the portal tracts. In primary biliary cirrhosis, the predominant serum immunoglobulin that is raised is IgM, while in autoimmune hepatitis it is IgG.

Serum autoantibodies

- *Antimitochondrial antibody* (AMA) is found in the serum in over 95% of patients with primary biliary cirrhosis (p. 373). Many different AMA subtypes have been described, depending on their antigen specificity. AMA is demonstrated by an immunofluorescent technique and is neither organ- nor species-specific. Some subtypes are occasionally found in autoimmune hepatitis and other autoimmune diseases.
- *Nucleic, smooth muscle (actin), liver/kidney microsomal antibodies* can be found in the serum in high titre in patients with autoimmune hepatitis. These antibodies can be found in the serum in other autoimmune conditions and other liver diseases.
- *Antinuclear cytoplasmic antibodies* (ANCA) are present in primary sclerosing cholangitis.

Bromsulphthalein (BSP) clearance test

This is now very rarely performed. The liver normally clears BSP from the blood. The level of BSP in the blood after an intravenous injection of BSP is a sensitive guide to hepatocellular damage. A second recirculation peak occurs in the congenital hyperbilirubinaemia of the Dubin–Johnson syndrome. Anaphylactic reactions may occur.

Urine tests

Dipstick tests are available for bilirubin and urobilinogen. Bilirubinuria is due to the presence of conjugated (soluble) bilirubin. It is found in the jaundiced patient with hepatobiliary disease; its absence implies that the jaundice is due to increased unconjugated bilirubin. Urobilinogen in the urine is, in practice, of little value but suggests haemolysis or hepatic dysfunction of any cause.

Imaging techniques

Ultrasound examination

This is a non-invasive, safe and relatively cheap technique. It involves the analysis of the reflected ultrasound beam detected by a probe moved across the abdomen. The normal liver appears as a relatively homogeneous structure. The gall bladder, common bile duct, pancreas, portal vein and other structures in the abdomen can be visualized. Abdominal ultrasound is useful in:

- a jaundiced patient (p. 349)
- hepatomegaly/splenomegaly
- the detection of gallstones (Fig. 7.6)
- focal liver disease – lesions > 1 cm
- general parenchymal liver disease
- assessing portal and hepatic vein patency
- lymph node enlargement.

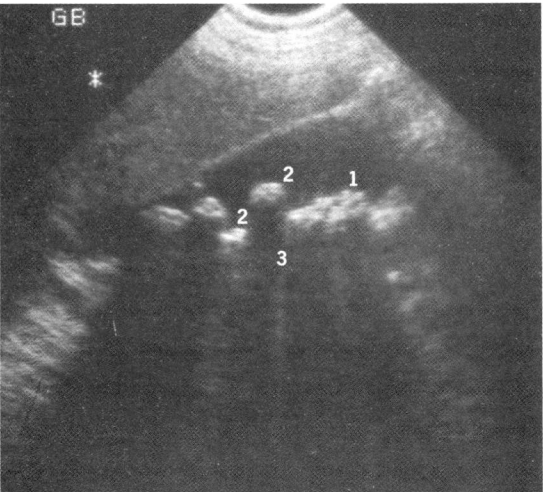

Fig. 7.6 **Gall bladder ultrasound with multiple echogenic gallstones causing well-defined acoustic shadowing.**
1, gall bladder; 2, gallstones; 3, echogenic shadow.

Other abdominal masses can be delineated and biopsies obtained under ultrasonic guidance. Colour Doppler ultrasound will demonstrate the vascularity of a lesion and the direction of blood flow in the portal and hepatic veins. The recent introduction of ultrasound contrast agents, most of which are based on the production of microbubbles within the flowing blood may enhance the vascularity within a lesion. Levovist allows abnormal circulation to be detected within liver nodules, allowing a more specific diagnosis of hepatocellular carcinoma.

Computed tomography (CT) examination

This technique is complementary to ultrasound, which should usually be performed first. It provides excellent visualization of the liver, pancreas, spleen, lymph nodes and lesions in the in the porta hepatis. CT allows assessment of the size, shape and density of the liver and can characterize focal lesions in terms of their vascularity. CT is more sensitive in detecting calcification than plain X-rays. Ultrasound is usually more valuable for lesions in the bile duct and gall bladder, CT has advantages in obese subjects.

Spiral CT involves rapid acquisition of a volume of data during or immediately after i.v. contrast injection. Data can thus be acquired in both arterial and portal venous phases of enhancement, enabling more precise characterization of a lesion and its vascular supply (Fig. 7.7). Retrospective analysis of data allows multiple overlapping slices to be obtained with no increase in the radiation dose. Multi-planar and three-dimensional reconstruction in the arterial phase can create a CT angiogram, often making formal invasive angiography unnecessary. CT also provides guidance for biopsy. In general lesions over 3 cm can usually be biopsied under ultrasound guidance, which is quicker and more cost-effective.

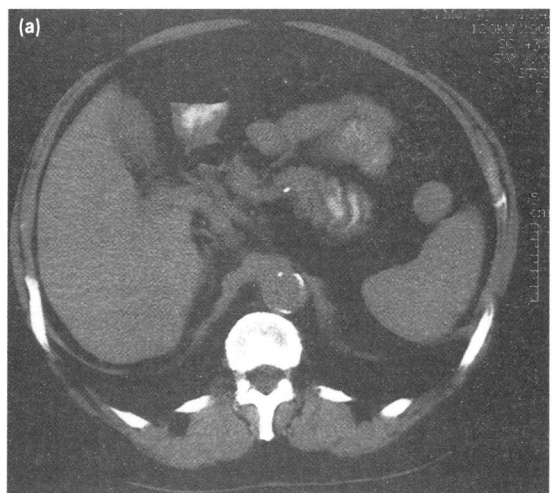

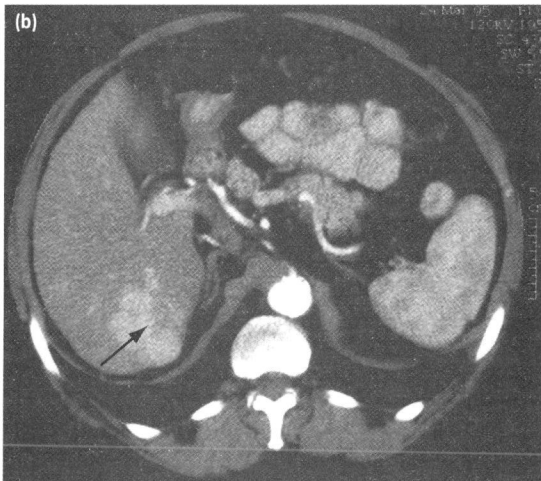

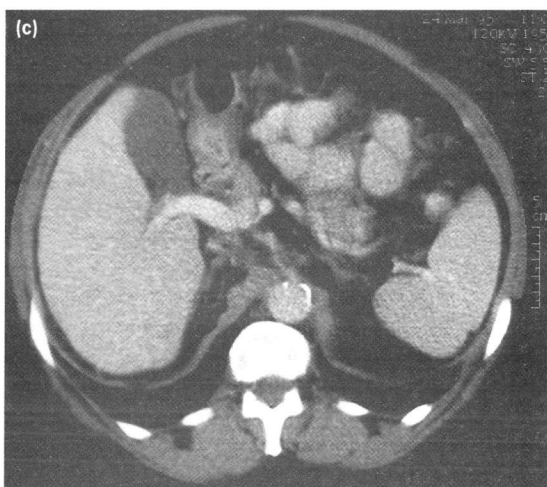

Fig. 7.7 **Use of contrast-enhanced spiral CT. (a)** Unenhanced, **(b)** arterial phase (note high density contrast in the aorta), and **(c)** portal venous phase scan through the right lobe of the liver. There is an irregular mass (arrow) in the posterior aspect of the right lobe of the liver which is only well seen on the early arterial phase enhanced scan **(b)**.

Magnetic resonance imaging (MRI)

(see also p. 1154)

MRI produces cross-sectional images in any plane within the body. Diffuse liver disease alters the T1 and T2 characteristics and MRI is probably the most sensitive investigation of focal liver disease. Other fat-suppression modes such as STIR allow good differentiation between haemangiomas and other lesions.

Magnetic resonance cholangiopancreatography (MRCP)

This technique involves the manipulation of a volume of data acquired by MRI. A heavily T2-weighted sequence enhances visualization of the 'water-filled' bile ducts and pancreatic ducts to produce high-quality images of ductal anatomy. This non-invasive technique is replacing diagnostic (but not therapeutic) ERCP (see below).

Plain X-rays of the abdomen

These are rarely requested but may show:

- gallstones – 10% contain enough calcium to be seen
- air in the biliary tree owing to its recent instrumentation, surgery or to a fistula between the intestine and the gall bladder
- pancreatic calcification
- rarely, calcification of the gall bladder (porcelain gall bladder).

Cholecystogram

This test is rarely required as it has been almost universally replaced by ultrasound but may be useful in a test of gall bladder function. Oral iopanoic acid is absorbed from the gut, conjugated in the liver, secreted in bile and concentrated in the gall bladder, which opacifies homogeneously. A fatty meal is given to make the gall bladder contract. The dye is excreted by the liver via the same mechanism as bilirubin, so that non-visualization will occur in the jaundiced patient and in the patient with liver disease.

Radionuclide imaging – scintiscanning

In a technetium-99m (^{99m}Tc) colloid scan, the colloid is injected intravenously to be taken up by the reticulo-endothelial cells of the liver and spleen. In chronic liver disease there is poor intake in the liver and most of the colloid is taken up in the spleen and bone marrow. Ultrasound has largely replaced this technique.

In a ^{99m}Tc-Iodida scan, technetium-labelled iododiethyl IDA is taken up by the hepatocytes and excreted rapidly into the biliary system. Its main uses are in the diagnosis of:

- acute cholecystitis
- jaundice due to either biliary atresia or hepatitis in the neonatal period.

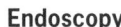

Endoscopy

Upper GI endoscopy

This is used for the diagnosis and treatment of varices, for the detection of portal hypertensive gastropathy, and for associated lesions such as peptic ulcers.

Endoscopic ultrasound (EUS)

In this technique, a small high-frequency ultrasound probe is mounted on the tip of an endoscope and placed by direct vision into the duodenum. The close proximity of the probe to the pancreas and biliary tree permits high-resolution ultrasound imaging. It allows accurate staging of small, potentially operable, pancreatic tumours and offers a less-invasive method for bile duct imaging. It has a high accuracy in detection of small neuro-endocrine tumours of the pancreas. EUS-guided fine-needle aspiration of tumours provides cytological/histological confirmation of malignancy.

Endoscopic retrograde cholangiopancreatography (ERCP)

This technique is used to outline the biliary and pancreatic ducts. It involves the passage of an endoscope into the second part of the duodenum and cannulation of the ampulla. Contrast is injected into both systems and the patient is screened radiologically. Contrast medium with a low iodine content of 1.5 mg/mL is used for the common bile duct so that gallstones are not obscured; a higher iodine content of 2.8 mg/mL is used for the pancreatic duct. In addition, other diagnostic and therapeutic procedures can be carried out:

- Common bile duct stones can be removed after balloon dilatation (if small) or diathermy cut to the sphincter has been performed to facilitate their withdrawal (p. 392). Sphincterotomy has a complication rate of 8–12%: acute pancreatitis in 5% of cases; severe haemorrhage in 2%, with an overall mortality of 0.5–1%. Endoscopic balloon dilatation preserves biliary sphincter function and appears safer.
- The biliary system can be drained by passing a tube (stent) through an obstruction, or placement of a nasobiliary drain.

The complication rate in diagnostic ERCP is 2–3%.

A raised serum amylase is often seen and pancreatitis is the most common complication. Cholangitis is also seen, and broad-spectrum antibiotics (e.g. 500 mg ciprofloxacin × 2) should be given prophylactically to all patients with suspected biliary obstruction, or a history of cholangitis.

Percutaneous transhepatic cholangiography (PTC)

Under a local anaesthetic, a fine flexible needle is passed into the liver. Contrast is injected slowly until a biliary radicle is identified and then further contrast is injected to outline the whole of the biliary tree. In patients with dilated ducts the success rate is near 100%. ERCP is the preferred first investigation because therapy (e.g. stone removal) can be undertaken at the same time.

In difficult cases the two techniques are sometimes combined, PTC showing the biliary anatomy above the obstruction, with ERCP showing the more distal anatomy. If an obstruction in the bile ducts is seen, a bypass stent can sometimes be inserted, draining either externally or, for long-term use, internally. Contra-indications are as for liver biopsy (see below). The main complications are bleeding and cholangitis with septicaemia, and prophylactic antibiotics should be given as for ERCP.

Angiography

This is performed by selective catheterization of the coeliac axis and hepatic artery. It detects the abnormal vasculature of hepatic tumours, but spiral CT has replaced this in many cases. The portal vein can be demonstrated with increased definition using subtraction techniques, and splenoportography (by direct splenic puncture) is rarely performed. In digital vascular imaging (DVI), contrast given intravenously or intra-arterially can be detected in the portal system using computerized subtraction analysis. Hepatic venous cannulation allows abnormal hepatic veins to be diagnosed in patients with Budd–Chiari syndrome and also serves as an indirect measurement of portal pressure. There is a 1:1 relationship of occluded (by balloon) hepatic venous pressure with portal pressure in patients with alcoholic or viral-related cirrhosis. The height of portal pressure has been shown to have prognostic value for survival and a reduced portal pressure 20% from baseline values has been associated with protection from rebleeding. Retrograde CO_2 portography is used when there is doubt about portal vein patency and can be combined with transjugular biopsy and hepatic venous pressure measurement.

Liver biopsy (see Practical box 7.1)

Histological examination of the liver is valuable in the differential diagnosis of diffuse or localized parenchymal disease. Liver biopsy can be performed on a day-case or overnight-stay basis. The indications and contraindications are shown in Table 7.2. The mortality rate is less than 0.02% when performed by experienced operators.

Liver biopsy guided by ultrasound or CT is often performed routinely, particularly when specific lesions need to be biopsied. Laparoscopy with guided liver biopsy is performed through a small incision in the abdominal wall under local anaesthesia (general anaesthesia is preferred in some centres). A transjugular approach is used when liver histology is essential for management but coagulation abnormalities prevent the percutaneous approach.

Needle biopsy of the liver

This should be performed only by experienced doctors and with sterile precautions. Patient consent must be obtained.

- The patient's coagulation status (prothrombin time, platelets) is checked.
- The patient's blood group is checked and serum saved for cross-matching.
- The patient lies on his back at the edge of the bed.
- The liver margins are delineated using percussion. *Alternatively* ultrasound examination can be used to confirm liver margins and position of the gall bladder.
- Local anaesthetic is injected at the point of maximum dullness in the mid-axillary line through the intercostal space during expiration. Anaesthetic (1% lidocaine (lignocaine), approximately 5 mL) should be injected down to the liver capsule.
- A tiny cut is made in the skin with a scalpel blade.
- A special needle (Menghini, Trucut or Surecut) is used to obtain the liver biopsy whilst the patient holds his breath in expiration.
- The biopsy is laid on filter paper and placed in 10% formalin. If a culture of the biopsy is required it should be placed in a sterile pot.
- The patient should be observed, with pulse and blood pressure measurements taken regularly for at least 6 h.

Most complications of liver biopsy occur within 24 hours (usually in the first 2 hours). They are often minor and include abdominal or shoulder pain which settles with analgesics. Minor intraperitoneal bleeding can occur, but this settles spontaneously. Rare complications include major intraperitoneal bleeding, haemothorax and pleurisy, biliary peritonitis, haemobilia and transient septicaemia. Haemobilia produces biliary colic, jaundice and melaena within 3 days of the biopsy.

FURTHER READING

Grant A, Neuberger J (1999) Guidelines on the use of liver biopsy in clinical practice. *Gut* **45** (Suppl 4).
Pratt D S, Kaplan MM (2000) Evaluation of abnormal liver enzyme results in asymptomatic patients. *New England Journal of Medicine* **342**: 1266–1274.
Saini S (1997) Imaging of the hepatobiliary tract. *New England Journal of Medicine* **336**: 1889–1894.

Symptoms of liver disease

Acute liver disease
This may be asymptomatic and anicteric. Symptomatic disease, which is often viral, produces generalized symptoms of malaise, anorexia and fever. Jaundice may appear as the illness progresses.

Table 7.2
Indications and contraindications for liver biopsy

Indications
Liver disease
  Unexplained hepatomegaly
  Some cases of jaundice
  Persistently abnormal liver biochemistry
  Occasionally in acute hepatitis
  Chronic hepatitis
  Cirrhosis
  Drug-related liver disease
  Infiltrations
  Tumours: primary or secondary
  Infections (e.g. tuberculosis)
  Storage disease (e.g. glycogen storage)
Screening relatives of patients with certain diseases
  (e.g. hereditary haemochromatosis)
Pyrexia of unknown origin

Usual contraindications to percutaneous needle biopsy
Uncooperative patient
Prolonged prothrombin time (by more than 3 s)
Platelets $< 80 \times 10^9$/L
Ascites
Extrahepatic cholestasis
Renal transplant

Chronic liver disease
Patients may be asymptomatic or complain of non-specific symptoms, particularly fatigue. Specific symptoms include:

- right hypochondrial pain due to liver distension
- abdominal distension due to ascites
- ankle swelling due to fluid retention
- haematemesis and melaena from gastrointestinal haemorrhage
- pruritus due to cholestasis – this is often an early symptom of primary biliary cirrhosis
- breast swelling (gynaecomastia), loss of libido and amenorrhoea due to endocrine dysfunction
- confusion and drowsiness due to neuropsychiatric complications (portosystemic encephalopathy).

Signs of liver disease

Acute liver disease
There may be few signs apart from jaundice and an enlarged liver. Jaundice is a yellow coloration of the skin and mucous membranes and is best seen in the conjunctivae and unexposed sclerae. In the cholestatic phase of the illness, pale stools and dark urine are present. Spider naevi and liver palms usually indicate chronic disease but they can occur in severe acute disease.

Chronic liver disease
The physical signs are shown in Figure 7.8. However, it is possible for the physical examination to be normal in patients with advanced chronic liver disease.

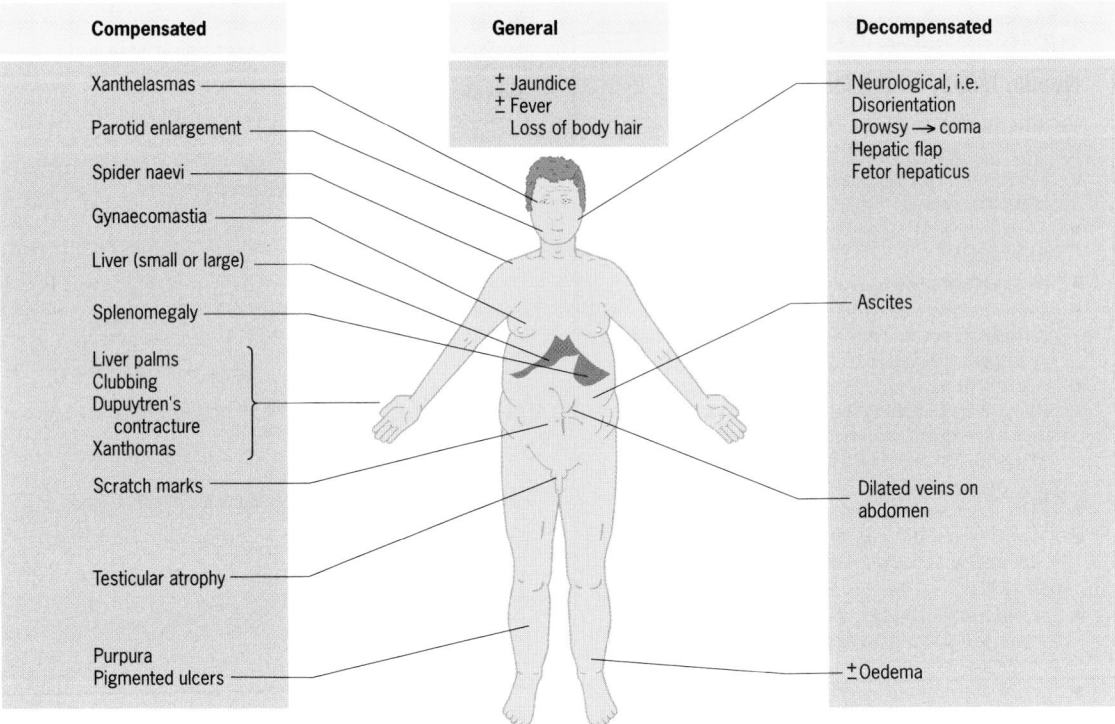

Fig. 7.8 **Physical signs in chronic liver disease.**

The skin

The chest and upper body may show spider naevi. These are telangiectases that consist of a central arteriole with radiating small vessels. They are found in the distribution of the superior vena cava (i.e. above the nipple line). They are also found in pregnancy. In haemochromatosis the skin may have a slate-grey appearance.

The hands may show palmar erythema, which is a non-specific change indicative of a hyperdynamic circulation; it is also seen in pregnancy, thyrotoxicosis or rheumatoid arthritis. Clubbing occasionally occurs, and a Dupuytren's contracture is often seen in alcoholic cirrhosis.

Xanthomas (cholesterol deposits) are seen in the palmar creases or above the eyes in primary biliary cirrhosis.

The abdomen

Initial hepatomegaly will be followed by a small liver in well-established cirrhosis. Splenomegaly is seen with portal hypertension.

The endocrine system

Gynaecomastia (occasionally unilateral) and testicular atrophy may be found in males. The cause of gynaecomastia is complex, but it is probably related to altered oestrogen metabolism or to treatment with spironolactone.

In decompensated cirrhosis, additional signs that can be seen are shown in Figure 7.8.

Jaundice

Jaundice (icterus) is detectable clinically when the serum bilirubin is greater than 50 μmol/L (3 mg/dL). The usual division of jaundice into prehepatic, hepatocellular and obstructive (cholestatic) is an oversimplification as in hepatocellular jaundice there is invariably cholestasis and the clinical problem is whether the cholestasis is intrahepatic or extrahepatic. Jaundice will therefore be considered under the following headings:

- haemolytic jaundice – increased bilirubin load for the liver cells
- congenital hyperbilirubinaemias – defects in conjugation
- cholestatic jaundice, including hepatocellular (parenchymal) liver disease and large duct obstruction.

Haemolytic jaundice

The increased breakdown of red cells (see p. 424) leads to an increase in production of bilirubin. The resulting jaundice is usually mild (serum bilirubin of 68–102 μmol/L or 4–6 mg/dL) as normal liver function can easily handle the increased bilirubin derived from excess haemolysis. Unconjugated bilirubin is not water-soluble and therefore will not pass into the urine; hence the term 'acholuric jaundice'. Urinary urobilinogen is increased.

The causes of haemolytic jaundice are those of haemolytic anaemia (p. 424). The clinical features depend on the cause; anaemia, jaundice, splenomegaly, gallstones and leg ulcers may be seen.

Investigations show features of haemolysis (p. 425). The level of unconjugated bilirubin is raised but the serum ALP, transferases and albumin are normal. Serum haptoglobulins are low. The differential diagnosis is from other forms of jaundice.

Congenital hyperbilirubinaemias (non-haemolytic)

Unconjugated

Gilbert's syndrome

This is the most common familial hyperbilirubinaemia and affects 2–7% of the population. It is asymptomatic and is usually detected as an incidental finding of a slightly raised bilirubin (17–102 µmol/L or 1–6 mg/dL) on a routine check. All the other liver biochemistry is normal and no signs of liver disease are seen. There is a family history of jaundice in 5–15% of patients. Hepatic glucuronidation is approximately 30% of normal, resulting in an increased proportion of bilirubin monoglucuronide in bile. Most patients have reduced levels of UDP-glucuronosyl transferase activity, the enzyme that conjugates bilirubin with glucuronic acid. Mutations occur in the gene encoding this enzyme with an expanded nucleotide repeat consisting of two extra bases in the upstream 5′ promoter element. This abnormality appears to be necessary for the syndrome, but is not in itself sufficient for the phenotypic expression of the syndrome.

The major importance of establishing this diagnosis is to inform the patient that this is not a serious disease and to prevent unnecessary investigations. The raised unconjugated bilirubin rises on fasting and during a mild illness. The reticulocyte count is normal, excluding haemolysis and no treatment is necessary.

Crigler–Najjar syndrome

This is very rare. Only patients with type II (autosomal dominant) with a decrease rather than absence (type I – autosomal recessive) of UDP-glucuronosyl transferase can survive into adult life. Mutation of the gene for UDP-glucuronosyl transferase has been demonstrated in the coding region. Liver histology is normal. Transplantation is the only effective treatment.

Conjugated

Dubin–Johnson (autosomal recessive) and *Rotor's* (possibly autosomal dominant) *syndromes* are due to defects in bilirubin handling in the liver. The prognosis is good in both. In the Dubin–Johnson syndrome there are mutations in both *MRP2* (p. 337) transporter genes.

The liver is black owing to melanin deposition.

Recurrent familial intrahepatic cholestasis (FICI) or benign recurrent intrahepatic cholestasis

This is rare. Recurrent attacks of acute cholestasis occur without progression to chronic liver disease. Jaundice, severe pruritus, steatorrhoea and weight loss develop. Serum γ-GT is normal. The gene has been mapped to the FICI locus, but the precise relation to cholestasis is unclear.

Progressive familial intrahepatic cholestasis syndromes

These are autosomal recessive. In *type 1*, with cholestasis in infancy (previously known as Byler's disease), γ-GT is normal. The gene is also on the FICI locus, but has been mapped to a region encoding P type ATPases. *Type 2* has been mapped to the bile salt export pump gene (*BSEP*). The protein is located in the canalicular domain of the plasma membrane of the hepatocyte. The phenotypic expression is frequently a presentation as a non-specific giant cell hepatitis progressing to cholestasis. *Type 3* is due to *PGY3* gene mutation leading to deficient canalicular phosphatidylcholine transport and thus toxic bile causing liver damage. Liver transplantation is the only cure for these syndromes.

Intrahepatic cholestasis of pregnancy

This has been associated with mutations in the genes of the progressive familial intrahepatic cholestasis syndromes. It is described on page 383.

FURTHER READING

Jansen PLM, Muller M (2000) The molecular genetics of familial intrahepatic cholestasis. *Gut* 47: 1–5.

Cholestatic jaundice (acquired)

This can be divided into extrahepatic and intrahepatic cholestasis. The causes are shown in Figure 7.9.

- Extrahepatic cholestasis is due to large duct obstruction of bile flow at any point in the biliary tract distal to the bile canaliculi.
- Intrahepatic cholestasis occurs owing to failure of bile secretion. A number of cellular mechanisms in cholestasis have been described in animal models, including inhibition of the Na$^+$–K$^+$-ATPase in the basolateral membranes, decreased fluidity of the sinusoidal plasma membrane, disruption of the microfilaments responsible for canalicular tone, and damage to the tight junctions. In addition, inflammatory change in ductular cells interferes with bile flow.

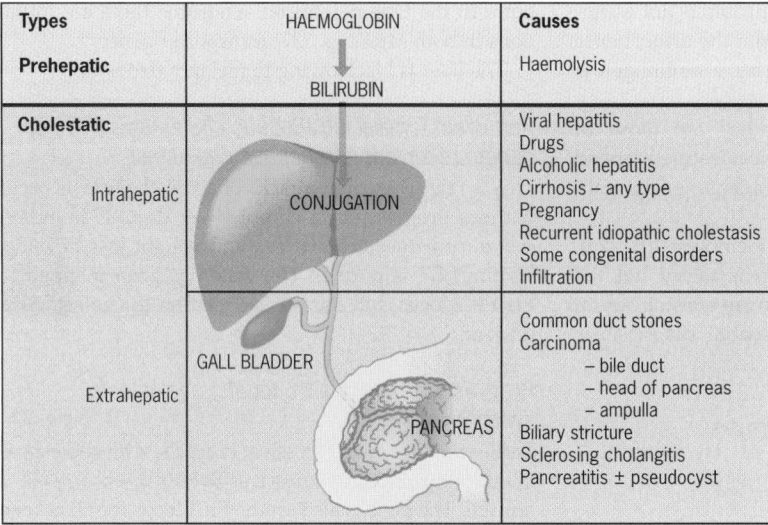

Types	HAEMOGLOBIN ↓ BILIRUBIN	Causes
Prehepatic		Haemolysis
Cholestatic		
Intrahepatic	CONJUGATION	Viral hepatitis Drugs Alcoholic hepatitis Cirrhosis – any type Pregnancy Recurrent idiopathic cholestasis Some congenital disorders Infiltration

Extrahepatic	GALL BLADDER
	PANCREAS
		Common duct stones
		Carcinoma
		  – bile duct
		  – head of pancreas
		  – ampulla
		Biliary stricture
		Sclerosing cholangitis
		Pancreatitis ± pseudocyst

Fig. 7.9 Causes of jaundice.

Clinically in both types there is jaundice with pale stools and dark urine, and the serum bilirubin is conjugated. However, intrahepatic and extrahepatic cholestatic jaundice must be differentiated as their clinical management is entirely different.

Differential diagnosis of jaundice

A careful history may give a clue to the diagnosis. Certain causes of jaundice are more likely in particular categories of people. For example, a young person is more likely to have hepatitis, so questions should be asked about drug and alcohol use, and sexual behaviour. An elderly person with gross weight loss is more likely to have a carcinoma. All patients may complain of malaise. Abdominal pain occurs in patients with biliary obstruction by gallstones and, sometimes with an enlarged liver there is pain resulting from distension of the capsule.

Questions should be appropriate to the particular situation, and the following aspects of the history should be covered.

- *Country of origin*. The incidence of hepatitis B virus (HBV) infection is increased in many parts of the world (p. 354).
- *Duration of illness*. A history of jaundice with prolonged weight loss in an older patient suggests malignancy. A short history, particularly with a prodromal illness of malaise, suggests a hepatitis.
- *Recent outbreak of jaundice*. An outbreak in the community suggests hepatitis A virus (HAV).
- *Recent consumption of shellfish*. This suggests HAV infection.
- *Intravenous drug abuse, or recent injections or tattoos*. These all increase the chance of HBV and hepatitis C virus (HCV) infection.
- *Male homosexuality*. This increases the chance of HBV infection.

- *Female prostitution*. This increases the chance of HBV infection.
- *Blood transfusion or infusion of pooled blood products*. Increased risk of HBV and HCV. In developed countries all donors are screened for HBV and HCV.
- *Alcohol consumption*. A careful history of drinking habits should be taken, although many patients often understate the actual amount they drink.
- *Drugs taken* (particularly in the previous 2–3 months). Many drugs cause jaundice (see p. 386).
- *Travel*. Certain areas have an increased risk of HAV infection as well as HEV infection (this has a high mortality in pregnancy).
- *Recent anaesthetics*. Halothane (see p. 386), enflurane, isoflurane, for example, may cause jaundice, particularly in those already sensitive to halogenated anaesthetics. The risk with desflurane appears remote.
- *Family history*. Patients with, for example, Gilbert's disease may have family members who get recurrent jaundice.
- *Recent surgery* on the biliary tract or for carcinoma.
- *Environment*. People engaged in recreational activities in rural areas, as well as farm and sewage workers, are at risk for leptospirosis.
- *Fevers or rigors*. These are suggestive of cholangitis or possibly a liver abscess.

Clinical features

The signs of acute and chronic liver disease should be looked for (p. 345). Certain additional signs may be helpful:

- **Hepatomegaly**. A smooth tender liver is seen in hepatitis and with extrahepatic obstruction, but a knobbly irregular liver suggests metastases. Causes of hepatomegaly are shown in Table 7.3.

Table 7.3
Causes of hepatomegaly

Apparent	Haematological
Low-lying diaphragm	Leukaemias
Reidel's lobe	Lymphoma
	Myeloproliferative disorders
Cirrhosis (early)	Thalassaemia
Inflammation	**Tumours: primary and**
Hepatitis	**secondary carcinoma**
Schistosomiasis	
Abscesses	**Venous congestion**
(pyogenic or amoebic)	Heart failure
	Hepatic vein occlusion
Cysts	
Hydatid	**Biliary obstruction**
Polycystic	**(particularly extrahepatic)**
Metabolic	
Fatty liver	
Amyloid	
Glycogen storage disease	

- **Splenomegaly**. This indicates portal hypertension in patients when signs of chronic liver disease are present. The spleen can also be 'tipped' occasionally in viral hepatitis.
- **Ascites**. This is found in cirrhosis but can also be due to carcinoma (particularly ovarian) and many other causes (see Table 7.14).

A palpable gall bladder can suggest a carcinoma of the pancreas obstructing the bile duct. Generalized lymphadenopathy suggests a lymphoma.

Cold sores may suggest a herpes simplex virus hepatitis

Investigations
Jaundice is not itself a diagnosis and the cause should always be sought. The two most useful tests are the viral markers for HAV, HBV and HCV (in high-risk groups), plus an ultrasound examination. Liver biochemistry confirms the jaundice and may help in the diagnosis.

An ultrasound examination should always be performed to exclude an extrahepatic obstruction, and to diagnose any features compatible with chronic liver disease except when hepatitis A is strongly suspected in a young patient. Ultrasound will demonstrate:

- the size of the bile ducts, which are dilated in extrahepatic obstruction (Fig. 7.10)
- the level of the obstruction
- the cause of the obstruction in virtually all patients with tumours and in 75% of patients with gallstones.

The pathological diagnosis of any mass lesion can be made by fine-needle aspiration cytology (sensitivity approximately 60%) or by needle biopsy using a spring-loaded device (sensitivity approximately 90%).

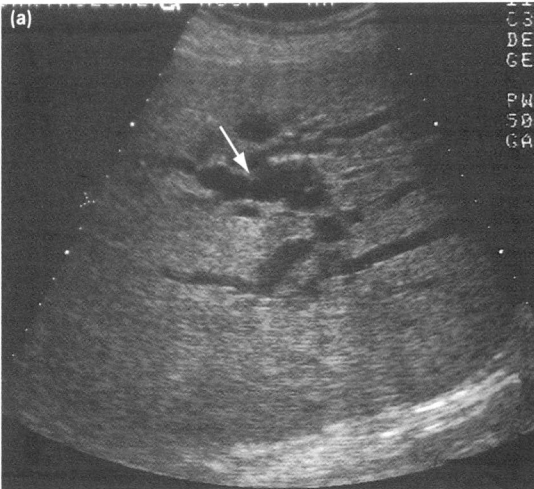

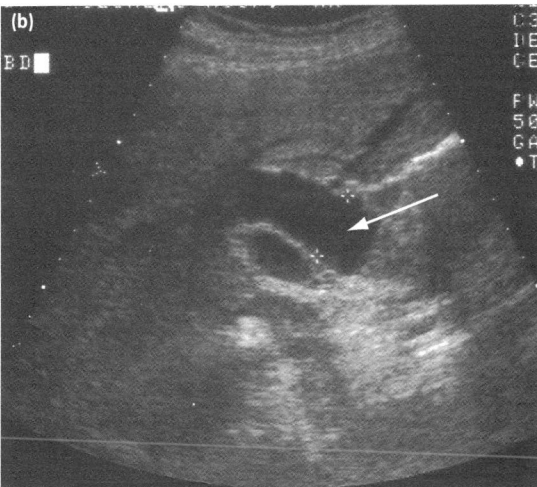

Fig. 7.10 **Liver ultrasound showing (a) dilated intrahepatic bile ducts (arrow), (b) common bile duct (arrow).** The normal bile duct measures 6 mm at the porta hepatis.

A flow diagram for the general investigation of the jaundiced patient is shown in Figure 7.11.

Liver biochemistry
In hepatitis, the serum AST or ALT tends to be high early in the disease with only a small rise in the serum ALP. Conversely, in extrahepatic obstruction the ALP is high with a smaller rise in aminotransferases. These findings cannot, however, be relied on alone to make a diagnosis in an individual case. The prothrombin time (PT) is often prolonged in long-standing liver disease, and the serum albumin is also low.

Haematological tests
In haemolytic jaundice the bilirubin is raised and the other liver biochemistry is normal (p. 346). A raised

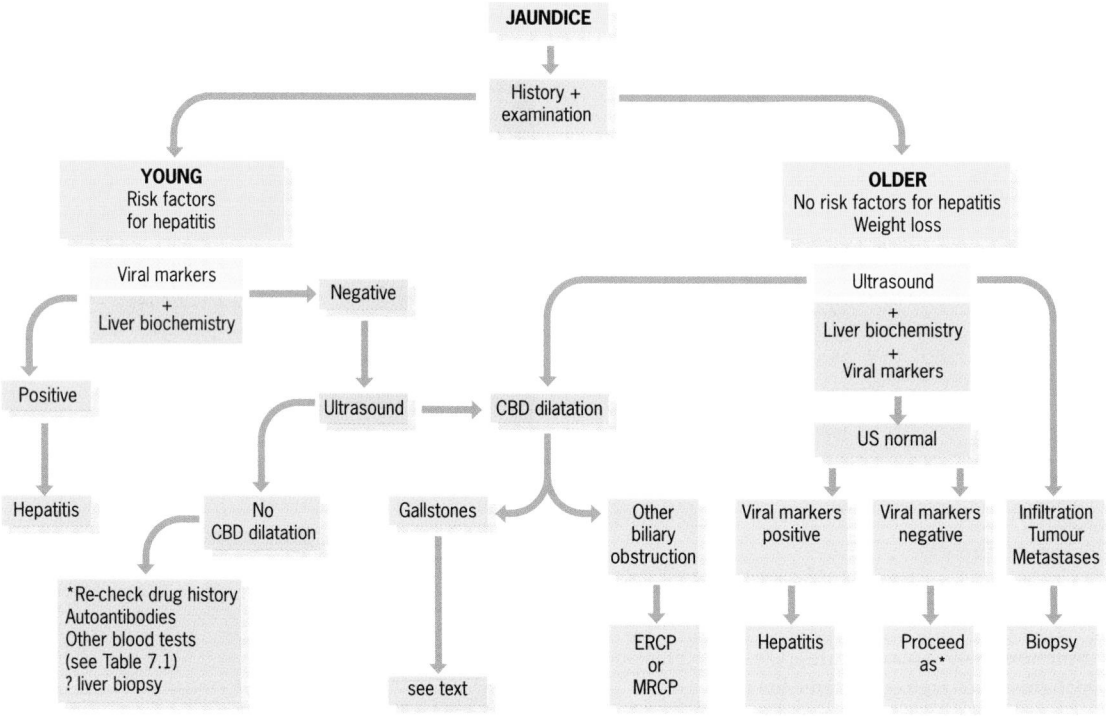

Fig. 7.11 **Approach to patient with jaundice.** ERCP, endoscopic retrograde cholangiopancreatography; CBD, common bile duct; US, ultrasound; MRCP, magnetic resonance cholangiopancreatography.

white cell count may indicate infection (e.g. cholangitis). A leucopenia often occurs in viral hepatitis, while abnormal mononuclear cells suggest infectious mononucleosis and a Monospot test should be performed.

Other blood tests

These include tests to exclude unusual causes of liver disease (e.g. cytomegalovirus antibodies), autoimmune antibodies, e.g. antimitochondrial antibodies (AMA) for the diagnosis of primary biliary cirrhosis, and α-fetoprotein for a hepatocellular carcinoma.

Acute hepatitis

Acute parenchymal liver damage can be caused by many agents (Fig. 7.12).

Pathology

Although some histological features are suggestive of the aetiological factor, most of the changes are essentially similar whatever the cause. Hepatocytes show degenerative changes (swelling, cytoplasmic granularity, vacuolation), undergo necrosis (becoming shrunken, eosinophilic Councilman bodies) and are rapidly removed. The distribution of these changes varies somewhat with the aetiological agent, but necrosis is usually

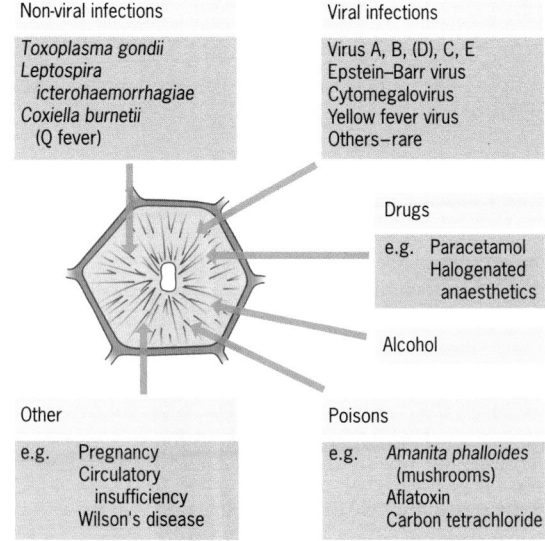

Fig. 7.12 **Some causes of acute parenchymal damage.**

maximal in zone 3. The extent of the damage is very variable between individuals affected by the same agent: at one end of the spectrum, single and small groups of hepatocytes die (spotty or focal necrosis), while at the other end there is multiacinar necrosis

Table 7.4
Some features of hepatitis viruses

	A	B	D	C	E
Virus	RNA	DNA	RNA	RNA	RNA
	27 nm	42 nm	36 nm (with HBsAg coat)	30–60 nm	27 nm
	Picorna	Hepadna	Unclassified	Flavi	Calici
Spread					
Faecal	Yes	No	No	No	Yes
Blood	Rare	Yes	Yes	Yes	No
Vertical	No	Yes	Rare	Occasional	No
Saliva	Yes	Yes	Yes	? No	?
Sexual	Rare	Yes	Yes (rare)	Occasional	No
Incubation	Short (2–3 weeks)	Long (1–5 months)	Long	Intermediate	Short
Age	Young	Any	Any	Any	Any
Carrier state	No	Yes	Yes	?	No
Chronic liver disease	No	Yes	Yes	Yes	No
Liver cancer	No	Yes	Rare	Yes	No
Mortality (acute)	< 0.5%	< 1%		< 1%	1–2% (pregnant women 10–20%)
Immunization:					
Passive	Normal immunoglobulin serum i.m. (0.04–0.06 mL/kg)	Hepatitis B immunoglobin (HBIg)	–	–	–
Active	Vaccine	Vaccine	HBV vaccine	–	–

involving a substantial part of the liver (massive hepatic necrosis) resulting in fulminant hepatic failure. Between these extremes there is limited confluent necrosis with collapse of the reticulin framework resulting in linking (bridging) between the central veins, the central veins and portal tracts, and between the portal tracts. The extent of the inflammatory infiltrate is also variable, but portal tracts and lobules are infiltrated mainly by lymphocytes. Other variable features include cholestasis in zone 3 and fatty change, the latter being prominent in hepatitis that is due to alcohol or certain drugs.

Management
This is discussed below under the individual aetiological factors.

Viral hepatitis

The differing features of the common forms of viral hepatitis are summarized in Table 7.4.

Hepatitis A
Hepatitis A virus (HAV)
HAV is a picornavirus, having the structure shown in Figure 7.13. It has a single serotype as only one epitope is immunodominant. It replicates in the liver, is excreted in bile and is then excreted in the faeces of infected persons for about 2 weeks before the onset of clinical illness and for up to 7 days after. The disease is maximally

(a) HAV virion

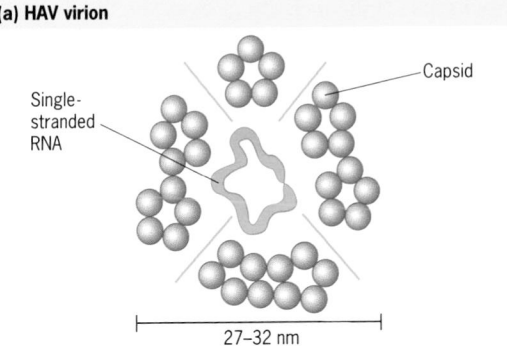

(b) HAV genome

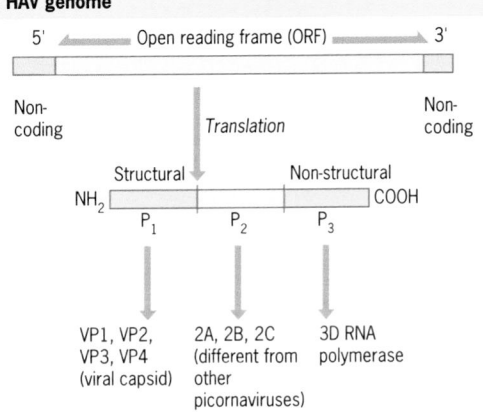

Fig. 7.13 **(a)** The hepatitis A (HAV) virion consists of four polypeptides (VP1–VP4) which form a tight protein shell, or capsid, containing the RNA. The major antigenic component is associated with VP1. **(b)** Arrangement of HAV genome.

infectious just before the onset of jaundice. HAV particles can be demonstrated in the faeces by electron microscopy.

Epidemiology

Hepatitis A is the most common type of viral hepatitis occurring world-wide, often in epidemics. The disease is commonly seen in the autumn and affects children and young adults. Spread of infection is mainly by the faeco-oral route and arises from the ingestion of contaminated food or water (e.g. shellfish). Overcrowding and poor sanitation facilitate spread. There is no carrier state. In the UK it is a notifiable disease.

Clinical features

The viraemia causes the patient to feel unwell with non-specific symptoms that include nausea, anorexia and a distaste for cigarettes. Many recover at this stage and remain anicteric.

After 1 or 2 weeks some patients become jaundiced and symptoms often improve. As the jaundice deepens, the urine becomes dark and the stools pale owing to intrahepatic cholestasis. The liver is moderately enlarged and the spleen is palpable in about 10% of patients. Occasionally, tender lymphadenopathy is seen, with a transient rash in some cases. Thereafter the jaundice lessens and in the majority of cases the illness is over within 3–6 weeks. Extrahepatic complications are rare but include arthritis, vasculitis, myocarditis and renal failure. A biphasic illness occasionally occurs, with the return of jaundice. Rarely the disease may be very severe with fulminant hepatitis, liver coma and death. The typical sequence of events after HAV exposure is shown in Figure 7.14.

Investigations

Liver biochemistry

In the prodromal stage the serum bilirubin is usually normal. However, there is bilirubinuria and increased urinary urobilinogen. A raised serum AST or ALT, which can sometimes be very high, precedes the jaundice.

In the icteric stage the serum bilirubin reflects the level of jaundice. Serum AST reaches a maximum 1–2 days after the appearance of jaundice, and may rise above 500 IU/L. Serum ALP is usually less than 300 IU/L.

After the jaundice has subsided, the aminotransferases may remain elevated for some weeks and occasionally for up to 6 months.

Haematological tests

There is leucopenia with a relative lymphocytosis. Very rarely there is a Coombs'-positive haemolytic anaemia or an associated aplastic anaemia. The prothrombin time (PT) is prolonged in severe cases. The erythrocyte sedimentation rate (ESR) is raised.

Viral markers: antibodies to HAV

IgG antibodies are common in the general population over the age of 50 years, but an anti-HAV IgM means an acute infection. In areas of high prevalence most children have antibodies by the age of 3 years following asymptomatic infection.

Other tests

Further tests are not necessary in the presence of an IgM antibody, but liver biochemistry must be followed to establish a return to normal levels.

Differential diagnosis

Clinically the differential diagnosis is from all other causes of jaundice – but in particular from other types of viral and drug-induced hepatitis.

Course and prognosis

The prognosis is excellent, with most patients making a complete recovery. The mortality in young adults is 0.1% but it increases with age. Death is due to fulminant hepatic necrosis. During convalescence, 5–15% of patients may have relapse of the hepatitis but this settles spontaneously. Occasionally a more severe jaundice with cholestasis will run a prolonged course of 7–20 weeks and is called 'cholestatic viral hepatitis'.

There is no reason to stop alcohol consumption other than for the few weeks when the patient is ill. Patients may complain of debility for several months following resolution of the symptoms and biochemical parameters. This is known as the post-hepatitis syndrome; it is a functional illness. Treatment is by reassurance. HAV hepatitis never progresses to chronic liver disease.

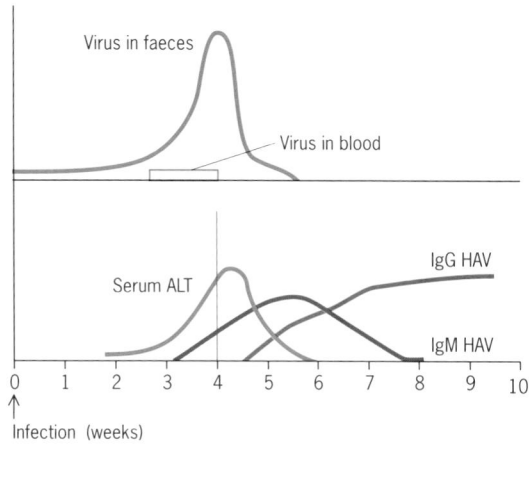

Fig. 7.14 HAV – sequence of events after exposure.

Treatment

There is no specific treatment, and rest and dietary measures are unhelpful. Corticosteroids have no benefit. Admission to hospital is not usually necessary.

Prevention and prophylaxis

Control of hepatitis depends on good hygiene. The virus is resistant to chlorination but is killed by boiling water for 10 minutes.

Active immunization

A formaldehyde-inactivated vaccine is given to people travelling frequently to endemic areas, patients with chronic liver disease, people with haemophilia, and workers in frequent contact with hepatitis cases (e.g. in residential institutions for patients with learning difficulties). Community outbreaks can be interrupted by vaccination. A single dose produces antibodies that persist for at least 1 year, when a booster is given. Immunity then can last for up to 10 years.

Passive immunization

Normal human immunoglobulin (0.04–0.06 mL/kg i.m.) gives protection for 3–4 months and is useful for persons who are occasionally at risk.

Hepatitis B

Hepatitis B virus (HBV)

The complete infective virion or Dane particle is a 42 nm particle comprising an inner core or nucleocapsid (27 nm) surrounded by an outer envelope of surface protein (HBsAg). This surface coat is produced in excess by the infected hepatocytes and can exist separately from the whole virion in serum and body fluid as 22 nm particles or 22 nm tubules.

HBsAg contains a major 'a' antigenic determinant as well as several subtypes: 'd', 'y', 'w' and 'r'. Combinations of these subdeterminants (e.g. adr, adw, ayw and ayr) are used in epidemiology for studying geographical patterns of infection.

The core or nucleocapsid is formed of core protein (HBcAg) containing incompletely double-stranded circular DNA and the DNA polymerase/reverse transcriptase. One strand is almost a complete circle and contains overlapping genes that encode both structural proteins (pre-S, surface (S), core (C)) and replicative proteins (polymerase and X). The other strand is variable in length (Fig. 7.15).

HBeAg is a protein formed via specific self-cleavage of the precore/core gene product which is secreted separately by the cell.

Pre-S_1 and pre-S_2 regions are involved in attachment to the specific HBV receptor on the hepatocyte. After penetration, the virus core is transported to the nucleus without processing, with transcription of HBV into mRNA taking place.

Translation into HBV proteins (Table 7.5) as well as replication of the genome takes place in the endoplasmic reticulum; they are then packaged together and exported from the cell. During the period of replication, the viral genome may integrate into the chromosomal DNA of the hepatocyte.

The HBV is not directly cytopathic and the liver damage produced is by the cellular immune response of the host. Specific failure of T cells to recognize HBV antigens leads to viral persistence.

Hepatitis B mutants

Mutations occur in the various reading frames of the HBV genome (see Fig. 7.15). These mutants can emerge in chronic HBV carriers or can be acquired by infection. Patients have HBsAg and HBV DNA but not the e antigen itself: anti-HBe is present in almost all cases. The

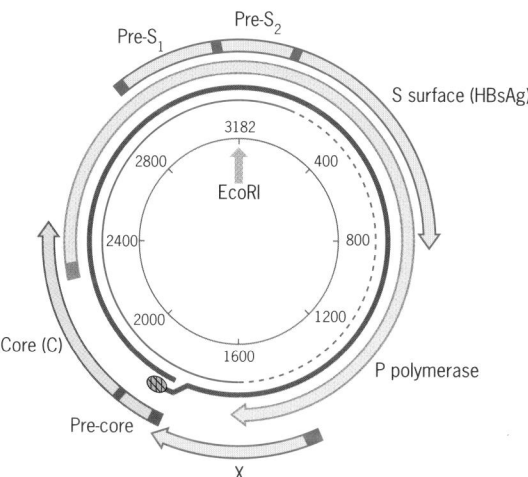

Fig. 7.15 Hepatitis B virus (HBV) genome. The viral DNA is partially double-stranded (red incomplete circle and blue circle). The long strand (blue) encodes seven proteins from four overlapping reading frames (S, surface (Pre-S_1, Pre-S_2, S); C, core (Pre C, C) P, polymerase (P) and X gene (X)). EcoRI restriction-enzyme-binding site is included as a reference point.

Table 7.5 HBV proteins	
HBV protein	**Clinical significance**
Core	Protein of core particle; kinase activity (role in replication?)
Pre-core (HBeAg)	Pre-core/core cleaves to HBeAg; good marker of active replication and role in inducing immunotolerance
Surface (HBsAg)	Envelope protein of HBV; basis of current vaccine
Pre-S_2	HBV binding and entry into hepatocytes
Pre-S_1	HBV binding and entry into hepatocytes
Polymerase	Viral replication
X protein	Trans-activation

amino acid sequence of the e antigen protein is almost identical to that of the core antigen which is involved in viral replication. Separate messenger RNAs have not been described for the two antigens, but HBeAg is initiated several nucleotides upstream of HBcAg. A guanosine (G) to adenosine (A) mutation in the precore region of the genome creates a stop codon (TAG) that prevents the production of HBeAg, but the synthesis of HBcAg is unaffected. Different mutants have also been seen following interferon or lamivudine therapy and in patients with fulminant and fatal hepatitis. Their existence means that serological markers such as the HBeAg are less useful in detecting infectivity and HBV DNA must be always measured.

Epidemiology

The hepatitis B virus is present world-wide and has infected more than 2000 million people. There are an estimated 300 million carriers. The UK and the USA have a low carrier rate (0.5%), but it rises to 10–15% in parts of Africa, the Middle and the Far East.

Spread of this virus is either by the intravenous route (e.g. by transfusion of infected blood or blood products, or by contaminated needles used by drug addicts, tattooists or acupuncturists), or by close personal contact, such as during sexual intercourse, particularly in male homosexuals. The virus can be found in semen and saliva. Vertical transmission from mother to child during parturition or soon after birth is the usual means of transmission world-wide. There is no evidence that HBV replicates in insect vectors but the virus has been detected in mosquitoes and bed bugs.

Clinical features

The sequence of events following acute HBV infection is shown in Figure 7.16. In many cases, however, the infection is subclinical. The clinical picture is the same as that found in HAV infection, although the illness may be more severe. In addition, a serum sickness-like immunological syndrome may be seen. This consists of rashes (e.g. urticaria or a maculopapular rash) and polyarthritis affecting small joints occurring in up to 25% of cases in the prodromal period. Fever is usual. Extrahepatic immune complex-mediated conditions such as an arteritis or glomerulonephritis are occasionally seen.

Investigations

These are generally the same as for hepatitis A.

Specific tests

The markers for HBV are shown in Table 7.6. HBsAg is looked for initially; if it is found, a full viral profile is then performed. In acute infection, as HBsAg may be cleared rapidly, anti-HBc IgM is diagnostic. HBV DNA is the most sensitive index of viral replication and is found without e antigen in hepatitis due to mutants.

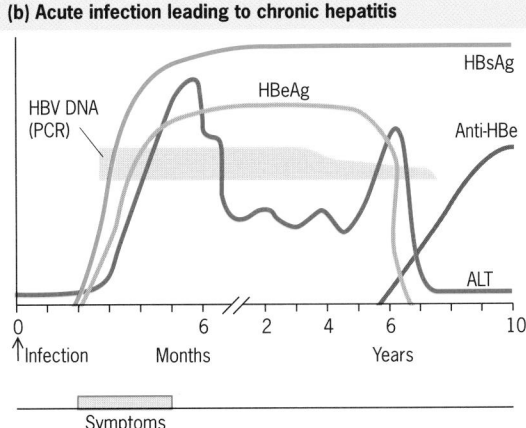

Fig. 7.16 Time course of the events and serological changes seen following infection with hepatitis B virus.

(a) Acute infection

Antigens

HBsAg appears in the blood from about 6 weeks to 3 months after an acute infection and then disappears.

HBeAg rises early and usually declines rapidly.

Antibodies

Anti-HBs appears late and indicates immunity.

Anti-HBc is the first antibody to appear and high titres of IgM anti-HBc suggest an acute and continuing viral replication. It persists for many months. IgM anti-HBc may be the only serological indicator of recent HBV infection in a period when HBsAg has disappeared and anti-HBs is not detectable in the serum.

Anti-HBe appears after the anti-HBc and its appearance relates to a decreased infectivity, i.e. a low risk.

(b) Acute infection leading to chronic hepatitis B

HBsAg persists and indicates a chronic infection (or carrier state).

HBeAg persists and correlates with increased severity and infectivity and the development of chronic liver disease. When anti-HBe develops (seroconversion) the Ag disappears and there is a rise in ALT.

HBV DNA suggests continual viral replication.

For **mutants** – see text.

Table 7.6
Significance of viral markers in hepatitis B

Antigens

HBsAg	Acute or chronic infection
HBeAg	Acute hepatitis B
	Persistence implies:
	continued infectious state
	development of chronicity
	increased severity of disease
HBV DNA	Implies viral replication
	Found in serum and liver

Antibodies

Anti-HBs	Immunity to HBV; previous exposure
Anti-HBe	Seroconversion
Anti-HBc	
IgM	Acute hepatitis B (high titre)
	Chronic hepatitis B (low titre)
IgG	Past exposure to hepatitis B (HBsAg-negative)

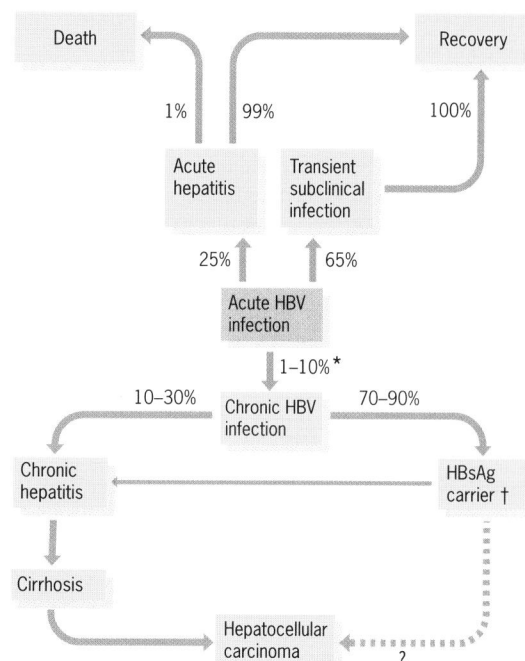

Fig. 7.17 Clinical course of hepatitis B infection. *, percentage variable world-wide; † have normal liver biochemistry – a minority, having acquired infection at birth or in childhood, are HBeAg and HBV-DNA-positive. They may develop hepatitis as the immune system recognizes infected hepatocytes.

Course

The majority of patients recover completely, fulminant hepatitis occurring in up to 1%. Some patients go on to develop chronic hepatitis (p. 360) and hepatocellular carcinoma (p. 384) or become asymptomatic carriers (Fig. 7.17). The outcome depends upon several factors, including the virulence of the virus and the immuno-competence and age of the patient as well as some genetic factors, while abnormalities in mannose-binding protein (p. 210) may alter host defence to HBV.

Treatment

There is no specific treatment apart from symptomatic therapy.

Prevention and prophylaxis

Prevention depends on avoiding risk factors, such as shared needles, multiple male homosexual partners, and prostitutes. Infectivity is highest in those with the e antigen and/or HBV DNA in their blood. These patients should be counselled about their infection. In develop-ing countries, blood and blood products are still a hazard. Standard safety precautions in laboratories and hospitals must be enforced strictly to avoid accidental needle punctures and contact with infected body fluids.

Passive and active immunization

Vaccination is universal in most developed countries as well as countries with high endemicity. In the UK, only the following at-risk groups are vaccinated:

- all healthcare personnel
- members of emergency and rescue teams
- morticians and embalmers
- children in high-risk areas
- people with haemophilia
- patients in some psychiatric units
- patients with chronic renal failure/on dialysis units

- long-term travellers
- homosexual and bisexual men and prostitutes
- intravenous drug abusers.

Combined prophylaxis (i.e. vaccination and immuno-globulin) should be given to:

- staff with accidental needle-stick injury
- all newborn babies of HBsAg-positive mothers
- regular sexual partners of HBsAg-positive patients, who have been found to be HBV-negative.

To adults give 500 IU of specific hepatitis B immuno-globulin (HBIG) (200 IU to newborns) and the vaccine i.m. at another site.

Active immunization

This is with a recombinant yeast vaccine produced by insertion of a plasmid containing the gene of HBsAg into a yeast.

Dosage regimen. Three injections (at 0, 1 and 6 months) are given into the deltoid muscle; this gives short-term protection in over 90% of patients. People who are over 50 years of age or clinically ill and/or immunocompromised (including those with HIV infec-tion or AIDS) have a poor antibody response; more frequent and larger doses are required. Antibody levels should be measured at 7–9 months after the initial dose in all at-risk groups. Antibody levels fall steadily after vaccination and booster doses may be required after approximately 3–5 years. It is not cost-effective to check antibody levels prior to active immunization. There are few side-effects from the vaccine; soreness at the site of injection may occur, with very occasionally a fever, rash or a 'flu-like' illness. Vaccines containing pre-S components which have a greater immunogenicity are being developed.

Chronic asymptomatic subjects with HBV

Following an acute HBV infection which may be subclinical, approximately 1–10% of patients will not clear the virus and most will become carriers of HBsAg. This occurs more readily with neonatal or childhood infection than when HBV is acquired in adult life. There is a vast geographical variation in the incidence of carriers. In the UK, asymptomatic carriers are usually discovered incidentally on blood tests, such as when they are screened for donating blood for transfusion or when attending genital medicine or antenatal clinics. Asymptomatic carriers have HBsAg in their serum and are HBeAg-negative, HBe antibody-positive with no HBV DNA in the serum. They have no evidence of active liver disease and are not highly infective. Most remain HBsAg-positive, but do not develop active liver disease; there is an annual spontaneous clearance rate of HBsAg of 1–2%.

There are also asymptomatic people who have the e antigen and HBV DNA in the serum. They may have normal liver function tests for many years; liver disease develops when the immune balance changes, and lymphocytes recognize infected hepatocytes causing hepatitis. These patients need to be followed up.

Hepatitis D

This is caused by the hepatitis D virus (HDV or delta virus). It is an incomplete RNA particle enclosed in a shell of HBsAg. It is unable to replicate on its own but is activated by the presence of HBV. It is particularly seen in intravenous drug abusers but can affect all risk groups for HBV infection. Active HBV synthesis is reduced by delta infection and patients are usually negative for HBeAg and HBV DNA. Hepatitis D viral infection can occur either as a co-infection with HBV or as a superinfection in an HBsAg-positive patient.

Co-infection of HDV and HBV is clinically indistinguishable from an acute icteric HBV infection, but a biphasic rise of serum aminotransferases may be seen. *Diagnosis* is confirmed by finding serum IgM anti-delta in the presence of IgM anti-HBc. IgM anti-delta appears at one week and disappears by 5–6 weeks (occasionally 12 weeks) when serum IgG anti-delta is seen. The infection may be transient but the clinical course is variable.

Superinfection results in an acute flare-up of previously quiescent chronic HBV infection. A rise in serum AST or ALT may be the only indication of infection. Diagnosis is by finding serum IgM anti-delta at the

same time as IgG anti-HBc; patients are usually negative for IgM anti-HBc.

Fulminant hepatitis can follow both types of infection but is more common after co-infection. HDV RNA in the serum and liver can be measured and is found in acute and chronic HDV infection.

Hepatitis C

Hepatitis C virus (HCV)

HCV is a single-stranded RNA virus of the Flaviviridae family. The RNA genome is approximately 10 Kb in length, encoding a polyprotein product consisting of structural (capsid and envelope) and non-structural viral proteins (Fig. 7.18). Comparisons of subgenomic regions, such as E1, NS4 or NS5, have allowed variants to be classified into at least six genotypes. Variability is distributed throughout the genome with the non-structural gene of different genotypes showing only 65–70% nucleotide sequence similarity. Genotypes 1a or 1b account for 70–80% of cases in the USA and Europe. There is a rapid change in envelope proteins, making it difficult to develop a vaccine. Antigens from the nucleocapsid regions have been used to develop enzyme-linked immunosorbent assays (ELISA). The current assay, ELISA-3, incorporates antigens NS3, NS4 and NS5 regions.

Epidemiology

HCV was identified in 1988 and was found to be responsible for 70–90% of post-transfusion hepatitis in all countries where blood was tested for HBV markers. The prevalence rate of infection in healthy blood donors is about 0.02% in Northern Europe, 1–3% in Southern Europe, possibly linked to intramuscular injections of vaccines or other medicines; 6% in Africa and with rates as high as 19% in Egypt, owing to parenteral antimony treatment for schistosomiasis. The virus is transmitted by blood and blood products and it is postulated that 80% of people with haemophilia in the UK may have been infected. The incidence in intravenous drug abusers is high, up to 90%. The low rate of HCV infection in high-risk groups, such as homosexuals, prostitutes and attendees at STI clinics, suggests a limited role

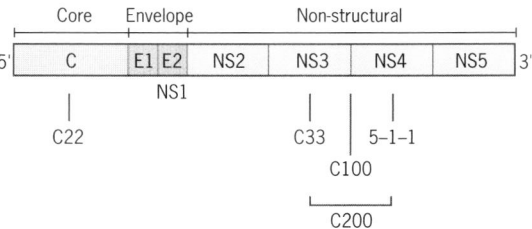

Fig. 7.18 Hepatitis C virus. Diagram showing a single-stranded RNA virus with viral proteins. C, core; NS, non-structural; E, envelope.

for sexual transmission. Vertical transmission from healthy mother to child can occur, but is very rare. Other routes of community-acquired infection (e.g. close contact) are unlikely. In 20% of cases the exact mode of transmission is unknown. An estimated 240 million people are infected with this virus world-wide.

Clinical features

Most acute infections are asymptomatic with about 10% of patients having a mild flu-like illness with jaundice and a rise in serum aminotransferases. Most patients will not be diagnosed until they present, years later, with evidence of abnormal transferase values at health checks or with chronic liver disease. Extrahepatic manifestations are seen, including arthritis, glomerulonephritis associated with cryoglobulinaemia, and porphyria cutanea tarda. There is a higher incidence of diabetes, and associations with lichen planus, sicca syndrome, and non-Hodgkin's lymphoma are under investigation.

Diagnosis

This is frequently by exclusion in a high-risk individual with negative markers for HAV, HBV and other viruses. A drug cause for hepatitis should be excluded if possible. HCV RNA can be detected 1 or 2 weeks after infection. Anti-HCV is usually positive 6 weeks from infection

Treatment (Fig. 7.19)

Interferon has been used in acute cases to prevent chronic disease. Needle-stick injuries must be followed and treated early if there is evidence of HCV viraemia.

Course

At least 85% of patients go on to develop chronic liver disease (p. 361). Cirrhosis develops in about 15–20% within 10–30 years and of these patients between 7% and 15% will develop hepatocellular carcinoma. The course is adversely affected by alcohol consumption which should be discouraged. Male patients and patients acquiring the infection over 40 years and those with genotype 1 or 4 have a more rapid development of fibrosis.

Hepatitis E

Hepatitis E virus (HEV) is an RNA virus (Calicivirus) which causes a hepatitis clinically very similar to hepatitis A. It is enterally transmitted, usually by contaminated water with 30% of dogs, pigs and rodents carrying the virus. Epidemics have been seen in many developing countries. It has a mortality from fulminant hepatic failure of 1–2% which rises to 20% in pregnant women. There is no carrier state and it does not progress to chronic liver disease. An ELISA for IgG and IgM anti-HEV is available for diagnosis, although this ELISA is not always reliable. HEV RNA can be detected in the serum or stools by PCR (polymerase chain reaction).

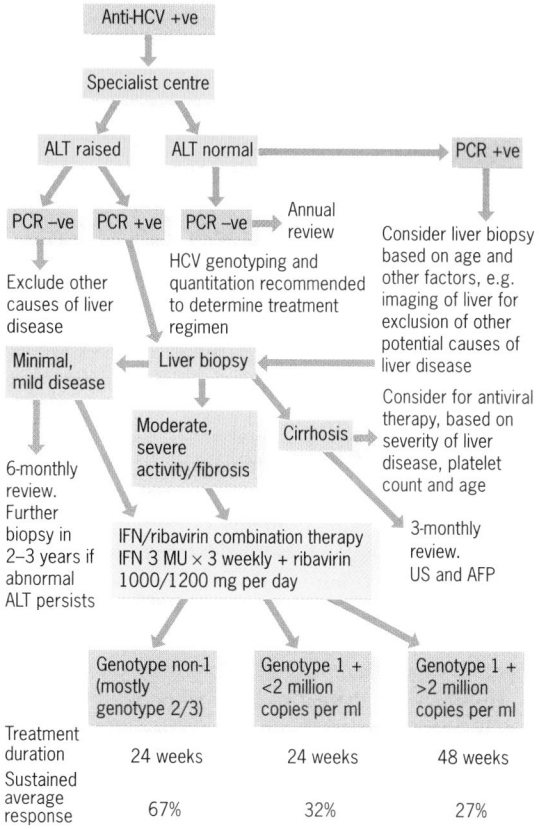

Fig. 7.19 Approach to a patient with hepatitis C. ALT, alanine aminotransferase; PCR, polymerase chain reaction. Adapted from Booth JCL, O'Grady J, Neuberger J (2001) Clinical guidelines for the management of hepatitis C. *Gut* **49** (Suppl 1): 1–21, with permission. **NB**: Pegylated interferon is now being used.

Prevention and control depend on good sanitation and hygiene; vaccination may soon be available.

Non-A–E hepatitis

Approximately 10–15% of acute viral hepatitides cannot be typed. GB agent (HGV hepatitis G virus) and TTV (transfusion-transmitted virus) agents have not been documented as causing disease in humans. Hepatitis non-A–E is the best term to label this cryptogenic group.

Fulminant hepatic failure (FHF)

This is defined as severe hepatic failure in which encephalopathy develops in under 2 weeks in a patient with a previously normal liver (occasionally in some patients with previous liver damage; e.g. D virus superinfection in a previous carrier of HBsAg and in Wilson's disease). Cases that evolve at a slower pace (2–12 weeks)

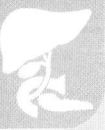

Table 7.7
Causes of fulminant hepatic failure

Viruses	**Toxins**
A, B, (D), E	*Amanita* poisoning
	Halohydrocarbons
Other viruses	
	Miscellaneous
Drugs (examples)	Wilson's disease
Analgesics (e.g. paracetamol)	Acute fatty liver of pregnancy
Monoamine oxidase inhibitors	Reye's syndrome
Halogenated anaesthetics	Budd–Chiari syndrome
Antituberculosis (e.g. isoniazid)	
Antiepileptic (e.g. valproate)	
'Social' drugs (e.g. 'Ecstasy')	

Box 7.1

Transfer criteria to specialized units for patients with acute liver injury

- INR > 3.0
- Presence of hepatic encephalopathy
- Hypotension after resuscitation with fluid
- Metabolic acidosis
- Prothrombin time (seconds) > interval (hours) from overdose (paracetamol cases)

are called subacute or subfulminant hepatic failure. FHF is a rare but often life-threatening syndrome that is due to acute hepatitis from any cause (Table 7.7). The causes vary throughout the world; the majority are due to viral hepatitis, but paracetamol overdose is commonly implicated in the UK (50% of cases). HCV does not cause FHF although exceptional cases have been reported from Japan.

Histologically there is multiacinar necrosis involving a substantial part of the liver. Severe fatty change is seen in pregnancy (p. 383), Reye's syndrome (p. 385), or following tetracycline administration intravenously.

Clinical features

Examination shows a jaundiced patient with a small liver and signs of hepatic encephalopathy. The mental state varies from slight drowsiness, confusion and disorientation (grades I and II) to unresponsive coma (grade IV) with convulsions. Fetor hepaticus is common, but ascites and splenomegaly are rare. Fever, vomiting, hypotension and hypoglycaemia occur. Neurological examination shows spasticity and extension of the arms and legs; plantar responses remain flexor until late. Cerebral oedema develops in 80% of patients with FHF but is far less common with subacute failure and its consequences of intracranial hypertension and brain herniation are the most common causes of death. Other complications include bacterial and fungal infections, gastrointestinal bleeding, respiratory arrest, renal failure (hepatorenal syndrome and acute tubular necrosis) and pancreatitis.

Investigations

There is hyperbilirubinaemia, high serum aminotransferases and low levels of coagulation factors, including prothrombin and factor V. Aminotransferases are not useful indicators of the course of the disease as they tend to fall along with the albumin with progressive liver damage. An EEG is sometimes helpful in grading the encephalopathy. Ultrasound will define liver size and any evidence of underlying liver pathology.

Treatment

There is no specific treatment, but patients should be managed in a specialized unit. Transfer criteria to such units are shown in Box 7.1. Supportive therapy as for hepatic encephalopathy is necessary (see p. 373). When signs of raised intracranial pressure (which is sometimes measured directly) are present, 20% mannitol (1 g/kg bodyweight) should be infused intravenously; this dose may need to be repeated. Dexametasone is of no value. Hypoglycaemia, hypokalaemia, hypomagnesaemia, hypophosphataemia and hypocalcaemia should be anticipated and corrected with 10% dextrose infusion (checked by 2-hourly Dextrostix testing), potassium, calcium, phosphate, and magnesium. Coagulopathy is managed with intravenous vitamin K, platelets, blood or fresh frozen plasma. Haemorrhage may be a problem and patients are given H_2-receptor antagonists to prevent gastrointestinal bleeding. Prophylaxis against bacterial and fungal infection is routine and suspected infection should be treated immediately with suitable antibiotics. Renal and respiratory failure should be treated as necessary. Liver transplantation has been a major advance for patients with FHF. It is difficult to judge the timing or the necessity for transplantation, but there are guidelines based on validated prognostic indices of survival (see below).

Course and prognosis

In mild cases (grades I and II encephalopathy with drowsiness and confusion), two-thirds of the patients will survive. The outcome of severe cases (grades III and IV encephalopathy with stupor or deep coma) is related to the aetiology. In special units, 70% of patients with paracetamol overdosage and grade IV coma survive, as do 30–40% patients with HAV or HBV hepatitis. Poor prognostic variables indicating a need to transplant the liver are shown in Box 7.2.

Acute hepatitis due to other viruses

Infectious mononucleosis (see also p. 49)

This is due to the Epstein–Barr (EB) virus. Mild jaundice associated with minor abnormalities of liver biochemistry

FURTHER READING

EASL International Consensus Conference on hepatitis C (1999) *Journal of Hepatology* **31** (Suppl 1).

Korzel MJ (1999) Cytokines in viral hepatitis. *Seminars in Liver Disease* **19**: 157–169.

Lau YNJ, Wright TL (1993) Molecular virology and pathogenesis of hepatitis B. *Lancet* **342**: 1335–1340.

Lee WM (1997) Hepatitis B virus infection. *New England Journal of Medicine* **337**: 1733–1745.

Murphy N, Wendon J (1999) Fulminant hepatic failure: treatment. In: McDonald H, Burroughs AK, Feagan B (eds) *Evidence Based Gastroenterology and Hepatology*. London: BMJ Books, 468–490.

Sarin SK, Okuda K (eds) (2002) *Hepatitis B and C*. Harcourt India Private Limited.

Skidmore SJ (1999) Factors in spread of hepatitis E. *Lancet* **354**: 1049–1050.

Zuckerman AJ (2000) Editorial. Effect of hepatitis B mutants on efficacy of vaccination. *Lancet* **355**: 1382–1383.

> **Box 7.2**
>
> **Poor prognostic variables in fulminant hepatic failure indicating a need for liver transplantation**
>
> **Non-paracetamol (three of following five)**
> - Drug or non-A–E hepatitis
> - Age < 10 and > 40 years
> - Interval from onset of jaundice to encephalopathy > 7 days
> - Serum bilirubin > 300 μmol/L
> - Prothrombin time > 50 s (or > 100 s in isolation)
>
> **Paracetamol**
> - Arterial pH < 7.3 (after resuscitation, 7.25 on *N*-acetylcysteine)
>
> Or
> - Serum creatinine > 300 μmol/L
> - PT > 100 s
> - Grade III–V encephalopathy

is extremely common, but 'clinical' hepatitis is rare. Hepatic histological changes occur within 5 days of onset; the sinusoids and portal tracts are infiltrated with large mononuclear cells but the liver architecture is preserved. A Paul–Bunnell or Monospot test is usually positive, and atypical lymphocytes are present in the peripheral blood. Treatment is of the symptoms.

Cytomegalovirus (CMV) (see also p. 49)
This can cause acute hepatitis, particularly in a patient with an impaired immune response. The virus may be isolated from the urine. The liver biopsy shows intranuclear inclusions and giant cells.

Yellow fever (see also p. 56)
This viral infection is carried by the mosquito *Aedes aegypti* and can cause acute hepatic necrosis. There is no specific treatment.

Herpes simplex (see also p. 46)
Very occasionally the herpes simplex virus causes a generalized acute infection, particularly in the immunosuppressed patient, and occasionally in pregnancy. Aminotransferases are usually massively elevated. Liver biopsy shows extensive necrosis. Aciclovir is used for treatment.

Other infectious agents

Abnormal liver biochemistry is frequently found in a number of acute infections. The abnormalities are usually mild and have no clinical significance.

Toxoplasmosis (see also p. 106)
This produces a clinical picture similar to that of infectious mononucleosis, with abnormal liver biochemistry, but the Paul–Bunnell test is negative.

Chronic hepatitis

Clinically this is defined as any hepatitis lasting for 6 months or longer. Chronic hepatitis is best classified according to the aetiology (Table 7.8):

- due to viral disease
- due to autoimmune disease
- drug-induced
- unknown cause.

Chronic viral hepatitis is the principal cause of chronic liver disease, cirrhosis and hepatocellular carcinoma in the world.

Pathology
Chronic inflammatory cell infiltrates comprising lymphocytes, plasma cells and sometimes lymphoid follicles are usually present in the portal tracts. The amount of inflammation varies from mild to severe. In addition, there may be:

- loss of definition of the portal/periportal limiting plate – interface hepatitis (the term 'interface hepatitis' is preferred to 'piecemeal necrosis' because the damage is due to apoptosis rather than necrosis)

Table 7.8
Causes of chronic hepatitis

Viral	Hereditary
Hepatitis B ± delta virus	α_1-Antitrypsin deficiency
Hepatitis C	Wilson's disease
Autoimmune	**Others**
	Inflammatory bowel disease
Drugs	– ulcerative colitis
(e.g. methyldopa, oxyphenisatin (withdrawn in UK), isoniazid, ketoconazole, nitrofurantoin)	Alcohol (rarely)

- lobular change, focal lytic necrosis, apoptosis and focal inflammation
- confluent necrosis
- fibrosis which may be mild, bridging (across portal tracts) or severe
- cirrhosis.

The overall severity of the hepatitis is judged by the degree of the hepatitis and inflammation (grading) and the severity of the fibrosis or cirrhosis (staging) using various scoring systems.

Terms such as 'chronic persistent' or 'chronic active' hepatitis should no longer be used.

Chronic hepatitis due to viral disease

Two main viruses (HBV and HCV) that cause chronic hepatitis (CH) can produce similar clinical features, biochemical abnormalities and histological characteristics, although some features are more suggestive of one virus than the other being involved.

Chronic hepatitis B infection

This is common in developing countries where vertical transmission still frequently occurs. In the UK it is mainly confined to high-risk groups (see p. 354) and immigrants from developing countries. The outcome of HBV infection is shown in Figure 7.17.

Pathogenesis

Cytotoxic T cells recognize the viral antigen via HLA class I molecules on the infected hepatocytes; Th1 responses (interleukin-2, gamma-interferon) are thought to be associated with the clearance of the virus and Th2 (interleukins 4, 5, 6, 10, 13) responses with the development of chronic infection and severity of the disease. Viral persistence in patients with a very poor cell-mediated response leads to a healthy carrier state. A better response, however, results in continuing hepatocellular damage with the development of CH.

Chronic HBV infection goes through a replicative and an integrated phase. In the former there is active viral replication with hepatic inflammation and the patient is highly infectious with HBeAg and HBV DNA positivity. At some stage the viral genome becomes integrated into the host DNA and the viral genes are then transcribed along with those of the host. At this stage, the level of HBV DNA in the serum is low and the patient is HBeAg-negative and HBe antibody-positive. The aminotransferases are now normal or only slightly elevated and liver histology shows little inflammation, often with cirrhosis. Hepatocellular carcinoma (HCC) develops in patients with this late-stage disease, but the mechanism is still unclear. Integration of the viral DNA

with the host-cell chromosomal DNA does appear to have a major role in carcinogenesis. There is evidence to implicate inactivation of p53-induced apoptosis by protein X (Table 7.5), allowing accumulation of abnormal cells and, eventually, carcinogenesis.

Clinical features and investigations

Chronic hepatitis is more frequent in men and it is often not preceded by an acute attack. The condition may be asymptomatic or may present as a mild, slowly progressive hepatitis; 50% present with established chronic liver disease. Clinical relapses occur, sometimes associated with seroconversion (see below) of HBeAg to anti-HBe or vice versa.

Investigations show a moderate rise in aminotransferases and a slightly raised ALP. The serum bilirubin is often normal. HBsAg and HBV DNA are found in the serum, usually with HBe antigen, unless a mutant virus is involved (see p. 353).

Histologically, there is a full spectrum of changes from near normal with only a few lymphocytes and interface hepatitis to a full-blown cirrhosis. HBsAg may be seen as a 'ground-glass' appearance in the cytoplasm on haematoxylin and eosin staining, and this can be confirmed on orcein staining or more specifically with immunohistochemical staining. HBcAg can also be demonstrated in hepatocytes by appropriate immunohistochemical staining.

Treatment

Patients with HBsAg, HBeAg and HBV DNA in the serum with abnormal serum aminotransferases and chronic hepatitis on liver biopsy should be treated. Patients with normal aminotransferases and those with decompensated liver disease should not be treated (see below).

The main aim of treatment is to eliminate the HBeAg and HBV DNA from the serum with consequent reduction in inflammatory necrosis of the hepatocyte. This seroconversion occurs spontaneously at a rate of 10–15% per year, and this varies in different countries.

In patients in whom HBeAg disappears, remission is usually sustained. The patient remains a carrier with HBsAg present, although some will eventually become HBsAg-negative.

Antiviral agents

Both interferon and lamivudine (p. 147) have been shown to be effective. Alpha-interferon is given in a dose of 5M units daily or 10M units three times weekly for 4–6 months. Drug treatment, which often causes transient elevation in aminotransferases, is sometimes accompanied by systemic symptoms, but treatment should be continued, unless these are severe. Pegylated interferon given once weekly is replacing alpha-interferon (p. 44).

Side-effects of treatment are many, with an acute flu-like illness occurring 6–8 hours after the first injection. This usually disappears after subsequent injections, but malaise, headaches and myalgia, are common and depression, diarrhoea, reversible hair loss and bone marrow depression and infection may occur. The platelet count should be monitored. These drug reactions occur in up to 30% of patients, and the dose may have to be lowered; in 10% the treatment has to be discontinued.

Overall, the response rate with disappearance of HBeAg is 25–40%. The success rate depends on factors shown in Table 7.9.

Those with chronic hepatitis with no HBeAg (i.e. a mutant HBV – see p. 353) generally do not respond to interferon, and HDV-infected patients only respond with prolonged high-dose courses; patients with concomitant HIV infection also have a poor response. Patients with decompensated liver disease often have severe side-effects and should not be routinely treated with this drug but could be treated with lamivudine.

Lamivudine 100 mg/day can be given orally and is well-tolerated. It appears more effective than interferon particularly in HBV-DNA-positive individuals who have acquired the infection perinatally or in childhood. However, there is a complication of a mutant escape virus (YMDD mutant – tyrosine, methionine, aspartate, aspartate) which in itself causes hepatitis, but usually less severe than that due to the wild type infection.

Duration of treatment, and combination with other antivirals is currently being assessed. Currently treatment is with alpha-interferon and lamivudine; the former for 4 months whilst the latter is continued for 1 year.

Table 7.9
Factors predictive of a sustained response to alpha-interferon in patients with chronic hepatitis

	Chronic hepatitis B	Chronic hepatitis C
Duration of disease	Short	Short
Liver biochemistry	High serum aminotransferase concentrations	
Histology	Active liver disease with fibrosis	Absence of cirrhosis or minimal amounts of hepatic fibrosis
Viral levels	Low HBV DNA levels Wild-type (HBeAg-positive) virus	Low HCV RNA levels Genotype 2 or 3 or absence of a high degree of genetic heterogenicity
Other	Absence of immunosuppression	Low hepatic iron stores Young age

Modified from Hoofnagle and Di Bisceglie (1997) The treatment of chronic viral hepatitis. *New England Journal of Medicine* **336**: 347–356.

Prognosis
The progression is slow and remission may occur. Established cirrhosis is associated with a poor prognosis. Primary liver cell carcinoma is a frequent association and is one of the most common carcinomas in HBV endemic areas such as the Far East.

Chronic hepatitis C infection (see also p. 356)
Pathogenesis
As with hepatitis B infection, cytokines in the Th2 phenotypes are profibrotic and lead to the development of chronic infection. A dominant CD4 Th2 response with a weak CD8 gamma-interferon response may lead to rapid fibrosis. Th1 cytokines are anti-fibrotic and thus a dominant CD4 Th1 and CD8 cytolytic response may cause less fibrosis. Variability may be related to the genetic phenotype; persistence of HCV infection has been shown to be associated with HLA-DRB1*0701 and DRB4*0101. Other factors also have an effect on the development of fibrosis (p. 357).

Clinical features
Patients with chronic hepatitis C infection are usually asymptomatic, the disease being discovered only following a routine biochemical test when mild elevations in the aminotransferases (usually ALT) are noticed (50%). The elevation in ALT may be minimal and fluctuating, and some patients have a persistently normal ALT (25%) – the disease being detected by checking HCV antibodies (e.g. in blood donors).

Despite this, severe chronic hepatitis (25%) and even cirrhosis can be present with only minimal elevation in aminotransferases, but progression is very uncommon in those with a persistently normal ALT. Those with severe inflammation may have fatigue. A few patients present with the symptoms and signs found in cirrhosis.

Diagnosis
This is made by finding HCV antibody in the serum using third-generation ELISA-3 tests. HCV RNA should be assayed using branched-chain DNA signal amplification; if this is negative (i.e. below the threshold of detection) HCV-RNA should be tested by PCR techniques. The viraemia is usually variable; less than 2×10^6 genome equivalents/mL signifies a greater likelihood of response to antiviral therapy.

The HCV genotype should be characterized, if possible, in patients who are to be given treatment (see below).

Liver biopsy is indicated if active treatment is being considered. The changes on liver biopsy are highly variable. Sometimes only minimal inflammation is detected, but in most cases the features of CH are present, as previously described (p. 359). Lymphoid follicles are often present in the portal tracts, and fatty change is frequently seen.

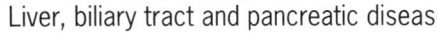

Treatment (Fig. 7.19)

Treatment is appropriate for patients with chronic hepatitis on liver histology who have HCV RNA in their serum and who have raised serum aminotransferases for more than 6 months. The presence of cirrhosis is not a contraindication, but therapeutic responses are less likely. Patients with decompensated cirrhosis should be considered for transplantation. The aim of treatment is to eliminate the HCV RNA from the serum in order to:

- stop the progression of active liver disease
- prevent the development of hepatocellular carcinoma.

Antiviral agents

Current therapy is combination therapy with recombinant alpha-interferon 2b (3M units three times a week) and ribavirin (10.6 mg/kg daily) in divided doses for 12 months if genotype 1; and 6 months for other genotypes. Efficacy is also determined by viral load with HCV RNA $> 2 \times 10^6$ genome equivalents per mL less likely to respond. Pegylated interferon (modified interferon with a polyethylene glycol tail), which only requires once-weekly injection is replacing recombinant interferon.

Side-effects (p. 361) are less than for the treatment of HBV infection because of the lower dose.

Monitoring results. The effects of treatment are monitored by measurement of the aminotransferases, with measurement of the HCV RNA at 4 months. If the aminotransferases remain abnormal and HCV RNA is present in the serum, treatment is stopped because a response to further treatment is then unlikely.

A sustained response is achieved in 28% at 12 months with genotype 1 and high viral load and 64% with genotype 2 or 3. Best results are obtained in patients with the predictive factors shown in Table 7.9. If PCR HCV-RNA remains negative 6 months after the end of treatment relapse is unlikely and histological progression is halted.

Patients with persistently normal aminotransferases are treated if they have abnormal histology.

Chronic D hepatitis

This is a relatively infrequent chronic hepatitis, but spontaneous resolution is rare. Between 60% and 70% of patients will develop cirrhosis and more rapidly than with HBV infection alone. In 15% the disease is rapidly progressive with development of cirrhosis in only a few years. The diagnosis is made by finding anti-delta antibody in a patient with chronic liver disease who is HBsAg-positive. It can be confirmed by finding HDV in the liver or HDV RNA in the serum by reverse transcription – polymerase reaction. Treatment is with alpha-interferon, usually at the high dose of 10M units three times weekly for 12 months, but response is poor. There are scanty data about the use of lamivudine.

Autoimmune hepatitis

This condition occurs most frequently in women. In Type I (see below) there is an association with other autoimmune diseases (e.g. pernicious anaemia, thyroiditis and Coombs'-positive haemolytic anaemia), and 60% of cases are associated with HLA, DR3, DR52a loci, HLADRB3*0101 and HLADRB*0401.

Pathogenesis

The cause is unknown. It is proposed, in a genetically predisposed person, that an environmental agent causes an autoimmune process to develop against liver antigens, producing a progressive necroinflammatory process which results in fibrosis and cirrhosis. In vitro observations have shown that there is a defect of suppressor (regulatory) T cells which may be primary or secondary. However, no clear mechanism causing the inflammation has been found.

Clinical features

There are two peaks in presentation. In the peri- and postmenopausal group, patients may be asymptomatic or present with fatigue, the disease being discovered by abnormalities in liver biochemistry or because of signs of chronic liver disease on routine examination. In the teenage and early twenties the disease often presents as an acute hepatitis with jaundice and very high aminotransferases, which do not improve with time. This age group often has clinical features of cirrhosis with hepatosplenomegaly, cutaneous striae, acne, hirsuties, bruises and, sometimes, ascites. An ill patient can also have features of an autoimmune disease with a fever, migratory polyarthritis, glomerulonephritis, pleurisy, pulmonary infiltration or fibrosing alveolitis.

There are overlap syndromes with primary biliary cirrhosis and primary sclerosing cholangitis.

Investigations
Liver biochemistry

The serum aminotransferases are high, with lesser elevations in the ALP and bilirubin. The serum γ-globulins are high, frequently twice normal, particularly the IgG.

Haematology

A mild normochromic normocytic anaemia with thrombocytopenia and leucopoenia is present, even before portal hypertension and splenomegaly. The prothrombin time is often high.

Autoantibodies

Three types of autoimmune hepatitis have been recognized:

- Type I with antibodies:
  (a) antinuclear
  (b) anti-smooth muscle (anti-actin).

- Type II with antibodies: anti-liver/kidney microsomal (anti-LKM1). The main target is cytochrome P4502D6 (CYP2D6) on liver cell plasma membranes.
- Type III with soluble liver antigen (this group probably is the same as type 1 and its existence is being debated).

Type II occurs most frequently in girls and young women.

Liver biopsy

This shows the changes of CH described previously. The amount of interface hepatitis is variable, but tends to be high in untreated patients. Lymphoid follicles are less often seen than in hepatitis C and plasma cell infiltration is frequent.

Approximately one-third of patients have cirrhosis at presentation.

Treatment

Prednisolone 30 mg is given daily for 2 weeks, followed by a slow reduction and then a maintenance dose of 10–15 mg daily; azathioprine (see p. 305) should be added, 1–2 mg/kg daily, as a steroid-sparing agent and in some patients as sole long-term maintenance therapy.

Course and prognosis

Steroid and azathioprine therapy induce remission in 80% of cases. The length of treatment is lifelong in most cases. Those with initial cirrhosis are more likely to relapse following treatment withdrawal and require indefinite therapy. Liver transplantation is performed if treatment fails, although the disease may recur.

Drug-induced chronic hepatitis

Many drugs can cause a CH which clinically bears many similarities to autoimmune hepatitis (see Table 7.8). Patients are often female, present with jaundice and hepatomegaly, have raised serum aminotransferases and globulin levels, LE cells and anti-LKM1 antibodies may be detected. Improvement follows drug withdrawal but exacerbations can occur with drug reintroduction.

Chronic alcoholic liver disease can occasionally have histological appearances more like a chronic hepatitis.

Chronic hepatitis of unknown cause

As more and more people are having routine blood tests, mild elevations in the serum aminotransferases and γGT are found. Many of these patients have no symptoms and no evidence of liver disease clinically. All known aetiological agents should be excluded (see above), as well as tests to exclude primary biliary cirrhosis, primary sclerosing cholangitis, Wilson's disease, haemochromatosis and α_1-antitrypsin deficiency.

Liver biopsy should be performed if the elevation in the aminotransferases continues for over a year, to confirm the presence of chronic hepatitis, although this is often unhelpful.

Steatohepatitis (non-alcoholic steatohepatitis – NASH)

The hallmark of this condition on liver biopsy is the association of an inflammatory infiltrate with fat. Often there is mild fibrosis, which may progress to cirrhosis. It is probable that this results from an insult causing oxidative stress which in turn leads to lipid perioxidation on top of a fatty liver – a double hit mechanism. Associated factors are obesity (particularly after jejuno-ileal bypass surgery), diabetes mellitus and raised blood lipids. Correction of these factors does not necessarily ameliorate the liver disease. Regular follow-up is warranted.

FURTHER READING

International Autoimmune Hepatitis Group report: review of criteria for diagnosis of autoimmune hepatitis (1999) *Journal of Hepatology* **31**: 929–938.

Ishak K, Baptista A, Bianchi L et al. (1995) Histological grading and staging of chronic hepatitis. *Journal of Hepatology* **22**: 696–699.

Kita H et al (2001) The lymphoid liver: considerations on pathways to autoimmune injury. *Gastroenterology* **120**: 1485–1501.

Krawitt EL (1996) Autoimmune hepatitis. *New England Journal of Medicine* **334**: 897–903.

Lauer GM, Walker BD (2001) Hepatitis C infection. *New England Journal of Medicine* **345**: 41–53.

Lok A (2000) Lamivudine therapy for chronic hepatitis B: is a longer duration of treatment better? *Gastroenterology* **119**: 263–266.

Manns MP, Strassburg CP (2001) Autoimmune hepatitis: clinical challenges. *Gastroenterology* **120**: 1502–1517.

Reid AE (2001) Non-alcoholic steatohepatitis. *Gastroenterology* **121**: 710-723.

Cirrhosis

Cirrhosis results from the necrosis of liver cells followed by fibrosis and nodule formation. The liver architecture is diffusely abnormal and this interferes with liver blood flow and function. This derangement produces the clinical features of portal hypertension and impaired liver cell function.

Aetiology

The causes of cirrhosis are shown in Table 7.10. Alcohol is now the most common cause in the West, but viral infection is the most common cause world-wide. With the identification of HCV, idiopathic (cryptogenic)

Table 7.10
Causes of cirrhosis

Common	Others
Alcohol	Biliary cirrhosis
Hepatitis B ± D	Primary
Hepatitis C	Secondary
? other viruses	Autoimmune hepatitis
	Hereditary haemochromatosis
	Hepatic venous congestion
	Budd–Chiari syndrome
	Wilson's disease
	Drugs (e.g. methotrexate)
	α_1-Antitrypsin deficiency
	Cystic fibrosis
	NASH, e.g. intestinal bypass operations for obesity
	Galactosaemia
	Glycogen storage disease
	Veno-occlusive disease
	Idiopathic (cryptogenic)

NASH, non-alcoholic steatohepatitis

cirrhosis is diagnosed less commonly. Young patients with cirrhosis must be investigated carefully as the cause may be treatable (e.g. Wilson's disease).

Pathogenesis

Chronic injury to the liver results in inflammation, necrosis and, eventually, fibrosis (Fig. 7.20). Fibrosis is initiated by activation of the stellate cells (see p. 336). Kupffer cells seem to have a role in their activation, but hepatocytes and other cells are probably involved. Stellate cells are activated by many cytokines and their receptors, reactive oxygen intermediates and other paracrine and autocrine signals.

In the early stage of activation the stellate cells become swollen and lose retinoids with upregulation of receptors for proliferative and fibrogenic cytokines,

such as platelet-derived growth factor (PDGF), and possibly transforming growth factor β_1 (TGF-β_1). TGF-β_1 is the most potent fibrogenic mediator identified so far.

In the space of Disse, the normal matrix is replaced by collagens, predominantly types 1 and 3, and fibronectin. Subendothelial fibrosis leads to loss of the endothelial fenestrations (ports), and this impairs liver function. Collagenases (matrix metalloproteinases, MMP) are able to degrade this collagen but are inhibited by tissue inhibitors of metalloproteinases (TIMPs) which are increased in human liver fibrosis. There is accumulating evidence that liver fibrosis is reversible.

Pathology

The characteristic features of cirrhosis are regenerating nodules separated by fibrous septa and loss of the normal lobular architecture within the nodules (Fig. 7.21a). Two types of cirrhosis have been described which give clues to the underlying cause:

- *Micronodular cirrhosis.* Regenerating nodules are usually less than 3 mm in size and the liver is

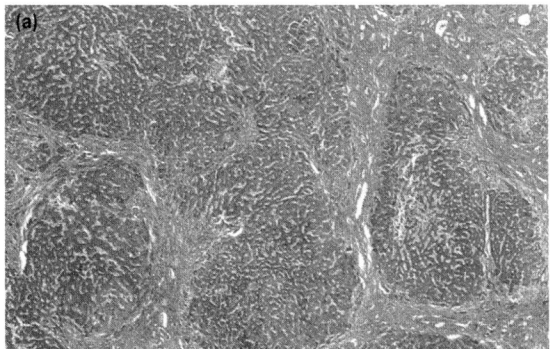

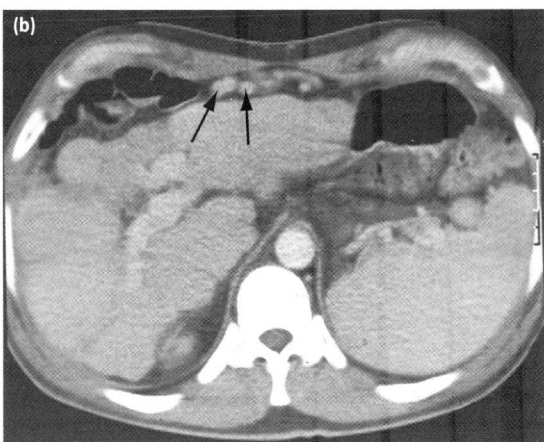

Fig. 7.21 **(a) Pathology of cirrhosis.** Histological appearance showing nodules of liver tissue of varying size surrounded by fibrosis. **(b) CT scan showing an irregular lobulated liver.** There is splenomegaly and enlargement of collateral vessels beneath the anterior abdominal wall (arrows) as a result of portal hypertension.

Fig. 7.20 **Pathogenesis of fibrosis.** Activation of the stellate cell is followed by proliferation of fibroblasts and the deposition of collagen.

Diagram labels (Fig. 7.20):
Normal liver — Formation of fibrosis
Endothelial cells
Sinusoid — Kupffer cell
Stellate cell — Collagen fibres
Subendothelial space of Disse
Hepatocytes
Activated stellate cells (devoid of retinoid droplets) — Damaged hepatocytes

involved uniformly. This type is often caused by ongoing alcohol damage or biliary tract disease.

- *Macronodular cirrhosis.* The nodules are of variable size and normal acini may be seen within the larger nodules. This type is often seen following previous hepatitis, such as HBV infection.

A mixed picture with small and large nodules is sometimes seen.

Symptoms and signs are described on page 345.

Investigations

These are performed to assess the severity and type of liver disease.

Severity

- **Liver function.** Serum albumin and prothrombin time are the best indicators of liver function: the outlook is poor with a level below 25 g/L. The prothrombin time is prolonged commensurate with the severity of the liver disease.
- **Liver biochemistry.** This can be normal depending on the severity of cirrhosis. In most cases there is at least a slight elevation in the serum ALP and serum aminotransferases. In decompensated cirrhosis all biochemistry is deranged.
- **Serum electrolytes.** A low sodium indicates severe liver disease due to a defect in free water clearance or to excess diuretic therapy.

In addition, serum α-fetoprotein if >400 ng/mL is strongly suggestive of the presence of a hepatocellular carcinoma.

Type

This can be determined by:

- viral markers
- serum autoantibodies
- serum immunoglobulins
- iron indices and ferritin
- copper, caeruloplasmin (p. 376)
- α_1-antitrypsin (p. 377).

Serum copper and serum α_1-antitrypsin should always be done in young cirrhotics. Total iron-binding capacity (TIBC) and ferritin should be measured to exclude hereditary haemochromatosis; genetic markers are also available.

Imaging

- **Ultrasound examination.** This can demonstrate changes in size and shape of the liver. Fatty change and fibrosis produce a diffuse increased echogenicity. In established cirrhosis there may be marginal nodularity of the liver surface and distortion of the arterial vascular architecture. The patency of the portal and hepatic veins can be evaluated. It is useful in detecting hepatocellular carcinoma.

- **CT scan** (see p. 342). Figure 7.21b shows hepatosplenomegaly and dilated collaterals seen in chronic liver disease. Arterial phase-contrast-enhanced scans are useful in the detection of hepatocellular carcinoma.
- **Endoscopy** is performed for the detection and treatment of varices, and portal hypertensive gastropathy.
- **MRI scan.** This is useful in the diagnosis of benign tumours such as haemangiomas. MR angiography can demonstrate the vascular anatomy and MR cholangiography the biliary tree. However, intrahepatic bile duct damage is poorly identified by current MR technology.

Liver biopsy

This is necessary to confirm the severity and type of liver disease. The core of liver often fragments and sampling errors may occur in macronodular cirrhosis. Special stains may be required for iron and copper, and various immunocytochemical stains can identify viruses, bile ducts and angiogenic structures. Chemical measurement of iron and copper are necessary to confirm diagnosis of iron overload or Wilson's disease.

Management

Management is that of the complications seen in decompensated cirrhosis. Patients should have 6-monthly ultrasound and serum α-fetoprotein measurements to detect the development of a hepatocellular carcinoma as early as possible (see p. 384), as all therapeutic strategies work best with small and single tumours.

There is no treatment that will arrest or reverse the cirrhotic changes although progression may be halted by correcting the underlying cause (see below). Patients with compensated cirrhosis should lead a normal life. The only dietary restriction is to reduce salt intake. Aspirin and NSAIDs should be avoided. Alcohol should be avoided, although if the cirrhosis is not due to alcohol and not due to viral hepatitis, small amounts not taken on a regular basis are probably not harmful.

Course and prognosis

This is extremely variable, depending on many factors, including the aetiology and the presence of complications. Poor prognostic indicators are given in Table 7.11. Development of any complication usually worsens the prognosis. In general, the 5-year survival rate is approximately 50%, but this also varies depending on the aetiology and the stage at which the diagnosis is made.

There are a number of prognostic classifications based on modifications of Child's grading (A, B and C). This is based on the presence of jaundice, ascites, encephalopathy and the level of serum albumin and prothrombin time. Patients with good liver function (Child's grade A) do better than patients with poor liver

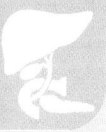

Table 7.11
Poor prognostic indicators in cirrhosis

Blood tests
Low albumin (< 28 g/L)
Low serum sodium (< 125 mmol/L)
Prolonged prothrombin time > 6 seconds
Raised creatinine > 160 µmol/L

Clinical
Persistent jaundice
Failure of response to therapy
Ascites
Haemorrhage from varices, particularly with poor liver function
Neuropsychiatric complications developing with progressive
  liver failure
Small liver
Persistent hypotension
Aetiology (e.g. alcoholic cirrhosis, if the patient continues drinking)

function (Child's grade C: albumin < 30 g/L, bilirubin > 50 µmol/L, and ascites).

Surgical procedures carry an overall operative mortality of 30% in non-bleeding cirrhotics. However, the range is from 10% in Child's grade A to 76% in grade C.

Liver transplantation

This is an established treatment for a number of liver diseases. Shortage of donors is a major problem in all developed countries. Indications include the following:

Acute liver disease. Patients with fulminant hepatic failure of any cause, including acute viral hepatitis (p. 358), may be considered.

Chronic liver disease. The indications for transplantation vary and the timing of the transplant is often difficult. All patients with end-stage (Child's grade C) cirrhosis should be considered and also those with debilitating symptoms.

- *Primary biliary cirrhosis.* Patients with this disease should be transplanted when their serum bilirubin rises above 100 µmol/L.
- *Chronic hepatitis B if HBV-DNA-negative.* Following transplantation, recurrence of the hepatitis can occur despite use of hepatitis B immunoglobulin and lamivudine, because of escape mutants (see p. 361).
- *Chronic hepatitis C.* In end-stage disease the 5-year prognosis of the graft is good, despite universal HCV reinfection. However, cirrhosis occurs in 10–20% at 5 years and there is progressive disease. Antiviral agents may delay this progression and trials are on-going.
- *Autoimmune hepatitis.* These are patients who have failed to respond to medical treatment or have major side-effects of corticosteroid therapy. It can reoccur.

- *Alcoholic liver disease.* Well-motivated patients who have stopped drinking without improvement of liver disease are offered a transplant.
- *Primary metabolic disorders.* Examples are Wilson's disease and α_1-antitrypsin deficiency.
- *Other conditions*, such as sclerosing cholangitis.

Contraindications

Absolute contraindications include active sepsis outside the hepatobiliary tree, malignancy outside the liver, liver metastases (except neuroendocrine), HIV infection, and if the patient is not psychologically committed.

Relative contraindications are mainly anatomical considerations that would make surgery more difficult, such as extensive splanchnic venous thrombosis. With exceptions, patients aged 65 years or over are not usually transplanted. In hepatocellular carcinoma the recurrence rate is high unless there are fewer than three small (< 3 cm) lesions, or a solitary nodule of < 5 cm.

Surgical procedure

Pretransplant work-up includes confirmation of the diagnosis, ultrasound and CT scanning, radiological demonstration of the hepatic arterial and biliary tree as well as assessment of cardiorespiratory and renal status. Because of the ethical and financial implications of this operation, regular psychosocial support is vital, and psychiatric counselling may be necessary in some cases.

The donor should be ABO-compatible. He or she should ideally be under 50 years of age and have no evidence of sepsis, malignancy, HIV, HBV or HCV infection. The liver is cooled and stored on ice; its preservation time can be up to 20 hours. The recipient operation takes approximately 8 hours and may require a large blood transfusion, but sometimes none at all.

The operative mortality is low. Most postoperative deaths occur in the first 3 months. Sepsis and haemorrhage can be serious complications. Opportunistic infections (see p. 33) are still a problem owing to immunosuppression. Various immunosuppressive agents have been used, but microemulsified ciclosporin, tacrolimus, azathioprine and steroids are the most common. A pretransplant serum creatinine above 160 µmol/L (2 mg/dL) is the best predictor of post-transplant death.

Rejection

Acute or cellular rejection is usually seen 5–10 days post-transplant; it can be asymptomatic but often there is a fever. Histologically, there is a pleomorphic portal infiltrate with prominent eosinophils, bile duct damage and endothelialitis of the blood vessels. This type of rejection responds to immunosuppressive therapy.

Chronic ductopenic rejection is seen from 6 weeks to 9 months post-transplant, with disappearing bile ducts (vanishing bile duct syndrome, VBDS) and an arteriopathy with narrowing and occlusion of the arteries. Early ductopenic rejection may rarely be reversed by immuno-suppression, but often requires retransplantation.

Graft-versus-host disease is extremely rare.

Prognosis

Elective liver transplantation in low-risk patients has a 90% 1-year survival. Five-year survivals are as high as 70–85% largely owing to the introduction of ciclosporin and tacrolimus. Patients require lifelong immunosuppression, although the doses can be reduced over time without significant problems.

Complications and effects of cirrhosis

These are shown in Table 7.12.

Portal hypertension

The portal vein is formed by the union of the superior mesenteric and splenic veins. The pressure within it is normally 5–8 mmHg with only a small gradient across the liver to the hepatic vein in which blood is returned to the heart via the inferior vena cava. Portal hypertension can be classified according to the site of obstruction:

- *prehepatic* – due to blockage of the portal vein before the liver
- *intrahepatic* – due to distortion of the liver architecture, which can be presinusoidal (e.g. in schistosomiasis) or postsinusoidal (e.g. in cirrhosis)
- *posthepatic* – due to venous blockage outside the liver (rare).

As portal pressure rises above 10–12 mmHg, the compliant venous system dilates and collaterals occur within the systemic venous system. The main sites of the collaterals are at the gastro-oesophageal junction, the rectum, the left renal vein, the diaphragm, the retroperitoneum and the anterior abdominal wall via the umbilical vein.

The collaterals at the gastro-oesophageal junction (varices) are superficial in position and tend to rupture. Portosystemic anastomoses at other sites seldom give rise to symptoms. Rectal varices are found frequently (30%) if carefully looked for and can be differentiated from haemorrhoids, which are lower in the anal canal.

Table 7.12
Complications and effects of cirrhosis

Portal hypertension and gastrointestinal haemorrhage
Ascites
Portosystemic encephalopathy
Renal failure
Hepatocellular carcinoma
Bacteraemias, infections
Malnutrition

Pathophysiology

Portal vascular resistance is increased in chronic liver disease. During liver injury, stellate cells are activated (see p. 336) and transform into myofibroblasts. In these cells there is de novo expression of the specific smooth muscle protein α-actin. Under the influence of mediators, such as endothelin, nitric oxide or prostaglandins, the contraction of these activated cells contributes to abnormal blood flow patterns and increased resistance to blood flow. In addition the balance of fibrogenic and fibrolytic factors is shifted towards fibrogenesis. This increased resistance leads to portal hypertension and opening of portosystemic anastomoses in both pre-cirrhotic and cirrhotic livers. Patients with cirrhosis have a hyperdynamic circulation. This is thought to be due to the release of mediators, such as nitric oxide and glucagon, which leads to peripheral and splanchnic vasodilatation. This effect is followed by plasma volume expansion due to sodium retention (see the discussion on ascites, p. 370), and this has a significant effect in maintaining portal hypertension.

Causes (see Table 7.13)

The most common cause is cirrhosis. Other causes include the following.

Prehepatic causes

Extrahepatic blockage is due to portal vein thrombosis. The cause is often unidentified, but some cases are due to portal vein occlusion secondary to congenital portal venous abnormalities or neonatal sepsis of the umbilical vein. Many are due to inherited defects causing pro-thrombotic conditions, e.g. factor V Leiden. Patients usually present with bleeding, often at a young age. They have normal liver function and, because of this, their prognosis following bleeding is excellent. The portal vein blockage can be identified by ultrasound or Doppler imaging. Splenectomy is only performed if there is isolated splenic vein thrombosis. Treatment is usually repeated endoscopic therapy or non-selective beta-blockade.

Table 7.13
Causes of portal hypertension

Prehepatic	Posthepatic
Portal vein thrombosis	Budd–Chiari syndrome
	Veno-occlusive disease
Intrahepatic	Right heart failure (rare)
Cirrhosis	Constrictive pericarditis
Hepatitis (alcoholic)	
Idiopathic non-cirrhotic	
portal hypertension	
Schistosomiasis	
Partial nodular transformation	
Congenital hepatic fibrosis	
Myelosclerosis	
(extramedullary haemopoiesis)	
Granulomata	

Intrahepatic causes

Although cirrhosis is the most common intrahepatic cause of portal hypertension, there are other causes:

- *Non-cirrhotic portal hypertension.* Patients present with portal hypertension and variceal bleeding but without cirrhosis. Histologically, the liver shows mild portal tract fibrosis. The aetiology is unknown, but arsenic, vinyl chloride and other toxic agents have been implicated. A similar disease is found frequently in India. The liver lesion does not progress and the prognosis is therefore good.
- *Schistosomiasis* with extensive pipe-stem fibrosis is a common cause world-wide, but is confined to endemic areas such as Egypt and Brazil. However, often there may be concomitant liver disease such as HCV infection.
- Other causes include congenital hepatic fibrosis, nodular regenerative hyperplasia, and partial nodular transformation. The last two conditions are rare. They share the common features of hyperplastic liver cell growth in the form of nodules, but in contrast to cirrhosis, fibrosis is typically absent. A wedge liver biopsy is usually required to establish the diagnosis. In none of these conditions are hormones implicated in aetiology or progression.

Posthepatic causes

Prolonged severe heart failure with tricuspid incompetence and constrictive pericarditis can both lead to portal hypertension. The Budd–Chiari syndrome is described on page 379.

Clinical features

Patients with portal hypertension are often asymptomatic and the only clinical evidence of portal hypertension is splenomegaly. Clinical features of chronic liver disease are usually present (see p. 345). Presenting features may include:

- haematemesis or melaena from rupture of gastro-oesophageal varices or portal hypertensive gastropathy
- ascites
- encephalopathy.

Variceal haemorrhage

Approximately 90% of patients with cirrhosis will develop gastro-oesophageal varices, over 10 years, but only one-third of these will bleed from them. Bleeding is likely to occur with large varices, red signs on varices (diagnosed at endoscopy) and in severe liver disease.

Management

Management can be divided into the active bleeding episode, the prevention of rebleeding, and prophylactic measures to prevent the first haemorrhage. Despite all the therapeutic techniques available, the prognosis

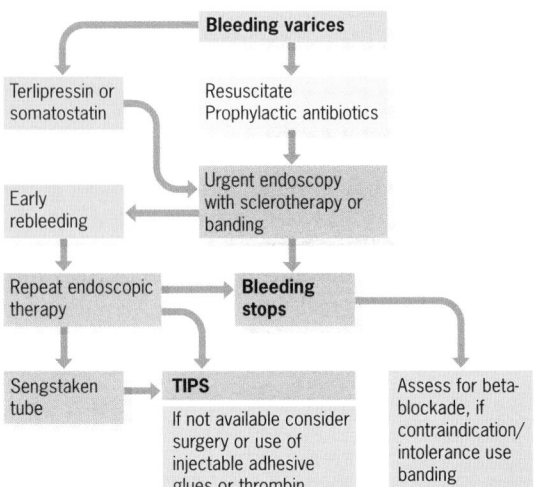

Fig. 7.22 **Management of gastrointestinal haemorrhage due to oesophageal varices.** TIPS, transjugular intrahepatic portosystemic shunt.

depends on the severity of the underlying liver disease, with an overall mortality from variceal haemorrhage of 25% – reaching 50% in Child's grade C.

Initial management of acute variceal bleeding
(Fig. 7.22)
See also the discussion of the general management of gastrointestinal haemorrhage on page 281.

Resuscitation

- Assess the general condition of the patient – pulse and blood pressure.
- Insert an intravenous line and obtain blood for grouping and crossmatching, haemoglobin, PT/INR, urea, electrolytes, creatinine, liver biochemistry and blood cultures.
- Restore blood volume with plasma expanders or, if possible, blood transfusion. These measures are discussed in more detail in the treatment of shock (p. 938). Prompt correction of hypovolaemia is necessary in patients with cirrhosis as their baroreceptor reflexes are diminished.

Urgent endoscopy

Endoscopy should be performed to confirm the diagnosis of varices (Fig. 7.23) and to exclude bleeding from other sites (e.g. gastric ulceration). Portal hypertensive (or congestive) gastropathy is the term used for chronic gastric congestion, punctate erythema and gastric erosions and is a source of bleeding. Varices may or may not be present. Propranolol (see below) is the best treatment for this.

Injection sclerotherapy or variceal banding

The varices should be injected with a sclerosing agent that may arrest bleeding by producing vessel thrombosis.

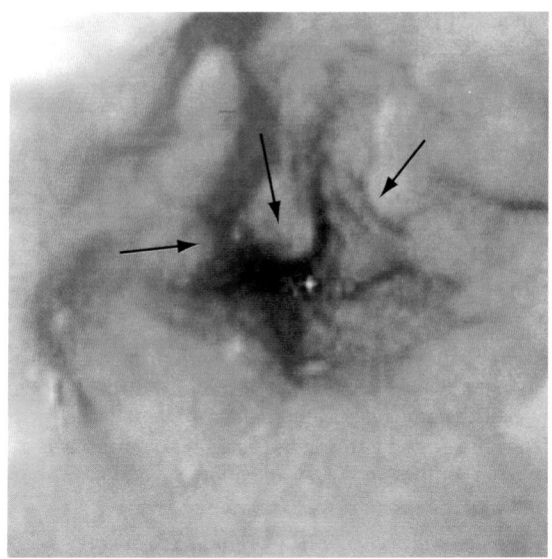

Fig. 7.23 Endoscopic picture of oesophageal varices.

A needle is passed down the biopsy channel of the endoscope and a sclerosing agent is injected into the varices. Alternatively, the varices can be banded by mounting a band on the tip of the endoscope, sucking the varix just into the end of the scope and dislodging the band over the varix using a trip-wire mechanism.

Acute variceal sclerotherapy and banding are the treatment of choice; they arrest bleeding in 80% of cases and reduce early rebleeding. Between 15% and 20% of bleeding comes from gastric varices and here results of endoscopic therapy are poor.

Other measures available

Vasoconstrictor therapy

The main use of this is for emergency control of bleeding whilst waiting for endoscopy and in combination with endoscopic techniques. The aim of vasoconstrictor agents is to restrict portal inflow by splanchnic arterial constriction.

- *Terlipressin*. This is the only vasoconstrictor which has been shown to reduce mortality, albeit in small trials. Dose is 2 mg 6-hourly, reducing to 1 mg 4-hourly after 48 hours if a prolonged dosage regimen is used. It should not be given to patients with ischaemic heart disease. The patient will complain of abdominal colic, will defecate and have facial pallor owing to the generalized vasoconstriction.
- *Somatostatin*. This drug has few side-effects. An infusion 250 µg/h (or perhaps 500 µg/h) appears to reduce bleeding, but has no effect on mortality. It should be used if there are contraindications to terlipressin, although the data on efficacy are less convincing than with terlipressin

Balloon tamponade

This procedure is used mainly to control bleeding if endoscopic therapy or vasoconstrictor therapy has failed or is contraindicated or if there is exsanguinating haemorrhage. The tube should be left in place for up to 12 hours and removed in the endoscopy room prior to the endoscopic procedure. The usual tube is a four-lumen Sengstaken–Blakemore. The tube is passed into the stomach and the gastric balloon is inflated with air and pulled back. It should be positioned in close apposition to the gastro-oesophageal junction to prevent the cephalad variceal blood flow to the bleeding point. The oesophageal balloon should be inflated only if bleeding is not controlled by the gastric balloon alone.

This technique is successful in up to 90% of patients and is very useful in the first few hours of bleeding. However, it can have serious complications such as aspiration pneumonia, oesophageal rupture and mucosal ulceration, which lead to a 5% mortality. The procedure is very unpleasant for the patient.

Additional management of acute episode

- *Prophylactic antibiotics*. These have been shown to reduce infection and reduce mortality. Both oral and intravenous quinolones have been used.
- *Measures to prevent encephalopathy*. Portosystemic encephalopathy (PSE) can be precipitated by a large bleed (since blood contains protein). The management is described on page 373.
- *Nursing*. Patients require high-dependency/intensive-care nursing. They should have nil by mouth until bleeding has stopped.
- *Sucralfate*. 1 g four times daily is given to reduce oesophageal ulceration following endoscopic therapy.

Management of an acute rebleed

Fifty per cent of patients rebleed within 10 days. The source of the rebleed should be established by endoscopy. It is sometimes due to an ulcer produced by previous sclerotherapy and this is difficult to manage. Management starts with repeat endoscopic therapy – once only to control rebleeding (further sessions of sclerotherapy or banding are not advisable). Consider a transjugular intrahepatic portocaval shunt (TIPS).

Transjugular intrahepatic portocaval shunt (TIPS)

In this technique, a guidewire is passed from the jugular vein into the liver and an expandable metal shunt is forced over it into the liver substance to form a channel between the systemic and portal venous systems. It reduces the hepatic sinusoidal and portal vein pressure by creating a total shunt, but without the risks of general anaesthesia and major surgery. TIPS is used in cases where the bleeding cannot be stopped after two sessions of endoscopic therapy within 5 days. It is useful in the short term, but recurrent portal hypertension owing to stent stenosis or thrombosis occurs.

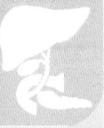

Emergency surgery

This is used when other measures fail or if TIPS is not available and, particularly, if the bleeding is from gastric fundal varices. Oesophageal transection and ligation of the feeding vessels to the bleeding varices is the most common surgical technique. Acute portosystemic shunt surgery (see below) is infrequently performed.

Prevention of recurrent variceal bleeding

Following an episode of variceal bleeding, the risk of recurrence is 60–80% over a 2-year period with an approximate mortality of 20% per episode. These facts justify the use of measures to prevent rebleeding.

Long-term measures

Endoscopic treatment. The use of repeated courses of banding at 2-weekly intervals leads to obliteration of the varices. This markedly reduces rebleeding, most occurring before the varices have been fully obliterated. Between 30% and 40% of varices return per year, so that follow-up endoscopy with ablation should be performed. Banding is superior to sclerotherapy.

Although a reduction in bleeding episodes occurs, the effect on survival is controversial and probably small. Complications include oesophageal ulceration, mediastinitis and rarely strictures.

Non-selective beta-blockade. Oral propranolol in a dose sufficient to reduce resting pulse rate by 25% has been shown to decrease portal pressure. Portal inflow is reduced by two mechanisms: by a decrease in cardiac output (β_1), and by the blockade of β_2 vasodilator receptors on the splanchnic arteries, leaving an unopposed vasoconstrictor effect. This has been shown to decrease the frequency of rebleeding, and is as effective as sclerotherapy and ligation as it also prevents bleeding from portal hypertensive gastropathy. It is the treatment of first choice, but a substantial number of patients have either contraindications or are intolerant of treatment.

Transjugular portosystemic stent shunts. These reduce rebleeding rates compared to endoscopic techniques but do not improve survival and increase encephalopathy. They are used if endoscopic or medical therapy fails.

Surgical procedures

Surgical portosystemic shunting is associated with an extremely low risk of rebleeding, but the diversion of portal blood away from the liver produces significant encephalopathy. Operative mortality is low in patients with Child's grade A (0–5%) but encephalopathy still occurs. Child's grade C has a very poor prognosis. The 'shunts' performed are usually an end-to-side portocaval anastomosis or a selective distal splenorenal shunt (Warren shunt), which maintains hepatic blood flow via the superior mesenteric vein. Devascularization procedures inducing oesophageal transection do not produce encephalopathy, and are used when there is splanchnic

venous thrombosis. Liver transplantation (p. 366) should always be considered when there is poor liver function.

Prophylactic measures

Patients with cirrhosis and varices, who have not bled, should be prescribed non-selective beta-blockers (e.g. propranolol). This reduces the chances of upper GI bleeding, may increase survival and is cost-effective. If there are contraindications or intolerance, banding may be an option.

Ascites

Ascites is the presence of fluid within the peritoneal cavity and is a common complication of cirrhosis of the liver. The pathogenesis of the development of ascites in liver disease is controversial, but is probably secondary to renal sodium and water retention. Several factors are involved.

- *Sodium and water retention* occur as a result of peripheral arterial vasodilatation and consequent reduction in the effective blood volume. Nitric oxide has been postulated as the putative vasodilator, although other substances (e.g. atrial natriuretic peptide and prostaglandins) may be involved. The reduction in effective blood volume activates various neurohumoral pressor systems such as the sympathetic nervous system and the renin–angiotensin system, thus promoting salt and water retention (Fig. 12.3).
- *Portal hypertension* exerts a local hydrostatic pressure and leads to increased hepatic and splanchnic production of lymph and transudation of fluid into the peritoneal cavity.
- *Low serum albumin* (a consequence of poor synthetic liver function) may further contribute by a reduction in plasma oncotic pressure.

In patients with ascites, urine sodium excretion rarely exceeds 5 mmol in 24 hours. Loss of sodium from extrarenal sites accounts for approximately 30 mmol in 24 hours. The normal daily dietary sodium intake may vary between 120 and 200 mmol, resulting in a positive sodium balance of approximately 90–170 mmol in 24 hours (equivalent to 600–1300 mL of fluid retained).

Clinical features

The abdominal swelling associated with ascites may accumulate over many weeks or as rapidly as a few days. Precipitating factors include a high sodium diet or the development of a hepatocellular carcinoma or splanchnic vein thrombosis. Mild generalized abdominal pain and discomfort are common but, if more severe, should raise the suspicion of spontaneous bacterial peritonitis (see below). Respiratory distress accompanies tense ascites, and also causes difficulty in eating.

The presence of fluid is confirmed by the demonstration of shifting dullness. Many patients will also have peripheral oedema. A pleural effusion (usually on the right side) may infrequently be found and is believed to arise from the passage of ascitic fluid through congenital defects in the diaphragm.

Investigations

A diagnostic aspiration of 10–20 mL of fluid should be obtained and the following performed:

- **Cell count**. A neutrophil count above 250 cells/mm^3 is indicative of an underlying (usually spontaneous) bacterial peritonitis.
- **Gram stain and culture** – for bacteria and acid-fast bacilli.
- **Protein**. The ascitic protein level enables a division into transudative and exudative ascites. For this division the serum albumin must be used as a reference point. An ascitic albumin of 11 g/L or more below the serum albumin level suggests a transudate. The level of ascitic protein provides an indirect estimate of opsonization capacity, and thereby the risk of developing spontaneous bacterial peritonitis. Patients at most risk are those with ascitic protein levels below 10 g/L.
- **Cytology** – for malignant cells.
- **Amylase** – to exclude pancreatic ascites.

The differential diagnosis of ascites is listed in Table 7.14.

Management

The aim is to both reduce sodium intake and increase renal excretion of sodium – and by doing so produce a net reabsorption of fluid from the ascites back into the circulating volume. The maximum rate at which ascites can be mobilized is 500–700 mL in 24 hours (see below). The management is as follows:

- Check serum electrolytes and creatinine at the start and every other day; weigh patient and measure urinary output daily.

Table 7.14

Causes of ascites divided according to the type of ascitic fluid

Straw-coloured	Chylous
Malignancy (most common cause)	Obstruction of main
Cirrhosis	lymphatic duct
Infective	(e.g. by carcinoma) –
Tuberculosis	chylomicrons are present
Following intra-abdominal	Cirrhosis
perforation – any bacteria	
may be found (e.g. *E. coli*)	**Haemorrhagic**
Spontaneous in cirrhotics	Malignancy
Hepatic vein obstruction	Ruptured ectopic pregnancy
(Budd–Chiari syndrome) –	Abdominal trauma
protein level high in fluid	Acute pancreatitis
Chronic pancreatitis	
Congestive cardiac failure	
Constrictive pericarditis	
Meigs' syndrome (ovarian tumour)	
Hypoproteinaemia,	
(e.g. nephrotic syndrome)	

- Bed rest alone will lead to a diuresis in a small proportion of people by improving renal perfusion, but in practice is not helpful.
- By dietary sodium restriction it is possible to reduce sodium intake to 40 mmol in 24 hours and still maintain an adequate protein and calorie intake with a palatable diet.
- Fluid restriction is probably not necessary unless the serum sodium is under 128 mmol/L (see below).
- The diuretic of first choice is the aldosterone antagonist spironolactone, staring at 100 mg daily. Chronic administration produces gynaecomastia; amiloride, 5–15 mg daily, is then substituted.

The aim of diuretic therapy should be to produce a net loss of fluid approaching 700 mL in 24 hours (0.7 kg weight loss or 1.0 kg if peripheral oedema is present). Although 60% of patients respond with this regimen, diuresis is often poor and the spironolactone can be increased gradually to 500 mg daily providing there is no hyperkalaemia. A loop diuretic, such as furosemide (frusemide) 20–40 mg or bumetanide 1 mg daily, may be added if response is poor. These loop diuretics have several potential disadvantages, including hyponatraemia, hypokalaemia and volume depletion.

Ascitic fluid is mobilized more slowly than interstitial fluid and diuretics should be given with great care in those without peripheral oedema.

Diuretics should be temporarily discontinued if a rise in serum creatinine level occurs, representing overdiuresis and hypovolaemia. Hyponatraemia occurring during therapy almost always represents haemodilution secondary to a failure to clear free water (usually a marker of reduced renal perfusion) and should be treated by stopping the diuretics if the sodium level falls below approximately 128 mmol/L as well as introducing water restriction. Diuretics should also be stopped if there is hyperkalaemia or the development of precoma.

Paracentesis

This is used to relieve symptomatic tense ascites. It is also used as a means of rapid therapy in patients with ascites and peripheral oedema, thus avoiding prolonged hospital stay. The main danger of this approach is the production of hypovolaemia as the ascites reaccumulates at the expense of the circulating volume. In patients with normal renal function and in the absence of hyponatraemia, this has largely been overcome by the administration of albumin (8 g per litre of ascitic fluid removed). In practice, up to 20 L can be removed over 4–6 hours. This procedure has more complications in end-stage cirrhosis or if the patient has renal failure.

Shunts

The introduction of a peritoneo-venous shunt – a catheter from the peritoneal cavity (subcutaneously) to the internal jugular vein, incorporating a one-way valve

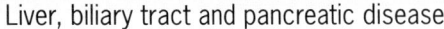
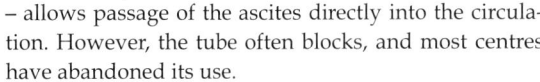
– allows passage of the ascites directly into the circulation. However, the tube often blocks, and most centres have abandoned its use.

A transjugular intrahepatic portocaval shunt (TIPS) is useful for resistant ascites providing there is inactive cirrhosis and minimal disturbance of renal function.

Spontaneous bacterial peritonitis (SBP)

This condition represents one of the more serious complications of ascites and occurs in approximately 8% of cirrhotics with ascites. The infecting organisms are believed to gain access to the peritoneum by haematogenous spread. The most frequently incriminated bacteria are *Escherichia coli*, *Klebsiella* and enterococci. The condition should be suspected in any patient with ascites with evidence of clinical deterioration. Features such as pain and pyrexia are frequently absent. Diagnostic aspiration should always be performed in patients with ascites (see above). A raised neutrophil count in ascites is alone sufficient evidence to start treatment immediately. A third-generation cephalosporin, such as cefotaxime or ceftazidime, is used and may be modified on the basis of culture results.

The prognosis is grave and depends on the severity of the liver disease. It has a 25% mortality and recurs in 70% of patients within a year. It is an indication for liver transplantation.

If the patient survives, an oral quinolone should be prescribed daily to prevent recurrence, and this prolongs survival. Although Gram-positive organisms are subsequently found to be a cause of SBP they are sensitive to third-generation cephalosporins.

Portosystemic encephalopathy

The term 'portosystemic encephalopathy' (PSE) refers to a chronic neuropsychiatric syndrome secondary to chronic liver disease. This condition occurs with cirrhosis, but a similar acute encephalopathy can occur in acute fulminant hepatic failure (see p. 358). PSE is seen in patients with portal hypertension that is due to spontaneous 'shunting', or in patients following a portosystemic shunt procedure, e.g. TIPS. Encephalopathy is potentially reversible.

Pathogenesis

The mechanism is unknown but several factors are thought to play a part. In cirrhosis, the blood bypasses the liver via the collaterals and the 'toxic' metabolites pass directly to the brain to produce the encephalopathy.

Many 'toxic' substances have been suggested as the causative factor, including ammonia, free fatty acids, mercaptans and accumulation of false neurotransmitters (octopamine) or activation of the γ-aminobutyric acid (GABA) inhibitory neurotransmitter system. Increased blood levels of aromatic amino acids (tyrosine and phenylalanine) and reduced branched-chain amino acids (valine, leucine and isoleucine) also occur. Nevertheless,

ammonia seems to have a major role, and ammonia-induced alteration of brain neurotransmitter balance – especially at the astrocyte–neurone interface – is the leading concept of the causation. Ammonia is produced by the breakdown of protein by intestinal bacteria, and a high blood ammonia is seen in most patients. The factors that can precipitate PSE are shown in Table 7.15.

Clinical features

An acute onset often has a precipitating factor (Table 7.15). The patient becomes increasingly drowsy and comatose.

Chronically, there is a disorder of personality, mood and intellect, with a reversal of normal sleep rhythm. These changes may be fluctuating and a history from a relative must be obtained. The patient is irritable, confused, disorientated and has slow slurred speech. General features include nausea, vomiting and weakness. Coma occurs as the encephalopathy becomes more marked, but there is always hyperreflexia and increased tone. Convulsions are so very rare that other causes must be looked for.

Signs include:

- fetor hepaticus (a sweet smell to the breath)
- a coarse flapping tremor seen when the hands are outstretched and the wrists hyperextended (asterixis)
- constructional apraxia, with the patient being unable to write or draw, for example, a five-pointed star
- decreased mental function, which can be assessed by using the serial-sevens test (see p. 1230). A trail-making test (the ability to join numbers and letters with a pen within a certain time – a standard psychological test for brain dysfunction) is prolonged and is a useful bedside test to assess encephalopathy.

Diagnosis is clinical. Routine liver biochemistry merely confirms the presence of liver disease, not the presence of encephalopathy.

Table 7.15

Factors precipitating portosystemic encephalopathy

High dietary protein
Gastrointestinal haemorrhage
Constipation
Infection, including spontaneous bacterial peritonitis
Fluid and electrolyte disturbance due to:
   diuretic therapy
   paracentesis
Drugs (e.g. any CNS depressant)
Portosystemic shunt operations, TIPS
Any surgical procedure
Progressive liver damage
Development of hepatocellular carcinoma

TIPS, transjugular intrahepatic portocaval shunt

Additional investigations:

- Electroencephalogram (EEG) shows a decrease in the frequency of the normal α-waves (8–13 Hz) to δ-waves of 1.5–3 Hz. These changes occur before coma supervenes.
- Visual evoked responses (see p. 1157) also detect subclinical encephalopathy.
- Arterial blood ammonia is occasionally useful in the differential diagnosis of the cause of the coma and to follow the course of the PSE, but is not readily available.

Management

Management consists of evacuation of the bowels and sterilizing the bowel. Restriction of protein intake is reserved for resistant cases.

Immediate management

- Identify and remove the possible precipitating cause, such as drugs with cerebral depressant properties, constipation or electrolyte imbalance due to overdiuresis.
- Give purgation and enemas to empty the bowels of nitrogenous substances. Lactulose (10–30 mL three times daily) is an osmotic purgative that reduces the colonic pH and limits ammonia absorption. Lactilol (β-galactoside sorbitol 30 g daily) is metabolized by colonic bacteria and is comparable in efficacy to lactulose. Hypernatraemia can result from water loss.
- Maintain nutrition with adequate calories, given if necessary via a fine-bore nasogastric tube, and do not restrict protein for more than 48 hours.
- Give antibiotics. Rifaximin is mainly unabsorbed and well tolerated long term. Metronidazole (200 mg four times daily) is also effective in the acute situation. Neomycin is now rarely used.
- Stop or reduce diuretic therapy.
- Give intravenous fluids as necessary (beware of too much sodium).
- Treat any infection.
- Increase protein in the diet to the limit of tolerance as the encephalopathy improves.

Course and prognosis

Acute encephalopathy, often seen in FHF, has a very poor prognosis as the disease itself has a high mortality. In cirrhosis, chronic PSE is very variable and the prognosis is that of the underlying liver disease. Very rarely an organic syndrome with cerebellar signs, or spastic paraparesis can develop in long-standing cases.

Renal failure (hepatorenal syndrome)

The hepatorenal syndrome occurs typically in a patient with advanced cirrhosis with jaundice and ascites. The urine output is low with a low urinary sodium concentration, a maintained capacity to concentrate urine (i.e. tubular function is intact) and an almost normal renal histology. The renal failure here is described as 'functional'. It is sometimes precipitated by overvigorous diuretic therapy, diarrhoea or paracentesis, but often no precipitating factor is found. Advanced cases may progress beyond the 'functional' stage to produce an acute tubular necrosis.

The mechanism is similar to that producing ascites. The initiating factor is thought to be extreme peripheral vasodilatation possibly due to nitric oxide, leading to an extreme decrease in the effective blood volume and hypotension (p. 670). This activates the homeostatic mechanisms, causing a rise in plasma renin, aldosterone, norepinephrine (noradrenaline) and vasopressin, leading to vasoconstriction of the renal vasculature. There is an increased preglomerular vascular resistance causing the blood flow to be directed away from the renal cortex. This leads to a reduced glomerular filtration rate and plasma renin remains high. Salt and water retention occur with reabsorption of sodium from the renal tubules.

A number of other mediators have been incriminated in the pathogenesis of the hepatorenal syndrome, in particular the eicosanoids. This has been supported by the precipitation of the syndrome by inhibitors of prostaglandin synthetase such as non-steroidal anti-inflammatory agents.

Diuretic therapy should be stopped and intravascular hypovolaemia corrected. Terlipressin has been used as a short-term measure with improvement, but the overall prognosis is poor. Studies of TIPS are in progress. Liver transplantation is the best option.

Primary hepatocellular carcinoma

This is discussed on page 384.

Types of cirrhosis

Alcoholic cirrhosis

This is discussed in the section on alcoholic liver disease (p. 378).

Primary biliary cirrhosis

Primary biliary cirrhosis (PBC) is a chronic disorder in which there is a progressive destruction of bile ducts, eventually leading to cirrhosis. Ninety per cent of those affected are women in the age range 40–50 years. It used to be rare but is now being diagnosed more frequently in its milder forms. The prevalence is approximately 7.5 per 100 000, with a marked increase in first-degree relatives. PBC has been called 'chronic non-suppurative destructive cholangitis'; this term is more descriptive of the early lesion and emphasizes that true cirrhosis occurs only in the later stages of the disease.

Aetiology

The aetiology is unknown, but immunological mechanisms may play a part. Serum antimitochondrial antibodies are found in almost all patients with PBC, and of the mitochondrial proteins involved, the antigen M2 is specific to PBC.

Five M2-specific antigens have been further defined using immunoblot techniques, of which the E2 component of the pyruvate dehydrogenase complex (PDC) is the major M2 autoantigen. The five antigens are a 72 kDa E2 subunit (PDC.E2), the 52 kDa protein X, the 50 kDa branched-chain 2-oxo-acid dehydrogenase complex (BCOADC.E2), the 48 kDa 2-oxo-glutarate dehydrogenase complex (OGDC.E2), and the 41 kDa E1 α-subunit of PDC.

The presence of AMA in high titre is unrelated to the clinical or histological picture and its role in pathogenesis is unclear.

It seems likely that an environmental factor acts on a genetically predisposed host. *E. coli* and other enterobacteria have been proposed as the triggering infective agent.

Although damage to bile ducts is a feature, antibodies to bile ductules are not specific to PBC. Biliary epithelium from patients with PBC expresses aberrant class II HLAs, but it is not known whether this expression is the cause or result of the inflammatory response. Cell-mediated immunity is impaired (demonstrated both in vitro and by skin testing), suggesting that sensitized T lymphocytes might be involved in producing damage. There may be a defect in immunoregulation, or a decrease in T suppressor cells which allows cytotoxic T cells to produce damage to the bile ducts. There is also evidence to suggest that lymphokine secretion and cell activation by T lymphocytes is impaired at the site of tissue destruction. There is an increased synthesis of IgM, thought to be due to a failure of the switch from IgM to IgG antibody synthesis.

Clinical features

Asymptomatic patients are discovered on routine examination or screening to have hepatomegaly, a raised serum alkaline phosphatase or autoantibodies.

Pruritus is often the earliest symptom, preceding jaundice by a few years. Fatigue may accompany pruritus particularly in progressive cases. When jaundice appears, hepatomegaly is usually found. In the later stages, patients are jaundiced with severe pruritus. Pigmented xanthelasma on eyelids or other deposits of cholesterol in the creases of the hands may be seen.

Associations

Autoimmune disorders (e.g. Sjögren's syndrome, scleroderma, rheumatoid arthritis) occur with increased frequency. Keratoconjunctivitis sicca (dry eyes and mouth) is seen in 70% of cases. Renal tubular acidosis and membranous glomerulonephritis occur.

Investigations

- **Mitochondrial antibodies** – measured routinely by ELISA (in titres >1:160) – are present in over 95% of patients; M2 antibody is specific. Other non-specific antibodies (e.g. antinuclear factor and smooth muscle) may also be present.
- **High serum alkaline phosphatase** is often the only abnormality in the liver biochemistry.
- **Serum cholesterol** is raised.
- **Serum IgM** may be very high.
- **Ultrasound** can show a diffuse alteration in liver architecture.
- **Liver biopsy** shows characteristic histological features of a portal tract infiltrate mainly of lymphocytes and plasma cells; approximately 40% have granulomas. Most of the early changes are in zone 1. Later, there is damage to and loss of small bile ducts with ductular proliferation. Portal tract fibrosis and, eventually, cirrhosis is seen.

Hepatic granulomas are not specific and are also seen in sarcoidosis, tuberculosis, schistosomiasis, drug reactions (e.g. phenylbutazone), brucellosis, parasitic infestation (e.g. strongyloidiasis) and other conditions.

Differential diagnosis

The classical picture presents little difficulty with diagnosis (high serum alkaline phosphatase and the presence of AMA); this can be confirmed by the characteristic features on liver biopsy. There is a group of patients with the histological changes of PBC, but the serology of autoimmune hepatitis (i.e. positive antinuclear and smooth muscle antibodies but negative AMA). This has been given the name of autoimmune cholangitis and responds to steroids and azathioprine.

In the jaundiced patient, extrahepatic biliary obstruction should be excluded by ultrasound and, if there is doubt about the diagnosis, ERCP (or MRCP) should be performed to make sure that the bile ducts are normal.

Treatment

Ursodeoxycholic acid (10–15 mg/kg) improves bilirubin and aminotransferase values. It is not clear if prognosis is altered. Symptoms are not improved. Steroids improve biochemical and histological disease but lead to osteoporosis.

Malabsorption of fat-soluble vitamins (A, D and K) occurs and supplementation is required when deficiency is detected and in the jaundiced patient prophylactically. Bisphosphonates are required for osteoporosis. Hyperlipidaemia should be treated (see p. 1109).

Pruritus is difficult to control, but colestyramine, one 4 g sachet three times daily, can be helpful, although it is unpalatable. Rifampicin as well as naloxone hydrochloride and naltrexone (opioid antagonists) have been shown to be of benefit in trials.

The lack of effective medical therapy has made PBC a major indication for orthotopic liver transplantation (p. 366).

Complications

The complications are those of cirrhosis. In addition, osteoporosis, and rarely osteomalacia and a polyneuropathy can also occur.

Course and prognosis

This is very variable. Asymptomatic patients and those presenting with pruritus will survive for more than 20 years. Symptomatic patients with jaundice have a more rapidly progressive course and die of liver failure or bleeding varices in approximately 5 years. Liver transplantation should therefore be offered when the serum bilirubin reaches 100 µmol/L. Transplantation has a 5-year survival of at least 80%.

Secondary biliary cirrhosis

Cirrhosis can result from prolonged (for months) large duct biliary obstruction. Causes include bile duct strictures, gallstones and sclerosing cholangitis. An ultrasound examination, followed by ERCP or PTC, is performed to outline the ducts and any remedial cause is dealt with.

Hereditary haemochromatosis

Hereditary haemochromatosis (HH) is an inherited disease characterized by excess iron deposition in various organs leading to eventual fibrosis and functional organ failure.

Prevalence and aetiology

HH is transmitted by an autosomal recessive gene with a prevalence in Caucasians of homozygotes (affected) of 1 in 400 and a heterozygote (carrier) frequency of 1 in 10. It is the most common single gene disorder in Caucasians. It is associated with HLA-A3 (72% versus 28% of the general population); in addition HLA-B14 is increased in France and HLA-B7 in Australia. The most common form of HH has been shown to be due to a mutation in a gene *HFE* – on the short arm of chromosome 6.

Between 83% and 90% of patients with overt HH are homozygous for the Cys 282 Tyr mutation. A second mutation (His 63 Asp; C 187G) occurs in about 25% of the population and is in complete linkage disequilibrium with Cys 282 Tyr. There is also a form of genetic haemochromatosis in Southern Europe, not associated with the above mutations.

Dietary intakes of iron and chelating agents (ascorbic acid) are probably also relevant. Iron overload may be present in alcoholics, but alcohol excess per se does not cause HH. There is a history of excess alcohol intake in 25% of patients.

Mechanism of damage. This is still unclear. The *HFE* gene may be involved in regulating the expression of other gene products including the divalent-cation transporter (DCTI) which is a mediator in intestinal iron absorption. Iron is taken up by the mucosal cells inappropriately, exceeding the binding capacity of transferrin; excess iron is then taken up by the liver and other tissues gradually over a long period. It seems likely that it is the iron itself that precipitates fibrosis.

Pathology

In symptomatic patients the total body iron content is 20–40 g, compared with 3–4 g in a normal person. The iron content is particularly increased in the liver and pancreas (50–100 times normal) but is also increased in other organs (e.g. the endocrine glands, heart and skin).

In established cases the liver shows extensive iron deposition and fibrosis. Early in the disease, iron is deposited in the periportal hepatocytes (in pericanalicular lysosomes). Later it is distributed widely throughout all acinar zones, biliary duct epithelium, Kupffer cells and connective tissue. Cirrhosis is a late feature.

Clinical features

The course of the disease depends on a number of factors, including sex, dietary iron intake, presence of associated hepatotoxins (especially alcohol) and genotype. Overt clinical manifestations occur more frequently in men; the reduced incidence in women is probably explained by physiological blood loss and a smaller dietary intake of iron. Most affected individuals present in the fifth decade. The classic triad of bronze skin pigmentation (due to melanin deposition), hepatomegaly and diabetes mellitus is only present in cases of gross iron overload.

Hypogonadism secondary to pituitary dysfunction is the most common endocrine feature. Deficiency of other pituitary hormones is also found, but symptomatic endocrine deficiencies, such as loss of libido, are very rare. Cardiac manifestations, particularly heart failure and arrhythmias, are common, especially in younger patients. Calcium pyrophosphate is deposited asymmetrically in both large and small joints (chondrocalcinosis) leading to an arthropathy. The exact relationship of chondrocalcinosis to iron deposition is uncertain.

Complications

Thirty per cent of patients with cirrhosis will develop primary hepatocellular carcinoma (HCC). HCC has only very rarely been described in non-cirrhotic patients in whom the excess iron stores have been removed. Early diagnosis is vital.

Investigations

Homozygotes

- **Serum iron** is elevated (> 30 µmol/L), with a reduction in the TIBC and complete or almost complete transferrin saturation (> 60%).

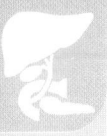
- **Serum ferritin** is elevated (usually >500 µg/L or 240 nmol/L).
- **Liver biochemistry** is often normal, even with established cirrhosis.

Heterozygotes

Heterozygotes may have normal biochemical tests or modest increases in serum iron transferrin saturation (>50%) or serum ferritin (usually >400 µg/L).

Liver biopsy

This can define the extent of tissue damage, assess tissue iron, and the hepatic iron concentration can be measured (>180 µmol/g dry weight of liver indicates haemochromatosis).

Mild degrees of parenchymal iron deposition in patients with alcoholic cirrhosis can often cause confusion with true homozygous HH. It is highly likely that many of this former group are heterozygotes for the haemochromatosis gene.

Magnetic resonance imaging

MRI shows dramatic reduction in the signal intensity of the liver and pancreas owing to the paramagnetic affect of ferritin and haemosiderin which profoundly shortens both the T1 and T2 relaxation times. In secondary iron overload (haemosiderosis) which involves the reticuloendothelial cells, the pancreas is spared – enabling distinction between these two conditions.

Treatment and management

Venesection

This prolongs life and may reverse tissue damage; the risk of malignancy still remains if cirrhosis is present. All patients should have excess iron removed as rapidly as possible. This is achieved using venesection of 500 mL performed twice-weekly for up to 2 years; i.e. 160 units with 250 mg of iron per unit, equals 40 g removed. During venesection, serum iron and ferritin and the mean corpuscular volume (MCV) should be monitored. These fall only when available iron is depleted. Three or four venesections per year are required to prevent reaccumulation of iron. Serum ferritin should remain within the normal range. Liver biopsy is useful to ensure removal of iron and to assess progress of hepatic disease.

Manifestations of the disease usually improve or disappear, except for diabetes, testicular atrophy and chondrocalcinosis. The requirements for insulin often diminish in diabetic patients. Testosterone replacement is often helpful.

Chelation therapy

In the rare patient who cannot tolerate venesection (because of severe cardiac disease or anaemia), chelation therapy with desferrioxamine either intermittently or continuously by infusion has been successful in removing iron.

Screening

In all cases of HH, all first-degree family members must be screened to detect early and asymptomatic disease. Serum ferritin is an excellent test with only occasional false-positives in hepatocellular necrosis and rare false-negatives in some family studies. Genetic markers are available for diagnosis.

In the general population, the serum iron and transferrin saturation are the best and cheapest tests available.

Wilson's disease (hepatolenticular degeneration)

Dietary copper is normally absorbed from the stomach and upper small intestine. It is transported to the liver loosely bound to albumin. Here it is incorporated into caeruloplasmin, a glycoprotein synthesized in the liver, and secreted into the blood. Copper is normally excreted in the bile.

Wilson's disease is a very rare inborn error of copper metabolism that results in copper deposition in various organs, including the liver, the basal ganglia of the brain and the cornea. It is potentially treatable and all young patients with liver disease must be screened for this condition.

Aetiology

It is an autosomal recessive disorder with a molecular defect within a copper-transporting ATPase encoded by a gene (designated *ATP7B*) located on chromosome 13. Over 60 mutations have been identified, the most frequent being His1070 Gly found in approximately 50% of cases in the USA and Europe. It occurs world-wide, particularly in countries where consanguinity is common. The basic problem is a failure of biliary excretion of copper. There is a low serum caeruloplasmin in over 80% of patients owing to poor synthesis, but the precise mechanism for the failure of copper excretion is not known.

Pathology

The liver histology is not diagnostic and varies from that of chronic hepatitis to macronodular cirrhosis. Stains for copper show a periportal distribution but this can be unreliable (see below). The basal ganglia are damaged and show cavitation, the kidneys show tubular degeneration, and erosions are seen in bones.

Clinical features

Children usually present with hepatic problems, whereas young adults have more neurological problems, such as tremor, dysarthria, involuntary movements and eventually dementia. The liver disease varies from episodes of acute hepatitis, especially in children, which can go on to fulminant hepatic failure to chronic hepatitis or cirrhosis.

Typical signs are of chronic liver disease with neurological signs of basal ganglia involvement (p. 1186). A specific sign is the Kayser–Fleischer ring, which is due to copper deposition in Descemet's membrane in the cornea. It appears as a greenish brown pigment at the corneoscleral junction just within the cornea. Identification of this ring frequently requires slit-lamp examination. It may be absent in young children.

Investigations
- **Serum copper and caeruloplasmin** are usually reduced but can be normal.
- **Urinary copper** is usually increased (100–1000 mg in 24 hours; normal levels < 40 mg in 24 hours).
- **Liver biopsy.** The diagnosis depends on measurement of the amount of copper in the liver, although high levels of copper are also found in the liver in chronic cholestasis. Measurement of ^{64}Cu incorporation into the liver may be helpful.
- **Haemolysis and anaemia** may be present.

Treatment
Lifetime treatment with penicillamine, 1–1.5 g daily, is effective in chelating copper. If treatment is started early, clinical and biochemical improvement can occur. Urine copper levels should be monitored and the drug dose adjusted downwards after 2–3 years. Serious side-effects of the drug occur in 10% and include skin rashes, leucopenia and renal damage. All siblings and children of patients should be screened and treatment given even in the asymptomatic if there is evidence of copper accumulation.

Prognosis
Early diagnosis and effective treatment have improved the outlook. Neurological damage is, however, permanent. Fulminant hepatic failure or decompensated cirrhosis should be treated by liver transplantation.

α_1-Antitrypsin deficiency (see also p. 864)
A deficiency of α_1-antitrypsin (α_1AT) is sometimes associated with liver disease and pulmonary emphysema (particularly in smokers). α_1AT is a glycoprotein, part of a family of *serine protease inhibitors*, or serpin, superfamily. α_1AT-deficiency is inherited as an autosomal dominant and 1 in 10 northern Europeans carries an abnormal gene.

The protein is a 394-amino acid 52 kDa acute phase protein that is synthesized in the liver and constitutes 90% of the serum α_1-globulin seen on electrophoresis. Its main role is to inhibit the proteolytic enzyme, neutrophil elastase.

The gene is located on chromosome 14. The genetic variants of α_1AT are characterized by their electrophoretic

mobilities as medium (M), slow (S) or very slow (Z). The normal genotype is protease inhibitor MM (PiMM), the homozygote for Z is PiZZ, and the heterozygotes are PiMZ and PiSZ. S and Z variants are due to a single amino acid replacement of glutamic acid at positions 264 and 342 of the polypeptide, respectively. This results in decreased synthesis and secretion of the protein by the liver as protein–protein interactions occur between the reactive centre loop of one molecule and the β-pleated sheet of a second (loop sheet polymerization).

How this causes liver disease is uncertain. It is postulated that the failure of secretion of the abnormal protein leads to an accumulation in the liver, causing liver damage.

Clinical features
The majority of patients with clinical disease are homozygotes with a PiZZ phenotype. Some may present in childhood and a few require transplantation. Approximately 10–15% of adult patients will develop cirrhosis, usually over the age of 50 years, and 75% will have respiratory problems. Approximately 5% of patients die of their liver disease. Heterozygotes (e.g. PiSZ or PiMZ) may develop liver disease, but the risk is small.

Investigations
- **Serum α_1-antitrypsin** is low, at 10% of the normal level in the PiZZ phenotypes, 60% of normal in the S variant.

On liver biopsy periodic acid–Schiff (PAS)-positive, diastase-resistant globules are seen in periportal hepatocytes. These can be shown to be α_1AT using specific antiserum. Fibrosis and cirrhosis can be present.

Treatment
There is no treatment apart from dealing with the complications of liver disease. Patients with hepatic decompensation should be considered for liver transplantation. Patients should be advised to stop smoking (see p. 865).

FURTHER READING

Arroyo V, Gines P, Gerbes AL et al. (1996) Definition and diagnostic criteria of refractory ascites and hepatorenal syndrome in cirrhosis. *Hepatology* **23**: 164–175.

Bacon BR (2001) Haemochromatosis: diagnosis and management. *Gastroenterology* **120**: 718–725.

Benyon RC, Iredale JP (2000) Is liver fibrosis reversible? *Gut* **46**: 443–446.

Carrell RW, Lomas DA (2002) Alpha-1 antitrypsin deficiency. *New England Journal of Medicine* **346**: 45–53.

Dagher L, Moore K (2001) The hepatorenal syndrome. *Gut* **49**: 729–737.

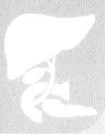

Garcia-Tsao G (2001) Current management of the complications of cirrhosis and portal hypertension. *Gastroenterology* **120**: 726–748.

Heathcote EJ (2000) Management of primary biliary cirrhosis. *Hepatology* **31**: 1005–1013.

Keefe F B (2001) Liver transplantation. *Gastroenterology* **120**: 749–762.

Major ME, Feinstone SM (1997) The molecular biology of hepatitis C. *Hepatology* **25**: 1527–1538.

Rees CJ, Hiubon M, Record CO (1997) Therapeutic modalities in portal hypertension. *European Journal of Gastroenterology and Hepatology* **9**: 9–11.

Riordan SM, Williams R (1997) Current concepts: treatment of hepatic encephalopathy. *New England Journal of Medicine* **337**: 473–479.

Rockey D (1997) The cellular pathogenesis of portal hypertension: stellate cell contractility, endothelin, and nitric oxide. *Hepatology* **25**: 2–5.

Alcoholic liver disease

This section gives the pathology and clinical features of alcoholic liver disease. The amounts needed to produce liver damage, alcohol metabolism, and other clinical effects of alcohol are described on page 250.

Ethanol is metabolized in the liver by two pathways (see p. 250), resulting in an increase in the NADH/NAD ratio. The altered redox potential results in increased hepatic fatty acid synthesis with decreased fatty acid oxidation, both events leading to hepatic accumulation of fatty acid that is then esterified to glycerides.

The changes in oxidation–reduction also impair carbohydrate and protein metabolism and are the cause of the centrilobular necrosis of the hepatic acinus typical of alcohol damage.

Acetaldehyde is formed by the oxidation of ethanol and its effect on hepatic proteins may well be a factor in producing liver cell damage. The exact mechanism of alcoholic hepatitis and cirrhosis is unknown, but since only 10–20% of people who drink heavily will suffer from cirrhosis, a genetic predisposition is proposed. Immunological mechanisms have also been proposed.

Alcohol can enhance the effects of toxic metabolites of drugs (e.g. paracetamol) on the liver, as it induces microsomal metabolism via the microsomal ethanol oxidizing system (MEOS) (p. 250).

Pathology

Alcohol can produce a wide spectrum of liver disease from fatty change to hepatitis and cirrhosis.

Fatty change

The metabolism of alcohol invariably produces fat in the liver, mainly in zone 3. This is minimal with small amounts of alcohol, but with larger amounts the cells become swollen with fat (steatosis) giving, eventually, a Swiss-cheese effect on haematoxylin and eosin stain. Steatosis can also be seen in obesity, diabetes, starvation and occasionally in chronic illness (p. 363). There is no liver cell damage. The fat disappears on stopping alcohol.

In some cases collagen is laid down around the central hepatic veins (perivenular fibrosis) and this can sometimes progress to cirrhosis without a preceding hepatitis. Alcohol directly affects stellate cells, transforming them into collagen-producing myofibroblast cells. Cirrhosis might then develop if there is an imbalance between degradation and production of collagen.

Alcoholic hepatitis

In addition to fatty change there is infiltration by polymorphonuclear leucocytes and hepatocyte necrosis mainly in zone 3. Dense cytoplasmic inclusions called Mallory bodies are sometimes seen in hepatocytes and giant mitochondria are also a feature. Mallory bodies are suggestive of, but not specific for, alcoholic damage as they can be found in other liver disease, such as Wilson's disease and PBC. If alcohol consumption continues, alcoholic hepatitis may progress to cirrhosis.

Alcoholic cirrhosis

This is classically of the micronodular type, but a mixed pattern may also be seen accompanying fatty change, and evidence of pre-existing alcoholic hepatitis may be present.

Clinical features
Fatty liver

There are often no symptoms or signs. Vague abdominal symptoms of nausea, vomiting and diarrhoea are due to the more general effects of alcohol on the gastrointestinal tract. Hepatomegaly, sometimes huge, can occur together with other features of chronic liver disease.

Alcoholic hepatitis

The clinical features vary in degree:

- The patient may be well, with few symptoms, the hepatitis only being apparent on the liver biopsy in addition to fatty change.
- Mild to moderate symptoms of ill-health, occasionally with mild jaundice, may occur. Signs include all the features of chronic liver disease. Liver biochemistry is deranged and the diagnosis is made on liver histology.
- In the severe case, usually superimposed on patients with alcoholic cirrhosis, the patient is ill, with jaundice and ascites. Abdominal pain is frequently present, with a high fever associated with the liver necrosis. On examination there is deep jaundice, hepatomegaly, sometimes splenomegaly, and ascites with ankle oedema. The signs of chronic liver disease are also present.

Alcoholic cirrhosis

This represents the final stage of liver disease from alcohol abuse. Nevertheless, patients can be very well with few symptoms. On examination, there are usually signs of chronic liver disease. The diagnosis is confirmed by liver biopsy.

Usually the patient presents with one of the complications of cirrhosis. In many cases there are features of alcohol dependency (see p. 1256) as well as evidence of involvement of other systems, such as polyneuropathy.

Investigations

Fatty liver

An elevated MCV often indicates heavy drinking. Liver biochemistry shows mild abnormalities with elevation of both serum aminotransferase enzymes. The γ-GT level is a sensitive test for determining whether the patient is taking alcohol. With severe fatty infiltration, marked changes in all liver biochemical parameters can occur. Ultrasound or CT will demonstrate fatty infiltration, as will liver histology.

Alcoholic hepatitis

Investigations show a leucocytosis with markedly deranged liver biochemistry with elevated:

- serum bilirubin
- serum AST and ALT
- serum alkaline phosphatase
- prothrombin time (PT).

A low serum albumin may also be found. Rarely, hyperlipidaemia with haemolysis (Zieve's syndrome) may occur.

The prolonged PT makes transjugular liver biopsy necessary.

Alcoholic cirrhosis

Investigations are as for cirrhosis in general.

Management and prognosis

General management

Patients should be advised to stop drinking. Delirium tremens (a withdrawal symptom) may be treated with diazepam. Intravenous thiamine should be given empirically to prevent Wernicke–Korsakoff encephalopathy. Bed rest with a diet high in protein and vitamin supplements is given. Dietary protein may have to be limited because of encephalopathy. Follow-up of patients with alcoholic liver disease shows, however, that – apart from highly motivated groups – most patients continue to drink alcohol.

Fatty liver

In all but the mildest cases the patient is advised to stop drinking alcohol; the fat will disappear and the liver biochemistry usually returns to normal. Small amounts of alcohol can be drunk subsequently as long as patients are aware of the problems and can control their consumption.

Alcoholic hepatitis

In severe cases the patient is confined to bed. Treatment for encephalopathy and ascites is commenced. Patients should be fed preferably via a fine-bore nasogastric tube or sometimes intravenously. Vitamins B and C should be given by injection. Corticosteroids should be given providing infection is absent, or following a course of antibiotics. Antifungal prophylaxis should also be used.

Patients are advised to stop drinking for life, as this is undoubtedly a precirrhotic condition. The prognosis is variable and, despite abstinence, the liver disease is progressive in many patients. Conversely, a few patients continue to drink heavily without developing cirrhosis.

In severe cases the mortality is at least 50%, and with a PT twice the normal, progressive encephalopathy and renal failure, the mortality approaches 90%.

Alcoholic cirrhosis

The management of cirrhosis is described on page 365. Again, all patients are advised to stop drinking for life. Abstinence from alcohol results in an improvement in prognosis, with a 5-year survival of 90%, but with continued drinking this falls to 60%. With advanced disease (i.e. jaundice, ascites and haematemesis) the 5-year survival rate falls to 35%, with most of the deaths occurring in the first year. Liver transplantation is being used widely in some countries with good survival figures.

A trial of abstention to establish if liver disease can improve is mandatory, but transplantation should not be denied if the patient continues to deteriorate.

Hepatocellular carcinoma is a complication particularly in men.

FURTHER READING

Lieber C (1995) Medical disorders of alcoholism. *New England Journal of Medicine* **133**: 1058–1065.
Tilg H, Diehl AM (2000) Cytokines in alcoholic steatohepatitis. *New England Journal of Medicine* **343**: 1467–1476.

Budd–Chiari syndrome

In this condition there is obstruction to the venous outflow of the liver owing to occlusion of the hepatic vein. In one-third of patients the cause is unknown, but specific causes include hypercoagulability states, such as polycythaemia vera, taking the contraceptive pill, or leukaemia. Other causes include occlusion of the hepatic vein owing to posterior abdominal wall sarcomas, renal or adrenal tumours, hepatocellular carcinoma, hepatic infections (e.g. hydatid cyst), congenital venous webs, radiotherapy, or trauma to the liver.

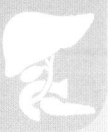

The acute form presents with abdominal pain, nausea, vomiting, tender hepatomegaly and ascites (a fulminant form occurs particularly in pregnant women). In the chronic form there is enlargement of the liver (particularly the caudate lobe), mild jaundice, ascites, a negative hepatojugular reflex, and splenomegaly with portal hypertension.

Investigations

Investigations show a high protein content in the ascitic fluid and characteristic liver histology with centrizonal congestion, haemorrhage, fibrosis and cirrhosis. Ultrasound, CT or MRI will demonstrate hepatic vein occlusion with diffuse abnormal parenchyma on contrast-enhancement, which spares the caudate lobe because of its independent blood supply and venous drainage. There may be compression of the inferior vena cava. Pulsed Doppler sonography or a colour Doppler are useful as they show abnormalities in the direction of flow in the hepatic vein. Investigations to identify a cause are also performed, such as blood tests and coagulation studies.

Differential diagnosis

A similar clinical picture can be produced by inferior vena caval obstruction, right-sided cardiac failure or constrictive pericarditis, and appropriate investigations should be performed.

Treatment

Ascites should be treated as well as any underlying cause (e.g. polycythaemia). Congenital webs should be treated radiologically or resected surgically. A side-to-side portocaval or splenorenal anastomosis may decompress the congested liver providing there is no caval obstruction, with considerable improvement in the clinical state of the patient. Liver transplantation is the treatment of choice for chronic Budd–Chiari syndrome and for the fulminant form, followed by lifelong anticoagulation. Transjugular intrahepatic portosystemic shunts (TIPS) instead of portocaval shunts are being increasingly used as caval compression does not prejudice the efficacy of TIPS.

Prognosis

The prognosis depends on the aetiology, but some patients can survive for several years.

Veno-occlusive disease

This is due to injury of the hepatic veins and presents clinically like the Budd–Chiari syndrome. It was originally described in Jamaica, where the ingestion of toxic pyrrolizidine alkaloids in bush tea (made from plants of the genera *Senecio*, *Heliotropium* and *Crotolaria*) caused damage to the hepatic veins. It can be seen in other parts of the world. It is also seen as a complication of chemotherapy and total body irradiation before allogeneic bone marrow transplantation. The development of veno-occlusive disease after transplantation carries a high mortality. Treatment is supportive with control of ascites and hepatocellular failure. TIPS has been used in a few cases.

Fibropolycystic diseases

These diseases are usually inherited and lead to the presence of cysts or fibrosis in the liver, kidney and occasionally the pancreas, and other organs.

Polycystic disease of the liver

In adults

This is inherited as an autosomal dominant and usually presents in middle age with abdominal swelling or right hypochondrial discomfort. It can also be detected by ultrasound scanning or may only be discovered at autopsy. There may or may not be hepatomegaly and bilateral irregular palpable polycystic kidneys. The cysts are of variable size and consist of thin-walled cavities containing clear fluid or altered blood. Liver function is normal and complications such as oesophageal varices are very rare. The prognosis is excellent and is often dependent on whether the kidneys are involved.

In children

Childhood polycystic disease is inherited in a different way from the adult type. It is an autosomal recessive condition presenting in the first few months of life. Renal involvement is common, with cystic changes in the renal tubules.

Congenital hepatic fibrosis

In this rare condition the liver architecture is normal but there are broad collagenous fibrous bands extending from the portal tracts. It is often inherited as an autosomal recessive condition but can also occur sporadically. It usually presents in childhood with hepatosplenomegaly, and portal hypertension is common. It may present later in life and can be misdiagnosed as cirrhosis. A wedge biopsy of the liver may be required to confirm the diagnosis. The outlook is good and the condition should be distinguished from cirrhosis. Patients who bleed do well after endoscopic therapy of varices or a portocaval anastomosis because of their good liver function.

Congenital intrahepatic biliary dilatation (Caroli's disease)

In this rare, non-familial disease there are saccular dilatations of the intrahepatic or extrahepatic ducts. It can present at any age (although usually in childhood) with fever, abdominal pain and recurrent attacks of cholangitis with Gram-negative septicaemia. Jaundice and portal hypertension are absent. Diagnosis is by ultrasound, PTC, ERCP or MRCP.

Solitary non-parasitic cysts
These are rare and probably a variant of polycystic disease.

Liver abscess

Pyogenic abscess
These abscesses are uncommon, but may be single or multiple. The most common cause was secondary to a portal pyaemia from intra-abdominal sepsis (e.g. appendicitis or perforations), but now in many cases the aetiology is not known. Biliary sepsis, particularly in the elderly, is a common cause. Other causes include trauma, bacteraemia and direct extension from, for example, a perinephric abscess.

The organism found most commonly is *E. coli*. *Streptococcus milleri* and anaerobic organisms such as *Bacteroides* are often seen. Other organisms include *Enterococcus faecalis*, *Proteus vulgaris* and *Staphylococcus aureus*. Often the infection is mixed. Failure to culture an organism may be due to previous antibiotic therapy or inadequate anaerobic culture.

Clinical features
Some patients are not acutely ill and present with malaise lasting several days or even months. Others can present with fever, rigors, anorexia, vomiting, weight loss and abdominal pain. In these patients a Gram-negative septicaemia with shock can occur. On examination there may be little to find. Alternatively, the patient may be toxic, febrile and jaundiced. In such patients, the liver is tender and enlarged and there may be signs of a pleural effusion or a pleural rub in the right lower chest.

Investigations
Patients are often investigated as a 'pyrexia of unknown origin' (PUO) and in the mild chronic case most investigations will be normal. Often the only clue to the diagnosis is a raised serum alkaline phosphatase.

- **Serum bilirubin** is raised in 25% of cases.
- **Normochromic normocytic anaemia** may occur, usually accompanied by a polymorphonuclear leucocytosis.
- **Serum alkaline phosphatase and ESR** are often raised.
- **Serum B_{12}** is very high, as vitamin B_{12} is stored in and subsequently released from the liver.
- **Blood cultures** are positive in only 30% of cases.

Imaging
Ultrasound is useful for detecting abscesses. A CT scan may be of value in complex and multiple lesions. A

chest X-ray will show elevation of the right hemidiaphragm with a pleural effusion in the severe case.

Management
Aspiration of the abscess should be attempted under ultrasound control. Antibiotics should initially cover Gram-positive, Gram-negative and anaerobic organisms until the causative organism is identified.

Further drainage via a large-bore needle under ultrasound control or surgically may be necessary if resolution is difficult or slow. The underlying cause must also be treated.

Prognosis
The overall mortality depends on the nature of the underlying pathology and has been reduced to approximately 16% with needle aspiration and antibiotics. A unilocular abscess in the right lobe has a better prognosis. Scattered multiple abscesses have a very high mortality, with only one in five patients surviving.

Amoebic abscess (see also p. 106)
This condition occurs world-wide and must be considered in patients travelling from endemic areas. *Entamoeba histolytica* (p. 106) can be carried from the bowel to the liver in the portal venous system. Portal inflammation results, with the development of multiple microabscesses and eventually single or multiple large abscesses.

Clinically the onset is usually gradual but may be sudden. There is fever, anorexia, weight loss and malaise. There is often no history of dysentery. On examination the patient looks ill and has tender hepatomegaly and signs of an effusion or consolidation in the base of the right side of the chest. Jaundice is unusual.

Investigations
These are as for pyogenic abscess, plus:

- **Serological tests for amoeba** (e.g. haemagglutination, amoebic complement-fixation test, ELISA). These are always positive, particularly if there are bowel symptoms, and remain positive after a clinical cure and therefore do not indicate current disease. A repeat negative test, however, is good evidence against an amoebic abscess.
- **Diagnostic aspiration of fluid** looking like anchovy sauce.

Treatment
Metronidazole 800 mg three times daily is given for 10 days. Aspiration is used in patients failing to respond, in multiple and large abscesses, and in those with abscesses in the left lobe of the liver.

Complications
Complications include rupture, secondary infection and septicaemia.

Other infections of the liver

Schistosomiasis (see also p. 115)

Schistosoma mansoni and *S. japonicum* affect the liver, but *S. haematobium* rarely does so. During their life cycle the ova reach the liver via the venous system and obstruct the portal branches, producing granulomas, fibrosis and inflammation but not cirrhosis.

Clinically there is hepatosplenomegaly and portal hypertension, which is particularly severe with *S. mansoni*.

Investigations show a raised serum alkaline phosphatase and ova can be found in the stools (centrifuged deposits) and in rectal and liver biopsies. Skin tests and other immunological tests often have false results and may also be positive because of past infection.

Treatment is with praziquantel, but fibrosis still remains with a potential risk of portal hypertension, characteristically pre-sinusoidal due to intense portal fibrosis.

Hydatid disease (see also p. 119)

Cysts caused by *Echinococcus granulosus* are single or multiple. They usually occur in the lower part of the right lower lobe. The cyst has three layers: an outside layer derived from the host, an intermediate laminated layer, and an inner germinal layer that buds off brood capsules to form daughter cysts.

Clinically there may be no symptoms or a dull ache and swelling in the right hypochondrium. Investigations show a peripheral eosinophilia in 30% of cases and usually a positive hydatid complement-fixation test or haemagglutination (85%). Plain abdominal X-ray may show calcification of the outer coat of the cyst. Ultrasound and CT scan demonstrate cysts and may show diagnostic daughter cysts within the parent cyst (Fig. 7.24).

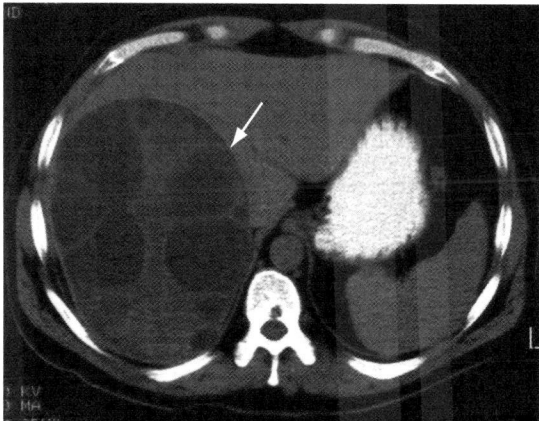

Fig. 7.24 CT scan of liver showing a large hydatid cyst (arrow) with 'daughter' cysts lying within it.

Fine-needle aspiration under ultrasound control with chemotherapeutic cover is now used therapeutically. Surgery can be performed with removal of the cyst intact if possible after first sterilizing the cyst with formalin or alcohol. Medical treatment (e.g. with albendazole, which penetrates into large cysts) can result in reduction of cyst size. Chronic calcified cysts can be left.

Complications include rupture, secondary infection and involvement of other organs. The prognosis without any complications is good, although there is always the risk of rupture. Preventative measures include deworming of pet dogs and prevention of pets from eating infected carcasses.

Acquired immunodeficiency syndrome (see also p. 134)

The liver is often involved but rarely causes significant morbidity or mortality. HIV itself is probably not the cause of the liver abnormalities. The following are seen:

- pre-existing/coincidental viral hepatitis (HBV, HCV, HDV)
- neoplasia: Kaposi's sarcoma and non-Hodgkin's lymphoma
- opportunistic infection (e.g. *Mycobacterium tuberculosis*, *M. avium-intracellulare*, *Cryptococcus*, *Candida albicans*, toxoplasmosis)
- drug hepatotoxicity
- sclerosing cholangitis (see p. 393).

Clinical hepatomegaly is common (60% of patients).

Liver disease in pregnancy

Liver function is not impaired in pregnancy. Any liver disease from whatever cause can occur incidentally and coincide with pregnancy. For example, viral hepatitis accounts for 40% of all cases of jaundice during pregnancy. Pregnancy does not necessarily exacerbate established liver disease, but it is uncommon for women with advanced liver disease to conceive.

The following changes take place:

- Plasma and blood volumes increase during pregnancy but the hepatic blood flow remains constant.
- The proportion of cardiac output delivered to the liver therefore falls from 35% to 29% in late pregnancy; drug metabolism can thus be affected.
- The size of the liver remains constant.
- Liver biochemistry remains unchanged apart from a rise in serum alkaline phosphatase from the placenta (up to three to four times) and a decrease in total protein owing to increased plasma volume.
- Triglycerides and cholesterol levels rise, and caeruloplasmin, transferrin, α_1-antitrypsin and fibrinogen levels are elevated owing to increased hepatic synthesis.

- Postpartum there is a tendency to hypercoagulability, and acute Budd–Chiari syndrome can occur.

There are a number of liver diseases that complicate pregnancy.

Hyperemesis gravidarum

Pathological vomiting during pregnancy can be associated with liver dysfunction and jaundice. Liver dysfunction resolves when vomiting subsides.

Intrahepatic cholestasis of pregnancy

This condition of unknown aetiology presents usually with pruritus alone in the third trimester. It has a familial tendency and there is a higher prevalence in Scandinavia, Chile and Bolivia.

Liver biochemistry shows a cholestatic picture with high serum ALP (up to four times normal) and raised aminotransferases which occasionally can be very high. The serum bilirubin is slightly raised with jaundice in 60% of cases. Liver biopsy is not indicated but would show centrilobular cholestasis.

Treatment is symptomatic with ursodeoxycholic acid 15 mg/kg. *Prognosis* is usually excellent for the mother but there is increased fetal loss and the condition resolves after delivery. Recurrent cholestasis may occur during subsequent pregnancies or with the ingestion of oestrogen-containing oral contraceptive pills.

Pre-eclampsia and eclampsia

Pre-eclampsia is characterized by hypertension, proteinuria and oedema occurring in the second or third trimester. Eclampsia is marked by seizures or coma in addition. Hepatic complications include subcapsular haematoma and infarction, and occasionally fulminant hepatic failure. The HELLP syndrome – a combination of haemolysis, elevated liver enzymes and a low platelet count – can occur in association with severe pre-eclampsia. In the HELLP syndrome, there is epigastric pain, nausea and vomiting, with jaundice in 5% of patients. Delivery is the best treatment for eclampsia.

Acute fatty liver of pregnancy (AFLP)

This is a rare, serious condition of unknown aetiology. There is an association between acute fatty liver and long-chain 3-hydroxylacyl-CoA-dihydroxyl (LCHAD) deficiency. The mechanism is unclear, but abnormal fatty acid metabolites produced by the homozygous or heterozygous fetus enter the circulation and overcome maternal hepatic mitochondrial oxidation systems in a heterozygote mother. It presents in the last trimester with symptoms of fulminant hepatitis – jaundice, vomiting, abdominal pain, occasionally haematemesis and coma.

Investigations show hepatocellular damage, hyperuricaemia, thrombocytopenia, and rarely DIC. CT scanning shows a low density of the liver owing to the high fat content. It can sometimes be difficult to differentiate from the HELLP syndrome and as LCHAD deficiency has also been shown in HELLP there is a view that there is a spectrum of HELLP to AFLP. Liver biopsy shows fine droplets of fat (microvesicles) in the liver cells with little necrosis, but is not necessary for diagnosis.

Immediate delivery of the child may save both baby and mother. Early diagnosis and treatment has reduced the mortality to less than 20%. Treatment is as for acute liver failure.

FURTHER READING

Koux TA, Olans LB (1996) Liver disease in pregnancy. *New England Journal of Medicine* 335: 569–576.

Liver tumours

The most common liver tumour is a secondary (metastatic) tumour (Fig. 7.25), particularly from the gastrointestinal tract, breast or bronchus. Clinical features are

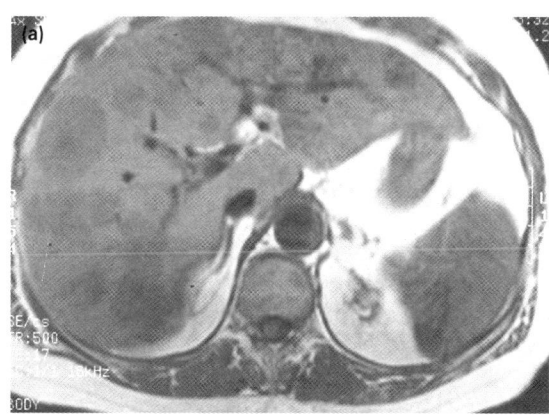

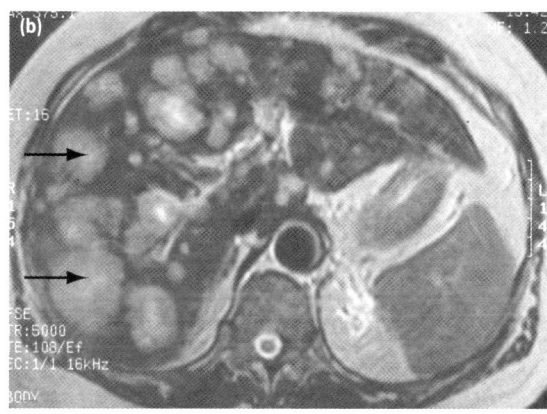

Fig. 7.25 **Liver MRI. (a)** T1- and **(b)** T2-weighted sequences showing multiple liver metastases. Structures of fluid density have high signal on T2 images. Note the central tumour necrosis in **(b)** (arrows).

variable but usually include hepatomegaly. Ultrasound is the primary investigation, with CT or MRI used when available; MRI is comparable to CT at detecting metastases. Primary liver tumours may be benign or malignant, but the most common are malignant.

Malignant tumours

Hepatocellular carcinoma (HCC)

Hepatocellular carcinoma (HCC) is one of the ten most common cancers world-wide, although it is uncommon in the West.

Aetiology

Carriers of HBV and HCV have an extremely high risk of developing HCC. In areas where HBV is prevalent, 90% of patients with this cancer are positive for the hepatitis B virus. Cirrhosis is present in over 80% of these patients. The development of HCC is related to the integration of viral DNA into the genome of the host hepatocyte (see p. 360). The risk of HCC in HCV is as high or higher than in HBV despite no viral integration. Primary liver cancer is also associated with other forms of cirrhosis, such as alcoholic cirrhosis and haemochromatosis. Males are affected more than females; this may account for the high incidence seen in haemochromatosis and low incidence in PBC. Other suggested aetiological factors are aflatoxin (a metabolite of a fungus found in groundnuts) and androgenic steroids, and there is a weak association with the contraceptive pill.

Pathology

The tumour is either single or occurs as multiple nodules throughout the liver. Histologically it consists of cells resembling hepatocytes. It can metastasize via the hepatic or portal veins to the lymph nodes, bones and lungs.

Clinical features

The clinical features include weight loss, anorexia, fever, an ache in the right hypochondrium, and ascites. The rapid development of these features in a cirrhotic patient is suggestive of HCC. On examination, an enlarged, irregular, tender liver may be felt. Increasingly due to surveillance, HCC is found without symptoms in cirrhotics.

Investigations

Serum α-fetoprotein may be raised, but is normal in at least a third of patients. Ultrasound scans show filling defects in 90% of cases. A liver biopsy, particularly under ultrasonic guidance may be performed for diagnosis, but is increasingly less used as imaging techniques show characteristic appearances and because seeding along the biopsy tract can occur.

Treatment and prognosis

Surgical resection is occasionally possible. Small tumours in patients with cirrhosis do well with liver transplantation. Chemotherapy and radiotherapy are unhelpful.

Survival, except in very selected groups, is seldom more than 6 months.

Prevention

Persistent HBV infection usually acquired after perinatal infection is a high risk factor for HCC in many parts of the world, such as South East Asia. Widespread vaccination against HBV is being used and this has shown a reduction in the annual incidence of HCC in Taiwan.

Cholangiocarcinoma

Cholangiocarcinomas can be extrahepatic (see p. 394) or intrahepatic. Intrahepatic adenocarcinomas arising from the bile ducts account for approximately 10% of primary tumours. They are not associated with cirrhosis or hepatitis B. In the Far East they may be associated with infestation with *Clonorchis sinensis* or *Opisthorchis viverrini*. The clinical features are similar to primary HCC except that jaundice is frequent with hilar tumours, and cholangitis is more frequent.

Surgical resection is rarely possible and patients usually die within 6 months. Transplantation is contraindicated.

Benign tumours

The most common benign tumour is a *haemangioma*. It is usually small and single but can be multiple and large. They are usually found incidentally on ultrasound, CT or MRI and have characteristic appearances. They require no treatment.

Hepatic adenomas are associated with oral contraceptives. They can present with abdominal pain or intraperitoneal bleeding. Resection is only required for symptomatic patients, or in those in whom discontinuation of the oral contraception does not result in shrinkage of the tumour.

FURTHER READING

Bruix J (1997) Treatment of hepatocellular carcinoma. *Hepatology* **25**: 259–262.

Miscellaneous conditions of the liver

Hepatic mitochondrial injury syndromes

These syndromes – in which there is mitochondrial damage with inhibition of β-oxidation of fatty acids – can be categorized as follows:

- *Genetic*, with abnormalities which include medium-chain acyl-coenzyme A dehydrogenase deficiency leading to microsteatosis.
- *Toxins* leading to liver failure include aflatoxin and cerulide (produced by *Bacillus cereus*) which causes food poisoning (see p. 74).
- *Drugs* (e.g. i.v. tetracycline, valproic acid and zidovudine) can produce a fatal microsteatosis.
- *Idiopathic*, the best known being fatty liver of pregnancy (p. 383) and Reye's syndrome. This condition, due to inhibition of β-oxidation and uncoupling of oxidative phosphorylation in mitochondria, leads in children to an acute encephalopathy and diffuse microvesicular fatty infiltration of the liver. Aspirin ingestion and viral infections have been implicated as precipitating agents. Mortality is about 50%, usually due to cerebral oedema.

Idiopathic adult ductopenia

This unexplained condition is characterized by pruritus and cholestatic jaundice. Histology of the liver shows a decrease in intrahepatic bile ducts in at least 50% of the portal tract, together with the features of cholestasis and marked fibrosis or cirrhosis. In most the disease is progressive and the only treatment is liver transplantation.

Indian childhood cirrhosis

This condition of children is seen in the Indian subcontinent. The cause is unknown. Eventually there is development of a micronodular cirrhosis with excess copper in the liver.

Hepatic porphyrias

These are dealt with on page 1119.

Cystic fibrosis (see also p. 871)

This disease affects mainly the lung and pancreas, but patients can develop fatty liver, cholestasis and cirrhosis. The aetiology of the liver involvement is unclear.

Drugs and the liver

Drug metabolism

The liver is the major site of drug metabolism. Drugs are converted from fat-soluble to water-soluble substances that can be excreted in the urine or bile. This metabolism of drugs is mediated by a group of mixed-function enzymes (p. 958).

Drug hepatotoxicity

Many drugs impair liver function and drugs should always be considered as a cause when mildly abnormal liver tests are found. Damage to the liver by drugs is usually classified as being either predictable (or dose-related) or non-predictable (not dose-related) (see p. 961).

This classification should not be used rigidly, as there is considerable overlap and many mechanisms may be involved in the production of damage.

Biochemical pathways

When a small amount of hepatotoxic drug whose effect is dose-dependent (e.g. paracetamol) is ingested, a large proportion of it undergoes conjugation with glucuronide and sulphate, whilst the remainder is metabolized by microsomal enzymes to produce toxic derivatives that are immediately detoxified by conjugation with glutathione. If larger doses are ingested, the former pathway becomes saturated and the toxic derivative is produced at a faster rate. Once the hepatic glutathione is depleted, large amounts of the toxic metabolite accumulate and produce damage (p. 985).

The 'predictability' of drugs to produce damage can, however, be affected by metabolic events preceding their ingestion. For example, chronic alcohol abusers may become more susceptible to liver damage because of the enzyme-inducing effects of alcohol, or ill or starving patients may become susceptible because of the depletion of hepatic glutathione produced by starvation. Many other factors such as environmental or genetic effects may be involved in determining the 'susceptibility' of certain patients to certain drugs.

Immunological mechanisms

These can be involved in the production of hepatic cell damage by certain drugs. The toxic metabolite produced by the microsomal enzymes may bind to the liver cell protein, thereby altering its antigenicity. The production of antibody against this will lead to immunologically mediated damage. An example of this mechanism is halothane- or enflurane-induced hepatic necrosis, which requires prior sensitization of the patient to these gases, although direct toxicity may also play a part.

Other pointers for the involvement of immunological mechanisms are the development of skin rashes, fever and arthralgia (serum-sickness syndrome) following ingestion of certain drugs. Eosinophilia and circulating immune complexes and antibodies may occasionally be detected.

Hepatitic damage

The type of damage produced by various drugs is shown in Table 7.16. The diagnosis of these conditions is usually by exclusion of other causes. Most reactions occur within 3 months of starting the drug. Monitoring liver biochemistry in patients on long-term treatment, such as antituberculosis therapy, is advisable. If a drug is suspected of causing hepatic damage it should be stopped immediately. Liver biopsy is of limited help in confirming the diagnosis, but occasionally hepatic eosinophilia or granulomas may be seen. Diagnostic challenge with subtherapeutic doses of the drug is sometimes required after the liver biochemistry has returned to normal, to confirm the diagnosis.

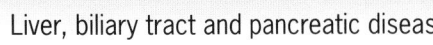

Table 7.16
Some drugs causing types of liver damage

Types of liver damage	Drugs	Types of liver damage	Drugs
Zone 3 necrosis	Carbon tetrachloride *Amanita* mushrooms Paracetamol Salicylates Piroxicam Cocaine	Chronic hepatitis	Methyldopa Nitrofurantoin Fenofibrate Isoniazid
Zone 1 necrosis	Ferrous sulphate	General hypersensitivity	Sulphonamides e.g. Sulfasalazine Co-trimoxazole Fansidar
Microvesicular fat	Sodium valproate Tetracyclines		Penicillins, e.g. Flucloxacillin
'Alcoholic' hepatitis (phospholipidosis)	Amiodarone Synthetic oestrogens Nifedipine		Ampicillin Amoxicillin Co-amoxiclav
Fibrosis	Methotrexate Other cytotoxic agents Arsenic Vitamin A Retinoids		NSAIDs e.g. Salicylates Diclofenac
			Allopurinol
Heparlobatum	Combination chemotherapy for metastatic breast cancer		Antithyroid e.g. Propylthiouracil Carbimazole
Vascular Sinusoidal dilatation	Contraceptive drugs Anabolic steroids Azathioprine		Quinine e.g. Quinidine
			Diltiazem
Pelioses hepatis	Oral contraceptives Anabolic steroids, e.g. Danazol Azathioprine		Anticonvulsants e.g. Phenytoin
		Canalicular cholestasis	Sex hormones Ciclosporin A
Veno-occlusive	Pyrrolizidine alkaloids (*Senecio* in bush tea) Cytotoxics – cyclophosphamide, azathioprine	Hepatocanalicular cholestasis	Chlorpromazine Haloperidol Erythromycin
Acute hepatitis	Isoniazid Rifampicin Methyldopa Atenolol Enalapril Verapamil Ketoconazole Cytotoxic drugs Clonazepam Disulfiram Niacin Volatile liquid anaesthetics, e.g. Halothane		Cimetidine/ranitidine Nitrofurantoin Imipramine Azathioprine Oral hypoglycaemics Dextropropoxyphene
		Ductular cholestasis	Benoxyprofen
		Biliary sludge	Ceftriaxone
		Sclerosing cholangitis	Hepatic arterial infusion of 5-fluorouracil
		Hepatic tumours	Pills with high hormone content (adenomas)
		Hepatocellular carcinoma	Contraceptive pill Danazol

NSAID, non-steroidal anti-inflammatory drug

Individual drugs

Paracetamol

In high doses paracetamol produces liver cell necrosis (see above). The toxic metabolite binds irreversibly to liver cell membranes. Overdosage is discussed on page 985.

Halothane and other volatile liquid anaesthetics

Halothane produces a hepatitis in patients having repeated exposures. The mechanism is thought to be a hypersensitivity reaction. An unexplained fever occurs approximately 10 days after the second or subsequent halothane anaesthetic and is followed by jaundice, typically with a hepatitic picture. Most patients recover spontaneously but there is a high mortality in severe cases. There are no chronic sequelae. Both enflurane and isoflurane also cause hepatotoxicity in those sensitized to halogenated anaesthetics but the risk is smaller than with halothane.

Steroid compounds
Cholestasis is caused by natural and synthetic oestrogens as well as methyltestosterone. These agents interfere with canalicular biliary flow and cause a pure cholestasis. Cholestasis is rare with the contraceptive pill because of the low dosage used. However, the contraceptive pill is associated with an increased incidence of gallstones, hepatic adenomas (rarely HCCs), the Budd–Chiari syndrome and peliosis hepatis. The latter condition, which also occurs with anabolic steroids, consists of dilatation of the hepatic sinusoids to form blood-filled lakes.

Phenothiazines
Phenothiazines (e.g. chlorpromazine) can produce a cholestatic picture owing to a hypersensitivity reaction. It occurs in 1% of patients, usually within 4 weeks of starting the drug. Typically it is associated with a fever and eosinophilia. Recovery occurs on stopping the drug.

Antituberculous chemotherapy
Isoniazid produces elevated aminotransferases in 10–20% of patients. Hepatic necrosis with jaundice occurs in a smaller percentage. The hepatotoxicity of isoniazid appears to be related to acetylator status, as the damage is due to the metabolites.

Rifampicin produces a hepatitis, usually within 3 weeks of starting the drug, particularly in patients on high doses.

Pyrazinamide produces abnormal liver biochemical tests and, rarely, liver cell necrosis.

Drug prescribing for patients with liver disease
The metabolism of drugs is impaired in severe liver disease (with jaundice and ascites) as the removal of many drugs depends on liver blood flow and the integrity of the hepatocyte. In general, therefore, the effect of drugs is prolonged by liver disease and also by cholestasis. This is further accentuated by portosystemic shunting, which diminishes the first-pass extraction of drugs. With hypoproteinaemia there is decreased protein binding of some drugs, and bilirubin competes with many drugs for the binding sites on serum albumin. In patients with portosystemic encephalopathy, care must be taken in prescribing drugs with a central depressant action.

FURTHER READING

Lee WM (1995) Drug-induced hepatotoxicity. *New England Journal of Medicine* **333**: 1118–1127.

Gall bladder and biliary system

The structure, formation and function of bile is discussed on page 337.

Gallstones

Prevalence of gallstones
Gallstones may be present at any age but are unusual before the third decade. The prevalence of gallstones is strongly influenced both by age and sex. There is a progressive increase in the presence of gallstones with age but the prevalence is two to three times higher in women than in men, although this difference is less marked in the sixth and seventh decade. At this age the prevalence ranges between 25–30%. There are considerable racial differences, gallstones being more common in Scandinavia, South America and Native North Americans.

Types of gallstones
Two principal types of gallstone disease occur. In the western world 80% of gallstones contain cholesterol. The second less frequent type of gallstone is 'pigment stones' being predominantly composed of calcium bilirubinate or polymer-like complexes with calcium and copper.

Cholesterol gallstones
The formation of cholesterol stones is the consequence of cholesterol crystallization from gall bladder bile. This is dependent upon three factors:

- cholesterol supersaturation of bile
- crystallization-promoting factors within bile
- motility of the gall bladder itself.

Cholesterol is derived partly from dietary sources, but in addition is synthesized within the liver. The rate-limiting step in cholesterol synthesis is beta-hydroxy-beta methyl glutaryl Co-A (HMG-CoA) reductase, which catalysis the first step, i.e. the conversion of acetate to mevalonate. The cholesterol formed is co-secreted with phospholipids into the biliary canaliculus as unilamellar vesicles. Cholesterol will only crystallize into stones when the bile is supersaturated with cholesterol relative to the bile salt and phospholipid content. This can occur as a consequence of excess cholesterol secretion into bile or because of a relative decrease in bile salt content. In some instances of cholesterol gallstones an increase in HMG-CoA reductase activity has been identified as the cause of the excess cholesterol secretion into bile. An alternative mechanism of supersaturation is a decreased bile salt content which may be genetically predetermined or occur as a consequence of bile salt loss (e.g. terminal ileal Crohn's disease).

Whilst cholesterol supersaturation of bile is essential for cholesterol stone formation, many individuals in whom such supersaturation occurs will never develop stones. It is the balance between cholesterol crystallizing and solubilizing factors that determine whether cholesterol will crystallize out of solution. A number of lipoproteins have been reported as putative crystallizing factors.

Gall bladder motility represents a further factor that may influence the cholesterol crystallization from supersaturated bile. There is evidence from animal models that gall bladder stasis leads to cholesterol crystallization mediated by hypersecretion of mucin.

Abnormalities of gall bladder motility have been suggested as factors in such circumstances as pregnancy, multiparity and diabetes as well as octreotide related gall bladder stones (p. 1034). Recognized risk factors for gallstones are shown in Table 7.17.

Bile pigment stones

The major component of pigment stones is calcium bilirubinate with less than 50% cholesterol content. The pathogenesis of pigment stones is entirely independent of cholesterol gallstones. There are two main types of pigment gallstones, black and brown.

Black pigment gallstones are composed of calcium bilirubinate and a network of mucin glycoproteins that interlace with salts such as calcium carbonate and/or calcium phosphate. These stones range in colour from deep black to very dark brown and have a glass-like cross-sectional surface on fracturing. Black pigment stones are seen in 40–60% of patients with haemolytic conditions such as sickle cell disease and hereditary spherocytosis in which there is chronic excess bilirubin production. However, the majority of pigment stones detected at the time of cholecystectomy are independent of excess haemolysis and are of unknown aetiology.

Brown stones are usually of a muddy hue and on cross-section seem to have alternating brown and tan layers. These stones are composed of calcium salts of fatty acids as well as calcium bilirubinate. They are almost always found in the presence of bile stasis and/or biliary infection. Brown stones are a common cause of recurrent bile duct stones following cholecystectomy

and may also be found in the intrahepatic ducts in circumstances of duct disease such as Caroli syndrome and primary sclerosing cholangitis. In the Far East such brown stones are identified both within the intra- and extrahepatic biliary tree and have been linked with chronic parasitic infection.

Clinical presentation of gallstones (Fig. 7.26)

The majority of gallstones are asymptomatic and remain so during a person's lifetime. Gallstones are increasingly detected as an incidental finding either at the time of abdominal radiography or ultrasound scanning. Over a 10- to 15-year period approximately 20% of these stones will be the cause of symptoms with 10% having severe complications (see below).

Biliary or gallstone colic

Biliary colic is the term used for the pain associated with the temporary obstruction of the cystic or common bile duct by a stone usually migrating from the gall bladder. Despite the term 'colic' the pain of stone-induced ductular obstruction is one of a severe but constant pain which has a crescendo characteristic. Many sufferers can relate the symptoms to over-indulgence with food, particularly when this has a high fat content. The most common time of day for such an episode is in the mid-evening and lasting until the early hours of the morning. The initial site of pain is usually in the epigastrium but there may be a right upper quadrant component. Radiation may occur over the right shoulder and right subscapular region. Nausea and vomiting frequently accompany the more severe attacks. The cessation of attack may be spontaneous after a number of hours or terminated by the administration of opiate analgesia. More protracted pain particularly when associated with fevers and rigors suggests secondary complications

Table 7.17
Risk factors for cholesterol gallstones

Increasing age	Drugs (e.g. contraceptive pill)
Sex (F > M)	Ileal disease or resection
Multiparity	Diabetes mellitus
Obesity	Acromegaly treated with octreotide
Rapid weight loss	Liver cirrhosis
Diet (e.g. high in animal fat)	

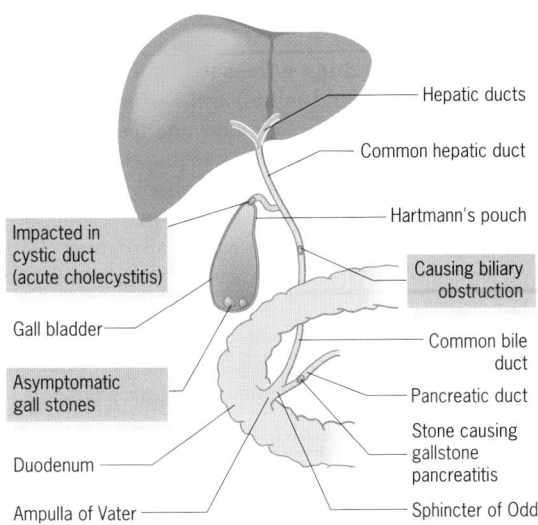

Fig. 7.26 Clinical presentation of gallstones.

such as cholecystitis, cholangitis or gallstone-related pancreatitis (see below).

Acute cholecystitis

The initial event in acute cholecystitis is obstruction to gall bladder emptying. In 95% of cases a gall bladder stone can be identified as the cause. Such obstruction results in an increase of gall bladder glandular secretion leading to progressive distension which in turn may compromise the vascular supply to the gall bladder. There is also an inflammatory response secondary to retained bile within the gall bladder. Infection is a secondary phenomena following the vascular and inflammatory events described above.

The initial clinical features of an episode of cholecystitis are similar to those of biliary colic described above. However, over a number of hours there is progression with severe localized right upper quadrant pain corresponding to parietal peritoneal involvement in the inflammatory process. The pain is associated with tenderness and muscle guarding or rigidity. Occasionally the gall bladder can become distended by pus (an empyema) and rarely an acute gangrenous cholecystitis develops which can perforate with generalized peritonitis.

Investigations

Biliary colic as a consequence of a stone in the neck of the gall bladder or cystic duct is unlikely to be associated with significant abnormality of laboratory tests. Acute cholecystitis is usually associated with a moderate leucocytosis and raised inflammatory markers (e.g. C-reactive protein).

- **The serum bilirubin, alkaline phosphatase and amino transferase** levels may be marginally elevated in the presence of cholecystitis alone even in the absence of bile duct obstruction. More significant elevation of the bilirubin and alkaline phosphatase is in keeping with bile duct obstruction.
- **An abdominal ultrasound scan** is the single most useful investigation for the diagnosis of gallstone-related disease (Fig. 7.27). Look for:
  - (a) *gallstones* within the gall bladder, particularly when these are obstructing the gall bladder neck or cystic duct
  - (b) *focal tenderness* over the underlying gall bladder
  - (c) *thickening of the gall bladder wall*. This may also be seen with hypoalbuminaemia, portal hypertension and acute viral hepatitis.

  Gallstones are a common finding in an ageing population and in the absence of specific symptoms great care should be taken as to whether the gallstones are responsible for the symptoms.
- **Iodida scintiscan** shows blockage of the cystic duct, with the bile duct but not the gall bladder being visualized. It is being replaced by ultrasound in most centres.

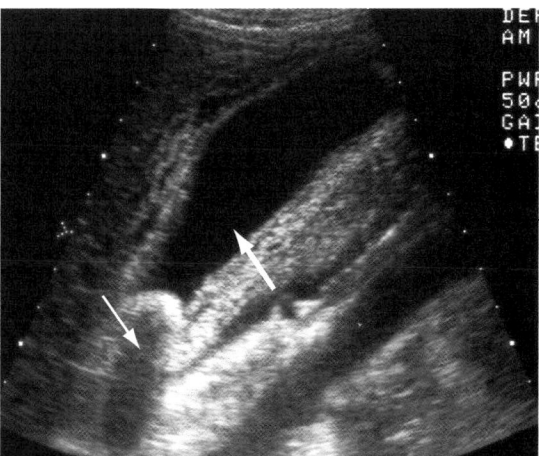

Fig. 7.27 **Ultrasound scan in a patient with acute cholecystitis.** There is a stone (casting an acoustic shadow – thin arrow) impacted in the gall bladder neck, with a distended gall bladder (thick arrow) and thickening and oedema of the gall bladder wall.

Differential diagnosis

With severe right upper quadrant pain acute cholecystitis is very likely. Acute pancreatitis, perforated peptic ulcer or intrahepatic abscess can give similar symptoms and signs. Conditions above the right diaphragm such as basal pneumonia as well as coronary insufficiency may on occasions mimic the clinical picture.

Colon spasm (see functional bowel disorders, p. 327) often presents with pain in the right hypochondrium; there is usually a history of recurrent episodes over a long period.

Other conditions that should be considered include atypical peptic ulcer disease and renal colic from the right kidney as well as low-grade pancreatitis.

Management of gall bladder stones

Cholecystectomy

Cholecystectomy is the treatment of choice for virtually all patients with *symptomatic* gall bladder stones. Cholecystectomy should not be performed in the absence of typical symptoms just because stones are found on investigation. The laparotomy approach to cholecystectomy has now been largely replaced by the laparoscopic technique. Postoperative pain is minimized with only a short period of ileus and the early ability to mobilize the patient. Laparoscopic cholecystectomy has been carried out on a day-care basis but more commonly requires a 48-hour admission. This has considerable cost benefits over open cholecystectomy, which is now reserved for a small proportion of patients with contraindications such as extensive previous upper abdominal surgery, ongoing bile duct obstruction or portal hypertension.

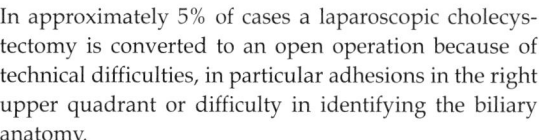

In approximately 5% of cases a laparoscopic cholecystectomy is converted to an open operation because of technical difficulties, in particular adhesions in the right upper quadrant or difficulty in identifying the biliary anatomy.

Acute cholecystitis. The initial management is conservative consisting of nil by mouth, intravenous fluids, opiate analgesia and intravenous antibiotics (e.g. cefotaxime).

Cholecystectomy is usually delayed for a few days to allow the symptoms to settle but can then be carried out quite safely in the majority of cases.

When the clinical situation fails to respond to this conservative management, particularly if there is increasing pain and fever, an empyema or gangrene of the gall bladder may have occurred. Urgent ultrasound is performed and urgent surgery will be required if these complications have developed.

Specific complications of cholecystectomy include a biliary leak either from the cystic duct or from the gall bladder bed. Injury to the bile duct itself occurs in up to 0.5% of laparoscopic operations and may have serious long-term sequelae in the form of biliary sepsis and secondary biliary liver injury.

Stone dissolution and shock wave lithotripsy

These *non-surgical techniques* for the management of gall bladder stones are infrequently used but are used in a highly selected group of patients who may not be fit for laparoscopic cholecystectomy.

Dissolution. Pure or near pure cholesterol stones can be solubilized by increasing the bile salt content of bile. Chenodeoxycholic acid and ursodeoxycholic acid are used. For dissolution to occur there must be a functioning gall bladder and optimally the stones should be almost pure cholesterol with a diameter of less than 10 mm. Using these criteria, only 20% of patients with gallstones will be eligible and even under such circumstances the time to achieve dissolution is often a matter of several months. There is also a high relapse rate when the drugs are discontinued. These limitations have restricted the application of this approach. Further benefit may be attained by the addition of an HMG-CoA reductase inhibitor (e.g. simvastatin) to a regimen of ursodeoxycholic acid. This will then combine reduced cholesterol content of bile as well an enhanced bile salt concentration but uses are still limited.

Extracorporeal shock wave lithotripsy. A shock wave can be directed either radiologically or by ultrasound on to gall bladder stones. This technique was highly successful but in only a restricted patient population. Fragmentation was limited to a small number of stones only and these had to be greater than 10 mm in diameter. The greater the calcium content of the stone the less likely the success of fragmentation. Gall bladder function has to be intact so the stone fragments can clear via the cystic duct.

The post-cholecystectomy syndrome

This refers to right upper quadrant pain often biliary in type which occurs a few months after the cholecystectomy but it may be delayed for a number of years. The patients often comment that the pain is identical to that for which the original operation was carried out. In many cases this syndrome is related to functional large bowel disease with colonic spasm at the hepatic flexure (hepatic flexure syndrome). In a few patients dysfunction of the sphincter of Oddi has been identified (the serum alkaline phosphatase is usually raised) and in such cases the abdominal pain responds to sphincterotomy.

Common bile duct stones

The classical features of common bile duct (CBD) stones are biliary colic, fever and jaundice (acute cholangitis). This triad is only present in the minority of patients. Abdominal pain is the most common symptom and has the typical features of biliary colic (see above). Jaundice is a variable accompaniment and is almost always preceded by abdominal pain. A patient with bile duct stones may experience sequential episodes of pain, only some of which are accompanied by jaundice. In contrast to malignant bile duct obstruction, the level of jaundice associated with CBD stones characteristically tends to fluctuate.

Fever is only present in a minority of cases but indicates biliary sepsis and sometimes an associated septicaemia. The presence of such biliary sepsis is a significant adverse prognostic factor.

A minority of patients with bile duct stones are discovered incidentally during imaging for gall bladder disease. Fifteen percent of patients undergoing cholecystectomy will have stones within the bile duct only detected at the time of operative cholangiography.

Physical examination

If the patient is examined between episodes there may be no abnormal physical finding. During a symptomatic episode the patient may be jaundiced with a fever and associated tachycardia. There may be tenderness in the right upper quadrant varying from mild to extremely severe.

More widespread abdominal tenderness extending from the epigastrium to the left upper quadrant, associated with distension, may indicate associated stone-related pancreatitis (see below).

Investigations
Laboratory tests
- *Full blood count* is usually normal in the presence of uncomplicated bile duct stones.
- *An elevated neutrophil count* as well as raised inflammatory markers (ESR and CRP) are frequent accompaniments of cholangitis.

- *The raised serum bilirubin* tends to be mild and often transient. Very high concentrations of bilirubin ($\cong 200$ μmol/L) almost always reflect complete bile duct obstruction.
- *Serum alkaline phosphatase and gamma glutamyl transpeptidase* are similarly elevated in proportion to the degree of hyperbilirubinaemia.
- *Aminotransferase levels* are usually mildly elevated but with complete bile duct obstruction they may rise to 10–15 times the normal value.
- *Serum amylase levels* are often mildly elevated in the presence of bile duct obstruction but are markedly so if stone-related pancreatitis has occurred.
- *Prothrombin time* may be prolonged if bile duct obstruction has occurred; this reflects decreased absorption of vitamin K.

Trans-abdominal ultrasound

This is the initial imaging technique of choice and in most cases the only imaging technique required.

Bile duct obstruction is characterized by dilatation of intrahepatic biliary radicals, which are usually easily detected by the ultrasound scan. It may, however, not be possible to identify the cause of obstruction. Stones situated in the distal common bile duct are poorly visualized by trans-abdominal ultrasound and up to 50% are missed. The detection of stones within the gall bladder

is poorly predictive as to the cause of bile duct obstruction. Asymptomatic gallstones are common (up to 15%) in patients in the cancer age group (65 years and older). Conversely, in 5–10% of patients with bile duct stones no calculi can be seen within the gall bladder.

Other imaging techniques

CT, usually with i.v. contrast is useful in patients (particularly obese) where the CBD pathology cannot be identified on ultrasound.

Magnetic resonance cholangiography (MRC) is an alternative non-invasive method for demonstrating the biliary tree (Fig. 7.28).

Endoscopic ultrasound scanning (Fig. 7.29) has enabled high-resolution imaging of the common bile duct, gall bladder and pancreas although unlike the preceding imaging techniques it is an invasive procedure. The endoscopic ultrasound probe can be brought into close proximity of the distal common bile duct and hence identify the majority of stones at this level.

This technique may be particularly useful for identifying small calculi (microcalculi).

Endoscopic retrograde cholangiography (ERC)

The endoscopic technique of ERC (p. 344) enables good visualization of the common bile duct. In experienced hands this will be successful in 98% of cases, providing good documentation of bile duct stones (Fig. 7.30). However microcalculi can still be missed.

ERC gives the therapeutic opportunity for sphincterotomy and stone extraction (see below).

Differential diagnosis

Cholangitis may occur independent of gallstones in conditions such as primary sclerosing cholangitis and Caroli's syndrome. On occasions cholangitis may accompany malignant bile duct obstruction. Jaundice may also accompany acute cholecystitis in the absence

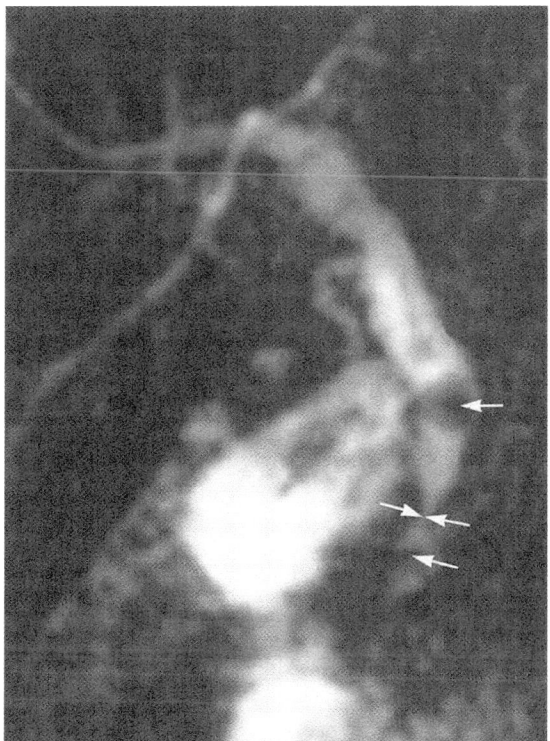

Fig. 7.28 **A magnetic resonance cholangiogram in a patient presenting with abdominal pain and jaundice.** This shows evidence of a distal common bile duct stricture (arrows) with a large gallstone proximal to this in the mid common bile duct (arrow).

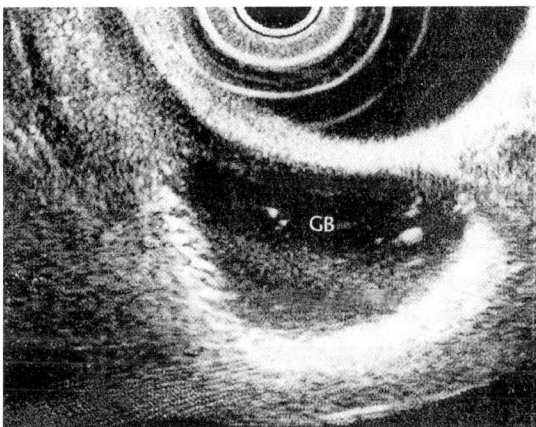

Fig. 7.29 **An endoscopic ultrasound scan** with the probe within the duodenum (upper margin of the figure) clearly demonstrating the gall bladder (GB) with multiple small stones within.

of bile duct stones. Common bile duct stones may produce pain but in the absence of jaundice, the differential diagnosis is that of biliary colic (see above).

Management

Acute cholangitis has a high morbidity and mortality particularly in the elderly age group. Successful management is dependent upon the introduction of intravenous antibiotics (e.g. i.v. cefotaxime), and urgent bile duct drainage is established by the use of the endoscopic retrograde approach (Fig. 7.30). Access to the bile duct is achieved by sphincterotomy and thereafter the bile duct stones can be removed either by balloon or basket catheters. In the severely ill patient a piece of plastic tubing (termed a stent) can be inserted into the bile duct to maintain bile drainage without the need to remove the stones, hence minimizing the time period to complete the procedure. The residual stones can then be removed endoscopically when the patient has recovered from the episode. In the presence of acute cholangitis surgical drainage has been associated with a high mortality and is now limited to those very few cases which cannot be managed by the endoscopic approach.

Endoscopic bile duct clearance is also the treatment of choice for patients with acute gallstone pancreatitis as well as patients who have retained common bile duct stones after a previous cholecystectomy.

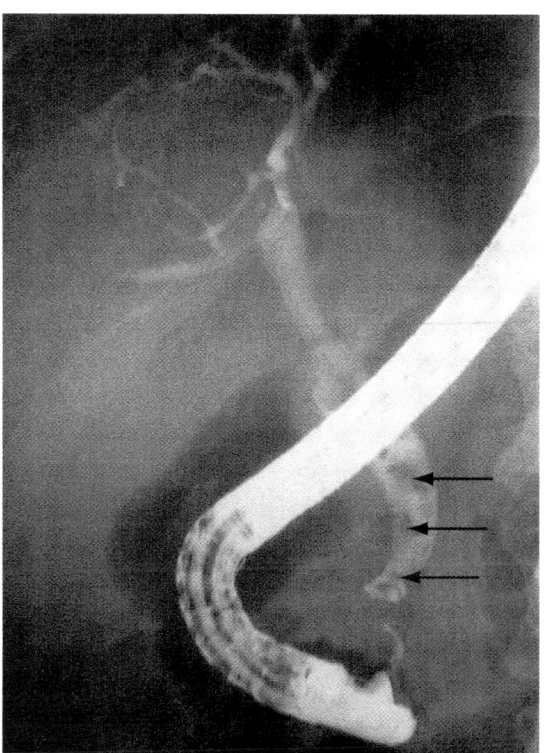

Fig. 7.30 An ERCP in a patient presenting with abdominal pain, jaundice and fever. Several stones can be seen within the dilated common bile duct (arrows).

Patients shown to have common bile duct stones as well as symptomatic gall bladder stones may be treated by two different approaches:

- *Laparoscopic cholecystectomy* which can also include exploration of the CBD via the cystic duct or by direct choledochotomy. By using these techniques the laparoscopist can extract stones from the common bile duct. This, however, prolongs the procedure, particularly in the presence of large stones or biliary sepsis.
- *Endoscopic approach* either immediately before or after the cholecystectomy. Removal of CBD stones by this method is the preferred way in the UK.

Complications of gallstones

- Acute cholecystitis and acute cholangitis have been discussed (p. 389).
- Gallstone-related pancreatitis is discussed on page 400.
- Gallstones can occasionally erode through the wall of the gall bladder into the intestine giving rise to a biliary enteric fistula. Passage of a gallstone through into the small bowel can give rise to an ileus or true obstruction.
- There is some evidence that gallstones are associated with an increased risk of adenocarcinoma of the gall bladder (p. 394).

Miscellaneous conditions of the biliary tract

Gall bladder

There are a number of non-calculous conditions of the gall bladder, some of which have been associated with symptoms.

Non-calculous cholecystitis

Almost 10% of gall bladders removed for biliary symptoms are shown to have chronic inflammation within the wall but an absence of gallstones. Such cases are described as non-calculous cholecystitis. In many instances the gall bladder inflammation is minor and of doubtful significance. In others the degree of inflammation is sufficient to account for the symptoms. In most cases the aetiology is not known but has been attributed to bile stasis as found in some diabetics as well as partial cystic duct obstruction.

Chemical inflammation of the gall bladder may also occur from reflux of pancreatic enzymes back into the biliary tree usually through the common channel at the ampulla of Vater.

Bacterial infection of the gall bladder has occasionally been recognized as a cause of chronic inflammation.

The decision to carry out cholecystectomy in the absence of defined gall bladder stones should be guided by the specific features of the history and whether there is evidence of diseased gall bladder wall on ultrasound scanning.

Cholesterolosis of the gall bladder

In cholesterolosis, cholesterol and other lipids are deposited in macrophages within the lamina propria of the gall bladder. These may be diffusely situated giving a granular appearance to the gall bladder wall or on occasions more discrete, giving a polypoid appearance (see below). Cholesterolosis of the gall bladder may coexist with gallstones but occurs independently. Some degree of cholesterolosis may be found in up to 25% of autopsies in an elderly population. It is doubtful whether this is a cause of symptoms.

Adenomyomatosis of the gall bladder

Adenomyomatosis is a gall bladder abnormality characterized by hyperplasia of the mucosa, thickening of the muscle wall and multiple intramural diverticulae (the so-called Rokitansky–Aschoff sinuses).

The condition is usually detected as an incidental finding during investigation for possible gall bladder disease. It has been suggested that this condition is secondary to increased intraluminal gall bladder pressure but this is not proven. Gallstones may frequently coexist but there is no evidence to support a direct relationship. It is unlikely that adenomyomatosis alone is a cause of biliary symptoms.

Chronic cholecystitis

There are no symptoms or signs that can conclusively be shown to be due to chronic cholecystitis. Symptoms attributed to this condition are vague, such as indigestion, upper abdominal discomfort or distension. There is no doubt that gallbladders studied histologically can show signs of chronic inflammation, and occasionally a small, shrunken gallbladder is found either radiologically or on ultrasound examination. However, these findings can be seen in asymptomatic people and therefore this clinical diagnosis should not be made. Most patients with chronic right hypochondrial pain suffer from functional bowel disease (p. 326).

Extrahepatic biliary tree

Primary sclerosing cholangitis

Primary sclerosing cholangitis (PSC) is a chronic cholestatic liver disease characterized by fibrosing inflammatory destruction of both the intra- and extra-hepatic bile ducts. In 75% of patients PSC is associated with inflammatory bowel disease (usually ulcerative colitis) but it is not unusual for the PSC to predate the onset of the inflammatory bowel disease. The causes are unknown but immunological mechanisms have been implicated. It is firmly established that genetic susceptibility to PSC is associated with the HLA A1-B8-DR3 haplotype. Seventy per cent of patients are men with an average age of onset of approximately 40 years.

With increasing screening of patients with inflammatory bowel disease PSC is detected at an asymptomatic phase with abnormal liver biochemistry, usually a raised serum alkaline phosphatase. Symptomatic presentation is usually with fluctuating pruritus, jaundice and cholangitis. The diagnosis is confirmed by a combination of endoscopic retrograde cholangiography (ERC), MRCP and liver biopsy. The cholangiogram characteristically shows both intra- and extrahepatic bile duct strictures, although either may be involved alone.

Liver histology shows inflammation of the intra-hepatic biliary radicals with considerable associated scar tissue classically described as being onion skin in appearance.

PSC is a slowly progressive lesion (symptoms and biochemical tests may fluctuate) ultimately leading to liver cirrhosis and associated decompensation. Cholangiocarcinoma is a well-recognized complication occurring in up to 20% of patients.

The only proven treatment is liver transplantation. The bile acid ursodeoxycholic acid has been evaluated extensively in PSC with some transient improvement in liver function but no evidence of proven long-term benefit.

Choledochal cyst

Congenital cystic disease of the bile ducts may occur at all levels of the biliary tree although the majority are extrahepatic. The dilatation may be saccular, diverticular or of fusiform configuration. The majority of symptomatic cases present in childhood with features of cholangitis. In adult life choledochal cysts may be a differential diagnosis in patients presenting with symptoms suggestive of bile duct stones. The cyst must be fully resected to avoid the recurrent biliary complications as well as averting the risk (approximately 15%) of subsequent bile duct cancer (cholangiocarcinoma).

Haemobilia

Haemobilia is the term used to describe bleeding into the biliary tree. This may be as a consequence of liver trauma or as a complication of liver surgery. Biopsy of the liver is also a well-recognized cause. The end result is a fistula between a branch of the hepatic artery and an intrahepatic bile duct.

Haemobilia may be a cause of significant gastro-intestinal blood loss and should be suspected when melaena is accompanied by right-sided upper abdominal pain and jaundice. However, the bleeding may occur

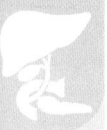

without any overt biliary symptoms. If the diagnosis is suspected bleeding may be managed by occlusion of the feeding artery by thrombosis performed radiologically. Some patients will require surgery to control the bleeding point.

Tumours of the biliary tract

Gall bladder polyps

Polyps of the gall bladder are a common finding, being seen in approximately 4% of all patients referred for hepatobiliary ultrasonography. The vast majority of these are small (less than 5 mm) and are non-neoplastic and are inflammatory in origin or composed of cholesterol deposits (see above). Adenomas are the most common benign neoplasm of the gall bladder. Only a proportion of these have a cancerous potential. The only reliable means of defining those at risks is by polyp size. Cholecystectomy is recommended for any polyp approximating to 1 cm in diameter or larger.

Primary cancer of the gall bladder

Adenocarcinoma of the gall bladder represents approximately 1% of all cancers. The mean age of occurrence is in the early sixties with a ratio of 3 women to 1 man. Gallstones have been suggested as an aetiological factor but this relationship remains unproven. Diffuse calcification of the gall bladder (porcelain gall bladder), considered to be the end stage of chronic cholecystitis has also been associated with cancer of the gall bladder and is an indication for early cholecystectomy. Adenomatous polyps of the gall bladder in excess of 1 cm in diameter are also recognized as premalignant lesions (see above).

Carcinoma of the gall bladder is often only detected at the time of planned cholecystectomy for gallstones and in such circumstances resection of an early lesion may be curative. Early lymphatic spread to the liver and adjacent biliary tract precludes curative resection in more advanced lesions. There are no proven chemotherapeutic agents for carcinoma of the gall bladder. A small proportion of cases are sensitive to radiotherapy but the overall 5-year survival is less than 5%.

Cholangiocarcinoma (see also p. 384)

Cancer of the biliary tree may be intra- or extrahepatic. These malignancies represent approximately 1% of all cancers. A number of associations have been identified such as that with choledochal cyst (see above), and chronic infection of the biliary tree with, for example, *Clonorchis sinensis*. There are also associations with autoimmune disease processes such as primary sclerosing cholangitis, and primary biliary cirrhosis. The bile duct malignancy usually presents with jaundice and may be suspected by imaging, initially ultrasound and thereafter spiral CT and in particular magnetic resonance cholangiopancreatography (MRCP). The disease spread is usually by local lymphatics or by local extension. Cholangiocarcinoma of the common bile duct may be resectable at presentation but local extension precludes such management in the majority of more proximal lesions. In the vast majority of cases treatment is palliative (see below).

Secondary malignant involvement of the biliary tree

Carcinoma of the head of the pancreas frequently presents with common bile duct obstruction and jaundice. Metastases to the bile ducts from distant cancers are uncommon. Melanoma is the most frequent neoplasm to do so.

Other carcinomas that have caused bile duct metastases, in order of frequency, are those arising in the lung, breast and colon as well as those from the pancreas (metastatic as compared to direct infiltration). Infiltration of the bile duct is not uncommon in disseminated lymphomatous disease.

Palliation of malignant bile duct obstruction

A small proportion of cholangiocarcinomas are surgically resectable, more commonly those in the distal bile duct as compared to the hilar region. All patients must be fully screened for operability using the imaging techniques described above. However, in the greater proportion of patients the treatment is palliative. The response to chemotherapy and radiation is poor in these tumours. Relief of bile duct obstruction has been shown to improve quality of life considerably and with pain control is the major end point of palliation. In recent years endoscopic techniques have allowed the insertion of stents into the biliary tree to re-established bile flow. The initial use of plastic stents has largely been replaced by self-expanding metal stents which have considerably longer periods of patency (Fig. 7.31). In the small proportion of patients in whom bile duct drainage is not possible endoscopically the percutaneous route offers an alternative method of stent placement.

FURTHER READING

Bree RL, Ralls PW, Balfe DM (2000) Evaluation of patients with acute right upper quadrant pain. American College of Radiology. ACR Appropriateness Criteria. *Radiology* **215** Suppl:153–157.

Dowling RH (2000) Review: pathogenesis of gallstones. *Alimentary Pharmacology and Therapeutics* 14 Suppl 2: 39–47.

Freeman ML, Nelson DB, Sherman S et al (1995) Complications of endoscopic biliary sphincterotomy. *New England Journal of Medicine* **225**: 909–917.

Grant AJ et al. (2002) Homing of mucosal lymphocytes to the liver in the pathogenesis of hepatic complications of inflammatory bowel disease. *Lancet* **359**: 150–157.

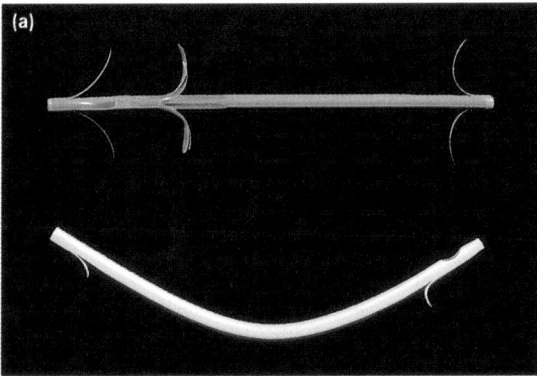

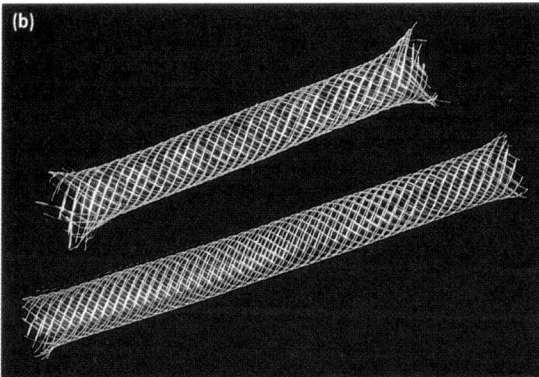

Fig. 7.31 Stents. (a) Plastic stents were the first means by which malignant bile duct obstruction could be relieved by the endoscopic approach. **(b)** The more recent introduction of self-expanding metal endoprostheses has provided more effective palliation.

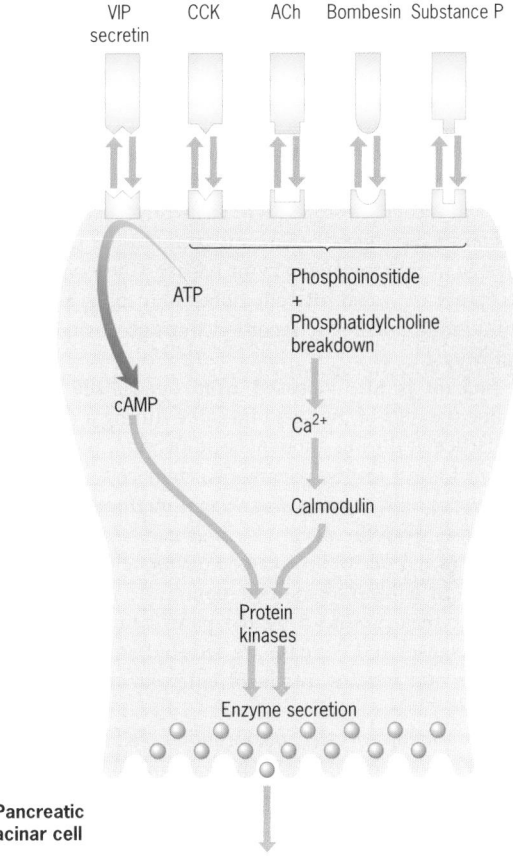

Fig. 7.32 Diagram showing stimulus–secretion coupling of pancreatic cell protein secretion. VIP, vasoactive intestinal polypeptide; CCK, cholecystokinin; ACh, acetylcholine.

The pancreas

Structure and function

Structure

The pancreas extends retroperitoneally across the posterior abdominal wall from the second part of the duodenum to the spleen. The head is encircled by the duodenum; the body, which forms the main bulk of the organ, ends in a tail that lies in contact with the spleen. The pancreas consists of exocrine and endocrine cells making up 98% of the human pancreas.

The pancreatic acinar cells are grouped into lobules forming the ductal system which eventually joins into the main pancreatic duct.

The main pancreatic duct has many tributary ductules and gradually tapers towards the tail of the pancreas. The main pancreatic duct itself usually joins the common bile duct to enter the duodenum as a short single duct at the ampulla of Vater.

Exocrine function

The pancreatic acinar cells are responsible for production of digestive enzymes. These include amylase, lipase, colipase, phospholipase and the proteases (trypsinogen and chymotrypsinogen). These enzymes are stored within the acinar cells in secretory granules and are released by exocytosis (Fig. 7.32).

After ingestion of a meal pancreatic exocrine secretion is regulated by cephalic, gastric, and intestinal stimuli. The *cephalic* phase is mediated by the central nervous system and is stimulated by behavioural cues related to the sight and smell of food. With ingestion of food, the *gastric* phase commences and in response to distension of the stomach a neural pathway involving the central nervous system stimulates pancreatic secretion. Both these phases are under vagal control.

Finally the presence of protein, fat and gastric acid within the small *intestine* further augments pancreatic secretion by both hormonal and neurotransmitter activity which produces local enteropancreatic control of secretion. Feedback regulatory events eventually terminate pancreatic secretion.

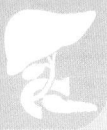
Cholecystokinin is produced in specialized gut endocrine cells (I cells) of the mucosa of the small intestine and is secreted in response to intraluminal food. It exerts its biological activity by binding to specific G-protein-coupled receptors on target cells in the pancreas. Activated G-proteins lead to the activation of phospholipases. This in turn leads to calcium release from intracellular stores, which in turn results in the fusion of the digestive enzyme granules to the apical plasma membrane and enzyme release. Cholecystokinin receptors on vagal afferent fibres may play a role in stimulating pancreatic secretion through a vago-vagal pathway.

Secretin is also released from specialized entero-endocrine cells of the small intestine during a meal and in particular during duodenal acidification. Secretin has a direct effect on the pancreatic acinar cells as well as the ductal cells. There is also a vagal-mediated secretory response. Secretin action is mediated via G-coupled receptors and calcium-mediated enzyme release. Secretin results in a bicarbonate-rich pancreatic secretion. Of the enzymes produced by the pancreatic acinar cells, the proteases and colipase are secreted as inactive precursors and require duodenal enterokinase to initiate activity.

Completion of the postprandial secretory phase involves both neural and hormonal control.

Central neuronal inhibition of pancreatic secretion acts through dopamine and somatostatin receptors mediated by noradrenergic nerves. The islet cell hormone pancreatic polypeptide is released from the pancreas in response to a meal and has an inhibitory effect upon acinar enzyme secretion both by a local effect and via central receptors.

Somatostatin, present within the pancreas, stomach and central nervous system, is released in response to food. Its effect is mediated both by direct pancreatic acinar inhibition and by a central nervous system effect. Two other mechanisms of inhibition have been described. Proteases within the duodenal lumen have a negative feedback on acinar secretion. Secondly, nutrients within the ileum inhibit pancreatic secretion by means of local hormone release (peptide YY and glucagon-like peptide) acting on the acinar cells themselves as well as centrally.

The endocrine pancreas

This consists of hormone-producing cells arranged in nests or islets (islets of Langerhans). The hormones produced are secreted directly into the circulation and there is no access to the pancreatic ductular system. There are *five main types of islet cell* corresponding to different secretory components. The beta-cells are the most common and are responsible for insulin production. The alpha-cells produce glucagon. The D cells produce somatostatin, PP-cells produce pancreatic polypeptide and enterochromaffin cells produce serotonin.

A number of other hormones have been identified within the endocrine pancreas including gastrin-releasing peptide, neuropeptide Y and galanin. These are believed to be neurotransmitters active in the neuro-gastrointestinal axis.

Investigations

Assessment of exocrine function

Overt fat malabsorption does not occur until approximately 85–90% of the function has been lost. This large reserve of pancreatic function means that any pancreatic function test based upon the measurement of either the pancreatic enzymes or their breakdown products is insensitive.

Duodenal sampling and pancreatic function tests

These tests rely upon the analysis of a duodenal aspirate following pancreatic stimulation.

The original test involved the oral administration of a specified meal (Lundh meal). Pancreatic stimulation is now achieved by intravenous secretin and cholecystokinin. The aspirate is assessed for pancreatic enzymes and bicarbonate production.

The procedure is time-consuming and requires a meticulous technique. There is a good correlation with moderate to severe pancreatic function loss, but not for mild damage.

Non-invasive test of pancreatic function

Serum biochemistry. Serum lipase, trypsin–trypsinogen and amylase can all be measured. Serum trypsin is the most useful although diminished levels are only detected after pancreatic insufficiency is clinically detectable by overt malabsorption. Their main use is in acute pancreatitis.

Faecal tests

- *Faecal fat estimation* (see p. 290).
- *Faecal chymotrypsin.* Recent refinements in the assay have revealed a good discriminatory capacity between those with normal and severely impaired pancreatic function. The test is not useful until severe impairment is present.
- *Faecal elastase.* This pancreatic specific enzyme is not degraded in the intestine and has high concentrations within the faeces. Diminished levels may be detected in moderate as well as severe pancreatic insufficiency and is probably more sensitive than other serum and faecal tests.

Oral pancreatic function tests

- *PABA-test.* Oral N-benzoyl-L-tyrosyl-p-aminobenzoic acid is hydrolized by chymotrypsin to release p-aminobenzoic acid (PABA), which is then absorbed, conjugated and excreted in the urine where it can be measured. The test is time-consuming but is specific for pancreatic insufficiency, with a 65–80% sensitivity.

- *Fluorescein dilaurate test.* Oral fluorescein dilaurate is digested by pancreatic esterase to release the fluorescein which is then absorbed and excreted in the urine. This test is relatively inexpensive and commercially available as the 'Pancreolauryl test'. This is highly sensitive and specific in severe pancreatic insufficiency but has only a 50% sensitivity in mild to moderate disease.

Clinical application of pancreatic function tests

Whilst the invasive duodenal aspiration tests represent the most sensitive and specific means of assessing pancreatic function, these are very rarely used outside specialized centres. The Pancreolauryl and PABA tests are non-invasive and are widely available but are only highly sensitive in the detection of severe pancreatic insufficiency. Recent evidence suggest that the faecal elastase test (in a commercially available form) may provide similar sensitivity and specificity and may represent the test of choice as a screening tool for pancreatic insufficiency, but again detection of mild disease is problematic.

Pancreatic imaging (see p. 342)

This can detect structural abnormalities even when functional tests are still within normal limits.

- A *plain abdominal radiograph* may show pancreatic calcification, particularly when alcohol is the aetiology.
- *Ultrasound* of the pancreas is a useful screening investigation for inflammation and neoplasia. Views may be limited by overlying bowel gas.
- *Spiral CT scan* with contrast enhancement is more reliable.
- *MRI scanning* represents an alternative to CT. Magnetic resonance cholangiopancreatography (MRCP) gives clear definition of the pancreatic duct as well as the biliary tree. Gallstones (including microcalculi) may also be identified in the biliary tree using MRI/MRCP.
- *Endoscopic ultrasound* is very useful for identifying distal common bile duct stones as well as a microcalculi either within the duct or within the gall bladder. Small space-occupying lesions may also be identified.
- *Endoscopic retrograde cholangiopancreatography (ERCP)* has been considered a gold standard modality for defining pancreatic disease. However, with improving imaging techniques ERCP is now more likely to be restricted to therapeutic intervention.

Summary. An initial transabdominal ultrasound supplemented by spiral CT provides sufficient diagnostic information for most inflammatory and neoplastic conditions of the pancreas. MRI and MRCP are now widely available and provide additional information,

particularly with respect to pancreatic ductular and biliary anatomy.

Endoscopic ultrasound is available in specialized centres if diagnostic information is still lacking.

Pancreatitis

Classification

Pancreatitis is divided into acute and chronic. By definition acute pancreatitis is a process that occurs on the background of a previously normal pancreas and can return to normal after resolution of the episode. In chronic pancreatitis there is continuing inflammation with irreversible structural changes.

In practice the differentiation between acute and chronic pancreatitis may be extremely difficult, particularly in the setting of recurrent acute episodes which may represent true acute pancreatitis or may be a manifestation of underlying chronic disease.

Acute pancreatitis

The causes of acute pancreatitis are listed in Table 7.18.

In the western world gallstones and alcohol account for the vast majority of episodes. Alcohol also has a high propensity to produce chronic pancreatitis (see below). The severity of the pancreatitis may range from mild and self-limiting to extremely severe with extensive pancreatic and peripancreatic necrosis as well as haemorrhage. In its most severe form the mortality rises to between 40–50%.

Pathogenesis

Mechanisms by which pancreatic necrosis occurs remain speculative. Any theory must take into account how a very diverse group of aetiological factors can produce the same end point. There is some suggestion that the final common pathway is a marked elevation of intracellular calcium which in turn leads to activation of

---

Table 7.18
Causes of pancreatitis

Acute	Chronic
Gallstones	Alcohol
Alcohol	Tropical (nutritional)
Infections	Hereditary
(e.g. mumps, Coxsackie B)	Trypsinogen and inhibitory
Pancreatic tumours	protein defects
Drugs (e.g. azathioprine,	Cystic fibrosis membrane
oestrogens, corticosteroids)	regulator defects
Iatrogenic	Idiopathic
(e.g. post-surgical, ERCP)	Trauma
Hyperlipidaemias	Hypercalcaemia
Miscellaneous	
Trauma	
Scorpion bite	
Cardiac surgery	
Idiopathic	

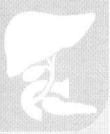

intracellular proteases. It is these activated enzymes which are responsible for cellular necrosis.

In the case of gallstone-related pancreatitis it is believed stones occlude the pancreatic drainage at the level of the ampulla leading to pancreatic ductular hypertension. Such ductular hypertension has been shown in animal models to increase cytosolic free ionized calcium. There is also evidence that alcohol interferes with calcium homeostasis in pancreatic acinar cells.

Clinical features

Acute pancreatitis is a differential diagnosis in any patient with upper abdominal pain. The pain usually begins in the epigastrium accompanied by nausea and vomiting. As inflammation spreads throughout the peritoneal cavity the pain becomes more intense. Involvement of the retroperitoneum frequently leads to back pain.

The patient may give a history of previous similar episodes or be known to have gallstones. An attack may follow an alcoholic binge. However, in many cases there are no obvious aetiological factors.

Physical examination at the time of presentation may show little more than a patient in pain with some upper abdominal tenderness but no systemic abnormalities. In more severe disease the patient may have a tachycardia, hypotension and be oliguric. Abdominal examination may show widespread tenderness with guarding as well as reduced or absent bowel sounds. Specific clinical signs that support a diagnosis of severe necrotizing pancreatitis include periumbilical (Cullen's sign) and flank bruising (Grey Turner's sign). In patients with a gallstone aetiology the clinical picture may also include the features of cholangitis, in particular jaundice (Table 7.19).

Diagnosis
Blood tests

- *Serum amylase level* is the standard laboratory test carried out to confirm the diagnosis. If this is measured within 24 hours of the onset of pain an elevation of three times the upper limit of normal is an extremely sensitive test. A number of other conditions may occasionally cause a very elevated amylase (see Table 7.20). Amylase levels gradually fall back towards normal over the next 3–5 days. With a late presentation the serum amylase level may give a false-negative result.
- *Urinary amylase* levels may be diagnostic as these remain elevated over a longer period of time.
- *Serum lipase levels* are also raised in acute pancreatitis and these remain elevated for a longer period of time than those of amylase. However, overall, the accuracy of serum lipase is not significantly greater than amylase and it is technically more difficult to measure.
- *Other baseline investigations* include a full blood count and CRP, urea and electrolytes, blood glucose, liver

Table 7.19
Complications of acute pancreatitis

Pancreatic	Systemic
Acute fluid collection	Metabolic
Necrosis	Malnutrition
Pseudocyst	Hypocalcaemia
Abscess	Hyperglycaemia
Ascites	Haematological
	Disseminated intravascular
Intestinal	coagulation
Paralytic ileus	Portal vein thrombosis
GI haemorrhage	Renal
	Acute renal failure
Hepatobiliary	Cardiovascular
Jaundice	Circulatory failure (shock)
Obstruction of CBD	Respiratory
Portal vein thrombosis	Hypoxic acute respiratory
	failure

Table 7.20
Elevations in serum amylase unrelated to pancreatitis

Leakage of upper gastrointestinal contents into the peritoneum
Upper gastrointestinal perforation
Biliary peritonitis
Intestinal infarction

Inherited abnormalities of amylase
Macroamylasaemia

biochemistry, plasma calcium and arterial blood gases. These are documented at presentation and then repeated at 24 and 48 hours and provide a basis for assessing the severity of an attack (see below).

Radiology
- An erect *chest X-ray* is mandatory to exclude gastroduodenal perforation, which also raises the serum amylase (Table 7.20). A supine abdominal film may show gallstones or pancreatic calcification.
- An *abdominal ultrasound scan* is used as a screening test to identify a possible biliary (gallstone) cause of pancreatitis. Gallstones are difficult to detect in the distal common bile duct but dilated intrahepatic ducts may be present in the presence of bile duct obstruction. Stones within the gall bladder are not sufficient to justify a diagnosis of gallstone-related pancreatitis. The ultrasound may also demonstrate pancreatic swelling and necrosis as well as peripancreatic fluid collections if present. In severe pancreatitis the pancreas may be difficult to visualize because of gas-filled loops of bowel.
- *Contrast-enhanced spiral CT scanning* is essential in all but the most mild attacks of pancreatitis. It detects the swelling of the pancreas and the presence of pancreatic necrosis and peripancreatic fluid collections (Fig. 7.33). The degree of pancreatic enhancement following contrast has been used as a means of assessing the extent of pancreatic injury.

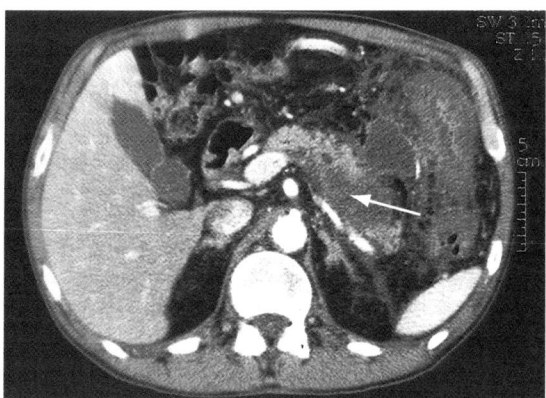

Fig. 7.33 **CT scan in patient with acute pancreatitis** showing necrosis of the pancreatic parenchyma (arrow) and a fluid collection extending outside the gland with inflammatory thickening of the colon.

- *MRI (MRCP)* is increasingly being used to assess the degree of pancreatic damage and also as a means of identifying gallstones within the biliary tree. MRI is particularly useful to differentiate between fluid and solid inflammatory masses.
- *ERCP* is used as a treatment measure to remove bile duct stones in the presence of gallstone-related pancreatitis (see below).

Assessment of disease severity

The majority of cases of acute pancreatitis are mild but approximately 25% run a more complicated course which may result in haemodynamic instability and multiple organ failure. The early prediction of such a severe attack allows appropriate monitoring and intensive care to be in place.

Early clinical assessment has been shown to have poor sensitivity for predicting a severe attack. Similarly individual laboratory tests have very limited value. To improve the predictive value multiple factors have been used to develop scoring systems (see Table 7.21). The Ranson and Glasgow scoring systems are based on such parameters and have been shown to have an 80% sensitivity for predicting a severe attack, although only after 48 hours following presentation. The acute physiology and chronic health evaluation score (APACHE) has been extensively adopted as a means of assessing the severity of a wide spectrum of illness (see Ch. 15). This scoring system appears to have a high sensitivity as early as 24 hours after onset of symptoms.

There is recent evidence that obesity predicts the outcome from an episode of pancreatitis. It is likely that the excessive adipose tissue is a substrate for activated enzyme activity. This will in turn generate an extensive inflammatory reaction.

Even modest obesity (basal metabolic index between 25–30) has an adverse affect. This is now being incorporated as an adverse factor in the APACHE score (p. 954) for acute pancreatitis.

Table 7.21
Factors during the first 48 hours that indicate severe pancreatitis and a poor prognosis

Age	> 55 years
WBC	$> 15 \times 10^9$/L
Blood glucose	> 10 mmol/L
Serum urea	> 16 mmol/L
Serum albumin	< 30 g/L
Serum aminotransferase	> 200 U/L
Serum calcium	< 2 mmol/L
Serum LDH	> 600 U/L
P_aO_2	< 8.0 kPa (60 mmHg)

LDH, lactate dehydrogenase

Treatment

The initial management of acute pancreatitis is similar, whatever the cause. The APACHE scoring system (modified by an obesity factor) should be carried out at the end of the first 24 hours after presentation to allow identification of the 25% of patients with a predicted severe attack. This should be repeated at 48 hours to identify a further subgroup who appear to be moving into the severe category. These patients should then be managed on a high-dependency or intensive care unit. Even patients outside of the severe category may require considerable supportive care.

Fluid losses in acute pancreatitis are often large requiring well-maintained intravenous access as well as a central line and urinary catheter to monitor circulating volume and renal function.

- *Nasogastric suction* prevents abdominal distension and vomitus and hence the risk of aspiration pneumonia.
- *Baseline arterial blood gases* determine the need for continuous oxygen administration.
- *Prophylactic antibiotics.* Broad-spectrum antibiotics, e.g. cefuroxime or imipenem, reduce the risk of infective complications and are given from the outset.
- *Analgesia requirements.* Pethidine and tramadol are the drugs of choice, usually administered by a patient control system. The morphine derivatives should be avoided because of their propensity to cause sphincter of Oddi contraction.
- *Feeding.* In patients with a severe episode there is little likelihood of oral nutrition for a number of weeks. Total parenteral nutrition has been associated with a high risk of infection and has been replaced by enteral nutrition. This is administered via a nasojejunal tube which is well tolerated and can maintain adequate nutritional input. The nasojejunal position of the feeding tube placed endoscopically overcomes the frequent problem of gastric paresis and there is less likelihood of pancreatic stimulation.

There has been a tendency to instigate total parenteral nutrition in such patients but this has been associated with a high risk of infection. There is now evidence to

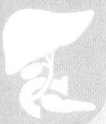

suggest that enteral nutrition administered via a naso-jejunal tube is well tolerated and can maintain adequate nutritional input. The nasojejunal position of the feeding tube overcomes the frequent problem of gastric paresis and there is less likelihood of pancreatic stimulation.

In a small proportion of patients multiorgan failure will develop in the first few days after presentation reflecting the extent of pancreatic necrosis. Such patients will require positive-pressure ventilation and often renal support. The mortality in this group is extremely high (in excess of 80%).

Gallstone-related pancreatitis

In patients with gallstone-related pancreatitis an ERCP, sphincterotomy and stone extraction may improve the outcome in all patients with cholangitis in association with acute pancreatitis. In the absence of cholangitis, sphincterotomy and stone extraction is only of proven benefit when the episode of pancreatitis is predicted as severe. In less severe cases of gallstone-related pancreatitis intervention can be deferred until full recovery is obtained (an approximate 6-week period).

Late complications of acute pancreatitis

Within the first 7 days the morbidity and mortality of acute pancreatitis reflects the systemic inflammatory response which in turn results in multiple organ failure. After this initial period the prognosis thereafter is most closely related to the extent of pancreatic necrosis. This can be most accurately assessed by contrast-enhanced CT, which should be carried out in all patients with severe disease after the first week. Extensive necrosis (greater than 50% of the pancreas) is associated with high risk of further complicated disease frequently requiring surgical intervention.

It is infection of the necrotic pancreas which is of most concern and which may rapidly lead to overwhelming sepsis. Prophylactic antibiotics have been used to prevent this but do not reliably do so. If there is evidence of incipient infection monitored by a rising neutrophil count and CRP level, an aspirate of the necrotic pancreas is taken and cultured. The vast majority of patients with a positive culture should be considered for surgical resection of the necrotic pancreas. In the most severe cases multiple operations are required to fully resect the areas of necrosis.

Peripancreatic fluid collections are common in the early stages of acute pancreatitis, the vast majority of which will resolve spontaneously.

Some fluid collections will be surrounded by granulation tissue producing the so-called *pseudocyst*. These by definition are not found until 6 weeks after the onset of the illness. The smaller pseudocysts (less then 6 cm in diameter) frequently resolve on their own but others may persist in the long term, giving rise to potential complications such as infection and intraperitoneal bleeding. Larger pseudocysts persisting for longer than 6 weeks are usually actively managed by either percutaneous (or endoscopic) drainage or by surgical intervention.

Long-term outcome

The vast majority of patients with a mild to moderate episode of acute pancreatitis will make a full recovery with no long-term sequelae. Recurrent episodes of pancreatitis may occur, particularly if there has been any long-term pancreatic ductular damage. Patients with more severe acute pancreatitis may become pancreatic insufficient both with respect to exocrine (malabsorption) and endocrine function (diabetes).

Chronic pancreatitis

Aetiology

In developed countries by far the most common cause of chronic pancreatitis is alcohol, accounting for 60–80% of cases (see Table 7.18).

In developing countries malnutrition and associated dietary factors have been implicated. In a small group of patients chronic pancreatitis has been shown to be hereditary, inherited as an autosomal dominant condition with variable penetrance. Almost all patients with cystic fibrosis (p. 402) have established chronic pancreatitis, usually from birth. Cystic fibrosis gene mutations have also been identified in patients with chronic pancreatitis but in whom there were no other manifestations of cystic fibrosis.

Obstruction of the pancreatic duct because of either a benign or malignant process may result in chronic pancreatitis. Controversy remains as to whether congenital abnormalities of the pancreatic duct such as pancreas divisum are aetiological factors.

Pathogenesis

A possible common pathway for pancreatic damage is the inappropriate activation of enzymes within the pancreas. This has been well demonstrated in the case of hereditary pancreatitis where genetic abnormalities of cationic trypsinogen and its inhibitory proteins have led to unopposed trypsin activity within the pancreas itself. Chronic alcohol intake is also believed to increase the level of trypsinogen relative to its inhibitor. Human trypsinogen has a propensity to autoactivate and any relative impairment or deficiency of inhibitor proteins will lead to unopposed enzyme activity and possible pancreatic damage.

It is believed that the intrapancreatic enzyme activity leads to the precipitation of proteins within the duct lumen in the form of plugs. These then form a nidus for calcification but are also the cause of ductal obstruction leading to ductal hypertension and further pancreatic damage. Cytokine activation and oxygen stress are thought to play a role in perpetuating this process.

Clinical features

Pain is the most common presentation of chronic pancreatitis and is usually epigastric and often radiating through into the back. The pattern of pain may be episodic with short periods of severe pain or chronic unremitting. Exacerbations of the pain may follow further alcohol excess although this is not a uniform relationship. During periods of abdominal pain anorexia is common and weight loss may be severe. This is particularly so in those patients with chronic unremitting symptoms.

Exocrine and endocrine insufficiency may develop at any time and occasionally malabsorption or diabetes are the presenting features in the absence of abdominal pain.

Jaundice secondary to common bile duct obstruction during its course through the fibrosed head of pancreas, may also occur and may be a presenting feature in a small proportion of patients.

Investigations

The extent to which investigations are required is dependent upon the clinical setting. In a patient with known alcohol abuse and typical pain few confirmatory tests are required.

- *Serum amylase and lipase* levels are rarely significantly elevated in established chronic pancreatitis.
- *Faecal elastase* level will be abnormal in the majority of patients with moderate to severe pancreatic disease.
- *PABA and Pancreolauryl tests* (see p. 396).
- *Transabdominal ultrasound scan* is used for initial assessment.
- *Contrast-enhanced spiral CT scan* provides a more detailed assessment. In the presence of pancreatic calcification and a dilated pancreatic duct the diagnosis of chronic pancreatitis can be easily established (Fig. 7.34). This may be much more difficult when these features are not present and in particular with an atypical presentation such as with steatorrhoea alone.
- *MRI with MRCP* is increasingly utilized to define more subtle abnormalities of the pancreatic duct which may be seen in non-dilated chronic pancreatitis.
- *Endoscopic ultrasound* is used in a small proportion of patients in whom the diagnosis is not confirmed with the above imaging or specifically for assessing complications of chronic pancreatitis including pseudocyst formation.
- *Diagnostic ERCP* has largely been replaced by MRCP.

Differential diagnosis

The differential diagnosis is that of pancreatic malignancy. Carcinoma of the pancreas can reproduce many of the symptoms and imaging abnormalities that are commonly seen with chronic pancreatitis. The diagnosis of malignancy should be considered in patients with a short history and in whom there is a localized ductular abnormality. Considerable difficulties may arise when a malignancy develops on the background of established chronic pancreatitis (the latter being a recognized premalignant lesion).

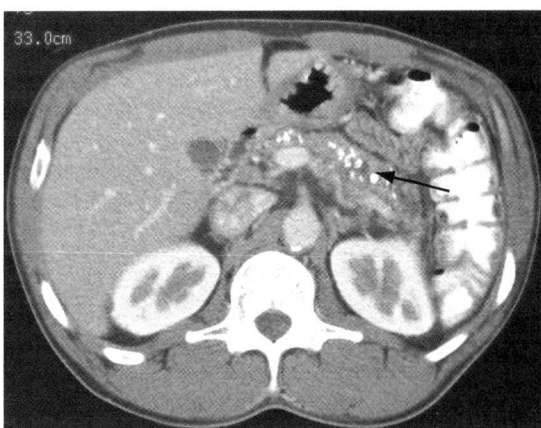

Fig. 7.34 Contrast-enhanced CT scan demonstrating multiple calcific densities (arrow) along the line of the main pancreatic duct in a patient with chronic pancreatitis.

High-quality imaging is able to define malignant features with a localized mass lesion, local invasion and lymph node enlargement. Endoscopic ultrasound may provide the most accurate assessment of a potential mass lesion.

Treatment

In patients with alcohol-related chronic pancreatitis long-term abstinence is likely to be of benefit although this has been difficult to prove.

Abdominal pain

For short-term flare-ups of pain a combination of a non-steroidal anti-inflammatory drug and an opiate (tramadol) is usually sufficient for symptomatic relief. In patients with chronic unremitting pain this may be inadequate and also risk opiate addiction.

Tricyclic antidepressants (e.g. amitriptyline) are used for chronic pain and reduce the need for opiates. Oral pancreatic enzyme supplements reduce pancreatic stimulation (by a negative-feedback mechanism) and hence the intensity of pain. Antioxidant use awaits evidence of benefit. Coeliac axis nerve block may produce good pain relief but is unreliable in its extent and duration of action.

In the majority of patients some spontaneous improvement in pain control occurs with time. After a 6- to 10-year period some 60% of patients will become pain-free. For patients with debilitating pain, surgical intervention is justified. Both duct drainage and limited resection procedures have been carried out with total or partial pain relief in approximately 80% of patients but with a mortality of 5%.

Other endoscopic techniques used to improve pancreatic drainage as well as managing intraductal stones have been tried with variable success.

Endocrine and exocrine insufficiency may occur. The steatorrhoea associated with pancreatic insufficiency may be large, with up to 30 mmol of fat lost

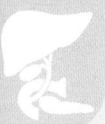
in the stool per 24 hours. This will usually respond well to pancreatic enzymes supplements. Current preparations are presented in the form of microspheres which reduce the problems of acid degradation in the stomach. An acid suppressor (H_2-receptor antagonist or proton pump inhibitor) is also given. Despite this, a proportion of patients continue to malabsorb usually reflecting the inadequate mixing of the pancreatic supplements with the food as well as the low pH in the duodenum secondary to inadequate pancreatic bicarbonate production.

The diabetes associated with pancreatic endocrine failure may be difficult to control with a rapid progression from oral hypoglycaemic agents to an insulin requirement. Brittle control is a common probably secondary to inadequate glucagon production from the damaged pancreas.

Complications

The most common structural complication of chronic pancreatitis is a pancreatic pseudocyst, which is where a fluid collection is surrounded by granulation tissue (see p. 400). These usually occur in relationship to a period of enhanced inflammatory activity within the pancreas giving abdominal pain but may develop silently during what would appear to be a stable phase. More acute presentations include intra- or retroperitoneal rupture, bleeding or cyst infection. The larger cyst may occlude nearby structures including the duodenum and the bile duct, thereby producing predictable symptoms. In patients in whom complications have occurred surgical management is almost always required. In pseudocysts less than 6 cm in diameter, spontaneous resolution can be anticipated. In larger cysts that have been present for a period in excess of 6 weeks, resolution is uncommon and the majority will require surgical or endoscopic drainage.

Ascites and occasionally pleural effusions can be a direct consequence of chronic pancreatitis when there has been disruption of the main pancreatic duct. The most important aspect of diagnosis is to suspect chronic pancreatitis as the cause, then an extremely high ascites or pleural fluid amylase will confirm the aetiology. Such disruptions of the main pancreatic duct will also require surgical intervention.

Cystic fibrosis (see pp. 180 and 871)

This common cause of pancreatic disease in childhood is inherited as an autosomal recessive. A specific gene mutation ΔF_{508} is present in 70% of cases. The gene(s) code for a membrane protein in epithelial cells which regulates chloride transport (the cystic fibrosis transmembrane regular CFTR). Defective transport of chloride across epithelial membranes leads to dehydrated secretions as water follows chloride movement. Pancreatic ducts become blocked by inspissated mucus secretion preventing enzyme production.

Clinical features and diagnosis

Clinical features and diagnostic tests are described on p. 871 in Chapter 14. Pancreatic function tests and imaging are described on p. 396.

Treatment

The main symptoms arising from pancreatic deficiency are steatorrhoea and malnutrition. Treatment is to improve nutrition and reduce steathorroea with pancreatic supplements. A high calorie intake (150% of recommended daily allowance) with vitamin supplements should be given. Pancreatic supplements which are enteric coated deliver a high enzyme concentration in the duodenum. Antacids or H_2 receptor antagonists are sometimes given to prevent inactivation by gastric juice. Fibrosing colonopathy with stricture formation has been reported in young children on these high-dose pancreatic preparations. Current recommendations are that the daily dose of lipase should not exceed 10 000 units of lipase per kg of body weight.

Carcinoma of the pancreas

The incidence of pancreatic cancer in the West has been estimated at approximately 9 cases per 100 000 and this has shown no tendency to increase over the last 20 years. Pancreatic cancer is now the fifth most common cause of cancer death in the western world. The incidence increases with age and the majority of cases occur in patients over the age of 60. Approximately 60% of patients with this condition are male. It has proved difficult to identify environmental risk factors but smoking is associated with a twofold increase. Other possible environmental factors include the petroleum product, naphthalamine. Chronic pancreatitis has been documented as a potential precancerous lesion. There is increasing evidence that pancreatic ductal adenocarcinoma is a result of accumulated genetic alterations. Subtle changes in an oncogene and both mutations and deletions of tumour suppressor genes are the most common forms of genetic alteration. The best known among the oncogenes is K-*ras*, present in 90% of human ductal adenocarcinomas. Other oncogenes include β-*catenin*. Tumour suppressor genes include *p16*, *p53* and *DPC4*.

Clinical picture

Pancreatic adenocarcinoma may be viewed clinically as two diseases – the lesions of the head and lesions of the body and tail.

Symptoms

Carcinoma of the head of pancreas or the *ampulla of Vater* tends to present earlier with obstruction to the bile duct as this passes through the head of pancreas giving jaundice. These more localized lesions are usually painless, although pain may become a feature with tumour progression. *Carcinoma localized to the body or tail* of the pancreas is much more likely to present with abdominal pain as well as non-specific symptoms such as anorexia and weight loss. The pain is often dull in character with radiation through into the back. A characteristic feature is partial relief of pain by sitting forward. Bile duct obstruction and jaundice may infrequently be a late phenomena.

Physical signs

With carcinoma of the head of pancreas the patient is jaundiced with the characteristic scratch marks secondary to cholestasis. In a proportion of cases the gall bladder will be palpable (Courvoisier's sign). A central abdominal mass may be palpable as well as hepatomegaly if metastatic disease is present. With carcinoma of the body and tail, there are often no physical signs.

Other presenting physical signs include thromboembolic phenomena, polyarthritis and skin nodules. The latter are secondary to localized fat necrosis and associated inflammation. These manifestations, distant to the tumour itself, have not been fully explained but may precede the overt presentation of pancreatic cancer by months to years.

Investigations

- *Transabdominal ultrasound* is the initial investigation in the majority of patients (Fig. 7.35a). In the presence of bile duct obstruction this will confirm dilated intrahepatic bile ducts as well as a mass in the head of the pancreas. Ultrasound is less reliable when the cancer is found in the body and tail of the pancreas because of overlying bowel gas, with a sensitivity of detection of 60%.
- *Contrast-enhanced spiral CT scan* should confirm the presence of a mass lesion (Fig. 7.35b).
- *CT scanning* is necessary prior to possible surgical resection with contrast providing vascular definition to exclude tumour invasion as well as local lymph node involvement and distant metastases. *Laparoscopy* is also used for pre-operative assessment.
- *ERCP* is usually restricted to palliative treatment but may provide a source of cytology to confirm the diagnosis when this is in question.
- *Percutaneous needle biopsy* is discouraged in potentially operable cases as this may be a source of tumour cell spread within the peritoneum. If palliative chemotherapy is considered, a histological diagnosis is essential prior to treatment.
- *MRI scanning and endoscopic ultrasound* are techniques that are useful in a small proportion of patients in whom the tumour has not been adequately defined.
- *Several tumour markers* have been evaluated for the diagnosis and monitoring of pancreatic cancer. The CA 19.9 has a high sensitivity (80%) but a high false-positive rate. The CA242 has a lower sensitivity (70%) but fewer false positives (less then 10%). In individual patients single values of these tumour

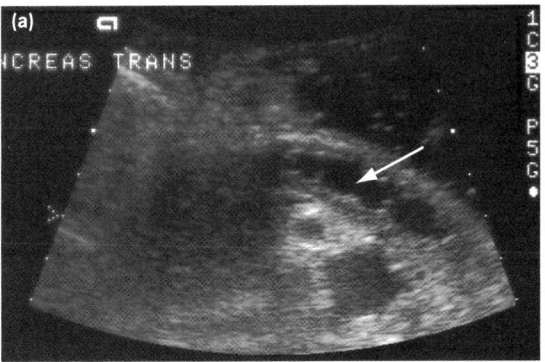

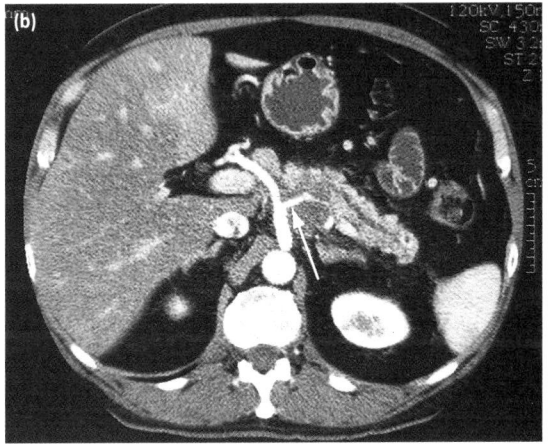

Fig. 7.35 (a) Ultrasound of the pancreas showing a tumour in the pancreatic head, with dilatation of the main pancreatic duct (arrow). (b) A contrast-enhanced CT scan showing a cancer of the body of the pancreas. There is retroperitoneal tumour extension enclosing the branches of the coeliac axis (arrow).

markers may be of little help but a progressive elevation over time is often diagnostic and in such circumstances tumour marker levels can be used to monitor response to treatment.

Differential diagnosis

The diagnosis of carcinoma of the pancreas should be considered in the presence of a wide spectrum of symptoms. The diagnosis should not be difficult in the presence of painless jaundice or epigastric pain radiating into the back with progressive weight loss.

Unfortunately many patients present with very minor symptoms including pain, change in bowel habit and weight loss. Pancreatic cancer may rarely present with recurrent episodes of typical acute pancreatitis.

Management

The 5-year survival rate for carcinoma of the pancreas is approximately 2% with surgical intervention representing the only chance of long-term survival. Approximately 20% of all cases have a localized tumour suitable for resection but in an elderly population many of these have co-morbid factors that preclude such major surgery. In the

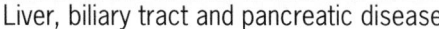

UK only 10% of all patients undergo a potential curable resection and only 25% of these will be alive at 5 years.

In the majority of cases the management is *palliative*. Jaundice is a debilitating complication often associated with severe pruritus but also the cause of non-specific malaise, lethargy and anorexia. Endoscopic placement of endoprostheses (stents) offers excellent palliation with a low associated procedural morbidity and mortality (p. 394). Palliative surgery has a role in duodenal obstruction (a complication seen in 10% of cases) but self-expanding metal stents can be placed across the duodenal obstruction.

Chemotherapy and radiotherapy have been used both as an adjuvant to possible curative surgery and as a primary treatment for unresectable pancreatic cancer. Clinical responses to treatment have been recognized but overall this approach has proved disappointing and may not be justified in the majority of patients who have a very short life-expectancy.

With disease progression, abdominal pain is a frequent complicating factor which may prove extremely difficult to treat.

This is best managed by experienced palliative care teams which offer a multidisciplinary approach. Endocrine and exocrine pancreatic failure occur and are managed as described on page 401.

Endocrine tumours of the pancreas

The islets of Langerhans (p. 396) have the capacity to synthesize more than one hormone. They also synthesize ectopic hormones that are not usually found in the pancreas such as gastrin, adrenocorticotrophin, vasoactive intestinal peptide and growth hormone. Whilst many pancreatic endocrine tumours are multihormonal, one peptide tends to predominate and is responsible for the clinical syndrome. Other tumours, whilst containing peptide hormone, are functionally inactive.

These tumours are rare with an incidence of less than 1 in 100 000 of the population. Insulinomas are the commonest variant and account for approximately 50% of cases, gastrinomas account for 20% and the rarer functioning tumours 5%. The remaining 25% are non-functioning tumours. Approximately 25% of islet cell tumours are associated with a multiple endocrine syndrome (type I) (see p. 1067). The majority of the endocrine pancreatic tumours are malignant in their behaviour.

Clinical syndromes

Insulinoma is described on page 1103.

A *gastrinoma* accounts for approximately 1 : 1000 cases of duodenal ulcer disease. This results from hypersecretion of gastric acid secondary to ectopic gastrin secretion within the endocrine pancreas (*Zollinger–Ellison*). Recurrent severe duodenal ulceration occurs with only a partial response to acid suppression. The diagnosis is confirmed by an elevated gastrin level. The gastrin-secreting tumour within the pancreas is often small and poorly defined by abdominal ultrasound or CT scanning. Endoscopic ultrasound is often required for diagnosis. It has been shown that the tumour takes up octreotide and this has been used as the substrate for a radiolabelled scan. High-dose proton pump inhibitors are used to suppress symptoms but the only curative approach is surgical resection of the primary tumour.

A *VIPoma* is an endocrine pancreatic tumour producing vasoactive intestinal polypeptide (VIP). This causes a severe secretory diarrhoea secondary to the stimulation of adenyl cyclase within the enterocyte (*Verner–Morrison syndrome*). The clinical syndrome is one of profuse watery diarrhoea, hypokalaemia and a metabolic acidosis. To produce the syndrome the tumours are usually in excess of 3 cm in diameter and can be readily detected by contrast-enhanced spiral CT scanning. The clinical syndrome can be controlled by either glucocorticoids, long-acting octreotide or lanreotide but the only definitive treatment is surgery.

Glucagonomas are rare alpha-cell tumours which are responsible for the syndrome of migratory necrolytic dermatitis, weight loss, diabetes mellitus, deep vein thrombosis, anaemia and hypoalbuminaemia. The diagnosis is made by measuring pancreatic glucagon in the serum. The tumours tend to be large at the time of presentation and are easily detectable by standard imaging techniques. Metastases are common at presentation but if the tumour is localized, pancreatic resection may be curative. Chemotherapy and octreotide therapy have been used for palliative therapy.

Non-functioning endocrine tumours usually present by the local mass effect with pain, weight loss and the occasional bile duct obstruction. At the time of presentation the tumours are frequently large with distant metastases. Curative resection is possible in only a small proportion. Palliative surgery may be indicated to alleviate mass-related symptoms.

FURTHER READING

Brand R (2001) The diagnosis of pancreatic cancer. *Cancer Journal* 7(4): 287–297.

Etemad B, Whitcomb DC (2001) Chronic pancreatitis: diagnosis, classification, and new genetic developments. *Gastroenterology* 120: 682–707.

Lowenfels AB, Lankisch PG, Maisonneuve P (2000) What is the risk of biliary pancreatitis in patients with gallstones? *Gastroenterology* 119(3): 879.

Sharma VK, Howden CW (1999) Metaanalysis of randomized controlled trials of endoscopic retrograde cholangiography and endoscopic sphincterotomy for the treatment of acute biliary pancreatitis. *American Journal of Gastroenterology* 94: 3211–3214.

Tamm E, Charnsangavej C (2001) Pancreatic cancer: current concepts in imaging for diagnosis and staging. *Cancer Journal* 7(4): 298–311.

Haematological disease

Introduction and general aspects

Blood consists of:

- red cells
- white cells
- platelets
- plasma, in which the above elements are suspended.

Plasma is the liquid component of blood, which contains soluble fibrinogen. Serum is what remains after the formation of the fibrin clot.

The formation of blood cells (haemopoiesis)

Haemopoiesis is the production of blood cells. The haemopoietic system includes the bone marrow, liver, spleen, lymph nodes and thymus. The turnover of cells is enormous; red cells survive 120 days, platelets around 7 days but granulocytes only 7 hours. The production of as many as 10^{13} new myeloid cells (all blood cells except for lymphocytes) per day in the normal healthy state obviously requires to be tightly regulated according to the needs of the body.

Blood islands are formed in the yolk sac in the third week of gestation and produce primitive blood cells which migrate to the liver and spleen. These organs are the chief sites of haemopoiesis from 6 weeks to 7 months, when the bone marrow becomes the main source of blood cells. The bone marrow is the only source of blood cells during normal childhood and adult life.

At birth, haemopoiesis is present in the marrow of nearly every bone. As the child grows the active red marrow is gradually replaced by fat (yellow marrow) so that haemopoiesis in the adult becomes confined to the central skeleton and the proximal ends of the long bones. Only if the demand for blood cells increases and persists do the areas of red marrow extend once again. Pathological processes interfering with normal haemopoiesis may result in resumption of haemopoietic activity in the liver and spleen, which is referred to as *extramedullary haemopoiesis.*

All blood cells are derived from pluripotent stem cells. The stem cell has two properties – the first is *self-renewal*, i.e. the production of more stem cells, and the second is its proliferation and differentiation into progenitor cells, committed to one specific cell line.

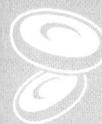

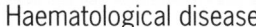

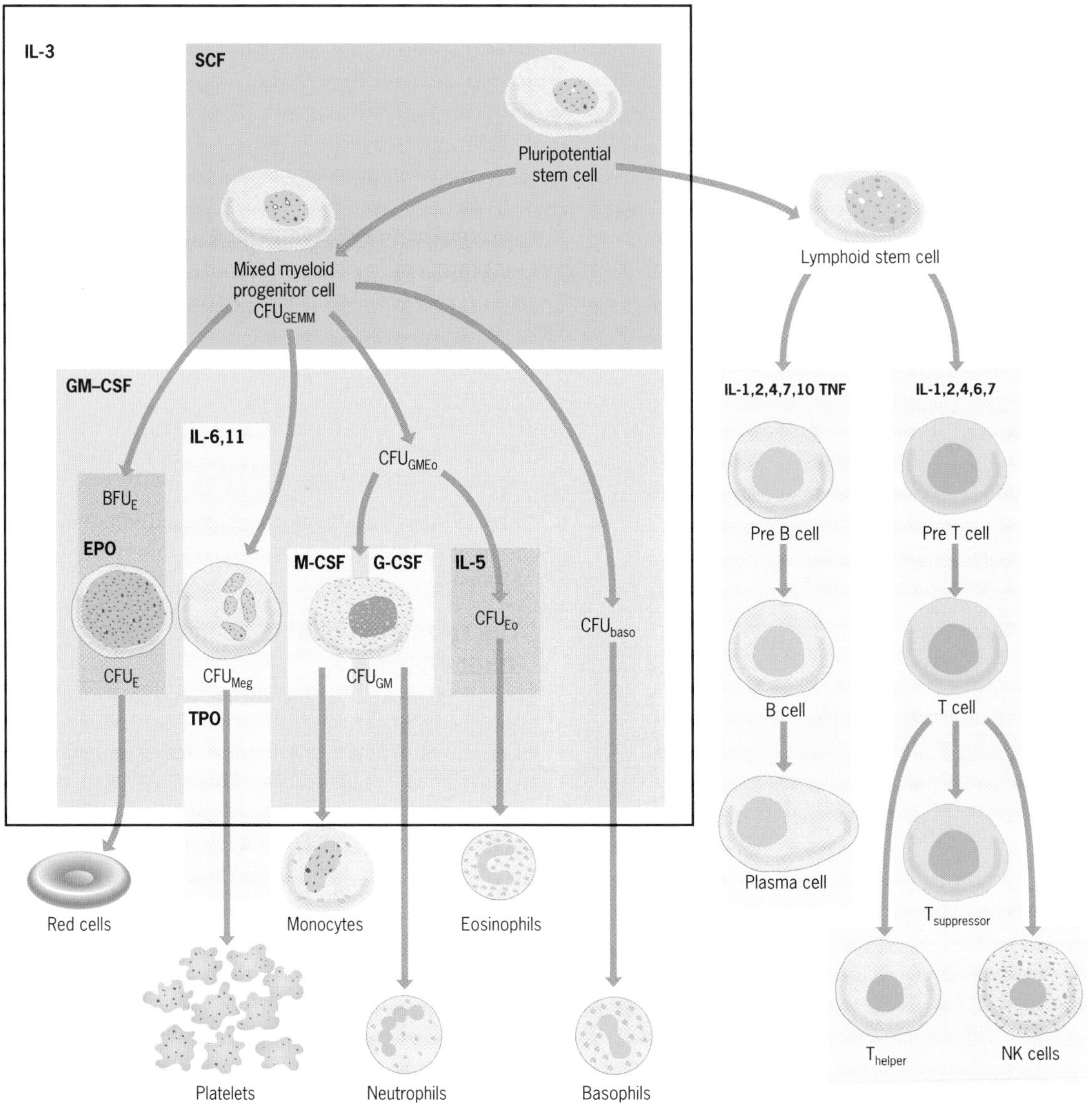

Fig. 8.1 **Role of growth factors in normal haemopoiesis.** Multiple growth factors act on stem cells and early progenitor cells. BFU, burst-forming unit; CFU, colony-forming unit; CSF, colony-stimulating factor; E, erythroid; Eo, eosinophil; EPO, erythropoietin; G, granulocyte; GEMM, mixed granulocyte, erythroid, monocyte, megakaryocyte; GM, granulocyte, monocyte; IL, interleukin; M, monocyte; Meg, megakaryocyte; SCF, stem cell (Steel) factor; TNF, tumour necrosis factor; TPO, thrombopoietin.

There are two major ancestral cell lines derived from the pluripotential stem cell: lymphocytic and myeloid (non-lymphocytic) cells (Fig. 8.1). The former gives rise to T and B cells. The myeloid stem cell gives rise to the progenitor CFU-GEMM (colony-forming unit, granulocyte–erythrocyte–monocyte–megakaryocyte). The progenitor cells such as CFU-GEMM cannot be recognized in bone marrow biopsies but are recognized by their ability to form colonies developing when haemopoietic cells are immobilized in a soft gel matrix. The CFU-GEMM can go on to lead to the formation of CFU-GM, CFU-Eo, and CFU-Meg, each of which can produce a

particular cell type (for example, neutrophils, eosinophils and platelets) under appropriate growth conditions. Haemopoiesis is under the control of growth factors and inhibitors, and the microenvironment of the bone marrow also plays an important role in its regulation.

Haemopoietic growth factors

Haemopoietic growth factors are glycoproteins which regulate the differentiation and proliferation of haemopoietic progenitor cells and the function of mature blood cells. They act on receptors expressed on haemopoietic cells at various stages of development to maintain the haemopoietic progenitor cells and to stimulate increased production of one or more cell lines in response to stresses such as blood loss and infection (Fig. 8.1).

The pluripotential stem cells are under the influence of a number of haemopoietic growth factors including interleukin-3 (IL-3), IL-6, IL-11 and stem cell factor (SCF, Steel factor). Colony stimulating factors (CSFs, the prefix indicating the cell type, see Fig. 8.1), as well as interleukins and erythropoietin (EPO) regulate the lineage committed progenitor cells. Thrombopoietin (TPO, which, like erythropoietin, is produced in the kidneys and the liver) along with IL-6 and IL-11 control platelet production. In addition to these factors stimulating haemopoiesis, other factors inhibit the process and include tumour necrosis factor (TNF) and transforming growth factor-β (TGF-β). Many of the growth factors are produced by activated T cells, monocytes and bone marrow stromal cells such as fibroblasts, endothelial cells and macrophages; these cells are also involved in inflammatory responses.

Many growth factors have been produced by recombinant DNA techniques and are being used clinically. Examples include G-CSF, which is used to accelerate haemopoietic recovery after chemotherapy and haemopoietic cell transplantation, and erythropoietin, which is used to treat anaemia in patients with chronic renal failure. Thrombopoietin is undergoing clinical trials in patients treated for malignant disease to reduce the need for platelet transfusions after intensive chemotherapy.

Peripheral blood

Automated cell counters are used to measure the level of haemoglobin (Hb) and the number and size of red cells, white cells and platelets (Table 8.1). Other indices can be derived from these values. The mean corpuscular volume (MCV) of red cells is the most useful of the indices and is used to classify anaemia (see p. 410).

The white cell count (WCC, or WBC, white blood count) gives the total number of circulating leucocytes, and many automated cell counters produce differential counts as well.

Normally, less than 2% of the red cells are reticulocytes. The reticulocyte count gives a guide to the erythroid activity in the bone marrow. An increased count is seen with haemorrhage or haemolysis, and during the response to treatment with a specific haematinic. A low count in the presence of anaemia indicates an inappropriate response by the bone marrow and may be seen in bone marrow failure (from whatever cause) or where there is a deficiency of a haematinic.

A carefully evaluated blood film is still an essential adjunct to the above, as definitive abnormalities of cells can be seen, and some examples are shown in Figure 8.8.

Erythrocyte sedimentation rate (ESR)

This is the rate of fall of red cells in a column of blood and is a measure of the acute phase response. The

Table 8.1
Normal values for peripheral blood

	Male	Female
Hb (g/dL)	13–18	11.5–15.5
PCV (haematocrit; L/L)	0.42–0.53	0.36–0.45
RCC (10^{12}/L)	4.5–6.0	3.9–5.
MCV (fl)	80–96	
MCH (pg)	27–33	
MCHC (g/dL)	32–35	
WBC (10^9/L)	4.0–11.0	
Platelets (10^9/L)	150–400	
ESR (mm/h)	< 20	
Reticulocytes (%)	0.5–2.5	

ESR, erythrocyte sedimentation rate; Hb, haemoglobin; MCH, mean corpuscular haemoglobin; MCHC, mean corpuscular haemoglobin concentration; MCV, mean corpuscular volume of red cells; PCV, packed cell volume; RCC, red cell count; WBC, white blood count.

pathological process may be immunological, infective, ischaemic, malignant or traumatic. A raised ESR reflects an increase in the plasma concentration of large proteins, such as fibrinogen and immunoglobulins. The proteins cause rouleaux formation, when cells clump together like a stack of coins, and therefore fall more rapidly. The ESR increases with age, and is higher in females than in males. It is low in polycythaemia vera, owing to the high red cell concentration, and increased in patients with severe anaemia.

Plasma viscosity

Plasma viscosity measurement is used instead of the ESR in many laboratories. As with the ESR, the level is dependent on the concentration of large molecules such as fibrinogen and immunoglobulins. There is no difference between levels found in males and females, and viscosity increases only slightly in the elderly. It is not affected by the level of Hb and the result may be obtained within 15 minutes.

C-reactive protein

C-reactive protein is a pentraxin, one of the proteins produced in the acute phase response (see Table 4.4). It is synthesized exclusively in the liver and rises within 6 hours of an acute event. It rises with fever (possibly triggered by IL-1, IL-6 and TNF-α and other cytokines) and in inflammatory conditions and after trauma. It follows the clinical state of the patient much more rapidly than does the ESR and is unaffected by the level of Hb, but it is less helpful than the ESR or plasma viscosity in monitoring chronic inflammatory diseases. Its measurement is easy and quick to perform using an immunoassay that can be automated. High-sensitivity assays have recently shown that increased levels predict future cardiovascular disease (p. 769).

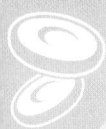

The red cell

Erythropoiesis

Red cell precursors pass through several stages in the bone marrow. The earliest morphologically recognizable cells are pronormoblasts. Smaller normoblasts result from cell divisions, and precursors at each stage progressively contain less RNA and more Hb in the cytoplasm. The nucleus becomes more condensed and is eventually lost from the late normoblast in the bone marrow, when the cell becomes a reticulocyte.

Reticulocytes contain residual ribosomal RNA and are still able to synthesize Hb. They remain in the marrow for about 1–2 days and are released into the circulation, where they lose their RNA and become mature red cells (erythrocytes) after another 1–2 days. Mature red cells are non-nucleated biconcave discs.

Nucleated red cells (normoblasts) are not normally present in peripheral blood, but are present if there is extramedullary haemopoiesis and in some marrow disorders (see leucoeryothroblastic anaemia, p. 452).

About 10% of erythroblasts die in the bone marrow even during normal erythropoiesis. Such ineffective erythropoiesis is substantially increased in some anaemias such as thalassaemia major and megaloblastic anaemia.

Erythropoiesis is controlled by the hormone erythropoietin. The gene for erythropoietin on chromosome 7 codes for a heavily glycosylated polypeptide of 165 amino acids. Erythropoietin has a molecular weight of 30 400 and is produced in the peritubular cells in the kidneys (90%) and in the liver (10%). Its production is regulated mainly by tissue oxygen tension. Production is increased if there is hypoxia from whatever cause – for example, anaemia or cardiac or pulmonary disease. Erythropoietin stimulates an increase in the proportion of bone marrow precursor cells committed to erythropoiesis, and CFU-E are stimulated to proliferate and differentiate. Increased 'inappropriate' production of erythropoietin is also seen in patients with renal disease and neoplasms in other sites resulting in polycythaemia (see Table 8.16).

Haemoglobin synthesis

Haemoglobin performs the main functions of red cells – carrying O_2 to the tissues and returning CO_2 from the tissues to the lungs. Each normal adult Hb molecule (Hb A) has a molecular weight of 68 000 and consists of two α and two β polypeptide chains ($\alpha_2\beta_2$) which have 141 and 146 amino acids respectively. Hb A comprises about 97% of the Hb in adults. Two other types, Hb A_2 ($\alpha_2\delta_2$) and Hb F ($\alpha_2\gamma_2$), are found in adults in small amounts (1.5–3.2% and < 1%, respectively).

Haemoglobin synthesis occurs in the mitochondria of the developing red cell (Fig. 8.2). The major rate-limiting step is the conversion of glycine and succinic acid to δ-aminolaevulinic acid (ALA) by ALA synthetase.

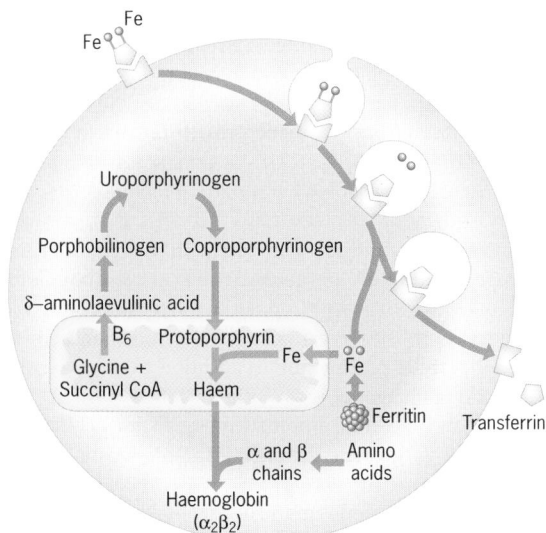

Fig. 8.2 Haemoglobin synthesis. Transferrin attaches to a surface receptor on developing red cells. Iron is released and transported to the mitochondria, where it combines with protoporphyrin to form haem. Protoporphyrin itself is manufactured from glycine and succinyl-CoA. Haem combines with α and β chains (formed on ribosomes) to make haemoglobin.

Vitamin B_6 is a coenzyme for this reaction, which is inhibited by haem and stimulated by erythropoietin. Two molecules of δ-ALA condense to form a pyrrole ring (porphobilinogen). These rings are then grouped in fours to produce protoporphyrins. Finally, iron is inserted to form haem. Haem is then inserted into the globin chains to form Hb. The structure of Hb is shown in Figure 8.3.

Haemoglobin function

The biconcave shape of red cells provides a large surface area for the uptake and release of oxygen and carbon dioxide. Haemoglobin becomes saturated with oxygen in the pulmonary capillaries where the partial pressure of oxygen is high and Hb has a high affinity for oxygen. Oxygen is released in the tissues where the partial pressure of oxygen is low and Hb has a low affinity for oxygen.

Adult haemoglobin (Hb A) consists of two α and two β globin chains. A haem group is bound to each globin chain; the haem group has a porphyrin ring with a ferrous atom which can reversibly bind one oxygen molecule. The haemoglobin molecule exists in two conformations, R and T. The T (tense) conformation of deoxyhaemoglobin is characterized by the globin units being held tightly together by electrostatic bonds (Fig. 8.4). These bonds are broken when oxygen binds to haemoglobin, resulting in the R (relaxed) conformation in which the remaining oxygen-binding sites are more exposed and have a much higher affinity for oxygen than in the T conformation. The binding of one oxygen molecule to deoxyhaemoglobin increases the

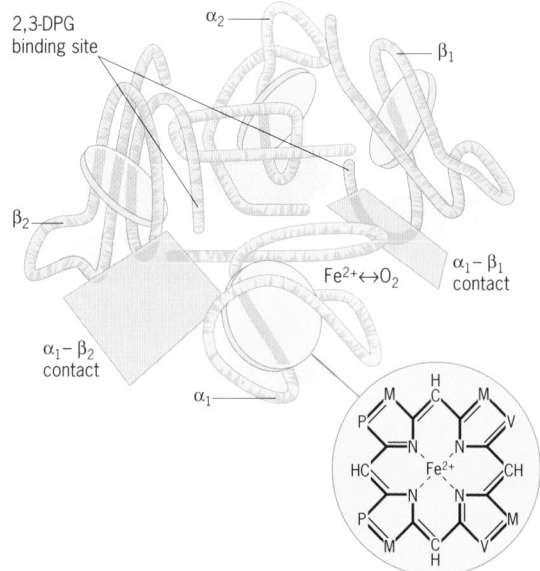

Fig. 8.3 **Model of the haemoglobin molecule showing α (pink) and β (blue) chains.** 2,3-DPG binds in the centre of the molecule and stabilizes the deoxygenated form by cross-linking the β chains (also see Fig. 8.4). M, methyl; P, propionic acid; V, vinyl.

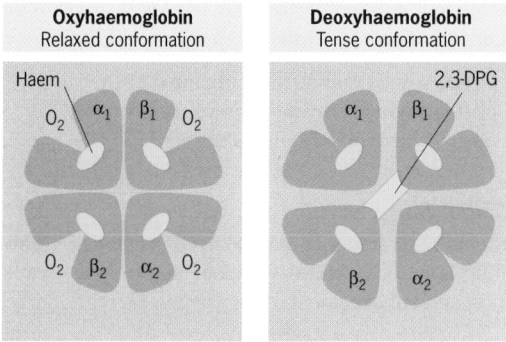

Fig. 8.4 **Oxygenated and deoxygenated haemoglobin molecule.** The haemoglobin molecule is predominantly stabilized by α–β chain bonds rather than α–α and β–β chain bonds. The structure of the molecule changes during O_2 uptake and release. When O_2 is released, the β chains rotate on the $α_1β_2$ and $α_2β_1$ contacts, allowing the entry of 2,3-DPG which causes a lower affinity of haemoglobin for O_2 and improved delivery of O_2 to the tissues. From Hoffbrand AV, Pettit JE (1993) *Essential Haematology*, 3rd edn. Oxford: Blackwell Scientific Publications, with permission.

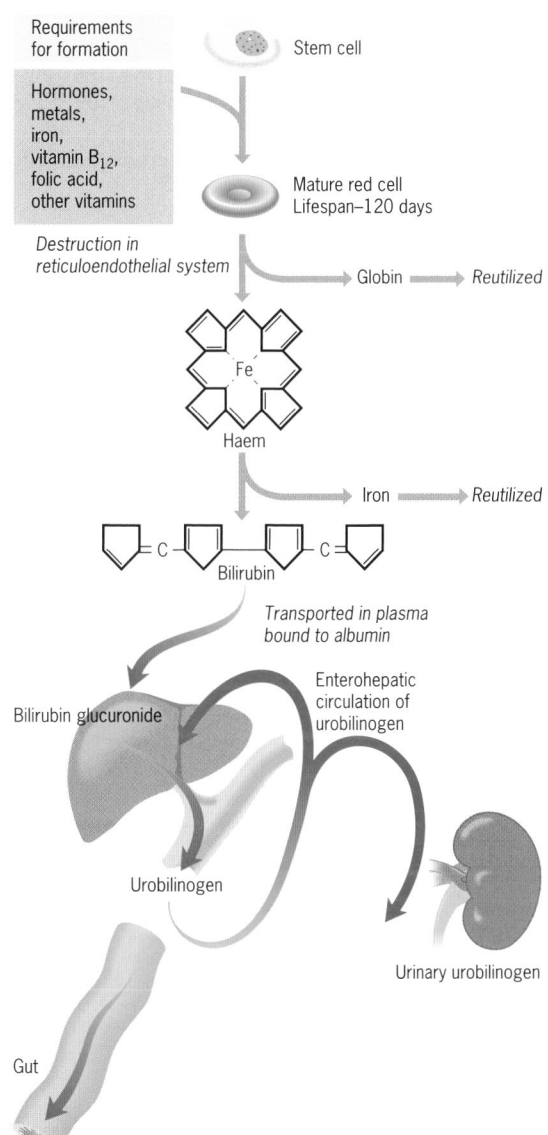

Fig. 8.5 **Red cell production and breakdown.**

oxygen affinity of the remaining binding sites – this property is known as 'cooperativity' and is the reason for the sigmoid shape of the oxygen dissociation curve. Haemoglobin is, therefore, an example of an allosteric protein. The binding of oxygen can be influenced by secondary effectors – hydrogen ions, carbon dioxide and red-cell 2,3-diphosphoglycerate (2,3-DPG). Hydrogen ions and carbon dioxide added to blood cause a reduction in the oxygen-binding affinity of haemoglobin (the Bohr effect) (Fig. 15.5). Oxygenation of haemoglobin

reduces its affinity for carbon dioxide (the Haldane effect). These effects help the exchange of carbon dioxide and oxygen in the tissues.

Red cell metabolism produces 2,3-DPG from glycolysis. 2,3-DPG accumulates because it is sequestered by binding to deoxyhaemoglobin. The binding of 2,3-DPG stabilizes the T conformation and reduces its affinity for oxygen. The P_{50} increases with 2,3-DPG concentrations, which increase when oxygen availability is reduced in conditions such as hypoxia or anaemia. The P_{50} is also raised with increasing body temperature, which may be beneficial during prolonged exercise. Haemoglobin regulates oxygen transport through the oxyhaemoglobin dissociation curve. When the primary limitation

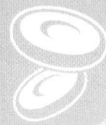

to oxygen transport is in the periphery, e.g. heavy exercise, anaemia, the P_{50} is increased to enhance oxygen unloading. When the primary limitation is in the lungs, e.g. lung disease, high altitude exposure, the P_{50} is reduced to enhance oxygen loading.

A summary of normal red cell production and destruction is given in Figure 8.5.

FURTHER READING

Haynes AP, Hunter AE, Russell NH (1996) The clinical use of haemopoietic growth factors. In: Brenner MK, Hoffbrand AV (eds) *Recent Advances in Haematology*, 8th edn. Edinburgh: Churchill Livingstone.

Heelzer D (1997) Hematopoietic growth factors: not whether, but when and where. *New England Journal of Medicine* **336**: 1822–1824.

Levin J (1997) Thrombopoietin: clinically realized? *New England Journal of Medicine* **336**: 434–436.

Lowe GDO (1994) Should plasma viscosity replace the ESR? *British Journal of Haematology* **86**: 6–11.

Pepys MB, Berger A (2001) The renaissance of C reactive protein. *British Medical Journal* **322**: 4–5.

Scott MA, Gordon MY (1995) In search of the haemopoietic stem cell. *British Journal of Haematology* **90**: 738–743.

Weatherall D, Provan D (2000) Red cells I: inherited anaemias. *Lancet* **355**: 1169–1175.

Anaemia

Anaemia is present when there is a decrease in the level of haemoglobin in the blood below the reference level for the age and sex of the individual (Table 8.1). Alterations in the level of Hb may occur as a result of changes in the plasma volume, as shown in Figure 8.6. A reduction in the plasma volume will lead to a spuriously

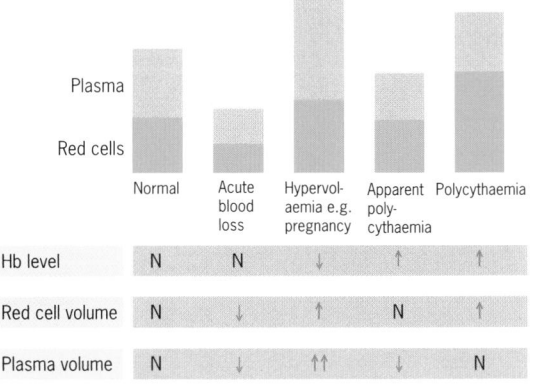

Fig. 8.6 Alterations of haemoglobin in relation to plasma.

high Hb – this is seen with dehydration and in the clinical condition of apparent polycythaemia (see p. 442). A raised plasma volume produces a spurious anaemia, even when combined with a small increase in red cell volume as occurs in pregnancy. After a major bleed, anaemia may not be apparent for several days until the plasma volume returns to normal.

The various types of anaemia, classified in terms of the red cell indices, particularly the MCV, are shown in Figure 8.7. There are three major types:

- hypochromic microcytic with a low MCV
- normochromic normocytic with a normal MCV
- macrocytic with a high MCV.

Clinical features

Patients with anaemia may be asymptomatic. A slowly falling level of Hb allows for haemodynamic compensation and enhancement of the oxygen-carrying capacity

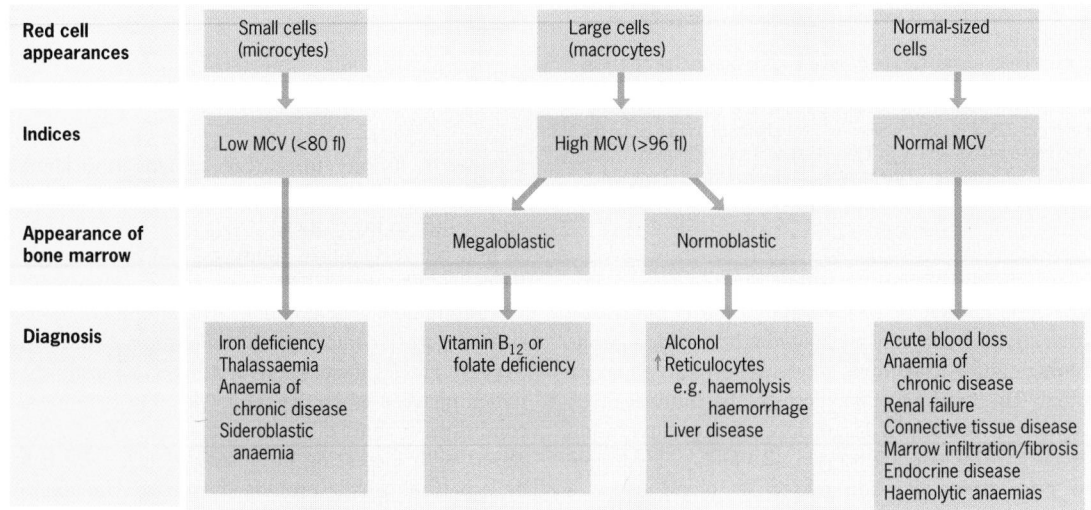

Fig. 8.7 **Classification of anaemia.** MCV, mean corpuscular volume.

of the blood. A rise in 2,3-DPG causes a shift of the oxygen dissociation curve to the right, so that oxygen is more readily given up to the tissues. Where blood loss is rapid, more severe symptoms will occur, particularly in elderly people.

Symptoms (all non-specific)

- Fatigue
- Headaches
- Faintness
  (the above three are all very common in the general population)
- Breathlessness
- Angina
- Intermittent claudication
- Palpitations.

Signs

- Pallor
- Tachycardia
- Systolic flow murmur
- Cardiac failure
- Rarely papilloedema and retinal haemorrhages after an acute bleed (can be accompanied by blindness).

Specific signs of the different types of anaemia will be discussed in the appropriate sections. Examples include:

- koilonychia – spoon-shaped nails seen in iron deficiency anaemia
- jaundice – found in haemolytic anaemia
- bone deformities – found in thalassaemia major

- leg ulcers – occur in association with sickle cell disease.

It must be emphasized that anaemia is not a diagnosis, and a cause must be found.

Investigations
Peripheral blood

A low haemoglobin should always be considered in relation to:

- the white blood cell (WBC) count
- the platelet count
- the reticulocyte count (as this indicates marrow activity)
- the blood film, as abnormal red cell morphology (see Fig. 8.8) may indicate the diagnosis.

Where two populations of red cells are seen, the blood film is said to be dimorphic. This may, for example, be seen in patients with 'double deficiencies' (e.g. combined iron and folate deficiency in coeliac disease, or following treatment of anaemic patients with the appropriate haematinic).

Bone marrow

Examination of the bone marrow is performed to further investigate abnormalities found in the peripheral blood (Practical box 8.1). Aspiration provides a film which can be examined by microscopy for the morphology of the developing haemopoietic cells. The trephine provides a core of bone which is processed as a histological

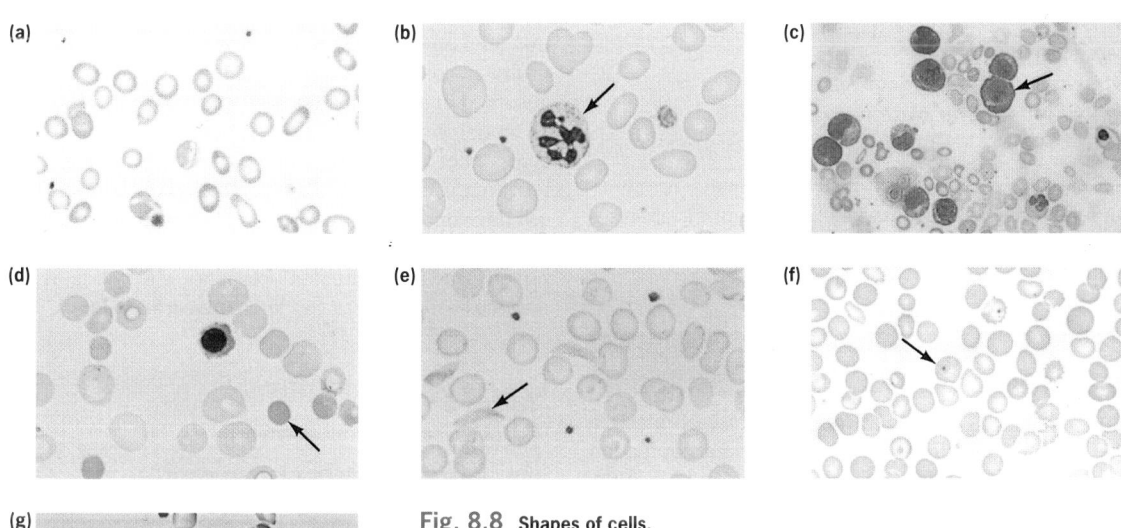

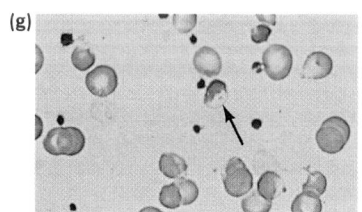

Fig. 8.8 Shapes of cells.
(a) Hypochromic microcytic cells.
(b) Macrocytes and a hypersegmented neutrophil (arrowed).
(c) Megaloblasts (arrowed) in the bone marrow.
(d) Spherocytes (arrowed), reticulocytes, polychromasias and a nucleated erythroblast.
(e) Sickle cells (arrowed) and target cells.
(f) Postsplenectomy film with Howell–Jolly bodies (arrowed), target cells and irregularly contracted cells.
(g) 'Blister' cells (arrowed) in G6PD deficiency.

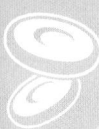

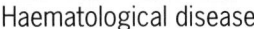

Practical box 8.1

Techniques for obtaining bone marrow

Aspiration
Site – usually iliac crest
Give local anaesthetic injection
Use special bone marrow needle (e.g. Salah)
Aspirate marrow
Make smear with glass slide
Stain with:
● Romanowsky technique
● Perls' reaction (acid ferrocyanide) for iron.

Trephine
Indications include:
● 'Dry tap' obtained with aspiration
● Better assessment of cellularity, e.g. aplastic anaemia
● Better assessment of presence of infiltration or fibrosis.

Technique
Site – usually posterior iliac crest
Give local anaesthetic injection
Use special needle (e.g. Jamshidi – longer and wider than
    for aspiration)
Obtain core of bone
Fix in formalin; decalcify – this takes a few days
Stain with:
● Haematoxylin and eosin
● Reticulin stain.

specimen and allows an overall view of the bone marrow architecture, cellularity and presence/absence of abnormal infiltrates. The following are assessed:

• cellularity of the marrow
• type of erythropoiesis (e.g. normoblastic or megaloblastic)
• cellularity of the various cell lines
• infiltration of the marrow
• iron stores.

Special tests may be performed: cytogenetic, immuno-logical, cytochemical markers, biochemical analyses (e.g. deoxyuridine suppression test), microbiological culture.

Microcytic anaemia

Iron deficiency is the most common cause of anaemia in the world affecting 30% of the world's population equivalent to 500 million people. This is because of the body's limited ability to absorb iron and the frequent loss of iron owing to haemorrhage. Although iron is abundant, most is in the insoluble ferric (Fe^{3+}) form, which has poor bioavailability. Free iron is toxic, and it is bound to various proteins for transport and storage.

The other causes of a microcytic hypochromic anaemia are anaemia of chronic disease, sideroblastic anaemia, and thalassaemia. In thalassaemia (p. 427) there is a defect in

globin synthesis, in contrast to the other three causes of microcytic anaemia where the defect is in the synthesis of haem.

Iron
Dietary intake
The average daily diet in the UK contains 15–20 mg of iron, although normally only 10% of this is absorbed. Absorption may be increased to 20–30% in iron deficiency and pregnancy.

Non-haem iron is mainly derived from cereals, which are commonly fortified with iron; it forms the main part of dietary iron. Haem iron is derived from haemoglobin and myoglobin in red or organ meats. Haem iron is better absorbed than non-haem iron, whose availability is more affected by other dietary constituents.

Absorption (Fig. 8.9 (a), (b))
This takes place in the duodenum and jejunum. The absorption of iron is a complex process; some of the factors influencing it are shown in Table 8.2. Haem iron is partly broken down to non-haem iron, but some haem iron is absorbed intact into mucosal cells.

Iron absorption occurs primarily in the duodenum. Non-haem iron is dissolved in the low pH of the stomach and reduced from the ferric to ferrous form by a brush border ferrireductase. Cells in duodenal crypts are able to sense the body's iron requirements and retain this information as they mature into cells capable of absorbing iron at the tips of the villi. A protein, divalent metal transporter 1 (DMT1), (formerly called divalent cation transporter [DCT1] or natural resistance-associated macrophage protein [NRAMP2]) transports iron (and other metals) across the apical (luminal) surface of the mucosal cells in the small intestine. Haem iron is absorbed in a separate less-well-characterized process.

Once inside the mucosal cell, iron may be transferred across the cell to reach the plasma, or be stored as ferritin; the body's iron status at the time the absorptive cell developed from the crypt cell is probably the crucial factor. Iron stored as ferritin will be lost into the gut lumen when the mucosal cells are shed; this is an important mechanism for regulating iron balance. The

Table 8.2
Factors influencing iron absorption

Haem iron is absorbed better than non-haem iron
Ferrous iron is absorbed better than ferric iron
Gastric acidity helps to keep iron in the ferrous state and
    soluble in the upper gut
Formation of insoluble complexes with phytate or phosphate
    decreases iron absorption
Iron absorption is increased with low iron stores and increased
    erythropoietic activity, e.g. bleeding, haemolysis, high altitude
There is a decreased absorption in iron overload, except in
    hereditary haemochromatosis, where it is increased

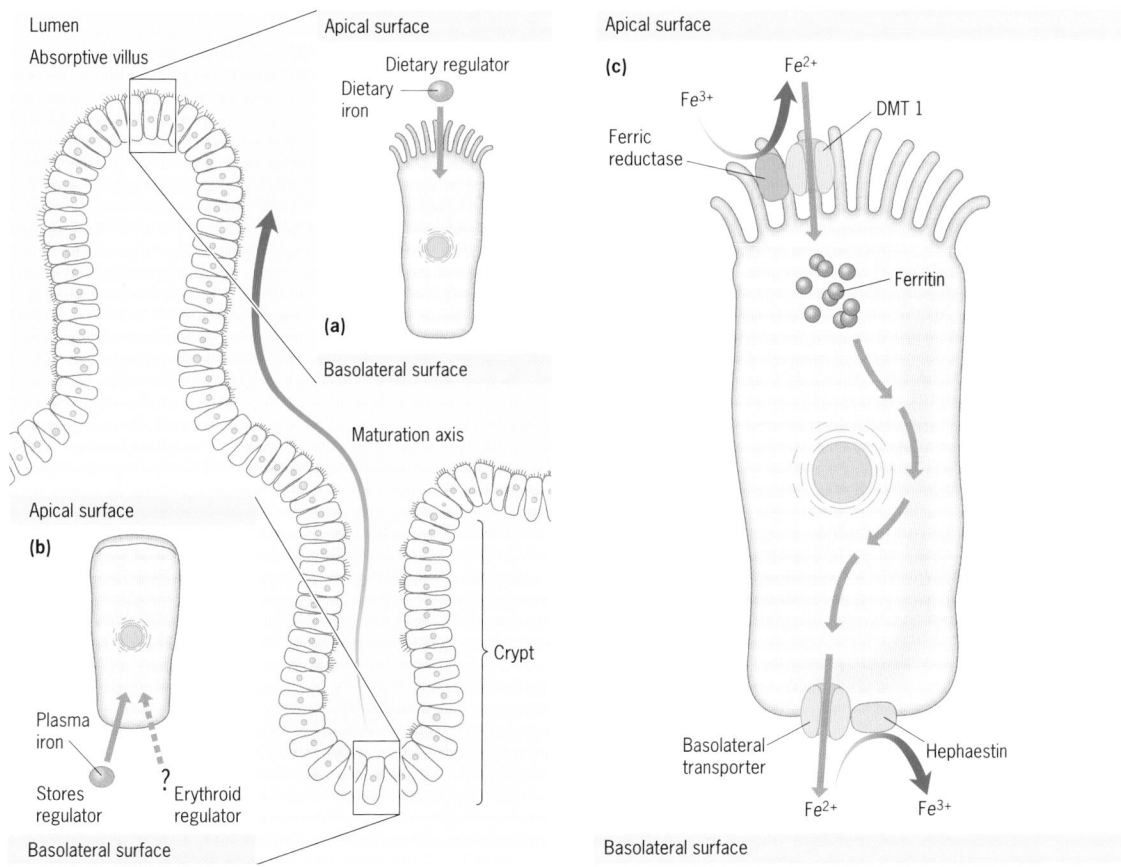

Fig. 8.9 (a), (b) Regulation of the absorption of intestinal iron. The iron-absorbing cells of the duodenal epithelium originate in the intestinal crypts and migrate toward the tip of the villus as they differentiate (maturation axis). Absorption of intestinal iron is regulated by at least three independent mechanisms. First, iron absorption is influenced by recent dietary iron intake (dietary regulator). After a large dietary bolus, absorptive cells are resistant to iron uptake for several days. Second, iron absorption can be modulated considerably in response to body iron stores (stores regulator). Third, an unidentified signal communicates the state of bone marrow erythropoiesis to the intestine (erythroid regulator). **(c) Iron transport across the intestinal epithelium.** Iron must cross two membranes to be transferred across the absorptive epithelium. Each transmembrane transporter is coupled to an enzyme that changes the oxidation state of iron. The apical transporter has been identified as divalent metal transporter 1 (DMT1). It acts in concert with a type of ferrireductase activity that has not yet been cloned. The basolateral transporter has not yet been identified. This transporter requires hephaestin, a ceruloplasmin-like molecule, for the transfer of iron to the plasma. On the basis of its structure, hephaestin is presumed to be a form of ferroxidase. In this diagram, hephaestin is depicted at the basolateral surface of the cell, although it has not yet been established that it functions in that location. Iron within enterocytes is stored as ferritin.

mechanism of transport of iron across the basolateral surface of mucosal cells is uncertain, but probably involves a transporter protein, Ireg1. This transporter protein requires an accessory, multicopper protein, hephaestin (see Fig. 8.9c).

The iron content of the body is kept within narrow limits and its loss and intake are normally finely balanced. Its absorption is closely related to the total iron stores of the body; in iron deficiency, absorption of iron may increase to 3–4 mg daily. The body is unable to excrete iron once it has been absorbed so the regulation of iron absorption is critical.

Iron absorption is regulated in several ways (see Fig. 8.9) by regulators called dietary, stores and erythroids.

Anaemias with increased rates of erythropoiesis do not cause equal increases in iron absorption; for example, conditions with 'ineffective erythropoiesis'

such as thalassaemia stimulate greater iron absorption than haemolytic anaemias such as hereditary spherocytosis and autoimmune haemolytic anaemia where red cell destruction occurs in the periphery.

Transport in the blood

The normal serum iron level is about 11–30 µmol/L; there is a diurnal rhythm with higher levels in the morning. Iron is transported in the plasma bound to transferrin, a β-globulin that is synthesized in the liver. Each transferrin molecule binds two atoms of ferric iron and is normally one-third saturated. Most of the iron bound to transferrin comes from macrophages in the reticuloendothelial system and not from iron absorbed by the intestine. Transferrin-bound iron becomes attached by specific receptors to erythroblasts and reticulocytes in the marrow and the iron is removed (see Fig. 8.2).

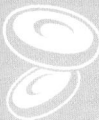

In an average adult male, 20 mg of iron, chiefly obtained from red cell breakdown in the macrophages of the reticuloendothelial system, is incorporated into Hb every day.

Iron stores

About two-thirds of the total body iron is in the circulation as haemoglobin (2.5–3 g in a normal adult man). Iron is stored in reticuloendothelial cells, hepatocytes and skeletal muscle cells (500–1500 mg). About two-thirds of this is stored as ferritin and one-third as haemosiderin in normal individuals. Small amounts of iron are also found in plasma (about 4 mg bound to transferrin), with some in myoglobin and enzymes.

Ferritin is a water-soluble complex of iron and protein. It is more easily mobilized than haemosiderin for Hb formation. It is present in small amounts in plasma.

Haemosiderin is an insoluble iron–protein complex found in macrophages in the bone marrow, liver and spleen. Unlike ferritin, it is visible by light microscopy in tissue sections and bone marrow films after staining by Perls' reaction.

Requirements

Each day 0.5–1.0 mg of iron is lost in the faeces, urine and sweat. Menstruating women lose 30–40 mL of blood per month, an average of about 0.5–0.7 mg of iron per day. Blood loss through menstruation in excess of 100 mL will usually result in iron deficiency as increased iron absorption from the gut cannot compensate for such losses of iron. The demand for iron also increases during growth (about 0.6 mg per day) and pregnancy (1–2 mg per day). In the normal adult the iron content of the body remains relatively fixed. Increases in the body iron content (haemochromatosis) are classified into:

- hereditary haemochromatosis (p. 375), where a mutation in the *HFE* gene causes upregulation of DMT1 and increased iron absorption
- secondary haemochromatosis (transfusion siderosis; see p. 429). This is due to iron overload in conditions where repeated transfusion is the only therapy.

Iron deficiency

Iron deficiency anaemia develops when there is inadequate iron for haemoglobin synthesis. A normal level of Hb is maintained for as long as possible after the iron stores are depleted; latent iron deficiency is said to be present during this period.

Causes
- Blood loss
- Increased demands such as growth and pregnancy
- Decreased absorption (e.g. postgastrectomy)
- Poor intake.

Most iron deficiency is due to blood loss, usually from the uterus or gastrointestinal tract. Premenopausal women are in a state of precarious iron balance owing to menstruation. Iron deficiency affects more than a quarter of the world's population, but isolated nutritional iron deficiency is rare in developed countries. The most common cause of iron deficiency world-wide is blood loss from the gastrointestinal tract resulting from hookworm infestation. The poor quality of the diet, predominantly containing vegetables, also contributes to the high prevalence of iron deficiency in developing countries. Even in developed countries, iron deficiency is not uncommon in infancy where iron intake is insufficient for the demands of growth. It is more prevalent in infants born prematurely or where the introduction of mixed feeding is delayed.

Clinical features
The symptoms of anaemia are described on page 411. Other clinical features occur as a result of tissue iron deficiency. These are mainly epithelial changes induced by the effect of inadequate iron in the cells:

- brittle nails
- spoon-shaped nails (koilonychia)
- atrophy of the papillae of the tongue
- angular stomatitis
- brittle hair
- a syndrome of dysphagia and glossitis (Plummer–Vinson or Paterson–Brown–Kelly syndrome; see p. 267).

The diagnosis of iron deficiency anaemia relies on a good clinical history with questions about dietary intake, regular self-medication with non-steroidal anti-inflammatory drugs (which may give rise to gastrointestinal bleeding), and the presence of blood in the faeces (which may be a sign of haemorrhoids or carcinoma of the lower bowel). In women, a careful enquiry about the duration of periods, the occurrence of clots and the number of sanitary towels or tampons (normal 3–5/day) used should be made.

Investigations
Blood count and film
A characteristic blood film is shown in Figure 8.8. The red cells are microcytic (MCV < 80 fl) and hypochromic (MCH < 27 pg). There is poikilocytosis (variation in shape) and anisocytosis (variation in size). Target cells are seen.

Serum iron and iron-binding capacity
The serum iron falls and the total iron-binding capacity (TIBC) rises in iron deficiency compared with normal. Iron deficiency is regularly present when the transferrin saturation (i.e. serum iron divided by TIBC) falls below 19% (Table 8.3).

Serum ferritin

The level of serum ferritin reflects the amount of stored iron, probably more accurately than the serum iron and iron-binding capacity, which are less frequently used to assess iron status now. The normal values for serum ferritin are 30–300 µg/L (11.6–144 nmol/L) in males and 15–200 µg/L (5.8–96 nmol/L) in females. In simple iron deficiency, a low serum ferritin confirms the diagnosis. However, ferritin is an acute-phase reactant, and levels increase in the presence of inflammatory or malignant diseases. In the majority of cases, the diagnosis of iron deficiency anaemia can be confirmed by measurement of either serum iron/TIBC or serum ferritin. In complex cases, for example where iron deficiency coexists with an inflammatory process or malignancy, measurement of both serum iron/TIBC and serum ferritin may be helpful.

Serum soluble transferrin receptor

The number of transferrin receptors increases in iron deficiency. The results of this immunoassay compares well with results from bone marrow aspiration at estimating iron stores.

This assay can help to distinguish between iron deficiency and anaemia of chronic disease (see Table 8.3), and may avoid the need for bone marrow examination even in complex cases.

Bone marrow

Erythroid hyperplasia with ragged normoblasts are seen in the marrow in iron deficiency. Staining using Perls' reaction (acid ferrocyanide) does not show the characteristic Prussian-blue granules of stainable iron in the bone marrow fragments or in the erythroblasts.

Examination of the bone marrow is not essential for the diagnosis of iron deficiency but it may be helpful in the investigation of complicated cases of anaemia, e.g. to determine if iron deficiency is present in a patient with anaemia of chronic disease.

Other investigations

These will be indicated by the clinical history and examination. Investigations of the gastrointestinal tract are often required to determine the cause of the iron deficiency (see p. 283).

Differential diagnosis

The presence of anaemia with microcytosis and hypo-chromia does not necessarily indicate iron deficiency. The most common other causes are thalassaemia, sideroblastic anaemia and anaemia of chronic disease, and in these disorders the iron stores are normal or increased. The differential diagnosis of microcytic anaemia is shown in Table 8.3.

Treatment

Iron deficiency is not a diagnosis per se. The correct management of iron deficiency is to find and treat the underlying cause, and to give iron to correct the anaemia and replace iron stores. The response to iron therapy can be monitored using the reticulocyte count and Hb level with an expected rise in haemoglobin of 1 g per week.

Oral iron is all that is required in most cases. The best preparation is ferrous sulphate (200 mg three times daily, a total of 180 mg ferrous iron) which is absorbed best when the patient is fasting. If the patient has side-effects such as nausea, diarrhoea or constipation, taking the tablets with food or reducing the dose using a preparation with less iron such as ferrous gluconate (300 mg twice daily, only 70 mg ferrous iron) is all that is usually required to reduce the symptoms. The use of expensive iron compounds, particularly the slow-release ones which release iron beyond its main sites of absorption, is unnecessary.

In developing countries, distribution of iron tablets is the main approach for the alleviation of iron deficiency. However, iron supplementation programmes have been ineffective, probably mainly because of poor compliance.

Table 8.3
Microcytic anaemia: the differential diagnosis

	Iron deficiency	Anaemia of chronic disease	Thalassaemia trait (α or β)	Sideroblastic anaemia
MCV	Reduced	Low normal or normal	Very low for degree of anaemia	Low in inherited type but often raised in acquired type
Serum iron	Reduced	Reduced	Normal	Raised
Serum TIBC	Raised	Reduced	Normal	Normal
Serum ferritin	Reduced	Normal or raised	Normal	Raised
Serum soluble transfer receptor	Increased	Normal	Normal or raised	Normal or raised
Iron in marrow	Absent	Present	Present	Present
Iron in erythroblasts	Absent	Absent or reduced	Present	Ring forms

TIBC, total iron binding capacity

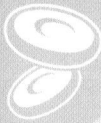
Oral iron should be given for long enough to correct the Hb level and to replenish the iron stores. This can take 6 months. The commonest causes of failure of response to oral iron are:

- lack of compliance
- continuing haemorrhage
- incorrect diagnosis, e.g. thalassaemia trait.

These possibilities should be considered before parenteral iron is used. However, parenteral iron is required by occasional patients, including those who have general intolerance of oral preparations even at low dose, those with severe malabsorption, and those who have chronic gastrointestinal diseases such as ulcerative colitis or Crohn's disease. Iron stores are replaced much faster with parenteral iron than with oral iron, but the haematological response is no quicker. Parenteral iron can be given as repeated deep intramuscular injections of iron–sorbitol or by slow intravenous infusion of iron–sucrose. To calculate the required dose of parenteral iron, the deficit in body iron should be estimated from the degree of anaemia and the patient's bodyweight.

Anaemia of chronic disease

One of the most common types of anaemia, particularly in hospital patients, is the anaemia of chronic disease, occurring in patients with chronic infections such as infective endocarditis and tuberculosis and osteomyelitis in developing countries, chronic inflammatory diseases such as rheumatoid arthritis, systemic lupus erythematosus (SLE) and polymyalgia rheumatica, and in patients with malignant disease. There is decreased release of iron from the bone marrow to developing erythroblasts, an inadequate erythropoietin response to the anaemia, and decreased red cell survival. The exact mechanisms responsible for these effects are not clear, but they seem to be mediated by inflammatory cytokines such as IL-1, tumour necrosis factor and interferons.

The serum iron and the TIBC are low, and the serum ferritin is normal or raised because of the inflammatory process. The serum soluble transferrin receptor level is normal (Table 8.3). Stainable iron is present in the bone marrow, but iron is not seen in the developing erythroblasts. Patients do not respond to iron therapy, and treatment is, in general, that of the underlying disorder. However, trials are being carried out with recombinant erythropoietin in rheumatoid arthritis with some success, and also in inflammatory bowel disease, where treatment in combination with oral iron produced an increase of more than 1 g/dL in more than 80% of patients after 12 weeks' therapy.

Sideroblastic anaemia

Sideroblastic anaemias are inherited or acquired disorders characterized by a refractory anaemia, a variable number of hypochromic cells in the peripheral blood,

Table 8.4
Classification of sideroblastic anaemia

Inherited
X-linked disease – transmitted by females

Acquired
Primary (one of the myelodysplastic syndromes, see p. 443)
Secondary
    Other types of myelodysplasia
    Myeloproliferative disorders
    Myeloid leukaemia
    Drugs, e.g. isoniazid
    Alcohol abuse
    Lead toxicity
    Other disorders, e.g. rheumatoid arthritis, carcinoma,
        megaloblastic and haemolytic anaemias, malabsorption

and excess iron and ring sideroblasts in the bone marrow. The presence of ring sideroblasts is the diagnostic feature of sideroblastic anaemia. There is accumulation of iron in the mitochondria of erythroblasts owing to disordered haem synthesis forming a ring of iron granules around the nucleus that can be seen with Perls' reaction. The blood film is often dimorphic; ineffective haem synthesis is responsible for the microcytic hypochromic cells. Sideroblastic anaemias are classified as shown in Table 8.4. A structural defect in δ-aminolaevulinic acid (ALA) synthetase, the pyridoxine-dependent enzyme responsible for the first step in haem synthesis (see Fig. 8.2), has been identified in one form of inherited sideroblastic anaemia. Primary acquired sideroblastic anaemia is one of the myelodysplastic syndromes (see p. 443).

Treatment

Some patients respond when drugs or alcohol are withdrawn, if these are the causative agents. In occasional cases, there is a response to pyridoxine. Treatment with folic acid may be required to treat accompanying folate deficiency.

Lead poisoning

The causes, clinical features and treatment are discussed on page 983. The characteristic haematological features include:

- *sideroblastic anaemia*, due to inhibition by lead of several enzymes involved in haem synthesis, including ALA synthetase
- *haemolysis*, which is usually mild, resulting from damage to the red cell membrane
- *punctate basophilia* (or basophilic stippling: the blood film shows red cells with small, round, blue particles), due to aggregates of RNA in red cells owing to inhibition by lead of pyrimidine-5-nucleotidase, which normally disperses residual RNA to produce a diffuse blue staining seen in reticulocytes on blood films (polychromasia).

FURTHER READING

Andrews NC (1999) Disorders of iron metabolism. *New England Journal of Medicine* **341**: 1986–1995.

Provan D, Weatherall D (2000) Red cells II: acquired anaemias. *Lancet* **355**: 1260–1268.

Spivak JL (2000) The blood in systemic disorders. *Lancet* **355**: 1707–1712.

Normocytic anaemia

Normocytic, normochromic anaemia is seen in anaemia of chronic disease, in some endocrine disorders (e.g. hypopituitarism, hypothyroidism and hypoadrenalism) and in some haematological disorders (e.g. aplastic anaemia and some haemolytic anaemias) (see Fig. 8.7). In addition, this type of anaemia is seen acutely following blood loss.

Macrocytic anaemias

These can be divided into megaloblastic and non-megaloblastic types, depending on bone marrow findings.

Megaloblastic anaemia

Megaloblastic anaemia is characterized by the presence in the bone marrow of erythroblasts with delayed nuclear maturation because of defective DNA synthesis (megaloblasts). Megaloblasts are large and have large immature nuclei. The nuclear chromatin is more finely dispersed than normal and has an open stippled appearance (see Fig. 8.8). A characteristic abnormality of white cells, giant metamyelocytes, is frequently seen in megaloblastic anaemia. These cells are about twice the size of normal cells and often have twisted nuclei. Megaloblastic changes occur in:

- vitamin B_{12} deficiency or abnormal vitamin B_{12} metabolism
- folic acid deficiency or abnormal folate metabolism
- other defects of DNA synthesis, such as congenital enzyme deficiencies in DNA synthesis (e.g. orotic aciduria), or resulting from therapy with drugs interfering with DNA synthesis (e.g. hydroxycarbamide (hydroxyurea), azathioprine, azidothymidine – AZT)
- myelodysplasia due to dyserythropoiesis.

Haematological values

Anaemia may be present. The MCV is characteristically > 96 fl unless there is a coexisting cause of microcytosis when there may be a dimorphic picture with a normal/low average MCV. The peripheral blood film shows macrocytes with hypersegmented polymorphs with six or more lobes in the nucleus (see Fig. 8.8). If severe, there may be leucopenia and thrombocytopenia.

Biochemical basis of megaloblastic anaemia

The key biochemical problem common to both vitamin B_{12} and folate deficiency is a block in DNA synthesis owing to an inability to methylate deoxyuridine monophosphate to deoxythymidine monophosphate, which is then used to build DNA (Fig. 8.10). The methyl group is supplied by the folate coenzyme, methylene tetrahydrofolate.

Deficiency of folate reduces the supply of this coenzyme; deficiency of vitamin B_{12} also reduces its supply by slowing the demethylation of methyltetrahydrofolate (methyl THF) and preventing cells receiving tetrahydrofolate for synthesis of methylene tetrahydrofolate polyglutamate.

Other congenital and acquired forms of megaloblastic anaemia are due to interference with purine or pyrimidine synthesis causing an inhibition in DNA synthesis.

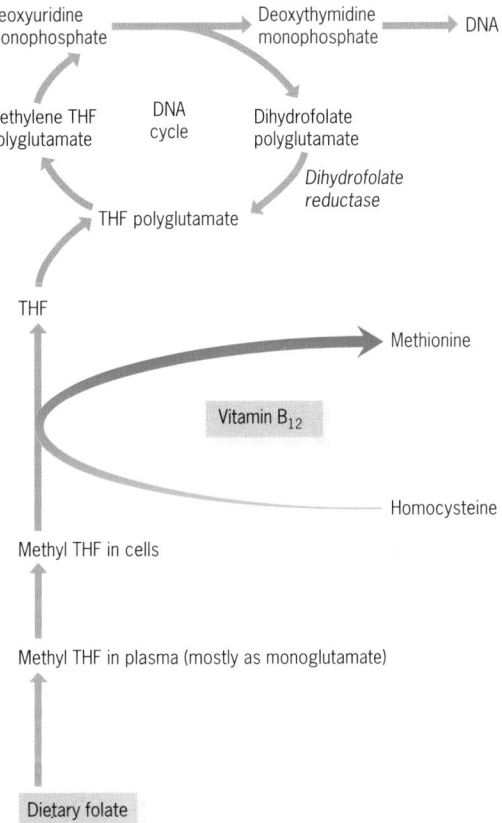

Fig. 8.10 Biochemical basis of megaloblastic anaemia. The metabolic relationship between vitamin B_{12} and folate and their role in DNA synthesis. THF, tetrahydrofolate.

Deoxyuridine suppression test

This is a useful method for rapidly determining the nature and severity of the vitamin B_{12} or folate deficiency in severe or complex cases of megaloblastic anaemia.

Tritiated thymidine is added to the patient's bone marrow in vitro. In a normoblastic marrow, the thymidine requirement is supplied by the methylation of deoxyuridine and this 'suppresses' the requirement for preformed tritiated thymidine to less than 5%. In a megaloblastic marrow, however, much more tritiated thymidine is used (5–50%). If the addition of B_{12} corrects the abnormality, it suggests that B_{12} is the cause of the deficiency. The addition of folate corrects the abnormality in both vitamin B_{12} and folate deficiency.

Vitamin B_{12}

Vitamin B_{12} is synthesized by certain microorganisms, and humans are ultimately dependent on animal sources. It is found in meat, fish, eggs and milk, but not in plants. Vitamin B_{12} is not usually destroyed by cooking. The average daily diet contains 5–30 µg of vitamin B_{12}, of which 2–3 µg is absorbed. The average adult stores some 2–3 mg, mainly in the liver, and it may take 2 years or more after absorptive failure before B_{12} deficiency develops, as the daily losses are small (1–2 µg).

Structure and function

Cobalamins consist of a planar group with a central cobalt atom (corrin ring) and a nucleotide set at right-angles (Fig. 8.11). Vitamin B_{12} was first crystallized as cyanocobalamin, but the main natural cobalamins have deoxyadenosyl-, methyl- and hydroxocobalamin groups attached to the cobalt atom.

The main function of B_{12} is the methylation of homocysteine to methionine with the demethylation of methyl THF polyglutamate to THF. THF is a substrate for folate polyglutamate synthesis.

Deoxyadenosylcobalamin is a coenzyme for the conversion of methylmalonyl CoA to succinyl CoA. Measurement of methylmalonic acid in urine was used as a test for vitamin B_{12} deficiency but it is no longer carried out routinely.

Absorption and transport

Vitamin B_{12} is liberated from protein complexes in food by gastric enzymes and then binds to a vitamin B_{12}-binding protein ('R' binder) related to plasma *transcobalamin I* (TC I), derived from saliva. Vitamin B_{12} bound to 'R' binder is released by pancreatic enzymes and becomes bound to intrinsic factor.

Intrinsic factor is a glycoprotein with a molecular weight of 45 000. It is secreted by gastric parietal cells along with H^+ ions. It combines with vitamin B_{12} and carries it to specific receptors on the surface of the mucosa of the ileum. Vitamin B_{12} enters the ileal cells and intrinsic factor remains in the lumen. Vitamin B_{12} is transported from the enterocytes to the bone marrow

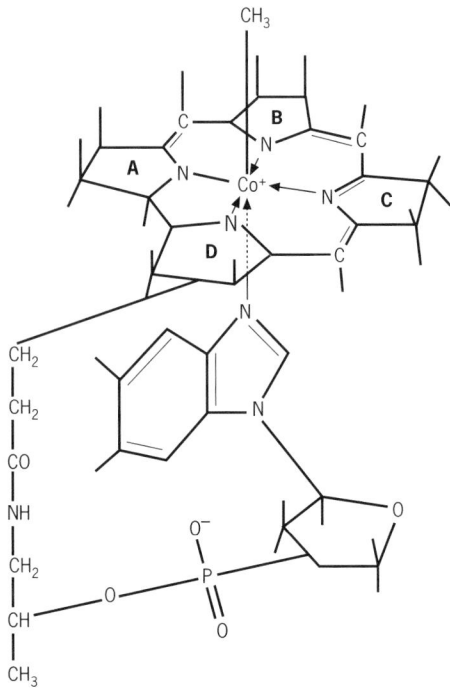

Fig. 8.11 Methylcobalamin structure. This is the main form of vitamin B_{12} in the plasma.

and other tissues by the glycoprotein *transcobalamin II* (TC II). Although TC II is the essential carrier protein for vitamin B_{12}, the amount of B_{12} on TC II is low; it has a rapid clearance and is able to deliver cobalamin to all cells of the body. Vitamin B_{12} in plasma is mainly bound to TC I (70–90%), but the functional role of this protein is unknown. About 1% of an oral dose of B_{12} is absorbed 'passively' without the need for intrinsic factor, mainly through the duodenum and ileum.

Vitamin B_{12} deficiency

There are a number of causes of B_{12} deficiency and abnormal B_{12} metabolism (Table 8.5). The most common cause of vitamin B_{12} deficiency in adults is pernicious anaemia. Malabsorption of vitamin B_{12} because of pancreatitis, coeliac disease or treatment with metformin is mild and does not usually result in significant vitamin B_{12} deficiency.

Pernicious anaemia

Pernicious anaemia (PA) is a condition in which there is atrophy of the gastric mucosa with consequent failure of intrinsic factor production and vitamin B_{12} malabsorption.

Pathogenesis of pernicious anaemia

This disease is common in the elderly, with 1 in 8000 of the population aged over 60 years being affected in

Table 8.5
Vitamin B$_{12}$ deficiency and abnormal B$_{12}$ metabolism: further causes (see text)

Low dietary intake	Abnormal metabolism
Vegans	Congenital transcobalamin II deficiency
Impaired absorption	Nitrous oxide (inactivates B$_{12}$)
Stomach	
Pernicious anaemia	
Gastrectomy	
Congenital deficiency of intrinsic factor	
Small bowel	
Ileal disease or resection	
Bacterial overgrowth	
Tropical sprue	
Fish tapeworm (*Diphyllobothrium latum*)	

the UK. It can be seen in all races, but occurs more frequently in fair-haired and blue-eyed individuals, and those who have the blood group A. It is more common in females than males.

There is an association with other autoimmune diseases, particularly thyroid disease, Addison's disease and vitiligo. Approximately one-half of all patients with PA have thyroid antibodies. There is a higher incidence of gastric carcinoma with PA than in the general population; the incidence in PA is 1–3%.

Parietal cell antibodies are present in the serum in 90% of patients with PA – and also in many older patients with gastric atrophy. Conversely, intrinsic factor antibodies, although found in only 50% of patients with PA, are specific for this diagnosis. Two types of intrinsic factor antibodies are found: a blocking antibody, which inhibits binding of intrinsic factor to B$_{12}$, and a precipitating antibody, which inhibits the binding of the B$_{12}$–intrinsic factor complex to its receptor site in the ileum.

B$_{12}$ deficiency may rarely occur in children from a congenital deficiency or abnormality of intrinsic factor, or as a result of early onset of the adult autoimmune type.

Pathology
Gastritis (see p. 277) affecting the fundus is present with plasma cell and lymphoid infiltration. The parietal and chief cells are replaced by mucin-secreting cells. There is achlorhydria and absent secretion of intrinsic factor. The histological abnormality can be improved by corticosteroid therapy, which supports an autoimmune basis for the disease.

Clinical features
The onset of PA is insidious, with progressively increasing symptoms of anaemia. Patients are sometimes said to have a lemon-yellow colour owing to a combination of pallor and mild jaundice caused by excess breakdown of haemoglobin because of ineffective erythropoiesis in the bone marrow. A red sore tongue (glossitis) and angular stomatitis are sometimes present.

The neurological changes, if left untreated, can be irreversible. These neurological abnormalities occur only with very low levels of serum B$_{12}$ (less than 60 ng/L) and occasionally occur in patients who are not clinically anaemic. The classical neurological features are those of a polyneuropathy progressively involving the peripheral nerves and the posterior and eventually the lateral columns of the spinal cord (subacute combined degeneration), page 1216. Patients present with symmetrical paraesthesiae in the fingers and toes, early loss of vibration sense and proprioception, and progressive weakness and ataxia. Paraplegia may result. Dementia and optic atrophy also occur from vitamin B$_{12}$ deficiency.

Investigations
- **Haematological findings** show the features of a megaloblastic anaemia as described on page 417.
- **Bone marrow** shows the typical features of megaloblastic erythropoiesis (Fig. 8.8), although it is frequently not performed in cases of straightforward macrocytic anaemia and a low serum vitamin B$_{12}$.
- **Serum bilirubin** may be raised as a result of ineffective erythropoiesis. Normally a minor fraction of serum bilirubin results from premature breakdown of newly formed red cells in the bone marrow. In many megaloblastic anaemias, where the destruction of developing red cells is much increased, the serum bilirubin can be increased.
- **Serum vitamin B$_{12}$** is usually well below 160 ng/L, which is the lower end of the normal range. Serum vitamin B$_{12}$ can be assayed using radioisotope dilution or immunological assays.
- **Serum folate level** is normal or high, and the red cell folate is normal or reduced owing to inhibition of normal folate synthesis.

Absorption tests
The absorption of B$_{12}$ can be measured using the Schilling test (Practical box 8.2). This test may give a falsely low result if there is an incomplete 24-hour collection of urine or if renal function is impaired. An alternative to the Schilling test is whole-body counting where a radioactive dose of B$_{12}$ is given orally and the total body activity is measured. The level of radioactivity is counted no less than 7 days later to measure how much vitamin B$_{12}$ has been retained. A normal result is retention of 50% or more of the 1 mg dose of radioactive B$_{12}$. Vitamin B$_{12}$ absorption tests are performed only occasionally when the underlying cause of the B$_{12}$ deficiency is not obvious.

Gastrointestinal investigations
In PA there is marked gastric atrophy with achlorhydria. Intubation studies can be performed to confirm this but

Practical box 8.2

Schilling test

Part 1

- Give 1 µg ^{58}Co-B_{12} orally to fasting patient.
- Give 1000 µg B_{12} (non-radioactive) by intramuscular injection to saturate B_{12}-binding proteins and to flush out ^{58}Co-B_{12}.
- Collect urine for 24 hours.
- Normal subjects excrete more than 10% of the radioactive dose.

Part 2

Repeat part 1 with oral intrinsic factor capsules.

Result

- If excretion now normal, diagnosis is pernicious anaemia or gastrectomy.
- If excretion is still abnormal, lesion is in the terminal ileum or there is bacterial overgrowth.
- Vitamin B_{12} malabsorption due to bacterial overgrowth may be corrected by antibiotic therapy.

are rarely carried out in routine practice. Endoscopy or barium meal examination of the stomach is performed only if gastric symptoms are present.

Differential diagnosis

Vitamin B_{12} deficiency must be differentiated from other causes of megaloblastic anaemia, principally folate deficiency, but usually this is quite clear from the blood level of these two vitamins.

Pernicious anaemia should be distinguished from other causes of vitamin B_{12} deficiency (see Table 8.5). Any disease involving the terminal ileum or bacterial overgrowth in the small bowel can produce vitamin B_{12} deficiency (see p. 291). Gastrectomy can lead, in the long term, to vitamin B_{12} deficiency. Vegans are strict vegetarians and eat no meat or animal products. A careful dietary history should be obtained.

Treatment

See below.

Folic acid

Folic acid monoglutamate is not present in nature but is the parent compound of folates, which are polyglutamates (extra glutamic acid residues).

Folates are present in food as polyglutamates in the reduced dihydrofolate or tetrahydrofolate forms (Fig. 8.12), with methyl (CH_3), formyl (CHO) or methylene (CH_2) groups attached to the pteridine part of the molecule. Polyglutamates are broken down to monoglutamates in the upper gastrointestinal tract, and during

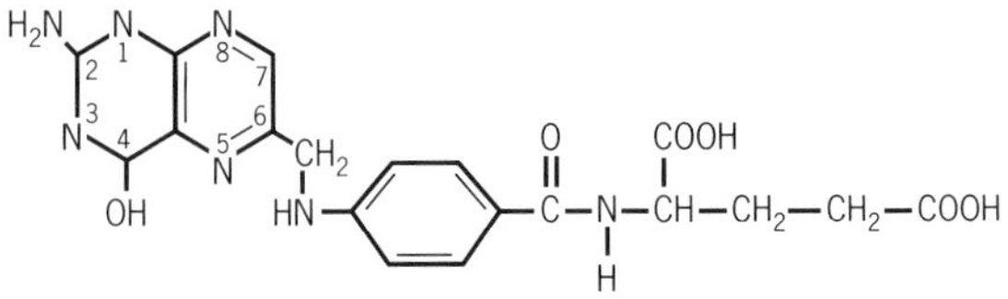

Fig. 8.12 Folic acid structure. This is formed from three building blocks as shown. Tetrahydrofolate has additional hydrogen atoms at positions 5, 6, 7 and 8.

the absorptive process these are converted to methyl THF monoglutamate, which is the main form in the serum. The methylation of homocysteine to methionine requires both methylcobalamin and methyl THF as coenzymes. This reaction is the first step in which methyl THF entering cells from the plasma is converted into folate polyglutamates. Intracellular polyglutamates are the active forms of folate and act as coenzymes in the transfer of single carbon units in amino acid metabolism and DNA synthesis (see Fig. 8.10).

Dietary intake

Folate is found in green vegetables such as spinach and broccoli, and offal, such as liver and kidney. Cooking causes a loss of 60–90% of the folate. The minimal daily requirement is about 100 µg.

Folate deficiency

The causes of folate deficiency are shown in Table 8.6. The main cause is poor intake, which may occur alone or in combination with excessive utilization or malabsorption. The body's reserves of folate, unlike vitamin B_{12}, are low (about 10 mg). On a deficient diet, folate deficiency develops over the course of about 4 months, but folate deficiency may develop rapidly in patients who have both a poor intake and excess utilization of folate (e.g. patients in intensive care units).

Clinical features

Patients with folate deficiency may be asymptomatic or present with symptoms of anaemia or of the underlying cause. Glossitis can occur. Unlike with B_{12} deficiency, neuropathy does not occur. Although there is no simple relationship between maternal folate status and fetal abnormalities, folic acid supplements at the time of conception and in the first 12 weeks of pregnancy reduce the incidence of neural tube defects. A high incidence of a partial deficiency in a key enzyme in folate metabolism, methyl THF reductase, has been found in parents of fetuses with neural tube defects. The 5% of individuals with this abnormality have increased levels of homocysteine (Fig. 8.10), which may be the mechanism underlying the increased incidence of neural tube defects.

Table 8.6
Causes of folate deficiency

Nutritional (major cause)

Poor intake
Old age
Poor social conditions
Starvation
Alcohol excess (also causes
    impaired utilization)

Poor intake due to anorexia
Gastrointestinal disease, e.g.
    partial gastrectomy, coeliac
    disease, Crohn's disease
Cancer

Antifolate drugs
Anticonvulsants
    Phenytoin
    Primidone
Methotrexate
Pyrimethamine
Trimethoprim

Excess utilization

Physiological
Pregnancy
Lactation
Prematurity

Pathological
Haematological disease
    with excess red cell
    production,
    e.g. haemolysis
Malignant disease with
    increased cell turnover
Inflammatory disease
Metabolic disease,
    e.g. homocystinuria
Haemodialysis or
    peritoneal dialysis

Malabsorption
Occurs in small bowel
    disease, but the effect
    is minor compared with
    that of anorexia

Investigations
The haematological findings are those of a megaloblastic anaemia as discussed on page 417.

Blood measurements
Serum and red cell folate are assayed by radioisotope dilution or immunological methods. Normal levels of serum folate are 4–18 µg/L (5–63 nmol/L). The amount of folate in the red cells is a better measure of tissue folate; the normal range is 160–640 µg/mL.

Further investigations
In many cases of folate deficiency the cause is not obvious from the clinical picture or dietary history. Occult gastrointestinal disease should then be suspected and appropriate investigations, such as jejunal biopsy, should be performed (p. 289).

Treatment and prevention of megaloblastic anaemia
Treatment depends on the type of deficiency. Blood transfusion is not indicated in chronic anaemia; indeed, it is dangerous to transfuse elderly patients, as heart failure may be precipitated. Folic acid may produce a haematological response in vitamin B_{12} deficiency but may aggravate the neuropathy. Large doses of folic acid alone should not be used to treat megaloblastic anaemia unless the serum vitamin B_{12} level is known to be normal. In severely ill patients, it may be necessary to treat with both folic acid and vitamin B_{12} while awaiting serum levels.

Treatment of vitamin B_{12} deficiency
Hydroxocobalamin 1000 µg can be given intramuscularly to a total of 5–6 mg over the course of 3 weeks; 1000 µg is then necessary every 3 months for the rest of the patient's life. Clinical improvement may occur within 48 hours and a reticulocytosis can be seen some 2–3 days after starting therapy, peaking at 5–7 days. Improvement of the polyneuropathy may occur over 6–12 months, but long-standing spinal cord damage is irreversible. Hypokalaemia can occur and, if severe, supplements should be given. Iron deficiency often develops in the first few weeks of therapy. Hyperuricaemia occurs but clinical gout is uncommon. In patients who have had a total gastrectomy or an ileal resection, vitamin B_{12} should be monitored; if low levels occur, prophylactic vitamin B_{12} injections should be given.

Intramuscular B_{12} has been traditionally used for treating pernicious anaemia, although it is known that about 1% of large doses of B_{12} are absorbed through a passive, intrinsic factor-independent mechanism. Treatment with oral B_{12}, even using large doses, has been previously discounted because of concerns about unpredictable absorption and compliance. However, there is renewed interest in using oral B_{12}; doses of 2000 µg daily have been shown to be as effective in treating pernicious anaemia as the intramuscular regimen described above. Compliance with an oral daily regimen may be a problem, particularly in elderly patients, and at present only 50 µg tablets are available. The use of sublingual nuggets of B_{12} (2 × 1000 µg daily) has been suggested to be an effective and more convenient option.

Treatment of folate deficiency
Folate deficiency can be corrected by giving 5 mg of folic acid daily; the same haematological response occurs as seen after treatment of vitamin B_{12} deficiency. Treatment should be given for about 4 months to replace body stores. Any underlying cause, e.g. coeliac disease, should be treated.

Prophylactic folic acid (400 µg daily) is recommended for all women planning a pregnancy. Many authorities also recommend prophylactic administration of folate throughout pregnancy. Whether this can be achieved by increased consumption of foods with a high folate content or whether women should take folate supplements is under debate. The US Food and Drugs Administration has introduced a requirement for the fortification with folic acid of grain products such as bread, flour and rice (p. 238).

Women who have had a child with a neural tube defect should have 5 mg folic acid before and during a subsequent pregnancy.

Prophylactic folic acid is also given in chronic haematological disorders where there is rapid cell turnover. A dose of 5 mg each week is probably sufficient.

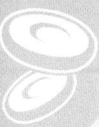
Macrocytosis without megaloblastic changes

A raised MCV with macrocytosis on the peripheral blood film can occur with a normoblastic rather than a megaloblastic bone marrow.

A common *physiological* cause of macrocytosis is pregnancy, and a newborn may also suffer.

Common *pathological* causes are:

- alcohol excess
- liver disease
- reticulocytosis
- hypothyroidism
- some haematological disorders (e.g. aplastic anaemia, sideroblastic anaemia, pure red cell aplasia)
- drugs (e.g. cytotoxics – azathioprine)
- spurious (agglutinated red cells measured on red cell counters)
- cold agglutinins due to autoagglutination of red cells (see p. 437) (the MCV decreases to normal with warming of the sample to 37°C).

In all these conditions, normal serum levels of vitamin B_{12} and folate will be found. The exact mechanisms in each case are uncertain, but in some there is increased lipid deposition in the red cell membrane.

An increased number of reticulocytes leads to a raised MCV because they are large cells.

Alcohol is a frequent cause of a raised MCV in an otherwise normal individual. A megaloblastic anaemia can also occur in people who abuse alcohol; this is due to a toxic effect of alcohol on erythropoiesis or to dietary folate deficiency.

FURTHER READING

Chanarin I, Metz J (1997) Diagnosis of cobalamin deficiency: the old and the new. *British Journal of Haematology* **97**: 695–700.

Elia M (1998) Oral or parenteral therapy for B_{12} deficiency. *Lancet* **352**: 1721–1722.

Mills JL (2000) Fortification of foods with folic acid. *New England Journal of Medicine* **342**: 1442–1445.

Toh BH, van Driel IR, Gleeson PA (1997) Pernicious anaemia. *New England Journal of Medicine* **337**: 1441–1448.

Wickramsinghe SN (1997) Folate and vitamin B_{12} deficiency and supplementation. *Prescribers' Journal* **37**: 88–95.

Anaemia due to marrow failure (aplastic anaemia)

Aplastic anaemia is defined as pancytopenia with hypocellularity (aplasia) of the bone marrow; there are no leukaemic, cancerous or other abnormal cells in the peripheral blood or bone marrow. It is an uncommon but serious condition that may be inherited but is more commonly acquired.

Aplastic anaemia is due to a reduction in the number of pluripotential stem cells (see Fig. 8.1) together with a fault in those remaining or an immune reaction against them so that they are unable to repopulate the bone marrow. Failure of one cell line may occur, resulting in isolated deficiencies such as the absence of red cell precursors in pure red cell aplasia. Evolution to myelodysplasia, paroxysmal nocturnal haemoglobinuria (PNH) or acute myeloblastic leukaemia occurs in some cases, probably owing the emergence of an abnormal clone of haemopoietic cells.

Causes

A list of causes of aplasia is given in Table 8.7. Immune mechanisms are probably responsible for most cases of idiopathic acquired aplastic anaemia and play a part in at least the persistence of many secondary cases. Activated cytotoxic T cells in blood and bone marrow are responsible for the bone marrow failure.

Many drugs may cause marrow aplasia, including cytotoxic drugs such as busulfan and doxorubicin, which are expected to cause transient aplasia as a consequence of their therapeutic use. However, some individuals develop aplasia due to sensitivity to non-cytotoxic drugs such as chloramphenicol, gold, carbimazole, chlorpromazine, phenytoin, tolbutamide, non-steroidal anti-inflammatory agents, and many others which have been reported to cause occasional cases of aplasia.

Congenital aplastic anaemias are rare. Fanconi's anaemia is inherited as an autosomal recessive and is associated with skeletal, renal and central nervous system abnormalities. It usually presents between the ages of 5 and 10 years.

Clinical features

The clinical manifestations of marrow failure from any cause are anaemia, bleeding and infection. Bleeding is

Table 8.7
Causes of aplastic anaemia

Primary
Congenital, e.g. Fanconi's anaemia
Idiopathic acquired (67% of cases)

Secondary
Chemicals, e.g. benzene
Drugs
    chemotherapeutic
    idiosyncratic reactions
Insecticides
Ionizing radiation
Infections:
    viral, e.g. hepatitis, EBV, HIV, Parvovirus
    other, e.g. tuberculosis
Paroxysmal nocturnal haemoglobinuria

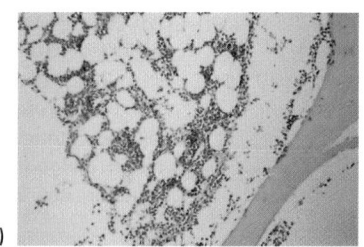 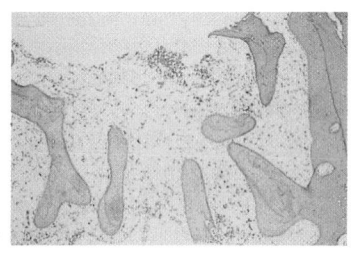

Fig. 8.13 Bone marrow trephine biopsies in low-power view. **(a)** Normal cellularity. **(b)** Hypocellularity in aplastic anaemia.

(a)　　　　　　　**(b)**

often the predominant initial presentation of aplastic anaemia with bruising with minimal trauma or blood blisters in the mouth. Physical findings include ecchymoses, bleeding gums and epistaxis. Mouth infections are common. Lymphadenopathy and hepatosplenomegaly are rare in aplastic anaemia.

Investigations

The laboratory diagnosis is made on the basis of:

- pancytopenia
- the virtual absence of reticulocytes
- a hypocellular or aplastic bone marrow with increased fat spaces (Fig. 8.13).

Differential diagnosis

This is from other causes of pancytopenia (Table 8.8). A bone marrow trephine is essential for assessment of the bone marrow cellularity.

Treatment and prognosis

The treatment of aplastic anaemia depends on providing supportive care while awaiting bone marrow recovery and specific treatment to accelerate marrow recovery.

The main danger is infection and stringent measures should be undertaken to avoid this (see also p. 483). Any suspicion of infection in a severely neutropenic patient should lead to immediate institution of broad-spectrum parenteral antibiotics. Supportive care including transfusions of red cells and platelets should be given as necessary. The cause of the aplastic anaemia must be eliminated if possible.

Table 8.8
Causes of pancytopenia

Aplastic anaemia (see Table 8.7)
Drugs
Megaloblastic anaemia
Bone marrow infiltration or replacement
　Hodgkin's and non-Hodgkin's lymphoma
　Acute leukaemia
　Myeloma
　Secondary carcinoma
　Myelofibrosis
Hypersplenism
Systemic lupus erythematosus
Disseminated tuberculosis
Paroxysmal nocturnal haemoglobinuria
Overwhelming sepsis

The course of aplastic anaemia can be variable, ranging from a rapid spontaneous remission to a persistent increasingly severe pancytopenia, which may lead to death through haemorrhage or infection. The most reliable determinants for the prognosis are the number of neutrophils, reticulocytes, platelets, and the cellularity of the bone marrow.

A bad prognosis (i.e. severe aplastic anaemia) is associated with the presence of two of the following three features:

- neutrophil count of $< 0.5 \times 10^9/L$
- platelet count of $< 20 \times 10^9/L$
- reticulocyte count of $< 40 \times 10^9/L$.

In severe aplastic anaemia, there is a very poor outcome without treatment. Bone marrow transplantation is the treatment of choice for patients under 50 years of age who have an HLA-identical sibling donor, which gives a 75–90% chance of long-term survival and restoring the blood count to normal. Patients over the age of 50 are not eligible for bone marrow transplantation whether an HLA-identical donor is available or not, because of the high risk of graft-versus-host disease as a complication of bone marrow transplantation. Immunosuppressive therapy is used for patients without HLA-matched siblings and those over the age of 50 years; antilymphocyte globulin (ALG) and ciclosporin are used alone or in combination. ALG alone produces a haematological recovery in 50–60% of cases and this is increased to 80% in patients also receiving ciclosporin.

Use of a second course of antilymphocyte globulin produces responses in about 50–60% of these cases.

For patients failing to respond to immunosuppression, bone marrow transplantation using unrelated donors is an option, but the results are poor (5-year survival of only 30%) owing to a high incidence of graft rejection, graft-versus-host disease and viral infections.

Levels of haemopoietic growth factors (Fig. 8.1) are normal or increased in most patients with aplastic anaemia, and are ineffective as primary treatment.

Androgens (e.g. oxymethalone) are sometimes useful in patients not responding to immunosuppression and in patients with moderately severe aplastic anaemia.

Steroids have little activity in severe aplastic anaemia but are used for serum sickness due to ALG. They are also used to treat children with congenital pure red cell aplasia (Diamond–Blackfan syndrome). Adult pure red cell aplasia is associated with a thymoma in 30% of cases and thymectomy may induce a remission. It may also be associated with autoimmune disease or may be idiopathic. Steroids and ciclosporin are effective treatment in some cases.

FURTHER READING

Marsh JCW, Gordon-Smith EC (1998). Treatment options in severe aplastic anaemia. *Lancet* **351**: 1830–1831.
Young NS, Maciejewski J (1997) The pathophysiology of acquired aplastic anaemia. *New England Journal of Medicine* **336**: 1365–1372.

Haemolytic anaemias: an introduction

Haemolytic anaemias are caused by increased destruction of red cells. The red cell normally survives about 120 days, but in haemolytic anaemias the red cell survival times are considerably shortened.

Breakdown of normal red cells occurs in the macrophages of the bone marrow, liver and spleen (see Fig. 8.5).

Consequences of haemolysis

Shortening of red cell survival does not always cause anaemia as there is a compensatory increase in red cell production by the bone marrow. If the red cell loss can be contained within the marrow's capacity for increased output, then a haemolytic state can exist without anaemia (*compensated haemolytic disease*). The bone marrow can increase its output by six to eight times by increasing the proportion of cells committed to erythropoiesis (*erythroid hyperplasia*) and by expanding the volume of active marrow. In addition, immature red cells (*reticulocytes*) are released prematurely. These cells are larger than mature cells and stain light blue on a peripheral blood film (the description of this appearance on the blood film is *polychromasia*). Reticulocytes may be counted accurately as a percentage of all red cells on a blood film using a supravital stain for residual RNA (e.g. new methylene blue).

Sites of haemolysis

Extravascular haemolysis

In most haemolytic conditions red cell destruction is extravascular. The red cells are removed from the circulation by macrophages in the reticuloendothelial system, particularly the spleen.

Intravascular haemolysis

When red cells are rapidly destroyed within the circulation, haemoglobin is liberated (Fig. 8.14). This is initially bound to plasma haptoglobins but these soon become saturated.

Excess free plasma Hb is filtered by the renal glomerulus and enters the urine, although small amounts are reabsorbed by the renal tubules. In the renal tubular cell, Hb is broken down and becomes deposited in the cells as *haemosiderin*. This can be detected in the spun sediment of urine using Perls' reaction. Some of the free plasma Hb is oxidized to *methaemoglobin*, which dissociates into *ferrihaem* and globin. *Plasma haemopexin* binds ferrihaem; but if its binding capacity is exceeded, ferrihaem becomes attached to albumin, forming *methaemalbumin*. On spectrophotometry of the plasma, methaemalbumin forms a characteristic band; this is the basis of *Schumm's test*.

The *liver* plays an important role in removing Hb bound to haptoglobin and *haemopexin* and any remaining free Hb.

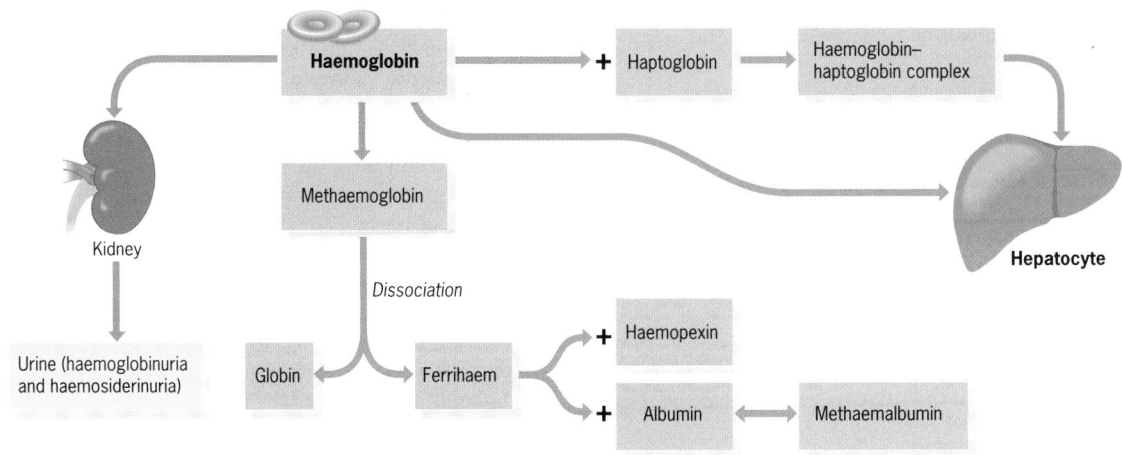

Fig. 8.14 The fate of haemoglobin in the plasma following haemolysis.

Evidence for haemolysis

Increased red cell breakdown leads to:

- elevated serum bilirubin (unconjugated)
- excess urinary urobilinogen (resulting from bilirubin breakdown in the intestine, Fig. 8.5)
- reduced plasma haptoglobin
- raised serum lactic dehydrogenase (LDH).

Increased red cell production leads to:

- reticulocytosis
- erythroid hyperplasia of the bone marrow.

There may be evidence of abnormal red cells in some haemolytic anaemias:

- spherocytes (see Fig. 8.8)
- sickle cells (see Fig. 8.8)
- red cell fragments.

Demonstration of shortened red cell life-span

Red cell survival can be estimated from ^{51}Cr-labelled red cells but is rarely performed.

Intravascular haemolysis

This is suggested by raised levels of plasma Hb, haemosiderinuria, very low or absent haptoglobins, and the presence of methaemalbumin (positive Schumm's test).

Table 8.9
Causes of haemolytic anaemia

Inherited	Acquired
Red cell membrane defect	*Immune*
Hereditary spherocytosis	Autoimmune
Hereditary elliptocytosis	(see Table 8.15)
	Warm
Haemoglobin abnormalities	Cold
Thalassaemia	Alloimmune
Sickle cell disease	Haemolytic transfusion
	reactions
Metabolic defects	Haemolytic disease of
Glucose-6-phosphate	the newborn
dehydrogenase deficiency	After allogeneic bone
Pyruvate kinase deficiency	marrow or organ
	transplantation
Miscellaneous	Drug-induced
Infections, e.g. malaria,	
mycoplasma	*Non-immune*
Clostridium welchii,	Acquired membrane defects
generalized sepsis	Paroxysmal nocturnal
Drugs and chemicals causing	haemoglobinuria
damage to the red cell	Mechanical
membrane or oxidative	Microangiopathic
haemolysis	haemolytic anaemia
Hypersplenism	Valve prosthesis
Burns	March haemoglobinuria
	Secondary to systemic disease
	Renal and liver failure

Various laboratory studies will be necessary to determine the exact type of haemolytic anaemia present. The causes of haemolytic anaemias are shown in Table 8.9.

Inherited haemolytic anaemia

Red cell membrane defects

The normal red cell membrane consists of a lipid bilayer crossed by integral proteins with an underlying lattice of proteins (or cytoskeleton), including spectrin, actin, ankyrin and protein 4.1, attached to integral proteins (Fig. 8.15).

Hereditary spherocytosis (HS)

HS is the most common inherited haemolytic anaemia in northern Europeans, affecting 1 in 5000. It is inherited in an autosomal dominant manner, but in 25% of patients neither parent is affected and it is presumed that HS has occurred by spontaneous mutation. HS is due to a defect in the red cell membrane, resulting in the cells losing part of the cell membrane as they pass through the spleen, possibly because the lipid bilayer is inadequately supported by the cytoskeleton. The surface-to-volume ratio decreases, and the cells become spherocytic. Spherocytes are more rigid and less deformable than normal red cells. They are unable to pass through the splenic microcirculation and they die.

Several defects in the cell membrane have been identified in HS. The best characterized is a deficiency in the structural protein spectrin, but quantitative defects in other membrane proteins have been identified (Fig. 8.15). The abnormal red cell membrane in HS is associated functionally with an increased permeability to sodium, and this requires an increased rate of active transport of sodium out of the cells which is dependent on ATP produced by glycolysis.

Clinical features

The condition may present with jaundice at birth. However, the onset of jaundice can sometimes be delayed for many years and some patients may go through life with no symptoms and are detected only during family studies. The patient may eventually develop anaemia, splenomegaly and ulcers on the leg. As in many haemolytic anaemias, the course of the disease may be interrupted by aplastic, haemolytic and megaloblastic crises. Aplastic anaemia usually occurs after infections, particularly with parvovirus, whereas megaloblastic anaemia is the result of folate depletion owing to the hyperactivity of the bone marrow. Chronic haemolysis leads to the formation of pigment gallstones (see p. 388).

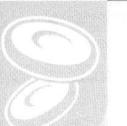

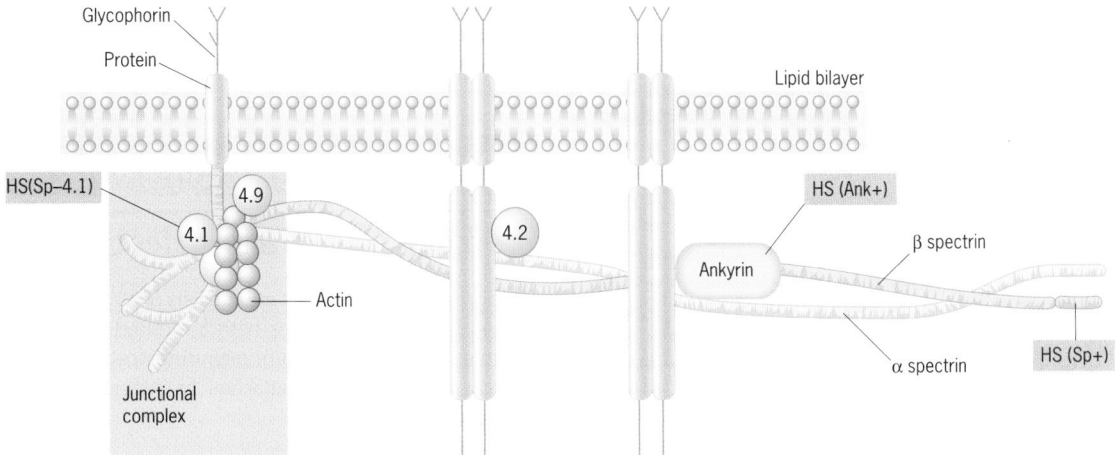

Fig. 8.15 **Red cell membrane showing the sites of the principal defects in hereditary spherocytosis (HS).** HS (Ank+), ankyrin deficiency; HS (Sp+), spectrin deficiency; HS (Sp-4.1) abnormal spectrin/protein 4.1 binding.

Investigations

- **Anaemia.** This is usually mild, but occasionally can be severe.
- **Blood film**. This shows spherocytes and reticulocytes
- **Haemolysis** is evident (e.g. the serum bilirubin and urinary urobilinogen will be raised).
- **Osmotic fragility**. When red cells are placed in solutions of increasing hypotonicity, they take in water, swell, and eventually lyse. Spherocytes tolerate hypotonic solutions less well than do normal biconcave red cells. Osmotic fragility tests are infrequently carried out in routine practice, but may be useful to confirm a suspicion of spherocytosis on a blood film.
- **Direct antiglobulin (Coombs') test** is negative in spherocytosis, virtually ruling out autoimmune haemolytic anaemia where spherocytes are also commonly present.

Treatment

The spleen, which is the site of cell destruction, should be removed in all but the mildest cases. The decision about splenectomy in symptomless patients is difficult, but a raised bilirubin and especially the presence of gallstones should encourage splenectomy.

It is best to postpone splenectomy until after childhood, as sudden overwhelming fatal infections, usually due to encapsulated organisms such as pneumococci, may occur (see p. 444). Splenectomy should be preceded by pneumococcal and Hib immunization and followed by lifelong penicillin prophylaxis (see p. 444).

Following splenectomy, the spherocytosis is reduced and the Hb level usually returns to normal as the red cells are no longer destroyed.

Folate deficiency often occurs in chronic haemolysis with rapid cell turnover. Folate levels should be monitored, or folic acid can be given prophylactically.

Hereditary elliptocytosis

This disorder of the red cell membrane is inherited in an autosomal dominant manner and has a prevalence of 1 in 2500 in Caucasians. The red cells are elliptical owing to spectrin and other protein abnormalities. Clinically it is a similar condition to HS but milder. Only a minority of patients have anaemia and only occasional patients require splenectomy. Rarely hereditary spherocytosis or elliptocytosis may be inherited in a homozygous fashion giving rise to a severe haemolytic anaemia sometimes necessitating splenectomy in early childhood.

Hereditary stomatocytosis

Stomatocytes are red cells in which the pale central area appears slit-like. Their presence in large numbers may occur in a hereditary haemolytic anaemia associated with a membrane defect, but excess alcohol intake is also a common cause.

Haemoglobin abnormalities

Normal haemoglobin

Normal adult Hb (Hb A) has two polypeptide globin chains, the α and β chains (Table 8.10), which have 141 and 146 amino acids respectively. These are folded so that haem molecules can be held within the fold and are yet able to combine reversibly with oxygen.

In early embryonic life, haemoglobins Gower 1, Gower 2 and Portland predominate (Fig. 8.16). Later, fetal haemoglobin (Hb F), which has two α and two γ chains,

Table 8.10
Some types of haemoglobin

	Haemoglobin	Structure	Comment
Normal	A	$\alpha_2\beta_2$	Comprises 97% of adult haemoglobin
	A_2	$\alpha_2\delta_2$	Comprises 2% of adult haemoglobin
			Elevated in β-thalassaemia
	F	$\alpha_2\gamma_2$	Normal haemoglobin in fetus from 3rd to 9th month
			Increased in β-thalassaemia
			Comprises <1% of haemoglobin in adult
Abnormal chain production	H	β_4	Found in α-thalassaemia
			Biologically useless
	Barts	γ_4	Comprises 100% of haemoglobin in homozygous α-thalassaemia
			Biologically useless
Abnormal chain structure	S	$\alpha_2\beta_2{}^S$	Substitution of valine for glutamic acid in position 6 of β chain
	C	$\alpha_2\beta_2{}^C$	Substitution of lysine for glutamic acid in position 6 of β chain

is produced. There is increasing synthesis of β chains from 13 weeks of gestation and at term there is 80% Hb F and 20% Hb A. The switch from Hb F to Hb A occurs after birth when the genes for γ chain production are further suppressed and there is rapid increase in the synthesis of β chains. The exact mechanism responsible for the switch remains unknown. There is little Hb F produced (normally less than 1%) from 6 months after birth. The β chain is synthesized just before birth and Hb A_2 ($\alpha_2\delta_2$) remains at a level of about 2% throughout adult life.

Globin chains are synthesized in the same way as any protein (see Ch. 3). Four globin chain genes are required to control α-chain production (Fig. 8.16). Two are present on each haploid genome (genes derived from one parent). These are situated close together on chromosome 16. The genes controlling the production of ε, γ, δ and β chains are close together on chromosome 11. The globin genes are arranged on chromosomes 16 and 11 in the order in which they are expressed.

Abnormal haemoglobins

Abnormalities occur in:

- globin chain production (e.g. thalassaemia)

- structure of the globin chain (e.g. sickle cell disease)
- combined defects of globin chain production and structure, e.g. sickle cell β-thalassaemia.

Genetic defects in haemoglobin are the most common of all genetic disorders.

The thalassaemias

The thalassaemias (Greek *thalassa* = sea) affect people throughout the world (Fig. 8.17). Normally there is balanced (1 : 1) production of α and β chains. The defective synthesis of globin genes in thalassaemia leads to 'imbalanced' globin chain production, leading to precipitation of globin chains within the red cell precursors and resulting in ineffective erythropoiesis. Precipitation of globin chains in mature red cells leads to haemolysis.

β-Thalassaemia

In homozygous β-thalassaemia, either no normal β chains are produced (β^0), or β-chain production is very

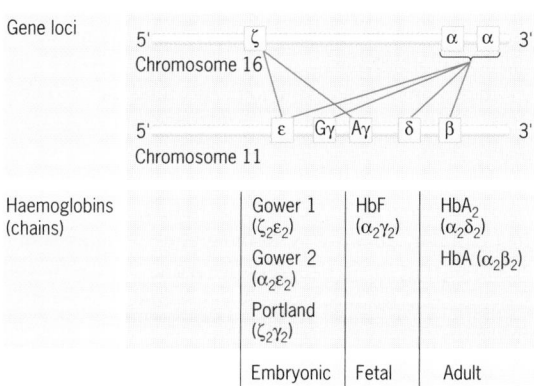

Fig. 8.16 Loci of genes on chromosomes 16 and 11 and the combination of various chains to produce different haemoglobins.

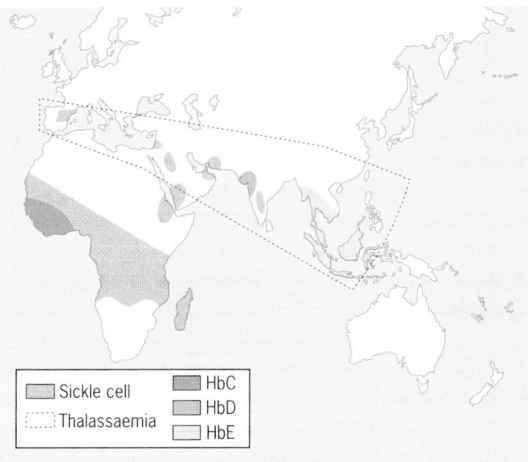

Fig. 8.17 Major haemoglobin abnormalities: geographical distribution.

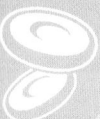

Table 8.11
Thalassaemia: findings in β-, δβ- and γδβ-thalassaemias

Type of thalassaemia	Findings in homozygote	Findings in heterozygote
β^+	Thalassaemia major Hb A + F + A$_2$	Thalassaemia minor Hb A$_2$ raised
β^0	Thalassaemia major Hb F + A$_2$	Thalassaemia minor Hb A$_2$ raised
δβ	Thalassaemia intermedia Hb F only	Thalassaemia minor Hb F 5–15% Hb A$_2$ normal
δβ (**Lepore**)	Thalassaemia major or intermedia Hb F and Lepore	Thalassaemia minor Hb Lepore 5–15% Hb A$_2$ normal

Adapted with permission from Weatherall DJ (1996) Disorders of the synthesis of function of haemoglobin. In Weatherall DJ, Ledingham JGG, Warrell DA (eds) *Oxford Textbook of Medicine*. Oxford: Oxford University Press.

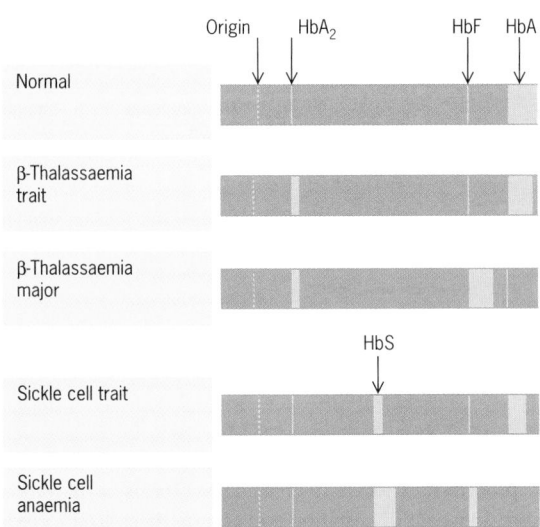

Fig. 8.18 Patterns of haemoglobin electrophoresis.

reduced (β^+). There is an excess of α chains, which precipitate in erythroblasts and red cells causing ineffective erythropoiesis and haemolysis. The excess α chains combine with whatever β, δ and γ chains are produced, resulting in increased quantities of Hb A$_2$ and Hb F and, at best, small amounts of Hb A. In heterozygous β-thalassaemia there is usually symptomless microcytosis with or without mild anaemia. Table 8.11 shows the findings in the homozygote and heterozygote for the common types of β-thalassaemia.

Molecular genetics

The molecular errors accounting for over 200 genetic defects leading to β-thalassaemia have been characterized. Unlike α-thalassaemia, the defects are mainly point mutations rather than gene deletions. The mutations result in defects in transcription, RNA splicing and modification, translation via frame shifts and nonsense codons producing highly unstable β-globin which cannot be utilized.

Clinical syndromes

Clinically, β-thalassaemia can be divided into the following:

- thalassaemia minor (or trait), the symptomless heterozygous carrier state
- thalassaemia intermedia, with moderate anaemia, rarely requiring transfusions
- thalassaemia major, with severe anaemia requiring regular transfusions.

Thalassaemia minor (trait)

This common carrier state (heterozygous β-thalassaemia) is asymptomatic. Anaemia is mild or absent. The red cells are hypochromic and microcytic with a low MCV and MCH, and it may be confused with iron deficiency. However, the two are easily distinguished as in thalassaemia trait the serum ferritin and the iron stores are normal (see Table 8.3). Hb electrophoresis usually shows a raised Hb A$_2$ and often a raised Hb F (Fig. 8.18). Iron should not be given to these patients unless they develop coincidental iron deficiency.

Thalassaemia intermedia

Thalassaemia intermedia includes patients who are symptomatic with moderate anaemia (Hb 7–10 g/dL) and who do not require regular transfusions. That is, it is more severe than in β-thalassaemia trait but milder than in transfusion-dependent thalassaemia major.

Thalassaemia intermedia may be due to a combination of homozygous mild β^+- and α-thalassaemia, where there is reduced α-chain precipitation and less ineffective erythropoiesis and haemolysis. The inheritance of hereditary persistence of Hb F with homozygous β-thalassaemia also results in a milder clinical picture than unmodified β-thalassaemia major because the excess α chains are partially removed by the increased production of γ chains.

Patients may have splenomegaly and bone deformities. Recurrent leg ulcers, gallstones and infections are also seen.

Thalassaemia major (Cooley's anaemia)

Most children affected by homozygous β-thalassaemia present during the first year of life with:

- failure to thrive and recurrent bacterial infections
- severe anaemia from 3–6 months when the switch from γ- to β-chain production should normally occur
- extramedullary haemopoiesis that soon leads to hepatosplenomegaly and bone expansion, giving rise to the classical thalassaemic facies (Fig. 8.19a).

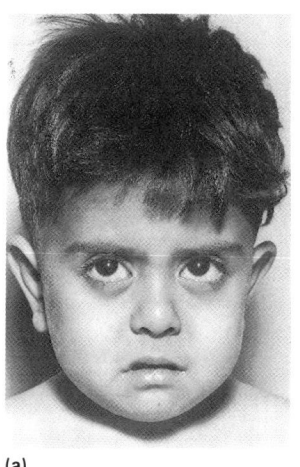

(a)

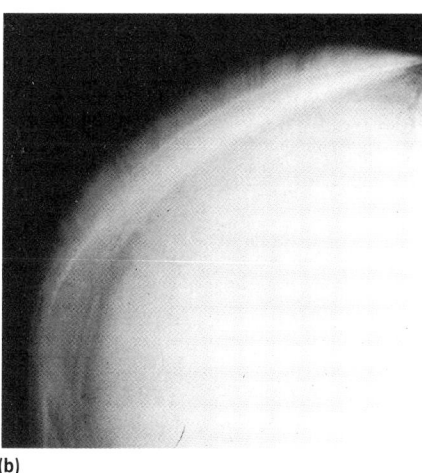

(b)

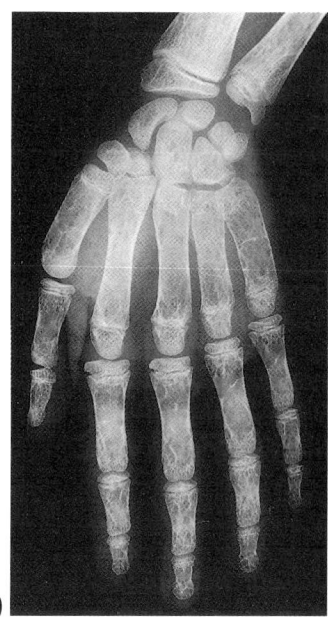

(c)

Fig. 8.19 **Thalassaemia.** **(a)** A child with thalassaemia, showing the typical facial features. **(b)** Skull X-ray of a child with β-thalassaemia, showing the 'hair on end' appearance. **(c)** X-ray of hand, showing expansion of the marrow and a thinned cortex.

Skull X-rays in these children show the characteristic 'hair on end' appearance of bony trabeculation as a result of expansion of the bone marrow into cortical bone (Fig. 8.19b). The expansion of the bone marrow is also shown in an X-ray of the hand (Fig. 8.19c).

The classic features of untreated thalassaemia major are only observed in patients from countries without good blood transfusion support.

Management

The aims of treatment are to suppress ineffective erythropoiesis, prevent bony deformities and allow normal activity and development. Long-term folic acid supplements are required, and regular transfusions should be given to keep the Hb above 10 g/dL. Blood transfusions may be required every 4–6 weeks.

If transfusion requirements increase, splenectomy should be considered, although this is usually delayed until after the age of 6 years because of the risk of infection. Prophylaxis against infection is required for patients undergoing splenectomy (see p. 444).

Iron overload caused by repeated transfusions (transfusion haemosiderosis) may lead to damage to the endocrine glands, liver, pancreas and the myocardium by the time patients reach adolescence. The iron-chelating agent of choice remains desferrioxamine, although it has to be administered parenterally. Unfortunately, there are no satisfactory oral iron-chelating agents. Desferrioxamine is given as an overnight subcutaneous infusion on 5–7 nights each week. Ascorbic acid 200 mg daily is given, along with desferrioxamine as it increases the urinary excretion of iron in response to desferrioxamine.

With current therapy, normal growth and sexual development occur but compliance may be a problem, especially in teenagers. Intensive treatment with desferrioxamine has been reported to reverse damage to the heart in patients with severe iron overload, but excessive doses of desferrioxamine may cause cataracts, retinal damage and nerve deafness. Infection with *Yersinia enterocolitica* occurs in iron-loaded patients treated with desferrioxamine. Iron overload should be periodically assessed by measuring the serum ferritin and by measurement of hepatic iron stores.

Bone marrow transplantation has been used in young patients with HLA-matched siblings. It has been successful in cases in good clinical condition with a mortality of less than 5%, but there is a high mortality (> 50%) in patients in poor condition with iron overload and liver dysfunction.

Prenatal diagnosis and gene therapy are discussed on page 186.

α-Thalassaemia
Molecular genetics

In contrast to β-thalassaemia, α-thalassaemia is often caused by gene deletions, although mutations also occur. The gene for α chains is duplicated on both chromosomes 16 i.e. there are four genes. Deletion of one α-chain gene (α^+) or both α-chain genes (α^0) on each chromosome 16 may occur (Table 8.12). The former is the most common of these abnormalities.

If all four genes are absent (deletion of both genes on both chromosomes), there is no α-chain synthesis and only Hb Barts (γ_4) is present. Hb Barts cannot carry oxygen and is incompatible with life (Tables 8.10 and 8.12). Infants are either stillborn at 28–40 weeks or die very shortly after birth. They are pale, oedematous and have enormous livers and spleens – a condition called hydrops fetalis.

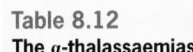

Table 8.12
The α-thalassaemias

Gene deletion			Haemoglobin type	Clinical picture
4 genes	α^0	$--/--$	Hb Barts (γ_4)	Hydrops fetalis
3 genes	α^0	$--/-\alpha$	Hb H (β_4)	Moderate anaemia Splenomegaly
2 genes	α^0	$--/\alpha\,\alpha$ or $-\alpha/-\alpha$	Some Hb H bodies Hb A	Mild anaemia α-Thalassaemia trait
1 gene	α^+	$-\alpha/\alpha\,\alpha$	'Normal'	α-Thalassaemia trait

If three genes are deleted, there is moderate anaemia (Hb 7–10 g/dL) and splenomegaly (Hb H disease). The patients are not usually transfusion-dependent. Hb A, Hb Barts and Hb H (β_4) are present. Hb A_2 is normal or reduced.

If two genes are deleted (α-thalassaemia trait) there is microcytosis with or without mild anaemia. Hb H bodies may be seen on staining a blood film with brilliant cresyl blue. With one gene deletion the blood picture is usually normal.

Globin chain synthesis studies for the detection of a reduced ratio of α to β chains may be necessary for the definitive diagnosis of α-thalassaemia trait.

Less commonly, α-thalassaemia may result from genetic defects other than deletions, for example mutations in the stop codon producing an α chain with many extra amino acids (Hb Constant Spring).

Sickle syndromes

The most important structural abnormality of the Hb chain is sickle cell haemoglobin (Hb S). Hb S results from a single-base mutation of adenine to thymine which produces a substitution of valine for glutamine at the sixth codon of the β-globin chain. In the homozygous state (*sickle cell anaemia*) both genes are abnormal (Hb SS), whereas in the heterozygous state (*sickle cell trait*, Hb AS) only one chromosome carries the gene. As the synthesis of Hb F is normal, the disease usually does not manifest itself until the Hb F decreases to adult levels at about 6 months of age.

The disease occurs mainly in Africans (25% carry the gene) but is also found in India, the Middle East and southern Europe (see Fig. 8.17).

Pathogenesis

Deoxygenated Hb S molecules are insoluble and polymerize. The flexibility of the cells is decreased and they become rigid and take up their characteristic sickle appearance (see Fig. 8.8). This process is initially reversible but, with repeated sickling, the cells eventually lose their membrane flexibility and remain in the sickle form. Sickling can produce:

- a shortened red cell survival
- impaired passage of cells through the microcirculation leading to obstruction of small vessels and tissue infarction.

Sickling is precipitated by infection, dehydration, cold, acidosis or hypoxia. In many cases the cause is unknown, but adhesion proteins on activated endothelial cells may play a role, particularly in vaso-occlusion. Hb S releases its oxygen to the tissues more easily than does normal Hb (see Fig. 15.5), and patients therefore feel well despite being anaemic except during crises or complications.

Sickle cell anaemia

The condition varies from a mild asymptomatic disorder to a severe haemolytic anaemia and recurrent severe painful crises. The condition may present in childhood with anaemia and mild jaundice. The hand-and-foot syndrome due to infarcts of small bones is quite common in children and may result in digits of varying lengths.

In the older patient, vaso-occlusive problems occur owing to sickling in the small vessels of any organ, mimicking many medical and surgical emergencies.

Typical infarctive *sickle crises* include:

- bone pain (most common)
- chest – pleuritic pain
- cerebral – hemiparesis, fits
- kidney – papillary necrosis causing haematuria, renal tubular defect resulting in lack of concentration of the urine
- spleen – painful infarcts
- penis – priapism
- liver – pain with abnormal biochemistry.

Attacks of pain with low-grade fever last from a few hours to a few days. In a given patient the degree of anaemia is usually stable, and during a crisis Hb does not fall unless there is one or more of the following:

- *Aplasia* – due to decreased erythropoiesis, associated with viral infections, particularly parvovirus.
- *Acute sequestration* – the liver and spleen become engorged with sickle cells.

- *Haemolysis* – due to drugs, acute infection or associated G6PD deficiency.

Long-term problems
- *Susceptibility to infections*, particularly to *Streptococcus pneumoniae*, which can cause a fatal meningitis or pneumonia. Osteomyelitis can occur in necrotic bone, often due to *Salmonella*.
- *Chronic leg ulcers*, due to ischaemia.
- *Gallstones*: pigment stones from persistent haemolysis.
- *Aseptic necrosis of bone*, particularly of the femoral heads.
- *Blindness*, due to retinal detachment and/or proliferative retinopathy.
- *Chronic renal disease.*

Investigations
- **Blood count**: the level of Hb is in the range 6–8 g/dL with a high reticulocyte count (10–20%).
- **Blood films** can show features of hyposplenism (see Fig. 8.8).
- **Sickling** of red cells on a blood film can be induced in the presence of sodium metabisulphite.
- **Sickle solubility test**: a mixture of Hb S in a reducing solution such as sodium dithionite gives a turbid appearance because of precipitation of Hb S, whereas normal Hb gives a clear solution. A number of commercial kits such as Sickledex are available for this rapid screening for the presence of Hb S, for example before surgery in appropriate ethnic groups and in the A&E department.
- **Hb electrophoresis** (see Fig. 8.18) is always needed to confirm the diagnosis. There is no Hb A, 80–95% Hb SS, and 2–20% Hb F.
- **The parents** of the affected child will show features of sickle cell trait.

Management
The 'steady state' anaemia requires no treatment. Precipitating factors (see above) should be avoided or treated quickly. The complications requiring inpatient management are shown in Table 8.13.

Acute attacks require supportive therapy with intravenous fluids, oxygen, antibiotics and adequate analgesia. Prophylaxis is given to prevent pneumococcal infection and *Haemophilus influenzae* type B (see p. 444). Folic acid is given to pregnant women and those with severe haemolysis.

The acute sickle chest syndrome is the commonest cause of death of adults with sickle cell disease. It is caused by infection, fat embolism from necrotic bone marrow or pulmonary infarction due to sequestration of sickle cells. It comprises shortness of breath, chest pain, hypoxia, and new chest X-ray changes due to consolidation. The presentation may be gradual or very rapid, leading to death in a few hours. Initial

---

Table 8.13

Complications requiring inpatient management

Pain uncontrolled by non-opiate analgesia
Swollen painful joints
Central nervous system deficit
Acute sickle chest syndrome or pneumonia
Mesenteric sickling and bowel ischaemia
Splenic or hepatic sequestration
Cholecystitis
Renal papillary necrosis resulting in colic or severe haematuria
Hyphema and retinal detachment

From Davies SC, Oni L (1997) Management of patients with sickle cell disease. *British Medical Journal* **315**: 656–660.

---

management is with pain relief, inspired oxygen, antibiotics and exchange transfusion to reduce the amount of Hb S to < 20%; occasionally ventilation may be necessary.

Regular transfusions are given only if there is severe anaemia or if patients are having frequent crises in order to suppress the production of Hb S. Before elective operations and during pregnancy, repeated transfusions may be used to reduce the proportion of circulating Hb S to less than 20% to prevent sickling. Exchange transfusions may be necessary in patients with severe or recurrent crises, or before emergency surgery. Transfusion and splenectomy may be life-saving for young children with splenic sequestration.

Hydroxycarbamide (hydroxyurea) is the first drug which has been widely used as therapy for sickle cell anaemia. Hydroxycarbamide acts by increasing Hb F concentrations but the reduction in neutrophils may also help. Hydroxycarbamide has been shown in trials to reduce the episodes of pain, the acute chest syndrome, and the need for blood transfusions.

Bone marrow transplantation has been used to treat sickle cell anaemia although in fewer numbers than for thalassaemia. Children and adolescents younger than 16 years of age who have severe complications (strokes, recurrent chest syndrome, or refractory pain) and have an HLA-matched donor are the best candidates for transplantation.

Prognosis
Some patients with Hb SS die in the first few years of life from either infection or episodes of sequestration. However, there is marked individual variation in the severity of the disease and some patients have a relatively normal life-span with few complications.

Sickle cell trait
These individuals have no symptoms unless extreme circumstances cause anoxia, such as flying in non-pressurized aircraft or problems with anaesthesia. Sickle cell trait protects against *Plasmodium falciparum* malaria (see p. 100), and consequently the sickle gene has been seen as an example of a balanced polymorphism (where the

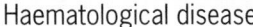
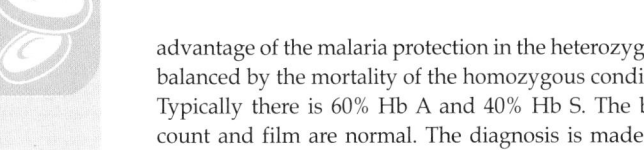

advantage of the malaria protection in the heterozygote is balanced by the mortality of the homozygous condition). Typically there is 60% Hb A and 40% Hb S. The blood count and film are normal. The diagnosis is made by a positive sickle test or by Hb electrophoresis (see Fig. 8.18).

Other structural globin chain defects

There are many Hb variants (e.g. Hb C, D), many of which are not associated with clinical manifestations.

Hb C disease may be associated with Hb S (Hb SC disease). The clinical course is similar to that with Hb SS, but there is an increased likelihood of thrombosis, and in particular this may lead to life-threatening episodes of thrombosis in pregnancy, and retinopathy.

Combined defects of globin chain production and structure

Abnormalities of Hb structure (e.g. Hb S, C) can occur in combination with thalassaemia. The combination of β-thalassaemia trait and sickle cell trait (sickle cell β-thalassaemia) resembles sickle cell anaemia (Hb SS) clinically. Hb E is the most common Hb variant in South East Asia, and the second most prevalent haemoglobin variant world-wide. Hb E heterozygotes are asymptomatic; the haemoglobin level is normal, but red cells are microcytic. Homozygous Hb E causes a mild microcytic anaemia, but the combination of heterozygosity for Hb E and β-thalassaemia produces a variable anaemia which can be as severe as β-thalassaemia major.

Prenatal diagnosis of severe haemoglobin abnormalities

Of the offspring of parents who both have either β-thalassaemia or sickle cell trait, 25% will have β-thalassaemia major or sickle cell anaemia, respectively. Recognition of these heterozygous states in parents and family counselling provides a basis for antenatal diagnosis.

If a pregnant woman is found to have a haemoglobin defect, her partner should be tested. Antenatal diagnosis is offered if both are affected as there is a risk of a severe fetal Hb defect, particularly β-thalassaemia major. Fetal DNA analysis can be carried out using amniotic fluid, chorionic villus or fetal blood samples. Abortion is offered if the fetus is found to be affected. Chorionic villus biopsy has the advantage that it can be carried out in the first trimester, thus avoiding the need for second trimester abortions.

Gene therapy

The ultimate corrective therapy for severe Hb abnormalities would be gene therapy. This might involve inserting normal Hb genes into the patient's haemopoietic cells in vitro and then transplanting these cells back into the patient after ablative treatment had been given to remove the abnormal bone marrow. However, numerous problems remain to be overcome before gene therapy for Hb defects becomes a practical option; for example the haemoglobin genes would need to be expressed in a regulated fashion in the correct tissues, i.e. bone marrow.

Metabolic disorders of the red cell

Red cell metabolism

The mature red cell has no nucleus, mitochondria or ribosomes and is therefore unable to synthesize proteins. Red cells have only limited enzyme systems but they are of major importance in maintaining the viability and function of the cells. In particular, energy is required in the form of ATP for the maintenance of the flexibility of the membrane and the biconcave shape of the cells to allow passage through small vessels, and for regulation of the sodium and potassium pumps to ensure osmotic equilibrium. In addition, it is essential that Hb be maintained in the reduced state.

The enzyme systems responsible for producing energy and reducing power are (Fig. 8.20):

- the glycolytic (Embden–Meyerhof) pathway, in which glucose is metabolized to pyruvate and lactic acid with production of ATP
- the hexose monophosphate (pentosephosphate) pathway, which provides reducing power for the red cell in the form of NADPH.

About 90% of glucose is metabolized by the former and 10% by the latter. The importance of the hexose monophosphate shunt is that it maintains glutathione (GSH) in a reduced state. Glutathione is necessary to combat oxidative stress to the red cell, and failure of this mechanism may result in:

- rigidity due to cross-linking of spectrin, which decreases membrane flexibility (see Fig. 8.15) and causes 'leakiness' of the red cell membrane
- oxidation of the Hb molecule, producing methaemoglobin and precipitation of globin chains as Heinz bodies localized on the inside of the membrane; these bodies are removed from circulating red cells by the spleen.

2,3-DPG is formed from a side-arm of the glycolytic pathway (see Fig. 8.20). It binds to the central part of the Hb tetramer, fixing it in the low-affinity state (see Fig. 8.4). A decreased affinity with a shift in the oxygen dissociation curve to the right enables more oxygen to be delivered to the tissues (see Fig. 15.5).

In addition to the G6PD and pyruvate kinase deficiencies described below, there are a number of rare enzyme deficiencies that need specialist investigation.

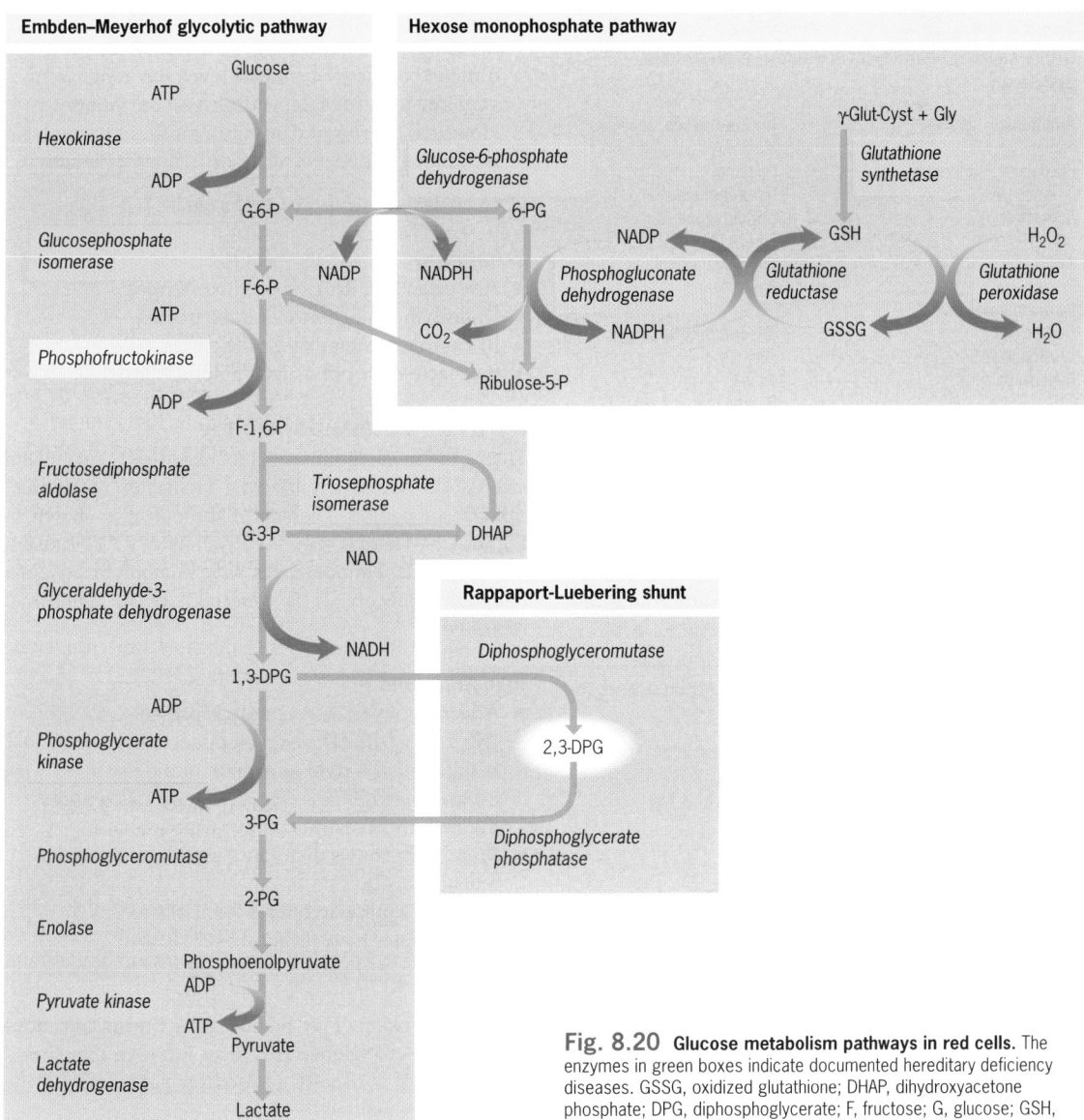

Fig. 8.20 Glucose metabolism pathways in red cells. The enzymes in green boxes indicate documented hereditary deficiency diseases. GSSG, oxidized glutathione; DHAP, dihydroxyacetone phosphate; DPG, diphosphoglycerate; F, fructose; G, glucose; GSH, reduced glutathione; P, phosphate; PG, phosphoglycerate.

Glucose-6-phosphate dehydrogenase (G6PD) deficiency

The enzyme G6PD holds a vital position in the hexose monophosphate shunt (Fig. 8.20), oxidizing glucose-6-phosphate to 6-phosphoglycerate with the reduction of NADP to NADPH. The reaction is necessary in red cells where it is the only source of NADPH, which is used via glutathione to protect the red cell from oxidative damage. G6PD deficiency is a common condition that presents with a haemolytic anaemia and affects millions of people throughout the world, particularly in Africa, around the Mediterranean, the Middle East (around 20%) and South East Asia (up to 40% in some regions).

The gene for G6PD is localized to chromosome Xq28 near the factor VIII gene. The deficiency is more common in males than females. However, female heterozygotes can also have clinical problems due to lyonization, whereby because of random X-chromosome inactivation female heterozygotes have two populations of red cells – a normal one and a G6PD-deficient one.

There are over 400 structural types of G6PD, and mutations are mostly single amino acid substitutions. The most common types with normal activity are called type B⁺, which is present in almost all Caucasians and about 70% of black Africans, and type A⁺, which is present in about 20% of black Africans. There are many variants with reduced activity but only two are common. In the African, or A⁻ type, the degree of deficiency is mild and more marked in older cells. Haemolysis is self-limiting as the young red cells newly produced by

433

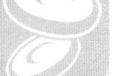
Table 8.14
Drugs causing haemolysis in glucose-6-phosphate deficiency

Analgesics, such as:
Aspirin
Phenacetin (withdrawn in the UK)
Acetanilide

Antimalarials, such as:
Primaquine
Pyrimethamine
Quinine
Chloroquine
Pamaquine

Antibacterials, such as:
Most sulphonamides
Dapsone
Nitrofurantoin
Nitrofurazone
Furazolidone
Chloramphenicol
Ciprofloxacin

Miscellaneous drugs, such as:
Vitamin K
Probenecid
Nalidixic acid
Quinidine
Dimercaprol
Phenylhydrazine

the bone marrow have nearly normal enzyme activity. However, in the Mediterranean type, both young and old red cells have very low enzyme activity. After an oxidant shock the Hb level may fall precipitously; death may follow unless the condition is recognized and the patient is transfused urgently.

Clinical syndromes
- Acute drug-induced haemolysis (Table 8.14)
- Favism (ingestion of fava beans)
- Chronic haemolytic anaemia
- Neonatal jaundice
- Infections and acute illnesses will also precipitate haemolysis in patients with G6PD deficiency.

The clinical features are due to rapid intravascular haemolysis with symptoms of anaemia, jaundice and haemoglobinuria.

Investigations
- **Blood count** is normal between attacks.
- **During an attack** the blood film may show irregularly contracted cells, bite cells (cells with an indentation of the membrane), blister cells (cells in which the Hb appears to have become partially detached from the cell membrane; see Fig. 8.8), Heinz bodies (best seen on films stained with methyl violet) and reticulocytosis.
- **Haemolysis** is evident (see p. 425).
- **G6PD deficiency** can be detected using several screening tests, such as demonstration of the decreased ability of G6PD-deficient cells to reduce dyes. The level of the enzyme may also be directly assayed. There are two diagnostic problems. Immediately after an attack the screening tests may be normal (because the oldest red cells with least

6GPD activity are destroyed selectively). Secondly, the diagnosis of heterozygous females may be difficult because the enzyme level may range from very low to normal depending on lyonization. However, the risk of clinically significant haemolysis is minimal in patients with borderline G6PD activity.

DNA analysis may also be performed.

Treatment
- Any offending drugs should be stopped.
- Underlying infection should be treated.
- Blood transfusion may be life-saving.
- Splenectomy is not usually helpful.

Pyruvate kinase deficiency
This is the most common defect of red cell metabolism after G6PD deficiency, affecting thousands rather than millions of people. The site of the defect is shown in Figure 8.20. There is reduced production of ATP causing rigid red cells. Homozygotes have haemolytic anaemia and splenomegaly. It is inherited as an autosomal recessive.

Investigations
- **Anaemia** of variable severity is present (Hb 5–10 g/dL). The oxygen dissociation curve is shifted to the right as a result of the rise in intracellular 2,3-DPG (Fig. 15.5), and this reduces the severity of symptoms due to anaemia.
- **Blood film** shows distorted ('prickle') cells and a reticulocytosis.
- **Pyruvate kinase activity** is low (affected homozygotes have levels of 5–20%).

Treatment
Blood transfusions may be necessary during infections and pregnancy. Splenectomy may improve the clinical condition and is usually advised for patients requiring frequent transfusions.

FURTHER READING

Bunn HF (1997) Pathogenesis and treatment of sickle cell disease. *New England Journal of Medicine* **337**: 762–769.
Mason PJ (1996) New insights into G6PD deficiency. *British Journal of Haematology* **94**: 585–591.
Platt OS (2000) The acute chest syndrome of sickle cell disease. *New England Journal of Medicine* **342**: 1904–1907.
Serjeant GR (1997) Sickle cell disease. *Lancet* **350**: 725–730.
Weatherall DJ, Provan AB (2000) Red cells I: inherited anaemias. *Lancet* **355**: 1169–1175.
Weatherall DJ (1997) The thalassaemias. *British Medical Journal* **314**: 1675–1678.

Acquired haemolytic anaemia

These anaemias may be divided into those due to immune, non-immune, or other causes (see Table 8.9).

Causes of immune destruction of red cells
- Autoantibodies
- Drug-induced antibodies
- Alloantibodies.

Causes of non-immune destruction of red cells
- Acquired membrane defects (e.g. paroxysmal nocturnal haemoglobinuria – see p. 439)
- Mechanical factors (e.g. prosthetic heart valves, or microangiopathic haemolytic anaemia – see p. 440).

It may also be secondary to systemic disease (e.g. renal and liver disease).

Miscellaneous causes
- Various toxic substances can disrupt the red cell membrane and cause haemolysis (e.g. arsenic, and products of *Clostridium welchii*).
- Malaria frequently causes anaemia owing to a combination of a reduction in red cell survival and reduced production of red cells.
- Hypersplenism (p. 444) results in a reduced red cell survival, which may also contribute to the anaemia seen in malaria.

- Extensive burns result in denaturation of red cell membrane proteins and reduced red cell survival.
- Some drugs (e.g. dapsone, sulfasalazine) cause oxidative haemolysis with Heinz bodies in normal subjects.
- Some ingested chemicals (e.g. weedkillers such as sodium chlorate) may cause severe oxidative haemolysis leading to acute renal failure.

Autoimmune haemolytic anaemias

Autoimmune haemolytic anaemias (AIHA) are acquired disorders resulting from increased red cell destruction due to red cell autoantibodies. These anaemias are characterized by the presence of a positive direct antiglobulin (Coombs') test, which detects the autoantibody on the surface of the patient's red cells (Fig. 8.21).

AIHA is divided into 'warm' and 'cold' types, depending on whether the antibody attaches better to the red cells at body temperature (37°C) or at lower temperatures. The major features and the causes of these two forms of AIHA are shown in Table 8.15. In warm AIHA, IgG antibodies predominate and the direct antiglobulin test is positive with IgG alone, IgG and complement, or complement only. In cold AIHA, the antibodies are usually IgM. They easily elute off red cells, leaving complement which is detected as C3d.

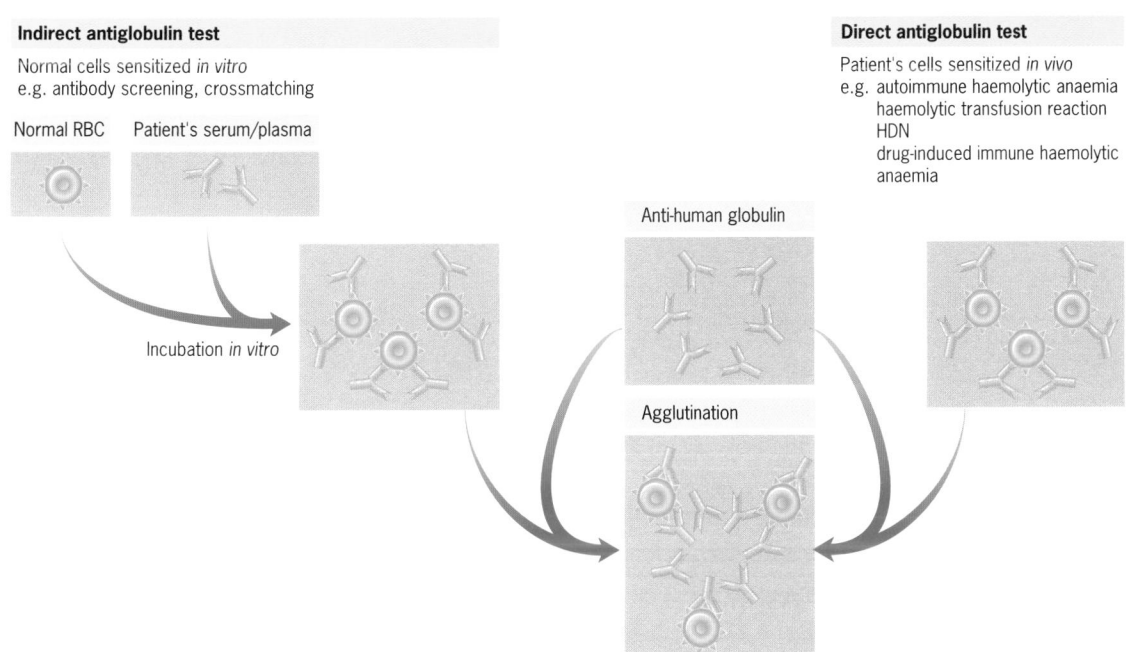

Indirect antiglobulin test

Normal cells sensitized *in vitro*
e.g. antibody screening, crossmatching

Normal RBC   Patient's serum/plasma

Incubation *in vitro*

Direct antiglobulin test

Patient's cells sensitized *in vivo*
e.g. autoimmune haemolytic anaemia
   haemolytic transfusion reaction
   HDN
   drug-induced immune haemolytic anaemia

Anti-human globulin

Agglutination

Fig. 8.21 Antiglobulin (Coombs') tests. The anti-human globulin forms bridges between the sensitized cells causing visible agglutination. The direct test detects patients' cells sensitized in vivo. The indirect test detects normal cells sensitized in vitro. HDN, haemolytic disease of newborn.

Table 8.15
Causes and major features of autoimmune haemolytic anaemias

	Warm	Cold
Temperature at which antibody attaches best to red cells	37°C	Lower than 37°C
Type of antibody	IgG	IgM
Direct Coombs' test	Strongly positive	Positive
Causes of primary conditions	Idiopathic	Idiopathic
Causes of secondary condition	Autoimmune disorders, e.g. systemic lupus erythematosus	Infections, e.g. infectious mononucleosis, *Mycoplasma pneumoniae*, other viral infections (rare)
	Lymphomas	Lymphomas
	Chronic lymphatic leukaemia	Paroxysmal cold haemoglobinuria (IgG)
	Hodgkin's disease	
	Carcinomas	
	Drugs, e.g. methyldopa	

Immune destruction of red cells

IgM or IgG red cell antibodies which fully activate the complement cascade cause lysis of red cells in the circulation (intravascular haemolysis).

IgG antibodies frequently do not activate complement and the coated red cells undergo extravascular haemolysis (Fig. 8.22). They are either completely phagocytosed in the spleen through an interaction with Fc receptors on macrophages, or they lose part of the cell membrane through partial phagocytosis and circulate as spherocytes until they too become sequestered in the spleen. Some IgG antibodies partially activate complement, leading to deposition of C3b on the red cell surface, and this may enhance phagocytosis as macrophages also have receptors for C3b.

Non-complement-binding IgM antibodies are rare and have little or no effect on red cell survival. IgM antibodies which partially rather than fully activate complement cause adherence of red cells to C3b receptors on macrophages, particularly in the liver, although this is an ineffective mechanism of haemolysis. Most of the red cells are released from the macrophages when C3b is cleaved to C3d and then circulate with C3d on their surface.

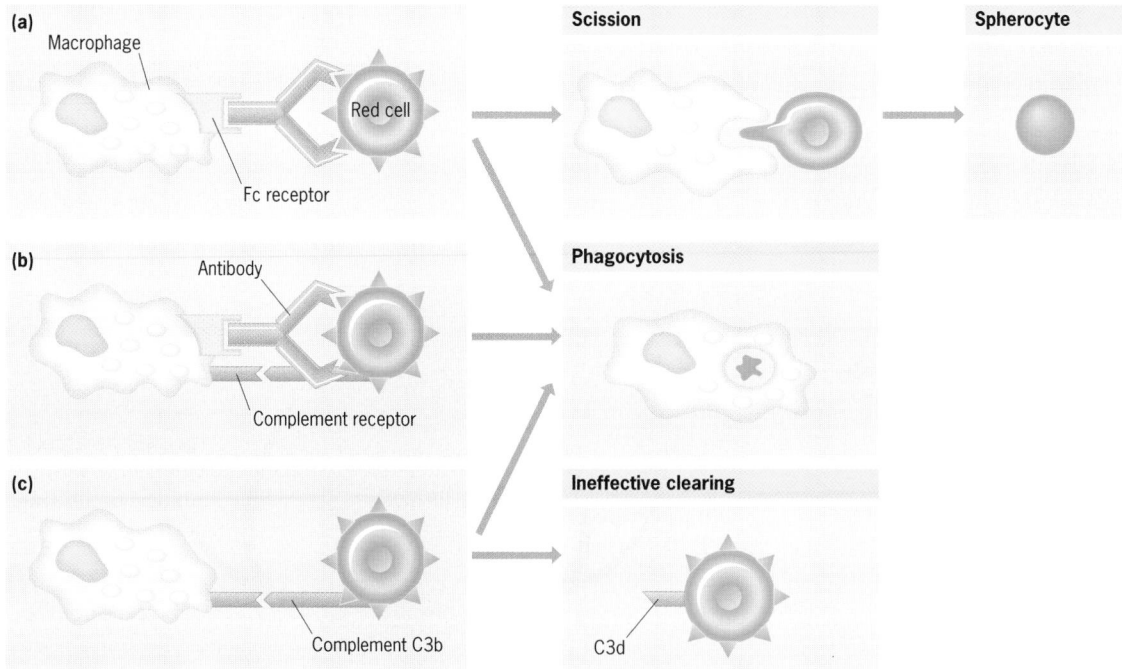

Fig. 8.22 Extravascular haemolysis is due to interaction of antibody-coated cells with cells in the reticuloendothelial system, predominantly in the spleen. (a) Spherocytosis results from partial phagocytosis. **(b)** Complete phagocytosis may occur and this is enhanced if there is complement as well as antibody on the cell surface. **(c)** Cells coated with complement only are ineffectively removed and circulate with C3d or C3b on their surface.

'Warm' autoimmune haemolytic anaemias

Clinical features

These anaemias may occur at all ages and in both sexes, although they are most frequent in middle-aged females. They can present as a short episode of anaemia and jaundice but they often remit and relapse and may progress to an intermittent chronic pattern. The spleen is often palpable. Infections or folate deficiency may provoke a profound fall in the haemoglobin level.

In more than 30% of cases, the cause remains unknown. These anaemias may be associated with lymphoid malignancies or diseases such as rheumatoid arthritis and SLE or drugs (Table 8.15).

Investigations

- **Haemolytic anaemia** is evident (see p. 425).
- **Spherocytosis** is present as a result of red cell damage.
- **Direct antiglobulin test** is positive, with either IgG alone (67%), IgG and complement (20%), or complement alone (13%) being found on the surface of the red cells.
- **Autoantibodies** may have specificity for the Rh blood group system (e.g. for the e antigen).
- **Autoimmune thrombocytopenia** and/or neutropenia may also be present (Evans' syndrome).

Treatment and prognosis

Corticosteroids (e.g. prednisolone in doses of 1mg/kg daily) are effective in inducing a remission in about 80% of patients. Steroids reduce both production of the red cell autoantibody and destruction of antibody-coated cells. Splenectomy may be necessary if there is no response to steroids or if the remission is not maintained when the dose of prednisolone is reduced. Other immunosuppressive drugs, such as azathioprine and cyclophosphamide, may be effective in patients who fail to respond to steroids and splenectomy.

'Cold' autoimmune haemolytic anaemias

Normally, low titres of IgM cold agglutinins reacting at 4°C are present in plasma and are harmless. At low temperatures these antibodies can attach to red cells and cause their agglutination in the cold peripheries of the body. In addition, activation of complement may cause intravascular haemolysis when the cells return to the higher temperatures in the core of the body.

After certain infections (such as *Mycoplasma*, cytomegalovirus, Epstein–Barr virus (EBV)) there is increased synthesis of polyclonal cold agglutinins producing a mild to moderate transient haemolysis.

Chronic cold haemagglutinin disease (CHAD)

This usually occurs in the elderly with a gradual onset of haemolytic anaemia owing to the production of monoclonal IgM cold agglutinins. After exposure to cold the patient develops an acrocyanosis similar to Raynaud's (see p. 831) as a result of red cell autoagglutination.

Investigations

- **Red cells** agglutinate in the cold or at room temperature. Agglutination is sometimes seen in the sample tube after cooling but is more easily seen on the peripheral blood film made at room temperature. The agglutination is reversible after warming the sample. The agglutination may cause a spurious increase in the MCV (see p. 422).
- **Direct antiglobulin test** is positive with complement alone.
- **Monoclonal IgM antibodies** with specificity for the Ii blood group system, usually for the I antigen but occasionally for the i antigen.

Treatment

The underlying cause should be treated, if possible. Patients should avoid exposure to cold. Treatment with steroids, alkylating agents and splenectomy is usually ineffective.

Paroxysmal cold haemoglobinuria (PCH)

This is a rare condition associated with common childhood infections, such as measles, mumps and chickenpox. Intravascular haemolysis is associated with polyclonal IgG complement-fixing antibodies. These antibodies are biphasic, reacting with red cells in the cold in the peripheral circulation, with lysis occurring due to complement activation when the cells return to the central circulation. The antibodies have specificity for the P red cell antigen. The lytic reaction is demonstrated in vitro by incubating the patient's red cells and serum at 4°C and then warming the mixture to 37°C (Donath–Landsteiner test). Haemolysis is self-limiting but supportive transfusions of warmed blood may be necessary.

Drug-induced immune haemolytic anaemia

The interaction between a drug and red cell membrane may produce a composite antigenic structure (or neoantigen), provoking two types of antibodies:

- *Drug-dependent antibodies*, which bind to both the drug and the cell membrane but not to either separately. Clinically there is usually severe complement-mediated intravascular haemolysis, which resolves quickly after withdrawal of the drug.
- *Drug-independent antibodies*, which are induced by a subtle alteration of the red cell membrane. Such antibodies react with red cells in vitro in the absence of the drug and are indistinguishable from 'true' autoantibodies. There is extravascular haemolysis and the clinical course tends to be more protracted.

This concept for drug-induced immune haemolytic anaemia probably also applies to drug-induced thrombocytopenia and neutropenia.

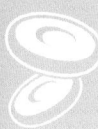

Alloimmune haemolytic anaemia

Antibodies produced in one individual react with the red cells of another. This situation occurs in haemolytic disease of the newborn, haemolytic transfusion reactions (see p. 447) and after allogeneic bone marrow, renal, liver or cardiac transplantation when donor lymphocytes transferred in the allograft ('passenger lymphocytes') may produce red cell antibodies against the recipient and cause haemolytic anaemia.

Haemolytic disease of the newborn (HDN)

HDN is due to fetomaternal incompatibility for red cell antigens. Maternal alloantibodies against fetal red cell antigens pass from the maternal circulation via the placenta into the fetus, where they destroy the fetal red cells. Only IgG antibodies are capable of transplacental passage from mother to fetus.

The most common type of HDN is that due to ABO incompatibility, where the mother is usually group O and the fetus group A.

HDN due to ABO incompatibility is usually mild and exchange transfusion is rarely needed. HDN due to RhD incompatibility has become much less common in developed countries following the introduction of anti-D prophylaxis (see below). HDN may be caused by antibodies against antigens in many blood group systems (e.g. other Rh antigens such as c and E, and Kell, Duffy and Kidd – see p. 445).

Sensitization occurs as a result of passage of fetal red cells into the maternal circulation (which most readily occurs at the time of delivery), so that first pregnancies are rarely affected. However, sensitization may occur at other times, for example after a miscarriage, ectopic pregnancy or blood transfusion, or due to episodes during pregnancy which cause transplacental bleeding such as amniocentesis, chorionic villus sampling and threatened miscarriage.

Clinical features

These vary from a mild haemolytic anaemia of the newborn to intrauterine death from 18 weeks' gestation with the characteristic appearance of hydrops fetalis (hepatosplenomegaly, oedema and cardiac failure).

Kernicterus occurs owing to severe jaundice in the neonatal period, where the unconjugated (lipid-soluble) bilirubin exceeds 250 µmol/L and bile pigment deposition occurs in the basal ganglia. This can result in permanent brain damage, choreoathetosis, and spasticity. In mild cases it may present as deafness.

Investigations

Routine antenatal serology

All mothers should have their ABO and RhD groups determined and their serum tested for atypical antibodies after attending the antenatal booking clinic. Tests for red cell antibodies should be repeated at 28 weeks' gestation.

If an antibody is detected, its blood group specificity should be determined and the mother should be retested at least monthly. A rising antibody titre of IgG antibodies or a history of HDN in a previous pregnancy is an indication for referral to a specialist unit to determine the need for amniocentesis (to assess the level of bilirubin in the amniotic fluid) or fetal blood sampling to determine the severity of HDN and to guide further management.

Ultrasound

This shows changes in the fetal blood flow and cardiac function caused by compensated anaemia and can be demonstrated in utero before hydrops develops. Fetal DNA may be obtained by amniocentesis, chorionic villous sampling, or fetal blood sampling; recently, it has been shown that soluble fetal DNA in maternal plasma can be used for this purpose avoiding an invasive procedure.

At the birth of an affected infant

A sample of cord blood is obtained. This shows:

- anaemia with a high reticulocyte count
- a positive direct antiglobulin test
- a raised serum bilirubin.

Treatment

Management of the baby

In mild cases, phototherapy may be used to convert bilirubin to water-soluble biliverdin. Biliverdin can be excreted by the kidneys and this therefore reduces the chance of kernicterus.

In more severely affected cases, exchange transfusion may be necessary to replace the infant's red cells and to remove bilirubin. Indications for exchange transfusion include:

- a cord Hb of < 12 g/dL (normal cord Hb is 13.6–19.6 g/dL)
- a cord bilirubin of > 60 µmol/L
- a later bilirubin of > 300 µmol/L
- a rapidly rising bilirubin level.

Further exchange transfusions may be necessary to remove the unconjugated bilirubin.

The blood used for exchange transfusions should be ABO-compatible with the mother and infant, lack the antigen against which the maternal antibody is directed, be fresh (no more than 5 days from the day of collection), and be CMV-seronegative to prevent transmission of cytomegalovirus.

A severely affected fetus may need intrauterine blood transfusions carried out in a special unit.

An advance in the antenatal management of RhD alloimmunized women is the development of molecular methods for fetal RhD blood grouping in women with partners heterozygous for RhD. RhD negative fetuses, who will be unaffected, can be distinguished from RhD positive fetuses, who may be severely affected and require intensive monitoring.

Prevention of RhD immunization in the mother

Anti-D should be given after delivery when all of the following are present:

- the mother is RhD negative
- the fetus is RhD positive
- there is no maternal anti-D detectable in the mother's serum; i.e. the mother is not already immunized.

The dose is 500 i.u. of IgG anti-D intramuscularly within 48 hours of delivery. *The Kleihauer test* is used to assess the number of fetal cells in the maternal circulation. A blood film prepared from maternal blood is treated with acid, which elutes Hb A. Hb F is resistant to this treatment and can be seen when the film is stained with eosin. If large numbers of fetal red cells are present in the maternal circulation, a higher or additional dose of anti-D will be necessary.

It may be necessary to give prophylaxis to RhD-negative women at other times when sensitization may occur, for example after an ectopic pregnancy, threatened miscarriage or amniocentesis. The dose of anti-D is 250 i.u. before 20 weeks' gestation and 500 i.u. after 20 weeks.

Of previously non-immunized RhD-negative women carrying RhD-positive fetuses, 1–2% are immunized by the time of delivery. *Antenatal prophylaxis* with administration of anti-D to RhD-negative women at 28 and 34 weeks' gestation has been shown to reduce the incidence of immunization in some studies. Antenatal prophylaxis is already used in some centres, and it has been recommended that all RhD-negative women should be given antenatal anti-D in the UK. Monoclonal anti-D could in principle replace polyclonal anti-D which is collected from RhD-negative women immunized in pregnancy and deliberately immunized RhD-negative males, but it is likely to be some years before trials have been completed and it is available in sufficient quantity.

FURTHER READING

Bowman JM (1998) RhD hemolytic disease of the newborn. *New England Journal of Medicine* **339**: 1775–1779.

Joint Working Party of the British Blood Transfusion Society and the Royal College of Obstetricians and Gynaecologists (1999) Guidelines for the use of anti-D immunoglobulin for Rh prophylaxis. *Transfusion Medicine* **9**: 93–97.

Urbaniak SJ, Greiss MA (2000) RhD haemolytic disease of the newborn. *Blood Reviews* **14**: 44–61.

Non-immune haemolytic anaemia

Paroxysmal nocturnal haemoglobinuria (PNH)

This is a rare acquired red cell defect in which a clone of red cells is particularly sensitive to destruction by activated complement. These cells are continually haemolysed intravascularly. Platelets and granulocytes are also affected and there may be thrombocytopenia and neutropenia.

The underlying defect is an inability of PNH cells to make glycerylphosphatidylinositol (GPI), which anchors surface proteins such as delay accelerating factor (DAF; CD55) and membrane inhibitor of reactive lysis (MIRL; CD59) to cell membranes. DAF and MIRL and other proteins are involved in complement degradation, and in their absence the haemolytic action of complement is not regulated. The molecular basis of PNH has been found to be mutations in the *pig*-A (phosphatidylinositol glycan protein A) gene responsible for synthesis of the GPI anchor.

Clinical features

Patients present with haemolysis which may be precipitated by infection, iron therapy or surgery. Characteristically only the urine voided at night and in the morning on waking is dark in colour, although the reason for this phenomenon is not clear. In severe cases all urine samples are dark. Urinary iron loss may be sufficient to cause iron deficiency.

Some patients present insidiously with signs of anaemia and recurrent abdominal pains.

Venous thrombotic episodes are very common, and unusual and severe thromboses may occur, for example in hepatic (Budd–Chiari syndrome), mesenteric or cerebral veins. The cause of the increased predisposition to thrombosis is not known, but may be due to complement-mediated activation of platelets deficient in CD55 and CD59.

Investigations

- **Intravascular haemolysis** is evident (see p. 425).
- **Flow cytometric analysis** of red cells with anti-CD55 and anti-CD59 has replaced the Ham's test.
- **Bone marrow** is sometimes hypoplastic despite haemolysis.

Treatment and prognosis

There is no specific treatment for PNH. It is a chronic disorder requiring supportive measures such as blood transfusions, which are necessary for patients with severe anaemia. Leucocyte-depleted blood should be used in order to prevent transfusion reactions resulting in complement activation and acceleration of the haemolysis.

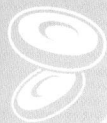

Long-term anticoagulation may be necessary for patients with recurrent thrombotic episodes. In patients with bone marrow failure, treatment options include immunosuppression with antilymphocyte globulin or ciclosporin, or bone marrow transplantation. Bone marrow transplantation has been successfully carried out using either HLA-matched sibling donors in patients under the age of 50 or matched unrelated donors in patients under the age of 25.

The course of PNH is variable. PNH may transform into aplastic anaemia or acute leukaemia, but it may remain stable for many years and the PNH clone may even disappear, which must be taken into account if considering potentially dangerous treatments such as bone marrow transplantation. The median survival is 10–15 years.

Gene therapy will perhaps be possible in the future.

Mechanical haemolytic anaemia

Red cells may be injured by physical trauma in the circulation. Direct injury may cause immediate cell lysis or may be followed by resealing of the cell membrane with the formation of distorted red cells or 'fragments'. These cells may circulate for a short period before being destroyed prematurely in the reticuloendothelial system.

The causes of mechanical haemolytic anaemia include:

- damaged artificial heart valves
- march haemoglobinuria, where there is damage to red cells in the feet associated with prolonged marching or running
- microangiopathic haemolytic anaemia (MAHA), where fragmentation of red cells occurs in an abnormal microcirculation caused by malignant hypertension, eclampsia, haemolytic uraemic syndrome, thrombotic thrombocytopenic purpura, vasculitis or disseminated intravascular coagulation.

FURTHER READING

Hillmen P, Lewis SM, Bessler M, Luzzatto L, Dacie JV (1995) Natural history of paroxysmal nocturnal haemoglobinuria. *New England Journal of Medicine* **333**: 1253–1258.

Hillmen P, Richards SJ (2000) Implications of recent insights into the pathophysiology of paroxysmal nocturnal haemoglobinuria. *British Journal of Haematology* **108**: 470–479.

Myeloproliferative disorders

In these disorders there is uncontrolled clonal proliferation of one or more of the cell lines in the bone marrow, namely erythroid, myeloid and megakaryocyte lines.

Myeloproliferative disorders include polycythaemia vera (PV), essential thrombocythaemia (ET), myelofibrosis and chronic myeloid leukaemia (CML). These disorders are grouped together as there can be transition from one disease to another; for example PV can lead to myelofibrosis. They may also transform to acute myeloblastic leukaemia. The non-leukaemic myeloproliferative disorders (PV, ET and myelofibrosis) will be discussed in this section. Chronic myeloid leukaemia is described on page 493.

Polycythaemia

Polycythaemia (or erythrocytosis) is defined as an increase in haemoglobin, PCV and red cell count. PCV is a more reliable indicator of polycythaemia than is Hb, which may be disproportionately low in iron deficiency. Polycythaemia can be divided into absolute erythrocytosis where there is a true increase in red cell volume, or relative erythrocytosis where the red cell volume is normal but there is a decrease in the plasma volume (see Fig. 8.6).

Absolute erythrocytosis is due to primary polycythaemia (PV) or secondary polycythaemia. Secondary polycythaemia is due to either an appropriate increase in red cells in response to anoxia, or an inappropriate increase associated with tumours, such as a renal carcinoma. The causes of polycythaemia are given in Table 8.16.

Primary polycythaemia: polycythaemia vera

PV is a clonal stem cell disorder in which there is an alteration in the pluripotent progenitor cell leading to excessive proliferation of erythroid, myeloid and megakaryocytic progenitor cells. This is due to a failure of apoptosis as a result of deregulation of the *Bcl-x* gene, which is known to oppose programmed cell death (p. 162).

Table 8.16
Causes of polycythaemia

Primary	Due to an inappropriate
Polycythaemia vera	*increase in erythropoietin:*
	Renal disease–renal cell
Secondary	carcinoma, Wilms' tumour
	Hepatocellular carcinoma
Due to an appropriate	Adrenal tumours
increase in erythropoietin:	Cerebellar haemangioblastoma
High altitude	Massive uterine fibroma
Lung disease	
Cardiovascular disease	**Relative**
(right-to-left shunt)	Stress or spurious polycythaemia
Heavy smoking	Dehydration
Increased affinity of	Burns
haemoglobin, e.g. familial	
polycythaemia	

Clinical features

The onset is insidious. It usually presents in patients aged over 60 years with tiredness, depression, vertigo, tinnitus and visual disturbance. It should be noted that these symptoms are also common in the normal population over the age of 60 and consequently PV is easily missed. These features, together with hypertension, angina, intermittent claudication and a tendency to bleed, are suggestive of PV.

Severe itching after a hot bath or when the patient is warm is common. Gout due to increased cell turnover may be a feature, and peptic ulceration occurs in a minority of patients. Thrombosis and haemorrhage are the major complications of PV.

The patient is usually plethoric and has a deep dusky cyanosis. Injection of the conjunctivae is commonly seen. The spleen is palpable in 70% and is useful in distinguishing PV from secondary causes. The liver is enlarged in 50% of patients.

Investigations

- **Hb and PCV** are increased. The WBC is raised in about 70% of cases of PV and the platelet count is elevated in about 50%.
- **Bone marrow** shows erythroid hyperplasia and increased numbers of megakaryocytes.
- **Red cell volume** measured using ^{51}Cr-labelled red cells is increased (> 36 mL/kg in males and 32 mL/kg in females).
- **Plasma volume** shows normal or increased values (normal range is 45 ± 5 mL/kg).
- **Serum uric acid** levels may be raised.
- **Leucocyte alkaline phosphatase** (LAP) score is usually high.
- **Serum vitamin B$_{12}$ and vitamin B$_{12}$-binding protein** transcobalamin I (TC I) levels may be high, although these are not routinely measured.

Differential diagnosis

An increase in the red cell volume should be established. Raised WBC and platelet counts with splenomegaly makes a diagnosis of PV very likely. The principal secondary causes can often be excluded by the history and examination, but a renal ultrasound, an arterial P_{O_2} and carboxyhaemoglobin levels are usually performed.

The serum erythropoietin level is not diagnostic but may be helpful in distinguishing PV from secondary polycythaemia. In PV the level is low or normal, whereas in secondary polycythaemia the level may be raised, as expected, but also can be normal.

Course and management

Treatment is designed to maintain a normal blood count and to prevent the complications of the disease, particularly thromboses and haemorrhage. *Treatment* is aimed at keeping the PCV below 0.45 L/L and the platelet count below 400×10^9/L. There are three types of specific treatment:

- **Venesection.** This will successfully relieve many of the symptoms of PV. Iron deficiency limits erythropoiesis. Venesection is often used as the sole treatment and other therapy is reserved to control the thrombocytosis.
- **Chemotherapy.** Continuous or intermittent treatment with hydroxycarbamide (hydroxyurea) is used frequently because of the ease of controlling thrombocytosis and general safety in comparison to the alkylating agents such as busulfan, which carry an increased risk of acute leukaemia. Low-dose intermittent busulfan may be more convenient for elderly people, and this must be weighed against the potential risk of long-term complications.
- **Radioactive ^{32}P.** One dose may give control for up to 18 months, but the administration of ^{32}P carries an increased risk of transformation to acute leukaemia. ^{32}P is confined to the over-70 years age group.

General treatment

Allopurinol is given to block uric acid production. The pruritus is lessened by avoiding very hot baths. H$_1$-receptor antagonists have largely proved unsuccessful in relieving distressing pruritus, but H$_2$-receptor antagonists such as cimetidine are occasionally effective.

It should be noted that patients with uncontrolled PV have a high operative risk; 75% of patients have severe haemorrhage following surgery and 30% of these patients die. Polycythaemia should be controlled before surgery. In an emergency, reduction of the haematocrit by venesection and appropriate fluid replacement must be carried out.

Prognosis

PV develops into myelofibrosis in 30% of cases and into acute myeloblastic leukaemia in 5% as part of the natural history of the disease.

Secondary polycythaemias

The causes of these are shown in Table 8.16. The treatment is that of the precipitating factor; for example, renal or posterior fossa tumours need to be resected. Heavy smoking can produce as much as 10% carboxyhaemoglobin and this can produce polycythaemia because of a reduction in the oxygen-carrying capacity of the blood. Complications of secondary polycythaemia are similar to those seen in PV, including thrombosis, haemorrhage and cardiac failure, but the complications due to myeloproliferative disease such as progression to myelofibrosis or acute leukaemia do not develop. Venesection may be symptomatically helpful in the hypoxic patient, particularly if the PCV is above 0.55 L/L.

'Relative' or 'apparent' polycythaemia (Gaisböck's syndrome)

This condition was originally thought to be stress-induced. The red cell volume is normal but, as the result of a decreased plasma volume, there is a relative polycythaemia. 'Relative' polycythaemia is more common than PV and occurs in middle-aged men, particularly in smokers who are obese and hypertensive. The condition may present with cardiovascular problems such as myocardial or cerebral ischaemia. For this reason, it may be justifiable to venesect the patient. Smoking should be stopped.

Essential thrombocythaemia (ET)

ET is closely related to PV. The platelet count is usually $> 1000 \times 10^9/L$. It presents with bruising, bleeding and cerebrovascular symptoms. Initially splenic hypertrophy may be seen but, as the condition progresses, recurrent thromboses owing to the increased number of platelets reduce the size of the spleen and it may atrophy.

ET should be distinguished from secondary thrombocytosis that is seen in haemorrhage, connective tissue disorders, malignancy, after splenectomy and in other myeloproliferative disorders.

Treatment is with hydroxycarbamide (hydroxyurea) or busulfan to control the platelet count at less than $400 \times 10^9/L$.

α-Interferon is also effective but it is expensive and is administered by subcutaneous injection. ET may eventually transform into PV, myelofibrosis or acute leukaemia, but the disease may not progress for many years.

Myelofibrosis (myelosclerosis)

The terms myelosclerosis and myelofibrosis are interchangeable. There is clonal proliferation of stem cells and myeloid metaplasia in the liver, spleen and other organs. There is increased fibrosis in the bone marrow caused by hyperplasia of abnormal megakaryocytes which release fibroblast-stimulating factors such as platelet-derived growth factor. In about 25% of cases there is a preceding history of PV.

Clinical features

The disease presents insidiously with lethargy, weakness and weight loss. Patients often complain of a 'fullness' in the upper abdomen due to splenomegaly. Severe pain related to respiration may indicate perisplenitis secondary to splenic infarction, and bone pain and attacks of gout can complicate the illness. Bruising and bleeding occur because of thrombocytopenia or abnormal platelet function. Other physical signs include anaemia, fever and massive splenomegaly (for other causes, see p. 444).

Investigations

- **Anaemia** with leucoerythroblastic features is present (p. 452). Poikilocytes and red cells with characteristic tear-drop forms are seen. The WBC count may be over $100 \times 10^9/L$, and the differential WBC count may be very similar to that seen in CML; later leucopenia may develop.
- **The platelet count** may be very high but, in later stages, thrombocytopenia occurs.
- **Bone marrow aspiration** is often unsuccessful and this gives a clue to the presence of the condition. A bone marrow trephine is necessary to show the markedly increased fibrosis. Increased numbers of megakaryocytes may be seen.
- **The Philadelphia chromosome** is absent; this helps to distinguish myelofibrosis from most cases of CML.
- **The LAP score** is normal or high.
- **A high serum urate** is present.
- **Low serum folate** levels may occur owing to the increased haemopoietic activity.

Differential diagnosis

The major diagnostic difficulty is the differentiation of myelofibrosis from CML as in both conditions there may be marked splenomegaly and a raised WBC count with many granulocyte precursors seen in the peripheral blood. The main distinguishing features are the appearance of the bone marrow and the absence of the Philadelphia chromosome in myelofibrosis.

Fibrosis of the marrow, often with a leucoerythroblastic anaemia, can also occur secondarily to leukaemia or lymphoma, tuberculosis or malignant infiltration with metastatic carcinoma, or to irradiation.

Treatment

This consists of general supportive measures such as blood transfusion, folic acid, analgesics and allopurinol. Drugs such as hydroxycarbamide (hydroxyurea) and busulfan are used to reduce metabolic activity and high WBC count and platelet levels; hydroxycarbamide is the most common drug used. Chemotherapy and radiotherapy are used to reduce splenic size. If the spleen becomes very large and painful, and transfusion requirements are high, it may be advisable to perform splenectomy. Splenectomy may also result in relief of severe thrombocytopenia.

Prognosis

Patients may survive for 10 years or more; median survival is 3 years. Death may occur in 10–20% of cases from transformation to acute myeloblastic leukaemia. The most common causes of death are cardiovascular disease, infection and gastrointestinal bleeding.

Myelodysplasia

Myelodysplasia (MDS) describes a group of acquired bone marrow disorders that are due to a defect in stem cells. They are characterized by increasing bone marrow failure with quantitative and qualitative abnormalities of all three myeloid cell lines (red cells, granulocyte/monocytes and platelets). The natural history of MDS is variable, but there is a high morbidity and mortality owing to bone marrow failure, and transformation into acute myeloblastic leukaemia occurs in about 30% of cases. There are a number of different types of MDS:

- refractory anaemia (RA)
- refractory anaemia with ringed sideroblasts (> 15% ringed sideroblasts – RARS)
- refractory anaemia with an excess of blasts (blasts 5–20% – RAEB)
- refractory anaemia with an excess of blasts in transformation (blasts 20–30%) (RAEB-T)
- chronic myelomonocytic leukaemia (CMML).

Clinical and laboratory features

MDS occurs mainly in the elderly and presents with symptoms of anaemia, infection or bleeding due to pancytopenia. Serial blood counts show evidence of increasing bone marrow failure with anaemia, neutropenia, monocytosis and thrombocytopenia, either alone or in combination. In CMML, monocytes are $> 1 \times 10^9/L$ and the WBC count may be $> 100 \times 10^9/L$.

The bone marrow usually shows increased cellularity despite the pancytopenia. Dyserythropoiesis is present, and granulocyte precursors and megakaryocytes also have abnormal morphology. Ring sideroblasts are present in all types. In RAEB and RAEB-T, the number of blasts in the bone marrow is increased, and the prognosis is worse than in those types with a normal number of blast cells (< 5%).

Management

Patients with < 5% blasts in the bone marrow are usually managed conservatively with red cell and platelet transfusions and antibiotics for infections, as they are needed. Haemopoietic growth factors (e.g. erythropoietin, G-CSF) may be useful in some patients.

Patients with > 5% blasts have a less favourable prognosis, and a number of treatment options are available:

- **Supportive care** only is suitable for elderly patients with other medical problems.
- **'Gentle' chemotherapy** (low-dose or single-agent) may be useful in patients with high WBC counts.
- **Intensive chemotherapy** schedules used for acute myeloblastic leukaemia (see p. 492) may be tried in patients under the age of 60, but the remission rate is less, and prolonged pancytopenia may occur owing to poor haemopoietic regeneration because of the defect in stem cells.
- **Bone marrow transplantation** offers the hope of cure in the small proportion of MDS patients who are under the age of 50 and who have an HLA-identical sibling or an unrelated HLA-matched donor.

FURTHER READING

Provan D (1997) Myelodysplastic syndromes. *Prescribers' Journal* **37**: 17–23.

Provan D, Weatherall D (2000) Red cells II: acquired anaemias. *Lancet* **355**: 1260–1268.

Schwartz RC (1998) Polycythaemia vera – chance, death and mutability. *New England Journal of Medicine* **338**: 613–615.

Tefferi A (2000) Myelofibrosis with myeloid metaplasia. *New England Journal of Medicine* **342**: 1255–1265.

The spleen

The spleen is the largest lymphoid organ in the body and is situated in the left hypochondrium. There are two anatomical components:

- the red pulp, consisting of sinuses lined by endothelial macrophages and cords (spaces)
- the white pulp, which has a structure similar to lymphoid follicles.

Blood enters via the splenic artery and is delivered to the red and white pulp. During the flow the blood is 'skimmed', with leucocytes and plasma preferentially passing to white pulp. Some red cells pass rapidly through into the venous system while others are held up in the red pulp.

Functions

Sequestration and phagocytosis. Normal red cells, which are flexible, pass through the red pulp into the venous system without difficulty. Old or abnormal cells are damaged by the hypoxia, low glucose and low pH found in the sinuses of the red pulp and are therefore removed by phagocytosis along with other circulating foreign matter. Howell–Jolly and Heinz bodies and sideroblastic granules have their particles removed by 'pitting' and are then returned to the circulation. IgG-coated red cells are removed through their Fc receptors by macrophages.

Extramedullary haemopoiesis. Pluripotential stem cells are present in the spleen and proliferate during severe haematological stress, such as in haemolytic anaemia or thalassaemia major.

Immunological function. About 25% of the body's T lymphocytes and 15% of B lymphocytes are present in the spleen. The spleen shares the function of production of antibodies with other lymphoid tissues.

Blood pooling. Up to one-third of the platelets are sequestrated in the spleen and can be rapidly mobilized. Enlarged spleens pool a significant percentage (up to 40%) of the red cell mass.

Splenomegaly

Causes

A clinically palpable spleen can have many causes.

- Infection:
  (a) acute – e.g. septic shock, infective endocarditis, typhoid, infectious mononucleosis
  (b) chronic – e.g. tuberculosis and brucellosis
  (c) parasitic – e.g. malaria, kala-azar and schistosomiasis.
- Inflammation: rheumatoid arthritis, sarcoidosis, SLE.
- Haematological: haemolytic anaemia, haemoglobinopathies and the leukaemias, lymphomas and myeloproliferative disorders.
- Portal hypertension: liver disease.
- Miscellaneous: storage diseases, amyloid, primary and secondary neoplasias, tropical splenomegaly.

Massive splenomegaly is seen in myelofibrosis, chronic myeloid leukaemia, chronic malaria, kala-azar or, rarely, Gaucher's disease.

Investigation is that of the primary disorder. The spleen can be visualized by ultrasound or CT scanning. Splenic function can be assessed with isotope scanning.

Hypersplenism

This can result from splenomegaly due to any cause. It is commonly seen with splenomegaly due to haematological disorders, portal hypertension, rheumatoid arthritis (Felty's syndrome) and lymphoma. Hypersplenism produces:

- pancytopenia
- haemolysis due to sequestration and destruction of red cells in the spleen
- increased plasma volume.

Treatment is often dependent on the underlying cause, but splenectomy is sometimes required for severe anaemia or thrombocytopenia.

Splenectomy

Splenectomy is performed mainly for:

- trauma
- autoimmune thrombocytopenic purpura (p. 459)
- haemolytic anaemias (p. 426)
- hypersplenism.

Problems after splenectomy

An immediate problem is an increased platelet count (usually $600–1000 \times 10^9/L$) for 2–3 weeks. Thromboembolic phenomena may occur. In the longer term there is an increased risk of overwhelming infections, particularly pneumococcal infections.

Prophylaxis against infection after splenectomy or splenic dysfunction

All patients should be educated about the risk of infection and the importance of early recognition and treatment. They should be given an information leaflet and should carry a card to alert health professionals to their risk of overwhelming infection.

Pneumococcal immunization should be given 2–3 weeks before splenectomy. It is effective if the types of pneumonia are reflected in the polysaccharides contained in the serum. The vaccination may need to be repeated in 5–10 years. The currently available polyvalent vaccine contains purified capsular polysaccharide from the 23 most prevalent serotypes. *Haemophilus influenzae* type B vaccine should also be given to those who have not previously been immunized. Meningococcal immunization is not routinely recommended, except for travellers to areas where there is an increased risk of infection. Long-term prophylactic penicillin (e.g. penicillin V 500 mg 12-hourly) is recommended.

Postsplenectomy haematological features

- *Thrombocytosis* persists in about 30% of cases.
- *The WBC count* is usually normal but there may be a mild lymphocytosis and monocytosis.
- *Abnormalities in red cell morphology* are the most prominent changes and include Howell–Jolly bodies, Pappenheimer bodies (contain sideroblastic granules), target cells and irregular contracted red cells (see Fig. 8.8). Pitted red cells can be counted.

Splenic atrophy

This is seen in sickle cell disease due to infarction. It is also seen in coeliac disease, in dermatitis herpetiformis, and occasionally in ulcerative colitis and essential thrombocythaemia. Postsplenectomy haematological features are seen.

FURTHER READING

British Committee for Standards in Haematology (1996) Guidelines for the prevention and treatment of infection in patients with an absent or dysfunctional spleen. *British Medical Journal* **312**: 430–434.

Blood transfusion

The cells and proteins in the blood express antigens which are controlled by polymorphic genes; that is, a specific antigen may be present in some individuals but not in others. A blood transfusion may immunize the recipient against donor antigens that the recipient lacks (alloimmunization), and repeated transfusions increase the risk of the occurrence of alloimmunization. Similarly, the transplacental passage of fetal blood cells during pregnancy may alloimmunize the mother against fetal antigens inherited from the father. Antibodies stimulated by blood transfusion or pregnancy, such as Rhesus antibodies, are termed *immune* antibodies and are usually IgG, in contrast to *naturally occurring* antibodies, such as ABO antibodies, which are made in response to environmental antigens present in food and bacteria and which are usually IgM.

Blood groups

The blood groups are determined by antigens on the surface of red cells; more than 400 blood groups have been found. The ABO and Rh systems are the two most important blood groups, but incompatibilities involving many other blood groups (e.g. Kell, Duffy, Kidd) may cause haemolytic transfusion reactions and/or haemolytic disease of the newborn (HDN).

ABO system

This blood group system involves naturally occurring IgM anti-A and anti-B antibodies which are capable of producing rapid and severe intravascular haemolysis of incompatible red cells.

The ABO system is under the control of a pair of allelic genes, *H* and *h*, and also three allelic genes, *A*, *B* and *O*, producing the genotypes and phenotypes shown in Table 8.17. The A, B and H antigens are very similar in structure; differences in the terminal sugars determine their specificity. The *H* gene codes for enzyme *H*, which attaches fucose to the basic glycoprotein backbone to form H substance, which is the precursor for A and B antigens (Fig. 8.23).

The *A* and *B* genes control specific enzymes responsible for the addition to H substance of N-acetyl-galactosamine for Group A and D-galactose for Group B. The *O* gene is amorphic and does not transform H substance and therefore O is not antigenic. The A, B and H antigens are present on most body cells. These antigens are also found in soluble form in tissue fluids such as saliva and gastric juice in the 80% of the population who possess secretor genes.

Rh system

There is a high frequency of development of IgG RhD antibodies in RhD-negative individuals after exposure

Table 8.17
The ABO system: antigens and antibodies

Phenotype	Genotype	Antigens	Antibodies	Frequency UK (%)
O	OO	None	Anti-A and anti-B	44
A	AA or AO	A	Anti-B	45
B	BB or BO	B	Anti-A	8
AB	AB	A and B	None	3

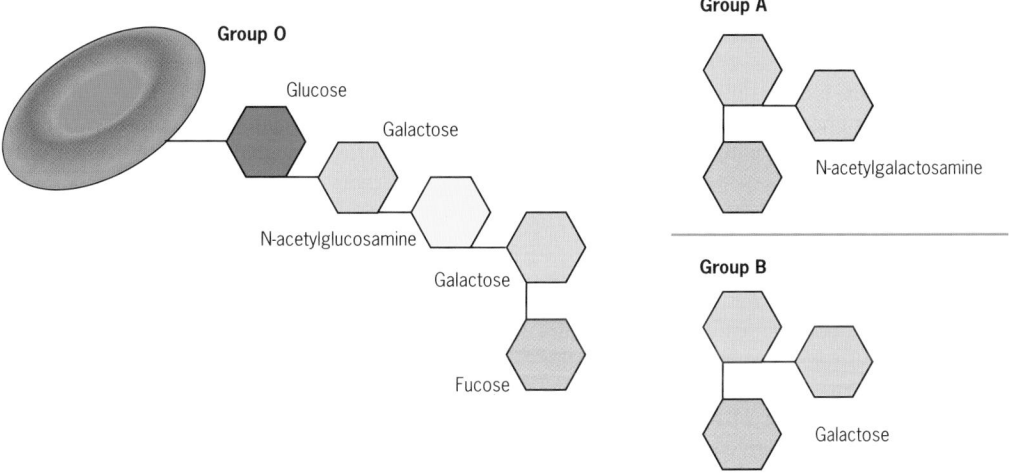

Fig. 8.23 **Sugar chains in the ABO blood group system.** Reproduced from Fricker J (1996) Conversion of red blood cells to group O. *Lancet* **347**: 680, © The Lancet Ltd. 1996.

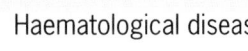

to RhD-positive red cells. The antibodies formed are of major importance in causing HDN and haemolytic transfusion reactions.

This system is coded by allelic genes, *C* and *c*, *E* and *e*, *D* and no *D*, which is signified as *d*; they are inherited as triplets on each chromosome, one from each pair of genes (i.e. *CDE*/*cde*). The presence of the d antigen has not been demonstrated and the presence or absence of the D antigen determines whether an individual is characterized as RhD positive or negative.

Procedure for blood transfusion

The safety of blood transfusion depends on meticulous attention to detail at each stage leading to and during the transfusion. Avoidance of simple errors involving patient and blood sample identification at the time of collection of the sample for crossmatching and at the time of transfusion would avoid most serious haemolytic transfusion reactions, almost all of which involve the ABO system.

Pretransfusion compatibility testing

This involves a number of steps, outlined below.

Blood grouping

The ABO and RhD groups of the patient are determined.

Antibody screening

The patient's serum or plasma is screened for atypical antibodies that may cause a significant reduction in the survival of the transfused red cells. The patient's serum or plasma is tested against red cells from at least two group O donors, expressing a wide range of red cell antigens, for detection of IgM red cell alloantibodies (using a direct agglutination test of cells suspended in saline) and IgG antibodies (using an indirect antiglobulin test, see p. 435). About 10% of patients have a positive antibody screening result, in which case, further testing is carried out using a comprehensive panel of typed red cells to determine the blood group specificity of the antibody (clinically significant red cell antibodies are detected in about 20% of patients with positive antibody screens).

Selection of donor blood and crossmatching

Donor blood of the same ABO and RhD group as the patient is selected. Matching for additional blood groups is carried out for patients with clinically significant red cell antibodies (see below), for patients who are likely to be multitransfused and at high risk of developing antibodies, e.g. sickle cell disease, and many centres routinely provide c-negative and Kell-negative blood for women of child-bearing age to minimize the risk of alloimmunization and subsequent HDN.

Crossmatching procedures

Patients without atypical red cell antibodies. The full crossmatch involves testing the patient's serum or plasma against the donor red cells suspended in saline in a direct agglutination test, and also using an indirect antiglobulin test. In some hospitals the *serological crossmatch* has been omitted as the negative antibody screen makes it highly unlikely that there will be any incompatibility with the donor units. A greater risk is that of a transfusion error involving the collection of the patient sample or a mix-up of samples in the laboratory. Laboratories can use the blood bank computer to check its records of the patient and the donor units and authorize the release of the donor units if a number of criteria are met (*computer or electronic crossmatching*), including:

- The system is automated for ABO and RhD grouping and antibody screening including positive sample identification and electronic transfer of results.
- The antibody screening procedure conforms to national recommendations.
- The patient's serum or plasma does not contain clinically significant red cell antibodies.
- The release of ABO incompatible blood must be prevented by conformation of laboratory computer software to the following requirements:
  (a) the issue of blood is not allowed if the patient has only been grouped once
  (b) the issue of blood is not allowed if the current group does not match the historical record
  (c) the system must not allow the reservation and release of units which are ABO incompatible with the patient.
- The laboratory must assure the validity of the ABO and RhD group of the donor blood either by written verification from the National Blood Service or confirmatory testing in the laboratory; the National Blood Service now guarantees that the blood group information is correct.

Alternatively, the crossmatch can be shortened to an immediate spin crossmatch where the patient's serum or plasma is briefly incubated with the donor red cells, followed by centrifugation and examination for agglutination; this rapid crossmatch is an acceptable method of excluding ABO incompatibility in patients known to have a negative antibody screen.

Patients with atypical red cell antibodies. Donor blood should be selected that lacks the relevant red cell antigen(s), as well as being the same ABO and RhD group as the patient. A full crossmatch should always be carried out.

Several other systems for blood grouping, antibody screening and crossmatching are available to hospital transfusion laboratories. They do not depend on agglutination of red cells in suspension, but rather on the differential passage of agglutinated and unagglutinated red cells through a column of dextran gel matrix (e.g. DiaMed, and Ortho Biovue systems), or on the capture of antibodies by red cells immobilized on the surface of a microplate well (e.g. Capture-R solid phase system).

Blood ordering

Elective surgery

Many hospitals have guidelines for the ordering of blood for elective surgery (maximum surgical blood ordering schedules). These are aimed at reducing unnecessary crossmatching and the amount of blood that eventually becomes outdated. Many operations in which blood is required only occasionally for unexpectedly high blood loss can be classified as 'group and save'; this means that, where the antibody screen is negative, blood is not reserved in advance but can be made available quickly if necessary, using serum or plasma saved in the laboratory. If a patient has atypical antibodies, compatible blood should always be reserved in advance.

Emergencies

There may be insufficient time for full pretransfusion testing. The options include:

1. Blood required immediately – use of 2 units of O RhD negative blood ('emergency stock'), to allow additional time for the laboratory to group the patient.
2. Blood required in 10–15 minutes – use of blood of the same ABO and RhD groups as the patient.
3. Blood required in 45 minutes – most laboratories will be able to provide fully crossmatched blood within this time.

Complications of blood transfusion (see Table 8.18)

In the United States, it has been mandatory to report transfusion-associated deaths to the Food and Drug Administration since 1975; such reports have provided useful data which have contributed to efforts to improve the safety of blood transfusion. Similar reporting schemes under the term 'haemovigilance' have been set up in other countries, including the Serious Hazards of Transfusion (SHOT) scheme which produced its first report in the UK in 1997. Errors from collection and administration were the commonest at 51%, with laboratory errors occuring in 36%. Errors from prescription sampling at request were 10%, with blood centre errors only being 3%. Figure 8.24 shows the reports to SHOT in 1998/99, indicating that 'incorrect blood component

Table 8.18
Complications of blood transfusion

Immunological	Non-immunological
Alloimmunization	*Transmission of infection*
Incompatibility	Viruses – HAV, HBV, HCV
Red cells	– HIV
Immediate haemolytic transfusion reactions	– CMV, EBV, HTLV-1
Delayed haemolytic transfusion reactions	Parasites – malaria, trypanosomiasis, toxoplasmosis
Leucocytes and platelets	Bacteria
Non-haemolytic (febrile) transfusion reactions	Prion – CJD
Post-transfusion purpura	*Circulatory failure* due to volume overload
Poor survival of transfused platelets and granulocytes	*Iron overload* due to multiple transfusions (see p. 429)
Graft-versus-host disease	*Massive transfusion* of stored blood may cause bleeding and electrolyte changes
Lung injury (TRALI)	*Physical damage* due to freezing or heating
Plasma proteins	*Thrombophlebitis*
Urticarial and anaphylactic reactions	*Air embolism*

transfused' was the most frequent error. Death was also attributed to other complications of blood transfusion including transfusion-associated lung injury (TRALI), transfusion-associated graft-versus-host disease (TA-GvHD), and bacterial infection of blood components.

Immunological complications

Alloimmunization

Blood transfusion carries a risk of alloimmunization to the many 'foreign' antigens present on red cells, leucocytes, platelets and plasma proteins. Alloimmunization may also occur during pregnancy – to fetal antigens inherited from the father and not shared by the mother.

Alloimmunization does not usually cause clinical problems with the first transfusion but these may occur with subsequent transfusions. There may also be delayed consequences of alloimmunization, such as HDN and rejection of tissue transplants.

Incompatibility

This may result in poor survival of transfused cells, such as red cells and platelets, and also in the harmful effects of antigen–antibody reaction.

Haemolytic transfusion reactions

Immediate reaction. This is the most serious complication of blood transfusion and is usually due to ABO incompatibility. There is complement activation by the antigen–antibody reaction, usually caused by IgM

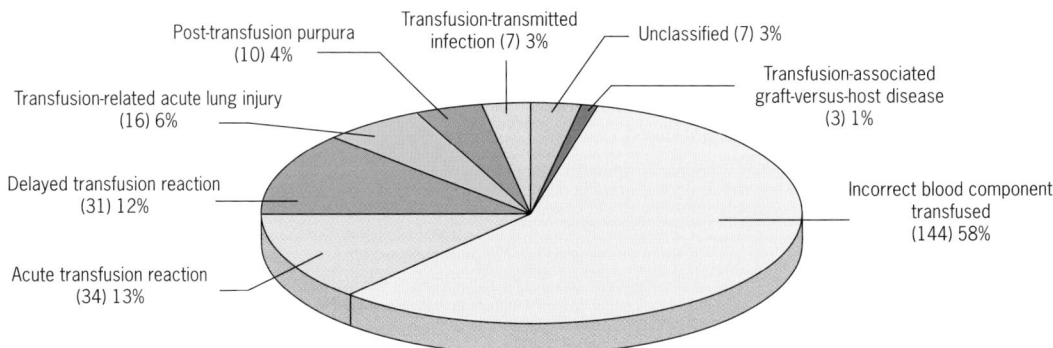

Fig. 8.24 Overview of 252 cases for which initial report forms were received by the Serious Hazards of Transfusion (SHOT) scheme in 1998/99.

antibodies, leading to rigors, lumbar pain, dyspnoea, hypotension, haemoglobinuria and renal failure. The initial symptoms may occur a few minutes after starting the transfusion. Activation of coagulation may also occur and bleeding due to disseminated intravascular coagulation (DIC) is a bad prognostic sign. Emergency treatment may be needed to maintain the blood pressure and renal function.

Diagnosis

This is confirmed by finding evidence of haemolysis (e.g. haemoglobinuria), and incompatibility between donor and recipient. All documentation should be checked to detect errors such as:

- failure to check the identity of the patient when taking the sample for compatibility testing (i.e. sample from the wrong patient)
- mislabelling the blood sample with the wrong patient's name
- simple labelling or handling errors in the laboratory
- errors in the collection of blood leading to delivery of the wrong blood to the ward/theatre
- failure to perform proper identity checks before the blood is transfused (i.e. blood transfused to the wrong patient).

The serious consequences of such failures emphasize the need for meticulous checks at all stages in the procedure of blood transfusion.

Investigations

To confirm where the error occurred, blood grouping should be carried out on:

- the patient's original sample (used for the compatibility testing)
- a new sample taken from the patient after the reaction
- the donor units.

At the first suspicion of any serious transfusion reaction, the transfusion should always be stopped and the donor units returned to the blood transfusion laboratory with a new blood sample from the patient to exclude a haemolytic transfusion reaction.

Delayed reaction. This may occur in patients alloimmunized by previous transfusions or pregnancies. The antibody level is too low to be detected by pretransfusion compatibility testing, but a secondary immune response occurs after transfusion, resulting in destruction of the transfused cells, usually by IgG antibodies.

Haemolysis is usually extravascular as the antibodies are IgG, and the patient may develop anaemia and jaundice about a week after the transfusion, although most of these episodes are clinically silent. The blood film shows spherocytosis and reticulocytosis. The direct antiglobulin test is positive and detection of the antibody is usually straightforward.

Non-haemolytic (febrile) transfusion reactions

Febrile reactions are a common complication of blood transfusion in patients who have previously been transfused or pregnant. The usual causes are the presence of leucocyte antibodies in an alloimmunized recipient acting against donor leucocytes in red cell concentrates leading to release of pyrogens, or the release of cytokines from donor leucocytes in platelet concentrates. Typical signs are flushing and tachycardia, fever (> 38°C), chills and rigors. Aspirin may be used to reduce the fever, although it should not be used in patients with thrombocytopenia. The general introduction of leucocyte-depleted blood in the UK, to minimize the risk of transmission of variant Creutzfeldt–Jakob disease (vCJD) by blood transfusion (see below), is expected to markedly reduce the incidence of febrile reactions.

Potent leucocyte antibodies in the plasma of donors, who are usually multiparous women, may cause severe pulmonary reactions (called transfusion-related acute lung injury or TRALI) characterized by dyspnoea, fever, cough, and shadowing in the perihilar and lower lung fields on the chest X-ray.

Urticaria and anaphylaxis

Urticarial reactions are often attributed to plasma protein incompatibility, but in most cases, they are unexplained. They are common but rarely severe; stopping or slowing the transfusion and administration of chlorphenamine (chlorpheniramine) 10 mg i.v. are usually sufficient treatment.

Anaphylactic reactions (see p. 961) occasionally occur; severe reactions are seen in patients lacking IgA who produce anti-IgA that reacts with IgA in the transfused blood. The transfusion should be stopped and epinephrine (adrenaline) 0.5 mg i.m. and chlorphenamine (chlorpheniramine) 10 mg i.v. should be given immediately; endotracheal intubation may be required. Patients who have had severe urticarial or anaphylactic reactions should receive either washed red cells, autologous blood, or blood from IgA-deficient donors for patients with IgA deficiency.

Non-immunological complications

Transmission of infection

The incidence of transmission of HBV and HCV is about 1 in 200 000 units transfused for each virus. Other viruses which may cause post-transfusion hepatitis include CMV and EBV, and there are likely to be other as yet unidentified viruses capable of causing post-transfusion hepatitis.

In the UK the incidence of transmission of HIV by blood transfusion is extremely low – probably under 1 in 3 million units transfused. Prevention is based on self-exclusion of donors in 'high-risk' groups and testing each donation for anti-HIV.

Testing for anti-HTLV-1 (see p. 62) is not carried out in the UK as it is in other countries, notably Japan and the United States. Only about 1 in 20 000 donors are seropositive, and there is a low risk of developing disease after infection because of the long incubation period.

There is an increased risk of viral transmission from coagulation factor concentrates prepared from large pools of plasma. However, these are now subjected to measures for inactivating viruses – such as treatment with heat, solvents and detergents.

The problem of viral transmission in relation to blood transfusion is still a major issue in the developing world.

Transfusion-transmitted syphilis is now very rare in the UK. Spirochaetes do not survive for more than 72 hours in blood stored at 4°C, and each donation is tested using the *Treponema pallidum haemagglutination assay* (TPHA).

Bacterial contamination of blood components is potentially a very serious event, and although rare it is one of the most frequent causes of death associated with transfusion after haemolytic transfusion reactions. Some organisms such as *Yersinia enterocolitica* can proliferate in red cell concentrates stored at 4°C, but platelet concentrates stored at 22°C are a more frequent cause of this problem. Several systems have been proposed to reduce the risk of bacterial contamination, including automated culture systems and bacterial antigen detection systems, but none are currently in routine use.

There is much concern about the rise of transmitting the prion protein causing vCJD (p. 63) by transfusion, although no proven case has been reported. This protein is associated with lymphocytes and has been found in tonsillar material. For this reason, universal leucocyte depletion of blood has been implemented in the UK since 1999. This also has other beneficial effects such as the reduction in incidence of post-operative infections. UK donor plasma is not now used for the manufacture of medicinal products; imported plasma from the US is used instead.

While stringent measures are being taken to minimize the risk of transfusion-transmitted infection in the UK, it may never be possible to guarantee that donor blood is absolutely 'safe'. The current approach to the safety of blood components and plasma in the UK is extremely cautious, but no absolute guarantee of safety.

Immunosuppression

Ever since observations were made of the favourable effect of transfusion on survival of subsequent renal allografts, the basis of transfusion-induced immuno-modulation has been the subject of debate. It is assumed that allogeneic leucocytes are required to cause transfusion-induced immunosuppression, but the underlying mechanisms remain uncertain. There has been considerable interest in other clinical effects caused by transfusion-induced immunosuppression, such as post-operative infection and tumour recurrence.

Strategies for avoiding or reducing the use of blood transfusion

Concerns about the safety of transfusion have led to increased interest in strategies for avoiding or reducing the use of donor blood. Consideration should be given to factors in the patient's past medical history or drug therapy indicating an increased risk of excessive blood loss, and attempting to correct them prior to surgery, for example discontinuing antiplatelet and anticoagulant drugs, if possible, several days before surgery. Anaemia, if present, should be investigated and treated appropriately in advance of elective surgery. Intraoperative measures include the use of meticulous surgical and anaesthetic techniques, a cautious use of anticoagulants during surgery and the use of drugs to enhance haemostasis, e.g. aprotinin.

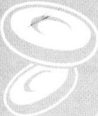

A comprehensive strategy for avoiding transfusion of donor blood also includes the employment of strict criteria (or 'triggers') for the use of blood components and blood products and consideration of autologous transfusion.

Artificial haemoglobin solutions and other blood substitutes are now in clinical trial. They have a short intravascular half-life, and are likely to find their initial clinical application in trauma and surgery.

Autologous transfusion

An alternative to using blood from volunteer donors is to use the patient's own blood. Interest in autologous transfusion was stimulated mainly by concern about transmission of infection, especially HIV, by blood transfusion. There are three types of autologous transfusion:

- *Predeposit*. The patient donates 2–5 units of blood at approximately weekly intervals before elective surgery.
- *Preoperative haemodilution*. One or two units of blood are removed from the patient immediately before surgery and retransfused to replace operative losses.
- *Blood salvage*. Blood lost during or after surgery may be collected and retransfused. Several techniques of varying levels of sophistication are available. The operative site must be free of bacteria, bowel contents and tumour cells.

There has been little demand for autologous transfusion in the UK as blood is generally perceived as being 'safe'. In addition, there are considerable costs in setting up a hospital-based predeposit autologous transfusion service, which would benefit only a minority of patients. In developing countries, however, autologous blood and blood from relatives is increasingly being used.

Blood, blood components and blood products

Most blood collected from donors is processed as follows:

- **Blood components**, such as red cell and platelet concentrates, fresh frozen plasma (FFP) and cryoprecipitate, are prepared from a single donation of blood by simple separation methods such as centrifugation and are transfused without further processing.
- **Blood products**, such as coagulation factor concentrates, albumin and immunoglobulin solutions, are prepared by complex processes using the plasma from many donors as the starting material (UK donor plasma not used).

In most circumstances it is preferable to transfuse only the blood component or product required by the patient (component therapy) rather than use whole blood. This is the most effective way of using donor blood, which is a scarce resource, and reduces the risk of complications from transfusion of unnecessary components of the blood.

Whole blood

The average volume of blood withdrawn is 470 mL taken into 63 mL of anticoagulant. Blood stored at 4°C has a 'shelf-life' of 5 weeks when at least 70% of the transfused red cells should survive normally. Whole blood is rarely used even for acute blood loss; packed cells or red cell concentrates plus crystalloid or colloid solutions are acceptable alternatives.

Red cell concentrates

Virtually all the plasma is removed and is replaced by about 100 mL of an optimal additive solution, such as SAG-M, which contains sodium chloride, adenine, glucose and mannitol. The mean volume is about 330 mL. The PCV is about 0.57 L/L, but the viscosity is low as there are no plasma proteins in the additive solution, and this allows fast administration if necessary. All blood components (red cell and platelet concentrates, and plasma) are now leucocyte-depleted in the UK by filtration within 48 hours of collection of the donor blood.

Washed red cell concentrates

These are preparations of red cells suspended in saline, produced by cell separators to remove all but traces of plasma proteins. They are used in patients who have had severe recurrent urticarial or anaphylactic reactions.

Platelet concentrates

These are prepared either from whole blood by centrifugation or by plateletpheresis of single donors using cell separators. They may be stored for up to 5 days at 22°C. They are used to treat bleeding in patients with severe thrombocytopenia, and prophylactically to prevent bleeding in patients with bone marrow failure.

Granulocyte concentrates

These are prepared from single donors using cell separators. They are used for patients with severe neutropenia with definite evidence of bacterial infection where antibiotic therapy has failed. They are rarely used, although there is interest in increasing the numbers of granulocytes collected by treating donors with G-CSF and steroids.

Fresh frozen plasma

FFP is prepared by freezing the plasma from 1 unit of blood at −30°C within 6 hours of donation. The volume is approximately 200 mL. FFP contains all the coagulation factors present in fresh plasma and is used mostly for replacement of coagulation factors in acquired coagulation factor deficiencies.

Cryoprecipitate

This is obtained by allowing the frozen plasma from a single donation to thaw at 4–8°C and removing the supernatant. The volume is about 20 mL and it is stored at −30°C. It contains factor VIII:C, von Willebrand factor (vWF) and fibrinogen. It is no longer used for the treatment of haemophilia A and von Willebrand's disease because of the greater risk of virus transmission compared with virus-inactivated coagulation factor concentrates. It may be useful in DIC and other conditions where the fibrinogen level is very low.

Factor VIII and IX concentrates

These are freeze-dried preparations of specific coagulation factors prepared from large pools of plasma. They are used for treating patients with haemophilia and von Willebrand's disease, where recombinant coagulation factor concentrates are unavailable. Recombinant coagulation factor concentrates, where they are available, are the treatment of choice for patients with inherited coagulation factor deficiencies (see p. 462).

Albumin

There are two preparations:

- *Human albumin solution 4.5%*, previously called plasma protein fraction (PPF), contains 45 g/L albumin and 160 mmol/L sodium. It is available in 50, 100, 250 and 500 mL bottles.
- *Human albumin solution 20%*, previously called 'salt-poor' albumin, contains approximately 200 g/L albumin and 130 mmol/L sodium and is available in 50 and 100 mL bottles.

Human albumin solutions are generally considered to be inappropriate fluids for acute volume replacement or for the treatment of shock because they are no more effective in these situations than synthetic colloid solutions such as polygelatins (Gelofusine) or hydroxyethyl starch (Haemaccel). However, albumin solutions are indicated for treatment of acute severe hypoalbuminaemia and as the replacement fluid for plasma exchange. The 20% albumin solution is particularly useful for patients with nephrotic syndrome or liver disease who are fluid overloaded and resistant to diuretics. Albumin solutions should not be used to treat patients with malnutrition or chronic renal or liver disease.

Normal immunoglobulin

This is prepared from normal plasma. It is used in patients with hypogammaglobulinaemia, to prevent infections, and in patients with immune thrombocytopenia.

Specific immunoglobulins

These are obtained from donors with high titres of antibodies. Many preparations are available, such as anti-D, anti-hepatitis B, and anti-varicella zoster.

FURTHER READING

Goodnough LT, Brecher ME, Kanter MH, Aubuchon JP (1999) Transfusion medicine: blood transfusion. *New England Journal of Medicine* **340**: 438–447.

Goodnough LT, Brecher ME, Kanter MH, Aubuchon JP (1999) Transfusion medicine: blood conservation. *New England Journal of Medicine* **340**: 525–532.

Klein HG (2000) The prospect for red cell substitutes. *New England Journal of Medicine* 342: 1666–1668.

Murphy MF, Pamphilon D (eds) (2001) *Practical Transfusion Medicine*. Oxford: Blackwell Science.

Turner M (1999) The impact of new-variant Creutzfeldt–Jakob disease on blood transfusion practice. *British Journal of Haematology* **106**: 842–850.

The white cell (see also Ch. 4)

The five types of leucocytes found in peripheral blood are neutrophils, eosinophils and basophils (which are all called *granulocytes*) and lymphocytes and monocytes. The development of these cells is shown in Figure 8.1.

Neutrophils

The earliest morphologically identifiable precursors of neutrophils in the bone marrow are myeloblasts, which are large cells constituting up to 3.5% of the nucleated cells in the marrow. The nucleus is large and contains 2–5 nucleoli. The cytoplasm is scanty and contains no granules. Promyelocytes are similar to myeloblasts but have some primary cytoplasmic granules, containing enzymes such as myeloperoxidase. Myelocytes are smaller cells without nucleoli but with more abundant cytoplasm and both primary and secondary granules. Indentation of the nucleus marks the change from myelocyte to metamyelocyte. The mature neutrophil is a smaller cell with a nucleus with 2–5 lobes with predominantly secondary granules in the cytoplasm which contain lysozyme, collagenase and lactoferrin.

Peripheral blood neutrophils are equally distributed into a circulating pool and a marginating pool lying along the endothelium of blood vessels. In contrast to the prolonged maturation time of about 10 days for neutrophils in the bone marrow, their half-life in the peripheral blood is extremely short, only 6–8 hours. In response to stimuli (e.g. infection, corticosteroid therapy) neutrophils are released into the circulating pool from both the marginating pool and the marrow. Immature white cells are released from the marrow when a rapid response (within hours) occurs in acute infection (described as a 'shift to the left' on a blood film).

Function

The prime function of neutrophils is to ingest and kill bacteria, fungi and damaged cells. Neutrophils are attracted to sites of infection or inflammation by chemotaxins. Recognition of foreign or dead material is aided by coating of particles with immunoglobulin and complement (opsonization) as neutrophils have Fc and C3b receptors (see p. 195). The material is ingested into vacuoles where it is subjected to enzymic destruction, which is either oxygen-dependent with the generation of hydrogen peroxide (myeloperoxidase) or oxygen-independent (lysosomal enzymes and lactoferrin).

Neutrophil leucocytosis

A rise in the number of circulating neutrophils to $> 10 \times 10^9$/L occurs in bacterial infections or as a result of tissue damage. This may also be seen in pregnancy, during exercise and after corticosteroid administration (Table 8.19). With any tissue necrosis there is a release of various soluble factors, causing a leucocytosis. Interleukin-1 is also released in tissue necrosis and causes a pyrexia. The pyrexia and leucocytosis accompanying a myocardial infarction are a good example of this and may be wrongly attributed to infection.

A leukaemoid reaction (an overproduction of white cells, with many immature cells) may occur in severe infections, tuberculosis, malignant infiltration of the bone marrow and occasionally after haemorrhage or haemolysis.

In leucoerythroblastic anaemia, nucleated red cells and white cell precursors are found in the peripheral blood. Causes include marrow infiltration with metastatic carcinoma, myelofibrosis, osteopetrosis, myeloma, lymphoma, and occasionally severe haemolytic or megaloblastic anaemia.

Neutropenia and agranulocytosis

Neutropenia is defined as a circulatory neutrophil count below 1.5×10^9/L. A virtual absence of neutrophils is called agranulocytosis. The causes are given in Table 8.20. It should be noted that black patients may have somewhat lower neutrophil counts. Neutropenia caused by viruses is probably the most common type. Chemotherapy and radiotherapy predictably produce neutropenia; many other drugs have been known to produce an idiosyncratic cytopenia and a drug cause should always be considered.

Clinical features

Infections may be frequent, often serious, and are more likely as the neutrophil count falls. An absolute neutrophil count of less than 0.5×10^9/L is regarded as 'severe' neutropenia and may be associated with life-threatening infections such as pneumonia and septicaemia. A characteristic glazed mucositis occurs in the mouth, and ulceration is common.

Investigations

The blood film shows marked neutropenia. The appearance of the bone marrow will indicate whether the neutropenia is due to depressed production or increased destruction of neutrophils. Neutrophil antibody studies may be performed if an immune mechanism is suspected.

Treatment

Antibiotics should be given as necessary to patients with acute severe neutropenia (see p. 483).

If the neutropenia seems likely to have been caused by a drug, all current drug therapy should be stopped. Recovery of the neutrophil count usually occurs after about 10 days. G-CSF (see p. 407) is used to decrease the period of neutropenia after chemotherapy and haemopoietic transplantation. It is also used successfully in the treatment of chronic neutropenia.

Steroids and high-dose intravenous immunoglobulin are used to treat patients with severe autoimmune neutropenia and recurrent infections, and G-CSF has produced responses in some cases.

Table 8.19
Neutrophil leucocytosis

Bacterial infections
Tissue necrosis, e.g. myocardial infarction, trauma
Inflammation, e.g. gout, rheumatoid arthritis
Drugs, e.g. corticosteroids, lithium
Haematological
    Myeloproliferative disease
    Leukaemoid reaction
    Leucoerythroblastic anaemia
Physiological, e.g. pregnancy, exercise
Malignant disease, e.g. bronchial, breast, gastric
Metabolic, e.g. renal failure, acidosis
Congenital, e.g. leucocyte adhesion deficiency, hereditary neutrophilia

---

Table 8.20
Causes of neutropenia

Acquired
Viral infection
Severe bacterial infection, e.g. typhoid
Felty's syndrome
Immune neutropenia – autoimmune, autoimmune neonatal neutropenia
Pancytopenia from any cause, including drug-induced marrow aplasia (see p. 423)
Pure white cell aplasia

Inherited
Ethnic (neutropenia is common in black races)
Kostmann's syndrome (severe infantile agranulocytosis)
Cyclical (genetic defect with neutropenia every 2–3 weeks)
Others, e.g. Schwachman–Diamond syndrome, dyskeratosis congenita, Chédiak–Higashi syndrome

Eosinophils

Eosinophils are slightly larger than neutrophils and are characterized by a nucleus with usually two lobes and large cytoplasmic granules that stain deeply red. The eosinophil plays a part in allergic responses (p. 194) and in the defence against infections with helminths and protozoa.

Eosinophilia is said to occur when the number of eosinophils is $> 0.4 \times 10^9/L$ in the peripheral blood. It is associated with a wide variety of disorders. The causes of eosinophilia are listed in Table 8.21.

Basophils

The nucleus of basophils is similar to that of neutrophils but the cytoplasm is filled with large black granules. The granules contain histamine, heparin and enzymes such as myeloperoxidase. The physiological role of the basophil is not known. Binding of IgE causes the cells to degranulate and release histamine and other contents involved in acute hypersensitivity reactions.

Basophils are usually few in number ($< 1 \times 10^9/L$) but are significantly increased in myeloproliferative disorders.

Monocytes

Monocytes are slightly larger than neutrophils. The nucleus has a variable shape and may be round, indented or lobulated. The cytoplasm contains fewer granules than neutrophils. Monocytes are precursors of tissue macrophages and spend only a few hours in the blood but can continue to proliferate in the tissues for many years.

A monocytosis ($> 0.8 \times 10^9/L$) may be seen in chronic bacterial infections such as tuberculosis or infective endocarditis, chronic neutropenia and patients with myelodysplasia, particularly chronic myelomonocytic leukaemia.

Lymphocytes

Lymphocytes form nearly half the circulating white cells. They descend from pluripotential stem cells. Circulating lymphocytes are small cells, a little larger than red cells, with a dark-staining central nucleus. There are two main types: T and B lymphocytes (see p. 199).

Lymphocytosis (lymphocyte count $> 5 \times 10^9/L$) occurs in response to viral infections, particularly EBV, CMV and HIV, and chronic infections such as tuberculosis and toxoplasmosis. It also occurs in chronic lymphocytic leukaemia and in some lymphomas.

FURTHER READING

Stock W, Hoffman R (2000) White blood cells 1: non-malignant disorders. *Lancet* **355**: 1351–1356.

Haemostasis and thrombosis

The integrity of the circulation is maintained by blood flowing through intact vessels lined by endothelial cells. Injury to the vessel wall exposes collagen and together with tissue injury sets in motion a series of events leading to haemostasis.

Haemostasis

Haemostasis is a complex process depending on interactions between the vessel wall, platelets and coagulation and fibrinolytic mechanisms. The formation of the haemostatic plug is shown in Figure 8.25.

Vessel wall

The vessel wall is lined by endothelium which, in normal conditions, preserves the circulation by preventing platelet adhesion and thrombus formation. This property is partly due to its negative charge but also to:

1. thrombomodulin and heparan sulphate expression
2. synthesis of prostacyclin (PGI_2) and nitric oxide (NO), which cause vasodilatation and inhibit platelet aggregation
3. production of plasminogen activator.

Table 8.21
Causes of eosinophilia

Parasitic infestations, such as:	**Pulmonary disorders,** such as:
Ascaris	Bronchial asthma
Hookworm	Tropical pulmonary
Strongyloides	eosinophilia
	Allergic bronchopulmonary
Allergic disorders, such as:	aspergillosis
Hayfever (allergic rhinitis)	Churg–Strauss syndrome
Other hypersensitivity	
reactions, including drug	**Malignant disorders,**
reactions	such as:
	Hodgkin's disease
Skin disorders, such as:	Carcinoma
Urticaria	Eosinophilic leukaemia
Pemphigus	
Eczema	**Miscellaneous,** such as:
	Hypereosinophilic syndrome
	Sarcoidosis
	Hypoadrenalism
	Eosinophilic gastroenteritis

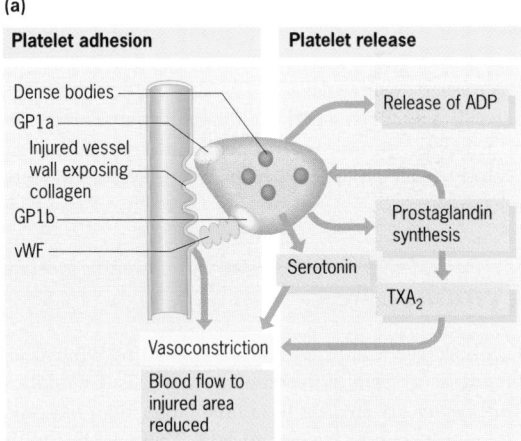

(a)

Platelet adhesion

Platelet release

Dense bodies
GP1a
Injured vessel wall exposing collagen
GP1b
vWF

Release of ADP

Prostaglandin synthesis

Serotonin

TXA$_2$

Vasoconstriction

Blood flow to injured area reduced

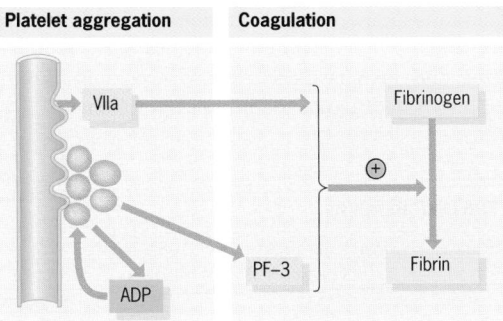

(b)

Platelet aggregation

Coagulation

VIIa

Fibrinogen

$\oplus$

PF–3

Fibrin

ADP

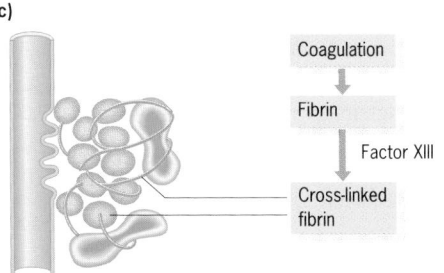

(c)

Coagulation

Fibrin

Factor XIII

Cross-linked fibrin

Fig. 8.25 **Formation of the haemostatic plug: sequential interactions between the vessel wall, platelets and coagulation factors.**

(a) Contact of platelets with collagen, either via the platelet receptor GPIb and factor vWF in plasma, or directly via GPIa, activates platelet prostaglandin synthesis which stimulates release of ADP from the dense bodies. Vasoconstriction of the vessel occurs as a reflex and by release of serotonin and thromboxane A$_2$ (TXA$_2$) from platelets.

(b) Release of ADP from platelets induces platelet aggregation and formation of the platelet plug. The coagulation pathway is stimulated leading to formation of fibrin.

(c) Fibrin strands are cross-linked by factor XIII and stabilize the haemostatic plug by binding platelets and red cells. PF-3, platelet factor-3.

Injury to vessels causes reflex vasoconstriction, while endothelial damage results in loss of antithrombotic properties, activation of platelets and coagulation and inhibition of fibrinolysis (Fig. 8.25).

Platelets

Platelet adhesion to collagen is dependent on platelet membrane receptors, glycoprotein Ia (GPIa), which binds directly to collagen, and glycoprotein Ib (GPIb), which binds to von Willebrand factor (vWF) in the plasma, and vWF in turn adheres to collagen. Following adhesion, platelets undergo a shape change from a disc to a sphere, spread along the subendothelium and release the contents of their cytoplasmic granules, i.e. the dense bodies (containing ADP and serotonin) and the α-granules (containing platelet-derived growth factor, platelet factor 4, β-thromboglobulin, fibrinogen, vWF and other factors).

The release of ADP leads to a conformational change in the fibrinogen receptor, the glycoprotein IIb–IIIa complex (GPIIb–IIIa), on the surfaces of adherent platelets, allowing it to bind to fibrinogen (see also Fig. 8.33). Fibrinogen then binds platelets into activated aggregates (platelet aggregation) and further platelet release occurs. A self-perpetuating cycle of events is set up leading to formation of a platelet plug at the site of the injury.

Further platelet membrane receptors, e.g. P2Y$_{12}$, are exposed during aggregation, providing a surface for the interaction of coagulation factors; this platelet activity is referred to as platelet factor 3 (PF-3). The presence of thrombin encourages fusion of platelets, and fibrin formation reinforces the stability of the platelet plug.

Central to normal platelet function is platelet prostaglandin synthesis, which is induced by platelet activation and leads to the formation of TXA$_2$ in platelets (Fig. 8.26). Thromboxane (TXA$_2$) is a powerful vasoconstrictor and also lowers cyclic AMP levels and initiates the platelet release reaction.

Prostaglandin I$_2$ (PGI$_2$) is synthesized in vascular endothelial cells and opposes the actions of TXA$_2$. It produces vasodilatation and increases the level of cyclic AMP, preventing platelet aggregation on the normal vessel wall as well as limiting the extent of the initial platelet plug after injury.

Coagulation and fibrinolysis

The coagulation cascade involves a series of enzymatic reactions leading to the conversion of soluble plasma fibrinogen to fibrin clot (Fig. 8.27). Roman numerals are used for most of the factors, but I and II are referred to as fibrinogen and prothrombin respectively; III, IV and VI are redundant. The active forms are denoted by 'a'.

The coagulation factors are primarily synthesized in the liver and are either enzyme precursors (factors XII, XI, X, IX and thrombin) or cofactors (V and VIII), except for fibrinogen, which is degraded to form fibrin.

Coagulation pathway

This enzymatic amplification system is traditionally divided into 'extrinsic' and 'intrinsic' pathways. This concept remains very useful for the interpretation of

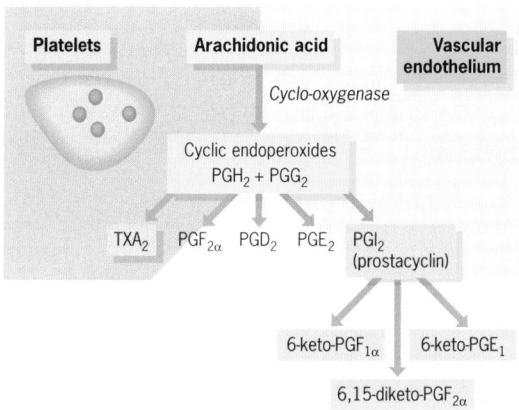

Fig. 8.26 Prostaglandin synthesis.

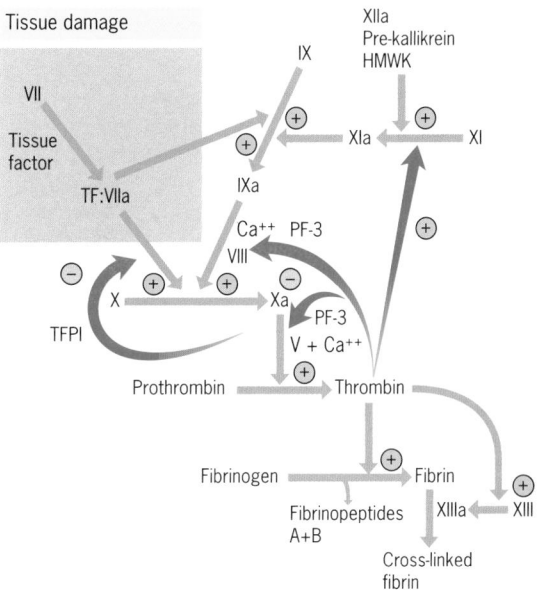

Fig. 8.27 Coagulation cascade. The pathway in vivo begins with activation of factor IX by factor VIIa. The factor XII and pre-kallikrein reactions are probably only relevant in vitro. Factor XI is activated by thrombin in vivo. HMWK, high-molecular-weight kininogen; TFPI, tissue factor pathway inhibitor.

clinical laboratory tests (see p. 456) but is an oversimplification. Coagulation is initiated by binding of activated factor VII (VIIa) in plasma to tissue factor (TF), a glycoprotein which is expressed on the surface of cells which are exposed after injury. The complex of VIIa and tissue factor (TF:VIIa) activates factor X but this reaction is opposed by tissue factor pathway inhibitor (TFPI), and the main role of TF:VIIa in vivo is to activate factor IX (Fig. 8.27). Activated factor IX then works with factor VIII to initiate the crucial activation of factor X. (It is this reaction which amplifies the generation of thrombin and which fails in haemophilia A and B. Factor XI is activated in vivo by thrombin and makes a limited contribution to haemostasis so that factor XI deficiency results in a rather mild bleeding disorder.)

Activated factor X induces the conversion of prothrombin to thrombin. Thrombin hydrolyses the peptide bonds of fibrinogen, releasing fibrinopeptides A and B, and allowing polymerization between fibrinogen molecules to form fibrin. At the same time, thrombin, in the presence of calcium ions, activates factor XIII, which stabilizes the fibrin clot by cross-linking adjacent fibrin molecules. The presence of thrombin helps in the activation of factors XI, V, VIII and XIII (and protein C).

Factor VIII consists of a molecule with coagulant activity (VIII:C) associated with von Willebrand factor, whose function is to stabilize factor VIII:C and to promote platelet–endothelial interaction. VIII:C is a single-chain protein with a molecular weight of about 350 000. vWF is a glycoprotein with a molecular weight of about 200 000 which readily forms multimers in the circulation with molecular weights of up to 20×10^6. The high-molecular-weight multimeric forms of vWF are the most effective in promoting platelet function.

Limitation of coagulation
Coagulation is limited to the site of injury by removal of activated coagulation factors by rapid blood flow at the periphery of the damaged area, by plasma inhibitors of activated coagulation factors, and by fibrinolysis.

Antithrombin. Antithrombin (AT), a member of the serine protease inhibitor (serpin) superfamily, is a potent inhibitor of coagulation. It inactivates the serine proteases by forming stable complexes with them, and its action is greatly potentiated by heparin.

Activated protein C. This is generated from its vitamin K-dependent precursor by the action of thrombin; thrombin activation of protein C is enhanced when thrombin is bound to thrombomodulin, which is an endothelial cell receptor (Fig. 8.28). Activated protein C destroys factor V and factor VIII, reducing further thrombin generation.

Protein S. This is a cofactor for protein C which acts by enhancing binding of activated protein C to the phospholipid surface. It circulates bound to C4b binding protein but some 30–40% remains unbound and active (free protein S).

Other inhibitors. Other natural inhibitors of coagulation include α_2-macroglobulin, α_1-antitrypsin and α_2-antiplasmin.

Fibrinolysis
Fibrinolysis, which helps to restore vessel patency, also occurs in response to vascular damage. In this system (Fig. 8.29), an inactive plasma protein – plasminogen – is converted to plasmin by plasminogen activators derived from the plasma or blood cells (intrinsic activation) or the tissues (extrinsic activation).

Plasmin is a serine protease which breaks down fibrinogen and fibrin into fragments X, Y, D and E,

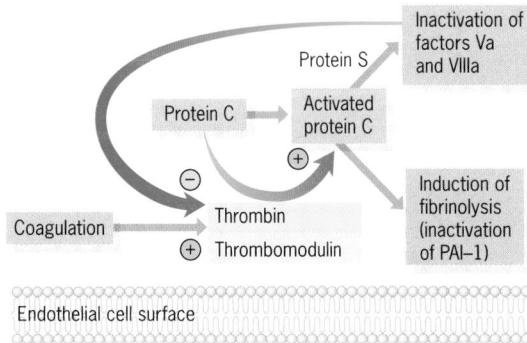

Fig. 8.28 **Activation of protein C.** PAI-1, plasminogen activator inhibitor 1.

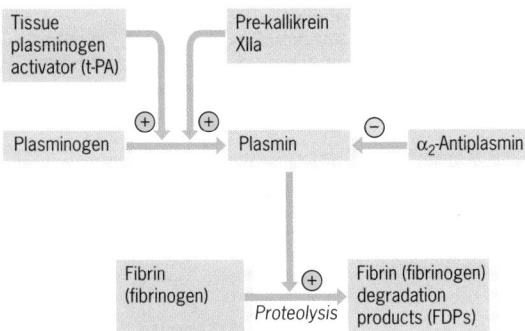

Fig. 8.29 **Fibrinolytic system.**

collectively known as fibrin (and fibrinogen) degradation products (FDPs). Degradation of cross-linked fibrin yields D-dimer and D-dimer-E fragments. Plasmin is also capable of breaking down coagulation factors such as factors V and VIII.

The fibrinolytic system is activated by the presence of fibrin. Plasminogen is specifically adsorbed to fibrin and fibrinogen by lysine-binding sites. However, little plasminogen activation occurs in the absence of fibrin, as fibrin also has a specific binding site for plasminogen activators, whereas fibrinogen does not (Fig. 8.30).

The major plasminogen activator is tissue-type plasminogen activator (t-PA); vascular endothelium is the major source of t-PA in plasma. Its release is stimulated by a number of mediators, including thrombin. Another plasminogen activator is urokinase, synthesized in the kidney and released into the urogenital tract. Intrinsic plasminogen activators such as factor XII and pre-kallikrein are of minor physiological importance.

t-PA is inactivated by plasminogen activator inhibitor-1 (PAI-1). Activated protein C inactivates PAI-1 and therefore induces fibrinolysis (Fig. 8.28). Inactivators of plasmin such as α_2-antiplasmin (Fig. 8.30) and thrombin-activatable fibrinolysis inhibitor (TAFI) also contribute to the regulation of fibrinolysis.

Investigation of bleeding disorders

Although the precise diagnosis of a bleeding disorder may depend on laboratory tests, much information may be obtained from the history and physical examination:

- **Is there a generalized haemostatic defect?**
  Supportive evidence for this includes bleeding from multiple sites, spontaneous bleeding, and excessive bleeding after injury.
- **Is the defect inherited or acquired?** A family history of a bleeding disorder should be sought. Severe inherited defects usually become apparent in infancy, while mild inherited defects may only come to attention later in life, for example with excessive bleeding after surgery, childbirth, dental extractions or trauma. Some defects are revealed by routine coagulation screens which are performed before surgical procedures.
- **Is the bleeding suggestive of a vascular/platelet defect or a coagulation defect?**

Vascular/platelet bleeding is characterized by easy bruising and spontaneous bleeding from small vessels. There is often bleeding into the skin. The term purpura includes both petechiae, which are small skin haemorrhages varying from pinpoint size to a few millimetres in diameter and which do not blanch on pressure, and ecchymoses, which are larger areas of bleeding into the skin. Bleeding also occurs from mucous membranes especially the nose and mouth.

Coagulation disorders are typically associated with haemarthroses and muscle haematomas, and bleeding after injury or surgery. There is often a short delay between the precipitating event and overt haemorrhage or haematoma formation.

Laboratory investigations

- **Blood count and film** show the number and morphology of platelets and any blood disorder such as leukaemia or lymphoma. The normal range for the platelet count is $150–400 \times 10^9/L$.
- **Bleeding time** measures platelet plug formation in vivo. It is determined by applying a sphygmomanometer cuff to the arm and inflating it to 40 mmHg. Two 1 mm deep, 1 cm long incisions are made in the forearm with a template. Each wound is blotted every 30 s and the time taken for bleeding to stop is recorded, normally between 3 and 10 minutes. Prolonged bleeding times are found in patients with platelet function defects and there is a progressive prolongation with platelet counts less than $80 \times 10^9/L$. The bleeding time should not be performed at low platelet counts.
- **Coagulation tests** are performed using blood collected into citrate, which neutralizes calcium ions and prevents clotting.

(a) Conversion of plasminogen to plasmin

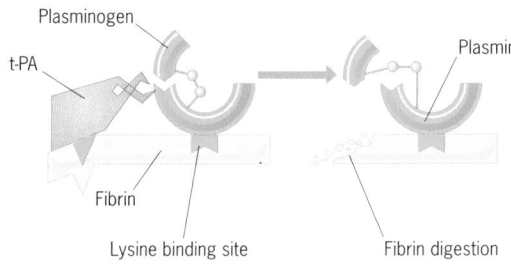

(b) Plasmin α₂–antiplasmin complex

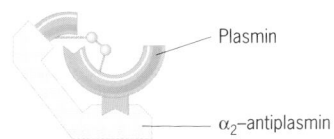

Fig. 8.30 **Fibrinolysis.** **(a)** The conversion of plasminogen to plasmin by plasminogen activator (t-PA) occurs most efficiently on the surface of fibrin, which has binding sites for both plasminogen and t-PA. **(b)** Free plasmin in the blood is rapidly inactivated by α_2-antiplasmin. Plasmin generated on the fibrin surface is partially protected from inactivation. The lysine-binding sites on plasminogen are important for the interaction between plasmin(ogen) and fibrin and between plasmin and α_2-antiplasmin.

The *prothrombin time* (PT) (also see p. 469) is measured by adding tissue thromboplastin in the form of animal brain extract, or a recombinant equivalent, and calcium to the patient's plasma ('extrinsic' system). The normal PT is 16–18 s, and it is prolonged with abnormalities of factors VII, X, V, II or I, liver disease, or if the patient is on warfarin.

The *activated partial thromboplastin time* (APTT) is also sometimes known as the PTT with kaolin (PTTK). It is performed by adding a surface activator (such as kaolin), phospholipid (as platelet substitute) and calcium to the patient's plasma ('intrinsic' system). The normal APTT is 30–50 s depending on the exact methodology, and it is prolonged with deficiencies or inhibitors to one or more of the following factors: XII, XI, IX, VIII, X, V, II or I (but not factor VII) (see Fig. 8.27).

The *thrombin time* (TT) is performed by adding thrombin to the patient's plasma. The normal TT is about 12 s, and it is prolonged with fibrinogen deficiency, dysfibrinogenaemia (normal level of fibrinogen but abnormal function) or inhibitors such as heparin or FDPs.

Correction tests can be used to differentiate prolonged times in the PT, APTT and TT due to various coagulation factor deficiencies and inhibitors of coagulation. Prolonged PT, APTT or TT because of coagulation factor deficiencies are corrected by addition of normal plasma to the patient's plasma; no correction of an abnormal result after the addition of normal plasma is suggestive of the presence of an inhibitor of coagulation.

Factor assays are used to confirm coagulation defects, especially where a single inherited disorder is suspected.

Special tests of coagulation will often be required to confirm the precise haemostatic defect. Such tests include estimation of fibrinogen and FDPs, platelet function tests such as platelet aggregation and tests of the fibrinolytic pathway which include the euglobulin clot lysis time (ELT) and assays of plasminogen, t-PA and PAI-1. The ELT involves precipitation by acidification of the euglobulin fraction of plasma, which contains fibrinogen, plasminogen and plasminogen activators but excluding α_2-antiplasmin. The euglobulin fraction is clotted with thrombin and the time taken for lysis of the fibrin clot is a measure of fibrinolytic activity; the normal range is 60–270 minutes. Factor XIII can be estimated by a clot stability screening test or by direct assay.

Vascular disorders

The vascular disorders (Table 8.22) are characterized by easy bruising and bleeding into the skin. Bleeding from mucous membranes sometimes occurs but the bleeding

Table 8.22
Vascular disorders

Congenital	**Allergic**
Hereditary haemorrhagic telangiectasia	Henoch–Schönlein purpura
(Osler–Weber–Rendu disease)	Autoimmune disorders (SLE, rheumatoid arthritis)
Connective tissue disorders (Ehlers–Danlos syndrome, osteogenesis	
imperfecta, pseudoxanthoma elasticum, Marfan's syndrome)	**Drugs**
	Steroids
	Sulphonamides
Acquired	
Severe infections:	
Septicaemia	**Others**
Meningococcal infections	Senile purpura
Measles	Easy bruising syndrome
Typhoid	Scurvy
	Factitious purpura

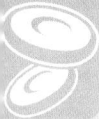
is rarely severe. Laboratory investigations including the bleeding time are normal. The vascular disorders include the following.

Hereditary haemorrhagic telangiectasia is a rare disorder with autosomal dominant inheritance. Dilatation of capillaries and small arterioles produces characteristic small red spots that blanch on pressure in the skin and mucous membranes, particularly the nose and gastrointestinal tract. Recurrent epistaxis and chronic gastrointestinal bleeding are the major problems and may cause chronic iron deficiency anaemia.

Easy bruising syndrome is a common benign disorder occurring in otherwise healthy women. It is characterized by bruises on the arms, legs and trunk with minor trauma, possibly due to skin vessel fragility. It may give rise to the suspicion of a serious bleeding disorder.

Senile purpura and purpura due to steroids are both due to atrophy of the vascular supporting tissue.

Purpura due to infections is mainly caused by damage to the vascular endothelium. The rash of meningococcal septicaemia is particularly characteristic (p. 78).

Henoch–Schönlein purpura (p. 605) occurs mainly in children. It is a type III hypersensitivity reaction that is often preceded by an acute upper respiratory tract infection. Purpura is mainly seen on the legs and buttocks. Abdominal pain, arthritis, haematuria and glomerulonephritis also occur. Recovery is usually spontaneous, but some patients develop renal failure.

Episodes of inexplicable bleeding or bruising may represent abuse, either self-inflicted or caused by others. These various forms of artificial or factitious purpura are expressions of severe emotional or psychiatric disturbances.

Platelet disorders

Bleeding due to thrombocytopenia or abnormal platelet function is characterized by purpura and bleeding from mucous membranes. Bleeding is uncommon with platelet counts above $50 \times 10^9/\text{L}$, and severe spontaneous bleeding is unusual with platelet counts above $20 \times 10^9/\text{L}$ (Table 8.23).

Thrombocytopenia

This is caused by reduced platelet production in the bone marrow or excessive peripheral destruction of platelets (Table 8.24). The underlying cause may be revealed by history and examination but a bone marrow examination will show whether the numbers of megakaryocytes are reduced, normal or increased, and will provide essential information on morphology. Specific laboratory tests may be useful to confirm the presence of such conditions as paroxysmal nocturnal haemoglobinuria (PNH) or systemic lupus erythematosus (SLE).

In patients with thrombocytopenia due to failure of production, no specific treatment may be necessary but the underlying condition should be treated if possible.

Table 8.23
The platelet count in platelet disorders

$> 500 \times 10^9/\text{L}$	Haemorrhage or thrombosis
$500–100 \times 10^9/\text{L}$	No clinical effect
$100–50 \times 10^9/\text{L}$	Moderate haemorrhage after injury
$50–20 \times 10^9/\text{L}$	Purpura may occur
	Haemorrhage after injury
$< 20 \times 10^9/\text{L}$	Purpura common
	Spontaneous haemorrhage from mucous membranes
	Intracranial haemorrhage (rare)

By permission of Richardson D, Colvin B (2000) *Medicine* 28(2): 29

Table 8.24
Causes of thrombocytopenia

Impaired production	Excessive destruction
Bone marrow failure	**Immune**
Megaloblastic anaemia	AITP
Leukaemia	Secondary immune (SLE, CLL,
Myeloma	viruses, drugs, e.g. heparin)
Myelofibrosis	Alloimmune neonatal
Solid tumour infiltration	thrombocytopenia
Aplastic anaemia	Post-transfusion purpura
drugs	
chemicals	**Sequestration**
viruses	Hypersplenism
paroxysmal nocturnal	
haemoglobinuria	**Dilutional**
	Massive transfusion
	Other
	Disseminated intravascular coagulation
	Thrombotic thrombocytopenic purpura
	Haemolytic uraemic syndrome

Where the platelet count is very low or the risk of bleeding is very high, then platelet concentrate administration is indicated.

Autoimmune (idiopathic) thrombocytopenic purpura (AITP)

Thrombocytopenia is due to immune destruction of platelets. The antibody-coated platelets are removed following binding to Fc receptors on macrophages. There are two distinct clinical syndromes.

Acute AITP

Acute AITP is usually seen in children, often following a viral infection, and acute development of platelet autoantibodies is probably responsible for the shortened platelet survival.

Chronic AITP

Chronic AITP is characteristically seen in adult women. It is usually idiopathic but may occur in association with other autoimmune disorders such as SLE, thyroid disease and autoimmune haemolytic anaemia (Evans' syndrome), in patients with chronic lymphocytic leukaemia and solid tumours, and after infections with viruses such as HIV. Platelet autoantibodies are detected in about 60–70% of patients, and are presumed to be present, although not detectable, in the remaining patients; the antibodies often have specificity for platelet membrane glycoproteins IIb/IIIa and/or Ib.

Clinical features

Major haemorrhage is rare and is seen only in patients with severe thrombocytopenia. Easy bruising, purpura, epistaxis and menorrhagia are common. Physical examination is normal except for evidence of bleeding. Splenomegaly is rare.

Investigation

The only blood count abnormality is thrombocytopenia. Normal or increased numbers of megakaryocytes are found in the bone marrow, which is otherwise normal. The detection of platelet autoantibodies is not essential for confirmation of the diagnosis, which often depends on exclusion of other causes of excessive destruction of platelets.

Treatment

Acute AITP in children usually remits spontaneously. Treatment in the acute phase with steroids or high-dose intravenous immunoglobulin is required only when the platelet count is < 20 × 10⁹/L and there is bleeding. *Chronic AITP.* Spontaneous remissions are rare.

The main aims of treatment are to reduce the production of platelet autoantibodies and the removal of antibody-coated platelets. Initial treatment is with prednisolone, 40–60 mg daily in adults, with cautious reduction of the dose after remission has occurred.

Twenty per cent of patients have a complete response and require no further treatment; 60% have a partial response, and half of these have little bleeding associated with mild or moderate thrombocytopenia (platelet count 30–100 × 10⁹/L). They may require small doses of steroids, such as prednisolone 5–15 mg daily, or no further treatment. The other half of the partial responders eventually relapse and require splenectomy, as do the 20% of patients who failed to respond to steroids at all.

There is a 90% response rate to splenectomy, although about 30% of responders eventually relapse. Some of these refractory patients may respond to immunosuppressive drugs such as azathioprine, cyclophosphamide or vincristine or to danazol, which is a non-virilizing androgen. Splenectomy should be avoided in young children because of the subsequent risk of severe pneumococcal infection (see p. 444). In older adults splenectomy is also unattractive and many patients respond adequately to immunosuppressive drugs alone.

Intravenous infusion of high-dose immunoglobulin produces a rapid rise in the platelet count owing to blockade of Fc receptors on macrophages in the spleen. The increase in platelet count is usually transient but may be useful in patients with acute haemorrhage and in preparing patients with chronic AITP for surgery. Anti-D has also been used and found to be effective in some cases.

Transfused platelets survive no longer than the patient's own platelets but may sometimes be beneficial in patients with life-threatening bleeding, when emergency splenectomy may be justified.

Other immune thrombocytopenias

Drugs cause immune thrombocytopenia by the same mechanisms as described for drug-induced immune haemolytic anaemia (p. 437). The same drugs may be responsible for immune haemolytic anaemia, thrombocytopenia or neutropenia in different patients.

Heparin-induced thrombocytopenia. See p. 469.

Fetomaternal alloimmune thrombocytopenia is due to fetomaternal incompatibility for platelet-specific antigens, usually for HPA-1a (human platelet alloantigen) and is the platelet equivalent of haemolytic disease of the newborn (HDN). The mother is HPA-1a-negative and produces antibodies which destroy the HPA-1a-positive fetal platelets.

Thrombocytopenia is self-limiting after delivery, but platelet transfusions may be required initially to prevent or treat bleeding associated with severe thrombocytopenia; platelets may be prepared from HPA-1a-negative volunteers or the mother herself. Severe bleeding such as intracranial haemorrhage may also occur in utero. Antenatal treatment of the mother – with platelet transfusions given directly to the fetus by ultrasound-guided needling of the umbilical vessels – has been effective in preventing haemorrhage in severely affected cases.

Post-transfusion purpura (PTP) is rare, occurring 2–12 days after a blood transfusion. PTP is associated with a platelet-specific alloantibody, usually anti-HPA-1a in an HPA-1a-negative individual. PTP almost invariably occurs in females who have been previously immunized by pregnancy or blood transfusion. The cause of the destruction of the patient's own platelets is not well understood, but they may be destroyed as 'bystanders' during the acute immune response to HPA-1a. PTP is self-limiting, but high-dose intravenous immunoglobulin may limit the period of thrombocytopenia.

Thrombotic thrombocytopenic purpura (TTP) (p. 611)
TTP is a rare, but very serious condition, in which platelet destruction leads to profound thrombocytopenia. There is a characteristic symptom complex of florid purpura, fever, fluctuating cerebral dysfunction and haemolytic anaemia with red cell fragmentation, often accompanied by renal failure. The coagulation screen is usually normal but lactic dehydrogenase (LDH) levels are markedly raised as a result of haemolysis.

The underlying cause is not fully understood but TTP seems to be due to endothelial damage associated with the presence in the circulation of very-high-molecular-weight multimers of von Willebrand factor (vWF) which accumulate owing to the absence of a protease which is normally responsible for vWF degradation. This absence is due to mutations in the *ADAMTS 13* gene. In some cases there is a true deficiency of the protease while in others an immune response appears to reduce protease activity temporarily. The related condition of haemolytic uraemic syndrome (HUS), in which renal failure is a prominent feature, probably has a different cause. TTP is associated with pregnancy, oral contraceptives, systemic lupus erythematosus, infection and drug treatment, including the use of ticlopidine and clopidogrel, but many cases have no obvious cause.

Treatment consists of plasma exchange using cryo-precipitate-depleted FFP (cryo-poor supernatant) or solvent detergent-treated FFP, both of which contain reduced amounts of high-molecular-weight vWF multi-mers. It is also thought that FFP supplies the missing protease. Most patients are also treated with prednisone 1 mg/kg daily and low-dose aspirin 75 mg daily is often given as the platelet count rises above 50×10^9/L. Platelet concentrates are contraindicated.

The untreated condition has a mortality of up to 90% but modern management has reduced this figure to about 10%. Recurrent and relapsing TTP occurs, often associated with a persistent lack of vWF protease. Disease activity is monitored by measuring the platelet count and serum LDH.

Platelet function disorders

These are usually associated with excessive bruising and bleeding and, in some of the acquired forms, with thrombosis. The platelet count is normal or increased and the bleeding time is prolonged. The rare inherited defects of platelet function require more detailed investigations such as platelet aggregation studies and factor VIII:C and vWF assays, if von Willebrand's disease is suspected.

Inherited types of platelet dysfunction
- *Glanzmann's thrombasthenia* – lack of the platelet membrane glycoprotein IIb/IIIa complex resulting in defective fibrinogen binding and failure of platelet aggregation.
- *Bernard–Soulier syndrome* – lack of platelet membrane glycoprotein Ib, the binding site for factor vWF. This causes a failure of platelet adhesion and moderate thrombocytopenia.
- *Storage pool disease* – lack of the storage pool of dense bodies, causing poor platelet function.

Acquired types of platelet dysfunction
- Myeloproliferative disorders
- Uraemia and liver disease
- Paraproteinaemias

- Drug-induced, such as by aspirin or other platelet inhibitory drugs.

If there is serious bleeding or if the patient is about to undergo surgery, drugs with antiplatelet activity should be withdrawn and any underlying condition should be corrected if possible. In patients with renal failure, the haematocrit should be increased to greater than 0.30 and the use of desmopressin (DDAVP) may be helpful. Platelet transfusions may be required if these measures are unsuccessful or if the risk of bleeding is high.

Thrombocytosis

The platelet count may rise above 400×10^9/L as a result of:

- splenectomy
- Hodgkin's disease and other malignancies
- inflammatory disorders such as rheumatoid arthritis, ulcerative colitis and Crohn's disease
- major surgery.

Thus thrombocytosis is part of the acute phase reaction, although following splenectomy platelet numbers are also elevated because of the loss of a major site of platelet destruction.

Essential thrombocythaemia, a myeloproliferative disorder which is described on page 442, and other myeloproliferative conditions such as polycythaemia vera (PV) and chronic myeloid leukaemia (CML) may also be associated with a high platelet count.

A persistently elevated platelet count can lead to arterial or venous thrombosis. It is usual to treat the underlying cause of the thrombocytosis but a small dose of aspirin (75 mg) is also sometimes given. In myeloproliferative disease there is also a paradoxical risk of abnormal bleeding and specific action to reduce the platelet count, usually with hydroxycarbamide (hydroxyurea), is often taken.

Inherited coagulation disorders

Coagulation disorders may be inherited or acquired. The inherited disorders are uncommon and usually involve deficiency of one factor only. The acquired disorders occur more frequently and almost always involve several coagulation factors; they are considered in the next subsection.

In inherited coagulation disorders, deficiencies of all factors have been described. Those leading to abnormal bleeding are rare, apart from haemophilia A (factor VIII deficiency), haemophilia B (factor IX deficiency) and von Willebrand's disease.

Haemophilia A

In haemophilia A, the level of factor VIII:C is reduced but the level of factor vWF is normal (see Fig. 8.31). The

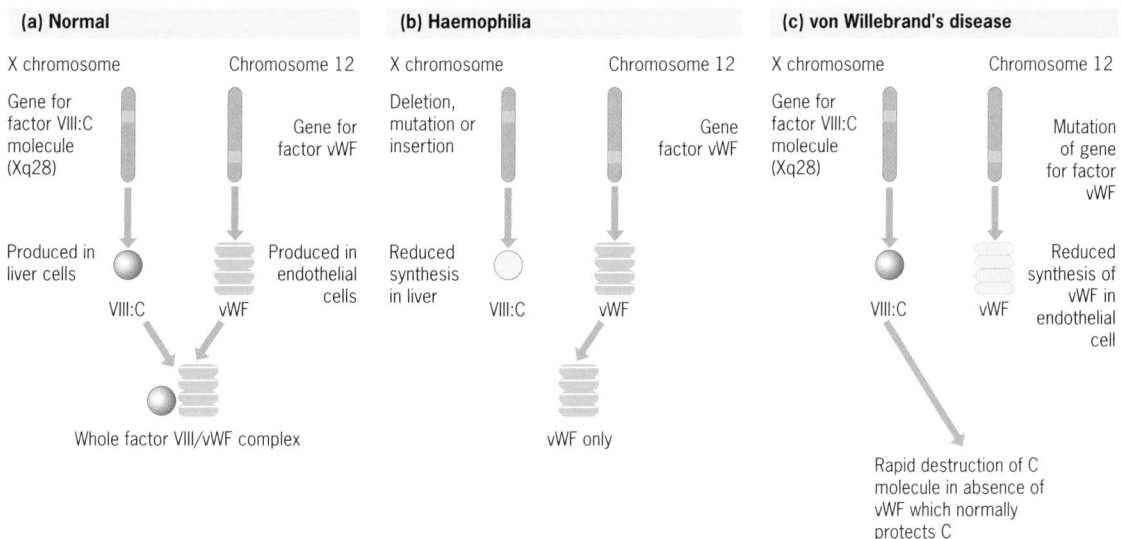

Fig. 8.31 (a) Normal factor VIII synthesis. (b) Haemophilia A showing defective synthesis of factor VIIIc. (c) von Willebrand's disease showing reduced synthesis of vWF.

Table 8.25
Blood changes in haemophilia A, von Willebrand's disease and vitamin K deficiency

	Haemophilia A	von Willebrand's disease	Vitamin K deficiency
Bleeding time	Normal	↑	Normal
PT	Normal	Normal	↑
APTT	↑+	↑±	↑
VIII:C	↓++	↓	Normal
vWF	Normal	↓	Normal

prevalence of haemophilia A is about 1 in 5000 of the male population. It is inherited as an X-linked disorder. If a female carrier has a son, he has a 50% chance of having haemophilia, and a daughter has a 50% chance of being a carrier. All daughters of people with haemophilia are carriers and the sons are normal.

The human factor VIII gene is enormous, constituting about 0.1% of the X chromosome, encompassing 186 kilobases of DNA. Various genetic defects have been found, including deletions, duplications, frameshift mutations and insertions. In approximately 50% of families with severe disease, the defect is an inversion. There is a high mutation rate, with one-third of cases being apparently sporadic with no family history of haemophilia.

Clinical and laboratory features
The clinical features depend on the level of factor VIII:C.

- *Levels of less than 1%* are associated with frequent spontaneous bleeding from early life.
  Haemarthroses are common and may lead to joint deformity and crippling if adequate treatment is not

given. Bleeding into muscles is also common, and intramuscular injections should be avoided.
- *Levels of 1 to 5%* are associated with severe bleeding following injury and occasional apparently spontaneous episodes.
- *Levels above 5%* produce mild disease, usually with bleeding only after injury or surgery. It should be noted that patients with mild haemophilia can still bleed badly once haemostasis has failed. Diagnosis in this group is often delayed until quite late in life.

The most frequent natural cause of death in patients with severe haemophilia is cerebral haemorrhage, but since the mid-1980s AIDS has been dominant following HIV transmission to many patients by coagulation factor concentrates between 1979 and 1985. In addition hepatic failure and hepatocellular carcinoma due to hepatitis C infection are increasingly common.

The main laboratory features of haemophilia A are shown in Table 8.25. The abnormal findings are a prolonged APTT and a reduced level of factor VIII:C. The PT, bleeding time and vWF level are normal.

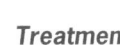

Treatment

Bleeding is treated by administration of factor VIII concentrate by intravenous infusion.

- *Minor bleeding*: the factor VIII:C level should be raised to 20–30%.
- *Severe bleeding*: the factor VIII:C should be raised to at least 50%.
- *Major surgery*: the factor VIII:C should be raised to 100% preoperatively and maintained above 50% until healing has occurred.

Factor VIII has a half-life of 12 hours and therefore must be administered at least twice daily to maintain the required therapeutic level. Continuous infusion is sometimes used to cover surgery. Factor VIII concentrate is freeze-dried and may be stored in domestic refrigerators at 4°C. This allows it to be administered by the patient immediately after bleeding has started, reducing the likelihood of chronic damage to joints and the need for inpatient care.

Recombinant factor VIII concentrate is now well established as the treatment of choice for people with haemophilia, but economic constraints and limited production capacity for recombinant factors have resulted in many previously treated patients still being offered treatment with plasma-derived concentrates.

The majority of severely affected patients are given prophylaxis three times per week from early childhood in an attempt to prevent permanent joint damage.

Synthetic vasopressin (DDAVP) – intravenous, subcutaneous or intranasal – produces a rise in factor VIII:C proportional to the initial level of factor VIII. It avoids the complications associated with blood products and is useful for treating bleeding episodes in mild haemophilia and as prophylaxis before minor surgery. It is ineffective in severe haemophilia.

People with haemophilia should be registered at comprehensive care centres (CCC), which take responsibility for their full medical care, including social and psychological support. Each person with haemophilia carries a special medical card giving details of the disorder and its treatment.

Complications

At least 10% of people with haemophilia have antibodies to factor VIII:C. These inhibitors develop most commonly in severely affected patients with no detectable VIII:C. Management of such patients may be very difficult, and even extremely high doses of factor VIII may not produce a rise in the plasma level of factor VIII:C. Purified porcine factor VIII may not cross-react with the patient's antibody. Some factor IX concentrates contain activated factors, which may 'bypass' the inhibitor and stop the bleeding. Recombinant factor VIIa also has this bypassing potential and shows great promise as an agent for treating patients with inhibitors. There is a growing interest in immune tolerance induction, especially in the management of recently developed inhibitors in young people. Similar strategies, including immunosuppression and immunoabsorption, have been described.

The risk of viral transmission has been virtually eliminated in developed countries by excluding high-risk blood donors, testing all donations for HBsAg, HCV and HIV antibodies, and by including steps to inactivate viruses during the preparation of plasma-derived concentrate.

Hepatitis A and B vaccination is offered routinely to all patients with haemophilia and von Willebrand's disease. The clinical consequences of haemophilia patients infected with HIV are similar to other HIV-infected patients (see p. 134), except that Kaposi's sarcoma does not occur. A number of patients with hepatitis C will progress to develop chronic liver disease and cirrhosis but antiviral therapy is becoming increasingly effective in this condition (see p. 362).

The use of recombinant factor VIII eliminates any residual risk of transfusion-transmitted infection, and it is safe and effective; but there is a similar incidence of inhibitor development as with plasma-derived factor VIII. The limited supply of recombinant factor VIII and its high cost are responsible for the continued use of both plasma-derived and recombinant products.

Carrier detection and antenatal diagnosis

Determination of carrier status in females begins with the gathering of detailed information from the family and coagulation factor assays. Female carriers usually have a factor VIII level of about 50% of normal, but the exact value is very variable, partly because of lyonization. Owing to this process early in embryonic life (that is, random inactivation of one chromosome – see p. 171), some carriers have very low levels of factor VIII while others will have normal levels. Carriers could be diagnosed with reasonable confidence if the level of factor VIII:C was 50% or less of that expected from the level of factor vWF measured at the same time, but often no clear-cut answer was provided by this method. Carrier detection can be carried out using molecular genetic testing, either by direct detection of mutations within the factor VIII gene or by tracking of the abnormal gene using DNA polymorphisms within the factor VIII gene as markers of the abnormal gene.

Antenatal diagnosis may be carried out by molecular analysis of fetal tissue obtained by chorionic villus biopsy at 9–11 weeks' gestation.

Haemophilia B (Christmas disease)

Haemophilia B is caused by a deficiency of factor IX. The inheritance and clinical features are identical to haemophilia A, but the incidence is only about 1 in 30 000 males. The gene is smaller at 34 kilobases and the half-life of the factor is longer at 18 hours. Haemophilia

B is treated with factor IX concentrates, recombinant factor IX now being available, and prophylactic doses are given twice a week. DDAVP is ineffective.

von Willebrand's disease (vWD)

In vWD, there is defective platelet function as well as factor VIII:C deficiency, and both are due to a deficiency or abnormality of vWF (see Fig. 8.31). vWF plays a role in platelet adhesion to damaged subendothelium as well as stabilizing factor VIII:C in plasma (see p. 455).

The vWF gene is located on chromosome 12 and numerous mutations of the gene have been identified. vWD has been classified into three types:

- *Type 1* is characterized by a mild reduction in vWF and is inherited as an autosomal dominant.
- *Type 2* is due to a decrease in the proportion of high-molecular-weight multimers, and it too is inherited as an autosomal dominant.
- *Type 3* is recessively inherited and patients have barely detectable levels of factor vWF (and therefore also of factor VIII:C). Their parents are often phenotypically normal.

Many subtypes have also been described, such as type 2B where increased vWF avidity for platelets causes mild thrombocytopenia and type 2N where there is an abnormal vWF binding site for VIII:C.

Clinical features. These are variable. Type 1 and type 2 patients usually have mild clinical features. Bleeding follows minor trauma or surgery, and epistaxis and menorrhagia often occur. Haemarthroses are rare. Type 3 patients have more severe bleeding but rarely experience the joint and muscle bleeds seen in haemophilia A.

Characteristic laboratory findings are shown in Table 8.25. These also include defective platelet aggregation with ristocetin.

Treatment depends on the severity of the condition and may be similar to that of mild haemophilia, including the use of DDAVP where possible. Intermediate purity factor VIII or von Willebrand factor concentrates should be used to treat bleeding or to cover surgery in patients who require replacement therapy especially in type 3 (severe) disease. Cryoprecipitate should be avoided because of the greater risk of transfusion-transmitted infection, since cryoprecipitate is not a virally inactivated product.

Acquired coagulation disorders

Vitamin K deficiency (see also p. 234)

Vitamin K is necessary for the γ-carboxylation of glutamic acid residues on coagulation factors II, VII, IX and X and on proteins C and S. Without it, these factors cannot bind calcium and form complexes with PF-3 to carry out their normal functions.

Deficiency of vitamin K may be due to:

- *inadequate stores*, as in haemorrhagic disease of the newborn and severe malnutrition (especially when combined with antibiotic treatment) (see p. 234)
- *malabsorption of vitamin K*, a fat-soluble vitamin, which occurs in cholestatic jaundice owing to the lack of intraluminal bile salts
- *oral anticoagulant drugs*, which are vitamin K antagonists.

The PT and APTT are prolonged (see Table 8.25) and there may be bruising, haematuria and gastrointestinal or cerebral bleeding. Minor bleeding is treated with phytomenadione (vitamin K_1) 10 mg intravenously. Some correction of the PT is usual within 6 hours but it may not return to normal for 2 days.

Newborn babies have low levels of vitamin K, and this may cause minor bleeding in the first week of life (*classical haemorrhagic disease of the newborn*). Vitamin K deficiency may also cause *late haemorrhagic disease of the newborn*, which occurs 2–26 weeks after birth and may result in severe bleeding such as intracranial haemorrhage. Most infants with these syndromes have been exclusively breast-fed, and both conditions may be prevented by administering 1 mg i.m. vitamin K to all neonates. There had been some concern that the administration of intramuscular vitamin K is associated with the development of cancer in childhood, but further studies provide no evidence for this association.

Liver disease

Liver disease may result in a number of defects in haemostasis:

- *Vitamin K deficiency*. This occurs owing to intrahepatic or extrahepatic cholestasis.
- *Reduced synthesis*. Reduced synthesis of coagulation factors may be the result of severe hepatocellular damage. The use of vitamin K does not improve the results of abnormal coagulation tests, but it is generally given to ensure that a treatable cause of failure of haemostasis has not been missed.
- *Thrombocytopenia*. This results from hypersplenism due to splenomegaly associated with portal hypertension or from folic acid deficiency.
- *Functional abnormalities*. Functional abnormalities of platelets and fibrinogen are found in many patients with liver failure.
- *Disseminated intravascular coagulation*. DIC (see below) may occur in acute liver failure.

Disseminated intravascular coagulation (DIC)

There is widespread generation of fibrin within blood vessels, owing to activation of coagulation by release of procoagulant material, and by diffuse endothelial damage or generalized platelet aggregation. Activation of leucocytes, particularly monocytes causing expression of tissue factor and the release of cytokines, may play a role in the development of DIC.

There is consumption of platelets and coagulation factors and secondary activation of fibrinolysis leading to production of fibrin degradation products (FDPs), which may contribute to the coagulation defect by inhibiting fibrin polymerization (Fig. 8.32). The consequences of these changes are a mixture of initial thrombosis followed by a bleeding tendency due to consumption of coagulation factors and fibrinolytic activation.

Causes of DIC

These include:

- malignant disease
- septicaemia (e.g. Gram-negative and meningococcal)
- haemolytic transfusion reactions
- obstetric causes (e.g. abruptio placentae, amniotic fluid embolism)
- trauma, burns, surgery
- other infections (e.g. falciparum malaria)
- liver disease
- snake bite.

Clinical features

The underlying disorder is usually obvious. The patient is often acutely ill and shocked. The clinical presentation of DIC varies from no bleeding at all to profound haemostatic failure with widespread haemorrhage. Bleeding may occur from the mouth, nose and venepuncture sites and there may be widespread ecchymoses.

Thrombotic events may occur as a result of vessel occlusion by fibrin and platelets. Any organ may be involved, but the skin, brain and kidneys are most often affected.

Investigations

The diagnosis is often suggested by the underlying condition of the patient.

Severe cases with haemorrhage.

- The PT, APTT and TT are usually very prolonged and the fibrinogen level markedly reduced.
- High levels of FDPs, including D-dimer are found owing to the intense fibrinolytic activity stimulated by the presence of fibrin in the circulation.
- There is severe thrombocytopenia.
- The blood film may show fragmented red blood cells.

Mild cases without bleeding. Increased synthesis of coagulation factors and platelets may result in normal PT, APTT, TT and platelet counts, although FDPs will be raised.

Treatment

The underlying condition is treated and this may be all that is necessary in patients who are not bleeding.

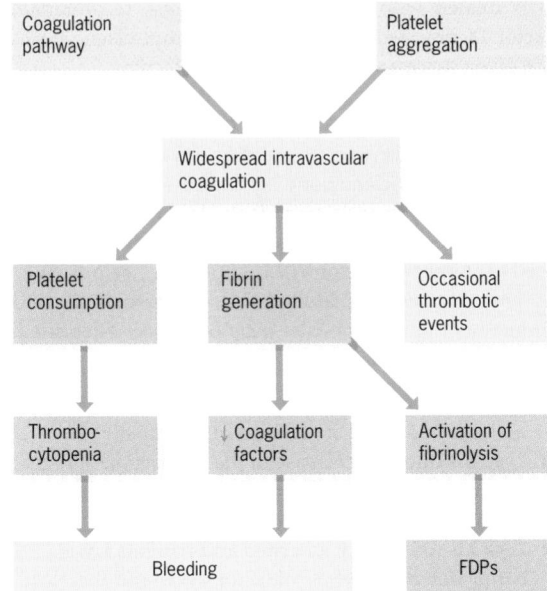

Fig. 8.32 Disseminated intravascular coagulation. FDP, fibrin degradation products.

Maintenance of blood volume and tissue perfusion is essential. Transfusions of platelet concentrates, FFP, cryoprecipitate and red cell concentrates is indicated in patients who are bleeding. The use of heparin to prevent intravascular coagulation is rarely indicated. Inhibitors of fibrinolysis such as tranexamic acid should not be used in DIC as dangerous fibrin deposition may result. There is growing interest in the use of antithrombin and/or protein C concentrates in selected cases.

Excessive fibrinolysis

Activation of fibrinolysis occurs in DIC as a secondary event in response to intravascular deposition of fibrin. It may also occur during surgery involving tumours of the prostate, breast, pancreas and uterus owing to release of tissue plasminogen activators. Such primary hyperfibrinolysis is very rare.

The clinical picture is similar to DIC with widespread bleeding. Laboratory investigations are also similar with a prolonged PT, APTT and TT, a low fibrinogen level, and increased FDPs, although fragmented red cells and thrombocytopenia are not seen, since disseminated coagulation is not present.

If the diagnosis is certain, fibrinolytic inhibitors such as ε-aminocaproic acid (EACA) or tranexamic acid should be considered. If DIC cannot be excluded, it is safer to treat as for DIC.

Massive transfusion

Few platelets and reduced levels of factors V and VIII are found in stored blood, although there are adequate amounts of the other coagulation factors. During massive transfusion (defined as transfusion of a volume of blood equal to the patient's own blood volume within 24 hours, e.g. approximately 10 units in an adult), the platelet count and PT and APTT should be checked at intervals. Transfusion of platelet concentrates and FFP should be considered if thrombocytopenia or defective coagulation are thought to be contributing to continued blood loss. Other problems of massive transfusion are described on page 939.

Inhibitors of coagulation

In addition to the factor VIII:C alloantibodies that are found in at least 10% of people with severe haemophilia A, factor VIII:C autoantibodies arise occasionally in patients with autoimmune disorders such as SLE, in elderly patients, and sometimes after childbirth. There can be severe bleeding. The antibodies sometimes disappear spontaneously, but treatment with plasma exchange, high-dose intravenous immunoglobulin and immunosuppressive drugs may be required in addition to any replacement therapy with factor concentrates (see above).

Lupus anticoagulants (p. 560) are autoantibodies directed against phospholipids (anti-phospholipid antibodies). They are found in about 10% of patients with SLE and also occur in otherwise healthy individuals. They lead to prolongation of phospholipid-dependent coagulation tests, particularly the APTT, but do not inhibit coagulation factor activity. Bleeding does not occur unless there is coexistent severe immune thrombocytopenia. The main clinical problems are thrombosis and recurrent miscarriages (p. 560).

Thrombosis

A thrombus is defined as a solid mass formed in the circulation from the constituents of the blood during life. Fragments of thrombi (emboli) may break off and block vessels downstream. Thromboembolic disease is much more common than abnormal bleeding; nearly half of adult deaths in England and Wales are due to coronary artery thrombosis, cerebral artery thrombosis or pulmonary embolism.

A thrombus results from a complex series of events involving coagulation factors, platelets, red blood cells and the vessel wall.

Arterial thrombosis

This usually occurs in association with atheroma, which tends to form at areas of turbulent blood flow such as the bifurcation of arteries. Platelets adhere to the damaged vascular endothelium and aggregate in response to ADP and TXA_2 to form a 'white thrombus'. The growth of the platelet thrombus is limited at its margins by PGI_2 and NO. Plaque rupture leads to the exposure of blood containing factor VIIa to tissue factor within the plaque

which may trigger blood coagulation and lead to thrombus formation. This results in complete occlusion of the vessel or embolization that produces distal obstruction. The risk factors for arterial thrombosis are related to the development of atherosclerosis (see p. 766).

Arterial thrombi may also form in the heart, as mural thrombi in the left ventricle after myocardial infarction, in the left atrium in mitral valve disease, or on the surfaces of prosthetic valves.

Venous thrombosis

Unlike arterial thrombosis, venous thrombosis often occurs in normal vessels. Major causes are stasis and hypercoagulability. The majority of venous thrombi occur in the deep veins of the leg, originating around the valves as 'red thrombi' consisting mainly of red cells and fibrin. The propagating thrombus is formed of fibrin and platelets and is particularly liable to embolize. Chronic venous obstruction following thrombosis in the deep veins of the leg frequently results in a permanently swollen limb and may lead to ulceration (post-phlebitic syndrome).

Risk factors for venous thrombosis in patients in hospital are shown in Table 8.26. Elevated levels of many blood coagulation factors have been associated with an increased risk of thrombosis but the clinical relevance of some of these findings has yet to be established. Both arterial and venous thrombosis may occur with changes in blood cells such as polycythaemia, thrombocythaemia and sickle cell anaemia, and with coagulation abnormalities (thrombophilia; see below).

The clinical features and diagnosis of venous thrombosis are discussed on page 832.

Table 8.26
Risk factors of venous thromboembolism

Patient factors	Disease or surgical procedure
Age	Trauma or surgery, especially of
Obesity	pelvis, hip or lower limb
Varicose veins	Malignancy
Long air travel	Cardiac failure
Immobility (bed rest > 4 days)	Recent myocardial infarction
Pregnancy and puerperium	Infection
Previous deep vein thrombosis	Inflammatory bowel disease
or pulmonary embolism	Nephrotic syndrome
Thrombophilia,	Polycythaemia
Antithrombin deficiency	Thrombocythaemia
Protein C or S deficiency	Paroxysmal nocturnal
Resistance to activated	haemoglobinuria
protein C (caused by	Sickle cell anaemia
factor V Leiden variant)	
Prothrombin gene variant	
Homocysteinaemia	
Antiphospholipid antibody	

This table was first published in the BMJ (Verstraete M (1997) Fortnightly review: prophylaxis of venous thromboembolism. *BMJ* **314**: 123–125) and is reproduced by permission of the BMJ.

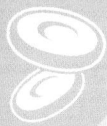

Thrombophilia

Thrombophilia is a term describing inherited or acquired defects of haemostasis leading to a predisposition to venous or arterial thrombosis. It should be considered in patients with:

- recurrent venous thrombosis
- venous thrombosis for the first time under age 40 years
- an unusual venous thrombosis such as mesenteric or cerebral vein thrombosis
- unexplained neonatal thrombosis
- recurrent miscarriages
- arterial thrombosis in the absence of arterial disease.

Coagulation abnormalities

Evidence has accumulated on the importance of a number of factors predisposing to thrombosis:

Factor V Leiden

Factor V Leiden is formed by a single nucleotide substitution (G1619A-arg506gln) in the factor V gene and this eliminates the site in the factor V protein which is cleaved by activated protein C. Factor V is a cofactor for thrombin generation (see Fig. 8.27) and the failure of activated protein C to inactivate factor V (see Fig. 8.28) results in a tendency to thrombosis. Factor V Leiden is found in 3–5% of healthy individuals in the West and in about 20% of patients with venous thrombosis.

The risk of venous thrombosis is increased in women with factor V Leiden who are pregnant or taking oral contraceptives. Consideration has been given to screening for the defect before prescribing oral contraceptives or during pregnancy. However, such a policy would be costly and might deny oral contraception to a substantial number of women who would then be at an increased risk of pregnancy, and therefore thrombosis. In addition, the use of oral anticoagulants in pregnancy carries a risk of fatal maternal bleeding, which may equal the risk of death due to postpartum thrombosis, and the fetus is also at risk of complications from the use of oral anticoagulants (see p. 469).

Prothrombin variant

A mutation in the 3′ untranslated region of the prothrombin gene has been described (G20210A). This variant is associated with elevated levels of prothrombin and a two- to threefold increase in the risk of venous thrombosis. There is an interaction with factor V Leiden and contraceptive pill use or pregnancy. The prevalence is 2% in Caucasian populations, 6% in unselected patients with thrombosis and about 18% in families with unexplained thrombophilia.

Antithrombin deficiency

This deficiency can be inherited as an autosomal dominant. Many variations have been described that lead to a conformational change in the protein. It can also be acquired following trauma, with major surgery and with the contraceptive pill. Low levels are also seen in severe proteinuria (e.g. the nephrotic syndrome). Recurrent thrombotic episodes occur starting at a young age in the inherited variety. Patients are relatively resistant to heparin as antithrombin is required for its action.

Protein C and S deficiency

These autosomal dominant conditions result in an increased risk of venous thrombosis, often before the age of 40 years. Homozygous protein C or S deficiency causes neonatal purpura fulminans, which is fatal without immediate replacement therapy.

Antiphospholipid antibody

See pages 560 and 465.

Investigations

Haemostatic screening tests

- **Full blood count** including platelet count
- **Coagulation screen** including a fibrinogen level.

These tests will detect erythrocytosis, thrombocytosis, and dysfibrinogenaemia and the possible presence of a lupus anticoagulant.

Testing for specific causes of thrombophilia

- **Assays** for naturally occurring anticoagulants such as AT, protein C and protein S
- **Assay** for activated protein C resistance and molecular testing for factor V Leiden and the prothrombin variant
- **Screen for a coagulation factor** inhibitor including a lupus anticoagulant (and anticardiolipin antibodies) (see p. 560)
- **Fibrinolytic pathway tests** (see p. 457).

Prevention and treatment of arterial thrombosis

Attempts to prevent or reduce arterial thrombosis are directed mainly at minimizing factors predisposing to atherosclerosis. Treatment of established arterial thrombosis includes the use of antiplatelet drugs and thrombolytic therapy.

Antiplatelet drugs

Platelet activation at the site of vascular damage is crucial to the development of arterial thrombosis, and this can be altered by the following drugs (Table 8.27):

- *Aspirin* inhibits the enzyme cyclo-oxygenase (see Fig. 8.26), resulting in reduced platelet production of TXA_2. It is widely used in cardiovascular disease.
- *Dipyridamole* – which inhibits platelet phosphodiesterase, causing an increase in cyclic AMP with potentiation of the action of PGI_2 – has been used widely as an antithrombotic agent, but there is little evidence that it is effective.

Table 8.27
Drugs used in the treatment of thrombotic disorders

Antiplatelet	Anticoagulant
Aspirin	Heparin
Dipyridamole	unfractionated
Ticlopidine	low molecular weight
Clopidogrel	Hirudins
IIb/IIIa inhibitors, e.g. abciximab,	Warfarin
eptifibatide, tirofiban	

Thrombolytic
Streptokinase
Single-chain urokinase-type plasminogen activator (scu-PA)
Tissue-type plasminogen activator (rt-PA or alteplase)
Reteplase

- *Ticlopidine* – blocks ADP-mediated platelet aggregation and transformation of the platelet fibrinogen receptor into a high-affinity form. It is a potential substitute for aspirin but its use has been associated with granulocytopenia and also, paradoxically, with thrombotic thrombocytopenic purpura (TTP).
- *Clopidogrel* – affects the ADP-dependent activation of the glycoprotein IIb/IIIa complex. It is similar to ticlopidine but has fewer side-effects. Recent trials support its use in acute coronary syndromes (p. 773).
- *Glycoprotein IIb/IIIa receptor antagonists* block a receptor on the platelet for fibrinogen and von Willebrand factor (Fig. 8.33). Three classes have been described:
  (a) murine–human chimeric antibodies (e.g. abciximab)
  (b) synthetic peptides (e.g. eptifibatide)
  (c) synthetic non-peptides (e.g. tirofiban).

They have been used as an adjunct in invasive coronary intervention and as primary medical

therapy in coronary heart disease. Excessive bleeding has been a problem and research continues to establish the optimum dose, the best combination with other drug treatments and the full range of clinical indications for these agents.

The indications for and results of antiplatelet therapy are discussed in the appropriate sections.

Thrombolytic therapy

Streptokinase

Streptokinase is a purified fraction of the filtrate obtained from cultures of haemolytic streptococci. It forms a complex with plasminogen, resulting in a conformational change which activates other plasminogen molecules to form plasmin. Streptokinase is given as an infusion of 1.5 million units over 1 hour in acute myocardial infarction. Laboratory monitoring of such short-term thrombolytic therapy is not necessary.

Streptokinase is antigenic and the development of streptococcal antibodies precludes repeated use. Activation of plasminogen is indiscriminate so that both fibrin in clots and free fibrinogen are lysed, leading to low fibrinogen levels and the risk of haemorrhage.

Urokinase

Urokinase is produced naturally by the kidney. It cleaves plasminogen directly to produce plasmin.

Tissue-type plasminogen activator (t-PA)

Tissue-type plasminogen activator (alteplase, reteplase) and single-chain urokinase-type plasminogen activator (scu-PA) are produced using recombinant gene technology. They were claimed to be relatively 'clot-specific' (i.e. to have a greater affinity for fibrin-bound plasminogen than circulating plasminogen), and therefore to cause less systemic fibrinolysis and bleeding than streptokinase. However, the use of these newer thrombolytic

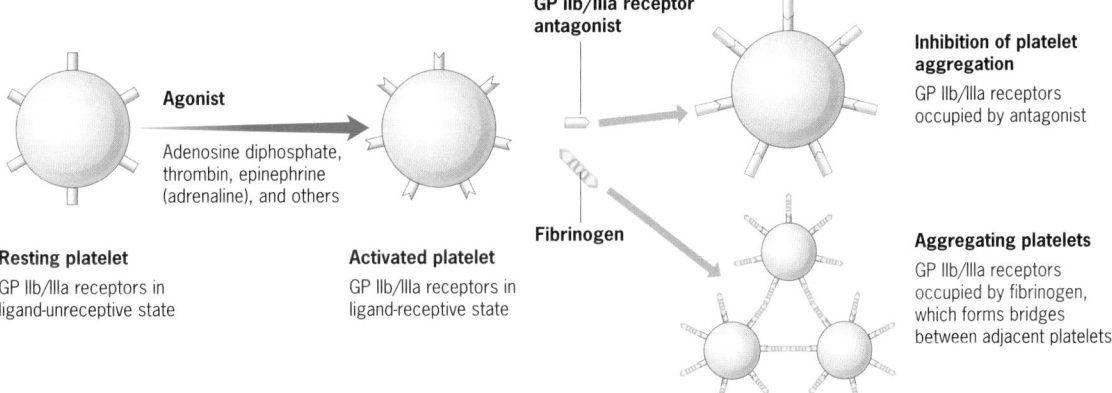

Fig. 8.33 The role of glycoprotein IIb/IIIa in platelet aggregation and the inhibition of platelet aggregation by inhibitors of glycoprotein IIb/IIIa receptors. Modified from Lefkovits J, Plow EF, Topol EJ (1995) *New England Journal of Medicine* **332**: 1554, with permission.

agents has not yet been shown to produce fewer bleeding episodes than does streptokinase. An accelerated dosage schedule of t-PA seems to produce a more rapid restoration of coronary flow.

Indications

The use of thrombolytic therapy in myocardial infarction is discussed on page 777. The combination of aspirin with thrombolytic therapy produces better results than thrombolytic therapy alone. The extent of the benefit depends on how quickly treatment is given, which is also true for cerebral infarction (p. 1168).

The main risk of thrombolytic therapy is bleeding. Treatment should not be given to patients who have had recent bleeding, uncontrolled hypertension or a haemorrhagic stroke, or surgery or other invasive procedures within the previous 10 days.

Prevention and treatment of venous thromboembolism

Venous thromboembolism is a common problem after surgery, particularly in high-risk patients such as the elderly, those with malignant disease and those with a history of previous thrombosis (Table 8.28). The incidence is also high in patients confined to bed following trauma, myocardial infarction or other illnesses. The prevention and treatment of venous thrombosis includes the use of anticoagulants.

Anticoagulants

Heparin

Heparin is not a single substance but a mixture of polysaccharides. Commercially available unfractionated heparin consists of components with molecular weights varying from 5000 to 35 000 with an average of about 13 000. It was extracted initially from liver – hence its name – but it is now prepared from porcine gastric mucosa.

Heparin has an immediate effect on coagulation by potentiation of the formation of irreversible complexes between antithrombin and activated serine protease coagulation factors (thrombin, XIIa, XIa, Xa, IXa and VIIa).

Low-molecular-weight heparins (LMW heparins)

These are produced by enzymatic or chemical degradation of standard heparin, producing fractions with molecular weights in the range of 2000–8000. Potentiation of thrombin inhibition (anti-IIa activity) requires a minimum length of the heparin molecule with an approximate molecular weight of 5400, whereas the inhibition of factor Xa requires only a smaller heparin molecule with a molecular weight of about 1700.

LMW heparins have the following properties:

- Bioavailability is better than that of unfractionated heparin.
- They have greater activity against factor Xa than against factor IIa, suggesting that they may produce an equivalent anticoagulant effect to standard heparin but have a lower risk of bleeding, although this has not generally been confirmed. In addition, LMW heparins cause less inhibition of platelet function.
- They have a longer half-life than standard heparin and so can be given as a once-daily subcutaneous injection instead of every 8–12 hours.
- They produce little effect on tests of overall coagulation, such as the APTT at doses recommended for prophylaxis. They are not fully neutralized by protamine.

Table 8.28

Classification of risk of deep vein thrombosis and pulmonary embolism for hospital patients

Low risk (proximal vein thrombosis 0.4%; fatal pulmonary embolism < 0.2%)
Patients < 40 years undergoing major surgery (> 30 minutes) with no other risk factors
Patients undergoing minor surgery (< 30 minutes) with no other risk factors
Patients with minor trauma or illness with no thrombophilia but history of deep vein thrombosis or previous pulmonary embolism

Medium risk (proximal vein thrombosis 2–4%; fatal pulmonary embolism 0.2–0.5%)
Major general, urological, gynaecological, cardiothoracic, vascular or neurological surgery in patients > 40 years or with one or more other risk factor(s)
Major acute medical illness such as myocardial infarction, heart failure, chest infection, cancer or inflammatory bowel disease
Major trauma
Minor surgery, trauma or illness in patients with previous deep vein thrombosis, pulmonary embolism or thrombophilia
Plastercast immobilization of the leg in patients with minor injury

High risk (proximal vein thrombosis 10–20%; fatal pulmonary embolism 1–5%)
Fracture or major orthopaedic surgery of pelvis, hip or leg
Major pelvic or abdominal surgery for cancer
Major surgery, trauma or illness in patients with previous deep vein thrombosis, pulmonary embolism or thrombophilia
Leg paralysis
Critical leg ischaemia or major leg amputation

Verstraete M (1997) Fortnightly review: prophylaxis of venous embolism *BMJ*; **314**:124, with permission of the BMJ.

LMW heparins are widely used for antithrombotic prophylaxis of high-risk surgical patients and for the treatment of established thrombosis (see p. 832).

The main complication of all heparin treatment is bleeding. This is managed by stopping heparin. Very occasionally it is necessary to neutralize unfractionated heparin with protamine. Other complications include osteoporosis with prolonged therapy and thrombocytopenia.

Heparin-induced thrombocytopenia (HIT) HIT is an uncommon complication of heparin therapy and usually occurs 5–14 days after first heparin exposure. It is due to an immune response directed against heparin/platelet factor 4 complexes. All forms of heparin have been implicated but the problem occurs less often with LMW heparins. A separate and unimportant immediate thrombocytopenia has also been described.

HIT is paradoxically associated with severe thrombosis and when diagnosed all forms of heparin must be discontinued, including heparin flush. Unfortunately the diagnosis can be difficult to make because patients on heparin are often very sick and may be thrombocytopenic for many other reasons. Laboratory tests based on bioassay or immunoassay are available but are neither sensitive nor specific and management decisions often have to be made before results are available.

It is usually necessary to continue some form of anticoagulation in patients with HIT and the choice lies between the heparinoid danaparoid and the new antithrombin hirudin. The introduction of warfarin should be covered by one of these agents as warfarin alone may be ineffective or even exacerbate thrombosis as protein C levels fall.

Hirudin

Two recombinant forms of hirudin, Lepirudin and Desirudin, are available. Lepirudin is used for the management of HIT. Hirudins act directly on thrombin and can be monitored by the use of the APTT. They are excreted by the kidney and must be used with caution in renal failure. Desirudin is used in the prophylaxis of DVT.

Oral anticoagulants

These act by interfering with vitamin K metabolism. There are two types of oral anticoagulants, the coumarins and indanediones. The coumarin warfarin is most commonly used because it has a low incidence of side-effects other than bleeding.

The dosage is controlled by PT tests. Thromboplastin reagents for PT testing are derived from a variety of sources and give different PT results for the same plasma. It is standard practice to compare each thromboplastin with an international reference preparation so that it can be assigned an international sensitivity index (ISI). The international normalized ratio (INR) is the ratio of the patient's PT to a normal control when using

---

Box 8.1

Indications for oral anticoagulation and target INR (British Society for Haematology 1998)

Target INR

2.5 Pulmonary embolism, proximal and calf deep vein thrombosis, recurrence of venous thromboembolism when no longer on warfarin therapy, symptomatic inherited thrombophilia, atrial fibrillation, cardioversion, mural thrombus, cardiomyopathy.

3.5 Recurrence of venous thromboembolism while on warfarin therapy, antiphospholipid syndrome, mechanical prosthetic heart valve, coronary artery graft thrombosis.

---

the international reference preparation. Therapeutic ranges using the INR for oral anticoagulation in various conditions are shown in Box 8.1.

Each laboratory can use a chart adapted to the ISI of their thromboplastin to convert the patient's PT to the INR. Suitably selected control plasmas can also be used to achieve the same objective. The use of this system means that PT tests on a given plasma sample using different thromboplastins result in the same INR and that anticoagulant control is comparable in different hospitals across the world.

Contraindications to the use of oral anticoagulants are seldom absolute and include:

- severe uncontrolled hypertension
- non-thromboembolic strokes
- peptic ulceration (unless cured by *Helicobacter pylori* eradication)
- severe liver and renal disease
- pre-existing haemostatic defects
- non-compliance.

Oral anticoagulants should be avoided in pregnancy because they are teratogenic in the first trimester and may be associated with fetal haemorrhage later in pregnancy. When anticoagulation is considered essential in pregnancy, specialist advice should be sought. Self-administered subcutaneous heparin should be used as an alternative, although this may not be as effective for women with prosthetic cardiac valves.

Many drugs interact with warfarin (see Ch. 16). More frequent PT testing should accompany changes in medication, which should occur with the full knowledge of the anticoagulant clinic.

An increased anticoagulant effect due to warfarin (Emergency box 8.1) is usually produced by one of the following mechanisms.

- drugs causing a reduction in the metabolism of warfarin, including tricyclic antidepressants, cimetidine, sulphonamides, phenothiazines and amiodarone

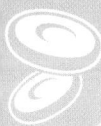

Emergency box 8.1

Management of bleeding and excessive oral anticoagulation (modified from British Society for Haematology 1998)

INR > 3.0 < 6.0 (target INR 2.5)	(1) reduce warfarin dose or stop
INR > 4.0 < 6.0 (target INR 3.5)	(2) restart warfarin when INR < 5.0
INR > 6.0 < 8.0 no bleeding or minor bleeding	(1) stop warfarin (2) restart when INR < 5.0
INR > 8.0, no bleeding or minor bleeding	(1) stop warfarin (2) restart warfarin when INR < 5.0 (3) if other risk factors for bleeding give 0.5–2.5 mg of vitamin K (oral)
Major bleeding	(1) stop warfarin (2) give prothrombin complex concentrate 50 units/kg or FFP 15 ml/kg (3) give 5 mg of vitamin K (oral or i.v.)

If unexpected bleeding occurs investigate the possibility of a local anatomical cause.

- drugs such as clofibrate and quinidine which increase the sensitivity of hepatic receptors to warfarin
- drugs interfering with vitamin K absorption (such as broad-spectrum antibiotics and colestyramine) which also potentiate the action of warfarin
- displacement of warfarin from its binding site on serum albumin by drugs such as sulphonamides (this is not usually responsible for clinically important interactions)
- drugs that inhibit platelet function (such as aspirin) which increase the risk of bleeding
- alcohol excess, cardiac failure, liver or renal disease, hyperthyroidism and febrile illnesses which result in potentiation of the effect of warfarin.

A decreased anticoagulant effect due to warfarin. This is usually produced by drugs that increase the clearance of warfarin by induction of hepatic enzymes that metabolize warfarin, such as rifampicin and barbiturates.

Prophylaxis to prevent venous thromboembolism

Prophylactic measures to prevent venous thrombosis during surgery are aimed at procedures for preventing stasis, such as early mobilization, elevation of the legs, compression stockings, and possibly calf-muscle stimulation and passive calf-muscle exercises during surgery, and methods for preventing hypercoagulability, usually using heparin.

- *Low-risk patients* (Table 8.28) require no specific measures other than early mobilization.
- *Moderate-risk patients* should receive specific prophylaxis with low-dose heparin at a dose of 5000 units subcutaneously every 8–12 hours until the patient is ambulatory or a standard dose LMW heparin such as enoxaparin 20 mg (2000 i.u.) subcutaneously daily. No laboratory monitoring is required.
- In *high-risk patients*, such as patients undergoing total hip replacement, LMW heparin once daily, such as enoxaparin 40 mg (4000 i.u.), has been shown to be more effective than standard low-dose heparin in preventing thrombosis. There is recent evidence to suggest that it is most effective when administered for a total of 1 month postoperatively rather than merely during the admission for surgery.

LMW heparin is replacing standard low-dose heparin for all surgical prophylaxis and is increasingly used for medical prophylaxis.

Treatment of established venous thromboembolism

The aim of anticoagulant treatment is to prevent further thrombosis and pulmonary embolization while resolution of venous thrombi occurs by natural fibrinolytic activity. Anticoagulation is started with heparin as it produces an immediate anticoagulant effect. There is no evidence that it is necessary to use heparin for any longer than it takes for simultaneously administered warfarin to produce an anticoagulant effect (INR 2.5) usually about 3–4 days (see Box 8.2).

LMW heparin (e.g. tinzaparin 175 units/kg daily) is equally effective and as safe as unfractionated heparin in the immediate treatment of deep vein thrombosis and pulmonary embolism. This creates the opportunity for treatment of venous thromboembolism without admission to hospital in compliant patients without coexisting risk factors for haemorrhage.

Anticoagulation (with warfarin approximately 3–9 mg daily for 6 weeks) is sufficient for patients after their first thrombosis provided there are no persisting risk factors. Long-term treatment should be given to patients with repeated episodes or continuing risk factors. Outpatient anticoagulation is best supervised in anticoagulant clinics. Patients are issued with national booklets for recording INR results and anticoagulant doses.

The role of thrombolytic therapy in the treatment of venous thrombosis is not established. It is sometimes used in patients with massive pulmonary embolism and in patients with extensive deep venous thrombi.

For the above conditions it is necessary to give a bolus dose of streptokinase, 250 000 units over 30 minutes, to inactivate antibodies formed by previous streptococcal infection, followed by a continuous infusion,

Box 8.2

Use of unfractionated heparin

- Obtain objective evidence of thrombosis using e.g. venography, ultrasound imaging or pulmonary ventilation/perfusion scanning as soon as possible (see p. 805).
- Perform a coagulation screen and platelet count before starting treatment to exclude a pre-existing haemostatic effect.
- Give an intravenous loading dose of 5000 units of standard heparin (except in severe pulmonary embolism when 10 000 units should be given).
- Heparinization should be continued with either:
  (a) an intravenous infusion of 1000–2000 units per hour, or
  (b) subcutaneous injections of 15 000 units every 12 hours.
- The dose of intravenous or subcutaneous heparin is adjusted by laboratory monitoring 4–6 hours after the dose of heparin to prolong the APTT to between 1.5 and 2.5 times the control value. Monitoring should be carried out at least once each day.
- Administer warfarin 5–10 mg (depending on the size and age of the patient) at the time the heparin is started. Give the same dose the next day and check the INR on the third day.
- Heparin is stopped when the INR reaches the therapeutic range (usually 2.5) and the dose of warfarin is adjusted to maintain the INR in the therapeutic range.

For LMW heparin use fixed dosage according to data sheet. Monitoring of LMW heparin is not usually necessary.

approximately 100 000 units every hour for 12–72 hours. The dose of streptokinase is adjusted to maintain the TT between two and four times the control value.

Thrombolytic therapy should be followed by anticoagulation with heparin for a few days and then by oral anticoagulants for a few months to prevent rethrombosis.

FURTHER READING

British Society for Haematology (1998) Guidelines on oral anticoagulation, 3rd edn. *British Journal of Haematology* **101**: 374–387.
Dahlback B (2000) Blood coagulation. *Lancet* **355**: 1627–1632.
Di Stefano V et al. (1999) The risk of recurrent deep venous thrombosis among heterozygous carriers of both factor V Leiden and the G20210A prothrombin mutation. *New England Journal of Medicine* **341**: 801–806.
Diuguid DL (1997) Oral anticoagulant therapy for venous thromboembolism. *New England Journal of Medicine* **336**: 433–434.
Gerhardt A et al. (2000) Prothrombin and factor V mutations in women with a history of thrombosis during pregnancy and the puerperium. *New England Journal of Medicine* **342**: 374–380.
George JN (2000) Platelets. *Lancet* **355**: 1531–1539.

Greaves M (2000) Heparin-induced thrombocytopenia and thrombosis. *Prescribers' Journal* **40**: 59–64.
Hirsch J, Weitz JI (1999) New antithrombotic agents. *Lancet* **353**: 1431–1436.
Holmes DR (1997) Preventing coronary stenosis and complications. *New England Journal of Medicine* **336**: 1748–1749.
Karpatkin S (1997) Autoimmune (idiopathic) thrombocytopenic purpura. *Lancet* **349**: 1531–1536.
Kyrle PA et al. (2000) High plasma levels of factor VIII and the risk of recurrent venous thromboembolism. *New England Journal of Medicine* **343**: 457–462.
Levi M, ten Cate H (1999) Disseminated intravascular coagulation. *New England Journal of Medicine* **341**: 586–592.
Lip GYH, Lowe GDO (1996) Antithrombotic treatment of atrial fibrillation. *British Medical Journal* **312**: 45–49.
Moake JL (1995) Thrombotic thrombocytopenic purpura. *Thrombosis and Haemostasis* **74**: 240–245.
Schafer AI (1996) Low-molecular-weight heparin: an opportunity for home treatment of venous thrombosis. *New England Journal of Medicine* **334**: 724–725.
Topol EJ, Byzova TV, Plow EF (1999) Platelet GP IIb-IIIa blockers. *Lancet* **353**: 227–231.

CHAPTER BIBLIOGRAPHY

Bain BJ (1995) *Blood Cells: A Practical Guide*. Oxford: Blackwell Science.
Bain BJ (1996) *A Beginner's Guide to Blood Cells*. Oxford: Blackwell Science.
Beutler E, Lichtman MA, Coller BS, Kipps TJ, Seligsohn U (2001) *Williams Hematology*, 6th edn. New York: McGraw-Hill.
Bloom AL, Forbes CD, Thomas DP, Tuddenham EGD (1994) *Haemostasis and Thrombosis*, 2nd edn. Edinburgh: Churchill Livingstone.
Brenner MK, Hoffbrand AV (1996) *Recent Advances in Haematology*, vol 8. London: Churchill Livingstone.
Hoffbrand AV, Pettit J, Moss P (2001) *Essential Haematology*, 4th edn. Oxford: Blackwell Science.
Hoffbrand AV, Pettit J (2000). *Atlas of Clinical Haematology*, 3rd edn, Edinburgh: Churchill Livingstone.
Issitt PD, Anstee DJ (1998) *Applied Blood Group Serology*, 4th edn. Durham, North Carolina: Montgomery Scientific Publications.
Murphy MF, Pamphilon D (2001) *Practical Transfusion Medicine*. Oxford: Blackwell Science.
Nathan DG, Oski SH (1997) *Hematology of Infancy and Childhood*, 5th edn. W.B. Saunders: Edinburgh.
Petz LD, Swisher SN, Kleinman S, Spence RK, Strauss RG (1996) *The Clinical Practice of Transfusion Medicine*, 3rd edn. New York: Churchill Livingstone.
Provan D, Gribben J (2000) *Molecular Haematology*. Oxford: Blackwell Science.
Provan D, Henson A (1997) *The ABC of Clinical Haematology*. London: BMJ Publications.
Weatherall D, Clegg J (2001) *The Thalassaemia Syndromes*, 4th edn. Oxford: Blackwell Science.

Medical oncology including haematological malignancy

The term 'malignant disease' encompasses a wide range of illnesses, including common ones such as lung, breast and colon cancer (Table 9.1), as well as rare ones, like the acute leukaemias. Malignant disease is widely prevalent and, in the West, almost a third of the population will develop cancer at some time during their life. It is second only to cardiovascular disease as the cause of death. Although the mortality of cancer is still high, many advances have been made, both in terms of treatment, and in understanding the biology of the disease at the molecular level.

Treatment may be given with curative or palliative intent, depending upon the evidence from continuing clinical trials. For many people, the word 'cancer' implies certain death, although this is clearly not always the case. Physicians have an obligation to be honest with their patients, combining realism about the prognosis with compassion and understanding so that they can take an informed part in treatment decisions.

Table 9.1
Epidemiology of cancer by site of origin in England and Wales

Type	Percentage of all cancers	Percentage of cancer deaths	Sex ratio M : F
Oral cavity/ pharynx	1	1.1	2.1 : 1
Oesophagus	2.2	3.6	2 : 1
Stomach	5	5.8	2.4 : 1
Large bowel	11.6	11.3	1.4 : 1
Pancreas	2.7	4.2	1.5 : 1
Lung	16.8	23.7	3.5 : 1
Melanoma	1.5	0.8	0.6 : 1
Other skin	12.2	0.3	1.7 : 1
Breast	11.1	9.6	0.01 : 1
Cervix	1.8	1.2	
Uterus	1.5	0.7	
Ovary	2.3	2.7	
Prostate	5	6.2	
Bladder	4.6	3.4	3.8 : 1
Kidney	1.6	1.8	2.2 : 1
Brain	1.3	1.8	1.5 : 1
Non-Hodgkin's lymphoma	2.4	2.6	1.5 : 1
Myeloma	1.1	1.5	1.5 : 1
Leukaemias	2.1	2.1	1.7 : 1

Cancers < 1% have been excluded
Derived from Doll R, Peto P (1996) In: *Oxford Textbook of Medicine*.
Oxford: Oxford University Press

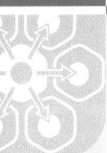
Aetiology and epidemiology

In most patients the cause of their cancer remains unknown and is probably multifactorial. Several environmental factors have, however, been identified as being associated with the development of malignancy.

Tobacco

The incidence of lung cancer in both men and women has increased dramatically in the last 25 years. The association of smoking with lung cancer is now indisputable and causative mechanisms have been identified: cigarette tobacco is responsible for one-third of all deaths from cancer in the UK. Smoking not only causes lung cancer, it is also associated with cancer of the mouth, larynx, oesophagus and bladder. As a consequence of public health campaigns, cigarette consumption in the UK is now beginning to decrease in men but not yet in women, in whom the incidence of lung cancer is still rising.

Alcohol

Alcohol is associated with cancers of the upper respiratory and gastrointestinal tracts (Table 9.2), but it also interacts with tobacco in the aetiology of these tumours. It may be associated with an increased risk of breast cancer.

Diet

Dietary factors have been attributed to account for a third of cancer deaths, although it may be difficult to differentiate these from other epidemiological factors. For example, the incidence of stomach cancer is particularly high in the Far East, while breast and colon cancers are more common in the western, economically more developed countries. Many associations have been observed without a causative mechanism being identified between the incidence of cancer and the consumption of dietary fibre, red meat, saturated fats, salted fish, vitamin E, vitamin A and many others. Food and its role in the causation of gastrointestinal cancer are discussed in Chapter 5.

Ultraviolet light

Ultraviolet light is known to increase the risk of skin cancer (basal cell, squamous cell and melanoma). The incidence of melanoma is therefore particularly high in the white Anglo-Celtic population of Australia, New Zealand and South Africa, where exposure to UV light is combined with a genetically predisposed population.

Occupational factors

In 1775, Percival Pott described the association between carcinogenic hydrocarbons in soot and the development of scrotal epitheliomas in chimney sweeps. Subsequently, other chemicals have been found to be carcinogenic.

The principal causes are asbestos (lung and pleural cancer), ionizing radiation (any cancer), and combustion of fossil fuels releasing polycyclic hydrocarbons (skin, lung, bladder cancers). Organic chemicals such as benzene may cause molecular abnormalities associated with the development of myeloid leukaemia.

Infectious agents

Viruses are known to cause cancer in animals. A great deal of time and money has therefore been expended in trying to establish whether they can also cause human cancer. The geographical distribution of a rare malignancy may suggest that it might be caused by, or associated with, an infective agent. For example, a specific type of T-cell leukaemia, seen almost exclusively in the residents from the southern island of Japan and in the West Indies, is caused by infection with the retrovirus, HTLV-1 (human T-cell leukaemia virus) which is endemic in these areas.

Less convincing evidence on causation is available for the association between hepatocellular carcinoma and infection with hepatitis B and C, and Epstein–Barr virus (EBV) with Burkitt's lymphoma and nasopharyngeal carcinoma. Patients with HIV infection or immunosuppression from organ transplantation have an increased incidence of EBV-related lymphoma and herpesvirus 8 associated Kaposi's sarcoma. The incidence of cervical cancer is increasing amongst younger women in association with human papilloma virus infection. Early sexual activity and multiple sexual partners have both been found to be associated with increased risk.

Table 9.2

Some causative factors associated with the development of cancer at various sites

Smoking	Mouth, pharynx, oesophagus, larynx, lung, bladder, lip
Ultraviolet light	Skin, lip
Alcohol	Mouth, pharynx, larynx, oesophagus, colorectal
Drugs (alkylating agents)	Bladder, bone marrow
Asbestos	Lung, mesothelium
Oestrogens	Endometrium, vagina, breast
Androgens	Prostate
Vinyl chloride	Liver (angiosarcoma)
Polycyclic hydrocarbons	Skin, lung, bladder, myeloid leukaemia
Aromatic amines	Bladder
Aflatoxin	Liver
Biological agents:	
Hepatitis B virus	Liver (hepatocellular carcinoma)
Hepatitis C virus	Liver (hepatocellular carcinoma)
Schistosoma japonicum	Bladder
Helicobacter pylori	Stomach
Human T cell leukaemia virus	Leukaemia

Bacterial infection with *Helicobacter pylori* is recognized as predisposing to the development of gastric cancer and gastric lymphoma, while *Schistosoma japonicum* infection predisposes to the development of squamous carcinomas in the bladder.

Drugs

Oestrogens have been implicated in the development of both vaginal and endometrial carcinoma. Alkylating agents and radiotherapy given, for example, for Hodgkin's disease (see later) are themselves associated with an increased incidence of secondary acute myelogenous leukaemia (AML) and bladder cancer. More recently the epipodophyllotoxin, etoposide, has also been shown to be associated with the development of secondary AML.

Geographical distribution

The incidence of specific tumours varies with geographical location. England, Scotland and Wales have the highest death rate from malignant disease in the world, mainly because of the very high incidence of lung cancer due to smoking. Breast, colon and prostatic cancer have a relatively low incidence in Asian countries, while liver cancer occurs world-wide but is rare in Europe and North America. Similarly, stomach cancer is particularly prevalent in Japan.

Environmental factors have been clearly implicated. For example, subsequent generations of people moving from countries with a low incidence to those with a high incidence of breast or colon cancer acquire the cancer incidence of the country to which they have moved. This suggests that for these specific cancers, environmental factors are more important than genetic ones.

The biology of cancer

Most human neoplasms are monoclonal in origin, i.e. they arise from genetic mutations within a single affected cell; however, over subsequent divisions heterogeneity develops through the accumulation of further abnormalities. The genes most commonly affected can be characterized as those controlling cell cycle check points, DNA repair and DNA damage recognition, apoptosis, differentiation, and growth signalling. Proliferation may continue at the expense of differentiation, which together with the failure of apoptosis leads to tumour formation with the accumulation of abnormal cells varying in size, shape and nuclear morphology as viewed down the light microscope.

The *kinetics* of cancer cell growth appear to be exponential; however, the doubling times of human tumours are enormously variable. Mutations are common in the genes controlling a series of intracellular proteins, such as the cyclins and cyclin-dependent kinases (p. 157), and oncogenes products such as c-*myc*, and the *ras* proteins

(see Cancer genetics, p. 182) that regulate proliferation. Proliferation may also be abnormal due to defects in the nuclear enzyme telomerase, contact with other cells, nutrient supply or cytokine signalling. Telomerase is an enzyme that prevents the normal shortening of DNA with each cell division that leads to senescence. Persistent telomerase activity helps to maintain the neoplastic state in cancer cells.

Epithelial growth factor (EGF) and its receptors are overexpressed in many human epithelial tumours, constitutively switching on unrestrained growth of these tumours. Transforming growth factor-β (TGF-β), a cytokine which has effects on extracellular matrix proteins, angiogenesis (see below) and immune effector cells, is also often overexpressed in tumour cells, and defects in TGF-β signalling are often found in cancer cells.

Apoptosis and growth

Tumour cell death may also be dysregulated. Normal cells usually die by an active and tightly regulated process known as apoptosis, or 'programmed cell death' (p. 162). Apoptosis can occur in response to a number of physiological or pathological stimuli (tumour necrosis factor, fas ligand, and DNA-damaging cytotoxic drugs) and is mediated within the cell by a family of proteins known as caspases. Caspase activity is, in turn, regulated by intracellular inhibitors such as the *Bcl-2* family of proteins and the inhibitor of apoptosis proteins (IAPs). Disturbances in the normal balance of these various proteins have been identified which favour survival of tumour cells over their normal counterparts. An example is the upregulation of the *Bcl-2* protein in follicular non-Hodgkin's lymphoma.

Tumour immunology

Tumour cells are usually not recognized and killed by the immune system. There are two main causes. The first is failure to express molecules such as HLA and costimulatory B7 molecules which are required for activation of cytotoxic, or 'killer', T lymphocytes, since expression of these 'costimulatory' molecules following gene transfection may augment an immune response. Secondly, tumours may also actively secrete immunosuppressive cytokines and cause a generalized immunosuppression, leading for example to the reactivation of latent herpes zoster in shingles associated with malignancy.

Angiogenesis

For many tumours, there is a progressive slowing of the rate of growth as the tumours become larger. This occurs for many reasons, but outgrowing the blood supply is paramount. New vessel formation (angiogenesis) is stimulated by a variety of peptides produced both by tumour cells and by host inflammatory cells, such as the vascular endothelial growth factors (VEGFs), basic fibroblast growth factor (bFGF) and

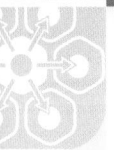

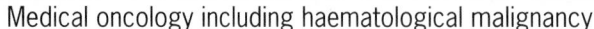

angiopoietin 2. Inhibition of angiogenesis is a potentially novel method of cancer therapy, as new vessel formation within and around tumours not only provides the cancer with nutrients and oxygen, but permits haematogenous spread, or metastasis.

Invasion and metastasis

Cancers spread by both local invasion and by metastasis in vessels of the blood or lymphatic systems. Infiltration into surrounding tissues is associated with loss of cell–cell cohesion. Cohesion is mediated by active homotypic cell adhesion molecules (CAMs). The cadherin molecules are transmembrane glycoproteins able to mediate cellular attachment. Epithelial cadherin (E-cadherin) is expressed by many carcinomas and loss of E-cadherin expression is associated with an increase in invasion of the tumour.

Invasion is partly determined by the balance of activators to inhibitors of proteolysis. Secretion of proteolytic enzymes, including the matrix metalloproteinases (particularly the collagenases), occurs from adjacent fibroblasts owing to failure of production of tissue inhibitors. The balance between the expression and activity of the matrix metalloproteinases (MMPs) and their tissue inhibitors (TIMPs) is important for tumour growth, invasion, metastasis and angiogenesis. Some TIMPs may regulate cell proliferation and survival of cancer cells independently of MMP activity.

Dissemination of tumour cells occurs when they enter the vascular and lymphatic vessels. Here they must survive host-defence mechanisms so as to spread throughout the body. The disseminated cancer cells lodge in distant sites, partly by chance, but also because of specific interactions between receptors/ligands found on endothelial cells and on tumour cells. This may account for the specific pattern of metastases with certain tumours; for example, breast tumours frequently metastasize to long bones.

The attachment of tumour cells to the endothelial cells is partly through adhesion molecules. Integrins are transmembrane heterodimeric glycoproteins formed by non-covalent association of α and β chains. These molecules are normally responsible for cell-substrate adhesion. Patterns of integrin expression in tumours are complex but, nevertheless, certain tumours demonstrate upregulation of specific integrins, such as the alpha v family, during tumour progression, and this may allow migration of tumour cells through the extracellular matrix substrate and invasion through the basement membrane and formation of a metastatic deposit. Integrins also act as receptors for signals regulating gene expression and apoptosis.

Cancer genetics

The development of cancer is associated with a fundamental genetic change within the cell. Evidence for the genetic origin of cancer is based on the following:

- Some cancers show a familial predisposition.
- Most known carcinogens act through induced mutations.
- Susceptibility to some carcinogens depends on the ability of cellular enzymes to convert them to a mutagenic form.
- Genetically determined traits associated with a deficiency in the enzymes required for DNA repair are associated with an increased risk of cancer.
- Some cancers are associated with chromosome 'instability' because of deficiencies in mismatch repair genes.
- Many malignant tumours represent clonal proliferations of neoplastic cells.
- Many tumours contain well-described cytogenetic abnormalities, which involve mutated or abnormally regulated oncogenes and tumour suppressor genes with transforming activity in cell lines.

Mutations may occur in the germline and therefore be present in every cell in the body, or they may occur by somatic mutation in response, for example, to carcinogens, and therefore be present only in the cells of the tumour.

Expression of the mutation and hence carcinogenesis will depend upon the penetrance (due to level of expression and presence of other genetic events) of the gene and whether the mutated allele has a dominant or recessive effect. There are a small group of autosomal dominant inherited mutations such as *RB* (in retinoblastoma) and a small group of recessive mutations (Table 9.3). Carriers of the recessive mutations are at risk of developing cancer if the second allele becomes mutated, leading to 'loss of heterozygosity' within the tumour although this is seldom sufficient as carcinogenesis is a multistep process.

Malignant transformation may result from a gain in function as cellular proto-oncogenes become mutated, (e.g. *ras*), amplified (e.g. *HER2*), or translocated (e.g. *BCR-ABL*). However, these mutations are insufficient to cause malignant transformation by themselves. Alternatively, there may be a loss of function of tumour suppressor genes that normally suppress growth and differentiation. A third mechanism involves alterations in the genes controlling the transcription of the oncogenes or tumour suppressor genes (e.g. p. 183) (Tables 9.3 and 9.4).

DNA repair

Some relatively rare autosomal recessive diseases associated with abnormalities of DNA repair predispose to the development of cancer (Table 9.3).

Patients with xeroderma pigmentosum have a defect in their ability to repair DNA damage caused by ultraviolet light and by some chemicals, leading to a high incidence of skin cancer. The ataxia telangiectasia mutation results in an increased sensitivity to ionizing

Table 9.3
Familial cancer syndromes

	Tumour suppressor gene	Neoplasms
Autosomal dominant		
Retinoblastoma	RB1	Eye
Wilms' tumour	WT1	Kidney
Li–Fraumeni	p53	Sarcoma/brain/leukaemia
Neurofibromatosis type 1	NF1	Neurofibromas
Familial adenomatous polyposis (FAP)	APC	Colon
Hereditary non-polyposis colon cancer (HNPCC)	MLH1 and MSH2	Colon, endometrium
Breast ovary families	BRCA1 and BRCA2	Breast/ovary
Melanoma	p16	Skin
Von Hippel–Lindau	VHL	Renal cell carcinoma and haemangioblastoma
Autosomal recessive		
Xeroderma pigmentosa	XP	Skin
Ataxia telangiectasia	AT	Leukaemia, lymphoma
Fanconi's anaemia	FA	Leukaemia, lymphoma
Bloom's syndrome	BS	Leukaemia, lymphoma

Table 9.4
Acquired/somatic mutations and proto-oncogenes

Point mutation

ras	Pancreatic cancer

DNA amplification

myc	Neuroblastoma
HER2	Breast cancer

Chromosome translocation

BCR-ABL	CML, AML, ALL
PML-RAR	APML
EWS	Ewing's sarcoma
IGH-bcl2	Follicular lymphoma

Abbreviations: CML, chronic myeloid leukaemia; AML, acute myeloid leukaemia; ALL, acute lymphoblastic leukaemia; APML, acute promyelocytic leukaemia

accounts for most cases of familial breast cancer and over half of ovarian cancers. BRCA1 and 2 proteins bind to the DNA repair enzyme Rad51 to make it functional in repairing DNA breaks. Mutations in the *BRCA* genes will lead to accumulation of unrepaired mutations in tumour-suppressor genes and crucial oncogenes.

- *Neurofibromatosis.* Inactivation of the *NF1* gene will lead to constitutive activation of *ras* proteins.
- *Multiple-endocrine-adenomatosis syndromes* (p. 1067). Multiple endocrine neoplasia type 2 (MEN2) is now thought to be associated with mutations in the *RET* proto-oncogene on chromosome 10 and as such is the exception to all the other syndromes which involve tumour suppressor genes.

radiation and an increased incidence of lymphoid tumours. An increased susceptibility to lymphoid malignancy is also seen in Bloom's syndrome and Fanconi's anaemia. It is not known why these chromosome-break syndromes predispose to tumours of lymphatic tissue.

The following are examples of cancer syndromes that exhibit dominant inheritance (Table 9.3):

- *Retinoblastoma*, an eye tumour found in young children. It occurs in both hereditary (40%) and non-hereditary (60%) forms. The 40% of patients with the hereditary form have a germline mutation on the long arm of chromosome 13 that predisposes to retinoblastoma. In addition to the latter, children inheriting this mutation at the so-called *RB1* locus are at risk for developing other tumours, particularly osteosarcoma.
- *Breast and ovarian cancer.* Two genes have been identified – *BRCA1* and *BRCA2*. A strong family history along with germline mutation of these genes

FURTHER READING

Murphy RM (2001) Chemokines and the molecular basis of cancer metastases. *New England Journal of Medicine* **345**: 833–835.
Pedersen-Bjergaard J (2001) Molecular cytogenetics in cancer. *Lancet* **357**: 491–492.
Stewart AK, Schuh AC (2000) White cells 2: impact of understanding the molecular basis of haematological malignant disorders on clinical practice. *Lancet* **355**: 1447–1453.
Wylie AH, Bellamy CO, Bubb VJ et al (1999) Apoptosis and carcinogenesis. *British Journal of Cancer* **80**; 51: 34–37.

The diagnosis of malignancy

Most common cancers (but not the haematological cancers) start as focal microscopic clones of transformed cells, and diagnosis only becomes likely once sufficient tumour bulk has accumulated to cause symptoms or signs. In order to try to make an earlier diagnosis and increase the curative possibilities, an increasing number of screening programmes are being investigated which target the asymptomatic or preinvasive stages of the cancer.

Increasingly, genetic screening is being used to target screening to those at most risk of developing cancer. To be successful in improving individual and population survival, this strategy is dependent upon finding tests that are sufficiently sensitive and specific, detection methods that identify cancer before it has spread, and curative treatment that is practical, consistent with maintenance of a normal lifestyle and quality of life, and is affordable.

Symptoms of cancer

Patients present with tumour site-specific symptoms, e.g. pain, and signs, e.g. a mass, ulceration or bleeding, which readily identify the primary site of the cancer. On the other hand, many may seek medical attention when more systemic and non-specific symptoms occur such as weight loss, fatigue, and anorexia. These usually indicate a more advanced stage of the disease except in some paraneoplastic and ectopic endocrine syndromes (see below). Other patients are only diagnosed upon the discovery of established metastases such as the back pain of metastatic prostatic cancer or the liver enlargement of metastatic gastrointestinal cancer.

Other indirect effects of the cancer manifest as paraneoplastic syndromes (Box 9.1) that are often associated with specific types of cancer and are reversible with treatment of the cancer. *Autoimmune syndromes* occur through antibodies with cross-reactivity between tumour antigens and normal tissues such as the acetylcholine release sites in the Lambert–Eaton myasthenic syndrome associated with small-cell lung cancer (p. 1233).

Cancer-associated immunosuppression can lead to reactivation of latent infections such as herpes zoster.

The *coagulopathy of cancer* may present with thrombophlebitis, deep venous thrombosis and pulmonary emboli, particularly in association with cancers of pancreas, stomach and breast.

Cachexia of advanced cancer is due to release of chemokines such as tumour necrosis factor (TNF), while other symptoms are related to peptide or hormone release, e.g. carcinoid or Cushing's syndrome, syndrome of inappropriate antidiuretic hormone (SIADH) release.

Physical examination

A general examination should be performed to include:

- main symptomatic areas, e.g. site, size of mass and associated lymphadenopathy
- precursor lesions, e.g. solar keratosis, dysplastic naevi
- general signs, e.g. jaundice, clubbing
- functional capacity (Table 9.6).

Histology

The diagnosis of cancer may be suspected by both patient and doctor but advice about treatment can usually only be given on the basis of a tissue diagnosis. This may be obtained by surgical biopsy or on the basis of cytology (e.g. lung cancer diagnosed by sputum cytology or cervix cancer diagnosed on the basis of a cervical smear). Malignant lesions can be distinguished morphologically from benign by the pleomorphic nature of the cells, increased numbers of mitoses, nuclear abnormalities in size, chromatin pattern and nucleolar organization, and evidence of invasion into surrounding tissues.

The degree of differentiation (or conversely of anaplasia) of the tumour has prognostic significance: generally speaking, more differentiated tumours have a better prognosis than poorly differentiated ones. Immunocytochemistry, using monoclonal antibodies against tumour antigens, is very helpful in differentiating between lymphoid and epithelial tumours and between some subsets of these, for example T and B cell lymphomas, germ cell tumours, prostatic tumours, neuroendocrine tumours, melanomas, sarcomas. However, many adenocarcinomas and squamous carcinomas do not bear any distinctive immunohistochemical markers that are diagnostic of their primary site of origin.

Tests for genetic markers in tissue sections employ fluorescent in situ hybridization (FISH, p. 175) to look for characteristic chromosomal translocations, deletions or duplications (see genetic basis of cancer).

Staging

Before a decision about treatment can be made, not only the type of tumour but also its extent and distribution need to be established. Various 'staging investigations' are therefore performed before a treatment decision is made. To be useful clinically the staging system must subdivide the patients into groups of different prognosis which can guide treatment selection.

The staging systems vary according to the type of tumour and may be site specific (see Hodgkin's disease, p. 496), or the TNM (tumour, node, metastases) classification shown in Table 9.5 which can be applied to most common cancers.

Box 9.1

Paraneoplastic syndromes

- Autoimmune
- Immunosuppression
- Coagulopathy
- Carcinoid
- Cushing's
- SIADH

Table 9.5
TNM classification as used for lung cancer

T = extent of primary tumour; N = extent of regional lymph node involvement; M = presence of distant metastases

Tx	Positive cytology only
T1	< 3 cm diameter
T2	> 3 cm/extends to hilar region/invades visceral pleura/partial atelectasis
T3	Involvement of chest wall, diaphragm, pericardium, mediastinum, pleura, total atelectasis
T4	Involvement of heart, great vessels, trachea, oesophagus, malignant effusion
N1	Peribronchial, ipsilateral hilar lymph node involvement
N2	Ipsilateral mediastinal
N3	Contralateral mediastinal, scalene or supraclavicular
M0	No distant metastases
M1	Metastases present

Table 9.6
Eastern Cooperative Oncology Group (ECOG) performance status scale

Status	Description
0	Asymptomatic, fully active and able to carry out all predisease performance without restrictions
1	Symptomatic, fully ambulatory but restricted in physically strenuous activity and able to carry out performance of a light or sedentary nature, e.g. light housework, office work
2	Symptomatic, ambulatory and capable of all self-care but unable to carry out any work activities. Up and about more than 50% of waking hours: in bed less than 50% of day
3	Symptomatic, capable of only limited self-care, confined to bed or chair more than 50% of waking hours, but not bedridden
4	Completely disabled. Cannot carry out any self-care. Totally bedridden

Performance status

In addition to anatomical staging, the person's age and general state of health need to be taken into account when planning treatment. The latter has been called 'performance status' and is of great prognostic significance for all tumour types (Table 9.6). Performance status reflects the effects of the cancer on the patient's functional capacity.

Tumour markers

Tumour markers are intracellular proteins or cell surface glycoproteins released into the circulation and detected by immunoassays. None are totally specific for cancer and it is rather that their inappropriate expression marks the presence of a cancer. They can, however, be useful in the serial monitoring of response to treatment, as they can be quite sensitive to changes in the tumour burden (Table 9.7).

Table 9.7
Tumour markers

α-Fetoprotein	Hepatocellular carcinoma, and non-seminomatous germ cell tumours of the gonads
β-Human chorionic gonadotrophin (β-HCG)	Choriocarcinomas, germ cell tumours and lung cancers
Prostate-specific antigen (PSA)	Carcinoma of prostate
Carcinoma embryonic antigen (CEA)	e.g. gastrointestinal cancers
CA-125	e.g. ovarian cancer
CA-19-9	e.g. gastrointestinal cancers particularly pancreatic cancer
CA-15-3	e.g. breast cancer

Cancer treatment

Aims of treatment

Cancer treatment requires the cooperation of a multi-disciplinary team to coordinate the delivery of the appropriate treatment (surgery, chemotherapy, radiotherapy and biological/endocrine therapy), supportive and symptomatic care, and psychosocial support. While all members will have the patient's care as their central concern, someone, often the oncologist, has to take responsibility for the coordination of the many professionals involved. Central to this endeavour is the involvement of the patient through education as to the nature of their disease and the treatment options available. An informed choice can then be made, even if in the end it is simply to abide by the decisions made by the professionals. Good communication embodies a humane approach which preserves hope at an appropriate level through empathy and understanding of the patient's position. Our patients offer us a privileged entry to their lives at a time of crisis, which can provide a powerful, positive and adaptive response when handled with sensitivity and respect. It can also provide us, their carers, with a humbling and yet sustaining illumination of the human condition.

Curing cancer

For most solid tumours local control is possible but not sufficient for cure because of the presence of systemic (microscopic) disease, while haematological cancers are usually disseminated from the outset. Improvement in the rate of cure of most cancers is thus dependent upon earlier detection and effective systemic treatment. The likelihood of cure of the systemic disease depends upon the type of cancer, its chemo-/hormonal sensitivity, and tumour bulk (microscopic or clinically detectable).

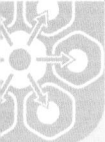

A few rare cancers are so chemosensitive in adults that even bulky metastases can be cured, e.g. leukaemia, lymphoma, gonadal germ cell tumours, and choriocarcinoma. For most common solid tumours such as breast and colorectal cancer, there is no current cure of bulky (clinically detectable) metastases, but micrometastatic disease treated by adjuvant chemotherapy (see below) after surgery can be cured in 10–20% of patients.

Palliation

When cure is no longer possible, palliation, i.e. relief of tumour symptoms and prolongation of life, is possible in many cancers in proportion to their chemo- and radiosensitivity. There is on average a 2–18 months prolongation in median life expectancy with current treatments for solid tumours and up to 5–8 years for some leukaemias and lymphomas, with those with the most responsive tumours experiencing the greatest benefit. The development of more effective chemotherapeutic drugs and better supportive care such as antiemetics has done much to reduce the side-effects of chemotherapy and to improve the cost/benefit ratio for the patient receiving palliative treatment. In addition, through early assessment during treatment, it is possible to stop if there is no evidence of benefit within 6–8 weeks of starting so as to minimize exposure to toxic and unsuccessful treatment.

Measuring response to treatment

A measurable response to treatment can serve as a useful early surrogate marker when assessing whether to continue a given treatment for an individual patient. It is also useful in early clinical trials, when investigating whether new treatments will be worth investing the resources for randomized trials.

Response to treatment can be subjective or objective. A subjective response is one perceived by the patient in terms of, for example, relief of pain and dyspnoea, or improvement in appetite, weight gain or energy. Such subjective response is a major aim of most palliative treatments. Quantitative measurements of these subjective symptoms form a part of the assessment of response to chemotherapy, especially in those situations where cure is not possible and where the aim of treatment is to provide prolongation of good-quality life. In these circumstances, measures of quality of life enable an estimate of the balance of benefit and side-effects to be made.

Objective response to treatment is measured either as a complete response, which is a complete disappearance of all detectable disease clinically and radiologically or partial response, which is conventionally defined as more than a 50% reduction in the size of the tumour. The terms used to evaluate the responses of tumours are given in Box 9.2. The term 'remission' is often used synonymously with 'response' which if complete means

Box 9.2

Definitions of response

Complete response	Complete disappearance of all detectable disease
Partial response	More than 50% reduction in the product of the bidimensional diameters of the tumour
Stable disease	No change, or < 50% reduction and < 25% increase
Progressive disease	Increase in size of tumour by at least 25% at any site

an absence of detectable disease without necessarily implying a cure of the cancer.

Oncological emergencies

- *Superior vena caval obstruction* can arise from any upper mediastinal mass but is most commonly associated with lung cancer. The patient presents with difficulty breathing and/or swallowing, with stridor, a swollen, oedematous facies and venous congestion. Treatment is with immediate steroids, anticoagulation and mediastinal radiotherapy or chemotherapy. Some tumours, e.g. lymphomas and germ cell tumours, are so sensitive to chemotherapy that this is preferred to radiotherapy as the masses are likely to be both large and associated with more disseminated disease elsewhere. An early decision is necessary on the patient's likely prognosis, as ventilatory support may be required until treatment has had time to relieve the obstruction.
- *Spinal cord compression* (p. 1206) needs to be rapidly diagnosed and urgent treatment arranged to salvage as much functional capacity as possible. Early neurological signs may be incomplete, more subjective than objective and gradual in onset. MR scanning is the investigation of choice and treatment should begin with high-dose steroids followed by surgical decompression and radiotherapy to the affected vertebrae to achieve the best disease control and palliation.
- *Neutropenic sepsis* (p. 483).
- *Acute hypercalcaemia* presents with vomiting, confusion, constipation and oliguria and should initially be treated by resuscitation with intravenous fluids until a saline diuresis is established, followed by i.v. pamidronate (Emergency box 18.2).
- *Raised intracranial pressure* due to intracerebral metastases presents classically with headache, nausea and vomiting. However, for many there is a slower onset with non-specific symptoms such as drowsiness or mental deterioration. Treatment is by high-dose steroids and investigation by MRI as to

whether surgery is appropriate or chemotherapy and radiotherapy are required.

- *Hyperviscosity* affects those with a very high haematocrit (> 50), white cell count (> 100×10^9/L) or platelet cell count (> 1000×10^9/L) from untreated acute leukaemia, polycythaemia or myeloma protein production, especially if the latter is IgM. Treatment is by venesection or leucophoresis and plasmapheresis followed by chemotherapy treatment for the underlying malignancy.

Adjuvant therapy for solid tumours

This is defined as treatment given in the absence of macroscopic evidence of metastases, to patients at risk of recurrence from micrometastases.

Micrometastatic spread by lymphatic or haematological dissemination often occurs early in the development of the primary tumour, and can be demonstrated by molecular biological methods capable of detecting the small numbers (1 in 10^6) of circulating cells. Studies correlating prognosis with histological features of the primary cancer, e.g. differentiation or presence of early metastatic invasion of blood vessels or regional lymph nodes, have led to an increasing ability to predict which patients are at high risk of local or distant recurrence from micrometastatic disease.

Trials of treatment with local radiotherapy or systemic endocrine, biological (e.g. interferon) or chemotherapy treatments have shown a significant improvement in survival in common adult cancers such as breast, bowel, prostate, head and neck, cervical cancer, choriocarcinoma and gonadal germ cell cancers. Central to these studies has been the careful selection of patients according to defined risk criteria, and the reduction of treatment toxicity to reach a balanced risk/benefit ratio. Absolute improvements in survival of 5–10% and relative risk reductions in the order of 12–25% (dependent upon the pre-existing risk) have been achieved in common epithelial cancers such as bowel, breast and prostate with greater absolute improvements of 25% in the more sensitive germ cell tumours.

While these improvements currently translate into many lives saved from common diseases at a public health level, the majority who receive such treatment do not benefit because they were already cured, or because the cancer is resistant to the treatment. Better tests in the future will identify those with the micrometastases who really need treatment. On an individual patient basis the decision on whether adjuvant treatment will be worthwhile must include consideration of other factors such as the patient's life expectancy, concurrent medical conditions, and lifestyle priorities.

Treatment of malignancy in sanctuary sites

A 'sanctuary site' is the term used to indicate that metastatic disease has involved a site that is not accessible to conventional drug therapy. An example of this is leukaemic infiltration of the meninges in children with acute lymphoblastic leukaemia. Because of the blood–brain barrier, agents such as vincristine and prednisolone do not enter the subarachnoid space in sufficient quantity to eliminate all the leukaemic cells, and are therefore ineffective in preventing the development of meningeal infiltration. In order to treat these cells, intrathecal chemotherapy and/or cranial irradiation are required.

Principles of chemotherapy

Chemotherapy employs systemically administered drugs that directly damage cellular DNA (and RNA). It kills cells by promoting apoptosis and sometimes frank necrosis. There is a narrow therapeutic window between effective treatment of the cancer and normal tissue toxicity, because the drugs are not cancer specific (unlike some of the biological agents), and the increased proliferation in cancers is not much greater than in normal tissues (see tumour growth and failure of apoptosis). The dose and schedule of the chemotherapy is limited by the normal tissue tolerance, especially in those more proliferative tissues of the bone marrow and gastrointestinal tract mucosa. All tissues can be affected, however, depending upon the pharmacokinetics of the drug and affinity for particular tissues (e.g. heavy metal compounds for kidneys and nerves).

The therapeutic effect on the cancer is achieved by a variety of mechanisms which seek to exploit differences between normal and transformed cells. While most of the drugs have been derived in the past by empirical testing of many different compounds, e.g. alkylating agents, the new molecular biology is leading to renewed attempts to target particular genetic defects in the cancer (see tyrosine kinase inhibitors for CML, p. 494).

Toxicity to normal tissue can be limited in some instances by supplying growth factors such as granulocyte colony-stimulating factor (G-CSF) or by the infusion of stem cell preparations to diminish myelotoxicity. The use of more specific biological agents with relatively weak pro-apoptotic effects in combination with the general cytotoxics may also improve the therapeutic ratio (see trastuzumab and breast cancer, p. 487).

Most tumours rapidly develop resistance to single agents given on their own. For this reason the principle of intermittent combination chemotherapy was developed. Several drugs are combined together, chosen on the basis of differing mechanisms of action and non-overlapping toxicities. These drugs are given over a period of a few days followed by a rest of a few weeks, during which time the normal tissues have the opportunity for regrowth. If the normal tissues are more proficient at DNA repair than the cancer cells, it may be possible to deplete the tumour while allowing the

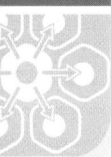

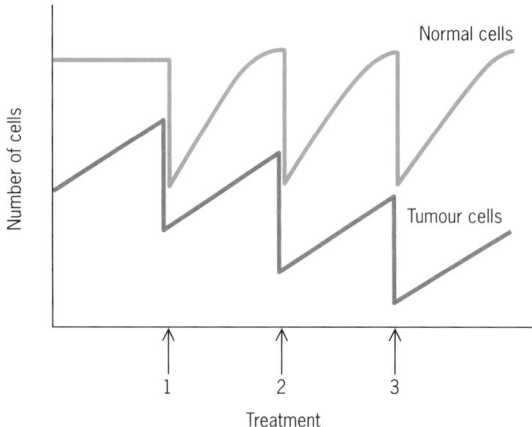

Fig. 9.1 Effects of multiple courses of cytotoxic chemotherapy.

Table 9.8
Chemotherapy: cytotoxic drugs

DNA damaging
Free radicals – alkylators, e.g. cyclophosphamide
DNA cross-linking – platinum, e.g. cisplatin, carboplatin

Antimetabolites
Thymidine synthesis, e.g. 5-fluorouracil, methotrexate and mercaptopurine

DNA repair inhibitors
Topoisomerase inhibitors – epipodophyllotoxins, e.g. etoposide; campothecins, e.g. irinotecan
DNA intercalation – anthracyclines, e.g. doxorubicin

Antitubulin
Tubulin binding – alkaloids, e.g. vincristine, vinorelbine
Taxanes – e.g. paclitaxel, docetaxel

restoration of normal tissues between chemotherapy cycles (Fig. 9.1).

In many experimental tumours it has been shown that there is a log–linear relationship between drug dose and number of cancer cells killed and that the maximum effective dose is very close to the maximum tolerated dose at which dose-limiting toxicity is reached. With a chemosensitive tumour, relatively small increases in dose may have a large effect on tumour cell kill. It is therefore apparent that where cure is a realistic option the dose administered is critical and may need to be maintained despite toxicity. In situations where cure is not a realistic possibility and palliation is the aim, a sufficient dose to exceed the therapeutic threshold, but not cause undue toxicity, is required as the short-term quality of life becomes a more important consideration.

Classification of cytotoxic drugs (Table 9.8)
DNA damaging
Alkylating agents
The alkylating agents such as cyclophosphamide act by covalently binding alkyl groups, and their major effect is to cross-link DNA strands, interfering with DNA synthesis and causing strand breaks. Despite being among the earliest cytotoxic drugs developed, they maintain a central position in the treatment of cancer. Common alkylating agents include cyclophosphamide, chlorambucil and busulfan.

Platinum compounds
Cisplatin, carboplatin and oxaliplatin cause interstrand cross-links of DNA and are often regarded as nonclassical alkylating agents. They have transformed the treatment of testicular cancer and have a major role against many other tumours, including lung, ovarian and head and neck cancer. Toxicity, as for other heavy metals, includes renal and peripheral nerve damage.

Antimetabolites
Antimetabolites are usually structural analogues of naturally occurring metabolites that interfere with normal synthesis of nucleic acids by falsely substituting purines and pyrimidines in metabolic pathways. Antimetabolites can be divided into:

- *Folic acid antagonist*, e.g. methotrexate. This is structurally very similar to folic acid and binds preferentially to dihydrofolate reductase, the enzyme responsible for the conversion of folic acid to folinic acid. It is used widely in the treatment of solid tumours and haematological malignancies, and also has a role as an immunosuppressant in non-malignant conditions such as rheumatoid arthritis.
- *Pyrimidine antagonists*, e.g. 5-fluorouracil, cytosine arabinoside (cytarabine) and gemcitabine. 5-Fluorouracil consists of a uracil molecule with a substituted fluorine atom. It acts by blocking the enzyme thymidylate synthetase which is essential for pyrimidine synthesis. 5-Fluorouracil has a major role in the treatment of solid tumours, particularly gastrointestinal cancers. Cytosine arabinoside is used almost exclusively in the treatment of acute myeloid leukaemia where it remains the backbone of therapy while its analogue gemcitabine is proving useful in a number of solid cancers such as lung and ovary.
- *Purine antagonists*, e.g. 6-mercaptopurine and 6-thioguanine, which are both used almost exclusively in the treatment of acute leukaemia.

DNA repair inhibitors
Epipodophyllotoxins
These are semisynthetic derivatives of podophyllotoxin, which is an extract from the mandrake plant. Etoposide is a drug used in a wide range of cancers and works by producing DNA strand breaks by acting on the enzyme topoisomerase II. Topoisomerase I inhibitors such as irinotecan and topotecan have also proved active against a variety of solid tumours. Both these enzymes allow unwinding and uncoiling of supercoiled DNA.

Cytotoxic antibiotics

These drugs such as doxorubicin and bleomycin act by intercalating adjoining nucleotide pairs on the same strand of DNA and by inhibiting DNA repair. They have a wide spectrum of activity in haematological and solid tumours. Doxorubicin is one of the most widely used of all cytotoxic drugs but has cumulative toxicity to the myocardium, while bleomycin has particular toxicity for the lungs.

Antitubulin agents

Vinca alkaloids

Drugs such as vincristine, vinblastine and vinorelbine act by binding to tubulin and inhibiting microtubule formation (see p. 158). They are used in the treatment of haematological and non-haematological cancers. They are associated with neurotoxicity due to their anti-microtubule effect.

Taxanes

Paclitaxel is isolated from the bark of the western Yew. Docetaxel is a semisynthetic taxane. They bind to tubulin dimers and prevent their assembly into microtubules, and are active drugs against many cancers such as ovarian, breast and lung cancer. Taxanes can cause neurotoxicity and hypersensitivity reactions and patients should be premedicated with steroids, H_1 and H_2 histamine antagonists prior to treatment.

Side-effects of chemotherapy

Chemotherapy carries many potentially serious side-effects and should be used only by trained practitioners. The four most common side-effects are vomiting, hair loss, tiredness and myelosuppression (Table 9.9). Side-effects are much more directly dose related than anti-cancer effects and it has been the practice to give drugs at doses close to their maximum tolerated dose, although this is not always necessary to achieve their maximum anticancer effect.

Table 9.9
Side-effects of chemotherapy

Common
Nausea and vomiting
Hair loss
Myelosuppression
Mucositis
Fatigue

Drug-specific
Cardiotoxicity, e.g. anthracyclines
Pulmonary toxicity, e.g. bleomycin
Neurotoxicity, e.g. platinum, vinca alkaloids, taxanes
Nephrotoxicity, e.g. platinum
Skin plantar–palmar dermatitis, e.g. 5-fluorouracil
Sterility, e.g. alkylating agents
Secondary malignancy, e.g. alkylating agents, epipodophyllotoxins

Nausea and vomiting

The severity of this common side-effect varies with the cytotoxic and can be eliminated in 75% of patients by using modern antiemetics. Nausea and vomiting are particular problems with platinum analogues and with doxorubicin. A stepped policy with antiemetics such as metoclopramide and domperidone or the 5-HT$_3$ serotonin antagonists (ondansetron and granisetron) combined with dexamethasone should be used to match the emetogenic potential of the chemotherapy.

Hair loss

Many but not all cytotoxic drugs are capable of causing hair loss. Scalp cooling can sometimes be used to reduce hair loss but in general this side-effect can only be avoided by selection of drugs where this is possible. Hair always regrows on completion of chemotherapy.

Bone marrow suppression and immunosuppression

Suppression of the production of red blood cells, white blood cells and platelets occurs with most cytotoxic drugs and is a dose-related phenomenon. Severely myelosuppressive chemotherapy may be required if treatment is to be given with curative intent despite the potential for rare but fatal infection or bleeding. Anaemia and thrombocytopenia are managed by red cell or platelet transfusions but white cell transfusions have not been successful until the advent of peripheral blood stem cell harvesting (see below).

Neutropenic patients are at high risk of bacterial and fungal infection often from enteric bowel flora. Those with a fever $> 37°C$ and less than 0.5×10^9 neutrophils/L are managed by the immediate introduction of broad-spectrum antibiotics intravenously for the treatment of infection (Box 9.3). Initial empirical therapy should be reviewed following microbiological results. Haemopoietic

---

Box 9.3

Febrile neutropenia treatment

Resuscitation with intravenous fluids to restore circulatory function, e.g. urine output, followed by cultures of blood, urine, sputum and stool and empirical antibiotics:

- Commonly require antibiotics including activity against pseudomonas, e.g. ceftazidine or ticacillin with gentamycin
- May require antibiotics against *Staph. aureus* especially with indwelling venous access lines, e.g. flucloxacillin or vancomycin.

If the patient deteriorates clinically and/or temperature still elevated after 48 hours, change antibiotics according to culture results or empirically increase Gram-negative and Gram-positive cover.

- Consider adding treatment for opportunistic infections if fever not responding to broad-spectrum antibiotics, e.g.
  amphotericin – fungus
  high-dose co-trimoxazole – pneumocystis
  clarithromycin – mycoplasma.

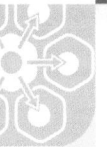

growth factors and peripheral blood stem cells can reduce the duration of neutropenia significantly, benefiting patients at high risk of infectious complications.

Mucositis

This common side-effect reflects the sensitivity of the mucosa to antimitotic agents. Treatment is with antiseptic and anticandidal mouthwash and, if severe, fluid and antibiotic support, as the mouth is a portal for entry of enteric organisms.

Cardiotoxicity

This is a rare side-effect of chemotherapy, usually associated with anthracyclines such as doxorubicin. It is dose-related and can largely be prevented by restricting the cumulative total dose of anthracyclines within the safe range (equivalent to 450 mg/m² body surface area cumulative doxorubicin dose).

Neurotoxicity

This occurs predominantly with the plant alkaloids, taxanes and platinum analogues (but not carboplatin). It is dose-related and cumulative. Chemotherapy is usually stopped before the development of a significant polyneuropathy, which once established is only partially reversible. Vincristine must never be given intrathecally as the neurological damage is progressive and fatal.

Nephrotoxicity

Platinum analogues (except carboplatin), methotrexate and ifosfamide (an alkylating agent) can potentially cause renal damage. This can usually be prevented by maintaining an adequate diuresis during treatment.

Sterility

Some anticancer drugs, particularly alkylating agents, may cause sterility, which may be irreversible. In males the storage of sperm prior to chemotherapy is an important consideration when chemotherapy is given with curative intent. In females it may be possible to collect oocytes to be fertilized in vitro and cryopreserved as embryos. Cryopreservation of ovarian tissue and retrieval of viable oocytes for subsequent fertilization is currently still experimental.

Secondary malignancies

Anticancer drugs have mutagenic potential and the development of secondary malignancies, predominantly acute leukaemia, is an uncommon but particularly unwelcome long-term side-effect in patients otherwise cured of their primary malignancies. The alkylating agents and epipodophyllotoxins are particularly implicated in this complication.

Drug resistance

Drug resistance is one of the major obstacles to curing cancer with chemotherapy. Some tumours have an inherently low level of resistance to currently available treatment and are often cured. These include gonadal germ cell tumours, Hodgkin's disease and childhood acute leukaemia. Solid tumours such as small-cell lung cancer initially appear to be chemosensitive, with the majority of patients responding, but most patients eventually relapse with resistant disease. In other tumours such as melanoma the disease is largely chemoresistant from the start.

It is thought that most resistance occurs as a result of genetic mutation and becomes more likely as the number of tumour cells increases. It has also been shown that anticancer drugs can themselves increase the rate of mutation to resistance. Resistance to cytotoxic drugs is often multiple and is then known as multidrug resistance (MDR), e.g. resistance to doxorubicin is often associated with resistance to vinca alkaloids and epipodophyllotoxins, and is mediated through increased expression of P-glycoprotein (a 170 kDa membrane phosphoglycoprotein), which mediates the efflux of cytotoxic drugs out of the cells. Many other mechanisms may also be involved in resistance to chemotherapy, such as the upregulation of anti-apoptotic proteins Bcl-2 and Bax.

High-dose therapy and autologous stem cell transplantation

Most anticancer drugs have a sigmoid dose–response relationship which suggests that, up to a point, a higher dose of a cytotoxic drug will induce a greater response. However, increasing cytotoxic drug doses is often not possible, owing to toxicity. For many chemotherapeutic agents the toxicity which limits the dose is bone marrow failure. If haemopoietic progenitor cells are collected and stored by cryopreservation prior to administration of high doses of chemotherapy, these can be returned as an intravenous infusion immediately after the chemotherapy has been completed and will restore haemopoiesis. This is the principle behind autologous haemopoietic stem cell transplantation (Box 9.4).

Haemopoietic stem cells may be collected from bone marrow, or more frequently by leucophoresis from peripheral blood following administration of the growth factor granulocyte colony-stimulating factor (G-CSF) These cells are then re-infused after an intensive, myeloablative chemotherapy regimen, sometimes also involving total body irradiation. This approach has been particularly effective in overcoming apparent drug resistance in relapsed leukaemias and lymphomas.

Box 9.4

Autologous haemopoietic stem cells

- Increased in peripheral blood by cytotoxics plus G-CSF
- Collected by leucophoresis
- Infused to restore normal haematopoiesis

However, there are problems. Not all cancers are any more responsive to high doses of chemotherapy than they are to conventional doses. Second, it may not be possible to collect haemopoietic progenitor cells from some patients, and those cells which are collected may be contaminated with tumour cells and lead to relapse of the primary malignancy. Third, even rescue with haemopoietic progenitor cells results in a period of severe cytopenia lasting around 2 weeks, with associated morbidity. Fourth, there is a long period of immuno-suppression for 6–12 months following the transplant, resulting in an increased risk of life-threatening opportunistic infections. Nevertheless, the procedure remains effective treatment for many patients with haematological malignancies, and clinical trials in other tumours continue.

Allogeneic haemopoietic transplantation

This combines treatment of the underlying malignancy by high doses of chemotherapy and/or radiotherapy, with the transplantation of donor haemopoietic cells to reconstitute the bone marrow and immune system (Box 9.5). It is thought that the engraftment of the donor immune system, with antitumour activity (graft versus tumour), is primarily responsible for the increased effectiveness of this approach. In general, ideal donors are fully matched at the major HLA antigens. Thus siblings are more likely to be found to be potential donors than unrelated volunteers. Some degree of HLA antigen mismatch may be tolerated in children, but is problematic in adults. Allogeneic transplantation has been successfully used in acute and chronic leukaemias, and myeloma.

Recently, it has been possible to engraft a donor immune system to achieve an anticancer effect with lesser doses of chemotherapy, in a procedure known as a 'non-myeloablative transplant' for previously untreatable cancers. Conventional and non-myeloablative procedures are complicated by the toxicity of 'graft-versus-host disease', an immune reaction of the donor cells against normal host organs, which can affect 30–50% of transplant recipients and is potentially fatal in some cases. Immunosuppression, both from conditioning therapy and from the immunosuppressive drugs given to prevent graft-versus-host disease, results in a high incidence of opportunistic infections. Mortality therefore from allogeneic stem cell transplantation is a major problem, with 20–40% at risk of dying from the procedure, depending on the age and status of the recipient, and the degree of HLA compatibility of the donor (see also Immunotherapy).

FURTHER READING

Loblaw DA, Laperriere NJ (1998) Emergency treatment of malignant extradural spinal cord compression. *Journal of Clinical Oncology* **16**: 13–24.

Pizzo PA (1999) Fever in immunocompromised patients. *New England Journal of Medicine* **341**: 893–900.

Principles of endocrine therapy

It has long been known that oestrogen is capable of stimulating the growth of breast and endometrial cancers, and androgens the growth of prostate cancer. Removal of these growth factors by manipulation of the hormonal environment may result in apoptosis and regression of the cancer. Endocrine therapy can be curative in a proportion of patients treated for micrometastatic disease in the adjuvant setting for breast and prostate cancer and provides a minimally toxic non-curative (palliative) treatment in advanced/metastatic disease. The presence of detectable cellular receptors for the hormone markedly increases the likelihood that the therapy will be effective. The binding of hormone to receptor and translocation of the hormone–receptor complex into the nucleus, where it binds to specific hormone-responsive transcription factors on the DNA, is shown diagrammatically in Figure 9.2.

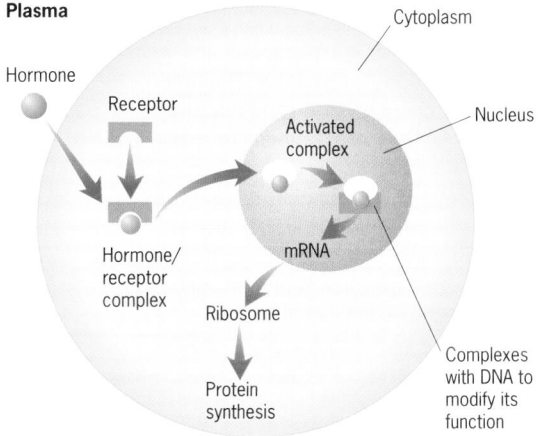

Fig. 9.2 Mechanism of the interaction between a steroid hormone and its receptor. This interaction modifies DNA activity and hence cell growth and replication.

> ### Box 9.5
>
> #### Allogeneic haemopoietic stem cells
>
> - Infused to restore normal haematopoiesis
> - Provide potent graft-versus-cancer immunotherapy
> - Morbidity from opportunistic infection and graft-versus-host (normal tissues) effects

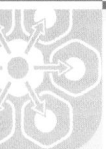
Oestrogens and progestogens

About one-third of patients with breast cancer have receptors for oestrogens and progesterones. Hormonal manipulation includes the use of tamoxifen, which blocks oestrogen receptors, and the reduction of endogenous oestrogen by oophorectomy or 'medical oophorectomy' via pituitary downregulation using a gonadotrophin-releasing hormone (GnRH) analogue such as goserilin. In patients with advanced metastatic breast cancer, oestrogen deprivation causes tumour regression in 30% of unselected women and in more than 60% of those with oestrogen-receptor-positive tumours for a median duration of 20 months.

In the adjuvant setting, ovarian ablation or tamoxifen results in a 25% reduction in relative risk of dying from metastatic disease, which is maintained for in excess of 20 years after only 5 years of postoperative treatment.

Progestogens have a direct effect in breast tumour cells as well as effects on the pituitary/ovarian and adrenal axis and can be as effective as tamoxifen. In postmenopausal women, androgens are synthesized by the adrenal glands and converted in subcutaneous fat to estrone by the enzyme aromatase. Aromatase inhibitors, for example anastrozole, reduce circulating oestrogen levels and oestrogen synthesis in tumour cells and have recently shown even greater efficacy than tamoxifen in the treatment of metastatic breast cancer in the post-menopausal woman.

Endometrial cancers have receptors for both oestrogens and progestogens. Approximately 20% of receptor-positive metastases will regress for a median 20 months with synthetic progestogens such as medroxyprogesterone acetate but paradoxically tamoxifen has little effect. Trials to date with adjuvant progestogens have not been successful in increasing survival.

Androgens

In advanced prostate cancer, androgen deprivation induces regression in 70% of cases for a median duration of 24 months. GnRH agonists, e.g. goserilin, and orchidectomy, are equally effective; however, androgen receptor blockers such as flutamide are less so. Combinations of goserilin and flutamide may be used in the initial phase of treatment to avoid a disease flare from the initial agonist action of GnRH analogues, but prolonged combination therapy has been no more effective than goserilin alone. In the adjuvant setting, the addition of androgen deprivation to prostatic radiotherapy or surgery has improved survival and continues to be investigated.

Principles of biological therapy

This term encompasses a wide range of treatments, most of which are thought to act by indirect anticancer mechanisms rather than by a direct cytotoxic effect. The group includes a range of protein molecules from small peptide chemokines, larger cytokines, to complex antibody molecules made available by genetically engineering the production of large quantities by microbial and eukaryotic cell cultures. There is great potential for the continuing expansion of this field.

Interferons

Interferons are naturally occurring cytokines that mediate the cellular immune response. They have many actions in treatment of malignant disease with both antiproliferative activity, and stimulation of humoral and cell-mediated immune responses to the tumour that can result in an antitumour effect if the host effector mechanisms are present and fully competent.

Alpha-interferon (IFN-α) has been used against several malignancies to treat established disease such as melanoma, renal cell cancer and chronic myeloid leukaemia. In the latter, it results in a reduction in the number of Philadelphia (Ph) chromosome-positive cells in at least 50% of patients, with total elimination in 10%. Cytogenetic response has been shown to result in prolongation of survival, but interferon is not curative. Interferon has also been used to maintain remission after cytotoxic treatment by suppressing microscopic residual disease, e.g. myeloma. In renal cell cancer alpha-interferon has a low (10–15%) but significant anticancer effect and prolongation of survival.

Treatment with IFN has side-effects due to its foreign protein nature, most commonly flu-like symptoms which tend to diminish with time, and fatigue which generally does not and can be treatment limiting. In addition the drug has to be given as a subcutaneous injection over long periods of time, although conjugation with polyethylene glycol (PEG interferon) has led to a reduction in frequency of injection and severity of side-effects.

Interleukins

Originally described for their activity in modulating leucocyte activation, these cytokines have widespread activity in coordinating cellular activity in many organs. Current therapeutic interest has been mainly concentrated on interleukin-2, a recombinant protein used to activate T cell responses, often in conjunction with interferon-stimulated B cell activation. Antitumour activity has been observed in renal cell cancer and melanoma with responses in 10–20% of patients, occasionally for prolonged periods. Toxicity is common; acutely this includes the capillary leak syndrome with hypotension, whilst pulmonary oedema, autoimmune thyroiditis and vitiligo occur later.

Haemopoietic growth factors

Granulocyte (G-CSF) and granulocyte/macrophage colony-stimulating factor (GM-CSF) are the recombinant human cytokines used:

- to reduce the duration of neutropenia following chemotherapy
- with or without chemotherapy, to stimulate the proliferation of haemopoietic progenitor cells in the marrow so that they enter the circulation and can be collected from the peripheral blood to support high-dose chemotherapy treatment (see p. 484) as an alternative to bone marrow transplantation.

Monoclonal antibodies

Monoclonal antibodies directed against tumour cell surface antigens are used in patients when they are 'humanized' by being genetically engineered as a chimera comprising a human constant region with the murine heavy and light chains of the antigen-combining site to reduce formation of blocking human anti-mouse antibodies. Uses include:

- *In vitro,* in conjunction with complement, they are used to deplete autologous bone marrow of tumour cells in patients with leukaemia and lymphoma receiving high-dose treatment with autologous haemopoietic progenitor cell support.
- *In vitro* in immunoadsorption columns to select the CD34-positive (stem cell) fraction from peripheral blood progenitor cell or autologous bone marrow collections, to support high-dose treatment in haematological and other malignancies.
- *In vivo,* as treatment for B cell non-Hodgkin's lymphoma (e.g. anti-CD20 surface antigen). Tumour cell lysis occurs by both complement and antibody-dependent cellular cytotoxicity.
- *As a carrier molecule* to target toxins or radioisotopes to the tumour cells, e.g. anti-CD20 conjugated to radioactive iodine is being used as treatment for non-Hodgkin's lymphoma.
- *Monoclonal antibodies* (trastazumab) against the Her2/Neu or C-erbB2 antigen, a member of the epidermal growth factor receptor family, have both direct anti-breast cancer activity in clinical trials and increase the apoptotic response to cytotoxics. This leads to improved survival of patients receiving concomitant chemotherapy for metastatic breast cancer.

Immunotherapy

It has long been recognized that the cellular immune system is a powerful weapon against cancer. Activation of the immune system using bacille Calmette–Guérin (BCG) for bladder cancer or interleukin-2 for renal cancer induces responses in 60% and 10% of patients respectively. More recently, immunotherapy has become more refined. Firstly, certain antigens that are specific to cancer cells, such as sequences of tumour immuno-globulin from B cell lymphomas or melanoma antigens have been used as tumour vaccines. Antigen-presenting cells (dendritic cells) from the patient can be genetically engineered to present both antigen and cytokines such as interleukin-2 or granulocyte macrophage colony-stimulating factor, and clinical responses have been observed. Another approach has used dendritic cells to further improve the vaccination strategy by engineering them to display the full range of HLA and B7 co-stimulatory molecules.

The use of non-myeloablative haemopoietic stem cell and donor lymphocyte infusions, while losing some of the specificity, has produced the strongest evidence for the efficacy of immunotherapy at the risk of the greatest toxicity.

Gene therapy

Antisense oligonucleotides are short sequences of DNA bases which specifically inhibit complementary sequences of either DNA or RNA. As a result, they can be generated against genetic sequences which are specific for tumour cells. Their clinical development has been hampered by poor uptake by tumour cells and rapid degradation by natural endonucleases. However, one antisense sequence directed against the *Bcl-2* onco-gene has been shown to have an antitumour effect in patients with non-Hodgkin's lymphoma and others are likely to follow. Creation of reliable vectors for the trans-fection of tumour cells in vivo still forms a major barrier to the greater application of this modality.

Intracellular signal inhibitors

The recognition that many cancer cells are transformed by the activity of the protein products of oncogenes has led to the search for peptides or other compounds which inhibit these proteins, or their intracellular signal pathways. An example is the tyrosine kinase inhibitor STI571, which specifically inhibits the fusion oncoprotein *BCR-ABL.* This compound is an extremely effective treatment for chronic myeloid leukaemia, a disease char-acterized by the presence of the *BCR-ABL* fusion protein. Many other similar molecules, inhibiting enzymes involved in cell cycling or cytokine signalling, are in pre-clinical or early clinical development. Examples include farnesyl transferase inhibitors, which inhibit ras proteins, inhibitors of the platelet-derived growth factor receptor, and drugs which inhibit matrix metalloproteinases.

Principles of radiation therapy

Radiation delivers energy to tissues, causing ionization and excitation of atoms and molecules. The biological effect is exerted through the generation of single- and double-strand DNA breaks, inducing apoptosis of cells as they progress through the cell cycle, and through the generation of short-lived free radicles, particularly from oxygen, which damage proteins and membranes.

The most commonly used form of radiotherapy is *external beam* or *teletherapy* from a linear accelerator

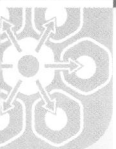
source which provides X-rays, the energy of which is transmitted as photons. Cobalt-60 generators can also provide gamma rays and high-energy photons.

Brachytherapy is the use of radiation sources in close contact with the tissue to provide intense exposure over a short distance to a restricted volume.

Systemic radionuclides, e.g. iodine-131, or radioisotope-labelled monoclonal antibodies and hormones can be administered by intravenous or intracavitary routes to provide radiation targeted to particular tissue uptake via surface antigens or receptors.

The radiation dose is measured in grays (Gy), where 1 gray = 1 joule absorbed per kilogram of absorbing tissue and 1 centigray = 1 rad. The biological effect is dependent upon the dose rate, duration, volume irradiated, and the tissue sensitivity. Sensitivity to photon damage is greatest during the G_2–M phase of the cell cycle and is also dependent upon the DNA repair capacity of the cell. Fractionation is the delivery of the radiation dose in increments separated by at least 4–6 hours to try to exploit any advantage in DNA repair between normal and malignant cells. Radiation dose is thus described by three factors:

- total dose in cGy
- number of fractions
- time for completion.

Most treatments are delivered in 150–200 cGy fractions daily for 5 days per week, although a regimen of two fractions daily (hyperfractionation) has improved survival benefit in a recent lung cancer trial.

The radiation effect will also depend upon the intensity of the radiation source measured as the linear energy transfer or frequency of ionizing events per unit of path, which is subject to the inverse square law as the energy diminishes with the distance from the source.

The generation of free radicles depends upon the degree of oxygenation/hypoxia in the target tissues. This can affect the biological effect by up to threefold and is the subject of continuing research for hypoxic cell sensitizers.

The depth of penetration of biological tissues by the photons depends upon the energy of the beam. Low-energy photons from an 85 kV source are suitable for superficial treatments while high-energy 35 MeV sources produce a beam with deeper penetration, less scatter both at the initial skin boundary (skin sparing) and at the margins of the beam, and less absorption by bone. Superficial radiation may be also delivered by electron beams from a linear accelerator that has had the target electrode that generates the X-rays removed.

Radiotherapy treatment planning involves both detailed physics of the applied dose and knowledge of the biology of the cancer and whether the intention is to treat the tumour site alone, or include the likely loco-regional patterns of spread. Normal tissue tolerance will determine the extent of the side-effects and a balanced decision

Table 9.10
Curative radiotherapy treatment

Primary modality
Retina
CNS
Skin
Oropharynx and larynx
Oesophagus
Cervix and vagina
Prostate
Lymphoma

Adjuvant to primary surgery
Lung
Breast
Uterus
Bladder
Rectum
Testis seminoma
Sarcoma

Box 9.6

Palliative benefits of radiotherapy

- Pain relief, e.g. bone metastases
- Reduction of headache and vomiting of raised intracranial pressure from CNS metastases
- Relief of obstruction of bronchus, oesophagus, ureter, and lymphatics
- Preservation of skeletal integrity from metastases in weight-bearing bones
- Reversal of neurological impairment from spinal cord or optic nerve compression by metastases

---

is made according to the curative or palliative intent of the treatment and the likely early or late side-effects.

The cancers for which radiotherapy is usually employed as primary curative when the tumour is anatomically localized are listed in Table 9.10 along with those in which radiotherapy has curative potential when used in addition to surgery (adjuvant radiotherapy). Palliative treatments are frequently used to provide relief of symptoms to improve quality if not duration of survival (Box 9.6).

Side-effects of radiotherapy

Radiotherapy side-effects may occur early within days to weeks of treatment when they are usually self-limiting but associated with general systemic disturbance (Table 9.11). The side-effects will depend upon tissue sensitivity, fraction size and treatment volume and are managed with supportive measures until normal tissue repair occurs. The toxicity may also be enhanced by exposure to other radiation-sensitizing agents, especially some cytotoxics, e.g. bleomycin, actinomycin, anthracyclines, cisplatin and 5-fluorouracil.

Later side-effects occur from months to years later, unrelated to the severity of the acute effects because of

Table 9.11
Side-effects of radiotherapy

Acute side-effects
Anorexia, nausea, malaise
Mucositis, e.g. oesophagitis, diarrhoea
Alopecia
Myelosuppression

Late side-effects

Skin	Ischaemia, ulceration
Bone	Necrosis, fracture
Mouth	Xerostomia, sialitis, ulceration
Bowel	Stenosis, fistula, diarrhoea
Bladder	Cystitis
Vagina	Dyspareunia, stenosis
Lung	Fibrosis
Heart	Pericardial fibrosis, cardiomyopathy
CNS	Myelopathy
Gonads	Infertility, menopause

their different mechanism. Late effects reflect both the loss of slowly proliferating cells and a local endarteritis which produces ischaemia and proliferative fibrosis.

Growth may be arrested if bony epiphyses are not yet fused and are irradiated, leading to distorted skeletal growth in later life.

Secondary malignancies following radiotherapy typically appear 10–20 years after the cure of the primary cancer. Haematological malignancies tend to occur sooner than the solid tumours from the irradiated tissues. The latter are very dependent upon the status of the tissue at the time of treatment, e.g. the pubertal breast is up to 300 times more sensitive to malignant transformation than the breast tissues of a woman in her thirties. Treatment of these secondary cancers can be successful providing there is normal bone marrow to reconstitute the haemopoietic system or the whole tissue at risk (e.g. thyroid after mantle radiotherapy for lymphoma) can be resected.

FURTHER READING

Gregor A (2000) How to improve effects of radiation and control its toxicity. *Annals of Oncology* **11**; 53: 231–234.

Haematological malignancies

Leukaemia, lymphoma and myeloma constitute only a small proportion of all malignancies. They are generally responsive to treatment so that many patients with acute leukaemia, Hodgkin's disease or high-grade non-Hodgkin's lymphoma can be cured. However, most people with haematological malignancy still die as a consequence of the disease, or because of complications of treatment.

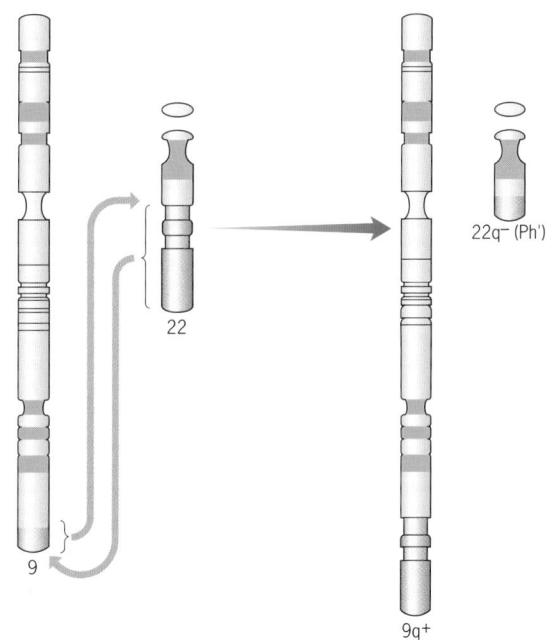

Fig. 9.3 The Philadelphia chromosome (Ph). The long arm (q) of chromosome 22 has been shortened by the reciprocal translocation with chromosome 9.

The leukaemias

These are rare diseases with an annual overall incidence of 5 per 100 000. Acute lymphoblastic leukaemia (ALL) is predominantly a disease of childhood, whereas acute myelogenous leukaemia (AML) is more frequently seen in older adults, as are the chronic leukaemias (see Classification below).

Genetic abnormalities in leukaemia
Studies of the genetic abnormalities in leukaemia have provided a paradigm for the investigation of other cancers. The inherited predisposition may be expressed any time from in utero in twin studies to later in adult life.

Leukaemic cells often have a somatically acquired cytogenetic abnormality, which may often be of prognostic, as well as diagnostic, importance. The first non-random chromosomal abnormality to be described was the Philadelphia (Ph) chromosome which is associated with chronic myeloid leukaemia (CML) in 97% of cases. The Ph chromosome is also found in ALL, the incidence in the latter illness increasing with age. The translocation is shown schematically in Figure 9.3. The Ph chromosome is an abnormal chromosome 22, resulting from a reciprocal translocation between part of the long arm of chromosome 22 and chromosome 9. The resulting karyotype is described as t(9;22)(q34;q11). The molecular consequences of the translocation are that part of the Abelson proto-oncogene (c-*ABL*) normally present on chromosome 9 is translocated to chromosome 22, where it

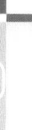

Table 9.12
Cytogenetic and molecular abnormalities in leukaemia and lymphoma

Cytogenetic rearrangement	Gene(s) involved	Diseases affected
Reciprocal translocations giving rise to fusion oncogenes		
T(9;22)	BCR-ABL	CML, AML, ALL
T(15;17)	PML-RAR	APML
Inv16	CBFb-MYH11	AML
T(6;9)	DEK-CAN	AML
T(8;21)	AML1-ETO	AML
T(1;19)	E2A-PBX1	ALL
T(12;21)	TEL-AML1	ALL
Reciprocal rearrangements upregulating proto-oncogenes		
T(8;14)	myc	Burkitt's lymphoma
T(11;14)	Bcl-1/PRAD (cyclinD1)	Mantle cell NHL
T(14;18)	Bcl-2	Follicular NHL
T(3;14)	Bcl-6	Large cell NHL
T(4;11)	MLL gene	ALL
T(4;14)	FGFR3	Myeloma
T(14;16)	c-MAF	Myeloma

Abbreviations: CML, chronic myeloid leukaemia; AML, acute myeloid leukaemia; APML, acute promyelocytic leukaemia; ALL, acute lymphoblastic leukaemia; CLL, chronic lymphoblastic leukaemia; NHL, non-Hodgkin's lymphoma; MDS, myelodysplastic syndrome

Table 9.13
The World Health Organization classification of acute leukaemia

a. AML (acute myeloid leukaemia)
1. AML with recurrent cytogenetic abnormalities (includes acute promyelocytic leukaemia with t(15;17) or variants)
2. AML with multi-lineage dysplasia (usually secondary to a pre-existing myelodysplastic syndrome)
3. Therapy-related AML
4. AML – other (including minimally differentiated AML)
5. Acute biphenotypic leukaemia (acute leukaemia expressing both lymphoid and myeloid phenotype)

b. ALL (acute lymphoblastic leukaemia)
1. Precursor B acute lymphoblastic leukaemia
2. Burkitt cell leukaemia
3. Precursor T acute lymphoblastic leukaemia

From Harris NL et al. (1999) *Journal of Clinical Oncology* **17**: 3835–3849

p. 493). Other genetic and cytogenetic abnormalities are often seen in leukaemic cells (Table 9.12).

Classification

The characteristics of leukaemic cells can be assessed by light microscopy, expression of cytosolic enzymes and expression of surface antigens. These will reflect the lineage and degree of maturity of the leukaemic clone. Thus, leukaemia can be divided on the basis of the speed of evolution of the disease into acute or chronic. Each of these is then further subdivided into myeloid or lymphoid, according to the cell type involved (Table 9.13).

- acute myelogenous leukaemia (AML)
- acute lymphoblastic leukaemia (ALL)
- chronic myeloid leukaemia (CML)
- chronic lymphocytic leukaemia (CLL).

comes into juxtaposition with a region of chromosome 22 named the 'breakpoint cluster region' (BCR). The translocation creates a hybrid transcription unit consisting of the 5′ end of the *BCR* gene and the c-*ABL* proto-oncogene.

The new 'fusion' gene is capable of being expressed as a chimeric messenger RNA which has been identified in cells from patients with CML. When translated, this produces a fusion protein that has tyrosine kinase activity and enhanced phosphorylating activity compared with the normal protein, resulting in altered cell growth, stromal attachment and apoptosis. The breakpoint differs in CML and Ph-positive ALL, leading to the production of two different tyrosine kinase proteins with molecular weights of 210 kD and 190 kD respectively. It is unclear whether the presence of *BCR-ABL* is sufficient for the development of the disease. It has recently been shown that normal subjects can carry low levels of the *BCR-ABL* fusion gene in their blood without developing leukaemia. New drugs, e.g. Glivec, have been successfully developed to target this aberrant tyrosine kinase and offer new opportunities for cancer-specific therapy.

Almost all patients with acute promyelocytic leukaemia (APML), a subtype of acute myelogenous leukaemia, have the t(15;17) reciprocal translocation, which occurs at the q25 band on chromosome 15 and the q22 band on chromosome 17. The breakpoint on chromosome 17 occurs in the gene encoding the retinoic acid receptor, fusing it with part of the *PML* gene. This is to some extent the explanation for the responsiveness of patients with APML to all-*trans*-retinoic acid (ATRA, see

Acute leukaemias

Clinical features

The symptoms and signs of acute leukaemia are a consequence of bone marrow failure:

- symptoms of anaemia, such as tiredness, weakness, shortness of breath on exertion
- repeated fever, infections and abscesses
- bruising and/or bleeding, especially oral mucosa, retina and lower limbs
- occasionally, lymph node enlargement and/or symptoms relating to enlargement of the liver and spleen.

Investigations

The definitive diagnosis is made on the basis of a peripheral blood film and a bone marrow aspirate, often with a bone marrow biopsy. Additional investigations such as cytogenetic analysis and immunophenotyping

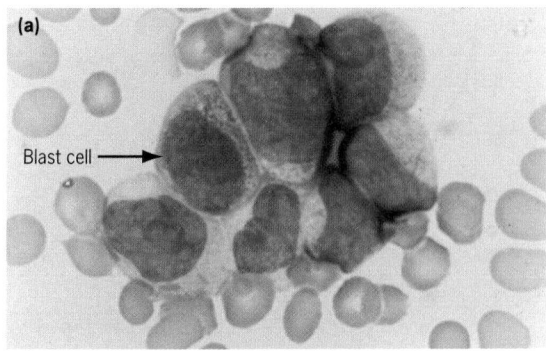

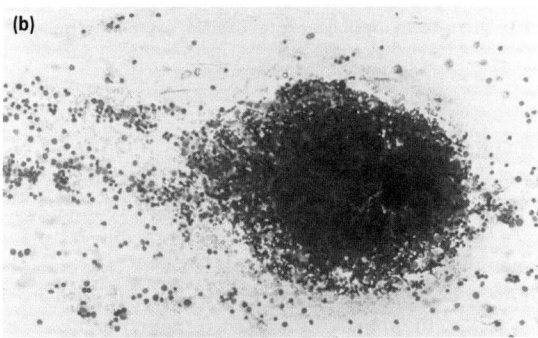

Fig. 9.4 **(a) Peripheral blood film showing characteristic blast cells.** The arrow points to the abnormal blast cell. **(b) Bone marrow aspirate** showing particle with increased cellularity. Courtesy of Dr Manzoor Mangi.

of the leukaemic blast cells are necessary for confirming the diagnosis, subclassifying the disease and attributing an accurate prognosis.

- Blood count typically shows a low haemoglobin (Hb) and often a raised white cell count, but this can be decreased or normal if there are not many circulating blast cells. The platelet count is usually low.
- Peripheral blood film shows characteristic leukaemic blast cells (Fig. 9.4).
- Bone marrow aspirate shows increased cellularity with abnormal lymphoid or myeloid blast cells (Fig. 9.4).

Acute myeloid leukaemia is distinguished by the presence of granules and 'Auer rods' in the cytoplasm, the presence of enzymes such as myeloperoxidase, expression of myeloid antigens (CD13, CD33) and the presence of typical cytogenetic abnormalities (see Table 9.12). Once identified, it can be subdivided into good risk, standard risk or poor risk depending on the cytogenetic and/or molecular genetic abnormalities (see above). Acute myeloid leukaemias arising as a result of prior chemotherapy or radiotherapy, or arising out of a background of another myeloproliferative disease, are usually referred to as 'secondary AML'. These leukaemias often carry complex chromosomal abnormalities which are associated with a poorer prognosis.

Acute lymphoblastic leukaemia may be identified by morphology, but the diagnosis is confirmed and the disease subclassified according to expression of lymphoid antigens. Most cases of ALL are derived from B cells, and will express the CD10 antigen. They can be divided into 'precursor B lymphoblastic leukaemia' and 'Burkitt cell leukaemia' (Table 9.13). The distinction between ALL and lymphoblastic lymphoma is arbitrary; ALL is defined as the presence of greater than 30% lymphoblasts in the bone marrow. Some cases of ALL express T cell antigens. In children, cytogenetic abnormalities such as hyperdiploidy or the presence of t(1;19) are of prognostic significance.

General principles of management

The decision to treat a patient with curative intent will depend on the person's age, their general state of health, the time-point in the course of the illness (presentation or recurrence), and the person's wishes. The use of intensive combination chemotherapy may, for example, be inappropriate in an older person. The diagnosis, its implications, treatment options and the likely outcome of such treatment, together with its side-effects, need to be explained to the patient and to their family. People often find it difficult to assimilate all of this information on one occasion; it is therefore essential to give them the opportunity to ask questions, particularly as circumstances change. Before starting treatment, the following points must be considered.

- *Anaemia and thrombocytopenia* need to be corrected by the administration of blood and platelets.
- *Infection* should be treated with intravenous antibiotics.
- *Leukaemic blast cells* can infiltrate the brain and lungs, resulting in coma and respiratory failure respectively. If the blast cell count in the peripheral blood is very high ($>100 \times 10^9/\text{L}$) the patient may need leucophoresis to prevent sludging of the capillary beds. Blood is collected from a vein and centrifuged so as to remove leukaemic cells, and the red cells and plasma are then returned to the patient via another vein. Leucophoresis can be life-saving.
- *Hyperuricaemia* can be treated or prevented by the administration of allopurinol, a xanthine oxidase inhibitor.
- *Tumour-lysis syndrome.* In certain types of leukaemia, chemotherapy causes such a rapid necrosis of the neoplastic cells (e.g. B cell and T cell ALL) that patients may develop a 'tumour lysis' syndrome when chemotherapy is given. This is characterized by hypercalcaemia and high serum levels of phosphate and potassium.

  This is a potentially life-threatening situation and difficult to treat once it has happened. It can usually be prevented by making sure that chemotherapy is not started until the uric acid level is normal and by diuresis established with intravenous fluids. Patients

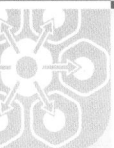

may require haemodialysis to correct severe metabolic imbalance.

- *Supportive care.* In what follows, specific treatments for the different types of leukaemia will be mentioned only briefly because regimens are evolving continually. Good 'supportive care' (with antibiotics and blood products) is virtually as important as the specific combination of drugs used. Patients with acute leukaemia should therefore be treated in specialist centres where the medical and nursing staff are familiar with the management of neutropenia and thrombocytopenia.

Acute myelogenous leukaemia (AML)

AML is a potentially curable disease in 30% of patients under 60 years old. The aim of treatment is to restore the bone marrow to normal and the patient to a normal state of health – complete remission (CR).

Treatment

Treatment has traditionally been regarded as being in two parts: remission induction and post-remission/ consolidation therapy. This is because at the point of complete remission – when there is no morphologically detectable leukaemia – there are still 10^8 or 10^9 leukaemic blast cells detectable using molecular biological markers.

Remission induction therapy usually includes an anthracycline drug such as daunorubicin or doxorubicin (or a newer analogue such as idarubicin), given in conjunction with cytosine arabinoside (cytarabine) with or without another drug such as etoposide. The patient needs to stay in hospital for about 4 weeks in the first instance owing to the risk of infection and bleeding consequent upon neutropenia and thrombocytopenia. Subsequent cycles of treatment are given as much as possible on an outpatient basis.

There is much debate as to the best post-remission therapy. Options include:

- further cycles of chemotherapy, the same as that given to induce remission
- chemotherapy different from that given to induce remission, particularly high doses of cytosine arabinoside.
- myeloablative therapy with allogeneic/autologous bone marrow transplantation (BMT) (see p. 484).

The use of bone marrow transplantation in standard-risk AML is controversial and depends on the interpretation of data from clinical trials that have been completed, as well as the results from studies that are still underway. In general, higher doses of cytosine arabinoside result in improved leukaemia-free survival but have unacceptable toxicity in older patients. A proportion of patients who do not receive a bone marrow transplant to consolidate their first remission may receive one if their disease relapses.

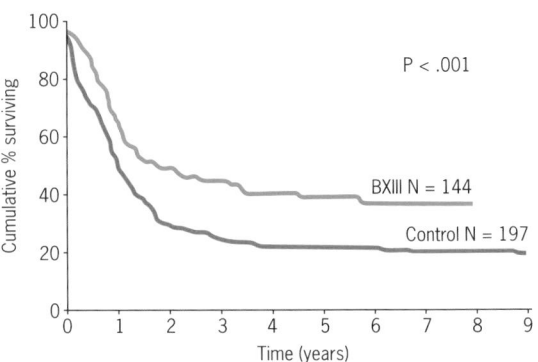

Fig. 9.5 **Acute myelogenous leukaemia: overall survival with or without myeloblative therapy** (from Rohatiner AZS et al (2000) *Annals of Oncology* **11**: 1007–1015 with permission).

Results of treatment

With modern combination chemotherapy, approximately 70–80% of people aged under 60 years will enter complete remission and return to normal health; for older patients around 50–60% can expect to achieve remission. However, within 1–3 years the disease will recur in at least 60%, the remainder almost certainly having been cured. Treatment has generally become more intensive over the last 25 years with a concomitant improvement in overall survival. Survival curves for patients treated during three consecutive time periods are shown in Figure 9.5.

Treatment at recurrence

Second remissions are more difficult to achieve and are rarely durable. The decision to treat a person at recurrence will therefore again depend on the patient's overall situation and his or her wishes. In younger patients, provided that second remission can be achieved, cure is still a possibility for a proportion, using myeloablative therapy with allogeneic/autologous haemopoietic progenitor cell support.

In older patients the options are further intensive combination chemotherapy or a palliative approach. The aim of palliation is to keep the person as well as possible for as long as possible with supportive measures such as blood transfusions, antibiotics, and the judicious use of orally administered drugs such as hydroxycarbamide (hydroxyurea) to help lower the number of circulating leukaemic cells.

Acute promyelocytic leukaemia (APML)

Acute promyelocytic leukaemia is associated with the chromosome translocation t(15;17). It warrants separate mention because of its specific association with disseminated intravascular coagulation (DIC). Patients may present with severe bleeding which worsens when treatment is started, as the leukaemic blast cells break down, leading to further consumption of clotting factors and platelets. This may be due to the abnormally high surface expression of the protein annexin II, which accelerates the activation of plasmin, a fibrinolytic plasma protein.

Treatment of APML

Active DIC can be managed by infusion of regular platelet transfusions and maintenance of the fibrinogen level with fresh frozen plasma as the chemotherapy is given. The administration of all-*trans*-retinoic acid (ATRA) is standard in all patients. ATRA differentiates the leukaemic cells of APML into mature granulocytes, which ameliorates both the DIC and the marrow failure associated with the disease. Chemotherapy is usually given without cytarabine and patients are kept on oral ATRA maintenance for 1 year after post-remission therapy has been completed.

Provided remission can be achieved, patients with APML have a somewhat better prognosis overall than patients with other subtypes of AML.

Acute lymphoblastic leukaemia

This is predominantly a disease of children. Overall, 90% of children respond to treatment and 60–70% are cured. The results in adults are not as good, with only approximately 30% being cured.

Treatment

The principles of initial treatment are the same as those for AML, the aim being to return the bone marrow to normal and the person to a good state of health. Cyclical combination chemotherapy comprising vincristine, prednisolone, L-asparaginase and an anthracycline such as doxorubicin forms the basis of most treatment regimens. Other drugs such as cyclophosphamide and/or cytosine arabinoside are also being used increasingly in both adults and children considered to be at high risk for recurrence. Care is taken over the cumulative dose of anthracycline administered to younger children owing to concerns over long-term cardiotoxicity.

The sequence of treatment, however, differs somewhat from that in AML because ALL has a propensity for involvement of the central nervous system (CNS). Thus, treatment includes prophylactic intrathecal drugs (a lumbar puncture is performed under local anaesthetic and methotrexate or cytosine arabinoside injected into the cerebrospinal fluid), with or without prophylactic radiotherapy to the cerebral meninges. Most patients also receive oral maintenance therapy for 2–3 years. The sequence of treatment is shown in Figure 9.6.

Treatment at recurrence

A proportion of patients are cured with the initial therapy. In the rest the disease recurs and ultimately proves fatal unless second remission can be achieved, and followed by high-dose treatment and some form of

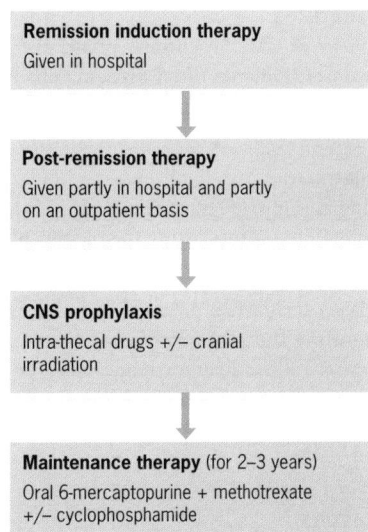

Fig. 9.6 Treatment regimen for acute lymphoblastic leukaemia.

transplant procedure. With such treatment, a further 20–30% of patients will survive long term.

Recurrence occurs most frequently in bone marrow and is associated with a worse prognosis if it occurs while the person is on maintenance therapy. Recurrence can also appear in the CNS and in the testes, requiring local as well as systemic therapy.

Chronic leukaemias

Chronic myeloid leukaemia (CML)

CML accounts for around 20% of all leukaemias. It is almost exclusively a disease of adults. The peak age for presentation is 40–60 years. The illness has a progressive clinical course which starts with a chronic phase of 3–4 years' duration. This evolves into an accelerated phase which may be manifest by increasing fever, weight loss, increasing splenomegaly, anaemia, thrombocytopenia and refractory leucocytosis with increasing numbers of blast cells. Cytogenetic abnormalities in addition to the standard t(9;22) may be acquired as the disease progresses.

The duration of the accelerated phase is variable though blastic transformation usually supervenes within a few months. Unlike de novo acute leukaemia, the blastic phase of CML is characterized by the development of acute leukaemia which may be myeloid (80%) or lymphoid (20%) in origin. The blastic phase is generally refractory to treatment, the median survival being less than 6 months. Less frequently, CML transforms into myelofibrosis, death ensuing from bone marrow failure.

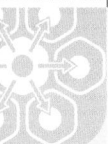

Clinical features

The *symptoms* of CML in chronic phase are usually of insidious onset. Patients often present when a routine blood count is performed for other reasons. Symptoms may be:

- anaemia
- sweating at night, fever, weight loss
- abdominal discomfort owing to splenic enlargement.

Symptoms of leucostasis from a high white cell count, e.g. blurred vision, headaches, or rarely, in males, priapism.

The signs are those of anaemia, with splenomegaly. In leucostasis retinal haemorrhages may be observed at fundoscopy. Their detection is important as leuco-phoresis should be performed as a matter of urgency (see AML).

Investigations

- **Blood count.** Hb is low or normal. WCC is raised with, characteristically, the whole spectrum of myeloid precursors, including a few blast cells visible on the blood film.
- **Platelet count.** This may be low, normal or raised.
- **Bone marrow aspirate.** This shows a hypercellular marrow with an increase in myeloid precursors. On cytogenetic analysis, the Ph chromosome t(9;22) is present in most patients (Fig. 9.7).

Expression of the *BCR-ABL* oncogene can be detected by reverse transcriptase polymerase chain reaction (RT-PCR) in all patients; if it is absent, the diagnosis is called into doubt.

Differential diagnosis

The differential diagnosis of CML can be divided into (a) reactive neutrophilia and (b) other myeloproliferative disease, such as primary proliferative polycythaemia (polycythaemia vera), or atypical CML. The presence of splenomegaly, absence of infection or cancer, or white cell count greater than $100 \times 10^9/L$, together with typical blood and bone marrow appearances, usually point towards malignancy rather than a reactive process.

Treatment

Alpha-interferons have been shown to induce haemato-logical remission in the majority of patients with CML and cytogenetic remission in about 10%. A further pro-portion of patients will have a reduction in the number of Ph chromosome-containing cells, which has been shown to be associated with prolongation of survival. The problems with IFN treatment are (a) that it has to be given by subcutaneous injection and (b) that at the relatively high doses needed to induce a meaningful cytogenetic response, most people experience side-effects (lack of energy and fatigue) which may make it hard to continue with the treatment. Preparations of interferon conjugated to polyethylene glycol (p. 486) reduce the

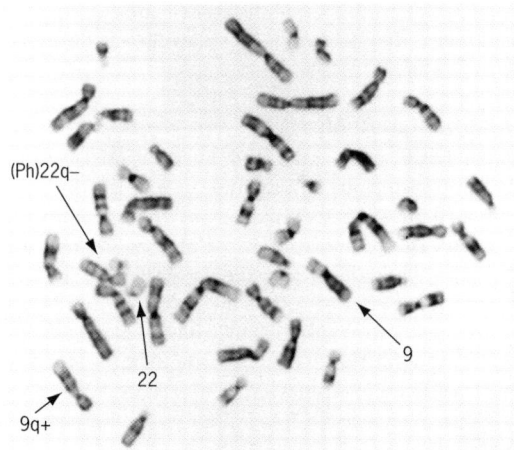

Fig. 9.7 Philadelphia chromosome. This is formed by a reciprocal translocation of part of the long arm (q) of chromosome 22 to chromosome 9. It is seen in 90–95% of patients with chronic granulocytic leukaemia. The karyotype is expressed as 46XX, (9;22)(q34;q11).

need for daily injections and hence toxicity. STI571, a tyrosine kinase inhibitor with specificity for *BCR-ABL*, has shown impressive efficacy in early clinical trials.

Myeloablative therapy supported by allogeneic BMT can be curative but the approach is limited by donor availability, the age of the patient, and the morbidity and mortality of the transplant procedure (see below). With the development of national and international donor panels, younger patients should now be considered for high-dose treatment with matched unrelated donor marrow. The use of high-dose treatment supported by autologous peripheral blood progenitor cells is also being evaluated, as is the use of non-myeloablative allo-geneic transplants (p. 484).

Chronic lymphocytic leukaemia (CLL)

CLL is characterized by an uncontrolled proliferation and accumulation of mature B lymphocytes (although T cell CLL does occur). The symptoms are a conse-quence of bone marrow failure and immunosuppres-sion: anaemia, infection and bleeding. A proportion of patients may remain asymptomatic and never need any treatment, dying of an unrelated cause. However, in the remainder, the disease can usually be kept under control for 9–10 years, infection being the predominant cause of death. Occasionally, CLL evolves into a high-grade large-cell non-Hodgkin's lymphoma (so-called 'Richter's transformation'). This usually responds very poorly to treatment.

Two different staging classifications are in use (Table 9.14). They are useful because they correlate closely with prognosis. The median survival of patients with stage 0 (or stage A) CLL is over 10 years, compared with 5 years for patients presenting with stages III or IV (or stage C) disease.

Table 9.14
The Rai and Binet staging systems for chronic lymphocytic leukaemia*

System and stage	Risk	Manifestations	Percent of patients	Median survival	Recommended treatment
Rai staging system					
0	Low	Lymphocytosis	31	>10	Watch and wait
I	Intermediate	Lymphadenopathy	35	9	Treat only with progression[†]
II	Intermediate	Splenomegaly, lymphadenopathy, or both	26	7	Treat only with progression[†]
III	High	Anaemia, organomegaly, or both	6	5	Treatment indicated in most cases
IV	High	One or more of the following: anaemia, thrombocytopenia and organomegaly	2	5	Treatment indicated in most cases
Binet staging system					
A	Low	Lymphocytosis, < 3 lymphoid areas enlarged[‡]	63[§]	>10	Watch and wait
B	Intermediate	≥ 3 Lymphoid areas enlarged[‡]	30	7	Treatment indicated in most cases
C	High	Anaemia, thrombocytopenia or both	7	5	Treatment indicated in most cases

* Lymphocytosis is present in all stages of the disease
[†] Progression is defined by weight loss, fatigue, fever, massive organomegaly and a rapidly increasing lymphocyte count
[‡] Enlarged lymphoid areas may include the cervical, axillary and inguinal lymph nodes; the spleen or liver may be enlarged
[§] Stage A includes all patients with Rai stage 0 disease, two-thirds of patients with Rai stage I disease and one-third of those with Rai stage II
From Dighiero G, Binet JL (2000) *New England Journal of Medicine* **343**: 1800

Clinical features

In asymptomatic patients, the diagnosis is often a chance finding on the basis of a blood count done for a quite different reason.

The *symptoms and signs* are:

- recurrent infections resulting from neutropenia and reduced immunoglobulin levels
- symptoms of anaemia, which may develop rapidly in the context of haemolysis (often precipitated by infection)
- painless lymph node enlargement and splenomegaly.

Investigations
Blood count:

- **Hb**: low or normal
- **WCC**: $> 15 \times 10^9/L$ of which at least 40% are lymphocytes
- **Platelets**: low or normal
- **Serum immunoglobulins**: low or normal
- **Coombs' test**: positive if haemolysis is occurring.

The diagnosis is usually made by the peripheral blood appearances, which usually show typical CLL small lymphocytes. Confirmation is provided by immunophenotyping, which shows co-expression of the CD5 and CD19 antigen. Cytogenetic abnormalities involving chromosomes 12 or 14 may be observed, and may have prognostic importance.

Treatment
The disease may remain stable for several years. There is no advantage in starting treatment before there is a clinical indication, such as anaemia, recurrent infections, bleeding, 'bulky' lymphadenopathy or increasing

splenomegaly. Chlorambucil is most often used, with or without prednisolone. Treatment is given intermittently, as and when necessary. Chlorambucil may be effective repeatedly. Haemolysis is a life-threatening situation and is treated in the first instance by high-dose steroids. The purine analogue fludarabine can achieve CR in some patients as opposed to just response. However, such remissions are not durable, and it remains to be seen whether fludarabine should be used as initial therapy instead of chlorambucil. Bone marrow transplantation for CLL is currently experimental.

Hairy cell leukaemia (HCL)
HCL is a clonal proliferation of abnormal B (or very rarely T) cells which, as in CLL, accumulate in the bone marrow and spleen. It is a rare disease of late middle age. The bizarre name relates to the appearance of the cells on a blood film – they have an irregular outline owing to the presence of filament-like cytoplasmic projections.

Clinical features are similar to CLL.

Treatment
The drug 2-chloroadenosine acetate (2-CDA) has been shown to have specific activity in this illness, complete remission often being achieved with just one cycle of treatment. The remissions sometimes last for several years and patients can be re-treated. Alpha-interferon, and the purine analogue deoxycoformycin, are also effective.

Prolymphocytic leukaemia
Prolymphocytic leukaemia is another rare disorder, often mistaken for CLL. It may be of B or of T cell lineage. It is characterized by bone marrow failure

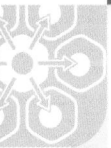

(anaemia, neutropenia and thrombocytopenia) and – as in HCL – splenomegaly. Treatment generally comprises chlorambucil as for CLL, although splenectomy may be indicated and fludarabine can be useful.

FURTHER READING

Dightero G, Binet JL (2000) When and how to treat chronic lymphatic leukaemia. *New England Journal of Medicine* **343**: 1799–1801.

Faderl S et al (1999) The biology of chronic myeloid leukaemia. *New England Journal of Medicine*. **341**: 164–172

Goldman JM, Melo JV (2001) Targeting the BCR-ABL tyrosine kinase in chronic lymphatic leukaemia. *New England Journal of Medicine* **344**: 1084–1086.

Leukaemia Series. *The Lancet*, starting January 1997.

Kersey JH (1997) Fifty years of the biology and therapy of childhood leukemia. *Blood* **90**: 4243–4251.

Rohatiner A, Lister TA (1996) Acute myelogenous leukemia in adults. In: Henderson ES, Lister TA, Greaves MF (eds) *Leukemia*. Philadelphia: WB Saunders, p. 479.

The myelodysplastic syndromes (MDS)

These are a heterogeneous group of myeloid disorders characterized by abnormal morphology and maturation in the bone marrow. They are much more common in older subjects, and often occur in response to bone marrow damage or acquired genetic rearrangement. MDS is as common as acute myeloid leukaemia and is being recognized with increasing frequency. They are described in detail on page 443.

The lymphomas

Lymphomas represent abnormal proliferations of B or T cells and are currently classified on the basis of histological appearance into:

- Hodgkin's disease
- non-Hodgkin's lymphomas.

The distinction between lymphoid leukaemias and lymphomas is not always clear. Often the same disease may be referred to as either lymphoma or leukaemia depending on whether it presents primarily in the lymph nodes or the blood and bone marrow. The World Health Organization classification of lymphoid neoplasms has helped to address some of these issues (see Table 9.17).

Hodgkin's disease (HD)

With modern treatment (radiotherapy, chemotherapy or both), HD is now curable in the majority of patients. The choice of treatment is determined largely by the distribution and extent of disease. The staging is shown in Table 9.15. The Ann Arbor staging classification has been modified to take into account the volume of lymph node masses and the use of modern imaging techniques such as CT scanning.

Clinical features

The symptoms and signs are:

- lymph node enlargement, most often of the cervical nodes (other causes are shown in Table 9.16); these are usually painless
- enlargement of the spleen/liver
- 'B' symptoms: fever, drenching night sweats, weight loss of >10% bodyweight (see Table 9.15)

Table 9.15

Staging classification of Hodgkin's disease (modified Ann Arbor classification)*, †

I	Involvement of a single lymph node region (I) or a single extralymphatic organ or site (IE)
II	Involvement of two or more lymph node regions on the same side of the diaphragm (II) or one or more lymph node regions plus an extralymphatic site (IIE)
III	Involvement of lymph node regions on both sides of the diaphragm (III) (the spleen is included in stage III, e.g. splenic involvement plus cervical lymph node enlargement = stage III)
IV	Involvement of one or more extralymphatic organs, e.g. lung, liver, bone, bone marrow, with or without lymph node involvement

* All stages are subclassified as A (asymptomatic) or B (fever, night sweats and loss of > 10% of bodyweight)

† Bulky disease (a lymph node mass > 10 cm in diameter, or if involving the mediastinum a mass greater than one-third of the intrathoracic diameter at the level of T10) is denoted by the suffix X

Table 9.16

Differential diagnosis of cervical lymph node enlargement

Infections	**Primary lymph node malignancies**
Acute	Hodgkin's disease
Pyogenic infections	Non-Hodgkin's lymphoma
Infective mononucleosis	Chronic lymphocytic leukaemia
Toxoplasmosis	Acute lymphoblastic leukaemia
Cytomegalovirus infection	
Infected eczema	**Secondary malignancies**
Cat scratch fever	Nasopharyngeal
Acute childhood exanthema	Thyroid
	Laryngeal
Chronic	Lung
Tuberculosis	Breast
Syphilis	Stomach
Sarcoidosis	
HIV infection	**Miscellaneous**
	Kawasaki's syndrome
Connective tissue disorders	
Rheumatoid arthritis	
Drug reactions	
Phenytoin	

other constitutional symptoms, such as pruritus, fatigue, anorexia and, occasionally, alcohol-induced pain at the site of enlarged lymph nodes

symptoms due to involvement of other organs (e.g. lung, bone, liver).

Investigations

- **Blood count** may be normal, or there can be a normochromic, normocytic anaemia.
- **Erythrocyte sedimentation rate** (ESR) is usually raised.
- **Liver biochemistry** is abnormal if the liver is involved.
- **Uric acid** is normal or raised.
- **Chest X-ray** may show mediastinal widening, with or without lung involvement.
- **CT scans** may show involvement of intrathoracic, abdominal or pelvic lymph nodes.
- **Bone marrow aspirate and trephine biopsy** may show involvement in patients with advanced disease. This is unusual at initial presentation.
- **Lymph node biopsy** is required for a definitive diagnosis. Classically, Sternberg–Reed cells are

present, together with a characteristic admixture of lymphocytes and histiocytes (Fig. 9.8). The Sternberg–Reed cell is usually a clonal, malignant B lymphocyte. Other cells in the lymph node may represent an immune reaction to the disease. Cytokine secretion, particularly interleukin-5, is increased and may account for many of the clinical features associated with Hodgkin's disease.

A typical chest X-ray and CT scan in one patient are shown in Figure 9.9.

Treatment

Initially, treatment is nearly always given with curative intent and consists of radiotherapy, cyclical combination chemotherapy or both. The choice of treatment will depend predominantly on:

- stage
- sites of involvement
- the 'bulk' of lymph node masses
- the presence or absence of 'B' symptoms (Table 9.15).

Stages IA and IIA

The majority of patients are treated with radiotherapy, provided that all the involved sites can be encompassed within a radiation field. Patients with a large mediastinal mass are usually given chemotherapy first, otherwise too much lung tissue would be irradiated with potential long-term damage. Radiotherapy is given subsequently.

Although radiotherapy is highly effective treatment for HD and does not cause some of the side-effects associated with chemotherapy (see p. 483), it is recognized that there is an increased risk of breast cancer in patients treated with high doses of radiotherapy to the mediastinum. There is also concern about potential impairment of cardiac function following irradiation of the mediastinum. In addition, up to 30% of patients with localized Hodgkin's disease may relapse following radiotherapy. As a result, adjuvant chemotherapy regimens are under evaluation.

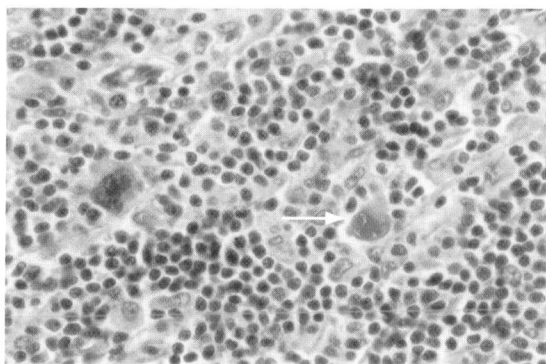

Fig. 9.8 **Histological appearance of Hodgkin's disease.** There is a background rich in small lymphocytes and histiocytes together with scattered mononuclear Hodgkin's cells and a classical binucleate Sternberg–Reed cell (arrow) to the right of centre. Courtesy of Dr AJ Norton.

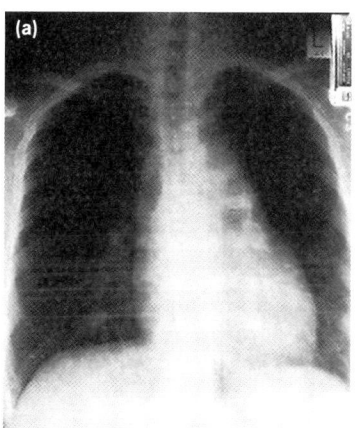

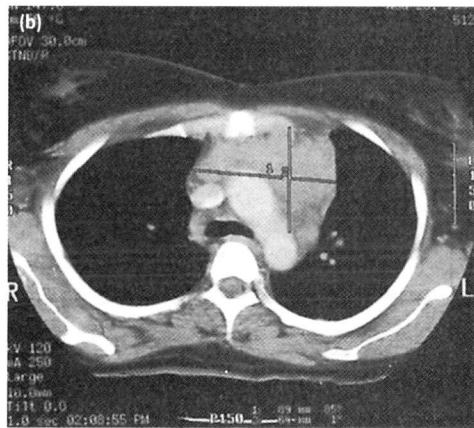

Fig. 9.9 **(a) Chest X-ray of a large mediastinal mass that is due to Hodgkin's disease. (b) CT scan of the same patient.** The mass is indicated here by crossed lines.

Stages IIB, IIIA/B and IVA/B

Treatment comprises combination chemotherapy in the first instance, with subsequent radiotherapy to sites of 'bulky' disease to reduce the risk of local recurrence.

New regimens designed to minimize the long-term effects experienced with the old chemotherapy regimens have been developed. The amount of alkylating agent is reduced with the addition of drugs such as doxorubicin leading to less infertility and second malignancies. The emphasis has been on using alternating, non-cross-resistant drug combinations, given as cycles of treatment (e.g. 4-weekly for 6 months).

Treatment for HD can usually be given on an outpatient basis and most people are able to lead a reasonably normal life while having treatment. The prognosis correlates closely with stage (Fig. 9.10). However, survival of patients in whom recurrence occurs is inferior to that of those who remain in continuous remission (Fig. 9.11).

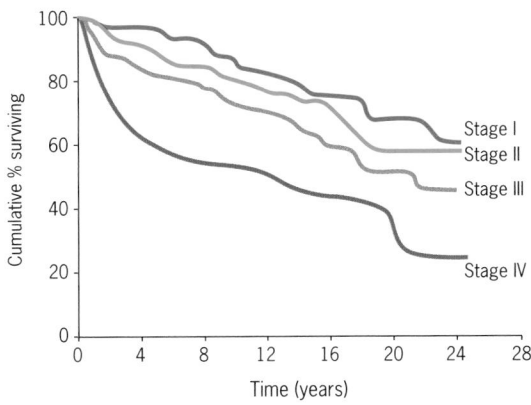

Fig. 9.10 Survival in Hodgkin's disease related to stage at presentation.

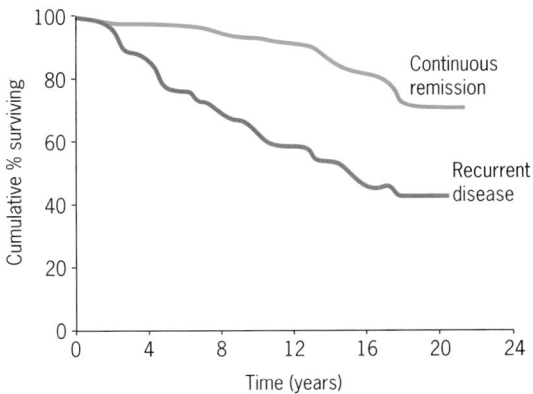

Fig. 9.11 Survival of patients with Hodgkin's disease. From Oza AM et al. (1993) Patterns of survival in patients with Hodgkin's disease: long follow-up in a single centre. From Oza AM et al. (1993) *Annals of Oncology* **4**: 385–392, with permission.

Prognosis at recurrence

Failure to achieve an initial complete or almost complete response, and recurrence within 1 year, are both associated with a very poor prognosis. Similarly, patients who develop recurrent HD more than once will almost certainly die of HD eventually. The use of myeloablative therapy with peripheral blood progenitor cell support is now being evaluated in these situations; it seems to be curative in up to 50% of subjects and has now been adopted as standard practice in western Europe. In contrast, patients who develop recurrent HD (e.g. within the abdomen) a few years after receiving radiotherapy for localized, supradiaphragmatic disease can be given combination chemotherapy and still be cured. Allogeneic transplantation for Hodgkin's disease remains experimental.

FURTHER READING

Rosenberg SA, Canellos GP (1998) Hodgkin's disease. In: Canellos GP, Lister TA, Sklar JL (eds) *The Lymphomas.* Philadelphia: WB Saunders, p. 305.

Non-Hodgkin's lymphomas (NHL)

The term 'non-Hodgkin's lymphoma' encompasses many different histological subtypes. Subdivision of the lymphomas into '*low grade*' and '*high grade*' reflects the rate at which the cells are dividing and thus the clinical progression of the disease. Paradoxically, high-grade lymphomas (those in which the cells are dividing quickly) are potentially curable, whereas low-grade lymphomas are generally considered to be incurable with conventional therapy, although patients may live for a number of years and respond to treatment several times. A further subdivision is made on the basis of B or T cell origin. Most NHLs are of B cell phenotype, although T cell tumours are increasingly being recognized.

Several different histological classifications of the non-Hodgkin's lymphomas have been suggested. The most widely used until recently was the Kiel classification, which was then superseded by the REAL (Revised European American Lymphoma Classification) and, latterly, by the proposed WHO classification (Table 9.17) following additional cytogenetic and immunochemical information.

Cytogenetic features

Burkitt's lymphoma was the first tumour in which a cytogenetic change was shown to involve the translocation of a specific gene. The most frequent change is a translocation between chromosomes 8 and 14 in which the *myc* oncogene moves from chromosome 8 to

Table 9.17
WHO classification of lymphoid neoplasms other than ALL

Name	Behaviour
1. Mature B cell neoplasms	
B cell CLL/small lymphocytic lymphoma	Indolent
B cell prolymphocytic leukaemia	Indolent
Lymphoplasmacytoid lymphoma	Indolent
Splenic marginal zone lymphoma (with or without villous lymphocytes)	Indolent
Hairy cell leukaemia	Indolent
Myeloma	Variable
MALT lymphoma	Indolent
Follicular lymphoma	Indolent
Mantle cell lymphoma	Variable
Diffuse large B cell lymphoma	Aggressive
Burkitt's lymphoma	Aggressive
2. Mature T cell neoplasms	
T cell prolymphocytic leukaemia	Variable
ATLL (HTLV1-associated lymphoma/leukaemia)	Variable
Mycosis fungoides	Indolent
Other indolent leukaemia/lymphomas	Indolent
Anaplastic large cell lymphoma	Aggressive
Angioimmunoblastic T cell lymphoma	Aggressive
Peripheral T cell lymphomas not otherwise classified	Usually aggressive

Hodgkin's disease

Nodular lymphocyte-predominant Hodgkin's lymphoma

Classical Hodgkin's disease
    Nodular sclerosis HD
    Lymphocyte-rich HD
    Mixed cellularity HD
    Lymphocyte-depleted HD

From Harris NL et al. (1999) *Journal of Clinical Oncology* **17**: 3835–3849

---

a position near the constant region of the immunoglobulin heavy chain gene on chromosome 14, resulting in upregulation of *myc*. Similar rearrangements involving the light chain loci are seen in the alternative Burkitt's lymphoma translocations between chromosome 8 and either chromosome 2 or 22. Other somatic cytogenetic abnormalities associated with human lymphoma are the t(14;18) in follicular lymphoma, involving upregulation of the *Bcl-2* gene, or the upregulation of cyclin D1 as a result of t(11;14) in mantle cell lymphoma.

Clinical features (Box 9.7)

Most patients present with peripheral lymph node enlargement, with or without systemic symptoms. NHL may also involve mediastinal, intra-abdominal and pelvic lymph nodes with resulting symptoms. They may involve only an extranodal site, such as part of the gastrointestinal tract, lung, brain or testis. Extranodal presentation is more common in NHL than in Hodgkin's disease.

Box 9.7

Lymphoma subtypes

Low grade	High grade
Middle-aged/older people	Any age group
Bone marrow infiltration common	Bone marrow infiltration uncommon
Incurable with conventional chemotherapy	Potentially curable

Investigations

- **Full blood count.** Anaemia, an elevated white cell count or thrombocytopenia are suggestive of bone marrow infiltration.
- **Urea and electrolytes.** Patients may have renal impairment as a consequence of ureteric obstruction secondary to intra-abdominal or pelvic lymph node enlargement.
- **Liver biochemistry.** This may be abnormal if there is hepatic involvement.
- **Chest X-ray**, **CT scans** of chest, abdomen and pelvis.
- **Bone marrow aspirate** and trephine biopsy.
- **Lymph node biopsy** (or Trucut needle biopsy, often under radiological guidance, in the case of surgically inaccessible nodes). It is essential for modern classification to submit the lymphoid tissue to immunophenotyping and cytogenetic/molecular analysis.

Treatment

As in Hodgkin's disease, treatment will depend on the extent and distribution of disease as well as on the histological subtype. Patients with localized indolent lymphoma may enter very long-term remissions with radiotherapy alone. It is not clear whether this is synonymous with cure. Those with more extensive disease require systemic therapy.

Low-grade lymphomas
Follicular lymphoma

This is often regarded as the paradigm for low-grade lymphomas. Repeated remissions can usually be achieved with relatively simple treatment, such as with the alkylating agent, chlorambucil. The response rates both at presentation, and at first and second recurrence, are approximately 75%, with a median survival of 9 years. Most patients are able to lead a normal life for most of this time. However, the disease remains incurable with conventional therapy. Several promising new approaches such as fludarabine-containing regimens, myeloablative therapy with peripheral blood progenitor cell (PBPC) support, and immunologically mediated treatments, such as antibodies to B cell antigens (e.g. CD20) or cellular immunotherapy, are therefore being investigated.

Lymphoplasmacytoid (LPC) lymphoma

This is generally a disease of older adults. The majority of patients present with advanced disease, the bone marrow frequently being involved. There may be a circulating paraprotein, often IgM but occasionally IgG. The prognosis for patients with LPC lymphoma is worse than that for patients with equivalent-stage follicular lymphoma, with a median survival of 5 years.

Mantle cell lymphoma

Again, this is predominantly a disease of older people. Most present with advanced disease, bone marrow infiltration being almost invariable. Gastrointestinal tract involvement is quite frequently seen. Although patients do respond to treatment as for follicular lymphoma, the median survival is less than 4 years. Morphologically it may be difficult to distinguish from small lymphocytic lymphoma, but may be defined by expression of the CD23 antigen in association with CD5 and CD19, and by the upregulation of PRAD/cyclin D1. The huge difference in prognosis between the two diseases underlines the importance of immunological and molecular evaluation of haematological malignancies.

High-grade lymphomas

High-grade lymphomas may be of B or T cell origin; the majority are diffuse large cell in the older REAL classification. Chemotherapy is given with curative intent. Achievement of remission is a prerequisite for cure. Treatment usually comprises an anthracycline (e.g. doxorubicin) given with cyclophosphamide, vincristine (Oncovin) and prednisolone (CHOP). Variations on the theme of CHOP have since been tried but, thus far, none has been shown to be superior. Between 60% and 70% of patients respond to treatment and about 40% overall are cured. The treatment is myelosuppressive and therefore, particularly in older patients, the main problem is potentially fatal infection.

An *International Prognostic Index* has been derived on the basis of outcome for a large number of patients treated at centres world-wide. When adjusted for age, the index shows four factors to correlate with survival (Box 9.8).

Patients who have two or all of the prognostic factors at presentation have a worse prognosis. New approaches are therefore being evaluated in this subgroup whose outlook with CHOP is generally poor. Combination with rituximab shows benefit.

Recurrent high-grade lymphoma has a grave prognosis. However, a proportion of patients who respond to further chemotherapy at recurrence can still be cured with myeloablative therapy with autologous haemopoietic progenitor cell support.

Burkitt's lymphoma

Burkitt's lymphoma is a high-grade lymphoma which was first described in children in West Africa who presented with a jaw tumour (Fig. 9.12), extranodal abdominal involvement and ovarian tumours. This type of lymphoma is endemic in West Africa where there is also a high incidence of Epstein–Barr virus (EBV) infection (p. 50). These are also areas where malaria is common and it has been suggested that the virus is carried from person to person by mosquitoes. Most patients have antibodies to EBV in their serum. The tumour is associated with a chromosome change, most commonly t(8;14). A lymphoma pathologically identical to African Burkitt's lymphoma also occurs in the United States and in Europe in adults. However, in these patients it is not usually associated with EBV, but the cytogenetic changes are the same. This disease is usually referred to as 'sporadic' Burkitt's lymphoma. The distinction from Burkitt cell ALL is made purely on the degree of infiltration of the bone marrow, irrespective of nodal and extranodal involvement. It is a very aggressive tumour; however, with modern intensive chemotherapy regimens, Burkitt's lymphoma can now be cured in most patients, particularly in children.

FURTHER READING

Hecht JL, Aster JL (2000) Molecular biology of Burkitt's lymphoma. *Journal of Clinical Oncology* **10**: 3707–3721.
Magrath IT (ed) (1997) *The Non-Hodgkin Lymphomas*, 2nd edn. Oxford: Oxford University Press.

> **Box 9.8**
>
> **Prognostic factors for non-Hodgkin's lymphoma**
>
> - Histology
> - Stage (stage III or IV)
> - Increased serum lactate dehydrogenase (LDH)
> - Performance status

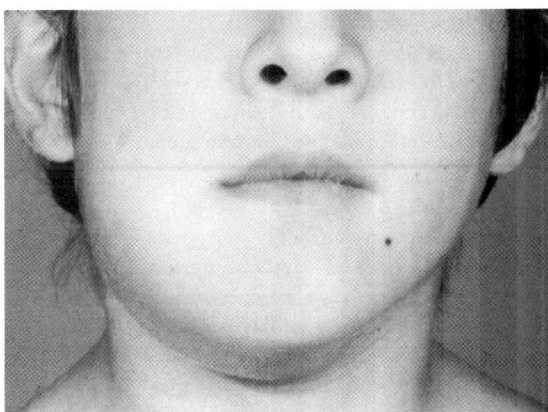

Fig. 9.12 **A child with Burkitt's lymphoma.**

Myeloma

Myeloma is part of a spectrum of diseases characterized by the presence of a paraprotein in the serum that can be demonstrated as a monoclonal band on protein electrophoresis. The paraprotein is produced by abnormal, proliferating plasma cells that produce, most often, IgG or IgA and rarely IgD. The paraproteinaemia may be associated with excretion of light chains in the urine, which are either kappa or lambda; the excess light chains have for many years been known as Bence Jones protein.

Clinical features

Myeloma is a disease of the elderly, the median age at presentation being 60 years. It is a complex illness which represents the interrelationship between:

- *bone destruction*, often causing fractures of long bones or vertebral collapse (which can cause spinal cord compression), and hypercalcaemia
- *bone marrow infiltration* resulting in anaemia, neutropenia and thrombocytopenia, together with production of the paraprotein which may (rarely) result in symptoms of hyperviscosity
- *renal impairment* owing to a combination of factors – deposition of light chains, hypercalcaemia, hyperuricaemia and (rarely) in patients who have had the disease for some time, deposition of amyloid.

Box 9.9 shows life-threatening complications and their management.

All of this is further complicated by a reduction in the normal immunoglobulin levels, contributing to the tendency for patients with myeloma to have recurrent infections.

Diagnosis

In order to make a diagnosis of myeloma, patients must have two out of three diagnostic features:

- paraprotein or Bence Jones protein
- radiological evidence of lytic lesions
- an increase in bone marrow plasma cells.

Anaemia and renal failure at presentation used to be the two factors associated with a very poor prognosis, 50% of patients dying within 9 months. The availability of renal dialysis has reduced the impact of renal failure. In patients without these features at presentation, the median survival with treatment is of the order of 2 years. The serum β_2-microglobulin level carries independent prognostic significance, as does the clinical stage of the disease at presentation. Staging is performed according to the Durie–Salmon criteria into three stages, with stage I being the earliest and stage III the most advanced. With conventional treatment, the median

survival for patients with myeloma may be 3–4 years. Younger patients receiving more intensive therapy may live longer.

Box 9.9

Life-threatening complications of myeloma

- Renal impairment – often a consequence of hypercalcaemia – requires urgent attention and patients may need to be considered for long-term peritoneal or haemodialysis.
- Hypercalcaemia should be treated by rehydration and use of bisphosphonates such as pamidronate.
- Spinal cord compression due to myeloma is treated with dexamethasone, followed by radiotherapy to the lesion delineated by a magnetic resonance imaging (MRI) scan.
- Hyperviscosity due to high circulating levels of paraprotein may be corrected by plasmapheresis.

Symptoms

- Bone pain – most commonly backache owing to vertebral involvement.
- Symptoms of anaemia.
- Recurrent infections.
- Symptoms of renal failure.
- Symptoms of hypercalcaemia.
- Rarely, symptoms of hyperviscosity (p. 502) and bleeding resulting from thrombocytopenia.

Investigations

- **Full blood count.** Hb is normal or low. WCC is normal or low. The platelet count is normal or low.
- **ESR.** This is almost always high.
- **Blood film.** There may be rouleaux formation as a consequence of the paraprotein.
- **Urea and electrolytes.** There may be evidence of renal failure (see above).
- **Serum calcium** is normal or raised.
- **Serum alkaline phosphatase** is usually normal.
- **Total protein** is normal or raised.
- **Serum albumin** is normal or low.
- **Serum protein electrophoresis** characteristically shows a monoclonal band.
- **Uric acid** is normal or raised.
- **Skeletal survey.** This may show characteristic lytic lesions, most easily seen in the skull (Fig. 9.13).
- **24-hour urine** – for assessment of light-chain excretion.
- **Bone marrow aspirate** shows characteristic infiltration by plasma cells (Fig. 9.14).

Treatment

Corrective and supportive care

Patients with myeloma may present with a number of symptomatic and life-threatening complications.

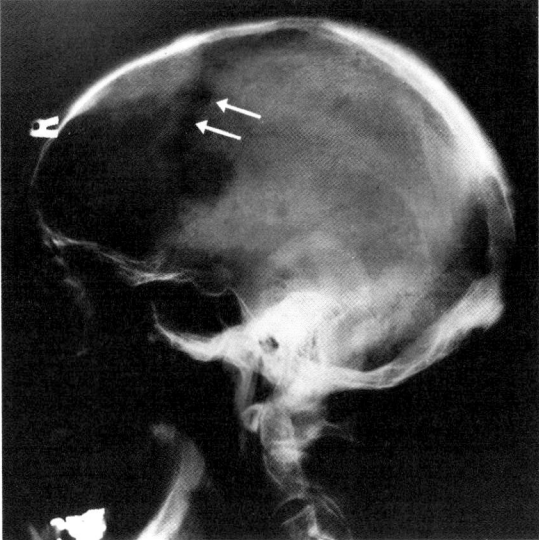

Fig. 9.13 **Myeloma affecting the skull.** Note the rounded lytic translucencies produced by infiltration of the skull with myeloma cells.

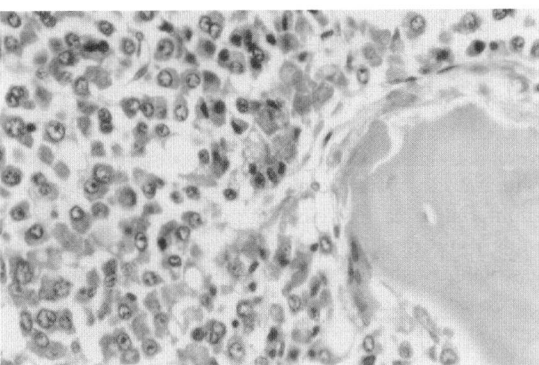

Fig. 9.14 **Multiple myeloma.** Histology shows replacement of the medullary cavity by abnormal plasma cells with some binucleate forms. A residual bony trabeculum is present towards the right. Courtesy of Dr AJ Norton.

- Anaemia should be corrected and infection treated.
- Bone pain can be helped most quickly by radiotherapy.
- Pathological fractures may also be prevented by prompt orthopaedic surgery with pinning of lytic bone lesions seen on the skeletal survey.

Myeloma is generally regarded to be incurable; no known therapy, including allogeneic bone marrow transplantation, is associated with indefinite remission. There is some debate as to whether patients with stage I myeloma should be treated with chemotherapy, or whether they should merely be monitored. Chemotherapy with melphalan has not been shown to improve survival of stage I disease, but may prevent the onset of debilitating complications such as fractures. Patients with bony lesions, bone marrow failure and renal impairment should receive chemotherapy immediately.

The use of alkylating agents (melphalan or cyclophosphamide) given in conjunction with prednisolone has improved the median survival of patients with advanced stage myeloma from 7 months to 2.5 years. More intensive doxorubicin-containing regimens may improve response rates, and might improve survival. High-dose melphalan supported by autologous BMT or PBPC support in younger patients seems to result in longer periods of remission. Adjuvant interferon therapy following both standard chemotherapy and high-dose melphalan have been shown to prolong remission, but may not significantly improve overall survival.

More recently, thalidomide has been shown to prolong remissions in myeloma. The mechanism of action is unclear, and studies continue. In addition, bony complications may be reduced in patients in 'plateau phase' by long-term administration of bisphosphonates.

The natural history of myeloma without therapy is to progress inexorably. Chemotherapy rarely eradicates the disease, but may induce a period of freedom from disease progression, known as the plateau phase. Relapse from plateau phase is inevitable after a number of months or years, and although further therapy is possible, it becomes less effective.

Waldenström's macroglobulinaemia

This is a type of lymphoplasmacytoid lymphoma. Patients tend to be older men and present with peripheral lymph node enlargement and symptoms that are due to bone marrow infiltration. The illness is associated with a paraprotein (IgM) which is responsible for symptoms of hyperviscosity.

Clinical features

- Symptoms of hyperviscosity (headaches, visual disturbance).
- General malaise and weight loss.
- Lymph node enlargement.
- Symptoms of anaemia.
- A tendency to bleed.

Investigations

- **Blood count.** Hb is normal or low. WCC is normal or low. Platelet count is normal or low.
- **ESR.** This is usually raised.
- **Blood film** usually shows rouleaux formation.
- **Bone marrow aspirate** usually shows infiltration with lymphoplasmacytoid cells.
- **Protein electrophoresis** shows an IgM paraprotein (> 20 g/L).

Treatment

Alkylating agents and, in younger patients, more intensive doxorubicin-containing regimens produce clinically significant responses but recurrence is inevitable. In patients in whom hyperviscosity is the main problem, regular plasmapheresis can be helpful. Death results from progressive bone marrow infiltration and infection.

Monoclonal gammopathy of undetermined significance (MGUS)

This is characteristically seen in older people; a paraprotein is found in the blood but the level is low (<2 g/L). Patients may be quite asymptomatic and the paraprotein detected as a result of investigations for some quite different reason. The blood count is usually normal and there is no renal impairment or bone destruction. In such patients, no specific treatment is required but they should be followed up regularly because they may later develop myeloma or lymphoma. Around 14–20% of patients with MGUS progress to myeloma. In many of these an immunoglobulin gene rearrangement can be detected in the B cells before myeloma develops, suggesting that MGUS is a clonal, premalignant disorder.

FURTHER READING

Bataille R, Harousseau J-L (1997) Multiple myeloma. *New England Journal of Medicine* **336**: 1657–1664.

Common solid tumour treatment

Some examples follow for the most common solid tumours in adults, and for some that are less common but illustrative of particular principles of medical treatment.

Lung cancer (p. 910)

This is the most common cancer in males, and the second most frequent in females (after breast cancer). It is also the most preventable cancer because over 90% is directly related to cigarette smoking.

Treatment

For practical purposes lung cancer can be divided into *small-cell cancer*, comprising about 20%, and *non-small-cell cancer*, comprising the other 80% of cases. Patients with non-small-cell lung cancer should be considered for surgery although only a quarter will be operable and only a quarter of those will be cured. Radiotherapy may provide useful palliation in inoperable patients and very good symptom relief in metastatic disease. Chemotherapy can palliate 25% of patients with platinum-containing regimens.

In small-cell lung cancer the disease has almost always disseminated by the time of diagnosis and surgery is thus inappropriate. Compared to non-small-cell lung cancer, this tumour is very chemosensitive and radiosensitive and approximately three-quarters of patients will respond to combination chemotherapy (e.g. etoposide and cisplatin) with good relief of symptoms and modest prolongation of life. A small proportion of small-cell lung cancer patients with limited disease will be cured. In patients with extensive disease, chemotherapy can still provide good symptomatic relief. As in non-small-cell lung cancer, radiotherapy can provide very useful palliative relief and may be used to treat the brain prophylactically in patients potentially cured of their systemic disease.

Breast cancer

Breast cancer is the most common cancer in women who do not smoke. The screening programme with mammography every 3 years from the age of 55 and improvements in multimodality treatment have improved overall survival and rates of cure, while breast-conserving surgery has greatly ameliorated the psychosexual impact of the disease.

Symptoms and signs

Most women present with a painless increasing mass which may also be associated with nipple discharge, skin tethering, ulceration and, in inflammatory cancers, oedema and erythema.

Investigations

The triple assessment of any symptomatic breast mass by palpation, radiology (mammography and ultrasound) and fine needle aspiration cytology is currently the most reliable way to differentiate breast cancer from the 15 times more common benign breast masses. Assessment should be carried out in a dedicated one-stop clinic able to provide the appropriate support and referral accordingly. Staging is both surgical with respect to tumour size and axillary lymph node status and, in advanced disease, by investigation of common sites of metastasis by chest X-ray, bone scan and liver scan. At present only 20% of patients are diagnosed with no evidence of microscopic nodal metastases.

Early breast cancer
Local treatment

Surgery with wide local excision and breast conservation, or mastectomy with or without reconstruction, and axillary dissection is dictated by the location and extent of the breast mass, and patient preferences. Radiotherapy is given to the conserved breast after wide local excision to reduce local recurrence, and after mastectomy if there are risk factors such as proximity to surgical margins or lymph node metastases, to complete the local control measures. Adjuvant radiotherapy reduces the risk of local recurrence by 25% and improves survival by 3%.

Adjuvant systemic treatment

Tamoxifen adjuvant therapy immediately following surgery for oestrogen and/or progesterone receptor-positive disease has reduced the relative risk of women

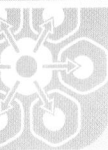

Box 9.10

Poor prognostic factors for breast cancer

- Young age
- Pre-menopausal
- Tumour size
- High tumour grade
- Oestrogen and progesterone receptor negative
- Positive nodes

Box 9.11

Clinical features that increase the likelihood of response to endocrine treatment for metastatic disease

- Oestrogen or progesterone receptor positive (60% vs 10% response in estrogen receptor (ER) negative disease)
- Long interval (more than 2 years) from initial surgery to time of relapse

dying from breast cancer by about 25%. A meta-analysis of all randomized trials of adjuvant therapy in breast cancer has shown that for premenopausal women with axillary lymph node metastases or other high-risk features (Box 9.10) adjuvant chemotherapy, most commonly with cyclophosphamide and 5-fluorouracil plus methotrexate or doxorubicin, for 6 months reduces the absolute death rate by about 10% and the relative risk of death by 20%. Ovarian ablation is equally effective as chemotherapy and when it occurs as a result of chemotherapy may explain some of its benefits. The effects of tamoxifen and chemotherapy are additive.

For postmenopausal women with oestrogen and/or progesterone receptor-positive disease, adjuvant tamoxifen given for 5 years reduces the risk of death from breast cancer by a similar 25%. Current trials have showed a small additive effect from adjuvant chemotherapy in addition to tamoxifen; however, in postmenopausal women in whom the cancer is receptor negative, chemotherapy can produce a similar relative risk reduction as at a younger age. The combined effects of radiotherapy together with the chemotherapy and tamoxifen is to halve the risk of dying of their cancer for appropriately selected patients.

Advanced breast cancer

Patients with established metastatic disease may require endocrine therapy, chemotherapy or radiotherapy. The treatment is not curative but may be of great palliative benefit and consistent often with many years of good-quality life. Little additional benefit has been gained by adding endocrine and chemotherapy together, although recently the addition of anti-HER2 antibodies to chemotherapy has produced a modest survival advantage. In general therefore, the serial use of intermittent courses of the different hormonal and chemotherapies seems most consistent with maintaining a good quality life for as long as possible.

Endocrine therapy

Women who have high levels of oestrogen receptors and progesterone receptors in their tumour have a greater chance of responding to endocrine treatments. In addition, certain clinical features can predict the likelihood of responding to hormonal manipulations (Box 9.11).

Table 9.18
Endocrine therapy of metastatic breast cancer

For premenopausal patients
(a) Suppression of ovarian function by means of oophorectomy, radiation-induced ovarian ablation or a GnRH analogue, e.g. Goserelin
(b) Anti-oestrogen, tamoxifen
(c) Progesterone

For postmenopausal patients
(a) Tamoxifen
(b) Progesterone
(c) Aromatase inhibitors (e.g. anastrozole)

Endocrine therapy is usually tried first in those patients who have characteristics suggesting they are likely to respond and who do not have immediately life-threatening disease. Remission lasts on average 2 years and is consistent with an excellent quality of life. When relapse occurs, further treatment with alternative agents may produce another remission. A range of hormonal manipulations is available (see also Principles of endocrine therapy, p. 485) (Table 9.18).

Chemotherapy

Chemotherapy is considered for patients who are unlikely to respond to hormonal treatment or who fail to respond to endocrine therapy or who require a rapid response if at risk of, for example, liver or respiratory failure. If chosen carefully, chemotherapy can provide good-quality palliation and prolongation of life. The most common regimens used include:

- CMF (cyclophosphamide, methotrexate, 5-fluorouracil)
- MM (mitoxantrone (mitozantrone) and methotrexate)
- doxorubicin and cyclophosphamide
- paclitaxel or docetaxel used as single agents or in combination with an anthracycline where initial cytotoxic chemotherapy has failed or is inappropriate (National Institute for Clinical Excellence, NICE, guidelines)
- vinorelbine.

There is very little difference in efficacy between the different regimens for metastatic disease with response rates varying from 40–60% for median duration of 8 months. The addition of docetaxel or trastuzumab to doxorubicin however have improved survival in metastatic breast cancer in recent years. The regimens do differ in toxicity with MM being one of the least toxic. The multiple regimens provide the possibility of avoiding drug resistance over several episodes of treatment interspersed with treatment-free periods so that the disease can be palliated often for several years.

Gastrointestinal cancer

Surgery is the primary treatment for localized gastrointestinal cancer, and provides definitive diagnosis and staging with cure of localized disease. Although many patients still present with metastases (most commonly in the liver), surgery may still be appropriate to relieve obstructive symptoms.

Upper gastrointestinal cancers

Oesophageal squamous cancer (p. 268)
In early-stage squamous cell carcinoma of the oesophagus, surgery is the treatment of choice. In patients who are inoperable, radiotherapy is given as the primary treatment. Chemotherapy, comprising 5-fluorouracil and cisplatin, given concurrently with radiotherapy, improves the cure rate to a similar level to that of surgery and is an alternative primary therapy.

Oesophageal and gastric adenocarcinoma (p. 277)
Early detection and surgery with curative potential is possible in only a minority of cases so that the overall survival at 5 years is only 5%. Attempts to improve this with adjuvant therapies show some promise with concurrent chemo-radiotherapy but this is quite toxic and will need confirmatory trials.

Colorectal cancer (p. 316)
Treatment
Surgery with total mesocolon/rectal excision offers the best rates of local control. The likelihood of cure can be related to the TNM or Duke's stage, i.e. extent of local invasion or lymph node involvement. Adjuvant radiotherapy for rectal cancers, preferably preoperatively, reduces local relapse rates, while adjuvant chemotherapy significantly improves survival of colorectal patients at high risk of relapse, i.e. with lymph node involvement (absolute increase in survival 5%, relative risk reduced by 12%).

Metastatic gastrointestinal cancers

Once detectable metastases are present, the opportunities for curative treatment are very limited. Palliation of advanced or recurrent gastrointestinal adenocarcinomas can be achieved in approximately 30% of patients for a median of 6–8 months with low-toxicity regimens of 5-fluorouracil and folinic acid chemotherapy as measured by tumour response and/or improved quality of life. New drugs such as irinotecan and oxaliplatin have been shown to both increase the response rate and prolong survival when combined with 5-FU at the cost of increased toxicity and are therefore the subject of ongoing trials.

Two special presentations deserve mention: local (anastamotic) recurrence in the colon or rectum may still be able to be curatively resected, and isolated liver metastases are amenable to local treatment such as resection, laser or cryo-ablation with up to 20% long-term survivors in carefully selected series.

Epithelial ovarian cancer

Epithelial ovarian cancer comprises 80% of all ovarian cancers, the remainder being of germ cell or stromal origin.

Symptoms and signs
Ovarian cancer typically causes few specific symptoms, sometimes there is a sensation of a pelvic mass which may become (acutely) painful, often there is only vague abdominal distension and epigastric discomfort.

Investigation
Pelvic examination should be complemented by a transvaginal ultrasound and serum CA125. Magnetic resonance imaging is currently the best imaging technique for the pelvis.

Treatment
Surgery (with total abdominal hysterectomy, bilateral salpingo-oophorectomy and omentectomy) has a major role in the treatment of ovarian cancer in all stages. For patients in whom the disease is confined to the ovary, the surgery can be curative in 80–90% if the histology is well to moderately differentiated. For patients with poorly differentiated or more advanced disease, with spread throughout the peritoneal cavity, surgery still has a major role in staging the patient and improving survival, as it has been shown that the response to chemotherapy, and survival, is much enhanced if the tumour is able to be surgically debulked to leave only small amounts (> 1 cm) of metastatic disease.

The most important drugs used to treat ovarian cancer are cisplatin and its analogue carboplatin, which is associated with fewer side-effects. Response is achieved in approximately two-thirds of patients. Paclitaxel has been shown to improve the survival of many patients when added to a platinum-based treatment such that the median survival following combination treatment of advanced metastatic disease is approximately 3 years. Up to 30% of those with metastatic disease may be alive after 5 years, although this falls to 5–10% if the cancer is not able to be debulked at operation or has spread outside the peritoneal cavity.

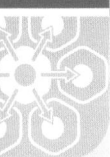
Prostate cancer

The second most common lethal cancer in males, it is almost unknown before the age of 40 and becomes increasingly common with age so that almost 70% of men are affected by the age of 80. However, for many it may be an irrelevant and coincidental finding as it will not be the cause of their death, especially if it is very well differentiated (low Gleason Score 1–4).

Serum prostate-specific antigen (PSA) tumour marker plus transrectal ultrasound with biopsy of the prostate and bone scan with pelvic CT or MRI scan is used to stage the disease. Interpretation of serum PSA must take into account the normal values, which rise with age, and the possible non-malignant causes of an increased PSA such as hyperplasia and inflammation.

Treatment

The frequency with which a finding of prostate cancer in the elderly is irrelevant to their health, has limited the usefulness of screening tests for the early detection of prostate cancer using the serum marker prostate-specific antigen (PSA).

The decision to treat early-stage prostate cancer can only be taken therefore in the full context of the patient's life expectations and co-morbid conditions. Surgical cure can be achieved by radical prostatectomy with nerve-sparing techniques, reducing the risks of impotence and incontinence. Radical radiotherapy may also offer long-term disease control, though with similar risks. Adjuvant treatment with androgen-deprivation therapy by monthly depot injections of a gonadotrophin-releasing hormone analogue such as goserelin or leuprorelin, or by orchidectomy, improves the survival of patients given local therapy, but at the cost of impotence.

Metastatic prostate cancer with either local or often skeletal spinal spread is rapidly and effectively palliated in 70% of patients by androgen deprivation. The median duration of response is 2 years and alternative treatments, e.g. chemotherapy, have yet to find a role outside of clinical trials. Radiotherapy provides a very effective palliation of painful skeletal metastases and can be delivered systemically by intravenous bone-seeking strontium-labelled bisphosphonate for patients with multiple affected sites.

Testicular and ovarian germ cell tumours

Germ cell tumours are the most common cancers in men aged 15–35 years but comprise only 1–2% of all cancers. They are much less common in women. There are two main histological types, seminoma (dysgerminoma in women) and teratoma. Teratomas may comprise varying proportions of mature and immature elements. Germ cell tumours may rarely occur in extragonadal sites in the midline from pituitary, mediastinum or retroperitoneum but should be treated in a similar manner.

Symptoms and signs

Most men present with a testicular mass which is often painful, some with symptoms of metastases to the para-aortic lymph nodes with back pain. In women the mass presents with vague pelvic mass symptoms but at a younger age than the more common epithelial ovarian cancers.

Investigations

Ultrasound of the testicle or ovary with serum tumour markers α-fetoprotein (AFP) and β-human chorionic gonadotrophin (β-HCG) and lactic dehydrogenase (LDH) followed by CT scan or MRI scan for distant metastases. Surgery for men is by the inguinal approach to avoid spillage of highly metastatic tumour in the scrotum. Surgery for diagnosis and staging stage I disease should be conservative in women with preservation of fertility because of the efficacy of chemotherapy.

Treatment
Seminomas

Seminomas are the least common of these tumours and are very radiosensitive and chemosensitive. Seminomas are associated with a raised serum LDH but only rarely a mildly raised HCG and never a raised AFP. Stage I disease limited to the gonad is associated with a 30% risk of recurrence. Adjuvant therapy with either modality leads to greater than 95% cure in early-stage disease but chemotherapy with single agent cisplatin or carboplatin does not have the long-term risks of secondary malignancy associated with radiotherapy. Combination chemotherapy (e.g. cisplatin, etoposide and bleomycin) will cure 90% of those with metastatic disease.

Teratomas

The risk of relapse with stage I disease varies from 5–40% depending upon the histological degree of differentiation and local invasion. Adjuvant chemotherapy for those at moderate to high risk (e.g. cisplatin, etoposide and bleomycin) leads to a 95% cure rate. Metastatic disease commonly involves para-aortic lymph nodes and lungs but may spread rapidly especially if there are trophoblastic (HCG-producing) elements present. HCG can be associated with gynaecomastia and can be tested for in any young male with rapidly progressive disease with a urinary pregnancy test to enable rapid institution of potentially life-saving treatment. About 80% of teratomas will express either HCG or AFP and almost all with metastatic disease will be associated with an elevation of the less-specific serum marker lactate dehydrogenase (LDH). Chemotherapy cure for metastatic teratoma varies from over 90% for those with small-volume to 40% for those with large-volume metastases.

Although approximately 20% of men will be infertile due to azoospermia at the time of diagnosis, the majority of the remainder will retain their fertility after chemotherapy and be able to father normal children. Similarly most women retain their fertility, although less is known about the association with infertility at presentation owing to the much lower frequency of germ cell tumours in women.

Cancer of unknown primary

Patients presenting with the symptoms of their metastases without a clinically obvious primary after investigation represent a common clinical problem and comprise 5–10% of patients in a specialist oncological centre. As a result of several systematic studies, some with post-mortem follow-up, the following guidance should aid the choice of appropriate investigation and treatment.

Diagnosis

Diagnosis requires histology first and foremost as it will lead to the identification of several distinct groups.

1. *Squamous cancers* – mostly presenting in the lymph nodes of the cervical region, 80% will be associated with an occult head and neck primary, the remainder arising from the lung. Inguinal nodes point usually to a primary of the genital tract or anal canal. Treatment with radiotherapy and chemotherapy may have curative potential.
2. *Poorly differentiated or anaplastic cancers* – this important group will contain the majority of the curable cancers such as high-grade lymphomas and germ cell tumours identifiable by their immunocytochemistry and tumour markers. Treatment and prognosis is as outlined in the respective primary sites.
3. *Adenocarcinomas* form the majority, and their investigation should be guided by the desire to identify the most treatable options and the knowledge that the largest proportion will have arisen from the lung or pancreas with relatively poor treatment prospects (Box 9.12). Investigations should therefore comprise a chest X-ray and abdominal CT scan with, in men, serum PSA and rectal ultrasound to identify prostate cancers, and in women, mammography to identify occult breast cancer, and pelvic CT or MRI scan to identify ovarian cancer. Tumour markers for other solid cancers, although highly sensitive, are too non-specific to be useful as diagnostic aids in this situation.

Box 9.12

Adenocarcinoma of unknown primary: primary sites with major treatment benefits

- Breast, e.g. isolated axillary lymphadenopathy
- Ovary, e.g. peritoneal carcinomatosis
- Prostate, e.g. pelvic lymphadenopathy

Treatment

Particular presentations of note in women are the isolated axillary lymph node metastasis, which should be treated as for lymph-node-positive breast cancer, and malignant ascites, which often warrants a trial of chemotherapy as for epithelial ovarian cancer, with the prognosis for those responding to the therapeutic trial being similar to disease of known primary origin. Otherwise, prognosis is generally poor with a median survival of 3 months from diagnosis. Therefore extensive investigation is not warranted when the diagnosis yield of, for example, gastrointestinal endoscopy is less than 5%. Patients presenting with other isolated nodal metastases do have a significantly better prognosis than the majority with visceral and/or bone metastases and may warrant more extensive investigation. For men the occasional occult prostatic cancer found from a raised serum PSA offers better palliative treatment prospects, otherwise decisions need to be based on the pattern of metastatic spread, fitness or performance status and a discussion of palliative aims with the patient.

FURTHER READING

Bosl GJ, Motzer RJ (1997). Testicular germ cell cancer. *New England Journal of Medicine* **337**: 242–253.
Hortobaggi GN (1998). Treatment of breast cancer. *New England Journal of Medicine* **339**: 974–984.

Palliative medicine and symptom control

Palliative care may be defined as the active, total care of patients whose disease is no longer responsive to curative treatment. The goal of this care is to achieve the best possible quality of life for patients and their families by controlling physical symptoms as well as recognizing psychological, social and spiritual problems. Death is accepted as a normal process, which should neither be hastened nor postponed and the need to provide a support system for the family in bereavement is also recognized.

Many symptoms suffered in incurable illness have a complex aetiology in which the physical component may be overlaid by psychosocial issues. For such patients considerable input from a multidisciplinary team of specialist palliative care professionals may be needed to resolve the symptoms. There is now good evidence that integration of palliative care and anti-tumour management early in the course of disease will reduce long-term distress and difficulty in symptom management. This view moves away from the traditional concentration on the provision of palliative care at the end of life.

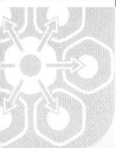

The most appropriate first step in providing care in complex situations is often to deal with physical symptoms.

Pain

The symptom most feared by cancer patients is pain, although only two-thirds suffer significant pain throughout the course of their disease. Those patients who suffer pain may present with several pains of differing aetiology, with cancer being directly responsible for about 70%. Pain may be related to associated problems such as rapid weight loss or pressure sores, or may have a separate, non-malignant cause, such as arthritis. The principles of pain relief are careful assessment and diagnosis of the cause of pain, use of analgesics according to the analgesic ladder, and regular review of the effectiveness of the prescribed drugs (Fig. 9.15).

The analgesic ladder

The cancer pain relief programme of the World Health Organization groups drugs into three main classes:

1. non-opioid drugs, such as paracetamol or aspirin and other non-steroidal anti-inflammatory medications
2. weak opioid drugs, such as codeine, dextropropoxyphene and combinations of codeine with paracetamol
3. strong opioid drugs, such as morphine and diamorphine.

The analgesic ladder states that, if optimal use of a drug from the non-opioid class (e.g. 1000 mg of paracetamol 6-hourly) does not result in satisfactory pain relief, the prescription should be increased up one step to a weak opioid. If the equivalent of codeine 60 mg 4-hourly is not sufficient to control pain, the patient will require a strong opioid. Adjuvant, co-analgesic drugs may be added to each step of the ladder.

Strong opioid drugs

Morphine is the drug of choice and in most circumstances should be given regularly by mouth. The dose can be tailored to the individual patient's needs by the addition of 'as required' doses; morphine has no ceiling analgesic effect. A suitable starting dose of morphine is 10 mg 4-hourly, or 5 mg if the patient is elderly or frail. Patients with renal failure will have impaired excretion of morphine metabolites; they should receive a single dose of morphine and be carefully observed for the return of pain in order to determine the approximate rate of excretion of the metabolites.

If a 10 mg dose of morphine relieves the pain but the relief does not last for 4 hours, a 50% increase in the dose should be made (i.e. 10, 15, 20, 30, 45, 60, 90, 120, 180 mg) until satisfactory pain control is achieved.

When the patient's 24-hour morphine requirement has been established, the prescription may be converted to a *controlled-release preparation*. There are now both 12-hour and 24-hour release preparations available. The appropriate dose may be calculated by simple addition. For example:

20 mg morphine elixir 4-hourly
= 120 mg morphine per day
= 60 mg twice-daily of a 12-hour preparation
or 120 mg daily of a 24-hour preparation.

If the patient is unable to take oral medication because of nausea or vomiting, gastrointestinal obstruction or altering levels of consciousness, the opioid should be given rectally or parentally. For cancer patients who need long-term analgesia, continuous subcutaneous infusion is the preferred route. Diamorphine is used in this situation because of its greater solubility. By subcutaneous or intramuscular injection, diamorphine is approximately twice as potent as morphine orally. Hence the conversion from oral morphine may be calculated as follows:

30 mg oral morphine 4-hourly
= 180 mg morphine per day
= 90 mg diamorphine subcutaneously over 24 hours.

Side-effects. *Constipation* caused by analgesic drugs is almost universal. The prescription of a stimulant laxative such as co-danthrusate 1–3 capsules at night should be mandatory at the same time as morphine is started. No tolerance develops to this side-effect and laxative medication must be continued as long as analgesics are prescribed.

Nausea or vomiting may occur in 30–60% of patients first started on morphine. However, for those who have worked up the analgesic ladder and who have no other cause for vomiting, the prescription of an 'as required'

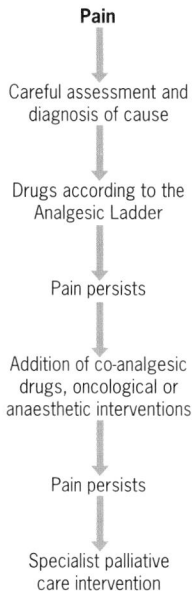

Pain
↓
Careful assessment and diagnosis of cause
↓
Drugs according to the Analgesic Ladder
↓
Pain persists
↓
Addition of co-analgesic drugs, oncological or anaesthetic interventions
↓
Pain persists
↓
Specialist palliative care intervention

Fig. 9.15 **Management of cancer pain.**

centrally acting antiemetic is usually sufficient. Tolerance will develop to this side-effect, usually within 4–5 days.

Confusion, nightmares and hallucinations occur in a small percentage of patients. Tolerance to these side-effects does not develop and a change of opiate drug is usually required.

Pain not responsive to opioids

Not all cancer pains are relieved by opioids. In some situations the addition of co-analgesic drugs will result in improved pain control. An increasing number of different classes of drugs have been used in this setting. Some of the most common include the following.

Non-steroidal anti-inflammatory drugs used in addition to a weak or strong opioid for bone pain. Published studies have most frequently used naproxen (500 mg twice-daily) but there is no clear evidence of any one drug being superior in effect. It may be that idiosyncratic side-effects require a trial of a different NSAID.

Pains of nerve destruction called dysaesthetic or deafferentation pain are generally only marginally improved by strong opiates. Several classes of drug, including *steroids*, have been found to be helpful in reducing the symptoms. In cases of constant burning dysaesthesia, the *tricyclic antidepressants* are helpful. Amitriptyline 10 mg at night increasing incrementally to 75–100 mg is usually sufficient (compare with the doses required for mood elevation) and the response, if achieved, can be expected in about a week. *Anticonvulsant* drugs are useful in the management of lancinating, neuropathic pains. Carbamazepine starting at a dose of 100 mg twice-daily is most commonly used, but sodium valproate 300 mg twice-daily may cause fewer adverse side-effects. Gabapentin is of benefit in some forms of neuropathic pain.

In addition to drugs, many other techniques such as radiotherapy, anaesthetic and neurosurgical intervention, are employed for the treatment of specific pains.

Regular review of the patient is necessary to achieve optimal pain control. Pain is a complex experience unique to each individual and its perception is modulated by the psychosocial and spiritual situation of the patient. If pain is proving difficult to control, it will be necessary to pay further attention to these other significant factors.

Gastrointestinal symptoms

Anorexia, malaise and weakness are among the most frequently troublesome symptoms in advanced cancer. Endogenously produced cytokines (e.g. tumour necrosis factor and interleukins) are mediators of the anorexia/cachexia syndrome. There is at present no specific therapy, but the approach to treatment depends on adequate management of associated symptoms. Care should be given to addressing the psychological distress caused by a change in body image, with attention to nutrition including dietary advice and the judicious use of steroids.

Nausea and vomiting occur in up to two-thirds of cancer patients in the last 6 weeks of life. The approach to treatment should be similar to that required for pain, involving careful assessment and diagnosis of the cause. It may, however, be more difficult to reach a diagnosis and a somewhat empirical approach to treatment is often adopted. In order to ensure adequate absorption of the antiemetic, parenteral administration, preferably by the subcutaneous route, may be helpful for the first 24–48 hours.

Antiemetics are classified according to their affinities for neurotransmitter receptor sites. A gastrokinetic dopamine antagonist such as metoclopramide 10 mg every 6–8 hours would be helpful in vomiting related to upper gastrointestinal tract stasis or to liver metastases. Metoclopramide should be avoided in cases of intestinal obstruction as it increases peristalsis in the upper bowel. Centrally acting antiemetics such as the phenothiazines, e.g. prochlorperazine 10 mg 8-hourly, cyclizine 50 mg 8-hourly, or the dopamine antagonist butyrophenone, haloperidol 1.5 mg 8-hourly are the drugs of choice in vomiting caused by drugs or metabolic disturbance. As with the prescription of analgesics, antiemetics will be most effective if prescribed on a regular rather than 'as-required' basis.

Bowel obstruction

Bowel obstruction may present acutely or in a more chronic manner and the cause is often multifactorial. A small number of patients may benefit from surgical intervention, so it is important that consideration be given to this modality of treatment in every case. Most patients will not be suitable for surgery and can be managed medically. The active medical management of malignant bowel obstruction includes:

- the relief of intestinal colic using an antispasmodic such as hyoscine butylbromide 60–80 mg daily; loperamide is sometimes helpful
- treating continuous pain with adequate analgesia such as diamorphine
- treating vomiting if nausea is a problem with a centrally acting antiemetic such as cyclizine 150 mg daily or haloperidol 5–10 mg daily.

It will be necessary to administer all of these medicines parenterally and the subcutaneous route is most appropriate.

Evidence suggests that the use of corticosteroids or the somatostatin analogue octreotide may shorten the length of episodes of obstruction. Octreotide also reduces the volume of fluids secreted into the bowel, thus reducing the volume of nasogastric aspirate or vomit.

Patients may be allowed to drink and eat low-residue diets which are mostly absorbed in the proximal gastrointestinal tract. It is usually possible, with adequate

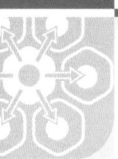
mouth care, to prevent a sensation of thirst and routine parenteral fluids are not required. A few patients with intractable vomiting due to a high intestinal block may benefit from continuous nasogastric aspiration or gastrostomy drainage.

Respiratory symptoms

Respiratory symptoms, in particular breathlessness, cause great distress to patients and their carers. Management is based on an accurate diagnosis of the cause and active treatment of all potentially reversible situations. Infections should be treated, pleural and pericardial effusions drained and symptomatic anaemic patients transfused. Radiotherapy, cytotoxic agents and local laser therapy or stent insertions may relieve specific areas of bronchial tree obstruction. The place of oxygen in managing breathlessness is not clear, but it may be helpful in patients with correctable hypoxia.

The sensation of breathlessness and a cycle of respiratory panic may be partially relieved by the prescription of regular benzodiazepines. Regular doses of short-acting opioids 5–20 mg 4-hourly are also helpful, as they are postulated to have a local as well as a central effect. Nebulization of a morphine solution may reduce the sensation of breathlessness in a proportion of patients.

Persistent unproductive cough is a very troublesome symptom. Opiates, codeine, methadone or morphine elixir are helpful as antitussive agents. Antitumour therapy may be required to alleviate pressure on a large airway. Nebulized local anaesthetic may also be helpful in the prevention of cough.

Other physical symptoms

Patients with cancer may develop a large number of physical symptoms. These may be related directly to the presence of the tumour (e.g. vaginal blood loss from a cervix carcinoma) or to the treatment received (e.g. lymphoedema of the arm following breast surgery and radiotherapy). Management of these symptoms will be specific and may require the intervention of other specialists.

Patients may also develop symptoms as a reflection of their debility, such as pressure sores, urinary incontinence, jaundice or recurrent infections. These symptoms may be managed according to the overall expectations and requirements of the patient and their family. These situations of multiple symptomatology in frail patients put considerable demands on the expertise and creativity of clinicians as they present a great challenge for the maintenance of the best possible quality of life.

Psychological symptoms

Effective communication with all patients and their families is a fundamental tenet of clinical practice but is particularly important in the stressful situations which surround fatal disease. Basic communication skills include allowing time for the patient to talk, using language which is appropriate to the circumstances, being prepared to repeat information, and being aware that both the patient and the family may receive bad news by blocking or denying it. It is important to remember that it is not always necessary to have an answer or a solution to every problem that is presented, but that considerable support may be given by sympathetic listening.

Care of cancer patients should be designed to allow them to spend as much time as possible in their own homes. Effective liaison between the cancer centre, the palliative care team and the primary healthcare team is essential to ensure total care. It is especially important to avoid misinterpretation of any information that may be given regarding treatment and prognosis.

Approximately 60% of cancer patients will die in general hospital wards under the care of the physician or surgeon who first diagnosed their tumour, although many are being transferred to hospice care. It is therefore important that every clinician develops some basic skills in symptom control and the ability to recognize those patients who require more specialist intervention. Caring for this group of patients demands detailed attention to alleviating physical symptoms and the establishment of a secure environment for the patient and family to obtain information and support.

The practice of specialist palliative medicine has traditionally been confined to patients with cancer, although most services now cover HIV and AIDS and some of the rapidly fatal neurological diseases. These are all conditions in which the clinical situation is changing rapidly and where difficult symptoms exist. There are undoubtedly patients with non-malignant disease such as end-stage renal or cardiac failure who would benefit from a similar multidisciplinary approach to their care. Expansion of specialist palliative medicine into non-malignant situations is currently being actively considered. The patient-orientated principles of palliative medicine can, however, be usefully applied throughout all medical practice.

FURTHER READING

Hardy J (2000) Sedation in terminally ill patients. *Lancet* **356**: 1866–1867

Kaye P (1997) *Tutorials in Palliative Medicine.* Northampton: EPL Publications.

Randall F, Downie RS (1996) *Palliative Care Ethics – A Good Companion.* Oxford: Oxford Medical Publications.

Twycross RG, Lack SA (1990) *Therapeutics in Terminal Cancer*, 2nd edn. Edinburgh: Churchill Livingstone.

Rheumatological and musculoskeletal disorders

Many common locomotor problems are short-lived and self-limiting or settle with a course of simple analgesia and/or physical treatment, for example, physiotherapy or osteopathy. Nonetheless, they represent 20–30% of the workload of the primary care physician. Recognition and appropriate early treatment of many painful rheumatic conditions may help reduce the incidence of chronic pain disorders. Early recognition and subsequent treatment of inflammatory arthritis by specialist multidisciplinary teams leads to better symptom control and prevents long-term joint damage and disability. A wide selection of pamphlets offer helpful advice for patients and their use should be encouraged. Most of the musculoskeletal diseases are seen world-wide, although the prevalence of individual conditions varies.

The normal joint

There are two types of joints – synovial and fibrocartilaginous.

Synovial joints (Fig. 10.1)
These include the ball-and-socket joints (e.g. hip) and the hinge joints (e.g. interphalangeal).

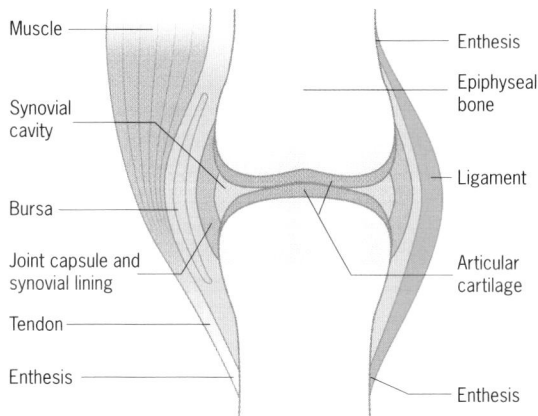

Fig. 10.1   The synovial joint.

They possess a cavity and permit the opposed cartilaginous articular surfaces to move painlessly over each other. Movement is restricted to a required range, and stability is maintained during use. The load is distributed across the surface, thus preventing damage by overloading or disuse.

Synovium and synovial fluid

Normal synovium is a few cells thick and vascular. Its surface is smooth and non-adherent and is permeable to proteins and crystalloids. As there are no macroscopic gaps, it is able to retain normal joint fluid even under pressure. The surface layer comprises macrophages and fibroblast-like cells. The fibroblasts release hyaluronan into the joint space, which helps to retain fluid in the joint. Synovial fluid is a highly viscous fluid secreted by the synovial cells and has a similar consistency to plasma. Glycoproteins ensure a low coefficient of friction between the cartilaginous surfaces. The synovium and synovial fluids also line tendon sheaths and bursae.

Fibrocartilaginous joints

These include the intervertebral discs, the sacroiliac joints, the pubic symphysis and the costochondral joints.

Juxta-articular bone

The bone which abuts a joint (epiphyseal bone) differs structurally from the shaft (metaphysis). It is highly vascular and comprises a light framework of mineralized collagen enclosed in a thin coating of tougher, cortical bone. The ability of this structure to withstand pressure is low and it collapses and fractures when the normal intra-articular covering of hyaline cartilage is worn away – as, for example, in osteoarthritis (OA). Loss of surface cartilage also leads to the abnormalities of bone growth and remodelling typical of OA (see p. 533).

Hyaline cartilage

This forms the articular surface and is avascular. It relies on diffusion from synovial fluid for its nutrition. It is rich in type II collagen that forms a meshwork enclosing giant macromolecular aggregates of proteoglycan. These heterogeneous macromolecules comprise protein chains (aggrecans) to which are attached side-chains of the carbohydrates keratan and chondroitin sulphate. These molecules retain water in the structure by producing a dynamic tension between the retaining force of the collagen matrix and the expansive effect of osmotic pressure. Intermittent pressure from 'loading' of the joint is essential to normal cartilage function and encourages movement of water, minerals and nutrients between cartilage and synovial fluid. Chondrocytes secrete collagen and proteoglycans and are embedded in the cartilage. They migrate towards the joint surface along with the matrix they produce.

Ligaments and tendons

These structures stabilize joints. Ligaments are variably elastic and this contributes to the degree of stiffness or laxity of joints (see p. 571). Tendons are inelastic and transmit muscle power to bones. The joint capsule is formed by intermeshing tendons and ligaments. The point where a tendon or ligament joins a bone is called an *enthesis* and may be the site of inflammation.

Components of extracellular matrix

All connective tissues contain an extracellular matrix of macromolecules – collagens, elastins, non-collagenous glycoproteins and proteoglycans in addition to cells, e.g. fibroblasts.

Collagens

Collagens consist of three polypeptide chains (alpha chains) wound into a triple helix These alpha chains contain repeating sequences of *Gly–x–y* triplets, where *x* and *y* are often prolyl and hydroxyprolyl residues. Collagen fibres show considerable genetic heterogeneity, with the genes on at least 12 chromosomes. The majority of collagen in the body is type I – the major component of bone, tendon, ligament, skin, sclera, cornea, blood vessels and the hollow organs. Types III, V and VI are also present in most tissues although little collagen type III is found in bone or cartilage. Other types of collagen are tissue specific, i.e. types II, IX, X and XI are found in hyaline cartilage, type IV in basement membrane and type VII in anchoring structures at junctions between epithelium and mesenchyme. There are several classes of collagen genes, based on their protein structures, and abnormalities of these may lead to specific diseases (see p. 585).

Elastin

Elastin is an insoluble protein polymer and is the main component of elastic fibres. Tropoelastin, its precursor, is synthesized by vascular smooth muscle cells and skin fibroblasts. Cross-linkages with desmosine and isodesmosine are specific to elastin fibres.

Glycoproteins

Fibronectin is the major non-collagenous glycoprotein in the extracellular matrix. Its molecule contains a number of functional domains, or cell recognition sites that bind ligands and are involved in cellular adhesion. A synthetic peptide sequence (*Arg–Gly–Asp*), which mimics some of the functions of fibronectin, is also found in other adhesion proteins (e.g. vitronectin, laminin and collagen type VI). Fibronectin plays a major role in tissue remodelling. Its production is stimulated by interferon-gamma and by transforming growth factor-beta and inhibited by tumour necrosis factor and interleukin-1.

Proteoglycans

These proteins contain glycosaminoglycan side-chains and are of variable form and size. Many have been identified at different sites in connective tissue, e.g. aggrecan, biglycan, fibromodulin, decorin (in extracellular matrix), syndecan, CD44, fibroglycan (on cell surfaces), cerebroglycan (in brain), serglycan (in intracellular tissues) and perglycan (in basement membranes). Their function is to bind extracellular matrix together, retain soluble molecules in the matrix and assist with cell binding. Abnormalities of any of these structures may lead to periarticular or articular symptoms and/or predispose to the development of arthritis.

Joint sensation

The ligaments, periosteum, synovial tissue and capsule of the joint are richly supplied by blood vessels and nerves. Pain usually derives from inflammation of these sites because the synovial membrane is relatively insensitive.

Clinical approach to the patient

Box 10.1 shows rheumatological terms.

Taking a musculoskeletal history

The following questions are helpful in assessing the problem and making a diagnosis. A history, taken carefully, can often lead to a diagnosis. Pattern recognition is the key to accurate diagnosis in rheumatic diseases.

Pain

- *Where is it? Is it localized or generalized?* The pattern of joint involvement is an important clue to the diagnosis (e.g. distal interphalangeal joints in osteoarthritis).
- *Is it arising from joints, the spine, muscles or bone?* Soft tissue lesions and inflamed joints are locally tender.
- *Could it be referred from another site?* Joint pain is localized but may radiate distally – shoulder to upper arm; hip to thigh and knee.

Box 10.1

Terms used in rheumatology

Monarticular	One joint involved
Polyarticular	Many joints involved (usually more than four)
Oligoarticular or pauciarticular	Two, three or four joints involved
Migratory	Arthritis moving from joint to joint
Arthralgia	Joint pain without swelling
Seropositive	Rheumatoid-factor positive
Seronegative	Rheumatoid-factor negative

- *Is it constant, intermittent or episodic? How severe is it – aching or agonizing?* For example, the pain of gout, or of septic arthritis in a previously fit, non-immunocompromised patient is agonizing. Joint pain lasting a day or so may indicate palindromic rheumatism, whilst longer bouts of a few days are typical of untreated gout. Constant pain, especially pain at night, may be due to an underlying malignancy.
- *Are there aggravating or precipitating factors?* For example:
  Mechanical problems are made worse by activity and eased by rest.
  Inflammatory joint pain and pain from the spine are worse after rest and improve with activity.
  Trauma is a common cause of musculoskeletal pain.
- *Are there any associated neurological features?* Numbness, pins and needles and/or loss of power suggest 'nerve' pain. Consider carpal tunnel syndrome (see p. 1213), a spinal problem such as disc prolapse (p. 1218) or spondylosis (p. 1218), or neurological disease. Nerve root pain, such as that due to a disc prolapse, reflects the anatomical distribution of the affected root.

Stiffness

- *Is it generalized or localized?* Spine or joint stiffness is common after injury.
- *Does it affect the limb girdles or periphery?*
- *Is it worse in the morning and relieved by activity?* Joints that are stiff for more than 15 minutes each morning are usually inflamed – think of rheumatoid arthritis (RA) (see p. 537) or another cause of inflammatory arthritis. Spinal stiffness and pain which is much worse in the morning may indicate ankylosing spondylitis (p. 548), especially in patients in their twenties or thirties. Shoulder and pelvic girdle stiffness and pain, which are worse in the morning in a patient over 55 years, may be polymyalgia rheumatica (p. 565).

Swelling

- *Is it of one joint, or of several?* Look for symmetry or asymmetry, and/or a peripheral or proximal pattern; these are important clues to the type of arthritis. Rheumatoid arthritis is typically polyarticular. An acute monarthritis may be due to trauma, gout (in a middle-aged male) or sepsis (fever or immunosuppression).
- *Is it constant or episodic?*
- *Are episodes of swelling short-lived, or longer?*
- *Is there associated inflammation (redness and warmth)?*

Gender

Gout (see p. 552), reactive arthritis (p. 550) and ankylosing spondylitis (p. 548) are more common in men. Rheumatoid arthritis and other autoimmune connective tissue diseases are more common in women.

Age

- *Is the person young, middle-aged or older? Injury is common in young people but can occur at any age.*
- *How old was the patient when the problem first started?* Osteoarthritis (see p. 533) and polymyalgia rheumatica (p. 565) rarely affect the under-fifties. Rheumatoid arthritis starts most commonly in women aged 20–50 years.

General health

- *Is there any associated ill-health or other worrying feature, such as weight loss or fever?* Systemic illness is a common feature of many rheumatic diseases. If there is weight loss and/or fever, think of autoimmune rheumatic disease, sepsis (joint infection may be due to septicaemia and is a medical emergency) or malignancy.
- *Are there other associated medical conditions that may be relevant?* Psoriasis (see p. 1287) or inflammatory bowel disease is associated with asymmetrical arthritis. Charcot's joints (p. 1098) are seen in diabetics.

Medication

Could a drug be a cause? Diuretics may precipitate gout in men and older women. Hormone replacement therapy or the oral contraceptive pill may precipitate systemic lupus erythematosus (SLE) (p. 557). Steroids can cause avascular necrosis. Some drugs cause a lupus-like syndrome (p. 559).

Race

Is this relevant? Sickle cell disease causes joint pain in young black Africans, but osteoporosis (see p. 578) is uncommon in older black Africans.

Past history

Have there been any similar episodes or is this the first? Are there any clues from previous medical conditions? Gout is recurrent; the episodes settle without treatment in about 10 days. Acute episodes of palindromic rheumatism may predate the onset of rheumatoid arthritis (see p. 537).

Family history

Does anyone in the family have a similar problem or another related disorder? Osteoarthritis may be familial. Seronegative spondarthritis (see p. 547) is seen in families with a history of arthritis, psoriasis, ankylosing spondylitis or inflammatory bowel disease. Autoimmunity has a familial tendency.

Occupational history

What job does the patient do? This can be a factor in soft tissue problems and osteoarthritis (e.g. in heavy labourers and dancers). Work-related problems are becoming more common and are complained of more.

Psychosocial history

- *Has there been an injury for which a legal case for compensation is pending?*
- *Has there been any recent major stress in family or working life? Could these be relevant?* Stress rarely causes rheumatic disease but may precipitate a flare-up of inflammatory arthritis. Stress also tends to reduce a person's ability to cope with pain or disability. Remember that the diagnosis of a chronic arthritis has a major influence on the lifestyle of the patient and their family. The extent of disability should be noted.

Extent of disability

The World Health Organization describes the impact of disease on an individual in terms of:

- *Impairment:* any loss or abnormality of psychological or anatomical structure or function
- *Disability:* any restriction or lack of ability to perform an activity in the manner or within the range considered normal for a human being
- *Handicap:* a disadvantage for an individual resulting from an impairment or disability that limits or prevents the fulfilment of a role that is normal for that individual.

The patient's own perception of limitation must be taken into account during assessment, as well as the impact of physical causes due to disease. Subjective and objective assessments must be made. Quality of life (QoL) involves physical and psychosocial factors. The aim of treatment is to reduce or cure physical and/or psychological disease and to reduce the impact of any impairment or disability on the individual. A variety of different standard questionnaires can be used to assess pain, disease impact and outcome (e.g. Health Assessment Questionnaire (HAQ), Arthritis Impact Measurement Scale (AIMS)).

Examination of the joints

Always observe a patient, looking for disabilities, as he or she walks into the room and sits down. General and neurological examinations are often necessary. Guidelines for rapid examinations of the limbs and spine are shown in Practical box 10.1.

Examining an individual joint involves three stages – looking, feeling and moving:

- *Appearance.* Look at it for swelling, rash or erythema, muscle wasting, deformity such as a distal bone displaced laterally as in knock knees (genu valgus) or bowed legs (genu varus), fixed flexion or hyperextension, loss of normal range and lack of fluidity of movement, and any pain caused by movement.

Practical box 10.1

Rapid examinations of the limb and spine

Rapid examination of the upper limbs
- *Raise arms sideways to the ears (abduction). Reach behind neck and back.* Difficulties with these movements indicate a shoulder or rotator cuff problem.
- *Hold the arms forward, with elbows straight and fingers apart, palm up and palm down.* Fixed flexion at the elbow indicates an elbow problem. Examine the hands for swelling, wasting and deformity.
- *Place the hands in the 'prayer' position with the elbows apart.* Flexion deformities of the fingers may be due to arthritis, flexor tenosynovitis or skin disease. Painful restriction of the wrist limits the person's ability to move the elbows out with the hands held together.
- *Make a tight fist.* Difficulty with this indicates a loss of flexion or grip. Grip strength can be measured.

Rapid examination of the lower limbs
- *Ask the patient to walk* a short distance away from and towards you, and to stand still. Look for abnormal posture or stance.
- *Ask the patient to stand on each leg.* Severe hip disease causes the pelvis on the non-weight-bearing side to sag (positive Trendelenburg test).
- *Watch the patient stand and sit*, looking for hip and/or knee problems.

- *Ask the patient to straighten and flex each knee.*
- *Ask the patient to place each foot in turn on the opposite knee with the hip externally rotated.* This tests for painful restriction of hip or knee. Abnormal hips or knees must be examined lying.
- *Move each ankle up and down.* Examine the ankle, medial arch and toes whilst standing.

Rapid examination of the spine
Stand behind the patient.
- *Ask the patient to (a) bend forwards to touch the toes with straight knees, (b) extend backwards, (c) flex sideways, and (d) look over each shoulder, flexing and extending and side-flexing the neck.* Observe abnormal spinal curves – scoliosis (lateral curve), kyphosis (forward bending) or lordosis (backward bending). A cervical and lumbar lordosis and a thoracic kyphosis are normal. Muscle spasm is worse whilst standing and bending. Leg length inequality leads to a scoliosis which decreases on sitting or lying (the lengths are measured lying).
- *Ask the patient to lie supine.* Examine any restriction of straight-leg raising (see disc prolapse, p. 524).
- *Ask the patient to lie prone.* Examine for anterior thigh pain during a femoral stretch test (flexing knee whilst prone), which indicates a high lumbar disc problem.
- *Palpate* the spine and buttocks for tender areas.

- *Feel* it for tenderness, warmth (indicates inflammation) and swelling which may be due to fluid, soft tissue or bone. Common descriptors are 'fluctuant' (fluid), 'firm' or 'boggy' (swelling of the synovium), and 'hard' (bony).
- *Movement.* Move it to assess the passive range of movement (e.g. flexion, extension, abduction, adduction and rotation), any instability, or the production of pain and crepitus (grating) seen with cartilage damage. The normal range varies between individuals. Comparing right with left and asking the patient about any change in range help to assess whether the endpoints are normal or not. A slightly more thorough screening examination of the locomotor system, known by the acronym GALS (global assessment of the locomotor system) has been devised.

X-ray of the joint often forms an integral part of the examination.

Investigations

Investigations are unnecessary in many of the common regional musculoskeletal problems and osteoarthritis (OA); the diagnosis is clear from the history and examination findings. Tests help to exclude another condition and to reassure the patient or their primary care physician.

Useful blood screening tests

- **Full blood count**
  Haemoglobin. Normochromic, normocytic anaemia occurs in chronic inflammatory and autoimmune diseases. Hypochromic, microcytic anaemia indicates iron deficiency, often due to non-steroidal anti-inflammatory drug (NSAID) induced gastrointestinal bleeding.
  White cell count. Neutrophilia is seen in bacterial infection (e.g. septic arthritis). It also occurs with corticosteroid treatment. Lymphopenia occurs with viral illnesses or active systemic lupus erythematosus (SLE). Neutropenia may reflect drug-induced bone marrow suppression. Eosinophilia is seen in the Churg–Strauss syndrome (p. 901).
  Platelets. Thrombocythaemia occurs with chronic inflammation. Thrombocytopenia is seen in drug-induced bone marrow suppression.
- **Erythrocyte sedimentation rate (ESR) and C-reactive protein (CRP).** An increase reflects inflammation. Plasma viscosity is also raised in inflammatory disease and measured in some laboratories in place of the sedimentation rate.
- **Bone and liver biochemistry.** A raised serum alkaline phosphatase may indicate liver or bone disease. A rise in liver enzymes is seen with drug-induced toxicity. For other investigations of bone, see page 577.

Table 10.1
Conditions in which rheumatoid factor is found in the serum

Rheumatoid arthritis (70%)

Other autoimmune rheumatic diseases
Systemic lupus erythematosus (25%)
Sjögren's syndrome (90%)
Systemic sclerosis (30%)
Polymyositis/dermatomyositis (50%)
Juvenile idiopathic arthritis (some forms)

Viral infections
Hepatitis
Infectious mononucleosis

Chronic infections
Tuberculosis
Leprosy
Infective endocarditis
Syphilis

Hyperglobulinaemias
Chronic liver disease
Sarcoidosis
Cryoglobulinaemia

Normal population
Elderly
Relatives of patients with RA

Table 10.2
Conditions in which serum antinuclear antibodies are found (Hep-2 cells as substrate)

Systemic lupus erythematosus (95%)
Systemic sclerosis (95%)
Sjögren's syndrome (80%)
Polymyositis and dermatomyositis (40%)
Rheumatoid arthritis (30%)
Juvenile idiopathic arthritis (variable incidence)

Other diseases
Autoimmune hepatitis (100%)
Drug-induced lupus (100%)
Myasthenia gravis (50%)
Diabetes mellitus (25%)
Normal population (8%)

Other blood and urine tests

- *Protein electrophoretic strip and urinary Bence Jones protein* – to exclude myeloma as a cause of a raised ESR.
- *Serum uric acid* – for gout.
- *Antistreptolysin-O titre* – in rheumatic fever.

Serum autoantibody studies

Rheumatoid factors (RFs)

IgM rheumatoid factors are detected by agglutination tests using IgG-coated latex particles (the Rose–Waaler test) or sensitized sheep red cells (sheep cell agglutination test or SCAT). They are antibodies (usually IgM, but occasionally IgG or IgA) against the Fc portion of IgG and are detected in 70% of patients with rheumatoid arthritis (RA), but are not diagnostic. A high titre in early RA indicates a poor prognosis. Positive titres occasionally predate the onset of RA. Titres may fluctuate. RFs are detected in many autoimmune rheumatic disorders (e.g. SLE), in chronic infections, and in asymptomatic older people (Table 10.1).

Antinuclear antibodies (ANAs)

These are detected by indirect immunofluorescent staining of fresh-frozen sections of rat liver or kidney or Hep-2 cell lines. Different patterns reflect a variety of antigenic specificities that occur with different clinical pictures (e.g. speckled, nucleolar or anticentromere patterns), and are detected in many autoimmune diseases. ANA is used as a screening test for SLE, but low titres occur in RA and chronic infections and in normal individuals, especially the elderly (Table 10.2).

The following patterns are seen:

- anti-DNA/histone (homogeneous) antibodies suggest active SLE
- anticentromere antibodies suggest systemic sclerosis.

Anti-double-stranded-DNA (dsDNA) antibodies

These are usually detected by a precipitation test (Farr assay), by ELISA, or by an immunofluorescent test using *Crithidia luciliae* (which contains double-stranded DNA). They are diagnostic of active SLE but may be negative in mild or inactive disease. High titres of IgG anti-dsDNA indicate a poor prognosis and are specific to SLE. Anti-single-stranded DNA antibodies are non-specific.

Anti-extractable nuclear antigen (ENA) antibodies

These produce a speckled ANA fluorescent pattern and can be distinguished by ELISA:

- anti-Ro (SS-A) – SLE + Sjögren's
- anti-La (SS-B) – Sjögren's
- anti-Sm – SLE
- anti-U1-RNP – a range of diseases, including SLE, overlap syndrome.

Anti Jo-1 antibodies

These antibodies to the enzyme histidyl tRNA synthetase block its amino-acylation and are found in polymyositis and dermatomyositis.

Topoisomerase 1 (ScL-70) antibodies

These are seen in systemic sclerosis.

Anti-neutrophil cytoplasmic antibodies (ANCAs)

These are detected on fixed human neutrophils. Two major ANCA patterns are recognized:

- proteinase 3 (PR3-ANCA), formerly called cytoplasmic or cANCA
- myeloperoxidase (MPO-ANCA), formerly called perinuclear or pANCA.

PR3-ANCA is present in up to 90% of serum from patients with Wegener's granulomatosis. MPO-ANCA is found in up to 60% of other vasculitides, such as microscopic polyarteritis (polyangiitis) and Churg–Strauss syndrome. An MPO-ANCA is found in inflammatory bowel disease and rheumatic disease, which is not associated with vasculitis.

Antiphospholipid antibodies
These are detected in the antiphospholipid syndrome and SLE.

Polymerase antibodies 1, 2 and 3.
These are measured in systemic sclerosis (see p. 561).

Immune complexes
Immune complexes are infrequently measured, largely because of variability between assays and difficulty in interpreting their meaning. Assays based on the polyethylene glycol precipitation method (PEG) or C1q binding are available commercially.

Complement
Low complement levels indicate consumption and suggest an active disease process in SLE.

Joint aspiration (Practical box 10.2)
Examination of joint (or bursa) fluid is used mainly to diagnose septic, reactive or crystal arthritis. The nature of the fluid is an indicator of the level of inflammation. Clear fluid indicates little inflammation in the joint, whereas translucent or opaque fluid indicates increasing cellularity and underlying inflammation. Purulent fluid is seen in septic arthritis, but crystal arthritis and reactive arthritis may also produce a highly cellular effusion. The procedure is often undertaken in combination with injection of a corticosteroid. Aspiration alone is therapeutic in crystal arthritis.

Diagnostic imaging and visualization
- **X-rays** can be diagnostic in certain conditions (e.g. rheumatoid arthritis), but remember the following points:
  (a) In acute low back pain, X-rays are indicated only if the pain is persistent, recurrent, associated with neurological symptoms or signs, or worse at night. They should also be performed if the pain is associated with such symptoms as fever or weight loss, which might indicate a more sinister underlying pathology.
  (b) Radiological changes are common in older people and may not indicate symptomatic osteoarthritis or spondylosis.

Practical box 10.2

Joint aspiration

This is a sterile procedure which should be carried out in a clean environment

1. Decide on the site to insert the needle and mark it.
2. Clean the skin and your hands scrupulously; remove rings and wristwatch. Gloves are not obligatory, but many prefer to use them.
3. Draw up local anaesthetic (and corticosteroid if it is being used) and then use a new needle.
4. Warn the patient, insert the needle, injecting local anaesthetic as it advances and, if a joint effusion is suspected, attempt to aspirate as you advance it.
5. If fluid is obtained, change syringes and aspirate fully.
6. Examine the fluid in the syringe and decide whether or not to proceed with a corticosteroid injection.
7. Cover the injection site and advise the patient to rest the affected area for a few days. Warn the patient that the pain may increase initially but to report urgently if this persists beyond a few days, if the swelling worsens, or if they become febrile, since this might indicate an infected joint.

  (c) X-rays are of little diagnostic value in early inflammatory arthritis but are useful as a baseline from which to judge later change.
- **Ultrasound (US)** is particularly useful for periarticular structures, soft tissue swellings and tendons. It is increasingly used to examine the shoulder and other structures during movement. This visualizes shoulder impingement syndrome (see p. 520). US can be used to guide local injections. Quantitative ultrasound of the heel may prove a convenient and portable means of assessing bone density.
- **Magnetic resonance imaging (MRI)** shows bone changes and intra-articular structures in striking detail. It is more sensitive than X-rays in the early detection of articular disease. It is the investigation of choice for most spinal disorders but is inappropriate in uncomplicated mechanical low back pain. Gadolinium injection enhances inflamed tissue.
- **Computerized axial tomography (CT)** is useful for detecting changes in calcified structures.
- **Bone scintigraphy** utilizes radionuclides, usually ^{99m}Tc, and detects abnormal bone turnover and blood circulation and, although non-specific, helps in detecting areas of inflammation, infection or malignancy. It is best used in combination with other anatomical imaging techniques, although tomographic bone scintigraphy is increasingly becoming more accurate.
- **DXA scanning** uses very low doses of X-irradiation to measure bone density and is used in the screening and monitoring of osteoporosis.

Box 10.2

Examination of synovial fluid

The fluid can be examined directly in a clear syringe or sterile pot. The characteristics of synovial fluid show a trend from clear to purulent which indicates roughly the type of arthritis.

Colour	Diagnosis	WCC per mm³
Clear, yellow and viscous	OA	< 3000
Translucent and thin Very cloudy	RA Seronegative arthritis Reiter's disease Crystal arthritis	3000–40 000
Purulent	Sepsis	750 000

Polarized light microscopy with a red filter needs to be undertaken by an expert.

- Gout – negatively birefringent, needle-shaped crystals of sodium urate
- Pyrophosphate arthropathy (pseudogout) – rhomboidal, weakly positively birefringent crystals of calcium pyrophosphate

Gram staining is essential if septic arthritis is suspected and may identify the organism immediately. Joint fluid should be cultured and antibiotic sensitivities requested.

RA, rheumatoid arthritis; OA, osteoarthritis

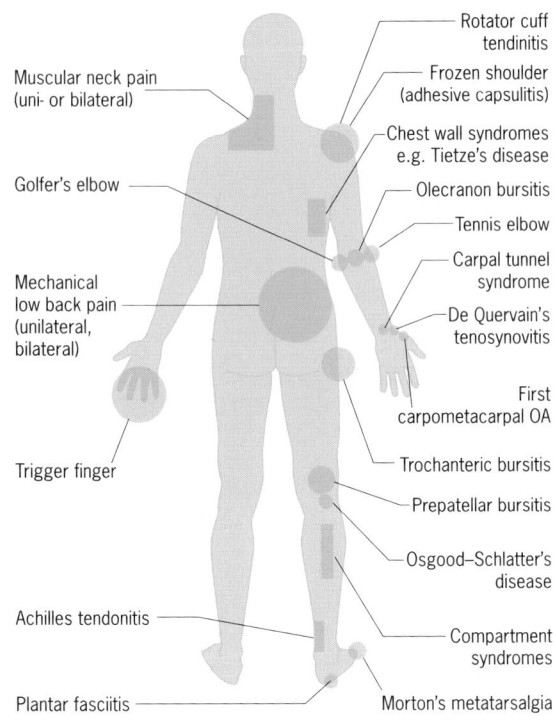

Fig. 10.2 Common regional musculoskeletal problems.

- **Arthroscopy** is a direct means of visualizing a joint, particularly the knee or shoulder. Biopsies can be taken, surgery performed in certain conditions (e.g. repair or trimming of meniscal tears), and loose bodies removed.

Examination of synovial fluid

This is described in Box 10.2.

FURTHER READING

Bellamy N (1998) Principles of outcome assessment. In: Klippel JH, Dieppe PA (eds) *Rheumatology*, 2nd edn. London: Mosby, Section 3, Ch. 14: 1–10.

Doherty M, Dacre J, Dieppe P, Snaith M (1992) The 'GALS' locomotor screen. *Annals of the Rheumatic Diseases* **51**: 1165–1169.

Morrow J, Nelson L, Watts R, Isenberg D (1999) *Autoimmune Rheumatic Diseases*, 2nd edn. Oxford: Oxford Medical Publications.

Common regional musculoskeletal problems (Fig. 10.2)

Analgesic and anti-inflammatory drugs used for treatment of musculoskeletal problems are discussed on page 531.

Pain in the neck and shoulder

(Table 10.3)

Mechanical or muscular neck pain (shoulder girdle pain)

Unilateral or bilateral muscular-pattern neck pain is common and usually self-limiting. It can follow injury, falling asleep in an awkward position, or prolonged keyboard working.

Worry and stress also cause muscle tension and lead to chronic neck pain, which is often burning in quality. Spondylosis (see p. 1218) seen on X-ray increases after the age of 40 years, but it is not always causal, as the pain often settles whilst the radiological changes persist. Spondylosis can, however, cause stiffness and increases the risk of mechanical or muscular neck pain. Muscle spasm can be palpable, is tender and may lead to abnormal neck posture (e.g. acute torticollis). Muscular-pattern neck pain is not localized but affects the trapezius muscle, the C7 spinous process, the paracervical musculature, or all three. It is also called shoulder girdle pain. Pain often radiates to the occiput but rarely beyond the tip of the shoulder. It is commonly associated with unilateral or bilateral tension headaches; pain radiating over the head to the temple and eye, described as like a pressure or tight band. These features are also seen in fibromyalgia (see p. 530).

Table 10.3
Pain in the neck and shoulder

Trauma (for example, a fall)
Mechanical or muscular neck pain
Whiplash injury
Disc prolapse – nerve root entrapment (p. 1212)
Ankylosing spondylitis
Shoulder lesions
    Rotator cuff tendonitis
    Calcific tendonitis or bursitis
    Impingement syndrome or rotator cuff tear
    Adhesive capsulitis (true 'frozen' shoulder)
    Inflammatory arthritis or osteoarthritis
Polymyalgia rheumatica
Fibromyalgia
Chronic (work-related) upper limb pain syndrome
Tumour

Table 10.4
Cervical nerve root entrapment – symptoms and signs

Nerve root	Sensory changes	Reflex loss	Weakness
C5	Lateral arm	Biceps	Shoulder abduction Elbow flexion
C6	Lateral forearm	Biceps	Elbow flexion
	Thumb and index finger	Supinator	Wrist extension
C7	Middle finger	Triceps	Elbow extension
C8	Medial forearm Little and ring fingers	None	Finger flexion
T1	Medial upper arm	None	Finger ab- and adduction

Treatment

Patients are given short courses of analgesic therapy along with reassurance and explanation. Physiotherapists can help to relieve spasm and pain, teach exercises and relaxation techniques, and improve posture. An occupational therapist can advise about the ergonomics of the workplace if the problem is work-related (see p. 530).

Nerve root entrapment

This is caused by an acute cervical disc prolapse or pressure on the root from spondylotic osteophytes narrowing the root canal.

Acute cervical disc prolapse presents with unilateral pain in the neck, radiating to the interscapular and shoulder regions. This diffuse, aching dural pain is followed by sharp, electric shock-like pain down the arm, in a nerve root distribution, often with pins and needles, numbness, weakness and loss of reflexes (see Table 10.4).

Cervical spondylosis occurs in the older patient with posterior osteophytes compressing the nerve root and causing root pain (see Fig. 20.27), commonly in C5/C6 or C6/C7; it is seen on oblique radiographs of the neck. An MRI scan shows facet joint OA and any associated disc prolapse clearly.

Treatment

A support collar, rest, analgesia and sedation are used as necessary. Patients should be advised not to carry heavy items. MRI is the investigation of choice if surgery is being considered or the diagnosis is uncertain (Fig. 10.3). A cervical root block administered under direct vision by an experienced pain specialist may relieve pain while the disc recovers. Neurosurgical referral is essential if the pain persists or if the neurological signs of weakness or numbness are severe or bilateral. Bilateral root pain is a neurosurgical emergency because a central disc prolapse may compress the cervical spinal cord.

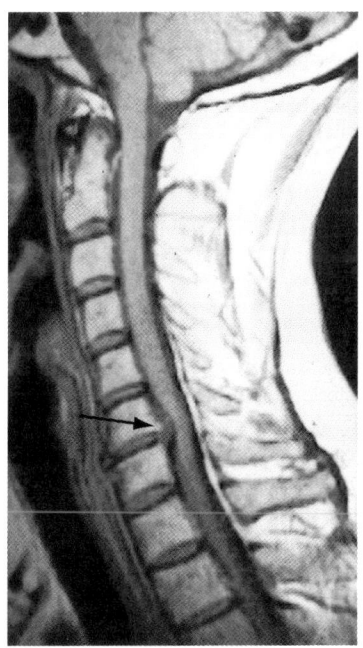

Fig. 10.3 MRI of cervical spine, showing a large central disc prolapse impinging on the spinal cord (arrow) at the C6/7 level.

Whiplash injury

Whiplash injury results from acceleration–deceleration forces applied to the neck, usually in a road traffic accident when a person wearing a seat belt has their car struck from behind. X-rays are rarely helpful but are essential to exclude a fracture. Delayed recovery depends in part upon the severity of the initial injury. A simple decision plan based on clinical criteria helps to distinguish those most at risk and who warrant radiography. There is a low probability of serious bony injury if there is no midline cervical tenderness, no focal neurological deficit, normal alertness, no intoxication and no painful distracting injury. CT scans are reserved for those with bony injury. MRI scans occasionally show severe soft tissue injury. Whiplash injuries commonly lead to litigation.

Whiplash injury is a common cause of chronic neck pain, although most people recover within a few weeks or months. The pattern of chronic neck pain is often complex, involving pain in the neck, shoulder and arm. Headache, dizziness, and loss of memory and poor concentration sometimes accompany this. The subjective nature of these symptoms has led to controversy about their cause. The problem is more commonly seen in industrialized countries. It has often been suggested that the syndrome is caused in part by the prospect of financial compensation. This may not be wholly conscious and may be contributed to in part by the conflictive nature of the compensation process. There appears to be a direct relationship between poor prognosis and potential for compensation – elimination of compensation for pain and suffering due to this type of injury may lead to an improved prognosis.

Treatment is with reassurance (as the patient may be very anxious), analgesia, a short-term collar and physiotherapy. Pain may take a few weeks or months to settle and the patient should be warned of this.

Pain in the shoulder

The shoulder is a shallow joint with a large range of movement. The humeral head is held in place by the rotator cuff (Fig. 10.4) which is part of the joint capsule. It comprises the tendons of infraspinatus and teres minor posteriorly, supraspinatus superiorly and teres major and subscapularis anteriorly. The rotator cuff (particularly supraspinatus) prevents the humeral head blocking against the acromion during abduction; the deltoid pulls up and the supraspinatus pulls in to produce a turning moment and permit the greater tuberosity to glide under the acromion without impingement.

Pain in the shoulder can sometimes be due to problems in the neck. The differential diagnosis of this is shown in Box 10.3. Although the term 'frozen shoulder' is commonly used for any painful stiff shoulder, true frozen shoulder (adhesive capsulitis) is uncommon – see below. A painful, stiff shoulder can result from rotator cuff lesions and is also seen following hemiplegia, chest or breast surgery or myocardial infarction. Painful shoulders may also be the initial presentation of RA, less commonly a seronegative spondarthritis, and of polymyalgia rheumatica in the elderly.

Rotator cuff (supraspinatus) tendonitis
This is a common cause of painful restriction of the shoulder at all ages. It follows trauma in 30% of cases and is bilateral in under 5%. The pain radiates to the upper arm and is made worse by arm abduction and elevation, which are often limited. The pain is often worse during the middle of the range of abduction, reducing as the arm is raised fully and the painful part of the tendon rotates through to the proximal side of the

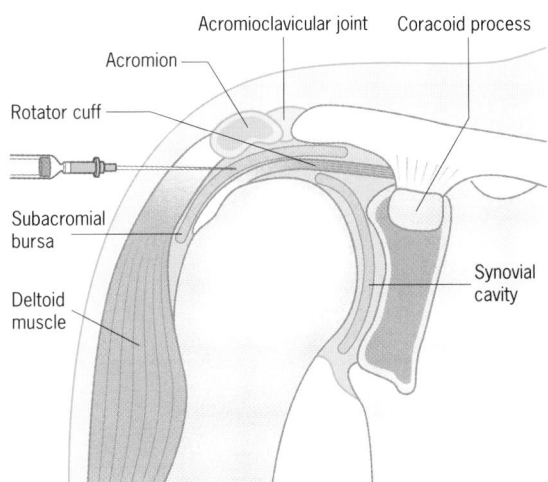

Fig. 10.4 The shoulder region, showing site of injection and subacromial space.

Box 10.3

Differential diagnosis of 'shoulder' pain

- Rotator cuff tendonitis pain is worse at night and radiates to the upper arm.
- Painful shoulders produce secondary muscular neck pain.
- Muscular neck pain (also known as shoulder girdle pain) does not radiate to the upper arm.
- Cervical nerve root pain is usually associated with pins and needles or neurological signs in the arm.

---

acromion – a so-called painful arc syndrome. When examined from behind, the scapula rotates earlier during elevation. Passive elevation reduces impingement and is less painful. Severe pain virtually immobilizes the joint, although some rotation is retained (cf. adhesive capsulitis). There is also painful spasm of the trapezius. X-rays are necessary only when rotator cuff tendonitis is persistent or the diagnosis is uncertain.

Treatment
Analgesics or NSAIDs may suffice, but severe pain responds to an injection of corticosteroid (Fig. 10.4). Patients should be warned that 10% will develop worse pain for 24–48 hours after injection. Seventy per cent improve over 5–20 days and mobilize the joint themselves. Physiotherapy helps persistent stiffness but further injections may be needed.

Calcific tendonitis and bursitis
Calcium pyrophosphate deposits in the tendon are visible on X-ray, but they are not always symptomatic. The pathogenesis is unclear, although the part of the tendon affected is likely to be affected by relative ischaemia. The deposit is usually just proximal to the greater tuberosity.

It may lead to acute or chronic recurrent shoulder pain and restriction of movement. A local corticosteroid injection may help and ultrasound treatment may help to resolve the calcification. Aspiration of the deposit under X-ray control may be required for persistent pain. Rarely arthroscopic removal is necessary.

Shedding of crystals into the subacromial bursa causes severe pain and shoulder restriction. The shoulder feels hot and is swollen, and an X-ray will show a diffuse opacity in the bursa. The differential diagnosis of calcific bursitis is gout, pseudogout or septic arthritis.

Aspiration and injection with corticosteroid can help.

Torn rotator cuff

This is caused by trauma in the young but also occurs spontaneously in the elderly and in rheumatoid arthritis (RA). It prevents active abduction of the arm, but patients learn to initiate elevation using the unaffected arm. Once elevated, the arm can be held in place by the deltoid muscle. In younger people, the tear is repaired surgically but this is rarely possible in the elderly or in RA. Repeated trauma of the cuff between humerus and acromion/acromioclavicular joint causes osteophyte and cyst formation.

Shoulder impingement syndrome causes pain and crepitus on abduction and rotation.

Adhesive capsulitis (true 'frozen' shoulder)

This is uncommon. Severe shoulder pain is associated with complete loss of all shoulder movements, including rotation. High doses of NSAIDs and intra-articular injections of corticosteroids are helpful. Once the pain settles, a manipulation under anaesthetic is advisable. When untreated, it recovers in 1–2 years.

Pain in the elbow

Pain in the elbow can be due to epicondylitis, inflammatory arthritis or occasionally osteoarthritis.

Epicondylitis

Two common sites where the insertions of tendons into bone become inflamed (*enthesitis*) are the insertions of the wrist extensor tendon into the lateral epicondyle ('tennis elbow') and the wrist flexor tendon into the medial epicondyle ('golfer's elbow'). Both are usually unrelated to either sporting activity.

There is local tenderness. Pain radiates into the forearm on using the affected muscles – typically, holding a heavy bag in tennis elbow or carrying a tray in golfer's elbow. Pain at rest also occurs.

Treatment

Advise rest and arrange review by a physiotherapist. A local injection of corticosteroid at the point of maximum tenderness is helpful when the pain is severe. Avoid

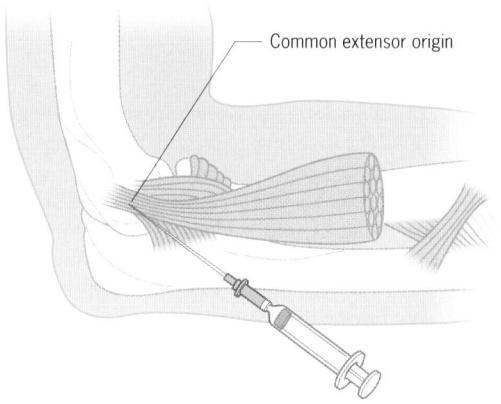

Fig. 10.5 **Injection for tennis elbow.**

the ulnar nerve when injecting golfer's elbow (Fig. 10.5). Both conditions settle spontaneously eventually, but occasionally become disabling.

Pain in the hand and wrist (Table 10.5)

Hand pain is commonly caused by injury or repetitive work-related use. When associated with pins and needles or numbness it suggests a neurological cause arising at the wrist, elbow or neck. Pain and stiffness that are worse in the morning are due to tenosynovitis or inflammatory arthritis. The distribution of hand pain often indicates the diagnosis.

Tenosynovitis

The finger flexor tendons run through a series of synovial sheaths and under loops which hold them in place. Inflammation occurs with repeated or unaccustomed use, or in inflammatory arthritis when the thickened sheaths are often palpable.

Flexor tenosynovitis causes finger pain when gripping and stiffness of the fingers in the morning. Occasionally

Table 10.5
Pain in the hand and wrist – causes

All ages	Older patients
Trauma/fractures	Nodal OA
Tenosynovitis	DIPs (Heberden's nodes)
Flexor with/without triggering	PIPs (Bouchard's nodes)
Dorsal	First carpometacarpal joint
De Quervain's	Trauma – scaphoid fracture
Carpal tunnel syndrome	Pseudogout
Ganglion	Gout
Inflammatory arthritis	Acute
Raynaud's syndrome (p. 831)	Tophaceous
Chronic regional pain	
Type I (p. 531)	

DIPs, PIPs = distal and proximal interphalangeal joints

a tendon causes a trigger finger, when the finger remains flexed after gripping and has to be pulled straight. A tendon nodule is palpable, usually in the palm.

Dorsal tenosynovitis is less common except in rheumatoid arthritis. The swelling is on the back of the hand and wrist.

De Quervain's tenosynovitis causes pain and swelling around the radial styloid where the abductor policis longus tendon is held in place by a retaining band. There is local tenderness, and the pain at the styloid is worsened by flexing the thumb into the palm.

Treatment
Therapeutic ultrasound helps some people. Usually corticosteroid is injected alongside the tendon under low pressure (not into the tendon itself). Occasionally surgery is needed.

Other conditions causing pain
Carpal tunnel syndrome
This is due to thickened tendons or synovitis in the carpal tunnel and is discussed on page 1213. The history is usually typical and diagnostic with the patient waking with numbness, tingling and pain in a median nerve distribution. The pain radiates to the forearm. The fingers feel swollen but usually are not. It is also seen during the last trimester of pregnancy.

Treatment is with a splint to hold the wrist in dorsiflexion overnight. This relieves the symptoms and is diagnostic; used nightly for several weeks it may produce full recovery. If it does not, a corticosteroid injection into the carpal tunnel helps in about 70% of cases, although it may recur. Persistent symptoms or nerve damage requires nerve conduction studies and surgical decompression of the carpal tunnel.

Inflammatory arthritis
This may present with pain, swelling and stiffness of the hands. In RA the wrists, proximal interphalangeal (PIP) joints and metacarpophalangeal (MCP) joints are affected symmetrically. In psoriatic arthritis and Reiter's disease a finger may be swollen (dactylitis) or the distal interphalangeal (DIP) joints are affected asymmetrically.

Nodal osteoarthritis
This affects the DIP and less commonly PIP joints, which are initially swollen and red. The inflammation and pain settle but bony swellings remain. There is often a strong family history and it rarely presents before 50 years of age. Reassurance and local treatment are all that is needed.

First carpometacarpal osteoarthritis
This causes pain at the base of the thumb when gripping, or painless stiffness at the base of the thumb.

Scaphoid fractures
These cause pain in the anatomical snuff box. They may not be seen immediately on X-ray. Untreated scaphoid fractures eventually cause pain because of failed union.

Ganglion
A ganglion is a jelly-filled, often painless swelling caused by a partial tear of the joint capsule. The wrist is a common site. Treatment is not essential as many resolve or cause little trouble. They rarely respond to injection, and surgical excision is possibly the best option.

Dupuytren's contracture
This is a painless, palpable fibrosis of the palmar aponeurosis, with fibroblasts invading the dermis. It causes puckering of the skin and gradual flexion of the affected fingers, usually the ring and little fingers. It is more common in males, Caucasians, in diabetes mellitus and in those who abuse alcohol. It is associated with Peyronie's disease of the penis – a painful inflammatory disorder of the corpora cavernosa, leading eventually to painless fibrosis and angulation of the penis during erection. Plastic surgical release of the contracture is restricted to those with severe deformity of the fingers.

Pain in the lower back

Low back pain is a common symptom. It is often traumatic and work-related, although lifting apparatus and other mechanical devices are used to avoid it. Episodes are generally short-lived and self-limiting, and patients attend a physiotherapist or osteopath more often than a doctor. Chronic back pain is the cause of 14% of long-term disability in the UK. The causes are listed in Table 10.6, and the management of back pain is summarized in Box 10.4.

Investigations
- **Spinal X-rays** are required only if the pain is associated with certain 'red flag' symptoms or signs, which indicate a high risk of more serious underlying problems:
  (a) starts before the age of 20 or after 50 years
  (b) is persistent and a serious cause is suspected
  (c) is worse at night or in the morning, when an inflammatory arthritis (e.g. ankylosing spondylitis), infection or a spinal tumour may be the cause
  (d) is associated with a systemic illness, fever or weight loss
  (e) is associated with neurological symptoms or signs.
- **MRI** is preferable to **CT** scanning when neurological signs and symptoms are present.

Table 10.6
Pain in the back (lumbar region) – causes

Mechanical
Trauma
Muscular and ligamentous pain
Fibrositic nodulosis
Postural back pain (sway back)
Lumbar spondylosis
Facet joint syndrome
Lumbar disc prolapse
Spinal and root canal stenosis
Spondylolisthesis
Disseminated idiopathic skeletal hyperostosis (DISH)
Fibromyalgia (see p. 530)

Inflammatory
Infective lesions of the spine
Ankylosing spondylitis/sacroiliitis (see p. 548)

Metabolic
Osteoporotic spinal fractures
Osteomalacia (see p. 584)
Paget's disease (see p. 582)

Neoplastic (see p. 572)
Metastases
Multiple myeloma
Primary tumours of bone
Referred pain

- **Bone scans** are useful in infective and malignant lesions but are also positive in degenerative lesions.
- **Full blood count, ESR and biochemical tests** are required only when the pain is likely to be due to malignancy, infection or a metabolic cause.

Mechanical low back pain

Mechanical low back pain starts suddenly, may be recurrent and is helped by rest. Mechanical back pain is often precipitated by an injury and may be unilateral or bilateral. It is usually short-lived.

Examination

The back is stiff and a scoliosis may be present when the patient is standing. Muscular spasm is visible and palpable and causes local pain and tenderness. It lessens when sitting or lying. Patients with spondylosis on X-ray probably have an increased risk of developing mechanical back pain but changes are often absent in the young and may be coincidental in the elderly. Pain relief and physiotherapy are helpful. The patient needs to be re-educated in lifting and shown exercises to prevent recurrent attacks of chronic pain. Once a patient has presented to a general practitioner with low back pain, although the episode itself is usually self-limiting, there is a significantly increased risk of further back pain episodes. Risk factors for recurrent back pain include female sex, increasing age, pre-existing chronic widespread pain (fibromyalgia) and such psychosocial factors as high levels of psychological distress, poor

self-rated health and dissatisfaction with employment. Chronic low back pain is a major cause of disability and time off work and is reduced by appropriate early management.

Spinal movement occurs at the disc and the posterior facet joints, and stability is normally achieved by a complex mechanism of spinal ligaments and muscles. Any of these structures may be a source of pain. An exact anatomical diagnosis is difficult, but some typical syndromes are recognized (see below). They are often associated with radiological spondylosis (see p. 1218).

Postural back pain develops in individuals who sit in poorly designed, unsupportive chairs.

Fibrositic nodulosis

This causes unilateral or bilateral low back pain, radiating to the buttock and upper posterior thigh. There are tender nodules in the upper buttock and along the iliac crest. Such nodules are relevant only if they are tender and associated with pain. They are probably traumatic. Local, intralesional corticosteroid injections help.

Postural back pain and sway back of pregnancy

Low back pain is common in pregnancy and reflects altered spinal posture and increased ligamentous laxity. There is usually a hyperlordosis on examining the patient standing. Weight control and pre- and postnatal exercises are helpful, and the pain usually settles after delivery. Analgesics and NSAIDs are best avoided during pregnancy and breast-feeding. Epidurals during delivery are not associated with an increased incidence of subsequent back pain. Poor posture causes a similar syndrome in the non-pregnant owing to obesity or muscular weakness. Poor sitting posture at work is an important cause of chronic low back pain.

Lumbar spondylosis

The fundamental lesion in spondylosis is in an intervertebral disc, a fibrous joint whose tough capsule inserts into the rim of the adjacent vertebrae. This capsule encloses a fibrous outer zone and a gel-like inner zone. The disc allows rotation and bending.

Changes in the discs may start in teenage years or early twenties and increase with age. The gel changes chemically, breaks up, shrinks and loses its compliance. The surrounding fibrous zones develop circumferential or radial fissures. In the majority this is initially asymptomatic but visible on MRI as decreased hydration. Later the discs become thinner and less compliant. These changes cause circumferential bulging of the intervertebral ligaments.

Reactive changes develop in adjacent vertebrae; the bone becomes sclerotic and osteophytes form around the rim of the vertebra (Fig. 10.6). The most common sites of lumbar spondylosis are L5/S1 and L4/L5. Disc prolapse through an adjacent vertebral endplate to produce a Schmorl's node on X-ray is painless but may accelerate disc degeneration.

Spondylosis may be symptomless, but it can cause:

- episodic mechanical spinal pain
- progressive spinal stiffening
- facet joint pain
- acute disc prolapse, with or without nerve root irritation
- spinal stenosis
- spondylolisthesis.

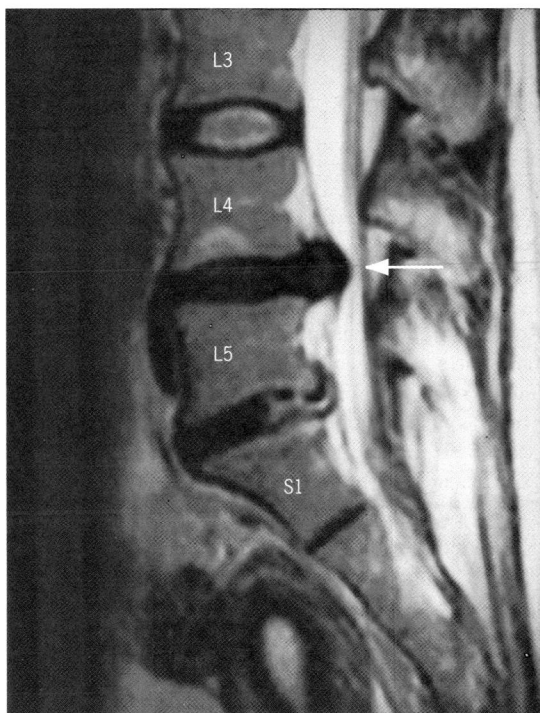

Fig. 10.6 **MRI of lumbar spine**, showing a central disc prolapse at the L4/L5 level (arrow). The signal from the L4/L5 and L5/S1 discs indicates dehydration, while the L3/L4 signal appearance is normal.

Facet joint syndrome

Lumbar spondylosis also causes secondary osteoarthritis of the facet joints. Pain is typically worse on bending backwards and when straightening from flexion. It is lumbar in site, unilateral or bilateral and radiates to the buttock. Diagnostic local anaesthetic injections into the joints (under X-ray vision) can be followed by a corticosteroid injection. The long-term value of this is unclear but many patients find the procedure helpful. Physiotherapy to reduce hyperlordosis and reducing weight are helpful.

Acute lumbar disc prolapse

The central disc gel may extrude into a fissure in the surrounding fibrous zone and cause acute pain and muscle spasm, which in turn leads to a forwards and sideways tilt when standing. These events are often self-limiting. A disc prolapse occurs when the extrusion extends beyond the limits of the fibrous zone (Fig. 10.6). The weakest point is posterolateral, where the disc may impinge on emerging spinal nerve roots in the root canal.

The episode starts dramatically during lifting, twisting or bending and produces a typical combination of low back pain and muscle spasm, and severe, lancinating pains, paraesthesia, numbness and neurological signs in one leg (rarely both). The back pain is diffuse, usually unilateral and radiates into the buttock. The muscle spasm leads to a scoliosis that reduces when lying down. The nerve root pain develops with, or soon after, the onset. The site of the pain and other symptoms is determined by the root affected (Table 10.7). A central high lumbar disc prolapse may cause spinal cord compression and long tract signs (i.e. upper motor neurone). Below L2/L3 it produces lower motor neurone lesions.

On examination, the back often shows a marked scoliosis and muscle spasm. The lying, straight-leg-raising test is positive in a lower lumbar disc prolapse – raising the straight leg beyond 30 degrees produces pain in the leg; slight limitation or pain in the back limiting the movement is not significant. Pain in the affected leg

Table 10.7
Lumbar nerve root entrapment – symptoms and signs

Nerve root	Sensory changes	Reflex loss	Weakness	Usual disc prolapse
L2	Front of thigh	None	Hip flexion/ adduction	L2/3
L3	Inner thigh and knee	Knee	Knee extension	L2/3
L4	Inner calf	Knee	Knee extension	L3/4
L5	Outer calf Upper, inner foot	None	Inversion of foot Dorsiflexion of toes	L4/5
S1	Posterior calf Lateral border of foot	Ankle	Plantar flexion of foot	L5/S1

produced by a straight raise of the other leg suggests a large or central disc prolapse. Look for perianal sensory loss, which might indicate a cauda equina lesion – a neurosurgical emergency. An upper lumbar disc prolapse produces a positive femoral stretch test – pain in the anterior thigh when the knee is flexed in the prone position.

Treatment

Advise a short period (2–3 days) of bed rest – lying flat for a lower disc but semi-reclining for a high lumbar disc – and prescribe analgesia and muscle relaxants. Once the pain is tolerable, encourage the patient to mobilize and refer to a physiotherapist for exercises and preventative advice. An X-ray-guided epidural or nerve root canal injection by a pain specialist reduces pain, although the evidence that it speeds resolution or prevents surgery is unclear. Caudal epidural injections are less effective than lumbar ones but technically easier. Resuscitation equipment must be available for these procedures. Referral to a surgeon for possible micro-discectomy or hemilaminectomy is necessary if the neurological signs are severe, if the pain persists and is severe for more than 6–10 weeks, or if the disc is central. If bladder or anal sphincter tone is affected it becomes a neurosurgical emergency. Chemical discolysis is still being evaluated.

Spinal and root canal stenosis

Progressive loss of disc height, OA of the facet joints, posterolateral osteophytes and hypertrophy of the ligamentum flavum all contribute to root canal stenosis. This causes nerve root pain or spinal root claudication – pain and paraesthesiae in a root distribution brought on by walking and relieved slowly by rest. The associated sensory symptoms, slow recovery when the patient rests and presence of normal foot pulses distinguish this from peripheral arterial claudication.

Spinal canal stenosis at more than one level is often associated with a congenitally narrow spinal canal. It causes buttock and bilateral leg pain, paraesthesiae and numbness when walking. Rest helps, as does bending forwards, a manoeuvre that opens the spinal canal. Specialist surgical advice is necessary.

Spondylolisthesis

This occurs in adolescents and young adults when bilateral congenital pars interarticularis defects cause instability and permit the vertebra to slip, with or without preceding injury. Rarely a cauda equina syndrome with loss of bladder and anal sphincter control and saddle-distribution anaesthesia develops (p. 1219). It is diagnosed radiologically. Low back pain in adolescents warrants investigation, and spondylolisthesis requires orthopaedic assessment. It needs careful monitoring during the growth spurt.

A degenerative spondylolisthesis may also develop in older people with lumbar spondylosis.

Diffuse idiopathic skeletal hyperostosis (DISH)

DISH (Forrestier's disease) affects the spine and extraspinal locations. It is an enthesopathy, causing bony overgrowths and ligamentous ossification and is characterized by flowing calcification over the antero-lateral aspects of the vertebrae. The spine is stiff but not always painful, despite the dramatic X-ray changes. Ossification at muscle insertions around the pelvis produces radiological 'whiskering'. Similar changes occur at the patella and in the feet.

Treatment is with analgesics or NSAIDs for pain, and exercise to retain movement and muscle strength.

Osteoporotic crush fracture of the spine

Osteoporosis is asymptomatic but leads to an increased risk of fracture of peripheral bones, particularly neck of femur and wrist, and thoracic or lumbar vertebral crush fractures. Such vertebral fractures develop without trauma, after minimal trauma, or as part of a major accident. They may develop painlessly or cause agonizing localized pain that radiates around the ribs and abdomen. Multiple fractures lead to an increased thoracic kyphosis ('widow's stoop'). The diagnosis is confirmed by X-rays, showing loss of anterior vertebral body height and wedging, with sparing of the vertebral end-plates and pedicles (Fig. 10.7).

Treatment

Advise bed rest and analgesia until the severe pain subsides over a few weeks, then gradual mobilization. It may warrant hospitalization. There may be some residual pain. Bone density measurement and preventative treatment of osteoporosis are essential (see p. 580).

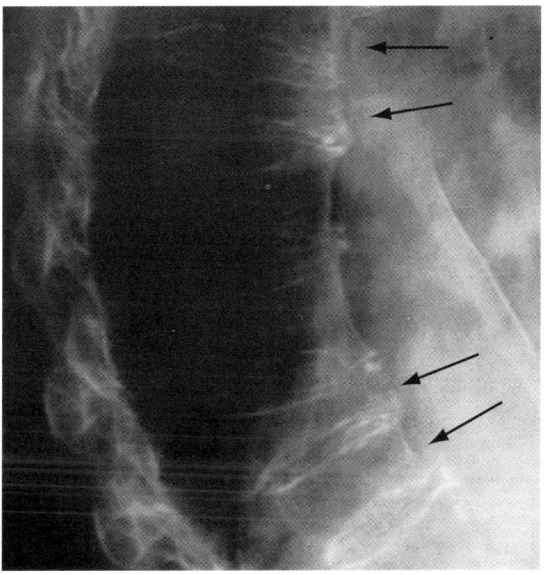

Fig. 10.7 X-ray of mid-thoracic spine, showing severe osteoporosis with multiple crush fractures (arrows) and biconcave vertebrae (typically the bone is difficult to see because of its porotic nature).

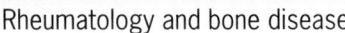
Ankylosing spondylitis (see also p. 548)

Buttock pain and low-back stiffness in a young adult suggests ankylosing spondylitis, especially if it is worse at night and in the morning.

Pain in the hip (Table 10.8)

'Hip' refers to a wide area between the upper buttock, trochanter and groin. It is useful to ask the patient to point to the site of pain and its field of radiation. Pain arising from the hip joint itself is felt in the groin, lower buttock and anterior thigh, and may radiate to the knee. Occasionally and inexplicably, hip arthritis causes pain only in the knee.

Osteoarthritis (OA) (see also p. 533)

OA is the most common cause of hip joint pain in a person over the age of 50 years. It causes pain in the buttock and groin on standing and walking. Stiff hip movements cause difficulty in putting on a sock and may produce a limp.

Trochanteric bursitis

This may be due to trauma or unaccustomed exercise, but sometimes has an unknown cause. It occurs in inflammatory arthritis. The pain over the trochanter is worse going up stairs and when abducting the hip, and the trochanter is tender to lie on. A local corticosteroid injection onto the surface of the trochanter is helpful.

Meralgia paraesthetica (see also p. 1213)

This causes numbness and burning dysaesthesia (increased sensitivity to light touch) over the anterolateral thigh and may be precipitated by a sudden increase in weight.

Fracture of the femoral neck

This usually occurs after a fall, occasionally spontaneously. There is pain in the groin and thigh, weight-bearing is painful or impossible, and the leg is shortened and externally rotated. Occasionally a fracture is not displaced and remains undetected. X-rays are diagnostic. Anyone with a hip fracture, especially after minimal trauma, should be reviewed for osteoporosis (see p. 578).

Avascular necrosis (osteonecrosis) of the femoral head

This is uncommon but occurs at any age. There is severe hip pain. X-rays are diagnostic after a few weeks, when a well-demarcated area of increased bone density is visible. In the femur this lies at the upper pole of the femoral head. The affected bone may collapse. Early, the X-ray is normal but bone scintigraphy or MRI demonstrate the lesion. Risk factors include treatment with corticosteroids or heparin, exposure to high barometric pressures (divers and tunnellers), excessive alcohol consumption, and sickle cell disease.

Table 10.8
Pain in the hip – causes

Hip region problems	Main sites of pain
Osteoarthritis of hip	Groin, buttock, front of thigh to knee
Trochanteric bursitis	Lateral thigh to knee
Meralgia paraesthetica	Anterolateral thigh to knee
Referred from back	Buttock
Facet joint pain	Buttock and posterior thigh
Fracture of neck of femur	Groin and buttock
Inflammatory arthritis	Groin, buttock, front of thigh to knee
Sacroiliitis (AS)	Buttock(s)
Avascular necrosis	Groin, buttock
Polymyalgia rheumatica	Buttocks, lumbar spine

AS, ankylosing spondylitis

Inflammatory arthritis of the hip

This produces pain in the groin and stiffness, which are worse in the morning. Rheumatoid arthritis (RA) rarely presents with hip pain, although the hip is involved eventually in severe RA. Ankylosing spondylitis and other seronegative spondarthritides cause inflammatory hip arthritis in younger people.

Polymyalgia rheumatica (see also p. 565)

Bilateral hip, buttock and thigh pain and stiffness that are worse in the morning in an elderly patient may be attributable to polymyalgia rheumatica.

Pain in the knee (Table 10.9)

The knee depends on ligaments and quadriceps muscle strength for stability. It is frequently injured, particularly during sports. Trauma or overuse of the knee leads to a variety of peri- and intra-articular problems. Some are self-limiting, others require physiotherapy, local corticosteroid injections or surgery.

The knee is also a common site of inflammatory arthritis and osteoarthritis. Minor radiographic changes of osteoarthritis (see p. 534) are common in the over-fifties and often coincidental, the cause of the pain being periarticular. Knee pain should not be attributed to osteoarthritis until other causes have been excluded. Symptomatic osteoarthritis of the knee correlates poorly with the severity of the radiological changes.

Common periarticular knee lesions
Medial knee pain

There may be medial or lateral ligament strain, but the medial ligament is more commonly affected. There is pain at the ligament's insertion into the upper medial tibia, which is worsened by standing or stressing the affected ligament.

Anserine bursitis causes pain and localized tenderness 2–3 cm below the posteromedial joint line in the upper part of the tibia at the site of the bursa. It occurs in obese women, often with valgus deformities, and in breast-stroke swimmers.

Treatment is with physiotherapy and a local corticosteroid injection.

Anterior knee pain

Anterior knee pain is common in adolescence. In many cases no specific cause is found despite careful investigation. This is called 'anterior knee pain syndrome' and settles with time. Isometric quadriceps exercises and avoidance of high heels both help the condition. Patient and parents often need firm reassurance. Abnormal patellar tracking may be a cause and need surgical treatment.

Pre- and infrapatellar bursitis are caused by unaccustomed kneeling ('housemaid's knee'). There is local pain, tenderness and fluctuant swelling. Avoidance of kneeling and a local corticosteroid injection are helpful. Septic bursitis can occur.

Chondromalacia patellae is diagnosed arthroscopically. The retropatellar cartilage is fibrillated. In most cases the pain settles eventually. When there is patellar misalignment it may need surgery, as does recurrent patellar dislocation in adolescent girls.

Osgood–Schlatter's disease causes pain and swelling over the tibial tubercle. It is a traction apophysitis of the patellar tendon and occurs in enthusiastic teenage sports players.

Hypermobility of joints causes joint pain (see also p. 571).

Common intra-articular traumatic lesions of the knee

Torn meniscus

The menisci are partially attached fibrocartilages that stabilize the rounded femoral condyles on the flat tibial plateaux. In the young they are resilient but this decreases with age. They can be torn by a twisting injury, commonly in sports that involve twisting and bending or the use of a studded boot. The history is usually diagnostic. There is immediate medial or lateral knee pain and dramatic swelling within a few hours. The affected side is tender. If the tear is large the knee may lock flexed. The immediate treatment is to apply ice to the knee. MRI demonstrates the tear (Fig. 10.8). In most circumstances, especially in active sportsmen, early arthroscopic repair or trimming of the torn meniscus is essential. Surgical intervention reduces recurrent pain, swelling and locking but not the risk of secondary osteoarthritis. The long-term benefit of repairing tears is not yet known. Post-surgical quadriceps exercises aid a return to sport.

Torn cruciate ligaments

Torn cruciate ligaments account for around 70% of knee haemarthroses in young people. They often coexist with a meniscal tear. Partial cruciate tears are difficult to diagnose clinically. On flexing the knee to 90 degrees, a torn anterior cruciate allows the tibia to be pulled forwards on the femur. MRI is the investigation of choice. Such injuries need urgent orthopaedic referral. There is a significant incidence of secondary OA.

Table 10.9
Pain in the knee

Trauma and overuse
  Periarticular problems
    Anterior knee pain or medial knee pain
    Internal derangements – meniscal tears or cruciate ligament tears

Osteoarthritis

Inflammatory arthritis
  Acute monarthritis
    Gout, pseudogout, Reiter's disease or septic arthritis
  Pauciarticular (< 4 joints)
    Seronegative spondarthritis or atypical rheumatoid arthritis
  Polyarticular
    Rheumatoid arthritis

Popliteal (Baker's) cyst/ruptured cyst

Osteochondritis dissecans

Hypermobility syndrome

Referred from hip joint

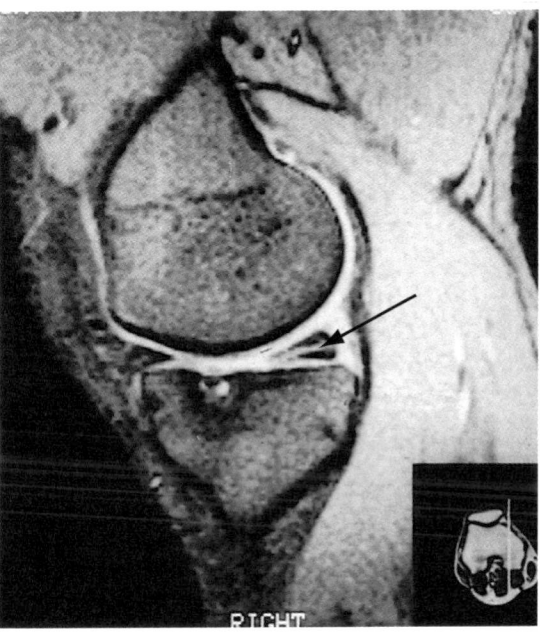

Fig. 10.8 MRI of a knee, showing a complete tear of the posterior horn of the medial meniscus, extending to its lower surface (arrow).

Osteochondritis dissecans

This occasionally causes knee pain and swelling in adolescents and young adults, more commonly males. It is probably traumatic, possibly with hereditary predisposing factors. A fragment of bone and its attached cartilage detach by shearing, most commonly from the lateral aspect of the medial femoral condyle.

There is aching pain after activity and, if the fragment becomes loose, locking or 'giving way' occurs. The lesion is seen on a tunnel-view X-ray, but MRI is more sensitive, especially if the fragment is undisplaced. Undisplaced lesions are treated with rest, then isometric quadriceps exercises. Loose fragments can be fixed arthroscopically or removed. A similar lesion affecting the lateral femoral condyle occurs in older people.

Knee joint effusions

An effusion of the knee causes swelling, stiffness and pain. The pain is more severe with an acute onset and with increasing inflammation due to stretching of the capsule that contains the pain receptors. A full clinical history and examination must include a past medical, family and drug history.

Inflammatory arthritis affects the knees and causes warmth and swelling. An acute inflammatory monoarthritis of the knee is a common presentation of a seronegative spondarthritis and occasionally is the first sign of RA.

Monarthritis of the knee, associated with severe pain and marked redness, may be due to septic arthritis, or gout in the middle-aged male, or to gout or pseudogout in an older male or female. A cool, clear, viscous effusion is seen in elderly patients with moderate or severe symptomatic OA.

Examination

A large and tense effusion is easily seen and felt on each side of the patella and in the suprapatellar pouch, and is fluctuant. The effusion delays the patella tapping against the femur when it is pressed firmly and quickly (the 'patellar tap' sign). Small effusions also demonstrate the 'bulge' sign when the patient is lying with the quadriceps relaxed. For this, apply a gentle sweeping pressure, first to the medial side of the joint and then, watching the medial dimple, to the lateral side. Slightly delayed bulging of the medial dimple indicates fluid in the joint.

Investigations

These are (a) blood biochemistry, and (b) aspiration and examination of the knee effusion. The basic technique of aspiration is described in Practical box 10.2 on page 517.

If there is a flexion deformity, externally rotate the leg or support the knee. Stand on the side opposite the joint and insert the needle between the patella, just proximal to its mid point, and the medial femoral condyle. Angle the needle slightly backwards and inject small volumes of local anaesthetic, advancing until aspiration detects fluid. Then change the syringe for a larger one and aspirate as much fluid as possible. Examine the fluid (see Box 10.2, p. 518) and decide whether to inject corticosteroid or arrange microbiological tests.

Haemarthrosis of the knee

This is caused by:

- trauma – meniscal, cruciate or synovial lining tear
- clotting or bleeding disorders, such as haemophilia, sickle cell disease or von Willebrand's disease.

Popliteal cyst (Baker's cyst)

In approximately 5% of patients with a knee effusion, a swollen, painful popliteal cyst develops. This is usually due to a bursa (usually the semimembranosus bursa), which in some individuals has a valve-like connection to the knee. This allows the effusion to flow into the bursa but not back. Occasionally there is a synovial herniation through the posterior joint capsule. The cyst is best seen and felt in the popliteal fossa with the patient standing.

Ruptured popliteal cyst

A popliteal cyst may rupture if the patient is mobile, particularly on standing up quickly or climbing stairs. Fluid escapes into the soft tissue of the popliteal fossa and upper calf, causing sudden and severe pain, swelling and tenderness of the upper calf. Dependent oedema of the ankle develops and the knee effusion reduces dramatically in size and may be undetectable.

A history of previous knee problems and the sudden onset of pain and tenderness high in the calf suggest a ruptured cyst rather than a deep vein thrombosis (DVT). However, the diagnosis is often missed and treated inappropriately with anticoagulants. A diagnostic ultrasound examination distinguishes a ruptured cyst from a DVT (see p. 832). Analgesics or NSAIDs, rest with the leg elevated, and aspiration and injection with corticosteroids into the knee joint are required.

Pain in the foot and heel (Table 10.10)

The feet are subjected to extreme pressures by weight-bearing and inappropriate shoes. They are commonly painful. Broad, deep, thick-soled shoes are essential for sporting activities, prolonged walking or standing, and in people with congenitally flat or arthritic feet.

There are two common types of foot deformity:

- flat feet stress the ankle and throw the hindfoot into a valgus (everted) position – a flat foot is rigid and inflexible
- high-arched feet place pressure on the lateral border and ball of the foot.

Table 10.10
Pain in the foot and heel – causes

Structural (flat (pronated) or high arched (supinated))
Hallux valgus/rigidus (± OA)
Metatarsalgia
Morton's neuroma
Stress fracture
Inflammatory arthritis
    Acute, monarticular – gout
    Chronic, polyarticular – RA
    Chronic, pauciarticular – seronegative spondarthritis
Tarsal tunnel syndrome
Heel pain

Plantar fasciitis	Below heel
Plantar spur	Below heel
Achilles tendonitis/bursitis	Behind heel
Sever's disease	

Arthritis of ankle/subtaloid joints

The foot is affected by a variety of inflammatory arthritic conditions. After the hand, the foot joints are the most commonly affected by rheumatoid arthritis. The diagnosis depends upon careful assessment of the distribution of the joints affected, the pattern of other joint problems, or by finding the associated condition (e.g. psoriasis, see p. 1287).

Hallux valgus

The great toe migrates laterally. In the congenital form the first metatarsal is displaced medially (metatarsus primus varus). The shape of modern shoes causes later onset of hallux valgus. It is a common complication of RA.

Hallux rigidus

Osteoarthritis of the first MTP joint in a normally aligned or valgus joint causes hallux rigidus – a stiff, dorsiflexed and painful great toe. Careful choice of footwear and the help of a podiatrist suffice for most cases, but some require surgery.

Metatarsalgia

This is common, especially in women who wear high heels, after trauma and in those with hammer toes. The ball of the foot is painful to walk and stand on. Callosities and pressure-induced bursae develop under the metatarsal heads. Rheumatoid arthritis causes misalignment of the metatarsal bones and severe metatarsalgia.

Treatment is with podiatry and the wearing of appropriate shoes. Surgery is occasionally needed, particularly in the rheumatoid forefoot.

Morton's metatarsalgia is due to a neuroma, usually between the third and fourth toes. It causes pain, burning and numbness in the adjacent surfaces of the affected toes when walking. It is helped by wearing wider, cushioned-soled shoes.

Stress (march) fractures

These cause sudden, severe weight-bearing pain in the distal shaft of the fractured metatarsal bone. They occur after unaccustomed walking or with new shoes. There is local tenderness and swelling, but initially X-rays are normal and diagnosis delayed. A radioisotope bone scan reveals the fracture earlier than X-rays. Reduced weight-bearing for a few weeks usually suffices.

Tarsal tunnel syndrome

This is an entrapment neuropathy of the posterior tibial nerve as it rounds the medial malleolus. It produces burning, tingling and numbness of the toes, sole and medial arch. The nerve is tender below the malleolus and, when tapped, produces a shock-like pain (Tinel's sign). A local steroid injection under the retinaculum, between the medial malleolus and calcaneum, is helpful.

Pain under the heel

Plantar fasciitis is an enthesitis at the insertion of the tendon into the calcaneum. It produces localized pain when standing and walking, and tenderness in the midline. It occurs alone or in seronegative spondarthritis.

Plantar spurs are traction lesions at the insertion of the plantar fascia in older people and are usually asymptomatic. They become painful after trauma.

Calcaneal bursitis is a pressure-induced (adventitious) bursa that produces diffuse pain and tenderness under the heel. Compression of the heel pad from the sides is painful, which distinguishes it from plantar fascia pain.

Whatever the cause, the pain is always worse in the morning as soon as weight is placed on the foot.

All of these lesions are treated with heel pads, and reduced walking; these are often self-limiting. A splint at night to hold the foot dorsiflexed and to stretch the plantar fascia is preferable to a local corticosteroid injection in plantar fasciitis. When an injection is necessary, a medial approach is used, rather than through the heel pad, under a posterior tibial nerve block.

Pain behind the heel and leg

Sever's disease is a traction apophysitis of the Achilles tendon in young people (cf. Osgood–Schlatter's disease p. 571).

Achilles tendonitis is an *enthesitis* at the insertion of the tendon into the calcaneum. This is traumatic or it can complicate seronegative spondarthritis. Raising the shoe heel reduces pain. Occasionally a low-pressure corticosteroid injection near the enthesis is necessary.

Partial tear of the Achilles tendon causes a painful, tender swelling a few centimetres above its insertion. Advise against walking barefoot and jumping. Therapeutic ultrasound is helpful. (Caution – a local injection may cause the tendon to rupture.)

Achilles' bursitis lies clearly anterior to the tendon and can be safely injected with corticosteroid.

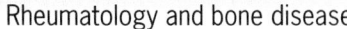

Compartment syndromes

The muscles of the lower leg are enclosed in fascial compartments, with little room for expansion to occur. Compartment syndromes can be acute and severe, such as following exercise.

In the *anterior tibial syndrome* there is severe pain in the front of the shin, occasionally with foot drop. Immediate surgical decompression to prevent muscle necrosis is sometimes required.

Chronic compartment syndrome produces pain in the lower leg that is aggravated by exercise and may therefore be mistaken for a vascular or neurological disorder.

Pain in the chest

Musculoskeletal conditions are sometimes a cause of chest pain. An example is Tietze's disease. In this condition, pain arises from the costosternal junctions. It is usually unilateral and affects one, two or three ribs. There is local tenderness, which helps to make the diagnosis. The condition is benign and self-limiting. It often responds well to anti-inflammatory drugs. Other causes of chest wall pain include rib fractures due to trauma or osteoporosis or a malignant deposit.

Chronic pain syndromes

(see also p. 1235)

Chronic pain syndromes are difficult to manage. Psychological factors are at least as important as inflammation or damage in determining a patient's perception of pain. It is essential to be objective and non-judgmental when dealing with them, discussing physical, psychological and social factors without assuming which is primary. Chronic pain syndromes are difficult to explain scientifically and it is all too easy for a doctor to 'blame' the patient for this lack of explanation. Some chronic pain states may be caused partly by the process of litigation that may follow an injury.

Any chronic painful condition can change the way a person copes. Some people with chronic diseases or chronic pain cope well, but others adopt coping strategies and patterns of behaviour which make things worse. They become anxious, depressed or socially isolated, and their quality of life is reduced. In chronic pain syndromes patients need help to lead a more normal life despite their pain, and are best referred to a specialist, multidisciplinary pain service.

Psychological states such as depression and anxiety produce physical symptoms, of which one is pain, while people with frank physical diseases are often understandably anxious and depressed.

Fibromyalgia (fibrositis syndrome)

'Fibromyalgia' (p. 1235) is a useful diagnosis of exclusion although it is not universally accepted as a diagnosis. Patients value a name to explain symptoms previously dismissed or attributed simply to psychological or social problems. A typical feature of fibromyalgia is tender trigger points. The tenderness is not 'all over', a point which distinguishes it from anxiety states. The patient is usually a middle-aged, middle-class woman who struggles on with her work and/or housework despite the pain. Such individuals are difficult to live with and there is often family discord. Many patients have sleep disturbances, so they awake unrefreshed and have poor concentration.

The pain is a widespread, unremitting, aching discomfort. There are often other health problems, such as chronic fatigue syndrome (see below), irritable bowel syndrome, premenstrual syndrome, tension headache, anxiety and depression; doctors sometimes inappropriately label them 'heart sink' patients. The patient's frustration is compounded by the fact that most tests are normal, and they fear doctors believe it is 'all in their mind'.

Treatment

A sympathetic approach is appropriate, with reassurance for the patient that fibromyalgia often improves and is not inevitably disabling. Encouragement should be given to undertake a graded aerobic exercise regimen. When depression is present, it should be treated, but potentially addictive anxiolytic agents are best avoided. A behavioural psychologist may persuade the person to pace their life more effectively and to cope better, although patients often resist referral for psychological help.

Drugs

Analgesics or NSAIDs help in some cases but are best used intermittently.

Low doses of sedative antidepressant drugs, such as amitriptyline or dosulepin (dothiepin), help when taken a few hours before bedtime. It should be explained that these doses are analgesic and not antidepressant, and their side-effects should be outlined.

Trigger-point injections with local anaesthetic, corticosteroids or acupuncture are sometimes helpful.

Oral corticosteroids are not helpful.

Chronic fatigue syndrome

Diffuse muscular pain and stiffness is common in this condition, which is described on page 1234.

Chronic (work-related) upper-limb pain syndrome

This name is preferred to 'repetitive strain injury' (RSI). The predominant symptoms are pain in all or part of one or both arms. A specific lesion, such as tennis elbow or carpal tunnel syndrome, or muscular-pattern neck pain often develops first, and early recognition and treatment may prevent chronicity. After a variable period, the pain becomes more diffuse and no longer simply work-related, and there is often severe distress. It is seen in keyboard workers and others who perform the same task without breaks for prolonged periods, and in musicians. When it arises at work, it is often at a time of changing work practices, shortage of staff or disharmony. Middle managers find it difficult to deal with and this compounds the stress.

It is seen throughout the developed world. It peaked in incidence in Australia in the 1970s and 1980s but has largely disappeared there, apparently because of changes in work practices, improvements in early medical management, changes in workers' compensation legislation, and reduced media discussion of the problem.

Treatment

If possible there should be a brief period off work and a gradual return to activity once the pain has settled. Cautious use of analgesia and NSAIDs, with physiotherapy, is helpful during the initial phase to prevent a vicious circle developing.

A review of working practices and the positioning of screen, keyboard and chair are essential, as is support of the patient by their manager. Musicians are helped by expert advice on playing technique and should reduce playing times temporarily, but not stop completely.

Temporomandibular pain dysfunction syndrome

This is a disorder of the temporomandibular joint associated with nocturnal tooth grinding or abnormalities of bite. It particularly occurs in anxious people. It gives rise to pain in one or both temporomandibular joints.

Dental correction of the bite helps a few but when no dental cause is found, low-dose tricyclic antidepressant therapy is used. Many patients are exposed to much unnecessary dental treatment.

Reflex sympathetic dystrophy (RSD), Sudek's atrophy or chronic regional pain syndrome type I

This is defined as 'a complex disorder or group of disorders that may develop as a consequence of trauma affecting the limbs, with or without obvious nerve lesions'. It may also develop after central nervous system lesions (e.g. strokes), or without cause. It occurred in 1.5% of soldiers injured in Vietnam. Its features are pain and other sensory abnormalities, including hyperaesthesia, autonomic vasomotor dysfunction, leading to abnormal blood flow and sweating, and motor system abnormalities. This leads to structural changes of superficial and deep tissues (trophic changes). Not all components need be present. The sensory, motor

and sympathetic nerve changes are not restricted to the distribution of a single nerve and may be remote from the site of injury. The early phase – with pain, swelling and increased skin temperature – is difficult to diagnose but potentially reversible.

After a period of weeks or months, a second, still painful, dystrophic phase develops, characterized by articular stiffness, cold skin and trophic changes, often with localized osteoporosis.

A late phase involves continued pain, skin and muscle atrophy, and muscle contractures, and is extremely disabling.

Diagnosis is initially clinical – a high index of suspicion and recognizing the unusual distribution of the pain. A three-phase bone scan shows diffuse or patchy increase in uptake in the affected limb in all three phases: early (a few seconds – arterial); middle (a few minutes – soft tissue); and late (several hours – mineral). The bone phase abnormalities appear early and well before demineralization is seen on X-ray. There is never loss of joint space, which distinguishes the appearances from the periarticular osteoporosis of inflammatory joint disease.

Treatment

Management is difficult and the problem often very disabling. Early diagnosis, effective pain relief and general care of the patient are essential. NSAIDs and corticosteroids are used in the early phase, together with active exercise of the limb. Calcitonin may also help at this stage. If pain persists despite initial treatment, a phentolamine test is used to test for evidence of sympathetically maintained pain (i.v. infusion of up to 40 mg with careful cardiac monitoring). If this is positive, a stellate ganglion block is used for upper limb and a sympathetic chain block for lower limb involvement. Guanethidine (an alpha-blocking agent) or lidocaine (lignocaine) administered to the limb under tourniquet is also useful. Referral to a pain management clinic is advisable.

Chronic regional pain syndrome type 2 is discussed on page 1150.

FURTHER READING

Jayson MIV (ed) (1992) *The Lumbar Spine and Back Pain*, 4th edn. London: Churchill Livingstone.
Yassi A (1997) Repetitive strain injuries. *Lancet* **349**: 943–947.

Analgesic and anti-inflammatory drugs for musculoskeletal problems

The key to using drugs, particularly in chronic disorders and the elderly, is to balance risk and benefit and

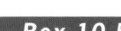
Box 10.5

Analgesics and NSAIDs

Analgesics (in order of potency)
Advise that they be taken *only* if needed. Maximum doses are indicated here.

Paracetamol	500–1000 mg	6-hourly
Paracetamol with codeine	1–2 tablets	6-hourly
Paracetamol with dextropropoxyphene	1–2 tablets	Every 6–8 hours
Paracetamol with dihydrocodeine	1–2 tablets	Every 6–8 hours
Dihydrocodeine	30–60 mg	Every 6–8 hours

Non-steroidal anti-inflammatory drugs (NSAIDs)
Always to be taken with food. Use slow-release preparations in inflammatory conditions or if more regular pain control is needed. Examples:

Ibuprofen	200–400 mg	Every 6–8 hours
Ibuprofen slow release	600–800 mg	Every 1–3 days
Diclofenac	25–50 mg	8-hourly
Diclofenac slow release	75–100 mg	1–2 daily
Celecoxib*	200 mg	1–2 daily

*An example of a COX-2 specific NSAID

constantly to review their appropriateness. Box 10.5 shows the main drugs available.

Simple and compound analgesic agents

Simple agents such as paracetamol, aspirin, or codeine compounds (or combination preparations), used when necessary or regularly, relieve pain and improve function. Sleep may also be improved. Side-effects are relatively infrequent, although drowsiness and constipation occur with codeine preparations, especially in the elderly.

Stronger analgesics, such as dihydrocodeine or morphine derivatives, should be used only with severe pain.

Non-steroidal anti-inflammatory drugs (NSAIDs)

NSAIDs have anti-inflammatory and centrally acting analgesic properties. They inhibit cyclo-oxygenase (COX), a key enzyme in the formation of prostaglandins, prostacyclins and thromboxanes (see Fig. 14.32). There are two specific cyclo-oxygenase enzymes: COX-1, the constitutive form, and COX-2, the form mainly induced by inflammation. Most of the older NSAIDs block both enzymes but with variable specificity; their therapeutic effect depends on blocking COX-2 and their side-effects mainly on blocking COX-1.

COX-1 is a constitutive enzyme present in many normal tissues. Inhibition of the enzyme by NSAIDs produces side-effects caused, for example, by the loss of gastric mucosal protection and a decrease in renal blood flow.

COX-2 is induced in response to pro-inflammatory cytokines and is not found in most normal tissues. It is associated with oedema and the nociceptive and pyretic effects of inflammation. COX-2 appears to be constitutive in the kidney. COX 2-specific NSAIDs are available.

Uses

- *Short courses* of NSAIDs are used occasionally in osteoarthritis and spondylosis, even when there is minimal inflammation. They are commonly used in musculoskeletal pain but simple analgesia is often more appropriate.
- *In crystal synovitis*, NSAIDs have a true anti-inflammatory effect (see p. 553).
- *In chronic inflammatory synovitis*, NSAIDs do not alter the chronic inflammatory process, nor decrease the risk of joint damage, but they do reduce pain and stiffness.
- Slow-release preparations are useful for *inflammatory arthritis* and when more constant pain control is needed.
- NSAID gels have no proven role in chronic arthritis.

Side-effects

The most common side-effects of standard, COX non-specific NSAIDs are indigestion or skin rashes. Gastric erosions and peptic ulceration with perforation and bleeding also occur. Proton-pump inhibitors are probably the best drugs to protect those at high risk from serious gastrointestinal events. H_2 blockers and prostaglandin-E_2 analogues also help as gastroprotective agents. The value of prostaglandin analogues is limited by their tendency to cause nausea and diarrhoea. In the elderly, NSAIDs may cause gastric mucosal damage and gastrointestinal bleeding without warning symptoms, thereby causing significant morbidity and mortality. They may also reduce renal function, especially in the elderly.

COX-2 specific NSAIDs produce fewer gastrointestinal side-effects (6% compared to 16% in one trial) but renal complications and fluid retention still occur. Their role in arthritis is being evaluated. They are advised on health-economic grounds as first line treatment for 'at-risk' patients and those over 65 years (NICE guidelines). Their higher cost is a disadvantage, but may be offset if it proves safe to avoid the co-prescription of gastroprotective agents, even in individuals with previous peptic ulceration or other indicators of increased risk of ulceration, and if fewer major gastrointestinal complications requiring hospitalization result.

FURTHER READING

Fitzgerald GA, Patrono C (2001) The coxibes, selective inhibitors of cyclooxygenase-2. *New England Journal of Medicine* **345**: 433–442.

Lipsky PE (2001) The role of COX-2 specific inhibitors in clinical practice. *American Journal of Medicine* **110, suppl 3A**: 1S–2S.

Osteoarthritis (OA)

Osteoarthritis is a disease of synovial joints characterized by cartilage loss with an accompanying periarticular bone response. There is no simple definition of OA as
it requires consideration of three overlapping areas –
pathological changes, radiological features and clinical
consequences. Pathologically, there is an alteration in
cartilage structure, radiologically there are osteophytes
and joint space narrowing, and clinically some patients
complain of pain and disability.

Epidemiology

Osteoarthritis is the most common type of arthritis. The
prevalence increases with age, and most people over 60
years will have some radiological evidence of it. It
occurs world-wide, although OA of the hip is less common in black Africans and Chinese populations than in
Caucasians. Most epidemiological studies have been
based on radiological evidence, which is much more
frequent than symptomatic OA. Women over 55 years
are affected more commonly than are men of a similar
age. There is a familial pattern of inheritance with
distal interphalangeal joint involvement as the hallmark
(nodal OA) and also with primary generalized OA.
OA has a variable distribution (Fig. 10.9). The resulting
disabilities have major socio-economic resource implications, particularly in the developed world.

Aetiology

Genes that encode collagen type II have been proposed
as candidate genes for familial OA. Osteoarthritis is the
result of active, sometimes inflammatory but potentially
reparative processes rather than the inevitable result of
trauma and ageing. Focal destruction of the articular
cartilage is the common pathological feature. The spectrum of OA ranges from atrophic disease in which cartilage destruction occurs without any subchondral bone
response, to hypertrophic disease in which there is massive new bone formation at the joint margins.

Cartilage is a matrix of collagen fibres (mainly type II,
see p. 585), enclosing a mixture of proteoglycans
and water. Proteoglycans are present mainly as large
molecular aggrecans, which consist of a protein core
with attached chondroitin sulphate and keratan sulphate
chains. The gene for human aggrecan has been cloned,
and polymorphisms of the gene have been correlated
with OA of the hand in older men.

Cartilage is smooth-surfaced and shock-absorbing.
Under normal circumstances there is a dynamic balance
between cartilage degradation by wear and its production by chondrocytes. Early in the development of OA
this balance is lost and, despite increased synthesis of
extracellular matrix, the cartilage becomes oedematous.
Focal erosion of cartilage develops. Chondrocytes die and,
although repair is attempted from adjacent cartilage, the

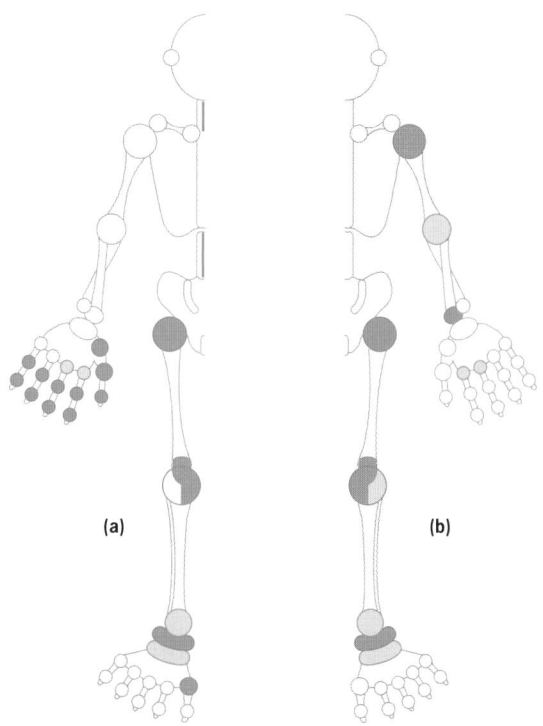

Fig. 10.9 **Typical distribution of affected joints in (a)
primary generalized OA and (b) pyrophosphate arthropathy.**
●, more commonly affected; ○, less commonly affected.

process is disordered. Eventually the synthesis of extracellular matrix fails and the surface becomes fibrillated
and fissured. Cartilage ulceration exposes underlying
bone to increased stress, producing microfractures and
cysts. The bone attempts repair but produces abnormal
sclerotic subchondral bone and overgrowths at the joint
margins, called *osteophytes* (Fig. 10.10). There is some
secondary inflammation.

Pathogenesis

Several mechanisms have been suggested for the pathogenesis:

- Matrix loss is caused by the action of matrix
  metalloproteinases such as collagenase (MMP-1)
  gelatinase (MMP-2) and stromelysin (MMP-3). These
  are secreted by chrondrocytes in an inactive form.
  Extracellular activation then leads to the
  degradation of collagen and proteoglycans.
- Tissue inhibitors of metalloproteinases (TIMPs)
  regulate the MMPs. Disturbance of this regulation
  may lead to increased cartilage degradation and
  contribute to the development of OA.
- There is synovial inflammation in OA, producing
  interleukin-1 (IL-1) and tumour necrosis factor
  (TNF-α). These cytokines stimulate
  metalloproteinase production and IL-1 inhibits
  type II collagen production.

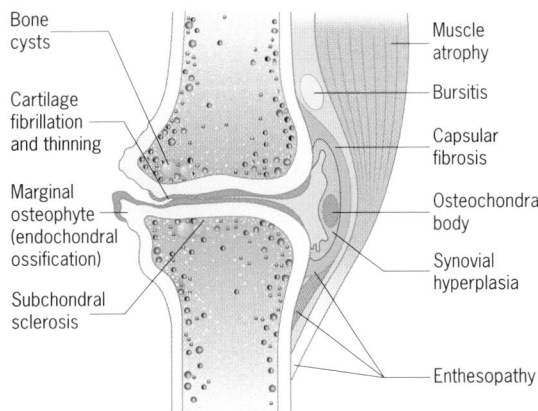

Bone cysts

Cartilage fibrillation and thinning

Marginal osteophyte (endochondral ossification)

Subchondral sclerosis

Muscle atrophy

Bursitis

Capsular fibrosis

Osteochondral body

Synovial hyperplasia

Enthesopathy

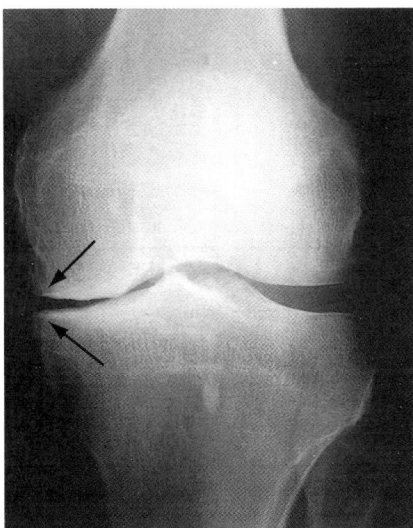

Fig. 10.10 **Diagram and X-ray of a knee**, showing early osteoarthritis. There is a medial compartment narrowing owing to cartilage thinning with subarticular sclerosis and marginal osteophyte formation (arrows).

- Growth factors, including insulin-like growth factor (IGF-1) and transforming growth factor (TGF-β), are involved in collagen synthesis, and their deficiency may play a role in impairing matrix repair.
- Mutations in the gene for type II collagen (COL2A1) have been associated with early polyarticular OA.
- Twin studies suggest a strong hereditary element underlying OA, and further studies may reveal genetic markers for the disease. The influence of genetic factors is estimated at 35–65%.
- In the Caucasian population there is an inverse relationship between the risk of developing OA and osteoporosis.
- A large population study has suggested that a high intake of vitamin C and other antioxidants may reduce the risk of OA. The lack of antioxidants is thought to contribute to many ageing processes.

> ### Box 10.6
>
> **Factors predisposing to osteoarthritis**
>
> - *Obesity* – Predicts later risk of radiological and symptomatic OA in population studies.
> - *Heredity* – Familial tendency to develop nodal and generalized OA.
> - *Gender* – Polyarticular OA is more common in women; a higher prevalence after the menopause suggests a role for sex hormones.
> - *Hypermobility* (see p. 571) – Increased range of joint motion and reduced stability lead to OA.
> - *Osteoporosis* – There is reduced risk of OA.
> - Other diseases – See Table 10.11.
> - *Trauma* – A fracture through any joint. Meniscal and cruciate ligament tears cause OA of the knee.
> - *Congenital joint dysplasia* – Alters joint biomechanics and leads to OA. Mild acetabular dysplasia is common and leads to earlier onset of hip OA.
> - *Joint congruity* – Congenital dislocation of the hip or a slipped femoral epiphysis or Perthes' disease; osteonecrosis of the femoral head (see p. 571) in children and adolescents causes early-onset OA.
> - *Occupation* – Miners develop OA of the hip, knee and shoulder, cotton workers OA of the hand, and farmers OA of the hip.
> - *Sport* – Repetitive use and injury in some sports causes a high incidence of lower-limb OA.

- In women, weight-bearing sports produce a two- to threefold increase in risk of OA of the hip and knee.
- In men, there is an association between hip OA and certain occupations – farming and labouring.
- Obesity is a risk factor for developing OA in later life.

The term primary OA is sometimes used when there is no obvious known predisposing factor.

Box 10.6 shows some of the predisposing factors for the development of OA, whilst Table 10.11 shows other conditions that sometimes cause secondary arthritis.

Clinical features

Osteoarthritis affects many joints, with diverse clinical patterns. Hip and knee OA is the major cause of disability. Early OA is rarely symptomatic unless accompanied by a joint effusion, whilst advanced radiological and pathological OA is not always symptomatic.

Some flare-ups are due to inflammation but are not associated with an increased ESR or CRP. Focal synovitis is caused by fragments of shed bone or cartilage. Radiological OA is usually, but not inevitably, progressive. This progression may be stepwise or continual. Radiological improvement is uncommon but has been observed, suggesting that repair is possible.

Table 10.11
Causes of osteoarthritis

Primary OA	No known cause
Secondary OA	Pre-existing joint damage
	Rheumatoid arthritis
	Gout
	Seronegative spondarthritis
	Septic arthritis
	Paget's disease
	Avascular necrosis, e.g. corticosteroid therapy
	Metabolic disease
	Chondrocalcinosis
	Hereditary haemochromatosis
	Acromegaly
	Systemic diseases
	Haemophilia – recurrent haemarthrosis
	Haemoglobinopathies, e.g. sickle cell disease
	Neuropathies
	Mechanical factors
	Trauma and meniscal/cruciate tears
	Joint hypermobility
	Joint dysplasia

Symptoms
- Joint pain
- Joint gelling (stiffening and pain after immobility)
- Joint instability
- Loss of function.

Signs
- Joint tenderness
- Crepitus on movement
- Limitation of range of movement
- Joint instability
- Joint effusion and variable levels of inflammation
- Bony swelling
- Wasting of muscles.

Clinical subsets
Localized OA
Nodal OA (Table 10.12)

The joints are usually affected one at a time over several years, with the distal interphalangeal joints (DIPs) being more often involved than the proximal interphalangeal joints (PIPs). The onset may be painful and associated with tenderness, swelling and inflammation and impairment of hand function. The inflammation often occurs around the female menopause. PIP-predominant nodal OA has a superficial similarity to early rheumatoid arthritis. Even if a weakly positive rheumatoid factor is found, it is of no significance. The inflammatory phase settles after some months or years, leaving painless bony swellings posterolaterally — Heberden's nodes (DIPs) and Bouchard's nodes (PIPs), along with stiffness and deformity (Fig. 10.11). Functional impairment is slight for most, although PIP osteoarthritis restricts gripping more than DIP involvement. On X-ray, the nodes are marginal osteophytes and there is joint space loss.

Table 10.12
Features of nodal OA

Familial
Has a higher incidence in women
Typical pattern of polyarticular involvement of the hand joints
Develops in late middle age
Has a generally good long-term functional outcome
Associated with OA of the knee, hip and spine

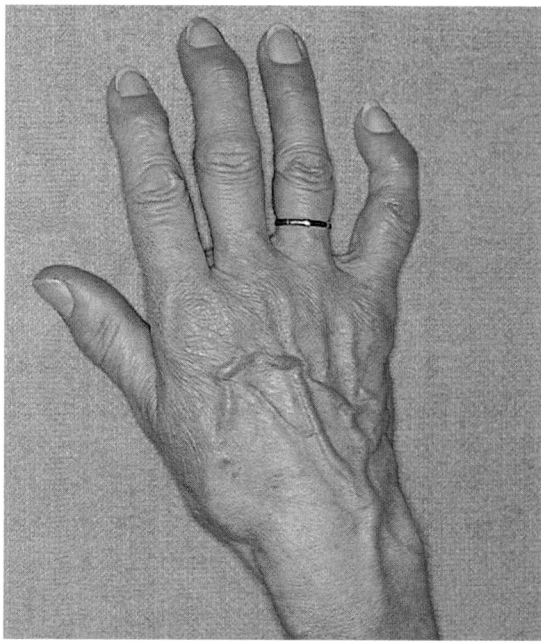

Fig. 10.11 Severe nodal osteoarthritis. The DIP joints demonstrate Heberden's nodes. The index finger DIP joint is deformed and unstable. The thumb is adducted and the bony swelling of the first carpometacarpal joint is clearly shown –'the squared hand of nodal OA'.

Carpometacarpal and metacarpophalangeal OA of the thumb coexist with nodal OA and cause pain, which decreases as the joint stiffens. The 'squared' hand in OA is caused by bony swelling of the carpometacarpal joint and fixed adduction of the thumb. Function is rarely severely compromised.

Polyarticular hand OA is associated with a slightly increased frequency of OA at other sites.

Hip OA

Hip OA affects 7–25% of white adult Caucasians but is significantly less common in black African populations. There are two major subgroups defined by the radiological appearance. The most common is *superior-pole hip OA*, where joint space narrowing and sclerosis predominantly affect the weight-bearing upper surface of the femoral head and adjacent acetabulum. This is most common in men and unilateral at presentation, although both hips may become involved because the disease is progressive. Less commonly, *medial cartilage loss occurs*. This is most common in women and associated with hand involvement (nodal, generalized OA, NGOA), and is usually bilateral.

Knee OA

The prevalence of knee OA is 40% in individuals aged over 75 years. It is commoner in women than men. There is a strong relationship with obesity. The disease is generally bilateral and strongly associated with *polyarticular OA of the hand* in elderly women. The medial compartment is most commonly affected and leads to a varus (bow-legged) deformity. There is often also retropatellar OA. Previous trauma, meniscal and cruciate ligament tears and obesity are risk factors for developing knee OA.

Primary generalized OA

This is less common than nodal OA of the hands but is usually seen in combination. It is also called 'nodal generalized OA' (NGOA). It predominantly affects women. The other joints affected are the knees, first MTP and hip joints, and spondylosis. There is a female preponderance and a strong familial tendency. NGOA is associated with immune complex deposition and may have an autoimmune cause. Its onset is often sudden and severe.

Erosive OA

This is rare. The DIPs and PIPs are inflamed and equally affected. In contrast to nodal OA, the functional outcome is poor. Radiologically, there are marked subchondral cysts. Erosive OA may develop into RA and may not be a true subset of OA.

Crystal-associated OA

This is most commonly seen with calcium pyrophosphate deposition in the cartilage (chondrocalcinosis). *Chondrocalcinosis* increases in frequency with age, but is usually asymptomatic. The joints most commonly affected are the knees (hyaline cartilage and fibrocartilage) and wrists (triangular fibrocartilage). There is patchy linear calcification on X-ray (Fig. 10.12).

A chronic arthropathy (pseudo-OA) occurs, predominantly in elderly women with severe chondrocalcinosis. There is a florid inflammatory component and marked osteophyte and cyst formation visible on X-rays. The joints affected differ from NGOA – affecting predominantly the knees, then wrists and shoulders, but also elbows, ankles and hips. Chondrocalcinosis is associated with pseudogout, an acute crystal-induced arthritis (see p. 554).

A rare, rapidly destructive arthritis in elderly women, affecting shoulders, hips and knees, is associated with finding crystals of calcium apatite in a bloody joint effusion. The outlook is poor and joints require early surgical replacement.

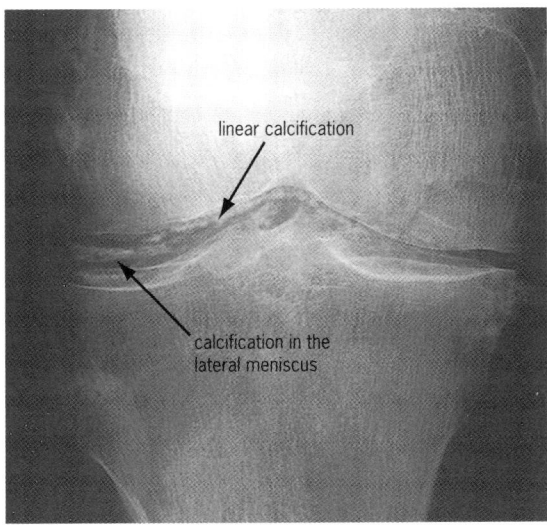

Fig. 10.12 Chondrocalcinosis of the knee. Note the linear calcification in the hyaline cartilage and calcification of the lateral meniscus (plus mild secondary OA).

Investigations in OA

- **Blood tests.** There is no specific test; the ESR and CRP are normal. Rheumatoid factor and antinuclear antibodies are negative.
- **X-rays** are abnormal only when the damage is advanced.
- **MRI** can demonstrate early cartilage changes.
- **Arthroscopy** can reveal early fissuring and surface erosion of the cartilage.

Treatment

The guiding principle is to treat the symptoms and disability, not the radiological appearances; depression and poor quadriceps strength are better predictors of pain than is radiological severity in OA of the knee. Education of the individual about the disease and its effects reduces pain, distress and disability and increases compliance with treatment. Psychological or social factors alter the impact of the disease.

Physical measures

Weight loss and exercises for strength and stability are useful. Hydrotherapy helps, especially in lower-limb OA. Local heat, ice packs, massage and rubifacients or local NSAID gels are all used, although the value of NSAID gels is probably marginal.

Complementary medicine is commonly used and, despite lack of scientific evidence, little is lost in trying it since a number of patients do seem to be helped.

Medication

Balance the potential benefit against potential side-effects. Drugs usually should be used only in severe disease. Patients should be prescribed short courses of simple analgesics before NSAIDs (see Box 10.5). NSAIDs should be used intermittently. It has been suggested that some NSAIDs may increase the cartilage damage, while others are 'chondroprotective', but these claims remain unproven.

Intra-articular corticosteroid injections produce short-term improvement when there is a painful joint effusion. Frequent injections into the same joint should be avoided.

The role of chondroitin sulphate and glycosaminoglycan (sold as food supplements) is still under investigation and unproven.

Surgery

Total replacement arthroplasty has transformed the management of severe OA. The safety of hip and knee replacements is now equal, with a complication rate of about 1%; loosening, and late blood-borne infection are the most serious. These slight but definite risks make it essential that the patient is certain that surgery is wanted, when all else has been tried. For the vast majority, a total hip or knee replacement reduces pain and stiffness and greatly increases function.

Other surgical procedures include realignment osteotomy of the knee or hip, excision arthroplasty of the first MTP and base of the thumb, and fusion of a first MTP joint.

FURTHER READING

Cicuttini F, Spector TD (1998) Osteoarthritis. *Medicine* **26**(6): 68–71.

Creamer P, Hocberg MC (1997) Osteoarthritis. *Lancet* **350**: 503–508.

Doherty M (2001) Risk factors for progression of knee osteoarthritis. *Lancet* **358**: 775–776.

Inflammatory arthritis

Inflammatory arthritis includes a large number of arthritic conditions in which the predominant feature is synovial inflammation. This disparate group includes postviral arthritis, rheumatoid arthritis, seronegative spondarthritis, crystal arthritis and Lyme arthritis. The diagnosis of these conditions is helped by the pattern of joint involvement (Table 10.13), along with any nonarticular disease; a past and family history may be helpful. The distribution of the affected joints (symmetrical or asymmetrical; large or small) as well as the periodicity of the arthritis (single acute, relapsing, chronic and progressive) may also help in the diagnosis.

Certain nonarticular diseases – for example, psoriasis, iritis, inflammatory bowel disease, non-specific urethritis or recent dysentery – may suggest a seronegative

Table 10.13
Pattern of joint involvement in inflammatory arthritis

Diseases presenting as an inflammatory monarthritis
Crystal arthritis, e.g. gout, pseudogout
Septic arthritis
Palindromic rheumatism
Traumatic ± haemarthrosis
Arthritis due to juxta-articular bone tumour
Occasionally, psoriatic, reactive, rheumatoid may present as monarthritis

Diseases presenting as an inflammatory polyarthritis
Rheumatoid arthritis
Reactive arthritis
Seronegative arthritis associated with psoriasis or ankylosing spondylitis
Postviral arthritis
Lyme arthritis
Enteropathic arthritis
Arthritis associated with erythema nodosum

spondarthritis. There may be evidence of recent viral illness (rubella, hepatitis B or parvovirus), of rheumatic fever, or of a tick bite and skin rash (Lyme disease). In early arthritis it may not be possible to make a specific diagnosis until the disease has evolved.

There is a distinct genetic separation of rheumatoid-pattern synovitis and the seronegative group; RA (p. 538) is associated with a genetic marker in the class II major histocompatibility genes, whilst seronegative spondarthritis shares certain alleles in the B locus of class I MHC genes, usually B27 (see p. 204).

In general the pain and stiffness of inflammatory arthritis are worse in the morning and after rest. This early-morning exacerbation may last several hours, in contrast to the much shorter post-rest gelling of OA. Inflammatory markers (ESR and CRP) are often raised in inflammatory arthritis, and there is often a normochromic normocytic anaemia. Specific types of arthritis are discussed below.

Rheumatoid arthritis (RA)

Rheumatoid arthritis is a chronic symmetrical polyarthritis of unexplained cause. It is a systemic disorder characterized by chronic inflammatory synovitis of mainly peripheral joints. Its course is extremely variable and it is associated with nonarticular features.

Aetiology and pathogenesis

- *Geographical.* RA has a world-wide distribution and affects 0.5–3% (depending on the definition) of the population. It is a significant cause of disability and mortality and carries a high socio-economic cost.
- *Age.* RA presents from early childhood (when it is rare) to late old age. The most common age of onset is between 30 and 50 years.

- *Gender*. Women before the menopause are affected three times more often than men. After the menopause the frequency of onset is similar between the sexes, suggesting an aetiological role for sex hormones. The use of oral contraceptives may delay the onset of RA but does not reduce the risk of developing it.
- *Familial*. The disease is familial but sporadic. In occasional families it affects several generations. It is estimated to account for 60% of disease susceptibility.
- *HLA types*. There is a strong association between susceptibility to RA and certain HLA haplotypes. HLA-DR4, which occurs in 50–75% of patients, correlates with a poor prognosis. The possession of a specific pentapeptide (QK/RAA) in the third allelic hypervariable region of HLA-DRβ-1 increases susceptibility. Combined with a positive rheumatoid factor it identifies individuals with a 13 times greater risk for developing bone erosions in early disease.

Immunology

The chronic synovial inflammation may be caused by ongoing *T cell activation* or may be maintained by the local production of rheumatoid factors and *continuous stimulation of macrophages* via IgG Fc receptors. Considering the extent of synovial inflammation and lymphocytic infiltration, there are only minimal amounts of the factors produced by T cells (interferon and interleukin-2 and -4). Conversely, the cytokines (IL-1, IL-8, TNF-α, granulocyte macrophage colony-stimulating factor) and chemokines produced by macrophages (macrophage inflammatory protein (MIP) and monocyte chemoattractant protein (MCP)) and fibroblasts (producing IL-6) are abundant. The relevance of these findings is unclear.

CD4-specific antibodies, when used therapeutically, produce a specific helper T-cell lymphopenia but do not significantly alter the disease, raising the possibility that T cells are less important.

Temporary B cell ablation (a technique used for treating B cell lymphomas) induces remission, reinforcing the central place of rheumatoid factor production in maintaining the chronic inflammation of RA.

Antibodies to TNF-α or specific blocking agents produce marked short-term improvement in synovitis, indicating the pivotal role of TNF-α in the chronic synovitis (see p. 546). They also reduce the malaise felt in active RA.

Synovial fibroblasts have high levels of the *adhesion molecule*, vascular cell adhesion molecule (VCAM-1), a molecule which supports B lymphocyte survival and differentiation, and of decay accelerating factor (DAF), a factor that prevents complement-induced cell lysis. These molecules may facilitate the formation of ectopic lymphoid tissue in synovium.

High-affinity antibodies are not a feature of RA unlike other autoimmune diseases. *The triggering antigen* remains unclear, although it is suggested that the glycosylation pattern of immunoglobulins may be abnormal in RA and lead to their becoming potentially antigenic. There is little evidence that collagen type II is the triggering antigen, although it is a cause of arthritis in animal models of RA.

Bacterial or slow virus infections have been implicated but are unproven. It has been suggested that an immune response to any pathogen is to produce autoantibodies by B cell clonal expansion. In susceptible individuals such clones may persist.

Pathology

Rheumatoid arthritis is typified by widespread persisting synovitis (inflammation of the synovial lining of joints, tendon sheaths or bursae). The cause of this is unclear, but the production of rheumatoid factors (RFs, see p. 539) by plasma cells in the synovium and the local formation of immune complexes play a part. In RA, the normal synovium becomes greatly thickened to the extent that it is palpable as a 'boggy' swelling around the joints and tendons. There is proliferation of the synovium into folds and fronds, and it is infiltrated by a variety of inflammatory cells, including polymorphs, which transit through the tissue into the joint fluid, and lymphocytes and plasma cells. There are disorganized lymphoid follicles that are responsive to exogenous antigens. The normally sparse surface layer of lining cells becomes hyperplastic and thickened (Fig. 10.13). There is marked vascular proliferation. Increased permeability of blood vessels and the synovial lining layer leads to joint effusions that contain lymphocytes and dying polymorphs. Activated lymphocytes and macrophages in the synovium produce a rich mixture of cytokines, including interleukins, prostaglandins and tumour necrosis factor alpha.

The hyperplastic synovium spreads from the joint margins on to the cartilage surface. This 'pannus' of inflamed synovium damages the underlying cartilage by blocking its normal route for nutrition and by the direct effects of cytokines on the chondrocytes. The cartilage becomes thinned and the underlying bone exposed. Local cytokine production and joint disuse combine to cause juxta-articular osteoporosis during active synovitis.

Fibroblasts from the proliferating synovium also grow along the course of blood vessels between the synovial margins and the epiphyseal bone cavity and damage the bone. This is shown by MRI to occur in the first 3–6 months following onset of the arthritis, and before the diagnostic, ill-defined juxta-articular bony 'erosions' appear on X-ray (Fig. 10.14). This early damage may justify the introductions of DMARDs (see p. 544) within 3–6 months of onset of the arthritis. Low-dose steroids

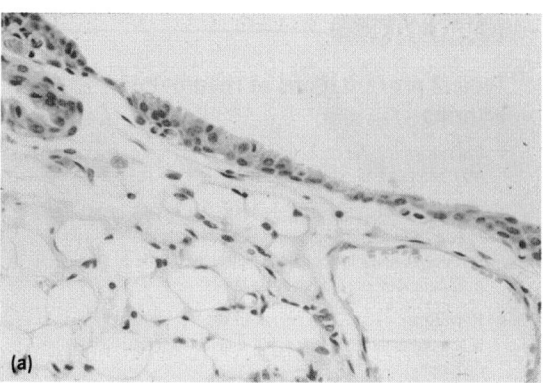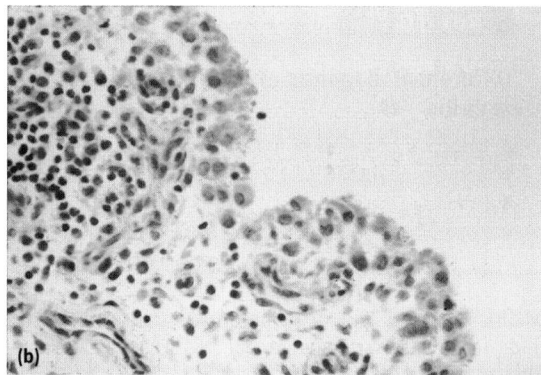

Fig. 10.13 **Histological appearance of RA synovium.** **(a)** Normal synovium. **(b)** Synovial appearances in established RA, showing marked hypertrophy of the tissues with infiltration by lymphocytes and plasma cells. From Shipley M (1993) *Colour Atlas of Rheumatology*, 3rd edn. Wolfe Mosby, with permission.

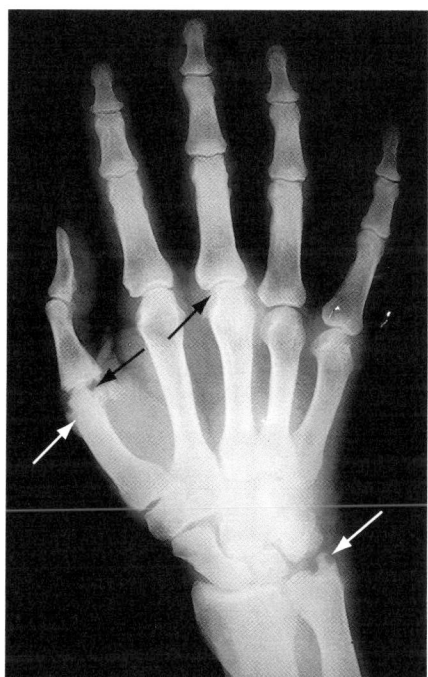

Fig. 10.14 **X-ray of early RA**, showing typical erosions at the thumb and middle MCP joints and at the ulnar styloid.

delay and anti-TNF-α agents halt or reverse erosion formation. Erosions lead to a variety of deformities and contribute to long-term disability.

Rheumatoid factors (RFs)

These are circulating autoantibodies, which have the Fc portion of IgG as their antigen. The nature of the antigen means that they self-aggregate into immune complexes and thus activate complement and stimulate inflammation, causing chronic synovitis. Transient production of RFs is an essential part of the body's normal mechanism for removing immune complexes, but in RA they show a much higher affinity and their production is persistent

and occurs in the joints. They may be of any immunoglobulin class (IgM, IgG or IgA), but the most common tests employed clinically detect IgM rheumatoid factor. Around 70% of patients with polyarticular RA have IgM rheumatoid factor in the serum.

The term seronegative RA is used for patients in whom the standard tests for IgM rheumatoid factor are persistently negative. They tend to have a more limited pattern of synovitis.

IgM rheumatoid factor is not diagnostic of RA, nor does its absence rule the disease out; but it is a useful predictor of prognosis. A persistently high titre in early disease implies more persistently active synovitis, more joint damage and greater disability eventually, and justifies earlier use of DMARDs.

Clinical features of RA

Typical presentation

The most typical presentation of rheumatoid arthritis (approximately 70% of cases) begins as a slowly progressive, symmetrical, peripheral polyarthritis, evolving over a period of a few weeks or months. Women are affected three times more often than men are. The patient is usually in her thirties or fifties, but the disease can occur at any age. Less commonly (15%) a rapid onset can occur over a few days (or explosively overnight) with a severe symmetrical polyarticular involvement, but surprisingly these patients often have a better prognosis. A worse than average prognosis (with a predictive accuracy of about 80%) is indicated by being female, a gradual onset over a few months, and a positive IgM rheumatoid factor, and/or anaemia within 3 months of onset. The differential diagnosis of early RA is shown in Box 10.7.

Symptoms and signs

The majority of patients complain of pain and stiffness of the small joints of the hands (metacarpophalangeal,

Differential diagnosis of early rheumatoid arthritis

- Postviral arthritis – rubella, hepatitis B or parvovirus
- Seronegative arthritis
- Polymyalgia rheumatica
- Acute nodal osteoarthritis (PIPs and DIPs involved)

Typical presentations of rheumatoid arthritis

- **Palindromic** – Monarticular attacks lasting 24–48 hours; 50% progress to other types of RA.

- **Transient** – A self-limiting disease, lasting less than 12 months and leaving no permanent joint damage. Usually seronegative for IgM rheumatoid factor. Some of these may be undetected postviral arthritis.

- **Remitting** – There is a period of several years during which the arthritis is active but then remits, leaving minimal damage.

- **Chronic, persistent** – The most typical form, it may be seropositive or seronegative for IgM rheumatoid factor. The disease follows a relapsing and remitting course over many years. Seropositive patients tend to develop greater joint damage and long-term disability. They warrant earlier and more agressive treatment with disease-modifying agents.

- **Rapidly progressive** – The disease progresses remorselessly over a few years and leads rapidly to severe joint damage and disability. It is usually seropositive, has a high incidence of systemic complications and is difficult to treat.

MCP), proximal and distal interphalangeal (PIP, DIP) and feet (metatarsophalangeal, MTP). The wrists, elbows, shoulders, knees and ankles are also affected. In most cases many joints are involved, but 10% present with a monarthritis of the knee or shoulder or with a carpal tunnel syndrome. The hips are rarely affected early in the disease.

The patient feels tired and unwell and the pain and stiffness are significantly worse in the morning and may improve with gentle activity.

The joints are usually warm and tender with some joint swelling. There is limitation of movement and muscle wasting. Deformities develop as the disease progresses. Nonarticular features develop (see below).

Other presentations

The presentation and progression of RA is variable. Presentations are shown in Box 10.8. Relapses and remissions occur either spontaneously or in response to drug therapy. In some patients the disease remains active, producing progressive joint damage. Rarely the process may cease ('burnt-out RA').

A *seronegative, limited synovitis* initially affects the wrists more often than the fingers and has a less symmetrical joint involvement. It has a better long-term prognosis, but some cases progress to severe disability. This form can be confused with psoriatic arthropathy, which has a similar distribution. There may be a family history of psoriasis or the patient may develop psoriasis later.

Palindromic rheumatism is unusual (5%) and consists of short-lived (24–48 h) episodes of acute monarthritis. The joint becomes acutely painful, swollen and red, but resolves completely. Further attacks occur in the same or other joints. About 50% go on to develop typical chronic rheumatoid synovitis after a delay of months or years. The rest remit or continue to have acute episodic arthritis. The detection of IgM rheumatoid factor predicts conversion to chronic, destructive synovitis.

Complications (Table 10.14)
Septic arthritis
This is a serious complication with significant morbidity and mortality. The joint (or joints) may be hot and inflamed with accompanying fever and a neutrophil leukocytosis in the blood. However, these signs are often absent, and any effusion, particularly of sudden onset, should be aspirated. *Staphylococcus aureus* is the

Table 10.14
Complications of rheumatoid arthritis

Complications of the condition
Ruptured tendons
Ruptured joints (Baker's cysts)
Joint infection
Spinal cord compression (atlanto-axial or upper cervical spine)
Amyloidosis (rare)

Side-effects of therapy
Dyspepsia
Gastrointestinal bleeding
Perforation
Anaemia
Renal impairment
Bone marrow hypoplasia

most common organism. Treatment is with systemic antibiotics (see p. 555) and drainage.

Amyloidosis (see p. 1119)
Amyloidosis is found in a very small number of people with severe rheumatoid arthritis. RA is the most common cause of secondary amyloidosis. Primary amyloidosis causes a polyarthritis that resembles RA in distribution and is also often associated with carpal tunnel syndrome and subcutaneous nodules.

Joint involvement in RA
Hands and wrists
The impact of RA on the hands is severe. In early disease the fingers are swollen, painful and stiff. Inflamed flexor

tendon sheaths increase functional impairment and may cause carpal tunnel syndrome. Joint damage causes a variety of typical deformities. Most typical is a combination of ulnar drift and palmar subluxation of the MCPs (Fig. 10.15). This leads to unsightly deformity, but function may be remarkably good once the patient has learned to adapt, and pain is controlled. Fixed flexion (buttonhole or boutonnière deformity) or fixed hyperextension (swan-neck deformity) of the PIP joints impairs hand function.

Swelling and dorsal subluxation of the ulnar styloid lead to wrist pain and may cause rupture of the finger extensor tendons, leading in turn to a sudden onset of finger drop of the little and ring fingers predominantly, which needs urgent surgical repair.

Shoulders

RA commonly affects the shoulders. Initially the symptoms mimic rotator cuff tendonitis (see p. 520) with a painful arc syndrome and pain in the upper arms at night. As the joints become damaged more global stiffening occurs. Late in the disease rotator cuff tears are common (see p. 521) and interfere with dressing, feeding and personal toilet.

Elbows

Synovitis of the elbows causes swelling and a painful fixed flexion deformity. In late disease flexion may be lost and severe difficulties with feeding result, especially combined with shoulder, hand and wrist deformities.

Feet

One of the earliest manifestations of RA is painful swelling of the MTP joints. The foot becomes broader and a hammer-toe deformity develops. Exposure of the metatarsal heads to pressure by the forwards migration of the protective fibrofatty pad (Fig. 10.16) causes pain. Ulcers may develop over the metatarsal heads and the dorsum of the toes. Mid- and hindfoot RA causes a flat medial arch and loss of flexibility of the foot. The ankle often assumes a valgus position. Appropriate broad, deep shoes are essential but rarely wholly adequate, and walking is often painful and limited. Podiatry helps and surgery may be required.

Knees

Massive synovitis and knee effusions occur, but respond well to aspiration and steroid injection (see p. 528). A persistent effusion increases the risk of popliteal cyst formation and rupture (see p. 528). In later disease, erosion of cartilage and bone causes loss of joint space on X-ray and damage to the medial and/or lateral and/or retropatellar compartments of the knees. Depending on the pattern of involvement, the knees may develop a varus or valgus deformity. Secondary OA follows. Total knee replacement is often the only way to restore mobility and relieve pain.

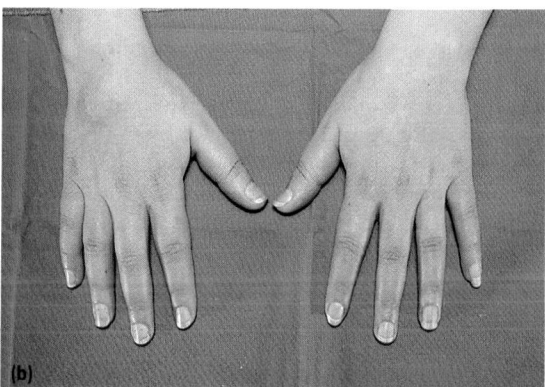

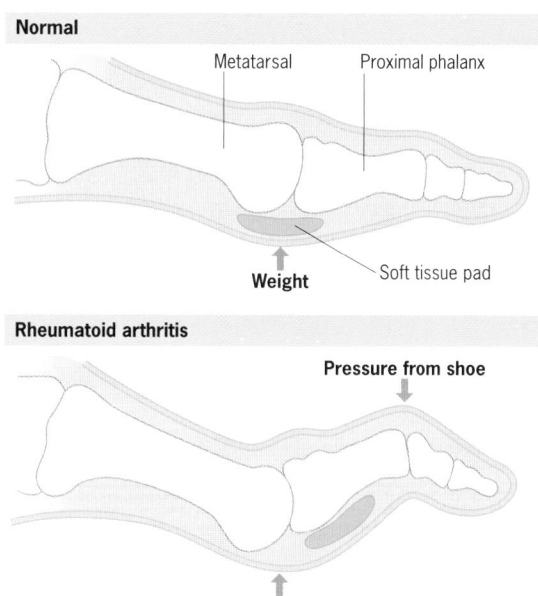

Fig. 10.15 **(a) Characteristic hand deformities in RA.**
(b) Early rheumatoid arthritis – dorsal tenosynovitis of the right wrist and small joints of both hands with spindling of the fingers.

Fig. 10.16 **The toes in RA**, showing exposure of the metatarsal heads with forward migration of the soft tissue pad.

Hips

The hips are rarely affected in early RA and are less commonly affected than the knees at all stages of the disease. Pain and stiffness are accompanied by radiological loss of joint space and juxta-articular osteoporosis. The latter may permit medial migration of the acetabulum (protrusio acetabulae). Later, secondary OA develops. Hip replacement is usually necessary.

Cervical spine

Painful stiffness of the neck in RA is often muscular, but it may be due to rheumatoid synovitis affecting the synovial joints of the upper cervical spine and the bursae which separate the odontoid peg from the anterior arch of the atlas and from its retaining ligaments. This synovitis leads to bone destruction, damages the ligaments and causes atlantoaxial or upper cervical instability. Subluxation and local synovial swelling may damage the spinal cord, producing pyramidal and sensory signs. MRI is the best way of visualizing this, but lateral flexed and extended neck X-rays can demonstrate instability. In late RA, difficulty walking which cannot be explained by articular disease, weakness of the legs or loss of control of bowel or bladder may be due to spinal cord compression and is a neurosurgical emergency. Image the cervical spine in flexion and extension in patients with RA before surgery or upper gastrointestinal endoscopy to check for instability and reduce the risk of cord injury during intubation.

Other joints

The temporomandibular, acromioclavicular, sternoclavicular, cricoarytenoid and any other synovial joint can be affected.

Nonarticular manifestations (Fig. 10.17)

Soft tissue surrounding joints

Subcutaneous nodules are firm, intradermal and generally occur over pressure points, typically the elbows, the finger joints and the Achilles tendon. They occur on the sacrum and occiput in bed-bound patients. They may ulcerate and become infected, but usually resolve when the disease comes under control. The nodules can be removed surgically or injected with corticosteroids if causing a problem. They tend to recur. Histologically there is a necrotic centre surrounded by rows of activated macrophages. This resembles synovitis without a synovial space.

The olecranon and other bursae may be swollen (*bursitis*).

Tenosynovitis of affected flexor tendons in the hand can cause a trigger finger. Swelling of the extensor tendon sheath over the dorsum of the wrist is common.

Muscle wasting around joints is common. Muscle enzyme concentrations are normal; myositis is extremely rare. Corticosteroid-induced myopathy may occur.

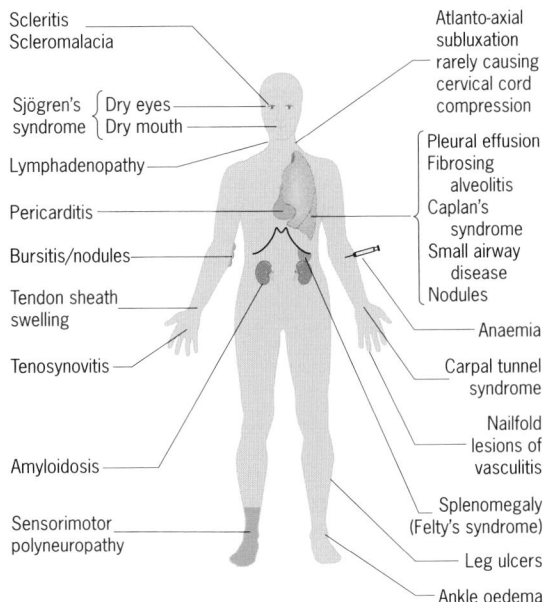

Fig. 10.17 Nonarticular manifestations of RA.

Lungs (see also p. 900)

Peripheral, intrapulmonary nodules are usually asymptomatic but may cavitate. When pneumoconiosis is present (Caplan's syndrome), large cavitating lung nodules develop.

Other manifestations are:

- serositis causing pleural effusion
- pleural nodules
- fibrosing alveolitis
- obstructive bronchiolitis.

Vasculitis

Vasculitis (see p. 564) is caused by immune complex deposition in arterial walls. Smoking is a risk factor. Other manifestations are:

- nail-fold infarcts due to cutaneous vasculitis
- widespread cutaneous vasculitis with necrosis of the skin (seen in patients with very active, strongly seropositive disease)
- mononeuritis multiplex (p. 564)
- bowel infarction due to necrotizing arteritis of the mesenteric vessels (this may be indistinguishable from polyarteritis nodosa).

The heart and peripheral vessels

Clinical pericarditis is rare. In strongly seropositive RA, echocardiogram or post-mortem studies, however, show that 30–40% of patients have pericardial involvement. Constrictive pericarditis is very rare.

Endocarditis and myocardial disease are rarely seen clinically, although found at post-mortem in approximately 20% of cases. These are secondary to the vasculitis.

Raynaud's syndrome may occur (see p. 831).

The nervous system

Neuropathies, either mononeuritis multiplex or a sensory loss in a glove and stocking pattern, are due to vasculitis of the vasa nervorum. Compression neuropathies such as carpal or tarsal tunnel syndrome are due to local synovial hypertrophy. Atlanto-axial subluxation can cause serious neurological abnormalities.

The eyes

Scleritis and episcleritis occur in severe, seropositive disease and produce painful red lesions in the eye. Scleritis may lead to perforation of the eye (scleromalacia perforans) and requires active treatment with local and systemic corticosteroids.

Sicca syndrome causes dry mouth and eyes (see Sjögren's syndrome, p. 564).

The kidneys

Amyloidosis causes the nephrotic syndrome and renal failure. Presentation is with proteinuria. It occurs rarely in severe, long-standing rheumatoid disease and is due to the deposition of highly stable serum amyloid A protein (SAP) in the intercellular matrix of a variety of organs. SAP is an acute-phase reactant, produced normally in the liver. It is rare and proteinuria in RA is more commonly due to DMARDs.

The spleen, lymph nodes and blood

Felty's syndrome is splenomegaly and neutropenia in a patient with RA. Leg ulcers or sepsis are complications. HLA-DRW4 is found in 95% of patients, compared with 70% of patients with RA alone.

The lymph nodes may be palpable, usually in the distribution of affected joints. There may be peripheral lymphoedema of the arm or leg.

Anaemia is almost universal and is usually the normochromic normocytic anaemia of chronic disease. It may be iron-deficient owing to gastrointestinal blood loss from NSAID ingestion, or rarely, haemolytic (Coombs' positive). There may be a pancytopenia due to hypersplenism in Felty's syndrome or as a complication of DMARD treatment. A high platelet count occurs with active disease.

Diagnosis and investigations

The diagnosis relies on the clinical features described above. The American College of Rheumatology (ACR) criteria are shown in Box 10.9 and are useful for

---

> ### Box 10.9
>
> **Criteria for the diagnosis of rheumatoid arthritis (American College of Rheumatology, 1987 revision)**
>
> - Morning stiffness > 1 hour ⎤
> - Arthritis of three or more joints ⎟ For 6 weeks
> - Arthritis of hand joints and wrists ⎟ or more
> - Symmetrical arthritis ⎦
> - Subcutaneous nodules
> - A positive serum rheumatoid factor
> - Typical radiological changes (erosions and/or periarticular osteopenia)
>
> Four or more criteria are necessary for diagnosis.

---

epidemiological and investigative studies but are unhelpful in early disease.

Initial investigations include:

- **Blood count.** Anaemia may be present. The ESR and/or CRP are raised in proportion to the activity of the inflammatory process and are useful in monitoring treatment.
- **Serology.** Rheumatoid factor is present in approximately 70% of cases and ANA at low titre in 30%.
- **X-rays** of the affected joint(s) to establish a baseline. Only soft tissue swelling is seen in early disease. MRI demonstrates early erosions.
- **Aspiration of the joint** if an effusion is present. The aspirate looks cloudy owing to white cells. In a suddenly painful joint septic arthritis should be suspected (see p. 555).

Other investigations will depend on the clinical picture as outlined above. In severe disease extensive imaging of joints may be required. MRI is the technique of choice, especially for the knee.

Management of RA (Box 10.10)

The diagnosis of RA inevitably causes concern and fear in the patient and requires a lot of explanation and reassurance. The doctor and therapist should retain a positive approach and remind the patient that most will continue to lead a more or less normal life despite their arthritis, with the help of drugs; 25% will recover completely. The earliest years are often the most difficult. It is important to try to keep people at work during this phase. Uncertainty about when the disease will remit and flare, when and if drugs will work, and whether they may produce side-effects, makes planning from day to day difficult. People learn to adjust remarkably but this takes time and support. A rheumatology unit

---

Box 10.10

Management of rheumatoid arthritis

- Establish the diagnosis clinically.
- Use NSAIDs and analgesics to control symptoms.
- Try to induce remission with i.m. depot methylprednisolone 80–120 mg if synovitis persists beyond 6 weeks.
- If synovitis recurs, refer to a rheumatologist to start sulfasalazine or methotrexate. Give a second dose of i.m. depot methylprednisolone.
- Refer for physiotherapy and general advice through a specialist team.
- If there is no significant improvement in 6–12 weeks as measured by less pain, less morning stiffness and reduced acute-phase response, consider a combination of methotrexate and sulfasalazine.
- If no better, consider an alternative agent, such as gold, D-penicillamine or leflunamide.
- If still no better, consider anti-TNF-α therapy.

---

will have a team, including doctors, specialist nurses and physiotherapists, to help the patient learn to cope. Leaflets give helpful advice, as do local patient groups.

Drug therapy

There is no curative agent available for RA. Symptoms are controlled with analgesia and NSAIDs. Recent data support the use of DMARDs early in the disease to prevent the long-term irreversible damaging effects of inflammation of the joints.

Non-steroidal anti-inflammatory drugs (NSAIDs)

Most patients with RA are unable to cope without an NSAID to relieve night pain and morning stiffness. NSAIDs do not reduce the underlying inflammatory process. They all act on the cyclo-oxygenase (COX) pathway (see Fig. 14.32) but newer drugs are more specific for blocking the COX-2 enzyme (p. 532). The individual response to NSAIDs varies greatly. It is desirable therefore to try several different drugs for a particular patient in order to find the best (see Box 10.5). Each compound should be given for at least a week. Start with an inexpensive NSAID with few side-effects and with which you are familiar. Regular doses are needed to be effective. The major side-effects of NSAIDs are discussed on page 532. If gastrointestinal side-effects are prominent, a COX-2 specific NSAID should be used. Slow-release preparations (e.g. slow-release diclofenac, 75 mg, taken after supper), or a suppository at bedtime, usually work well and can be given in addition to daytime therapy if necessary. For additional relief a simple analgesic is taken as required (e.g. paracetamol or a combination of dextropropoxyphene and paracetamol). Many patients need night sedation.

Disease-modifying anti-rheumatic drugs

(Table 10.15)

DMARDs, which mainly act through cytokine inhibition, reduce inflammation, as reflected by a reduction of joint swelling, a fall in the plasma acute phase reactants and slowing of the development of joint erosions and irreversible damage. Their beneficial effect is not immediate (hence 'slow-acting agents') and may be partial or transient. The problem with all DMARDs is that their effect is often only partial, achieving between 20 and 50% improvement by ACR criteria for disease remission. Drugs which achieve 70% improvement are required. Nonetheless there is good evidence that DMARDs control symptoms and signs of joint inflammation and that their withdrawal leads to a flare. Methotrexate, sulfasalazine, leflunamide and ciclosporin have all been shown to reduce the rate of progressive joint damage in early and late disease.

Generally DMARDs are used after symptomatic treatment, but in seropositive patients with a poor prognosis they should be used early, before the appearance of erosions on X-rays of hands and feet. The early use of depot injections of a corticosteroid at 6–12 weeks may induce remission. Studies of early RA suggest that intervention with DMARDs at 6 weeks to 6 months improves the outcome. The use of combinations of three or four drugs (steroids, methotrexate, sulfasalazine and hydroxychloroquine) in early RA (the inverted pyramid approach), reducing the number of agents once remission has been achieved, is more controversial and its long-term efficacy is yet to be proven. Toxicity appears to be reduced with such combinations, possibly because inflammation is controlled effectively. It is important not to overtreat people who are not going to develop erosions. Most prognostic assessments in early disease are only 80% accurate for risk of erosion and clinical judgement retains a central place in managing RA. DMARDs are usually prescribed by a rheumatologist (Table 10.15).

Sulfasalazine

This is a combination of sulfapyridine and 5-amino-salicylic acid. Sulfapyridine is probably the active component. It is well tolerated and for many is the first-choice DMARD. It produces a response in about half the patients in the first 3–6 months. Serious side-effects are rare, being mainly leukopenia and thrombocytopenia.

Methotrexate

This is considered by many to be the drug of choice, although care needs to be taken in those who are planning a family. It is given at an initial weekly dose of 2.5–7.5 mg orally, increased up to 15–25 mg if necessary. It is well tolerated and this therapy can be introduced early in the disease. Oral folic acid should be given in addition to reduce side-effects, although it may marginally reduce efficacy. Full blood counts and liver

Table 10.15
Disease-modifying anti-rheumatic drugs (DMARDs)

Drug	Dose	Side-effects	Monitoring
Sulfasalazine enteric coated	500 mg daily after food, increasing to 2–3 g daily	Nausea Skin rashes and mouth ulcers Neutropenia and/or thrombocytopenia Abnormal liver biochemistry	Initial, fortnightly, then 4-monthly Initial, monthly, then 4-monthly
Methotrexate	2.5 mg increasing to 25 mg weekly, orally or s.c.	Nausea, mouth ulcers and diarrhoea Abnormal liver biochemistry Neutropenia and/or thrombocytopenia Renal impairment Pulmonary fibrosis (rare)	Initial, fortnightly, then monthly Initial, weekly, then monthly Initial, then every 3–6 months Baseline chest X-ray
Sodium aurothiomalate	10 mg test dose i.m., then 20–50 mg weekly Monthly with improvement	Skin rashes and mouth ulcers Neutropenia and/or thrombocytopenia Renal impairment	Initial and with each injection Test urine for blood/protein weekly
Leflunamide	100 mg daily for 1–3 days, then 20 (or 10) mg daily	Diarrhoea Neutropenia and/or thrombocytopenia Abnormal liver biochemistry Alopecia Hypertension	Initial, then fortnightly; monthly at 6 months Initial, then fortnightly; monthly at 6 months
Hydroxychloroquine	200–400 mg daily, reduce to 5 days/week	Skin rashes Corneal deposits Retinal damage (very rare before 6 years therapy)	Test visual fields at 6 months and fundoscopy if abnormal
D-penicillamine	125 mg, increasing slowly to 500–1000 mg daily before food	Nausea or loss of taste Skin rashes and mouth ulcers Neutropenia and/or thrombocytopenia Renal impairment Lupus-like syndrome	Initial, fortnightly, then monthly Test urine for blood/protein weekly
TNF-α blockade Etanercept and infliximab	For use in specialist centres – central registry of patients		
Less commonly used			
Azathioprine	25 mg, increasing to 150 mg daily (max. 2.5 mg/kg/day)	Nausea Neutropenia and/or thrombocytopenia Abnormal liver biochemistry	Initial, then weekly, then monthly Initial, then monthly
Ciclosporin	2.5 mg/kg/day for 6 weeks, then 4 mg/kg/day. Reduce if creatinine doubles or BP rises	Renal impairment Hypertension	Initial, then fortnightly, then monthly Initial, then fortnightly, then monthly

biochemistry should be monitored carefully. It usually works within 1–2 months. More patients remain on this agent than on most other DMARDs, indicating that it is effective and has relatively few side-effects.

Gold

Sodium aurothiomalate is given by deep intramuscular injection. A test dose of 10 mg is followed by weekly doses of 50 mg until response occurs, usually in about 3 months. If there is no remission after a total dose of 1 g, treatment should be stopped. If a response is obtained, the interval between injections is increased to 4 weeks, continued for up to 5 years. With relapse the dose frequency is again increased. Side-effects occur in a third of patients on i.m. gold. Rare side-effects include pulmonary fibrosis, colitis, polyneuropathy and cholestatic jaundice. Gold-induced glomerulonephritis can occur, particularly in patients who are HLA-DR3 positive, and routine urinalysis for proteinuria is performed. Auranofin, an oral gold preparation, is rarely used. It has fewer side-effects but lower efficacy.

D-penicillamine

This has to be given *before food* and for at least 3 months before improvement occurs. Penicillamine should not be continued if there is no improvement within 1 year. If proteinuria exceeds 2 g/24 h the drug must be stopped. Loss of taste is reversible. Other rare side-effects include a lupus erythematosus-like syndrome and a myasthenia gravis-like syndrome.

Antimalarials

Hydroxychloroquine is well tolerated. It is used alone in mild disease or as an adjunct to other DMARDs. Retinopathy is the most serious side-effect, but this is rare before 6 years of treatment. Patients should have 6-monthly checks of macular function with an Amsler chart as retinopathy is irreversible.

Leflunamide

This new DMARD exerts an immunomodulatory effect by preventing pyrimidine production in proliferating lymphocytes through blockade of the enzyme dihydro-orotate dehydrogenase. Most cells are able to bypass this blockade but T cells cannot – thus it has a specific effect to block clonal expansion of T cells by slowing progression through the maturation phases G to S1. It is 80% absorbed by mouth and there is no significant interaction with food. It has a long half-life of 4–28 days. The loading dose is 100 mg daily for one to three days, then 20 mg daily (10 mg if diarrhoea is a problem). The main side-effects are diarrhoea, nausea, alopecia and rash. Diarrhoea diminishes with time. Blood monitoring is obligatory. Its onset of action is 4 weeks compared with 6 weeks for methotrexate. The initial response is similar to sulfasalazine but improvement continues and is better sustained at 2 years. Leflunamide works in some patients who have failed to respond to methotrexate or it can be administered with methotrexate to enhance the response. It is probably more effective when given without folate supplements. It may need a washout of 2 years before attempting to become pregnant so is best avoided in premenopausal women.

Corticosteroids

The use of oral corticosteroids has a number of problems (Box 10.11). They are powerful disease-controlling drugs, but are avoided in the long term because side-effects are inevitable. Early intensive short-term regimens are used in some centres. Others use doses of 5–7.5 mg as maintenance therapy. There is some evidence that increased physical activity because of better symptom control reduces the risk of osteoporosis. Corticosteroids are also invaluable to patients with severe disease with extra-articular manifestations such as vasculitis.

Intra-articular injections with semicrystalline steroid preparations have a powerful but sometimes only short-lived effect.

Intramuscular depot injections (40–120 mg depot methylprednisolone) help to control severe disease flares, or can be used before a holiday or other important life event, but should be used with caution and also infrequently.

Tumour necrosis factor (TNF-α) blockers

The recent availability of agents that block TNF-α is beginning to alter the traditional use of DMARDs. Etanercept is a fully humanized p75 TNF-α receptor IgG1 fusion protein given by subcutaneous injection. Around 65% of patients respond well. Some develop an injection reaction. Infliximab is a monoclonal antibody against TNF-α and is given intravenously. Infliximab is co-prescribed with methotrexate to prevent loss of efficacy because of antibody formation. Both products

---

Box 10.11

Problems associated with the use of corticosteroids

- Patients are increasingly anxious about the use of corticosteroids because of adverse publicity about their potential side-effects. This must be discussed frankly and the risks of not treating them be described and balanced against the risks of the drug itself.
- Patients must be warned to avoid sugars and saturated fats and to eat less because of the risk of weight gain.
- The skin becomes thin and easily damaged.
- Monitor for diabetes and hypertension.
- Cataract formation may be accelerated.
- Osteoporosis develops within 6 months on doses above 7.5 mg daily, and hormone replacement therapy and/or calcium and vitamin D and bisphosphonate are used (see p. 578).

slow or halt erosion formation in up to 70% of patients with RA and produce healing in a few. Patients often comment that their malaise and tiredness improve in a manner that is not seen with other DMARDs. If the short-term studies (2–3 years) are reproducible and long-term side-effects do not emerge, this will represent a major therapeutic advance in the treatment of RA and juvenile idiopathic arthritis. There is no evidence to date of increased tumour development. Some people become ANA positive and develop a reversible lupus-like syndrome. Reactivation of old TB may occur. These agents are extremely expensive when compared with traditional DMARDs and their use will cause funding problems for most healthcare systems even if they save costs in the longer term by reducing disability and the need for hospitalization and surgery. Their use should be restricted to specialist centres, and patients should be included in long-term cohort studies to unequivocally prove efficacy and to search for potential serious late-onset side-effects.

Drugs used less commonly

Azathioprine at a maximum dose of 2.5 mg/kg and cyclophosphamide 1–2 mg/kg have been used, usually when other DMARDs have been ineffective. They are often used when extra-articular features are severe, particularly with vasculitis. They are also used in patients who have been treated with corticosteroids and who have developed the severe side-effects of those agents. Ciclosporin 2.5–4 mg/kg is used for active rheumatoid arthritis when conventional therapy has been ineffective. Side-effects include a rise in creatinine level and hypertension.

Physical measures

Patients with RA need constant advice and support from physiotherapists and nurse specialists, especially while they are learning to adjust. A combination of rest for active arthritis and exercises to maintain joint range and muscle power is essential. Exercise in a hydrotherapy pool is popular and effective. Advice about managing activities of daily living despite the arthritis, and about gadgets, seating or structural changes in the home or at work are helpful.

Surgery

This should be considered carefully in the long-term approach to patient management. Its main objectives are prophylactic, to prevent joint destruction and deformity, and reconstructive, to restore function.

Single-joint disease can be treated by surgical synovectomy to reduce the bulk of inflamed tissue and prevent damage. Excision arthroplasty of the ulnar styloid reduces pain and the risk of extensor tendon damage. Excision arthroplasties of the metatarsal heads reduce metatarsal pain and relieve pressure points. The major surgical advance has been the development of total replacement arthroplasty of the hip, knee, finger joints, elbows and shoulders. Such procedures need careful planning and preparation, and the expected outcomes and risks should be explained to the patient.

FURTHER READING

Choy EHS, Panayi GS (2001) Cytokine pathways and joint inflammation in rheumatoid arthritis. *New England Journal of Medicine* **344**: 907–916.

Klippel J H (2000) Biological therapy for rheumatoid arthritis. *New England Journal of Medicine* **343**: 1640–1641.

Lee DM, Weinblatt ME (2001) Rheumatoid arthritis. *Lancet* **358**: 903–911.

Madhok R, Capell H (1999) Outstanding issues in the use of disease-modifying agents in RA. *Lancet* **353**: 257–258.

Pisetsky DS (2000) Editorial. Tumor necrosis factor blockers in rheumatoid arthritis. *New England Journal of Medicine* **342**: 810–811.

Smolen JS et al. (1999) Efficacy and safety of leflunamide in active RA. *Lancet* **353**: 259–266.

Seronegative spondarthritides

This awkward title describes a group of conditions affecting the spine and peripheral joints, which cluster in families and are linked to certain type 1 HLA antigens (Table 10.16).

The joint involvement is more limited than that seen in RA and its distribution is different. There are associated extra-articular and genetic features. These diseases occasionally present in childhood.

Histologically the synovitis itself is difficult to distinguish from that of RA, but there is no production of rheumatoid factors – hence 'seronegative'. Inflammation of the enthesis (junction of ligament or tendon and bone) and joint ankylosis develop more commonly than in RA. All are associated with an increased frequency of sacroiliitis and an increased frequency of HLA-B27.

Aetiology

The common aetiological thread of these disorders is their striking association with HLA-B27, particularly ankylosing spondylitis (AS). This was the first demonstrated disease association of any HLA type (B27 is

Table 10.16
Seronegative spondarthritides

Ankylosing spondylitis (AS)
Psoriatic arthritis
Reactive arthritis
    Sexually acquired (Reiter's disease)
    Post-dysenteric reactive arthritis
Enteropathic arthritis (ulcerative colitis/Crohn's disease)

present in > 90% of Caucasians with AS but only 8% of controls). Its aetiological relevance remains unclear. The role of class I HLA antigens in pathogenesis is supported by the fact that HLA-B27 transgenic mice spontaneously develop arthritis, skin, gut and genitourinary lesions.

There are clues that infections play a role, possibly by molecular mimicry, with parts of the organism which are structurally similar to the HLA molecule triggering cross-reactive antibody formation. This is unproven. AIDS is increasing the prevalence of reactive arthritis and spondylitis in sub-Saharan Africa even in the absence of HLA-B27. The explanation for this changing epidemiology is unclear.

The types of arthritis that follow a precipitating infection are called reactive arthritis (p. 550).

The specialized immune systems of the gut and genitourinary mucous membranes may also play a causal role, perhaps reacting to local infections or to antigens which cross the damaged mucosa.

Ankylosing spondylitis (AS)

This is an inflammatory disorder of the back affecting mainly young adults. The frequency of AS in different populations is roughly paralleled by the incidence of HLA-B27; Africans and Japanese have a low incidence of both HLA-B27 and ankylosing spondylitis, while the North American Haida Indians have a high incidence of both. There are at least 11 subtypes of HLA-B27 (B*2701–B*2711). Some appear to increase risk; others have a protective role. Twin studies indicate a much higher disease concordance in HLA-B27-positive monozygotic twins than in dizygotic twins. Other genetic loci appear to be involved. The disease occurs in men and women (2.5 : 1). It is milder in women so men are more likely to present with symptoms of the disease (in a ratio of 4 : 1). There is lymphocyte and plasma cell infiltration and local erosion of bone at the attachments of the intervertebral and other ligaments. This heals with new bone (syndesmophyte) formation.

Clinical features

Episodic inflammation of the sacroiliac joints in the late teenage years or early twenties is the first manifestation of AS. Pain in one or both buttocks and low back pain and stiffness are typically worse in the morning and relieved by exercise. Initially the diagnosis is often missed because the patient is asymptomatic between episodes and radiological abnormalities are absent. Retention of the lumbar lordosis during spinal flexion is an early sign. Later, paraspinal muscle wasting develops. Spinal stiffness can be measured by Schoeber's test – a tape measure is placed in the midline 10 cm above the dimples of Venus. Any movement of a marker at 15 cm during flexion is recorded. A reading of less than

---

> ### Box 10.12
>
> **Nonarticular problems in seronegative spondarthritides**
>
> - Uveitis, in all types.
> - Cutaneous lesions in reactive arthritis (keratoderma blenorrhagica), histologically identical to pustular psoriasis.
> - Nail dystrophy, in psoriasis and reactive arthritis.
> - Aortitis, occasionally in AS and reactive arthritis.

5 cm implies spinal stiffness. Individuals may be able to touch the floor with a stiff back if they have good hip movements but serial movement of the finger tip to floor distance highlights any change. Non-spinal complications (uveitis or costochondritis) suggest the diagnosis (Box 10.12). Costochondral junction inflammation causes anterior chest pain and measurable reduction of chest expansion.

Peripheral joint involvement is asymmetrical and affects a few, predominantly large joints. Hip involvement leads to fixed flexion deformities of the hips and further deterioration of the posture. Young teenage boys occasionally present with a lower-limb monarthritis, which predates the development of spinal symptoms (see p. 570).

Acute anterior uveitis is strongly associated with HLA-B27 in AS and related diseases and is occasionally the presenting complaint. Severe eye pain, photophobia and blurred vision are an emergency. Patients with AS should be asked to report eye pain and redness immediately.

Investigations

- **Blood.** The ESR and CRP are usually raised.
- **HLA testing** is rarely of value because of the high frequency of HLA-B27 in the population, but may give supporting evidence in a difficult case.
- **X-rays.** The medial and lateral cortical margins of both sacroiliac joints lose definition owing to erosions and eventually become sclerotic (Fig. 10.18). The earliest radiological appearances in the spine are blurring of the upper or lower vertebral rims at the thoracolumbar junction (best seen on a lateral X-ray) and caused by an enthesitis at the insertion of the intervertebral ligaments. These changes may eventually affect the whole spine. Persistent inflammatory enthesitis causes bony spurs (syndesmophytes). Syndesmophytes are more vertically oriented than the beak-like osteophytes of spondylosis and the disc is preserved, unlike in spondylosis (see p. 1218). Syndesmophytes cause bony ankylosis and permanent stiffening. The sacroiliac joints eventually fuse, as may the costovertebral joints, reducing chest expansion.

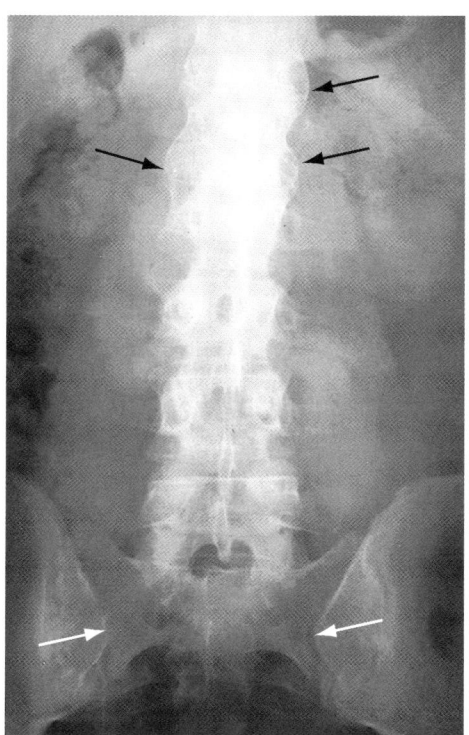

Fig. 10.18 **X-ray of ankylosing spondylitis.** The sacroiliac joints are eroded and show marginal sclerosis (white arrows). There is bridging syndesmophyte formation at the thoracolumbar junction (black arrows).

Calcification of the intervertebral ligaments and fusion of the spinal facet joints and syndesmophytes leads to what is often called a 'bamboo' spine (Fig. 10.19).

Treatment

The key to effective management of AS is early diagnosis so that a regimen of preventative exercises is started before syndesmophytes have formed. Morning exercises aim to maintain spinal mobility, posture and chest expansion. Failure to control pain and to encourage regular spinal and chest exercises leads to an irreversible dorsal kyphosis and wasted paraspinal muscles. This, along with stiffening of the cervical spine, makes forward vision difficult.

When the inflammation is active, the morning pain and stiffness are too severe to permit effective exercise. An evening dose of a long-acting or slow-release NSAID or an NSAID suppository improves sleep, pain control and exercise compliance. Peripheral arthritis and enthesitis are managed with NSAIDs or local steroid injections. Sulfasalazine or methotrexate may help the peripheral arthritis but there is little evidence that they control spinal disease.

Most patients with AS are HLA-B27 positive and they should be made aware that they risk passing the gene to 50% of their children. HLA-B27 positive offspring then have a 30% risk of developing AS.

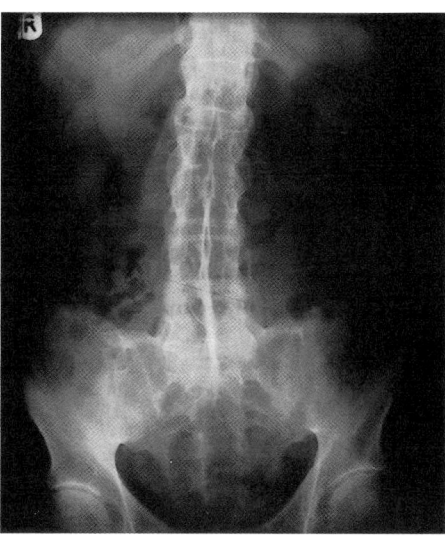

Fig. 10.19 **X-ray of bamboo spine in ankylosing spondylitis.** In advanced disease there is calcification of the interspinous ligaments and fusion of the facet joints as well as syndesmophytes at all levels. The sacro-iliac joints fuse.

Prognosis

With exercise and pain relief, the prognosis is excellent and over 80% of patients are fully employed. The back may be stiff, but disability is minimal unless the hips are involved.

Psoriatic arthritis (see also p. 1287)

The term 'psoriatic arthritis' describes a variety of different patterns of arthritis and enthesitis seen in people with psoriasis or with a family history of psoriasis. Five to eight per cent of individuals with psoriasis develop one of several different patterns of arthritis for which there is no serological marker. Activated CD4+ T lymphocytes appear to cause the lesions. Different subtypes of activated lymphocyte migrate to skin or joint, accounting for the skin and joint disease flaring at different times. There is compelling evidence that this is a reaction to organisms, such as group A streptococci, producing an autoimmune response in psoriatic skin plaques. These activated T lymphocytes release cytokines (interleukin 1, TNF-β and interferon).

Clinical features

The arthritis is typically more limited in distribution and less severe than in RA. The skin disease can be mild and may develop after the arthritis.

The most typical pattern of joint involvement in psoriasis is distal interphalangeal arthritis. It is unsightly, but rarely disabling, and there is often adjacent nail dystrophy. Cutaneous lesions, interphalangeal joint synovitis and tenosynovitis causing a 'sausage' finger or toe

549

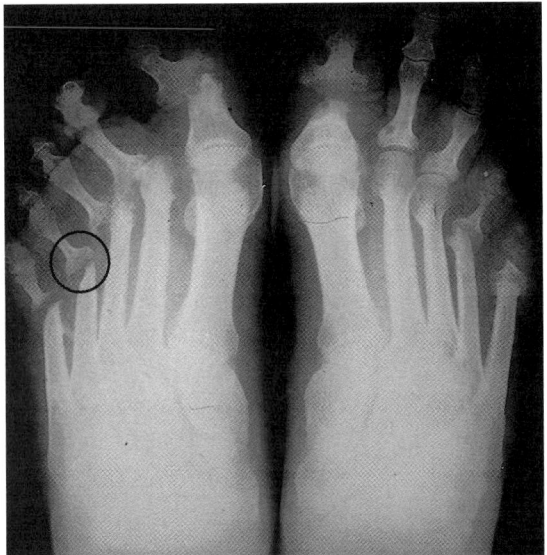

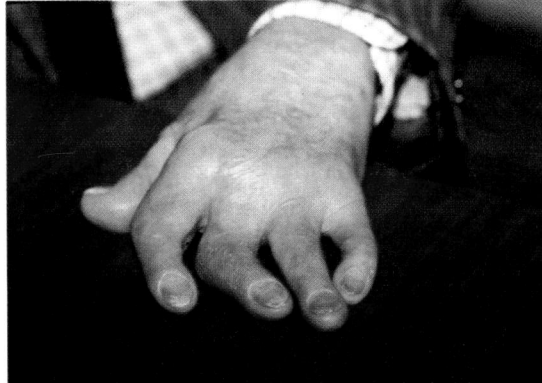

Fig. 10.21 Hand showing psoriatic arthritis mutilans. All the fingers are shortened and the joints unstable, owing to underlying osteolysis.

Fig. 10.20 X-ray of psoriatic arthritis. There is osteolysis of the metatarsal heads and central erosion of the proximal phalanges to produce the 'pencil in cup' appearance (circle). All the lesser toes are subluxed.

(dactylitis) are seen in pauciarticular psoriatic arthritis (and in reactive arthritis).

A seronegative symmetrical polyarthritis similar to rheumatoid arthritis also occurs.

Radiologically, psoriatic arthritis is erosive but the erosions are central in the joint, not juxta-articular, and produce a 'pencil in cup' appearance (Fig. 10.20).

Arthritis mutilans affects about 5% of patients with psoriatic arthritis and causes marked periarticular osteolysis and bone shortening ('telescopic' fingers) (Fig. 10.21), in which, despite the deformity, pain may be mild and function often surprisingly good.

Individuals with psoriasis may develop unilateral or bilateral sacroiliitis and typical AS, but with early involvement of the neck; only 50% are HLA-B27 positive.

Treatment and prognosis

NSAIDs and/or analgesics help the pain but they can occasionally worsen the skin lesions. Local synovitis responds to intra-articular corticosteroid injections.

In milder, polyarticular cases, sulfasalazine slows the development of joint damage.

When the disease is severe, methotrexate or ciclosporin is given because they control both the skin lesions and the arthritis. Early studies suggest that anti-TNF-α agents, e.g. etanercept (see p. 546) are highly effective for severe skin and joint disease. Corticosteroids orally may destabilize the skin disease and are best avoided.

The prognosis for the joint involvement is generally better than in RA.

Reactive arthritis

Reactive arthritis is a sterile synovitis, which occurs following an infection (see also post-streptococcal arthritis, p. 571).

Seronegative spondarthritis develops in 1–2% of patients after an acute attack of dysentery, or a sexually acquired infection – non-specific urethritis (NSU) in the male, non-specific cervicitis in the female. In male patients who are HLA-B27 positive the relative risk is 30–50. Being HLA-B27 positive is not obligatory, however. Women are less commonly affected.

Aetiology

A variety of organisms can be the trigger, including some strains of *Salmonella* or *Shigella* spp. in bacillary dysentery. *Yersinia enterocolitica* causes diarrhoea and a reactive arthritis. In NSU the organisms are *Chlamydia trachomatis* or *Ureaplasma urealyticum*.

Bacterial antigens or bacterial DNA have been found in the inflamed synovium of affected joints, suggesting that this persistent antigenic material is driving the inflammatory process. Other environmental factors may explain why even in susceptible individuals, repeated infections do not necessarily produce a reactive arthritis. The methods by which HLA-B27 increases susceptibility to reactive arthritis may include:

- T cell receptor repertoire selection
- molecular mimicry causing autoimmunity against HLA-B27 and/or other self antigens
- mode of presentation of bacteria-derived peptides to T lymphocytes.

These are not mutually exclusive.

There are other organisms which also trigger reactive arthritis, but which have a different genetic basis; see post-streptococcal arthritis (p. 571), gonococcal arthritis (p. 555) and brucellosis (p. 556). In these, the borderline

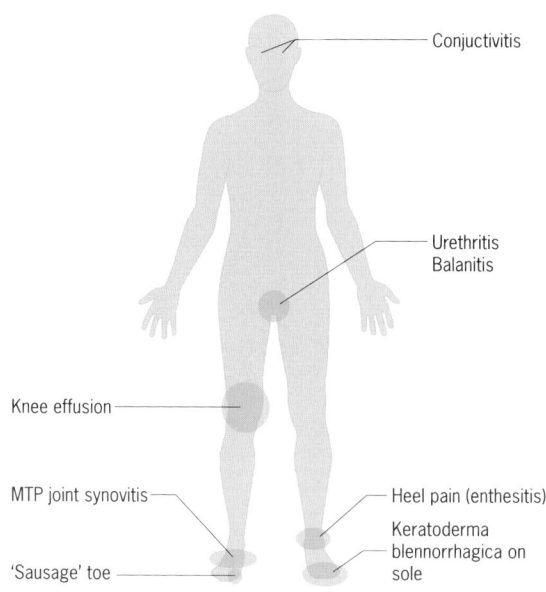

Conjuctivitis

Urethritis
Balanitis

Knee effusion

MTP joint synovitis

'Sausage' toe

Heel pain (enthesitis)

Keratoderma
blennorrhagica on
sole

Fig. 10.22 Clinical features of reactive arthritis.

between reactive arthritis and septic arthritis is more indistinct and they can cause both.

Clinical features (Fig. 10.22)

The arthritis is typically an acute, asymmetrical, lower-limb arthritis, occurring a few days to a couple of weeks after the infection. The arthritis may be the presenting complaint if the infection is mild or asymptomatic. Enthesitis is common, causing plantar fasciitis or Achilles tendonitis (see p. 529). Seventy per cent recover fully within 6 months but many have a relapse.

In susceptible individuals with reactive arthritis, sacroiliitis and spondylitis may also develop. Acute anterior uveitis may complicate more severe or relapsing disease but is not synchronous with the arthritis.

The skin lesions resemble psoriasis:

- *Circinate balanitis* in the uncircumcised male causes painless superficial ulceration of the glans penis. In the circumcised male the lesion is raised, red and scaly. Both heal without scarring.
- *Keratoderma blenorrhagica* – the skin of the feet and hands develops painless, red and often confluent raised plaques and pustules histologically similar to pustular psoriasis.
- *Nail dystrophy* may occur.

Other features

These include:

- bilateral conjunctivitis occurs in 30%
- the classically described triad of Reiter's disease – urethritis, arthritis and conjunctivitis.

Treatment

There is some evidence that treating persisting infection with antibiotics will alter the course of the arthritis, once it has developed. Cultures should be taken and any infection treated. Sexual partners may require specialist advice about and treatment for sexually acquired diseases.

Pain responds well to NSAIDs and local corticosteroid injections. The majority of individuals with reactive arthritis have a single attack which settles, but a few develop a disabling relapsing and remitting arthritis. Relapsing cases are sometimes treated with sulfasalazine or methotrexate (see Table 10.15).

Enteropathic arthritis associated with inflammatory bowel disease

Enteropathic synovitis occurs in approximately 10–15% of patients with ulcerative colitis and Crohn's disease (see p. 302). The link between the bowel disease and the inflammatory arthritis is not clear. Selective mucosal leakiness may expose the individual to antigens that trigger synovitis.

The arthritis is asymmetrical and predominantly affects lower-limb joints. An HLA-B27-associated sacroiliitis or spondylitis is seen in 5% of patients with inflammatory bowel disease and is independent of disease activity. The joint symptoms may predate the development of bowel disease and lead to its diagnosis.

Remission of ulcerative colitis or total colectomy usually leads to remission of the joint disease, but arthritis may persist even in well-controlled Crohn's disease.

Treatment

The inflammatory bowel disease should be treated (see p. 304). In all cases of enteropathic arthritis, the joint disease should be managed symptomatically with NSAIDs, although they may make diarrhoea worse. A monoarthritis is best treated by intra-articular corticosteroids. Sulfasalazine is frequently prescribed as this may help both bowel and joint disease.

FURTHER READING

Nuki G (1998) Ankylosing spondylitis, HLA B27, and beyond. *Lancet* **351**: 767–769.

Crystal arthritis

Aetiology

Two main types of crystal account for the majority of crystal-induced arthritis. They are sodium urate and calcium pyrophosphate and are distinguished by their

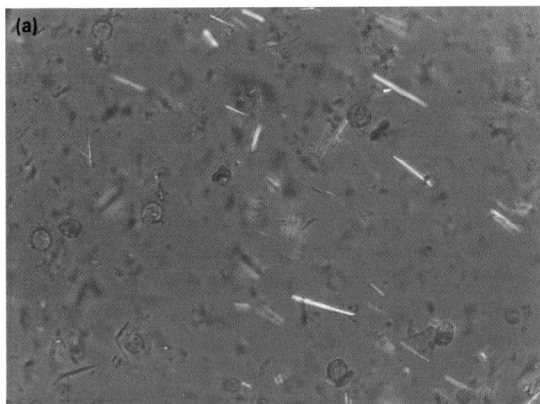

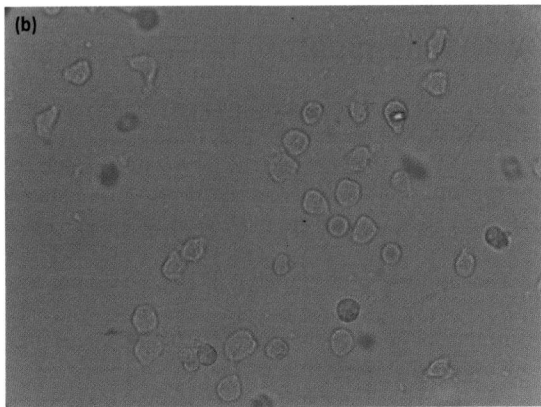

Fig. 10.23 **(a) Needle-shaped urate crystals**, viewed under polarized light with a red filter. **(b) A small intracellular pyrophosphate crystal**, viewed under polarized light with a red filter.

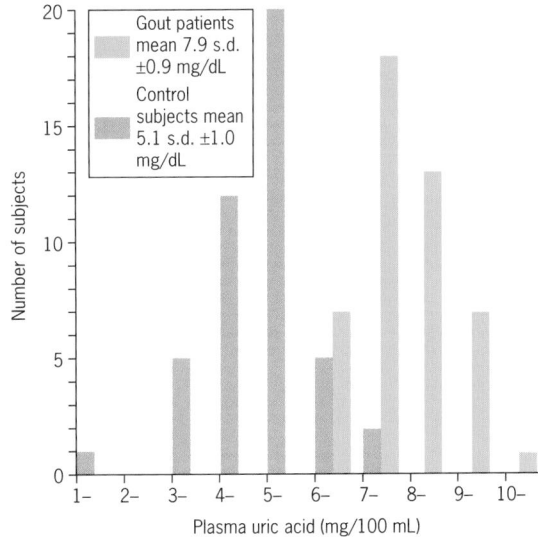

Fig. 10.24 **Serum uric acid levels in normals and in patients with gout.** 7.9 mg/dL is equivalent to 474 µmol/L, 5.1 mg/dL is equivalent to 306 µmol/L. From Snaith ML, Scott JT (1977) *Annals of Rheumatic Disease*, with permission.

different shapes and refringence properties under polarized light with a red filter (Fig. 10.23). Rarely crystals of calcium apatite (see p. 536) or cholesterol cause acute synovitis.

Neutrophils ingest the crystals and release pro-inflammatory enzymes from their phagosomes into the joint, thus triggering complement activation and attracting more neutrophils. Crystals may be found in asymptomatic joints. Why they initiate an attack is unclear. In pseudogout (p. 554), crystal shedding from the cartilage causes an attack.

Gout and hyperuricaemia

Gout is an inflammatory arthritis associated with hyperuricaemia.

Epidemiology

The prevalence of gout in Europe and the USA is approximately 0.2%, although hyperuricaemia in this population occurs in about 5%. The prevalence of gout is increasing and is mainly seen in developed countries. Gout develops in men more than women (10 : 1) and

rarely occurs before young adulthood (when it suggests a specific enzyme defect), and seldom in premenopausal females. Hyperuricaemia is common in certain ethnic groups (e.g. Maoris).

Uric acid levels start to rise after puberty and are higher in men than women until the female menopause. There is a normal distribution of serum uric acid in the population with a skewed distribution at the upper end of the range. Hyperuricaemia is defined as a serum uric acid level greater than two standard deviations from the mean (420 µmol/L in males, 360 µmol/L in females).

Most people with hyperuricaemia are asymptomatic. The range for gouty individuals is higher than for normals, but the curves overlap (Fig. 10.24). Serum uric acid levels increase with age, obesity, a high-protein diet, a high alcohol consumption, combined hyperlipidaemia, diabetes mellitus, ischaemic heart disease and hypertension. There is often a family history of gout.

Pathogenesis

Causes of hyperuricaemia are shown in Table 10.17. In many patients with gout there is no obvious cause, and in these patients there is often both increased production and decreased excretion of urate. Hyperuricaemia is the major determinant for developing gout.

Uric acid levels in the blood depend on the balance between purine synthesis and the ingestion of dietary purines, and the elimination of urate by the kidney and intestine. The body pool is about 1000 mg and 60% is turned over daily.

Uric acid synthesis. Uric acid is the last step in the breakdown pathway of purines. The last two steps, the conversion of hypoxanthine to xanthine and

Table 10.17
Causes of hyperuricaemia

Impaired excretion of uric acid
Chronic renal disease (clinical gout unusual)
Drug therapy, e.g. thiazide diuretics, low-dose aspirin
Hypertension
Lead toxicity
Primary hyperparathyroidism
Hypothyroidism
Increased lactic acid production from alcohol, exercise, starvation
Glucose-6-phosphatase deficiency (interferes with renal excretion)

Increased production of uric acid
Increased purine synthesis de novo due to:
   Hypoxanthine–guanine–phosphoribosyl transferase (HGPRT)
     reduction (an X-linked inborn error causing the
     Lesch–Nyhan syndrome)
   Phosphoribosyl–pyrophosphate synthetase overactivity
   Glucose-6-phosphatase deficiency with glycogen storage
     disease type 1 (patients who survive develop
     hyperuricaemia due to increased production as well as
     decreased excretion)
Increased turnover of purines due to:
   Myeloproliferative disorders, e.g. polycythaemia vera
   Lymphoproliferative disorders, e.g. leukaemia
   Others, e.g. carcinoma, severe psoriasis

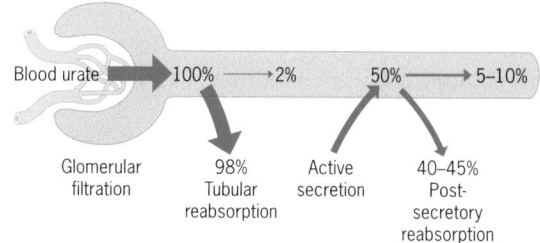

Fig. 10.25 Urate renal transport. The net result is that about 5–10% of the glomerular load is excreted in the urine under normal circumstances.

Box 10.13

Hyperuricaemia causes four clinical syndromes

- Acute urate synovitis – gout
- Chronic polyarticular gout
- Chronic tophaceous gout
- Urate renal stone formation (p. 627)

---

of xanthine to uric acid, are catalysed by the enzyme xanthine oxidase.

Uric acid excretion (Fig. 10.25). Uric acid is completely filtered by the glomerulus; 98–100% is then reabsorbed in the proximal tubule and 50% is secreted by the distal tubule. Some post-secretory reabsorption also takes place. Low-dose aspirin blocks urate secretion. High-dose aspirin also blocks its reabsorption, leading to increased net excretion. Ninety per cent of patients with gout have impaired excretion of urate, 10% have increased production also and in less than 1% an inborn error of metabolism leads to purine overproduction. One-third of uric acid is eliminated in the faeces.

Clinical features

Hyperuricaemia causes four clinical syndromes (Box 10.13).

Acute gout presents typically in a middle-aged male with sudden onset of agonizing pain, swelling and redness of the first MTP joint. The attack occurs at any time, but may be precipitated by too much food or alcohol, by dehydration or by starting a diuretic. Untreated attacks last about 7 days. Recovery is typically associated with desquamation of the overlying skin. In 25% of attacks, a joint other than the great toe is affected.

In *severe attacks,* overlying crystal cellulitis makes gout difficult to distinguish clinically from infective cellulitis. A family or personal history of gout and the finding of a raised serum urate suggest the diagnosis but, if in doubt, blood and other cultures should be taken.

Chronic polyarticular gout is unusual, except in elderly people on long-standing diuretic treatment, in renal failure, or occasionally in men who have been started on treatment with allopurinol too soon after an acute attack.

Chronic tophaceous gout (see p. 554).

Investigations

The clinical picture is often diagnostic, as is the rapid response to NSAIDs.

- **Joint fluid microscopy** is the most specific and diagnostic test but is technically difficult.
- **Serum urate** is usually raised (> 600 μmol/L). If it is not, recheck it several weeks after the attack, as the level falls immediately after an acute attack. Acute gout never occurs with a serum uric acid in the lower half of the normal range.
- **Serum urea and creatinine** are monitored for signs of renal impairment.

Treatment

The use of NSAIDs in high doses rapidly reduces the pain and swelling. Initial doses, taken with food, are:

- naproxen: 750 mg immediately, then 500 mg every 8–12 hours
- diclofenac: 75–100 mg immediately, then 50 mg every 6–8 hours
- indometacin: 75 mg immediately, then 50 mg every 6–8 hours.

After 24–48 hours, reduced doses are given for a further week. *Caution*: NSAIDs may cause renal impairment. In individuals with renal impairment or a history of peptic ulceration, alternative treatments include:

- colchicine: 1000 mg immediately, then 500 mg every 6–12 hours, but this causes diarrhoea
- corticosteroids: intramuscular or intra-articular depot methylprednisolone.

Dietary advice

The first attacks may be separated by many months or years and are managed symptomatically. Individuals should be advised to reduce their alcohol intake, especially beer, which is high in purines. A diet which reduces total calorie and cholesterol intake and avoids such foods as offal, some fish and shellfish and spinach, all of which are rich sources of purines, is advised. This can reduce serum urate by 15% and delay the need for drugs that reduce serum urate levels.

Treatment with agents that reduce serum urate levels

Only when the attacks are frequent and severe, despite dietary changes, or associated with renal impairment or tophi, or when the patient finds NSAIDs or colchicine difficult to tolerate should allopurinol or a uricosuric agent be used. They should *never* be started within a month of an acute attack and always be started under cover of a course of NSAID or colchicine for the first 2–4 weeks before and 4 weeks after starting allopurinol.

Allopurinol (300–600 mg) blocks the enzyme xanthine oxidase, which converts xanthine into urate (see Fig. 15.11). It reduces serum urate levels rapidly and is relatively non-toxic but should be used at low doses (50–100 mg) in renal impairment. Skin rashes are the most common side-effect. Bone marrow suppression is very rare. Allopurinol may induce acute gout when it is first introduced.

Uricosuric agents (probenecid, 0.5–1 g 12-hourly) increase urate excretion and are used in individuals who are allergic to allopurinol. They should not be used in renal failure or in patients with urate stones. They may be given in combination with allopurinol in severe tophaceous gout with high urate loads.

Chronic tophaceous gout

Individuals with very high levels of urate can present with different clinical pictures. In chronic tophaceous gout, sodium urate forms smooth white deposits (tophi) in skin and around joints. They may occur on the ear lobe, the fingers or the Achilles tendon. Large deposits are unsightly and ulcerate. There is chronic joint pain and sometimes superimposed acute gouty attacks.

Periarticular deposits lead to a halo of radio-opacity and clearly defined ('punched out') bone cysts on X-ray.

Tophaceous gout is often associated with renal impairment and/or the long-term use of diuretics. There may be acute or chronic urate nephropathy or renal stone formation. Whenever possible, stop the diuretics or change to less urate-retaining ones, such as bumetamide.

FURTHER READING

Emerson BT (1996) The management of gout. *New England Journal of Medicine* **334**: 445–450.

Pseudogout (pyrophosphate arthropathy)

Calcium pyrophosphate deposits in hyaline and fibro-cartilage produce the radiological appearance of chondrocalcinosis (see p. 538). Shedding of crystals into a joint precipitates acute synovitis which resembles gout, except that it is more common in elderly women and usually affects the knee or wrist. The attacks are often very painful. In young people it may be associated with haemochromatosis, hyperparathyroidism, Wilson's disease or alkaptonuria.

Diagnosis

The diagnosis is made by detecting rhomboidal, weakly positively birefringent crystals in joint fluid, or deduced from the presence of chondrocalcinosis on X-ray. The joint fluid looks purulent. Septic arthritis must be excluded and joint fluid should be sent for culture.

The attacks may be associated with fever and a raised white blood cell count.

Treatment

Aspiration of the joint reduces the pain dramatically but it is usually necessary to use an NSAID or colchicine, as for gout. If infection can be excluded, an intra-articular injection of a corticosteroid helps.

Infections of joints and bones

Joints may become infected by direct injury or by blood-borne infection from an infected skin lesion or other site.

Chronically inflamed joints (e.g. in rheumatoid arthritis) are more prone to infection than are normal joints. Individuals who are immunosuppressed, by AIDS or by immunosuppressive agents, are particularly at risk, as are the elderly and those who abuse alcohol. Artificial joints are also potential sites for infection.

Septic arthritis

The organism that most commonly causes septic arthritis is *Staphylococcus aureus*. Other organisms include streptococci, other species of staphylococcus, *Neisseria gonorrhoeae*, *Haemophilus influenzae* in children, and these and other Gram-negative organisms in the elderly or complicating RA.

Clinical features

Suspected septic arthritis is a medical emergency. In young and previously fit people, the joint is hot, red, swollen, and agonizingly painful and held immobile by muscle spasm. In the elderly and immunosuppressed and in RA the clinical picture is less dramatic, so a high index of suspicion is needed to avoid missing treatable but potentially severely destructive septic arthritis.

Investigations

- **Aspirate** the joint and send the fluid for urgent Gram staining and culture. The fluid is usually frankly purulent. The culture techniques should include those for gonococci and anaerobes.
- **Blood cultures** are often positive.
- **Leucocytosis** is usual, unless the person is severely immunosuppressed.
- **X-rays** are of no value in diagnosis.

Treatment

This should be started immediately on diagnosis because joint destruction occurs in days. The joint should be immobilized initially and then physiotherapy started early to prevent stiffness and muscle wasting. Intravenous antibiotics should be given for a week. It is usual to give two antibiotics to which the organism is sensitive for 6 weeks, then one for a further 6 weeks orally.

Empirical treatment in septic arthritis

This is started before the results of culture are obtained. Discuss the case with a microbiologist. Intravenous flucloxacillin 1–2 g is given 6-hourly, plus fusidic acid 500 mg orally 8-hourly. If the patient is allergic to penicillin, replace flucloxacillin with erythromycin 1 g i.v. 6-hourly or clindamycin 600 mg i.v. 8-hourly. In immunosuppressed patients, flucloxacillin 1–2 g i.v. 6-hourly plus gentamicin (to cover Gram-negative organisms) should be used. Change the antibiotics if the organism is not sensitive. Drainage of the joint and arthroscopic joint washouts are helpful in relieving pain.

Prognosis

Surgical drainage may be required if there is joint destruction and osteomyelitis. Patients can start weight-bearing as soon as the inflammation subsides. Resolution of the septic arthritis with complete recovery can occur in a few days or weeks. It may lead to secondary osteoarthritis (see p. 535).

Specific types of bacterial arthritis

Gonococcal arthritis

This is the most common cause of a septic arthritis in previously fit young adults, more commonly affecting women and homosexual men.

Initially the patient becomes febrile and develops characteristic pustules on the distal limbs. Polyarthralgia and tenosynovitis are common at this stage and about 40% have a gonococcaemia. This phase settles and blood cultures usually become negative. Later, large-joint mon- or pauciarticular arthritis may follow. Culture is usually positive from the genital tract, although the joint fluid may be sterile. It is not clear whether this is simply a septic arthritis – although it responds rapidly to antibiotics – or whether there is also a reactive element to bacterial lipopolysaccharide.

Treatment consists of oral penicillin, ciprofloxacin or doxycycline for 2 weeks, and joint rest.

Tuberculous arthritis

Around 1% of patients with tuberculosis develop joint and/or bone involvement. It occurs as the primary disease in children. In adults, it is usually due to haematogenous spread from secondary pulmonary or renal lesions. The onset is insidious and diagnosis often delayed.

The organism invades the synovium or intervertebral disc. There are caseating granulomas and rapid destruction of cartilage and adjacent bone. Some patients develop a reactive polyarthritis (Poncet's disease).

A hip or knee (30%) is most commonly affected, but around 50% develop spinal disease. The patient is febrile, has night sweats, is anorexic and loses weight. The usual risk factors for tuberculosis apply – debility, alcohol abuse or immunosuppression. HIV-positive/AIDS patients are at particular risk.

Investigations should include culture of fluid, and culture and biopsy of the synovium. *M. tuberculosis* is the usual organism, but atypical mycobacteria are occasionally implicated. A chest X-ray should be performed. Initially joint or spinal X-rays may be normal but joint-space reduction and bone destruction develop rapidly if treatment is delayed. MRI shows the abnormality earlier in the spine and MRI-guided biopsy from the affected disc is necessary to obtain cultures.

Treatment is as for tuberculosis (see p. 895). The joint should be rested and the spine immobilized in the acute phase.

Meningococcal arthritis

This may complicate a meningococcal septicaemia and presents as a migratory polyarthritis. Organisms can only rarely be cultured from the joint and most cases are due to immune complex deposition. Treatment is with penicillin.

Infective endocarditis

This may present with arthralgia, polymyalgia rheumatica-like symptoms or an infective arthritis. It is discussed on page 793.

Lyme arthritis

A person with Lyme disease (see p. 81) develops a fever and headache, and an expanding, erythematous rash called erythema chronicum migrans. About 25% of cases develop an acute pauciarticular arthritis. This usually resolves but 20% of untreated cases go on to develop a chronic arthritis. It is unclear whether this and other late manifestations are due to chronic infection or are antibody-induced.

Diagnosis is by the detection of IgM antibodies against the spirochete *Borrelia burgdorferi*.

Treatment with antibiotics (amoxicillin or doxycycline) is highly effective in early disease. The response of chronic arthritis to antibiotic treatment may be delayed for months.

Brucellosis

Brucellosis (see p. 80) has a world-wide distribution. The most common cause of chronic brucellosis and of arthritis is *Brucella melitensis*. There is usually a peripheral mon- or oligoarticular arthritis, which may be septic or reactive. Arthritis is more common in chronic infections of more than 6 months.

Syphilitic arthritis

Congenital syphilis (see p. 126) can cause an acute painful epiphysitis or osteochondritis sometimes associated with para-articular swelling in the first few weeks of life. Later, at age 8–16 years, painless effusion of the knees may occur (Clutton's joints).

In acquired syphilis, arthralgia and arthritis occur in the secondary stage. Charcot's (neuropathic) joints usually involve the knees in tabes dorsalis (see p. 1196).

Actinomycetes infection

Actinomycetes (see p. 91) can affect the mandible or vertebrae.

Arthritis in viral disease

A transient polyarthritis or arthralgia can occur before, during or after many viral illnesses. These include infectious mononucleosis, chickenpox, mumps, adenovirus, parvovirus B19, hepatitis B, arboviral infections and HIV. In most of these it is due to a direct toxic effect or immune complex deposition.

In *rubella* (see p. 54) the virus can occasionally be isolated from the joint. This arthritis occurs most commonly in up to 50% of young adult females a few days after rubella infection (6% of men). It is a symmetrical polyarthritis involving the MCP or PIP joints most commonly, but many joints can be affected. It closely resembles rheumatoid arthritis. IgM rubella antibodies are present. It resolves within a few weeks in most cases. A mild arthritis occurs rarely 2–4 weeks after rubella vaccination.

Parvovirus B19 causes an acute, self-limiting arthritis and is associated with erythema infectiosum ('slapped cheek disease').

In *hepatitis B infection* (see p. 352) a sudden symmetrical polyarticular arthritis of the small joints of the hands occurs in approximately one-third of patients, often in the prodromal phase and mostly resolving before the onset of jaundice. Hepatitis C causes type II mixed cryoglobulinaemia (see p. 357).

Arbovirus infections (see p. 55) which are endemic in many parts of the world give rise to an arthralgia and/or arthritis. For example, the Ross River virus has caused an epidemic polyarthritis in Australia and the South Pacific; it involves the small joints of the hands and clears in 2–4 weeks. Other viral infections causing epidemic arthritis include chikungunya (see p. 55) and O'nyong-nyong (p. 55).

Musculoskeletal aspects of infection with human immunodeficiency virus (HIV) and acquired immunodeficiency syndrome (AIDS)

The clinical features seen in these patients are due to a number of causes such as opportunistic infections and drug therapy and are not usually caused directly by HIV. Infective arthritis seen in these immunosuppressed patients often has minimal symptoms and signs. Some of the newer antiviral agents cause an acute arthritis, possibly because of crystallization in the joint.

Arthralgia is common in AIDS. There is a seronegative, predominantly lower-limb arthritis, similar to psoriasis or Reiter's disease. Spondylitis also occurs. Avascular necrosis, possibly associated with corticosteroids or alcohol, is seen.

Nonarticular diseases such as Sjögren's- and lupus-like syndromes, systemic vasculitis of the necrotizing and hypersensitivity types (see p. 564), and myositis also occur.

Fungal infection

Fungal infections of joints occur rarely. Bone abscesses may be seen. Destructive joint lesions can also occur with blastomycosis. A benign polyarthritis accompanied by erythema nodosum occasionally occurs in coccidioidomycosis and histoplasmosis. Culture of purulent synovial fluid and skin tests for fungi may help the diagnosis.

Bone infections

Acute and chronic osteomyelitis

Osteomyelitis can be due either to metastatic haematogenous spread (e.g. from a boil) or to local infection. Malnutrition, debilitating disease and decreased immunity may play a part in the pathogenesis.

Staphylococcus is the organism responsible for 90% of cases of acute osteomyelitis. Other organisms include *Haemophilus influenzae* and salmonella; infection with the latter may occur as a complication of sickle cell anaemia. Diagnosis and treatment within a few days carries a good prognosis. Delayed treatment leads to chronic osteomyelitis. In chronic osteomyelitis sinus formation is usual. There is often fever and pain. Subacute osteomyelitis is associated with a chronic abscess within the bone (Brodie's abscess). Symptoms may be limited to local pain.

Treatment of osteomyelitis is with immobilization and antibiotic therapy with flucloxacillin and fusidic acid. Surgical drainage and removal of dead bone (sequestrum) may be possible but recurrence is common.

Tuberculous osteomyelitis

This is usually due to haematogenous spread from a reactivated primary focus in the lungs or gastrointestinal tract. The disease starts in intra-articular bone. The spine is commonly involved (Pott's disease), with damage to the bodies of two neighbouring vertebrae leading to vertebral collapse and acute angulation of the spine (gibbus). Later an abscess forms ('cold abscess'). Pus can track along tissue planes and discharge at a point far from the affected vertebra. Symptoms consist of local pain and later swelling if pus has collected. Systemic symptoms of malaise, fever and night sweats occur.

Treatment is as for pulmonary tuberculosis (see p. 895) together with immobilization.

FURTHER READING

Goldenberg DL (1998) Septic arthritis. *Lancet* **351**: 197–202.

Autoimmune diseases (connective tissue disorders)

Autoimmune diseases are conditions in which the immune system damages specific organs or causes systemic ill-health. Organ-specific autoimmune diseases include Graves' disease, Hashimoto's thyroiditis, pernicious anaemia and insulin-dependent diabetes mellitus. In most of the autoimmune rheumatic diseases it is thought that self-antigens provide the drive, although the trigger may yet prove to be exogenous. They are clinically diverse but are unified by the detection of non-organ-specific autoantibodies in the serum and various tissues. Rheumatoid arthritis (RA, see p. 537) is the most common autoimmune rheumatic disease.

Some of the diseases in this section, e.g. systemic lupus erythematosus (SLE), polymyositis and dermatomyositis and systemic sclerosis are discussed because of their similar pathophysiology. They are sometimes referred to as connective tissue disorders.

Systemic lupus erythematosus (SLE) and lupus-like diseases

SLE is an inflammatory, multisystem disorder with arthralgia and rashes as the most common clinical features, and cerebral and renal disease as the most serious problems.

Epidemiology

SLE occurs world-wide but the prevalence varies from country to country, with the most common prevalence of 1 : 250 being in African American women. It is about nine times as common in women than in men, with a peak age of onset between 20 and 40 years.

Aetiology

The cause is unknown but there are several predisposing factors:

- *Heredity.* There is a higher concordance rate in monozygotic twins (up to 25%) compared to dizygotic twins (3%). First-degree relatives have a 3% chance of developing the disease, but approximately 20% have autoantibodies.
- *Genetics.* There is an increased frequency of HLA-B8 and DR3 in Caucasians. There is a stronger association with HLA-DR2 in Japanese lupus patients.
- *Complement.* There is an inherited deficiency of C2 and C4 (which are in linkage disequilibrium with HLA-DR3 and DR2). A functional deficiency of C_1q has been suggested.
- *Sex hormone status.* Premenopausal women are most frequently affected. In addition, SLE has been seen in males with Klinefelter's syndrome (XXY) (see p. 174). In New Zealand mice, a lupus-like disease is ameliorated by oophorectomy or treatment with male hormones.

Immunological factors

Loss of 'self'-tolerance has several consequences:

- *B cell activation* results in increased autoantibody (mainly IgG) production to a variety (up to 2000) of antigens (nuclear, cytoplasmic and plasma membrane), e.g. ANA, anti-dsDNA.
- Development of and failure to remove *immune complexes* from the circulation leads to deposition of

complexes in the tissue, causing vasculitis and disease (e.g. glomerulonephritis). Immune complexes also form in situ, e.g. kidney glomerular basement membrane.

- There is impaired *T cell regulation* of the immune response.
- There is *abnormal cytokine production* (IL-1 and IL-2), although its exact role in the pathogenesis is unknown. IL-6 and IL-10 levels are often raised.
- *TNF-α promoters* have also been linked to SLE.

Environmental triggers

Drugs such as hydralazine, methyldopa, isoniazid, D-penicillamine and minocycline can induce lupus not associated with anti-dsDNA (see below). Flare-ups can be induced by the contraceptive pill and hormone replacement therapy (HRT). Ultraviolet light is another well-recognized trigger, probably via increased apoptosis (see below).

A viral agent causing SLE is a possible aetiological factor leading to the production of antibodies to nuclear material.

Pathogenesis

Although much interest has been focused on immunological abnormalities in relation to lupus, there seems from most reports to be little wrong with the process itself but rather a failure to clear apoptotic material efficiently. Nuclear constituents, e.g. DNA and histones, are released from these cells and their inefficient removal may lead to their being present in excess and possibly in some altered form. The nuclear material is then taken up by antigen-presenting cells and presented to T cells which in turn stimulate B cells to produce antibodies directed against nuclear antigens, e.g. Ro, La. The formation of some of these autoantibodies is due to proteases such as granzyme B which are active during apoptosis. Different subsets of autoantibodies may be related to the different clinical patterns.

Pathology

SLE is characterized by a widespread vasculitis affecting capillaries, arterioles and venules. Fibrinoid (an eosinophilic amorphous material) is found along blood vessels and tissue fibres. The synovium of joints may be oedematous and also contain fibrinoid deposits which contain immune complexes. Haematoxylin bodies (rounded blue homogeneous haematoxylin-stained deposits) are seen in inflammatory infiltrates and are thought to result from the interaction of antinuclear antibodies and cell nuclei.

The pathology of lesions in other organs is described in the appropriate chapters.

Clinical features

SLE is extremely variable in its manifestations and most of the clinical features are due to the consequences of

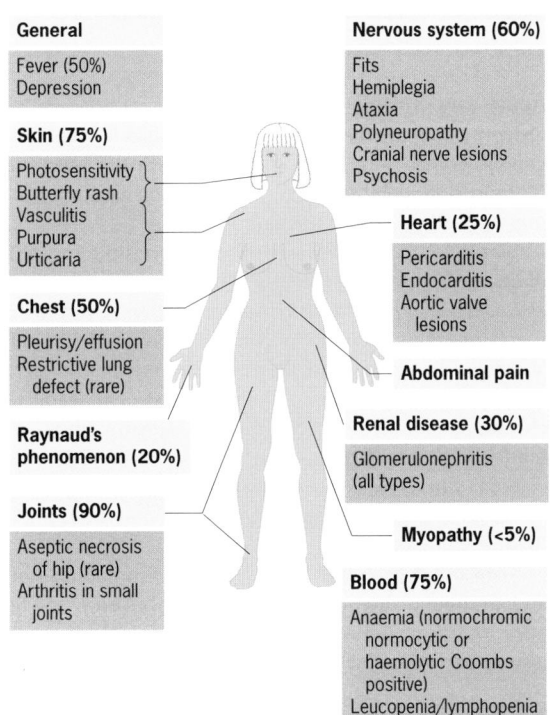

Fig. 10.26 Clinical features of systemic lupus erythematosus (SLE).

vasculitis. Mild cases may present only with arthralgia and fatigue, and can be difficult to diagnose (Fig. 10.26).

General features

Fever is common in exacerbations, occurring in up to 50% of cases. Patients complain of marked malaise and tiredness.

The joints and muscles

Joint involvement is the most common clinical feature (≥ 90%). Patients often present with symptoms that sound like RA with small joints being involved in a symmetrical fashion. Joints are painful but characteristically appear clinically normal, although sometimes there is slight soft-tissue swelling surrounding the joint. Deformity because of joint capsule and tendon contraction is rare, as are bony erosions. Rarely major joint deformity resembling RA (known as Jaccoud's arthropathy) may be seen. Aseptic necrosis affecting the hip or knee is a rare complication of the disease.

Myalgia is present in up to 50% of patients but a true myositis in < 5%.

The skin (see p. 1299)

This is affected in 75% of cases. Erythema, in a 'butterfly' distribution on the cheeks of the face and across the bridge of the nose (see Fig. 22.25) is characteristic. Vasculitic lesions on the finger tips and around the nail

558

folds, purpura and urticaria occur. In one-third of cases there is photosensitivity, and prolonged exposure to sunlight can lead to exacerbations of the disease. Livedo reticularis, palmar and plantar rashes, pigmentation and alopecia may be seen. Raynaud's phenomenon (see p. 831) is common and may precede the development of arthralgia and other clinical problems by years.

Immunofluorescence of 'normal' skin, obtained on biopsy, will show immunoglobulin and complement deposition at the dermo–epidermal junction (known as the positive band test).

Discoid lupus is described on page 1299.

The lungs (see p. 900)
Up to 60% of patients will have lung involvement sometime during the course of the disease. Recurrent pleurisy and pleural effusions (exudates) are the most common manifestations and often are bilateral. Pneumonitis and atelectasis may be seen; eventually a restrictive lung defect develops with loss of lung volumes and raised hemidiaphragms. Rarely, pulmonary fibrosis occurs.

The heart and cardiovascular system
The heart is involved in 25% of cases. Pericarditis, with small pericardial effusions detected by echocardiography, is common. A mild myocarditis also occurs giving rise to arrhythmias. Aortic valve lesions and a cardiomyopathy can rarely be present. A non-infective endocarditis involving the mitral valve (Libman–Sacks syndrome) is very rare. Raynaud's, vasculitis, arterial and venous thromboses can occur.

The kidneys
These invariably show histological changes, but clinical renal involvement occurs in approximately 30% of cases. Histological changes range from minimal-change nephropathy to crescentic glomerulonephritis. Proteinuria (> 1 g per 24 h) is common. Hypertension may occur owing to progression to either the nephrotic syndrome or renal failure.

The nervous system
Involvement of the nervous system occurs in up to 60% of cases and symptoms may fluctuate. There may be a mild depression but occasionally more severe psychiatric disturbances occur. Epilepsy, migraines, cerebellar ataxia, aseptic meningitis, cranial nerve lesions, cerebrovascular disease or a polyneuropathy may be seen. These lesions are due to vasculitis or immune-complex deposition.

The eyes
Retinal vasculitis can cause infarcts (cytoid bodies) which appear as hard exudates, and haemorrhages. There may be episcleritis, conjunctivitis or optic neuritis, but blindness is uncommon. Secondary Sjögren's syndrome may be seen in about 15% of cases.

The gastrointestinal system
SLE causes gastrointestinal symptoms, of which mouth ulcers are the commonest and may be a presenting feature. Mesenteric vasculitis can produce inflammatory lesions involving the small bowel (infarction or perforation). Liver involvement is unusual, although lupoid antibodies are described in autoimmune hepatitis. Pancreatitis is uncommon.

Lupus variants
Chronic discoid lupus is a benign variant of the disease, in which skin involvement is often the only feature, although systemic abnormalities may occur with time. The rash is characteristic and appears on the face as well-defined erythematous plaques that progress to scarring and pigmentation (see p. 1299). Subacute cutaneous lupus erythematosus, a rare variant, is described on page 1299.

Drug-induced SLE is usually characterized by arthralgia and mild systemic features, rashes and pericarditis, but seldom renal or cerebral disease. It usually disappears when the drug causing it is stopped. Hydralazine and procainamide are the most likely causes, but other drugs have occasionally been implicated.

Overlap syndrome is discussed on page 564.

Antiphospholipid syndrome (see below) was originally described in SLE and the presence of antiphospholipid antibodies partially accounts for the increased tendency to thrombosis.

Investigations
- **Blood:**
  - (a) *A full blood count* usually shows a leucopenia, lymphopenia and/or thrombocytopenia. An autoimmune haemolytic anaemia may occur. The ESR is raised in proportion to the disease activity. In contrast, the CRP is normal.
  - (b) *Serum antinuclear antibodies* (ANA) are positive in almost all cases. Double-stranded DNA (dsDNA) binding is specific for SLE, although it is only present in 50% of cases, particularly those with severe systemic involvement (e.g. renal disease). Antinucleosome antibodies predate anti-dsDNA antibodies. Antibodies to RNA (ss and ds) anti-Ro and anti-La can also be detected.
  - (c) *Rheumatoid factor* is positive in 25% of the patients.
  - (d) *Serum complement levels* are reduced during active disease.
  - (e) *Anticardiolipin antibodies* are present in 35–45% of the patients.
  - (f) *Serological tests for syphilis* – a third of patients have a false-positive test for syphilis owing to the anticardiolipin antibody.
  - (g) *Immunoglobulins* are raised (usually IgG and IgM).
- **Histology.** Characteristic histological and immunofluorescent abnormalities are seen in biopsies from, for example, the kidney and skin.

- **Diagnostic imaging.** CT scans of the brain sometimes show infarcts or haemorrhage with evidence of cerebral atrophy. MR can detect lesions in white matter which are not seen on CT. However, it can be very difficult to distinguish true vasculitis from small thrombi.

Management

The disease and its management should be discussed, pointing out that the prognosis is much improved though patients are advised to avoid excessive exposure to sunlight and should reduce cardiovascular risk factors.

Drug therapy should be used for active disease. There is no evidence that treatment in remission alters the progression of the disease.

- Arthralgia, arthritis, fever and serositis all respond well to standard doses of NSAIDs.
- Antimalarial drugs (chloroquine or hydroxychloroquine) (see Table 10.15) help mild skin disease, fatigue and arthralgias that cannot be controlled with NSAIDs.
- Corticosteroids orally or as high-dose intravenous boluses and/or immunosuppressive drugs such as azathioprine or cyclophosphamide are essential for more severe disease (glomerulonephritis, vasculitis, cerebral disease or blood dyscrasias) and when the symptoms are poorly controlled.
- Newer therapies include anti-CD40 ligand monoclonal antibodies which are undergoing clinical trials.

Course and prognosis

An episodic course is characteristic, with exacerbations and complete remissions that may last for long periods. These remissions may occur even in patients with renal disease.

A chronic course is occasionally seen. Earlier estimates of the mortality in SLE were exaggerated; 10-year survival rate is about 90%. In most cases the pattern of the disease becomes established in the first 10 years; if serious problems have not developed in this time, they are unlikely to do so. The arthritis is usually intermittent. Chronic progressive destruction of joints as seen in RA and OA occurs rarely, but a few patients develop deformities such as ulnar deviation.

Pregnancy and SLE

Fertility is usually normal except in severe disease and there is no major contraindication to pregnancy. Barrier methods of contraception rather than the pill are advisable. Recurrent miscarriages occur and these may be associated with antiphospholipid antibodies. Remission and exacerbations can occur during pregnancy with frequent exacerbations of the disease postpartum. The patient's usual treatment should be continued during pregnancy. Hypertension must be controlled. With severe renal disease and high antiphospholipid antibodies, fetal mortality is high (> 25%).

Antiphospholipid syndrome

The antiphospholipid syndrome is associated with autoantibodies which have specificity for negatively charged phospholipids. The terms lupus anticoagulant and anticardiolipin are used to describe these antibodies. A small proportion of these patients have SLE. Recurrent arterial and venous thromboses and miscarriages are the hallmark of the syndrome. The paradoxical association between a prothrombotic state and the presence of autoantibodies with in-vitro anticoagulant effects is not fully understood. However, β_2-glycoprotein (β_2GP1), also known as apolipoprotein H, has been identified as the target for both anticardiolipin antibodies and lupus anticoagulant.

Clinical features

Arterial and venous thromboses

Approximately 20% of strokes occurring under the age of 45 years are thought to be due to the antiphospholipid syndrome. Thromboses of different types occur and cause other features of the disease, including the Budd–Chiari syndrome and Addison's disease.

Abortions

Twenty-seven per cent of women who have had more than two abortions have the anticardiolipin syndrome. Antiphospholipid antibodies reduce the levels of annexin V, a protein with potent anticoagulant activity found in the placenta and vascular endothelium.

Other features

These include:

- thrombocytopenia
- chorea, migraine and epilepsy
- valvular heart disease
- cutaneous manifestations (e.g. livedo reticularis)
- positive Coombs' test.

The syndrome may also be important in the development of accelerated atheroma.

Investigations

Anticardiolipin antibodies (detected by ELISA) are diagnostic. Lupus anticoagulant antibodies are found in coagulation assays and these antibodies, directed against β_2GP1, can be detected by ELISA. The ESR is usually normal and antinuclear antibodies are usually negative.

Treatment

Anticoagulants are used. Small doses of aspirin are suitable in mild cases, warfarin in severe cases. Heparin and aspirin are given in early pregnancy, however, because warfarin is toxic to the fetus.

Systemic sclerosis (scleroderma) (see p. 1298)

Systemic sclerosis (SSc) is a multisystem disease of unknown cause. It is the most deadly of the sclero-derma-related disorders. It is related to but different from localized scleroderma, which is a skin and soft tissue disorder, not an organ-based disease.

SSc occurs world-wide with no racial differences. The incidence of SSc is 10/million population per year with a 3:1 male to female ratio. The peak incidence is between 30 and 50 years of age. It is rare in children.

Environmental risk factors for scleroderma-like disorders include exposure to vinyl chloride, silica dust, adulterated rape seed oil and trichlorethylene. Drugs such as bleomycin may also produce a similar picture. Familial cases have been described, but concordance in twins is rare.

Pathology and pathogenesis

Figure 10.27 shows the pathogenic interaction and mechanisms in systemic sclerosis.

Vascular features

An early lesion is widespread vascular damage involving small arteries, arterioles and capillaries. There is initial endothelial cell damage with release of cytokines including endothelin-1, the latter causing vasoconstriction. There is continued intimal damage with increasing vascular permeability, leading to cellular activation, activation of adhesion molecules (E selectin, VCAM, ICAM-1) (Table 4.2), with migration of cells into the extracellular matrix. Migrating lymphocytes are IL-2-producing cells, expressing surface antigens such as CD3, CD4 and CD5 (Table 4.7). All these factors

cause release of other mediators (e.g. interleukin-1, -4, -6 and -8, TGF-β and PDGF) (Table 4.5) with activation of fibroblasts.

The damage to small blood vessels also produces widespread obliterative arterial lesions and subsequent chronic ischaemia.

Fibrotic features

Fibroblasts synthesize increased quantities of collagen types I and III, as well as fibronectin and glycosaminoglycans, producing fibrosis in the lower dermis of the skin as well as the internal organs.

Humoral immunity

Humoral immunity is also involved because at least 80% of patients have antinuclear antibodies (see below).

Clinical features

Raynaud's phenomenon

Raynaud's phenomenon is seen in almost 100% of cases and can precede the onset of the full-blown disease by many years.

Limited cutaneous scleroderma (LcSSc) – 60% of cases

This usually starts with Raynaud's phenomenon many years (up to 15) before any skin changes. The skin involvement is limited to the hands, face, feet and forearms. The skin is tight over the fingers and often produces flexion deformities of the fingers. Involvement of the skin of the face produces a characteristic 'beak'-like nose and a small mouth (microstomia). Painful digital ulcers and telangiectasia with dilated nail-fold capillary loops are seen. Digital ischaemia may lead to gangrene. Gastrointestinal tract involvement is common in this group. Pulmonary hypertension develops in 10–15% of this group and pulmonary interstitial disease may occur.

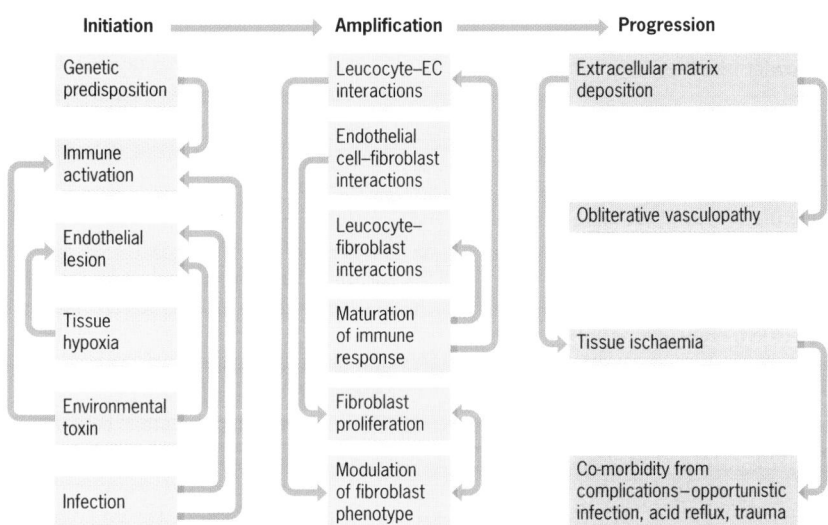

Fig. 10.27 **Pathogenic mechanisms in systemic sclerosis.** EC, endothelial cell.

The CREST syndrome (Calcinosis, Raynaud's phenomenon, Esophageal involvement, Sclerodactyly and skin changes in the fingers, Telangiectasia) was the term previously used to describe this syndrome.

Diffuse cutaneous scleroderma (DcSSc) – 40% of cases (see also p. 1298)

Initially oedematous in onset, skin sclerosis rapidly follows. Raynaud's phenomenon usually starts just before or concomitant with the oedema.

Diffuse swelling and stiffness of the fingers is rapidly followed by more extensive sclerosis which can involve most of the body in the severest cases. Later the skin becomes atrophic.

Early involvement of other organs occurs with general symptoms of lethargy, anorexia and weight loss.

- Heartburn, reflux or dysphagia due to oesophageal involvement are almost invariable and anal incontinence occurs in many patients. Malabsorption from bacterial overgrowth due to dilatation and atony of the small bowel is not infrequent, and more rarely dilatation and atony of the colon occurs. Pseudo-obstruction is a known complication.
- Renal involvement may be acute or chronic. Acute hypertensive renal crisis used to be the most common cause of death in systemic sclerosis. ACE inhibitors and better care along with dialysis and renal transplantation have changed this.
- Lung disease, both fibrosis and pulmonary hypertension (PHT), contribute significantly to mortality in SSc. PHT can be isolated or secondary to fibrosis and high plasma levels of endothelin-1 are seen.
- Myocardial fibrosis leads to arrhythmias and conduction defects. Pericarditis is found occasionally.

Sometimes these systemic features occur without skin involvement (*scleroderma sine scleroderma*). Overlap syndromes with additional features of SLE, RA or inflammatory muscle disorder occur.

Investigations

- **Full blood count.** A normocytic, normochromic anaemia may occur and a microangiopathic haemolytic anaemia is seen in some patients with renal disease.
- **Urea and electrolytes.**
- **Autoantibodies:**
  (a) *In LcSSc:* speckled, nucleolar or anticentromere antibodies (ACAs) occur in 70–80% of cases.
  (b) *In DcSSc:* there are antitopoisomerase-1 antibodies in 30% of cases, and anti-RNA polymerase (I, II and III) antibodies in 20–25%.
  (c) *Rheumatoid factor* is positive in 30%.
- **Urine.** Microscopy and, if there is proteinuria, a 24-hour urine collection for protein and creatinine clearance.

- **Imaging:**
  (a) CXR – used to exclude other pathology, changes in cardiac size and established lung disease
  (b) Hands – deposits of calcium around fingers (in severe cases, erosion and absorption of the tufts of the distal phalanges)
  (c) Barium swallow – for impaired oesophageal motility.
  (d) High-resolution CT – to demonstrate fibrotic lung involvement.
- Other investigations of gastrointestinal tract (e.g. see Fig. 6.4), lung, renal and cardiac as appropriate.

Management

Treatment should be organ-based in order to try to control the disease. Currently there is no cure.

- Education, counselling and family support are essential.
- Regular exercises and skin lubricants may limit contractures.
- Raynaud's may be improved by hand warmers, oral vasodilators (calcium-channel blockers, ACE inhibitors) and parenteral vasodilators (prostacyclin analogues and calcitonin gene-related peptide). Lumbar and digital sympathectomy may help.
- Oesophageal symptoms can be improved by proton-pump inhibitors and prokinetic drugs.
- Symptomatic malabsorption requires nutritional supplements and rotational antibiotics (see p. 294).
- Renal involvement requires intensive control of hypertension. First drug of choice is an ACE inhibitor.
- Intravenous prostacyclin may be helpful. High-dose corticosteroids have no place in the management of scleroderma and may precipitate renal crisis.
- Pulmonary hypertension is treated with oral vasodilators, oxygen, warfarin, i.v. prostacyclin; endothelin-receptor antagonists are being tried.
- Pulmonary fibrosis is currently treated with immunosuppression.
- No effective anti-fibrotic therapies are yet of proven efficacy.

Prognosis

In limited cutaneous scleroderma the disease is often milder, with much less severe internal organ involvement and a 70% 10-year survival. Pulmonary hypertension is a significant but later cause of death. This is in contrast to diffuse disease (55% 10-year survival) where organ involvement is often severe and many patients die of pulmonary, cardiac and/or renal involvement.

Localized forms of scleroderma occur either in patches (morphoea, p. 1298) or linear forms. These are more commonly seen in children and adolescents and do not convert into systemic forms.

Polymyositis (PM) and dermatomyositis (DM)

Polymyositis is a rare disorder of unknown cause, in which the clinical picture is dominated by inflammation of striated muscle, causing proximal muscle weakness. When the skin is involved it is called 'dermatomyositis'. These are rare disorders (incidence 2–10/million population per annum) and occur in all races and at all ages. The aetiology is unknown, although viruses (e.g. Coxsackie, rubella, influenza) have been implicated and persons with HLA-B8/DR3 appear to be genetically predisposed.

Clinical features

The clinical subsets are:

- adult polymyositis
- adult dermatomyositis
- adult polymyositis, dermatomyositis with malignancies
- PM/DM in association with other connective tissue diseases
- childhood DM.

Adult polymyositis

Women are effected three times more commonly than men.

The onset can be insidious, over months, but can be acute. General malaise, weight loss and fever can develop during the acute phase.

The major feature of polymyositis is proximal muscle weakness which is progressive. There is wasting of the shoulder and pelvic girdle muscles with weakness. Pain and tenderness are uncommon features. Involvement of pharyngeal, laryngeal and respiratory muscles can lead to dysphagia, dysphonia and respiratory failure. The changes can occur at a frightening speed but are often less rapid. Patients have difficulty squatting, going up stairs, rising from a chair, raising their hands above the head and holding their head up.

Respiratory muscles are affected in severe disease (especially those with anti-Jo-1 antibodies) and patients may require ventilation. Dysphagia is seen in about 50% owing to oesophageal muscle involvement. Arthralgia is seen in about 25% but is mild and Raynaud's phenomenon occurs in some patients.

Adult dermatomyositis

This is also more common in women.

Cutaneous features include a heliotrope (purple) discoloration of the eyelids and periorbital oedema. Scaly, purple-red raised vasculitic patches occur over the extensor surfaces of joints and fingers (collodion patches). Ulcerative vasculitis and calcinosis of the subcutaneous tissue occurs in 25% of cases. Muscle weakness is common. Myalgia, polyarthritis and Raynaud's phenomenon occur in this group. In the long term, muscle fibrosis and contractures of joints occur.

Childhood dermatomyositis

This most commonly affects children between the ages of 4 and 10 years. The typical rash of dermatomyositis is usually accompanied by muscle weakness. Muscle atrophy, subcutaneous calcification and contractures may be widespread and severe. Ulcerative skin vasculitis is common and recurrent abdominal pain due to vasculitis is also a feature.

Associated with other connective tissue diseases

There is an association with other autoimmune rheumatic diseases (e.g. SLE, RA and systemic sclerosis) with their associated clinical features such as deforming arthritis, malar rash and skin sclerosis.

Association with malignancies

The incidence remained uncertain until 1992 when a large study concluded a relative risk of cancer of 2.4 for male and 3.4 for female patients and a wide variety of cancers have been reported. The onset and clinical picture does not differ from that of typical DM/PM. The associated cancer may not become apparent for 2–3 years, and recurrent or refractory dermatomyositis should prompt a search for occult malignancy.

There is also an association with malignancy (e.g. lung, ovary, breast, stomach), which can predate the onset of myositis. This occurs particularly in males with dermatomyositis.

Investigations

- Serum creatine phosphokinase (CPK), aminotransferases and aldolase are usually raised and are useful guides to the activity of the disease.
- **The ESR** is raised in about 5% of cases.
- **Serum autoantibody studies.** Antinuclear antibody testing is commonly positive in patients with dermatomyositis. Rheumatoid factor is present in up to 50% and many myositis-specific antibodies (MSAs) have been recognized and correlate with certain subsets. Antibodies to Jo-1 (antibodies to histidyl tRNA synthetase) are predictive of pulmonary fibrosis but are rarely seen in patients with dermatomyositis.
- **Electromyography** (EMG) shows a typical triad of changes with myositis: spontaneous fibrillation potentials at rest; polyphasic or short-duration potentials on voluntary contraction; and salvos of repetitive potentials on mechanical stimulation of the nerve.
- **Fine needle muscle biopsy** shows fibre necrosis and regeneration in association with an inflammatory cell infiltrate with lymphocytes around the blood vessels and between muscle fibres.
- **MRI** can be used to target abnormal muscle.

- **Screening for malignancy** is usually limited to relatively non-invasive investigation such as CXR mammography, pelvic/abnormal ultrasound, urine microscopy and a search for circulating tumour markers.

Treatment

Bed rest is usually helpful but must be combined with an exercise programme. Prednisolone is the mainstay of treatment; 0.5–1.0 mg/kg bodyweight as initial therapy given for at least 1 month after myositis has become clinically and enzymatically inactive. Tapering of steroids must be slow. Early intervention with steroid-sparing agents such as methotrexate, azathioprine, ciclosporin, cyclophosphamide and mycophenolate mofetil is common. Intravenous immunoglobulin therapy (IVIG) is helpful in some recalcitrant cases.

Sjögren's syndrome and keratoconjunctivitis sicca

The syndrome of dry eyes (keratoconjunctivitis sicca) in the absence of rheumatoid arthritis or any of the autoimmune diseases is known as 'primary Sjögren's syndrome'. There is an association with HLA B8 DR3. Dryness of the mouth, skin or vagina may also be a problem. Salivary and parotid gland enlargement is seen.

Associated systemic features include:

- arthralgia and occasional non-progressive polyarthritis, like that seen in SLE (but much less common)
- Raynaud's phenomenon
- dysphagia and abnormal oesophageal motility as seen in systemic sclerosis (but less common)
- other organ-specific autoimmune disease, including thyroid disease, myasthenia gravis, primary biliary cirrhosis and autoimmune hepatitis
- renal tubular defects (uncommon) causing nephrogenic diabetes insipidus and renal tubular acidosis
- pulmonary diffusion defects and fibrosis
- polyneuropathy, fits and depression
- vasculitis
- increased incidence of non-Hodgkin's B cell lymphoma.

Pathology and investigations

Biopsies of the salivary gland or of the lip show a focal infiltration of lymphocytes and plasma cells.

- **Schirmer tear test.** This is a standard strip of filter paper placed on the inside of the lower eyelid; wetting of < 10 mm in 5 minutes indicates defective tear production.
- **Rose Bengal staining** of the eyes shows punctate or filamentary keratitis.

- **Laboratory abnormalities.** These include raised immunoglobulin levels, circulating immune complexes and many autoantibodies. Rheumatoid factor is usually positive. Antinuclear antibodies are found in 60–70% of cases and antimitochondrial antibodies in 10%. Anti-Ro (SSA) antibodies are found in 70%, compared with 10% of cases of RA and secondary Sjögren's syndrome. This antibody is of particular interest because it can cross the placenta and cause congenital heart block.

Treatment is with artificial tears and saliva-replacement solutions.

'Overlap' syndromes

Patients may present with varied clinical and serologic features not within the accepted boundaries of a single disease entity but sufficiently differentiated to fit more than one diagnosis. This is termed 'overlap syndrome'. These syndromes are rare. The combination includes:

- RA and SLE
- SSc, PM and/or SLE.

Mixed connective tissue disease was a term coined in the 1970s to describe patients with high-titre nRNP antibodies. Its existence as a separate disease is in question.

Systemic inflammatory vasculitis

Vasculitis is an inflammation of the vessel wall. The classification remains controversial, but is usually based on the type of artery affected (Fig. 10.28 and Table 10.18). There is some overlap and some cases are difficult to classify, partly because in many conditions there is always some vasculitis histologically. An alternative classification is shown in Table 22.14. Table 10.19 shows other infective and non-infective conditions in which a vasculitis is seen.

The disorders are characterized by inflammation in or through a blood vessel wall, with fibrinoid necrosis with or without granuloma formation. Histologically there are several different patterns: necrotizing vasculitis; giant cell arteritis; and granulomatous angiitis. The clinical manifestations are due to ischaemic necrosis and vary with the size and type of blood vessel affected. The vasculitides are systemic diseases which affect the skin and musculoskeletal, renal and gastrointestinal systems. Skin lesions are palpable and commonly urticarial. Many types of systemic non-autoimmune vasculitis are associated with antineutrophilic cytoplasmic antibody (ANCA, see p. 608).

- *Large vessel* refers to the aorta and its major tributaries.
- *Medium vessel* refers to medium and small-sized arteries and arterioles.

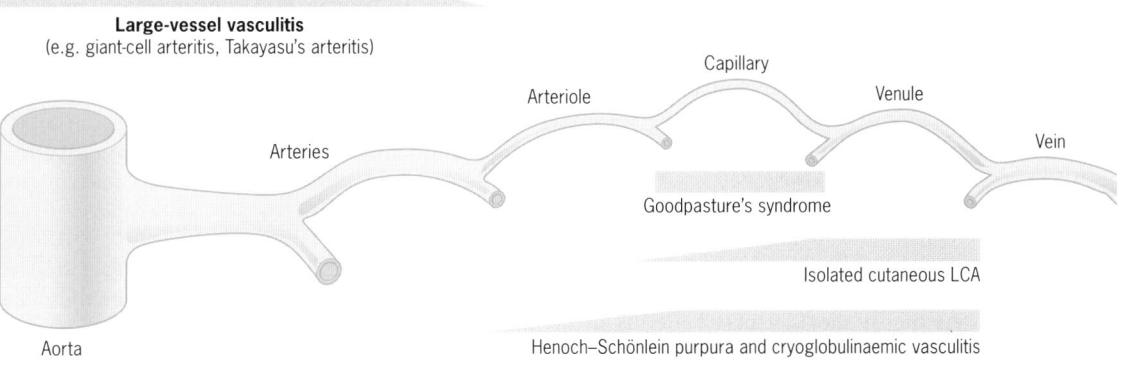

Small-vessel vasculitis
(e.g. microscopic polyangiitis, Wegener's granulomatosis)

Medium-sized-vessel vasculitis
(e.g. polyarteritis nodosa, Kawasaki's disease)

Large-vessel vasculitis
(e.g. giant-cell arteritis, Takayasu's arteritis)

Capillary

Arteriole

Venule

Arteries

Vein

Goodpasture's syndrome

Isolated cutaneous LCA

Aorta

Henoch–Schönlein purpura and cryoglobulinaemic vasculitis

Microscopic polyangiitis, Wegener's granulomatosis, and Churg–Strauss syndrome

Fig. 10.28 **Sites of vascular involvement by vasculitides.** From Jeanette JC and Falk RJ (1997) *New England Journal of Medicine* **337**: 1512–1523. Copyright © 1997 Massachussetts Medical Society. All rights reserved.

Table 10.18
Types of systemic vasculitis

Non-infective

Large	Giant cell arteritis	
	Takayasu's arteritis	
Medium	Classical polyarteritis nodosum (PAN)	
	Kawasaki's disease	
Small	Microscopic polyangiitis	
	Wegener's granulomatosis	ANCA associated
	Churg–Strauss syndrome	
	Henoch–Schönlein purpura	
	Cutaneous leucocytoclastic angiitis	
	Essential cryoglobulinaemia	

Table 10.19
Other conditions associated with vasculitis
(see also Table 10.18)

Infective	e.g. Subacute infective endocarditis
Non-infective	Vasculitis with rheumatoid arthritis
	Systemic lupus erythematosus
	Scleroderma
	Polymyositis/dermatomyositis
	Drug-induced Behçet's disease
	Goodpasture's syndrome
	Hypocomplementaemia
	Serum sickness
	Paraneoplastic syndromes
	Inflammatory bowel disease

- *Small vessel* refers to small arteries (ANCA-associated disease only), arterioles, venules and capillaries.

Large vessel vasculitis

Polymyalgia rheumatica (PMR) and giant cell (temporal) arteritis are systemic illnesses of the elderly. Both are associated with the finding of a giant cell arteritis on temporal artery biopsy.

Polymyalgia rheumatica (PMR)

PMR causes a sudden onset of severe pain and stiffness of the shoulders and neck, and of the hips and lumbar spine; a limb girdle pattern. These symptoms are worse in the morning lasting from 30 minutes to several hours. The clinical history is usually diagnostic and the patient is always over 50 years.

Patients develop systemic features of tiredness, fever, weight loss, depression and occasionally nocturnal sweats if it is not diagnosed and treated early. A differential diagnosis is shown in Box 10.14.

Symptom patterns in some muscle disorders

- **Polymyositis** – proximal muscle ache and weakness
- **Polymyalgia rheumatica** – proximal morning stiffness and pain
- **Myopathy** – weakness, but no pain or stiffness

Investigation of PMR

- **A raised ESR and/or CRP** is a hallmark of this condition. It is rare to see PMR without an acute-phase response. If it is absent, the diagnosis should be questioned and the tests repeated a few weeks later before treatment is started.
- **Serum alkaline phosphatase and γ-glutamyltranspeptidase** may be raised.
- **Anaemia** (mild normochromic, normocytic) is often present.
- **Temporal artery biopsy** shows giant cell arteritis in 10–30% of cases, but is not usually performed.

Giant cell arteritis (GCA)

GCA is inflammatory granulomatous arteritis of large arteries which occurs in association with PMR. It affects only the over-fifties. The patient may have current PMR, a history of recent PMR, or be on treatment for PMR. It may present with the symptoms of GCA which are:

- severe headaches, usually unilateral temporal or occipital
- tenderness of the scalp (combing the hair may be painful) or of the temple
- claudication of the jaw when eating
- tenderness and swelling of one or more temporal or occipital arteries
- systemic manifestations – severe malaise, tiredness and fever.

Involvement of the ophthalmic arteries causes sudden painless temporary or permanent visual loss. Occasionally GCA presents as a potentially treatable cerebrovascular episode. If a person with PMR on treatment develops unilateral severe headaches, GCA should be considered. Nevertheless, remember that tension headaches are common.

Investigation of GCA

- **ESR** is usually raised (in the region of 50–120 mm/h) and the CRP very high.
- **Liver biochemistry.** Abnormalities occur, as in PMR.
- **A temporal artery biopsy** from the affected side is the definitive diagnostic test. This should be taken before, or within 7 days of starting, high doses of corticosteroids. Start the drug first if the patient is very ill, in severe pain or has experienced visual loss or stroke. The lesions are patchy and the whole length of the biopsy must be examined.

The histological features of GCA are:

- intimal hypertrophy
- inflammation of the intima and sub-intima
- breaking up of the internal elastic lamina
- giant cells in the internal elastic lamina.

Treatment of PMR or GCA

Corticosteroids produce a dramatic reduction of symptoms within 24–48 hours of starting treatment, provided the dose is adequate. This should reduce the risk of patients with PMR developing GCA. NSAIDs are less effective and should not be used.

In GCA, corticosteroids are obligatory because they significantly reduce the risk of irreversible visual loss and other focal ischaemic lesions, but much higher doses are needed. Both diseases settle after between 12 and 36 months of treatment in about 75% of patients, but the remaining 25% continue to require low doses of corticosteroids for years. Starting doses of prednisolone are:

- **PMR**: 10–15 mg prednisolone as a single dose in the morning
- **GCA**: 60–100 mg prednisolone, usually in divided doses.

With GCA it is best to start at the higher dose, as the response is more dramatic and diagnostic. The dose should then be reduced gradually in weekly or monthly steps. While the dose is above 20 mg the step reductions are 5 mg, reducing the evening doses first. Between 20 mg and 10 mg the reduction can be in 2.5 mg steps, but below 10 mg the rate should be slower and the steps each of 1 mg.

Dose reduction (and increases when necessary) are titrated against the response or recurrence of symptoms and a fall or rise in the ESR or CRP.

Bone prophylaxis to avoid osteoporosis should be used.

Takayasu's arteritis

This is a granulomatous inflammation of the aorta and its major branches and is discussed on page 831.

Medium-sized vessel vasculitis

Polyarteritis nodosa (PAN)

Classic PAN is a rare condition which, unlike other vasculitic diseases, usually occurs in middle-aged men. It is accompanied by severe systemic manifestations, and its occasional association with hepatitis B antigenaemia suggests a vasculitis secondary to the deposition of immune complexes. Pathologically, there is fibrinoid necrosis of vessel walls with microaneurysm formation, thrombosis and infarction.

Clinical features

These include fever, malaise, weight loss and myalgia. These initial symptoms are followed by dramatic acute features that are due to organ infarction.

- *Neurological* – mononeuritis multiplex is due to arteritis of the vasa nervorum.
- *Abdominal* – pain due to arterial involvement of the abdominal viscera, mimicking acute cholecystitis, pancreatitis or appendicitis. Gastrointestinal haemorrhage occurs because of mucosal ulceration.
- *Renal* – presents with haematuria and proteinuria. Hypertension and acute/chronic renal failure occur.
- *Cardiac* – coronary arteritis causes myocardial infarction and heart failure. Pericarditis may occur.
- *Skin* – subcutaneous haemorrhage and gangrene occur. A persistent livedo reticularis is seen in chronic cases. Cutaneous and subcutaneous palpable nodules occur, but are uncommon.
- *Lung* – involvement is rare.

Investigations and treatment
- **Blood count**. Anaemia, leucocytosis and a raised ESR occur.
- **Biopsy** material from an affected organ shows features listed above.
- **Angiography**. Demonstration of microaneurysms in hepatic, intestinal or renal vessels if necessary.
- **Other investigations** as appropriate (e.g. ECG and abdominal ultrasound), depending on the clinical problem. ANCA is positive only rarely in classic PAN.

Treatment is with corticosteroids, usually in combination with immunosuppressive drugs such as azathioprine.

Kawasaki's disease

This is an acute systemic vasculitis involving medium-sized vessels, affecting mainly children under 5 years of age. It is very frequent in Japan, suggesting an infective aetiology, but none has been demonstrated. It occurs world-wide and is also seen in adults.

Clinical features and treatment

The clinical features are:

- fever lasting 5 days or more
- bilateral conjunctival congestion 2–4 days after onset
- dryness and redness of the lips and oral cavity 3 days after onset
- acute cervical lymphadenopathy accompanying the fever
- polymorphic rash involving any part of the body
- redness and oedema of the palms and soles 2–5 days after onset.

Five of these six features should be present to make the diagnosis, or four of six if coronary aneurysms can be seen on two-dimensional echocardiography or angiography.

Cardiovascular changes in the acute stage include pancarditis and coronary arteritis leading to aneurysms or dilatation. Other features include diarrhoea, albuminuria, aseptic meningitis and arthralgia and, in most, there is a leucocytosis, thrombocytosis and a raised CRP.

Treatment is with high-dose intravenous gammaglobulin, which prevents the coronary artery disease, followed after the acute phase by aspirin 200–300 mg daily.

Small vessel vasculitis

This can be separated into those that are positive or negative for antineutrophilic cytoplasmic antibody (ANCA). The role of these antibodies in the pathogenesis is unclear, but there is a correlation between ANCA titres and disease activity. ANCAs are specific for antigens in neutrophil granules and monocyte lysosomes. There are two types (see p. 608):

- antimyeloperoxidase (anti-MPO)
- antiproteinase-3 (anti-PR-3).

Neutrophils activated by ANCA may lead to endothelial injury by interaction between the neutrophils and cytokine-activated endothelium which precedes the vasculitic lesions.

The clinical features and diagnosis of small vessel vasculitis are shown in Table 10.20.

ANCA-positive vasculitis
- Wegener's granulomatosis – see page 901.
- Churg–Strauss granulomatosis – see page 901.
- Microscopic polyangiitis – see page 901.

ANCA-negative small-vessel vasculitis
This includes Henoch–Schönlein purpura – see pages 570 and 605.

Cutaneous leucocytoclastic angiitis
This is the characteristic acute purpuric lesion which histologically involves the dermal post-capillary venules. This lesion affects only the skin and should be differentiated from similar lesions produced in systemic vasculitis. The purpura may be accompanied by arthralgia and glomerulonephritis. Hepatitis C infection is common and may be an aetiological agent. The condition can also be caused by drugs such as sulphonamides and penicillin.

Treatment of small cell vasculitis
Small vessel vasculitis may be self-limiting and requires little treatment. Aggressive therapy with corticosteroids and immunosuppressive agents is required for severe disease.

Table 10.20
Diagnosis and clinical features of small vessel vasculitis

	Wegener's granulomatosis	Churg–Strauss syndrome	Microscopic polyangiitis	Henoch–Schönlein purpura	Cryoglobulinaemic vasculitis
Features					
ANCA (in blood) – PR3	90%	+	+	–	–
– MPO	–	60%	60%		
Necrotizing granulomas	+	+	–	–	–
Cryoglobulins (in blood and vessels	–	–	–	–	–
IgA immune deposits (mainly)	–	–	–	+	–
Asthma and eosinophilia	–	+	–	–	–
Organs involved					
Skin	40	60	40	90	90
Kidneys	80	45	90	50	55
Lungs	90	70	50	< 5	< 5
ENT	90	50	35	< 5	< 5
Musculoskeletal	60	50	60	75	70
Neurological	20	70	30	10	40
Gastrointestinal	50	50	50	60	30

Modified from Jeanette JC, Falk RJ (1997) Small vessel vasculitis. *New England Journal of Medicine* **337**: 1512–1523

Behçet's disease

Behçet's disease is an inflammatory disorder of unknown cause. There is a striking geographical distribution, it being most common in Turkey, Iran and Japan. The prevalence per 100 000 is 10–15 in Japan and 80–300 in Turkey. There is a link to the HLA-B55 allele, with a relative risk of 5–10; this association is not seen in patients in the USA and Europe.

Clinical features

The cardinal clinical feature is recurrent oral ulceration. The international criteria for diagnosis require oral ulceration and any two of the following: genital ulcers, defined eye lesions, defined skin lesions, or a positive skin pathergy test (see below). Oral ulcers can be aphthous or herpetiform. The eye lesions include an anterior or posterior uveitis or retinal vascular lesions. Cutaneous lesions consist of erythema nodosum, pseudofolliculitis and papulopustular lesions.

Other manifestations include a self-limiting peripheral mon- or oligoarthritis affecting knees, ankles, wrists and elbows; gastrointestinal symptoms of diarrhoea, abdominal pain and anorexia; pulmonary and renal lesions; a brainstem syndrome, organic confusional states and a meningoencephalitis. All the common manifestations are self-limiting except for the ocular attacks. Repeated attacks of uveitis can cause blindness.

The pathergy reaction is highly specific to Behçet's disease. Skin injury, by a needle prick for example, leads to papule or pustule formation within 24–48 hours. An intradermal injection of urate crystals is also used.

Treatment

Corticosteroids, immunosuppressant agents and ciclosporin-A are used for chronic uveitis and the rare neurological complications. Colchicine helps erythema nodosum and joint pain.

FURTHER READING

Black CM (1997) Systemic sclerosis. In: Klippel JH, Dieppe PA (eds) *Management in Rheumatology*, 2nd edn. London: Mosby, Section 7, Ch. 11: 1–10.
Callen JP (2000) Dermatomyositis. *Lancet* **355**: 53–57.
CME Section (2001) Rheumatological and immunological disorders. *Clinical Medicine* 1(1): 7–20.
Denton CP, Black CM (2000) Scleroderma and related disorders: therapeutic aspects. *Baillière's Clinical Rheumatology* **14**(1): 17–35.
Pickering MC, Haskard DP (2000) Behçet's syndrome. *Journal of the Royal College of Physicians London* **24**: 169–177.
Sakane T, Takeno M, Suzuki N, Inaba G (1999) Behçet's disease. *New England Journal of Medicine* **341**: 1284–1291.
Scott DGI, Watts RA (2000) Systemic vasculitis: epidemiology, classification and environmental factors. *Annals of Rheumatology* **59**: 161–163.

Differential diagnosis of rheumatic complaints in the elderly (Fig. 10.29)

Musculoskeletal problems
These are common at all ages. In the elderly, pain arises from a combination of age-related changes and injury.

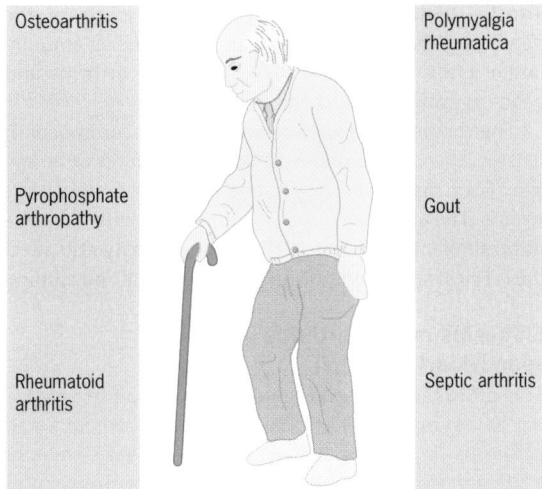

Fig. 10.29 The differential diagnosis of arthritis in the elderly.

Back and neck pain (see pp. 518 and 522)

These are commonly associated with spondylosis on X-ray and are more likely to be associated with such complications as spinal stenosis or nerve root claudication. Look for locally tender areas, which might be injected. Mechanical back pain may be worse in the morning, especially when spondylosis is severe or there is marked deformity; there is a normal ESR and CRP, which distinguishes this from polymyalgia rheumatica. Rarely elderly women present with previously undiagnosed ankylosing spondylitis.

Osteoporotic fractures

Osteoporotic fractures of the spine cause acute pain or deformity and subsequent postural back pain. The acute pain may warrant a period of bed rest (see p. 580). The management of such problems in the elderly is the same as for younger people but a response to treatment is less predictable. Advice about posture, exercise and general fitness is important but must be tempered by the patient's general health.

Symptomatic osteoarthritis (see p. 534)

This increases with increasing age and is uncommon below the age of 50 years. It is necessary to look for possible reversible causes of pain and disability, such as periarticular lesions or a joint effusion. Caution about drug treatment is necessary because of the increased risk of side-effects in older patients. Joint replacement surgery has transformed the outlook for many older people with OA by offering pain control and increased mobility and independence.

Rheumatoid arthritis

RA may present in the elderly as a dramatic onset of symmetrical polyarthritis. This has a reasonable prognosis and responds well to low doses of prednisolone and other drug therapy. RA in the older patient may mimic polymyalgia rheumatica; the synovitis becomes apparent as the corticosteroid dose is reduced. Treat with DMARDs as for RA in order to reduce the corticosteroid dose.

Polymyalgia rheumatica and giant cell arteritis

These must be recognized and treated. Failure to respond to adequate doses of prednisolone should trigger a search for an alternative disease, such as RA, vasculitis, infection or malignancy.

Chondrocalcinosis

This increases with increasing age and is seen on over 40% of knee X-rays in the over-80s. It may produce a variety of arthritic conditions (see p. 536).

Pseudogout

This is an important cause of acute monarthritis of the wrist or knee in older people. It responds well to aspiration and injection and to intra-articular corticosteroids or oral NSAIDs.

Gout

True gout causes acute monarthritis in the elderly but may also present as a polyarticular inflammatory arthritis, especially in elderly women on long-term diuretic treatment, or as tophaceous gout (p. 554).

Septic arthritis

Septic arthritis in the elderly and frail produces articular symptoms, and signs that may be muted. The patient usually has septicaemia and the best way to ensure its recognition is to retain it in the differential diagnosis of all musculoskeletal presentations in unwell, elderly people.

Treatment

In all cases the management is similar to that described in the main part of the chapter, but special care should be taken to reduce doses of medication where possible and to think about possible adverse drug effects or interactions.

Arthritis in children

Joint and limb pains are common in children but arthritis is fortunately rare. Babies and young children may present with immobility of a joint or a limp, but the diagnosis can be extremely difficult. Figure 10.30 summarizes the differential diagnosis.

For chronic conditions the child and family often need a great deal of support from physiotherapists, occupational therapists, psychologists, teachers, social workers and orthopaedic surgeons. These are best obtained in specialist paediatric centres.

Juvenile idiopathic arthritis		Other conditions
Systemic arthritis Oligoarthritis (persistent) Oligoarthritis (extended) Polyarticular arthritis (rheumatoid-factor positive) Polyarticular arthritis (rheumatoid-factor negative) Juvenile spondyloarthro-pathy Psoriatic arthritis Unclassified	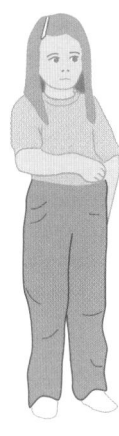	Henoch–Schönlein purpura Infections, e.g. tuberculosis, septic arthritis, viral arthritis Rheumatic fever Hypermobility syndrome Leukaemia Sickle cell disease SLE and other autoimmune connective tissue disease Transient synovitis of the hip

Fig. 10.30 The differential diagnosis of arthritis in children.

Juvenile idiopathic arthritis (JIA)

Systemic arthritis

Still's disease (which accounts for 10% of cases of JIA) affects boys and girls equally up to 5 years of age; then girls are more commonly affected. Adult-onset Still's disease is extremely rare.

Clinical features include a high, swinging, early-evening pyrexia, an evanescent pink maculopapular rash with arthralgia and arthritis, myalgia and generalized lymphadenopathy. Hepatosplenomegaly and pericarditis and pleurisy occur. The differential diagnoses include malignancy, in particular leukaemia and neuroblastoma, and infection. Laboratory tests show a high ESR and CRP, neutrophilia and thrombocytosis. Autoantibodies are negative.

Oligoarthritis (persistent)

This is the most common form of JIA (50–60%) but is still a relatively uncommon condition. It affects, by definition, four or fewer joints – especially knees, ankles and wrists – often in an asymmetrical pattern. It affects mainly girls, with a peak age of 3 years. The prognosis is generally good with most going into remission. Uveitis (often with a positive ANA) occurs and requires regular screening by a 3-monthly slit-lamp examination. Blindness can occur if it is untreated. Prognosis is generally good, with remission occurring eventually in most patients.

Oligoarthritis (extended)

In approximately 25% of patients oligoarthritis extends to affect many more joints after around 6 months. This form of arthritis can be very destructive.

Polyarticular JIA

The rheumatoid factor-positive form occurs in older girls, usually over 8 years. It is a systemic disease; the arthritis commonly involves the small joints of the hands, wrists, ankles and feet initially, and eventually larger joints. It can be a very destructive arthritis and needs aggressive treatment.

The rheumatoid factor-negative form is commoner. It usually affects girls under 12 years but can occur at any age. They may be ANA positive, with a risk of chronic uveitis. The arthritis is often asymmetrical, with a distribution similar to that seen in RF-positive. It may also affect the cervical spine, temporomandibular joints and elbows.

Enthesitis-related arthritis (juvenile spondyloarthropathy)

This affects teenage and younger boys, mainly producing an asymmetrical arthritis of lower-limb joints and enthesitis. It is associated with HLA-B27 and a risk of acute anterior uveitis. It is the childhood equivalent of adult ankylosing spondylitis but spinal involvement is rare in childhood. Approximately one in three develop spinal disease in adulthood.

Psoriatic arthritis

This may occur in children and is similar in pattern to the adult form. The arthritis may be very destructive. Psoriasis may develop long after the arthritis but is found commonly in a first-degree relative.

Treatment of JIA

JIA should always be referred to a specialist paediatric rheumatology unit with the facilities to assess and design treatment programmes which aim to prevent long-term disability. These units also need facilities for rehabilitation, education and surgical intervention. NSAIDs reduce pain and stiffness but disease-modifying agents such as methotrexate and ciclosporin are often essential to control severe disease. Corticosteroids may be required in systemic disease but risk causing growth suppression; intravenous pulsed methylprednisolone or high-dose methotrexate helps reduce this risk. Etanercept (p. 546) is of benefit in polyarticular JIA. Aspirin may be a cause of Reye's syndrome and should not be used under the age of 12 years.

Prognosis

Up to 50% of children develop long-term disability; 25% may continue to have active arthritis into adult years. Death may be due to infection or systemic disease with pericarditis or amyloidosis.

Other types

Henoch–Schönlein purpura (see also p. 605)

This is the commonest systemic vasculitis seen in children. IgA immune complexes deposit in the small vessels. It often occurs after upper respiratory tract infections. Other manifestations include lower limb purpura, a transient non-migratory polyarthritis, and abdominal pain. Fifty per cent of these patients will have haematuria and proteinuria, due to a glomerulonephritis; treatment of this is discussed on page 606. The prognosis is excellent, although 1% develop chronic renal damage.

Rheumatic fever

Rheumatic fever still occurs occasionally in developed countries but is more common in developing countries. Its incidence was declining before the antibiotic era, probably because of improvements in public health, possibly combined with declining virulence of the organism. It predominantly affects children aged 4–15 years, with a peak at 7–8 years. It may affect adults. It is triggered by the group-A beta-haemolytic *Streptococcus*, and the diagnosis depends upon a positive culture of this organism and/or raised antistreptolysin-O antibody titres. Not all streptococci produce ASO–DNAase B but other streptococcal antigens may be detected. The major complications are carditis and chorea and are caused by cross-reactive antibodies with sarcolemma or neural tissue. They develop in the 1–5 weeks after the initial infection. Clinical features are described on page 79.

The fever is persistent but rarely as high as in Still's disease (see above) and the temperature often remains above normal. The arthritis affects larger joints and migrates between joints, each being affected for a few days at a time. This is unlike Still's disease, where arthritis is usually much more persistent in each affected joint. A child may not volunteer a history of sore throat and the carditis may be silent. Isolated arthritis is the presenting symptom in 14–42%. The disease is easily missed if not included in the differential diagnosis of acute childhood arthritis.

Treatment includes bed rest during the acute phase with paracetamol and high-dose NSAIDs for fever and arthritis. The original streptococcal infection is treated and prophylactic penicillin offered until 20 years of age. Corticosteroids may be needed in some patients with carditis.

Hypermobility syndrome

Five to ten per cent of children are hypermobile. A proportion of them will develop various musculoskeletal complaints in early childhood, such as late walking, flat feet, or nocturnal leg pains, possibly due to hypermobile ankles and knees suffering recurrent sprains and strains after exercise. Joint effusions, subluxation, dislocation and ligamentous injuries may occur throughout childhood. Low back pain may develop in affected adolescents. There may be some risk of the early development of osteoarthritis in adulthood. More severe hypermobility is also seen in the Ehlers–Danlos and Marfan's syndromes (see pp. 585 and 803).

Treatment is with exercise directed at improving the strength of muscles that cross affected joints, as well as overall fitness and endurance. It may be necessary to reduce or change sporting and other activities.

Miscellaneous conditions

Some children develop *idiopathic musculoskeletal pain* that can become chronic. Management of these children requires exclusion of the causes shown in Figure 10.30, but without performing unnecessary laboratory investigations. *Nocturnal musculoskeletal pains* are episodic and may be associated with hypermobility. They may be called 'growing pains'. They often last 15–30 minutes and awaken the child from sleep, and may require physiotherapy and analgesics, together with advice and support to the parents.

Osteochondritis can affect the ossification centre of the ends of bones. A typical condition is *Osgood–Schlatter disease*, which is characterized by localized pain and swelling over the tibial tubercle or at the patellar tendon insertion. It is usually seen in athletic teenagers and responds to local treatment and changes of sporting activities. *Sever's disease* is an osteochondritis of the insertion of the Achilles tendon into the calcaneum.

Perthes' disease is an idiopathic, possibly avascular, necrosis of the proximal femoral epiphysis, of unknown aetiology. It presents as a painless limp, usually in boys aged 3–12 years, and is occasionally bilateral. If severe it may require surgical correction.

Transient synovitis of the hip causes painful limitation of movement, usually of one hip, after an upper respiratory infection in young children. Although the symptoms usually resolve within a few weeks, it is important to exclude other more serious causes of hip pain. Septic arthritis can be excluded by culture of the hip aspirate.

FURTHER READING

Woo P, Wedderburn LR (1998) Juvenile chronic arthritis. *Lancet* **351**: 969–973.

Rheumatological problems seen in other diseases

Gastrointestinal and liver disease

- *Enteropathic synovitis* – see page 551.
- *Autoimmune hepatitis* (see p. 362) may be accompanied by an arthralgia similar to that seen in systemic lupus erythematosus. Joint pain occurs in a bilateral, symmetrical distribution, with the small joints of the hands being prominently affected. Joints usually look normal but sometimes there is a slight soft-tissue swelling. These patients often have positive tests for antinuclear antibodies.

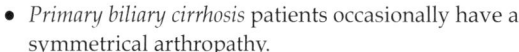
- *Primary biliary cirrhosis* patients occasionally have a symmetrical arthropathy.
- *Hereditary haemochromatosis* is associated with arthritis in 50% of cases; this is often the first sign of the disease and chondrocalcinosis is common.
- *Whipple's disease* (see p. 295) is accompanied by fever and arthralgia.

Malignant disease

It is not uncommon for malignant diseases to present with musculoskeletal symptoms. Bone pain may be due to multiple myeloma, lymphoma, a primary tumour of bone or secondary deposits. The pain is typically unremitting, worse at night and there are other clinical clues such as weight loss or ill-health. Secondary gout occurs in conditions such as chronic myeloid leukaemia.

Neoplastic disease of bone

Malignant tumours of bone are shown in Table 10.21. The most common tumours are metastases from the bronchus, breast and prostate. Metastases from kidney and thyroid are less common. Primary bone tumours are rare and usually seen only in children and young adults.

Symptoms are usually related to the anatomical position of the tumour, with local bone pain. Systemic symptoms (e.g. malaise and pyrexia) and aches and pains occur and are occasionally related to hypercalcaemia (see p. 1060). The diagnosis of metastases can often be made from the history and examination, particularly if the primary tumour has already been diagnosed. Symptoms from bony metastases may, however, be the first presenting feature.

Investigations

Skeletal isotope scans show bony metastases as 'hot' areas before radiological changes occur.

- **X-rays** may show metastases as osteolytic areas with bony destruction. Osteosclerotic metastases are characteristic of prostatic carcinoma.

Table 10.21
Malignant neoplasms of bone

Metastases (osteolytic)
Bronchus
Breast
Prostate (often osteosclerotic as well)
Thyroid
Kidney

Multiple myeloma

Primary bone tumours (rare; seen in the young) e.g.
Osteosarcomas
Fibrosarcomas
Chondromas
Ewing's tumour

- **Serum alkaline phosphatase** (from bone) is usually raised.
- **Hypercalcaemia** is seen in 10–20% of patients with malignancies. It is associated chiefly with metastases, but can also result from ectopic parathormone or parathyroid hormone-related protein secretion.
- **Prostate specific antigen** (PSA) and serum acid phosphate is raised in the presence of prostatic metastases.

Treatment

Treatment is usually with analgesics and anti-inflammatory drugs. Local radiotherapy to bone metastases relieves pain and reduces the risk of pathological fracture. Some tumours respond to chemotherapy, others are hormone-dependent and respond to hormonal therapy. Occasionally pathological fractures require internal fixation.

Hypertrophic pulmonary osteoarthropathy

Hypertrophic osteoarthropathy is most often associated with carcinoma of the bronchus. It is a non-metastatic complication and may be the presenting feature of the disease. It occurs only rarely with other conditions that also cause clubbing. It is seen most often in middle-aged men, who present with pain and swelling of the wrists and ankles. Other joints are involved occasionally.

The diagnosis is made on the presence of clubbing of the fingers, which is usually gross, and periosteal new bone formation along the shafts of the distal ends of the radius, ulna, tibia and fibula on X-ray. A chest X-ray usually shows the malignancy.

Treatment should be directed at the underlying carcinoma; if this can be removed, the arthropathy disappears. NSAIDs relieve the symptoms.

Paraneoplastic polyarthritis

This is seen with carcinoma of the breast in women and of the lung in men, and also with renal cell carcinoma. The neoplasm may be occult at onset and the diagnosis is then difficult to make.

Skin disease
Psoriatic arthritis

This is discussed on page 549.

Erythema nodosum

This can be due to several conditions (e.g. sarcoidosis) and is accompanied by arthritis in over 50% of cases. The knees and ankles are particularly affected, being swollen, red and tender. The arthritis subsides, along with the skin lesions, within a few months. Treatment is with NSAIDs or occasionally steroids.

Neurological disease

Neuropathic joints (Charcot's joints) are joints damaged by trauma as a result of the loss of the protective pain sensation. They were first described by Charcot in relation to tabes dorsalis. They are also seen in syringomyelia, diabetes mellitus and leprosy. The site of the neuropathic joint depends upon the localization of the pain loss:

- in tabes dorsalis, the knees and ankles are most often affected
- in diabetes mellitus, the joints of the tarsus are involved
- in syringomyelia, the shoulder is involved.

Neuropathic joints are not painful, although there may be painful episodes associated with crystal deposition. Presentation is usually with swelling and instability. Eventually severe deformities develop.

The characteristic finding is a swollen joint with abnormal but painless movement. This is associated with neurological findings that depend upon the underlying disease (e.g. dissociated sensory loss in syringomyelia or polyneuropathy in diabetes). X-ray changes are characteristic, with gross joint disorganization and bony distortion.

Treatment is symptomatic. Surgery may be required in advanced cases.

Blood disease

Arthritis due to haemarthrosis is a common presenting feature of *haemophilia* (see p. 461). Attacks begin in early childhood in most cases and are recurrent. The knee is the most commonly affected joint but the elbows and ankles are sometimes involved. The arthritis can lead to bone destruction and disorganization of joints. Apart from replacement of factor VIII, affected joints require initial immobilization followed by physiotherapy to restore movement and measures to prevent and correct deformities.

Sickle cell crises (p. 430) are often accompanied by joint pain that particularly affects the hands and feet in a bilateral, symmetrical distribution. Affected joints usually look normal but are occasionally swollen. This condition may also be complicated by avascular necrosis (see p. 526) and by salmonella osteomyelitis.

Arthritis can also occur in acute leukaemia; it may be the presenting feature in childhood. The knee is particularly affected and is very painful, warm and swollen. Treatment is directed at the underlying leukaemia. Arthritis may also occur in chronic leukaemia, with leukaemic deposits in and around the joints.

Individuals with thalassaemia major (see p. 428) are living longer and are presenting with back pain due to premature disc degeneration, secondary spondylosis and crush fractures due to osteoporosis. There is marked discal calcification.

Endocrine and metabolic disorders

Hypothyroid patients may complain of pain and stiffness of proximal muscles, resembling polymyalgia rheumatica. They may also have carpal tunnel syndrome. Less often, there is an arthritis accompanied by joint effusions, particularly in the knees, wrist and small joints of the hands and feet. These problems respond rapidly to thyroxine.

Hyperparathyroidism may be complicated by chondrocalcinosis and acute pseudogout.

In *acromegaly*, arthralgia occurs in about 50% of patients. It particularly affects the small joints of the hands and knees. There may be carpal tunnel syndrome.

In *Cushing's disease*, back pain is common.

Joint disorders related to *diabetes mellitus* are described on page 1100.

Familial hypercholesterolaemia is associated with oligo- or polyarthritis usually with tendon xanthomata. Arthritis also occurs in combined hyperlipidaemia.

Miscellaneous arthropathies

Familial Mediterranean fever (FMF)

FMF is inherited as an autosomal recessive condition and occurs in certain ethnic groups, particularly Arabs, Turks, Armenians and Sephardic Jews. The gene, called *MEFV*, has been localized to chromosome 16. It encodes for pyrin or marenostrin, which activate the biosynthesis of a chemotactic-factor inactivator in neutrophils. Failure to produce this leads to FMF attacks.

These are characterized by recurrent attacks of fever, arthritis and serositis. Abdominal or chest pain due to peritonitis or pleurisy occurs. The arthritis is usually monarticular and attacks last up to 1 week. The condition may be mistaken for palindromic rheumatism, but such attacks are not usually accompanied by fever

The diagnosis can be made by PCR, if available, but usually it is based on the clinical picture and exclusion of other conditions.

Treatment regularly with colchicine 1000–1500 µg daily can usually prevent the attacks. In general the disorder is benign but in 25% of cases renal amyloidosis develops.

Sarcoidosis (see also p. 897)

The most common type of arthritis is that associated with erythema nodosum, which occurs in 20% of cases of sarcoidosis at or soon after the onset of the disease. The most useful diagnostic test is a chest X-ray, which shows hilar lymphadenopathy in 80% of cases.

Other patterns of arthritis occur later in the disease. These include a transient rheumatoid-like polyarthritis and an acute monarthritis that can be mistaken for gout.

Treatment is with NSAIDs, but if these fail to control the symptoms, corticosteroids are usually very effective.

Osteochondromatosis

In this condition, foci of cartilage form within the synovial membrane. These foci become calcified and then ossified (osteochondromas). They may give rise to loose bodies within the joint. The condition occurs in a single joint of a young adult and X-rays are usually diagnostic.

Treatment involves removal of loose bodies and synovectomy.

Pigmented villonodular synovitis

This is characterized by exuberant synovial proliferation that occurs either in joints or in tendon sheaths. The main manifestation in joints is recurrent haemarthrosis. It may produce progressive local bone destruction but a malignant form is seen.

Treatment is synovectomy or radiotherapy. In tendon sheaths, the condition gives rise to a nodular mass that requires excision.

Relapsing polychondritis

Relapsing polychondritis is a rare inflammatory condition of cartilage. It occurs equally in males and females, usually the elderly. Tenderness, inflammation and eventual destruction of cartilage occur, mainly in the ear, nose, larynx or trachea. A seronegative polyarthritis occurs, as well as episcleritis and evidence of a vasculitis (e.g. glomerulonephritis). The diagnosis is clinical with laboratory evidence of acute inflammation.

Treatment involves corticosteroids and immunosuppressive agents.

Diseases of bone

Bone is a specialized connective tissue, serving three major functions:

- *mechanical* – providing structure and muscular attachment for movement
- *metabolic* – as a reserve of calcium and phosphate
- *protective* – enclosing bone marrow and vital organs.

Structure and physiology

Long bones (e.g. femur, tibia, humerus) and flat bones (e.g. skull, scapula, mandible) have different embryological templates, with cortical and trabecular bone in varying proportions (Fig. 10.31).

- *Cortical (compact) bone* forms the shaft (diaphysis) of long bones and the outer shell of flat bones. It has mainly mechanical and protective functions.
- *Trabecular (cancellous) bone* is found at the end of long bones (epiphysis) and inside the cortex of flat bones, consisting of a network of interconnecting trabecular plates and rods. It is the major site of bone remodelling and resorption for mineral homeostasis.
- *Woven bone* lacks the organized structure of cortical or cancellous bone. It is the first bone laid down in fracture repair, and also appears in Paget's disease.

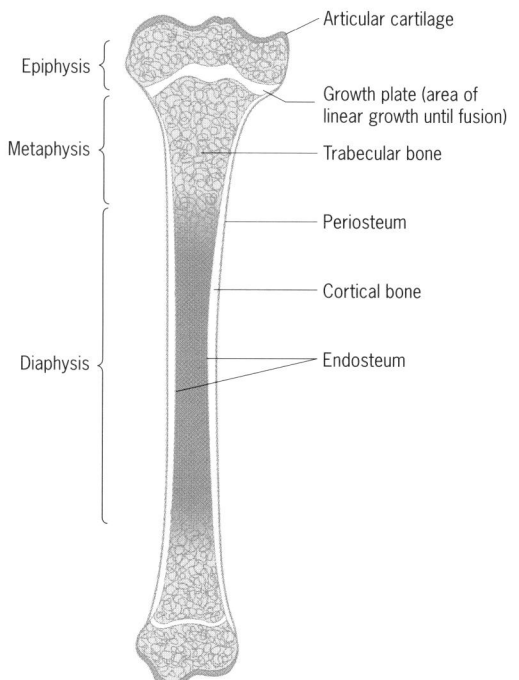

Fig. 10.31 **Diagram of a longitudinal section of a growing long bone.**

Bone comprises cells and a matrix of organic (mainly protein) and inorganic (mineral) elements.

Matrix components

Type I collagen confers structure and resistance to tensile stress, forming parallel lamellae in trabecular bone. In cortical bone, concentric lamellae form around blood vessels in Haversian canals which communicate via transverse (Volkmann's) canals. Non-collagenous proteins (NCPs) including osteocalcin, osteopontin and fibronectin regulate mineralization and remodelling. Calcium and phosphate are the primary minerals forming hydroxyapatite and other unique crystals, giving bone its resistance to compressive forces.

Bone cells

Osteocytes

These small, flattened cells act as transducers of mechanical stress in bone, their cytoplasmic processes communicating with other osteocytes and projecting through the osteoid seam to active osteoblasts.

Osteoblasts

Derived from local mesenchymal stem cells, osteoblasts cluster along the bone surface and synthesize bone matrix (osteoid) and regulate its mineralization, after which a large proportion of the redundant osteoblasts are removed, some lining the surface or becoming embedded in newly mineralized bone as osteocytes. Osteoblasts are also critical in the regulation of osteoclast function through production of stimulatory RANK-L (the *l*igand for *r*eceptor *a*ctivator of *n*uclear factor *k*appa-B) and the inhibitory factor osteoprotegerin (OPG). Osteoblasts are rich in alkaline phosphatase and express many receptors, including those for glucocorticoids, parathyroid hormone (PTH), vitamin D_3 (1,25-$(OH)_2D_3$), oestrogen, prostaglandins, interleukins and transforming growth factor (TGF)-β.

Osteoclasts

Osteoclasts develop from haemopoietic stem cells of the macrophage/monocyte lineage. They express receptors for colony-stimulating factor-1 (M-CSF), RANK-L and calcitonin, but not for PTH. They attach to bone, forming a ruffled border to create a series of extracellular lysosomal compartments. Hydrogen ions are secreted into this space, the acid environment dissolving the crystals and exposing the matrix which is then degraded by cysteine protease enzymes (e.g. cathepsin K) functioning at their optimal pH.

Bone growth and remodelling

Longitudinal growth occurs at the epiphyseal growth plate (between the epiphysis and metaphysis). Cartilage is produced by chondrocytes and ossified until skeletal maturity at 18–21 years of age when the epiphysis

and metaphysis fuse. Damage to the growth plate will impair growth.

In adults bone is continually being remodelled by basic multicellular units (Fig. 10.32). Osteocytes communicate mechanical strain to osteoblasts on the bone surface via cytoplasmic projections. The osteoblast responds to this or to other signals (parathyroid hormone, dihydroxy-vitamin D_3, cytokines or growth factors by increasing RANK-L (the **l**igand for **r**eceptor **a**ctivator of **n**uclear factor **k**appa B) and M-CSF (macrophage colony stimulating factor), and reducing osteoprotegerin. This promotes osteoclast formation from circulating monocyte precursors and directs osteoclasts to the area of bone to be resorbed. Unknown inhibitory signals limit osteoclast recruitment and activity. Macrophages remove apoptotic osteoclasts and prepare the resorbed surface (the cement line). Growth factors drive osteoblast formation from local stem cells (*coupling* of resorption and formation), producing osteoid which is mineralized to form new bone. On completing the cycle (about 120 days), remodelling is *balanced* if there has been no net change in the amount of bone.

Hormone regulation of bone

In addition to the hormones regulating calcium homeostasis (below), other hormones influencing bone turnover include:

- *Insulin and growth hormone*, acting via insulin-like growth factor (IGF)-1, increase bone matrix synthesis and mineralization

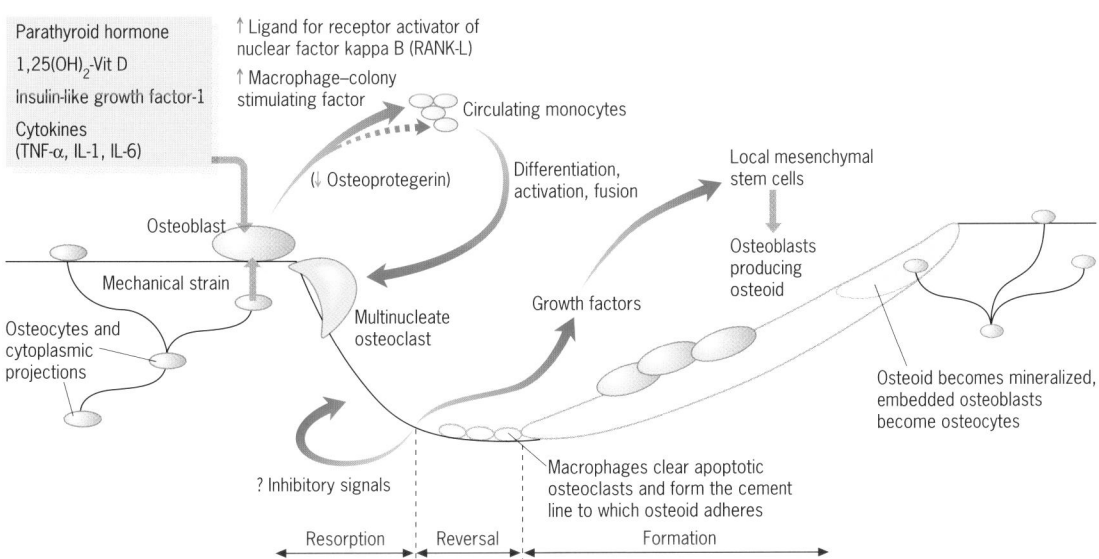

Fig. 10.32 A diagram of bone remodelling, representing a cross-section of a groove in a flat area of bone at a single time-point. (Resorption and formation in fact occur simultaneously at different points along the groove or tunnel.) On the left, the multinucleate osteoclast is resorbing bone at the groove's apex, in response to increased RANK-L and M-CSF (and reduced osteoprotegerin) from adjacent osteoblasts which have been activated by hormones, cytokines or by osteocytes under mechanical strain. Macrophages appear in the osteoclasts' wake, clearing apoptotic cells (reversal) and preparing the resorbed bone surface as a 'cement line'. Growth factors released from the bone stimulate differentiation of local stem cells to osteoblasts that form new bone, completing the cycle. TNF, tumour necrosis factor; IL, interleukin.

- *Oestrogens and the selective oestrogen receptor modulators* (SERMs), which act on the oestrogen receptor (see Osteoporosis, p. 581), and possibly androgens, inhibit bone resorption indirectly by reducing levels of IL-1 and -6 and of TGF-β.

FURTHER READING

Bland R (2000) Steroid hormone receptor expression and action in bone. *Clinical Science* **98**: 217–240.
Suda T et al. (1999) Modulation of osteoclast differentiation and function by the new members of the tumor necrosis factor receptor and ligand families. *Endocrinology Reviews* **20**: 345–357.

Calcium homeostasis and its regulation

Calcium homeostasis is regulated by the effects of PTH and 1,25-$(OH)_2D_3$ on gut, kidney and bone. Calcium-sensing receptors are present in the parathyroid gland, kidney, brain and other organs.

Calcium absorption and distribution (Fig. 10.33)

Daily calcium consumption, primarily from dairy foods, should ideally be around 20–25 mmol (800–1000 mg). Dietary calcium deficiency is rarely a significant cause of bone disease because proportional absorption can increase in response to low intake. Absorption is reduced by vitamin D deficiency and sometimes by generalized malabsorption.

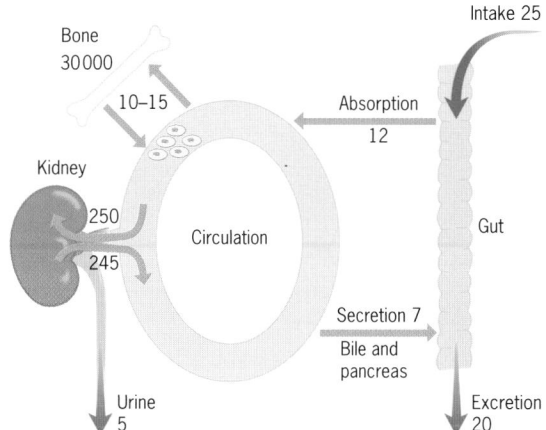

Fig. 10.33 **Calcium exchange in the normal human.**
The fluxes are shown in mmol per day.

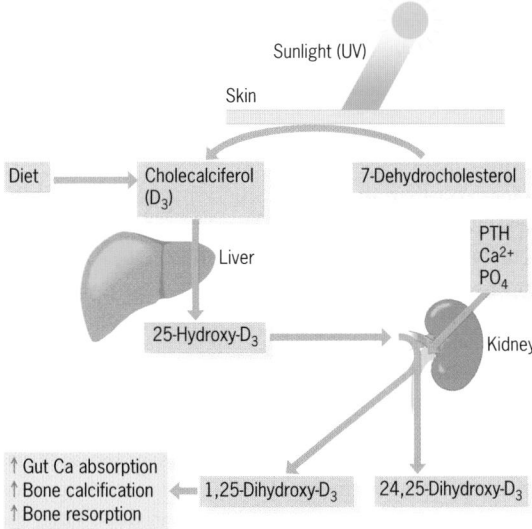

Fig. 10.34 **The metabolism and actions of vitamin D.**
PTH, parathyroid hormone.

Vitamin D metabolism (Fig. 10.34)

The primary source of Vitamin D in humans is photoactivation (in the skin) of 7-dehydrocholesterol to cholecalciferol, converted in the liver to 25-hydroxycholecalciferol (25-$(OH)D_3$) and further converted by the kidney tubule enzyme, 1α-hydroxylase, to the active metabolite 1,25-dihydroxycholecalciferol (1,25-$(OH)_2D_3$). (This step can occur in lymphomatous and sarcoid tissue, resulting in the hypercalcaemia that may complicate these diseases.) A less active metabolite, 24,25-$(OH)_2D_3$, is formed if vitamin D supplies are adequate. Regulation of this enzyme is by PTH, phosphate and by feedback inhibition by 1,25-$(OH)_2D_3$.

Parathyroid hormone (PTH)

PTH, an 84-amino-acid hormone, is secreted from the chief cells of the parathyroid glands (normally situated posterior to the thyroid, but occasionally elsewhere in the neck or mediastinum). PTH increases renal phosphate excretion, and increases plasma calcium by:

- increasing osteoclastic resorption of bone (occurring rapidly)
- increasing intestinal absorption of calcium (a slow response)
- increasing synthesis of 1,25-$(OH)_2D_3$
- increasing renal tubular reabsorption of calcium.

Hypomagnesaemia can suppress the normal PTH response to hypocalcaemia.

Thyroid hormones

Calcitonin is produced by thyroid C cells. Total thyroidectomy (absent calcitonin) or medullary carcinoma of the thyroid (excess calcitonin) have no significant skeletal effects. Plasma calcitonin levels do, however, rise with increasing serum calcium, and calcitonin inhibits osteoclastic bone resorption and increases the renal excretion of calcium and phosphate. It may be used in treating osteoporosis or hypercalcaemia.

Excess thyroxine (T_4) and triiodothyronine (T_3) cause increased bone turnover, hypercalcaemia and bone loss, while hypothyroidism leads to growth delay.

Investigation of bone and calcium disorders (Fig. 10.35)

Total plasma calcium (normal range 2.2–2.6 mmol/L) About 40% is ionized and physiologically relevant; the remainder is complexed or protein-bound, particularly to albumin. Ionized calcium is difficult to measure and not routinely assessed. Total plasma calcium can be approximately corrected for protein binding by adding or subtracting 0.02 mmol/L for every gram per litre of a simultaneous albumin level below or above 40 g/L. For critical measurements, samples should be taken in the fasting state and without a tourniquet (the latter may increase local plasma protein concentration).

Plasma phosphate (normal range 0.8–1.4 mmol/L) Phosphate is essential to most biological systems. As renal phosphate reabsorption is decreased by PTH, primary hyperparathyroidism is associated with low levels of plasma phosphate. High levels are found in renal failure or in hypoparathyroidism.

PTH measurements
The PTH assay measures the intact PTH molecule. Interpretation requires a simultaneous calcium measurement. Urinary cyclic adenosine monophosphate (cAMP) concentration reflects the bioactivity of PTH, but is not commonly measured.

25-hydroxyvitamin D
Together with PTH levels, and allowing for seasonal variation (higher in summer with increased sunlight), measurement may be useful where hypovitaminosis D or interaction with antiepileptic drugs is suspected in hypocalcaemia, or in hypercalcaemia where excess ingestion of vitamin D is of concern. Measurements of $1,25\text{-}(OH)_2D_3$ are seldom helpful clinically.

Urinary calcium (normal range 2.5–7.5 mmol/24 h) This is increased where renal tubular resorption of calcium is decreased, or in hypercalcaemia. An exception to the latter is familial hypocalciuric hypercalcaemia, where urinary calcium excretion is inappropriately normal in the face of hypercalcaemia. The main role of urinary calcium assay is in the investigation of renal calculi.

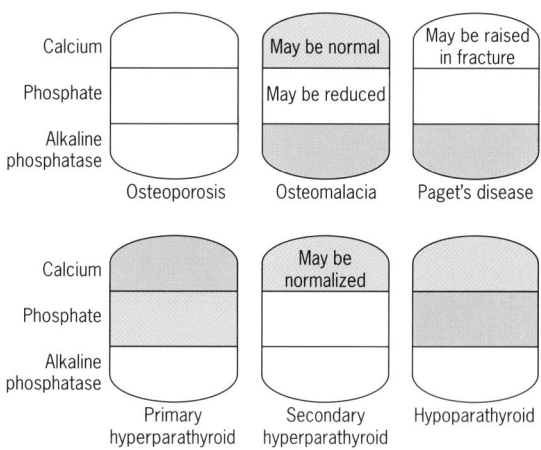

Fig. 10.35 Changes in serum calcium, phosphatase and alkaline phosphatase in main bone disorders. Shading represents increased (red), reduced (blue) or normal (white) levels.

Markers of bone formation
- *Alkaline phosphatase* is derived from liver, bone, kidney (and placenta). Bone-specific alkaline phosphatase is synthesized by osteoblasts; serum levels are raised in the growing child and in certain bone diseases (Fig. 10.35).
- *Serum osteocalcin* levels do not always parallel bone-specific alkaline phosphatase levels.
- *Type I collagen propeptides* are by-products of collagen synthesis. Carboxyterminal propeptide of collagen I (P1CP) is the most commonly used, though its diagnostic value is still disputed.

Markers of bone resorption
- *Pyridinoline or deoxypyridinoline cross-links of collagen* are produced by collagen degradation, and excreted in urine. Deoxypyridinoline is bone-specific, and both are more sensitive than urinary hydroxyproline.
- *N-terminal and C-terminal cross-linked telopeptides* also reflect bone resorption and may alter more rapidly in response to disease or treatment.

Diagnostic imaging
- *Plain radiographs* identify fracture, tumours and infections. Features characteristic of specific metabolic bone diseases may be seen (see separate sections).
- *Radionuclide scans.* Technetium-99m-labelled methylene bisphosphonate uptake is predominantly dependent on blood flow, detecting increased bone activity in cases of fracture, infection, metastases or in metabolic bone disease with greater sensitivity than X-rays.
- *Magnetic resonance imaging* allows detailed assessment of subchondral and other bone areas.

Table 10.22
Indications for DEXA scan

Radiographic osteopenia or vertebral deformity
Loss of height or thoracic kyphosis
Hypogonadism
Previous fragility fracture
Glucocorticoid therapy
Body mass index < 19 (kg/m^2)
Maternal history of hip fracture
Diseases associated with osteoporosis (Table 10.23)

Variations in technique (T1, T2, STIR (which suppresses the high signal from fat in bone marrow)) offer specific diagnostic or prognostic information, for example in suspected avascular necrosis.

Bone density measurements

- *Conventional radiographs* are relatively insensitive for detecting osteopenia.
- *Dual energy X-ray absorptiometry* (DXA) measures areal bone density (mineral per surface area rather than a true volumetric density), usually of the lumbar spine and proximal femur. It is precise, accurate, uses low doses of radiation and is the gold standard in osteoporosis diagnosis (Table 10.22).
- *Quantitative CT scanning* allows true volumetric assessment, and distinction between trabecular and cortical bone. However, it is more expensive, requires higher radiation than other techniques, and to date offers no clinical advantage.
- *Quantitative ultrasound* of the calcaneum. Difficulties with measurement reproducibility, and inconsistency comparing different devices have limited its routine use, though its use is likely to increase in the future.

Bone biopsy

A core of bone is removed (from cortex to cortex at the iliac crest) with a trephine, and the non-decalcified specimen is examined for indices of bone turnover and remodelling. A fluorochrome (usually oral tetracycline) is given for 2 days, on two occasions 10 days apart. The rate of uptake of this marker on the mineralization front is demonstrated by comparing the two fluorescence bands. It is decreased in osteomalacia.

Osteoporosis

Definition and incidence

Osteoporosis is defined as 'a disease characterized by low bone mass and micro-architectural deterioration of bone tissue, leading to enhanced bone fragility and an increase in fracture risk'. Bone is normally mineralized but is deficient in quantity, quality and structural integrity (Fig. 10.36).

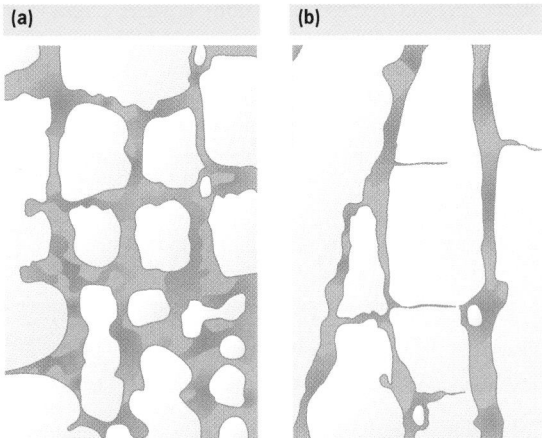

Fig. 10.36 **The microarchitecture of (a) normal and (b) osteoporotic bone.** There is thinning and a loss of trabecular plates.

The World Health Organization (WHO) defines osteoporosis as a bone density more than 2.5 standard deviations (SDs) below the young adult mean value (T-score < –2.5). Values between 1 and 2.5 SDs below the young adult mean are termed 'osteopenia'.

As the risk of fracture increases exponentially with age (Fig. 10.37(a)), changing population demographics will increase the burden of disease (currently costing almost £1 billion annually in the UK). The lifetime risk of hip fracture for a white woman at age 50 is around 15%, 5% for men, with equal risks around 11–13% for Colles' or vertebral fractures. Of those surviving to 80 years of age, 30% of women and 15% of men will suffer a hip fracture. Caucasian and Asian races are particularly at risk.

Pathogenesis

The changes in bone mass with age are shown in Figure 10.37(b). After a peak around 30 years of age, there is a gradual decline in men, whereas in women, accelerated loss occurs in the 10 years following the menopause.

Bone mass therefore depends on peak mass attained and on the rate of loss later in life. Genetic factors are the single most significant influence on peak bone mass but are polygenic, including polymorphisms in the genes for collagen type IA1, vitamin D receptor and oestrogen receptor. Nutritional factors, sex hormone status and physical activity also affect the peak mass attained.

Risk factors associated with increased bone loss may be considered as endogenous or exogenous (Table 10.23).

- Endogenous factors include ethnicity, female gender, advancing age, family history of fracture.
- Exogenous factors are hypogonadism (male or female), glucocorticoid treatment, low body mass index, previous fracture, smoking, immobilization, excess alcohol; vitamin D and calcium deficiencies are particularly relevant in the elderly.

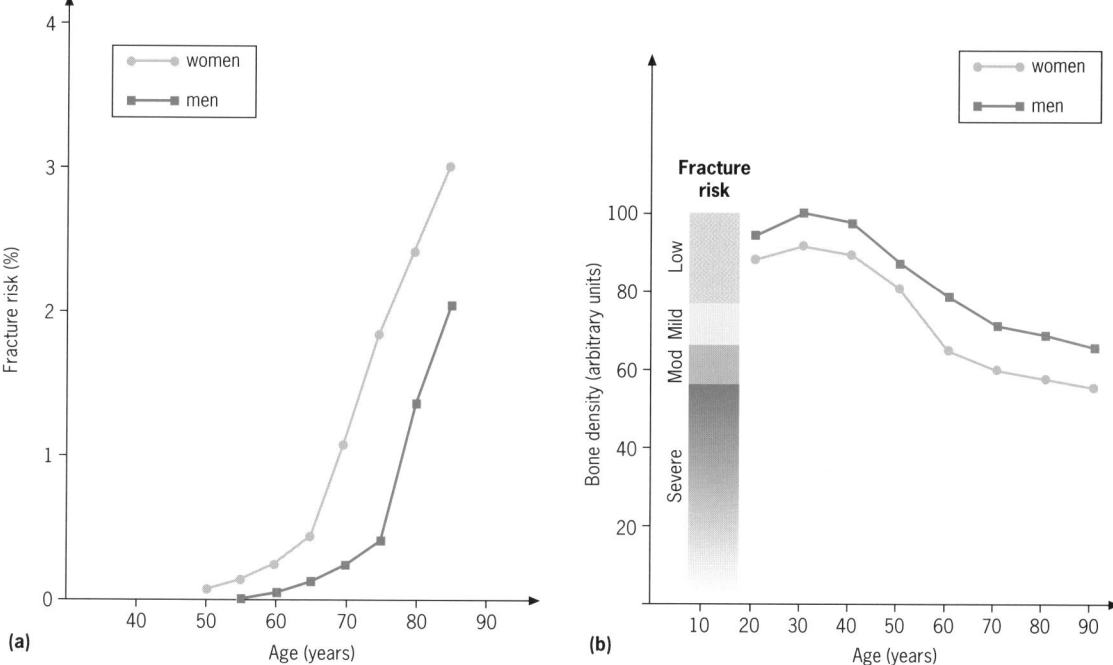

Fig. 10.37 **Features of osteoporosis according to age and sex. (a)** The risk of hip fracture. **(b)** Schematic diagram showing the decrease in bone density with increasing age, along with an increased fracture risk.

Table 10.23
Risk factors for osteoporosis

Risk factors	Diseases
Female sex	*Endocrine*
Increasing age	Cushing's syndrome
Early menopause	Hyperparathyroidism
(including ovariectomy)	Hypogonadism
Caucasians and Asians	(including orchidectomy)
Slender habitus	Acromegaly
Lack of exercise/immobility	Type I diabetes mellitus
Smoking	*Joint*
Family history	Rheumatoid arthritis
Excess alcohol	*Other*
Nutrition (very low calcium	Chronic renal failure
diet, high protein intake	Chronic liver disease
for a long time)	Mastocytosis
	Anorexia nervosa
Drug therapy	Inflammatory bowel disease
Corticosteroids	Coeliac disease
Heparin	
Ciclosporin	
Cytotoxics	

Hyperparathyroidism, hyperthyroidism, inflammatory bowel or joint diseases, chronic liver or renal disease increase the risk of osteoporosis.

Environment (e.g. poor lighting, uneven floor surface), neuromuscular and cardiovascular disease and commonly prescribed drugs (diuretics, sedatives, anxiolytics) are often overlooked causes of falls in the elderly which contribute considerably to fracture risk.

Not all causes of osteoporosis affect bone architecture in the same way. An early consequence of oestrogen deficiency (possibly transient) is reduced osteoclast apoptosis. Increased numbers of basic multicellular units (BMUs) appear, with increased resorption depth exceeding the synthetic capacity of osteoblasts, causing a loss of resistance to fracture not entirely reflected by measured BMD. Hyperparathyroidism and hyperthyroidism are also associated with increased turnover. In older patients, reduced formation is more significant than increased resorption. Glucocorticoid-induced osteoporosis (GIO) is initially associated with a high-turnover state, though chronic use is associated with reduced bone formation and low turnover.

Clinical features

Fracture is the only cause of symptoms in osteoporosis. Sudden onset of severe pain in the spine resolving over 6 weeks suggests vertebral crush fracture. However, only about one in three vertebral fractures are symptomatic. Pain from mechanical derangement, increasing kyphosis, height loss and abdominal protuberance follow crushed vertebrae. Colles' fracture, with the classical dinner-fork deformity, typically follows a fall on an outstretched arm. Fractures of the neck of the femur usually occur in older patients falling on their side or back. Other causes of low-trauma fractures must not be overlooked, including metastatic disease and myeloma. New vertebral fractures often require bed rest for 1–2 weeks with strong analgesia (e.g. meptazinol) and transcutaneous electrical nerve stimulation (TENS) may be helpful. Muscle relaxants (e.g. diazepam 2 mg three times daily), subcutaneous calcitonin (50 IU daily) or a single intravenous infusion of pamidronate (60–90 mg) are useful for pain relief, and physiotherapy helps restore confident mobilization. Non-spinal fractures should be treated by conventional orthopaedic means.

Investigations

If fracture suspected

Plain radiographs usually show a fracture and may reveal previous asymptomatic vertebral fractures. Where plain films are normal, fractures (especially of pelvis or vertebrae) may be detected by bone scintigraphy. A metastatic lesion may be distinguished from an osteoporotic fracture by pedicle destruction or if associated with multiple scintigraphic lesions.

Bone density

A DXA scan provides a T-score reflecting fracture risk which may influence treatment decisions (Fig. 10.38). Indications are given in Table 10.22. Because of osteophytes and vertebral deformity, spinal values should be interpreted with caution in the elderly.

Associated disease and risk factors

Investigations to exclude other diseases or identify contributory factors associated with osteoporosis are particularly necessary in men (Table 10.23).

Prevention and treatment (Box 10.15)

Predisposing lifestyle factors should be addressed, and those at significant risk can be identified for DXA.

- *Diet* should include at least 1000 mg of calcium daily (ideally 1500 mg postmenopausally) and 400–800 IU of vitamin D. As calcium is always given to the patients in clinical trials, benefits of the trial drug assume adequate calcium intake.
- *Exercise.* Thirty minutes of weight-bearing exercise three times a week may be beneficial to bone, though not a universal finding in all studies.
- *Smoking cessation.* Smoking accelerates bone loss and may negate the beneficial effect of oestrogen therapy, possibly by accelerating oestrogen metabolism.
- *Reduce falls.* Physiotherapy and assessment of home safety may be required. Hip protectors for elderly patients in residential care reduced fracture risk by 60%.

Those requiring 7.5 mg of prednisolone or equivalent for 6 months or more should be assessed for coexisting risks (age, previous fracture, hormone status); preventative treatment (usually bisphosphonate) is advocated for those with additional risks. DXA results guide treatment for other patients.

The evidence base for secondary prevention (reducing fracture risk in those with osteoporosis) varies considerably. Adequately powered randomized controlled trials, with fracture as endpoint, exist for alendronate, risedronate, raloxifene and combined calcium/vitamin D.

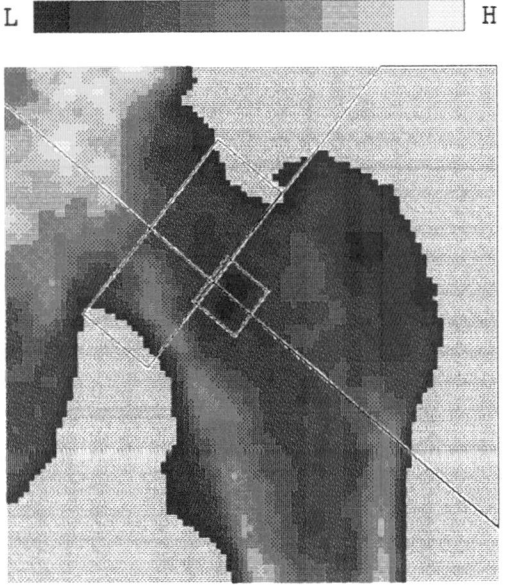

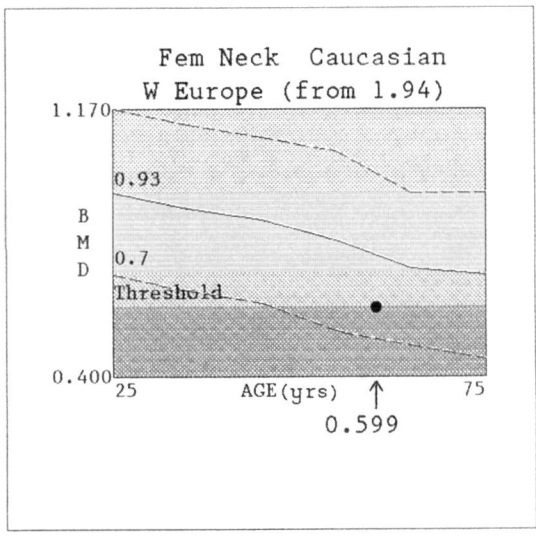

Fig. 10.38 **DXA scan of the left femoral neck in a 60-year-old Caucasian female (height 153.1 cm, weight 59.8 kg) with osteoporosis.** On the right-hand graph the black dot indicates the patient's BMD (0.599), which is below the threshold level. BMD, bone mass density. Courtesy of Wellington Regional Bone Density Service.

Suggested management of osteoporosis*

1. Evaluate all aspects of fracture risk (age, race, family history, mobility, falls).
2. Consider specific guidelines, e.g. for corticosteroid users.
3. Lifestyle advice – exercise, smoking, alcohol, calcium intake.

If previous fracture (vertebral, Colles' or hip): bisphosphonate.

If no previous fracture:

- Premenopausal women and men:
  - Identify and treat cause/contributory factors
  - Bisphosphonate (caution in women in child-bearing years)
- Amenorrhoeic women (e.g. athletes, anorexia) and postmenopausal osteoporosis:
  - If menopausal symptoms, HRT
  - If HRT poorly tolerated or used for > 10 years, and without menopausal symptoms, SERM or bisphosphonate
  - If no menopausal symptoms, bisphosphonate (SERM or calcitriol if not tolerated)
- Older men/women (70+) particularly if in institutional care:
  - Vitamin D and calcium
  - Consider hip protectors.

SERM, selective estrogen receptor modulator. Scott et al (2000). Guidelines for gastrointestinal disease, see p. 299.

* See text and Royal College of Physicians' guidelines (in list of further reading) for discussion.

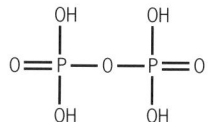

Fig. 10.39 Comparative structures of bisphosphonates and pyrophosphate.

(hip, forearm) in postmenopausal women. If there are also significant menopausal symptoms, it is a good choice. However, HRT needs to be used lifelong for sustained benefit in bone. The balance of benefits (reduced fractures) and adverse effects (on breast, endometrium, thrombosis) is complex. In addition, many women are dissatisfied with breakthrough bleeding, though 'no-bleed' preparations are available.

- *Raloxifene* is the first available selective oestrogen-receptor modulator (SERM) for osteoporosis. It has no stimulatory effect on endometrium but activates oestrogen receptors in bone (i.e. physiologically similar to HRT). It prevents BMD loss at spine and hip in postmenopausal women, though fracture rates were only reduced in the spine. It also reduced the incidence of oestrogen-receptor-positive breast carcinoma by 90% over 3 years. Leg cramps and flushing occur more commonly than with HRT, the risk of thromboembolic complications being comparable.
- *Androgens* should be given to hypogonadal men, though prostatic hypertrophy may sometimes be a limiting factor, and PSA should be normal. (Bisphosphonates are also useful in men.)
- *Combination therapy of calcium with vitamin D* is necessary in the elderly, particularly those in residential care.

Strategies used less commonly
These include:

- *Combination therapies*, particularly of HRT or SERM and a bisphosphonate, are currently being evaluated.
- *Calcitriol* ($1,25\text{-}(OH)_2D_3$) produces improvement in bone density, reducing vertebral and non-vertebral fractures, and may be an option where bisphosphonate and HRT are not tolerated. Serum calcium level must be regularly checked.
- *Calcitonin.* Nasal or subcutaneous calcitonin may be used; vertebral fracture rates may be reduced, though there is no clear evidence of benefit at other sites.
- *Fluoride.* Fluoride has been shown to increase bone density, but there is concern about the quality of the bone formed and it is not currently recommended.
- Parathyroid hormone therapy is being assessed.

Observational data support the use of hormone replacement therapy.

- *Bisphosphonates*, analogues of normal bone pyrophosphate (Fig. 10.39) adhere to hydroxyapatite and inhibit osteoclasts. The amino-bisphosphonates possibly interfere with a mevalonate pathway of prenylation involved in regulating osteoclast function. *Alendronate* increases bone mass at hip and spine, and reduces the incidence of fractures at vertebral, hip and other sites, particularly in women who have already sustained a vertebral fracture. *Risedronate* is broadly similar. The effect of *etidronate* on bone density is similar to that of alendronate, though studies have been underpowered to demonstrate the same degree of reduction in fracture risk. Etidronate is given cyclically, alternating 2 weeks of the drug with 76 days of calcium supplement. The optimal duration of bisphosphonate therapy is unknown, and studies of intermittent therapy are under way. Prolonged suppression of bone turnover may have adverse effects, and it is currently advised to reassess treatment after 3–5 years.
- *Hormone replacement therapy* (HRT) reduces BMD loss and fracture risk at vertebral and other sites

FURTHER READING

Compston JE (ed) (2000) Osteoporosis. *Baillière's Best Practice and Research* **14**(2): 171–329.

Dawson-Hughes B (2001) Bone loss accompanying medical therapies. *New England Journal of Medicine* **345**: 989–991.

Eastell R et al. (1998) UK consensus group management of glucocorticoid induced osteoporosis: an update. *Journal of Internal Medicine* **244**: 271–292.

Royal College of Physicians (2000) *Osteoporosis: Clinical Guidelines for Prevention and Treatment. Update on Pharmacological Interventions and an Algorithm for Management.* London: Royal College of Physicians.

Paget's disease

Osteitis deformans or Paget's disease is a focal disorder of bone remodelling. The initial event of excessive resorption is followed by a compensatory increase in new bone formation, increased local bone blood flow and fibrous tissue in adjacent bone marrow. Ultimately, new bone exceeds resorption but is structurally abnormal.

Epidemiological studies are difficult because most patients are asymptomatic. Most often seen in Europe and particularly in northern England, it affects men and women (2 : 3) over age 40 years. Incidence approximately doubles per decade thereafter, with up to 10% radiologically affected by the age of 90. A positive family history is noted in about 14%.

Aetiology and pathogenesis

A gene predisposing to Paget's disease has been identified on chromosome 18q. Intracellular inclusions in the osteoclasts in a pagetic lesion are believed to be paramyxovirus nucleocapsid (e.g. canine distemper virus, measles or respiratory syncitial virus). However, similar microfilaments are seen in other bone disorders, and theories of a viral aetiology in Paget's remain contentious. Altered expression of *c-fos* (an oncogene) is one suggested mechanism linking viral infection with the pathogenic changes in osteoclasts, which are more numerous and contain an increased number of nuclei (up to 100), and produce increased amounts of IL-6 and TNF-α (promoting resorption) and of osteogenic growth factors. These osteoclasts are also hyper-responsive to $1,25\text{-}(OH)_2D_3$. Increased osteoclastic bone resorption is followed by formation of woven bone. While mineralization is normal, this bone is softer, leading to deformity and increased fracture risk. Unaffected bone remains normal throughout life (i.e. Paget's disease does not spread, but can become symptomatic at previously silent sites).

Clinical features (Fig. 10.40)

Most (60–80%) patients with radiologically identified Paget's disease are entirely asymptomatic. Diagnosis often follows the finding of an asymptomatic elevation of serum alkaline phosphatase, or a plain X-ray performed for other indications. The disease may involve one bone (monostotic, in 15%) or many (polyostotic). The most common sites in order of frequency are pelvis, lumbar spine, femur, thoracic spine, sacrum, skull, tibia.

Symptoms can include:

- bone pain, most often in the spine or the pelvis
- joint pain when an involved bone is close to a joint, leading to cartilage damage and osteoarthritis
- deformities, in particular bowed tibia and skull changes
- complications from:
  (a) nerve compression (deafness from VIIIth cranial nerve; also cranial nerves II, V, VII; spinal stenosis, hydrocephalus)
  (b) increased bone blood flow (myocardial hypertrophy and high-output cardiac failure)
  (c) pathological fractures
- osteogenic sarcoma in pagetic bone (fewer than 1% of cases, but a 30-fold increased risk compared with non-pagetic patients).

Investigations

- **X-ray** features vary from predominantly lytic lesions (osteoporosis circumscripta in the skull is characteristic), through a mixed phase, to a mainly sclerotic phase of bone expansion, thickening of trabeculae and loss of distinction between cortex and trabeculae (dedifferentiation).
- **Bone scans** show the extent of skeletal involvement, but are unable to distinguish between Paget's disease and sclerotic metastatic carcinoma (especially breast and prostate).
- **Increased serum alkaline phosphatase** (may exceed 1000 U/L) with normal serum calcium and phosphate, reflects increased bone turnover. Levels may be normal with limited or monostotic Paget's. Levels are reduced with treatment and are a marker of relapse. Mild hypercalcaemia follows immobilization only when there is very extensive disease.
- **Other markers of bone resorption and formation** (p. 577) are not commonly used in practice, though offering increased sensitivity over serum alkaline phosphatase for diagnosis and assessing response to treatment.

Treatment

Bisphosphonates are the mainstay of treatment. New bone formed after treatment is lamellar, not woven (reflecting a normalization of bone turnover rather than a direct effect on osteoblasts). In addition to treating symptomatic patients (the minority), studies to date indicate that treatment of asymptomatic lesions is appropriate if there is a significant risk of potential complications, e.g. fracture in weight-bearing long bones or the spine,

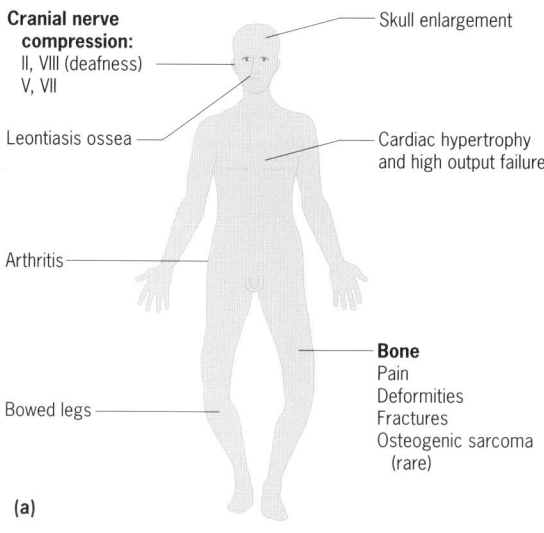

Cranial nerve
compression:
II, VIII (deafness)
V, VII

Skull enlargement

Leontiasis ossea

Cardiac hypertrophy
and high output failure

Arthritis

Bowed legs

Bone
Pain
Deformities
Fractures
Osteogenic sarcoma
(rare)

(a)

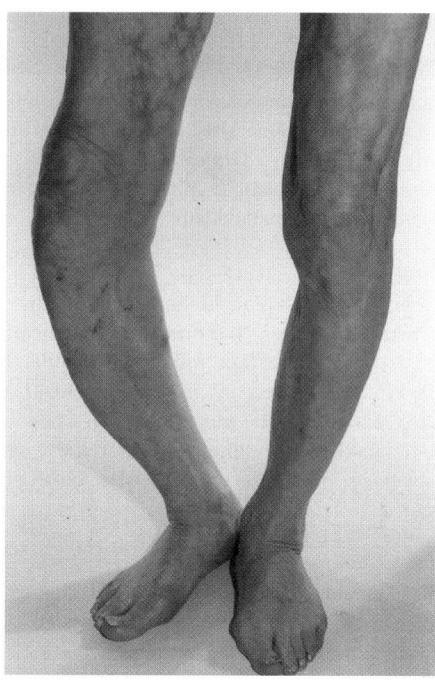

(b)

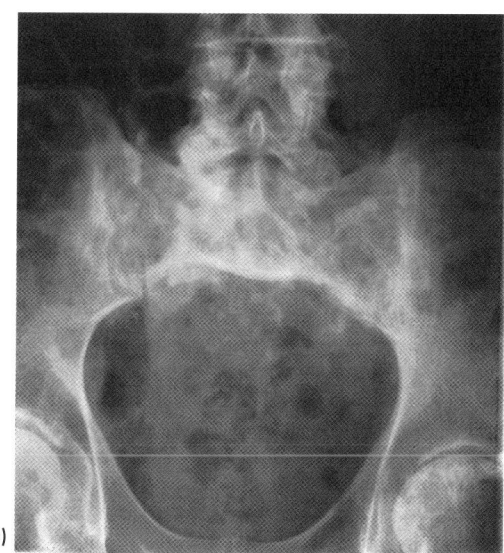

(c)

Fig. 10.40 **Paget's disease.** **(a)** Clinical features. **(b)** The tibia, showing bowing caused by increased bone growth. **(c)** X-ray appearance of the pelvis, showing osteolytic and osteosclerotic lesions.

achieved 50–70% reduction in serum alkaline phosphatase in trials, maintained for up to 18 months in over 80% of patients, it is not currently licensed for this indication. Risedronate (30 mg/day) appears to normalize alkaline phosphatase within 3 months, with long-term efficacy comparable to that of alendronate.

In bisphosphonate resistance, alkaline phosphatase levels fail to fall to the same extent, or rise again more quickly after repeated treatment with the same drug. Changing to a different bisphosphonate is effective in overcoming this unexplained finding.

Surgery

Joint replacement or osteotomy is sometimes necessary to correct deformity or pain due to (secondary) degenerative joint disease. Intra-articular injection of lidocaine (lignocaine) can be useful to differentiate joint or bone disease. Neurosurgery may be required where there is spinal disease. Osteosarcoma usually requires amputation, though wide excision and limb-salvage can be successful at distal sites.

nerve entrapment or deafness with skull involvement, and treatment before orthopaedic procedures in involved bone (to reduce vascularity).

Intravenous bisphosphonates

Intravenous pamidronate (single or repeated infusions – regimens vary considerably) is highly efficacious, but can be associated with a first-dose reaction characterized by 'flu-like' symptoms including a transient pyrexia over 24–48 hours. (Zoledronate and ibandronate offer shorter infusion times and rapid normalization of alkaline phosphatase but the clinical value of this remains to be shown, and these agents are not currently licensed for this indication.)

Oral bisphosphonates

Tiludronate is indicated for the treatment of Paget's disease. While alendronate (40 mg daily for 6 months)

FURTHER READING

Lyles KW et al (2001) A clinical approach to diagnosis and management of Paget's disease of bone. *Journal of Bone and Mineral Research* **16**: 1379–1387.

Rickets and osteomalacia

Rickets (in children) and osteomalacia (in adults) result from inadequate mineralization of bone matrix (osteoid). They are two clinical manifestations of the same disease which is usually caused by a defect in vitamin D availability or metabolism.

Pathology

In children the growth plate is elongated with distortion of the arrangement of chondrocytes. Calcification is delayed and vascularization impaired. In adults, osteomalacia is characterized by increased osteoid width (> 15 µm) and delayed mineralization assessed by double-tetracycline labelling. Unmineralized osteoid may cover up to 100% of trabecular bone surface (normal < 27%).

Aetiology (Table 10.24)

Vitamin D deficiency is usually due to inadequate sunlight exposure (Fig. 10.35), particularly in Asian women in Western countries whose clothing covers their skin, and whose diet may contain only small amounts of vitamin D. The elderly who are immobile and housebound similarly are not exposed to sunlight. Anticonvulsant therapy may affect vitamin D metabolism; these drugs are also toxic to osteoblasts. Malabsorption of vitamin D rarely occurs in gastrointestinal disease.

Chronic renal failure results in reduced 1α-hydroxylation of 25-(OH)D$_3$. Mutations in the *p450c1* α gene (chromosome 12) cause 1α-hydroxylase deficiency, also known as *vitamin D-dependent rickets type I*, an autosomal recessive disease. In *type II vitamin D-dependent rickets* there is a defect in the intracellular 1,25-(OH)$_2$D$_3$ receptor. X-linked hypophosphataemic rickets resulting in lower-limb deformities and stunted growth rate in

affected males is caused by mutations in the *PEX* gene (see Ch. 12). In the Fanconi syndrome and in renal tubular acidosis, osteomalacia can develop, mainly because of the continuous phosphaturia.

Osteomalacia has been associated with many mesenchymal tumours which are believed to produce a humoral factor 'phosphatonin' which increases phosphate excretion. Treatment of the tumour results in remineralization.

Clinical features

Adult osteomalacia may produce vague symptoms of bone or muscle pain and tenderness. Fractures are rare and usually asymptomatic. Occasionally a marked proximal myopathy leads to a characteristic 'waddling' gait. Deformity is uncommon. In modern practice many cases are detected biochemically in high-risk patients, especially those with gastrointestinal disease or surgery, before clear symptoms are present. Occasionally, tetany or other hypocalcaemic features may occur.

At birth, neonatal rickets may present as craniotabes (thin deformed skull). In the first few years of life there may be widened epiphyses at the wrists and beading at the costochondral junctions, producing the 'rickety rosary', or a groove in the rib cage (Harrison's sulcus). In older children, lower limb deformities are seen. A myopathy also occurs.

Investigations

- **Increased serum alkaline phosphatase**, indicating increased osteoblast activity, is the most common abnormality (note: alkaline phosphatase is elevated during skeletal growth).
- **Plasma calcium** is low or normal, in association with secondary hyperparathyroidism and a raised PTH.
- **Serum phosphate** may be low, owing to increased PTH-dependent phosphaturia, though this is variable.
- **Serum 25-hydroxyvitamin D$_3$** is usually low (exceptions being vitamin-D-resistant rickets).
- **X-rays** are often normal in adults, but may show defective mineralization, especially in the pelvis, long bones and ribs, with 'Looser's zones' – linear areas of low density surrounded by sclerotic borders.
- **Iliac crest biopsy** with double tetracycline labelling (see above) is occasionally necessary if biochemical tests are equivocal.

Treatment

Treatment should be directed towards correction of the cause where possible, with increase in dietary vitamin D intake and sunlight exposure.

Multiple formulations of vitamin D and its metabolites are available. When deficiency is nutritional, 'replacement' doses are needed (400–800 IU daily). Much higher 'pharmacological' doses (up to 40 000–100 000 IU) may be needed in patients with gastrectomy, malabsorp-

---

Table 10.24
Causes of rickets and osteomalacia

Vitamin D deficiency
Inadequate synthesis in skin
Low dietary intake
Malabsorption
    Coeliac disease
    Intestinal resection
    Chronic cholestasis, e.g. primary biliary cirrhosis

Renal disease
Chronic renal failure
Renal osteodystrophy
Bone disease due to dialysis
Tubular disorders, e.g. renal tubular acidosis, Fanconi's syndrome

Miscellaneous
Multiple myeloma
Vitamin-D-dependent rickets types I and II
X-linked hypophosphataemia (vitamin-D-resistant rickets)
Mesenchymal tumours

tion, liver disease or hypoparathyroidism. However, some patients respond to more conventional doses. Experts should initiate such treatment and all patients receiving pharmacological doses of vitamin D should have their serum calcium measured regularly; excessive dosage presents with the features of hypercalcaemia, often with nausea and vomiting.

Prevention

Health education to ensure a balanced diet, adequate exposure to sunlight and, where appropriate in high-risk individuals or communities, dietary vitamin D supplementation are all important aspects of prevention.

Skeletal dysplasias

These include a large group of heterogeneous disorders of bone and connective tissue.

Collagen defects

Collagen is responsible for many of the structural, tensile and load-bearing properties in the various tissues where it is found. The structure of collagen is discussed on page 512. Twenty-eight dispersed genes encode for more than 16 different types of collagen:

- The fibrillar collagens, e.g. types I, II, III, V and XI, are encoded by COL1A1–2, COL2A1, COL3, COL5, COL11. Mutations of these genes produce osteogenesis imperfecta and Ehlers–Danlos syndrome.
- Basement membrane collagen, type IV, is encoded by COL4A1–5. Mutations lead to Alport's disease (see p. 607).
- Fibril-associated collagens with interrupted triple helices (FACIT), e.g. types IX, XII and XIV, are encoded by COL9, COL12.
- Filament producing collagen type VI is encoded by COL6A1, 2, 3.
- Network-forming collagens types VIII and X are encoded by COL8A1, COL10A1.
- Anchoring fibril collagen, e.g. type VII, is encoded by COL7A1. Mutations of this gene produce epidermolysis bullosa (p. 1304).

Ehlers–Danlos syndrome

This is a heterogeneous group of disorders of collagen. Ten different types have been recognized with varying degrees of skin fragility, skin hyperextensibility and joint hypermobility. Types I, II and III are inherited in an autosomal dominant fashion; the biochemical basis is unknown. No abnormalities in COL1A1, COL1A2 and COL2A1 genes have been found.

Type IV is also autosomal dominant and involves arteries, the bowel and uterus, as well as the skin. Mutations in COL3A1 gene produce abnormalities in structure, synthesis or secretion of type III collagen.

Type VI is a recessively inherited disorder and results from a mutation in the gene that encodes lysyl hydroxylase.

Type VII is an autosomal dominant disorder where there is a defect in the conversion of procollagen to collagen; COL1A1 and COL1A2 mutations delete the N-proteinase cleavage sites.

Other forms of Ehlers–Danlos are very rare and their defects have not been elucidated. The clinical features are described on page 1311.

Osteogenesis imperfecta (fragilitas ossium, brittle bone syndrome)

This is a heterogeneous group of mainly autosomally dominant inherited disorders. In the majority there are mutations in the genes encoding the chains in type I collagen, i.e. COL1A1, COL1A2. There are four types, distinguished by the very variable clinical pictures ranging from death in the perinatal period (type II), severe bone deformity (type III), to a normal lifespan (types I and IV).

The major clinical feature is very fragile and brittle bones but other collagen-containing tissues are also involved, such as tendons, the skin and the eyes. Osteogenesis imperfecta tarda (type I) has mild bony deformities, blue sclerae, defective dentine, early-onset deafness, hypermobility of joints, and heart valve disorders. More severe forms present with multiple fractures and gross deformities. Prognosis is variable, depending on the severity of the disease.

Osteochondrodysplasia

There are over 150 variants some, but not all, due to mutations in the COL2A1 gene that encodes type II collagen. Many types have not yet been clearly identified. All show abnormalities of the vitreous humour of the eye and abnormalities of articular cartilage, both of which have abundant type II collagen.

Miscellaneous defects

Osteopetrosis (marble bone disease)

This condition may be inherited in either an autosomal dominant or an autosomal recessive manner; the recessive type is severe and the dominant type is mild. In addition, another recessive form associated with renal tubular acidosis is due to carbonic anhydrase II deficiency.

In the severe form, bone density is increased throughout the skeleton but bones tend to fracture easily. Involvement of the bone marrow leads to a leuco-erythroblastic anaemia. There is mental retardation and early death.

In the mild form there may be only X-ray changes, but fractures and infection can occur. The acid phosphate level is raised.

Marfan syndrome

This is described on page 803.

585

Fibroblast growth factor receptor defect

Achondroplasia ('dwarfism') is diagnosed in the first years of life. The disease is inherited in an autosomal dominant manner and is caused by a defect in the fibroblast growth factor receptor-3 gene. The trunk is of normal length but the limbs are very short and broad. The vault of the skull is enlarged, the face is small and the nose bridge is flat. Intelligence is normal.

FURTHER READING

Favus MJ (ed.) (2000) *Primer on the Metabolic Bone Diseases and Disorders of Mineral Metabolism*, 4th edn. Philadelphia: Lippincott Raven, American Society for Bone and Mineral Research.

Scriver CR, Beaudet AL, Sly WS, Valle D (2000). *The Metabolic Basis of Inherited Disease*, 8th edn. New York: McGraw Hill.

Anatomy

The kidneys are paired organs, 11–14 cm in length in adults (approximately equivalent to the length of three vertebral bodies), 5–6 cm in width and 3–4 cm in depth. Each kidney weighs approximately 150 g. The kidneys lie retroperitoneally on either side of the vertebral column at the level of T12 to L3. The right kidney lies approximately 1.5 cm lower than the left owing to the presence of the liver. Each kidney moves about 3 cm downwards on inspiration and upwards on expiration. The renal parenchyma comprises an outer cortex and an inner medulla. The functional unit of the kidney is the nephron of which each contains about one million. Each nephron is made up of a glomerulus, proximal tubule, loop of Henle, distal tubule and collecting duct.

The renal capsule and ureters are innervated via T10–12 and L1 nerve roots and renal pain is felt over the corresponding dermatomes.

Arterial blood is supplied to the kidneys via the renal arteries, which branch off the abdominal aorta, and venous blood is conveyed to the inferior vena cava via the renal veins. Approximately 25% of humans possess dual or multiple renal arteries on one or both sides. The left renal vein is longer than the right and for this reason the left kidney, where possible, is usually chosen for live donor transplant nephrectomy. The renal artery undergoes a series of divisions within the kidney forming successively the interlobar arteries, which run radially to the corticomedullary junction, arcuate arteries, which run circumferentially along the corticomedullary junction, and interlobular arteries which run radially through the renal cortex towards the surface of the kidney. Afferent glomerular arterioles arise from the interlobular arteries to supply the glomerular capillary bed, which drains into efferent glomerular arterioles. Efferent arterioles from the outer cortical glomeruli drain into a peritubular capillary network within the renal cortex and thence into increasingly large and more proximal branches of the renal vein. By contrast, blood from the juxtamedullary glomeruli passes via the vasa recta in the medulla and then turns back towards the area of the cortex from which the vasa recta originated. Vasa recta possess fenestrated walls, which facilitates movement of diffusible substances. The collecting ducts merge in the inner medulla to form the ducts of Bellini, which empty at the apices of the papillae into the calyces. The calyces, in common with the renal pelvis, ureter and bladder are lined with transitional cell epithelium.

The glomerulus comprises three main cell types: (1) endothelial cells which are fenestrated with 500–1000 Å pores; (2) epithelial cells, visceral and parietal; (3) mesangial cells. Mesangial cells are believed to be related to macrophages of the reticuloendothelial system and have a phagocytic function. They also secrete the mesangial matrix of the glomerulus. The glomerular capillary basement membrane lies between the endothelial and the visceral epithelial cells. The latter put out multiple long foot processes (podocytes) which interdigitate with those of adjacent epithelial cells. Together the endothelial cells, basement membrane and epithelial cells form the filtration barrier or sieve.

The renal tubules are lined by epithelial cells, which are cuboidal except in the thin limb of the loop of Henle where they are flat. Proximal tubular cells differ from other cells of the system in possession of a luminal brush border. The cortical portion of the collecting tubules contains two cell types with different functions, namely principal cells and intercalated cells (see p. 691). Fibroblast-like cells in the renal cortical interstitium have been identified and shown to produce erythropoietin in response to hypoxia.

The juxtaglomerular apparatus comprises the macula densa, the extraglomerular mesangial mesangium and the terminal portion of the afferent glomerular arteriole (which contains renin-producing granular cells) together with the proximal portion of the efferent arteriole. The macula densa is a plaque of cells containing large, tightly packed cell nuclei (hence the name macula densa) within the thick ascending limb of the loop of Henle. This anatomical arrangement is such as to allow changes in the renal tubule to influence behaviour of the adjacent glomerulus.

Renal function (see also Ch. 12)

The kidneys' principal role is the elimination of waste material and the regulation of the volume and composition of body fluid (Table 11.1). The kidneys have a unique system involving the free ultrafiltration of water and non-protein-bound low-molecular-weight compounds from the plasma and the selective reabsorption and/or excretion of these as the ultrafiltrate passes along the tubule.

A conventional diagrammatic representation of the nephron is shown in Figure 11.1a and a physiological version in Figure 11.1b.

An essential feature of renal function is that a large volume of blood – 25% of cardiac output or approximately 1300 mL per minute – passes through the two million glomeruli.

A hydrostatic pressure gradient of approximately 10 mmHg (a capillary pressure of 45 mmHg minus 10 mmHg of pressure within Bowman's space and 25 mmHg of plasma oncotic pressure) provides the driving force for ultrafiltration of virtually protein-free and fat-free fluid across the glomerular capillary wall into Bowman's space and so into the renal tubule (Fig. 11.2).

The ultrafiltration rate (glomerular filtration rate; GFR) varies with age and sex but is approximately 120–130 mL/min per 1.73 m² surface area in adults. This means that each day ultrafiltration of 170–180 L of water and unbound small-molecular-weight constituents of blood occurs. The 'need' for this high filtration rate relates to the elimination of compounds present in relatively low concentration in plasma (e.g. urea). If these large volumes of ultrafiltrate were excreted unchanged as urine, it would be necessary to ingest huge amounts of water and electrolytes to stay in balance. This is avoided by the selective reabsorption of water, essential electrolytes and other blood constituents, such as glucose and amino acids, from the filtrate in transit along the nephron. Thus, 60–80% of filtered water and sodium are reabsorbed in the proximal tubule along with virtually all the potassium, bicarbonate, glucose and amino acids (Fig. 11.1b). Further water and sodium chloride are reabsorbed more distally, and fine tuning of salt and water balance is achieved in the distal and collecting tubules under the influence of aldosterone and antidiuretic hormone (ADH). The final urine volume is thus 1–2 L daily. Calcium, phosphate and magnesium are also selectively reabsorbed in proportion to the need to maintain a normal electrolyte composition of body fluids.

The urinary excretion of some compounds is more complicated. For example, potassium is freely filtered at the glomerulus, almost completely absorbed in the proximal tubule, and excreted in the distal tubule and collecting ducts. An important clinical consequence of this is that the ability to eliminate unwanted potassium is less dependent on GFR than is the elimination of urea or creatinine. Other compounds filtered and reabsorbed or excreted to a variable extent include urate and many organic acids, including many drugs or their metabolic breakdown products. The more tubular secretion of a compound occurs, the less dependent is elimination on the GFR; penicillin and cefradine are examples of compounds secreted by the tubules.

Table 11.1
Functions of the kidney

Excretory
Excretion of waste products, drugs

Regulatory
Control of body fluid volume and composition

Endocrine
Production of erythropoietin, renin, prostaglandins, endothelins

Metabolic
Metabolism of vitamin D, small-molecular-weight proteins

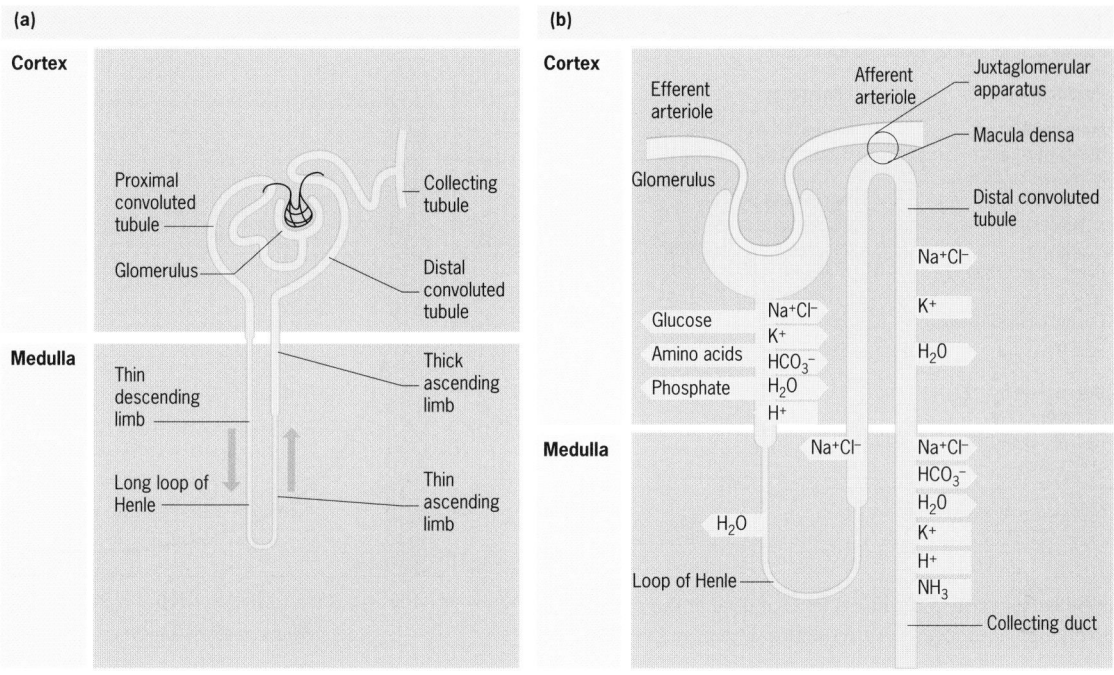

Fig. 11.1 (a) Principal parts of the nephron. (b) Sites of removal or addition of electrolytes from or into tubular fluid.
Note: The descending limb is permeable to water and impermeable to sodium, whereas in the ascending limb the permeabilities are reversed.

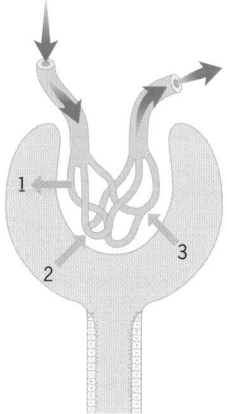

Fig. 11.2 Pressures controlling glomerular filtration.
1, capillary hydrostatic pressure (45 mmHg); **2**, hydrostatic pressure in Bowman's space (10 mmHg); **3**, plasma protein oncotic pressure (25 mmHg). Arrows (1, 2, 3) indicate the direction of a pressure gradient.

Urine concentration and the countercurrent system

Urine is concentrated by a complex interaction between the loops of Henle, the medullary interstitium, medullary blood vessels (vasa recta) and the collecting tubules (see p. 668). The proposed mechanism of urine concentration is termed 'the countercurrent mechanism'. The countercurrent hypothesis states that a small difference in osmotic concentration at any point between fluid flowing

in opposite directions in two parallel tubes connected in a hairpin manner is multiplied many times along the length of the tubes. Tubular fluid moves from the renal cortex towards the papillary tip of the medulla via the proximal straight tubule and the thin descending limb of the loop of Henle which is permeable to water and impermeable to sodium. The tubule then loops back towards the cortex so that the direction of the fluid movement is reversed in the ascending limb, which is impermeable to water but permeable to sodium. This results in a large osmolar concentration difference between the corticomedullary junction and the hairpin loop at the tip of the papilla, and hence countercurrent multiplication. There is an analogy with heat exchangers.

Acid–base balance

Tubular function is also critical to the control of acid–base balance. Thus, filtered bicarbonate is largely reabsorbed and hydrogen ions are excreted mainly buffered by phosphate (see p. 691).

Glomerular filtration rate

In health the GFR remains remarkably constant owing to intrarenal regulatory mechanisms. In disease, with a reduction in intrarenal blood flow, damage to or loss of glomeruli, or obstruction to the free flow of ultrafiltrate along the tubule, the GFR will fall and the ability to eliminate waste material and to regulate the volume and composition of body fluid will decline. This will be

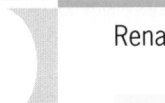

Table 11.2
Factors influencing serum urea levels

Production	Elimination
Increased by	**Increased by**
High-protein diet	Elevated GFR, e.g. pregnancy
Increased catabolism	
Surgery	**Decreased by**
Infection	Glomerular disease
Trauma	Reduced renal blood flow
Corticosteroid therapy	Hypotension
Tetracyclines	Dehydration
Gastrointestinal bleeding	Urinary obstruction
Cancer	Tubulointerstitial nephritis
Decreased by	
Low-protein diet	
Reduced catabolism, e.g. old age	
Liver failure	

GFR, glomerular filtration rate

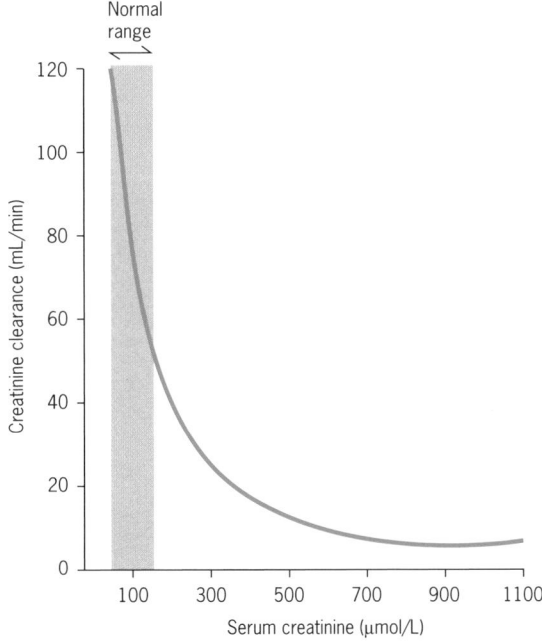

Fig. 11.3 **Creatinine clearance versus serum creatinine.**
Note that the serum creatinine does not rise above the normal range until there is a reduction of 50–60% in the glomerular filtration rate (creatinine clearance).

manifest as a rise in the blood level of urea or the plasma level of creatinine and in a reduction in measured GFR.

Uraemia

The concentration of urea or creatinine in blood or plasma represents the dynamic equilibrium between production and elimination. In healthy subjects there is an enormous reserve of renal excretory function, and serum urea and creatinine do not rise above the normal range until there is a reduction of 50–60% in the GFR. Thereafter, the level of urea depends both on the GFR and the production rate (Table 11.2). The latter is heavily influenced by protein intake and tissue catabolism. The level of creatinine is much less dependent on diet but is more related to age, sex and muscle mass. Once it is elevated, serum creatinine is a better guide to GFR than urea and, in general, measurement of serum creatinine is a good way to monitor further deterioration in the GFR.

It must be re-emphasized that a normal serum urea or creatinine is not synonymous with a normal GFR.

Measurement of the glomerular filtration rate

Measurement of the GFR is necessary to define the exact level of renal function. It is essential when the serum (plasma) urea or creatinine is within the normal range.

Inulin clearance – the gold standard of physiologists – is not practical or necessary in clinical practice. The most widely used measurement is the creatinine clearance (Fig. 11.3).

The use of creatinine clearance is dependent on the fact that daily production of creatinine (principally from muscle cells) is remarkably constant and little affected by protein intake. Serum creatinine and urinary output thus vary very little throughout the day. This permits the use of 24-hour urine collections, which reduce collection errors, and the measurement of a single serum creatinine value during the 24 hours (Practical box 11.1).

✚ *Practical box 11.1*

To obtain a timed 24-hour urine collection and to measure creatinine clearance

1 Empty the bladder at the beginning of the collection period. Discard the urine. Note the time.

2 Collect *all* urine passed (including overnight) during the subsequent 24 hours.

3 Exactly 24 hours after commencement of collection, empty the bladder. Urine thus voided is to be included in collection.

Measurement of creatinine clearance

● Urine is collected over 24 hours for measurement of urinary creatinine; a 24-hour collection diminishes collection errors.

● A plasma level of creatinine is measured sometime during the 24-hour period.

● Given the rate of urine flow (*V*), the urine (*U*) and plasma (*P*) concentrations of creatinine, clearance is obtained from the formula:

$$\frac{U \times V}{P} \times 100$$

where *U* and *P* are measured in mmol/L, and *V* is measured in mL per minute.

● Normal ranges: men 90–140 mL/min, women 80–125 mL/min.

Creatinine excretion is, however, by both glomerular filtration and tubular secretion, although at normal serum levels the latter is relatively small. As most laboratory methods for measurement of serum creatinine give slight overestimates, the calculation of clearance fortuitously gives a value close to that of inulin.

With progressive renal failure, creatinine clearance may overestimate GFR but, in clinical practice, this is seldom important. Certain drugs – for example cimetidine, trimethoprim, spironolactone and amiloride – reduce tubular secretion of creatinine, leading to a rise in serum creatinine and a fall in measured clearance.

Given these observations, creatinine clearance, nevertheless, is a reasonably accurate measure of GFR in those situations in which it is most required – normal or near normal renal function.

Where urine collections are difficult (e.g. with ileal conduits) or deemed inaccurate, the GFR may be measured by the single injection of compounds such as [^{51}Cr]EDTA (ethylenediaminetetraacetic acid), [^{99m}Tc]DTPA (diethylenetriaminepentaacetic acid) or [^{125}I]iothalamate, their excretion being primarily by glomerular filtration. Following intravenous injection of the compound, three blood samples are obtained at 2, 3 and 4 hours (or rather longer intervals if the patient is oedematous or if renal failure is suspected). The GFR may then be calculated from the slope of the exponential fall in blood level of the compound.

Urea clearance is not an accurate measure of GFR, particularly when urine flow rate is low, and should not be used as a measure of GFR.

Tubular function

The major function of the tubule is the selective reabsorption or excretion of water and various cations and anions to keep the volume and electrolyte composition of body fluid normal (see Ch. 12).

The active reabsorption from the glomerular filtrate of compounds such as glucose and amino acids also takes place. Within the normal range of blood concentrations these substances are completely reabsorbed by the proximal tubule. However, if blood levels are elevated above the normal range, the amount filtered (filtered load = GFR × plasma concentration) may exceed the maximal absorptive capacity of the tubule and the compound 'spills over' into the urine. Examples of this occur with hyperglycaemia in diabetes mellitus or elevated plasma phenylalanine in phenylketonuria.

Conversely, inherited or acquired defects in tubular function may lead to incomplete absorption of a normal filtered load, with loss of the compound in the urine (a lowered 'renal threshold'). This is seen in renal glycosuria, in which there is a genetically determined defect in tubular reabsorption of glucose. It is diagnosed by demonstrating glycosuria in the presence of normal blood glucose levels. Inherited or acquired defects in the tubular reabsorption of amino acids, phosphate, sodium, potassium and calcium also occur, either singly or in combination. Examples include cystinuria and the Fanconi syndrome (see p. 1116). Tubular defects in the reabsorption of water result in nephrogenic diabetes insipidus. Under normal circumstances, antidiuretic hormone induces an increase in the permeability of water in the collecting tubules by attachment to receptors with subsequent activation of adenyl cyclase. This then activates a protein kinase, which induces preformed cytoplasmic vesicles containing water channels (termed 'aquaporins') to move to and insert into the tubular luminal membrane. This allows water entry into tubular cells down a favourable osmotic gradient. Water then crosses the basolateral membrane and enters the bloodstream. When the effect of ADH wears off, water channels return to the cell cytoplasm.

Investigation of tubular function in clinical practice
Proximal tubular function

Five tests of proximal tubular function are employed in clinical practice:

- *Hypokalaemia* in the face of a normal or increased urinary potassium excretion (> 40 mmol in 24 hours) is indicative of proximal tubular failure of potassium reabsorption. Other explanations such as treatment with thiazide diuretics or hyperaldosteronism must be ruled out.
- *Hypophosphataemia* is attributed to a proximal tubular abnormality provided alternative explanations, such as the use of gut phosphorus binders and primary hyperparathyroidism, can be ruled out.
- *Glycosuria* in the absence of hyperglycaemia.
- *Generalized aminoaciduria.*
- *Proteins derived from tubular cells*, such as β$_2$-microglobulin, are reabsorbed in the proximal nephron. If proteinuria is present, and urine electrophoresis shows the characteristic 'tubular' as distinct from 'glomerular' pattern (i.e. albumin), a proximal tubular defect is demonstrated.

Distal tubular function

Two tests of distal tubular function are commonly applied in clinical practice: measurement of urinary concentrating capacity in response to water deprivation, and measurement of urinary acidification. These tests are dealt with on pages 695 and 1058.

Endocrine function

Renin–angiotensin system (see also p. 1064)
The juxtaglomerular apparatus is made up of specialized arteriolar smooth muscle cells that are sited on the

afferent glomerular arteriole as it enters the glomerulus (see Fig. 11.1b). These cells secrete renin, which converts angiotensinogen in blood to angiotensin I. Renin release is controlled by:

- pressure changes in the afferent arteriole
- sympathetic tone
- chloride and osmotic concentration in the distal tubule via the macula densa (Fig. 11.1b)
- local prostaglandin release.

Angiotensin II is generated from angiotensin I by angiotensin-converting enzyme (ACE). Angiotensin II is both a vasoconstrictor and the most important stimulus for the release of aldosterone by the adrenal cortex. It also modifies intrarenal blood flow (see p. 669).

Endothelins

The endothelins ET-1, ET-2 and ET-3 are a family of potent vasoactive peptides that also influence cell proliferation and epithelial solute transport. They do not circulate but act locally. The genes for two of the receptors ET_A and ET_B have been cloned. The vascular actions are mediated by both these receptors, whilst the tubular transport and interstitial proliferative actions are mediated by ET_B. Intrarenal levels of ET-1 are raised in acute and chronic renal disease.

Erythropoietin (see also p. 407)

Erythropoietin is a glycoprotein produced principally by fibroblast-like cells in the renal interstitium and is the major stimulus for erythropoiesis. Loss of renal substance, with decreased erythropoietin production, results in a normochromic, normocytic anaemia. Conversely, erythropoietin secretion may be increased, with resultant polycythaemia, in patients with polycystic renal disease, benign renal cysts or renal cell carcinoma.

Recombinant human erythropoietin has been biosynthesized and is available for clinical use, particularly in patients with renal failure (see p. 650).

Prostaglandins

Prostaglandins are unsaturated fatty acid compounds synthesized from cell membrane phospholipids (see Fig. 14.32). They exert their main effects in close proximity to the site of production. The main prostaglandins synthesized in the kidney are PGE_2 (the main renal medullary prostaglandin), PGF_2, PGD_2, prostacyclin (PGI_2, the main renal cortical prostaglandin) and thromboxane A_2.

Prostaglandins are important in the maintenance of renal blood flow and glomerular filtration rate in the face of reductions induced by vasoconstrictor stimuli such as angiotensin II, catecholamines and α-adrenergic stimulation. In the presence of renal underperfusion, inhibition of prostaglandin synthesis by non-steroidal anti-inflammatory drugs results in a further reduction in GFR, sometimes sufficiently severe as to cause acute renal failure. Renal prostaglandins also have a natriuretic renal tubular effect and antagonize the action of antidiuretic hormone. Renal prostaglandins do not regulate salt and water excretion in normal subjects, but in some circumstances, such as chronic renal failure, prostaglandin-induced vasodilatation is important in maintaining renal blood flow. Patients with chronic renal failure are thus vulnerable to further deterioration in renal function on exposure to non-steroidal anti-inflammatory drugs, as are elderly patients in many of whom renal function is compromised by renal vascular disease and/or the effects of ageing upon the kidney.

Kallikrein–kinin system

The role of this system is not fully understood but it too probably plays a part in the control of the distribution of renal blood flow and in salt and water excretion.

The natriuretic-peptide family (see also p. 1065)

Atrial natriuretic peptide (ANP) mRNA has been found in many tissues, but most abundantly in the cardiac atria. Two other peptides derived from different precursor molecules encoded by different genes have been isolated. These are brain natriuretic peptide (BNP) and C-natriuretic peptide (CNP). Confusingly, BNP is found in highest concentration in myocardial tissue, whereas CNP is found predominantly in the brain. ANP and BNP have mainly natriuretic and vasorelaxant properties, whereas CNP is not natriuretic. Natriuretic peptide receptors have been cloned for each of the peptides. Natriuretic peptides are cleaved by the enzyme neutral endopeptidase, although this is not the only mechanism of clearance. The affinity of the enzyme for BNP is much less than that for ANP and CNP.

Collectively, natriuretic peptides counterbalance the effects of the renin–angiotensin–aldosterone system. In response to volume expansion and pressure overload of the heart, plasma ANP and BNP concentrations increase, and one or both of them antagonize the effects of angiotensin II on the vascular tone, aldosterone secretion, renal tubular sodium reabsorption and vascular cell growth. Intravenous infusion of ANP is followed by a marked natriuresis with a rise in glomerular filtration rate and a fall in blood pressure. Concentrations are elevated in heart failure and renal failure, and a possible therapeutic role for these actions in such conditions has been explored. Currently, interest focuses mainly on the use of neutral endopeptidase inhibitors in the promotion of a salt and water diuresis. Plasma CNP concentrations change little with cardiac overload, and the main role of this peptide appears to be the regulation of vascular tone.

Vitamin D metabolism (see also p. 576)

Naturally occurring vitamin D requires hydroxylation in the liver and again by a 1α-hydroxylase enzyme in the kidney to produce the powerfully metabolically active 1,25-dihydroxycholecalciferol (1,25-$(OH)_2D_3$). Reduced 1α-hydroxylase activity in diseased kidneys results in relative deficiency of 1,25-$(OH)_2D_3$. As a result, gastrointestinal calcium absorption is reduced and bone mineralization impaired. Receptors for 1,25-$(OH)_2D_3$ exist in the parathyroid glands and reduced occupancy of the receptors by the vitamin alters the set-point for release of parathyroid hormone (PTH) in response to a given decrement in plasma calcium concentration. Gut calcium malabsorption, which induces a tendency to hypocalcaemia, and relative lack of 1,25-$(OH)_2D_3$, contribute therefore to the hyperparathyroidism seen regularly in patients with renal impairment, even of modest degree.

Protein and polypeptide metabolism

The kidney is a major site for the catabolism of many small-molecular-weight proteins and polypeptides, including many hormones such as insulin, PTH and calcitonin. In renal failure the metabolic clearance of these substances is reduced and their half-life is prolonged. This accounts, for example, for the reduced insulin requirements of diabetic patients as their renal function declines.

FURTHER READING

Hendry BM, James AF (1997) Endothelin antagonists in renal disease. *Lancet* **350**: 381–382.

Wilkins MR, Redondo J, Brown LA (1997) The natriuretic-peptide family. *Lancet* **349**: 1307–1311.

Tests for renal disease or malfunction

Renal disease is suspected if there are:

- symptoms referable to the urinary tract
- hypertension
- an elevated serum urea or creatinine concentration
- abnormalities on urinalysis.

The urine

Appearance

This is of little value in the differential diagnosis of renal disease except in the diagnosis of haematuria. Overt 'bloody' urine is usually unmistakable but should be checked using dipsticks (Stix testing). Very concentrated urine may also appear dark or smoky. Other causes of discoloration of urine include cholestatic jaundice, haemoglobinuria, drugs such as rifampicin, use of fluorescein or methylthioninium chloride (methylene blue), and ingestion of beetroot. Discoloration of urine after standing for some time occurs in porphyria, alkaptonuria and in patients ingesting the drug L-dopa. In patients with frequency or dysuria the passage of crystal-clear urine usually indicates that significant bacteriuria is absent.

Volume

In health, the volume of urine passed is primarily determined by diet and fluid intake. In temperate climates it lies within the range 800–2500 mL per 24 hours. The minimum amount passed to stay in fluid balance is determined by the amount of solute – mainly urea and electrolytes – being excreted and the maximum concentrating power of the kidneys. On a normal diet, some 800 mOsm of solute are passed daily. Since the maximum urine concentration is approximately 1200 mOsm/kg, the minimum volume of urine obligated by excretion of 800 mOsm of solute would thus be approximately 650 mL (Table 11.3). Fluid intake is generally greater than this, so that larger volumes of more dilute urine are passed. A diet rich in carbohydrate and fat and low in protein and salt results in a lower solute excretion and as little as 300 mL of urine per day may be required. Conversely, a high-salt, high-protein intake obligates a larger urine flow and, via the thirst mechanism, a higher fluid intake. The appropriateness of a given daily urine output must therefore be related to factors such as diet, body size and fluid intake.

In disease, impairment of concentrating ability requires increased volumes of urine to be passed, given the same daily solute output (Table 11.3). An increased solute output, such as in glycosuria or increased protein

Table 11.3
Relationship between diet, kidney function and urine volume

Diet	Approximate solute output (mOsmol per 24 h)	Minimum urine volume required to excrete solute load (mL per 24 h)	
		With normal urine concentration (maximum 1200 mOsm/kg)	In disease (impaired urine concentration – maximum 300 mOsm/kg)
Normal	800	667	2667
High-protein/salt	1200	1000	4000
Low-protein/salt	360	300	1200

catabolism following surgery or associated with sepsis, also demands increased urine volumes.

The maximum urine output depends on the ability to produce a dilute urine. Intakes of 10 or even 20 L daily can be tolerated by normal humans but, given a daily solute output of 800 mOsm, require the ability to dilute to 80 and 40 mOsm/kg, respectively. Where diluting ability is impaired, the ability to excrete large volumes of ingested water is also impaired.

Oliguria

Oliguria, usually defined as the excretion of less than 300 mL of urine per day, may be 'physiological', as in patients with hypotension and hypovolaemia, where urine is maximally concentrated in an attempt to conserve water. More often, it is due to intrinsic renal disease or obstructive nephropathy (see p. 632).

Anuria (no urine) suggests urinary tract obstruction until proved otherwise; bladder outflow obstruction must always be considered first.

Polyuria

Polyuria is a persistent, large increase in urine output, usually associated with nocturia. It must be distinguished from frequency of micturition with the passage of small volumes of urine. Documentation of fluid intake and output may be necessary. Polyuria is the result of an excessive (hysterical) intake of water, an increased excretion of solute (as in hyperglycaemia and glycosuria), or a defective renal concentrating ability or failure of production of ADH.

Specific gravity and osmolality

Urine specific gravity is a measure of the weight of dissolved particles in urine, whereas urine osmolality reflects the number of such particles. Usually the relationship between the two is close. An exception exists when a relatively small number of relatively large particles are present in urine, such as in multiple myeloma. Measurement of urine specific gravity or osmolality is required only under limited circumstances, such as the differential diagnosis of oliguric renal failure or the investigation of polyuria or inappropriate ADH secretion.

Urinary pH

Measurement of urinary pH is unnecessary except in the investigation and treatment of renal tubular acidosis (see p. 695).

Chemical (Stix) testing

Routine Stix testing of urine for blood, protein and sugar is obligatory in all patients suspected of having renal disease.

Blood

Haematuria may be overt, with bloody urine, or microscopic and found only on chemical testing. Currently used Stix tests for blood are very sensitive, being positive if two or more red cells are visible under the high-power field of a light microscope. Indeed, the test is too sensitive, sometimes giving positive results in normal individuals. A further disadvantage is that Stix testing cannot distinguish between blood and free haemoglobin. A positive Stix test must always be followed by microscopy of fresh urine to confirm the presence of red cells and so exclude the relatively rare conditions of haemoglobinuria or myoglobinuria. In females with a positive Stix test result for blood, it is essential to enquire whether the patient is menstruating. Bleeding may come from any site within the urinary tract (Fig. 11.4):

- *Overt bleeding from the urethra* is suggested when blood is seen at the start of voiding and then the urine becomes clear.
- *Blood diffusely present* throughout the urine comes from the bladder or above.
- *Blood only at the end of micturition* suggests bleeding from the prostate or bladder base.

Careful urine microscopy is mandatory as the presence of red-cell casts is diagnostic of bleeding from the kidney itself, most often due to glomerulonephritis. In the absence of red-cell casts, further investigations, such as urine cytology, intravenous urography and cystoscopy, are required to define the site of bleeding. Renal biopsy may be required (see p. 600).

Protein

Proteinuria is one of the most common signs of renal disease. Detection is now primarily by Stix testing. Most reagent strips can detect a concentration of 100 mg/L or more in urine. They react primarily with

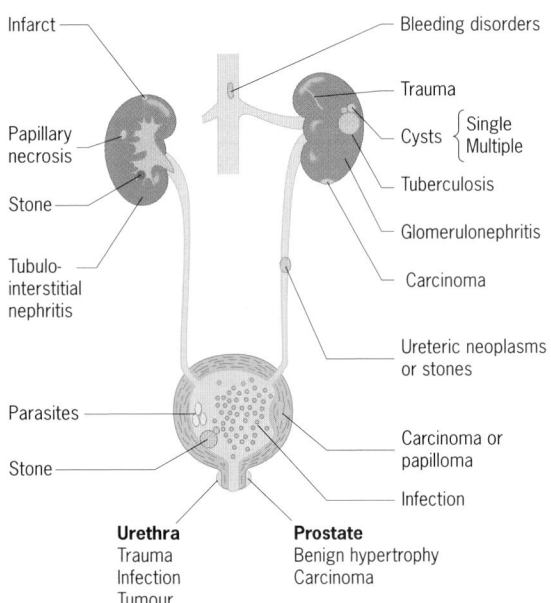

Fig. 11.4 Sites and causes of bleeding from the urinary tract.

albumin and are relatively insensitive to globulin and Bence Jones proteins.

If proteinuria is confirmed on repeated Stix testing, protein excretion in 24-hour urine collections should be measured (but see below). Normal values for urinary protein excretion are dependent on the laboratory methods used and in particular whether or not the method measures Tamm–Horsfall glycoprotein, which is a normal constituent of urine. Results must therefore take account of the laboratory's normal reference range. Given this caveat, healthy adults excrete approximately 60–100 mg of protein daily but up to 150–200 mg daily is within the acceptable range. Slightly higher values – up to 300 mg daily – may be excreted by adolescents. Pyrexia, exercise and adoption of the upright posture all increase urinary protein output. Proteinuria, while occasionally benign, always requires further investigation.

Postural proteinuria. This term is used to refer to proteinuria present on dipstick testing which becomes undetectable after a period of hours lying flat. Typically, a negative dipstick result is obtained on the first urine passed on rising in the morning, whereas subsequent specimens give a positive result. This is regarded by many – including some insurance companies – as a benign condition. Renal biopsy sometimes discloses glomerular abnormalities but progressive renal failure is rare.

Microalbuminuria

The term microalbuminuria is an unfortunate one since the albumin referred to is of normal molecular size and weight. Normal individuals excrete less than 30 µg of albumin per minute (43 mg in 24 hours). Dipsticks, however, detect albumin only in a concentration around 100 mg/L (150 mg per 24 hours if urine volume is normal). An increase in albumin excretion between these two levels – so-called microalbuminuria – is now known to be an early indicator of diabetic glomerular disease. It is widely used as a predictor of the development of nephropathy in diabetics and may be extended to other conditions.

For example, the majority of patients with systemic lupus erythematosus but without overt renal disease have microalbuminuria and some ultimately develop clinically evident glomerulonephritis. By contrast, patients with minimal-change nephropathy (see p. 604) after remission have normal albumin excretion.

Timed 24-hour urinary excretion rates provide the most precise measure of microalbuminuria. However, in clinical practice it is more convenient to test for microalbuminuria using random urine samples in which albumin concentration is related to urinary creatinine concentration. Kits are now available to test for microalbuminuria.

Glucose

Renal glycosuria is uncommon, so that a positive test for glucose always requires exclusion of diabetes mellitus.

Bacteriuria

Dipsticks are available for testing for bacteriuria based on the detection of nitrite produced from the reduction of urinary nitrate by bacteria and also for the detection of leucocyte esterase, an enzyme specific for neutrophils. Although each test on its own has limitations, a positive reaction with both tests has a high predictive value for urinary tract infection (p. 618).

Microscopy

An unspun sample of urine may be examined by placing a drop on a slide using a pipette, covering with a coverslip and examining by low-power and higher-power microscopy. Phase-contrast microscopy is a helpful additional tool. Frequently, a spun-urine sample is examined. Urine is centrifuged, the supernatant is discarded and an aliquot of the residuum placed on a glass slide employing a Pasteur pipette. Quantitation of white cells or red cells expressed per high-power field by this method is inaccurate.

Urine microscopy should be carried out in all patients suspected of having renal disease. Care must be taken to obtain a 'clean' sample of mid-stream urine (Practical box 11.2). The presence of numerous skin squames suggests a contaminated, poorly collected sample that cannot be properly interpreted.

If a clean sample of urine cannot be obtained, suprapubic aspiration is required in suspected urinary tract infections.

Most urines are examined by microscopy in hospital practice by microbiology laboratory technicians who

---

✚ Practical box 11.2

Collection of mid-stream specimens of urine

Female
1 The patient's bladder should be full ('desperate to go')
2 The patient removes underpants and stands over the toilet pan.
3 The labia are separated using the left hand.
4 The vulva is cleansed front to back with sterile swabs.
5 The patient voids downward into the toilet and continues until 'half-done'.
6 Without stopping the urine flow, the sterile container is plunged into the stream of urine with the right hand. Only a small volume is required.
7 The patient then completes voiding into the toilet.

Male
1 The patient's bladder should be full.
2 The foreskin, if present, is retracted.
3 The glans penis is cleaned with a sterile swab.
4 The patient voids into the toilet until 'half-done'.
5 Without stopping the urine flow, the sterile container is plunged into the stream of urine.
6 The patient then completes voiding into the toilet.

must process large numbers of such urines each day. Best results are obtained in nephrological practice if microscopy is carried out by the physician caring for the patient.

White cells

The presence of 10 or more white blood cells (WBCs) per cubic millimetre in fresh unspun mid-stream urine samples is abnormal and indicates an inflammatory reaction within the urinary tract. Most commonly it is due to urinary tract infection (UTI), but it may also be found in sterile urine in patients during antibiotic treatment of urinary infection or within 14 days of treatment. Sterile pyuria also occurs in patients with stones, tubulointerstitial nephritis, papillary necrosis, tuberculosis, and interstitial cystitis.

Red cells

The presence of one or more red cells per cubic millimetre in unspun urine samples results in a positive Stix test for blood and is abnormal. It is claimed that red cells of glomerular origin can be identified by their dysmorphic appearance, especially on phase-contrast microscopy, but the method is subject to observer error and has not gained wide acceptance.

Casts (see Fig. 11.5)

These cylindrical bodies, which are moulded ('cast') in the shape of the distal tubular lumen, may be hyaline, granular or cellular. Hyaline casts and fine granular casts represent precipitated protein and may be seen in normal urine, particularly after exercise. More coarsely granular casts occur with pathological proteinuria in glomerular and tubular disease. Red-cell casts – even one – always indicate renal disease. If red cells degenerate, a rusty coloured 'haemoglobin' granular cast is seen. White cell casts may be seen in acute pyelonephritis. They may be confused with the tubular cell casts that occur in patients with acute tubular necrosis.

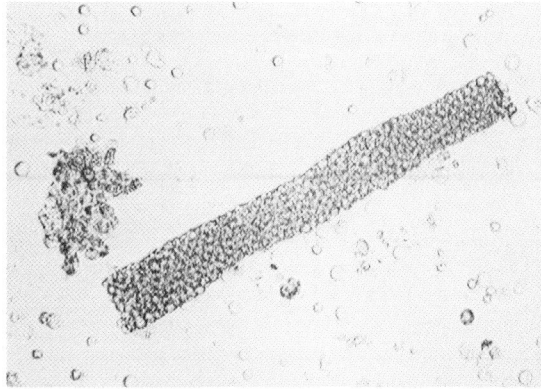

Fig. 11.5 **Red-cell cast.** Note aggregation of red cells as a 'cast' of the tubule.

Bacteria

The demonstration of bacteria on Gram staining of the centrifuged deposit of a clean-catch mid-stream urine sample is highly suggestive of urinary infection and can be of value in the immediate differential diagnosis of UTI. If accompanied by pyuria it may be accepted as evidence of UTI in the ill and febrile patient and treatment should be initiated.

Urine for quantitative culture (see p. 618) must always be obtained prior to starting antibiotic treatment in order to confirm the diagnosis and to allow definition of bacterial antibiotic sensitivities.

Stix testing for blood or protein is of no value in the diagnosis of UTI, as both are absent from the urine of many patients with bacteriuria.

Quantitative tests of renal function

The use of serum urea, creatinine and GFR as measures of renal function is discussed on page 590. Quantification of proteinuria, including the investigation of selective proteinuria, is discussed on page 613. Other quantitative tests of disturbed renal function are described under the relevant disorders.

Imaging techniques

Plain X-ray

A plain radiograph of the abdomen is always taken prior to urography. Its main value is to identify renal calcification or radiodense calculi in the kidney, renal pelvis, line of the ureters or bladder (Fig. 11.6). Care must be taken in viewing the X-ray in order not to miss calculi obscured by bowel shadows or bone. Renal size and outline are best assessed during excretion urography or by ultrasound. If bowel gas overlying the kidney renders exclusion of calcification and calculi impossible, plain renal tomograms will often resolve the matter.

Excretion urography

Excretion urography, also known as intravenous urography (IVU) or intravenous pyelography (IVP) still plays a role in renal diagnosis, especially in patients with haematuria and stone disease, but has in part been replaced by ultrasonography. A plain X-ray film of the urinary tract is obtained to check for urinary tract calcification. An organic iodine-containing contrast medium is then given intravenously. A small proportion of patients will have an 'allergic' reaction to contrast medium. With modern low-osmolality contrast media the risk is relatively low (e.g. 1% develop bronchospasm or urticaria, less than 0.003% develop more severe

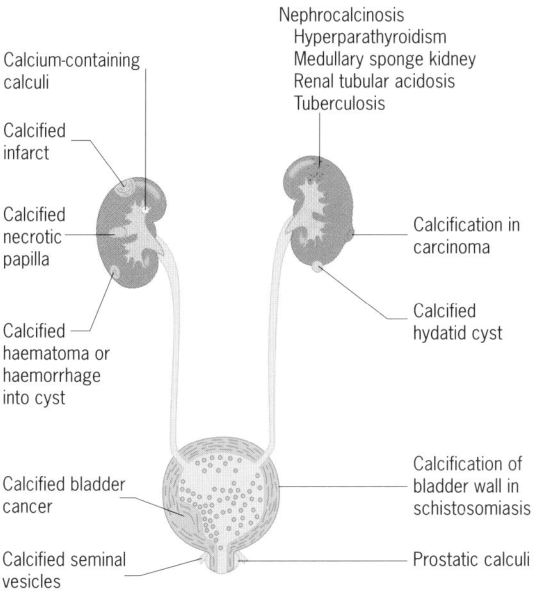
Nephrocalcinosis
Hyperparathyroidism
Medullary sponge kidney
Renal tubular acidosis
Tuberculosis
Calcium-containing calculi
Calcified infarct
Calcified necrotic papilla
Calcified haematoma or haemorrhage into cyst
Calcification in carcinoma
Calcified hydatid cyst
Calcified bladder cancer
Calcification of bladder wall in schistosomiasis
Calcified seminal vesicles
Prostatic calculi

Fig. 11.6 Calcification in the renal tract. Calculi can occur at any site.

complications such as cardiac arrhythmias and convulsions and the mortality is of the order 1 in 200 000). Patients who have had a previous contrast medium reaction, who have asthma or a history of allergy requiring medical treatment should receive steroid prophylaxis before contrast medium (e.g. prednisolone 30 mg 12 hours and 2 hours before contrast medium). Contrast media do not cause renal damage in normovolaemic patients with normal renal function, but may be nephrotoxic in patients with impaired renal function, especially when this results from diabetic nephropathy (p. 1095).

The contrast medium is rapidly excreted by glomerular filtration and a film at the end of the injection shows opacification of the renal parenchyma (the nephrogram). The kidneys usually have smooth outlines and measure 11–14 cm in length in adults, with the two sides differing by less than 2 cm. An irregular renal outline may be caused either by scars or masses. A small kidney indicates chronic disease either of the renal parenchyma or vasculature.

If there is no dilatation of the pelvicalyceal systems suggesting obstruction on a film obtained 5 minutes after contrast medium injection, a compression band is applied to the lower abdomen for 5 minutes to cause distension of the upper tracts. The film with compression in place is used to assess the pelvicalyceal system for calyceal clubbing, filling defects or cavities.

When the compression band is removed, a full-length abdominal film is obtained to show the ureters and bladder. A further full-length film after voiding is used to evaluate emptying of the pelvicalyceal systems and ureters as well as bladder emptying.

Ultrasonography

Ultrasonography of the kidneys and bladder has the advantage over X-ray techniques of avoiding ionizing radiation and intravascular contrast medium. In renal diagnosis it is the method of choice for:

- renal measurement
- checking for pelvicalyceal dilatation as an indication of renal obstruction when chronic renal obstruction is suspected; in suspected acute ureteric obstruction either intravenous urography or unenhanced spiral CT are the methods of choice
- characterizing renal masses as cystic or solid
- diagnosing polycystic kidney disease
- detecting intrarenal and/or perinephric fluid (e.g. pus, blood)
- demonstrating renal arterial perfusion (using Doppler techniques)
- detecting renal vein thrombosis (using Doppler techniques).

Ultrasonography of the distended bladder is used to measure bladder wall thickness and to check for bladder tumours and stones. A scan obtained after voiding allows bladder emptying to be assessed.

The disadvantages of using ultrasonography to assess the urinary tract are:

- It does not show detailed pelvicalyceal anatomy.
- It does not fully visualize the normal adult ureter.
- It may miss small renal calculi and does not detect the majority of ureteric calculi. A plain abdominal film should usually be obtained to improve the detection of calculi if ultrasonography is to be the only imaging method used.
- It is operator-dependent.

In patients with suspected benign prostatic hypertrophy, examination of the bladder before and after voiding, with measurement of the prostate, and examination of the kidneys to check for pelvicalyceal dilatation suffice. If prostate cancer is suspected, more detailed examination of the prostate with a transrectal transducer, usually with transrectal prostate biopsy, is necessary.

Computed tomography (CT)

Computed tomography is used mainly as a second-line imaging method in the urinary tract, but increasingly as a first-line investigation in cases of suspected ureteric colic. The spiral technology allows collection of imaging data from a volume of tissue rather than slice by slice. This has both improved image resolution and allowed reconstruction of the imaging data in a variety of planes. CT is used:

- to characterize renal masses which are indeterminate at ultrasonography
- to stage renal tumours

- to detect 'lucent' calculi; low-density calculi which are lucent on plain films (e.g. uric acid stones) are well seen on CT
- to evaluate the retroperitoneum for tumours, retroperitoneal fibrosis (periaortitis) and other causes of ureteric obstruction
- to assess severe renal trauma
- to visualize the renal arteries and veins
- to stage bladder and prostate tumours; MR is, however, increasingly used to stage prostate cancer.

The use of spiral unenhanced CT in suspected uteric colic permits diagnosis of causes of pain other than calculi more readily than does urography.

Magnetic resonance imaging (MRI)

MRI is another second-line imaging method which is used:

- to characterize renal masses not characterized by CT
- to stage renal, prostate and bladder cancer
- to demonstrate the renal arteries.

Antegrade pyelography (Fig. 11.7)

Antegrade pyelography involves percutaneous puncture of a pelvicalyceal system with a needle and the injection of contrast medium to outline the pelvicalyceal

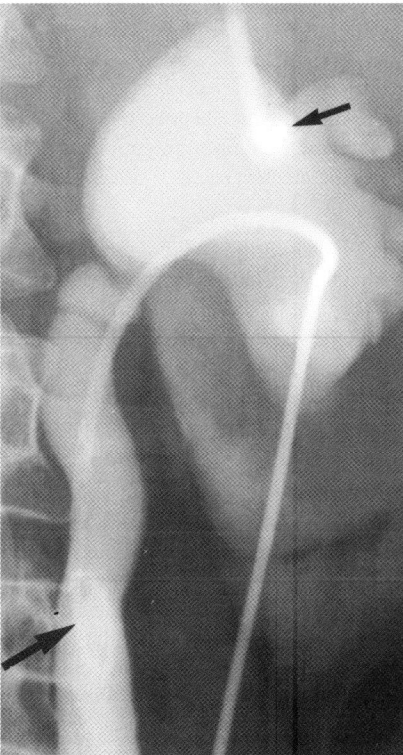

Fig. 11.7 Antegrade pyelography via percutaneous catheter (small arrow) of obstructed system. Percutaneous drainage catheter (large arrow) has been inserted.

system and ureter to the level of obstruction. It is used when ultrasonography has shown a dilated pelvicalyceal system in a patient with suspected obstruction. Antegrade pyelography is the preliminary to percutaneously placing of a drainage catheter in the obstructed pelvicalyceal system (percutaneous nephrostomy).

Retrograde pyelography

Following cystoscopy, preferably under screening control, a catheter is either impacted in the ureteral orifice or passed a short distance up the ureter, and contrast medium is injected. Retrograde pyelography is mainly used to investigate lesions of the ureter and to define the lower level of ureteral obstruction shown on excretion urography or ultrasound plus antegrade studies. It is invasive, commonly requires a general anaesthetic, and may result in the introduction of infection.

Micturating cystourethrography (MCU)

This involves catheterization and the instillation of contrast medium into the bladder. The catheter is then removed and the patient screened during voiding to check for vesicoureteric reflux and to study the urethra and bladder emptying. It is used primarily in children with recurrent infection (see p. 619) and in adults with disturbed bladder function, when it may be combined with urodynamic studies of bladder pressure and urethral flow.

MCU is not an appropriate part of the investigation of the adult female with recurrent bacterial cystitis if the IVU, including an after-micturition bladder film, is normal. This is because vesicoureteric reflux and urinary tract infection cause renal scarring and calyceal distortion in early life, but reflux tends to disappear by the time adulthood is reached. If reflux is detected in an adult with normal renal anatomy, it is thought not to induce kidney damage later. The absence of reflux in an adult does not therefore exclude the diagnosis of chronic atrophic pyelonephritis (reflux nephropathy) and reflux if present in an adult with normal renal anatomy does not require surgical intervention. Therefore, whatever the finding on micturating cystourethrography, management is not altered.

The presence or absence of vesicoureteric reflux may also be investigated by scintigraphy (see below).

Aortography or renal arteriography

Conventional or digital subtraction angiography (DSA) is used. The latter allows the use of smaller doses of contrast medium which can be injected via a central venous catheter (venous DSA) or via a fine transfemoral arterial catheter (arterial DSA). Angiography is mainly used to define extrarenal or intrarenal arterial disease. Arteriography is still the 'gold standard' method of renal artery imaging but magnetic resonance angiography and spiral CT angiography are being used increasingly (Fig. 11.8).

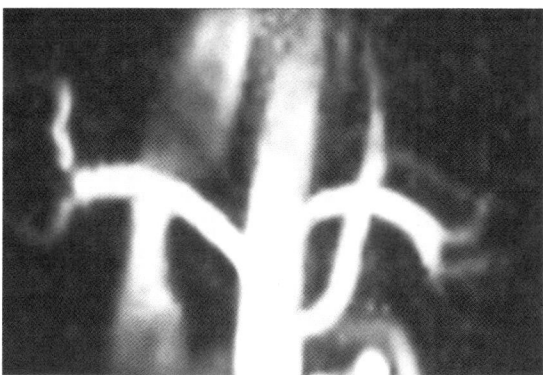

Fig. 11.8 **Magnetic resonance angiogram of normal renal arteries.**

Venography is only used occasionally to exclude renal vein thrombosis. In most instances this can be done less invasively with Doppler ultrasonography, CT or MRI.

Renal scintigraphy

Renal scintigraphy using a gamma camera is divided into:

- *dynamic studies* in which the function of the kidney is examined serially over a period of time, most often using a radiopharmaceutical excreted by glomerular filtration
- *static studies* involving imaging of tracer that is taken up and *retained* by the renal tubule.

Dynamic scintigraphy

The radiopharmaceutical technetium-labelled diethylenetriaminepentaacetic acid, [^{99m}Tc]DTPA is excreted by glomerular filtration. ^{123}I-labelled ortho-iodohippuric acid (Hippuran) is both filtered and secreted by the tubules. Mercaptoacetyltriglycine (MAG3) labelled with technetium (^{99m}Tc) is excreted by renal tubular secretion and is increasingly employed. Following venous injection of a bolus of tracer, emissions from the kidney can be recorded and stored on computer for analysis of time–activity curves. Analogue images can also be generated at intervals as the study proceeds. This information allows examination of blood perfusion of the kidney, uptake of tracer as a result of glomerular filtration, transit of tracer through the kidney, and the outflow of tracer-containing urine from the collecting system.

Renal blood flow

Dynamic studies can be used to investigate patients in whom renal artery stenosis is suspected as a cause for hypertension and in patients with severe oliguria (post-traumatic, post-aortic surgery, or after a kidney transplant) to establish whether, and to what extent, there is renal perfusion. In patients with unilateral renal artery stenosis there is, typically, a slowed and reduced uptake of tracer with delay in reaching a peak. Studies carried out before and after administration of an ACE inhibitor may demonstrate a fall in uptake that is suggestive

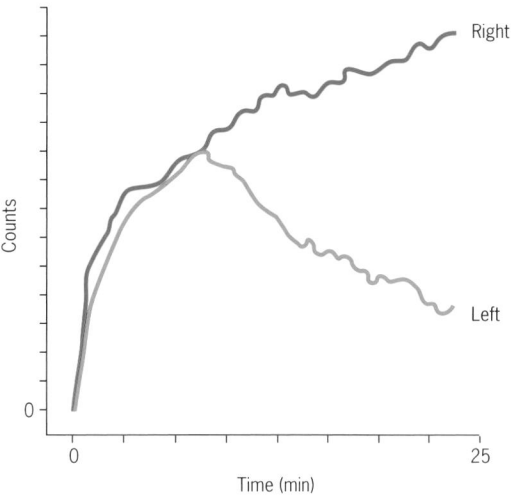

Fig. 11.9 **Dynamic scintigram.** Note the progressive rise of the right kidney curve to a plateau (in contrast to the normal left kidney curve) owing to urinary tract obstruction on the right side.

of functional arterial stenosis. Both false-positive and false-negative results occur with this test and renal arteriography remains the 'gold standard' in the diagnosis of main renal artery stenosis. In patients with total renal artery occlusion, no kidney uptake of tracers is observed.

Investigation of obstruction

Renal scintigraphy provides functional evidence of obstruction. After injection of, for example, (^{99m}Tc)MAG3 a rise in resistance to flow in the pelvis or ureter prolongs the parenchymal transit of tracer and there is usually a delay in emptying the pelvis. On whole-kidney renograms, the time–activity curve fails to fall after an initial peak, or continues to rise (Fig. 11.9). These activity–time curves do not alone enable a distinction to be made between obstructive nephropathy, in which parenchymal transit time is prolonged, and retention of tracer within a large, baggy, low-pressure, unobstructed pelvis, where the parenchymal transit time is normal. Parenchymal transit times must therefore be measured through renographic data analysis to make this distinction. Whereas obstructive nephropathy is associated with prolonged transit of tracer through the renal parenchyma, a normal parenchymal transit time with delayed outflow indicates a non-obstructed dilated pelvis.

When the possibility of obstruction is suspected, a dynamic renal scintigram is performed with diuresis. Furosemide (frusemide) (0.5 mg/kg, adult dose 40 mg) is given intravenously about 18–20 minutes into the study. Time–activity curves show an immediate fall after the injection of furosemide in the normal and in the absence of obstruction. In the presence of obstruction, the retention of activity in the pelvis persists, the activity–time curve fails to fall or falls to a lesser extent than the previous rate of rise of the activity–time curve.

A decision as to whether conservative surgery or nephrectomy should be carried out in unilateral obstruction is facilitated by renographic assessment of the contribution of each kidney.

Bladder emptying

At the end of dynamic studies, bladder emptying may be investigated and any postmicturition residual urine measured. Vesicoureteric reflux may be observed, although the sensitivity for detection of this is low. Increased sensitivity can be obtained by direct isotope cystography when a dilute isotope solution is instilled into the bladder by catheter.

Glomerular filtration rate

This is discussed on page 584.

Static scintigraphy

This is usually performed using [^{99m}Tc]DMSA (dimercaptosuccinic acid), which is taken up by tubular cells. Uptake is proportional to renal function.

Relative renal function

Function is normally evenly divided between the kidneys, with a range of 45–55%. Static studies are particularly useful in unilateral renal disease, where the relative uptake of the two kidneys can be calculated.

Kidney visualization

Normal kidneys show a uniform uptake with a smooth renal outline. Scars can be identified as photon-deficient 'bites'. Static scintigraphy is of considerable value in identifying ectopic kidneys or 'pseudotumours' of the kidneys (i.e. normally functioning renal tissue abnormally placed within the kidney).

Localization of infection

The use of citrate labelled with gallium-67 or isotopically labelled leucocytes that are taken up by inflammatory tissue may be of value in defining localized infection, such as renal abscesses or infection within a renal cyst.

Transcutaneous renal biopsy

(Practical box 11.3)

Indications for and contraindications to transcutaneous renal biopsy are shown in Table 11.4.

The biopsies are carried out under ultrasound control using a spring-loaded biopsy needle. Native renal biopsy material must be examined by conventional histochemical staining, by electron microscopy, and by immunoperoxidase or immunofluorescence staining. Light microscopy will suffice for some renal transplant biopsies.

The complications of transcutaneous renal biopsy are shown in Table 11.5.

Table 11.4
Renal biopsy

Indications
Nephrotic syndrome (with some exceptions)
Unexplained renal failure with normal-sized kidneys
Failure to recover from assumed reversible acute renal failure
Diagnosis of systemic disease with renal involvement, such as sarcoidosis, amyloidosis
   (occasional indication only)
Asymptomatic proteinuria or haematuria
   (very occasional indication – justified only if knowledge of prognosis is essential)

Contraindications
Uncooperative patient
Single kidney (with the exception of transplant kidney, when biopsy is acceptable)
Small kidneys (technically difficult, histology hard to interpret, prognosis cannot be altered)
Haemorrhagic disorders (unless correctable temporarily or permanently, e.g. by factor VIII administration in haemophilia)
Gross obesity or oedema (technical difficulties)
Uncontrolled hypertension

Table 11.5
Complications of transcutaneous renal biopsy

Macroscopic haematuria – about 20%
Pain in the flank, sometimes referred to shoulder tip
Perirenal haematoma
Arteriovenous aneurysm formation – about 20%, almost always of no clinical significance
Profuse haematuria demanding blood transfusion – 1–3%
Profuse haematuria demanding occlusion of bleeding vessel at angiography or nephrectomy – approximately 1 in 400
Introduction of infection
The mortality rate is about 0.1%

 Practical box 11.3

Transcutaneous renal biopsy

Before biopsy
1 A coagulation screen is performed. It must be normal.
2 The serum is grouped and saved for crossmatching.
3 The patient is given a full explanation of what is involved.

During biopsy
1 The patient lies prone with a hard pillow under the abdomen.
2 The kidney is localized by ultrasound.
3 Local anaesthetic is injected along the biopsy track.
4 The patient holds a breath when the biopsy is performed.

After biopsy
1 A pressure dressing is applied to the biopsy site and the patient rests in bed for 24 hours.
2 The fluid intake is maximized to prevent clot colic.
3 The pulse and blood pressure are checked regularly.
4 The patient is advised to avoid heavy lifting or gardening for 2 weeks.

FURTHER READING

Birnbaumer M et al. (1992) Molecular cloning of the receptor for human antidiuretic hormone. *Nature* **357**: 333–335.

Chantler C, Barrett TM (1972) Estimation of the glomerular filtration rate from the plasma clearance of 51-chromium EDTA. *Archives of Disease in Childhood* **47**: 613–617.

Marples D (2000) Water channels: who needs them? *Lancet* **355**: 1571–1572.

Wrong O, Davies HEF (1959) The excretion of acid in renal disease. *Quarterly Journal of Medicine* **28**: 259–313.

Glomerular diseases

Glomerulonephritides

Glomerulonephritis is the third most common cause of end-stage renal disease (after diabetes and hypertension) in Europe and the USA, accounting for some 10–15% of such patients.

Glomerulonephritis is a general term for a group of disorders in which:

- there is primarily an immunologically mediated injury to glomeruli, although renal interstitial damage is a regular accompaniment
- the kidneys are involved symmetrically
- secondary mechanisms of glomerular injury come into play following an initial immune insult (see below)
- the renal lesion may be part of a generalized disease (e.g. systemic lupus erythematosus, SLE).

Pathogenesis

Pathogenetic mechanisms include:

- deposition or in situ formation of immune complexes
- deposition of antiglomerular basement membrane antibody (fewer than 5% of glomerulonephritides)
- deposition of an immunoglobulin of atypical configuration in glomeruli, as in IgA nephropathy.

These pathogenetic mechanisms activate secondary mechanisms that produce glomerular damage.

Immune complex nephritis

Circulating antigen–antibody complexes (see p. 214) are deposited in the kidney, or complexes are formed locally when circulating free antigen has become trapped in the glomerulus. The nature of the antigen involved in the complex formation is important in many instances.

The antigen may be exogenous or endogenous:

- exogenous (e.g. bacterial) – for example, a nephritogenic Lancefield group A β-haemolytic streptococcus can cause glomerulonephritis in previously healthy individuals

- endogenous – for example, patients with SLE may form antibodies to host DNA, leading to a glomerulonephritis.

Harmful immune complexes can also occur when there is impaired host ability to produce appropriate antibody. Certain strains of black mice regularly develop glomerulonephritis as a result of an impaired ability to produce antibody of appropriate quality or quantity, and it is likely that there are human counterparts of this phenomenon. There is an association between HLA markers and certain nephritides. For example, in Europe there is an increased prevalence of the HLA-A1 B8 DR3 haplotype in patients with membranous glomerulonephritis.

Impaired ability on the part of the host to clear immune complexes from the circulation and deficiencies in the complement system are each associated with an increased incidence of glomerulonephritis.

Antiglomerular basement membrane (anti-GBM) antibody

The major component of the glomerular basement membrane is type 4 collagen (COLIV). This collagen molecule is a heterotrimer containing paired polypeptide α chains (see p. 585).

Anti-GBM antibodies are autoantibodies that bind mainly to the non-collagenous domain of the α-3 chain type IV collagen (COLIVα3). This antigenic target is also present in alveolar basement membrane, which accounts for the association of both lung haemorrhage and glomerulonephritis (Goodpasture's syndrome, p. 605). Anti-GBM antibodies are of IgG type.

Secondary mechanisms of glomerular injury

Several events can be triggered by the above immunological insults:

- complement activation
- fibrin deposition
- platelet aggregation
- inflammation with inflammatory cytokine mechanisms and free oxygen radical-induced damage.

Immune complex or anti-GBM antibody deposition trigger these mechanisms to varying degrees, resulting in an increase in capillary permeability and glomerular damage.

In experimentally induced glomerulonephritis in animals, prior anticoagulation, prevention of complement activation, and depletion of polymorphonuclear leucocytes have all been shown to reduce the severity of the induced glomerular injury. However, in humans presenting with most forms of glomerulonephritis these measures do not help.

T-cell dysfunction may play a part in the production of lesions when immune complexes are not seen.

Causes

In the majority of patients with immune complex-mediated glomerulonephritis, the cause is unknown; i.e. the nature of the antigen involved is not determined. Antigen derived from viruses, bacteria, parasites, drugs and from the host may be involved (Table 11.6). The reasons for the development of anti-GBM antibody are not known; viral or solvent damage to alveolar capillary basement membrane, rendering it antigenic, has been suggested as a possible cause.

Pathology

Macroscopic appearances

In *acute* glomerulonephritis, the kidneys are normal in size or enlarged and oedematous, and the surface of the kidney may show punctate haemorrhages.

In long-standing progressive *chronic* glomerulonephritis the kidneys may be normal in size or small with finely granular cortical scarring.

Microscopic appearances

Different immunological insults may induce similar or identical histological changes. For example, the immune complex-mediated glomerulonephritis in mumps is not distinguishable from that following β-haemolytic streptococcal infection. Conversely, different histological responses may occur in the same disease process in different individuals (e.g. in SLE, see below).

The histological response to immune complex deposition probably depends on the size of the complexes, their rate of deposition, and the efficiency of host clearance mechanisms.

Renal tissue, obtained at transcutaneous renal biopsy, is examined by the following processes:

- *light microscopy* – to assess the extent and histological type of disease
- *electron microscopy* – to define the type of disease and to correlate with immunofluorescence; e.g. to see the exact sites of deposits
- *immunofluorescence* – to assess the type of immunological injury (immunoperoxidase methods may also be applied).

All three methods of examination are necessary for proper histopathological assessment.

Immune complex deposition results in a diffuse granular pattern of staining, with IgG, IgM, IgA, components of the complement system and, in addition, fibrin and fibrinogen all present (Fig. 11.10).

The presence of anti-GBM antibody produces a smooth linear pattern of staining for IgG on immunofluorescence (Fig. 11.11).

Types

There is not a complete correlation between the histopathological types of glomerulonephritides and the

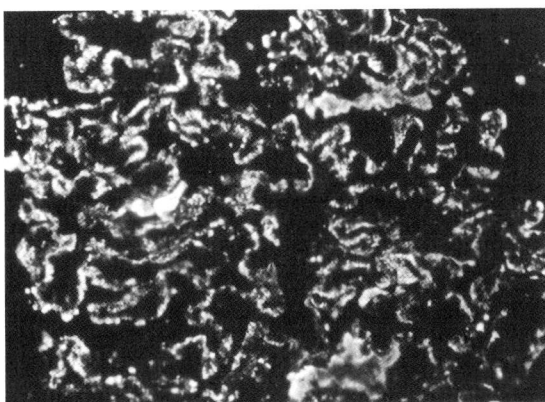

Fig. 11.10 Immunofluorescence, showing immune complex deposition in a diffuse granular pattern.

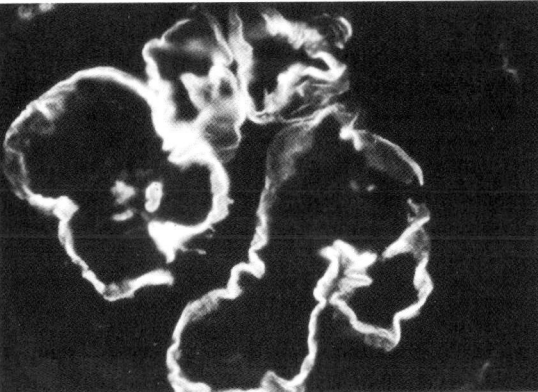

Fig. 11.11 Immunofluorescence, showing antiglomerular basement membrane antibody (anti-GBM) deposition in a linear pattern typical of Goodpasture's syndrome.

Table 11.6

Some causes of immune complex-mediated glomerulonephritis

Viruses
Mumps
Measles
Hepatitis B and C
Epstein–Barr
Coxsackie
Varicella
HIV

Bacteria
Lancefield group A
  β-haemolytic streptococci
Streptococcus viridans
  (infective endocarditis)
Staphylococci
Treponema pallidum
Gonococci
Salmonella

Parasites
Plasmodium malariae
Schistosoma
Filariasis

Host antigens
DNA (systemic lupus
  erythematosus)
Cryoglobulin
Malignant tumours

Drugs
Penicillamine

clinical features of disease. Table 11.7 shows the most common associations.

Proliferative glomerulonephritis

Proliferative changes occur in many immune complex-mediated nephritides and also in anti-GBM nephritis. There are the following subtypes.

Diffuse proliferative glomerulonephritis

All the glomeruli are similarly affected. Figure 11.12 shows the typical histological changes, and a normal glomerulus is shown for comparison in Figure 11.13. Immunofluorescence shows granular deposits of immunoglobulin and C3. This type of glomerulonephritis, presenting as an acute nephritis, is commonly seen after a streptococcal infection (see below). Immune complexes are seen as electron-dense deposits on electron microscopy (Fig. 11.14).

Focal segmental glomerulonephritis

Only some of the glomeruli here show proliferative changes whilst others are normal; hence the term 'focal'. The affected glomeruli show segmental involvement of the tufts; i.e. changes are present in one or more parts of the glomerulus.

This condition may occur as a primary renal disease, but it is also seen in SLE, subacute infective endocarditis, with infected atrioventricular shunts (shunt nephritis), and in disorders with IgA deposits (e.g. Henoch–Schönlein purpura and IgA nephropathy). A severe focal necrotizing form is seen in microscopic polyangiitis and Wegener's granulomatosis. Special subtypes (IgA nephropathy and focal glomerulosclerosis) are discussed below.

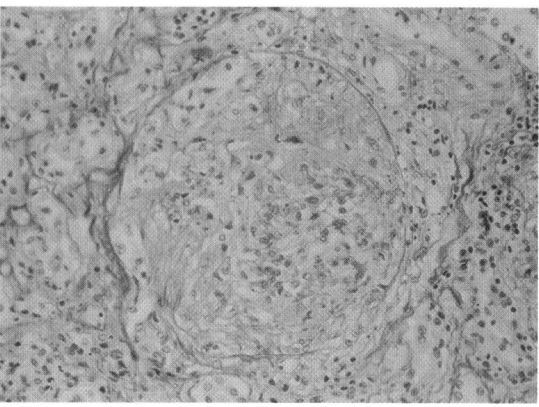

Fig. 11.12 **A glomerulus showing proliferative glomerulonephritis.** The glomerulus is swollen, packed with cells, and bulges into the opening of the proximal tubule. There is proliferation of the endothelial and mesangial cells, and polymorphonuclear leucocytes are present.

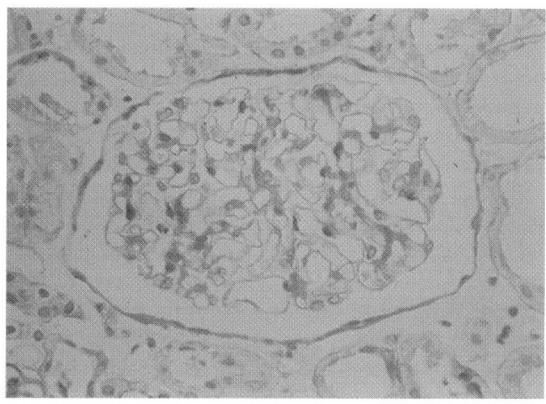

Fig. 11.13 A normal glomerulus.

Table 11.7
Correlation between the histological type of glomerulonephritis and the clinical picture

Histological type	Most common clinical presentation
Proliferative glomerulonephritis	
Diffuse	Acute nephritic syndrome
Focal segmental	Haematuria, proteinuria
With crescent formation (rapidly progressive glomerulonephritis)	Progressive renal failure
Mesangiocapillary (membranoproliferative)	Haematuria, proteinuria, acute nephritic or nephrotic syndrome
Membranous glomerulonephritis	Nephrotic syndrome in adults
Minimal-change nephropathy	Nephrotic syndrome, especially in children
IgA nephropathy	Asymptomatic haematuria
Focal glomerulosclerosis	Proteinuria or nephrotic syndrome

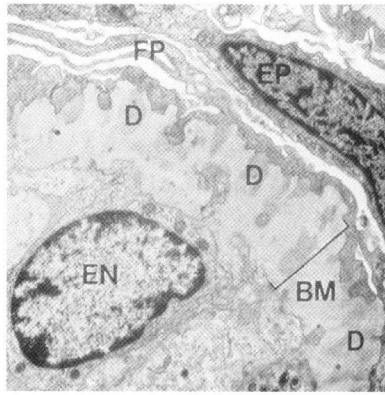

Fig. 11.14 **Electron micrograph, showing immune complex-mediated glomerulonephritis.** BM, basement membrane; D, electron-dense deposits (antigen–antibody complexes); EN, endothelial cell; EP, epithelial podocyte; FP, foot process.

Proliferative glomerulonephritis with crescent formation (rapidly progressive glomerulonephritis; RPGN) or crescentic glomerulonephritis

The term 'crescent' is applied to an aggregate of macrophages and epithelial cells in Bowman's space (Fig. 11.15). Crescents are associated with severe damage to the glomerular tuft and are seen in occasional glomeruli in several types of glomerulonephritis. However, if most glomeruli show crescents the glomerulonephritis is usually placed in this subtype, as clinical progression to renal failure is rapid.

This condition is seen in both immune complex- and anti-GBM antibody-mediated nephritis. It particularly occurs in microscopic polyangiitis, Wegener's granulomatosis and Goodpasture's syndrome.

Mesangiocapillary (membranoproliferative) glomerulonephritis (MCGN)

In *type 1* there is mesangial cell proliferation, with mainly subendothelial immune complex deposition and apparent splitting of the capillary basement membrane, giving a 'tram-line' effect. It may be idiopathic or may occur with shunt nephritis. It can be associated with persistently reduced plasma levels of C3 and normal levels of C4. In some cases hepatitis B and C infection is present and appears to be an aetiological factor.

In *type 2* there is mesangial cell proliferation with electron-dense, linear intramembranous deposits that usually stain for C3 only. This type may be idiopathic or may occur after measles. Partial lipodystrophy (loss of subcutaneous fat in various parts of the body) may be seen. MCGN affects young adults. Patients present with haematuria, proteinuria, the nephrotic syndrome or renal failure. Most patients eventually go on to develop renal failure over several years.

Membranous glomerulonephritis

Thickening of the capillary basement membrane because of immune complex deposition is the main feature of this disease (Fig. 11.16). In the majority of patients the antigenic component of the complex is unknown. Associations include SLE (where the antigen is host DNA), malignancy of the bowel and bronchus (tumour-derived antigen), penicillamine therapy and hepatitis B infection. *Plasmodium malariae* is a common cause in the tropics. A strong association with HLA-DR3 has been found.

This condition occurs mainly in adults, predominantly in males. Patients present with proteinuria or frank nephrotic syndrome. Approximately one-third of patients develop end-stage renal failure within 10–20 years of diagnosis. Younger patients, females and those with asymptomatic proteinuria of modest degree at the time of presentation do best. Spontaneous remission occurs in about one-third of patients, particularly females.

Uncertainty exists as to the place of corticosteroid and immunosuppressive treatment with, for example, chlorambucil, cyclophosphamide or azathioprine in the treatment of membranous glomerulonephritis. Interpretation of controlled trial data in unselected patients with the condition has proved difficult owing to the fact that a significant proportion of patients are destined to do well without specific treatment. There is an increasingly strong consensus (supported by meta-analysis of trial data) that patients with a poor prognosis (those with heavy proteinuria and progressive renal impairment) do benefit from such treatment.

Minimal-change glomerular lesion (minimal-change nephropathy)

This is not a true glomerulonephritis (the suffix 'itis' suggests the presence of inflammation and inflammatory change in glomeruli is not seen in this condition). It is included here for convenience. In this condition the glomeruli appear normal on light microscopy. The only abnormality seen on electron microscopy is fusion of the foot processes of epithelial cells (podocytes). This is a

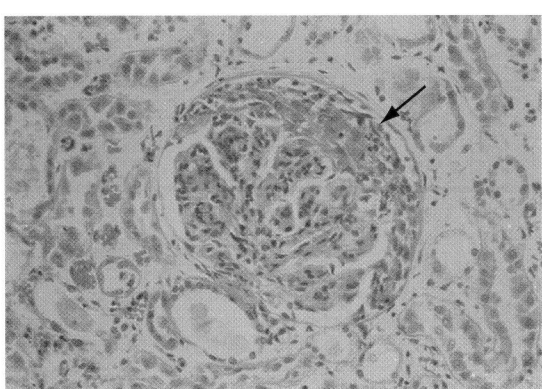

Fig. 11.15 Crescentic glomerulonephritis. Note the 'epithelial' crescent at the periphery of the glomerulus (arrow).

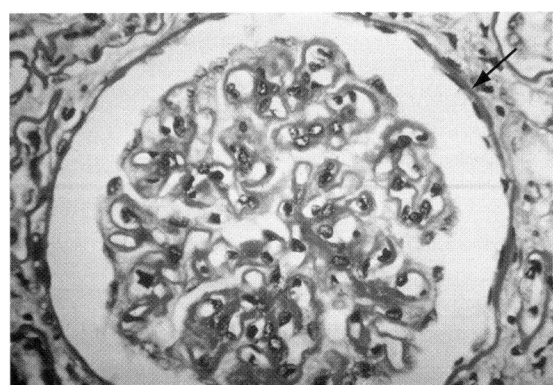

Fig. 11.16 Membranous glomerulonephritis showing thickened basement membrane (arrow).

non-specific finding and is seen in many conditions associated with proteinuria.

Neither immune complexes nor anti-GBM antibody can be demonstrated by immunofluorescence. However, the immunological pathogenesis of this condition is suggested by three factors:

- its response to steroids and immunosuppressive drugs
- its occurrence in Hodgkin's disease, with remission following successful treatment
- patients with the condition and family members having a higher incidence of asthma and eczema; remission following desensitization or antigen avoidance has been described.

A suggested explanation for the proteinuria is the production by T lymphocytes of a factor that increases glomerular permeability to protein.

Minimal-change nephropathy is most common in children, particularly males, accounting for the large majority of cases of nephrotic syndrome in childhood. The condition accounts for 20–25% of cases of adult nephrotic syndrome. It is often regarded as a condition which does not lead to chronic renal failure (but see focal sclerosis below).

Specific treatment is with corticosteroids, cyclophosphamide and ciclosporin (see p. 657).

IgA nephropathy

This is the most common form of glomerulonephritis seen world-wide, having replaced poststreptococcal glomerulonephritis in this respect. The disease consists of focal proliferative glomerulonephritis with mesangial deposits of IgA. In some cases IgG, IgM and C3 may also be seen in the glomerular mesangium. The disease may be a result of an exaggerated bone marrow and tonsillar IgA_1 immune response to viral or other antigens associated with an abnormality in O-linked glycosylation in the hinge region of the IgA_1 molecule. Such abnormal IgA_1 molecules may bind to other IgA_1 molecules or to fibronectin forming macromolecular aggregates which are cleared slowly from the circulation and become trapped passively in the glomerular mesangium.

IgA nephropathy tends to occur in children and young males. They present with asymptomatic microscopic haematuria or recurrent macroscopic haematuria sometimes following an upper respiratory or gastrointestinal viral infection. Proteinuria occurs and 5% can be nephrotic. The prognosis is usually good especially in those with normal blood pressure, normal renal function and absence of proteinuria at presentation. Surprisingly, recurrent macroscopic haematuria is a good prognostic sign although this may be due to 'lead-time bias' (p. 278), patients with overt haematuria coming to medical attention at an earlier stage of their illness.

Meta-analysis has not confirmed initial evidence suggesting a beneficial effect of fish oil. Claims of benefit have been made for corticosteroid treatment with or without immunosuppressive drugs but a meta-analysis of controlled trials provides no convincing evidence that benefit exceeds the risks of treatment. Approximately 20% of patients develop renal failure 20 years from the time of diagnosis. Mesangial IgA deposits are commonly found in the allografts of transplanted patients but loss of graft function as a result is uncommon.

Henoch–Schönlein syndrome

This clinical syndrome comprises a characteristic skin rash, abdominal colic, joint pain and glomerulonephritis. The rash is of purpuric type and the synonym Henoch–Schönlein purpura is often used. It occurs at all ages and in both sexes, but is mainly a disease of early childhood. Males are twice as often affected as females. A recent history of infection, often respiratory, is common. The disease is rare in adults. Serum concentrations of IgA are increased in about half the patients during the first 3 months of the disease and IgA-containing immune complexes have been detected in serum in a high proportion of cases. The renal lesion is a focal segmental proliferative glomerulonephritis, sometimes with mesangial hypercellularity. Epithelial crescents may be present. Immunoglobulin deposition, mainly of IgA, is seen in the glomerular mesangium and to a lesser extent in the capillary walls on immunofluorescence. IgG, IgM and components of the complement system may also be detectable. Electron-dense deposits, presumably immune complexes, are seen in the mesangium and subendothelial position on electron microscopy. No treatment is of proven benefit.

Goodpasture's syndrome (see also p. 403)

This rare condition is mediated by anti-GBM antibody (p. 601). It presents with recurrent haemoptysis and a severe progressive proliferative, often crescentic, glomerulonephritis. There is a strong association with HLA-DR2. Lung haemorrhage, which occurs more commonly in cigarette smokers, responds to repeated plasma exchange (which removes the anti-GBM antibody) combined with immunosuppressive therapy with cytotoxic drugs and corticosteroids. The effect of this treatment upon the glomerulonephritis is less clearcut; when oliguria occurs or serum creatinine rises above 600–700 µmol/L, renal failure is almost always irreversible.

Clinical features

Glomerulonephritis presents in one of four ways:

- asymptomatic proteinuria and/or microscopic haematuria
- acute nephritic syndrome (see below)
- nephrotic syndrome (p. 611)
- chronic renal failure (p. 642).

Asymptomatic proteinuria and/or microscopic haematuria is discovered incidentally, for example at a routine medical examination. Some causes of haematuria are shown in Figure 11.4. Overt haematuria may occur after exercise.

Investigations

Since false-positives are often obtained using Stix methods, the presence of significant proteinuria must be demonstrated by measuring the 24-hour urinary output of protein on two consecutive occasions (see p. 594).

Urine microscopy is performed to look for haematuria. A positive Stix test for blood may result from haematuria or haemoglobinuria. These can be differentiated on microscopy since red cells are seen only in patients with haematuria. Red cell morphology may provide a guide to diagnosis (see p. 596).

Further investigations will include:

- **urine microscopy** for red-cell casts
- **assessment of renal function** by estimation of serum urea, creatinine and endogenous creatinine clearance
- **renal imaging**, initially by excretion urography.

Acute nephritic syndrome

This comprises:

- haematuria (macroscopic or microscopic) – red-cell casts are typically seen on urine microscopy
- proteinuria
- hypertension
- oedema (periorbital, leg or sacral)
- oliguria
- uraemia.

Clinical features

In classical poststreptococcal glomerulonephritis the patient, usually a child, will have suffered a streptococcal infection 1–3 weeks before the onset of the acute nephritic syndrome. Streptococcal tonsillitis or pharyngitis, otitis media or cellulitis may be responsible.

The infecting organism is a Lancefield group A β-haemolytic streptococcus of a nephritogenic type. The latent interval between the infection and development of symptoms and signs of renal involvement reflects the time taken for immune complex formation and deposition and glomerular injury to occur.

Investigations

A list of investigations is given in Table 11.8.

If the clinical diagnosis of a nephritic illness is clear-cut (e.g. in poststreptococcal glomerulonephritis), renal imaging and renal biopsy are usually unnecessary. A biopsy is required if the diagnosis is uncertain, if the clinical features are unusual, or if renal failure is rapidly progressive, suggesting the presence of crescentic glomerulonephritis (RPGN).

Table 11.8
Investigation of acute nephritic syndrome

Investigations	Positive findings
Urine microscopy	Red cells, red-cell casts
Serum urea	May be elevated
Serum creatinine	May be elevated
Culture (throat swab, discharge from ear, swab from inflamed skin)	Nephritogenic organism – not always
Antistreptolysin-O titre	Elevated in poststreptococcal nephritis
C3 and C4 levels	May be reduced
Antinuclear antibody	Present in significant titre in systemic lupus erythematosus
ANCA	Positive in vasculitis
Anti-GBM	Positive in Goodpasture's syndrome
Cryoglobulins	Increased in cryoglobulinaemia
Creatinine clearance	Reduced
Urinary protein output	Increased
Chest X-ray	Cardiomegaly, pulmonary oedema (not always)
Renal imaging	Usually normal
Renal biopsy	Glomerulonephritis

Management

In the majority of patients with glomerulonephritis, neither corticosteroid nor immunosuppressive therapy is of benefit. The same applies to treatment with agents that alter coagulation and platelet function. Important exceptions to this general rule include glomerulonephritis complicating SLE, systemic vasculitides such as microscopic polyangiitis and Wegener's granulomatosis, Goodpasture's syndrome and some forms of rapidly progressive crescentic glomerulonephritis (see later), and probably idiopathic membranous nephropathy with progressive renal impairment.

As spontaneous remissions usually occur in acute glomerulonephritis, the aim of management is to prevent patients dying from pulmonary oedema, uraemia or hypertensive encephalopathy while awaiting improvement in renal function.

Hospital admission is advisable for all children with oliguria and marked hypertension; levels of blood pressure that are of no risk to adults may be associated with hypertensive fits in the young.

Otherwise, hospital admission is not mandatory, provided the general practitioner is able to visit daily to examine the patient and check blood pressure. Blood for measurement of urea or serum creatinine concentrations should be taken every few days.

Management in hospital

Most patients require:

- daily recording of fluid intake and output
- daily weighing (as a check on change in body fluid status)
- regular measurement of blood pressure.

Strict bed rest is unnecessary unless the patient feels ill, is severely hypertensive or has pulmonary oedema.

Dietary protein restriction is required only if severe uraemia occurs, but salt restriction is always necessary. In oliguric patients, fluid restriction is necessary to maintain body weight at a level at which severe hypertension, pulmonary congestion and gross oedema are prevented.

Mild-to-moderate hypertension and oedema may respond to salt restriction and diuretic therapy (e.g. furosemide (frusemide) given orally or parenterally). Other hypotensive agents may be required. β-Adrenergic receptor-blocking therapy should be used with caution for hypertension as it may precipitate pulmonary oedema in those on the brink of heart failure.

The prognosis in immune complex-mediated glomerulonephritis is improved if the antigen responsible can be eradicated. In patients with poststreptococcal glomerulonephritis, a course of penicillin should be given.

Management of life-threatening complications

Hypertensive encephalopathy (p. 1167)
In this condition the priorities are to maintain the airway and to reduce the blood pressure using a parenteral agent such as intravenous sodium nitroprusside or hydralazine. Fits should be controlled with parenteral diazepam (10 mg i.v.), but this may induce respiratory depression so facilities for resuscitation must be available.

Pulmonary oedema
This should be treated in the usual way (see p. 765). Because of the renal failure, high doses of potent diuretics such as furosemide (frusemide) given parenterally are required. If this fails to produce a diuresis, salt and water are removed osmotically by peritoneal dialysis, by haemofiltration, or by ultrafiltration during haemodialysis (see p. 653).

Severe uraemia
Peritoneal dialysis, haemodialysis or haemofiltration will be required pending recovery of the renal function.

Outbreak of poststreptococcal glomerulonephritis in a closed community
Prophylactic penicillin (phenoxymethyl penicillin 500 mg daily) should be given to all individuals at risk, provided they are not allergic to penicillin. If one member of a family living in overcrowded conditions develops the disorder, other members should be treated prophylactically. Evidence in support of long-term penicillin prophylaxis after the development of glomerulonephritis is lacking.

Prognosis
Poststreptococcal glomerulonephritis. The prognosis in children is excellent. A small number of adults develop hypertension and/or renal impairment later in life. Therefore in older patients, an annual blood pressure check, and less frequently an estimation of serum creatinine, is a reasonable precaution, even after apparent complete recovery.

Acute glomerulonephritis of unknown cause. The prognosis is less good and the need for follow-up is correspondingly greater.

Systemic vasculitides and progressive crescentic glomerulonephritis occurring in isolation. The prognosis is often poor and severe renal failure with oliguria and hypertension often occurs within a few weeks or months of the onset of the illness. This group of conditions constitute a nephrological emergency since specific treatment is beneficial (see p. 641).

Other glomerular disorders

Focal segmental glomerulosclerosis (FSGS)
This is a disease of unknown aetiology. It is particularly prone to recur in kidneys transplanted into affected individuals, sometimes within days of transplantation. A circulating factor may be involved. It presents as proteinuria or nephrotic syndrome and is usually resistant to steroid therapy. All age groups are affected.

On light microscopy, segmental glomerulosclerosis is seen, which later progresses to global sclerosis. The deep glomeruli at the corticomedullary junction are affected first. These may be missed on transcutaneous biopsy, leading to a mistaken diagnosis of a minimal-change glomerular lesion. In addition, some believe that a pathogenetic link exists between minimal-change nephropathy and focal glomerulosclerosis, and that a proportion of cases classified as having the former condition develop progressive renal impairment. Immunofluorescence may show deposits of C3 and IgM in affected portions of the glomerulus, but non-specific fixation to damaged tissue, rather than immune complex deposition, may well be the explanation for this.

About 50% of patients progress to end-stage renal failure within 10 years of diagnosis.

AIDS-associated nephropathy
A number of renal lesions have been described in association with HIV infection. These include glomerulonephritis of various histological types and the haemolytic uraemic syndrome. The most common histological abnormality is a focal glomerulosclerosis. A characteristic 'collapsed' appearance of glomeruli is often seen on light microscopy but is not unique to the condition. When renal failure supervenes, the prognosis is poor. Antiretroviral agents may result in stabilization of renal function (p. 148).

Familial glomerular diseases
Alport's syndrome
Alport's syndrome is a rare condition characterized by hereditary nephritis with haematuria, progressive renal failure and high-frequency nerve deafness. It is

principally expressed in males and both X-linked (mutation in COLIVα5 gene) and dominant modes of inheritance have been described. Some 15% of cases may have ocular abnormalities such as bilateral anterior lenticonus and macular and perimacular retinal flecks. In families with leiomyomas there is an additional mutation in the COLIVα6 gene. The disease is progressive and accounts for some 5% of cases of end-stage renal failure in childhood or adolescence. Anti-GBM antibody does not adhere normally to the glomerular basement membrane of affected individuals.

Congenital nephrotic syndrome
This syndrome is rare.

Thin glomerular basement membrane disease
The condition is inherited as an autosomal dominant and typically presents with microscopic haematuria. The diagnosis is made by renal biopsy when thinning and splitting of the glomerular capillary basement membrane is seen on electron microscopy. The condition is much commoner than previously believed, having been underdiagnosed owing to limited use of electron microscopy and technical difficulty in reliable measurement of glomerular basement membrane width. The prognosis for renal function is usually, but not invariably, good. No treatment is of known benefit.

FURTHER READING

Couser WG (1999) Glomerulonephritis. *Lancet* **353**: 1509–1513.

Feehally J (1997) IgA nephropathy: a disorder of IgA production? *Quarterly Journal of Medicine* **90**: 387–390.

Gaskin G (1997) Management of rapidly progressive glomerulonephritis. *Journal of the Royal College of Physicians* **31**: 15–18.

Mason PD (1997) The treatment of minimal change nephropathy and focal segmental glomerulosclerosis. *Journal of the Royal College of Physicians* **31**: 137–141.

Monnens LAH (2001) Thin glomerular basement membrane disease. *Kidney International* **60**: 799–800.

The kidney in systemic disease

Glomerulonephritis as a part of systemic vasculitis

Systemic lupus erythematosus (lupus glomerulonephritis) (see also p. 557)
The disease is much more common in females than in males and in black rather than white individuals. All varieties of histological abnormality are seen, ranging from a minimal-change lesion to crescentic glomerulonephritis. The World Health Organization classification of histological types is:

- Type I – Normal on light microscopy
- Type II – Mesangial change, whether seen on light microscopy or detectable only by immunological staining and/or electron microscopy
- Type III – Focal proliferative
- Type IV – Diffuse proliferative
- Type V – Membranous.

Serial renal biopsies show that in approximately 25% of patients, histological appearances alter from one histological classification to another during the interbiopsy interval. The prognosis is better in patients with Types I and V.

Pregnancy is associated with significant risk to the lupus patient, not only owing to hypertension and premature delivery, but also to more rapid progression of the glomerular lesion following delivery.

Whilst corticosteroid therapy improves the extrarenal manifestations of SLE, evidence is lacking that this treatment alters the renal prognosis. Both azathioprine and cyclophosphamide improve renal function, but long-term studies suggest that cyclophosphamide is better. There is no proof that intravenous 'pulse' cyclophosphamide treatment is safer or more efficacious than continuous oral therapy. Mycophenolate mofetil with prednisolone has recently been shown to be effective.

The indications for treatment vary. Those whose urine sediment contains many red cells and red-cell casts and those in whom renal function is impaired or is observed to deteriorate are strong candidates for treatment. A histological diagnosis should be obtained before commencing such potentially hazardous treatment.

Systemic vasculitides (see also p. 564)
In this group of disorders there is considerable overlap between individual varieties. The common feature is an immunologically mediated inflammation of vessels of varying size. Arthralgia or arthritis and a characteristic vasculitic rash (Fig. 11.17) may be present.

A major advance in understanding has followed the discovery of autoantibodies directed against constituents of the cytoplasm of normal human granulocytes and monocytes in patients with systemic vasculitis. Antineutrophil cytoplasmic antibodies (ANCA) are now established as a marker for vasculitides involving the kidney with or without signs of systemic disease. Two forms of ANCA can be demonstrated, proteinase-3 PR3-ANCA and myeloperoxidase MPO-ANCA. Binding of PR3-ANCA to neutrophils in indirect immunofluorescence assays produces a granular cytoplasmic stain – hence the use of the old term 'cytoplasmic c-ANCA'. MPO-ANCA produces a perinuclear stain – hence the old term 'perinuclear p-ANCA'. If ELISA and indirect immunofluorescence techniques are combined, diagnostic specificity is 99%.

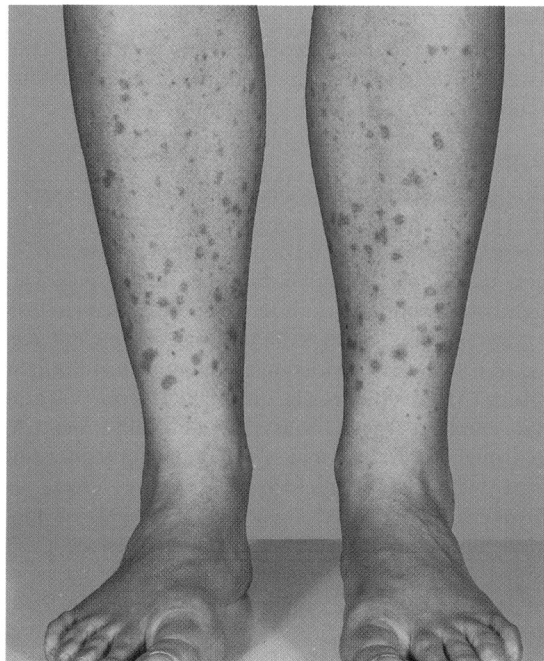

Fig. 11.17 Vasculitic rash.

PR3-ANCA positivity is found in the large majority of patients with active Wegener's granulomatosis and in up to 50% of patients with microscopic polyangiitis. Anti-MPO positivity is present in the majority of patients with idiopathic crescentic glomerulonephritis and in a variable number of cases of microscopic polyangiitis. Testing for antineutrophil cytoplasmic antibodies should be accompanied by appropriate tests of autoantibodies directed against DNA and the glomerular basement membrane antigen. The simultaneous occurrence of ANCA and anti-GMB antibody is well documented; such patients tend to follow the natural history of Goodpasture's disease. Whether ANCA is only a marker of disease or whether it takes part in the pathogenic process is undetermined. ANCA levels can be measured by enzyme-linked immunosorbent assay (ELISA) and variations in the ANCA titre have been used in the assessment of disease activity.

Polyarteritis nodosa (PAN) (see also p. 566)
Classical PAN is a multisystem disorder. Aneurysmal dilatation of medium-sized arteries may be seen on renal arteriography. The condition is more common in men and in the elderly and, typically, the patient is ANCA-negative. Hypertension and haematuria occur and renal failure is common.

Microscopic polyangiitis
In this condition, crescentic glomerulonephritis without immune complex deposition occurs with both PR3- and MPO-ANCA positivity. The lungs may be involved but granulomata are not seen.

Hepatitis B infection appears to be an aetiological factor in some cases.

Wegener's granulomatosis (see also p. 901)
In this condition, glomerulonephritis occurs together with necrotizing granulomatous lesions affecting the nasopharynx, lungs and kidneys. The necrotizing glomerular lesions do not appear to be due to immune complex deposition. PR3-ANCA positivity is the rule.

Treatment
The sooner treatment is instituted the more chance there is of recovery of renal function. Corticosteroids and cyclophosphamide are of benefit: pulsed high-dose methylprednisolone and plasmapheresis may reverse advanced disease. Once remission has been achieved, azathioprine or mycophenolate mofetil may be substituted for cyclophosphamide. Relapse after complete cessation of immunosuppressive therapy has been observed relatively frequently, and there is now a consensus that long-term, albeit relatively low-dose, immunosuppression is appropriate. Long-term follow-up of patients is mandatory. Intravenous immunoglobulin therapy shows promise in the treatment of severe and drug-resistant cases.

Cryoglobulinaemic renal disease
Cryoglobulins are immunoglobulins which precipitate reversibly in the cold. Three types are recognized.

In *type 1*, the cryoprecipitable immunoglobulin is a single monoclonal type, as is found in multiple myeloma and lymphoproliferative disorders.

Types 2 and 3 cryoglobulinaemias are mixed types. In each, a polyclonal IgG antigen is bound to an antiglobulin. In type 2, the antiglobulin component, which is usually of the IgM class, is monoclonal, while in type 3 it is polyclonal. Glomerular disease is more common in type 2 than type 3 cryoglobulinaemia. In approximately 30% of these 'mixed' cryoglobulinaemias, no underlying or associated disease is found (essential cryoglobulinaemia). Recognized associations include viral infections (hepatitis B and C, cytomegalovirus, Epstein–Barr infection), fungal and spirochaetal infections, malaria, infective endocarditis and autoimmune diseases (SLE, rheumatoid arthritis and Sjögren's syndrome).

Glomerular pathological changes include the following:

- There is endocapillary proliferation caused by leucocyte, mainly monocyte, infiltration.
- There are large, amorphous, PAS-positive, Congo-red-negative deposits within glomerular capillary lumina and on the inner side of the glomerular capillary membrane. On electron microscopy these have an amorphous or fibrillar appearance and appear to be composed of cryoglobulin.

- There is glomerular basement membrane thickening. There is an interstitial mononuclear leucocyte infiltration without much interstitial fibrosis. Vasculitis of small and medium-sized arteries may be present.

Presentation is usually in the fourth or fifth decades of life and women are more frequently affected than men. The majority of reported cases have been from Mediterranean countries. Systemic features include purpura, arthralgia, leg ulcers, Raynaud's phenomenon, evidence of systemic vasculitis, a polyneuropathy, and hepatic involvement. The glomerular disease presents typically as asymptomatic proteinuria, microscopic haematuria or both, but presentation with an acute nephritic syndrome or features of renal impairment also occurs.

Serological investigation reveals a reduction in concentration of early complement components with an elevation of later components.

Spontaneous remission occurs in about one-third of cases and approximately one-third pursue an indolent course. About 10–20% of patients progress to end-stage renal failure over several years. Corticosteroid and/or immunosuppressive therapy with cyclophosphamide may be of benefit, but evaluation of the efficacy of treatment is difficult owing to the rarity of the disease and the occurrence of spontaneous remissions. Intensive plasma exchange or cryofiltration has been used in selected cases.

Renal involvement in other diseases

Diabetes mellitus
Renal disease is a major complication of diabetes; it is discussed on page 1095.

Systemic sclerosis (see also p. 561)
Interlobular renal arteries are affected with intimal thickening, and fibrinoid changes occur in afferent glomerular arterioles. Glomerular changes are non-specific. The pathogenesis is unknown and neither steroid nor immunosuppressive therapy is of value. Serum ANCA is not present. Treatment with ACE-inhibitor drugs is of benefit, reducing proteinuria and in some cases halting or even partially reversing decline in renal function. 'Scleroderma renal crisis' is a term applied to rapid loss of renal function owing to rapid progression of renal microvascular disease in this condition. Early ACE inhibitor treatment may be of benefit, as may continuous intravenous infusion of prostacyclin. ACE inhibitors oppose the angiotensin II-induced vasoconstriction. The vasodilatory action of prostacyclin is responsible for its effectiveness.

Amyloidosis
The kidney is often affected in amyloidosis (see p. 1118). Presentation is with asymptomatic proteinuria, nephrotic syndrome or renal failure.

Pathology
On light microscopy, eosinophilic deposits are seen in the mesangium, capillary loops and arteriolar walls. Staining with Congo red renders these deposits pink and they show green birefringence under polarized light. Immunofluorescence is unhelpful, but on electron microscopy the characteristic fibrils of amyloid can be seen. Amyloid consisting of immunoglobulin light chains (AL amyloid) can be distinguished from the protein found in secondary amyloid (amyloid protein A, AA amyloid). AL amyloid is found in disorders associated with lymphoproliferative diseases such as myeloma, Waldenström's macroglobulinaemia or non-Hodgkin's lymphoma. It is also present in cases of so-called primary amyloidosis where an abnormal clone of cells is presumed to be responsible, although at present not identifiable. AA amyloid is found following long-standing inflammatory conditions such as suppurative infections, rheumatoid arthritis and familial Mediterranean fever.

Diagnosis and treatment
The diagnosis can often be made clinically when features of amyloidosis are present elsewhere. On imaging, the kidneys are often large. Renal biopsy is necessary in doubtful cases.

Treatment of the underlying cause should be undertaken. In primary amyloid, treatment also used in myeloma such as corticosteroids and melphalan and bone marrow transplantation may be of benefit. The success of dialysis and kidney transplantation is dependent upon the extent of amyloid deposition in extrarenal sites, especially the heart.

Haemolytic uraemic syndrome (HUS)
HUS is characterized by intravascular haemolysis with red-cell fragmentation (microangiopathic haemolysis), thrombocytopenia and acute renal failure. The syndrome often follows a febrile illness, particularly gastroenteritis or upper respiratory tract infection. A few particular strains of pathogenic *Escherichia coli*, notably strain O157, have been isolated in many cases and in outbreaks of the disease. It has been suggested that infection triggers endothelial damage and that derangements of the haemostatic coagulation system then occur in susceptible individuals. Recurrent episodes of HUS have been described in the same individual, and familial forms of the disease (with both recessive and dominant inheritance) exist. It is suggested that the non-induced diarrhoeal form of HUS may be a complement-driven illness related to deficiency of complement factor H. Fibrin deposition is seen in the vascular

endothelium, particularly in the renal arterioles and glomerular capillaries. Most children recover spontaneously, although a proportion never recover normal renal function or, having apparently done so, develop hypertension and renal impairment in later years. Mortality rates are higher in the elderly as was demonstrated during the *E. coli* O157-associated outbreak of haemolytic uraemic syndrome in Scotland in 1996/97.

Treatment with heparin, inhibitors of platelet aggregation, synthetic prostacyclins, infusion of fresh-frozen plasma and plasma exchange have been employed, but controlled trials of treatment are lacking. It has been proposed that antibiotic treatment of *E. coli* O157 infections increases the risk of development of HUS.

Thrombotic thrombocytopenic purpura (TTP) (p. 459)

TTP is characterized by the presence of widespread hyaline thrombi in small vessels. Young adults are most commonly affected. Microangiopathic haemolysis, renal failure and evidence of neurological disturbance are characteristically found. It is now believed that the pathogenesis of TTP differs from that of HUS. In TTP only, there is deficiency of (or the presence of auto-antibody to) the protease enzyme which cleaves von Willebrand factor. Controlled trials are lacking but there is a consensus that repeated plasma exchange is beneficial in TTP. Infusion of fresh plasma may also be of benefit. Some patients with TTP have underlying SLE or polyangiitis.

Multiple myeloma

Acute renal failure is relatively common in myeloma, occurring in 2–8% of affected individuals. Histological appearances may be simply those of acute tubular necrosis; tubular blockage by Tamm–Horsfall glycoprotein, light chains and immunoglobulin may be apparent. Dehydration and the administration of intravenous or intra-arterial contrast medium to the volume-depleted patient with myeloma predispose to the development of acute renal failure.

In myeloma, free κ and λ light chains are excreted. Blockage of tubules by casts composed in part at least of light chains, and their toxic effects upon tubular cells, account for the proteinuria and chronic renal impairment associated with 'myeloma kidney'. Renal amyloid deposition often complicates myeloma, accounting both for proteinuria – sometimes of nephrotic proportions – and chronic renal failure.

Hypercalcaemia, renal sepsis and (rarely) urinary tract obstruction due to bulky myeloma deposits are further causes of renal impairment in myelomatosis.

Idiopathic fibrillary glomerulopathy

In this rare condition, characteristic microfibrillary structures are seen on electron microscopy in the absence of overt myeloma or amyloidosis. No treatment is known to be of benefit, although isolated instances of apparent response to corticosteroid and immuno-suppressive therapy have been reported.

Contrast nephropathy

In patients with impaired renal function, iodinated radiological contrast media may be nephrotoxic, possibly by causing renal vasoconstriction and by a direct toxic effect upon renal tubules. The effect is dose-dependent and therefore more commonly seen in procedures which require large amounts of contrast media such as angiography with or without angioplasty. In many patients the effect is mild, transient, fully reversible and of no clinical significance. The risk and severity of contrast nephropathy is amplified by the presence of hypovolaemia and renal impairment, especially if due to diabetic nephropathy. Diabetes per se is not a risk factor.

Prevention involves minimization as far as possible of the dose of contrast employed and use of low-osmolality contrast medium. The only proven preventative measure is prevention of hypovolaemia before administration of contrast. Pre-hydration with intravenous saline is of proven benefit. A popular regimen involves infusion of 1 litre of saline during the 12 hours before and 12 hours after contrast exposure. Care must be taken to avoid volume overload in susceptible patients. Recent evidence that acetylcysteine may be of benefit in preventing worsening of pre-existing renal impairment following intravenous contrast requires confirmation.

When deterioration in renal function occurs after intra-arterial injection of contrast (for example, after coronary angiography) it may be difficult to differentiate the effects of contrast-induced damage from those of atheromatous embolization (see p. 624). The latter carries a worse prognosis.

FURTHER READING

Baker CSR, Baker LRI (2001) Prevention of contrast nephropathy after cardiac catheterization. *Heart* **85**: 361–362.

Hawkins PN, Wootton R, Pepys MB (1990) Metabolic studies of radioiodinated serum amyloid P component in normal subjects and patients with systemic amyloidosis. *Journal of Clinical Investigation* **86**: 1862–1869.

Jennette JC, Falk RJ (1997) Small vessel vasculitis. *New England Journal of Medicine* **337**: 1512–1523.

Savage COS, Harper L, Adu T (1997) Primary systemic vasculitis. *Lancet* **349**: 553–558.

Nephrotic syndrome

The nephrotic syndrome consists of heavy urinary protein loss, hypoalbuminaemia and oedema. Hyper-cholesterolaemia is almost always present.

Pathophysiology

Urinary protein loss of the order 3–5 g daily or more in an adult is required to cause hypoalbuminaemia. In children, proportionately less proteinuria results in hypoalbuminaemia.

The normal dietary protein intake in the UK is of the order 70 g daily and the normal liver can synthesize albumin at a rate of 10–12 g daily. How then does a urinary protein loss of the order of 3–5 g daily result in hypoalbuminaemia? The explanation appears to be that in normal individuals there is some catabolism within the kidney of albumin filtered at the glomeruli. In nephrotic patients with heavy proteinuria, catabolism is substantially increased, limiting the amount of protein appearing in the urine and concealing the extent of protein loss through the glomerulus.

The mechanism of the proteinuria is complex. It occurs partly because structural damage to the glomerular basement membrane leads to an increase in the size and number of pores, allowing passage of more and larger molecules. Electrical charge is also involved in glomerular permeability. Fixed negatively charged components are present in the glomerular capillary wall, which repel negatively charged protein molecules. Reduction of this fixed charge occurs in glomerular disease and appears to be an important factor in the genesis of heavy proteinuria.

Pathogenesis of oedema in hypoalbuminaemia

The pathogenesis of the oedema is incompletely understood. A conventional explanation is that a reduction in the concentration of osmotically active albumin molecules in the blood results in a reduction in the oncotic force that retains fluid within blood vessels, and salt and water escape into the extravascular compartment; i.e. oedema occurs. Such loss of salt and water results in a fall in blood volume and a reduction in pressure within afferent glomerular arterioles. This activates the renin–angiotensin–aldosterone system (see p. 670). The consequent hyperaldosteronism promotes sodium and water reabsorption in the distal nephron, increasing the tendency to oedema.

Unfortunately, this explanation does not fit the facts. Plasma renin activity in nephrotic patients is often normal and measured blood volume may be normal or high in nephrotic patients, even those without renal failure. Moreover, sodium retention by the kidney in minimal-change nephropathy has been shown to occur before the development of hypoalbuminaemia. Intrarenal mechanisms of salt retention are presumably involved in this situation.

Causes

All types of glomerulonephritis can produce the nephrotic syndrome. Although proliferative glomerulonephritis is more common than membranous disease, the latter is the most common form of glomerulonephritis to cause nephrotic syndrome in adults in the UK (Table 11.9).

Table 11.9
Causes of the nephrotic syndrome

All glomerulonephritides and minimal-change glomerular lesions
Systemic vasculitides, mainly systemic lupus erythematosus
Diabetic glomerulosclerosis
Amyloidosis
Drugs
Allergies

Minimal-change glomerular disease accounts for most cases of the nephrotic syndrome in childhood compared with approximately 20% of adult cases. In tropical areas, minimal change is present in fewer than 10% of nephrotic children owing to the high incidence of nephrotic syndrome due to infections such as malaria. Minimal-change disease does not progress to chronic renal failure (see p. 604).

Diabetic glomerular disease (p. 1095) can also cause the nephrotic syndrome. The histological lesion seen on light microscopy in diabetes may comprise amorphous nodular deposits (which are not immune complexes) in the glomeruli or a diffuse glomerulosclerosis. There is associated glomerular basement membrane thickening.

Diabetes is also a cause of renal papillary necrosis, but patients with this lesion alone do not have sufficiently heavy proteinuria to become nephrotic.

Drug reactions

Many drugs can cause sufficiently heavy proteinuria to result in the nephrotic syndrome. Penicillamine, which in all probability combines with a plasma protein to form an antigenic hapten, induces an immune complex-mediated membranous glomerulonephritis, as may high-dose captopril. Various metals, whether used therapeutically (e.g. gold) or in industry (e.g. mercury and cadmium), can induce proteinuria severe enough to cause the nephrotic syndrome.

Allergic reactions

Reactions to many allergens such as poison ivy, pollens, bee stings and cows' milk may be associated with the nephrotic syndrome, but evidence of a causal relationship is lacking in most cases.

Most lists of causes of the nephrotic syndrome include renal vein thrombosis, but this is probably a complication rather than a cause of the syndrome. It is particularly likely to complicate membranous glomerulonephritis. In nephrotic patients the blood is more coagulable than normal and the circulation may be sluggish owing to hypovolaemia, both of which are likely to induce thrombosis. Estimates of the incidence of this complication range from 5% to approximately 50% in nephrotic syndrome due to membranous glomerulonephritis.

Renal disorders not associated with the nephrotic syndrome

Proteinuria severe enough to cause the nephrotic syndrome is not a feature of reflux nephropathy (chronic atrophic pyelonephritis), chronic tubulointerstitial nephritis, renal tuberculosis, polycystic disease, or many other renal disorders.

Clinical features

The history may provide clues to the aetiology, such as exposure to a drug or allergen. Patients with a minimal-change lesion may give a history or family history of atopy. There may be a family history of renal disease.

Patients with heavy proteinuria may have noted that their urine has been frothy; the onset of the renal lesion can be timed from this observation.

Examination will reveal oedema; ascites may also be present, particularly in children. Genital oedema is sometimes seen. The oedema may involve the face (periorbital oedema) and arms. Neither elevation of the jugular venous pressure nor pulmonary oedema are features of the nephrotic syndrome, though either or both may be present if renal and/or cardiac failure are present in the nephrotic patient.

Features of the underlying disorder may be evident, such as the butterfly facial rash of SLE or the neuropathy and retinopathy associated with diabetes mellitus.

The following must be excluded:

- *primary cardiac failure* – here, the venous pressure is high, oedema is not usually present in the face, and the proteinuria is less severe
- *liver disease*, and other causes of hypoalbuminaemia (Table 11.10), with oedema and ascites.

Investigations

The presence of the nephrotic syndrome is established by measuring:

- **24-hour urinary protein** – usually more than 3–5 g daily in adults
- **serum albumin concentration** – usually less than 30 g/L.

Increased hepatic albumin synthesis is accompanied by increased cholesterol synthesis and there is an approximate reciprocal relationship between the serum albumin and the serum cholesterol concentration. Low-density lipoprotein (LDL) cholesterol concentrations are elevated,

---

Table 11.10
Causes of hypoalbuminaemia

Inadequate protein intake: protein–energy malnutrition
Failure of protein production: liver disease
Excessive protein loss: nephrotic syndrome, protein-losing enteropathy, extensive burns
Pregnancy

---

but high-density lipoprotein (HDL) cholesterol is usually normal. Hypertriglyceridaemia is present in about 50% of patients.

Renal function is assessed by measuring:

- **serum urea and creatinine**
- **creatinine clearance**, to determine the GFR.

Further investigations are required to elucidate the cause:

- *Microscopy* of the urine may show red cells and red-cell casts; the latter are virtually diagnostic of glomerulonephritis. Minimal-change lesions do not usually result in red cells or red-cell casts in the urine.
- *Throat swab* and serum ASO titre may show evidence of streptococcal infection.
- *Serum C3 complement* concentrations may be decreased in immune complex-mediated glomerulonephritis.
- *Presence of antinuclear antibody* may suggest SLE. A search for extractable nuclear antigens and/or antibody to double-stranded DNA should be made if antinuclear antibody is detected. A positive test for ANCA (see p. 608) will suggest a systemic vasculitis, and detection of anti-GBM antibody leads to the diagnosis of Goodpasture's syndrome.
- *Screening for hepatitis B surface antigen and hepatitis C antibody.*
- *Cryoglobulinaemia* can be detected if blood is taken and placed immediately in a water bath at 37°C before testing. Cold-precipitable globulins may be found, for example, when nephrotic syndrome is associated with a malignant lymphoproliferative disorder or hepatitis C infection.
- *Serum electrophoresis.* In the nephrotic syndrome there is always a reduced serum albumin, commonly with an increase in the α- and β-globulin fractions (Fig. 11.18) on serum electrophoresis. In myeloma, a monoclonal paraprotein band is present and there may be associated immune paresis with reduction in the concentration of one or more of IgG, IgA or IgM proteins. Abnormal protein constituents will be found on electrophoresis of urine. Ten per cent of patients with myeloma have renal amyloid deposition.
- *Raised blood glucose* indicates diabetes mellitus.
- *Selective protein clearance* may be measured. Blood and urine samples are taken at the same time; a timed urine collection is not required. The clearance of large-molecular-weight protein such as IgG is compared with that of a smaller molecule such as albumin or transferrin. A low ratio (selective protein leak) is found in minimal-change glomerulopathy, early diabetes and renal amyloidosis. Severe glomerulonephritides (e.g. diffuse proliferative glomerulonephritis with crescent formation) are more typically associated with an unselective protein leak. Overlap between the groups exists.

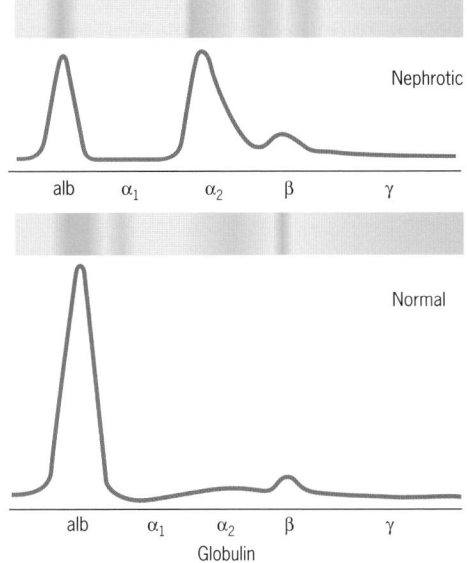

Fig. 11.18 **Serum electrophoresis in a normal person and in a patient with nephrotic syndrome.** Note the reduced albumin and increased α- and β-globulin in the nephrotic patient.

Measurement of selective protein clearance is unnecessary if renal biopsy is to be carried out. Its main use is in children in whom a minimal-change lesion is suspected. An unselective protein leak in such a child would bring this diagnosis into question and might prompt renal biopsy (see below).

Renal biopsy (see also p. 600)

Transcutaneous biopsy is performed to make a histological diagnosis when management will be affected, particularly when the major question is whether a steroid-sensitive minimal-change lesion is present or not. It is *not* indicated in three groups of patients:

- *in young children* (particularly males) who have a highly selective protein leak, no hypertension and no red cells or red-cell casts in the urine (the diagnosis is almost certain to be a minimal-change lesion, so a trial of steroids should be instituted first)
- *in long-standing, insulin-dependent diabetics* with associated retinopathy or neuropathy, since the diagnosis is in little doubt
- *in patients on drugs* such as penicillamine, which should be stopped first.

Management
General measures

Initial treatment should be with dietary sodium restriction and a thiazide diuretic (e.g. bendrofluazide). Unresponsive patients require furosemide (frusemide) 40–120 mg daily with the addition of amiloride (5 mg daily), but the serum potassium concentration should be monitored carefully. Nephrotic patients may malabsorb diuretics (as well as other drugs) owing to gut mucosal oedema. Resistance to oral diuretic treatment may demand parenteral administration for a time. Patients are sometimes hypovolaemic, and moderate oedema may have to be accepted in order to avoid postural hypotension.

A high-protein diet (approximately 80–90 g protein daily) confers no benefit and normal protein intake is advisable.

Infusion of albumin produces only a transient effect and is normally employed only in diuretic-resistant patients and those with oliguria and uraemia in the absence of severe glomerular damage, such as those with minimal-change nephropathy. Such infusion is combined with diuretic therapy. Diuresis, when once initiated in this way, often continues with diuretic treatment alone.

Specific measures

The aim is to reverse the abnormal urinary protein leak.

Minimal-change glomerular lesion

High-dose corticosteroid therapy with prednisolone 60 mg daily (dose corrected to a normal body surface area of 1.73 m^2) for 8 weeks corrects the urinary protein leak in more than 95% of children. Response rates in adults are significantly lower and response may occur only after many months of steroid therapy. Spontaneous remission also occurs and steroid therapy should, in general, be withheld if urinary protein loss is insufficient to cause hypoalbuminaemia or oedema.

In both children and adults, if remission lasts for 4 years after steroid therapy, further relapse is very rare. In children, approximately one-third do not subsequently relapse, but in the remainder further courses of corticosteroids are indicated. One-third of these patients relapse regularly on steroid withdrawal and in these patients remission is induced with steroid therapy once more and a course of cyclophosphamide 3 mg/kg daily is given for 6–8 weeks. This increases the likelihood of long-term remission. Steroid-unresponsive patients may also respond to cyclophosphamide. No more than two courses of cyclophosphamide should be prescribed in children because of the risk of side-effects, which include azoospermia.

An alternative to cyclophosphamide is ciclosporin, which is effective but must be continued long term to prevent relapse on stopping treatment. Excretory function and ciclosporin blood levels must be monitored carefully as ciclosporin is potentially nephrotoxic.

Membranous glomerulonephritis

This is discussed on page 604.

Other causes

Remission occurs if the underlying disease can be treated. In patients with SLE, treatment with steroids and cyclophosphamide or azathioprine usually induces long-term remission.

When the glomerular lesion causing the nephrotic syndrome progresses and the GFR declines, the degree of proteinuria often diminishes so that the hypoalbuminaemia and oedema improve.

Prevention, and management of complications
Venous thrombosis
Hypovolaemia and a hypercoagulable state predispose to venous thrombosis. The hypercoagulable state is due to loss of clotting factors (e.g. antithrombin) in the urine and an increased hepatic production of fibrinogen. Prolonged bed rest should therefore be avoided.

Once renal vein thrombosis has occurred, prolonged anticoagulation is required. Thromboembolism is exceptionally common in nephrotic syndrome due to membranous glomerulonephritis, and in the absence of any contraindication, long-term prophylactic anticoagulation is indicated.

Sepsis
Sepsis is an important cause of death in nephrotic patients. The increased susceptibility to infection is partly due to loss of immunoglobulin in the urine. Pneumococcal infections are particularly common and pneumococcal vaccine should be given.

Early detection and aggressive treatment of infections, rather than long-term antibiotic prophylaxis, is the best approach.

Oliguric renal failure
A low blood volume and hypotension may lead to underperfused kidneys. Acute tubular necrosis may therefore readily develop when renal ischaemia occurs from other complications such as blood loss or septicaemia. In some patients, uraemia appears to result from derangements in renal perfusion in the absence of hypotension.

Albumin infusion combined with mannitol or another diuretic may initiate a diuresis in oliguric renal failure.

Lipid abnormalities
It is suggested that these are responsible for an increase in the risk of myocardial infarction or peripheral vascular disease. Treatment of hypercholesterolaemia is best with an HMG-CoA reductase inhibitor (p. 1111).

FURTHER READING

Baker LRI (1995) Salt, water and the kidney. *Lancet* **346**: 133–134.

Oliveira DBG (1998) Membranous nephropathy: an IgG4-mediated disease. *Lancet* **351**: 617–671.

Orth SR, Ritz E (1998) The nephrotic syndrome. *New England Journal of Medicine* **338**: 1202–1211.

Ponticelli C et al. (1992) Methylprednisolone plus chlorambucil compared with methylprednisolone alone for treatment of idiopathic membranous nephropathy. *New England Journal of Medicine* **327**: 599–603.

Urinary tract infection

Urinary tract infection (UTI) is common in women, uncommon in men and of special importance in children. Recurrent infection causes considerable morbidity; if complicated, it can cause severe renal disease including end-stage renal failure. It is also a common source of life-threatening Gram-negative septicaemia.

Pathogenesis
Infection is most often due to bacteria from the patient's own bowel flora (Table 11.11). Transfer to the urinary tract may be via the bloodstream, the lymphatics or by direct extension (e.g. from a vesicocolic fistula), but is most often via the ascending transurethral route (Fig. 11.19). For the latter route, three important steps are involved.

First, the lower vagina and periurethral area is heavily colonized by uropathogenic bacteria. This is facilitated by the adhesion of bacteria to uroepithelial surfaces by pili or fimbriae present on the bacterial cell surface. Previous UTIs may also predispose to further colonization which may not be eliminated by treatment of the

Table 11.11
Organisms causing urinary tract infection in domiciliary practice

Organism	Approximate frequency (%)
Escherichia coli and other 'coliforms'	68+
Proteus mirabilis	12
*Klebsiella aerogenes**	4
*Enterococcus faecalis**	6
Staphylococcus saprophyticus or *epidermidis†*	10

* More common in hospital practice
† More common in young women (20–30%)

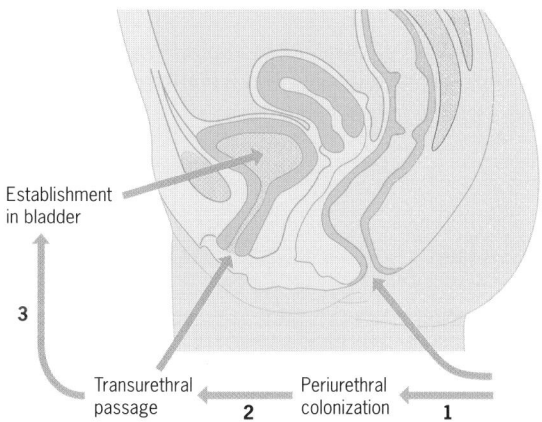

Fig. 11.19 Ascending infection of the urinary tract.

infection, initiating a vicious circle. Important factors contributing to colonization include use of a diaphragm and spermicidal jelly, hormone-deficient vaginal atrophy, and systemic antibiotic treatment for non-urinary tract infections. There is little evidence that personal hygiene affects colonization, but the use of bubble baths may be a contributory factor.

Second, bacteria are transferred along the urethra to the bladder. This step is facilitated by sexual intercourse or catheterization. Spontaneous transfer along the short female urethra is easy, while the longer male urethra protects against transfer of bacteria to the bladder; in addition, prostatic fluid has defensive bactericidal properties.

The third is the establishment and multiplication of bacteria within the bladder. Bladder urine is normally sterile, owing to defence mechanisms within the bladder. These include hydrokinetic and bladder mucosal factors and constituents of urine. A low flow rate and infrequent and poor bladder emptying predispose to infection.

Mucosal defence mechanisms are poorly understood. The establishment of infection may be facilitated by fimbriated bacteria adhering to the bladder uroepithelium or previous damage to this epithelium. A thin layer of mucopolysaccharide coats the transitional epithelial cells and prevents adhesion of bacteria. Loss or depletion of this layer because of previous infection, bladder trauma from catheterization or vigorous intercourse may predispose to infection.

The first phase in the development of UTI is the entry and establishment of bacteria within the bladder. Extension of infection up the ureters to the kidneys is relatively easy and is facilitated by vesicoureteric reflux and dilated hypotonic ureters. Once infection is established it can pass up or down the system quite readily.

Natural history
UTI is commonly an isolated, rather than a repeated event (Fig. 11.20).

Complicated versus uncomplicated infection
(Fig. 11.21)
It is necessary to distinguish between UTI occurring in patients with functionally normal urinary tracts and in those with abnormal tracts.

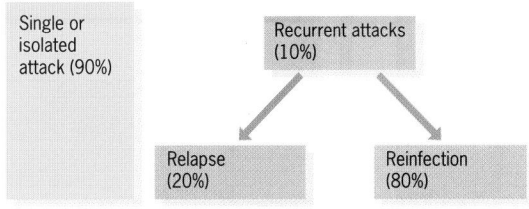

Fig. 11.20 The natural history of urinary tract infection.

Functionally normal urinary tracts (with normal excretion urography). Here, persistent or recurrent infection seldom results in serious kidney damage (uncomplicated UTI).

Abnormal urinary tracts. Tracts with stones, or associated diseases such as diabetes mellitus which themselves cause kidney damage, may be made worse with infection (complicated UTI). UTI, particularly with *Proteus*, may predispose to stone formation. The combination of infection and obstruction results in severe, sometimes rapid, kidney damage (obstructive pyonephrosis) and is an important cause of Gram-negative septicaemia.

Acute pyelonephritis
Localization studies have shown that distinguishing between upper and lower urinary tract infection on clinical grounds can be inaccurate. However, the combination of fever, loin pain and tenderness and significant bacteriuria is usually regarded as indicating bacterial infection of the kidney (acute pyelonephritis). Small renal cortical abscesses and streaks of pus in the renal medulla are often present. Histologically there is focal infiltration by polymorphonuclear leucocytes and many polymorphs in tubular lumina.

Although with antibiotics significant permanent kidney damage in adults with normal urinary tracts is rare, CT scanning, however, can show wedge-shaped areas of inflammation in the renal cortex (Fig. 11.22) and hence damage to renal function.

Reflux nephropathy
This was called chronic pyelonephritis or atrophic pyelonephritis and it results from a combination of:

* vesicoureteric reflux, and
* infection acquired in infancy or early childhood.

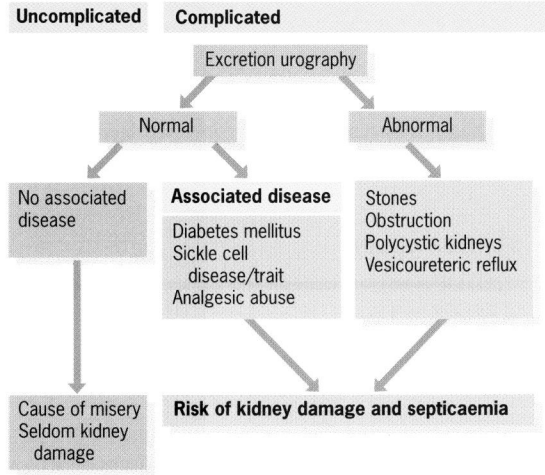

Fig. 11.21 Complicated versus uncomplicated urinary tract infection.

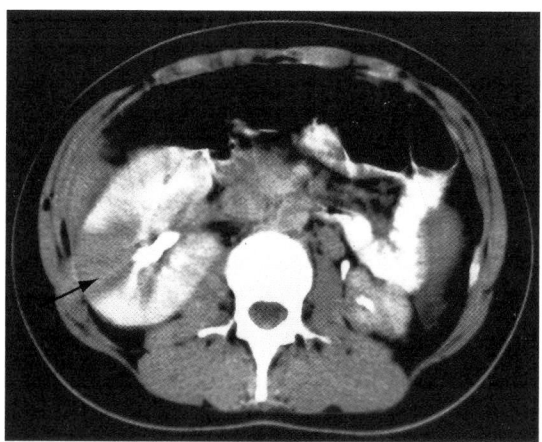

Fig. 11.22 CT scan showing a wedge-shaped area of renal cortical loss (arrow) following acute pyelonephritis.

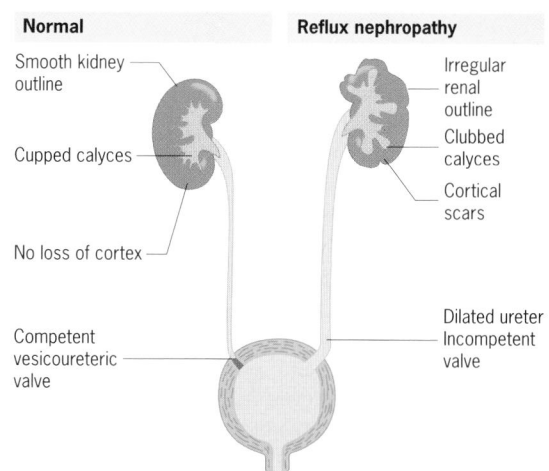

Fig. 11.23 Excretion urography findings in reflux nephropathy compared with normal.

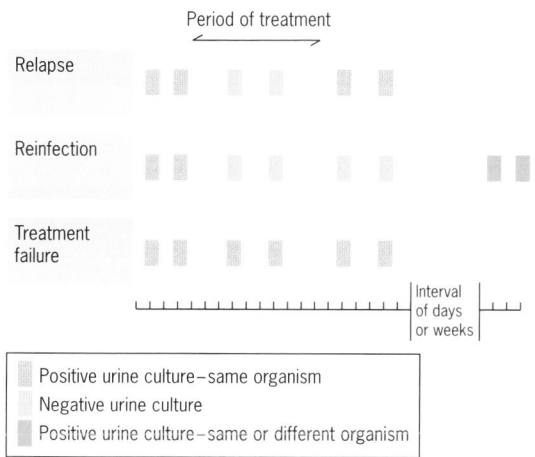

Fig. 11.24 A comparison of reinfection, relapse and treatment failure in urinary tract infection.

Normally the vesicoureteric junction acts as a one-way valve (Fig. 11.23), urine entering the bladder from above; the ureter is shut off during bladder contraction, thus preventing reflux of urine. In some infants and children – possibly even in utero – this valve mechanism is incompetent, bladder voiding being associated with variable reflux of a jet of urine up the ureter. A secondary consequence is incomplete bladder emptying, as refluxed urine returns to the bladder after voiding. This latter event predisposes to infection, and the reflux of infected urine leads to kidney damage.

Typically there is papillary damage, interstitial nephritis and cortical scarring in areas adjacent to 'clubbed calyces'. Diagnosis is based on excretion urography, which shows irregular renal outlines, clubbed calyces and a variable reduction in renal size. The condition may be unilateral or bilateral and affect all or part of the kidney.

Reflux usually ceases around puberty with growth of the bladder base. Damage already done persists and progressive renal fibrosis and further loss of function occurs in severe cases even though there is no further infection. This condition does not develop in the absence of reflux and does not begin in adult life. Adult females with bacteriuria and a normal urogram can be reassured that kidney damage due to reflux nephropathy will not develop. Chronic reflux nephropathy acquired in infancy predisposes to hypertension in later life and, if severe, is a relatively common cause of end-stage renal failure in childhood or adult life. Meticulous early detection and control of infection, with or without ureteral reimplantation to create a competent valve, can prevent further scarring and allow normal growth of the kidneys. No proof exists that reimplantation surgery confers benefit. Only one small adequately controlled trial of surgery plus medical treatment versus medical treatment alone is available. No benefit was observed in the operated group.

Reinfection versus relapsing infection

When UTI is recurrent it is necessary to distinguish between relapse and reinfection.

Relapse is diagnosed by recurrence of bacteriuria with the same organism within 7 days of completion of antibacterial treatment and implies failure to eradicate infection (Fig. 11.24). It usually occurs in conditions in which it is difficult to eradicate the bacteria, such as stones, scarred kidneys, polycystic disease or bacterial prostatitis.

Reinfection is when bacteriuria is absent after treatment for at least 14 days, usually longer, followed by recurrence of infection with the same or different organisms. This is not due to failure to eradicate infection, but is the result of reinvasion of a susceptible tract with new organisms. Approximately 80% of recurrent infections are due to reinfection.

Symptoms and signs

The most typical symptoms of UTI are:

- frequency of micturition by day and night
- painful voiding (dysuria)
- suprapubic pain and tenderness
- haematuria
- smelly urine.

These symptoms relate to bladder and urethral inflammation, commonly called 'cystitis', and suggest lower urinary tract infection. Loin pain and tenderness, with fever and systemic upset, suggest extension of the infection to the pelvis and kidney, known as pyelitis or pyelonephritis. However, localization of the site of infection on the basis of symptoms alone is unreliable.

UTI may also be present with minimal or no symptoms or may be associated with atypical symptoms such as abdominal pain, fever or haematuria in the absence of frequency or dysuria.

In small children, who cannot complain of dysuria, symptoms are often 'atypical'. The possibility of UTI must always be considered in the fretful, febrile sick child who fails to thrive.

Diagnosis

Diagnosis is based on quantitative culture of a clean-catch mid-stream specimen of urine and the presence or absence of pyuria. The criteria for the diagnosis of UTI, particularly in symptomatic women, are shown in Table 11.12. A diagnosis based on rigid adherence to a bacterial count of at least 10^5 organisms per millilitre of urine in symptomatic women is incorrect. Diagnosis of 'low count bacteriuria' ($\geq 10^2$ organisms) demands additionally the presence of pyuria. Many laboratories cannot report bacterial counts under 10^4 per mL. In doubtful cases of 'low count bacteriuria', and especially when recurrent, urine should be obtained by suprapubic aspiration when any growth of a uropathogenic organism is evidence of infection.

Table 11.12
Criteria for diagnosis of bacteriuria

Symptomatic young women
$\geq 10^2$ coliform organisms/mL urine plus pyuria
 (> 10 WCC/mm³)

OR

$\geq 10^5$ any pathogenic organism/mL urine

OR

any growth of pathogenic organisms in urine by
 suprapubic aspiration

Symptomatic men
$\geq 10^3$ pathogenic organisms/mL urine

Asymptomatic patients
$\geq 10^5$ pathogenic organisms/mL of urine on two occasions

---

Dipstick tests can be used to detect nitrites in urine. Most Gram-negative organisms reduce nitrates to nitrites and produce a red colour in the reagent square. False-negative results are common. Dipsticks that detect significant pyuria depend on the release of esterases from leucocytes. Dipstick tests *positive for both nitrite and leucocyte esterase* are *highly predictive* of acute infection.

Abacteriuric frequency or dysuria ('urethral syndrome')

Causes of truly abacteriuric frequency/dysuria include postcoital bladder trauma, vaginitis, atrophic vaginitis or urethritis in the elderly, and interstitial cystitis (Hunner's ulcer). In symptomatic young women with 'sterile pyuria', *Chlamydia* infection and tuberculosis must be excluded.

Interstitial cystitis is an uncommon but distressing complaint, most often affecting women over the age of 40 years. It presents with frequency, dysuria and often severe suprapubic pain. Urine cultures are sterile. Cystoscopy shows typical inflammatory changes with ulceration of the bladder base. The cause is unclear but it is commonly thought to be an autoimmune disorder. Various treatments are advocated with variable success. These include oral prednisolone therapy, bladder instillation of sodium cromoglicate and bladder stretching under anaesthesia.

Careful history-taking will identify a group with predominant frequency and passage of small volumes of urine who have 'irritable bladders', possibly consequent on previous UTI or conditioned by psychosexual factors. Such patients must be distinguished from those with frequency due to polyuria. Repeated courses of antibiotics in patients with genuine abacteriuric frequency or dysuria are quite inappropriate and detract from identifying the true nature of the problem.

Special investigations
Excretion urography

Excretion urography is not indicated in women with one or two isolated episodes of UTI if post-treatment urinalysis, including microscopy and urine culture, are normal. If there are further attacks or if post-treatment urinalysis is abnormal, excretion urography should be performed to identify or exclude anatomical or functional abnormalities predisposing to or complicating infection, such as impaired bladder emptying.

Excretion urography should be carried out in all males and children following a first proven episode of bacteriuria to identify complicating factors.

Plain abdominal X-rays and ultrasonography

Plain abdominal X-rays combined with ultrasonography can identify most renal stones, upper tract obstruction and renal scars, as well as define bladder emptying. This combination of imaging is especially valuable in patients presenting with acute pyelonephritis. Neither it nor DMSA scanning can define calyceal detail or ureteric anatomy, and cannot define conditions such as papillary necrosis or medullary sponge kidney which can affect the course and management of recurrent UTI. *Intravenous urography*, therefore, remains the investigation of first choice.

Micturating cystourethrography (MCU)

MCU is indicated in children with abnormal excretion urograms and may be required to evaluate abnormal bladder emptying at any age. Otherwise it is of no value in the management of UTI.

Cystoscopy

Cystoscopy in patients with known UTI has a very limited role. It is indicated only to investigate abnormal bladder or ureteral emptying, or haematuria in bacteriuric women over the age of 40 years, since bladder cancer becomes more common with age. It is more appropriately performed in abacteriuric frequency or dysuria to exclude bladder lesions such as carcinoma, tuberculosis or interstitial cystitis (Hunner's ulcer).

Treatment

Single isolated attack

Pretreatment urine culture is desirable but not mandatory. In primary care, a positive dipstick test for nitrite and leucocyte esterase is sufficient. Treatment is over 3–5 days with amoxicillin (250 mg three times daily), nitrofurantoin (50 mg three times daily), trimethoprim (200 mg twice daily) or an oral cephalosporin. The treatment regimen may be modified in light of the result of urine culture and sensitivity testing, and/or the clinical response. For resistant organisms the alternative drugs are co-amoxiclav or ciprofloxacin.

A high (2 L daily) fluid intake should be encouraged during treatment and for some subsequent weeks. Urinalysis, microscopy and culture should be repeated 5 days after treatment. 'Single-shot' treatment with 3 g of amoxicillin or 1.92 g of co-trimoxazole can be used for patients with bladder symptoms of less than 36 hours' duration who have no previous history of UTI.

If the patient is acutely ill with high fever, loin pain and tenderness (acute pyelonephritis), a broad-spectrum antibiotic is given intravenously, such as aztreonam, cefuroxime, ciprofloxacin or gentamicin (2–5 mg/kg daily in divided doses) switching to a further 7 days' treatment with oral therapy as symptoms improve. Intravenous fluids may be required to achieve a good urine output.

In patients presenting for the first time with high fever, loin pain and tenderness, urgent renal ultrasound examination is required to exclude an obstructed pyonephrosis. If this is present it should be drained by percutaneous nephrostomy.

Recurrent infection

Pretreatment and post-treatment urine cultures are mandatory to confirm the diagnosis and identify whether recurrent infection is due to relapse or reinfection.

In *relapse*, a search should be made for a cause (e.g. stones or scarred kidneys), and this should be eradicated if possible, for example by the removal of stones. Intense or prolonged treatment – intravenous or intramuscular aminoglycoside for 7 days or oral antibiotics for 4–6 weeks – is required. If this fails, long-term antibiotics are required.

Reinfection implies that the patient has a predisposition to periurethral colonization or poor bladder defence mechanisms. Contraceptive practice should be reviewed and the use of a diaphragm and spermicidal jelly discouraged. Atrophic vaginitis should be identified in postmenopausal women, who should be treated (see below). All patients must undertake prophylactic measures:

- a 2 L daily fluid intake
- voiding at 2- to 3-hour intervals with double micturition if reflux is present
- voiding before bedtime and after intercourse
- avoidance of bubble baths and other chemicals in bathwater
- avoidance of constipation, which may impair bladder emptying.

Evidence of impaired bladder emptying on excretion urography requires urological assessment. If UTI continues to recur, treatment for 6–12 months with low-dose prophylaxis (trimethoprim 100 mg, co-trimoxazole 480 mg, cefalexin 125 mg at night, or macrocrystalline nitrofurantoin) is required; it should be taken last thing at night when urine flow is low. An alternative for infrequent attacks is immediate self-treatment with a conventional antibiotic for 3–5 days. When infection is clearly related to coitus, a single dose of macrocrystalline nitrofurantoin following intercourse may reduce the total drug usage for prophylaxis. Intravaginal oestrogen therapy has been shown to produce a reduction in the number of episodes of UTI in postmenopausal women.

Urinary infections in the presence of an indwelling catheter

Colonization of the bladder by a urinary pathogen is common after a urinary catheter has been present for more than a few days. So long as the bladder catheter is in situ, antibiotic treatment is likely to be ineffective and will encourage the development of resistant organisms. Treatment is indicated only if the patient has symptoms or evidence of infection, and should be accompanied by replacement of the catheter. There may be a place for antibiotic treatment at the time of catheter removal. Bladder stones may form in patients with long-term indwelling catheters, further complicating the situation.

Infection by *Candida* is a frequent complication of prolonged bladder catheterization. Treatment should be reserved for patients with evidence of invasive infection or those who are immunosuppressed, and should consist of removal or replacement of the catheter and possibly intravesical antifungals.

Bacteriuria in pregnancy

The urine of pregnant women must always be cultured as 2–6% have asymptomatic bacteriuria. Whilst asymptomatic bacteriuria in the non-pregnant female seldom leads on to acute pyelonephritis and often does not require treatment, acute pyelonephritis frequently occurs in pregnancy under these circumstances. Failure to treat may thus result in severe symptomatic pyelonephritis later in pregnancy, with the possibility of premature labour. Asymptomatic bacteriuria, in the presence of previous renal disease, may predispose to pre-eclamptic toxaemia, anaemia of pregnancy, and small or premature babies. Therefore bacteriuria must always be treated and be shown to be eradicated. Reinfection may require prophylactic therapy. Tetracycline, trimethoprim, sulphonamides and 4-quinolones must be avoided in pregnancy. Amoxicillin and ampicillin, nitrofurantoin and oral cephalosporins may safely be used in pregnancy.

Bacterial prostatitis

Bacterial prostatitis is a relapsing infection which is difficult to treat. It presents as perineal pain, recurrent epididymo-orchitis and prostatic tenderness, with pus in expressed prostatic secretion. Treatment is for 4–6 weeks with drugs that penetrate the prostate, such as trimethoprim or ciprofloxacin. Long-term low-dose treatment may be required. Prostadynia (prostatic pain in the absence of active infection) may be a very persistent sequel to bacterial prostatitis. Amitriptyline and carbamazepine may alleviate the symptoms.

Renal carbuncle

Renal carbuncle is an abscess in the renal cortex caused by a blood-borne *Staphylococcus*, usually from a boil or carbuncle of the skin. It presents with a high swinging fever, loin pain and tenderness, and fullness in the loin. The urine shows no abnormality as the abscess does not communicate with the renal pelvis, more often extending into the perirenal tissue. Staphylococcal septicaemia is common. Diagnosis is by ultrasound or CT scanning. Treatment involves antibacterial therapy with flucloxacillin and surgical drainage.

Tuberculosis of the urinary tract

Tuberculous infection is once again on the increase world-wide. Particular dangers are posed by the reservoir of infection in susceptible HIV-infected individuals and by the emergence of drug-resistant strains. Tuberculosis of the urinary tract should be kept in mind in patients presenting with frequency, dysuria or haematuria, particularly in the Asian immigrant population of the UK. Cortical lesions result from haematogenous spread in the primary phase of infection. Most heal, but in some, infection persists and spreads to the papillae, with the formation of cavitating lesions and the discharge of mycobacteria into the urine. Infection of the ureters and bladder commonly follows, with the potential for the development of ureteral stricture and a contracted bladder. Rarely, cold abscesses may form in the loin. In males the disease may present with testicular or epididymal discomfort and thickening.

Diagnosis depends on constant awareness, especially in patients with sterile pyuria. Excretion urography may show cavitating lesions in the renal papillary areas, commonly with calcification. There may also be evidence of ureteral obstruction with hydronephrosis. Diagnosis of active infection depends on culture of mycobacteria from early-morning urine samples. The urogram may be normal in diffuse interstitial renal tuberculosis when diagnosis is made by renal biopsy. Some patients present with small unobstructed kidneys, when the diagnosis is easy to miss.

The treatment is as for pulmonary tuberculosis (see p. 895). Renal ultrasonography or excretion urography should be carried out 2–3 months after initiation of treatment as ureteric strictures may first develop in the healing phase.

Xanthogranulomatous pyelonephritis

This is an uncommon chronic interstitial infection of the kidney, most often due to *Proteus*, in which there is fever, weight loss, loin pain and a palpable enlarged kidney. It is usually unilateral and associated with staghorn calculi. CT scanning shows up intrarenal abscesses as lucent areas within the kidney. Nephrectomy is the treatment of choice; antibacterial treatment rarely, if ever, eradicates the infection.

Malakoplakia

This is a rare condition in which plaques of abnormal inflammatory tissue grow within the urinary tract in the presence of urinary infection. The histological appearances are characteristic. It is thought that the condition is caused by an acquired inability of macrophages to kill phagocytosed bacteria. Cholinergic agonists and ascorbic acid may improve macrophage function; ciprofloxacin penetrates the macrophage well and is the antibiotic of choice. Prolonged treatment may be needed.

Viral renal infections

Viruses are present in the urine in a wide range of common viral infections, but very few viruses cause significant renal disease. Secondary immune complex glomerulonephritis may result from chronic viral infections; for instance, membranous nephropathy complicating hepatitis B and cryoglobulinaemic mesangiocapillary glomerulonephritis complicating hepatitis C infection. The role of cytomegalovirus in renal disease is unclear. *Haemorrhagic fever with renal syndrome* is the name given to a spectrum of diseases caused by Hanta viruses (see p. 57); renal failure may be severe, and is caused by an acute haemorrhagic interstitial nephritis. Human immunodeficiency virus infection is associated both with focal glomerulosclerosis and with haemolytic uraemic syndrome, but the pathogenesis of these complications remains uncertain.

FURTHER READING

Cattell WR (ed) (1996) *Infections of the Kidney and Urinary Tract.* Oxford: Oxford University Press.
Nicolle LE (2000) Asymptomatic bacteriuria – important or not? *New England Journal of Medicine* **343**: 1037–1039.

Tubulointerstitial nephritis

Interstitial inflammation with tubular damage is a regular feature of bacterial pyelonephritis but it rarely, if ever, leads to severe chronic renal damage in the absence of reflux, obstruction or other complicating factors. Presentation may be with acute, often oliguric renal failure or more commonly as chronic slowly progressive renal disease.

Acute tubulointerstitial nephritis

Acute tubulointerstitial nephritis is most often due to a hypersensitivity reaction to drugs (Table 11.13), most commonly drugs of the penicillin family and non-steroidal anti-inflammatory drugs (NSAIDs). Patients present with fever, arthralgia, skin rashes and acute oliguric or non-oliguric renal failure. Many have eosinophilia and eosinophiluria. Renal biopsy shows an intense interstitial cellular infiltrate, often including eosinophils, with variable tubular necrosis.

Treatment involves withdrawal of offending drugs. High-dose steroid therapy (prednisolone 60 mg daily) is commonly given but its efficacy has not been proved. Patients may require dialysis for management of the acute renal failure. Most patients have good recovery of kidney function, but some may be left with significant interstitial fibrosis.

Chronic tubulointerstitial nephritis

The major causes of chronic tubulointerstitial nephritis are set out in Table 11.14. In many cases no cause is found.

The patient usually either presents with polyuria and nocturia, or is found to have proteinuria or uraemia. Proteinuria is usually slight (less than 1 g daily). Papillary necrosis with ischaemic damage to the papillae occurs in a number of interstitial nephritides, for example in analgesic abuse, diabetes mellitus, sickle cell disease or trait. The papillae can separate and be passed in the urine. Chronic tubulointerstitial nephritis may be associated with microscopic or overt haematuria or sterile pyuria, and occasionally a sloughed papilla may cause ureteric colic or produce acute ureteric obstruction. The radiological appearances must be distinguished from those of reflux nephropathy (Fig. 11.25).

Table 11.13
Common causes of acute tubulointerstitial nephritis

Penicilins	Cephalosporins
Sulphonamides	Rifampicin
Non-steroidal anti-inflammatory drugs	Diuretics: furosemide (frusemide), thiazides
Phenindione	Cimetidine
Allopurinol	Phenytoin

Table 11.14
Causes of chronic tubulointerstitial nephritis

Common	Uncommon
Reflux nephropathy	Alport's syndrome
Non-steroidal anti-inflammatory drugs	Balkan nephropathy
Diabetes	Irradiation
Sickle cell disease or trait	Sjögren's syndrome
Cadmium or lead intoxication	Hyperuricaemic nephropathy

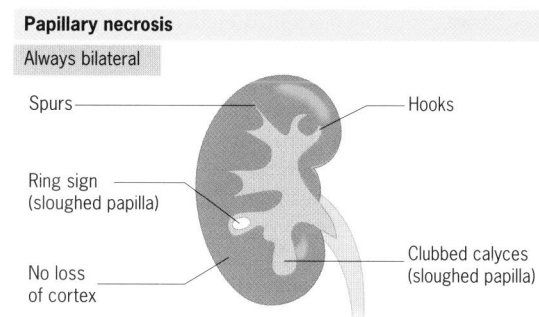

Papillary necrosis

Always bilateral

Spurs — Hooks

Ring sign (sloughed papilla)

No loss of cortex

Clubbed calyces (sloughed papilla)

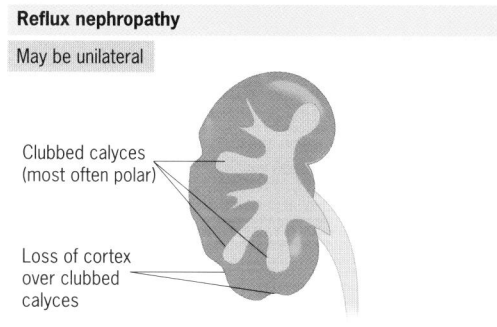

Reflux nephropathy

May be unilateral

Clubbed calyces (most often polar)

Loss of cortex over clubbed calyces

Fig. 11.25 A comparison of radiological appearances of papillary necrosis and reflux nephropathy.

Tubular damage to the medullary area of the kidney leads to defects in urine concentration and sodium conservation with polyuria and salt wasting. Fibrosis progressing into the cortex leads to loss of excretory function and uraemia.

Analgesic nephropathy

The chronic consumption of large amounts of analgesics (especially those containing phenacetin) and NSAIDs leads to chronic tubulointerstitial nephritis and papillary necrosis. COX II specific NSAIDs are still being evaluated. In Australia, the incidence of end-stage renal failure due to analgesic nephropathy has declined as 'over-the-counter' purchase of nephrotoxic analgesics has been reduced by legislation.

Clinical features

Analgesic nephropathy is twice as common in women as in men and presents typically in middle-age. Patients are often depressed or neurotic. Presentation may be with anaemia, chronic renal failure, symptoms of urinary infection (which may be difficult to eradicate), haematuria, or urinary tract obstruction (owing to sloughing of a renal papilla). Salt and water-wasting renal disease may occur.

Chronic analgesic abuse also predisposes to the development of uroepithelial tumours.

Management

The consumption of analgesics should be discouraged. If necessary, dihydrocodeine or paracetamol are reasonable alternative choices. This may result in the arrest of the disease and even in improvement in function.

UTI, hypertension (if present) and saline depletion will require appropriate management.

The development of flank pain or an unexpectedly rapid deterioration in renal function should prompt ultrasonography or urography to screen for urinary tract obstruction due to a sloughed papilla.

Balkan nephropathy

This is a chronic tubulointerstitial nephritis endemic in areas along the tributaries of the River Danube. Inhabitants of the low-lying plains which are subjected to frequent flooding and where the water supply comes from shallow wells are affected, whereas the disease does not occur in hillside villages where surface water provides the water supply.

Its cause is unknown. The disease is insidious in onset, with mild proteinuria progressing to renal failure in 3 months to 10 years. Patients exhibit a high incidence of uroepithelial tumours. There is no treatment.

Other forms of chronic tubulointerstitial nephritis

These are rare (see Table 11.14). Diagnosis of all forms depends on a careful history being taken, with special attention to drug-taking and industrial exposure to nephrotoxins. In patients with unexplained renal impairment with normal-sized kidneys, renal biopsy must always be undertaken to exclude a treatable interstitial nephritis.

Hyperuricaemic (gouty) nephropathy

Two patterns of renal disease have been described in patients with hyperuricaemia or hyperuricosuria:

- acute hyperuricaemic nephropathy
- uric acid stone formation (see p. 626).

There is no convincing evidence that chronic hyperuricaemia per se causes progressive renal failure, nor that allopurinol treatment improves renal function (see p. 554) There is one exception: a rare form of familial hyperuricaemia and gout occurring in adolescence is associated with renal impairment and allopurinol therapy both improves and protects kidney function.

Acute hyperuricaemic nephropathy

This is a well-recognized cause of acute renal failure in patients with marked hyperuricaemia that is due to lymphoproliferative or myeloproliferative disorders. It may occur prior to treatment but most often follows on commencement of treatment, when there is rapid lysis of malignant cells, release of large amounts of nucleoprotein and increased uric acid production. Renal failure is due to intrarenal and extrarenal obstruction caused by deposition of uric acid crystals in the collecting ducts, pelvis and ureters. The condition is manifest as oliguria or anuria with increasing uraemia. There may be flank pain or colic. Plasma urate levels are above 0.75 mmol/L and may be as high as 4.5 mmol/L. Diagnosis is based on the hyperuricaemia and the clinical setting. Ultrasound may demonstrate extrarenal obstruction due to stones, but a negative scan does not exclude this where there is coexistent intrarenal obstruction.

Prevention

Allopurinol 100–200 mg three times daily for 5 days is given prior to and continuing throughout treatment with radiotherapy or cytotoxic drugs. A high rate of urine flow must be maintained by oral or parenteral fluid and the urine kept alkaline by the administration of sodium bicarbonate 600 mg four times daily and acetazolamide 250 mg three times daily, since uric acid is more soluble in an alkaline than an acid medium.

Treatment

Allopurinol treatment should be commenced immediately and a forced alkaline diuresis attempted with intravenous 1.26% sodium bicarbonate plus acetazolamide (500 mg orally, then 250 mg three times daily). In severely oliguric or anuric patients, dialysis is required to lower the plasma urate, which allows urate to diffuse out of the obstructed collecting ducts into the peritubular capillaries. Percutaneous nephrostomy (see p. 598) may be required to relieve extrarenal obstruction caused by stones in the pelvis or ureters. Such stones may subsequently be passed spontaneously or may require surgical removal (p. 628).

FURTHER READING

Nickeleit V, Mihatsch MJ (1997) Uric acid nephropathy and end-stage renal disease: review of a non-disease. *Nephrology Dialysis and Transplantation* **12**: 1832–1838.

Hypertension and the kidney

Hypertension can be the cause or the result of renal disease. It is often difficult to differentiate between the two on clinical grounds. Routine tests as described on page 823 should be performed on all patients, but IVU is usually unnecessary. A guide to which patients should be fully investigated is given on page 1064.

Essential hypertension

Pathophysiology

In benign essential hypertension, arteriosclerosis of major renal arteries and changes in the intrarenal vasculature (nephrosclerosis) occur as follows:

- *In small vessels and arterioles*, intimal thickening with reduplication of the internal elastic lamina occurs and the vessel wall becomes hyalinized.
- *In large vessels,* concentric reduplication of the internal elastic lamina and endothelial proliferation produce an 'onion skin' appearance.
- *Reduction in size of both kidneys* may occur; this may be asymmetrical if one major renal artery is more affected than the other.
- *The proportion of sclerotic glomeruli* is increased compared with age-matched controls.

Deterioration in excretory function accompanies these changes, but severe renal failure is unusual in whites. In black Africans, by contrast, hypertension much more often results in the development of renal failure.

In accelerated, or malignant-phase hypertension:

- *Arteriolar fibrinoid necrosis* occurs, probably as a result of plasma entering the media of the vessel through splits in the intima. It is prominent in afferent glomerular arterioles.

- *Fibrin deposition* within small vessels is often associated with thrombocytopenia and red-cell fragmentation seen in the peripheral blood film (microangiopathic haemolytic anaemia).

Microscopic haematuria, proteinuria, usually of modest degree (1–3 g daily), and progressive uraemia occur. If untreated, fewer than 10% of patients survive 2 years.

Management

The management of benign essential and malignant hypertension is described on page 823.

If treatment is begun before renal impairment has occurred, the prognosis for renal function is good. Stabilization or improvement in renal function with healing of intrarenal arteriolar lesions and resolution of microangiopathic haemolysis occur with effective treatment of malignant-phase hypertension. Lifelong follow-up of the patient is mandatory.

Renal hypertension

Bilateral renal disease

Hypertension commonly complicates bilateral renal disease such as chronic glomerulonephritis, bilateral reflux nephropathy (chronic atrophic pyelonephritis of childhood), polycystic disease and analgesic nephropathy. Two main mechanisms are responsible:

- activation of the renin–angiotensin–aldosterone system
- retention of salt and water owing to impairment in excretory function, leading to an increase in blood volume and hence blood pressure.

The second of these assumes greater importance as renal function deteriorates.

Hypertension occurs earlier, is more common and tends to be more severe in patients with renal cortical disorders, such as glomerulonephritis, than in those with disorders affecting primarily the renal interstitium, such as reflux or analgesic nephropathy.

Management is described on page 823. Meticulous control of the blood pressure is necessary to prevent further deterioration of renal function secondary to vascular changes produced by the hypertension itself. There is good evidence that ACE-inhibitor drug treatment confers an additional reno-protective effect for a given degree of blood pressure control than other hypotensive drugs.

Unilateral renal disease

A small proportion of cases of hypertension are due to unilateral renal disease. The main causes are:

- *unilateral renal artery stenosis* due to fibromuscular hyperplasia (typically in young women) or atheroma in the elderly
- *unilateral reflux nephropathy* (atrophic pyelonephritis).

Mechanism of hypertension

Unilateral renal ischaemia results in a reduction in the pressure in afferent glomerular arterioles. This leads to an increase in the production and release of renin from the juxtaglomerular apparatus (see p. 1064) with a consequent increase in angiotensin II.

Physiological changes in renal artery stenosis

In unilateral renal artery stenosis, renal perfusion pressure is reduced and nephron transit time is prolonged on the side of the stenosis; salt and water reabsorption is therefore increased. As a result, urine from the ischaemic kidney is more concentrated but has a lower sodium concentration than urine from the contralateral kidney. Inulin, creatinine and *p*-aminohippuric acid (PAH) clearances are decreased on the ischaemic side.

Screening for unilateral renovascular disease

Radionuclide studies (see p. 599). These can demonstrate decreased renal perfusion on the affected side. In unilateral renal artery stenosis, a disproportionate fall in uptake of isotope on the affected side following administration of an ACE inhibitor such as captopril is suggestive of the presence of significant renal artery stenosis. A completely normal result renders the diagnosis unlikely.

Doppler ultrasound. This method is highly operator-dependent and has not to date proved reliable in routine clinical practice.

Magnetic resonance imaging. MRI can be used to visualize the renal arteries and a good – though not perfect – correlation between MRI findings and those of renal arteriography has been reported in several studies.

Helical ('spiral') CT scanning. This permits non-invasive imaging of the renal arteries. It is much less expensive than MRI but does expose the patient to ionizing radiation and to contrast injection and is less reliable than MRI.

Renal arteriography (see p. 598) remains the 'gold standard' investigation in the diagnosis of renal arterial disease. It is invasive and requires cannulation of the femoral artery. It involves the injection of contrast medium with the associated risk of contrast-induced kidney damage as well as cholesterol embolization (see p. 624).

Treatment

The aim of treatment is to correct hypertension and improve renal perfusion and excretory function. The options in renal artery stenosis include transluminal angioplasty to dilate the stenotic region, insertion of stents across the stenosis (sometimes the only endoscopic option when the stenosis occurs close to the origin of the renal artery from the aorta, rendering angioplasty technically difficult or impossible), reconstructive vascular surgery and nephrectomy. With good selection of patients, in more than 50% hypertension is cured or improved by intervention. Occasional dramatic improvements in renal function ensue but results are generally disappointing. No test can predict with satisfactory reliability the results of vascular surgery and many patients will do well on hypotensive therapy with or without surgery. ACE inhibitors must be avoided as hypotensive therapy as they can lead to acute renal failure in the presence of renal artery stenoses.

Unilateral atrophic pyelonephritis

In this condition, prediction of the outcome after nephrectomy is currently not possible. The case for nephrectomy is strengthened if isotope renography demonstrates the abnormal kidney to be making an insignificant contribution to overall excretory function, particularly if the patient is young and medical treatment has proved unsatisfactory. About one-third of patients with unilateral atrophic pyelonephritis benefit from nephrectomy.

FURTHER READING

Lewis EJ, Hunsicker LG, Bain RP, Rohde RD (1993) The effect of angiotensin-converting enzyme inhibition on diabetic nephropathy. *New England Journal of Medicine* **329**: 1456–1462.

Raine AEG (1996) Hypertension: its effects on the kidney. *Oxford Textbook of Medicine*. Oxford: Oxford University Press, pp. 3247–3250.

Ritz E, Mann JFE (2000) Renal angioplasty for lowering blood pressure. *New England Journal of Medicine* **342**: 1042–1043.

Safian RD, Textor SC (2001) Medical progress: renal artery stenosis. *New England Journal of Medicine* **343**: 431–442.

Other vascular disorders of the kidney

Renal artery occlusion

This occurs from thrombosis in situ usually in a severely damaged atherosclerotic vessel or more commonly from embolization. Both lead to renal infarction, resulting in a wide spectrum of clinical manifestations depending on the size of the artery involved. Occlusion of a small branch artery may produce no effect, but occlusion of larger vessels results in dull flank pain and varying degrees of renal failure.

Embolization may occur from the heart (e.g. in atrial fibrillation).

Cholesterol embolization

Showers of cholesterol-rich atheromatous material from ulcerated plaques may reach the kidney from the aorta and/or renal arteries, particularly after catheterization of the abdominal aorta or attempts at renal artery angioplasty. Anticoagulants and thrombolytic agents may also precipitate cholesterol embolization. Renal failure from cholesterol emboli may be acute or slowly progressive. Clinical features include fever, eosinophilia, back and abdominal pain, and evidence of embolization elsewhere, for example to the retina or digits. The diagnosis can be confirmed by renal biopsy. No treatment is of proven benefit.

Renal vein thrombosis

This is usually of insidious onset, occurring in the nephrotic syndrome, with a renal cell carcinoma, and in conditions associated with an increased risk of venous thrombosis (e.g. antithrombin deficiency or the presence of anticardiolipin antibodies).

FURTHER READING

Scoble JE (1997) Atherosclerosis and the kidney. *Journal of the Royal College of Physicians* **31**: 19–22.

Calculi and nephrocalcinosis

Renal and vesical calculi

Approximately 2% of the population in the UK have a urinary tract stone at any given time. A much higher prevalence of stone disease has been recorded elsewhere, notably in the Middle East. In the West, most stones occur in the upper urinary tract. The incidence of bladder stones has declined in the UK since the eighteenth and nineteenth centuries, whereas in some developing countries they are still common.

Most stones are composed of calcium oxalate and phosphate; these are more common in men (Table 11.15). Mixed infective stones, which account for about 15% of all calculi, are twice as common in women as in men. The overall male:female ratio of stone disease is 2:1.

Stone disease is frequently a recurrent problem. More than 50% of patients with a calculus will have formed a further stone or stones within 10 years. The risk of recurrence increases if a metabolic or other abnormality predisposing to stone formation is present and is not modified by treatment.

Aetiology

It is in a sense surprising that stones are not universal, since some constituents of urine are at times present in concentrations that exceed their maximum solubility in water. The presence of inhibitors of crystal formation in normal urine appears to be of importance in preventing stones.

Many stone-formers have no detectable metabolic defect, although microscopy of warm, freshly passed urine reveals both more and larger calcium oxalate crystals than are found in normal subjects. Factors predisposing to stone formation in these so-called 'idiopathic stone-formers' are:

- chemical composition of urine that favours stone crystallization
- production of a concentrated urine as a consequence of dehydration associated with life in a hot climate or work in a hot environment
- impairment of inhibitors that prevent crystallization in normal urine. Postulated inhibitors include inorganic magnesium, pyrophosphate and citrate. Organic inhibitors include glycosaminoglycans and nephrocalcin (an acidic protein of tubular origin). Tamm-Horsfall protein may have a dual role in both inhibiting and promoting stone formation.

Recognized causes of stone formation are listed in Table 11.16.

Hypercalcaemia

If the GFR is normal, hypercalcaemia almost invariably leads to hypercalciuria. The common causes of hypercalcaemia leading to stone formation are:

- primary hyperparathyroidism
- vitamin D ingestion
- sarcoidosis.

Of these, primary hyperparathyroidism (see p. 1060) is the most common cause of stones.

Hypercalciuria

This is by far the most common metabolic abnormality detected in calcium stone-formers.

Approximately 8% of men excrete in excess of 7.5 mmol of calcium in 24 hours. Calcium stone formation is more common in this group, but as the majority

---

Table 11.15
Type and frequency of renal stones in the UK

Type of renal stone	Approximate frequency (%)
Calcium oxalate usually with calcium phosphate	65
Calcium phosphate alone	15
Magnesium ammonium phosphate (struvite)	10–15
Uric acid	3–5
Cystine	1–2

Table 11.16
Causes of urinary tract stone formation

Dehydration	Infection
Hypercalcaemia	Cystinuria
Hypercalciuria	Renal tubular acidosis
Hyperoxaluria	Primary renal disease
Hyperuricaemia and	(polycystic kidneys,
hyperuricosuria	medullary sponge kidneys)
	Drugs

of even these individuals do not form stones the definition of 'pathological' hypercalciuria is arbitrary. A reasonable definition is 24-hour calcium excretion of more than 7.5 mmol in male stone-formers and more than 6.25 mmol in female stone-formers.

The kidney is the major site for plasma calcium regulation. Approximately 90% of the ionized calcium filtered by the kidney is reabsorbed. Renal tubular reabsorption is controlled largely by parathyroid hormone (PTH).

Approximately 65% of the filtered calcium is absorbed in the proximal convoluted tubule, 20% by the thick ascending limb of the loop of Henle, and 15% by the distal convoluted tubule and collecting ducts. The cells of the thick ascending limb express Ca^{2+}-sensing receptors. A high luminal calcium concentration is 'sensed' by these receptors and this triggers a series of events leading to reduced calcium reabsorption; conversely a low luminal concentration leads to avid calcium reabsorption and hypocalciuria.

Causes of hypercalciuria are:

- hypercalcaemia
- an excessive dietary intake of calcium
- excessive resorption of calcium from the skeleton, such as occurs with prolonged immobilization or weightlessness
- idiopathic hypercalciuria.

There are two main mechanisms of idiopathic hypercalciuria. The majority of patients with idiopathic hypercalciuria can be shown to have increased absorption of calcium from the gut. Dietary calcium restriction in this group markedly reduces urinary calcium excretion. A proportion of patients appear to have a renal tubular calcium leak with secondary compensatory hyperabsorption of calcium from the gut. Calcium restriction has less effect on urinary calcium excretion in this group.

Hyperoxaluria

The inborn errors of glyoxalate metabolism that cause increased endogenous oxalate biosynthesis are inherited in an autosomal recessive manner. In type I (primary hyperoxaluria) there is increased glycolate excretion as well as hyperoxaluria. In type II, L-glycerate excretion is increased. In both types, calcium oxalate stone formation occurs.

The prognosis is poor owing to widespread calcium oxalate crystal deposition in the kidneys. Renal failure typically develops in the late teens or early twenties. Successful liver transplantation has been shown to cure the metabolic defect in type I hyperoxaluria.

Much more common causes of mild hyperoxaluria are:

- excess ingestion of foodstuffs high in oxalate, such as spinach, rhubarb and tea
- dietary calcium restriction, with compensatory increased absorption of oxalate

- gastrointestinal disease (e.g. Crohn's), usually with an intestinal resection, associated with increased absorption of oxalate from the colon.

Dehydration secondary to fluid loss from the gut also plays a part in stone formation.

Hyperuricaemia and hyperuricosuria

Uric acid stones account for 3–5% of all stones in the UK, but in Israel the proportion is as high as 40%.

Uric acid is the end-point of purine metabolism. Hyperuricaemia (see p. 551) can occur as a primary defect in idiopathic gout, and as a secondary consequence of increased cell turnover, for example in myeloproliferative disorders. Increased uric acid excretion occurs in these conditions, and stones will develop in some patients. Some uric acid stone-formers have hyperuricosuria (> 4 mmol per 24 hours on a low-purine diet) without hyperuricaemia.

Dehydration alone may also cause uric acid stones to form. Patients with ileostomies are at particular risk both from dehydration and from the fact that loss of bicarbonate from gastrointestinal secretions results in the production of an acid urine (uric acid is more soluble in an alkaline than in an acid medium).

Some patients with calcium stones also have hyperuricaemia and/or hyperuricosuria; it is believed the calcium salts precipitate upon an initial nidus of uric acid in such patients.

Urinary tract infection

Mixed infective stones are composed of magnesium ammonium phosphate together with variable amounts of calcium. Such struvite stones are often large, forming a cast of the collecting system (staghorn calculus). They are believed to form as a result of infection of the urinary tract with organisms such as *Proteus mirabilis* that hydrolyse urea, with formation of the strong base ammonium hydroxide:

$$\begin{matrix} NH_2 \\ \diagdown \\ \diagup \\ NH_2 \end{matrix} C = O + HOH \rightleftharpoons 2NH_3 + CO_2$$

$$NH_3 + HOH \rightleftharpoons NH_4OH \rightleftharpoons NH_4^+ + OH^-$$

The availability of ammonium ions and the alkalinity of the urine favour stone formation. An increased amount of mucoprotein resulting from infection also creates an organic matrix on which stone formation can occur.

Cystinuria (see also p. 1116)

Cystinuria results in the formation of cystine stones. About 1–2% of all stones are composed of cystine.

Primary renal diseases

There is a moderate increase in prevalence of stone disease in patients with polycystic renal disease (see p. 658).

Medullary sponge kidney is another primary renal disorder associated with stones. In this congenital (though not inherited) condition there is dilatation of the collecting ducts with associated stasis and calcification (Fig. 11.26). Approximately 20% of these patients have hypercalciuria and a similar proportion have a renal tubular acidification defect.

The renal tubular acidoses, both inherited and acquired, are associated with nephrocalcinosis and stone formation, owing, in part at least, to the production of a persistently alkaline urine and reduced urinary citrate excretion.

Drugs

These can be associated with stone formation in three ways. Some drugs promote calcium stone formation (e.g. loop diuretics, antacids, glucocorticoids, theophylline, vitamins D and C, acetazolamide); some promote uric acid stones (e.g. thiazides, salicylates, allopurinol); and some precipitate into stones (e.g. indinavir, triamterine).

Aetiology of bladder stones

Bladder stones are endemic in some developing countries. The cause of this is unknown but dietary factors are probably important. Stones forming in the bladder do so as a result of:

- bladder outflow obstruction (e.g. urethral stricture, neuropathic bladder, prostatic obstruction)
- the presence of a foreign body (e.g. catheters, non-absorbable sutures).

Significant bacteriuria is usually found in patients with bladder stones. Some stones found in the bladder have been passed down from the upper urinary tract.

Pathology

Stones may be single or multiple and vary enormously in size from minute, sand-like particles to staghorn calculi or large stone concretions in the bladder. They may be located within the renal parenchyma or within the collecting system. Pressure necrosis from a large calculus may cause direct damage to the renal parenchyma and stones regularly cause obstruction, leading to hydronephrosis. They may ulcerate through the wall of the collecting system, including the ureter. A combination of obstruction and infection accelerates damage to the kidney.

Clinical features

Most people with urinary tract calculi are asymptomatic. Pain is the most common symptom and may be sharp or dull, constant, intermittent or colicky (Table 11.17).

When urinary tract obstruction is present, measures that increase urine volume, such as copious fluid intake or diuretics, including alcohol, make the pain worse. Physical exertion may cause mobile calculi to move, precipitating pain and, occasionally, haematuria. Calyceal colic – pain resulting from movement of stones within the calyces – is a real entity, but whether small calyceal calculi are the cause of backache or not is often difficult to decide.

Ureteric colic occurs when a stone enters the ureter and either obstructs it or causes spasm during its passage down the ureter. This is one of the most severe pains known. Radiation from the flank to the iliac fossa and testis or labium in the distribution of the first lumbar nerve root is common. Pallor, sweating and vomiting often occur and the patient is restless, tending to assume a variety of positions in an unsuccessful attempt

Table 11.17
Clinical features of urinary tract stones

Asymptomatic
Pain: renal colic
Haematuria
Urinary tract infection
Urinary tract obstruction

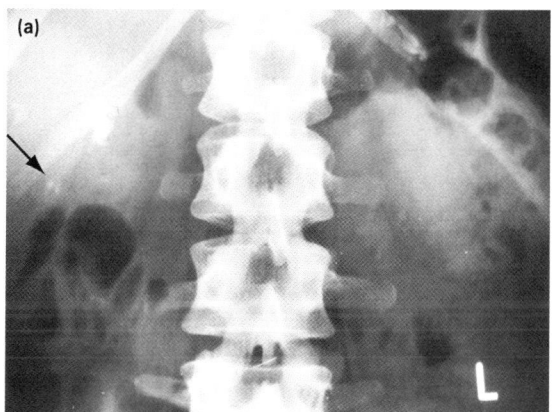
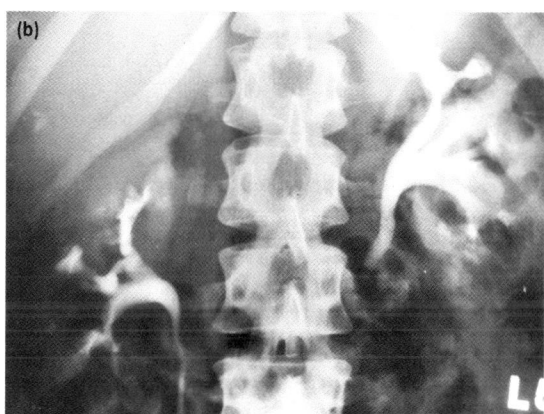

Fig. 11.26 Medullary sponge kidney. (a) Plain film showing 'spotty' calcification in the renal areas (arrow). **(b)** After injection of contrast, the calcification is shown to be small calculi in the papillary zones.

to obtain relief from the pain. Haematuria often occurs. Untreated, the pain of ureteric colic typically subsides after a few hours.

When urinary tract obstruction and infection are present, the features of acute pyelonephritis or of a Gram-negative septicaemia may dominate the clinical picture.

Vesical calculi associated with bladder bacteriuria may present with frequency, dysuria and haematuria; severe introital or perineal pain may occur if trigonitis is present. A calculus at the bladder neck or an obstruction in the urethra may cause bladder outflow obstruction, resulting in anuria and painful bladder distension.

A history of possible aetiological factors should be obtained, including:

- occupation and residence in hot countries likely to be associated with dehydration
- a history of vitamin D consumption
- gouty arthritis.

Calcified papillae may mimic ordinary calculi, so that causes of papillary necrosis such as analgesic abuse should be considered.

Physical examination should include a search for corneal or conjunctival calcification, gouty tophi and arthritis and features of sarcoidosis.

Investigations

These should include a mid-stream specimen of urine for culture and measurement of serum urea, electrolyte, creatinine and calcium levels.

Plain abdominal X-ray, and excretion urography, are the mainstay of diagnosis although unenhanced helical (spiral) CT is increasingly used in developed countries.

Advantages include speed (the examination takes 5–10 minutes), avoidance of contrast exposure and ability to diagnose non-renal causes of pain mimicking renal colic. There is an increased radiation dose. Renal tomography is still sometimes necessary. Ureteric stones can be missed by ultrasound.

Pure uric acid stones are radiolucent. Mixed infective stones in which organic matrix predominates are barely radiopaque. Calcium-containing and cystine stones are radiopaque. Calculi overlying bone are easily missed (Fig. 11.27). Staghorn calculi may be missed if the plain abdominal X-ray carried out before contrast injection during urography is not inspected (Fig. 11.28). Uric acid stones may present as a filling defect after injection of contrast medium (Fig. 11.29). Such stones are readily seen on CT scanning (Fig. 11.30).

Excretion urography is carried out during the episode of pain; a normal urogram excludes the diagnosis of pain due to calculous disease. The urographic appearances in a patient with acute left ureteric obstruction are shown in Figure 11.31. The urine of the patient should be passed through a sieve to trap any calculi passed for chemical analysis.

Management

Adequate analgesia should be given, such as intramuscular morphine 10–15 mg repeated as necessary. Alternatively an NSAID can be tried. A high fluid intake and, if feasible, increased physical activity are recommended but the efficacy of these measures is doubtful.

Stones less than 0.5 cm diameter usually pass spontaneously and can be left. Stones greater than 1 cm diameter usually require intervention.

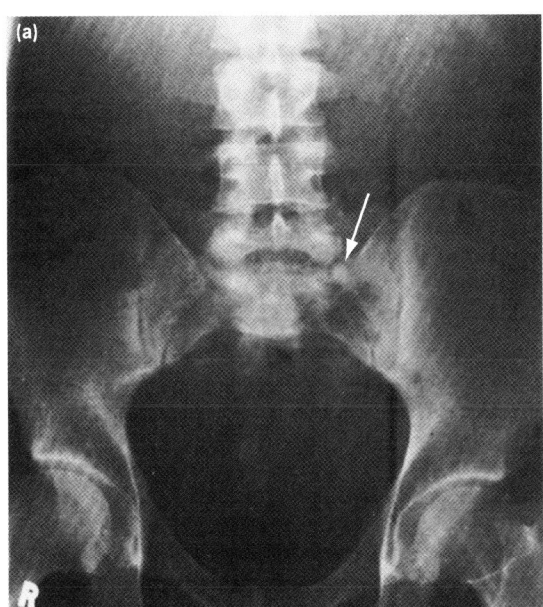
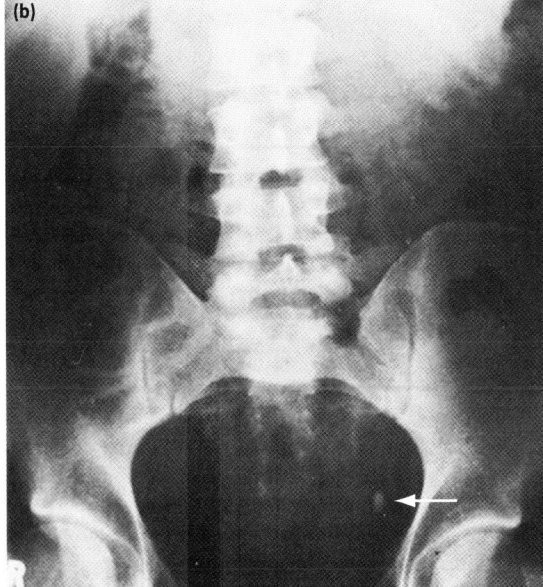

Fig. 11.27 X-rays showing calculus. (a) The calculus is overlying bone on the left (easily missed). **(b)** The same patient 1 week later: the calculus has descended and is easily seen in the pelvis of the left side (arrow).

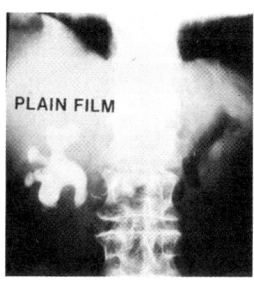
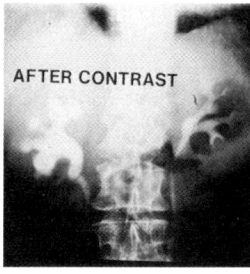

Fig. 11.28 Staghorn calculus. X-ray appearances before and after contrast on the right side are identical owing to a staghorn calculus in a non-functioning right kidney. A plain film may be confused with those taken after contrast injection.

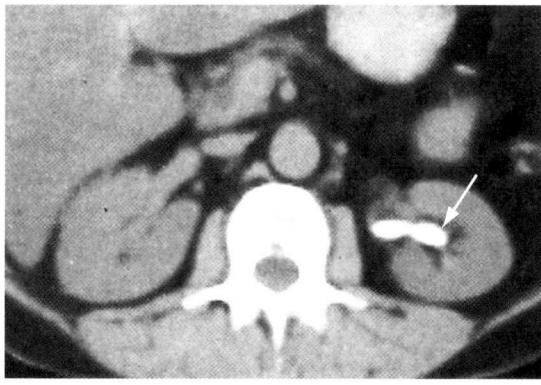

Fig. 11.30 CT scan, showing a uric acid stone, which appears as a bright lesion in the left kidney (arrow).

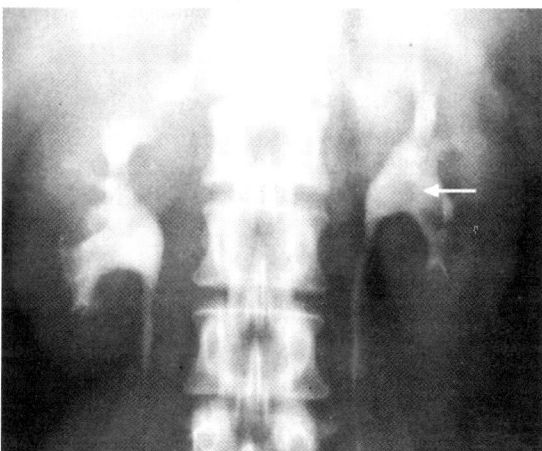

Fig. 11.29 Excretion urogram, showing a lucent filling defect (uric acid stone; arrow) in the left renal pelvis. The differential diagnosis includes a sloughed papilla and a transitional cell tumour.

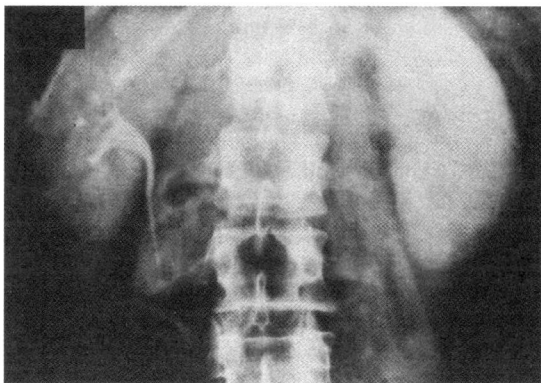

Fig. 11.31 X-ray, showing acute left ureteric obstruction. Note the increased density of the nephrogram and the absence of a pyelogram on the left side 15 minutes after contrast injection. From Weatherall DJ, Ledingham JGG, Warrell DA (eds) (1987) *Oxford Textbook of Medicine*, 2nd edn, by permission of Oxford University Press.

Persistent pain, frequent bouts of severe pain, or anuria, are indications for further therapy. Intervention is also required if a stone is not moving though causing only partial obstruction in the absence of infection. With the advent of percutaneous surgery and extracorporeal shock-wave lithotripsy (see below) there has developed a trend towards earlier intervention in such cases. Complete obstruction or the coexistence of UTI with partial obstruction should prompt even earlier intervention owing to the increased risk of permanent kidney damage in these circumstances.

Cutting operations (nephrolithotomy for renal calculi, pyelolithotomy for stones in the renal pelvis, and ureterolithotomy for ureteric stones) are avoided by using either percutaneous nephrolithotomy or extracorporeal shock-wave lithotripsy. In the former, stones in the calyces and renal pelvis are removed by creating a percutaneous track down to the collecting system followed by endoscopic removal along this track. In the latter, shock waves are focused upon the renal calculi, causing them to fragment. Most of the fragments then pass spontaneously via the urethra. Fragments that do not pass can be removed percutaneously.

Ureteric stones may be removed endoscopically or may be pushed up into the upper urinary tract, to allow percutaneous nephrolithotomy or extracorporeal shock-wave lithotripsy.

Large renal stones need to be reduced in bulk by percutaneous means before lithotripsy can be expected to be successful. Some staghorn calculi are best dealt with by open operation.

Bladder stones can be removed endoscopically. They may be dealt with by direct electrohydraulic disintegration at cystoscopy or may be gripped in a lithotrite and crushed, the stone fragments then being washed out. Open cystotomy is required for very large bladder stones.

Investigating the cause of stone formation

In an elderly patient who has had a single episode with one stone, only limited investigation is required. Younger patients and those with recurrent stone formation require detailed investigation.

- **An excretion urogram** is necessary to define the presence of a primary renal disease predisposing to stone formation.
- **Significant bacteriuria** may indicate mixed infective stone formation, but relapsing bacteriuria may be a consequence of stone formation rather than the original cause.
- **Chemical analysis** of any stone passed may be of great value and may be all that is required to make a diagnosis of cystinuria or uric acid stone formation.
- **Serum calcium concentration** should be estimated and corrected for serum albumin concentration (see p. 577). Hypercalcaemia, if present, should be investigated further (see p. 1061).
- **Serum urate concentration** is often, but not invariably, elevated in uric acid stone-formers.
- **A screening test for cystinuria** should be carried out by adding sodium nitroprusside to a random unacidified urine sample; a purple colour indicates that cystinuria may be present. Urine chromatography is required to define the diagnosis precisely.
- **Urinary calcium, oxalate and uric acid output** should be measured in two consecutive carefully collected 24-hour urine samples. After withdrawing aliquots for estimation of uric acid, it is necessary to add acid to the urine in order to prevent crystallization of calcium salts upon the walls of the collection vessel, which would give falsely low results for urinary calcium and oxalate.
- **Plasma bicarbonate** is low in renal tubular acidosis. The finding of a urine pH that does not fall below 5.5 in the face of metabolic acidosis is diagnostic of this condition (see p. 694).

Prophylaxis

The age of the patient and the severity of the problem affect both the need for and the type of prophylaxis.

Idiopathic stone-formers

Where no metabolic abnormality is present, the mainstay of prevention is maintenance of a high intake of fluid throughout the day and night. The aim should be to ensure a daily urine volume of 2–2.5 L, which requires a fluid intake in excess of this, substantially so in the case of those who live in hot countries or work in a hot environment. It is helpful to advise the patient that if his or her urine is deep yellow, fluid intake is inadequate. A large glass of water should be drunk before retiring for the night and on waking during the night if this occurs. Special dietary measures are not warranted, although avoidance of excessive consumption of calcium-rich dairy products seems sensible.

Idiopathic hypercalciuria

Severe dietary calcium restriction is inappropriate (see p. 626). Intake of milk, cheese, and white bread if this is fortified (as it is in the UK) with calcium and vitamin D is reduced. Vitamin D supplements should be avoided. Dietary calcium restriction results in hyperabsorption of oxalate, and so foods containing large amounts of oxalate should also be limited. The advice of a dietitian is helpful. A high fluid intake should be advised as for idiopathic stone-formers. Patients who live in a hard-water area may benefit from drinking softened water.

If hypercalciuria persists and stone formation continues, a thiazide is used (e.g. bendrofluazide 2.5 or 5 mg each morning). Thiazides reduce urinary calcium excretion by a direct effect on the renal tubule. They may precipitate diabetes mellitus or gout and worsen hypercholesterolaemia. Avoidance of excessive sodium intake is also advisable as sodium and calcium excretion are linked.

Mixed infective stones

Recurrent stones should be prevented by maintenance of a high fluid intake and meticulous control of bacteriuria. This will require long-term follow-up and may demand the use of long-term low-dose prophylactic antibacterial agents.

Uric acid stones

Dietary measures are probably of little value and are difficult to implement. Effective prevention can be achieved by the long-term use of the xanthine oxidase inhibitor allopurinol to maintain the serum urate and urinary uric acid excretion in the normal range. A high fluid intake should also be maintained. Uric acid is more soluble at alkaline pH and long-term sodium bicarbonate supplementation to maintain an alkaline urine is an alternative approach in those few patients unable to take allopurinol. However, alkalinization of the urine facilitates precipitation of calcium oxalate and phosphate.

Cystine stones

These can be prevented and indeed will dissolve slowly if there is obsessional attention to maintenance of a high fluid intake – 5 L of water must be drunk each 24 hours, and the patient must wake twice during the night to ingest 500 mL or more of water. Many patients cannot tolerate this regimen. An alternative, though potentially more troublesome, option is the long-term use of the chelating agent penicillamine; this causes cystine to be converted to the more soluble penicillamine–cysteine complex. Side-effects include drug rashes, blood dyscrasias and immune complex-mediated glomerulonephritis and are by no means uncommon. In addition, the drug is expensive. It is, however, especially effective in promoting dissolution of cystine stones already present.

Mild hyperoxaluria with calcium oxalate stones

A high fluid intake and dietary oxalate restriction are required.

Nephrocalcinosis

The term 'nephrocalcinosis' means diffuse renal paren-chymal calcification that is detectable radiologically (Fig. 11.32). The condition is typically painless. Hypertension and renal impairment commonly occur. The main causes of nephrocalcinosis are listed in Table 11.18.

Dystrophic calcification occurs following renal corti-cal necrosis. In hypercalcaemia and hyperoxaluria, deposition of calcium oxalate results from the high con-centration of calcium and oxalate within the kidney.

In renal tubular acidosis (see p. 693) failure of urinary acidification and a reduction in urinary citrate excretion both favour calcium phosphate and oxalate precipitation, since precipitation occurs more readily in an alkaline medium and the calcium-chelating action of urinary citrate is reduced.

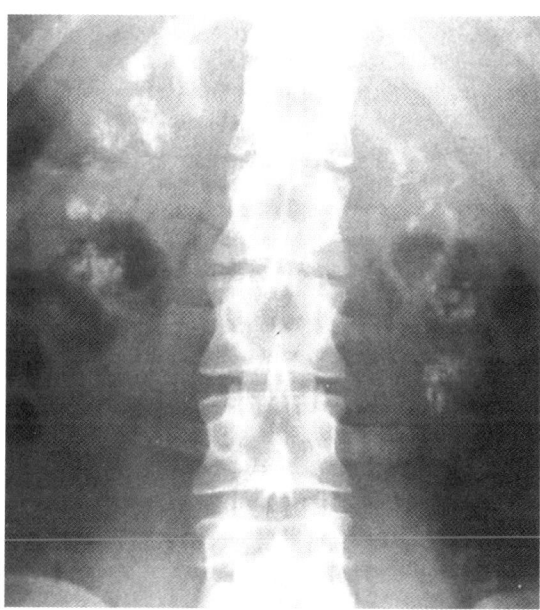

Fig. 11.32 X-ray of nephrocalcinosis.

Treatment and prevention of nephrocalcinosis consist of treatment of the cause.

FURTHER READING

Bihl G, Meyers A (2001) Recurrent renal stone disease – advances in pathogenesis and management. *Lancet* **358**: 651–656.
Borghi L et al. (2002) Comparison of two diets for the prevention of recurrent stones in idiopathic hypercalciuria. *New England Journal of Medicine* **346**: 77–84.
Danpure CJ (1994) Molecular and cell biology of primary hyperoxaluria type I. *Clinical Investigation* **72**: 725–727.

Urinary tract obstruction

The urinary tract may be obstructed at any point between the kidney and the urethral meatus. This results in dilatation of the tract above the obstruction. Dilatation of the renal pelvis is known as hydronephrosis.

Aetiology

Obstructing lesions may lie within the lumen, or in the wall of the urinary tract, or outside the wall, causing obstruction by external pressure. The major causes of obstruction are shown in Table 11.19. Overall, the

Table 11.18
Causes of nephrocalcinosis

Mainly cortical (rare)
Renal cortical necrosis (tram-line calcification)

Mainly medullary
Hypercalcaemia (primary hyperparathyroidism, hypervitaminosis D, sarcoidosis)
Renal tubular acidosis (inherited and acquired)
Primary hyperoxaluria
Medullary sponge kidney
Tuberculosis

Table 11.19
Causes of urinary tract obstruction

Within the lumen
Calculus
Blood clot
Sloughed papilla (diabetes; analgesia abuse; sickle cell disease or trait)
Tumour of renal pelvis or ureter
Bladder tumour

Within the wall
Pelviureteric neuromuscular dysfunction (congenital, 10% bilateral)
Ureteric stricture (tuberculosis, especially after treatment; calculus; after surgery)
Ureterovesical stricture (congenital; ureterocele; calculus; schistosomiasis)
Congenital megaureter
Congenital bladder neck obstruction
Neuropathic bladder
Urethral stricture (calculus; gonococcal; after instrumentation)
Congenital urethral valve
Pin-hole meatus

Pressure from outside
Pelviureteric compression (bands; aberrant vessels)
Tumours (e.g. retroperitoneal tumour or glands, carcinoma of colon)
Diverticulitis
Aortic aneurysm
Retroperitoneal fibrosis (periaortitis)
Accidental ligation of ureter
Retrocaval ureter (right-sided obstruction)
Prostatic obstruction
Tumours in pelvis (e.g. carcinoma of cervix)
Phimosis

frequency is the same in men and women. However, in the elderly, urinary tract obstruction is more common in men owing to the frequency of bladder outflow obstruction.

Pathophysiology

Obstruction with continuing urine formation results in:

- progressive rise in intraluminal pressure
- dilatation proximal to the site of obstruction
- compression and thinning of the renal parenchyma, eventually reducing it to a thin rim and resulting in a decrease in the size of the kidney.

Acute obstruction is followed by transient renal arterial vasodilatation succeeded by vasoconstriction, probably mediated mainly by angiotensin II and thromboxane A. Ischaemic interstitial damage mediated by free oxygen radicals and inflammatory cytokines compounds the damage induced by compression of the renal substance.

Clinical features

Symptoms of upper tract obstruction

Loin pain occurs which can be dull or sharp, constant or intermittent. It may be provoked by measures that increase urine volume and hence distension of the collecting system, such as a high fluid intake or diuretics, including alcohol.

Complete anuria is strongly suggestive of complete bilateral obstruction or complete obstruction of a single kidney.

Conversely, polyuria may occur in partial obstruction owing to impairment of renal tubular concentrating capacity. Intermittent anuria and polyuria indicates intermittent complete obstruction.

Infection complicating the obstruction may give rise to malaise, fever and septicaemia.

Symptoms of bladder outflow obstruction

Symptoms may be minimal. Hesitancy, narrowing and diminished force of the urinary stream, terminal dribbling and a sense of incomplete bladder emptying are typical features. The frequent passage of small volumes of urine occurs if a large volume of residual urine remains in the bladder after urination. Incontinence of such small volumes of urine is known as 'overflow incontinence' or 'retention with overflow'.

Infection commonly occurs, causing increased frequency, urgency, urge incontinence, dysuria and the passage of cloudy smelly urine. It may precipitate acute retention.

Signs

Loin tenderness may be present. An enlarged hydronephrotic kidney may be palpable. In acute or chronic retention the enlarged bladder may be felt or percussed.

Examination of the genitalia, rectum and vagina are essential, since prostatic obstruction and pelvic malignancy are common causes of urinary tract obstruction. However, the apparent size of the prostate on digital examination is a poor guide to the presence of prostatic obstruction.

Investigations

Routine blood and biochemical investigations may be abnormal; for example, there may be a raised serum urea or creatinine, hyperkalaemia, anaemia of chronic disease or blood in the urine. Nevertheless, the diagnosis of obstruction cannot be made on these tests alone and further investigations must be performed.

Ultrasonography (see p. 597)

This is a reliable means of ruling out upper urinary tract dilatation. Ultrasound cannot distinguish a baggy, low-pressure unobstructed system from a tense, high-pressure obstructed one, so that false-positive scans are seen. However, in the hands of an experienced observer, a normal scan does rule out urinary tract obstruction, except in very rare circumstances such as, for example, encasement of the kidney by fibrous or malignant tissue.

Radionuclide studies (see p. 599)

These have no place in the initial investigation of acute obstruction. Their main role in possible long-standing obstruction is to differentiate true obstructive nephropathy from retention of tracer in a baggy, low-pressure, unobstructed pelvicalyceal system.

Excretion urography

A plain film is necessary to detect calcification. However, calculi overlying bone are easily missed.

In recent unilateral obstruction, the affected kidney is enlarged and smooth in outline. The nephrogram is delayed owing to a reduction in the GFR. The calyces and pelvis fill with contrast medium later than on the normal side.

In time, the nephrogram on the affected side becomes denser than normal, owing to the prolonged nephron transit time, which allows greater than normal concentration of contrast medium within the tubules. Later, the site of obstruction may be seen, with dilatation of the system proximal to the level of the block (Fig. 11.33).

A full-length film should be taken after an attempt at bladder emptying by the patient. Complete emptying indicates either that no obstruction to bladder outflow exists or that intravesical pressure can be raised sufficiently to overcome it. Apparent bladder outflow impairment may be the result of nervousness or embarrassment on the part of the patient, or failure to carry out the X-ray before the bladder has refilled with contrast medium from above, or may be due to an atonic but non-obstructed bladder. Vesicoureteric reflux can result in contrast medium returning to the bladder from above, giving the appearance of a partially full bladder.

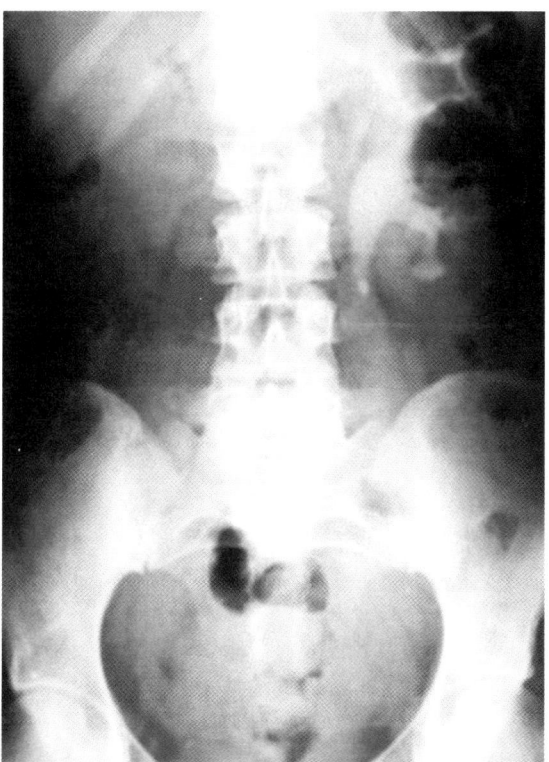

Fig. 11.33 X-ray taken 24 hours after injection of contrast, showing a delayed nephrogram and pyelogram on the left side and dilatation of the system to the level of the block. By this time contrast medium has disappeared from the normal right side.

Helical (spiral) CT scanning
This is used to outline in detail the cause of the obstruction.

Antegrade pyelography and ureterography
(see p. 598)
This defines the site and cause of obstruction. It can be combined with drainage of the collecting system by percutaneous needle nephrostomy.

Retrograde ureterography (see p. 598)
This is indicated if antegrade examination cannot be carried out or if there is the possibility of dealing with ureteric obstruction from below at the time of examination. The technique carries the risk of introducing infection into an obstructed urinary tract.

In obstruction due to neuromuscular dysfunction at the pelviureteric junction or retroperitoneal fibrosis, the collecting system may fill normally from below.

Cystoscopy, urethroscopy and urethrography
Obstructing lesions within the bladder and urethra can be seen directly by endoscopic examination.

Urethrography involves introducing contrast medium into the bladder by catheterization or suprapubic bladder puncture, and taking X-ray films during voiding to show obstructing lesions in the urethra. It is of particular value in the diagnosis of urethral valves and strictures.

Pressure–flow studies
Pressure changes within the bladder during filling and emptying can be recorded. Demonstration that a high voiding pressure is required to maintain urine flow is indicative of bladder outflow obstruction. This may be combined with video cystography and urethrography to define the site of obstruction.

Normally, while the bladder is being filled there is only a small pressure rise before the voluntary initiation of urination. Uninhibited contractions of the detrusor muscle during filling may be seen in upper motor neurone bladder neuropathy, such as occurs in multiple sclerosis. Less commonly, a neuropathic bladder may be 'hypotonic', readily accepting large volumes of fluid before the initiation of weak contractions at a low intravesical pressure. A common cause of such lower motor neurone bladder neuropathy is diabetes mellitus.

Pressure–flow and video studies may enable a logical decision to be taken as to whether surgery to relieve bladder outflow impairment should be carried out.

Treatment
Aims
Treatment involves:

- relieving the obstruction
- treating the underlying cause
- preventing and treating infection.

The ultimate aim of treatment is to relieve symptoms and to preserve renal function.

Temporary external drainage of urine by nephrostomy may be valuable, as this allows time for further investigation when the site and nature of the obstructing lesion is uncertain, doubt exists as to the viability of the obstructed kidney, or when immediate definitive surgery would be hazardous.

Recent, complete upper urinary tract obstruction demands urgent relief to preserve kidney function, particularly if infection is present.

In contrast, with partial urinary tract obstruction, particularly if spontaneous relief is expected – such as by passage of a calculus – there is no immediate urgency.

Surgical management
This depends on the cause of the obstruction (see below). Dialysis may be required in the ill patient prior to surgery.

Nephrectomy or nephroureterectomy is justified when obstruction is due to malignant disease or when it is judged that no worthwhile amount of renal excretory function will be conserved by, or will return after, relief of obstruction.

Permanent urinary diversion is required when the obstruction cannot be relieved; in such cases malignant disease is usually present. Ureteric anastomosis to an ileal conduit opening on to the abdominal wall is often a satisfactory method of diversion. In some patients, obstruction is best relieved by the insertion of indwelling catheters or stents into the ureter. An obstruction high in the urinary tract may require a permanent nephrostomy.

In obstruction due to untreatable malignant disease it is wise to consider carefully whether urinary diversion or stent insertion is justified, since this may exchange a pain-free death from renal failure for a painful one with malignant invasion of bones or nerves.

Diuresis usually follows relief of obstruction at any site in the urinary tract. Massive diuresis may occur following relief of bilateral obstruction owing to previous sodium and water overload and the osmotic effect of retained solutes combined with a defective renal tubular reabsorptive capacity (as in the diuretic phase of recovering acute tubular necrosis). This diuresis is associated with increased blood volume and high levels of atrial natriuretic peptide (ANP). Defective renal tubular reabsorptive capacity cannot be the sole mechanism of severe diuresis since this phenomenon is not observed following relief of unilateral obstruction. The diuresis is usually self-limiting, but a minority of patients will develop severe sodium, water and potassium depletion requiring appropriate intravenous replacement. In milder cases, oral salt and potassium supplements together with a high water intake are sufficient.

Specific causes of obstruction

Calculi
These are discussed on page 632.

Pelviureteric junction obstruction (Fig. 11.34)
This appears to result from a functional disturbance in peristalsis of the collecting system in the absence of mechanical obstruction. Surgical attempts at correction of the obstruction by open or percutaneous pyeloplasty are indicated in patients with recurrent loin pain and those in whom serial excretion urography, background-subtraction isotope renography or measurements of GFR indicate progressive kidney damage. Nephrectomy to remove the risk of developing pyonephrosis and septicaemia is indicated if long-standing obstruction has destroyed kidney function.

Obstructive megaureter
This childhood condition may become evident only in adult life. It results from the presence of a region of defective peristalsis at the lower end of the ureter adjacent to the ureterovesical junction. The condition is more common in males. It presents with UTI, flank pain or haematuria. The diagnosis is made on excretion urography or, if necessary, ascending ureterography.

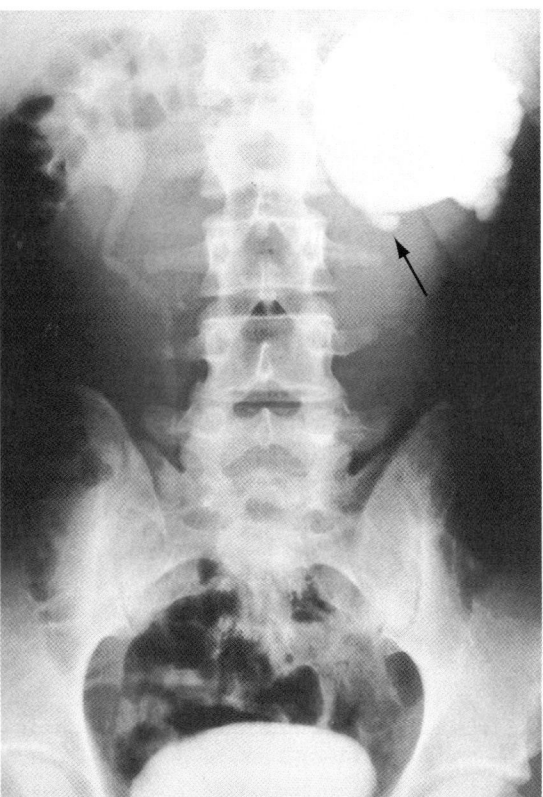

Fig. 11.34 X-ray, showing left pelviureteric junction obstruction (arrow).

Excision of the abnormal portion of ureter with reimplantation into the bladder is always indicated in children, and is indicated in adults when the condition is associated with evidence of progressive deterioration in renal function, bacteriuria that cannot be controlled by medical means, or recurrent stone formation.

Retroperitoneal fibrosis (chronic periaortitis)
In this condition the ureters become embedded in dense retroperitoneal fibrous tissue with resultant unilateral or bilateral obstruction. The condition may extend from the level of the second lumbar vertebra to the pelvic brim. The incidence of the condition in men is three times that in women. An autoallergic response to leakage of material, probably ceroid, derived from atheromatous plaques is considered to be the underlying cause of the condition. Recognized associations are with abdominal aortic aneurysm and prolonged exposure to the drug methysergide. The differential diagnosis includes retroperitoneal lymphoma or cancer.

Malaise, back pain, normochromic anaemia, uraemia and a raised erythrocyte sedimentation rate (ESR) are typical features. Excretion urography shows bilateral or unilateral ureteric obstruction commencing at the level of the pelvic brim. A periaortic mass may be seen on a CT scan (Fig. 11.35).

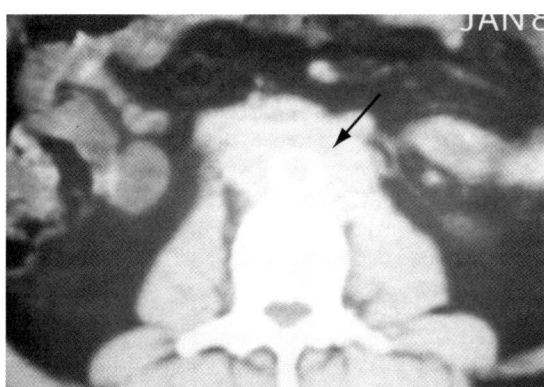

Fig. 11.35 Retroperitoneal fibrosis (periaortitis). Note the large mass surrounding the abdominal aorta on this CT scan (arrow).

Obstruction is relieved surgically by ureterolysis. Biopsy should be performed at operation to determine whether there is an underlying lymphoma or carcinoma. Corticosteroids are of benefit, and in bilateral obstruction in frail patients it may be best to free only one ureter and to rely upon steroid therapy to induce regression of fibrous tissue on the contralateral side, since bilateral ureterolysis is a major operation. In some patients, surgery alone or steroid therapy alone may suffice, but in the majority both surgery and subsequent corticosteroid therapy appear to be necessary. An alternative approach is to relieve obstruction by placement of a ureteric stent or stents, and to rely on corticosteroid therapy to induce regression of the periaortic mass, with later stent removal. A disadvantage is that an adequate biopsy of the mass – readily obtainable on open operation – is not easily obtained and regular (usually 6-monthly) changes of the stent or stents is required if the periaortic mass does not regress.

Response to treatment and disease activity are assessed by serial measurements of ESR and GFR supplemented by isotopic and imaging techniques including CT scanning. The latter method enables the size of the retroperitoneal mass to be assessed. Relapse after withdrawal of steroid therapy may occur and treatment may need to be continued for years. Long-term follow-up is mandatory.

Benign prostatic hypertrophy
Benign prostatic hypertrophy is a common cause of urinary tract obstruction. It is described on page 663.

Prognosis of urinary tract obstruction
The prognosis depends upon the cause and the stage at which obstruction is relieved. In obstruction, four factors influence the rate at which kidney damage occurs, its extent and the degree and rapidity of recovery of renal function after relief of obstruction. These are:

- whether obstruction is partial or complete
- the duration of obstruction

- whether or not infection occurs
- the site of obstruction.

Complete obstruction for several weeks will lead to irreversible or only partially reversible kidney damage. If the duration of complete obstruction is several months, total irreversible destruction of the affected kidney will result. Partial obstruction carries a better prognosis, depending upon its severity.

Bacterial infection coincident with obstruction rapidly increases kidney damage.

Obstruction at or below the bladder neck may induce hypertrophy and trabeculation of the bladder without a rise in pressure within the upper urinary tract, in which case the kidneys are protected from the effects of back-pressure.

FURTHER READING

Baker LRI (1996) Urinary tract obstruction. In: Weatherall DJ, Ledingham JGG, Warrell DA (eds) *Oxford Textbook of Medicine*. Oxford: Oxford University Press, pp. 3232–3247.

Ormond JK (1988) Bilateral ureteral obstruction due to envelopment and compression by an inflammatory process. *Journal of Urology* **59**: 1072–1079.

Parums DV, Mitchinson MJ (1990) Serum antibodies to oxidised LDL and ceroid in chronic periaortitis. *Archives of Pathology and Laboratory Medicine* **114**: 383–387.

Whitaker RH (1990) The diagnosis of upper urinary tract obstruction. *Postgraduate Medical Journal* **66** (Suppl 1): 25–30.

Drugs and the kidney

Drug-induced impairment of renal function
Prerenal
Impaired perfusion of the kidneys can result from drugs that cause:

- hypovolaemia – for example:
  - (a) potent loop diuretics such as furosemide (frusemide), especially in elderly patients
  - (b) renal salt and water loss, such as from hypercalcaemia induced by vitamin D therapy (since hypercalcaemia adversely affects renal tubular salt and water conservation)
- decrease in cardiac output, which impairs renal perfusion (e.g. beta-blockers)
- decreased renal blood flow (e.g. ACE inhibitors).

Renal
Several mechanisms of drug-induced renal damage exist and may coexist.

Acute tubular necrosis produced by direct nephrotoxicity. Examples include prolonged or excessive treatment with aminoglycosides (kanamycin, gentamicin, streptomycin), amphotericin B, cefaloridine, heavy metals or carbon tetrachloride. The combination of amino-glycosides or cefaloridine with furosemide (frusemide) is particularly nephrotoxic.

Acute tubulointerstitial nephritis (see p. 621) with interstitial oedema and inflammmatory cell infiltration. This cell-mediated hypersensitivity nephritis occurs with many drugs, including penicillins, particularly methicillin, sulphonamides and NSAIDs.

Chronic tubulointerstitial nephritis due to drugs. See page 621.

Immune complex-mediated glomerulonephritis. Examples include penicillamine.

Postrenal

Retroperitoneal fibrosis with urinary tract obstruction may result from the use of methysergide.

Use of drugs in patients with impaired renal function (Box 11.1)

Many aspects of drug handling are altered in patients with renal impairment.

Absorption

This may be unpredictable in uraemia as nausea and vomiting are frequently present.

Metabolism

Oxidative metabolism of drugs by the liver may be altered in uraemia. This is rarely of clinical significance.

The rate of drug metabolism by the kidney may be reduced as a result of two factors:

- *Reduced drug catabolism.* Insulin, for example, is in part catabolized by the normal kidney. In renal disease, insulin catabolism is reduced. The insulin requirements of diabetics decline as renal function deteriorates, for this reason.
- *Reduced conversion of a precursor to a more active metabolite,* such as the conversion of 25-hydroxycholecalciferol to the more active $1,25\text{-}(OH)_2D_3$. The 1α-hydroxylase enzyme responsible for this conversion is located in the kidney. In renal disease, production of the enzyme declines and deficiency of $1,25\text{-}(OH)_2D_3$ results.

Protein binding

Reduced protein binding of a drug potentiates its activity and increases the potential for toxic side-effects. Measurement of the total plasma concentration of such a drug can give misleading results. For example, the serum concentration of phenytoin required to produce an antiepileptic effect is much higher in normal individuals than in those with renal failure, since in the latter proportionately more drug is present in the free form.

Some patients with renal disease are hypoproteinaemic and reduced drug-binding to protein results. This is not the sole mechanism of reduced drug-binding in such patients. For example, hydrogen ions, which are retained in renal failure, bind to receptors for acidic drugs such as sulphonamides, penicillin and salicylates, thus enhancing their potential for causing toxicity.

Volume of distribution

Salt and water overload or depletion may occur in patients with renal disease. This affects the concentration of drug obtained from a given dose.

End-organ sensitivity

The renal response to drug treatment may be reduced in renal disease. For example, mild thiazide diuretics

---

Box 11.1

Safe prescribing in renal disease

Safe prescribing in renal failure demands knowledge of the clinical pharmacology of the drug and its metabolites in normal individuals and in uraemia. The clinician should ask the following questions when prescribing:

1 Is treatment mandatory? Unless it is, it should be withheld.

2 Can the drug reach its site of action?
For example, there is little point in prescribing the urinary antiseptic nitrofurantoin in renal failure since bacteriostatic concentrations will not be attained in the urine.

3 Is the drug's metabolism altered in uraemia?

4 Will accumulation of the drug or metabolites occur?
Even if accumulation is a potential problem owing to the drug or its metabolites being excreted by the kidneys, it is not necessarily an indication to change the drug given. The size of the loading dose will depend upon the size of the patient and is unrelated to renal function.
Avoidance of toxic levels of drug in blood and tissues subsequently requires the administration of normal doses of the drug at longer time intervals than usual or smaller doses at the usual time intervals.

5 Is the drug toxic?

6 Are the effective concentrations of the drug in biological tissues similar to the toxic concentrations? Should blood levels of the drug be measured?

7 Will the drug worsen the uraemic state by means other than nephrotoxicity, e.g. steroids, tetracycline?

8 Is the drug a sodium or potassium salt? These are potentially hazardous in uraemia.

Not suprisingly, adverse drug reactions are more than twice as common in renal failure as in normal individuals. Elderly patients, in whom unsuspected renal impairment is common, are particularly at risk. Careful attention to the above and careful titration of the dose of drugs employed should reduce this problem.

The dose may be titrated by:

- observation of its clinical effect, e.g. hypotensive agents
- early detection of toxic effects
- measurement of drug levels in the blood, e.g. gentamicin levels.

have little diuretic effect in patients with severe renal impairment.

Renal elimination
The major problem in the use of drugs in renal failure concerns the reduced elimination of many drugs normally excreted by the kidneys.

Water-soluble drugs such as gentamicin that are poorly absorbed from the gut, typically given by injection and are not metabolized by the liver, give rise to far more problems than lipid-soluble drugs such as propranolol, which are well absorbed and principally metabolized by the liver. Metabolites of lipid-soluble drugs, however, may themselves be water-soluble and potentially toxic.

Drugs causing uraemia by effects upon protein anabolism and catabolism
Tetracyclines, with the exception of doxycycline, have a catabolic effect and as a result the concentration of nitrogenous waste products is increased. They may also cause impairment of GFR by a direct effect. Corticosteroids have a catabolic effect and so also increase the production of nitrogenous wastes. A patient with moderate impairment of renal function may therefore become severely uraemic if given tetracyclines or corticosteroid therapy.

Drugs and toxic agents causing specific renal tubular syndromes include mercury, lead, cadmium and vitamin D.

Problem patients
Particular problems are presented by patients in whom renal function is altering rapidly, such as those with recovering acute tubular necrosis. In addition, drugs may be removed by dialysis and haemofiltration, which will affect the dosage required.

FURTHER READING
British Medical Association and Royal Pharmaceutical Society of Great Britain (2001) Renal impairment. In: *British National Formulary*, 42nd edn. Bath: Bath Press.
Golper TA (1991) Drug removal during continuous hemofiltration or hemodialysis. *Contributions to Nephrology* 93: 110–116.

Acute renal failure

The term 'renal failure' means failure of renal excretory function owing to depression of the glomerular filtration rate. This is accompanied to a variable extent by failure of erythropoietin production (see p. 592), vitamin D hydroxylation (p. 592), regulation of acid–base balance (p. 690) and regulation of salt and water balance and blood pressure (p. 592).

Definition
Acute renal failure means abrupt deterioration in parenchymal renal function which is usually, but not invariably, reversible over a period of days or weeks. In clinical practice, such deterioration in renal function is sufficiently severe to result in uraemia. Oliguria is usually, but not invariably, a feature. Acute renal failure may cause sudden, life-threatening biochemical disturbances and is a medical emergency. The distinction between acute and chronic renal failure may not be readily apparent in a patient presenting with uraemia. Patients with chronic renal impairment are not immune from the development of a superimposed acute-on-chronic renal failure under appropriate circumstances.

Renal failure results in reduced excretion of nitrogenous waste products of which urea is the most commonly measured. A raised serum urea concentration (uraemia) may conveniently be classified as: (i) prerenal, (ii) renal or (iii) postrenal. More than one category may be present in an individual patient. Other causes of altered serum urea and creatinine concentration are shown in Table 11.20.

Prerenal uraemia
In prerenal uraemia, there is impaired perfusion of the kidneys with blood. This results either from hypovolaemia, hypotension, impaired cardiac pump efficiency or vascular disease limiting renal blood flow, or combinations of these factors. Usually the kidney is able to maintain glomerular filtration close to normal despite wide variations in renal perfusion pressure and volume status – so-called 'autoregulation'. Further depression of renal perfusion leads to a drop in glomerular filtration and development of prerenal uraemia. Drugs which impair renal autoregulation, such as ACE inhibitors and NSAIDs, increase the tendency to develop prerenal uraemia. All causes of prerenal uraemia may lead to established parenchymal kidney damage and the development of acute renal failure. By definition, excretory function in prerenal uraemia improves once normal renal perfusion has been restored.

Table 11.20
Causes of altered serum urea and creatinine concentration other than altered renal function

	Decreased concentration	Increased concentration
Urea	Low protein intake Liver failure Sodium valproate treatment	Corticosteroid treatment Tetracycline treatment Gastrointestinal bleeding
Creatinine	Low muscle mass	High muscle mass Red meat ingestion Muscle damage (rhabdomyolysis) Decreased tubular secretion (e.g. cimetidine, trimethoprim therapy)

A number of criteria have been proposed to differentiate between prerenal and intrinsic renal causes of uraemia (Table 11.21).

- *Urine specific gravity and urine osmolality* are easily obtained measures of concentrating ability but are unreliable in the presence of glycosuria or other osmotically active substances in the urine.
- *Urine sodium* is low if there is avid tubular reabsorption, but may be increased by diuretics or dopamine.
- *Fractional excretion of sodium* (FE_{Na}), the ratio of sodium clearance to creatinine clearance, increases the reliability of this index but may remain low in some 'intrinsic' renal diseases, including contrast nephropathy and myoglobinuria.

Laboratory tests, however, are no substitute for careful clinical assessment. A history of blood or fluid loss, sepsis potentially leading to vasodilatation, or of cardiac disease may be helpful. Hypotension (especially postural), a weak rapid pulse and a low jugular venous pressure will suggest that the uraemia is prerenal. In doubtful cases, measurement of central venous pressure is often invaluable.

Management

If the prerenal uraemia is a result of hypovolaemia and hypotension, prompt replacement with appropriate fluid is essential to correct the problem and prevent development of ischaemic renal injury and acute renal failure. Since prerenal and renal uraemia may coexist, and fluid challenge in the latter situation may lead to volume overload with pulmonary oedema, careful clinical monitoring is vital. Blood pressure should be checked regularly and signs of elevated jugular venous pressure and of pulmonary oedema sought frequently. Central venous pressure monitoring is usually advisable (see p. 933). If the problem relates to cardiac pump insufficiency or occlusion of the renal vasculature, appropriate measures – albeit often unsuccessful – need to be taken.

Postrenal uraemia

Here, uraemia results from obstruction of the urinary tract at any point from the calyces to the external urethral orifice. The causes and presentation of urinary tract obstruction are dealt with on page 631. Screening for urinary tract obstruction is by renal ultrasonography. Urinary tract obstruction may present in an acute fashion (if obstruction of a single functioning kidney by, for example, a calculus occurs) but typically is of insidious onset.

Acute uraemia due to renal parenchymal disease
Causes

This is most commonly due to acute renal tubular necrosis (Table 11.22). *Other causes* include disease affecting the intrarenal arteries and arterioles as well as glomerular capillaries, such as a vasculitis (p. 568), accelerated hypertension, cholesterol embolism, haemolytic uraemic syndrome, thrombotic thrombocytopenic purpura (TTP), pre-eclampsia and crescentic glomerulonephritis. Acute tubulointerstitial nephritis (p. 621) may also cause acute renal failure. This also occurs when renal tubules are acutely obstructed by crystals, for example following sulphonamide therapy in a dehydrated patient (sulphonamide crystalluria) or after rapid lysis of certain malignant tumours following chemotherapy (acute hyperuricaemic nephropathy). Acute bilateral suppurative pyelonephritis or pyelonephritis of a single kidney can cause acute uraemia.

Acute tubular necrosis
Causes

Acute tubular necrosis (ATN) is common, particularly in hospital practice. It results most often from renal ischaemia but can also be caused by direct renal toxins including drugs such as the aminoglycosides, lithium and platinum derivatives (Table 11.22).

Kidneys appear to be particularly vulnerable to ischaemic injury when cholestatic jaundice is present, and more than one ischaemic factor appears to be

---

Table 11.21
Criteria for distinction between prerenal and intrinsic causes of renal dysfunction

	Prerenal	Intrinsic
Urine specific gravity	> 1.020	< 1.010
Urine osmolality (mOsm/kg)	> 500	< 350
Urine sodium (mmol/L)	< 20	> 40
$Fe_{Na} = \dfrac{U_{Na}}{P_{Na}} \times \dfrac{U_{Cr}}{P_{Cr}} \times 100$	< 1%	> 1%

FE, fractional excretion; P, plasma; U, urine; C, creatinine

Table 11.22
Some causes of acute tubular necrosis

Haemorrhage	Haemoglobinaemia (due to
Burns	haemolysis, e.g. in
Diarrhoea and vomiting,	falciparum malaria,
fluid loss from fistulae	'blackwater fever')
Pancreatitis	Hepatorenal syndrome
Diuretics	Radiological contrast agents
Myocardial infarction	Drugs, e.g. aminoglycosides,
Congestive cardiac failure	NSAIDs, ACE inhibitors,
Endotoxic shock	platinum derivatives
Snake-bite	Abruptio placentae
Myoglobinaemia	Pre-eclampsia and eclampsia

present in some situations. For example, disseminated intravascular coagulation complicating Gram-negative septicaemia and complications of pregnancy such as placental rupture, pre-eclampsia and eclampsia, may result in occlusion or partial occlusion of intrarenal vessels, exacerbating the ischaemic insult resulting from hypotension associated with the underlying condition.

Myoglobinaemia and haemoglobinaemia consequent upon muscle injury (rhabdomyolysis) complicating trauma, pressure necrosis or heroin use predispose to ATN, perhaps in part owing to occlusion of renal tubules by myoglobin and haemoglobin casts. In liver failure, acute renal failure appears to result from rapidly reversible vasomotor abnormalities within the kidney. A kidney removed from a patient with hepatic cirrhosis and liver failure dying with oliguric renal failure may function normally immediately after transplantation into a normal individual. Efferent glomerular arteriolar dilatation resulting from ACE-inhibitor drug therapy, with consequent lowering of glomerular filtration pressure, may cause acute deterioration in excretory function if renal arterial disease is also present. The effect is compounded by concomitant use of non-steroidal anti-inflammatory agents which reduce prostaglandin production, opposing this effect.

Factors postulated to be involved in the development of ATN include: (i) entry of calcium into cells with an increase in cytosolic cell calcium concentration; (ii) induction by hypoxia of nitric oxide synthases with increased production of nitric oxide; (iii) increased production of intracellular proteases such as calpain (fairly strong evidence exists that this mechanism operates in ciclosporin-induced nephrotoxicity); (iv) activation of phospholipase A_2 with increased production of free fatty acids and consequent damage to cell membranes; (v) cell injury resulting from reperfusion with blood after initial ischaemia; (vi) vasoconstriction; (vii) liberation of toxic endothelial factors; (viii) damage from the vasodilator effects of endotoxins; (ix) reduced prostaglandin production; (x) tubular obstruction by desquamated cells and casts.

The decline in the supply of oxygen and essential nutrients to tubular cells and the effect of various toxic factors results in patchy tubular cell necrosis with disruption of the cell membrane, denaturation of intracellular protein, lysosomal disruption and cell necrosis. Tubular cells have the capacity to regenerate rapidly and to reform the disrupted tubular basement membrane, which explains the reversibility of ATN. In established ATN renal blood flow is much reduced, particularly blood flow to the renal cortex.

Ischaemic tubular damage contributes to a reduction in glomerular filtration by a number of interrelated mechanisms:

- *glomerular contraction* reducing surface area available for filtration
- *reflex afferent arteriolar spasm*

- *'back leak' of filtrate* in the proximal tubule owing to loss of function of the tubular cells
- *obstruction of the tubule* by debris shed from ischaemic tubular cells.

The exact pathogenesis of acute renal tubular necrosis still remains unclear. Reduced glomerular filtration alone appears unlikely to provide a full explanation. In animal experiments of acute tubular necrosis, single-nephron GFR measurements during the acute oliguric phase indicate that GFR is reduced to only 20% of normal or thereabouts. GFR measured by clearance methods in humans with acute oliguric renal failure due to tubular necrosis are of course much lower than this.

Course and prognosis

The clinical course of acute renal failure associated with ATN is variable depending on the severity and duration of the renal insult. Oliguria is common in the early stages: non-oliguric renal failure is usually a result of a less severe renal insult. Recovery of renal function typically occurs after 7–21 days, although recovery is delayed by continuing sepsis. In the recovery phase, GFR may remain low while urine output increases, sometimes to many litres a day owing to defective tubular reabsorption of filtrate. The clinical course is variable and ATN may last for up to 6 weeks even after a relatively short-lived initial insult. Eventually renal function usually returns almost to normal or to normal, although exceptions exist (e.g. in renal cortical necrosis – see below). During the recovery phase the kidneys appear relatively insensitive to further insult, such as a recurrence of hypovolaemia.

The overall mortality of ATN is approximately 50% and significantly this has not changed in the last 30 years. This reflects in large measure the effect of the underlying illness on prognosis. An alteration in the case-mix of patients with acute renal failure now seen compared with 30 years ago is evident in the UK. ATN associated with septic abortion (which carries a good prognosis) is now rare, probably owing to legislative changes, whereas acute renal failure following, for example, major vascular and cardiac surgery in elderly patients is seen more often.

No treatment is, as yet, known which will reduce the duration of acute renal tubular necrosis once it has occurred. Claims that intravenous mannitol, furosemide (frusemide) or 'renal-dose' dopamine may do so are not supported by controlled trial evidence, and none of these treatments is without risk. No overall benefit has been proven from the use of the synthetic analogue of atrial natriuretic factor, anaritide, in reducing the duration of or mortality from ATN. However, oliguric patients did appear to do better whilst non-oliguric ones did worse when treated with this agent in a large clinical trial.

Whether a state of 'incipient' ATN exists in some patients with prerenal uraemia, and whether ATN can be prevented by administration of mannitol, furosemide (frusemide) or dopamine, also remain uncertain. Many nephrologists will administer one or more of these agents if correction of prerenal factors does not initiate a diuresis, but proof of benefit is lacking.

Clinical and biochemical features

These are the features of the causal condition together with features of rapidly progressive uraemia. The rate at which serum urea and creatinine concentrations increase is dependent upon the rate of tissue breakdown in the individual patient. This is increased in the presence of trauma, sepsis and following surgery. Hyperkalaemia is common, particularly following trauma to muscle and in haemolytic states. Metabolic acidosis is usual unless hydrogen ion loss by vomiting or aspiration of gastric contents is a feature. Hyponatraemia may be present owing to water overload if patients have continued to drink in the face of oliguria, or if overenthusiastic fluid replacement with 5% dextrose has been carried out. Pulmonary oedema owing to salt and water retention is not uncommon, particularly after inappropriate attempts to initiate a diuresis by infusion of normal saline without adequate monitoring of the patient's volume status. Hypocalcaemia due to reduced renal production of 1,25-dihydroxycholecalciferol and hyperphosphataemia due to phosphate retention are common.

Symptoms of uraemia such as anorexia, nausea, vomiting and pruritus develop, followed by intellectual clouding, drowsiness, fits, coma and haemorrhagic episodes. Epistaxes and gastrointestinal haemorrhage are relatively common. Severe infection may have initiated the acute renal failure or have complicated it owing to the impaired immune defences of the uraemic patient or ill-considered management, such as the insertion and retention of an unnecessary bladder catheter with complicating urinary tract infection and bacteraemia.

Investigation of the uraemic emergency

Investigations are aimed at defining whether the patient has acute or chronic uraemia, whether uraemia results from prerenal, renal or postrenal factors, and establishing the cause.

Acute or chronic uraemia?

The distinction between acute and chronic uraemia depends in part on the history, duration of symptoms and previous urinalysis or measurements of renal function.

A rapid rate of change of serum urea and creatinine with time suggests an acute process. A normochromic, normocytic anaemia suggests chronic disease, but anaemia may complicate many of the diseases which cause acute renal failure owing to a combination of haemolysis, haemorrhage and deficient erythropoietin production.

Ultrasound assessment of renal echogenicity and size is helpful. Small kidneys of increased echogenicity are diagnostic of a chronic process, although the reverse is not true; the kidney may remain normal in size in diabetes and amyloidosis, for instance.

Evidence of renal osteodystrophy (for example, digital subperiosteal erosions due to hyperparathyroid bone disease) is indicative of chronic disease.

Measurement of carbamylated haemoglobin (a product of non-enzymatic reaction between urea and haemoglobin, cf. glycosylated haemoglobin) is not widely employed.

Prerenal, renal or postrenal uraemia?

Bladder outflow obstruction is ruled out by insertion of a urethral catheter or flushing of an existing catheter, which should then be removed unless a large volume of urine is obtained. Absence of upper tract dilatation on renal ultrasonography will, with very rare exceptions, rule out urinary tract obstruction.

The distinction between prerenal and renal uraemia may be difficult. Assessment of the patient's volume status is essential and central venous pressure measurement may be extremely helpful. If volume status is low, appropriate corrective measures are indicated. If no diuresis ensues, acute intrinsic renal failure is present. Some believe that an infusion of furosemide (frusemide) or mannitol, or of 'renal-dose' dopamine ($1–3 \mu g/kg$ bodyweight per minute) may induce a diuresis in this situation and prevent progression from prerenal uraemia to established intrinsic renal failure. Proof that this is the case is lacking.

Other investigations

These include urinalysis, urine microscopy, particularly for red cells and red-cell casts (indicative of glomerulonephritis) and urine culture; measurement of serum urea, electrolytes, creatinine, calcium, phosphate, albumin, alkaline phosphatase and urate concentrations; full blood count and examination of the peripheral blood film; testing, where appropriate, of urine for free haemoglobin and myoglobin; coagulation studies; blood cultures and measurements of nephrotoxic drug blood levels.

Management

The aim of management of acute renal tubular necrosis is to keep the patient alive until spontaneous recovery of renal function occurs. Ideally patients should be managed by a nephrologist or intensivist with access to facilities for blood purification and fluid removal (see p. 642). Early specialist referral is advisable. Poor initial management and late referral result in the arrival in the specialist centre of a patient who is severely uraemic, acidotic and hyperkalaemic, with pulmonary oedema following overenthusiastic intravenous fluid administration and with a Gram-negative septicaemia complicating the presence of an unnecessary indwelling bladder catheter.

General measures

Good nursing and physiotherapy are vital. Regular oral toilet, chest physiotherapy and consistent documentation of fluid intake and output, and where possible measurement of daily bodyweight to assess fluid balance changes, all have a role. The patient should be confined to bed only if essential.

Emergency measures

Hyperkalaemia

This is a life-threatening complication owing to the risk of cardiac dysrhythmias, particularly ventricular fibrillation. Treatment is outlined in Chapter 12, Emergency box 12.1. Correction of acidosis with intravenous sodium bicarbonate will also reduce serum potassium concentration, but administration of sodium may be inappropriate if the patient is salt- and water-overloaded. Rapid correction of acidosis in a hypocalcaemic patient may also trigger tetany, since hydrogen ions displace calcium from albumin-binding sites, thus increasing the physiologically active calcium concentration in blood. Ion exchange resins are used to prevent subsequent hyperkalaemia rather than to deal with the acute emergency. In many patients, hyperkalaemia will be controlled only by dialysis or haemofiltration.

Pulmonary oedema

Unless a diuresis can be induced with intravenous furosemide (frusemide), dialysis or haemofiltration will be required.

Sepsis

Infections, when detected, should be treated promptly, bearing constantly in mind the need to avoid nephrotoxic drugs and to use drugs excreted by the kidneys with appropriate precautions such as alteration of drug dosage and monitoring of blood levels. Neither the use of prophylactic antibiotics nor barrier-nursing are considered appropriate.

Use of drugs

Great care must be exercised in the use of drugs (see p. 636).

Fluid and electrolyte balance

Twice daily clinical assessment is needed. In general, once the patient is euvolaemic, daily fluid intake should equal urine output plus losses from fistulae and from vomiting, plus an allowance of 500 mL daily for insensible loss. Febrile patients will require an additional allowance. Sodium and potassium intake should be minimized. If abnormal losses of fluid occur, for example in diarrhoea, additional fluid and electrolytes will be required. The development of signs of salt and water overload (peripheral oedema, basal crackles, elevation of jugular venous pressure) or of hypovolaemia should prompt reappraisal of fluid intake. Large changes in

daily weight reflecting change in fluid balance status should also prompt a reappraisal of the situation.

Diet

With rare exceptions, sodium and potassium restriction are appropriate. The place of dietary protein restriction is controversial. If it is hoped to avoid dialysis or haemofiltration, protein intake is sometimes restricted to approximately 40 g daily. This poses the risk of a negative nitrogen balance despite attempts to reduce endogenous protein catabolism by maintenance of a high energy intake in the form of carbohydrate and fat. Patients treated by blood purification techniques are more appropriately managed by providing 70 g protein daily or more. Hypercatabolic patients will require an even higher nitrogen intake to prevent negative nitrogen balance.

Routes of intake are, in preferred order, enteral by mouth, enteral by nasogastric tube, and parenteral. The last of these is, however, only necessary if vomiting or bowel dysfunction render the enteral route inappropriate.

Vitamin supplements are usually supplied. Vitamin D analogue therapy and pharmacological doses of erythropoietin are not employed routinely.

Dialysis and haemofiltration

The main indications for blood purification and/or excess fluid removal by these techniques are:

- symptoms of uraemia
- complications of uraemia, such as pericarditis
- severe biochemical derangement in the absence of symptoms (especially if a rising trend is observed in an oliguric patient and in hypercatabolic patients)
- hyperkalaemia not controlled by conservative measures
- pulmonary oedema
- severe acidosis
- for removal of drugs causing the acute renal failure, e.g. gentamicin, lithium, severe aspirin overdose.

The main options are peritoneal dialysis, intermittent haemodialysis combined with ultrafiltration, if necessary, intermittent haemofiltration, continuous arteriovenous or venovenous haemofiltration, and haemodiafiltration. For reasons that are incompletely understood, adverse cardiovascular effects are much less during haemofiltration than during haemodialysis. Continuous treatments are superior to intermittent ones in this respect.

Continuous treatments

Blood flow is achieved either by using the patient's own blood pressure to generate arterial blood flow through a filter or by the use of a blood pump to draw blood from the lumen of a dual-lumen catheter placed in the jugular, subclavian or femoral vein.

Continuous arteriovenous or venovenous haemofiltration (CAVH, CVVH) refers to the continuous removal of ultrafiltrate from the patient, usually at rates of up to 1000 mL/h, combined with simultaneous infusion of replacement solution. For instance, in a fluid-overloaded patient one might remove filtrate at 1000 mL/h and replace at a rate of 900 mL/h, achieving a net fluid removal of 100 mL/h.

Continuous haemodiafiltration (CAVHDF, CVVHDF) is a combination of haemofiltration and haemodialysis, involving both the net removal of ultrafiltrate from the blood and its replacement with a replacement solution, together with the countercurrent passage of dialysate (which may be identical to the replacement solution). Both the ultrafiltrate and the spent dialysate appear as 'waste'.

Acute renal failure in the intensive care unit

In the UK, increasing numbers of patients with acute renal failure are managed in the setting of an intensive care unit. Many such patients have multiorgan failure, sepsis or both, with associated cardiovascular instability. Continuous methods of blood purification and control of fluid balance, such as venovenous haemofiltration, are preferable to intermittent haemodialysis or peritoneal dialysis in such patients. Advantages include:

- much less disturbance of cardiovascular stability
- the ability to generate as much 'space' for fluid administration as is required, which can be adjusted flexibly to the needs of the patient (many patients require large volumes of fluid to be administered for nutritional and other reasons)
- the removal of potentially harmful substances such as inflammatory cytokines via the more porous membrane employed in haemofiltration.

Acute respiratory distress syndrome (ARDS) is not uncommon in patients with multiorgan failure, including acute renal failure, requiring intensive therapy. In such patients the wish to remove as much fluid from the patient as possible to reduce pulmonary congestion must be balanced against the need of organs, including the kidneys, for an adequate blood flow, if recovery is to occur.

Management of the recovery phase

Usually, after 1–3 weeks, renal function improves as evidenced by an increase in urine volume and improvement in serum biochemistry. Dialysis or haemofiltration, if they have been required, can be discontinued. A careful watch on clinical state, salt and water balance, and serum chemistry is required at this stage, particularly if a major diuretic phase develops owing to recovery of glomerular filtration at a time when renal tubular reabsorptive capacity for sodium, potassium and water remains impaired. Intravenous fluid replacement is sometimes required together with supplements of sodium chloride and potassium. Typically, the diuretic phase lasts for only a few days.

Acute cortical necrosis

Renal hypoperfusion results in diversion of blood flow from the cortex to the medulla, with a drop in GFR. Medullary ischaemic damage is largely reversible owing to the capacity of the tubular cells for regeneration. In contrast, glomerular ischaemic injury heals not with regeneration but with scarring – glomerulosclerosis. Prolonged cortical ischaemia may lead to irreversible loss of renal function termed 'cortical necrosis'. This may be patchy or complete. Any cause of acute tubular necrosis, if sufficiently severe or prolonged, may lead to cortical necrosis. This outcome is particularly common if acute renal failure has been accompanied by derangements of the vascular endothelial system or coagulation system, such as occurs in haemolytic uraemic syndrome and complications of pregnancy.

FURTHER READING

Forni LG, Hilton PJ (1997) Continuous haemofiltration in the treatment of acute renal failure. *New England Journal of Medicine* **336**: 1303–1309.

Hughes HD (1997) Editorial: Acute renal failure: the promise of new therapies. *New England Journal of Medicine* **336**: 870–871.

Klahr S, Muller SB (1998) Acute oliguria. *New England Journal of Medicine* **338**: 671–676.

Chronic renal failure

In the UK, the prevalence of chronic renal impairment is approximately 600 individuals per million population per year. The incidence of end-stage renal failure is of the order 200 per million population per year.

Chronic renal failure implies long-standing, and usually progressive, impairment in renal function. In many instances, no effective means are available to reverse the primary disease process. Exceptions include correction of urinary tract obstruction, immunosuppressive therapy for systemic vasculitis and Goodpasture's syndrome, treatment of accelerated hypertension, and correction of critical narrowing of renal arteries causing renal impairment. A good deal, however, can be done to slow the rate of deterioration in renal function otherwise to be expected (see p. 648). A list of causes of chronic renal failure is given in Table 11.23.

Wide geographical variations in the incidence of disorders causing chronic renal failure exist. For example, the most common cause of glomerulonephritis in sub-Saharan Africa is malaria. Schistosomiasis is a common cause of renal failure due to urinary tract obstruction in parts of the Middle East, including southern Iraq. These disorders are seen in the UK only in those who have resided in endemic areas. The incidence of end-stage

Table 11.23
Causes of chronic renal failure

Congenital and inherited disease
Polycystic kidney disease (adult and infantile forms)
Medullary cystic disease
Tuberose sclerosis
Oxalosis
Cystinosis
Congenital obstructive uropathy

Glomerular disease
Primary glomerulonephritides including focal glomerulosclerosis
Secondary glomerular disease (systemic lupus, polyangiitis, Wegener's granulomatosis, amyloidosis, diabetic glomerulosclerosis, accelerated hypertension, haemolytic uraemic syndrome, thrombotic thrombocytopenic purpura, systemic sclerosis, sickle cell disease)

Vascular disease
Hypertensive nephrosclerosis (common in black Africans)
Atherosclerotic main renal vascular disease
Small and medium-sized vessel vasculitis

Tubulointerstitial disease
Tubulointerstitial nephritis – idiopathic, due to drugs (especially nephrotoxic analgesics), immunologically mediated
Reflux nephropathy (chronic atrophic pyelonephritis)
Tuberculosis
Schistosomiasis
Nephrocalcinosis
Multiple myeloma (myeloma kidney)
Balkan nephropathy
Renal papillary necrosis (diabetes, sickle cell disease and trait, analgesic nephropathy)

Urinary tract obstruction
Calculous disease
Prostatic disease
Pelvic tumours
Retroperitoneal fibrosis
Schistosomiasis

renal failure varies between racial groups, as does the relative importance of different causes of chronic renal failure. For example, end-stage renal failure is three to four times as common in black Africans in the UK and USA as it is in whites, and hypertensive nephropathy is a much more frequent cause of end-stage renal failure in this group. The prevalence of diabetes mellitus and hence of diabetic nephropathy is higher in some Asian groups than in whites. The age group involved is also of relevance. For example, chronic renal failure due to atherosclerotic renal vascular disease is much more common in the elderly than in the young.

Clinical approach to the patient with chronic renal failure

History
Particular attention should be paid to:

- *duration of symptoms*
- *drug ingestion*, including non-steroidal anti-inflammatory agents, analgesic and other medications, and unorthodox treatments such as herbal remedies
- *previous medical and surgical history*, e.g. previous chemotherapy, multisystem diseases such as SLE
- *previous occasions* on which urinalysis or measurement of urea and creatinine might have been performed, e.g. pre-employment or insurance medical examinations, new patient checks
- *family history* of renal disease.

Symptoms
The early stages of renal failure are often completely asymptomatic, despite the accumulation of numerous metabolites. Serum urea and creatinine concentrations are measured in renal failure since methods for their determination are available and a rough correlation exists between urea and creatinine concentrations and symptoms. These substances are, however, in themselves not particularly toxic. The nature of the metabolites which are involved in the genesis of symptoms is unclear. Such metabolites must be products of protein catabolism (since dietary protein restriction may reverse symptoms associated with renal failure) and many of them must be of relatively small molecular size (since haemodialysis employing membranes which allow through only relatively small molecules improves symptoms). Little else is known with certainty.

Symptoms are common when the serum urea concentration exceeds 40 mmol/L, but many patients develop uraemic symptoms at lower levels of serum urea. Symptoms include:

- malaise, loss of energy
- loss of appetite
- insomnia
- nocturia and polyuria due to impaired concentrating ability (bed-wetting in children may be a result of nocturia rather than emotional disturbance)
- itching
- nausea, vomiting and diarrhoea
- paraesthesiae due to polyneuropathy
- 'restless legs' syndrome (overwhelming need to frequently alter position of lower limbs)
- bone pain due to metabolic bone disease
- paraesthesiae and tetany due to hypocalcaemia
- symptoms due to salt and water retention – peripheral or pulmonary oedema
- symptoms due to anaemia (see p. 411)
- amenorrhoea in women; erectile impotence in men.

In more advanced uraemia (serum urea >50–60 mmol/L), these symptoms become more severe, and CNS symptoms are common:

- mental slowing, clouding of consciousness, and seizures
- myoclonic twitching.

Severe depression of glomerular filtration can result in oliguria. This can occur with either acute renal failure or in the terminal stages of chronic renal failure.

However, even if the GFR is profoundly depressed, failure of tubular reabsorption may lead to very high urine volumes. For instance, a GFR of 5 mL per minute without any tubular reabsorption would produce a urine output of 300 mL per hour or over 7 L a day! Because tubular dysfunction always accompanies glomerular disease to some extent, the urine output is therefore not a useful guide to renal function.

Examination

There are few physical signs of uraemia per se. Findings include:

- *short stature* – in patients who have had chronic renal failure in childhood
- *pallor* – due to anaemia
- *increased photosensitive pigmentation* – which may make the patient look misleadingly healthy
- *brown discoloration of the nails*
- *scratch marks* due to uraemic pruritus
- *signs of fluid overload*
- *pericardial friction rub*
- *flow murmurs* – mitral regurgitation due to mitral annular calcification; aortic and pulmonary regurgitant murmurs due to volume overload
- *glove and stocking peripheral sensory loss* (rare).

The kidneys themselves are usually impalpable unless grossly enlarged as a result of polycystic disease, obstruction or tumour. Rectal and vaginal examination may disclose evidence of an underlying cause of renal failure, particularly urinary obstruction, and should always be performed.

In addition to these findings, there may be physical signs of any underlying disease which may have caused the renal failure, for instance:

- cutaneous vasculitic lesions in systemic vasculitides
- retinopathy in diabetes
- evidence of peripheral vascular disease
- evidence of spina bifida or other causes of neurogenic bladder.

An assessment of the central venous pressure, skin turgor, blood pressure both lying and standing and peripheral circulation should also be made. The major symptoms and signs of chronic renal failure are shown in Figure 11.36.

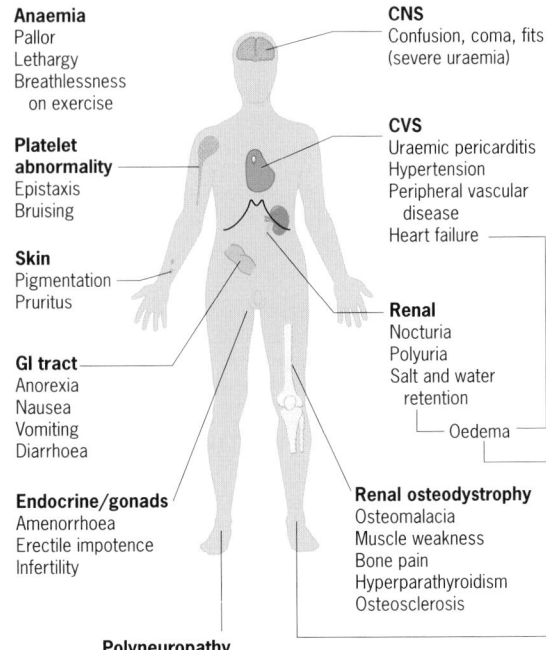

Anaemia
Pallor
Lethargy
Breathlessness
on exercise

Platelet abnormality
Epistaxis
Bruising

Skin
Pigmentation
Pruritus

GI tract
Anorexia
Nausea
Vomiting
Diarrhoea

Endocrine/gonads
Amenorrhoea
Erectile impotence
Infertility

Polyneuropathy

CNS
Confusion, coma, fits
(severe uraemia)

CVS
Uraemic pericarditis
Hypertension
Peripheral vascular
disease
Heart failure

Renal
Nocturia
Polyuria
Salt and water
retention

Oedema

Renal osteodystrophy
Osteomalacia
Muscle weakness
Bone pain
Hyperparathyroidism
Osteosclerosis

Fig. 11.36 **Symptoms and signs of chronic renal failure.** Oedema may be due to a combination of primary renal salt and water retention and heart failure.

Investigations

Urinalysis

- *Haematuria* may indicate glomerulonephritis, but other sources must be considered. Haematuria should not be assumed to be due to the presence of an indwelling catheter.
- *Proteinuria*, if heavy, is strongly suggestive of glomerular disease. Urinary infection may also cause proteinuria.
- *Glycosuria* with normal blood glucose is common in CRF.

Urine microscopy (see p. 595)

- *White cells* in the urine usually indicate active bacterial urinary infection, but this is an uncommon cause of acute renal failure; sterile pyuria suggests papillary necrosis (see p. 622) or renal tuberculosis.
- *Eosinophiluria* is strongly suggestive of allergic tubulointerstitial nephritis or cholesterol embolization.
- *Granular casts* are formed from abnormal cells within the tubular lumen, and indicate active renal disease.
- *Red-cell casts* are highly suggestive of glomerulonephritis.
- *Red cells in the urine* may be from anywhere between the glomerulus and the urethral meatus.

Urine biochemistry

- *24-hour creatinine clearance* is useful in assessing the severity of renal failure.

- *Measurements of urinary electrolytes* are unhelpful in chronic renal failure. The use of urinary sodium concentration in the distinction between prerenal and intrinsic renal disease is discussed on page 638.
- *Urine osmolality* is a measure of concentrating ability. A low urine osmolality is normal in the presence of a high fluid intake but indicates renal disease when the kidney should be concentrating urine, such as in hypovolaemia or hypotension.
- *Urine electrophoresis* is necessary for the detection of light chains, which can be present without a detectable serum paraprotein.

Serum biochemistry

- *Urea and creatinine.*
- *Electrophoresis* should be performed for myeloma.
- *Extreme elevations of creatine kinase* and a disproportionate elevation in serum creatinine and potassium compared to urea suggest rhabdomyolysis.

Haematology

- *Eosinophilia* suggests vasculitis, allergic tubulointerstitial nephritis, or cholesterol embolism.
- *Markedly raised viscosity or ESR* suggests myeloma or vasculitis.
- *Fragmented red cells and/or thombocytopenia* suggests intravascular haemolysis due to accelerated hypertension, haemolytic uraemic syndrome or thrombotic thrombocytopenic purpura.
- *Tests for sickle cell disease* should be performed when relevant.

Immunology

- *Complement components* may be low in active renal disease due to SLE, mesangiocapillary glomerulonephritis, poststreptococcal glomerulonephritis, and cryoglobulinaemia.
- *Autoantibody screening* is useful in detection of SLE (p. 559), scleroderma (p. 562), Wegener's granulomatosis and microscopic polyangiitis (p. 901), and Goodpasture's syndrome (p. 605).
- *Cryoglobulins* should be sought in patients with unexplained glomerular disease, particularly mesangiocapillary glomerulonephritis.

Microbiology/virology

- *Urine culture* should always be performed.
- *Early-morning urine samples* should be cultured if tuberculosis is possible.
- *Antibodies to streptococcal antigens* (ASOT, anti-DNAase B) should be sought if poststreptococcal glomerulonephritis is possible.
- *Antibodies to hepatitis B and C* may point to polyarteritis or membranous nephropathy (hepatitis B) or to cryoglobulinaemic renal disease (hepatitis C).
- *Antibodies to HIV* raise the possibility of HIV-associated renal disease.

- *Malaria* is a major cause of glomerular disease in the tropics.

Radiological investigation

- *Ultrasound*. Every patient should undergo ultrasonography (for renal size and to exclude hydronephrosis), and plain abdominal radiography and renal tomography to exclude low-density renal stones or nephrocalcinosis, which may be missed on ultrasound.
- *Intravenous urography* is seldom diagnostic in advanced renal disease.
- *CT* is useful for the diagnosis of retroperitoneal fibrosis and some other causes of urinary obstruction, and may also demonstrate cortical scarring.

Renal biopsy (see p. 600)

This should be considered in every patient with unexplained renal failure and normal-sized kidneys, unless there are strong contraindications. If rapidly progressive glomerulonephritis is possible, this investigation must be performed within 24 hours of presentation if at all possible, to guide immunosuppressive treatment.

Complications of chronic renal failure

Anaemia

Anaemia is present in the great majority of patients with chronic renal failure. Several factors have been implicated:

- *erythropoietin deficiency* (the most important)
- *bone marrow toxins* retained in renal failure
- *bone marrow fibrosis* secondary to hyperparathyroidism
- *haematinic deficiency* – iron, vitamin B_{12}, folate
- *increased red cell destruction*
- *abnormal red cell membranes* causing increased osmotic fragility
- *increased blood loss* – occult gastrointestinal bleeding, blood sampling, blood loss during haemodialysis or because of platelet dysfunction
- *ACE inhibitors* (may cause anaemia in chronic renal failure, probably by interfering with the control of endogenous erythropoietin release).

Red cell survival is reduced in renal failure. Increased red cell destruction may occur during haemodialysis owing to mechanical, oxidant and thermal damage.

Bone disease: renal osteodystrophy

The term 'renal osteodystrophy' embraces the various forms of bone disease which may develop alone or in

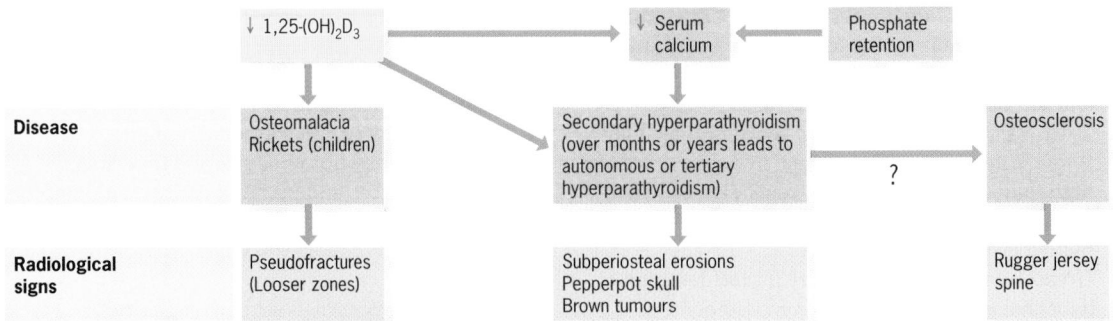

Fig. 11.37 **Pathogenesis and radiological features of renal osteodystrophy.**

combination in chronic renal failure – hyperparathyroid bone disease, osteomalacia, osteoporosis and osteosclerosis (Fig. 11.37). Covert renal osteodystrophy is present in many patients with moderate renal impairment and in almost all of those with end-stage renal failure.

Pathogenesis of bone disease

Decreased renal production of the 1α-hydroxylase enzyme results in reduced conversion of $25\text{-}(OH)_2D_3$ to the more metabolically active $1,25\text{-}(OH)_2D_3$. Receptors for this exist on the parathyroid glands, failure of occupancy of which leads to increased release of parathyroid hormone. 1,25-Dihydroxycholecalciferol deficiency also results in gut calcium malabsorption. Phosphate retention owing to reduced excretion by the kidneys also indirectly (and probably directly) results in an increase in PTH secretion and release. PTH promotes reabsorption of calcium from bone and increased proximal renal tubular reabsorption of calcium, and this opposes the tendency to develop hypocalcaemia induced by $1,25\text{-}(OH)_2D_3$ deficiency and phosphate retention. This 'secondary' hyperparathyroidism leads to increased osteoclastic activity, cyst formation and bone marrow fibrosis (osteitis fibrosa cystica). Radiologically, digital subperiosteal erosions and 'pepperpot skull' are seen. Long-standing secondary hyperparathyroidism ultimately leads to hyperplasia of the glands with autonomous or 'tertiary' hyperparathyroidism in which hypercalcaemia is present. Serum alkaline phosphatase concentration is raised in both secondary and tertiary hyperparathyroidism. Long-standing parathyroid hormone excess is also thought to cause increased bone density (osteosclerosis) seen particularly in the spine where alternating bands of sclerotic and porotic bone give rise to a characteristic 'rugger jersey' appearance.

$1,25\text{-}(OH)_2D_3$ deficiency and hypocalcaemia result in impaired mineralization of osteoid (osteomalacia). Such impaired mineralization also occurs when osteoblasts are inhibited by, for example, aluminium given as gut phosphorus binders, or accumulated in bone as a result of exposure to aluminium in source water used to make up dialysate for haemodialysis. In this situation, serum alkaline phosphatase concentration tends to be only slightly elevated.

The condition of 'adynamic bone disease' in which both bone formation and resorption are depressed (in the absence of aluminium bone disease or overtreatment with vitamin D), is recognized in patients with renal failure. The pathogenesis of this condition is unclear and it is not known whether it leads to an increased risk of fractures or other complications. No treatment is of proven benefit.

Many patients with chronic renal failure are found histologically to have mixed bone disease; that is, a combination of hyperparathyroidism and osteomalacia.

Skin disease

Pruritus (itching) is common in severe renal failure and is usually attributed in the main to retention of nitrogenous waste products of protein catabolism. Certainly, marked improvement often follows the institution of dialysis. Other causes of pruritus include:

- hypercalcaemia
- hyperphosphataemia
- elevated calcium × phosphate product
- hyperparathyroidism (even if calcium and phosphate levels are normal)
- iron deficiency.

In dialysis patients, inadequate dialysis is a cause of pruritus. Nevertheless, a significant number of dialysis patients who are well dialysed and in whom other causes of pruritus can be excluded suffer persistent itching. The cause is unknown and no effective treatment exists.

Many patients with renal failure suffer from dry skin for which simple aqueous creams are helpful. Eczematous lesions, particularly in relation to the region of an arteriovenous fistula, are relatively common. Chronic renal failure may also cause pseudoporphyria (cutanea tarda), a blistering photosensitive skin rash. This results from a decrease in hepatic uroporphyrinogen decarboxylase combined with a decreased clearance of porphyrins in the urine or by dialysis.

Gastrointestinal complications

These include:

- decreased gastric emptying and increased risk of reflux oesophagitis
- increased risk of peptic ulceration
- increased risk of acute pancreatitis
- constipation – particularly in patients on continuous ambulatory peritoneal dialysis (CAPD).

However, elevations of serum amylase of up to three times normal may be found in chronic renal failure without any evidence of pancreatic disease, owing to retention of high-molecular-weight forms of amylase normally excreted in the urine.

Metabolic abnormalities

Gout. Urate retention is a common feature of chronic renal failure. Treatment of asymptomatic hyperuricaemia does not (as once thought) protect against further deterioration in renal function. Treatment of clinical gout is complicated by the nephrotoxic potential of NSAIDs. Colchicine is useful in treatment of the acute attack, and allopurinol should be introduced later under colchicine cover to prevent further attacks. The dose of allopurinol should be reduced in renal impairment.

Insulin. Insulin is catabolized by and to some extent excreted via the kidneys. For this reason insulin requirements in diabetic patients decrease as renal failure progresses. By contrast, end-organ resistance to insulin is a feature of advanced renal impairment resulting in modestly impaired glucose tolerance when a standard glucose tolerance test is carried out. Insulin resistance may contribute to hypertension and lipid abnormalities.

Lipid metabolism abnormalities. These are common in renal failure, and include:

- impaired clearance of triglyceride-rich particles
- hypercholesterolaemia (particularly in advanced renal failure).

The situation is further complicated in end-stage renal disease, when regular heparinization (in haemodialysis), excessive glucose absorption (in CAPD) and immunosuppressive drugs (in transplantation) may all contribute to lipid abnormalities. Correction of lipid abnormalities by, for example, HMG-CoA reductase inhibitor therapy is used in renal failure patients, although without formal proof of benefit derived from prospective controlled trials. Evidence that such treatment is of benefit in lowering the risk of coronary events and death in asymptomatic middle-aged men with normal renal function (see p. 1111), and the high incidence of cardiovascular death in renal failure patients, has prompted an active approach to treatment of lipid abnormalities.

Endocrine abnormalities

These include:

- *hyperprolactinaemia*, which may present with galactorrhoea in men as well as women

- *increased luteinizing hormone* (LH) levels in both sexes, and abnormal pulsatility of LH release
- *decreased serum testosterone levels* (only seldom below the normal level); impotence and decreased spermatogenesis are common
- *absence of normal cyclical changes in female sex hormones*, resulting in oligomenorrhoea or amenorrhoea
- *complex abnormalities of growth hormone secretion and action*, resulting in impaired growth in uraemic children (pharmacological treatment with recombinant growth hormone and insulin-like growth factor is being studied)
- *abnormal thyroid hormone levels*, partly because of altered protein binding.

Sensitive assays for thyroid-stimulating hormone are the best way to assess thyroid function. True hypothyroidism occurs with increased frequency in renal failure. Posterior pituitary gland function is normal in renal failure.

Muscle dysfunction

Uraemia appears to interfere with muscle energy metabolism, but the mechanism is uncertain. Decreased physical fitness (cardiovascular deconditioning) also contributes.

Nervous system

Central nervous system

Severe uraemia causes an unusual combination of depressed cerebral function and decreased seizure threshold. However, convulsions in a uraemic patient are much more commonly due to other causes such as accelerated hypertension, thrombotic thrombocytopenic purpura, or drug accumulation. Asterixis, tremor and myoclonus are also features of severe uraemia.

Rapid correction of severe uraemia by haemodialysis leads to 'dialysis disequilibrium' owing to osmotic cerebral swelling. This can be avoided by correcting uraemia gradually by short, repeated haemodialysis treatments or by the use of peritoneal dialysis.

'Dialysis dementia' is a syndrome of progressive intellectual deterioration, speech disturbance, myoclonus and fits which is now known to be due to aluminium intoxication; it may be accompanied by aluminium bone disease and by microcytic anaemia. Low-grade aluminium exposure may also cause more subtle, subclinical deterioration in intellectual function. Prevention involves removal of aluminium from source water used to manufacture dialysis fluid, and restriction or avoidance of aluminium-containing gut-phosphorus binders. Treatment is with the chelating agent desferrioxamine.

Autonomic nervous system

Autonomic dysfunction is common in renal impairment. Findings include:

- increased circulating catecholamine levels associated with down-regulation of α-receptors

- impaired baroreceptor sensitivity
- impaired efferent vagal function.

Overactivity of the sympathetic nervous system in chronic renal failure is believed to play a part in the genesis of hypertension in this condition.

All of these abnormalities improve to some extent after institution of regular dialysis and resolve after successful renal transplantation.

Peripheral nervous system

Median nerve compression in the carpal tunnel is common, and usually due to β_2-microglobulin-related amyloidosis.

'Restless legs' syndrome is common in uraemia. Patients complain of an irresistible need to move their legs, often interfering with sleep. The syndrome is difficult to treat. Iron deficiency should be treated if present. Attention should be paid to adequacy of dialysis. Symptoms may improve with the correction of anaemia by erythropoietin. Clonazepam and codeine phosphate are sometimes useful. Renal transplantation cures the problem.

A polyneuropathy occurs in patients who are inadequately dialysed.

Cardiovascular disease

Life expectancy remains severely reduced compared with the normal population owing to a greatly increased (16-fold) incidence of cardiovascular disease, particularly myocardial infarction, cardiac failure, sudden cardiac death and stroke. Coronary artery calcification is more common in patients with end-stage renal failure than in normal individuals and it is highly likely that this contributes significantly to cardiovascular mortality.

Hypertension is a frequent complication of renal failure.

Cardiac hypertrophy is common. Risk factors include hypertension, anaemia (causing increased cardiac work), obesity and male sex.

Systolic and diastolic dysfunction are also common. Diastolic dysfunction is largely attributable to left ventricular hypertrophy and contributes to hypotension during fluid removal on haemodialysis. Systolic dysfunction may be due to:

- myocardial fibrosis
- abnormal myocyte function owing to uraemia
- calcium overload and hyperparathyroidism
- carnitine and selenium deficiency.

Successful renal transplantation improves some, but not all, of these abnormalities.

Left ventricular hypertrophy is a risk factor for early death in renal failure, as in the general population. Systolic dysfunction is also an important marker for early death in renal failure.

Vascular calcification is frequent in all sizes of vessel in renal failure. In addition to the classical risk factors for atherosclerosis, a raised calcium × phosphate product causes medial calcification. Hyperparathyroidism may also contribute independently to the pathogenesis by increasing intracellular calcium. Diffuse calcification of the myocardium is also common; the causes are similar.

There is no good evidence that dialysis per se results in accelerated atherosclerosis.

Pericarditis is common and occurs in two clinical settings:

- *Uraemic pericarditis* is a feature of severe, preterminal uraemia or of underdialysis. Haemorrhagic pericardial effusion and atrial arrhythmias are often associated. There is a danger of pericardial tamponade, and anticoagulants should be used with caution. Pericarditis usually resolves with intensive dialysis.
- *Dialysis pericarditis* occurs as a result of an intercurrent illness or surgery in a patient receiving apparently adequate dialysis.

Progression of chronic renal impairment

Once established, and whatever the initial cause, chronic renal impairment tends to progress inexorably to end-stage renal failure, although the rate of progression may depend upon the underlying nephropathy. Patients with chronic glomerular diseases tend to deteriorate more quickly than those with chronic tubulo-interstitial nephropathies. Hypertension and heavy proteinuria are bad prognostic indicators in this context. A non-specific renal scarring process common to renal disorders of different aetiologies may be responsible for progression. Angiotensin-converting enzyme gene polymorphism may in part account for varying rates of progression between individuals, possession of the DD phenotype carrying a poorer prognosis (see p. 768).

Animal experiments in which one kidney is removed and the other partially removed indicate that progressive loss of renal function follows the initial reduction in nephron mass. A rise in intraglomerular capillary pressure and adaptive glomerular hypertrophy under conditions of reduced nephron mass have been postulated as causes of glomerular scarring in this connection, as has proteinuria per se. Renal interstitial scarring also occurs and is likely to be of major importance. It is not widely appreciated that the prognosis for renal function in chronic glomerular disorders is judged more accurately by interstitial histological appearances than by glomerular morphology. The pathogenesis of progressive interstitial damage is currently uncertain. Slowing of deterioration in renal function in diabetic nephropathy by meticulous control of blood pressure and, in particular, the use of ACE inhibitors, has been proved in a large controlled clinical trial, as has the benefit of tight glycaemic control. In non-diabetics, excellent control of hypertension is of benefit, and ACE inhibitors (which reduce intraglomerular capillary pressure and proteinuria) have been shown to be of particular value. Dietary protein restriction is not of proven benefit in slowing progression. Many other possible approaches to the problem are currently under investigation.

Management of chronic renal failure

The underlying cause of renal disease should be treated aggressively wherever possible.

Blood pressure control
Blood pressure should be reduced to 130/80 mmHg or lower if the patient can tolerate this level of pressure. Adequate control may require a combination of drugs together with large doses of diuretics to correct sodium and water retention. In the absence of contraindications, initial regimens should consist of or include an ACE inhibitor (see above). Measurement of 24-hour ambulatory blood pressure provides a much more accurate guide to blood pressure control than occasional outpatient clinic recordings. The aim of management is to prevent or reverse left ventricular hypertrophy, which will itself be significantly underdiagnosed if reliance is placed only upon clinical examination and electrocardiography. Echocardiography is essential.

Hyperkalaemia
Hyperkalaemia often responds to dietary restriction of potassium intake. Drugs which cause potassium retention (see p. 685) should be stopped. Occasionally it may be necessary to prescribe ion-exchange resins to remove potassium in the gastrointestinal tract. Emergency treatment of severe hyperkalaemia is described on page 686.

Acidosis
Correction of acidosis helps to correct hyperkalaemia in chronic renal failure, and may also decrease muscle catabolism. Sodium bicarbonate supplements are often effective, but may cause oedema and hypertension owing to extracellular fluid expansion. Calcium carbonate, also used as a calcium supplement and phosphate binder, has a beneficial effect on acidosis.

Calcium and phosphate
Hypocalcaemia and hyperphosphataemia should be treated aggressively, preferably with regular (e.g. 3-monthly) measurements of serum PTH to assess how effectively hyperparathyroidism is being suppressed.

Recent studies indicate that most current assays for PTH also measure a fragment of the molecule that actually inhibits PTH action. Renal physicians have long recognized that suppression of PTH levels to below two or three times the upper limit of 'normal' carries a high risk of development of adynamic bone disease. This is the probable explanation. Dietary restriction of phosphate is seldom effective alone, because so many foods contain it. Oral calcium carbonate acts as a calcium supplement and also reduces bioavailability of dietary phosphate. Aluminium-containing gut phosphate binders have the disadvantage that absorption of aluminium poses the risk of aluminium bone disease and development of cognitive impairment. Recently, the polymer sevelamer has been introduced as a gut-phosphate binder and shows considerable promise. Treatment with calcitriol or a vitamin D analogue such as alfacalcidol in early renal impairment has no deleterious effect upon renal function provided hypercalcaemia is avoided. Treatment should probably not be started unless serum PTH level is three times or more the upper limit of normal, in order to prevent the development of adynamic bone disease (see p. 646). Vitamin D therapy has the disadvantage that it increases gut phosphate absorption and may therefore exacerbate hyperphosphataemia. H_2 antagonists decrease the effectiveness of phosphate binders.

Dietary restrictions
In advanced renal disease, reduction of protein intake lessens the amount of nitrogenous waste products generated, and this may delay the onset of symptomatic uraemia. Most patients with renal impairment will require a diet restricted in sodium and potassium. A minority of patients (particularly those with tubulo-interstitial disease) manifest impaired capacity to retain salt and water (salt-losing renal disease) and require a high salt intake and/or sodium supplement.

Prolonged dietary protein restriction should be avoided. It is preferable to commence renal replacement therapy a little earlier than to cause malnutrition. It may well be the best policy to commence dialysis when glomerular filtration rate reaches 10 ml per minute, smaller 'doses' of dialysis being employed initially.

Fluid intake
Fluid depletion and overload should be avoided. Maximum water excretion is approximately 500 mL per 24 hours per mL GFR. It follows that a patient with a GFR of 5 mL per minute cannot usually excrete more than 2.5 L daily. Dilutional hyponatraemia may occur if water intake exceeds the capacity to excrete the water load. Advice to maximize fluid intake in patients with chronic renal failure may thus be misplaced. Conversely, the large majority of patients with moderate chronic renal impairment do not need to restrict fluid intake.

Drug therapy

This should be minimized in patients with chronic renal impairment. Tetracyclines (with the possible exception of doxycycline) should be avoided in view of their antianabolic effect and tendency to worsen uraemia. Drugs excreted by the kidneys, such as gentamicin, should be prescribed with caution and drug levels monitored if feasible. Non-steroidal anti-inflammatory drugs should be avoided. Potassium-sparing agents, such as spironolactone and amiloride, pose particular dangers, as do artificial salt substitutes, all of which contain potassium.

Anaemia

The anaemia of erythropoietin deficiency can be treated with synthetic (recombinant) human erythropoietin, starting at a dose of 25–50 U/kg three times a week; subcutaneous administration is more effective than intravenous. Blood pressure, haemoglobin concentration and reticulocyte count are measured every 2 weeks and the dose adjusted to maintain a target haemoglobin of 10–12 g/dL.

Failure to respond to 300 U/kg weekly, or a fall in haemoglobin after a satisfactory response, may be due to iron deficiency, bleeding, malignancy or infection. The demand for iron by the bone marrow is enormous when erythropoietin is commenced. Recently available intravenous (rather than oral) iron supplements optimize response to treatment.

Partial correction of anaemia with erythropoietin improves quality of life, exercise tolerance, sexual function and cognitive function in dialysis patients, and leads to regression of left ventricular hypertrophy. Avoidance of blood transfusion also lessens the chance of sensitization to HLA antigens, which may otherwise be a barrier to successful renal transplantation.

The disadvantages of erythropoietin therapy are that it is expensive and causes a rise in blood pressure in up to 30% of patients, particularly in the first 6 months. Peripheral resistance rises in all patients, owing to loss of hypoxic vasodilatation and to increased blood viscosity. A rare complication is encephalopathy with fits, transient cortical blindness and hypertension. Other causes of anaemia should be looked for and treated appropriately (see p. 410).

Male impotence

Testosterone deficiency should be corrected. If vascular or neurological causes exist, intracavernosal injection prostaglandin therapy, the use of a vacuum device or the use of a penile prosthetic implant should be considered. The oral phosphodiesterase inhibitor sildenafil has been shown to be effective in a controlled trial in patients with end-stage renal failure. Known coronary artery disease (common in renal failure patients) and use of nitrates are contraindications to this treatment.

Early referral of patients with chronic renal failure

Patients with chronic renal impairment should be referred to a nephrologist with access to facilities for renal replacement therapy at an early stage since late referral has been shown to be associated with increased mortality and morbidity when such patients commence renal replacement therapy. Old age is no bar to referral in the reasonably fit elderly patient.

Referral should be arranged when serum creatinine reaches 350 mmol/L in non-diabetics and when it reaches 250 mmol/L in diabetics, who are more prone to require early dialysis owing to impaired cardiac function and consequent pulmonary oedema. Measures aimed at slowing progression of renal failure and limiting its complications can thus be optimized and sufficient time gained to plan replacement therapy if needed.

Patients need time to adjust to the demands of chronic renal failure and its treatment, and to absorb information. Management in the predialysis phase should take account of future needs for vascular access for haemodialysis. Veins required in the future for fashioning of an arteriovenous fistula should not be rendered useless by cannulation (Fig. 11.38).

If the patient opts for regular haemodialysis, fashioning of an arteriovenous fistula should be carried out well in advance of the need for dialysis, when serum creatinine is of the order 400–500 mmol/L in non-diabetics and at an even earlier stage in diabetics with poorer vasculature. Such fistulae require several weeks to mature and become usable for vascular access.

Renal replacement therapy

Approximately 100 white individuals per million population commence renal replacement therapy in the UK

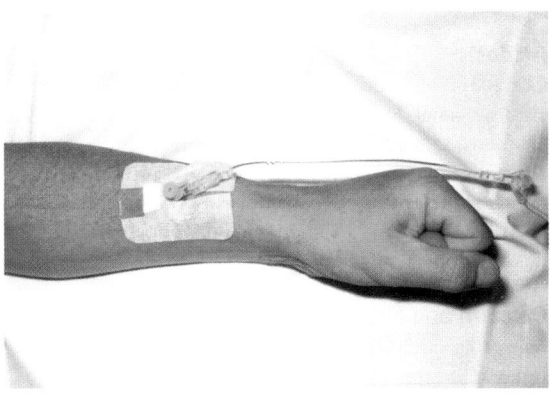

Fig. 11.38 Intravenous cannula in exactly the wrong place, in a right-handed patient with chronic renal impairment who will in future need a left (non-dominant arm) radiocephalic fistula.

each year. The corresponding figure in black Africans and Asians in the UK is three to four times higher, largely owing to diabetic and hypertensive nephropathy. The aim of all renal replacement techniques is to mimic the excretory functions of the normal kidney, including excretion of nitrogenous wastes, maintenance of normal electrolyte concentrations, and maintenance of a normal extracellular volume.

Haemodialysis

Basic principles

In haemodialysis, blood from the patient is pumped through an array of semipermeable membranes (the dialyser, often called an 'artificial kidney') which bring the blood into close contact with dialysate, flowing countercurrent to the blood. The plasma biochemistry changes towards that of the dialysate owing to diffusion of molecules down their concentration gradients (Fig. 11.39).

The dialysis machine comprises a series of blood pumps, with pressure monitors and bubble detectors and a proportionating unit, also with pressure monitors and blood leak detectors. Blood flow during dialysis is usually 200–300 mL per minute and the dialysate flow usually 500 mL per minute. The efficiency of dialysis in achieving biochemical change depends on blood and dialysate flow and the surface area of the dialysis membrane.

Dialysate is prepared by a proportionating unit which mixes specially purified water with concentrate,

resulting in fluid with the composition described in Table 11.24. Newer highly permeable synthetic membranes allow more rapid haemodialysis than with cellulose-based membranes (high-flux haemodialysis).

Access for haemodialysis

Adequate dialysis requires a blood flow of at least 200 mL per minute. The most reliable long-term way of achieving this is surgical construction of an arteriovenous fistula (Figs 11.40 and 11.41), using the radial or brachial artery and the cephalic vein. This results in distension of the vein and thickening ('arterialization') of its wall, so that after 6–8 weeks large-bore needles may be inserted to take blood to and from the dialysis machine.

Arteriovenous shunts are large-bore plastic cannulae surgically tied into a superficial artery and adjacent vein. These allow direct flow of arterial blood into the dialyser, which is then returned directly into a vein. Between dialysis sessions flow between artery and vein is restored by a plastic connector between the two cannulae, which lie outside the body, usually on the

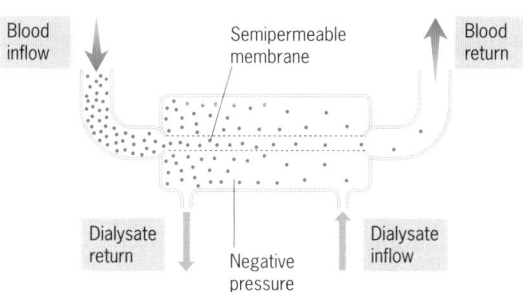

Fig. 11.39 Changes across a semipermeable dialysis membrane.

Table 11.24
Range of concentrations (mmol/L) in routinely available final dialysates used for haemodialysis

Sodium	130–145
Potassium	0.0–4.0
Calcium	1.0–1.6
Magnesium	0.25–0.85
Chloride	99–108
Bicarbonate	35–40
OR	
Acetate	35–40
Glucose	0–10

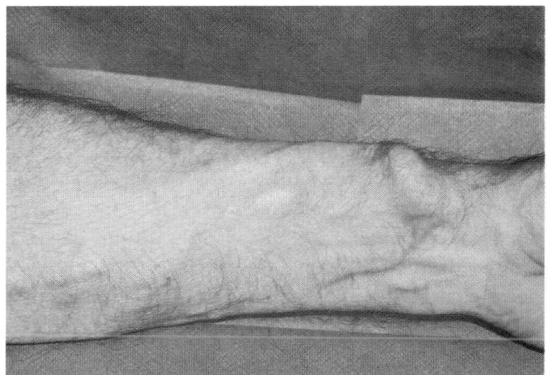

Fig. 11.40 Left forearm arteriovenous (radiocephalic) fistula.

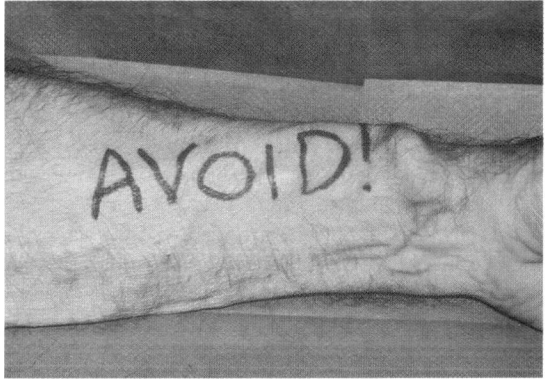

Fig. 11.41 One way of reminding the anaesthetic, nursing and surgical team about the presence of an existing arteriovenous fistula in a haemodialysis patient about to undergo surgery. In particular, the fistula should not be compressed during surgery to avoid thrombosis within it.

forearm. Disadvantages include a high rate of infection, thrombosis and the potential for disconnection which could result in exsanguination.

If dialysis is needed immediately, a large-bore double-lumen cannula may be inserted into a central vein – usually the subclavian, jugular or femoral. Semipermanent dual-lumen venous catheters may also be inserted with a skin tunnel to lessen the risk of infection. Nevertheless, the risk of local and systemic sepsis with such external devices is substantial and there is much associated morbidity and some increased risk of mortality. Stenosis of the subclavian vein is common when such devices are used and the jugular route is in general to be preferred.

Dialysis prescription

Dialysis must be tailored to an individual patient to obtain optimal results.

Dry weight

This is the weight at which a patient is neither fluid overloaded nor depleted. Patients are weighed at the start of each dialysis session and the transmembrane pressure adjusted to achieve fluid removal equal to the amount by which they exceed their dry weight.

The dialysate buffer

The dialysate buffer is usually acetate or bicarbonate. The sodium and calcium concentrations of the dialysate buffer are carefully monitored. A high dialysate sodium causes thirst and hypertension. A high dialysate calcium causes hypercalcaemia, whilst a low-calcium dialysate combined with poor compliance of medication with oral calcium carbonate and vitamin D may result in hyperparathyroidism.

Frequency and duration

Frequency and duration of dialysis are adjusted to achieve adequate removal of uraemic metabolites and to avoid excessive fluid overload between dialysis sessions. An adult of average size usually receives 4–5 hours' treatment three times a week. Twice-weekly dialysis is adequate only if the patient has considerable residual renal function.

Increasingly, short-duration dialysis using very biocompatible high-flux membranes is employed. Advantages include shorter duration of treatment and hence increased patient convenience. Disadvantages include higher cost of the membranes employed and, in all probability, higher prevalence of hypertension in such patients, requiring hypotensive medication. It should not be forgotten that normal kidneys work for 24 hours a day, 7 days a week, and that dialysis is a poor substitute for the natural state.

Underdialysis, which occurred in the USA in the 1980s, is associated with much increased patient morbidity and mortality. Adequate/optimal dialysis should be adjusted to individual patients' needs. All patients are anticoagulated (usually with heparin) during treatment as contact with foreign surfaces activates the clotting cascade. In the UK, a modest minority of patients manage self-supervised home haemodialysis.

Complications

Hypotension during dialysis is the major complication. Contributing factors include: an excessive removal of extracellular fluid, inadequate 'refilling' of the blood compartment from the interstitial compartment during fluid removal, abnormalities of venous tone, autonomic neuropathy, acetate intolerance (acetate acts as a vasodilator) and left ventricular hypertrophy.

Very rarely patients may develop anaphylactic reactions to ethylene oxide, which is used to sterilize most dialysers. Patients receiving ACE inhibitors are at risk of anaphylaxis if polyacrylonitrile dialysers are used.

Other potential, rare, complications include the hard-water syndrome (caused by failure to soften water resulting in a high calcium concentration prior to mixing with dialysate concentrate), haemolytic reactions and air embolism.

Adequacy of dialysis

Dialysis treatment is empirical since the size, number and nature of 'uraemic toxins' is unclear. The only true measure of adequacy is patient mortality and morbidity. Adequate nutrition of the patient is as important as (perhaps more important than) adequacy of dialysis in reducing morbidity and mortality.

Symptoms of underdialysis are non-specific and include insomnia, itching, fatigue despite adequate correction of anaemia, restless legs and a peripheral sensory neuropathy.

Adequacy of dialysis may be assessed by computerized calculation of urea kinetics, requiring measurement of the residual renal urea clearance, the rate of rise of urea concentration between dialysis sessions, and the reduction in urea concentration during dialysis. It is likely that duration of haemodialysis is important in itself in addition to the efficiency with which small molecules such as urea are cleared.

Haemodialysis is the most efficient way of achieving rapid biochemical improvement, for instance in the treatment of acute renal failure or severe hyperkalaemia. This advantage is offset by disadvantages such as haemodynamic instability, especially in acutely ill patients with multiorgan disease, and over-rapid correction of uraemia can lead to 'dialysis disequilibrium'. This is characterized by nausea and vomiting, restlessness, headache, hypertension, myoclonic jerking, and in severe instances seizures and coma owing to rapid changes in plasma osmolality leading to cerebral oedema.

These problems have led to the increasing adoption of gentler continuous methods for the treatment of acute renal failure (see below).

Haemofiltration

This involves removal of plasma water and its dissolved constituents (e.g. K^+, Na^+, urea, phosphate) by convective flow across a high-flux semipermeable membrane, and replacing it with a solution of the desired biochemical composition (Fig. 11.42). Lactate is used as buffer in the replacement solution because rapid infusion of acetate causes vasodilatation and bicarbonate may cause precipitation of calcium carbonate.

Haemofiltration can be used for both acute and chronic renal failure. High volumes need to be exchanged in order to achieve adequate small molecule removal; typically a 22 L exchange three times a week for maintenance treatment and 1 L per hour in acute renal failure. Financial costs of disposable items (such as filters and replacement fluid) are high and only a tiny minority of patients with end-stage renal failure are managed in this way. However, nursing costs are reduced when acute renal failure is managed in an intensive care unit setting since haemofiltration can be managed by ITU nursing staff rather than renal unit nurses.

Peritoneal dialysis

Peritoneal dialysis utilizes the peritoneal membrane as a semipermeable membrane, avoiding the need for extracorporeal circulation of blood. This is a very simple, low-technology treatment compared to haemodialysis. The principles are simple (Fig. 11.43).

- A tube is placed into the peritoneal cavity through the anterior abdominal wall.
- Dialysate is run into the peritoneal cavity, usually under gravity.
- Urea, creatinine, phosphate, and other uraemic toxins pass into the dialysate down their concentration gradients.
- Water (with solutes) is attracted into the peritoneal cavity by osmosis, depending on the osmolarity of the dialysate. This is determined by the dextrose content of the dialysate (Table 11.25).
- The fluid is changed regularly to repeat the process.

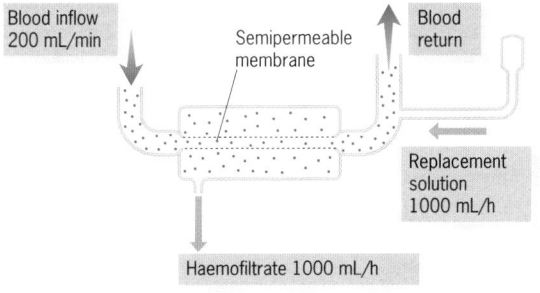

Fig. 11.42 **Principles of haemofiltration.**

Table 11.25
Range of concentrations (mmol/L) in routinely available CAPD dialysate*

Sodium	130–134
Potassium	0
Calcium	1.0–1.75
Magnesium	0.25–0.75
Chloride	95–104
Lactate	35–40
Glucose	77–236
Total osmolality	356–511 mOsmol/kg

*Glucose content is often expressed as g/dL of anhydrous glucose (e.g. 1.36% = 77 mmol/L). An even more hypertonic dialysate (6.36%) is available for acute (intermittent) peritoneal dialysis

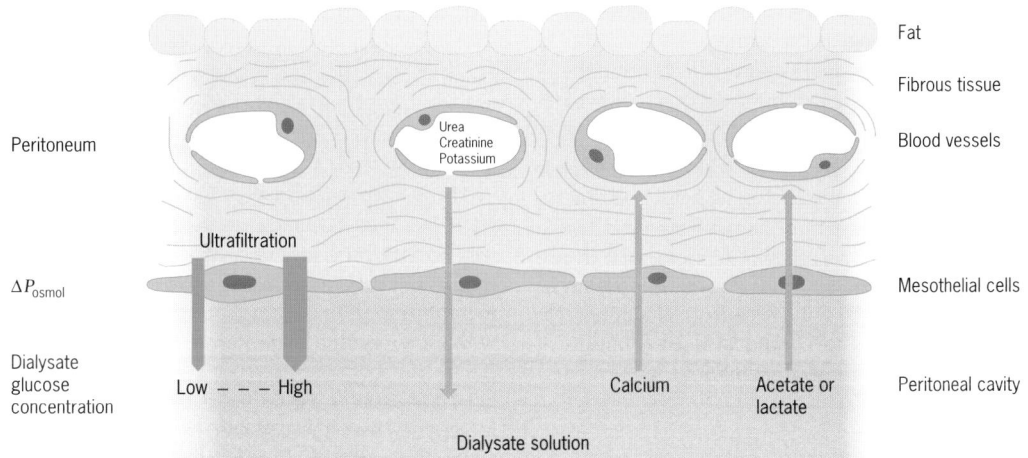

Fig. 11.43 **Principles of peritoneal dialysis.**

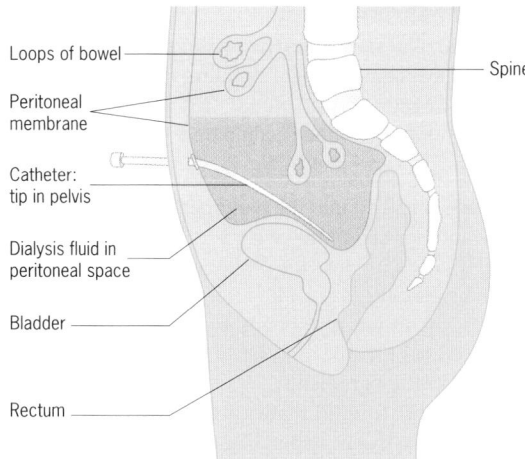

Loops of bowel

Peritoneal membrane

Catheter: tip in pelvis

Dialysis fluid in peritoneal space

Bladder

Rectum

Spine

Fig. 11.44 The siting of a Tenckhoff peritoneal dialysis catheter.

Chronic peritoneal dialysis requires insertion of a soft catheter, with its tip in the pelvis, exiting the peritoneal cavity in the midline and lying in a skin tunnel with an exit site in the lateral abdominal wall (Fig. 11.44).

This form of dialysis can be adapted in several ways.

- **Continuous ambulatory peritoneal dialysis (CAPD).** Dialysate is present within the peritoneal cavity continuously, except when dialysate is being exchanged. Dialysate exchanges are performed three to five times a day, using a sterile no-touch technique to connect 1.5–3 L bags of dialysate to the peritoneal catheter; each exchange takes 20–40 minutes. This is the technique most often used for maintenance peritoneal dialysis in patients with end-stage renal failure.
- **Nightly intermittent peritoneal dialysis (NIPD).** An automated device is used to perform exchanges each night while the patient is asleep. Sometimes dialysate is left in the peritoneal cavity during the day in addition, to increase the time during which biochemical exchange is occurring.
- **Tidal dialysis.** A residual volume is left within the peritoneal cavity with continuous cycling of smaller volumes in and out.

Osmotic removal of excess plasma water and solutes is achieved using hypertonic dialysate, which exerts an osmotic 'drag'. Depending on the patient's fluid intake and residual urine output, it may be necessary to use one or more hypertonic dialysate bags daily to achieve fluid balance in CAPD. Fluid overload is a relatively common problem in CAPD, and is due to failure of transport across the peritoneal membrane.

Complications
Peritonitis
Bacterial peritonitis is the most common serious complication of CAPD and other forms of peritoneal dialysis.

Table 11.26
Some causes of CAPD peritonitis*

	Approximate percentage of cases
Staphylococcus epidermidis	40–50
Escherichia coli, Pseudomonas and other Gram-negative organisms	25
Staphylococcus aureus	15
Mycobacterium tuberculosis	2
Candida and other fungal species	2

*In approximately 20%, no bacteria are found

Clinical presentations include abdominal pain of varying severity (guarding and rebound tenderness are unusual), and a cloudy peritoneal effluent – without which the diagnosis cannot be made. Microscopy reveals a neutrophil count of above 100 cells per mL. Nausea, vomiting, fever and paralytic ileus may be seen if peritonitis is severe. The incidence of CAPD-associated peritonitis has been much reduced (to about one episode every three patient years) by use of a Y-disconnect system in preference to previous methods.

CAPD peritonitis must be investigated with culture of peritoneal effluent. Empirical antibiotic treatment is started, with a spectrum which covers both Gram-negative and Gram-positive organisms. Antibiotics may be given by the oral, intravenous or intraperitoneal route; most centres rely on intraperitoneal antibiotics. Common causative organisms are listed in Table 11.26.

Staph. aureus peritonitis should lead to a search for nasal carriage of this organism and *Staph. epidermidis* peritonitis may indicate contamination from the patient's (or helper's) skin. Relapsing *Staph. epidermidis* peritonitis with an organism with the same antibiotic sensitivity pattern on each occasion may indicate that the Tenckhoff catheter has become colonized: often this is difficult to eradicate without replacement of the catheter under antibiotic cover.

Gram-negative peritonitis may complicate septicaemia from urinary or bowel infection. A mixed growth of Gram-negative and anaerobic organisms strongly suggests bowel perforation, and is an indication for laparotomy.

Fungal peritonitis often follows antibacterial treatment but may occur de novo. Clinical presentation is very variable. It is rare to be able to cure fungal peritonitis without catheter removal as well as antifungal treatment. Intraperitoneal amphotericin has been associated with the formation of peritoneal adhesions.

Infection around the catheter site
Infection where the catheter exits through the skin is relatively common. It should be treated aggressively (with systemic and/or local antibiotics) to prevent spread of the infection into the subcutaneous tunnel and

the peritoneum. The most common causative organisms are staphylococci.

Other complications

CAPD is often associated with constipation, which in turn may impair flow of dialysate in and out of the pelvis. Occasionally dialysate may leak through a diaphragmatic defect into the thoracic cavity, causing a massive pleural 'effusion'. The glucose content of the effusion is usually diagnostic, or the diagnosis may be made by instillation of methylthioninium chloride (methylene blue) with dialysate and the demonstration of a blue colour on pleural tap. Dialysate may also leak into the scrotum down a patent processus vaginalis.

Failure of peritoneal membrane function is a predictable complication of long-term CAPD, resulting in worsening biochemical exchange and decreased ultrafiltration with hypertonic dialysate. It is thought that this problem may be accelerated by excessive reliance on hypertonic dialysate to remove fluid.

Sclerosing peritonitis is a potentially fatal complication of CAPD. The cause is often unclear, but recurrent peritonitis, and exposure of the peritoneum to unphysiological high glucose concentrations, is responsible in most cases. Progressive thickening of the peritoneal membrane occurs in association with adhesions and strictures, turning the small bowel into a mass of matted loops and causing repeated episodes of small bowel obstruction. CAPD should be abandoned. Improvement may follow renal transplantation or treatment with prednisolone or azathioprine.

Contraindications

There are few absolute contraindications apart from unwillingness or inability on the patient's part to learn the technique.

Previous peritonitis causing peritoneal adhesions may make peritoneal dialysis impossible: but the extent of adhesions is difficult to predict, and it may be worth an attempted surgical placement of a dialysis catheter.

The presence of a stoma (colostomy, ileostomy, ileal urinary conduit) makes successful placement of a dialysis catheter extremely unlikely.

Active intra-abdominal sepsis, for instance due to diverticular abscesses, is an absolute contraindication to peritoneal dialysis although diverticular disease per se is not.

Abdominal hernias may often expand during CAPD as a result of increased intra-abdominal pressure, and should ideally be repaired before or at the time of CAPD catheter insertion.

Visual impairment may make it difficult for a patient to perform dialysate exchanges, but completely blind patients can be trained in the technique if adequately motivated.

Severe arthritis makes it difficult to perform the exchanges, but a large number of mechanical aids are available. Sterilization of connections by heat or ultraviolet light reduces the risk of peritonitis.

Adequacy of peritoneal dialysis

No consensus yet exists on how the adequacy of peritoneal dialysis should be measured and the optimum degree of removal of urea and other waste products to be obtained in unit time. Urea kinetic modelling may be employed, as with haemodialysis. However, it is increasingly appreciated that patient prognosis improves with greater degrees of waste product removal than were hitherto considered acceptable, and that peritoneal dialysis inadequacy is common when residual renal function declines to zero. With increasing time on treatment, adequacy may become impaired owing to alterations in the efficiency of the peritoneal membrane in transporting waste products, fluid and electrolytes. Under these circumstances conversion to haemodialysis is necessary.

Complications of long-term dialysis

Cardiovascular disease (see p. 643) and sepsis are the leading causes of death in long-term dialysis patients.

Causes of fatal sepsis include peritonitis complicating peritoneal dialysis and *Staph. aureus* infection (including endocarditis) complicating the use of indwelling access devices for haemodialysis.

Dialysis amyloidosis

This is the accumulation of amyloid protein (p. 1118) as a result of failure of clearance of β_2-microglobulin, a molecule of 11.8 kDa. This protein is the light chain of the class I HLA antigens and is normally freely filtered at the glomerulus but is not removed by cellulose-based haemodialysis membranes. Complement activation resulting from the use of cellulose-based membranes may increase the generation rate of the protein. The protein polymerizes to form amyloid deposits, which may cause median nerve compression in the carpal tunnel or a dialysis arthropathy – a clinical syndrome of pain and disabling stiffness in the shoulders, hips, hands, wrists and knees. β_2-Microglobulin-related amyloid may be demonstrated in the synovium. There is little inflammation and the pathogenesis is not well understood. Rapid improvement after renal transplantation is probably due to steroid therapy. Low-dose prednisolone alone can also cause an improvement. A change to a biocompatible synthetic membrane has also been reported to be of benefit: again, the mechanism for this improvement is not clear. Amyloid deposits can also cause pathological bone cysts and fractures, pseudotumours and gastrointestinal bleeding caused by amyloid deposition around submucosal blood vessels.

The extent of amyloid deposition is best assessed by nuclear imaging, either using [^{99m}Tc]DMSA, or, more specifically, by the use of radiolabelled serum amyloid P component.

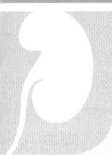

Surgery in patients with chronic renal failure

To reduce the risk of worsening renal failure and the risk of morbidity and mortality, the following measures are undertaken:

- Ensure that blood volume is normal, employing measurement of central venous pressure if necessary.
- Ensure an adequate diuresis in the perioperative period, using intravenous fluid infusion as necessary.
- Avoid hypotension, using inotropes if necessary.
- Delay surgery if hyperkalaemia (serum potassium >5.5 mmol/L) or fluid overload is present preoperatively until these have been corrected.
- Monitor urea, electrolyte and creatinine concentrations carefully. Serum potassium should be checked immediately postoperatively (or intraoperatively if surgery is prolonged) and 4–6 hours later, and urea, electrolyte and creatinine concentrations should be checked daily thereafter. If possible weigh the patient daily to monitor fluid balance.
- Prior mannitol infusion may reduce the risk of acute renal tubular necrosis in patients with extrahepatic cholestatic jaundice.
- The action of some anaesthetic agents such as muscle relaxants and opiates are prolonged in renal impairment. Appropriate precautions should be taken. Anaesthetic agents that are safe in renal failure and can be used without alteration in dosage include fentanyl, atropine, diazepam, isoflurane and nitrous oxide.

Patients near to end-stage renal failure who may be precipitated into the need for dialysis by surgery should be operated on only if essential. For example, coronary bypass surgery in a patient with a serum creatinine of 600 mmol/L should, if possible, be deferred until the patient is safely established on regular dialysis and is stable. All possible attempts should be made to avoid breaching the peritoneum in patients on CAPD or damaging an arteriovenous fistula in haemodialysis patients (see Fig. 11.41).

Transplantation

Successful renal transplantation offers the potential for almost complete rehabilitation in end-stage renal failure. It allows freedom from dietary and fluid restriction, anaemia and infertility are corrected, and the need for parathyroidectomy is reduced.

The technique involves the anastomosis of an explanted human kidney, usually either from a cadaveric donor or, less frequently, from a living close relative, on

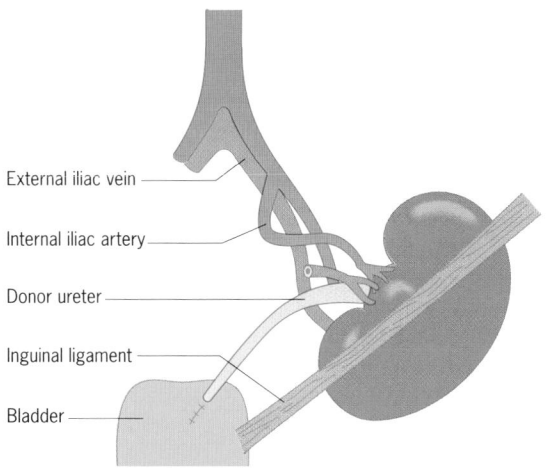

Fig. 11.45 Anatomy of a renal transplant operation.

to the iliac vessels of the recipient (Fig. 11.45). The donor ureter is placed into the recipient's bladder. Unless the donor is genetically identical (i.e. an identical twin), immunosuppressive treatment is needed, for as long as the transplant remains in place, to prevent rejection. Eighty per cent of grafts now survive for 5–10 years in the best centres, and 60% for 10–30 years.

Factors affecting success

ABO (blood group) compatibility between donor and recipient is required.

Matching donor and recipient for HLA type

Matching for HLA-DR antigens appears to have the most impact on survival, followed by the B and, least importantly, the A locus antigens. Complete compatibility at A, B and DR offers the best chance of success, followed by a single HLA mismatch (i.e. antigen possessed by the donor and not possessed by the recipient). The effect of further degrees of mismatching upon graft survival in first transplants is of modest degree. Nationwide matching schemes for kidneys retrieved from cadaver donors are in existence.

Adequate immunosuppressive treatment

See below.

The 'centre effect'

Graft survival is higher in those centres with extensive experience of management of transplant recipients.

The donor kidney

Cadaveric donation

Most countries allow the removal of kidneys and other organs from patients who have suffered irretrievable brain damage ('brainstem death') while their hearts are still beating (see p. 955).

Living related donation

A close relative may volunteer as a potential donor. A sibling donor may be HLA identical or share one or no haplotypes with the potential recipient. Most transplant centres accept one-haplotype matches as well as HLA-identical donors. Some avoid using child-to-parent donation unless the circumstances are exceptional. In the UK, donor age must be 18 years or more.

Potential living related donors are subjected to an intensive preoperative evaluation, including clinical examination and measurement of renal function, tests for carriage of hepatitis B, C, HIV and cytomegalovirus, and detailed imaging of renal anatomy with IVU and then arteriography, to be sure that transplantation will be technically feasible.

Unrelated living donors may be accepted provided no inducement (financial or otherwise) is involved. Paid live non-related donor transplantation is illegal in the UK.

Immunosuppression for transplantation

Long-term drug treatment for the prevention of rejection is employed in all cases apart from living related donation from an identical twin. Some degree of immunological tolerance does develop, and the risk of rejection is highest in the first 3 months after transplantation. In the early months rejection episodes occur in 30–50% of cadaver kidney recipients. Most are reversible. A combination of immunosuppressive drugs is usually used.

Corticosteroids. Corticosteroids have a non-specific immunosuppressive action. High-dose methylprednisolone is used as the primary treatment for acute rejection.

Azathioprine. Azathioprine prevents cell-mediated rejection by interfering with nucleic acid synthesis and preventing replication of lymphocytes. Adverse effects include suppression of red cell and platelet production, an increased incidence of infections (particularly viral), and hepatotoxicity.

Ciclosporin. Ciclosporin, a calcineurin inhibitor, prevents the activation of T lymphocytes in response to new antigens and is highly effective in preventing rejection, while leaving the functioning of the rest of the immune system largely intact. Its introduction has revolutionized organ transplantation. Disadvantages include high cost and nephrotoxicity. Even with careful adjustment of the dose in response to trough blood levels, renal function may be adversely affected.

Tacrolimus, also a calcineurin inhibitor, blocks T-cell activation by a mechanism very similar to that of ciclosporin but with fewer rejection episodes.

Mycophenolate mofetil is metabolized to mycophenolic acid and is supplanting azathioprine as an immunosuppressant, as trials have shown a reduction in rejection episodes.

Antilymphocyte and antithymocyte globulin. These are potent immunosuppressive agents. Antibodies may be polyclonal or monoclonal, derived from mouse, rabbit, horse, or 'humanized', and directed against any of a number of lymphocyte surface marker proteins, enabling neutralization or killing of lymphocytes with certain functions (e.g. T cells, activated T cells, cells expressing adhesion molecules, cells expressing the interleukin-2 receptor). Basiliximab is a chimeric (human and mouse) CD25 monoclonal antibody, which binds to IL-2 receptors inhibiting IL-2-driven proliferative responses. Recent trials have shown its safety, and when given prophylactically it reduces first-time rejection by 40%. The risk of long-term infections and virus-associated malignancy (e.g. lymphoma) remain to be evaluated.

Complications

Technical failures

There may be occlusion or stenosis of the arterial anastomosis, occlusion of the venous anastomosis, and urinary leaks owing to damage to the lower ureter, or defects in the anastomosis between ureter and recipient bladder.

Immunosuppression

- Corticosteroid therapy (see p. 1055) can lead to weight gain, 'mooning' of the face, skin striae, increased skin fragility with ecchymoses, diabetes, osteoporosis and fractures, particularly of the femoral neck owing to avascular necrosis of bone.
- Ciclosporin therapy can produce nephrotoxicity, rash, tremor, increased hairiness and diabetes.
- Tacrolimus therapy can lead to neurotoxicity and nephrotoxicity that appear to be greater than with ciclosporin. The incidence of drug-induced diabetes is much higher than with ciclosporin.
- Azathioprine therapy can lead to bone marrow depression and hepatotoxicity.

Both corticosteroid and ciclosporin treatment contribute to post-transplant hypertension. Ciclosporin and azathioprine may cause liver damage. Treatment with corticosteroids, ciclosporin and azathioprine alone or in combination increase the risk of skin tumours, including basal and squamous cell carcinomata. In white recipients, exposure to ultraviolet light should be minimized and sun-block creams employed. All immunosuppressive agents used, including antilymphocyte and antithymocyte globulin, increase the risk of infections, particularly opportunistic infections such as *Pneumocystis carinii* and cytomegalovirus infection. Malignancy, particularly lymphomas and skin cancers, may often be attributable to viral induction of malignancy.

Other complications

Recurrence of the disease which caused renal failure, although uncommon, may occur in specific diseases. Examples are primary oxalosis, mesangiocapillary glomerulonephritis, focal segmental glomerulosclerosis and Goodpasture's syndrome.

Other possibilities are that there may be de novo glomerulonephritis in the grafted kidney, or lipid abnormalities and a high risk of cardiovascular events.

Choice of renal replacement therapy

For many patients with end-stage renal failure a renal transplant is the treatment of choice, but because of the limited availability of donor organs many patients remain on dialysis for years whilst waiting for a transplant. Sensitization to HLA antigens, for instance by pregnancy, blood transfusion or a previous failed transplant, makes finding a compatible organ more difficult. In addition, there are a number of factors rendering patients less suitable for transplantation, such as:

- previous malignancy
- severe non-renal disease likely to limit survival and the degree of rehabilitation after transplantation
- vascular disease (especially in diabetes) rendering vascular anastomoses difficult and compromising blood flow to the lower limb.

Age in itself is no bar to transplantation, so policies which limit transplantation to, for example, the under-70 age group, are unjustified. An increase in the supply of donor organs is desirable.

Combined renal and pancreatic transplantation is appropriate in carefully selected patients with diabetes mellitus. When successful, the effect upon quality of life is often dramatic.

The choice between CAPD and haemodialysis is influenced by medical, social, psychological and other factors. Unless specific indications or contraindications exist, patients should be offered a free choice of modality of treatment.

FURTHER READING

Baigent C, Burbury K, Wheeler D (2000) Premature cardiovascular disease in chronic renal failure. *Lancet* **356**: 147–152.

El Nahas AE, Coles EA (1997) Progressive renal failure. *Journal of the Royal College of Physicians* **31**: 27–31.

GISEN Trial (1997) Randomized placebo-controlled trial of effect of ramipril on decline in glomerular filtration rate and risk of terminal renal failure in proteinuric, non-diabetic nephropathy. *Lancet* **349**: 1857–1863. Also, Editorial: 1852–1853.

Klahr S (1991) Chronic renal failure: management. *Lancet* **338**: 423–427.

Lewis H et al. (1993) The effect of angiotensin converting enzyme inhibitor on diabetic nephropathy. *New England Journal of Medicine* **329**: 1456–1462.

Lightstone L et al. (1995) High incidence of end-stage renal disease in Indo-Asians in the UK. *Quarterly Journal of Medicine* **88**: 191–195.

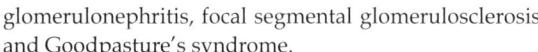

Cystic, congenital and familial disease

Cystic renal disease

Solitary or multiple renal cysts are common, especially with advancing age: 50% of those aged 50 years or more have one or more such cysts. They have no special significance except in the differential diagnosis of renal tumours (see p. 661). Such cysts are often asymptomatic and are found on excretion urography or ultrasound examination performed for some other reason. Occasionally they may cause pain and/or haematuria owing to their large size, or bleeding may occur into the cyst. Cystic degeneration (the formation of multiple cysts which enlarge with time) occurs regularly in the kidneys of patients with end-stage renal failure treated by dialysis and/or transplantation. Malignant tumour formation seems to be more common in such kidneys than in the general population.

Autosomal-dominant polycystic kidney disease

Autosomal-dominant polycystic kidney disease (ADPKD) is an inherited disorder usually presenting in adult life. It is characterized by the development of multiple renal cysts, variably associated with extrarenal (mainly hepatic and cardiovascular) abnormalities. ADPKD is by far the most common inherited nephropathy, with a prevalence rate ranging from 1:400 to 1:1000 in white populations. It accounts for 3–10% of all patients commencing regular dialysis in the West.

In about 85% of cases, the gene responsible (*PKD1*) has been located on chromosome 16. A second gene, *PKD2*, which has been mapped on chromosome 4, accounts for the vast majority of other cases. A third polycystic gene may exist. These genetic abnormalities are distinct from the autosomal recessive form of polycystic disease which is often lethal in early life. The protein corresponding to *PKD1* gene, polycystin I, appears to be an integral membrane glycoprotein involved in cell-to-cell and/or cell-to-matrix interaction. The protein corresponding to the *PKD2* gene appears to function as an ion channel or pore. Polycystin could act as the regulator of the *PKD2* channel activity. How mutations in *PKD1* and *PKD2* lead to cyst development and other abnormalities is unclear. It is hoped that elucidation of the mechanism involved may pave the way to intervention which prevents or, at any rate, arrests or slows the manifestations of the disease.

Clinical features

Clinical presentation may be at any age from the second decade. Presenting symptoms include:

- acute loin pain and/or haematuria owing to haemorrhage into a cyst, cyst infection or urinary tract stone formation

- loin or abdominal discomfort owing to the increasing size of the kidneys
- subarachnoid haemorrhage associated with berry aneurysm rupture
- complications of hypertension
- complications of associated liver cysts
- symptoms of uraemia and/or anaemia associated with chronic renal failure.

Erythraemia is a rare complication and presentation of ADPKD.

The natural history of the disease is one of progressive renal impairment, sometimes punctuated by acute episodes of loin pain and haematuria, and commonly associated with the development of hypertension. The rate of progression to renal failure is variable. The determinants of progression are both genetic and nongenetic. In the *PKD2* form, renal cysts develop more slowly and end-stage renal failure (ESRF) occurs 10–15 years later than in the *PKD1* form. Gender affects renal prognosis, males with ADPKD reaching end-stage renal failure 5–6 years earlier than females. There is a large variability in the age at ESRF within families, even between affected monozygotic twins.

Complications and associations
Pain
A minority of patients suffer chronic renal pain resistant to common analgesics, presumably owing to the pressure effect of large cysts. Surgical decompression of such cysts appears to be of benefit in about two-thirds of patients. Laparoscopic cyst decortication is a minimally-invasive alternative technique.

Cyst infection
The response to standard antibacterial therapy is often poor owing to poor penetration of conventional antibiotics across the cyst wall. Lipophilic antibiotics active against Gram-negative bacteria, such as co-trimoxazole and fluoroquinolones, penetrate into the cysts better and their use has greatly improved the treatment of this complication.

Renal calculi
These are diagnosed in about 10–20% of patients with ADPKD. Frequently they are composed of uric acid and hence radiolucent. Obstructing or painful stones are treated no differently than are stones in patients with normal urinary tracts. Percutaneous stone removal and extracorporeal lithotripsy may safely be employed.

Hypertension
Hypertension is an early and very common feature of ADPKD. Elevation of blood pressure, still within the normal range, is detectable in young affected individuals and is associated with an increase in left ventricular mass. It appears that left ventricular hypertrophy occurs

to a greater degree for a given rise in blood pressure in ADPKD compared with other renal disorders and with essential hypertension. Intrarenal activation of the renin–angiotensin system is, in all probability, of central importance in pathogenesis, and ACE inhibitors are logical first-line agents in treatment. Early control of blood pressure is essential as cardiovascular complications are a major cause of death in ADPKD.

Progressive renal failure
This is the most serious complication of ADPKD. At glomerular filtration rates below 50 mL per minute, the rate of decline in GFR averages 5 mL per minute each year, which is more rapid than in other primary renal disorders. The probability of being alive without requiring dialysis or transplantation by the age of 70 years is of the order 30%. Survival rates on regular haemodialysis and after renal transplantation in ADPKD are similar to those of patients with other primary renal diseases.

Hepatic cysts
Approximately 30% of patients have hepatic cysts and in a minority of patients massive enlargement of the polycystic liver is seen. Pain, infection of cysts and, more rarely, compression of the bile duct, portal vein or hepatic venous outflow may occur. Rarely, percutaneous drainage of painful cysts, laparoscopic fenestration or even partial hepatectomy may be necessary. Infected cysts may require drainage.

Intracranial aneurysm formation
About 8% of ADPKD patients have an asymptomatic intracranial aneurysm and the prevalence is twice as high in the subgroup of patients with a family history of such aneurysms or of subarachnoid haemorrhage. Such haemorrhage is preceded in from 20–40% of cases by premonitory headaches from a few hours up to 2 weeks before the onset of subarachnoid bleeding. Headache of sudden onset or unusual character or severity in a patient with ADPKD should prompt investigation. Contrast-enhanced spiral CT is the best investigation. Screening for intracranial aneurysm in ADPKD is currently recommended for patients aged 18–40 years who have a positive family history. Screening is performed either by magnetic resonance angiography or spiral CT.

Mitral valve prolapse
This is found in 20% of individuals with ADPKD, whereas it is present in only 2–3% of the general population.

Diagnosis
Physical examination commonly reveals large, irregular kidneys and possibly hepatomegaly. Definitive diagnosis is established by ultrasound examination (Fig. 11.46). However, such renal imaging techniques may be equivocal, especially in subjects under the age of 20 years.

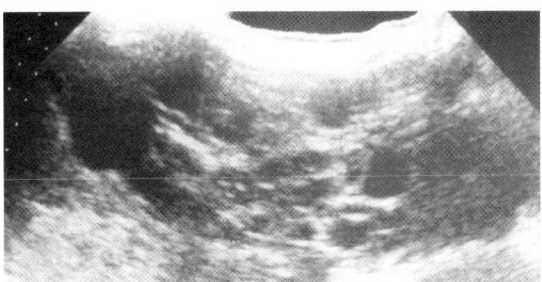

Fig. 11.46 Ultrasound scan of a polycystic kidney, showing an enlarged kidney with many cysts of varying size.

Screening

The children and siblings of patients with established ADPKD should, in general, be offered screening. Affected individuals should have regular blood pressure checks and should be offered genetic counselling. Screening by ultrasonography should not be carried out before the age of 20 years, as excluding the condition may be difficult and hypertension is unusual before this age. Even at age 20, renal ultrasonography may give a false-negative result. Gene linkage analysis can be utilized in many families.

Medullary cystic disease ('juvenile nephronophthisis')

Developing early in childhood, juvenile nephronophthisis is commonly inherited in an autosomal recessive manner. A similar condition developing later in childhood (medullary cystic disease) is inherited as an autosomal dominant trait, but sporadic cases occur in both conditions. Despite its name, the dominant histological finding is interstitial inflammation and tubular atrophy, with later development of medullary cysts. Progressive glomerular failure is a secondary consequence.

The dominant features are polyuria, polydipsia and growth retardation. Diagnosis is based on the family history and renal biopsy, the cysts rarely being visualized by imaging techniques.

Medullary sponge kidney

Medullary sponge kidney is an uncommon but not rare condition that usually presents with renal colic or haematuria. Although it is most often sporadic, a few affected families have been reported. The condition is characterized by dilatation of the collecting ducts in the papillae, sometimes with cystic change. In severe cases the medullary area has a sponge-like appearance. The condition may affect one or both kidneys or only part of one kidney. Cyst formation is commonly associated with the development of small calculi within the cyst. In about 20% of patients there is associated hypercalciuria or renal tubular acidosis (see p. 693). Hemihypertrophy of the skeleton has been described in this condition.

The diagnosis is made by excretion urography, which shows small calculi in the papillary zones with an increase in radiodensity around these following injection of contrast medium as the dilated or cystic collecting ducts are filled with contrast (see Fig. 11.26).

The natural history is one of intermittent colic with passage of small stones or haematuria. Renal function is usually well maintained and renal failure is unusual, except where obstructive nephropathy develops owing to the presence of stones in the pelvis or ureters.

Congenital abnormalities

Agenesis

Agenesis may be bilateral or unilateral. Unilateral agenesis ('solitary kidney') occurs in 1 in 1000 of the population. It is usually associated with compensatory hypertrophy of the single kidney and normal renal function. Save for the potential hazard of trauma to this solitary kidney, it has no clinical significance.

Hypoplasia

Renal hypoplasia (failed development) of one kidney is uncommon, and hypoplasia of both kidneys is rare. It may be difficult to distinguish unilateral renal hypoplasia from a small kidney because of renal artery stenosis, obstruction or reflux nephropathy in early life. Clinical interest in the condition most often arises in patients with hypertension, where the small kidney may be considered the cause. If the small kidney is shown by radioisotope studies to contribute no useful renal function, and if the hypertension has developed in a young subject or is difficult to control by medical treatment, nephrectomy should be undertaken.

Ectopic kidneys

Defects in embryological renal development may lead to ectopic or maldeveloped renal systems. At the risk of oversimplification, the kidneys may be thought of as developing in the embryo as one structure in the 'pelvic' area, migrating upwards and separating with growth. Failure in normal development may result in failure of the kidneys to migrate normally and indeed they may fail to separate. This results in a 'pelvic kidney' when one or both remain in the pelvis, a 'crossed ectopic kidney' when both have moved to the same side of the spine, a horseshoe or discoid kidney when there is partial (usually fusion of the lower poles) or total failure of separation.

In clinical practice the main problem associated with ectopic kidneys usually relates to impaired urinary drainage with secondary obstruction or stone formation. This may be compounded if infection supervenes, the poor drainage making eradication of infection difficult and predisposing to stone formation. Pelvic kidneys may interfere with parturition.

Renal tubular transport defects

Renal tubular transport defects include cystinuria, Hartnup disease, adult Fanconi syndrome, galactosaemia and fructosaemia. They are discussed in more detail on page 1116.

Animal experiments now suggest that X-linked hypophosphataemia ('vitamin D-resistant rickets'), formerly regarded as an intrinsic proximal renal tubular transport defect, results from the effect of a distant mediator upon renal tubular phosphate handling. A mouse model of X-linked hypophosphataemia exists and transplantation of a kidney from an affected animal into a normal bi-nephrectomized mouse does not confer a renal tubular phosphate leak on the recipient. Conversely, transplantation of a normal mouse kidney into a bi-nephrectomized mouse with X-linked hypophosphataemia does not correct the renal tubular phosphate leak.

Renal glycosuria

Renal glycosuria, in which there is glucose in the urine in subjects demonstrated to have normal blood glucose levels, who are not starved and who have no other urinary abnormality, is uncommon. Such patients have either a defect in the tubular threshold for reabsorption of glucose in the proximal tubule (a 'splayed' reabsorption curve) or a defect in the maximal tubular reabsorption of glucose. Both autosomal dominant and recessive inheritance have been postulated. It has no clinical significance except in the differential diagnosis of patients with diabetes mellitus or other tubular disorders such as the Fanconi syndrome.

FURTHER READING

Pirson Y (1996) Recent advances in the clinical management of autosomal-dominant polycystic kidney disease. *Quarterly Journal of Medicine* **89**: 803–806.

Tumours of the kidney and genitourinary tract

Malignant renal tumours

These comprise 1–2% of all malignant tumours, and the male/female ratio is 2:1.

Renal cell carcinoma

Renal cell carcinomas (previously called hypernephromas or Grawitz tumours) arise from proximal tubular epithelium. They are the most common renal tumour in adults. They rarely present before the age of 40 years, the average age of presentation being 55 years.

In von Hippel–Lindau disease, an autosomal dominant disorder, bilateral renal cell carcinomas are common and haemangioblastomas, phaeochromocytomas and renal cysts are also found. Polymorphic probes from chromosome 3p, the region implicated in renal cell carcinoma, have demonstrated genetic linkage between them and von Hippel–Lindau disease. It seems likely, therefore, that mutation of the same tumour suppressor gene may be responsible for both renal cell carcinoma and von Hippel–Lindau disease. Deletion of the short arm of chromosome 3 is the most consistent cytogenetic finding in sporadic tumours.

Pathology

The tumours may be solitary, multiple or occasionally bilateral. The tumour lies within the kidney but it may eventually penetrate the capsule. Macroscopically, its cut surface appears as a yellow mass, sometimes containing areas of haemorrhage and cystic degeneration. Local invasion of renal veins and spread to the opposite kidney may occur, as may metastasis to lymph nodes, liver, bone and lung (often as an apparently solitary metastasis). Renal cell carcinomas are highly vascular tumours. Microscopically most tumours are composed of large cells containing clear cytoplasm.

Clinical features

Patients present with haematuria, loin pain and a mass in the flank. Malaise, anorexia and weight loss (30%) may occur, and 5% of patients have polycythaemia (see p. 441). Thirty per cent of patients have hypertension due to secretion of renin by the tumour with anaemia due to depression of erythropoietin in approximately the same number. Pyrexia is present in about one-fifth of patients and approximately one-quarter present with metastases. Rarely, a left-sided varicocele may be associated with left-sided tumours that have invaded the renal vein and caused obstruction to drainage of the left testicular vein.

Diagnosis

Excretion urography will reveal a space-occupying lesion in the kidney; 10% of these show calcification.

Ultrasonography is used to demonstrate the solid lesion and to examine the patency of the renal vein and inferior vena cava. A renal cell carcinoma too small to cause displacement of the collecting system may be missed on excretion urography. Ultrasonography *and* excretion urography are required in the investigation of haematuria (whether microscopic or macroscopic) if one or other investigation carried out initially appears normal. Urography allows diagnosis of calculi and calyceal and other abnormalities which may be missed by ultrasound examination. CT scanning can also be used to identify the renal lesion and involvement of the renal vein or inferior vena cava. MRI is better than CT for tumour staging. Renal arteriography will reveal the

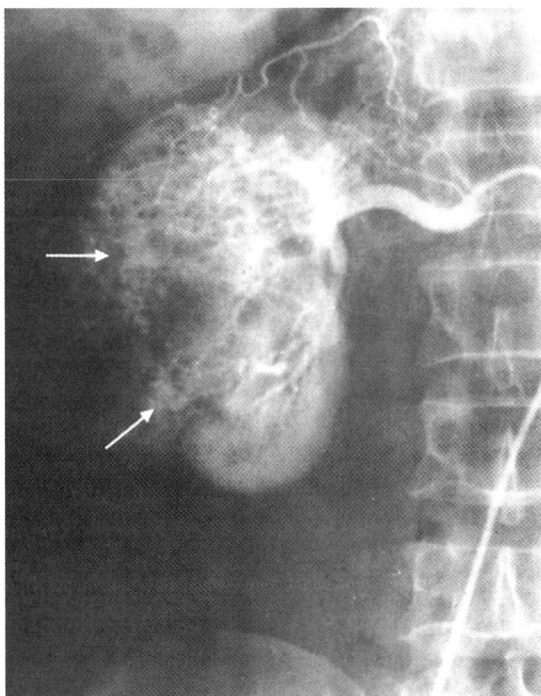

Fig. 11.47 **Renal arteriogram in a patient with renal cell carcinoma.** Note the abnormal tumour circulation.

tumour's circulation (Fig. 11.47) but is now seldom employed. Urine cytology for malignant cells is of no value. The ESR is usually raised. Liver biochemistry may be abnormal, returning to normal after surgery.

Treatment

Treatment is by nephrectomy unless bilateral tumours are present or the contralateral kidney functions poorly, in which case conservative surgery such as partial nephrectomy may be indicated. If metastases are present, nephrectomy may still be warranted since regression of metastases has been reported after removal of the main tumour mass. Severe flank pain may also demand nephrectomy despite the presence of metastases. Radiotherapy has no proven value. Medroxyprogesterone acetate is of some value in controlling metastatic disease. Treatment with interleukin-2 and α-interferon produces a remission in about 20% of cases. Recently, striking regression of metastases has been reported after non-myeloablative chemotherapy followed by allogeneic (sibling) peripheral blood stem-cell transplantation.

Prognosis

The prognosis depends upon the degree of differentiation of the tumour and whether or not metastases are present. The 5-year survival rate is 60–70% with tumours confined to the renal parenchyma, 15–35%, with lymph node involvement, and only approximately 5% in those who have distant metastases.

Nephroblastoma (Wilms' tumour)

This tumour is seen mainly within the first 3 years of life and may be bilateral. It presents as an abdominal mass, rarely with haematuria. Diagnosis is established by excretion urography followed by arteriography. A combination of nephrectomy, radiotherapy and chemotherapy has much improved survival rates, even in children, with metastatic disease. Overall, 5-year survival rate in UK children diagnosed between 1971 and 1985 was 79%.

Benign renal tumours

Renal adenoma

Benign adenomas are usually an incidental finding, presenting as a space-occupying lesion on excretion urography. They seldom cause symptoms. On urography they may be difficult to distinguish from a renal cell carcinoma.

Simple cysts

Simple cysts are common. They are discussed in more detail on page 658.

Differentiation of benign renal cyst from malignant tumour

If a space-occupying lesion is a chance finding on excretion urography in a patient with no relevant symptoms and no haematuria, ultrasonography should be carried out. If the lesion is transonic with no features suggesting a tumour, no further investigation is required. If haematuria has been present, a needle should be inserted into the transonic lesion and cyst fluid aspirated and examined for malignant cells. Contrast medium may be injected to delineate the walls of the cyst. Lesions shown to be solid or non-homogeneous on ultrasonography require further investigation by CT or MRI.

Urothelial tumours

The calyces, renal pelvis, ureter, bladder and urethra are lined by transitional cell epithelium. Transitional cell tumours account for about 3% of deaths from all forms of malignancy. Such tumours are uncommon below the age of 40 years, and the male/female ratio is 4:1. Bladder tumours are about 50 times as common as those of the ureter or renal pelvis.

Predisposing factors include:

- cigarette smoking
- exposure to industrial carcinogens such as β-naphthylamine and benzidine (workers in the chemical, cable and rubber industries are at particular risk)
- exposure to drugs (e.g. phenacetin, cyclophosphamide)

- chronic inflammation (e.g. schistosomiasis, usually associated with squamous carcinoma).

Presentation

Painless haematuria is the most common presenting symptom of bladder malignancy, although pain may occur owing to clot retention. Symptoms suggestive of UTI may develop in the absence of significant bacteriuria. In patients with bladder cancer, pain may also result from local nerve involvement.

Presenting symptoms may result from local metastases.

Transitional cell carcinomas in the kidney and ureter may present with haematuria. They may also give rise to flank pain, particularly if urinary tract obstruction is present.

Investigations

- **Cytological examination** of urine for malignant cells.
- **Excretion urography**.
- **Cystoscopy** if no evidence of upper urinary tract pathology has been found.

Cystoscopy may be omitted in men under 20 and women under 30 years if significant bacteriuria accompanies the haematuria and ceases following control of the infection, provided urine cytology and excretion urography are normal. With these exceptions, haematuria should always be investigated.

In cases where the tumour is not clearly outlined on excretion urography, abdominal CT scanning and/or retrograde ureterography may be helpful.

Treatment

Pelvic and ureteric tumours

These are treated by nephroureterectomy. Radiotherapy and chemotherapy appear to be of little or no value. Subsequently, cystoscopy should be regularly carried out, since about half the patients will develop bladder tumours.

Bladder tumours

Painless haematuria is the most common presentation. The diagnosis is made at cystoscopy. *Treatment* depends upon the stage of the tumour (in particular whether it has penetrated the bladder muscle) and its degree of differentiation. Treatment options include local cystodiathermy and/or resection with follow-up check cystoscopies/cytological examination of urine, cystectomy, radiotherapy, or local and systemic chemotherapy.

Prognosis

The prognosis ranges from a 5-year survival rate of 80–90% for lesions not involving bladder muscle to 5% for those presenting with metastases.

Diseases of the prostate gland

Benign enlargement of the prostate gland

Benign prostatic enlargement occurs most often in men over the age of 60 years. Such enlargement is much less common in Asian individuals. It is unknown in eunuchs. The aetiology of the condition is unknown.

Microscopically, hyperplasia affects the glandular and connective tissue elements of the prostate. Enlargement of the gland stretches and distorts the urethra, obstructing bladder outflow. The bladder musculature hypertrophies so that a higher than usual pressure is generated within the bladder in order to overcome the obstruction and allow voiding of urine. Bands of muscle fibre are seen at cystoscopy (trabeculation). Eventually the bladder becomes dilated and the muscle hypotonic. The sphincter mechanism at the vesicoureteric junction may be impaired and reflux of urine from the bladder into the ureters and upper urinary tract may occur.

Clinical features

Frequency of urination, usually first noted as nocturia, is a common early symptom. Difficulty or delay in initiating urination, with variability and reduced forcefulness of the urinary stream and post-void dribbling, are often present. Suprapubic pain occurs if bladder bacteriuria is present, if a bladder calculus has formed as a result of stagnation of urine within the bladder, or in acute retention of urine. Flank pain may accompany dilatation of the upper tracts. Acute retention of urine (see below) or retention with overflow incontinence may occur. Occasionally, severe haematuria results from rupture of prostatic veins or as a consequence of bacteriuria or stone disease. Occasional patients present with severe renal failure.

Abdominal examination for bladder enlargement together with examination of the rectum are essential. A benign prostate feels smooth. An accurate impression of prostatic size cannot be obtained on rectal examination.

Investigations

These should include urine culture, assessment of renal function by measuring serum urea and creatinine concentrations, measurement of prostate-specific antigen (markedly raised in prostatic cancer), a plain abdominal X-ray, and renal ultrasonography to define whether upper tract dilatation is present. Excretion urography is not usually necessary. The completeness of bladder emptying after an act of voiding can be assessed by ultrasonography or by inspection of the after-voiding radiograph carried out during excretion urography if this is performed. Cystourethroscopy is only essential in patients with haematuria.

Management and prognosis

Patients with mild-to-moderate symptoms should be managed by 'watchful waiting', because symptoms following therapy are sometimes greater than those with no therapy at all.

Patients with moderate prostatic symptoms can be treated medically. A number of drugs have been employed, including alpha-blockers such as tamsulosin. Finasteride is a competitive inhibitor of 5α-reductase, which is the enzyme involved in the conversion of testosterone to dihydrotestosterone. This is the androgen primarily responsible for prostatic growth and enlargement. Finasteride decreases prostatic volume with an increase in urine flow.

Deterioration in renal function or the development of upper tract dilatation requires surgery. Transurethral resection is usually successful unless the gland is very large. It carries a lower morbidity and mortality with a shorter stay in hospital than open prostatectomy. Microwave hyperthermia, balloon dilatation and prostatic stents are all being tried, but evidence from long-term randomized prospective controlled trials is not yet available. Very large glands require open transvesical prostatectomy.

In acute retention or retention with overflow, the first priorities are to relieve pain and to establish urethral catheter drainage. If urethral catheterization is impossible, suprapubic catheter drainage should be carried out. The choice of further management is then between immediate prostatectomy, a period of catheter drainage followed by prostatectomy, or the acceptance of a permanent indwelling suprapubic or urethral catheter.

Prostatic carcinoma

Prostatic carcinoma accounts for 7% of all cancers in men and is the fourth most common cause of death from malignant disease in men in England and Wales. Malignant change within the prostate becomes increasingly common with advancing age. By the age of 80 years, 80% of men have malignant foci within the gland, but most of these appear to lie dormant. Histologically, the tumour is an adenocarcinoma. Hormonal factors are thought to play a role in the aetiology.

Clinical features

In developed countries, most patients now present as a result of screening for prostate cancer by measurement of prostate-specific antigen (PSA). Presentation may be with symptoms of lower urinary tract obstruction or of metastatic spread, particularly to bone. The diagnosis may be made by the incidental finding of a hard irregular gland on rectal examination, or as an unexpected histological result after prostatectomy for what was believed to be benign prostatic hypertrophy.

Investigations

Investigations are as for benign enlargement of the prostate gland, supplemented by transrectal ultrasound of the prostate and prostatic biopsy. Prostate-specific antigen levels are unaffected by the presence of renal failure.

A histological diagnosis is essential before treatment is considered. This may be obtained by histological examination of biopsy material or material obtained at transurethral or open prostatectomy.

If metastases are present, serum prostate-specific antigen levels are usually markedly elevated (>16 µg/L); it is a myth that elevated levels occur as a result of rectal examination.

Ultrasonography and transrectal ultrasonography are of value in defining the size of the gland and staging any tumour present. The upper renal tracts can be examined by ultrasonography for evidence of dilatation. Bone metastases may appear as osteosclerotic lesions on X-ray or may be detected by isotopic bone scans.

Treatment

Microscopic, impalpable tumours can sometimes be managed expectantly. Treatment for disease confined to the gland is radical prostatectomy (provided the patient is fit for the procedure) or radiotherapy. Evidence is accumulating that radical prostatectomy is the treatment of choice in younger patients with poorly differentiated tumours. There have, however, been no controlled trials of this therapy and survival may be good without therapy. Locally extensive disease is managed with radiotherapy with or without androgen ablation therapy. Metastatic disease can be treated with orchidectomy, but many men refuse. Luteinizing hormone-releasing hormone (LHRH) analogues such as buserelin or goserelin are equally effective and preferred by many. Non-hormonal chemotherapy is unhelpful.

Prognosis

The duration of survival depends on the age of the patient and the degree of differentiation and extent of the tumour.

Screening

The value or otherwise of screening for prostate cancer is debated and the place, if any, of screening is unclear. Undoubtedly an annual measurement of prostate-specific antigen in asymptomatic men results in earlier diagnosis. It is not clear, however, that any benefit ensues in terms of increased survival; the financial cost of screening, emotional impact upon the patient of a positive result, and complications of treatment of any abnormality found have to be set against any possible benefit. Large-scale trials are in progress.

Testicular tumours

Testicular tumours, though uncommon, are the most common malignant disease in men between the ages of 29 and 34 years. All such tumours should nowadays be regarded as curable. Patient survival depends upon early diagnosis, accurate staging of the tumour and appropriate treatment and follow-up. The expertise of a specialist centre is invaluable.

More than 96% of testicular tumours arise from germ cells. Two main types of tumour exist:

- seminomas (about one-third)
- teratomas (about two-thirds).

Aetiology

The aetiology is unknown. The risk of malignant change is much greater in undescended testes and there is a history of orchidopexy in about 10% of patients. Previous testicular biopsy appears to be associated with an increased risk of malignant change.

Clinical features

Common presenting symptoms are:

- testicular swelling, which may be painless or painful
- symptoms from metastases.

Differential diagnosis

The differential diagnosis includes:

- epididymo-orchitis
- torsion
- chronic infection (e.g. tuberculosis, syphilitic gumma).

Investigations

Diagnosis may only be possible after surgical exploration of the testis through the groin. Scrotal exploration and scrotal testicular biopsy should be avoided owing to the high incidence of tumour implantation.

Staging of the tumour will require:

- chest X-ray to look for metastases
- estimation of α-fetoprotein and β-human chorionic gonadotrophin concentrations (tumour markers)
- abdominal CT scanning.

Treatment

Seminomas are radiosensitive, so tumours confined to the testis or with metastases below the diaphragm only are treated by radiotherapy. More widespread tumours require chemotherapy.

Teratomas are treated by orchidectomy if the growth is confined to the testis. Chemotherapy is required for more widespread disease (see p. 506).

FURTHER READING

Diasko JC, Lange PH (1997) Prostate cancer. *New England Journal of Medicine* **337**: 340–341.
Frydenberg M, Stricker PD, Kaye KW (1997) Prostate cancer diagnosis and management. *Lancet* **349**: 1681–1685.
Motzer RJ, Bander NH, Nanus DM (1996) Medical progress: renal cell carcinoma. *New England Journal of Medicine* **335**: 865–875.
Slavin S (2000) Cancer immunotherapy with alloreactive lymphocytes. *New England Journal of Medicine* **343**: 802–803.

Renal disease in the elderly

Renal disease and renal failure are common in the elderly. Acceptance of patients aged 65 years and over for renal replacement therapy approximately doubles the number of patients in whom renal replacement is initiated.

Renal failure in the elderly more often results from renal vascular disease or urinary tract obstruction than in younger age groups. In males, obstruction is most often due to benign or malignant prostatic enlargement, while in females it results from pelvic cancer.

Progressive sclerosis of glomeruli occurs with ageing and this, together with the development of atheromatous renal vascular disease, accounts for the progressive reduction in GFR seen with advancing years. A GFR of 50–60 mL per minute (about half the normal value for a young adult) may be regarded as 'normal' in patients in their eighties. The reduction in muscle mass often seen with ageing may mask this deterioration in renal function in that the serum creatinine concentration may be less than 0.12 mmol/L in an elderly patient whose GFR is 50 mL per minute or lower. The use of serum creatinine as a measure of renal function in the elderly must take this into account. This is especially so in the elderly when prescribing drugs whose excretion is in whole or in part by the kidney.

Urinary tract infections

UTIs are more common in the elderly, in whom impaired bladder emptying due to prostatic disease in males and neuropathic bladder – especially common in females – is frequently found. Symptoms may be atypical, the major complaints being incontinence, nocturia, smelly urine or vague change in well-being with little in the way of dysuria. Demonstration of significant bacteriuria in the presence of such symptoms requires treatment.

Urinary incontinence

This is one of the major disabilities of the elderly. Correctable factors, such as chronic constipation, diuretic therapy, infections and treatable bladder outflow impairment need to be excluded. Often there is a combination of factors including, for example, difficulty in getting to the toilet, and dementia. An expert and committed incontinence advisory and treatment service combining nursing and medical skills is invaluable for elderly patients with this distressing problem. Home visits to ensure the availability of commodes and toilets is essential. For established incontinence, catheterization may be necessary.

Incontinence and its treatment is a matter of major importance and by no means solely in the elderly.

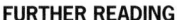

FURTHER READING

Consensus article: Assessment and treatment of urinary incontinence (2000) *Lancet* **355**: 2153–2158.

Fliser D, Franek E, Ritz E (1997) Renal function in the elderly: is the dogma of an inexorable decline of renal function correct? *Nephrology, Dialysis, Transplantation* **12**: 1553–1555.

Tropical nephrology

This chapter approaches nephrology from the perspective of a nephrologist practising in a developed Western country, the climate of which is temperate. Inevitably, an unbalanced view is therefore provided of nephrological problems world-wide. Wide geographical variations exist in the incidence and prevalence of diseases affecting the kidneys in developing and tropical countries.

For example, in some parts of southern Iraq the onset of macroscopic haematuria in pubescent males is regarded as almost a normal development – akin to the onset of menstruation in females – owing to the wide prevalence of infection with *Schistosoma haematobium*. In Nigeria, the most common causes of acute renal failure are typhoid and snake-bite, usually envenomation from a puff adder bite. In sub-Saharan Africa, malarial infection remains an extremely common cause of glomerulonephritis. In black Africans living in urban (as distinct from rural) areas, hypertension is exceptionally common, being characterized by relatively low levels of renin and normal levels of aldosterone in blood. Such hypertension has a particular predilection for inducing kidney damage and it is likely – although data are scant – that end-stage renal failure due to hypertensive nephropathy in urban blacks is extremely common.

Certainly in the UK and USA, end-stage renal failure is reached at about four times the rate in blacks compared with whites and hypertension is a major cause of this. It appears that less efficient renal excretion of sodium in blacks versus whites explains some of these observations. In rural sub-Saharan Africa, dietary salt intake is in general very low and in a hot country where sodium intake is low, reduced renal capacity to excrete sodium might well have been an evolutionary advantage. Exposure to a higher dietary salt intake in cities may well account, in part at least, for the high prevalence of hypertension in urban blacks.

The vast majority of black individuals reaching end-stage renal failure in sub-Saharan Africa die untreated since facilities for dialysis and transplantation are, by comparison with developed countries, minimal.

CHAPTER BIBLIOGRAPHY

Cameron JS, Davison AM, Grunfeld JP, Kerr DNS, Ritz E (eds) (1997) *Oxford Textbook of Clinical Nephrology*. Oxford: Oxford University Press.

Johnson RJ, Feehally J (2000) *Comprehensive Clinical Nephrology*. St Louis: Mosby

Schrier RW (ed) (1997) *Renal Electrolyte Disorders*, 5th edn. Philadelphia: Lippincott Raven.

Weatherall DJ, Ledingham JGG, Warrell JDA (eds) (1996) *Oxford Textbook of Medicine*, 3rd edn. Oxford: Oxford University Press.

Current Opinions in Nephrology and Hypertension is a monthly journal with review articles: each issue devoted to one or two topics.

Journal of Royal College of Physicians has a series on renal disease, starting Jan/Feb 1997.

Nephrology, Dialysis, Transplantation is the major European journal devoted to the subject, with review articles, editorial comments and original papers.

Water, electrolytes and acid–base balance

In health, the volume and biochemical composition of both extracellular and intracellular fluid compartments in the body remains remarkably constant. Many different disease states result in changes of control either of extracellular fluid volume, or of the electrolyte composition of extracellular fluid. An understanding of these abnormalities is therefore essential for the management of a wide range of clinical disorders.

Distribution and composition of body water

In normal persons, the total body water constitutes 50–60% of lean bodyweight in men and 45–50% in women. In a healthy 70 kg male, total body water is approximately 42 L. This is contained in three major compartments:

- the intracellular fluid (28 L, about 35% of lean bodyweight)
- the interstitial fluid that bathes the cells (9.4 L, about 12%)
- plasma (4.6 L, about 4–5%).

In addition, small amounts of water are contained in bone, dense connective tissue, and epithelial secretions, such as the digestive secretions and cerebrospinal fluid.

The intracellular and interstitial fluids are separated by the cell membrane; the interstitial fluid and plasma are separated by the capillary wall (Fig. 12.1). In the absence of solute, water molecules move randomly and in equal numbers in either direction across a permeable membrane. However, if solutes are added to one side of the membrane, the intermolecular cohesive forces reduce the activity of the water molecules. As a result, water tends to stay in the solute-containing compartment because there is less free diffusion across the membrane. This ability to hold water in the compartment can be measured as the osmotic pressure.

Osmotic pressure

Osmotic pressure is the primary determinant of the distribution of water between the three major compartments. The concentrations of the major solutes in these fluids differ, and each compartment has one solute that is primarily limited to that compartment and therefore determines its osmotic pressure: K^+ salts in the intracellular fluid (most of the cell Mg^{2+} is bound and

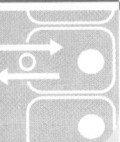
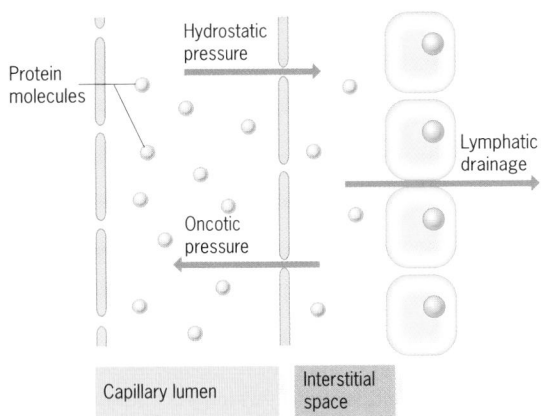

Fig. 12.1 Distribution of water between the vascular and extravascular (interstitial) spaces. This is determined by the equilibrium between hydrostatic pressure, which tends to force fluid out of the capillaries, and oncotic pressure, which acts to retain fluid within the vessel. The net flow of fluid outwards is balanced by 'suction' of fluid into the lymphatics, which returns it to the bloodstream. Similar principles govern the volume of the peritoneal and pleural spaces.

osmotically inactive), Na$^+$ salts in the interstitial fluid, and proteins in the plasma. Regulation of the plasma volume is somewhat more complicated because of the tendency of the plasma proteins to hold water in the vascular space by an oncotic effect which is in part counterbalanced by the hydrostatic pressure in the capillary that is generated by cardiac contraction (Fig. 12.1). The composition of intracellular and extracellular fluids is shown in Table 12.1.

A characteristic of an osmotically active solute is that it cannot freely leave its compartment. The capillary wall, for example, is relatively impermeable to plasma proteins, and the cell membrane is 'impermeable' to Na$^+$ and K$^+$ because the Na$^+$–K$^+$-ATPase pump largely restricts Na$^+$ to the extracellular fluid and K$^+$ to the intracellular fluid. By contrast, Na$^+$ freely crosses the capillary wall and achieves similar concentrations in the interstitium and plasma; as a result, it does not contribute to fluid distribution between these compartments.

Table 12.1
Electrolyte composition of intracellular and extracellular fluids

	Plasma (mmol/L)	Interstitial fluid (mmol/L)	Intracellular fluid (mmol/L)
Na$^+$	142	144	10
K$^+$	4	4	160
Ca^{2+}	2.5	2.5	1.5
Mg^{2+}	1.0	0.5	13
Cl$^-$	102	114	2
HCO$_3^-$	26	30	8
PO$_4^{2-}$	1.0	1.0	57
SO$_4^{2-}$	0.5	0.5	10
Organic acid	3	4	3
Protein	16	0	55

Similarly, urea crosses both the capillary wall and the cell membrane and is osmotically inactive. Thus, the retention of urea in renal failure does not alter the distribution of the total body water.

A conclusion from these observations is that body Na$^+$ stores are the primary determinant of the extracellular fluid volume. Thus the extracellular volume – and therefore tissue perfusion – are maintained by appropriate alterations in Na$^+$ excretion. For example, if Na$^+$ intake is increased, the extra Na$^+$ will initially be added to the extracellular fluid. The associated increase in extracellular osmolality will cause water to move out of the cells, leading to extracellular volume expansion. Balance is restored by excretion of the excess Na$^+$ in the urine.

Distribution of different types of replacement fluids

Figure 12.2 shows the relative effects of the addition of identical volumes of water, saline and colloid solutions on the compartments. Thus, 1 L of water given intravenously as 5% dextrose is distributed equally into all compartments, whereas the same amount of 0.9% saline remains in the extracellular compartment. The latter is thus the correct treatment for extracellular water depletion – sodium keeping the water in this compartment. The addition of 1 L of colloid with its high oncotic pressure stays in the vascular compartment and is the treatment for hypovolaemia.

Regulation of extracellular volume (Fig. 12.3)

The extracellular volume is determined by the sodium concentration. The regulation of extracellular volume is dependent upon a tight control of sodium balance which is exerted by normal kidneys. Renal Na$^+$ excretion varies directly with the effective circulating volume. In a 70 kg man, plasma fluid constitutes one-third of extracellular volume (4.6 L), of which 85% (3.9 L) lies in the venous side and only 15% (0.7 L) resides in the arterial circulation. The unifying hypothesis of extracellular volume regulation in health and disease proposed by Schrier states that the fullness of the arterial vascular compartment – or the so-called effective arterial blood volume (EABV) – is the primary determinant of renal sodium and water excretion. Thus effective arterial blood volume constitutes effective circulatory volume for the purposes of body fluid homeostasis. The fullness of the arterial compartment depends upon a normal ratio between cardiac output and peripheral arterial resistance. Thus diminished EABV is initiated by a fall in cardiac output or a fall in peripheral arterial resistance (an increase in the holding capacity of the arterial vascular tree). When the EABV is expanded, the urinary Na$^+$ excretion is increased and can exceed 100 mmol/L. In contrast, the urine can be rendered virtually free of Na$^+$ in the presence of EABV depletion and normal renal function.

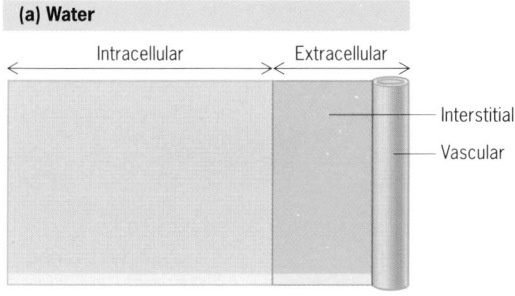

(a) Water

Intracellular | Extracellular

Interstitial
Vascular

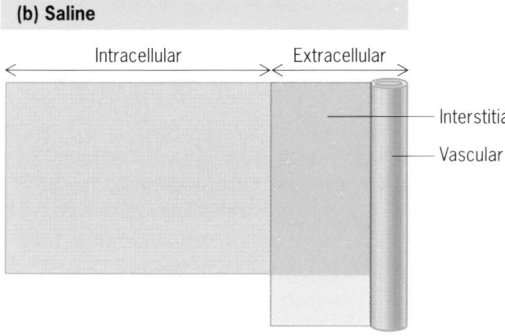

(b) Saline

Intracellular | Extracellular

Interstitial
Vascular

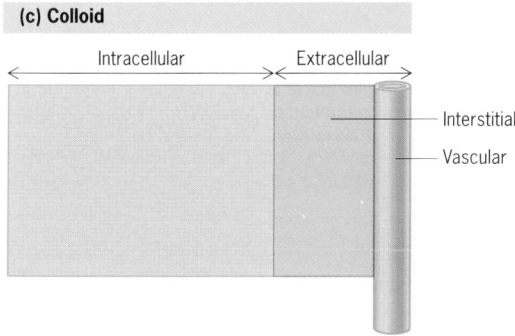

(c) Colloid

Intracellular | Extracellular

Interstitial
Vascular

Fig. 12.2 Relative effects of the addition of 1 L of (a) water, (b) saline 0.9%, and (c) a colloid solution.

These changes in Na$^+$ excretion can result from alterations both in the filtered load, determined primarily by the glomerular filtration rate (GFR), and in tubular reabsorption, which is affected by multiple factors. In general, it is changes in tubular reabsorption that constitute the main adaptive response to fluctuations in the effective circulating volume. How this occurs can be appreciated from Table 12.2, which depicts the sites and determinants of segmental Na$^+$ reabsorption. Although the loop of Henle and distal tubule make a major overall contribution to net Na$^+$ handling, transport in these segments primarily varies with the amount of Na$^+$ delivered; that is, reabsorption is flow-dependent. In comparison, the neurohumoral regulation of Na$^+$ reabsorption according to body needs occurs primarily in the proximal and collecting tubules.

Neurohumoral regulation of extracellular volume

This is mediated by volume receptors which sense changes in the EABV rather than alterations in the sodium concentration. These receptors are distributed in both the cardiovascular and renal tissues.

- *Extrarenal receptors.* These are located in the vascular tree in the left atrium and major thoracic veins, and in the carotid sinus body and aortic arch. These volume receptors respond to a slight reduction in effective circulating volume and result in increased sympathetic nerve activity and a rise in catecholamines. In addition, volume receptors in the cardiac atria control the release of a powerful natriuretic hormone – atrial natriuretic peptide (ANP) – from granules located in the atrial walls.
- *Intrarenal receptors.* Receptors in the walls of the afferent glomerular arterioles respond, via the juxtaglomerular apparatus, to changes in renal perfusion, and control the activity of the renin–angiotensin–aldosterone system (p. 1064). In addition, sodium concentration in the distal tubule and sympathetic nerve activity alter renin release from the juxtaglomerular cells. Prostaglandins I$_2$ and E$_2$ are also generated within the kidney in response to angiotensin II, acting to maintain glomerular filtration rate and sodium and water excretion, modulating the sodium-retaining effect of this hormone.

There is considerable evidence that high-pressure arterial receptors (carotid, aortic arch, juxtaglomerular apparatus) predominate over low-pressure volume receptors in volume control in mammals. The receptors distributed in the thoracic tissues (cardiac atria, right ventricle, thoracic veins, pulmonary vessels) are low-pressure volume receptors and their role in the volume regulatory system is marginal.

Aldosterone and possibly atrial natriuretic peptide (ANP) are responsible for day-to-day variations in Na$^+$ excretion, by their respective ability to augment and diminish Na$^+$ reabsorption in the collecting tubules. A salt load, for example, leads to an increase in the effective circulatory and extracellular volume, raising both renal perfusion pressure, and atrial and arterial filling pressure. The increase in the renal perfusion pressure reduces the secretion of renin, and subsequently that of angiotensin II and aldosterone, whereas the rise in atrial and arterial filling pressure increases the release of ANP. These factors combine to reduce Na$^+$ reabsorption in the collecting duct, thereby promoting excretion of excess Na$^+$. In contrast, in patients on low Na$^+$ intake or in those who become volume-depleted as a result of vomiting and diarrhoea, the ensuing decrease in effective volume enhances the activity of the renin–angiotensin–aldosterone system and reduces the secretion of ANP. The net effect is enhanced Na$^+$ reabsorption in the collecting tubules, which accounts for the appropriate fall in Na$^+$

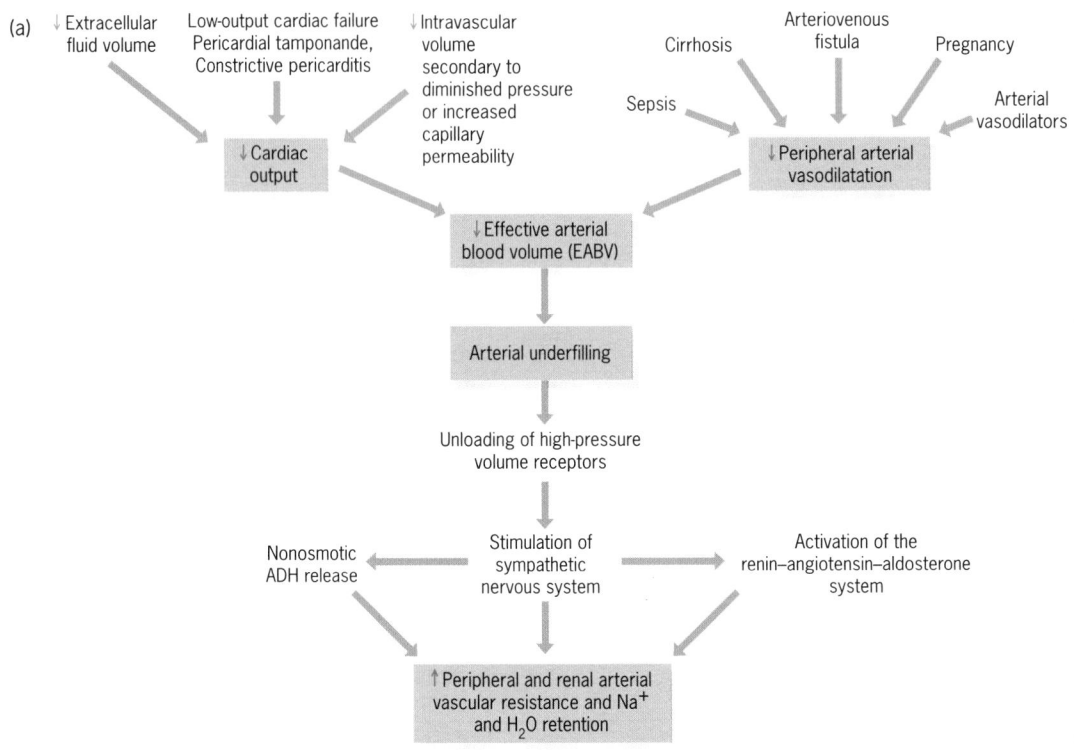

(a)

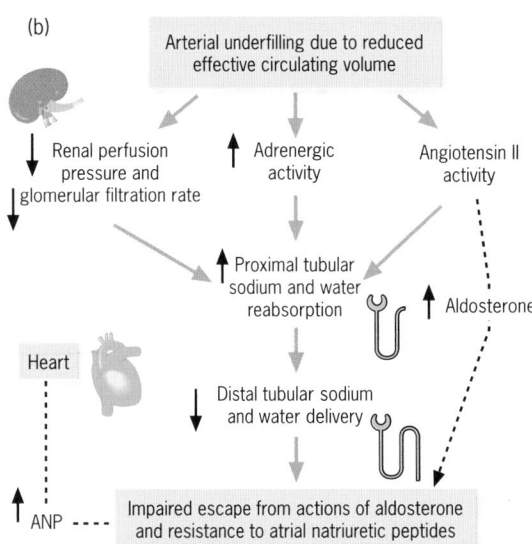

(b)

Fig. 12.3 (a) Sequence of events in which a decrease in cardiac output or peripheral arterial dilatation initiates renal sodium and water retention. (b) Mechanism of impaired escape from the actions of aldosterone and resistance to atrial natriuretic peptides (**ANP**). Modified from Schrier RW (1997) *Renal and Electrolyte Disorders*, 5th edn.

of antidiuretic hormone (ADH). The pressure natriuresis phenomenon may be the final defence against changes in the effective circulating volume. Marked persistent hypovolaemia leads to systemic hypotension and increased salt and water absorption in the proximal tubules and ascending limb of Henle. This process may be mediated by changes in renal interstitial hydrostatic pressure and local prostaglandin and nitric oxide production.

Volume regulation in oedematous conditions

Sodium and water are retained despite increased extracellular volume in oedematous conditions such as cardiac failure, hepatic cirrhosis and hypoalbuminaemia. Here the principal mediator of salt and water retention is the concept of arterial underfilling due to either reduced cardiac output or diminished peripheral arterial resistance. Arterial underfilling in these settings leads to reduction of pressure or stretch (i.e. 'unloading' of arterial volume receptors) which results in the activation of the sympathetic nervous system, activation of the renin–angiotensin–aldosterone system and nonosmotic

excretion in this setting. It tends to increase the extracellular volume towards normal.

With more marked hypovolaemia, a decrease in GFR and increase in proximal and thin ascending limb Na^+ reabsorption also contribute to Na^+ retention. This is brought about by enhanced sympathetic activity acting directly on kidneys and indirectly by stimulating the secretion of renin/angiotensin II and nonosmotic release

Table 12.2

Mechanisms of sodium transport in the various nephron segments

Tubule segment	Filtered Na$^+$ reabsorbed (%)	Major mechanism of luminal Na$^+$ entry	Major factors regulating transport
Proximal tubule	60–70	Na$^+$–H$^+$ exchange and cotransport of Na$^+$ with glucose, phosphate and other organic solutes	Angiotensin II Noradrenaline (norepinephrine)
Loop of Henle	20–25	Na$^+$–K$^+$–2Cl$^-$ cotransport	Flow dependent Pressure natriuresis mediated by nitric oxide
Distal tubule	5	Na$^+$–Cl$^-$ cotransport	Flow dependent
Collecting tubules	4	Na$^+$ channels	Aldosterone Atrial natriuretic peptide

release of antidiuretic hormone (ADH). These neurohumoral mediators promote salt and water retention in the face of increased extracellular volume. The common nature of the degree of arterial fullness and neurohumoral pathway in the regulation of extracellular volume in health and disease states forms the basis of Schrier's unifying hypothesis of volume homeostasis (Fig. 12.3a).

Mechanism of impaired escape from actions of aldosterone and resistance to ANP

The activity of the renin–angiotensin–aldosterone system in oedematous conditions such as cardiac failure, hepatic cirrhosis and hypoalbuminaemia is not only increased but also the action of aldosterone is more persistent than in normal subjects and patients with Conn's syndrome, who have increased aldosterone secretion (p. 1065). In normal subjects, high doses of mineralocorticoids initially increase renal sodium retention so that the extracellular volume is increased by 1.5–2 litres. However, renal sodium retention then ceases, sodium balance is re-established, and there is no detectable oedema. This escape from mineralocorticoid-mediated sodium retention explains why oedema is not a characteristic feature of primary hyperaldosteronism (Conn's syndrome). The escape is dependent on an increase in delivery of sodium to the site of action of aldosterone in the collecting ducts. The increased distal sodium delivery is achieved by high extracellular volume-mediated arterial overfilling. This suppresses sympathetic activity and angiotensin II generation, and increases cardiac release of ANP with resultant increase in renal perfusion pressure and GFR. The net result of these events is reduced sodium absorption in the proximal tubules and increased distal sodium delivery which overwhelms the sodium-retaining actions of aldosterone.

In patients with oedematous conditions such as cardiac failure, hepatic cirrhosis and hypoalbuminaemia escape from the sodium-retaining actions of aldosterone does not occur and therefore they continue to retain sodium in response to aldosterone. Accordingly they have substantial natriuresis when given spironolactone, which

blocks mineralocorticoid receptors. Alpha-adrenergic stimulation and elevated angiotensin II increase sodium transport in the proximal tubule, and reduced renal hypoperfusion and GFR further increase sodium absorption from the proximal tubules by presenting less sodium and water in the tubular fluid. Sodium delivery to the distal portion of the nephron, and thus the collecting duct, is reduced. Similarly, increased cardiac ANP release in these conditions requires optimum sodium concentration at the site of its action in the collecting duct for its desired natriuretic effects. Decreased sodium delivery to the collecting duct is therefore the most likely explanation for the persistent aldosterone-mediated sodium retention, absence of escape phenomenon and resistance to natriuretic peptides in these patients (Fig. 12.3b).

Regulation of water excretion

Body water homeostasis is effected by thirst and the urine concentrating and diluting functions of the kidney. These in turn are controlled by intracellular osmoreceptors, principally in the hypothalamus, to some extent by volume receptors in capacitance vessels close to the heart, and via the renin–angiotensin system. Of these, the major and best-understood control is via osmoreceptors. Changes in the plasma Na$^+$ concentration and osmolality are sensed by osmoreceptors that influence both thirst and the release of ADH (also called vasopressin) from the supraoptic and paraventricular nuclei.

ADH plays a central role in urinary concentration by increasing the water permeability of the normally impermeable cortical and medullary collecting tubules. The ability of ADH to increase the urine osmolality is related indirectly to transport in the ascending limb of the loop of Henle, which reabsorbs NaCl without water. This process, which is the primary step in the countercurrent mechanism, has two effects: it makes the tubular fluid dilute and the medullary interstitium concentrated. In the absence of ADH, little water is reabsorbed in the collecting tubules, and a dilute urine is excreted.

In contrast, the presence of ADH promotes water reabsorption in the collecting tubules down the favourable osmotic gradient between the tubular fluid and the more concentrated interstitium. As a result, there is an increase in urine osmolality and a decrease in urine volume.

The cortical collecting tubule has two cell types with very different functions:

- *Principal cells* (about 65%) have sodium and potassium channels in the apical membrane and, as in all sodium-reabsorbing cells, Na^+–K^+-ATPase pumps in the basolateral membrane.
- *Intercalated cells*, in comparison, do not transport NaCl, since they have a lower level of Na^+–K^+-ATPase activity. They appear to play a role in hydrogen and bicarbonate handling and in potassium reabsorption in states of potassium depletion.

The ADH-induced increase in collecting tubule water permeability occurs primarily in the principal cells. ADH acts on V2 (vasopressin) receptors located on the basolateral surface of principal cells, resulting in the activation of adenyl cyclase. This initiates a sequence of events in which a protein kinase is activated, leading to preformed cytoplasmic vesicles that contain unique water channels (called aquaporins) moving to and then being inserted into the luminal membrane. The water channels span the luminal membrane and permit water movement into the cells down a favourable osmotic gradient (Fig. 12.4). This water is then rapidly returned to the systemic circulation across the basolateral membrane. When the ADH effect has worn off, the water channels aggregate within clathrin-coated pits, from which they are removed from the luminal membrane by endocytosis and returned to the cytoplasm. A defect in any step in this pathway, such as attachment of ADH to its receptor or the function of the water channel, can cause resistance to the action of ADH and an increase in urine output. This disorder is called *nephrogenic diabetes insipidus*.

Plasma osmolality

In addition to influencing the rate of water excretion, ADH plays a central role in osmoregulation because its release is directly affected by the plasma osmolality. At a plasma osmolality of less than 275 mOsm/kg, which usually represents a plasma Na^+ concentration of less than 135–137 mmol/L, there is essentially no circulating ADH. As the plasma osmolality rises above this threshold, however, the secretion of ADH increases progressively.

Two simple examples will illustrate the basic mechanisms of osmoregulation, which is so efficient that the plasma Na^+ concentration is normally maintained within 1–2% of its baseline value.

Ingestion of a water load leads to an initial reduction in the plasma osmolality, thereby diminishing the release of ADH. The ensuing reduction in water reabsorption in

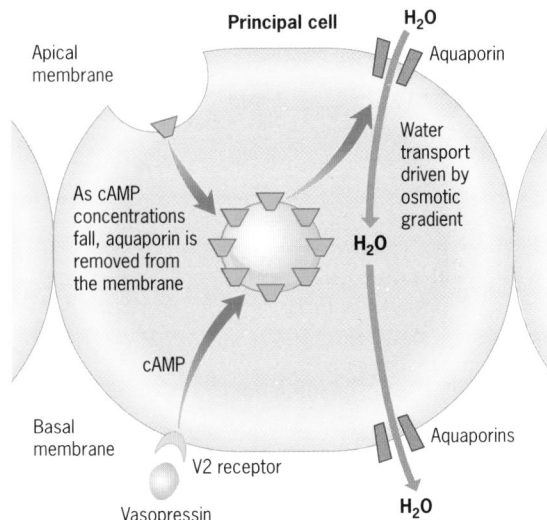

Fig. 12.4 Aquaporin-mediated water transport in the renal collecting duct. Stimulation of the vasopressin 2 receptor causes cAMP-mediated insertion of the aquaporin into the apical membrane, allowing water transport down the osmotic gradient. Adapted from Connolly DL, Shanahan CM, Weissberg PL (1996) *Lancet* **347**: 211.

the collecting tubules allows the excess water to be excreted in a dilute urine.

Water loss resulting from sweating is followed by, in sequence, a rise in both plasma osmolality and ADH secretion, enhanced water reabsorption, and the appropriate excretion of a small volume of concentrated urine. This renal effect of ADH minimizes further water loss but does not replace the existing water deficit. Thus, optimal osmoregulation requires an increase in water intake, which is mediated by a concurrent stimulation of thirst. The importance of thirst can also be illustrated by studies in patients with central diabetes insipidus, who are deficient in ADH. These patients often complain of marked polyuria, which is caused by the decline in water reabsorption in the collecting tubules. However, they do not typically become hypernatraemic, because urinary water loss is offset by the thirst mechanism.

Osmoregulation versus volume regulation

A common misconception is that regulation of the plasma Na^+ concentration is closely correlated with the regulation of Na^+ excretion. However, it is related to volume regulation, which has different sensors and effectors (volume receptors) from those involved in water balance and osmoregulation (osmoreceptors).

The roles of these two pathways should be considered separately when evaluating patients. A water load, for example, is rapidly excreted (in 4–6 hours) by inhibition of ADH release. This process is normally so efficient that volume regulation is not affected and there is no change in ANP release or in the activity of the renin–angiotensin–aldosterone system. Thus, a dilute urine is excreted, and there is little alteration in the excretion of Na^+. In contrast, the administration of iso-tonic saline causes an increase in volume but no change in plasma osmolality. In this setting, ANP secretion is increased, aldosterone secretion is reduced, and ADH secretion does not change. The net effect is the appropriate excretion of the excess Na^+ in a relatively iso-osmotic urine.

In some cases, both volume and osmolality are altered and both pathways are activated. For example, if a person with normal renal function eats salted potato chips and peanuts without drinking any water, the excess Na^+ will increase the plasma osmolality, leading to osmotic water movement out of the cells and increased extracellular volume. The rise in osmolality will stimulate both ADH release and thirst (the main reason why many restaurants and bars supply free salted foods), whereas the hypervolaemia will enhance the secretion of ANP and suppress that of aldosterone. The net effect is increased excretion of Na^+ without water.

This principle of separate volume and osmoregulatory pathways is also evident in the syndrome of inappropriate ADH secretion (SIADH). Patients with SIADH have impaired water excretion and hyponatraemia caused by the persistent presence of ADH; but the release of ANP and aldosterone is not impaired; thus, Na^+ handling remains intact. These findings have implications for the correction of the hyponatraemia in this setting and require restriction of water intake.

However, there is convincing evidence that ADH is also secreted by nonosmotic stimuli such as stress (e.g. surgery, trauma), markedly reduced effective circulatory volume (cardiac failure, hepatic cirrhosis), psychiatric disturbance, and nausea, irrespective of plasma osmolality. This is mediated by the effects of sympathetic overactivity on supraoptic and paraventricular nuclei. In addition to water retention, ADH release in these conditions promotes vasoconstriction owing to the activation of V1 (vasopressin) receptors distributed in the vascular tissue.

Regulation of cell volume

Maintenance of a constant volume in the face of extracellular and intracellular osmotic alterations is a critical problem faced by all cells. Most cells respond to swelling or shrinkage by activating specific metabolic or membrane-transport processes that return cell volume to its normal resting state. Within minutes after exposure to hypotonic solutions and resulting cell swelling, a common feature of many cells is the increase in plasma membrane potassium and chloride conductance. Although extrusion of intracellular potassium certainly contributes to a regulatory volume decrease, the role of chloride efflux itself is modest, given the relatively low intracellular chloride concentration. Indeed other intracellular osmolytes, such as taurine and other amino acids, are transported out of the cell to achieve a regulatory volume decrease. In contrast, these regulatory mechanisms are operative in reverse to protect cell volume under hypertonic conditions, as is the case in the renal medulla. The tubular cells at the tip of renal papillae, which are constantly exposed to an hypertonic extracellular milieu, maintain their cell volume on a long-term basis by actively taking up smaller molecules, such as betaine, taurine and myoinositol, and by synthesizing more sorbitol and glycerophosphocholine.

Increased extracellular volume

Increased extracellular volume occurs in numerous disease states. The physical signs depend on the distribution of excess volume and on whether the increase is local or systemic. According to Starling principles, distribution depends on:

- venous tone, which determines the capacitance of the blood compartment and thus hydrostatic pressure
- capillary permeability
- oncotic pressure – mainly dependent on serum albumin
- lymphatic drainage.

Depending on these factors, fluid accumulation may result in expansion of interstitial volume, blood volume, or both.

Clinical features

Peripheral oedema is caused by expansion of the extracellular volume by at least 2 L (15%). The ankles are normally the first part of the body to be affected, although the ankles may be spared in patients with lipodermatosclerosis (where the skin is tethered and cannot expand to accommodate the oedema). Oedema may be noted in the face, particularly in the morning. In a patient in bed, oedema may accumulate in the sacral area. Expansion of the interstitial volume also causes pulmonary oedema, pleural effusion, pericardial effusion and ascites. Expansion of the blood volume (overload) causes a raised jugular venous pressure, cardiomegaly, added heart sounds, basal crackles as well as a raised arterial blood pressure in certain circumstances.

Causes

Extracellular volume expansion is due to sodium chloride retention. Increased salt intake does not normally cause volume expansion because of rapid homeostatic mechanisms which increase salt excretion. However, a rapid intravenous infusion of a large volume of saline will cause volume expansion. Thus most causes of extracellular volume expansion are associated with renal sodium chloride retention.

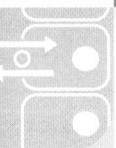

Heart failure

Reduction in cardiac output and the consequent fall in effective circulatory volume and arterial filling leads to activation of the renin–angiotensin–aldosterone system, nonosmotic release of ADH, and increased activity of the renal sympathetic nerves via volume receptors and baroreceptors (Fig. 12.3a). Sympathetic overdrive also indirectly augments ADH and renin–angiotensin–aldosterone response in these conditions. The cumulative effect of these mediators results in increased peripheral and renal arteriolar resistance and water and sodium retention. These factors result in extracellular volume expansion and increased venous pressure, causing oedema formation.

Hypoalbuminaemia

The major mechanism is loss of plasma oncotic pressure leading to loss of water from the vascular space to the interstitial space. Reduction in effective circulatory volume and the consequent fall in cardiac output and arterial filling leads to a chain of events as in cardiac failure (see above). These factors result in extracellular volume expansion and increased venous pressure, causing oedema formation. However, other factors may be involved. There is some evidence that the nephrotic syndrome itself alters renal sodium handling (see p. 612). Furthermore, a small group of patients do not manifest oedema with hypoalbuminaemia, the cause of which remains unclear.

Hepatic cirrhosis

The mechanism is again complex, but involves peripheral vasodilatation, possibly owing to increased nitric oxide generation resulting in reduced effective volume and arterial filling. This leads to an activation of a chain of events common to cardiac failure and other conditions with marked peripheral vasodilatation (Fig. 12.3a and b). The cumulative effect results in increased peripheral and renal resistance, water and sodium retention, and oedema formation.

Sodium retention

A decreased GFR decreases the renal capacity to excrete sodium. This may be acute, as in the acute nephritic syndrome (p. 606), or may occur as part of the presentation of chronic renal failure. In end-stage renal failure, extracellular volume is controlled by the balance between salt intake and its removal by dialysis.

Mild sodium retention can also be caused by oestrogens which have a weak aldosterone-like effect. This produces weight gain in the premenstrual phase.

Numerous other drugs may cause renal sodium retention, particularly in patients whose renal function is already impaired:

- *mineralocorticoids and liquorice* (the latter potentiates the sodium-retaining action of cortisol), which have aldosterone-like actions

- *NSAIDs* cause sodium retention in the presence of activation of the renin–angiotensin–aldosterone system by heart failure, cirrhosis and in renal artery stenosis. Selective inhibitors of COX-2 (p. 532) have a similar effect.

Substantial amounts of sodium and water may accumulate in the body without clinically obvious oedema or evidence of raised venous pressure. In particular, several litres may accumulate in the pleural space or as ascites; these spaces are then referred to as 'third spaces'. Bone may also act as a 'sink' for sodium and water.

Other causes of oedema

- Initiation of insulin treatment for type 1 diabetes and refeeding after malnutrition are both associated with the development of transient oedema. The mechanism is complex.
- Oedema may result from increased capillary pressure owing to relaxation of precapillary arterioles. The best example is the peripheral oedema caused by dihydropyridine calcium-channel blockers such as nifedipine.
- Oedema may be caused by increased interstitial oncotic pressure as a result of increased capillary permeability to proteins. This can occur as part of a rare complement-deficiency syndrome; with therapeutic use of interleukin-2 in cancer chemotherapy; or in ovarian hyperstimulation syndrome.

Idiopathic oedema of women

This, by definition, occurs in women without heart failure, hypoalbuminaemia, renal or endocrine disease. Oedema is intermittent and often worse in the premenstrual phase. The condition remits after the menopause. Patients complain of swelling of the face, hands, breasts and thighs, and a feeling of being bloated. Sodium retention during the day and increased sodium excretion during recumbency are characteristic; an abnormal fall in plasma volume on standing caused by increased capillary permeability to proteins may be the cause of this. The oedema may respond to diuretics, but returns when they are stopped. A similar syndrome of diuretic-dependent sodium retention can be caused by abuse of diuretics, for instance as part of an attempt to lose weight; but not all women with idiopathic oedema admit to having taken diuretics, and the syndrome was described before diuretics were introduced for clinical use.

Local increase in oedema

This does not reflect disturbances of extracellular volume control per se, but can cause clinical confusion. Examples are ankle oedema due to venous damage following thrombosis or surgery, ankle or leg oedema due to immobility, oedema of the arm due to subclavian thrombosis, and facial oedema due to superior vena caval obstruction. Local loss of oncotic pressure may result from increased capillary permeability to proteins, caused by inflammatory mediators such as histamine and interleukins (e.g. a bee sting). Lastly, local loss of lymphatic drainage causes lymphoedema (see p. 1311).

Treatment

The underlying cause should be treated where possible. Heart failure, for example, should be treated, and offending drugs such as NSAIDs withdrawn.

Sodium restriction has only a limited role, but is useful in patients who are resistant to diuretics. Sodium intake can easily be reduced to approximately 100 mmol daily; reductions below this are often difficult to achieve without affecting the palatability of food.

Manoeuvres which increase venous return stimulate salt and water excretion by effects on cardiac output and ANP release. This is the rationale for strict bed rest in congestive cardiac failure. Water immersion also causes redistribution of blood towards the central veins, but is seldom of practical use. Venous compression stockings or bandages may help to mobilize oedema in heart failure.

The mainstay of treatment is the use of diuretic agents, which increase sodium, chloride and water excretion in the kidney (Table 12.3). These agents act by interfering with membrane ion pumps which are present on numerous cell types; but most achieve specificity for the kidney by being secreted into the proximal tubule, resulting in much higher concentrations in the tubular fluid than in other parts of the body.

Clinical use of diuretics

Loop diuretics (see Fig. 12.5, p. 683)

These potent diuretics, which are used widely, are useful in the treatment of any cause of systemic extracellular volume overload. They stimulate excretion of both sodium chloride and water by blocking the sodium–potassium–2-chloride channel in the thick ascending limb of Henle and are useful in stimulating water excretion in states of relative water overload. They also act by causing increased venous capacitance, resulting in rapid clinical improvement in patients with left ventricular failure, preceding the diuresis. Unwanted effects include:

- urate retention causing gout
- hypokalaemia
- hypomagnesaemia
- decreased glucose tolerance
- allergic tubulo-interstitial nephritis and other allergic reactions
- myalgia – especially with bumetanide
- ototoxicity (due to an action on sodium pump activity in the inner ear) – particularly with furosemide (frusemide)
- interference with excretion of lithium, resulting in toxicity.

In most situations there is little to choose between the drugs in this class. Bumetanide has a better oral bioavailability than furosemide (frusemide), particularly in patients with severe peripheral oedema, and has more beneficial effects than furosemide on venous

Table 12.3
Types and clinical uses of diuretics

Class	Major action	Examples	Clinical uses	Potency
Loop diuretics	↓ Na^+ Cl^- K^+ cotransport in thick ascending limb	Furosemide (frusemide) Bumetanide Torasemide	Volume overload (CCF, nephrotic syndrome, CRF) Sodium-dependent hypertension Hypercalcaemia ?Acute renal failure SIADH	+++
Thiazide and related diuretics	↓ Na^+ Cl^- cotransport in early distal tubule	Bendroflumethiazide (bendrofluazide) Chlorthalidone Metolazone Indapamide	Hypertension Volume overload (CCF) Hypercalciuria	++
Potassium sparing	↓ Na^+ reabsorption (in exchange for K^+) in collecting duct	Aldosterone antagonist e.g. oral spironolactone or i.v. potassium canrenoate Others: Amiloride Triamterene	Hyperaldosteronism (primary and secondary) Bartter's syndrome Prevention of K^+ deficiency in combination with loop or thiazide Heart failure Cirrhosis with fluid overload	+
Carbonic anhydrase inhibitors	↓ Na^+ HCO_3^- reabsorption in proximal tubule ↓ Aqueous humour formation	Acetazolamide	Metabolic alkalosis Glaucoma	+

CCF, congestive cardiac failure; CRF, chronic renal failure; SIADH, syndrome of inappropriate antidiuretic hormone secretion

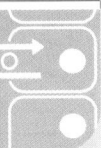

capacitance in left ventricular failure. It can cause severe muscle cramps when used in high doses.

Thiazide diuretics (see Fig. 12.6, p. 683)

These are weaker than loop diuretics. They act by blocking a sodium chloride channel in the distal convoluted tubule They cause relatively more urate retention, glucose intolerance and hypokalaemia than loop diuretics. They interfere with water excretion and may cause hyponatraemia, particularly if combined with amiloride or triamterene. This effect is clinically useful in diabetes insipidus. Thiazides reduce peripheral vascular resistance by mechanisms which are not completely understood but which do not appear to depend on their diuretic action, and are widely used in the treatment of essential hypertension. They are also used extensively in mild to moderate cardiac failure. Thiazides reduce calcium excretion. This effect is useful in patients with idiopathic hypercalciuria, but may cause hypercalcaemia. Numerous agents are available, with varying half-lives but little else to choose between them. Metolazone is not dependent for its action on glomerular filtration, and therefore retains its potency in renal impairment.

Potassium-sparing diuretics (see Fig. 12.7, p. 684)

These are relatively weak and are most often used in combination with thiazides or loop diuretics to prevent potassium depletion. They are of two types. Spironolactone, an aldosterone antagonist, competes with aldosterone in the collecting ducts, so reducing sodium absorption. Spironolactone is now increasingly used in patients with heart failure because it significantly reduces the mortality in these patients by antagonizing the fibrotic effect of aldosterone on the heart. Amiloride and triamterene inhibit sodium uptake by blocking epithelial sodium channels in the collecting duct and reduce renal potassium excretion by reducing lumen-negative transepithelial voltage.

Carbonic anhydrase inhibitors

These are relatively weak diuretics and are seldom used except in the treatment of glaucoma. They may cause metabolic acidosis and hypokalaemia.

Resistance to diuretics

Resistance may occur as a result of:

- poor bioavailability
- reduced GFR, which may be due to decreased circulating volume despite oedema (e.g. nephrotic syndrome, local causes of oedema) or intrinsic renal disease
- activation of sodium-retaining mechanisms, particularly aldosterone.

Intravenous administration may establish a diuresis. High doses of loop diuretics may be required to achieve adequate concentrations in the tubule if GFR is depressed.

However, the daily dose of furosemide (frusemide) must be limited to a maximum of 2 g for an adult, because of ototoxicity. *Intravenous albumin* solutions restore plasma oncotic pressure temporarily in the nephrotic syndrome and may allow mobilization of oedema.

Combinations of various classes of diuretics are extremely helpful in patients with resistant oedema. A loop diuretic plus a thiazide inhibits two major sites of sodium reabsorption; this effect may be further potentiated by addition of a potassium-sparing agent. Metolazone in combination with a loop diuretic is particularly useful in refractory congestive cardiac failure, because its action is less dependent on glomerular filtration. However, this potent combination can cause severe electrolyte imbalance.

Both aminophylline and dopamine increase renal blood flow and may be useful in refractory cardiogenic sodium retention.

Effects on renal function

All diuretics may increase plasma urea concentrations by increasing urea reabsorption in the medulla. Thiazides may also promote protein breakdown. In certain situations diuretics may also decrease GFR:

- Excessive diuresis may cause volume depletion and prerenal failure.
- Diuretics may cause allergic tubulo-interstitial nephritis.
- Thiazides may directly cause a drop in GFR; the mechanism is complex and not fully understood.

Decreased extracellular volume

Deficiency of sodium and water causes shrinkage both of the interstitial space and of the blood volume and may have profound effects on organ function.

Clinical features

Symptoms are variable. Thirst, muscle cramps, nausea and vomiting, and postural dizziness may occur. Severe depletion of circulating volume causes hypotension and impairs cerebral perfusion, causing confusion and eventual coma.

Signs can be divided into those due to loss of interstitial fluid and those due to loss of circulating volume.

- *Loss of interstitial fluid* leads to loss of skin elasticity ('turgor') – the rapidity with which the skin recoils to normal after being pinched. Skin turgor decreases with age, particularly at the peripheries. The turgor over the anterior triangle of the neck or on the forehead is a very useful sign in all ages.
- *Loss of circulating volume* leads to decreased pressure in the venous and (if severe) arterial compartments. Loss of up to 1 L of extracellular fluid in an adult may be compensated for by venoconstriction and may cause no physical signs. Loss of more than this causes the following:

Postural hypotension

Normally the blood pressure rises if a subject stands up, as a result of increased venous return due to venoconstriction (this maintains cerebral perfusion). Loss of extracellular fluid (underfill) prevents this and causes a fall in blood pressure. This is one of the earliest and most reliable signs of volume depletion, as long as the other causes of postural hypotension are excluded (Table 12.4).

Low jugular venous pressure

In hypovolaemic patients, the jugular venous pulsation can be seen only with the patient lying completely flat, or even head down, because the left atrial pressure is lower than 5 cmH$_2$O.

Peripheral venoconstriction

This causes cold skin with empty peripheral veins, which are difficult to cannulate just when the patient needs intravenous therapy the most! This sign is often absent in sepsis, where peripheral vasodilatation contributes to effective hypovolaemia.

Tachycardia

This is not always a reliable sign. Beta-blockers and other antiarrhythmics may prevent tachycardia, and hypovolaemia may activate vagal mechanisms and actually cause bradycardia.

Causes

Salt and water may be lost from the kidneys, from the gastrointestinal tract, or from the skin. Examples are given in Table 12.5.

In addition, there are a number of situations where signs of volume depletion occur despite a normal or increased body content of sodium and water.

- Septicaemia causes vasodilatation of both arterioles and veins, resulting in greatly increased capacitance of the vascular space. In addition, increased capillary permeability to plasma proteins leads to loss of fluid from the vascular space to the interstitium.
- Diuretic treatment of heart failure or nephrotic syndrome may lead to rapid reduction in plasma volume. Mobilization of oedema may take much longer.
- There may be inappropriate diuretic treatment of oedema (e.g. when the cause is local rather than systemic).

Investigations

Blood tests are in general not helpful in the assessment of extracellular volume. Plasma urea may be raised owing to increased urea reabsorption and, later, to pre-renal failure (when the creatinine rises as well), but this is very non-specific. Urinary sodium is low if the kidneys are functioning normally, but is misleading if the cause of the volume depletion involves the kidneys (e.g. diuretics, intrinsic renal disease). Urine osmolality is high in volume depletion (owing to increased water reabsorption), but may also often mislead.

The assessment of volume status is still best achieved by simple clinical observations which you should do yourself. Check:

- jugular venous pressure
- central venous pressure both basal and after intravenous fluid challenge
- serial weights of the patient
- postural changes in blood pressure
- a chest X-ray.

Treatment

The overriding principle is to aim to replace what is missing.

Haemorrhage

This involves the loss of whole blood. The rational treatment of acute haemorrhage is therefore the infusion of whole blood, or a combination of red cells and a plasma substitute. (Chronic anaemia causes salt and water retention rather than volume depletion by a mechanism common to conditions with peripheral vasodilatation.)

Table 12.4
Postural hypotension: some causes of a fall in blood pressure from lying to standing

Decreased circulating volume (hypovolaemia)	Interference with peripheral vasoconstriction by drugs
	Nitrates
Autonomic failure	Calcium-channel blockers
Diabetes	Alpha-adrenoreceptor blocking
Systemic amyloidosis	drugs
Shy–Drager syndrome	
Interference with autonomic function by drugs	**Prolonged bed rest (cardiovascular deconditioning)**
Ganglion blockers	
Tricyclic antidepressants	

Table 12.5
Causes of extracellular volume depletion

Haemorrhage	Renal losses
External	Diuretic use
Concealed, e.g. leaking	Impaired tubular sodium
aortic aneurysm	conservation
	Reflux nephropathy
Burns	Papillary necrosis
	Analgesic nephropathy
Gastrointestinal losses	Diabetes
Vomiting	Sickle cell disease
Diarrhoea	
Ileostomy losses	
Ileus	

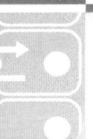

Loss of plasma

Loss of plasma, as occurs in burns or severe peritonitis, should be treated with human plasma or a plasma substitute (see p. 939).

Loss of water and electrolytes

Loss of water and electrolytes, as occurs with vomiting, diarrhoea, or excessive renal losses, should be treated by replacement of the loss. If possible, this should be done with oral water and sodium salts. These are available as slow sodium (600 mg, approximately 10 mmol of each Na^+ and Cl^- per tablet), the usual dose of which is 6–12 tablets per day with 2–3 L of water. It is used in mild or chronic salt and water depletion, such as that associated with renal salt wasting.

Sodium bicarbonate (500 mg, 6 mmol each of Na^+ and HCO_3^- per tablet) is used in doses of 6–12 tablets per day with 2–3 L of water. This is used in milder chronic sodium depletion with acidosis (e.g. chronic renal failure, post-obstructive renal failure, renal tubular acidosis). Sodium bicarbonate is less effective than sodium chloride in causing positive sodium balance.

Oral rehydration solutions are described in Box 2.9 (see p. 73). Intravenous fluids may sometimes be required (Table 12.6). Rapid infusion (e.g. 1000 mL per hour or even faster) is necessary if there is hypotension and evidence of impaired organ perfusion (e.g. oliguria, confusion); in these situations, plasma expanders (colloids) are often used in the first instance to restore an adequate circulating volume (see p. 939). Repeated clinical assessments are vital in this situation, usually complemented by frequent measurements of central venous pressure (see p. 933 in Ch. 15 for the management of shock). Severe hypovolaemia induces venoconstriction, which maintains venous return; over-rapid correction does not give time for this to reverse, resulting in signs of circulatory overload (e.g. pulmonary oedema) even if a total body ECF deficit remains. In less severe ECF depletion (such as in a patient with postural hypotension complicating acute tubular necrosis), the fluid should be replaced at a rate of 1000 mL every 4–6 hours, again with repeated clinical assessment. If all that is required is avoidance of fluid depletion during surgery, 1–2 L may be given over 24 hours, remembering that surgery is a stimulus to sodium and water retention and that over-replacement may be as dangerous as under-replacement. Regular monitoring by fluid balance charts, bodyweight and plasma biochemistry is mandatory.

Loss of water alone

This causes extracellular volume depletion only in severe cases, because the loss is spread evenly between all the compartments of body water. In the rare situations where there is a true deficiency of water alone, as in diabetes insipidus in a patient who is unable to drink (after surgery, for instance), the correct treatment is to give water.

If intravenous treatment is required, water is given as 5% dextrose, because pure water would lead to osmotic lysis of blood cells.

FURTHER READING

Brater DC (1998) Diuretic therapy. *New England Journal of Medicine* **339**: 387–395.

Connolly DL, Shanahan CM, Weissberg PL (1996) Water channels in health and disease. *Lancet* **347**: 210–212.

McManus LM, Churchwell KB, Strange K (1995) Regulation of cell volume in health and disease. *New England Journal of Medicine* **333**: 1260–1266.

Marples D (2000) Water channels: who needs them? Editorial. *Lancet* 355: 1571–1572.

Schrier RW (1992) A unifying hypothesis of body fluid regulation. *Journal of the Royal College of Physicians, London* **26**: 295–299.

Schrier RW, Abraham WT (1999) Hormones and hemodynamics in heart failure. *New England Journal of Medicine* **341**: 577–585.

Table 12.6
Intravenous fluids in general use for fluid and electrolyte disturbances

	Na^+ (mmol/L)	K^+ (mmol/L)	HCO_3^- (mmol/L)	Cl^- (mmol/L)	Indication (see footnote)
Normal plasma values	142	4.5	26	103	
Sodium chloride 0.9%	150	–	–	150	1
Sodium chloride 0.18% + glucose 4%	30	–	–	30	2
Glucose 5% + potassium chloride 0.3%	–	40	–	40	3
Sodium bicarbonate 1.26%	150	–	150	–	4

1. Volume expansion in hypovolaemic patients. Rarely to maintain fluid balance when there are large losses of sodium. The sodium (150 mmol/L) is greater than plasma and hypernatraemia can result. It is often necessary to add KCl 20–40 mmol/L.

2. Maintenance of fluid balance in normovolaemic, normonatraemic patients.

3. To replace *water*. Can be given with or without potassium chloride. May be alternated with normal saline as an alternative to (2).

4. For volume expansion in hypovolaemic, acidotic patients alternating with (1). Occasionally for maintenance of fluid balance combined with (2) in salt-wasting, acidotic patients. To induce forced alkaline diuresis, e.g. in severe salicylate poisoning.

Disorders of sodium concentration

These are best thought of as disorders of body water content. As discussed above, sodium content is regulated by volume receptors; water content is adjusted to maintain, in health, a normal osmolality and (in the absence of abnormal osmotically active solutes) a normal sodium concentration. Disturbances of sodium concentration are caused by disturbances of water balance.

Hyponatraemia

Hyponatraemia (Na < 135 mmol/L) is one of the most common abnormalities detected in biochemistry laboratories. It may be associated with normal extracellular volume (Table 12.7) and total body sodium content. The differential diagnosis of hyponatraemia depends on an assessment of extracellular volume.

Rarely, hyponatraemia may be a 'pseudo-hyponatraemia'. This occurs in hyperlipidaemia or hyperproteinaemia where there is a spuriously low measured sodium concentration, the sodium being confined to the aqueous phase but having its concentration expressed in terms of the total volume of plasma. In this situation, plasma osmolality is normal and therefore treatment of 'hyponatraemia' is unnecessary. Artefactual 'hyponatraemia' caused by taking blood from the limb into which fluid of low sodium concentration is being infused should be excluded!

Salt-deficient hyponatraemia

This is due to salt loss in excess of water; the causes are listed in Table 12.8. In this situation, ADH secretion is initially suppressed (via the hypothalamic osmoreceptors); but as fluid volume is lost, volume receptors override the osmoreceptors and stimulate both thirst and the release of ADH. This is an attempt by the body to defend circulating volume at the expense of osmolality.

With extrarenal losses and normal kidneys, the urinary excretion of sodium falls in response to the volume depletion, as does water excretion, leading to concentrated urine containing less than 10 mmol/L of sodium. However, in salt-wasting kidney disease, renal compensation cannot occur and the only physiological protection is increased water intake in response to thirst.

Clinical features

With sodium depletion the clinical picture is usually dominated by features of volume depletion (see p. 676). The diagnosis is usually obvious where there is a history of gut losses, diabetes mellitus or diuretic abuse.

Table 12.9 shows the potential daily losses of water and electrolytes from the gut. Losses due to renal or adrenocortical disease may be less easily identified and are suggested by a urinary sodium concentration of more than 20 mmol/L in the presence of clinically evident volume depletion.

Treatment

This is directed at the primary cause whenever possible.

In a healthy patient:

- give oral electrolyte–glucose mixtures (p. 73)
- increase salt intake with slow sodium 60–80 mmol.

In a patient with vomiting or severe volume depletion:

- give intravenous normal saline with potassium supplements
- correction of acid–base abnormalities is usually not required.

Hyponatraemia due to water excess (dilutional hyponatraemia)

This results from an intake of water in excess of the kidney's ability to excrete it. With normal kidney function, dilution hyponatraemia is uncommon even if

---

Table 12.7
Causes of hyponatraemia with normal extracellular volume

Abnormal ADH release	**Increased sensitivity to ADH**
Vagal neuropathy (failure of inhibition of ADH release)	Chlorpropamide
Deficiency of adrenocorticotrophic hormone (ACTH) or glucocorticoids (Addison's disease)	Tolbutamide
Hypothyroidism	**ADH-like substances**
Severe potassium depletion	Oxytocin
	1-Deamino-D-arginine vasopressin (DDAVP)
Syndrome of inappropriate antidiuretic hormone (see Table 18.36)	**Unmeasured osmotically active substances stimulating osmotic ADH release**
	Glucose
Major psychiatric illness	Alcohol
'Psychogenic polydipsia'	Mannitol
Nonosmotic ADH release?	Sick-cell syndrome
Antidepressant therapy	(leakage of intracellular ions)

Table 12.8
Causes of hyponatraemia with decreased extracellular volume

Gut	Kidney
Vomiting	Osmotic diuresis
Diarrhoea	(e.g. hyperglycaemia, severe uraemia)
Haemorrhage	Excessive use of diuretics
	Adrenocortical insufficiency
	Tubulo-interstitial renal disease
	Unilateral renal artery stenosis
	Recovery phase of acute tubular necrosis

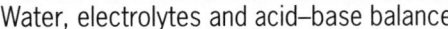

Table 12.9

Average concentrations and potential daily losses of water and electrolytes from the gut

	Na+ (mmol/L)	K+ (mmol/L)	Cl− (mmol/L)	Volume (mL in 24 hours)
Stomach	50	10	110	2500
Small intestine				
Recent ileostomy	120	5	110	1500
Adapted ileostomy	50	4	25	500
Bile	140	5	105	500
Pancreatic juice	140	5	60	2000
Diarrhoea	130	10–30	95	1000–2000+

a patient drinks approximately 1 L per hour. The most common iatrogenic cause is overgenerous infusion of 5% glucose into postoperative patients; in this situation it is exacerbated by an increased ADH secretion in response to stress. Some degree of hyponatraemia is usual in acute oliguric renal failure, while in chronic renal failure it is most often due to ill-given advice to 'push' fluids.

The most common presentation of hyponatraemia due to water excess is in patients with severe cardiac failure, hepatic cirrhosis or the nephrotic syndrome in which there is evidence of volume overload (Table 12.10). In all these conditions there is usually an element of reduced glomerular filtration rate with avid reabsorption of sodium and chloride in the proximal tubule. This leads to reduced delivery of chloride to the 'diluting' ascending limb of Henle's loop and a reduced ability to generate 'free water', with a consequent inability to excrete dilute urine. This is commonly compounded by the administration of diuretics that block chloride reabsorption and interfere with the dilution of filtrate either in Henle's loop (loop diuretics) or distally (thiazides).

Clinical features

Symptoms are common with dilutional hyponatraemia when this develops acutely. Symptoms rarely occur until the serum sodium is less than 120 mmol/L and are more usually associated with values around 110 mmol/L or lower. They are principally neurological and are due to the movement of water into brain cells in response to the fall in extracellular osmolality. Symptoms and signs of hyponatraemia are non-specific and include headache, confusion, and restlessness leading to drowsiness, myoclonic jerks, generalized convulsions, and eventually coma. Other features depend on the cause, such as signs of congestive cardiac failure or liver disease.

Table 12.10

Causes of hyponatraemia with increased extracellular volume

Heart failure
Liver failure
Oliguric renal failure
Hypoalbuminaemia

Investigations

No further investigation of hyponatraemia is usually necessary if it is associated with clinically detectable extracellular volume excess. The cause of hyponatraemia with apparently normal extracellular volume is usually less obvious, and this category requires careful investigations to:

- exclude Addison's disease
- exclude hypothyroidism
- consider 'syndrome of inappropriate ADH secretion' (SIADH) and drug-induced water retention.

It should be remembered that potassium and magnesium depletion potentiate ADH release and are causes of diuretic-associated hyponatraemia.

The syndrome of inappropriate ADH secretion is often over-diagnosed. Some causes are associated with a lower set point for ADH release, rather than completely autonomous ADH release; an example is chronic alcohol abuse.

Treatment

The underlying cause should be corrected where possible. Most cases are simply managed by restriction of water intake (to 1000 or even 500 mL per day) with review of diuretic therapy. Magnesium and potassium deficiency must be corrected. The use of hypertonic saline is restricted to patients with acute water retention in whom there are severe neurological signs, such as fits or coma. It should be given very slowly (not more than 70 mmol per hour), the aim being to increase the serum sodium to more than 125 mmol/L.

If hyponatraemia has developed slowly, as it does in the majority of patients, the brain will have adapted by decreasing intracellular osmolality. A rapid rise in extracellular osmolality, particularly if there is an 'overshoot' to high serum sodium and osmolality, will result in severe shrinking of brain cells and in the syndrome of 'central pontine myelinolysis', which may be fatal. Hypertonic saline must not be given to patients who are already fluid overloaded because of the risk of acute heart failure; in this situation, 100 mL of 20% mannitol may be infused in an attempt to increase renal water excretion.

Syndrome of inappropriate ADH secretion

This is described in Chapter 18.

Hypernatraemia

This is much rarer than hyponatraemia and nearly always indicates a water deficit. This may be due to (Table 12.11):

- impaired thirst or impaired conscious state
- pituitary diabetes insipidus (see p. 1057) (failure of ADH secretion)
- nephrogenic diabetes insipidus (failure of response to ADH)
- osmotic diuresis, e.g. diabetic ketoacidosis
- excessive loss of water through the skin or lungs.

Excessive administration of hypertonic sodium may also contribute, for example:

- excessive reliance on 0.9% (150 mmol/L) saline for volume replacement
- administration of drugs with a high sodium content (e.g. piperacillin)
- use of 8.4% sodium bicarbonate after cardiac arrest.

Hypernatraemia is always associated with increased plasma osmolality, which is a potent stimulus to thirst. None of the above cause hypernatraemia unless thirst sensation is abnormal or access to water limited. For instance, a patient with diabetes insipidus will maintain a normal serum sodium concentration by maintaining a high water intake until an intercurrent illness prevents this. Thirst is frequently deficient in elderly people, making them more prone to water depletion. Hypernatraemia may occur in the presence of normal, reduced or expanded extracellular volume, and does not necessarily imply that total body sodium is increased.

Clinical features

Symptoms of hypernatraemia are non-specific. Nausea, vomiting, fever and confusion may occur. A history of long-standing polyuria, polydipsia and thirst suggests diabetes insipidus. There may be clues to a pituitary cause. A drug history may reveal ingestion of nephrotoxic drugs. Assessment of extracellular volume status guides resuscitation. Mental state should be assessed. Convulsions occur in severe hypernatraemia.

Investigations

Simultaneous urine and plasma osmolality and sodium should be measured. Plasma osmolality is high in hypernatraemia. Passage of urine with an osmolality lower than that of plasma in this situation is clearly abnormal and indicates diabetes insipidus. In pituitary diabetes insipidus, urine osmolality will increase after administration of desmopressin; the drug (a vasopressin analogue) has no effect in nephrogenic diabetes insipidus. If urine osmolality is high this suggests either an osmotic diuresis due to an unmeasured solute (e.g. in parenteral feeding) or excessive extrarenal loss of water (e.g. heat stroke).

Treatment

Treatment is that of the underlying cause, for example:

- in ADH deficiency, replace ADH in the form of desmopressin, a stable nonpressor analogue of ADH
- remember to withdraw nephrogenic drugs where possible and replace water either orally or, if necessary, intravenously.

In severe (> 170 mmol/L) hypernatraemia, 0.9% saline (150 mmol/L) should be used initially. It is absolutely necessary to avoid too rapid a drop in serum sodium concentration; the aim is correction over 48 hours, as over-rapid correction may lead to cerebral oedema.

In less severe (e.g. > 150 mmol/L) hypernatraemia, the treatment is 5% dextrose or 0.45% saline; the latter is obviously preferable in hyperosmolar diabetic coma. Very large volumes – 5 L a day or more – may need to be given in diabetes insipidus.

If there is clinical evidence of volume depletion (see p. 676), this implies that there is a sodium deficit as well as a water deficit. Treatment of this is discussed on page 677.

Table 12.11
Causes of hypernatraemia

ADH deficiency Diabetes insipidus	**Osmotic diuresis** Total parenteral nutrition Hyperosmolar diabetic coma
Iatrogenic Administration of hypertonic sodium solutions	**PLUS** Deficient water intake
Insensitivity to ADH **(nephrogenic diabetes insipidus)** Lithium Tetracyclines Amphotericin B Acute tubular necrosis	

FURTHER READING

Adrogue HJ, Madias NE (2000) Hypernatremia. *New England Journal of Medicine* **342**: 1493–1499.

Adrogue HJ, Madias NE (2000) Hyponatremia. *New England Journal of Medicine* **342**: 1581–1589.

Cadnapaphornchai MA, Schrier RW (2000) Pathogenesis and management of hyponatremia. *American Journal of Medicine* **109**: 688–692.

Kumar S, Berl T (1998). Electrolyte quintet. Sodium. *Lancet* **352**: 220–228.

Disorders of potassium content and concentration

Regulation of serum potassium concentration

The usual dietary intake varies between 80 and 150 mmol daily, depending upon fruit and vegetable intake. Most of the body's potassium (3500 mmol in an adult man) is intracellular. Serum potassium levels are controlled by:

- uptake of K^+ into cells
- renal excretion
- extrarenal losses (e.g. gastrointestinal).

Uptake of potassium into cells is governed by the activity of the Na^+–K^+-ATPase in the cell membrane and by H^+ concentration.

Uptake is *stimulated* by:

- insulin
- β-adrenergic stimulation
- theophyllines.

Uptake is *decreased* by:

- α-adrenergic stimulation
- acidosis – K^+ exchanged for H^+ across cell membrane
- cell damage or cell death – resulting in massive K^+ release.

Renal excretion of potassium is increased by aldosterone, which stimulates K^+ and H^+ secretion in exchange for Na^+ in the collecting duct (see Fig. 12.7). Because H^+ and K^+ are interchangeable in the exchange mechanism, acidosis decreases and alkalosis increases the secretion of K^+. Aldosterone secretion is stimulated by hyperkalaemia and increased angiotensin II levels, as well as by some drugs, and this acts to protect the body against hyperkalaemia and against extracellular volume depletion. The body adapts to dietary deficiency of potassium by reducing aldosterone secretion. However, because aldosterone is also influenced by volume status, conservation of potassium is relatively inefficient, and significant potassium depletion may therefore result from prolonged dietary deficiency.

A number of drugs affect K^+ homeostasis by affecting aldosterone release (e.g. heparin, NSAIDs) or by directly affecting renal potassium handling (e.g. diuretics).

Normally only about 10% of daily potassium intake is excreted in the gastrointestinal tract. Vomit contains around 5–10 mmol/L of K^+, but prolonged vomiting may cause hypokalaemia by inducing sodium depletion, stimulating aldosterone, which increases renal potassium excretion. Potassium may be secreted by the colon, and diarrhoea contains 10–30 mmol/L of K^+; profuse diarrhoea can therefore induce marked hypokalaemia. Colorectal villous adenomas may rarely produce profuse diarrhoea and K^+ loss.

Hypokalaemia

Causes

The most common causes of chronic hypokalaemia are diuretic treatment (particularly thiazides) and hyperaldosteronism. Acute hypokalaemia is often caused by intravenous fluids without potassium and redistribution into cells. The common causes are shown in Table 12.12.

Rare causes

Bartter's syndrome

This consists of metabolic hypokalaemia, alkalosis, hypercalciuria, normal blood pressure, and elevated plasma renin and aldosterone. The primary defect in this disorder appears to be an impairment in sodium and chloride reabsorption in the thick ascending limb (Fig. 12.5). Mutation in the genes encoding either the sodium–potassium–2-chloride cotransporter (NKCC2) or the ATP-regulated potassium channel (ROMK) or kidney-specific basolateral chloride channel (CLC-Kb)

Table 12.12
Causes of hypokalaemia

Increased renal excretion	Reduced intake
Diuretics	Intravenous fluids without K^+
Thiazides	Dietary deficiency
Loop diuretics	
	Redistribution into cells
Increased aldosterone	β-Adrenergic stimulation
secretion	Acute myocardial infarction
Liver failure	Beta-agonists: e.g. fenoterol,
Heart failure	salbutamol
Nephrotic syndrome	Insulin treatment,
Cushing's syndrome	e.g. treatment of diabetic
Conn's syndrome	ketoacidosis
ACTH-producing tumours	Correction of megaloblastic
	anaemia, e.g. B_{12} deficiency
Exogenous	Alkalosis
mineralocorticoid	Hypokalaemic periodic paralysis
Corticosteroids	
Carbenoxolone	**Gastrointestinal losses**
Liquorice (potentiates renal	Vomiting
actions of cortisol)	Severe diarrhoea
	Purgative abuse
Renal disease	Villous adenoma
Renal tubular acidosis	Ileostomy or
types 1 and 2	uterosigmoidostomy
Renal tubular damage	Fistulae
(diuretic phase)	Ileus/Intestinal obstruction
Acute leukaemia	
Cytotoxic treatment	
Nephrotoxicity	
Amphotericin	
Aminoglycosides	
Release of urinary tract	
obstruction	
Bartter's syndrome	
Liddle's syndrome	
Gitelman's syndrome	

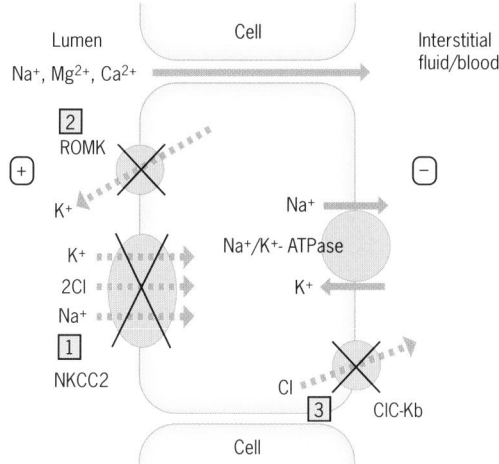

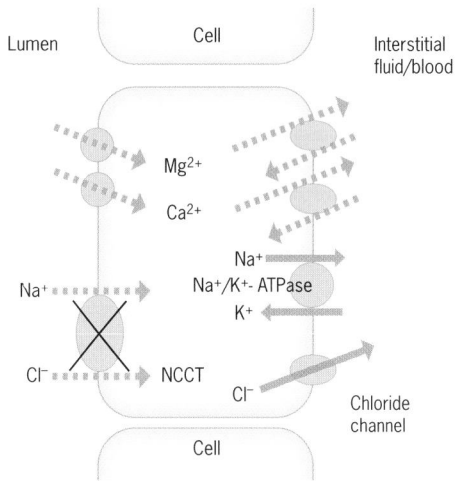

Fig. 12.5 Transport mechanisms in the thick ascending limb of Henle. Sodium chloride is reabsorbed in the thick ascending limb by the bumetanide-sensitive sodium–potassium–2-chloride cotransporter (NKCC2). The electroneutral transporter is driven by the low intracellular sodium and chloride concentrations generated by the Na^+–K^+-ATPase and the kidney-specific basolateral chloride channel (ClC-Kb). The availability of luminal potassium is rate-limiting for NKCC2, and recycling of potassium through the ATP-regulated potassium channel (ROMK – rat outer medulla K^+ channel) ensures the efficient functioning of the NKCC2 and generates a lumen-positive transepithelial potential.

Genetic studies have identified putative loss-of-function mutations in the genes encoding NKCC2 ①, ROMK ②, and ClC-Kb ③ in subgroups of patients with **Bartter's syndrome**. In contrast to the normal condition, loss of function of NKCC2 ① impairs reabsorption of sodium and potassium. Inactivation of the basolateral ClC-Kb ③ reduces transcellular reabsorption of chloride. Loss of function of any of these transporters will reduce the transepithelial potential and thus decrease the driving force for the paracellular reabsorption of cations. In most patients with Bartter's syndrome, urinary calcium excretion is increased.

Fig. 12.6 Transport mechanisms in the distal convoluted tubule. Under normal conditions, sodium chloride is reabsorbed by the apical thiazide-sensitive sodium–chloride cotransporter (NCCT) in the distal convoluted tubule. The electroneutral transporter is driven by the low intracellular sodium and chloride concentrations generated by the Na^+–K^+-ATPase and an as yet undefined basolateral chloride channel. In this nephron segment, there is an apical calcium channel and a basolateral sodium-coupled exchanger. Physiological evidence indicates that the mechanisms for the transport of magnesium are similar to those for calcium.

In **Gitelman's syndrome**, putative loss-of-function mutations in the sodium–chloride cotransporter (NCCT (**X**)) lead to decreased reabsorption of sodium chloride and increased reabsorption of calcium.

causes loss of function of these channels, with consequent impairment of sodium and chloride reabsorption. There is also an increased intrarenal production of prostaglandin E_2 which is secondary to sodium and volume depletion, hypokalaemia and the consequent neurohumoral response rather than a primary defect.

This tubular defect in sodium chloride transport is thought to initiate the following sequence, which is almost identical to that seen with chronic ingestion of a loop diuretic. The initial salt loss leads to mild volume depletion, resulting in activation of the renin–angiotensin–aldosterone system. The combination of hyperaldosteronism and increased distal flow (owing to the reabsorptive defect) enhances potassium and hydrogen secretion at the secretory sites in the collecting tubules, leading to hypokalaemia and metabolic alkalosis.

Diagnostic pointers include high urinary potassium and chloride despite low serum values as well as increased plasma renin (NB: in primary aldosteronism, renin levels are low). Hyperplasia of the juxtaglomerular apparatus is seen on renal biopsy (careful exclusion of diuretic abuse is necessary). Hypercalciuria is a common feature but magnesium wasting, though rare, may

also occur. Treatment is with combinations of potassium supplements, amiloride and indometacin or specific COX-2 inhibitor NSAID (p. 532).

Gitelman's syndrome

Gitelman's syndrome is a phenotype variant of Bartter's syndrome characterized by hypokalaemia, metabolic alkalosis, hypocalciuria, hypomagnesaemia, normal blood pressure, and elevated plasma renin and aldosterone. There are striking similarities between the Gitelman syndrome and the biochemical abnormalities induced by chronic thiazide diuretic administration. Thiazides act in the distal convoluted tubule to inhibit the function of the apical sodium–chloride cotransporter (NCCT) (Fig. 12.6). Analysis of the gene encoding the NCCT has identified loss of function mutations in Gitelman's syndrome.

Like Bartter's syndrome, defective NCCT function leads to increased solute delivery to the collecting duct, with resultant solute wasting, volume contraction and an aldosterone-mediated increase in potassium and hydrogen secretion. Unlike Bartter's syndrome, the degree of volume depletion and hypokalaemia is not sufficient to stimulate prostaglandin E_2 production. Impaired function of NCCT is predicted to cause hypocalciuria, as does thiazide administration. Impaired sodium reabsorption across the apical membrane coupled with continued intracellular chloride efflux across the basolateral membrane, causes the cell to

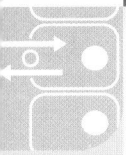

become hyperpolarized. This in turn stimulates calcium reabsorption via apical, voltage-activated calcium channels. Decreased intracellular sodium also facilitates calcium efflux via the basolateral sodium–calcium exchanger. The mechanism for urinary magnesium losses is not known. Treatment of Gitelman's syndrome consists of potassium and magnesium supplementation ($MgCl_2$) and a potassium-sparing diuretic. Volume resuscitation is usually not necessary, because patients are not dehydrated. Elevated prostaglandin E_2 excretion is not a feature of Gitelman's syndrome; therefore, NSAIDs are not indicated in this disorder.

Liddle's syndrome

This is characterized by potassium wasting, hypokalaemia and alkalosis, but is associated with low renin and aldosterone production, and high blood pressure. There is a mutation in the gene encoding for the amiloride-sensitive epithelial sodium channel in the distal tubule/collecting duct. This leads to constitutive activation of the epithelial sodium channel resulting in excessive sodium reabsorption with coupled potassium and hydrogen secretion. Unregulated sodium reabsorption across the collecting tubule results in volume expansion, inhibition of renin and aldosterone secretion and development of low renin hypertension (Fig. 12.7).

Therapy in Liddle's syndrome consists of sodium restriction along with amiloride or triamterene administration, both potassium-sparing diuretics which directly close the sodium channels. The mineralocorticoid antagonist spironolactone is ineffective, since the increase in sodium-channel activity is not mediated by aldosterone in this disorder.

Hypokalaemic periodic paralysis (p. 1224)

This condition may be precipitated by carbohydrate intake, suggesting that insulin-mediated potassium influx into cells may be responsible. This syndrome also occurs in association with hyperthyroidism in Chinese patients.

Clinical features

Hypokalaemia is usually asymptomatic, but severe hypokalaemia (< 2.5 mmol) may cause muscle weakness. Potassium depletion may also cause symptomatic hyponatraemia (see p. 679).

Hypokalaemia is associated with an increased frequency of atrial and ventricular ectopic beats. This association may not always be causal, because adrenergic activation (for instance after myocardial infarction) causes both hypokalaemia and increased cardiac irritability. Hypokalaemia in patients without cardiac disease is unlikely to lead to serious arrhythmias.

Hypokalaemia seriously increases the risk of digoxin toxicity by increasing binding of digoxin to cardiac cells, potentiating its action, and decreasing its clearance.

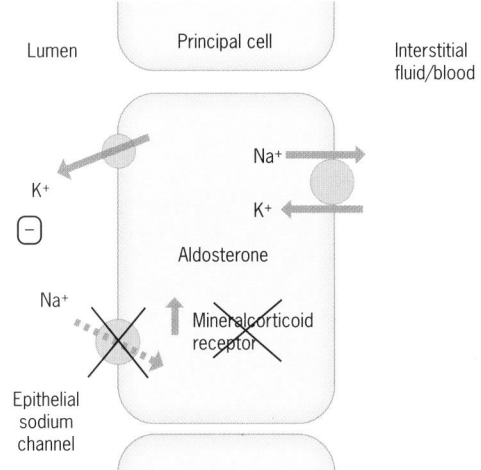

Fig. 12.7 **Aldosterone-regulated transport in the cortical collecting tubule.** Under normal conditions, the epithelial sodium channel is the rate-limiting barrier for the normal entry of sodium from the lumen into the cell. The resulting lumen-negative transepithelial voltage (indicated by the minus sign) drives potassium secretion from the principal cells and proton secretion from the α-intercalated cells (see Fig. 12.11).

In **Liddle's syndrome**, increased mutation in the gene encoding the epithelial sodium channel results in persistent unregulated reabsorption of sodium and increased secretion of potassium (not shown).

In **autosomal recessive pseudo-hypoaldosteronism type I**, loss-of-function mutations (**X**) in this gene inactivate the channel.

In **autosomal dominant pseudo-hypoaldosteronism type I**, mutation is in the gene encoding the mineralocorticoid regulation of the activity of the epithelial sodium channel. Either mechanism reduces the activity of the epithelial sodium channel, thus causing salt wasting and decreasing the secretion of potassium and protons.

Chronic hypokalaemia is associated with interstitial renal disease, but the pathogenesis is not completely understood.

Treatment

The underlying cause should be identified and treated where possible. Table 12.13 shows some examples.

Acute hypokalaemia may correct spontaneously. In most cases, withdrawal of oral diuretics or purgatives, accompanied by the oral administration of potassium supplements in the form of slow-release potassium or effervescent potassium, is all that is required. Intravenous potassium replacement is required only in conditions such as cardiac arrhythmias, muscle weakness or severe diabetic ketoacidosis when the potassium is < 2.5 mmol/L. When using intravenous therapy in the presence of poor renal function, replacement rates > 20 mmol per hour should be used only, with hourly monitoring of serum potassium and ECG changes.

The treatment of adrenal disorders is described on page 1066.

Failure to correct hypokalaemia may be due to concurrent hypomagnesaemia. Serum magnesium should be measured and any deficiency corrected.

Table 12.13
Treatment of hypokalaemia

Cause	Treatment
Dietary deficiency	Increase intake of fresh fruit/vegetables or oral potassium supplements (20–40 mmol daily)
	(Potassium supplements can cause gastrointestinal irritation)
Hyperaldosteronism, e.g. cirrhosis	Spironolactone
Thiazide therapy	Co-prescription of a potassium-sparing diuretic with a similar onset and duration of action
Intravenous fluid replacement	Add 20 mmol/L of K$^+$ with monitoring

Table 12.14
Causes of hyperkalaemia

Decreased excretion	Increased extraneous load
Renal failure*	Potassium chloride
Drug:* direct effect on potassium handling	Salt substitutes
Amiloride	Transfusion of stored blood*
Triamterene	
Spironolactone	**Spurious**
Aldosterone deficiency	*Increased in vitro release from abnormal cells:*
Hyporeninaemic hypoaldosteronism (RTA type 4)	Leukaemia
	Infectious mononucleosis
Addison's disease	Thrombocytosis
ACE inhibitors*	Familial pseudohyperkalaemia
NSAIDs	Haemolysis in syringe
Ciclosporin treatment	*Increased release from muscles:*
Heparin treatment	Vigorous fist clenching during phlebotomy
Acidosis*	
Gordon's syndrome	

Increased release from cells
(decreased Na$^+$–K$^+$-ATPase activity)
Acidosis
Diabetic ketoacidosis
Rhabdomyolysis/tissue damage
Tumour lysis
Succinylcholine (amplified by muscle denervation)
Digoxin poisoning
Vigorous exercise (α-adrenergic; transient)

*Common causes

Hyperkalaemia

Causes

Acute self-limiting hyperkalaemia occurs normally after vigorous exercise and is of no pathological significance. Hyperkalaemia in all other situations is due either to increased release from cells or to failure of excretion (Table 12.14). The most common causes are renal impairment and drug interference with potassium excretion. The combination of ACE inhibitors with potassium-sparing diuretics or NSAIDs is particularly dangerous.

Rare causes

Hyporeninaemic hypoaldosteronism

This is also known as type 4 renal tubular acidosis (see p. 693). Hyperkalaemia occurs here because of acidosis and hypoaldosteronism.

Pseudo-hypoaldosteronism type 1 (autosomal recessive and dominant types)

This is a disease of infancy apparently due to resistance to the action of aldosterone. It is characterized by hyperkalaemia and evidence of sodium wasting (hyponatraemia, extracellular volume depletion). Autosomal recessive forms result from loss of function because of mutations in the gene for epithelial sodium channel activity (opposite to Liddle's syndrome). This disorder involves multiple organ systems and is especially marked in the neonatal period. With aggressive salt replacement and control of hyperkalaemia, these children can survive and the disorder appears to become less severe with age. The autosomal dominant type is due to mutations affecting the mineralocorticoid receptor (Fig. 12.7). These patients present with salt wasting and hyperkalaemia but do not have other organ-system involvement.

Hyperkalaemic periodic paralysis (see p. 1224)

This is precipitated by exercise, and is caused by an autosomal dominant mutation of the skeletal muscle sodium channel gene.

Gordon's syndrome

This appears to be a mirror image of Bartter's syndrome (see p. 682), in which primary renal retention of sodium causes hypertension, volume expansion, low renin/aldosterone, hyperkalaemia and metabolic acidosis.

Suxamethonium and other depolarizing muscle relaxants

These cause release of potassium from cells. Induction of muscle paralysis during general anaesthesia may result in a rise of plasma potassium of up to 1 mmol/L. This is not usually a problem unless there is pre-existing hyperkalaemia.

Clinical features

Serum potassium of greater than 7.0 mmol/L is a medical emergency and is associated with ECG changes (Fig. 12.8). Severe hyperkalaemia may be asymptomatic and may predispose to sudden death from asystolic cardiac arrest. Muscle weakness is often the only symptom, unless

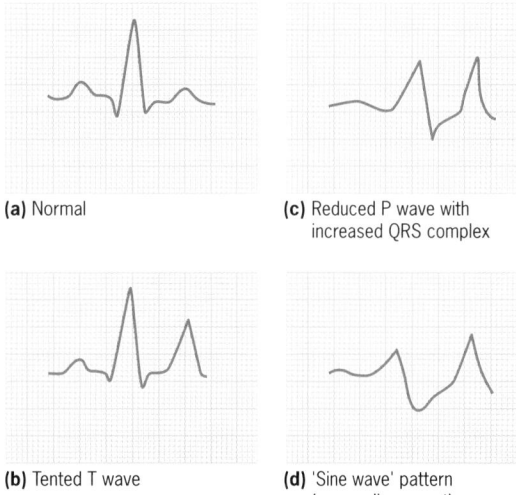

(a) Normal

(c) Reduced P wave with increased QRS complex

(b) Tented T wave

(d) 'Sine wave' pattern (pre-cardiac arrest)

Fig. 12.8 Progressive ECG changes with increasing hyperkalaemia.

Emergency box 12.1

Correction of hyperkalaemia

IMMEDIATE

Protect myocardium
10 mL of 10% calcium gluconate given in the presence of ECG change
Effect is temporary but dose can be repeated

Drive K⁺ into cells
Insulin 10 units + 50 mL of 50% glucose followed by regular checks of blood glucose and plasma K⁺
Repeat as necessary

and/or correction of severe acidosis (pH < 6.9) – NaHCO₃ (1.26%)

and/or salbutamol 0.5 mg in 100 mL of 5% glucose over 15 min (rarely used)

LATER

Deplete body K⁺ (to decrease plasma K⁺ over next 24 h)
Polystyrene sulphonate resins:
  15 g orally up to three times daily with laxatives
  30 g rectally followed 3–6 hours later by an enema
Haemodialysis or peritoneal dialysis

(as is commonly the case) the hyperkalaemia is associated with metabolic acidosis, causing Kussmaul respiration. Hyperkalaemia causes hyperpolarization of cell membranes, leading to decreased cardiac excitability, hypotension, bradycardia, and eventual asystole.

Treatment

Treatments for hyperkalaemia require both urgent measures to save lives and maintenance therapy to keep potassium down as summarized in Emergency box 12.1. The cause of the hyperkalaemia should be found and treated.

Calcium ions protect the cell membranes from the effects of hyperkalaemia but do not alter the potassium concentration. *Insulin* drives potassium into the cell, but must be accompanied by glucose to avoid hypoglycaemia. Regular measurements of blood glucose must be used for at least 6 hours after use of insulin in this situation, and extra glucose must be available for immediate use. Alternatively, glucose can be given (without insulin) as this stimulates endogenous insulin and avoids problems with hypoglycaemia.

Intravenous salbutamol has not yet found widespread acceptance and may cause disturbing muscle tremor at the doses required.

Correction of acidosis with hypertonic (8.4%) sodium bicarbonate causes volume expansion and should not be used; 1.26% is used with severe acidosis (pH < 6.9) (p. 696). *Gastric aspiration* will remove potassium and leads to alkalosis.

Ion-exchange resins (polystyrene sulphonate resins) are used as maintenance therapy to keep potassium down *after* emergency treatment. They make use of the ion fluxes which occur in the gut to remove potassium from the body, and are the only way short of dialysis of

removing potassium from the body. They may cause fluid overload (resonium contains Na⁺) or hypercalcaemia (calcium resonium).

In general, all of these measures are simply ways of buying time either to correct the underlying disorder or to arrange removal of potassium by dialysis, which is the definitive treatment for hyperkalaemia.

All of these measures may cause digoxin toxicity in patients receiving digoxin, in whom cardiac monitoring is essential.

FURTHER READING

Ackerman MJ, Clapham DE (1997) Ion channels – basic science and clinical disease. *New England Journal of Medicine* **336**: 1575–1586.

Amerlate I, Dawson KP (2000) Bartter's syndrome; an overview. *Quarterly Journal of Medicine* **93**: 207–215.

Gennari FJ (1998) Hypokalaemia. *New England Journal of Medicine* **339**: 451–458.

Halperin ML, Kamel KS (1998) Electrolyte quintet. Potassium. *Lancet* **352**: 135–140.

Disorders of magnesium concentration

Plasma magnesium levels are normally maintained within the range 0.7–1.1 mmol/L. Magnesium balance is a function of intake and excretion. The average daily magnesium intake is 15 mmol. One-third of this magnesium is absorbed, principally in the small bowel. In the healthy adult, there is no net gain or loss of magnesium from bone, so that balance is achieved by the urinary excretion of the net magnesium absorbed.

Primary disturbance of magnesium balance is uncommon, hypo- or hypermagnesaemia usually developing on a background of more obvious fluid and electrolyte disturbances. Disturbance in magnesium balance should always be suspected in association with other fluid and electrolyte disturbances when the patient develops unexpected neurological signs or symptoms.

Renal handling of magnesium

Magnesium transport differs from that of most other ions in that the proximal tubule is not the major site of reabsorption. Only 15–25% of the filtered magnesium is reabsorbed passively in the proximal tubule and 5–10% in the distal tubule. The major site of magnesium transport is the thick ascending limb of the loop of Henle, where 60–70% of the filtered load is reabsorbed (Fig. 12.5). Loop magnesium reabsorption varies with changes in the plasma magnesium concentration, which is the main physiological regulator of urinary magnesium excretion. Hypermagnesaemia inhibits loop transport, while hypomagnesaemia stimulates magnesium transport. Hypercalcaemia inhibits magnesium loop transport by an unknown mechanism.

Another factor that can influence loop magnesium transport is the rate of sodium chloride reabsorption. This effect is relatively unimportant in normal subjects, but decreased reabsorption and magnesium wasting can be induced by the administration of a loop diuretic (Fig. 12.5).

Hypomagnesaemia

This most often develops as a result of deficient intake, defective gut absorption, or excessive gut or urinary loss (Table 12.15). It can also occur with acute pancreatitis, possibly owing to the formation of magnesium soaps in the areas of fat necrosis. Calcium deficiency usually develops with hypomagnesaemia. The serum magnesium is usually < 0.7 mmol/L.

Clinical features

Symptoms and signs include irritability, tremor, ataxia, carpopedal spasm, hyperreflexia, confusional and hallucinatory states, and epileptiform convulsions. An ECG may show a prolonged QT interval, broad flattened T waves, and occasional shortening of the ST segment.

Treatment

This involves the withdrawal of precipitating agents such as diuretics or purgatives and the parenteral infusion of 50 mmol of magnesium chloride in 1 L of 5%

Table 12.15
Causes of hypomagnesaemia

Decreased magnesium absorption	Gut losses
Malabsorption (severe)	Prolonged nasogastric
Malnutrition	suction
Alcohol excess	Excessive purgation
	Gastrointestinal/
Increased renal excretion	biliary fistulae
Drugs	Severe diarrhoea
Loop diuretics	
Thiazide diuretics	**Miscellaneous**
Digoxin	Acute pancreatitis
Diabetic ketoacidosis	
Gitelman's syndrome (p. 1065)	
Hyperaldosteronism	
SIADH	
Alcohol excess	
Hypercalciuria	
1,25-(OH)-vitamin D_3 deficiency	
Drug toxicity	
Amphotericin	
Aminoglycosides	
Cisplatin	
Ciclosporin	

SIADH, syndrome of inappropriate antidiuretic hormone secretion

dextrose or other isotonic fluid over 12–24 hours. This should be repeated daily until the plasma magnesium level is normal.

Hypermagnesaemia

This primarily occurs in patients with acute or chronic renal failure given magnesium-containing laxatives or antacids. It can also be induced by magnesium-containing enemas. Mild hypermagnesaemia may occur in patients with adrenal insufficiency. Causes are given in Table 12.16.

Clinical features

Symptoms and signs relate to neurological and cardiovascular depression, and include weakness with hyporeflexia proceeding to narcosis, respiratory paralysis and cardiac conduction defects. Symptoms usually develop when the plasma magnesium level exceeds 2 mmol/L.

Treatment

Treatment requires withdrawal of any magnesium therapy. An intravenous injection of 10 mL of calcium gluconate 10% (2.25 mmol calcium) is given to antagonize the effects of hypermagnesaemia, along with dextrose and insulin (as for hyperkalaemia) to lower the plasma magnesium level. Dialysis may be required in patients with severe renal failure.

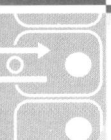

Table 12.16
Causes of hypermagnesaemia

Impaired renal excretion
Chronic renal failure
Acute renal failure

Increased magnesium intake
Purgatives, e.g. magnesium sulphate
Antacids, e.g. magnesium trisilicate

Haemodialysis with high [Mg^{2+}] dialysate

Table 12.17
Causes of hypophosphataemia

Redistribution	**Decreased intake/absorption**
Respiratory alkalosis	Dietary
Treatment of diabetic ketoacidosis	Malabsorption
	Vomiting
Carbohydrate administration after fasting	Gut phosphate binders, e.g. aluminium hydroxide
Cellular uptake syndrome	Vitamin D deficiency or resistance
After parathyroidectomy	Alcohol withdrawal
Renal losses	
Hyperparathyroidism	
Renal tubular defects	
Diuretics	

Disorders of phosphate concentration

Phosphate forms an essential part of most biochemical systems, from nucleic acids downwards. About 80% of all body phosphorus is within bone, plasma phosphate normally ranging from 0.80 to 1.40 mmol/L. Phosphate reabsorption from the kidney is decreased by parathyroid hormone (PTH); thus hyperparathyroidism is associated with low plasma levels of phosphate.

The regulation of plasma phosphate level is closely linked to calcium.

Hypophosphataemia

Significant hypophosphataemia (< 0.4 mmol/L) may occur in a number of clinical situations, owing to redistribution into cells, to renal losses, or to decreased intake (Table 12.17). It may cause:

- muscle weakness – diaphragmatic weakness, decreased cardiac contractility, skeletal muscle rhabdomyolysis
- a left-shift in the oxyhaemoglobin dissociation curve (reduced 2,3-diphosphoglycerate (2,3-DPG)) and rarely haemolysis
- confusion, hallucinations and convulsions.

Mild hypophosphataemia often resolves without specific treatment. However, diaphragmatic weakness may be severe in acute hypophosphataemia, and may impede weaning a patient from a ventilator. Interestingly, chronic hypophosphataemia (in X-linked hypophosphataemia) is associated with normal muscle power.

Hypophosphataemic (vitamin D resistant) rickets
This interesting disorder represents a set of abnormalities characterized by hypophosphataemia, elevated urinary phosphate excretion, rachitic bone changes and failure to respond to usual doses of vitamin D. It is commonly inherited as an X-linked dominant affecting both males and females. The gene locus was mapped to the short arm of the X chromosome. Mutations in patients with hypophosphataemic rickets were found in the gene designated PHEX (phosphate regulating gene with homologies to endopeptidases on the X chromosome). The pathophysiology of hypophosphataemic rickets is not fully elucidated but it is generally believed that PHEX expressed in bones and teeth binds with phosphate-regulating humoral factor, designated as phosphatonin.

Phosphatonin bound to PHEX acts on the sodium–phosphate cotransporter (NPT2) in the renal proximal tubules and promotes phosphate reabsorption. It also downregulates 24-hydroxylase activity, thus decreasing the degradation of 1,25-dihydroxyvitamin D. Loss of function owing to a mutation in the PHEX gene results in unbound phosphatonin. Unbound phosphatonin downregulates NPT2 and upregulates 24-hydroxylase activity. The consequence is inappropriate urinary phosphate excretion and increased degradation of 1,25-dihydroxyvitamin D (Fig. 12.9). Treatment includes combined therapy with phosphate supplementation and calcitriol (1,25-dihydroxyvitamin D) administration.

Treatment of acute hypophosphataemia, if warranted, is with intravenous phosphate at a maximum rate of 9 mmol every 12 hours, with repeated measurements of calcium and phosphate, as over-rapid administration of phosphate may lead to severe hypocalcaemia, particularly in the presence of alkalosis. Chronic hypophosphataemia can be corrected, if warranted, with oral effervescent sodium phosphate.

Hyperphosphataemia

Hyperphosphataemia is common in patients with chronic renal failure (see p. 644) (Table 12.18). Hyperphosphataemia is usually asymptomatic but may result in precipitation of calcium phosphate, particularly in the presence of a normal or raised calcium or of alkalosis. Uraemic itching may be caused by a raised

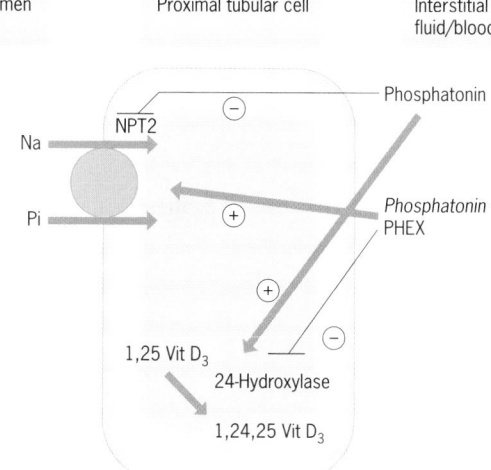

Lumen   Proximal tubular cell   Interstitial
                                                         fluid/blood

Fig. 12.9 **PHEX regulation of phosphate transport and vitamin D metabolism in the proximal tubule.** The hormone, phosphatonin, bound to PHEX (phosphate-regulating gene with homologies to endopeptidase on the X chromosome), is thought to stimulate phosphate reabsorption via the sodium–phosphate cotransporter (NPT2) and to retard the degradation of 1,25-dihydroxyvitamin D by downregulating 24-hydroxylase activity. PHEX appears to modify phosphatonin by an, as yet, undefined mechanism, probably at a site distant from the kidney. If PHEX is absent or non-functioning because of a mutation, an incorrectly processed phosphatonin is released into the circulation and causes renal phosphate wasting, as well as increased 1,25-dihydroxyvitamin D degradation. Modified from Rowe PSN (1998).

Table 12.18
Causes of hyperphosphataemia

Chronic renal failure
Phosphate-containing enemas
Tumour lysis
Myeloma-abnormal phosphate-binding protein
Rhabdomyolysis

calcium × phosphate product. Prolonged hyperphosphataemia causes hyperparathyroidism, and periarticular and vascular calcification.

Usually no treatment is required for acute hyperphosphataemia, as the causes are self-limiting. Treatment of chronic hyperphosphataemia is with gut phosphate binders and dialysis (see p. 649).

FURTHER READING

Rowe PSN (1998) The role of the PHEX gene in families with X-linked hypophosphataemic rickets. *Current Opinion in Nephrology and Hypertension* **7**: 367–376.
Weiseinger JR, Bellorin-Fort E (1998) Electrolyte quintet. Magnesium and phosphate. *Lancet* **352**: 391–396.

Acid–base disorders

The concentration of hydrogen ions in both extracellular and intracellular compartments is extremely tightly controlled, and very small changes may lead to major cell dysfunction. The blood pH is tightly regulated and is normally maintained at between 7.38 and 7.42. Any deviation from this range indicates a change in the hydrogen ion concentration [H^+] because blood pH is the negative logarithm of [H^+] (Table 12.19). The [H^+] at a physiological blood pH of 7.40 is 40 nmol/L. An increase in the [H^+] – a fall in pH – is termed acidaemia. A decrease in [H^+] – a rise in the blood pH – is termed alkalaemia. The disorders that cause these changes in the blood pH are acidosis and alkalosis, respectively.

Normal acid–base physiology

The normal adult diet contains 70–100 mmol of acid. Throughout the body, there are buffers that minimize any changes in blood pH that these ingested hydrogen ions might cause. Such buffers include intracellular proteins (e.g. haemoglobin) and tissue components (e.g. the calcium carbonate and calcium phosphate in bone) as well as the bicarbonate–carbonic acid buffer pair generated by the hydration of carbon dioxide. This buffer pair is clinically most important, in part because its contribution can be measured and because alterations in this buffer pair reveal changes in all other buffer systems. Bicarbonate ions (HCO_3^-) and carbonic acid (H_2CO_3) exist in equilibrium; and in the presence of carbonic anhydrase, carbonic acid dissociates to carbon dioxide and water, as expressed in the following equation:

$$H^+ + HCO_3^- \xrightleftharpoons{} H_2CO_3 \xrightleftharpoons[]{\substack{\text{carbonic} \\ \text{anhydrase}}} CO_2 + H_2O.$$

The addition of hydrogen ions drives the reaction to the right, decreasing the plasma bicarbonate concentration [HCO_3^-] and increasing the arterial carbon dioxide pressure ($P_a CO_2$). As shown in the following Henderson–

Table 12.19
Relationship between [H⁺] and pH

pH	[H⁺] (nmol/L)
6.9	126
7.0	100
7.1	79
7.2	63
7.3	50
7.4	40
7.5	32
7.6	25

Hasselbalch equation, a fall in the plasma $[HCO_3^-]$ increases $[H^+]$ and thus lowers blood pH:

$$[H^+] = 181 \times P_a co_2 / [HCO_3^-]$$

where $[H^+]$ is expressed in nmol per litre, $P_a CO_2$ in kilopascals, $[HCO_3^-]$ in mmol per litre, and 181 is the dissociation coefficient of carbonic acid. Alternatively the equation can be expressed as:

$$pH = pK + \log [HCO_3^-]/[H_2CO_3]$$

where $pK = 6.1$. Thus, the bicarbonate used in the buffering process must be regenerated to maintain normal acid–base balance.

Although the acidaemia stimulates an increase in ventilation, which blunts this change in pH, increased ventilation does not regenerate the bicarbonate used in the buffering process. Consequently, the kidney must excrete hydrogen ions to return the plasma $[HCO_3^-]$ to normal. Maintenance of a normal plasma $[HCO_3^-]$ under physiological conditions depends not only on daily regeneration of bicarbonate but also on reabsorption of all bicarbonate filtered across the glomerular capillaries.

Renal reabsorption of bicarbonate

The plasma $[HCO_3^-]$ is normally maintained at approximately 25 mmol/L. In individuals with a normal glomerular filtration rate (120 mL/min), about 4500 mmol of bicarbonate is filtered each day. If this filtered bicarbonate were not reabsorbed, the plasma $[HCO_3^-]$ would fall, along with blood pH. Thus, maintenance of a normal plasma $[HCO_3^-]$ requires that essentially all of the bicarbonate in the glomerular filtrate be reabsorbed (Fig. 12.10).

The proximal convoluted tubule reclaims 85–90% of filtered bicarbonate; in contrast, the distal nephron reclaims very little. This difference is caused by the greater quantity of luminal carbonic anhydrase in the proximal tubule than in the distal nephron. As a result of these quantitative differences, bicarbonate that escapes reabsorption in the proximal tubule is excreted in the urine.

Proximal tubular bicarbonate reabsorption is catalysed by the Na^+–K^+-ATPase pump located in the basolateral cell membrane. By exchanging peritubular potassium ions for intracellular sodium ions, the pump keeps the intracellular sodium concentration low, allowing sodium ions to enter the cell by moving down the sodium concentration gradient from the tubule lumen to the cell interior. Hydrogen ions are transported in the opposite direction (at the Na^+–H^+ antiporter), thereby maintaining electroneutrality. Before bicarbonate enters the proximal tubule, it combines with secreted hydrogen ions, forming carbonic acid. In the presence of luminal carbonic anhydrase, carbonic acid rapidly dissociates into carbon dioxide and water, which can then rapidly enter the proximal tubular cell. In the cell, carbon

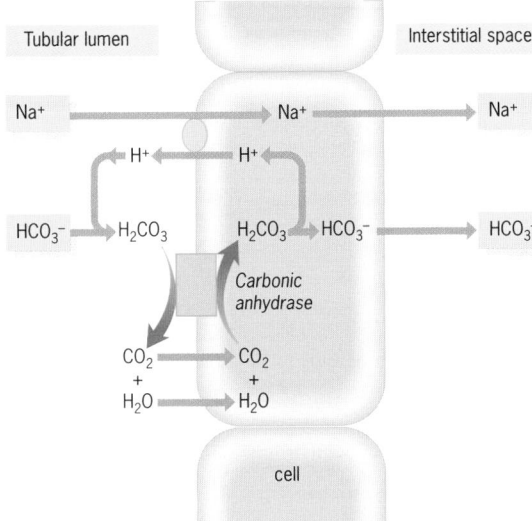

Fig. 12.10 Resorption of sodium bicarbonate in the renal (mainly proximal) tubule. Bicarbonate is reclaimed by the secretion of H^+ into the tubule in exchange for Na^+. This results in the formation of H_2CO_3, which is then broken down to CO_2. This is reabsorbed and converted back to H_2CO_3, which now dissociates into H^+ and HCO_3^-. The net result is reabsorption of Na^+ and HCO_3^-. This process is dependent on carbonic anhydrase within the cells and on the luminal surface of the tubular cell.

dioxide is hydrated, ultimately forming bicarbonate, which is then transported down an electrical gradient from the cell interior, across the membrane into the peritubular fluid, and into the blood. In this process, each hydrogen ion secreted into the proximal tubule lumen is reabsorbed and can be resecreted; there is no net loss of hydrogen ions or net gain of bicarbonate ions.

Renal excretion of [H+] (Fig. 12.11)

More acid is secreted into the proximal tubule (up to 4500 nmol of hydrogen ions each day) than into any other nephron segment. However, the hydrogen ions secreted into the proximal tubule are almost completely reabsorbed with bicarbonate; consequently, proximal tubular hydrogen ion secretion does not contribute significantly to hydrogen ion elimination from the body. The excretion of the daily acid load requires hydrogen ion secretion in more distal nephron segments.

Most dietary hydrogen ions come from sulphur-containing amino acids that are metabolized to sulphuric acid (H_2SO_4), which then reacts with sodium bicarbonate as follows:

$$H_2SO_4 + 2NaHCO_3 \rightarrow Na_2SO_4 + 2CO_2 + 2H_2O.$$

Excess sulphate is excreted in the urine, whereas excess hydrogen ions are buffered by bicarbonate and lower the plasma $[HCO_3^-]$. This fall in plasma $[HCO_3^-]$ leads to a slight decrease in the blood pH, although a smaller decrease in the blood pH than would have occurred if buffer were unavailable. The subsequent excretion of

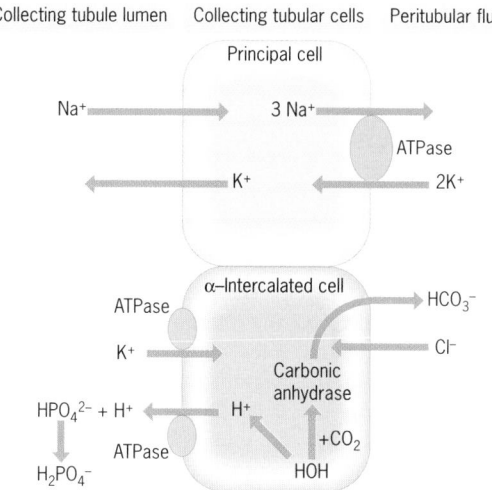

Collecting tubule lumen   Collecting tubular cells   Peritubular fluid

Fig. 12.11 **Renal excretion of H⁺.** Secretion of H⁺ from the cortical collecting tubule is indirectly linked to Na⁺ reabsorption. Intracellular potassium is exchanged for sodium in the principal cell. Aldosterone stimulates H⁺ secretion by entering the principal cell, where it opens Na⁺ channels in the luminal membrane and increases Na⁺–K⁺-ATPase activity. The movement of cationic Na⁺ into the principal cells then creates a negative charge within the tubule lumen. K⁺ moves from the electrochemical gradient and into the lumen. Aldosterone apparently also stimulates the H⁺-ATPase directly in the intercalated cell, further enhancing H⁺ secretion. When the urinary pH falls to 4.0–4.5, further H⁺ secretion by the alpha-intercalated cells ceases. The filtration of titratable acids (e.g. phosphoric acid) raises the intraluminal pH and permits this process to continue. Secreted H⁺ binds to the conjugate anion of a titratable acid (HPO_4^{2-}, in this case) and is excreted in the urine. The H⁺ to be secreted arises from the reassociation of H_2O and CO_2 in the presence of carbonic anhydrase; thus, a bicarbonate molecule is regenerated each time an H⁺ is eliminated in the urine.

hydrogen ions takes place primarily in the collecting tubule and results in the regeneration of 1 mmol of bicarbonate for every mmol of hydrogen ions excreted in the urine.

The collecting tubule has two types of cells:

- The principal cell with an aldosterone-sensitive Na⁺ absorption site. These cells reabsorb Na⁺ and H_2O and secrete K⁺ under the influence of aldosterone.
- The α-intercalated cell, which possesses the proton pump for the active secretion of hydrogen ions in exchange for reabsorption of K⁺ ions. Aldosterone increases H⁺ ion secretion.

Secretion of hydrogen ions from the cortical collecting tubule is indirectly linked to sodium reabsorption. Aldosterone has several facilitating effects on hydrogen ion secretion. Aldosterone opens sodium channels in the luminal membrane of the principal cell and increases Na⁺–K⁺-ATPase activity. The subsequent movement of cationic sodium into the principal cell creates a negative charge within the tubule lumen. Potassium ions from the principal cells and hydrogen ions from the α-intercalated cells move out from the cells down the electrochemical gradient and into the lumen. Aldosterone also

stimulates directly the H⁺-ATPase in the α-intercalated cell, further enhancing hydrogen ion secretion.

When hydrogen ions are secreted into the lumen of the collecting tubule, a tiny, but physiologically critical, fraction of these excess hydrogen ions remains in solution. Here, they increase the urinary [H⁺] and lower urinary pH below 4.0. Nevertheless, below this urine pH, inhibition of proton-secreting pumps such as H⁺-ATPase severely restricts kidney secretion of more hydrogen ions. Consequently, secretion of hydrogen ions depends on the presence of buffers in the urine that maintain the urine pH at a level higher than 4.0.

Buffer systems in acid excretion

Two buffer systems are important in acid excretion: the titratable acids such as phosphate and the ammonia system. Each system is responsible for excreting about half of the daily acid load of 50–100 mmol under physiological conditions (Fig. 12.11).

Titratable acid

A titratable acid is a filtered buffer substance having a conjugate anion that can be titrated within the pH range occurring physiologically in the urine. Phosphoric acid (pK_a 6.8) is the usual titratable urinary buffer. Hydrogen ions bind to the conjugate anions of the titratable acids and are excreted in the urine. For each hydrogen ion excreted in this form, a bicarbonate ion is regenerated within the cell and returned to the blood (Fig. 12.11).

Ammonium (NH_4^+)

Although half of dietary hydrogen ions are excreted as titratable acid and the other half as ammonium, in pathophysiological conditions the ammonia (NH_3) buffer system is far more important than titratable acids. In the setting of metabolic acidosis, titratable acids cannot increase significantly because availability of the titratable acid is fixed by the plasma concentration of the buffer and by the GFR. The ammonia buffer system, in contrast, can increase several hundred-fold when necessary. Consequently, impaired renal excretion of hydrogen ions is always associated with a defect in ammonium excretion (Fig. 12.12).

All ammonia used to buffer urinary hydrogen ions in the collecting tubule is synthesized in the proximal convoluted tubule. Glutamine is the primary source of ammonia. It undergoes deamination catalysed by glutaminase, resulting in α-ketoglutaric acid (see Fig. 12.12) and ammonia. Once formed, ammonia can diffuse into the proximal tubule lumen and become acidified, forming ammonium. Once in the proximal tubule lumen, ammonium flows along the tubule to the thick ascending limb of Henle's loop. Here, it is transported out of the tubule into the medullary interstitium. Ammonium then dissociates to ammonia, leading to a high interstitial ammonia concentration. Ammonia diffuses down its concentration gradient into the lumen of the collecting

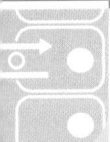

Proximal   Proximal tubular cell   Peritubular fluid
lumen tubule

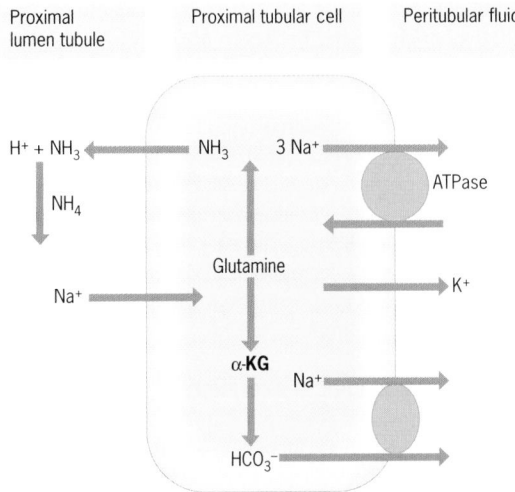

Fig. 12.12 **The ammonia buffering system in the kidney.** All ammonia used to buffer H^+ in the collecting tubule is synthesized in the proximal convoluted tubule, and glutamine is the main source of this ammonia. As glutamine is metabolized, α-ketoglutarate (α-KG) is formed, which ultimately breaks down to bicarbonate that is then secreted into the peritubular fluid at an Na^+–HCO_3^- cotransporter.

tubule. Here, it reacts with the hydrogen ions secreted by the collecting tubular cells to form ammonium. Because ammonium (NH_4) is not lipid-soluble, it is trapped in the lumen and excreted in the urine as ammonium chloride. Controversy still exists about whether glutamine metabolism in the liver plays a role in acid–base homeostasis.

Two conditions predominantly promote ammonia synthesis by the proximal tubular cell: systemic acidosis and hypokalaemia.

Causes of acid–base disturbance

Acid–base disturbance may be caused by:

- abnormal CO_2 removal in the lungs ('respiratory' acidosis and alkalosis)
- abnormalities in the regulation of bicarbonate and other buffers in the blood ('metabolic' acidosis and alkalosis).

Both may, and usually do, coexist. For instance, metabolic acidosis causes hyperventilation (via medullary chemoreceptors, see p. 838), leading to increased removal of CO_2 in the lungs and partial compensation for the acidosis. Conversely, respiratory acidosis is accompanied by renal bicarbonate retention, which could be mistaken for primary metabolic alkalosis. The situation is even more complex if a patient has both respiratory disease and a metabolic disturbance.

Diagnosis

Clinical history and examination usually point to the correct diagnosis. Table 12.20 shows the typical changes, but in complicated patients the acid–base nomogram

Table 12.20
Changes in arterial blood gases

	pH	P_aCO_2	HCO_3^-
Respiratory acidosis	N or ↓	↑↑	↑ (compensated)
Respiratory alkalosis	N or ↑	↓↓	↓ (slight)
Metabolic acidosis	N or ↓	↓	↓↓
Metabolic alkalosis	N or ↑	↑ (slight)	↑↑

(Fig. 12.13) is invaluable. The $[H^+]$ and P_aCO_2 are measured in arterial blood (for precautions see p. 945) as well as the bicarbonate. If the values from a patient lie in one of the bands in the diagram, it is likely that only one abnormality is present. If the $[H^+]$ is high (pH low) but the P_aCO_2 is normal, the intercept lies between two bands: the patient has respiratory dysfunction, leading to failure of CO_2 elimination, but this is partly compensated for by metabolic acidosis, stimulating respiration and CO_2 removal (this is the most common 'combined' abnormality in practice).

Respiratory acidosis and alkalosis

Respiratory acidosis

This is caused by retention of CO_2. The P_aCO_2 and $[H^+]$ rise. Renal retention of bicarbonate may partly compensate, returning the $[H^+]$ towards normal (see p. 690).

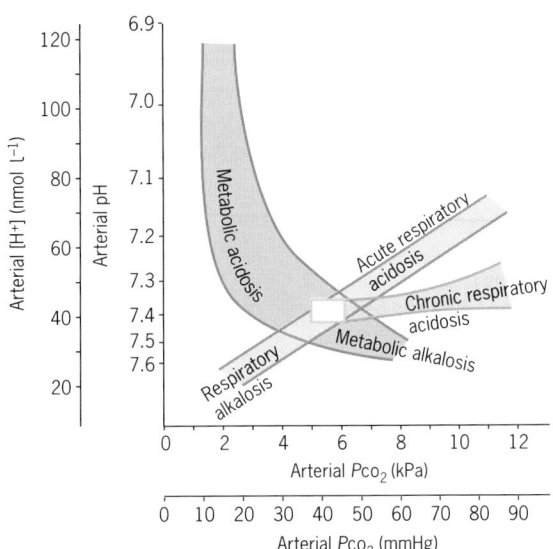

Fig. 12.13 **The Flenley acid–base nomogram.** This was derived from a large number of observations in patients with 'pure' respiratory or metabolic disturbances. The bands show the 95% confidence limits representing the individual varieties of acid–base disturbance. The central white box shows the approximate limits of arterial pH and P_{CO_2} in normal individuals.

Respiratory alkalosis

Increased removal of CO_2 is caused by hyperventilation, so there is a fall in P_aCO_2 and $[H^+]$ (see p. 838).

Metabolic acidosis

This is due to the accumulation of any acid other than carbonic acid and there is a primary decrease in the plasma $[HCO_3^-]$. Several disorders can lead to metabolic acidosis: acid administration, acid generation (e.g. lactic acidosis during shock or cardiac arrest), impaired acid excretion by the kidneys, or bicarbonate losses from the gastrointestinal tract or kidneys. From a diagnostic viewpoint, calculation of the plasma anion gap is extremely useful in narrowing this differential diagnosis.

The anion gap

The first step is to identify whether the acidosis is due to retention of H^+Cl^- or to another acid. This is achieved by calculation of the anion gap. The principles underlying this calculation are straightforward:

- The normal cations present in plasma are Na^+, K^+, Ca^{2+}, Mg^{2+}.
- The normal anions present in plasma are Cl^-, HCO_3^-, negative charges present on albumin, phosphate, sulphate, lactate, and other organic acids.
- The sums of the positive and negative charges are equal.
- Measurement of plasma $[Na^+]$, $[K^+]$, $[Cl^-]$ and $[HCO_3^-]$ is usually easily available.

$$\text{ANION GAP} = \{[Na^+] + [K^+]\} - \{[HCO_3^-] + [Cl^-]\}.$$

Because there are more unmeasured anions than cations, the normal anion gap is 10–18 mmol/L, although recent calculations with more sensitive methods place this at 6–12 mmol/L. Albumin normally makes up the largest portion of these unmeasured anions. As a result, a fall in the plasma albumin concentration from the normal value of about 40 g/L to 20 g/L may reduce the anion gap by as much as 6 mmol/L, because each 1 g/L of albumin has a negative charge of 0.2–0.28 mmol/L.

Metabolic acidosis with a normal anion gap

If the anion gap is normal in the presence of acidosis, this suggests that H^+Cl^- is being retained or that $Na^+HCO_3^-$ is being lost. Causes of a normal-anion-gap acidosis are given in Table 12.21. In these conditions, plasma bicarbonate decreases and is replaced by chloride to maintain electroneutrality. Consequently, these disorders are sometimes referred to collectively as hyperchloraemic acidoses.

Table 12.21

Causes of metabolic acidosis with a normal anion gap

Increased gastrointestinal bicarbonate loss	Decreased renal hydrogen ion excretion
Diarrhoea	Distal (type 1) renal tubular acidosis
Ileostomy	Type 4 renal tubular acidosis (aldosterone deficiency)
Ureterosigmoidostomy	
Increased renal bicarbonate loss	
Acetazolamide	**Increased HCl production**
Proximal (type 2) renal tubular acidosis	Ammonium chloride ingestion
Hyperparathyroidism	Increased catabolism of lysine, arginine
Tubular damage, e.g. drugs, heavy metals, paraproteins	

Renal tubular acidosis (RTA)

This term refers to systemic acidosis caused by impairment of the ability of the renal tubules to maintain acid–base balance. This group of disorders is uncommon and only rarely a cause of significant clinical disease. Renal tubular acidosis may be secondary to immunological, drug-induced or structural damage to the tubular cells, an inherited abnormality, or an isolated ('primary') abnormality. As with most disorders which are not well understood, the nomenclature is confusing.

Type 4 renal tubular acidosis

Also called 'hyporeninaemic hypoaldosteronism', this is probably the most common of these disorders. The cardinal features are hyperkalaemia and acidosis occurring in a patient with mild chronic renal insufficiency, usually caused by tubulo-interstitial disease (e.g. reflux nephropathy) or diabetes. Plasma renin and aldosterone are found to be low even after measures which would normally stimulate their secretion (Table 12.22). An identical syndrome may be caused by chronic ingestion of NSAIDs, which impair renin and aldosterone secretion. In the presence of acidosis, urine pH may be low. Treatment is with fludrocortisone, sodium bicarbonate, diuretics, or ion exchange resins to remove potassium, or some combination of these. Dietary potassium restriction alone is ineffective.

Type 3 renal tubular acidosis

This condition is vanishingly rare, and represents a combination of type 1 and type 2.

Type 2 ('proximal') renal tubular acidosis

This is very rare in adult practice (Table 12.23). It is caused by failure of sodium bicarbonate reabsorption in the proximal tubule. The cardinal features are acidosis, hypokalaemia, an inability to lower the urine

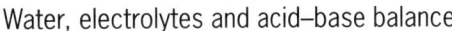
Table 12.22
Diagnosis of hyporeninaemic hypoaldosteronism (type 4 renal tubular acidosis)

Hyperkalaemia
(In the absence of drugs known to cause hyperkalaemia)
Low plasma bicarbonate and hyperchloraemia

Normal ACTH stimulation test

Low basal 24-hour urinary aldosterone

Subnormal response of plasma renin and plasma aldosterone to stimulation
Samples taken over 2 hours supine and again after 40 mg furosemide (frusemide) (80 mg if creatinine > 120 µmol/L) and 4 hours upright posture

Correction of hyperkalaemia by fludrocortisone 0.1 mg daily

Table 12.23
Causes of proximal renal tubular acidosis (type 2 RTA)

Cystinosis	**Vitamin D deficiency/ hyperparathyroidism**
Tyrosinaemia	
	Toxins and drugs
Wilson's disease	Carbonic anhydrase inhibitors
	Lead
Glycogen storage disease, type I	Cadmium
	Mercury
	Uranium
Pyruvate carboxylase deficiency	Copper
	Outdated tetracycline
Multiple myeloma	

Table 12.24
Causes of distal renal tubular acidosis (type 1 RTA)

Primary	**Drugs and toxins**
Idiopathic	Amphotericin B
	Lithium carbonate
Genetic	NSAIDs
Familial	Lead
Marfan's syndrome	
Ehlers–Danlos syndrome	**Autoimmune diseases**
Sickle cell anaemia	Sjögren's syndrome*
	Thyroiditis
Nephrocalcinosis	Autoimmune hepatitis
Chronic hypercalcaemia	Primary biliary cirrhosis
Medullary sponge kidney	Systemic lupus erythematosus
Hypergammaglobulinaemic states	**Renal transplant rejection***
Amyloidosis*	
Cryoglobulinaemia	
Chronic liver disease	

*May also cause proximal renal tubular acidosis

These abnormalities result in osteomalacia, renal stone formation and recurrent urinary infections. Osteomalacia is caused by buffering of H⁺ by Ca²⁺ in bone, resulting in depletion of calcium from bone. Renal stone formation is caused by hypercalciuria, hypocitraturia (citrate inhibits calcium phosphate precipitation), and alkaline urine (which favours precipitation of calcium phosphate).

Recurrent urinary infections are caused by renal stones. Treatment is with sodium bicarbonate, potassium supplements and citrate. Thiazide diuretics are useful by causing volume contraction and increased proximal sodium bicarbonate reabsorption. Diagnosis of renal tubular acidosis requires logical steps as summarized in Practical box 12.1.

Urinary anion gap
Another useful tool in the evaluation of metabolic acidosis with a normal anion gap is the urinary anion gap:

$$\text{URINARY ANION GAP} = \{\text{urinary } [Na^+] + \text{urinary } [K^+]\} - \text{urinary } [Cl^-].$$

This calculation can be used to distinguish the normal-anion-gap acidosis caused by diarrhoea (or other gastrointestinal alkali loss) from that caused by distal renal tubular acidosis. In both disorders, the plasma [K⁺] is characteristically low. In patients with renal tubular acidosis, urinary pH is always greater than 5.3.

Although excretion of urinary hydrogen ions in the patient with diarrhoea should acidify the urine, hypokalaemia leads to enhanced ammonia synthesis by the proximal tubular cells. Despite acidaemia, the excess urinary buffer increases the urine pH to a value above 5.3 in some patients with diarrhoea.

Whenever urinary acid is excreted as ammonium chloride, the increase in urinary chloride excretion

pH below 5.5 despite systemic acidosis, and the appearance of bicarbonate in the urine despite a subnormal plasma bicarbonate. This disorder normally occurs as part of a generalized tubular defect, together with other features such as glycosuria and amino-aciduria. Treatment is with sodium bicarbonate: massive doses may be required to overcome the renal 'leak'.

Type 1 ('distal') renal tubular acidosis
This is due to a failure of H⁺ excretion in the distal tubule (Table 12.24). It consists of:

- acidosis
- hypokalaemia (few exceptions)
- inability to lower the urine pH below 5.3 despite systemic acidosis
- low urinary ammonium production.

These features may be present only in the face of increased acid production; hence the need for an acid load test in diagnosis (Practical box 12.1). Other features include:

- low urinary citrate
- hypercalciuria.

Diagnosis of renal tubular acidosis

Plasma HCO_3^- < 21 mmol/L, urine pH > 5.3 = renal tubular acidosis

To differentiate between proximal (very rare) and distal (rare) requires bicarbonate infusion test

Plasma HCO_3^- > 21 mmol/L but suspicion of partial renal tubular acidosis (e.g. nephrocalcinosis associated diseases): **acid load test** required as follows

> Give 100 mg/kg ammonium chloride by mouth
> Check urine pH hourly and plasma HCO_3^- at 3 hours
> Plasma HCO_3^- should drop below 21 mmol/L unless the patient vomits
>> (in which case the test should be repeated with an antiemetic)
> If urine pH remains > 5.3 despite a plasma HCO_3^- of 21 mmol/L, the diagnosis is confirmed

Table 12.25

Causes of metabolic acidosis with an increased anion gap

Renal failure (sulphate, phosphate)

Accumulation of organic acids

Lactic acidosis
L-lactic
    Type A – anaerobic metabolism in tissues
        Hypotension/cardiac arrest
        Sepsis
        Poisoning – e.g. ethylene glycol, methanol
    Type B – decreased hepatic lactate metabolism
        Insulin deficiency (decreased pyruvate dehydrogenase activity)
        Metformin accumulation (chronic renal failure)
        Haematological malignancies
        Rare inherited enzyme defects
D-lactic (fermentation of glucose in bowel by abnormal bowel flora, complicating abnormal small bowel anatomy, e.g. blind loops)

Ketoacidosis
Insulin deficiency
Alcohol excess
Starvation

Exogenous acids
Salicylate

decreases the urinary anion gap. Thus, the urinary anion gap should be negative in the patient with diarrhoea regardless of the urine pH. On the other hand, although hypokalaemia may result in enhanced proximal tubular ammonia synthesis in distal renal tubular acidosis, the inability to secrete hydrogen ions into the collecting tubule in this condition limits ammonium chloride formation and excretion; thus, the urinary anion gap is positive in distal renal tubular acidosis.

Metabolic acidosis with a high anion gap

If the anion gap is increased, one may conclude that an unmeasured anion is present in increased quantities. This may be either one of the acids normally present in small, but unmeasured quantities, such as lactate, or an exogenous acid. Causes of a high-anion-gap acidosis are given in Table 12.25.

Lactic acidosis

Increased lactic acid production occurs when cellular respiration is abnormal, because of either a lack of oxygen in the tissues ('type A') or a metabolic abnormality, such as drug-induced ('type B') (Table 12.25). The most common cause in clinical practice is type A lactic acidosis, occurring in septic or cardiogenic shock. Significant acidosis can occur despite a normal blood pressure and P_aCO_2, owing to splanchnic and peripheral vasoconstriction. Acidosis worsens cardiac function and vasoconstriction further, contributing to a downward spiral and fulminant production of lactic acid.

Diabetic ketoacidosis (see p. 1088)

This is a high-anion-gap acidosis resulting from the accumulation of organic acids, acetoacetic acid and hydroxybutyric acid, owing to increased production and some reduced peripheral utilization.

Uraemic acidosis

Kidney disease may cause acidosis in several ways. Reduction in the number of functioning nephrons decreases the capacity to excrete ammonia and H^+ in the urine. In addition, tubular disease may cause bicarbonate wasting. Acidosis is a particular feature of those types of chronic renal failure in which the tubules are particularly affected, such as reflux nephropathy and chronic obstructive uropathy.

Chronic acidosis is most often caused by chronic renal failure, where there is a failure to excrete fixed acid. Up to 40 mmol of hydrogen ions may accumulate daily. These are buffered by bone, in exchange for calcium. Chronic acidosis is therefore a major risk factor for renal osteodystrophy and hypercalciuria.

Chronic acidosis has also been shown to be a risk factor for muscle wasting in renal failure, and may also contribute to the inexorable progression of some types of renal disease.

Uraemic acidosis should be corrected because of the effects of chronic acidosis on growth, muscle turnover and bones. Oral sodium bicarbonate 2–3 mmol/kg daily is usually enough to maintain serum bicarbonate above 20 mmol/L, but may contribute to sodium overload. Calcium carbonate improves acidosis and also acts as a phosphate binder and calcium supplement, and is commonly used. Acidosis in end-stage renal failure is usually fully corrected by adequate dialysis.

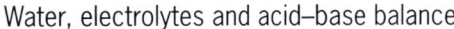
Mixed metabolic acidosis

Both types of acidosis may coexist. For instance, cholera would be expected to cause a normal-anion-gap acidosis owing to massive gastrointestinal losses of bicarbonate, but the anion gap is often increased owing to renal failure and lactic acidosis as a result of hypovolaemia.

Clinical features

Clinically the most obvious effect is stimulation of respiration, leading to the clinical sign of 'air hunger', or Kussmaul's sign. Interestingly, patients with profound hyperventilation may not complain of breathlessness, although in others it may be a presenting complaint.

Acidosis increases delivery of oxygen to the tissues by shifting the oxyhaemoglobin dissociation curve to the right, but it also leads to inhibition of 2,3-DPG production, which returns the curve towards normal (see Ch. 8). Cardiovascular dysfunction is common in acidotic patients, although it is often difficult to dissociate the numerous possible causes of this. There is no doubt that acidosis is negatively inotropic. Severe acidosis also causes venoconstriction, resulting in redistribution of blood from the peripheries to the central circulation, and increased systemic venous pressure, which may worsen pulmonary oedema caused by myocardial depression. Arteriolar vasodilatation also occurs, further contributing to hypotension.

Cerebral dysfunction is variable. Severe acidosis is often associated with confusion and fits, but numerous other possible causes are usually present.

As mentioned earlier, acidosis stimulates potassium loss from cells, which may lead to potassium deficiency if renal function is normal, or to hyperkalaemia if renal potassium excretion is impaired.

General treatment of acidosis

Treatment should be aimed at correcting the primary cause. In lactic acidosis caused by poor tissue perfusion ('type A'), treatment should be aimed at maximizing oxygen delivery to the tissues by protecting the airway, improving breathing and circulation. This usually requires inotropic agents, mechanical ventilation and invasive monitoring. In 'type B' lactic acidosis, treatment is that of the underlying disorder; e.g.

- insulin in diabetic ketoacidosis
- treatment of methanol and ethylene glycol poisoning with ethanol
- removal of salicylate by dialysis.

The question of whether severe acidosis should be treated with bicarbonate is extremely controversial. Severe acidosis ([H^+] > 100 nmol/L, pH < 7.0) is associated with a very high mortality, which makes many doctors keen to correct it. Since acidosis is known to impair cardiac contractility, it would seem sensible to correct acidosis with bicarbonate in a sick patient. However:

- Rapid correction of acidosis may result in tetany and fits owing to a rapid decrease in ionized calcium.
- Administration of sodium bicarbonate (8.4%) provides 1 mmol/mL of sodium, which may lead to extracellular volume expansion, exacerbating pulmonary oedema.
- Bicarbonate therapy increases CO_2 production and will therefore correct acidosis only if ventilation can be increased to remove the added CO_2 load.
- The increased amounts of CO_2 generated may diffuse more readily into cells than bicarbonate, worsening intracellular acidosis.

Administration of sodium bicarbonate (50 mmol, as 50 mL of 8.4% sodium bicarbonate intravenously) is still occasionally given during cardiac arrest and is often necessary before arrhythmias can be corrected. Correction of hyperkalaemia associated with acidosis is also of undoubted benefit. In other situations there is no clinical evidence to show that correction of acidosis improves outcome, but it is standard practice to administer sodium bicarbonate when [H^+] is above 126 nmol/L (pH < 6.9), using intravenous 1.26% (150 mmol/L) bicarbonate.

Metabolic alkalosis

Metabolic alkalosis is common, comprising half of all the acid–base disorders in hospitalized patients. This observation should not be surprising since vomiting, the use of diuretics, and nasogastric suction are common among hospitalized patients. The mortality associated with metabolic alkalosis is substantial; the mortality rate is 45% in patients with an arterial pH of 7.55 and 80% when the pH is greater than 7.65. Although this relationship is not necessarily causal, severe alkalosis should be viewed with concern.

Classification and definitions

Metabolic alkalosis has been classified on the basis of underlying pathophysiology (Table 12.26).

The most common group is due to chloride depletion which can be corrected without potassium repletion. The other major grouping is that due to potassium depletion, usually with mineralocorticoid excess. Metabolic alkalosis due to both potassium and chloride depletion also occurs.

Chloride may be lost from the gut, kidney or skin. The loss of gastric fluid rich in acid results in alkalosis because bicarbonate generated during the production of gastric acid returns to the circulation. In Zollinger–Ellison syndrome (p. 404) or pyloric stenosis these losses can be massive. Although sodium and potassium loss in the gastric juice is variable, the obligate urinary loss of these cations is intensified by bicarbonaturia, which occurs during disequilibrium.

Table 12.26
Causes of metabolic alkalosis

Chloride depletion
Gastric losses: vomiting, mechanical drainage, bulimia
Chloruretic diuretics: e.g. bumetanide, furosemide (frusemide), chlorothiazide, metolazone
Diarrhoeal states: villous adenoma, congenital chloridorrhoea
Cystic fibrosis (high sweat chloride)

Potassium depletion/mineralocorticoid excess
Primary aldosteronism
Secondary aldosteronism
Apparent mineralocorticoid excess
   Primary deoxycorticosterone excess: 11α- and 17α-hydroxylase deficiencies
   Drugs: liquorice (glycyrrhizic acid) as a confection or flavouring, carbenoxolone
   Liddle's syndrome
Bartter's and Gitelman's syndromes and their variants
Laxative abuse, clay ingestion

Hypercalcaemia states
Hypercalcaemia of malignancy
Acute or chronic milk–alkali syndrome

Others
Ampicillin, penicillin therapy
Bicarbonate ingestion: massive or with renal insufficiency
Recovery from starvation
Hypoalbuminaemia

Chloruretic agents all directly produce loss of chloride, sodium and fluid in the urine. These losses in turn promote metabolic alkalosis by several mechanisms:

- diuretic-induced increases in sodium delivery to the distal nephron enhance potassium and hydrogen ion secretion;
- extracellular volume contraction stimulates renin and aldosterone secretion, which blunts sodium losses but accelerates potassium and hydrogen ion secretion;
- potassium depletion augments bicarbonate reabsorption in the proximal tubule and
- stimulates ammonia production which in turn will increase urinary net acid excretion.

Urinary losses of chloride exceed those for sodium and are associated with alkalosis even when potassium depletion is prevented. The cessation of events that generate alkalosis is not necessarily accompanied by resolution of the alkalosis. A widely accepted hypothesis for the maintenance of alkalosis is chloride depletion rather than volume depletion. Although normal functioning of the proximal tubule is essential for bicarbonate absorption, the collecting tubule appears to be the major nephron site for altered electrolyte and proton transport in both maintenance and recovery from metabolic alkalosis. During maintenance, the α-intercalated cells in the cortical collecting duct do not secrete bicarbonate because insufficient chloride is available for bicarbonate

exchange. When chloride is administered and luminal or cellular chloride concentration increases, bicarbonate is promptly excreted and alkalosis is corrected.

Metabolic alkalosis in hypokalaemia is generated primarily by an increased intracellular shift of hydrogen ion causing intracellular acidosis. Potassium depletion is also associated with enhanced ammonia production with increased obligate net acid excretion. However, the role of intracellular acidosis is supported by the correction of the alkalosis by infusion of potassium without any suppression of renal net excretion. The correction is assumed to occur by the movement of potassium into and of hydrogen ion out of the cell, which titrates extracellular fluid bicarbonate.

Milk–alkali syndrome in which both bicarbonate and calcium are ingested produces alkalosis by vomiting, calcium-induced bicarbonate absorption and reduced GFR. Cationic antibiotics in high doses can cause alkalosis by obligatory bicarbonate loss in the urine.

Clinical features
The symptoms of metabolic alkalosis per se are difficult to separate from those of chloride, volume, or potassium depletion. Tetany (see p. 1063), apathy, confusion, drowsiness, cardiac arrhythmias and neuromuscular irritability are common when alkalosis is severe. The oxyhaemoglobin dissociation curve is shifted to the left. Respiration may be depressed.

Treatment
Chloride-responsive metabolic alkalosis. Although replacement of the chloride deficit is essential in chloride depletion states, selection of the accompanying cation – sodium, potassium or proton – is dependent on the assessment of extracellular fluid volume status (p. 677), the presence or absence of associated potassium depletion and degree and reversibility of any depression of GFR. If kidney function is normal, bicarbonate and base equivalents will be excreted with sodium or potassium and metabolic alkalosis will be rapidly corrected as chloride is made available.

If chloride and extracellular depletion coexist then isotonic saline solution is appropriate therapy.

In the clinical settings of fluid overload, saline is contraindicated. In such situations, intravenous use of hydrochloride acid or ammonium chloride can be considered. If GFR is adequate, the use of acetazolamide, which causes bicarbonate diuresis by inhibiting carbonic anhydrase, can also be considered. When the kidney is incapable of responding to chloride repletion, dialysis is necessary.

Chloride-resistant metabolic alkalosis. Metabolic alkalosis due to potassium depletion is managed by the correction of the underlying cause (see hypokalaemia). Mild to moderate alkalosis requires oral potassium chloride administration. However, the presence of cardiac arrhythmia or generalized weakness requires intravenous potassium chloride.

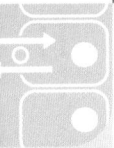

FURTHER READING

Adrogue HJ, Madias NE (1998) Management of life-threatening acid–base disorders. *New England Journal of Medicine* **338**: 26–34 and 107–111.

Atkinson DE, Bourke E (1987) Metabolic aspects of the regulation of systemic pH. *American Journal of Physiology* **252**: F947–F956.

Cameron et al. (eds) (1993) Water, electrolyte or acid–base disorders. In: *Oxford Textbook of Clinical Nephrology.* Oxford: Oxford University Press, pp. 867–917.

Schrier RW (eds) (1997) In *Renal and Electrolyte Disorders.* New York: Lippincott–Raven, pp. 1–240.

Case studies

Case 12.1

A 44-year-old patient with known chronic liver disease secondary to hepatitis B presented with marked exertional dyspnoea. Examination revealed: blood pressure 130/80, elevated JVP at 8 cm, bilateral pleural effusions, ascites and marked pitting pedal oedema. Investigations revealed: plasma sodium 136 mmol/L, potassium 3.6 mmol/L, bicarbonate 32 mmol/L, chloride 96 mmol/L, urinary sodium < 10 mmol/day, urinary potassium 60 mmol/day.

Question

(a) Explain the persistent retention of sodium in the face of salt and water overload?

Answer

(a) In cirrhosis, arterial vasodilatation due to nitric oxide overactivity leads to arterial underfilling. This is perceived by the pressure and volume receptors as hypovolaemia with consequent activation of the sympathetic system, nonosmotic release of ADH and activation of the renin–angiotensin–aldosterone system. These mediators lead to salt and water reduction (see Fig. 12.3a, p. 670).

Case 12.2

A 32-year-old patient was referred for investigation of refractory hypertension. His blood pressure was elevated at 210/110 with grade 3 hypertensive retinopathy despite taking beta-blockers, a calcium antagonist and an ACE

inhibitor. The rest of the examination was normal. Investigations revealed: sodium 148 mmol/L, potassium 3 mmol/L, bicarbonate 32 mmol/L, urea 4 mmol/L, glucose 4 mmol/L, urine dipstick negative for proteins.

Questions

(a) What is the likely diagnosis?

(b) What is the cause of absence of oedema in this patient?

Answers

(a) Conn's syndrome (p. 1065).

(b) This is due to the escape from the action of aldosterone. The escape is dependent on an increase in delivery of sodium to the site of aldosterone in the collecting duct. The increase in sodium delivery is achieved by high extracellular volume mediated arterial overfilling. This suppresses sympathetic activity and angiotensin II generation, and increases cardiac release of ANP with resultant increase in renal perfusion pressure and GFR. The net result of these events is reduced sodium absorption in the proximal tubules and increased sodium delivery, which overwhelms the sodium-retaining actions of aldosterone (see Fig. 12.3b, p. 670).

Case 12.3

A 62-year-old woman is found lying on the floor of her house. On examination she is bradycardic and peripherally shut down. ECG confirms sinus bradycardia with changes consistent with inferior myocardial infarction. Emergency electrolyte measurements revealed: sodium 136 mmol/L, potassium 4 mmol/L, bicarbonate 10 mmol/L, chloride 102 mmol/L, urea 7.5 mmol/L.

Question

(a) Comment on the biochemistry and how you will confirm your diagnosis?

Answer

(a) The biochemical picture is one of high-anionic-gap metabolic acidosis. In the presence of myocardial infarction and hypotension, the likely cause would be lactic acidosis. Measurement of plasma lactate (normally < 2 mmol/L) would confirm the diagnosis. Correction of the underlying cause will correct the acidosis by itself.

Case 12.4

The plasma biochemistry of a patient who presented with severe loin pain is as follows: sodium 138 mmol/L, potassium 2.5 mmol/L, urea 3.8 mmol/L, chloride 114 mmol/L, bicarbonate 14.5 mmol/L, urinary pH 6.5.

Questions
(a) What is the cause of this metabolic abnormality?
(b) What is the cause of the loin pain?

Answers
(a) Distal renal tubular acidosis (see the section on renal tubular acidosis).
(b) Nephrocalcinosis and renal colic due to renal stones are characteristic features of renal tubular acidosis.

Case 12.5

An 18-year-old boy was referred for the investigation of chronic fatigue syndrome. His mother comments that he is easily tired by sport and is not doing well at school. He is normotensive. Investigations revealed: sodium 145 mmol/L, potassium 2.8 mmol/L, bicarbonate 35 mmol/L, chloride 80 mmol/L, magnesium 0.6 mmol/L (normal range > 0.8 mmol/L), urea 5 mmol/L, glucose 5.2 mmol/L, urinary sodium excretion of 60 mmol and potassium excretion of 60 mmol/day.

Question
(a) What is the likely diagnosis?

Answer
(a) This patient has classic Gitelman's syndrome. It is similar to Bartter's but hypomagnesaemia favours Gitelman's syndrome.

Case 12.6

A 36-year-old woman with a past medical history of peptic ulceration presented with a history of 3 days of vomiting. She looked unwell and investigations revealed: haemoglobin 16.3 mmol/L, sodium 138 mmol/L, potassium 2.8 mmol/L, urea 14.3 mmol/L, pH 7.52, bicarbonate 36 mmol/L, chloride 75 mmol/L.

Questions
(a) What is the likely metabolic abnormality?
(b) What is the likely diagnosis?
(c) What is the pH of the patient's urine?

Answers
(a) This patient suffers from hypochloraemic metabolic alkalosis.
(b) The underlying cause is pyloric stenosis.
(c) The patient's urine is paradoxically acid, despite alkalosis.

Case 12.7

A 72-year-old man was admitted with a 3-week history of feeling unwell, poor appetite and diarrhoea. On examination, he was clearly dehydrated and had acidotic breathing. His blood pressure was 90/70; the postural drop to 60/30. He was frail. The rest of the general and system examination was unremarkable. The initial biochemistry revealed: sodium 121 mmol/L, potassium 1.9 mmol/L, chloride 83 mmol/L, bicarbonate 4 mmol/L, urea 90 mmol/L, creatinine 960 μmol/L, pH 7.1, P_{O_2} 15.7 kPa, P_{CO_2} 2.2 kPa, serum osmolality 334 mOsm/kg, urine osmolality 404 mOsm/kg, urinary sodium 2 mmol/L and potassium 28 mmol/L. He continued to pass between 50–80 mL of urine per hour.

Questions
(a) How would you describe the metabolic abnormality?
(b) What was the likely cause?
(c) Why did this patient remain polyuric in the face of severe dehydration?

Answers
(a) This patient suffers from volume depletion syndrome characterized by dehydration, hyperkalaemia, and hypochloraemic metabolic acidosis with high ionic gap. He has severe acute prerenal failure with normal urine output and dilute urine.
(b) The only single diagnosis which can explain this abnormality is secretory villous adenoma.
(c) His polyuria in the face of severe dehydration is due to nephrogenic diabetes insipidus secondary to chronic hypokalaemia. Hypokalaemia downregulates aquaporin II, which is essential for ADH-dependent water absorption from the collecting duct.

Cardiovascular disease

13

Essential anatomy, physiology and embryology of the heart

The cellular basis of myocardial contraction

Myocardial cells (myocytes) constitute about 75% of the heart mass but only about 25% of the cell number. Each cell, which is about 100 μm long, branches and interdigitates with adjacent cells. An intercalated disc permits electrical conduction to adjacent cells. Myocytes contain bundles of parallel myofibrils. Each myofibril is made up of a series of sarcomeres (Fig. 13.1). A sarcomere (which is the basic unit of contraction) is bound by two transverse Z lines, to each of which is attached a perpendicular filament of the protein actin. The actin filaments from each of the two Z bands overlap with thicker parallel protein filaments known as myosin. Actin and myosin filaments are attached to

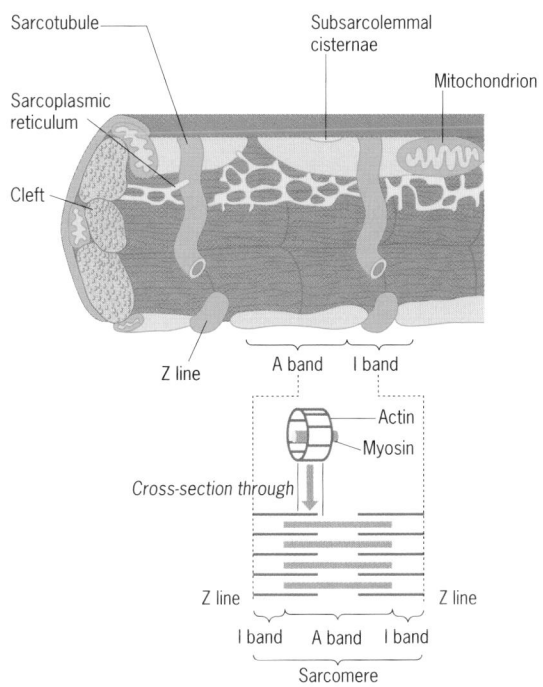

Fig. 13.1 **Schematic showing the structure of a myofibril within a myocyte.** The myofibrils are made up of a series of sarcomeres joined at the Z line.

each other by cross-bridges that contain ATPase, which breaks down adenosine triphosphate (ATP) to provide the energy for contraction. Two chains of actin molecules form a helical structure, with another molecule, tropomyosin in the grooves of the actin helix, and a further molecule, troponin, is attached to every seven actin molecules.

During cardiac contraction the length of the actin and myosin monofilaments does not change. Rather, the actin filaments slide between the myosin filaments when ATPase splits a high-energy bond of ATP. To supply the ATP, the myocyte (which cannot stop for a rest) has a very high mitochondrial density (35% of the cell volume). As calcium ions bind to troponin-C, the activity of troponin-I is inhibited, which induces a conformational change in tropomyosin. This event unlocks the active site between actin and myosin, enabling contraction to proceed. Calcium is made available during the plateau phase (phase 2) of the action potential (see Fig. 13.32, p. 736) by calcium ions entering the cell and by being mobilized from the sarcoplasmic reticulum. The force of cardiac muscle contraction ('inotropic state') is thus regulated by the influx of calcium ions into the cell through calcium channels (Fig. 13.2). T (transient) calcium channels open when the muscle is more depolarized, whereas L (long-lasting) calcium channels require less depolarization. The extent to which the sarcomere can shorten determines the stroke volume of the ventricle. It is maximally shortened in response to powerful inotropic drugs or severe exercise.

Starling's law of the heart

The contractile function of an isolated strip of cardiac tissue can be described by the relationship between the velocity of muscle contraction, the load that may be moved by the contracting muscle, and the extent to which the muscle is stretched before contracting. As with all other types of muscle, the velocity of contraction of myocardial tissue is reduced by increasing the load against which the tissue must contract. However, in the non-failing heart, prestretching of cardiac muscle improves the relationship between the force and velocity of contraction (Fig. 13.3).

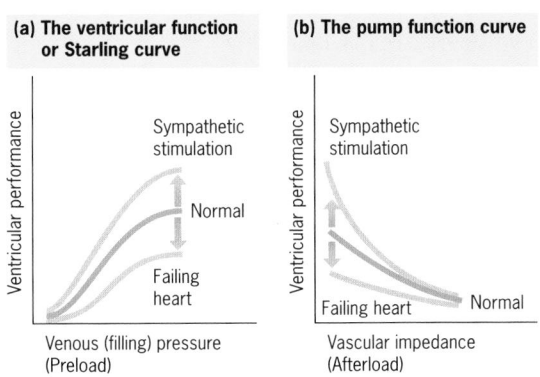

Fig. 13.3 **The Frank–Starling mechanism,** showing the effect on ventricular contraction of alteration in filling pressures and outflow impedance in the normal, failing and sympathetically stimulated ventricle.

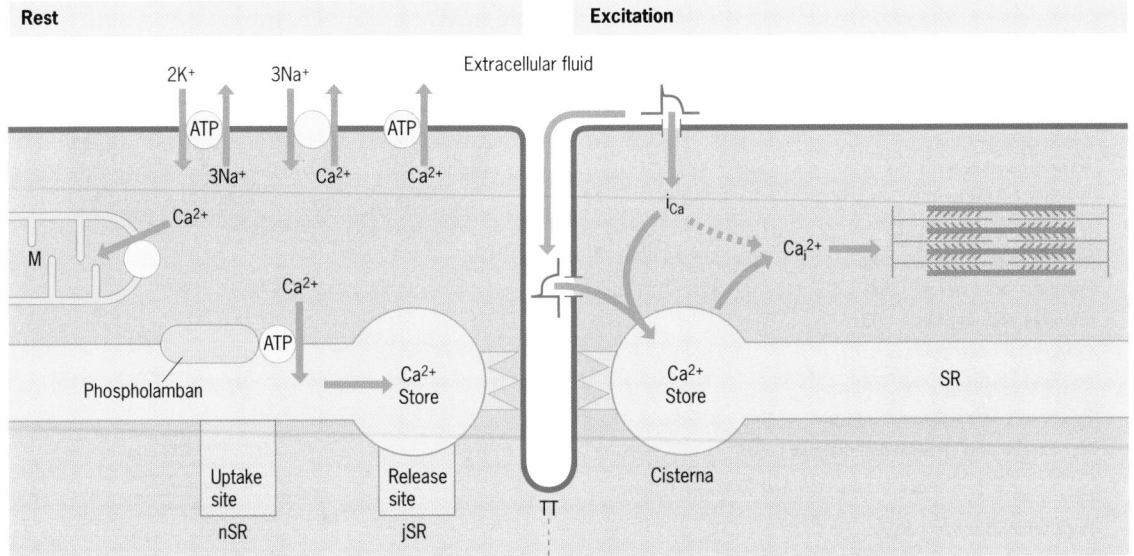

Fig. 13.2 **The calcium cycle.** *Right side – excitation.* Early plateau current i_{Ca} passes through L (long-lasting)-type, dihydropyridine-sensitive calcium channels in the surface and transverse tubule (TT) membrane. This Ca^{2+} activates nearby calcium-induced calcium-release channels, which form the 'feet' on the junctional sarcoplasmic reticulum (jSR). Release of stored Ca^{2+} follows. *Left side – rest.* Calcium pumps in network sarcoplasmic reticulum (nSR) restock the store, and are regulated by phospholamban. Na–Ca exchangers in the surface expel Ca^{2+}. Mitochondria (M) contribute to long-term buffering of intracellular Ca^{2+}. From Levick JR (2000) *Introduction to Cardiovascular Physiology*, 3rd edn by permission of Edward Arnold Limited.

This phenomenon was described in the intact heart as an increase of stroke volume (ventricular performance) with an enlargement of the diastolic volume (preload), and is known as 'Starling's law of the heart' or the 'Frank–Starling relationship'. It has been transcribed into more clinically relevant indices. Thus, stroke work (aortic pressure × stroke volume) is increased as ventricular end-diastolic volume is raised. Alternatively, within certain limits, cardiac output rises as pulmonary capillary wedge pressure increases. This clinical relationship is described by the ventricular function curve (Fig. 13.3), which also shows the effect of sympathetic stimulation.

The conduction system of the heart

Each natural heartbeat begins in the heart's pacemaker – the sinoatrial (SA) node. This is a crescent-shaped structure that is located around the medial and anterior aspect of the junction between the superior vena cava and the right atrium (Fig. 13.4). Progressive loss of the diastolic resting membrane potential is followed, when the threshold potential has been reached, by a more rapid depolarization of the sinus node tissue. This depolarization triggers depolarization of the atrial myocardium. The atrial tissue is activated like a 'forest fire', but the activation peters out when the insulating layer between the atrium and the ventricle – the annulus fibrosus – is reached. Controversy still exists about whether impulses from the SA node travel over specialized conducting 'pathways' or over ordinary atrial myocardium.

The depolarization continues to conduct slowly through the atrioventricular (AV) node. This is a small, bean-shaped structure that lies beneath the right atrial endocardium within the lower interatrial septum. The AV node continues as the His bundle, which penetrates the annulus fibrosus and conducts the cardiac impulse rapidly towards the ventricle. The His bundle reaches the crest of the interventricular septum and divides into the right bundle branch and the main left bundle branch.

The right bundle branch continues down the right side of the interventricular septum to the apex, from where it radiates and divides to form the Purkinje network, which spreads throughout the subendocardial surface of the right ventricle. The main left bundle branch is a short structure, which fans out into many strands on the left side of the interventricular septum. These strands can be grouped into an anterior superior division (the anterior hemibundle) and a posterior inferior division (the posterior hemibundle). The anterior hemibundle supplies the subendocardial Purkinje network of the anterior and superior surfaces of the left ventricle, and the inferior hemibundle supplies the inferior and posterior surfaces. Impulse conduction through the AV node is slow and depends on action potentials largely produced by slow transmembrane calcium flux. In the atria, ventricles and His–Purkinje system conduction is rapid and is due to action potentials generated by rapid transmembrane sodium diffusion.

Nerve supply of the cardiovascular system

Adrenergic nerves supply atrial and ventricular muscle fibres as well as the conduction system. β_1-Receptors predominate in the heart with both epinephrine (adrenaline) and norepinephrine (noradrenaline) having positive inotropic and chronotropic effects. β_2-Receptors predominate in the vascular smooth muscle and cause vasoconstriction. Cholinergic nerves from the vagus supply mainly the SA and AV nodes via M_2 muscarinic receptors. The ventricular myocardium is sparsely innervated by the vagus. Under basal conditions, vagal inhibitory effects predominate over the sympathetic excitatory effects, resulting in a slow heart rate.

β-Adrenergic stimulation and cellular signalling

β-Adrenergic stimulation enhances Ca^{2+} flux in the myocyte and thereby strengthens the force of contraction. Binding of catecholamines (e.g. norepinephrine (noradrenaline)) to the myocyte β_1-adrenergic receptor stimulates membrane-bound adenylate kinases. These enzymes enhance production of cyclic AMP that activates intracellular protein kinases, which in turn phosphorylate cellular proteins, including L-type calcium channels within the cell membrane. β-Adrenergic stimulation of the myocyte also enhances myocyte relaxation. The return of calcium from the cytosol to the sarcoplasmic reticulum (SR) is regulated by phospholamban (PL), a low-molecular-weight protein in the SR membrane. In its dephosphorylated state, PL inhibits Ca^{2+} uptake by the SR ATPase pump (Fig. 13.2). However, β_1-adrenergic activation of protein kinase phophorylates PL, and blunts its inhibitory effect. The subsequently greater uptake of calcium ions by the SR hastens Ca^{2+} removal from the cytosol and promotes myocyte relaxation. The increased cAMP activity also results in phosphorylation of troponin-I, an action that inhibits actin–myosin interaction, and further enhances myocyte relaxation. Production of SR proteins Ca^{2+} ATPase and phospholamban is also regulated by the thyroid hormone T_3 acting through changes in gene transcription.

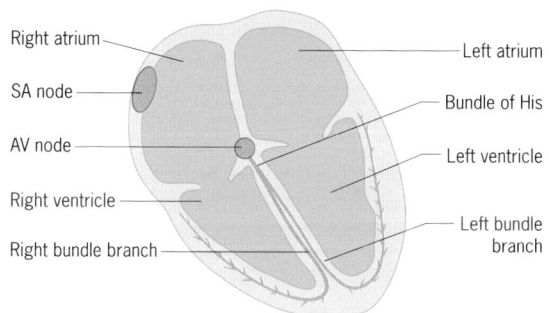

Fig. 13.4 **The normal cardiac conduction system.**
AV, atrioventricular; SA, sinoatrial.

(a)

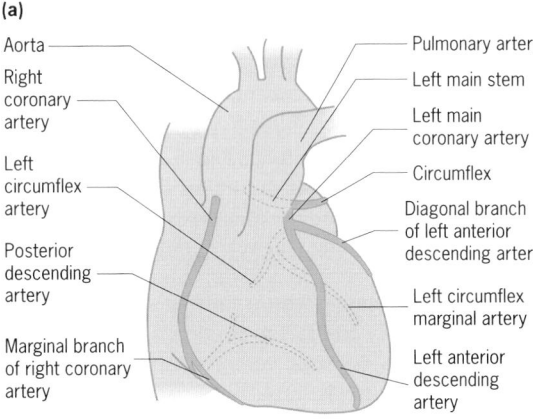

Aorta

Right coronary artery

Left circumflex artery

Posterior descending artery

Marginal branch of right coronary artery

Pulmonary artery

Left main stem

Left main coronary artery

Circumflex

Diagonal branch of left anterior descending artery

Left circumflex marginal artery

Left anterior descending artery

(b)

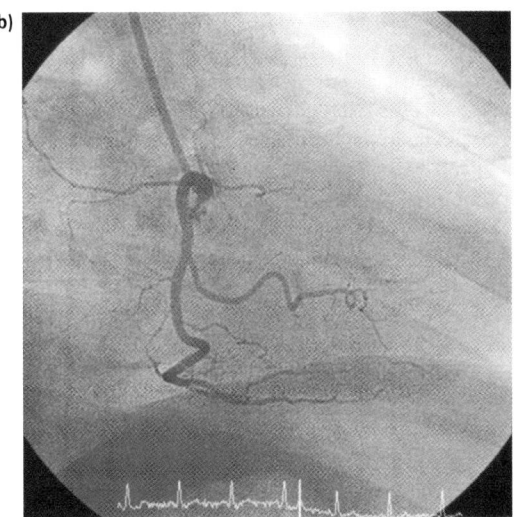

(c)

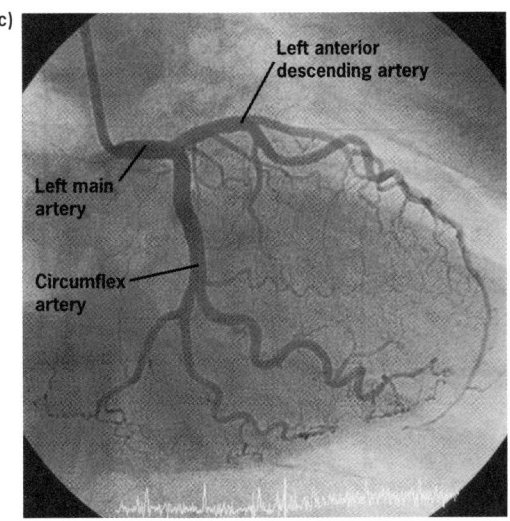

Left anterior descending artery

Left main artery

Circumflex artery

Fig. 13.5 (a) Diagram of the normal coronary arterial anatomy. (b) Angiogram of non-dominant right coronary system. (c) Angiogram of dominant left coronary system from the same patient. Right anterior oblique projection.

MAP kinases (p. 157)

The mitogen-activated protein (MAP) kinases are a family of serine–threonine kinases involved in numerous types of intracellular signalling. Mammalian MAP kinases can be divided into three families according to their structure and function:

(1) the extracellular signal-regulated kinases (ERK-1 and 2) are related to promotion of cell growth in response to growth factor receptor activation;

(2) the c-Jun N-terminal kinase/stress-activated protein kinases (JNK/SAPK), whose activation is associated with arrest of cell growth and apoptosis; and

(3) the p38 kinase, activation of which is associated with apoptosis in a variety of cell systems and may be related to JNK/SAPK activation.

The coronary circulation

The coronary arterial system (Fig. 13.5) consists of the right and left coronary arteries. These arteries branch from the aorta, arising immediately above two cusps of the aortic valve. These arteries are unique in that they fill during diastole, when not occluded by valve cusps and when not squeezed by myocardial contraction. The right coronary artery arises from the right coronary sinus and courses through the right side of the atrioventricular groove, giving off vessels that supply the right atrium and the right ventricle. The vessel usually continues as the posterior descending coronary artery, which runs in the posterior interventricular groove and supplies the posterior part of the interventricular septum and the posterior left ventricular wall.

Within 2.5 cm of its origin from the left coronary sinus, the left main coronary divides into the left anterior descending artery and the circumflex artery. The left anterior descending artery runs in the anterior interventricular groove and supplies the anterior septum and the anterior left ventricular wall. The left circumflex artery travels along the left atrioventricular groove and gives off branches to the left atrium and the left ventricle (marginal branches).

The sinus node and the AV node are supplied by the right coronary artery in about 60% and 90% of people, respectively. Therefore, disease in this artery may cause sinus bradycardia and AV nodal block. The majority of the left ventricle is supplied by the left coronary artery, so that stenosis in the left main artery is extremely dangerous; total obstruction of this vessel is rarely compatible with life.

Some blood from the capillary beds in the wall of the heart drains directly into the cavities of the heart by tiny veins, but the majority returns by veins which accompany the arteries, to empty into the right atrium via the coronary sinus.

An extensive lymphatic system drains into vessels that travel along the coronary vessels and then into the thoracic duct.

Functions of the vascular endothelium

The vascular endothelium is a cardiovascular endocrine organ, which occupies a strategic interface between blood and other tissues, and has many regulatory roles:

- modulation of immunoresponses
- regulation of vascular cell growth
- vasomotor control
- pro- and antithrombotic mechanisms.

Enzymes located on the endothelial surface control the level of circulating compounds, such as bradykinin, serotonin, angiotensin and adenine nucleotides. In addition, the endothelium releases substances which affect vascular tone and platelet function. Many endothelium-derived substances have been characterized and play a major role in the physiological control of the coronary circulation through the production of endothelium-derived relaxing and contracting factors. The most potent of these factors are nitric oxide (NO), prosta-cyclin (PGI_2) and endothelin.

NO is a rapidly diffusible gas with a half-life of only a few seconds; it is formed in endothelial cells from the amino acid L-arginine via the action of the enzyme NO synthase (NOS), which is controlled by cytoplasmic calcium/calmodulin (see Fig. 15.10). NO has immuno-logical and inflammatory functions and has a trans-mitter function in 'nitrergic' nerves in the central and peripheral nervous systems. Its cardiovascular effects protect against atherosclerosis, thrombosis and heart failure as well as contributing to the physiological control of blood pressure.

Nitric oxide release is triggered by shear stress (flow) and by several agonists. These include vasoconstrictors, e.g. endothelin I, angiotensin II, and drugs with mixed action, e.g. serotonin and α_2-agonists as well as rela-tively 'pure' endothelium-dependent vasodilators, e.g. acetylcholine, β_2-agonists, bradykinin and substance P. NO relaxes vascular smooth muscle and inhibits platelet function through activation of soluble guanylate cyclase, leading to an increase in the intracellular levels of cyclic 3,5-guanosine monophosphate. The potent vasomotor and antiplatelet properties of NO indicate a functional role of the endothelium in maintenance of adequate organ blood flow.

Endothelium-dependent coronary vasodilatation can be improved by a variety of interventions, including the use of agents such as angiotensin-converting enzyme inhibitors, β-hydroxymethylglutaryl-coenzyme A reduc-tase inhibitors (statins) and antioxidants. Among the non-pharmacological therapeutic options for patients with coronary artery disease, regular physical exercise improves endothelium-dependent vasodilatation both in epicardial and resistance vessels. The mechanism responsible for these effects suggest that endothelial cells respond to short-term increases in shear stress by producing vasodilator compounds such as prostacyclin and NO. The sustained increases in shear stress (regular physical exercise) elicit an adaptive response in endo-thelial cells that is manifested, in part, by increased expression of the enzyme that catalyses NO production. Alteration in sympathetic and parasympathetic cardiac control has been proven as a strong and independent predictor of cardiac death or ventricular arrhythmia in patients with cardiac disease. Recent evidence suggests that NO may act as a mediator in this pathway.

The normal endothelium is a non-thrombogenic sur-face, which under physiological circumstances does not react with platelets or blood constituents. NO inhibits platelet aggregation, adhesion and secretion. Several other factors contribute to the anti-aggregatory activity of the endothelium. Endothelial cells offer a negatively charged surface that repels the negatively charged platelets. Prostacyclin (PGI_2) is formed by the endothe-lial lining of blood vessels. It inhibits platelet aggrega-tion and formation of platelet-derived growth factors. In addition to their inhibitory effects on platelet function, prostacyclin and NO act together to antagonize pro-coagulant factors such as thrombin and thromboxane A_2.

Endothelin is a 21-amino-acid peptide, the secretion of which is stimulated by angiotensin II, vasopressin, and thrombin, and inhibited by increased shear stress. Endothelin promotes vasconstriction and hypertrophy of vascular smooth muscle, counteracting the effects of NO and PGI_2. An imbalance between these opposing forces is an early feature of hypertension and atheroma, where increased production of endothelin and reduced secretion of NO may contribute to the increased vascu-lar tone.

Other endothelium-derived compounds are also spe-cific antagonists to the procoagulant activity of thrombin. Endothelial cells generate specific thrombin inhibitors that remove thrombin from the circulation. Examples of these are thrombomodulin, a surface receptor, and heparin sulphate, a glycosaminoglycan, which activates antithrombin. Endothelium also modulates fibrinolysis by generation of fibrinolytic components.

The fetal circulation

In utero, the pulmonary circulation is largely unneces-sary because fetal blood is oxygenated by placental blood flow, a parallel and integral element in the sys-temic circulation. In the fetus, systemic venous blood returning to the right atrium is partly deflected through the foramen ovale to the left atrium. Blood that passes through the right ventricle is diverted from the pul-monary artery to the aorta through the ductus arteriosus. Thus, the systemic venous return, which is a mixture of oxygenated and deoxygenated blood, is mostly returned to the systemic arterial system.

At birth, inspiration dilates the pulmonary arterioles, resulting in a dramatic reduction of pulmonary vascular resistance. Blood therefore flows through the pul-monary circulation. The increased oxygen tension and reduced levels of prostaglandins trigger closure of the

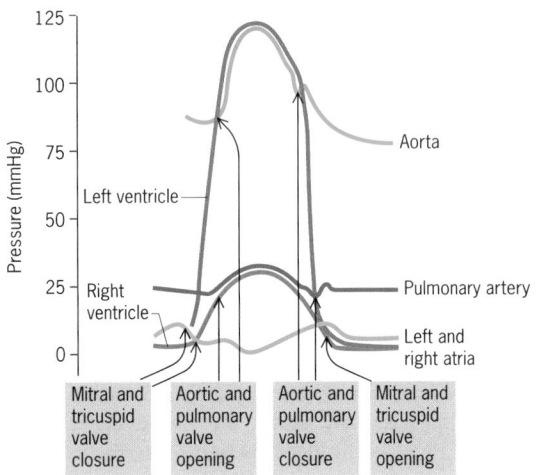

Fig. 13.6 **The cardiac cycle.**

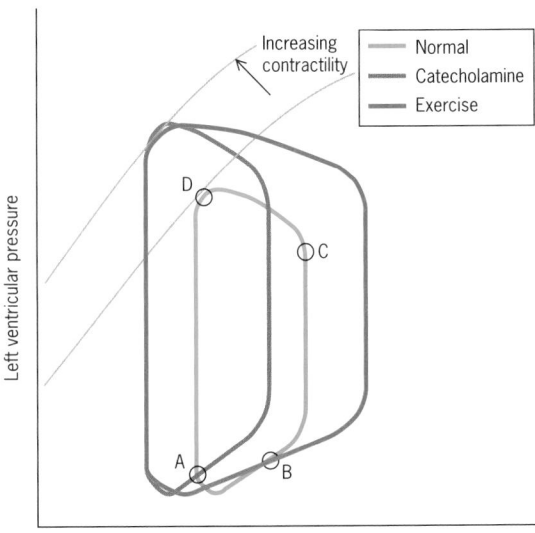

Fig. 13.7 **Pressure–volume loop.** AB, diastole-ventricular filling; BC, systole-isovolumetric ventricular contraction; CD, systole-ventricular emptying; DA, diastole-isovolumetric ventricular relaxation.

ductus arteriosus, and the reduced right atrial pressure and increasing left atrial pressure tend to close the foramen ovale. Thus, the circulation is divided into two separate circuits connected in series.

In the fetus the left and right heart both propel blood from the systemic veins to the systemic arteries; thus, severe abnormalities of the heart may not compromise fetal blood flow.

The cardiac cycle (Fig. 13.6)

The cardiac cycle consists of precisely timed rhythmic electrical and mechanical events that propel blood into the systemic and pulmonary circulations. The first event in the cardiac cycle is atrial depolarization (a P wave on the surface ECG) followed by right atrial and then left atrial contraction. Ventricular activation (the QRS complex on the ECG) follows after a short interval (the PR interval). Left ventricular contraction starts and shortly thereafter right ventricular contraction begins. The increased ventricular pressures exceed the atrial pressures, and close first the mitral and then the tricuspid valves. Until the aortic and pulmonary valves open, the ventricles contract with no change of volume (isovolumetric contraction). When ventricular pressures rise above the aortic and pulmonary artery pressures, the pulmonary valve and then the aortic valve open and ventricular ejection occurs. As the ventricles begin to relax, their pressures fall below the aortic and pulmonary arterial pressures, and aortic valve closure is followed by pulmonary valve closure. Isovolumetric relaxation then occurs. After the ventricular pressures have fallen below the right atrial and left atrial pressures, the tricuspid and mitral valves open.

The cardiac cycle can be graphically depicted as the relationship between the pressure and volume of the ventricle. This is shown in Figure 13.7, which illustrates the changing pressure–volume relationships in response to increased contractility and to exercise.

FURTHER READING

Chowdhary S, Townend JN (1999). Role of nitric oxide in the regulation of cardiovascular autonomic control. *Clinical Science* **97**: 5–17.

Hambrecht R et al. (2000). Effect of exercise on coronary endothelial function in patients with coronary artery disease. *New England Journal of Medicine* **342**: 454–460.

Klein I, Ojamaa K (2001) Thyroid hormone and the cardiovascular system. *New England Journal of Medicine* **344**: 501–509.

Levick JR (2000) *An Introduction to Cardiovascular Physiology*, 3rd edn. London: Arnold.

Vita JA, Keaney JK (2000) Exercise – toning up the endothelium? *New England Journal of Medicine* **342**: 503–505.

Xia Z et al. (1995) Opposing effects of ERK and JNK-p38 MAP kinases on apoptosis. *Science* 270: 1326–1331.

Symptoms of heart disease

Even severe heart disease may be asymptomatic. However, symptoms often include the following:

Dyspnoea

Dyspnoea is an abnormal awareness of breathlessness, and can be due to cardiac or respiratory causes. It occurs on exertion or may be present at rest. The New York Heart Association has graded this symptom (Table 13.1), but this classification, although often used, has been discontinued and is replaced by a very similar grading known as 'cardiac status' (Table 13.2).

Table 13.1
The New York Heart Association functional and therapeutic classification applied to dyspnoea

Grade 1   No breathlessness
Grade 2   Breathlessness on severe exertion
Grade 3   Breathlessness on mild exertion
Grade 4   Breathlessness at rest

Table 13.2
The New York Heart Association grading of 'cardiac status'

Grade 1   Uncompromised
Grade 2   Slightly compromised
Grade 3   Moderately compromised
Grade 4   Severely compromised

It is also clinically valuable to grade dyspnoea by the amount of physical exertion possible before breathlessness occurs – for example, climbing 14 stairs or walking 200 yards on the flat.

Left ventricular failure causes dyspnoea because of a rise of pressure in the left atrium and pulmonary capillaries leading to interstitial and alveolar oedema. This makes the lungs stiff (less compliant), which increases the amount of respiratory effort necessary to breathe. Usually a fast breathing rate (tachypnoea) is also present owing to stimulation of the pulmonary stretch receptors.

Dyspnoea on effort usually precedes other forms of breathlessness, such as orthopnoea or nocturnal dyspnoea. *Orthopnoea* is a form of breathlessness that occurs when the patient lies flat, and occurs because lying flat results in redistribution of blood, leading to an increased central and pulmonary blood volume. Recumbency also causes the abdominal contents to press up against the diaphragm. Both factors increase the difficulty of breathing. Patients usually cope with orthopnoea by propping themselves up with pillows.

Paroxysmal nocturnal dyspnoea (PND) occurs when there is an accumulation of fluid in the lungs (pulmonary oedema) at night. The mechanism is similar to orthopnoea, but because sensory awareness is depressed during sleep, severe interstitial and alveolar oedema can accumulate (see p. 764). The patient is woken from sleep fighting for breath, a dramatic and frightening experience. Sitting on the side of the bed or getting up may relieve the breathlessness. Sometimes the patient will get up and open a window to gasp for fresh air. Wheezing, due to bronchial endothelial oedema, is common (cardiac asthma), and a cough, often productive of frothy or blood-tinged sputum, usually occurs. Initially these episodes terminate spontaneously. Episodes of 'PND', often with coughing, can occur in asthma, but conventionally the term is reserved for cardiac problems.

Cheyne–Stokes respiration   (see also p. 1161)

In very severe heart failure, alternate hyperventilation and apnoea known as Cheyne–Stokes respiration may occur. This may also develop in the elderly without obvious heart failure. It is related to depression of the respiratory centre, as a consequence of poor cardiac output and cerebrovascular disease. This type of respiration is also seen after morphine administration.

Chest pain

Pain in the chest is the most common symptom associated with ischaemic heart disease.

Angina pectoris

Angina pectoris literally means a strangling sensation (angina) in the chest (pectoris). It is a gripping or crushing central chest pain (or discomfort) that may be felt around the whole chest or deep within the chest. The pain may radiate into the neck or jaw and, rarely, into the teeth, back or abdomen. It is associated with heaviness, paraesthesia or pain in one (usually the left) or both arms. It is typically provoked by exercise and is promptly relieved by rest. Angina of increasing frequency, or coming on at rest or unpredictably is called unstable (or crescendo) angina. A pain of similar distribution and type also occurs at rest in myocardial infarction (see p. 774). The mechanism of the pain is myocardial hypoxia secondary to inadequate coronary blood flow. Sharp pains over the heart are not usually angina.

Other causes of chest pain

The pain of pericarditis is felt in the centre of the chest and, like that of pleurisy, is aggravated by movement, posture, respiration and coughing, but may be relieved by sitting forwards. It is sharp and severe.

Central chest pain that radiates to the back is characteristic of a dissecting or enlarging aortic aneurysm (see p. 830) and can mimic the pain of myocardial infarction. A dissection must be excluded since the administration of a thrombolytic agent in this circumstance is catastrophic.

Left, submammary stabbing pain – known as 'precordial catch' – is usually associated with anxiety and is sometimes known as effort (Da Costa's) syndrome. Occasionally, cardiac conditions such as mitral valve prolapse cause similar pain. Central chest pain similar to angina can occur with oesophageal disease and can be difficult to differentiate (see p. 264). Other causes of chest pain are pulmonary embolism, pulmonary hypertension, costochondritis, pleurisy, pneumothorax and mediastinitis.

Palpitations

A palpitation is an increased awareness of the normal heartbeat or the sensation of slow or rapid heart rate or an irregular heart rhythm. The normal heartbeat is

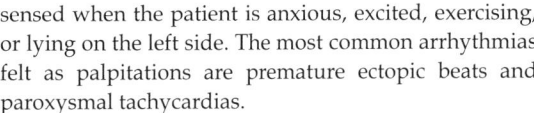

sensed when the patient is anxious, excited, exercising, or lying on the left side. The most common arrhythmias felt as palpitations are premature ectopic beats and paroxysmal tachycardias.

Premature beats

These are usually felt as 'missed beats' because the premature beat is followed by a pause before the next normal beat, which is rather forceful because of the longer diastolic filling period. Premature beats often occur in clusters and may cause the patient much anxiety.

Paroxysmal tachycardias

These start abruptly and may terminate equally suddenly. Often, however, the tachycardia slows before terminating and therefore seems to fade away. Paroxysmal atrial fibrillation is noticeably irregular, whereas other forms of paroxysmal supraventricular or ventricular tachycardia are regular. Paroxysms of rapid tachycardia, especially when prolonged, may be associated with syncope, presyncope, dyspnoea or chest pain. Palpitations can be graded in a similar way to the grading of dyspnoea or angina. Supraventricular tachycardias, such as atrial fibrillation or junctional tachycardias, may produce polyuria.

Some patients experience tachycardia on standing, associated with a mild drop in blood pressure and symptoms of dizziness or near syncope. These patients have a form of autonomic dysfunction termed the *postural orthostatic tachycardia syndrome* (POTS).

Bradycardias

An unduly slow heart rate may be appreciated as slow, regular, 'heavy' or forceful beats. Most often bradycardias are not felt as palpitations.

Syncope

Syncope can be due to many causes (see p. 1180), the most common of which is situational or vasovagal syncope. These attacks may be provoked by fright, anxiety, phobias or other situations such as micturition or coughing. The basic mechanism is vasodilatation leading to venous pooling followed by emptying of the heart. Vigorous contraction of the near-empty heart stimulates mechanoreceptors in the inferoposterior wall of the left ventricle. Consequent reflexes via the central nervous system lead to further vasodilatation and sometimes profound bradycardia. This is also known as 'neuro-cardiogenic' syncope (empty heart syndrome). Recent evidence also suggests that genetic or acquired deficits in norepinephrine (noradrenaline) inactivation (norepinephrine-transporter deficiency) may underlie hyper-adreneric states that lead to orthostatic intolerance. The episodes are usually associated with a prodome that consists of dizziness, nausea, sweating, ringing in the ears, a sinking feeling and yawning. Recovery occurs within a few seconds, particularly if the patient lies down.

Cardiovascular syncope is usually sudden and brief. The classical variety is known as a Stokes–Adams attack and is due to a disturbance of cardiac rhythm (e.g. a profound bradycardia related to complete heart block). Without warning, the patient falls to the ground, pale and deeply unconscious. The pulse is usually very slow or absent. After a few seconds the patient flushes brightly and recovers consciousness as the pulse quickens. If the period of unconsciousness is prolonged the patient may suffer a generalized convulsion but this is not usual. Often there are no sequelae, but patients may injure themselves during falls.

Postural hypotension is common in the elderly. There is inadequate reflex vasoconstriction on standing from the lying or sitting position, with a resultant pronounced blood pressure drop and reduced cerebral perfusion, which may cause the patient to collapse to the ground. There is no specific treatment, but vasodilating drugs (e.g. for hypertension or angina) should be avoided.

Carotid sinus syncope is an uncommon cause of syncope. It occurs when there is an exaggerated vagal response to stimulation of the carotid sinus. The resulting vasodilatation and bradycardia lead to dizziness and syncope.

Other causes of syncope due to heart disease can be grouped as cardiac arrhythmias or obstructive cardiac or vascular disease (Table 13.3).

Oedema

Heart failure results in salt and water retention. Retained fluid accumulates in the feet and ankles of ambulant patients and over the sacrum of bed-bound patients. The oedema associated with heart failure becomes progressively worse during the day and is often absent on initial rising as the fluid is reabsorbed on lying down. When severe, the calf and thigh may become oedematous and ascites or pleural effusion may develop.

Table 13.3
Cardiac causes of syncope

Arrhythmias
Ventricular tachycardia
Rapid supraventricular tachycardia
Sinus arrest
Atrioventricular block
Artificial pacemaker failure

Obstruction
Aortic/pulmonary stenosis
Hypertrophic obstructive cardiomyopathy
Fallot's tetralogy
Pulmonary hypertension/embolism
Atrial myxoma
Atrial thrombus
Defective prosthetic valve

Situational
Neurocardiogenic (vasovagal)
Postural hypotension

Systemic symptoms

Fatigue is a feature of heart failure, persistent cardiac arrhythmias and cyanotic heart disease. It is due to poor cerebral and peripheral perfusion and poor oxygenation. When severe cardiac disorders are not present, an active infection such as infective endocarditis may be responsible. However, disorders of most systems may produce this non-specific symptom. Drugs prescribed for angina or hypertension, particularly beta-blockers, may cause fatigue.

Weight loss and anorexia, which are features of chronic cardiac conditions such as heart failure, give rise to cardiac cachexia. Congestive cardiac failure can also cause abdominal symptoms such as nausea, vomiting and dyspepsia, due to engorgement of the visceral organs.

Examination of the cardiovascular system

Examination of the cardiovascular system is often waived in favour of awaiting results from further investigations, such as echocardiography. This is bad practice; confirmation of physical findings with the results of technical investigations helps to improve diagnostic skills.

General examination

General features of the patient's well-being should be noted as well as the presence of conjunctival pallor, obesity, jaundice and cachexia.

Clubbing (see also p. 845)

The most common cardiac cause of clubbing is congenital cyanotic heart disease, particularly Fallot's tetralogy. The incidence of subacute infective endocarditis and consequently clubbing due to this cause is now low, possibly reflecting improvements in diagnosis and treatment. Clubbing takes months to develop and is not seen in acute endocarditis or in neonates or infants with cyanotic heart disease. Clubbing in cor pulmonale is due to the underlying pulmonary disease (e.g. bronchiectasis or fibrosing alveolitis).

Splinter haemorrhages

These small, subungual linear haemorrhages are frequently due to trauma, but are also seen in infective endocarditis.

Cyanosis

This is a dusky blue discoloration of the skin (particularly at the extremities) or of the mucous membranes when the capillary oxygen saturation is less than 85%.

Central cyanosis is seen in the tongue and lips, and is due to desaturation of central arterial blood. This occurs in cardiac and respiratory disorders associated with shunting of deoxygenated venous blood into the systemic circulation, as in the presence of a right-to-left heart shunt.

Peripheral cyanosis is seen in the hands and feet, which are cold. A patient who is centrally cyanosed will also be peripherally cyanosed but isolated peripheral cyanosis occurs in conditions associated with peripheral vasoconstriction and stasis of blood in the extremities leading to increased peripheral oxygen extraction. Such conditions include congestive heart failure, circulatory shock, exposure to cold temperatures and abnormalities of the peripheral circulation.

The arterial pulse

A pulse is felt by compressing an artery against a bone. The first pulse to be examined is the right radial pulse. The timings of the left radial and femoral pulses are then compared with that of the right radial pulse. Delayed femoral pulsation occurs because of a proximal stenosis, particularly of the aorta (coarctation).

Pulse rate

The pulse rate should be between 60 and 80 beats per minute (b.p.m.) when an adult patient is lying quietly in bed. Young children may have higher pulse rates and athletes and elderly adults may have slower rates. The exact rate is often less important than the changes in heart rate observed over time (seen on a pulse chart). When the pulse is irregular, not all ventricular systolic beats may be detected by palpation of the radial pulse. Such apex–radial pulse deficits may be appreciated by counting the radial pulse whilst simultaneously listening to the heart beat with a stethoscope, and are commonly associated with atrial fibrillation and ventricular ectopy.

Rhythm

In normal subjects the pulse is regular except for a slight quickening in early inspiration and a slowing in expiration (sinus arrhythmia). Irregularities of the pulse rhythm are usually due to premature beats, intermittent heart block or atrial fibrillation.

Premature beats occur as occasional or repeated irregularities superimposed on a regular pulse rhythm. Similarly, intermittent heart block is revealed by occasional beats dropped from an otherwise regular rhythm. A more irregular pattern (irregularly irregular) of heart beats in which no pattern is recognizable occurs in atrial fibrillation. This irregular pattern persists when the pulse quickens in response to exercise, in contrast to pulse irregularity due to ectopic beats, which usually disappears on exercise. However, this is not a reliable way to distinguish ectopic beats from other causes of pulse irregularity.

Carotid pulse

Carotid pulsations are not normally apparent on inspection of the neck but may be visible (Corrigan's sign) in conditions associated with a large-volume pulse, including high output states (such as thyrotoxicosis, anaemia or fever) and in aortic regurgitation. The carotid pulse may also be visible when the carotid artery is aneurysmal or kinked. The amplitude and shape of the carotid pulse is normally examined by palpation of the right carotid artery. Light palpation should be used to detect the presence of a thrill.

A large-volume pulse may also be associated with the large stroke volume that is necessary if bradycardia is present. A 'collapsing' or 'waterhammer' pulse is a large volume pulse characterized by a short duration with a brisk rise and fall. This is best appreciated by palpating the axillary artery with the palmar aspect of four fingers whilst elevating the patients arm above the level of the heart. A collapsing pulse is characteristic of aortic valvular regurgitation or a persistent ductus arteriosus.

A small-volume pulse is seen in cardiac failure, shock and obstructive valvular or vascular disease. It may also be present during tachyarrhythmias. The pulse of aortic stenosis is not only small in volume but is slow in rising to a peak (plateau pulse) and is often associated with a notch on the upstroke (anacrotic pulse) or a systolic shudder or thrill (Fig. 13.8).

Other changes in arterial pulse

Paradoxical pulse (pulsus paradoxus)

Paradoxical pulse is a misnomer as it is actually an exaggeration of the normal pattern (Fig. 13.8). In normal subjects, the systolic pressure and the pulse pressure (the difference between the systolic and diastolic blood pressures) fall during inspiration. The normal fall of systolic pressure is less than 10 mmHg and this can be measured using a sphygmomanometer. It is due to increased pulmonary intravascular volume during inspiration. In severe airflow limitation (especially severe asthma) there is an increased negative intrathoracic pressure on inspiration which enhances the normal fall in blood pressure. In patients with cardiac tamponade, the fluid in the pericardium increases the intrapericardial pressure, thereby impeding diastolic filling of the heart. The normal inspiratory increase in venous return to the right ventricle is at the expense of the left ventricle, as both ventricles are confined by the accumulated pericardial fluid within the pericardial space. Paradox can occur through a similar mechanism in constrictive pericarditis but is less common.

Alternating pulse (pulsus alternans)

This is characterized by regular alternate beats that are weak and strong. It is a feature of severe myocardial failure and is due to the prolonged recovery time of damaged myocardium; it indicates a very poor prognosis. It is easily noticed when taking the blood pressure because the systolic pressure may vary from beat to beat by as much as 50 mmHg. Pulsus alternans may also occur when there is rapid, abnormal tachycardia. In this case it acts as a compensatory mechanism and does not indicate a poor prognosis. Pulsus alternans should be distinguished from a bigeminal pulse (see below).

Bigeminal pulse (pulsus bigeminus)

This is due to a premature ectopic beat following every sinus beat. The rhythm is not regular (Fig. 13.8) because every weak pulse is premature.

Pulsus bisferiens

This is a pulse that is found in hypertrophic obstructive cardiomyopathy and in mixed aortic valve disease (regurgitation combined with stenosis). The first systolic wave is the 'percussion' wave produced by the transmission of the left ventricular pressure in early systole. The second peak is the 'tidal' wave caused by recoil of the vascular bed. This normally happens in diastole (the dicrotic wave), but when the left ventricle empties slowly or is obstructed from emptying completely, the tidal wave occurs in late systole. The result is a palpable double pulse.

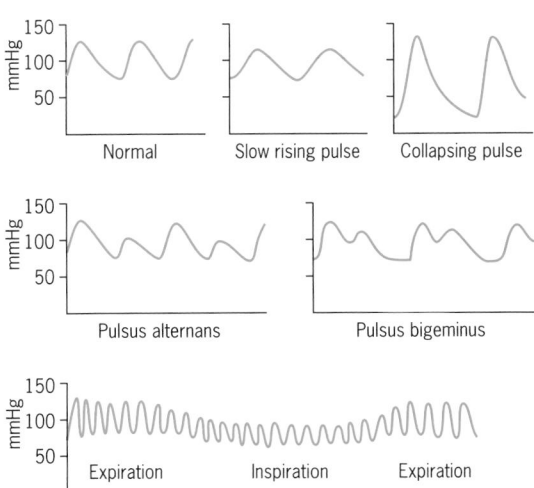

Fig. 13.8 **Various arterial waveforms.**

Blood pressure (Practical box 13.1)

The peak systemic arterial blood pressure is produced by transmission of left ventricular systolic pressure. Vascular tone and an intact aortic valve maintain the diastolic blood pressure. The normal blood pressure is discussed on page 818.

Practical box 13.1

Taking the blood pressure

1. The blood pressure is taken in the (right) arm with the patient relaxed and comfortable.

2. The sphygmomanometer cuff is wrapped around the upper arm with the inflation bag placed over the brachial artery.

3. The cuff is inflated until the pressure exceeds the arterial pressure – when the radial pulse is no longer palpable.

4. The diaphragm of the stethoscope is positioned over the brachial artery just below the cuff.

5. The cuff pressure is slowly reduced until sounds (Korotkoff sounds) can be heard (phase 1). This is the **systolic pressure**.

6. The pressure is allowed to fall further until the Korotkoff sounds become suddenly muffled (phase 4).

7. The pressure is allowed to fall still further-until they disappear (phase 5).

The **diastolic pressure** is usually taken as phase 5 because this phase is more reproducible and nearer to the intravascular diastolic pressure. The Korotkoff sounds may disappear (phase 2) and reappear (phase 3) between the systolic and diastolic pressures. Do not mistake phase 2 for the diastolic pressure or phase 3 for the systolic pressure.

Variations in blood pressure

The systolic blood pressure varies by up to 10 mmHg between the right and left brachial arteries. Standing usually causes a slight reduction of the systolic pressure (< 20 mmHg) and an increase in the diastolic blood pressure (< 10 mmHg). In postural (orthostatic) hypotension, a large postural fall of both the systolic and diastolic pressures is associated with dizziness. When an irregular heart rhythm such as atrial fibrillation is present, the blood pressure is variable. Because the blood pressure is normally liable to variation, it must be estimated on several occasions before it can be declared elevated.

Jugular venous pulse

There are no valves between the internal jugular vein and the right atrium. Observation of the column of blood in the internal jugular system is therefore a good measure of right atrial pressure. The external jugular cannot be relied upon because of its valves and because it may be obstructed by the fascial and muscular layers through which it passes; it can only be used if typical venous pulsation is seen, indicating no obstruction to flow.

Measurement of jugular venous pressure (JVP)

1. The patient is positioned at about 45° to the horizontal (between 30° and 60°), wherever the top of the venous pulsation can be seen in a good light.

2. The jugular venous pressure is measured as the vertical distance between the manubriosternal angle and the top of the venous column.

3. The normal jugular venous pressure is usually less than 3 cmH$_2$O, which is equivalent to a right atrial pressure of 8 cmH$_2$O when measured with reference to a point midway between the anterior and posterior surfaces of the chest. The venous pulsations are not usually palpable (except for the forceful venous distension associated with tricuspid regurgitation).

Hepatojugular reflux. Abdominal compression causes a temporary increase in central and hence jugular venous pressure. It is a simple way of confirming the venous nature of a pulsation in the neck.

An abnormally low jugular venous pressure cannot be measured clinically. Causes include haemorrhage and other forms of hypovolaemia.

Elevation of the jugular venous pressure occurs in heart failure. It is also produced by:

- constrictive pericarditis
- cardiac tamponade
- renal disease with salt and water retention
- overtransfusion or excessive infusion of fluids
- superior vena caval obstruction (but in this case pulsation is absent).

In constrictive pericarditis or cardiac tamponade, ventricular filling is reduced during inspiration because the ventricles are squeezed by the pericardial fluid or non-compliant pericardium, which tightens as the diaphragm descends. Thus, the level of venous pressure increases during inspiration (Kussmaul's sign). Other causes of an increased jugular pressure also distort the shape of the pressure wave and are considered below.

The jugular venous pressure wave

This consists of three peaks and two troughs (Fig. 13.9). The peaks are described as *a, c* and *v* waves and the troughs are known as *x* and *y* descents:

- The *a* **wave** is produced by atrial systole.
- The *x* **descent** occurs when the atrial contraction finishes.
- As the pressure falls there is a small transient increase that produces a positive deflection called the *c* **wave**. This is caused by transmission of the rapidly increasing right ventricular pressure before the tricuspid valve closes.
- The *v* **wave** develops as the venous return fills the right atrium during continued ventricular systole.
- The *y* **descent** follows the *v* wave when the tricuspid valve opens.

The *a* wave can be distinguished from the *v* wave by observing the venous pulse while palpating the carotid artery. The *a* wave occurs immediately before carotid pulsation and the *v* wave occurs simultaneously with carotid pulsation.

The main abnormalities of the shape of the jugular venous pressure wave are elevations of the *a* and v waves and steepness of the *y* descent (Fig. 13.9).

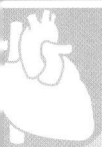
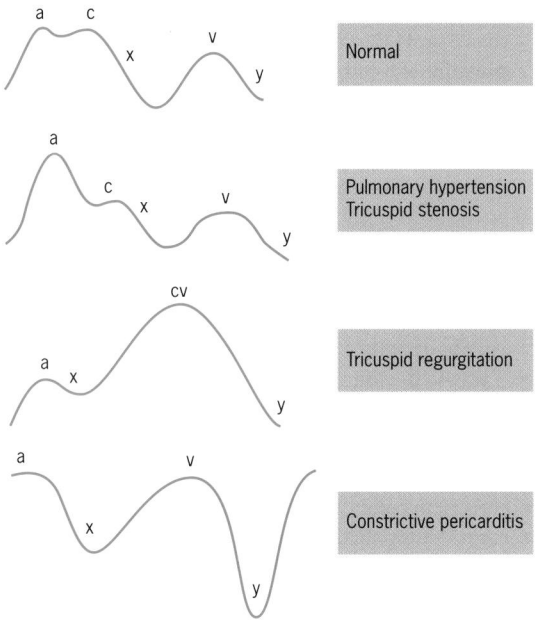

	Normal
	Pulmonary hypertension Tricuspid stenosis
	Tricuspid regurgitation
	Constrictive pericarditis

Fig. 13.9 Various jugular venous waveforms.

Large *a* waves

These are caused by increased resistance to ventricular filling, as seen with right ventricular hypertrophy due to pulmonary hypertension or pulmonary stenosis. They may also be caused by tricuspid stenosis, but this is unusual because patients with tricuspid stenosis are usually in atrial fibrillation and therefore do not have *a* waves.

A very large *a* wave occurs when the atrium contracts against a closed tricuspid valve; this is known as a 'cannon wave'. Cannon waves occur irregularly in complete heart block and in ventricular tachycardia. In both these situations there is atrioventricular dissociation, and by random chance there is occasional simultaneous atrial and ventricular contraction. In junctional rhythms the atria and ventricles usually contract simultaneously and rapid, regular cannon waves are produced.

Large *v* waves

Tricuspid regurgitation results in giant *v* waves (systolic waves) because the right ventricular pressure is transmitted directly to the right atrium and the great veins.

Steep *y* descent

Diastolic collapse of elevated venous pressure can occur in right ventricular failure but is more dramatic in constrictive pericarditis and tricuspid regurgitation. At the end of ventricular systole the elevated atrial pressure suddenly falls when the tricuspid valve opens. However, the ventricles are stiff and cannot be distended and therefore, the venous pressure rapidly rises again. This rapid fall and rise of the jugular venous pulse is known as Friedreich's sign.

Examination of the precordium

Inspection

Deformities should be looked for as they can mimic cardiac abnormalities. For example, pectus excavatum (funnel chest) or kyphoscoliosis may cause an ejection systolic murmur. The position of the apex beat and other cardiac pulsations should be noted; a left ventricular aneurysm may produce an eccentric and abnormal pulsation.

Palpation

The apex beat is defined as the most inferior and most lateral point of cardiac pulsation. It is usually felt just inside the mid-clavicular line at the level of the fourth or fifth left intercostal space. Cardiac enlargement, particularly left ventricular dilatation, displaces the apex beat to the left. The apex beat may also be displaced by a pneumothorax, pulmonary collapse or skeletal abnormalities such as scoliosis. The apex beat is normally just palpable and confined to a point that can be covered by one finger. There are several abnormal forms:

- **Tapping** is a sudden but brief cardiac impulse felt in mitral stenosis. This suggests that the anterior mitral valve leaflet is pliable.
- **Thrusting** (hyperdynamic) is vigorous but non-sustained pulsation typical of 'volume overload' due to mitral or aortic regurgitation.
- **Heaving** (sustained) is a vigorous and sustained pulsation due to 'pressure overload' as in aortic stenosis and systemic hypertension. There is often confusion about the terms thrusting and heaving.
- An **impalpable** apex occurs in emphysema, pleural effusion, obesity and pericardial effusion.
- **Double pulsation** – two apical pulsations with each heartbeat – may be felt in hypertrophic cardiomyopathy. This may be due to a palpable atrial impulse. A double apex can also be due to accentuated outward movement in late systole in a ventricular aneurysm.

A *sustained parasternal impulse* (heave) is elicited by pressing the outstretched hand flat against the sternum or against the costal cartilages just to the left of the sternum. It occurs because of right ventricular hypertrophy. An enlarged left atrium may also cause a parasternal heave. Left atrial pulsation can be distinguished from pulsation due to right ventricular hypertrophy because it occurs before the apex beat or carotid pulsation. Vigorous pulmonary artery pulsation may be appreciated by palpation in the second left interspace. This is usually due to pulmonary hypertension.

Thrills are palpable murmurs that are most easily appreciated with the flat or ulnar border of the hand rather than with the fingers. A thrill implies a definite abnormality. Systolic thrills in the aortic area are usually due to aortic stenosis, whereas at the apex a systolic thrill is due to mitral regurgitation. A diastolic thrill is usually caused by mitral stenosis; a diastolic thrill due to aortic regurgitation is uncommon.

Heart sounds that are very loud may also be palpated. In systemic hypertension the aortic second sound may be felt, and in pulmonary hypertension the pulmonary component of the second sound may be felt. Occasionally a third or fourth heart sound may be palpated.

Percussion

Percussion is not usually undertaken, but it may allow the approximate position and size of the heart to be determined.

Auscultation

The sounds best heard with the bell of the stethoscope are of low frequency, and those heard best with the diaphragm are of high frequency.

There are four traditional areas where the heart sounds and valvular murmurs are best heard:

- The **mitral area** or **apex** is the point at which the apex beat is felt. The first heart sound and mitral murmurs are loudest here, and aortic regurgitation and third and fourth left ventricular sounds are often heard best at this point.
- The **tricuspid area** is in the fourth interspace to the left of the sternum (left sternal edge). Not only is this close to the tricuspid valve but is also over the ventricles. Therefore, as well as the murmurs and sounds from the tricuspid valve, the murmurs of pulmonary and aortic regurgitation and third and fourth right ventricular sounds are also heard well here.
- The **pulmonary area** is in the second interspace just to the left of the sternum. This is the closest point to the pulmonary valve, where the murmur of pulmonary stenosis and the pulmonary component of the second heart sound are loudest.
- The **aortic area** is in the second intercostal space immediately to the right of the sternum. The aorta arches upwards and forwards from the aortic valve and the murmur of aortic stenosis is transmitted best to this area.

The sequence of cardiac auscultation is summarized in Table 13.4.

Heart sounds

The first heart sound

This is caused by the closure of the mitral and tricuspid valves and is best heard at the cardiac apex. The sound is usually single but may be slightly split. If split, this 'double' sound at the beginning of systole must be distinguished from the combination of the first heart sound with a fourth heart sound or with an ejection click.

The first heart sound is loud when the patient is thin and when the circulation is hyperdynamic (e.g. due to

Table 13.4
Summary of the auscultation procedure

The mitral, tricuspid, pulmonary and aortic areas should be auscultated in turn	**Sitting forward** Aortic diastolic murmur – tricuspid and mitral areas
Supine First heart sound – mitral area Second heart sound – pulmonary and aortic areas, during inspiration and expiration Third and fourth heart sounds – mitral and tricuspid areas Clicks, snaps – mitral and tricuspid areas Systolic murmurs – all four auscultation areas, also the neck, axilla and back	**Lying on the left side** Mitral diastolic murmur – mitral area (exactly over the apex beat) **During inspiration and expiration** – see Table 13.5 **Exercise, Valsalva manoeuvres** Can be used to accentuate murmurs

anaemia or thyrotoxicosis). The sound is also loud if the valve is still open when ventricular systole begins (e.g. in mitral stenosis).

A soft first heart sound occurs in patients with obesity, emphysema or pericardial effusion. It is also present when the valve leaflets are immobile (e.g. in severe calcific mitral stenosis), or when the leaflets are partly closed when systole begins, which occurs when the PR interval is long. A soft first heart sound also occurs when the valve does not close properly, as in mitral regurgitation. Heart failure and cardiogenic shock are also associated with a soft first heart sound.

The intensity of the first heart sound is variable when the relationship between atrial and ventricular systole is not constant (e.g. during ventricular tachycardia or complete heart block). When the PR interval is short the sound is loud, and when the PR interval is long the sound is soft.

The second heart sound

This is caused by the closure of the aortic and pulmonary valves. The pulmonary component of the second sound is heard only in the pulmonary area unless it is excessively loud. Left heart emptying is usually finished just before right heart emptying; therefore the pulmonary component of the second sound closely follows the aortic component. Inspiration results in increased venous return to the right heart, which further delays right heart emptying. The pulmonary sound is therefore delayed further on inspiration and the second heart sound becomes audibly split (Fig. 13.10). Splitting of the second heart sound on inspiration is known as normal or physiological splitting and is most commonly heard in children or young adults.

Reversed splitting of the second heart sound (when the aortic component follows the pulmonary component) is more marked on expiration. It is due to a delay in left heart emptying caused by aortic stenosis, left bundle

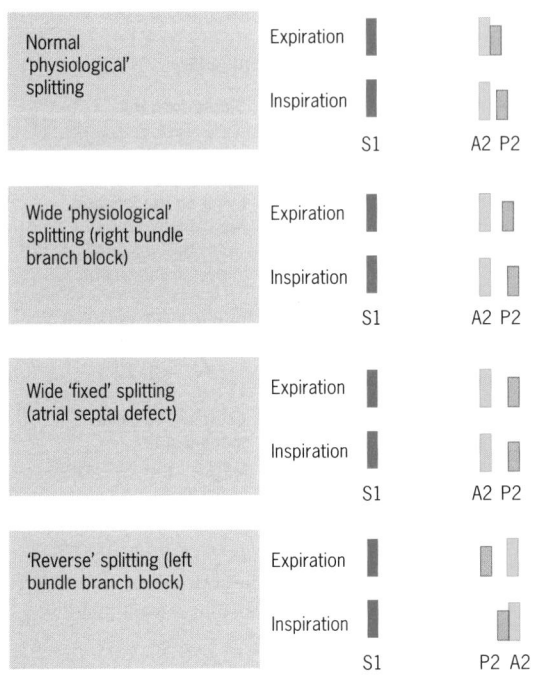

Fig. 13.10 **Variations of the second heart sound.** S1, first heart sound; A2, aortic component; P2, pulmonary component.

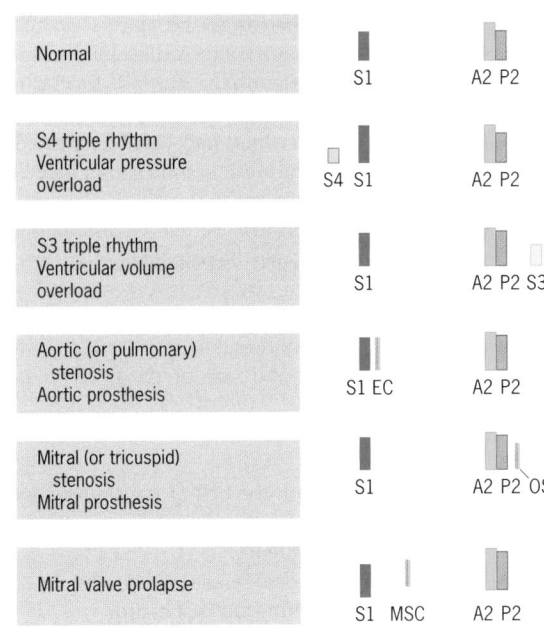

Fig. 13.11 **Normal and additional heart sounds and the conditions in which they are found.** A2, aortic component of the second sound; EC, ejection click; MSC, mid-systolic click; OS, opening snap; P2, pulmonary component of the second sound; S1, first heart sound; S3, third heart sound; S4, fourth heart sound.

branch block or left ventricular failure. Thus, when right heart emptying is delayed during inspiration, the two sounds move together, and when the right heart empties more quickly during expiration, the sounds move apart.

Wide splitting of the second heart sound is characteristic of conditions associated with delayed emptying of the right ventricle such as right bundle branch block or pulmonary stenosis. The second heart sound is also widely split in the presence of an uncomplicated atrial septal defect due to shunting of blood from the left to the right heart (and the presence of some degree of right bundle branch block in many cases). In such circumstances, the widely split second heart sound is also fixed owing to respiratory variation in shunting at the atrial level which counterbalances the normal respiratory variation in systemic venous return responsible for physiological splitting (see above).

The aortic second sound is louder in systemic hypertension and when a hyperdynamic circulation is present. It is soft in aortic stenosis because the valve is relatively immobile, and it is soft in cardiac failure because of low blood flow. Similarly, the pulmonary component of the second heart sound is loud in pulmonary hypertension and soft in pulmonary stenosis.

Additional heart sounds (Fig. 13.11)

Third and fourth heart sounds are additional diastolic heart sounds. The presence of a third or fourth sound produces a triple rhythm that, when associated with sinus tachycardia, sounds like a galloping horse – a gallop rhythm.

The third sound. A third heart sound is heard immediately after the second heart sound during the early, passive filling phase of ventricular diastole. This is due to rapid ventricular filling as soon as the mitral and tricuspid valves open. It is a normal finding in children and young adults when it is heard at the apex, especially in the left lateral position. In those over 40 years it represents heart failure or volume overload, for example due to mitral regurgitation.

The fourth sound. A fourth heart sound is heard immediately before the first sound and is associated with atrial contraction during the late, active filling phase of ventricular diastole. This is caused by the surge of ventricular filling that accompanies atrial systole. It may be a normal finding in an elderly subject, but in younger patients it usually indicates increased ventricular stiffness associated with hypertension, aortic stenosis or acute myocardial infarction.

Opening sounds. Normal heart sounds are associated with valvular closure but additional opening sounds may become audible in the presence of valvular abnormalities.

Systolic clicks. An ejection click occurs immediately after the first heart sound and is produced by the sudden opening of a deformed but mobile aortic or pulmonary valve. It is most commonly heard in association with a bicuspid aortic valve when it is easily heard throughout the respiratory cycle. A stenotic pulmonary valve also produces an ejection click, but this is best heard on expiration. A dilated aorta or pulmonary artery may also give rise to an ejection click. A mid-systolic click may also be associated with sudden prolapse of the mitral valve into the left atrium during ventricular systole. However, the auscultatory features of mitral valve prolapse are often somewhat inconsistent and wax and wane with time.

Opening snaps. A stenotic mitral or tricuspid valve may produce a high-frequency opening snap that occurs just after the second heart sound. It can be distinguished from a split second sound or a third sound by the site at which it is best heard, its higher frequency and its lack of respiratory variation.

Prosthetic sounds

Unlike native valves, mechanical prosthetic heart valves may produce loud clicks during both opening and closure. These prosthetic sounds may be muffled or absent if thrombus or vegetations impede valve movement.

Heart murmurs

Heart murmurs are caused by turbulent blood flow. Turbulence may be produced by a number of mechanisms including high blood flow through a normal valve or normal blood flow through an abnormal valve (or into a dilated chamber). Turbulence is also caused by the regurgitation of blood through a leaking valve. Murmurs produced by high-velocity blood flow (e.g. the systolic murmur of mitral regurgitation) are high frequency and are often described as 'blowing' in quality. The intensity of murmurs is determined by the blood velocity and volume, and by the distance of the source of the murmur from the stethoscope. Right-sided murmurs tend to become louder on inspiration because inspiration increases the venous return to the right heart.

Heart murmurs may occur with a normal or near-normal heart (innocent murmurs). They are usually soft and short, and occur early in systole. High cardiac output states (such as anaemia, thyrotoxicosis and pregnancy) may also produce 'flow murmurs' which are usually brief systolic ejection murmurs heard best at the left sternal edge or in the pulmonary area. These murmurs are believed to emanate from the pulmonary or aortic valve. Similar murmurs are heard in association with skeletal abnormalities such as kyphoscoliosis or funnel chest. A very small ventricular septal defect may also produce a short early systolic murmur, heard well at the left sternal edge. The murmur is short because contraction of the ventricle closes the small defect early in systole. Where doubt exists, the absence of any valvular pathology or structural cardiac abnormality in such cases should be confirmed by echocardiography.

Pathological murmurs are classified as systolic, diastolic or continuous (another functional classification divides systolic murmurs into ejection or regurgitant). Murmurs should be assessed carefully by systematic auscultation as summarized in Table 13.4. The intensity of cardiac murmurs can be graded: systolic 1–6 and diastolic 1–4 according to increasing loudness. Table 13.5 lists some common structural causes.

Systolic murmurs

Systolic murmurs occur synchronously with carotid pulsation. There are three main varieties of pathological systolic murmur:

- *Ejection mid-systolic murmurs* are heard separately from the first and second heart sounds. Their intensity rises then falls, being greatest in mid-systole.

Table 13.5
Some common structural causes of murmurs

Murmur	Position where murmur is best heard
Systolic	
Ejection (mid-)systolic	
Aortic stenosis	Aortic area, clavicles and carotids
Pulmonary stenosis }	Left sternal edge
Atrial septal defect }	on inspiration
Left (e.g. hypertrophic cardiomyopathy, HCM) and right (e.g. Fallot's tetralogy) outflow tract obstruction may also cause mid-systolic murmurs	
Pansystolic	
Mitral regurgitation (blowing)	Apex to axilla
Tricuspid regurgitation (low-pitched)	Left sternal edge
Ventricular septal defect (loud and rough)	Left sternal edge
Late systolic	
Dynamic outflow tract obstruction (HCM)	Accentuated on standing
Mitral valve prolapse	Apex
Coarctation of the aorta	Left sternal edge
Diastolic	
Mid-diastolic	
Mitral stenosis (low-frequency rumbling)	Apex, patient on left side, accentuated on exertion
Tricuspid stenosis	Left sternal edge, accentuated on inspiration
Austin Flint murmur	Apex
Early diastolic	
Aortic regurgitation (blowing, high-pitched)	Left sternal edge and apex, patient sitting forward and in expiration
Pulmonary regurgitation (blowing, variable pitch)	Right of sternum, louder on inspiration
Graham Steell in pulmonary hypertension (due to mitral stenosis)	Left sternal edge
Combined systolic and diastolic	
Patent ductus arteriosus	Left sternal edge
Aortic stenosis and regurgitation	

HCM, hypertrophic cardiomyopathy

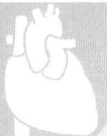

- *Pansystolic murmurs* extend from the first to the second heart sound and tend to be of constant intensity throughout the whole of systole.
- *Late systolic murmurs* are separated from the first sound but extend up to the second sound.

Diastolic murmurs

Diastolic murmurs are always associated with cardiac disease. They are of two types:

- *Mid-diastolic murmurs* usually arise from the mitral and tricuspid valves. In aortic regurgitation the flow of blood back into the left ventricle may partially close and obstruct the mitral valve, producing a mitral mid-diastolic murmur (Austin Flint murmur).
- *Early diastolic murmurs* usually result from aortic regurgitation and rarely from pulmonary regurgitation. These murmurs begin with the second heart sound and are blowing (high-pitched) in quality. Pulmonary hypertension secondary to mitral stenosis may lead to pulmonary valve regurgitation (Graham Steell murmur).

Continuous murmurs

A continuous murmur may occur because of a combination of systolic and diastolic murmurs, owing to connections between the aorta and pulmonary artery (e.g. in patent ductus arteriosus) or owing to arteriovenous anastomoses and collateral circulations (such as those associated with coarctation of the aorta). High venous flow, especially in young children, can produce a continuous venous hum in the neck. This is reduced by occluding the vein or by laying the child flat. Similarly, high mammary blood flow in pregnant or lactating women can produce a continuous murmur known as a 'mammary souffle'.

Extracardiac sounds

Bruits, usually due to arterial stenoses, are murmurs arising from a peripheral artery, including the distal aorta.

A *pericardial friction rub* is a scratching or crunching noise produced by the movement of inflamed pericardium. Since it is relatively high frequency, it is best heard with the diaphragm. It is most obvious in systole but may also be heard in early diastole or synchronously with atrial contraction. It should be listened for during both held inspiration and expiration.

FURTHER READING

Perloff JK (1990) *Physical Examination of the Heart and Circulation*, 2nd edn. Philadelphia: WB Saunders.
Shannon JR et al. (2000) Orthostatic and tachycardia associated with norepinephrine-transporter deficiency. *New England Journal of Medicine* **342**: 541–54.

Cardiac investigations

Chest X-ray

Ideally, this is taken in the postero-anterior (PA) direction at maximum inspiration with the heart close to the X-ray film to minimize magnification with respect to the thorax. A lateral may give additional information if the PA is abnormal. The cardiac structures and great vessels that can be seen on these X-rays are indicated in Figure 13.12.

Heart size

Heart size can be reliably assessed only from the PA chest film. The maximum transverse diameter of the heart is compared with the maximum transverse diameter of the thorax measured from the inside of the ribs (the cardiothoracic ratio).

The cardiothoracic ratio (CTR) is usually less than 50%, except in neonates, infants, athletes and patients with skeletal abnormalities such as scoliosis and funnel chest. A transverse cardiac diameter of more than 15.5 cm is abnormal. Pericardial effusion or cardiac dilatation causes an increase in the ratio.

A pericardial effusion produces a globular, sharp-edged shadow. This enlargement may occur quite suddenly and, unlike heart failure, there is no associated change in the pulmonary vasculature. The echocardiogram is more specific than the chest X-ray for the diagnosis of pericardial effusion, particularly because at least 250 mL of fluid must accumulate before X-ray changes are apparent.

Certain patterns of specific chamber enlargement may be seen on the chest X-ray:

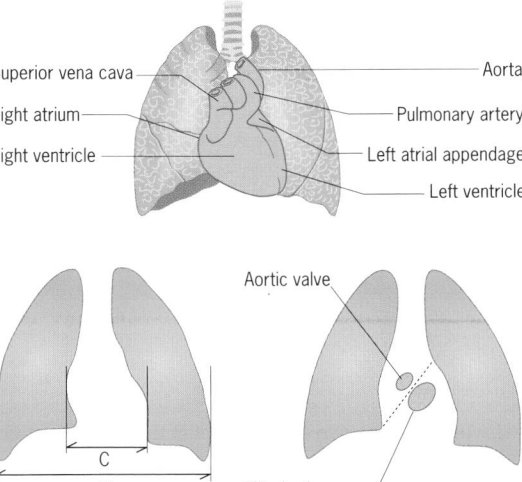

Fig. 13.12 **Diagrams to show the heart silhouette on the chest X-ray,** measurements of the cardiothoracic ratio (CTR) and the location of the cardiac valves. CTR = (C/T) × 100%; normal CTR < 50%.

Left atrial dilatation. This results in prominence of the left atrial appendage and a straightening or convex bulging of the upper left heart border, a double atrial shadow to the right of the sternum, and splaying of the carina because a large left atrium elevates the left main bronchus (Fig. 13.13). On a lateral chest X-ray an enlarged left atrium bulges backwards, impinging on the oesophagus.

Left ventricular enlargement. This results in an increase in the CTR and a smooth elongation and increased convexity of the left heart border. A left ventricular aneurysm may produce a distinct bulge or distortion of the left heart border.

Right atrial enlargement. This results in the right border of the heart projecting into the right lower lung field.

Right ventricular enlargement. This can be due to congenital heart disease. It results in an increase of the CTR and an upward displacement of the apex of the heart because the enlarging right ventricle pushes the left ventricle leftwards, upwards and eventually backwards. Differentiation of left from right ventricular enlargement may be difficult from the shape of the left heart border alone, but the lateral view shows enlargement anteriorly for the right ventricle and posteriorly for the left ventricle.

Ascending aortic dilatation or enlargement. This is seen as a prominence of the aortic shadow to the right of the mediastinum between the right atrium and superior vena cava.

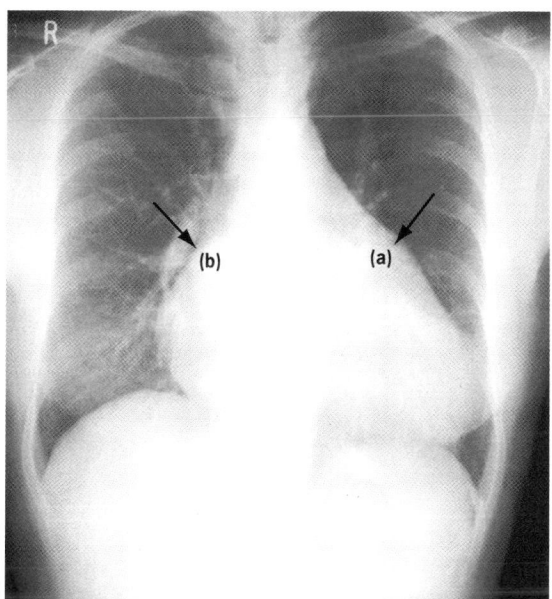

Fig. 13.13 **Plain PA chest X-ray taken from a patient with mixed mitral valve disease.** The left atrium is markedly enlarged (a). Note the large bulge on the left heart border (left atrium) and the 'double shadow' (border of the right and left atria) (b) on the right side of the heart. There is cardiac (left ventricular) enlargement due to mitral regurgitation.

Dissection of the ascending aorta. This is seen as a widening of the mediastinum, although it is often difficult to assess on an AP chest X-ray. A left-sided pleural effusion may be evident if the aneurysm is leaking or there may be blood around the apex of the lung ('capping').

Enlargement of the pulmonary artery. Enlargement of the pulmonary artery in pulmonary hypertension, pulmonary artery stenosis and left-to-right shunts produces a prominent bulge on the left-hand border of the mediastinum below the aortic knuckle.

Calcification

Calcification in the cardiovascular system occurs because of tissue degeneration. Calcification is visible on a lateral or a penetrated PA film, but is best studied by fluoroscopy or CT scanning. Various types of calcification can occur.

Pericardial calcification. This is seen as plaque-like opacities over the surface of the heart, but particularly concentrated in the atrioventricular groove. Such calcification often results from tuberculous pericarditis and may be associated with pericardial constriction.

Valvular calcification. This results from long-standing rheumatic or bicuspid aortic valve disease. On the lateral film, a calcified aortic valve is seen on or above a line joining the carina to the sternophrenic angle. Mitral valvular calcification is seen below and behind this line (see Fig. 13.12).

Myocardial calcification. This occurs after myocardial infarction, especially in association with a left ventricular aneurysm (Fig. 13.14).

Calcification of the aorta. Calcification of the aorta is a common, normal finding in patients over the age of 40 years and appears as a curvilinear opacity around the circumference of the aortic knuckle. Calcification in the ascending aorta usually denotes syphilitic aortitis, whereas in the descending aorta it is due to atheroma or, in the younger patient, to non-specific aortitis.

Coronary arterial calcification. Coronary arterial calcification, especially of the proximal left coronary artery, is associated with coronary atheroma but does not necessarily correspond to the site of maximal stenosis.

Lung fields

Pulmonary plethora results from left-to-right shunts (e.g. atrial or ventricular septal defects). It is seen as a general increase in the vascularity of the lung fields and as an increase in the size of hilar vessels (e.g. in the right lower lobe artery), which normally should not exceed 16 mm diameter.

Pulmonary oligaemia is a paucity of vascular markings and a reduction in the width of the arteries. It occurs in situations where there is reduced pulmonary blood flow, such as pulmonary embolism, severe pulmonary stenosis and Fallot's tetralogy.

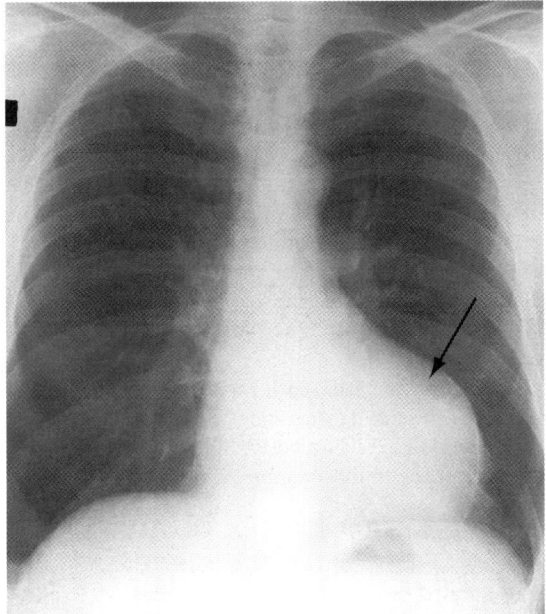

Fig. 13.14 **Plain PA chest X-ray demonstrating a cardiac silhouette with a 'bulge' (arrow) on the left lateral border.** This bulge is due to **aneurysm** formation of many years following a myocardial infarction. A thin line of calcification can be seen along the edge of this bulge.

Pulmonary arterial hypertension may result from pulmonary embolism, chronic lung disease or chronic left heart disease, such as shunts due to a ventricular septal defect or mitral valve stenosis. In addition to X-ray features of these conditions, the pulmonary arteries are prominent close to the hila but are very reduced in size (pruned) in the peripheral lung fields. This pattern is usually symmetrical.

Pulmonary venous hypertension occurs in left ventricular failure or mitral valve disease. Normal pulmonary venous pressure is 5–14 mmHg at rest. Mild pulmonary venous hypertension (15–20 mmHg) produces isolated dilatation of the upper zone vessels. Interstitial oedema occurs when the pressure is between 21 and 30 mmHg. This manifests as fluid collections in the interlobar fissures, interlobular septa (Kerley B lines) and pleural spaces. This gives rise to indistinctness of the hilar regions and haziness of the lung fields. Alveolar oedema occurs when the pressure exceeds 30 mmHg, appearing as areas of consolidation and mottling of the lung fields (Fig. 13.15) and pleural effusions. Patients with long-standing elevation of the pulmonary venous pressure have reactive thickening of the pulmonary arteriolar intima, which protects the alveoli from pulmonary oedema. Thus, in these patients the pulmonary venous pressure may increase to well above 30 mmHg before frank pulmonary oedema develops.

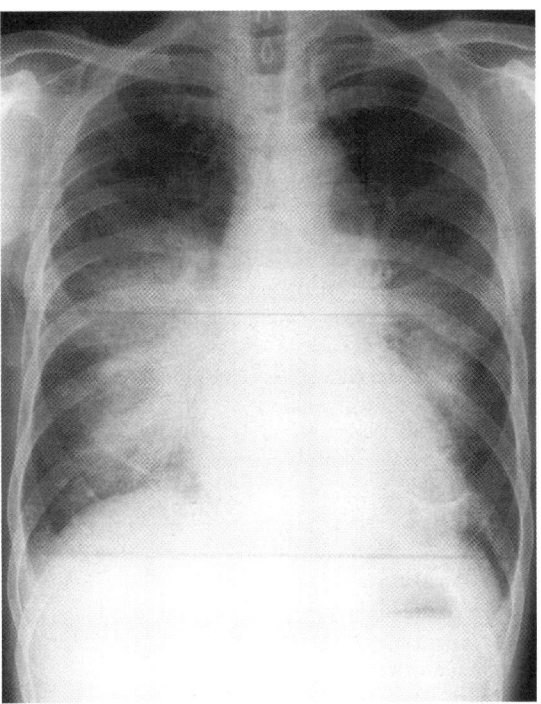

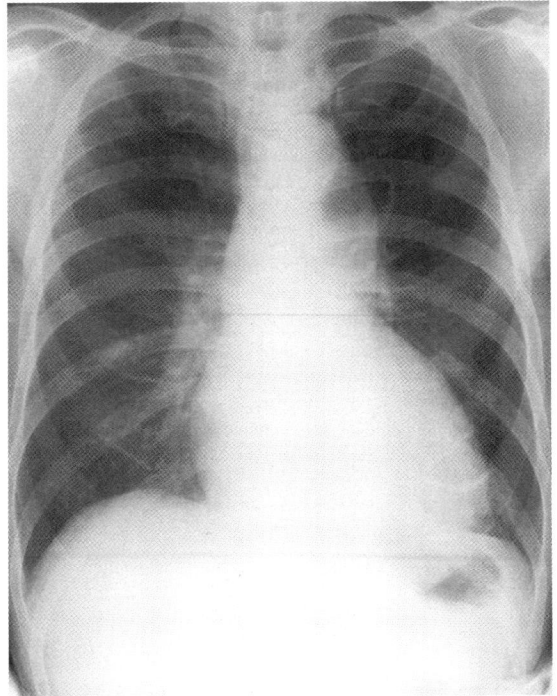

Fig. 13.15 **This pair of chest X-rays were taken from a patient before (left) and after (right) treatment of acute pulmonary oedema.** The chest X-ray taken when the oedema was present demonstrates hilar haziness, Kerley B lines, upper lobe venous engorgement and fluid in the right horizontal interlobar fissure. These abnormalities are resolved on the film taken after successful treatment.

Fluoroscopy

Fluoroscopy is an X-ray procedure used to observe the form and motion of deep structures of the body. It has been largely superseded by echocardiography. However, it is still essential for the insertion of cardiac catheters and pacemaker electrodes, and sometimes used to assess mechanical prosthetic valves.

Electrocardiography

The electrocardiogram (ECG) is a recording of the electrical activity of the heart. It is the vector sum of the depolarization and repolarization potentials of all myocardial cells (see Fig. 13.32). At the body surface these generate potential differences of about 1 mV and the fluctuations of these potentials create the familiar P–QRS–T pattern. At rest the intracellular voltage of the myocardium is polarized at –90 mV compared with that of the extracellular space. This diastolic voltage difference occurs because of the high intracellular potassium concentration, which is maintained by the sodium–potassium pump despite the free membrane permeability to potassium. Depolarization of cardiac cells occurs when there is a sudden increase in the permeability of the membrane to sodium. Sodium rushes into the cell and the negative resting voltage is lost (phase 0 in Fig. 13.32). The depolarization of a myocardial cell causes the depolarization of adjacent cells and, in the healthy heart, the entire myocardium is depolarized in a coordinated fashion. During repolarization, cellular electrolyte balance is slowly restored (phases 1, 2 and 3). Slow diastolic depolarization (phase 4) follows until the threshold potential is reached. Another action potential then follows.

The ECG is recorded from two or more simultaneous points of skin contact (electrodes). When cardiac activation proceeds towards the positive contact, an upward deflection is produced on the ECG. Correct representation of a three-dimensional spatial vector requires recordings from three mutually perpendicular (orthogonal) axes. The shape of the human torso does not make this easy, so the practical ECG records 12 projections of the vector, called 'leads' (Fig. 13.16 and Practical box 13.2).

＋ Practical box 13.2

ECG leads

Standard leads (bipolar) are derived:

Lead I	Right arm (–ve) to left arm (+ve)
Lead II	Right arm (–ve) to left leg (+ve)
Lead III	Left arm (–ve) to left leg (+ve)

Augmented leads (augmented bipolar) are derived:

AVR	Right arm (+ve) to left arm and left leg (–ve)
AVL	Left arm (+ve) to left leg and right arm (–ve)
AVF	Left leg (+ve) to left arm and right arm (–ve)

Chest leads (unipolar) are derived by connecting the V lead against the three extremity leads – the exploring electrodes are placed as follows:

V_1	4th intercostal space just to the right of the sternum
V_2	4th intercostal space just to the left of the sternum
V_3	Halfway between V_2 and V_4
V_4	5th intercostal space in the left mid-clavicular line
V_5	On same horizontal as V_4 in anterior axillary line
V_6	On same horizontal as V_4 in mid-axillary line

(a) The bipolar leads

(b) The augmented bipolar leads

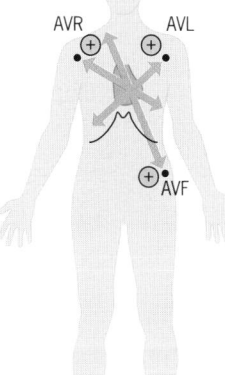

(c) The chest (unipolar) leads

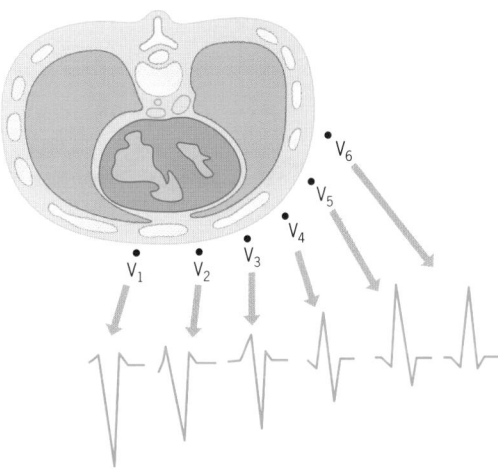

Fig. 13.16 **The connections or directions that comprise the 12–lead electrocardiogram.**

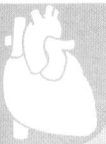

Cardiovascular disease

Six of the leads are obtained by recording voltages from the limbs (I, II, III, AVR, AVL and AVF). The other six leads record potentials between points on the chest surface and an average of the three limbs: RA, LA and LL. These are designated V_1–V_6 and aim to select activity from the right ventricle (V_1–V_2), interventricular septum (V_3–V_4) and left ventricle (V_5–V_6). Note that leads AVR and V_1 are oriented towards the cavity of the heart, leads II, III and AVF face the inferior surface, and leads I, AVL and V_6 face the lateral wall of the left ventricle. A V_4 on the right side of the chest (V_4R) is occasionally useful (e.g. for the diagnosis of right ventricular infarction).

Most ECG machines are simultaneous three-channel recorders with output either as a continuous strip or with automatic channel switching. Many ECG machines also analyse the recordings and print the analysis on the record. Usually the machine interpretation is correct, but many arrhythmias still defy automatic analysis.

The ECG waveform

The shape of the normal ECG waveform (Fig. 13.17) has similarities, whatever the orientation. The first deflection is caused by atrial depolarization, and it is a low-amplitude slow deflection called a *P wave*. The *QRS complex* reflects ventricular activation or depolarization and is sharper and larger in amplitude than the P wave. An initial downward deflection is called the *Q wave*. An initial upward deflection is called an *R wave*. The *S wave* is the last part of ventricular activation. The *T wave* is another slow and low-amplitude deflection that results from ventricular repolarization.

The atrial repolarization wave is not seen in a conventional ECG because it is low in voltage and is hidden by the QRS complex.

The *PR interval* is the length of time from the start of the P wave to the start of the QRS complex. It is the time taken for activation to pass from the sinus node, through the atrium, AV node and the His–Purkinje system to the ventricle.

The *QT interval* extends from the start of the QRS complex to the end of the T wave. This interval represents the time taken to depolarize and repolarize the ventricular myocardium.

The *ST segment* is the period between the end of the QRS complex and the start of the T wave. In the normal heart, all cells are depolarized by this phase of the ECG, i.e. the ST segment represents ventricular repolarization.

A normal ECG is shown in Figure 13.18, and the normal values for the electrocardiographic intervals are indicated in Table 13.6. Leads that face the lateral wall of the left ventricle have predominantly positive deflections, and leads looking into the ventricular cavity are usually negative. Detailed patterns depend on the size, shape and rhythm of the heart and the characteristics of the torso.

Cardiac vectors

At any point in time during depolarization and repolarization, electrical potentials are being propagated in different directions. Most of these cancel each other out

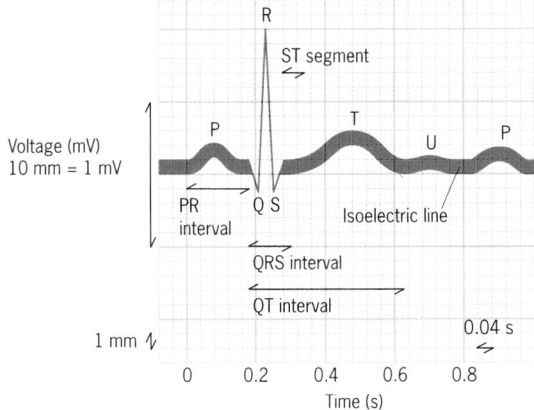

Fig. 13.17 The waves and elaboration of the normal electrocardiogram. From Goldman MJ (1976) *Principles of Clinical Electrocardiography*, 9th edn with permission of the McGraw–Hill Companies.

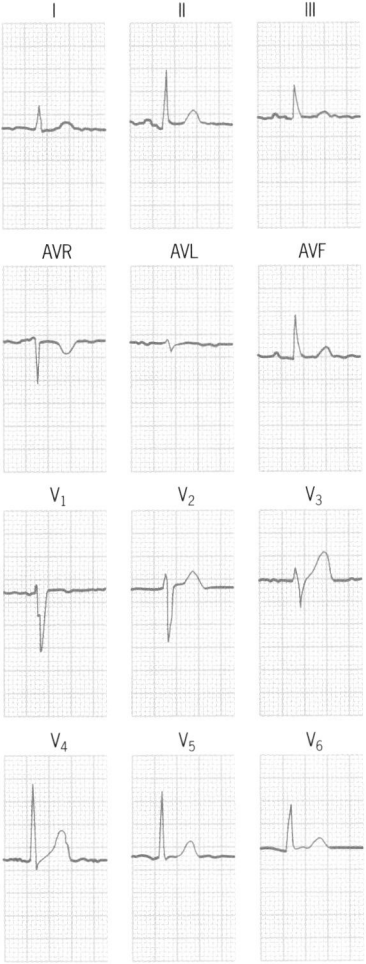

Fig. 13.18 A normal 12-lead electrocardiogram.

Table 13.6
Normal ECG intervals

P wave duration	≤ 0.12 s
PR interval	0.12–0.22 s
QRS complex duration	≤ 0.10 s
Corrected QT (QT$_c$)	≤ 0.44 s (male) ≤ 0.46 s (female)
$QT_c = \dfrac{QT}{\sqrt{RR\ interval}}$	(Bajett's correction)

and only the net force is recorded. This net force in the frontal plane is known as the cardiac vector.

The mean QRS vector can be calculated from the six standard leads (Fig. 13.19); it normally lies between −30° and +90°. Left axis deviation lies between −30° and −90° and right axis deviation between +90° and +150°. Calculation of this vector is useful in the diagnosis of some cardiac disorders.

Exercise electrocardiography

This is a technique used to assess the cardiac response to exercise. The ECG is recorded whilst the patient walks or runs on a motorized treadmill or cycles on a stationary cycle ergometer. Most exercise tests are performed according to a standardized method, e.g. the Bruce protocol. Recording an ECG *after* exercise is not an adequate form of stress test. Normally there is little change in the T wave or ST segment.

The patient's exercise capacity (the total time achieved) will depend on many factors; however, patients who can only exercise for less than 6 minutes generally have a poorer prognosis.

Myocardial ischaemia provoked by exertion results in ST segment depression (>1 mm) in leads facing the affected area. Although most abnormalities are detected in leads V$_5$ (anterior and lateral ischaemia) or AVF (inferior ischaemia), it is best to record a full 12-lead ECG. The form of ST segment depression provoked by ischaemia is characteristic: it is either planar or shows down-sloping depression (Fig. 13.20). Up-sloping depression is a non-specific finding. During an exercise test the blood pressure and rhythm responses to exercise are also assessed. Exercise normally causes an increase in heart rate and blood pressure. A sustained fall in blood pressure usually indicates severe coronary artery disease. A slow recovery of the heart rate to basal levels has also been reported to be a predictor of mortality.

Frequent premature ventricular depolarizations during the test are associated with a long-term increase in the risk of death from cardiovascular causes and further testing is required in these patients.

The usual indications and contraindications for the test are shown in Table 13.7. Its use in angina is described on page 769.

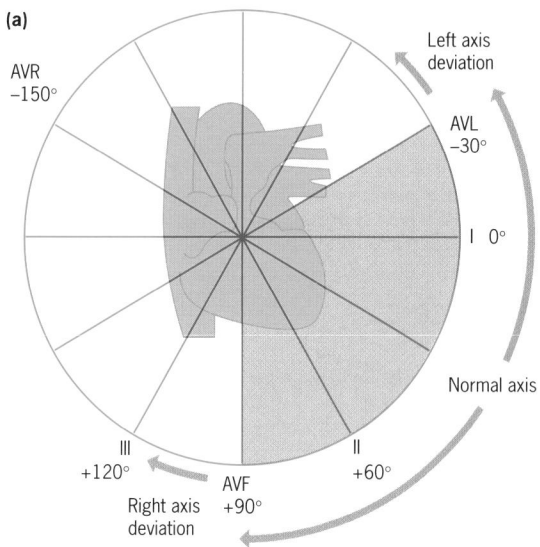

(a)

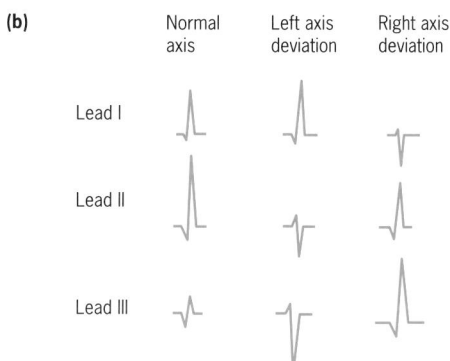

(b)

Fig. 13.19 **(a) The hexaxial reference system,** illustrating the six leads in the frontal plane, e.g. lead I is 0°, lead II is +60°, lead III is +120°. **(b) Calculating the direction of the cardiac vector.** In the first column the QRS complex with zero net amplitude (i.e. when the positive and negative deflections are equal) is seen in lead III. The mean QRS vector is therefore perpendicular to lead III and is either −150° or +30°. Lead I is positive, so the axis must be +30°, which is normal. In left axis deviation (second column) the main deflection is positive (R wave) in lead I and negative (S wave) in lead III. In right axis deviation (third column) the main deflection is negative (S wave) in lead I and positive (R wave) in lead III. The frontal plane QRS axis is normal only if the QRS complexes in leads I and II are predominantly positive.

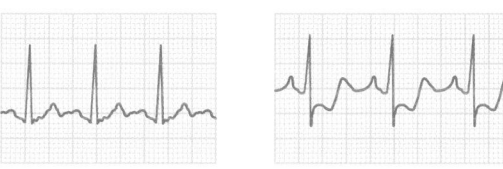

Fig. 13.20 **Electrocardiographic changes on exercise.** Left trace – at rest. Right trace – during exercise, showing positive ST segment depression.

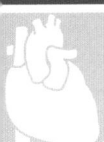

Table 13.7

Indications and contraindications for exercise electrocardiography

Indications
Investigation of chest pain
Evaluation of treatment of ischaemia
Provocation of arrhythmia
Assessment of exercise tolerance
Risk assessment after myocardial infarction
Assessment of pacemaker function

Contraindications
Recent myocardial infarction (within 1 week)
Unstable angina
Severe hypertrophic cardiomyopathy
Severe aortic stenosis
Malignant hypertension

Provided that adequate precautions are observed (doctor and resuscitation facilities available, continuous ECG and blood pressure monitoring), the mortality from exercise testing is less than 0.01%. Myocardial infarction occurs in less than 0.05%

24-hour ambulatory taped electrocardiography

This is a technique for recording transient changes such as a brief paroxysm of tachycardia, an occasional pause in the rhythm, or intermittent ST segment shifts. A conventional 12-lead ECG is recorded in less than a minute and usually samples less than 20 complexes. In a 24-hour period over 100 000 complexes are recorded. Such a large amount of data must be analysed by automatic or semi-automatic methods. This technique is called 'Holter' electrocardiography after its inventor.

Event recording, using a device called a cardiomemo, is another technique that may be used to record less frequent arrhythmias. The patient is provided with a pocket-sized device that can record and store a short segment of the ECG. The device may be kept for several days or weeks until the arrhythmia is recorded. Most units of this kind will also allow transtelephonic ECG transmission so that the physician can determine the need for treatment or the continued need for monitoring.

A very small event recorder can also be implanted subcutaneously, triggered by events or a magnet and interrogated by the physician.

Heart rate variability (HRV) can be assessed from a 24-hour ECG. HRV is decreased in some patients following myocardial infarction and represents an abnormality of autonomic tone or cardiac responsiveness. Low HRV is a major risk factor for sudden death and ventricular arrhythmias in patients discharged following myocardial infarction.

Ambulatory ECG recordings may also be used to monitor the level of the ST segment and to record transient ST segment depression.

Tilt testing

Patients with suspected neurocardiogenic (vasovagal) syncope should be investigated by upright tilt testing.

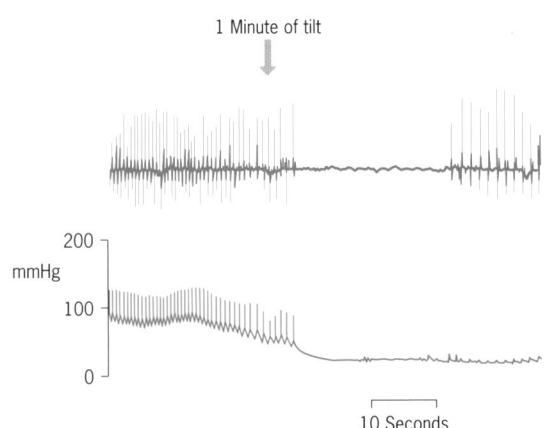

Fig. 13.21 **Tilt test.** The ECG (top trace) and arterial blood pressure recorded during a tilt test. After 1 minute of tilt, hypotension, bradycardia and syncope occur.

The patient is secured to a table which is tilted to +60° to the vertical for 45 minutes or more. The ECG and blood pressure are monitored throughout. If neither symptoms nor signs develop, isoprenaline may be slowly infused or glyceryl trinitrate inhaled and the tilt repeated. A positive test results in hypotension, sometimes bradycardia (Fig. 13.21) and presyncope/syncope, and supports the diagnosis of neurocardiogenic syncope. If symptoms and signs appear, placing the patient flat can quickly reverse them. The effect of treatment can be evaluated by repeating the tilt test, but it is not always reproducible.

Carotid sinus massage

Carotid sinus massage (see p. 741) may lead to asystole (>3 s) and/or a fall of blood pressure (>50 mmHg). This hypersensitive response occurs in many of the normal (especially elderly) population, but may also be responsible for loss of consciousness in some patients with carotid sinus syndrome (see p. 737). In one-third of cases carotid sinus massage is only positive when the patient is standing.

Echocardiography

Echocardiography uses echoes of ultrasound waves to map the heart and study its function. To provide detailed images, ultrasound wavelengths of 1 mm or less are used, which correspond to frequencies of 2 MHz (2 million cycles per second) or more. At such high frequencies, the ultrasound waves behave more like light and can be focused into a 'beam' and aimed at a particular region of the heart. The waves are generated in very short bursts or pulses a few microseconds long by a crystal transducer, which also detects returning echoes and converts them into electrical signals.

When the crystal transducer is placed on the body surface, the emitted ultrasound pulses encounter interfaces between various body tissues as they pass through the body. In crossing each interface, some of the wave energy is reflected, and if the beam path is approximately at right angles to the plane of the interface, the reflected waves return to the transducer as an echo. Since the velocity of sound in body tissues is almost constant (1550 m/s), the time delay for the echo to return measures the distance of the reflecting interface. Thus, if a single ultrasound pulse is transmitted, a series of echoes return, the first from the closest interface, and so on, until the distance becomes too great for further echoes to be detected.

To document in detail the motion patterns of individual structures, a technique called M-mode is used. The echo signals from a particular beam direction are recorded as a column of dots on a roll of photosensitive paper that is pulled past the cathode-ray tube display at constant speed. Stationary structures thus generate straight lines, the distances of which from the top of the paper indicate their depths, and movements, such as those of heart valves, are indicated by zigzag lines (Fig. 13.22c).

(a)

Recorder

Chest wall

LV

Aorta

LA

IVS

RVOT

Aorta

AMVC
PMVC

LA

Fig. 13.22 (a) Diagram showing the anatomy of the area scanned and a diagrammatic representation of the echocardiogram.

(b)–(e) Echocardiograms from a normal subject:
(b) *Two-dimensional long-axis view.*
(c) *M-mode recording* with the ultrasound beam directed across the left ventricle, just below the mitral valve.
(d) *Two-dimensional short-axis view* at the level of the tips of the papillary muscles.
(e) *Apical four-chamber view.* Note that the convention that shows the position of the transducer (the apex of the sector image) at the top of the paper causes the heart to appear 'upside down' in these views. AMVC, anterior mitral valve cusp; Ao, aorta; IVS, interventricular septum; LA, left atrium; LV, left ventricle; LV(d), LV(s), left ventricular end-diastolic and end-systolic dimensions; MV, mitral valve; PM, papillary muscle; PMVC, posterior mitral valve cusp; PVW, posterior ventricular wall; RA, right atrium; RV, right ventricle; RVOT, right ventricular outflow tract.

(b)

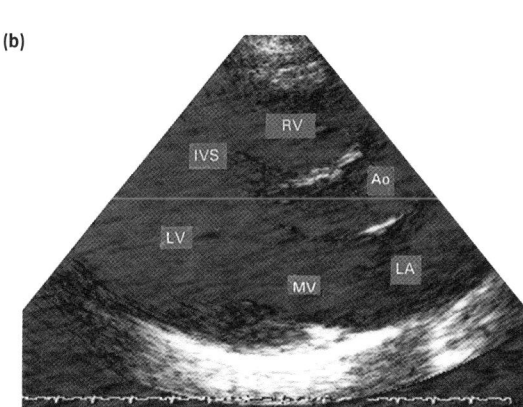

(c)

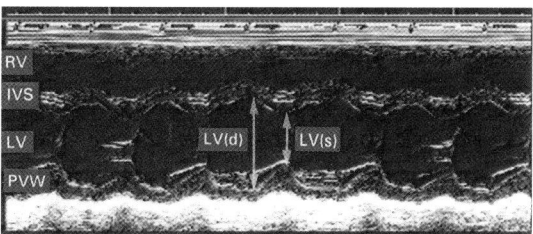

(d)

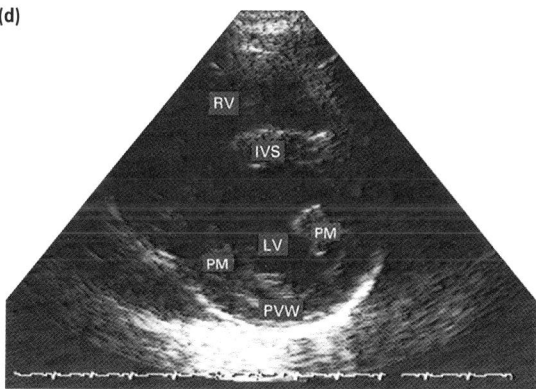

(e)

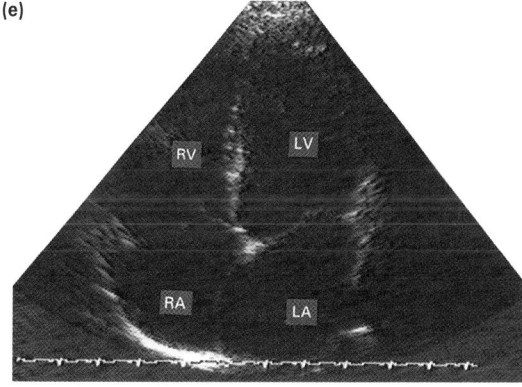

Calibration markers indicate depth at 1 cm intervals and lines along the edges of the paper show time intervals of 0.04 s. It is customary to add an ECG trace as an aid to identifying the phases of the heart cycle.

Alternatively a series of views from different positions can be obtained in the form of a two-dimensional image (cross-sectional 2-D echocardiography) (Fig. 13.22a, b and d). This method is useful for delineating anatomical structures.

The echocardiographic examination

Echocardiography is a 'non-invasive' procedure that causes the patient no discomfort and is harmless. A physician or technician performs the studies and a comprehensive examination takes 15–30 minutes.

The major problem of echocardiography is that the lungs and rib cage, both of which form impenetrable barriers to ultrasound in the adult subject, restrict access to the heart. Small 'windows' can usually be found in the third and fourth left intercostal spaces (termed left parasternal); just below the xiphoid process of the sternum (subcostal); and, with the subject turned to the left and exhaling, from the point where the apical beat is palpated (apical). By positioning the transducer successively over these sites and angling and rotating it to line up with the scan plane, a series of standard sectional views is obtained. In children, and some adults, the aortic arch can be visualized from a suprasternal position. *Transoesophageal echocardiography (TOE)* involves placing the inducer mounted on a flexible tube into the oesophagus. High-quality images can be obtained because of the close proximity of the heart. It is often used in infective endocarditis and aortic dissection.

The standard nomenclature for two-dimensional echocardiographic images is shown in Figure 13.22a. The left parasternal position gives access to the long-axis and short-axis planes. The apical approach gives a second view of the long-axis plane, but with the apex in the foreground, and also shows the four-chamber plane (Fig. 13.22e). Note that the convention of showing the transducer position at the top of the image results in these views being 'upside-down'.

M-mode recordings are obtained from the parasternal position to document motion patterns of the aorta, aortic valve and left atrium, the mitral valve, and the left and right ventricles (Fig. 13.22c).

The 1 cm calibration markers on M-mode recordings permit measurement of cardiac dimensions at any point in the cardiac cycle with an accuracy typically of ±2–3 mm.

Comparison of end-diastolic and end-systolic values allows some parameters of cardiac function to be derived. For example, the percentage reduction in the left ventricular cavity size ('shortening fraction' – SF) is given by:

$$SF = \frac{LVDD - LVSD}{LVDD} \times 100\%$$

where LVDD is left ventricular diastolic diameter and LVSD is left ventricular systolic diameter. The normal range is 30–45%.

The echocardiographic findings in particular conditions are discussed in relevant sections, but a brief overview is given below.

Valve stenosis. Congenitally abnormal aortic or pulmonary valves show a characteristic 'dome' shape in systole because the cusps cannot separate fully and a bicuspid configuration may be demonstrated. The presence of calcium in a valve gives rise to intense echoes that generate multiple, parallel lines on M-mode recordings. CW Doppler (p. 726) directed from the apex measures velocity of the jet crossing the diseased valve, from which the pressure gradient can be calculated (Fig. 13.23).

(a)

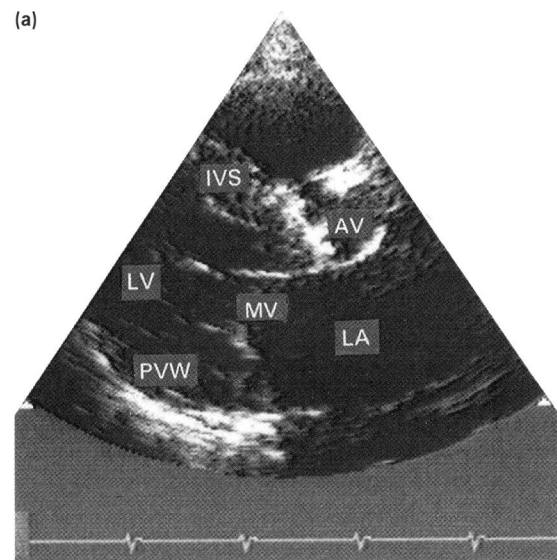

(b)

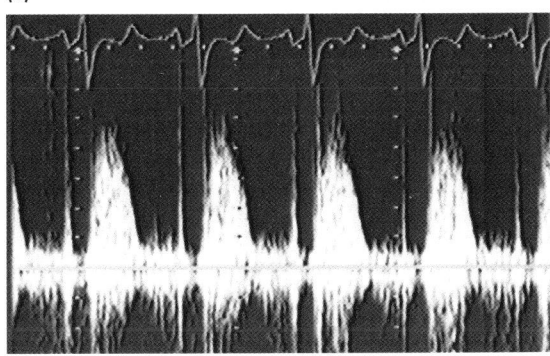

Fig. 13.23 **(a) Two-dimensional echocardiogram (long-axis view)** in a patient with **calcific aortic stenosis**. The calcium in the valve generates abnormally intense echoes. There is some evidence of the associated left ventricular hypertrophy. **(b) Continuous-wave (CW) Doppler signals** obtained from the right upper parasternal edge, where the high-velocity jet from the stenotic valve is coming towards the transducer. The peak jet velocity is 5 m/s, corresponding to a pressure gradient of 100 mmHg. AV, aortic valve; LA, left atrium; MV, mitral valve; LV, left ventricle; IVS, interventricular septum; PVW, posterior ventricular wall.

Mitral stenosis. The M-mode shows restriction and reversal of direction of the posterior leaflet motion (Fig. 13.24). A short-axis view shows the shape of the mitral orifice in diastole and its area can be measured directly from the image. Peak, mean and end-diastolic pressure gradients can be obtained from CW Doppler. Additional imaging views indicate the size of the left atrium, and may show the presence of left atrial thrombus.

Valve regurgitation. Doppler (see below) is extremely sensitive for detecting valve regurgitation and, indeed, demonstrates mild physiological regurgitation through the tricuspid and pulmonary valves in the majority of normal subjects. Angiography is still the gold standard for the evaluation of the regurgitation but echo can provide a good quantitative estimate and also determine the underlying cause such as rheumatic disease or *mitral valve prolapse.*

Aortic aneurysms and dissections. Dilatation of the aortic root can be measured accurately and the presence of a reflecting structure within the lumen of the aorta is strongly suggestive of an intimal flap associated with dissection. Transoesophageal views are particularly suitable for detecting pathology in the ascending and descending aorta. In many hospitals this is the investigation of first choice when aortic dissection is suspected.

Prosthetic heart valves. Each type of heart valve prosthesis has characteristic echocardiographic features. Irregularity or restriction of movement can be shown on M-mode recordings. The presence of stenosis or regurgitation may be documented by Doppler. Prosthetic valves cast acoustic shadows that obscure the area behind the valve. A transoesophageal approach is often used to inspect a prosthetic mitral valve for evidence of endocarditis or thrombosis.

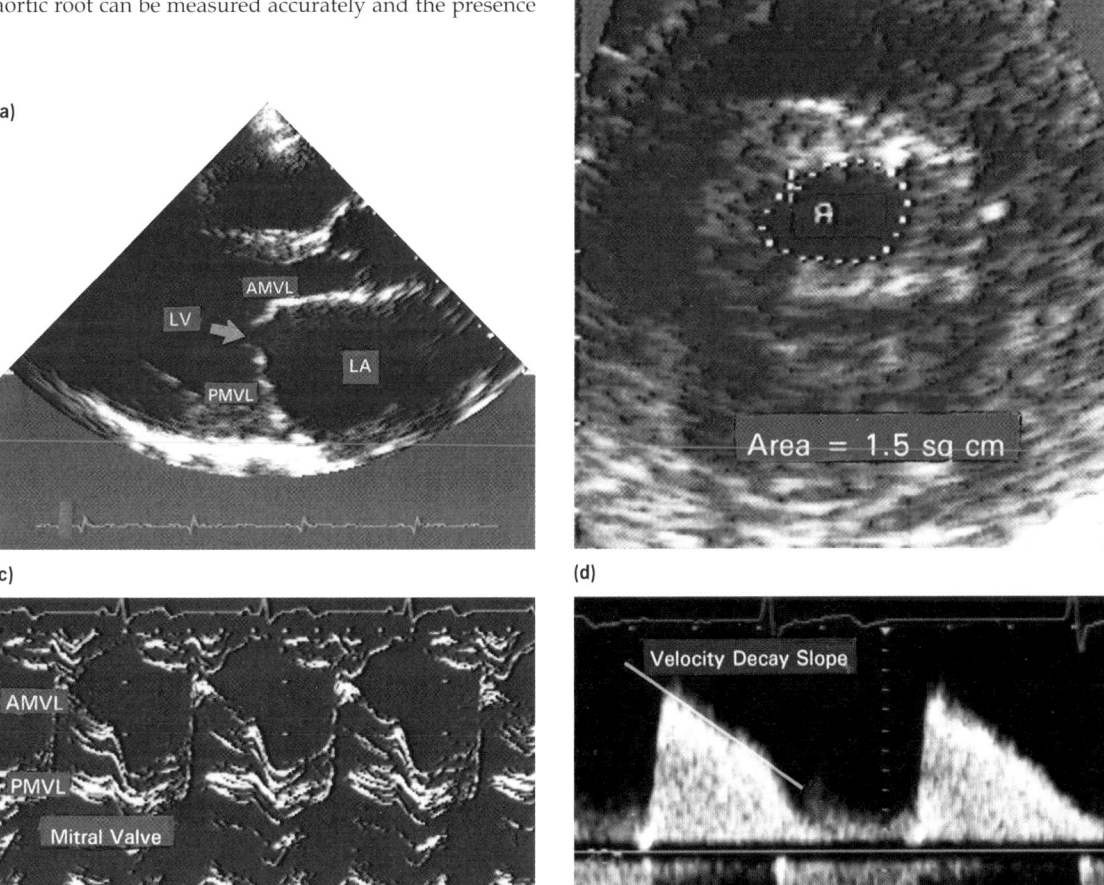

Fig. 13.24 **Echocardiograms in rheumatic mitral valve disease.** **(a)** *Two-dimensional long-axis view* showing enlarged left atrium and 'hooked' appearance of the mitral valve leaflets resulting from commissural fusion. **(b)** *Magnified short-axis view* showing the mitral valve orifice as seen from the direction of the arrow in (a). The orifice area can be planimetered to assess the severity; in this case it is 1.5 cm², indicating moderately severe disease. **(c)** *M-mode recording* of the mitral valve showing restricted motion of the thickened leaflets. **(d)** *Continuous-wave (CW) Doppler recording* showing slow rate of decay of flow velocity from the left atrium to the left ventricle during diastole. It is also possible to derive the valve orifice area from the velocity decay rate. LA, left atrium; LV, left ventricle, AMVL, PMVL, anterior and posterior mitral valve leaflets.

Infective endocarditis. Vegetations >2 mm can be detected (see Fig. 13.76, p. 796).

Cardiac failure. Left ventricular function and response to treatment is readily assessed and should be performed in all patients with heart failure.

Cardiomyopathies. Dilated cardiomyopathy is characterized by an enlarged, globular-shaped, thin-walled left ventricle with poor function and low stroke output shown by reduced movements of the valves (see Fig. 13.91, p. 812).

In hypertrophic cardiomyopathy (see Fig. 13.93, p. 813), the left ventricle is small, with a grossly thickened, immobile interventricular septum (asymmetric septal hypertrophy – ASH). There is a characteristic, though poorly understood, displacement of the mitral valve apparatus towards the septum in systole (systolic anterior motion – SAM). In restrictive cardiomyopathy LV diastolic function can be evaluated.

Pericardial effusion. Fluid in the pericardial cavity shows as an echo-free region between the myocardium and the intense echo of the parietal pericardium (Fig. 13.25).

Masses within the heart. Echocardiography is a sensitive method for detecting masses within the heart (see Fig. 13.88, p. 809).

Ischaemic disease. Coronary arteries cannot be imaged adequately using echo techniques, but images may be useful for the diagnosis of complications related to myocardial infarction, such as mitral papillary muscle rupture, tamponade or ventricular septal rupture.

In the postinfarction period, echocardiography and Doppler are used to diagnose left ventricular aneurysm, left ventricular thrombus, mitral regurgitation and pericardial effusion as well as to assess left ventricular function (ejection fraction).

Congenital heart disease. Echocardiography has largely replaced cardiac catheterization and angiography. The aim of the examination is first to establish the sequence of blood flow through the heart, and to define anatomical abnormalities as well to evaluate the postoperative status of the operated congenital heart patients.

Doppler echocardiography

Echocardiography imaging utilizes echoes from tissue interfaces. Using high amplification, it is also possible to detect weak echoes scattered by small targets, including those from red blood cells. If the blood is moving relative to the direction of the ultrasound beam, the frequency of the returning echoes will be changed according to the Doppler phenomenon. The Doppler shift frequency is directly proportional to the blood velocity.

Blood velocity data can be acquired and displayed in several ways.

Pulsed-wave (PW) Doppler extracts velocity data from the pulse echoes used to form a two-dimensional image and gives useful qualitative information. It can be thought of as a small intracardiac 'stethoscope' the location of which can be determined precisely. Doppler colour flow imaging uses one colour for blood flowing towards the transducer and another colour for blood flowing away. This technique allows the direction, velocity and timing of the flow to be measured with a simultaneous view of cardiac structure and function.

Continuous-wave (CW) Doppler collects all the velocity data from the path of the beam and analyses it to generate a spectral display. CW Doppler does not provide any depth information.

The outline of the envelope of the spectral display shows the value of peak velocity throughout the cardiac cycle. Normal velocities are of the order of 1 m/s for the normal aortic valve, but if there is an obstructive lesion, such as a stenotic valve, velocities of 5 m/s or more can occur. These velocities are generated by the pressure gradient that exists across the lesion. According to the Bernoulli equation:

$$\text{Pressure gradient} = 4 \times (\text{velocity})^2$$

This equation has been validated in a wide variety of clinical situations, including valve stenoses, ventricular septal defects and intraventricular obstruction as in hypertrophic cardiomyopathy. It is unnecessary to resort to invasive methods to measure intracardiac pressure gradients in many cases. Pulmonary systolic pressure and right ventricular diastolic pressure can be calculated using the Bernoulli equation.

Valvular stenosis or regurgitation can be assessed using PW or CW Doppler. The regurgitant fraction can be calculated. Cardiac output can also be calculated using the formula: CO = stroke volume × heart rate.

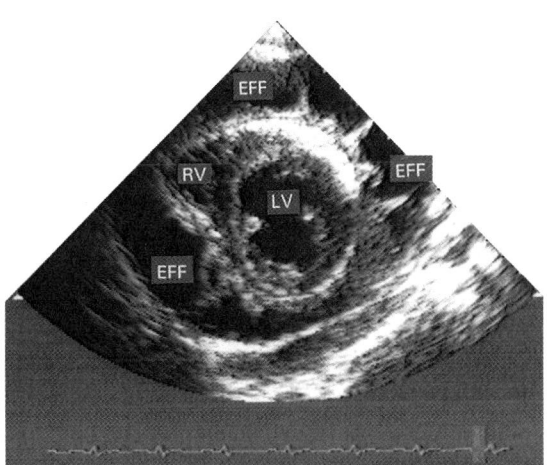

Fig. 13.25 Two-dimensional echocardiogram (short-axis view) from a patient with a large **pericardial effusion** associated with pulmonary tuberculosis. The exudate is seen between the visceral and parietal layers of the pericardium and would give a false impression of cardiomegaly on a chest X-ray. Note the multiple fibrous strands within the effusion, showing that it is consolidating and will probably lead to constriction of cardiac function. LV, left ventricle; RV, right ventricle; EFF, effusion.

Diastolic dysfunction of the LV can be detected using the mitral E/A wave ratio, the E wave deceleration time, the isovolumetric relaxation time and the pulmonary flow pattern.

Doppler will differentiate constrictive pericarditis from restrictive cardiomyopathy.

Colour Doppler is useful in determining valve regurgitation and septal defects.

Stress echo

Stress echocardiography is where alterations in wall motion are sought in response to alterations in cardiac work. Echo sequences are obtained at rest and then compared to gated sequences after stress. 'Stress' images are taken after exercise or following the administration of dobutamine, adenosine or dipyridamole (which may induce ischaemia).

Contrast echo

Intravenous contrast agents have been developed to improve the definition of the myocardium and to assess intramyocardial flow patterns.

Intracardiac and intravascular (coronary) ultrasound probes are now used to image intracardiac structures and coronary abnormalities. Prior to percutaneous transluminal coronary angioplasty (PTCA) atheroma morphology and plaque may be assessed before implanting a stent.

Nuclear imaging

Nuclear imaging may be used to detect myocardial infarction or to measure myocardial function, perfusion or viability, depending on the radiopharmaceutical used and the technique of imaging. These data are particularly valuable when used in combination.

Image type

Gamma cameras produce a planar image in which structures are superimposed as in a standard radiograph. Single-photon-emission computed tomography (SPECT) imaging uses similar raw data to construct tomographic images, just as a CT image is reconstructed from X-rays. This gives finer anatomical resolution, but is technically demanding. These methods may be used with any of the radiopharmaceuticals.

Myocardial perfusion and viability

Thallium-201 is rapidly taken up by the myocardium, so an image taken immediately after injection reflects the distribution of blood flow to the myocardium. Areas of ischaemia or infarction receive less ^{201}Tl and appear dark. Between 2 and 24 hours after injection, ^{201}Tl is redistributed so that all cardiac myocytes contain a comparable concentration. Images at this time show dark areas where the myocardium has infarcted, but normal density in ischaemic areas. Comparison of the early and late images is one method of predicting whether an ischaemic area of myocardium contains enough viable tissue to justify coronary bypass or angioplasty.

Technetium-99-labelled sestamibi (Fig. 13.26) is also taken up rapidly by cardiac myocytes, but does not undergo redistribution. When this substance is injected during exercise, its distribution in the myocardium reflects the distribution of blood at the time of the exercise, even if the image is taken several hours later. This is a sensitive method of detecting myocardial viability. Images produced following injection of ^{99m}Tc-sestamibi during exercise can be compared to images produced following injection at rest to decide which areas of ischaemia are reversible (p. 763). In patients unable to exercise, the heart can be stressed with drugs, e.g. dipyridamole or dobutamine.

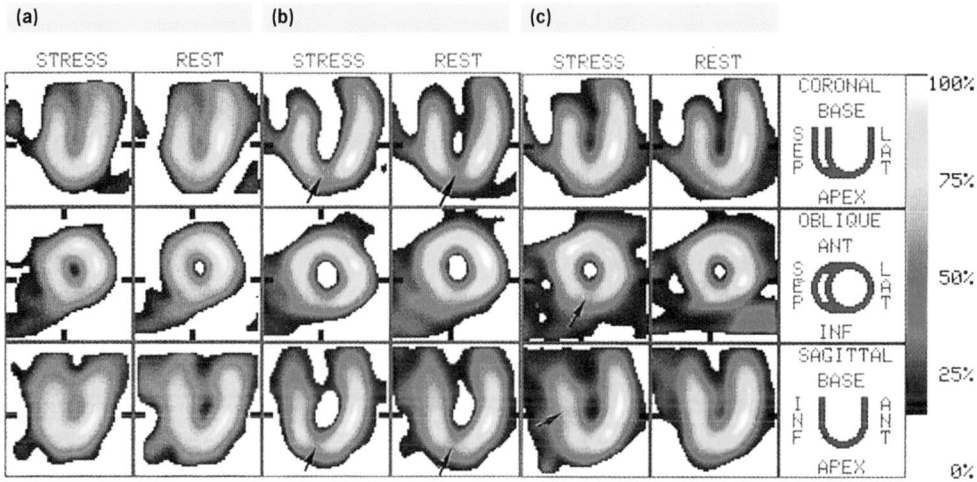

Fig. 13.26 Technetium-99-labelled sestamibi myocardial scintigram during stress and afterwards at rest in three patients. (a) Normal perfusion at rest and during stress. (b) Similar (fixed) defect at rest and during stress (arrow). This is due to a previous myocardial infarction. (c) Poor reperfusion in the inferior wall during stress which is largely resolved at rest owing to 'reversible ischaemia' (arrow).

Infarct imaging

Perfusion images produced using compounds labelled with ^{201}Tl or ^{99m}Tc-sestamibi show a myocardial infarction as a perfusion defect or 'cold spot'. These methods are sensitive for detecting and localizing the infarct, but give no information about its chronicity. [99m]Tc pyrophosphate is preferentially taken up by myocardium which has undergone infarction within the previous few days. Images are difficult to interpret because the isotope is also concentrated by bone and cartilage.

Radionuclide ventriculography

Two methods are used to obtain blood pool images:

- A *MUGA* (multigated acquisition) or equilibrium image is obtained by intravenous injection of ^{99m}Tc, which attaches to the patient's own red cells in vivo and which is therefore retained in the vascular space. Over 200 heart beats are imaged. Comparison of the study with the ECG allows systolic and diastolic points of the cycle to be identified.

- A *first-pass study* images the heart as a bolus of isotope makes a single pass through the circulation.

These techniques are complementary, but both outline the cardiac chambers, particularly the left ventricle, by imaging the isotope within the central circulation during systole and diastole. The percentage of the left ventricular volume ejected with each systole (the ejection fraction) can be measured accurately, and any section of the left ventricular wall that contracts abnormally (a wall motion defect) can be visualized (Fig. 13.27).

Positron emission tomography (PET)

This is an imaging technique based on detection of high-energy emissions caused by annihilation of positrons released from unstable isotopes. The uniqueness of PET imaging lies in its ability to image and quantify metabolic processes, receptor occupancy and blood flow. PET promises to be even more accurate than single-photon emission computed tomography (SPECT) for the detection of coronary artery disease. It may also provide an estimate of coronary blood flow as well as myocardial viability.

Cardiac catheterization

Cardiac catheterization is the introduction of a thin radiopaque tube (catheter) into the circulation. The right heart is catheterized by introducing the catheter into a peripheral vein (usually the right femoral or internal jugular vein) and advancing it through the right atrium and ventricle into the pulmonary artery. The pressures in the right heart chambers, and pulmonary artery can be measured directly. An indirect measure of left atrial pressure can be obtained by 'wedging' a catheter into the distal pulmonary artery (see p. 935). In this position

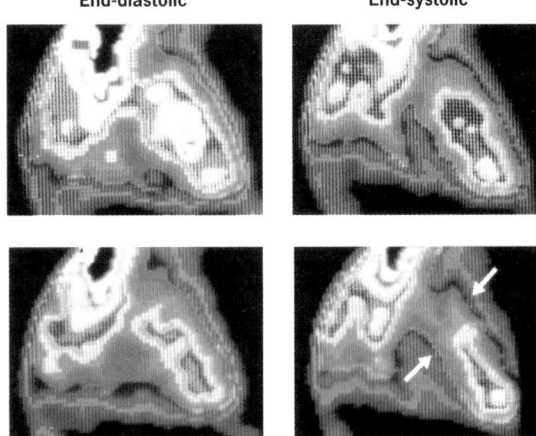

End-diastolic   **End-systolic**

Fig. 13.27 MUGA scan of patient with left ventricular aneurysm. End-diastolic and end-systolic images were recorded before administration of sublingual nitrate (above) and again after administration (below). The apical aneurysm is not altered by administration of nitrate, although the remainder of the left ventricle shows a reduced end-systolic size (arrows).

the pressure from the right ventricle is obstructed by the catheter and only the pulmonary venous and left atrial pressures are recorded.

Left heart catheterization is usually performed via the right femoral artery, although the brachial and radial arteries are sometimes used in patients with significant peripheral vascular disease. A pigtail catheter is advanced up the aorta and manipulated through the aortic valve into the left ventricle. Pressure tracings are taken from the left ventricular cavity. The end-diastolic pressure is invariably elevated in patients with left ventricular dysfunction. A power injection of radiopaque contrast material is used to opacify the left ventricular cavity (left ventriculography) and thereby assess left ventricular systolic function. Figure 13.28 presents a normal angiogram showing normal left ventricular function. The catheter is then withdrawn across the aortic valve into the aorta and the 'pullback' gradient across the valve is measured.

Aortography (a power injection into the aortic root) can be performed to assess the aortic root and the presence and severity of aortic regurgitation.

Specially designed catheters are then used to selectively engage the left and right coronary arteries and contrast cine-angiograms are taken in order to define the coronary circulation and identify the presence and severity of any coronary artery disease. Coronary angiography is described further on page 770.

During cardiac catheterization, blood samples may be withdrawn to measure the concentration of ischaemic metabolites (e.g. lactate) and the oxygen content. These estimations are used to gauge ischaemia, quantify intracardiac shunts, and measure cardiac output.

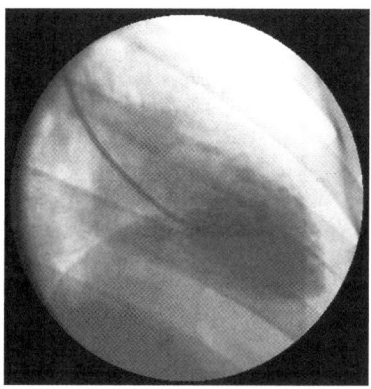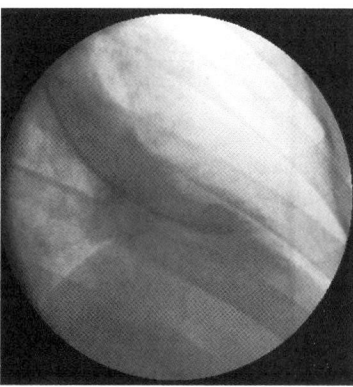

Fig. 13.28 Normal angiogram. Diastolic (left) and systolic (right) frames recorded after X-ray contrast was injected into the left ventricle (contrast left ventriculogram). Normal left ventricular function is demonstrated.

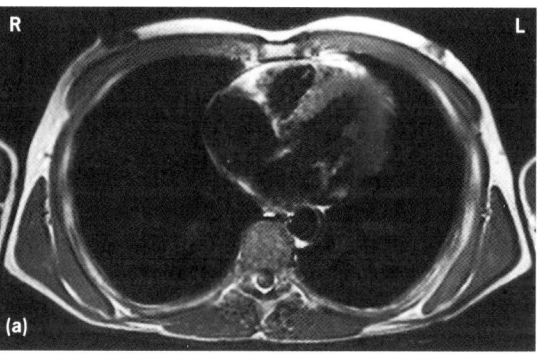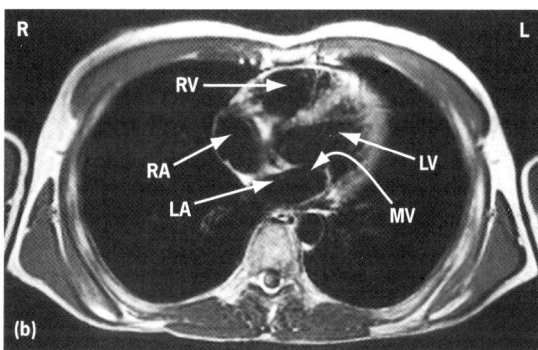

Fig. 13.29 Magnetic resonance image (MRI), showing a pair of axial images taken through the mid-thorax at the level of the mitral valve. **(a)** A view of end-systole. **(b)** Taken at end-diastole. Note the clear differentiation between the atria and ventricles. This is a normal study. LA, left atrium; LV, left ventricle; MV, mitral valve; RA, right atrium; RV, right ventricle.

Digital subtraction angiography

This technique permits the injection of small volumes of radiocontrast agents during cardiac catheterization with the production of computer-analysed high-quality angiograms.

Unfortunately, peripheral injection of contrast does not give adequate visualization of the coronary arteries, but aortic lesions can be visualized.

CT scanning

CT scanning is limited because an image must be obtained in approximately 50 ms to eliminate cardiac motion. Both conventional and spiral CT are used to image the thoracic aorta and mediastinum. CT involves ionizing radiation, requires intravascular contrast media and has been largely superseded by MRI. Electron-beam CT, which produces a faster beam image, has been developed, but is expensive.

Magnetic resonance imaging (MRI)

MRI is a non-invasive imaging technique that does not involve harmful radiation. A powerful magnetic field is used to line up the protons in the hydrogen atoms of the body, each of which can be thought of as a tiny magnet. A radiofrequency emission distorts this line-up, but when the radio waves are turned off, the atoms return to their previous position and give off energy. This energy can be reconstituted as an image.

Synchronization with the ECG allows cardiac images in systole and diastole to be obtained (Fig. 13.29). MRI is particularly useful in congenital heart disease, intracardiac masses and pericardial disease. It is also useful in imaging thoracic aneurysms either for surveillance or in the diagnosis of acute dissection. Apart from structure, images can also be obtained for flow velocity. Recently, contrast-enhanced MRI has been used in the assessment of myocardial viability.

FURTHER READING

Ashley E A, Myers J, Froelicher U (2000) Exercise testing in clinical medicine. *Lancet* **356**: 1592–1597.

Monaghan MJ (1990) *Practical Echocardiography and Doppler.* Chichester: John Wiley.

Pennell DJ, Prvulovich E (1995) *Nuclear Cardiology.* London: BPC Wheatons Ltd. British Nuclear Society.

Peterson KL, Nicol P (1996) *Cardiac Catheterization. Methods, Diagnosis and Therapy.* Philadelphia: WB Saunders.

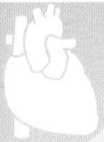

Therapeutic procedures

Cardiac resuscitation

Regardless of where cardiac arrest occurs it is essential that basic life support is initiated immediately. The longer the period of respiratory and circulatory arrest, the less the possibility of restoring healthy life. After 3 minutes there may be permanent cerebral dysfunction. Sudden unexpected cardiac arrest is relatively common in hospitals, and usually causes a great deal of excitement and panic. All medical students and doctors are fully conversant with basic procedures. An order of command should be established rapidly as organization and teamwork is the key to a successful outcome.

Basic life support (BLS)

The first step is to ensure the safety not only of the victim but also of the rescuer. The next is to ascertain the unresponsiveness of the victim. This is best achieved by both firmly shaking the victim and shouting into one ear. If no response is obtained help should be sought immediately prior to commencement of basic life support. As the likely cause of the unconsciousness is due to a breathing problem (e.g. trauma, drowning, choking, drug/alcohol intoxication or if the victim is an infant or child) then the rescuer should perform resuscitation for about 1 minute before going for help. Basic life support is easily remembered as A (airway), B (breathing) and C (circulation) (see Emergency box 13.1).

> **! Emergency box 13.1**
>
> **Basic life support** 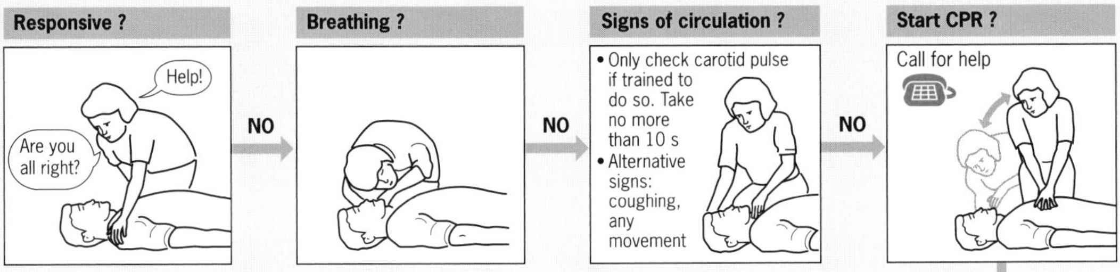 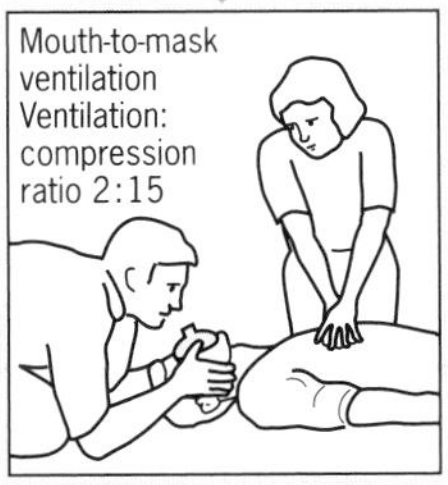
>
> | Responsive ? | | Breathing ? | | Signs of circulation ? | | Start CPR ? |
> |---|---|---|---|---|---|---|
> | Help! / Are you all right? | **NO** | | **NO** | • Only check carotid pulse if trained to do so. Take no more than 10 s • Alternative signs: coughing, any movement | **NO** | Call for help |
>
> Mouth-to-mask ventilation
> Ventilation: compression ratio 2:15
>
> CHECK RESPONSIVENESS — Shake and shout
>
> ↓
>
> OPEN AIRWAY — Head tilt/chin lift/jaw thrust
>
> ↓
>
> If breathing: recovery position   CHECK BREATHING
> • Look – for chest movement
> • Listen – for breath sounds
> • Feel – for expired air
>
> ↓
>
> BREATHE — Give 2 effective breaths
>
> ↓
>
> ASSESS 10 seconds only — Signs of a circulation
>
> ↓
>
> CIRCULATION PRESENT CONTINUE RESCUE BREATING
> Check circulation every minute
>
> NO CIRCULATION COMPRESS CHEST
> 100 per minute
> 15:2 ratio
>
> **Send or go for help as soon as possible according to guidelines**

Airway

Any loose obstruction (e.g. blood and mucus) in the mouth and pharynx should be quickly removed. Unless loose and/or ill-fitting, dentures should be left in place as they provide form and support to the oral cavity. Next the airway should be opened gently by flexing the neck and extending the head ('sniffing the morning air' position). This manoeuvre is not recommended if trauma is suspected. Any obstruction deep in the oral cavity/upper respiratory tract may require abdominal and or chest thrusts (Heimlich manoeuvre, see p. 861).

Breathing

Once a clear airway has been established the victim's breathing should be assessed. This is most effectively done by 'listening, feeling and looking'. With one's cheek close to the victim's mouth, breath sounds are felt and heard. At the same time a rise and fall of the chest and abdomen is observed. If there is no evidence of breathing, expired air respiration should be commenced. With the head of the victim tilted backwards (*head tilt*), the chin pulled forward (*chin lift*) or *jaw thrust* and the nostrils pinched firmly, the rescuer takes a deep breath and seals his/her lips around the mouth of the victim. Two effective breaths are given over 2 seconds each. Expired air respiration is the only method of artificial respiration that successfully ventilates the patient. If resistance to these puffs is experienced the airway needs to be reassessed and/or the head tilt and jaw lift corrected. It is essential to note that any reservations about initiating mouth to mouth resuscitation should NOT discourage the rescuer from proceeding to the next step (i.e. chest compressions).

Circulation

Cardiac arrest is usually accompanied by circulatory collapse. This is indicated by the absence of the carotid pulse, which lies lateral and posterior to the thyroid cartilage but medial to the medial border of sternocleidomastoid. The absence of a carotid pulse should be assessed for at least 10 seconds if you are trained to do so. Lay people are not trained to feel the carotid pulse. If absent, circulation is best established by external chest compression. The heel of one hand is placed over the lower half of the victim's sternum and the heel of the second hand is placed over the first with the fingers interlocked. The arms are kept straight and the sternum is rhythmically depressed by 2–5 cm at a rate of approximately 100 per minute. Chest compressions do not massage the heart. The thorax acts as a pump and the heart provides a system of one-way valves to ensure forward circulation. Respiratory and circulatory support is continued by providing two effective breaths for every 15 cardiac compressions (15 : 2 for one or two persons).

If possible, it is better to give compressions without interruption. This maintains adequate cerebral and coronary perfusion pressures. Ventilation can easily be achieved despite continued chest compression.

Advanced cardiac life support

By the time effective life support has been established, more help should have arrived and advanced cardiac life support can begin. This consists of ECG monitoring, endotracheal intubation and setting up an intravenous infusion in a large peripheral vein or a central vein. Immediate therapy includes defibrillation, oxygen and cardioactive drugs. It is not possible to recommend an exact sequence of management because it will depend on the arrival of skilled personnel and equipment and the nature of the cardiac arrest. However, as soon as possible the cardiac rhythm should be established. At first this is easily achieved by monitoring the ECG through the paddles of a defibrillator. Later, ECG monitoring can be set up. If the ECG shows ventricular fibrillation or if there is any doubt as to the nature of the rhythm (e.g. 'fine' VF may be confused with asystole), no time should be lost before defibrillating the patient. If initial defibrillation attempts are unsuccessful, time can then be spent intubating the patient and setting up an intravenous infusion whilst the circulation is supported by external chest compression. If there is any difficulty in intubating the patient, ventilation should be continued by means of an airway, a ventilating bag and oxygen. Intravenous epinephrine (adrenaline) results in vasoconstriction and increases the proportion of the cardiac output delivered to the brain.

There are two main mechanisms of sudden unexpected cardiac arrest (Box 13.1):

- ventricular fibrillation/ventricular tachycardia (VF/VT)
- non-VF/VT (asystole and pulseless electrical activity also known as electromechanical dissociation).

Box 13.1

Causes of unexpected cardiac arrest

Each year in the UK there are approximately 100 000 unexpected deaths occurring within 24 hours of the development of cardiac symptoms. About half of these deaths are almost instantaneous. There are several causes:

- cardiac arrhythmias (e.g. ventricular fibrillation)
- sudden pump failure (e.g. acute myocardial infarction)
- acute circulatory obstruction (e.g. pulmonary embolism)
- cardiovascular rupture (e.g. aortic dissection, myocardial rupture)
- vasomotor collapse (e.g. in pulmonary hypertension).

Most deaths are due to ventricular fibrillation or rapid ventricular tachycardia, and a small proportion are due to severe bradyarrhythmias. Coronary artery disease accounts for approximately 80% of the sudden cardiac death in western society. Transient ischaemia is suspected as the major trigger factor; however, only a small proportion of survivors have clinical evidence of acute myocardial infarction.

The principal difference in the management of these two groups of arrhythmias is the need for attempted defibrillation in those patients with VF/VT (see Fig. 13.30).

Three-quarters of arrests are due to ventricular fibrillation or rapid ventricular tachycardia. Only a very small proportion are due to electromechanical dissociation, and the remainder are due to asystole. In patients dying of other causes, such as terminal pneumonia, the heart rhythm is described as being agonal. This is characterized by an inexorable slowing and widening of the QRS complexes associated with falling blood pressure and cardiac output. This type of arrhythmia is very difficult to reverse and usually no attempt should be made because it is the result rather than the cause of death.

Arrests are treated in the following ways:

- *Ventricular fibrillation* is readily treated with defibrillation, antiarrhythmic drugs and epinephrine (adrenaline). Antiarrhythmic drugs, which are routinely employed, include intravenous lidocaine (lignocaine) and procainamide. A bolus dose of intravenous amiodarone may be of benefit in refractory VF/VT.
- *Asystole* is more difficult to treat but the heart may respond to atropine or epinephrine (adrenaline). If there is any sign of slow electromechanical activity (e.g. bradycardia with a weak pulse), emergency pacing should be used.
- *Electromechanical dissociation* is often due to a severe mechanical problem such as pericardial tamponade or massive pulmonary embolism. These conditions should be treated urgently. Toxic levels of cardiodepressant drugs, such as beta-blockers, may also cause electromechanical dissociation. If there is an antidote, such as epinephrine (adrenaline), it should be administered.

Figure 13.30 shows the treatments recommended by the European Resuscitation Council and the Resuscitation Council UK.

Defibrillation

This technique is used for the conversion of ventricular fibrillation into sinus rhythm. Electrical energy is discharged through two paddles placed on the chest wall. Initially 200 J is used for defibrillation.

The paddles are placed in one of two positions:

1. One paddle is placed to the right of the upper sternum and the other over the cardiac apex.
2. One paddle is placed under the tip of the left scapula and the other is placed over the anterior wall of the left chest.

Electrode jelly or electrolyte gel pads should be used to ensure good contact between the electrode paddles and the skin. Jelly smeared carelessly across the chest may cause short-circuits and arcing of the charge. All personnel should stand clear of the patient.

When the defibrillator is discharged, a high-voltage field envelopes the heart. This depolarizes the myocardium and allows an organized heart rhythm to emerge.

Biphasic defibrillators which require less energy are becoming available. Automated external defibrillators (AED) which recognize ventricular fibrillation automatically deliver a shock if indicated. These are now available in some public places.

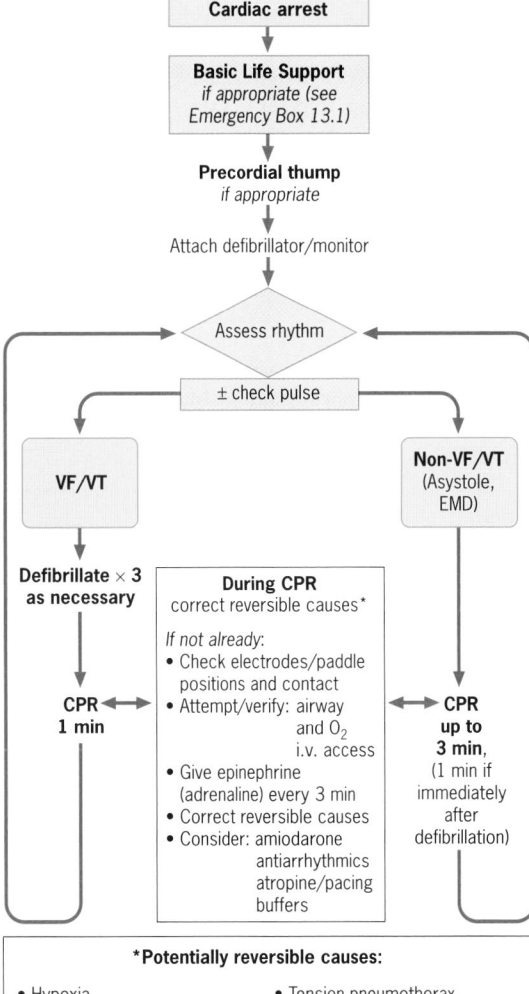

Fig. 13.30 **Universal advanced life-support algorithm**
Reproduced by permission of the European Resuscitation Council and Laerdal Medical Ltd. CPR, cardiopulmonary resuscitation; EMD, electromechanical dissociation; VF/VT, ventricular fibrillation/ventricular tachycardia.

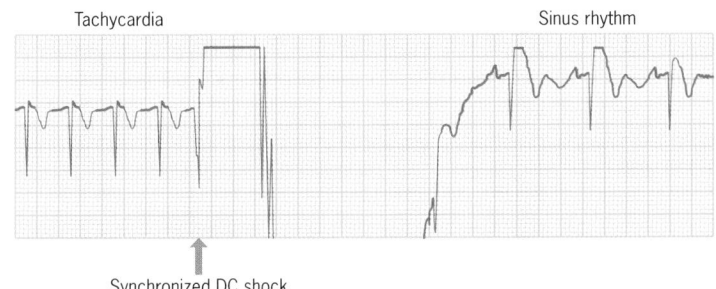

Tachycardia

Sinus rhythm

↑
Synchronized DC shock

Fig. 13.31 **DC-cardioversion of a supraventricular tachycardia to sinus rhythm.** The direct current shock is delivered synchronously with the QRS complex.

DC-cardioversion

Tachyarrhythmias that do not respond to medical treatment or that are associated with haemodynamic compromise (e.g. hypotension, worsening heart failure) may be converted to sinus rhythm by the use of a transthoracic electric shock. A short-acting general anaesthetic is used. Muscle relaxants are not usually given. When the arrhythmia has definite QRS complexes, the delivery of the shock should be timed to occur with the downstroke of the QRS complex (synchronization) (Fig. 13.31). This is the major difference between defibrillation and cardioversion, since a non-synchronized shock is used to defibrillate.

The usual indications for cardioversion are atrial fibrillation, atrial flutter, and sustained ventricular tachycardia. Occasionally, sustained junctional tachycardias may have to be DC-cardioverted to sinus rhythm.

If the arrhythmia, especially atrial fibrillation, has been present for more than a few days, it is necessary to anticoagulate the patient for 4 weeks before and 6 weeks after elective cardioversion to reduce the risk of embolization.

Digoxin toxicity may lead to ventricular arrhythmias or asystole following cardioversion. Therapeutic digitalization does not increase the risks of cardioversion, but it is conventional to omit digoxin several days prior to elective cardioversion in order to be sure that toxicity is not present.

Repeated cardioversion leads to an enzyme rise because of damage to the muscles of the chest wall. Specific cardiac enzymes increase very slightly because of myocardial damage produced by the shock.

Temporary pacing

Therapeutic cardiac pacing is employed in any patient with sustained symptomatic or haemodynamically compromising bradycardia. Bradycardias may be due to either a slow intrinsic heart rate (e.g. sinus node dysfunction) or heart block. *Prophylactic cardiac pacing* is employed in asymptomatic patients with either bradycardia or conduction abnormalities in whom the risk of progression to symptomatic bradycardia justifies such a strategy.

Transvenous pacing is the preferred method in patients with symptomatic bradycardias. In summary a thin (French gauge 5 or 6), bipolar pacing electrode wire is inserted via an internal jugular vein, a femoral vein or a subclavian vein and is positioned at the right ventricular apex using cardiac fluoroscopy. The energy needed for successful pacing (the pacing threshold) is assessed by reducing the energy until the pacemaker fails to stimulate the tissue (loss of capture). The output energy is then set at three times the threshold value to prevent inadvertent loss of capture. If the threshold increases above 5 V, the pacemaker-wire should be resited. A temporary pacemaker unit is almost always set to work 'on demand' – to fire only when a spontaneous beat has not occurred. The rate of temporary pacing is usually 60–80 per minute.

Transcutaneous pacing is the preferred method in selected patients with asymptomatic bradycardia or conduction abnormalities and may be life-saving for patients in whom a cardiac arrest is precipitated by bradycardia. In this method the myocardium is depolarized by current flow between two large adhesive electrodes positioned anteriorly and posteriorly on the chest wall. Transcutaneous pacing is uncomfortable for the conscious patient. However, it can usually be tolerated until a temporary transvenous pacemaker is inserted.

Permanent pacing

Permanent pacemakers are fully implanted in the body and connected to the heart by one or two electrode leads. The pacemaker is powered by solid-state lithium batteries, which usually last 5–10 years. Pacemakers are 'programmable' in that their operating characteristics (e.g. the pacing rate) can be changed by a programmer that transmits specific electromagnetic signals through the skin. The pacemaker leads are passed transvenously to the right heart chambers. Pacemakers are designed to both pace and sense either the ventricles or the atria or more commonly both chambers. A single chamber ventricular pacemaker is described as a 'VVI' unit because it paces the ventricle (V), senses the ventricle (V) and is inhibited (I) by a spontaneous ventricular signal. Occasionally (e.g. in symptomatic sinus bradycardia), an atrial pacemaker (AAI) may be implanted. Pacemakers that are connected to both the right atrium and ventricle ('dual chamber' pacemakers) are used to simulate the natural pacemaker and activation sequence of the heart. This form of pacemaker is called DDD because it paces the two (Dual) chambers, senses both (D) and reacts in two (D) ways – pacing in the same

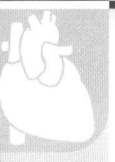
chamber is inhibited by spontaneous atrial and ventricular signals, and ventricular pacing is triggered by spontaneous atrial events. In addition, pacemakers may be 'rate responsive' (R). A rate-responsive pacemaker detects motion (level of vibration or acceleration), respiration, or changes in QT interval, and by employing one or more biosensors, changes its rate of pacing so that it is appropriate to the level of exertion.

The choice of pacemaker mostly depends on the underlying rhythm abnormality and the general condition of the patient. For example, complete heart block in patients with sinus rhythm should be treated with a dual-chamber device (p. 733) in order to maintain AV synchrony, whereas inactive or infirm patients may not benefit from the most sophisticated units.

Permanent pacemakers are inserted under local anaesthetic using fluoroscopy to guide the insertion of the electrode leads via the cephalic or subclavian veins. Perioperative prophylactic antibiotics are routinely prescribed. The pacemaker is usually positioned subcutaneously in front of the pectoral muscle. Following surgery, which usually takes 60–90 minutes, the patient rests in bed for 6–12 hours before being discharged. Patients may not drive for at least 1 week after implantation, and must inform the licensing authorities and their motor insurers.

Complications are few but include the following:

- *Infection.* When a pacemaker system is infected, antibiotic treatment is not sufficient and the pacemaker must usually be removed before antibiotics will subdue the infection. Another pacemaker is fitted later.
- *Erosion.* The pacemaker may erode through the skin. This is usually due to a low-grade infection. Mechanical factors may also be responsible.
- *Pocket haematoma.* Bleeding into the pacemaker pocket may result in significant pain, swelling, and on occasions wound breakdown and extrusion of the pulse generator. To avoid this complication warfarin is routinely stopped prior to pacemaker implantation and surgery is deferred in patients with an INR > 1.5.
- *Lead displacement.* In most cases the pacing lead is securely wedged into the trabeculae of the right ventricle. It takes approximately 6 weeks for the pacing lead to become firmly adherent to the myocardium. Most lead displacements occur early, typically within the first 24 hours. Routinely, a chest X-ray is performed and the pacing system is checked prior to hospital discharge. Lead displacement rarely occurs after 6 weeks but when it does it may lead to sudden loss of pacing and a recurrence of prepacing symptoms.
- *Electromagnetic interference.* This is not common with modern pacemakers. High-tension cables, high-energy radars, arc-welding equipment and some medical equipment, such as MRI machines and lithotripters, may transiently inhibit the output of a pacemaker or convert it to interference mode (continuous pacing despite an adequate underlying rhythm). Digital cellular telephones may cause similar problems, but only when the telephone is held in very close proximity to the pulse generator.

Pericardiocentesis

A pericardial effusion is an accumulation of fluid between the parietal and visceral layers of pericardium. Fluid is removed to relieve symptoms that are due to haemodynamic embarrassment or for diagnostic purposes.

Pericardial aspiration or pericardiocentesis is performed by inserting a needle into the pericardial space, usually via a subxiphisternal route under ultrasound guidance. If a large volume of fluid is to be removed, a wide-bore needle and cannula are inserted. The needle may be removed and the cannula left in situ to drain the fluid. Fluid that is removed is sent for chemical analysis, microscopy, including cytology, Gram-stain, and culture. If a reaccumulation of pericardial fluid is anticipated, the cannula may be left in place for several days or an operation can be performed to cut a window in the parietal pericardium (fenestration) or to remove a large section of the pericardium.

Right-heart bedside catheterization
(see Fig. 15.19)
Bedside catheterization of the pulmonary artery with a pulmonary artery balloon flotation catheter is performed in patients with:

- cardiac failure
- cardiogenic shock
- doubtful fluid status.

Intra-aortic balloon pumping

This is a technique used to assist temporarily the failing left ventricle. A catheter with a long sausage-shaped balloon at its tip is introduced percutaneously into the femoral artery and manipulated under X-ray control so that the balloon lies in the descending aorta just below the aortic arch. The balloon is rhythmically deflated and inflated with carbon dioxide gas. Using the ECG or intra-aortic pressure changes, the inflation is timed to occur during ventricular diastole to increase diastolic aortic pressure and consequently to improve coronary and cerebral blood flow. During systole the balloon is deflated, resulting in a reduction in the resistance to left ventricular emptying. Intra-aortic balloon pumping is used for circulatory support in the following acute situations:

- *Cardiogenic shock.* Balloon pumping is used to improve cardiac output when there is a transient or reversible depression of left ventricular function, such as in a patient with severe mitral valve regurgitation who is awaiting surgical replacement of the mitral valve, or in a patient with a ventricular septal defect that is due to septal infarction. It may also be used to support patients awaiting heart transplantation.

- *Unstable angina pectoris.* Balloon pumping is used to treat unstable angina pectoris by improving coronary flow and decreasing myocardial oxygen consumption by reducing the 'afterload'. This technique may be successful, even when medical therapy has failed. It is followed by early arteriography and appropriate definitive therapy such as surgery or coronary angioplasty.

Contraindications and complications

Balloon pumping should not be used when there is no remediable cause of cardiac dysfunction. It is also unsuitable in patients with aortic valve regurgitation or dissection of the aorta.

Complications of balloon pumping occur in about 20% of patients and include aortic dissection, leg ischaemia, emboli from the balloon, and balloon rupture. Embolic complications are reduced by anticoagulation with heparin.

FURTHER READING

De Latorre F et al (2001) European Resuscitation Council Guidelines. *Resuscitation* **48**: 211–221.
Eisenberg MS, Mengert TJ (2001) Cardiac resuscitation. *New England Journal of Medicine* **344**: 1304–1313.
Lockey AS, Nolan JP (2001) Cardiopulmonary resuscitation in adults. *British Medical Journal* **323**: 819–820.
Morley-Davis A, Cobbes M (1997) Cardiac pacing. *Lancet* **349**: 41–46.
Resuscitation Guidelines (2000) Resuscitation Council (UK).
Skinner DV (1996) *Cardiopulmonary Resuscitation*, 2nd edn. Oxford: OUP.

Email: enquiries@resus.org.uk (website: www.resus.org.uk).

Cardiac arrhythmias

An abnormality of the cardiac rhythm is called a cardiac arrhythmia. Such a disturbance of rhythm may cause sudden death, syncope, heart failure, dizziness, palpitations or no symptoms at all. There are two main types of arrhythmia:

- *Bradycardia:* the heart rate is slow (< 60 b.p.m.)
- *Tachycardia:* the heart rate is fast (> 100 b.p.m.).

Tachycardias are more symptomatic when the arrhythmia is fast and sustained. Tachycardias are subdivided into supraventricular tachycardias, which arise from the atrium or the atrioventricular junction, and ventricular tachycardias, which arise from the ventricles.

Some arrhythmias occur in patients with apparently normal hearts, and in others arrhythmias originate from scar tissue as a result of underlying structural heart disease. When myocardial function is poor, arrhythmias tend to be more symptomatic and are potentially life-threatening.

Sinus node function

The normal cardiac pacemaker is the sinus node (p. 703) and, like most cardiac tissue, it depolarizes spontaneously. Its rate of discharge is modulated by the autonomic nervous system. Normally the parasympathetic system predominates, resulting in slowing of the spontaneous discharge rate from approximately 100 to 70 b.p.m. A reduction of parasympathetic tone or an increase in sympathetic stimulation leads to tachycardia; conversely, increased parasympathetic tone and decreased sympathetic stimulation produces bradycardia. The sinus rate in women is slightly faster than in men. Normal sinus rhythm is characterized by P waves that are upright in leads I, II, III, and AVF of the ECG (see Fig. 13.18, p. 720), but are inverted in the cavity leads AVR and V_1 (see Fig. 13.33).

Sinus arrhythmia

Fluctuations of autonomic tone result in phasic changes of the sinus discharge rate. Thus, during inspiration, parasympathetic tone falls and the heart rate quickens, and on expiration the heart rate falls. This variation is normal, particularly in children and young adults. Typically sinus arrhythmia results in a regularly irregular pulse.

Sinus bradycardia

A sinus rate of less than 60 b.p.m. during the day or less than 50 b.p.m. at night is known as sinus bradycardia.

It is usually asymptomatic unless the rate is very slow. It is normal in athletes owing to increased vagal tone. Other causes may be divided into systemic or cardiac and are discussed under Bradycardias and heart block (p. 736).

Sinus tachycardia

Sinus rate acceleration to more than 100 b.p.m. is known as sinus tachycardia. Again, causes may be divided into systemic or cardiac and are discussed under Supraventricular tachycardias (p. 740).

Mechanisms of arrhythmia production

Abnormalities of automaticity, which could arise from a single cell, and abnormalities of conduction, which require abnormal interaction between cells, account for both bradycardia and tachycardia. Sinus bradycardia is a result of abnormally slow automaticity while bradycardia due to AV block is caused by abnormal conduction within the AV node or the distal AV conduction system. The mechanisms of tachycardia production are shown in Figure 13.32.

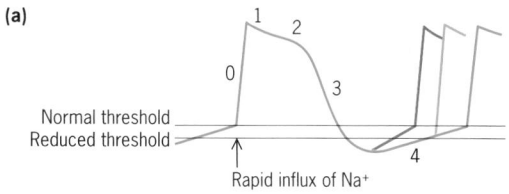

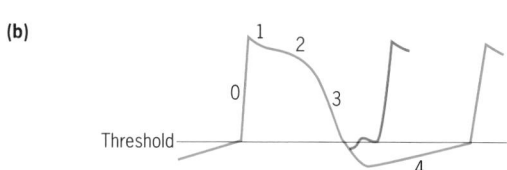

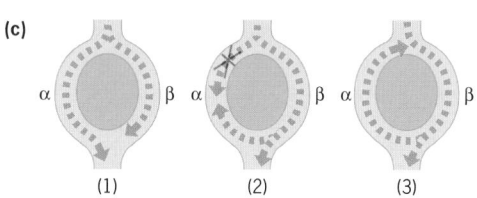

Fig. 13.32 Mechanisms of arrhythmogenesis. (a) and (b) **Action potentials** (i.e. the potential difference between intracellular and extracellular fluid) of ventricular myocardium after stimulation. **(a) Increased (accelerated) automaticity** due to reduced threshold potential or an increased slope of phase 4 depolarization (see p. 719). **(b) Triggered activity due to 'after' depolarizations** reaching threshold potential. **(c) Mechanism of circus movement or re-entry.** In panel (1) the impulse passes down both limbs of the potential tachycardia circuit. In panel (2) the impulse is blocked in one pathway (α) but proceeds slowly down pathway β, returning along pathway α until it collides with refractory tissue. In panel (3) the impulse travels so slowly along pathway β that it can return along pathway α and complete the re-entry circuit, producing a circus movement tachycardia.

Accelerated automaticity (Fig. 13.32a)

The normal mechanism of cardiac rhythmicity is slow depolarization of the transmembrane voltage during diastole until the threshold potential is reached and the action potential of the pacemaker cells takes off. This mechanism may be accelerated by increasing the rate of diastolic depolarization or changing the threshold potential. Such changes are thought to produce sinus tachycardia, escape rhythms and accelerated AV nodal (junctional) rhythms.

Triggered activity (Fig. 13.32b)

Myocardial damage can result in oscillations of the transmembrane potential at the end of the action potential. These oscillations may reach threshold potential and produce an arrhythmia. The abnormal oscillations can be exaggerated by pacing and by catecholamines and these stimuli can be used to trigger this abnormal form of automaticity. The atrial tachycardias produced by digoxin toxicity are due to triggered activity. The initiation of ventricular arrhythmia in the long QT syndrome (p. 747) may be caused by this mechanism.

Re-entry (or circus movements) (Fig. 13.32c)

The mechanism of re-entry occurs when a 'ring' of cardiac tissue surrounds an inexcitable core (e.g. in a region of scarred myocardium). Tachycardia is initiated if an ectopic beat finds one limb refractory (α) resulting in unidirectional block and the other limb excitable. Provided conduction through the excitable limb (β) is slow enough, the other limb (α) will have recovered and will allow retrograde activation to complete the re-entry loop. If the time to conduct around the ring is longer than the recovery times (refractory periods) of the tissue within the ring, circus movement will be maintained, producing a run of tachycardia. The majority of regular paroxysmal tachycardias are produced by this mechanism.

Bradycardias and heart block

Bradycardias may be due to failure of impulse formation (sinus bradycardia) or failure of impulse conduction from the atria to the ventricles (atrioventricular block).

Bradycardia

Sinus bradycardia

Sinus bradycardia may be due to extrinsic factors influencing a relatively normal sinus node or due to intrinsic sinus node disease. In addition the mechanism may be acute and reversible or chronic and degenerative. Common causes of sinus bradycardia include:

Extrinsic causes

- Hypothermia, hypothyroidism, cholestatic jaundice and raised intracranial pressure.
- Drug therapy with beta-blockers, digitalis and other antiarrhythmic drugs.
- Neurally mediated syndromes (see below).

Intrinsic causes

- Acute ischaemia and infarction of the sinus node (as a complication of acute myocardial infarction).
- Chronic degenerative changes such as fibrosis of the atrium and sinus node (sick sinus syndrome).

Sick sinus syndrome or sinoatrial disease is usually caused by idiopathic fibrosis of the sinus node. Other causes of fibrosis such as ischaemic heart disease, cardiomyopathy or myocarditis can also cause the syndrome. Patients develop episodes of sinus bradycardia or sinus arrest (Fig. 13.33) and commonly, due to diffuse atrial disease, experience paroxysmal atrial tachyarrhythmias (tachy–brady syndrome).

Neurally mediated syndromes

Neurally mediated syndromes are due to a reflex that may result in both bradycardia (sinus bradycardia, sinus arrest and AV block) and reflex peripheral vasodilatation. These syndromes usually present as syncope or presyncope (dizzy spells).

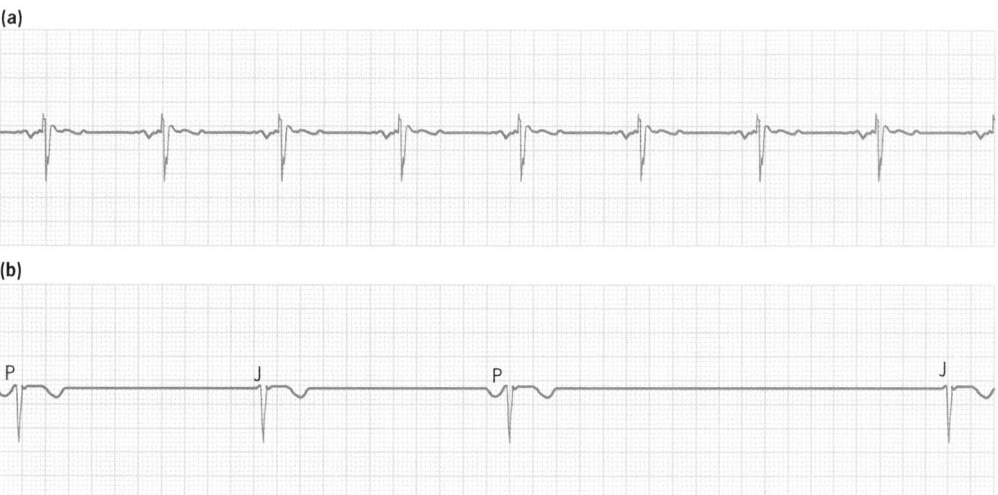

Fig. 13.33 **(a) An ECG showing normal sinus rhythm** (PR interval <0.2 s). P wave preceding each QRS complex. **(b) A patient with sick sinus syndrome.** This shows sinus arrest (only occasional sinus P waves) and junctional escape beats (J). P waves are inverted in the cavity leads that are shown here.

Carotid sinus syndrome occurs in the elderly and mainly results in bradycardia. Fainting in the carotid sinus syndrome is due to stimulation of the carotid sinus by turning the neck, wearing stiff collars or coughing.

Neurocardiogenic (vasovagal) syncope (syndrome) usually presents in young adults but may present for the first time in elderly patients. It results from a variety of situations (physical and emotional) that affect the autonomic nervous system. The efferent output may be predominantly bradycardic, predominantly vasodilatory or mixed.

Treatment

The management of sinus bradycardia is first to identify and if possible remove any extrinsic causes. Temporary pacing may be employed in patients with reversible causes until a normal sinus rate is restored and in patients with chronic degenerative conditions until a permanent pacemaker is implanted.

Treatment of chronic symptomatic sick sinus syndrome requires permanent pacing (AAI), with additional antiarrhythmic drugs to manage any tachycardia element. Thromboembolism is common in tachy–brady syndrome and patients should be anticoagulated unless there is a contraindication.

Patients with carotid sinus hypersensitivity (asystole >3 seconds), especially if symptoms are reproduced by carotid sinus massage, and in whom life-threatening causes of syncope have been excluded benefit from pacemaker implantation.

Treatment options in neurocardiogenic syndrome include avoidance, if possible, of situations known to cause syncope in a particular patient. Increased salt intake, compression of the lower legs with hose and drugs such as beta-blockers, alpha-agonists or myocardial negative inotropes (such as disopyramide) may

be helpful. In selected patients with 'malignant' neurocardiogenic syncope (syncope associated with injuries) permanent pacemaker therapy is helpful. These patients benefit from dual chamber pacemakers with a feature called 'rate drop response' which, once activated, paces the heart at a fast rate for a set period of time in order to prevent syncope.

Heart block

Heart block or conduction block may occur at any level in the conducting system. Block in either the AV node or the His bundle results in atrioventricular (AV) block, whereas block lower in the conduction system produces bundle branch block.

Atrioventricular block

There are three forms:

First-degree AV block

This is simple prolongation of the PR interval to more than 0.22 s. Every atrial depolarization is followed by conduction to the ventricles but with delay (Fig. 13.34).

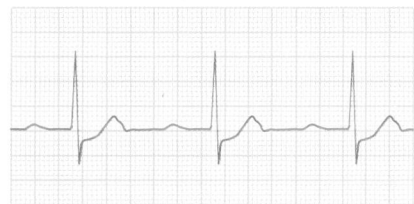

Fig. 13.34 **An ECG showing first-degree atrioventricular block** with a prolonged PR interval. In this trace coincidental ST depression is also present.

Second-degree AV block

This occurs when some P waves conduct and others do not. There are several forms (Fig. 13.35):

- *Mobitz I block* (Wenckebach block phenomenon) is progressive PR interval prolongation until a P wave fails to conduct. The PR interval before the blocked P wave is much longer than the PR interval after the blocked P wave.
- *Mobitz II block* occurs when a dropped QRS complex is not preceded by progressive PR interval prolongation.
- *2 : 1 or 3 : 1 (advanced) block* occurs when every second or third P wave conducts to the ventricles. This form of second-degree block is neither Mobitz I nor II.

Wenckebach AV block in general is due to block in the AV node whereas *Mobitz II block* signifies block at an infranodal level such as the His bundle. The risk of progression to complete heart block is greater and the reliability of the resultant escape rhythm is less with Mobitz II block. Therefore pacing is usually indicated in Mobitz II block whereas patients with Wenckebach AV block are usually monitored. Acute myocardial infarction produces a *second-degree heart block*. In inferior myocardial infarction, close monitoring and transcutaneous temporary backup pacing are all that is required. In anterior myocardial infarction, second-degree heart block is associated with a high risk of progression to *complete heart block*, and temporary pacing followed by permanent pacemaker implantation is usually indicated. *2 : 1 Heart block* may either be due to block in the AV node or at an infranodal level. Management depends on the clinical setting in which it occurs.

Third-degree (complete) AV block

Complete heart block occurs when all atrial activity fails to conduct to the ventricles (Fig. 13.36). In patients with complete heart block the aetiology needs to be established (Table 13.8) In this situation life is maintained by a spontaneous escape rhythm.

Narrow complex escape rhythm (< 0.125 QRS complex), implies that it originates in the His bundle and therefore that the region of block lies more proximally in the AV node. The escape rhythm occurs with an adequate rate (50–60 b.p.m.) and is relatively reliable.

Treatment depends on the aetiology. Recent-onset narrow-complex AV block due to transient causes may respond to intravenous atropine, but temporary pacing facilities should be available for the management of these patients. Chronic narrow-complex AV block requires permanent pacing if it is symptomatic or associated with heart disease and is usually advocated for isolated, congenital AV block, even if asymptomatic.

Broad complex escape rhythm (> 0.125), implies that the escape rhythm originates below the His bundle and therefore that the region of block lies more distally in the His–Purkinje system.

The resulting rhythm is slow (15–40 b.p.m.) and relatively unreliable. Dizziness and blackouts (Stokes–Adams

(a)

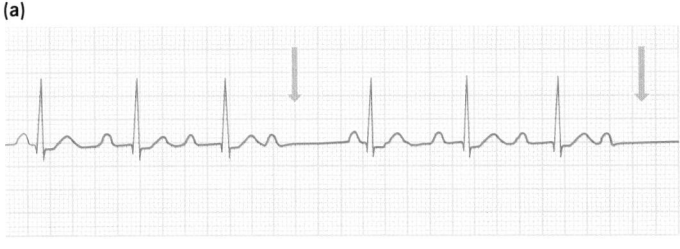

(b)

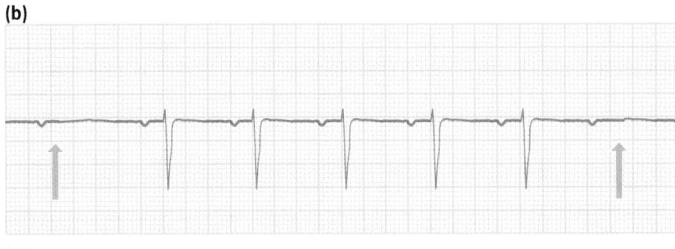

(c)

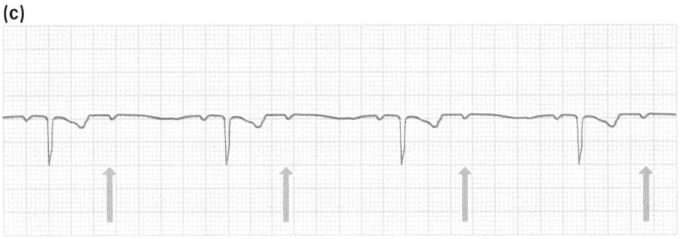

Fig. 13.35 Three varieties of second-degree atrioventricular (AV) block.

(a) *Wenckebach (Mobitz type I) AV block.* The PR interval gradually prolongs until the P wave does not conduct to the ventricles (arrow).

(b) *Mobitz type II AV block.* The P waves that do not conduct to the ventricles (arrows) are not preceded by gradual PR interval prolongation.

(c) *Two P waves to each QRS complex.* The PR interval prior to the dropped P wave is always the same. It is not possible to define this type of AV block as type I or type II Mobitz block and it is, therefore, a third variety of second-degree AV block (arrows show P waves).

(a)

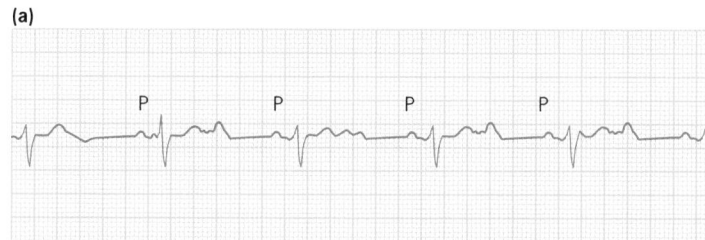

(b)

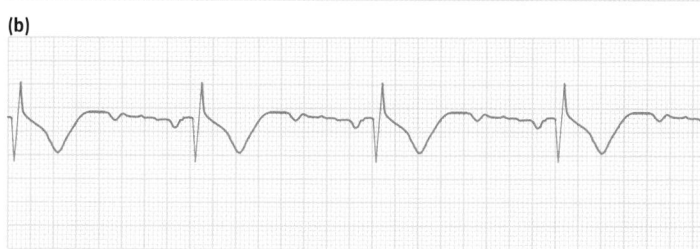

(c)

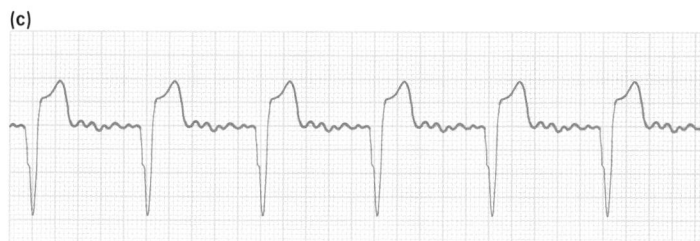

Fig. 13.36 **Three examples of complete heart block.**

(a) Congenital complete heart block. The QRS complex is narrow (0.08 s) and the QRS rate is relatively rapid (52 b.p.m.).

(b) Acquired complete heart block. The QRS complex is broad (0.13 s) and the QRS rate is relatively slow (38 b.p.m.).

(c) Drug-induced complete heart block in a patient with atrial fibrillation rather than sinus rhythm (note the undulating baseline but the regular and slow ventricular rate).

Table 13.8
Aetiology of complete heart block

Congenital
Autoimmune (e.g. maternal SLE)
Structural heart disease (e.g. transposition of the great vessels)

Idiopathic fibrosis
Lev's disease (progressive fibrosis of distal His–Purkinje system in elderly patients)
Lenegre's disease (proximal His–Purkinje fibrosis in younger patients)

Ischaemic heart disease
Acute myocardial infarct
Ischaemic cardiomyopathy

Non-ischaemic heart disease
Calcific aortic stenosis
Idiopathic dilated cardiomyopathy
Infiltrations (e.g. amyloidosis, sarcoidosis, neoplasia)

Cardiac surgery
e.g. following aortic valve replacement, CABS, VSD repair

Iatrogenic
Radiofrequency AV node ablation and pacemaker implantation

Drug-induced
e.g. digoxin, amiodarone

Infections
Endocarditis
Lyme disease
Chagas' disease

Connective tissue diseases
e.g. SLE, rheumatoid arthritis

Neuromuscular diseases
e.g. Duchenne muscular dystrophy

SLE, systemic lupus erythematosus; CABS,– coronary artery bypass surgery; VSD, ventricular septal defect

attacks) often occur. In the elderly, it is usually caused by degenerative fibrosis and calcification of the distal conduction system (Lev's disease). In younger patients, broad-complex AV block may be caused by ischaemic heart disease. Temporary pacing followed by permanent pacemaker implantation (p. 733) is indicated, as pacing considerably reduces the mortality from the condition, even when asymptomatic.

Bundle branch block

The His bundle gives rise to the right and left bundle branches. The left bundle subdivides into the anterior and posterior divisions of the left bundle. Various conduction disturbances can occur.

Bundle branch conduction delay. This produces trivial widening of the QRS complex (up to 0.11 s). It is known as incomplete bundle branch block.

Complete block of a bundle branch. This is associated with a wider QRS complex (0.12 s or more). The shape of the QRS depends on whether the right or the left bundle is blocked.

Right bundle branch block (an example is shown in Fig. 13.66, p. 780) produces late activation of the right ventricle. This is seen as deep S waves in leads I and V₆ and as a tall late R wave in lead V₁ (see Fig. 13.87, p. 807) (late activation moving towards right- and away from left-sided leads).

Left bundle branch block (Fig. 13.37) produces the opposite – a deep S wave in lead V₁ and a tall late R wave in leads I and V₆. Because left bundle branch conduction is normally responsible for the initial ventricular activation, left bundle branch block also produces abnormal Q waves.

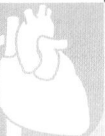

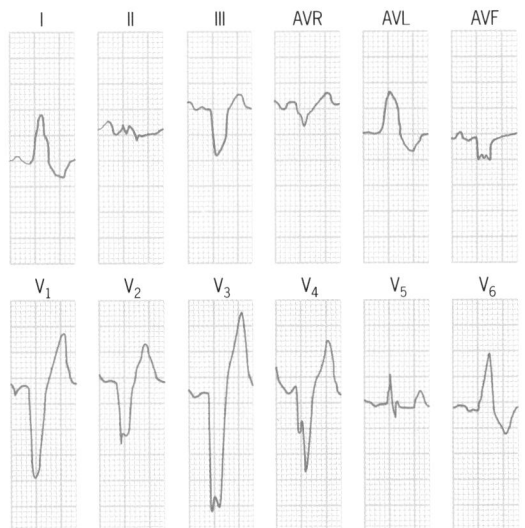

Fig. 13.37 **A 12-lead ECG showing left bundle branch block.** The QRS duration is greater than 0.12 s. Note the broad notched R waves with ST depression in leads I, AVL, and V₆, and the broad QS waves in V₁–V₃.

Table 13.9
Causes of right bundle branch block.
It is also a normal finding in 1% of young adults and 5% of elderly adults

Congenital heart disease	Myocardial disease
Atrial septal defect	Acute myocardial infarction
Fallot's tetralogy	Cardiomyopathy
Pulmonary stenosis	Conduction system fibrosis
Ventricular septal defect	
Pulmonary disease	
Cor pulmonale	
Recurrent pulmonary embolism	
Acute pulmonary embolism	
(transient)	

Table 13.10
Causes of left bundle branch block

Left ventricular outflow obstruction	Coronary artery disease
Aortic stenosis	Acute myocardial infarction
Hypertension	Severe coronary disease
	(two- to three-vessel disease)

Hemiblock. Delay or block in the divisions of the left bundle branch produces a swing in the direction of depolarization (electrical axis) of the heart. When the anterior division is blocked (left anterior hemiblock), the left ventricle is activated from inferior to superior. This produces a superior and leftwards movement of the axis (left axis deviation). Delay or block in the postero-inferior division swings the QRS axis inferiorly to the right (right axis deviation).

Bifascicular block (see Fig. 13.66). This is a combination of a block of any two of the following: the right bundle branch, the left anterosuperior division and the left posteroinferior division. Block of the remaining fascicle will result in complete AV block.

Clinical features
Bundle branch blocks are usually asymptomatic. Right bundle branch block causes wide but physiological splitting of the second heart sound. Left bundle branch block may cause reverse splitting of the second sound. Patients with intraventricular conduction disturbances may complain of syncope. This is due to intermittent complete heart block or to ventricular tachyarrhythmias. ECG monitoring and electrophysiological studies are needed to determine the cause of syncope in these patients.

Causes
Right bundle branch block occurs as an isolated congenital anomaly or is associated with cardiac or pulmonary conditions (Table 13.9). Right bundle branch block alone does not alter the electrical axis of the heart. Axis deviations signify right ventricular hypertrophy (RV overload)

or coexistent fascicular block. The combination of right bundle branch block with left axis deviation is associated with ostium primum atrial septal defects. In the rare Brugada syndrome, right bundle branch block with ST elevation in right precordial leads of the ECG leads to a high incidence of sudden death secondary to a ventricular tachyarrhythmia. It is due to a mutation in the gene that encodes for a sodium channel.

Complete left bundle branch block is often associated with extensive left ventricular disease. The most common causes are listed in Table 13.10 and are similar to those of complete heart block.

Supraventricular tachycardias

Supraventricular tachycardias (SVTs) arise from the atrium or the atrioventricular junction. Conduction is via the His–Purkinje system; therefore the QRS morphology during tachycardia is usually similar to that seen in the same patient during baseline rhythm. The causes of supraventricular tachycardia are listed in Table 13.11. Some of these are discussed in more detail below.

Acute management of SVTs
Short-term management of acute episodes of SVT usually involves both treating the tachycardia and diagnosing the underlying mechanism. Patients presenting with SVT and haemodynamic instability (e.g. hypotension, pulmonary oedema) require emergency cardioversion and stabilization. In patients who are stable, manoeuvres to help diagnose the arrhythmia mechanism, which in some cases are both therapeutic and diagnostic, should

Table 13.11
Causes of supraventricular tachycardia (SVT)

Tachycardia	ECG features	Comment
Sinus tachycardia	P wave morphology similar to sinus rhythm	Need to determine underlying cause
AV node re-entry tachycardia (AVNRT)	No visible P wave, or inverted P wave immediately before or after QRS complex	Commonest cause of palpitations in patients with normal hearts
AV reciprocating tachycardia (AVRT)	P wave visible between QRS and T wave complexes	Due to an accessory pathway. If pathway conducts in both directions, ECG during sinus rhythm may be pre-excited
Atrial fibrillation	Irregularly irregular RR intervals and absence of organized atrial activity	Commonest tachycardia in patients over 65 years
Atrial flutter	Visible flutter waves at 300/min (saw-tooth appearance) usually with 2:1 AV conduction	Suspect in any patient with regular SVT at 150/min
Atrial tachycardia	Organized atrial activity with P wave morphology different from sinus rhythm	Usually occurs in patients with structural heart disease
Multifocal atrial tachycardia	Multiple P wave morphologies (≥ 3) and irregular RR intervals	Rare arrhythmia; most commonly associated with significant chronic lung disease
Accelerated junctional tachycardia	ECG similar to AVNRT	Rare in adults

be employed. These consist of inducing transient AV block. Tachycardias that require AV conduction for their maintenance, atrioventricular nodal re-entry tachycardia (AVNRT) and atrioventricular reciprocating tachycardia (AVRT), are effectively terminated by inducing AV block. Supraventricular tachycardias that do not require AV conduction for their maintenance, namely, all tachycardias in Table 13.11 except AVNRT and AVRT, can be more easily diagnosed by examining a continuous ECG recording during transient induced heart block. An intense efferent vagal discharge commonly induces transient AV nodal heart block.

Carotid sinus massage (Practical box 13.3), and the Valsalva manoeuvre may be used to stimulate the vagal efferent discharge. Of these techniques, the Valsalva manoeuvre is the best and often easier for the patient to perform successfully. It should be undertaken when the patient is resting in the supine position (thus avoiding elevated background sympathetic tone). Several seconds after the release of strain, the resulting intense vagal effect may terminate a junctional re-entry tachycardia or may produce sufficient AV block to reveal an underlying atrial tachyarrhythmia. If physical manoeuvres have not been successful, intravenous adenosine (up to 0.25 mg/kg) should be tried. This is a very short-acting (half-life < 10 s) naturally occurring purine nucleoside that causes complete heart block for a fraction of a second following i.v. administration. It is highly effective at terminating 'junctional' tachycardias (AVNRT and AVRT) or unmasking underlying atrial activity. It rarely affects ventricular tachycardia. The side-effects of adenosine are very brief but include bronchospasm, flushing, chest pain and heaviness of the limbs. It is contraindicated in patients with a history of asthma. An alternative treatment is verapamil 10 mg i.v. over

 Practical Box 13.3

Carotid sinus massage

Carotid sinus massage is performed for three reasons:

- to break junctional tachycardia (AVNRT and AVRT) by blocking AV nodal conduction
- to reveal on the ECG the P wave pattern of an atrial arrhythmia by reducing the frequency of AV nodal conduction during the tachycardia so that the QRS complexes do not mask the artrial activity
- to test for carotid sinus hypersensitivity, which is a severe fall in blood pressure or heart rate in response to carotid sinus stimulation.

The carotid sinus is stimulated by firm rotary pressure of the carotid sinus against the transverse processes of the third cervical vertebrum. Provided that there is no carotid bruit, each carotid should be tried in turn. In general, right carotid pressure tends to slow the sinus rate and left carotid pressure tends to impair AV nodal conduction.

5–10 minutes (Fig. 13.38). Verapamil must not be given if beta-blockers have been previously administered or if the tachycardia presents with broad (> 0.12 s) QRS complexes. Patients with atrial fibrillation or atrial flutter in whom the exact duration is unknown or who have been in tachycardia for greater than 24–48 hours should, if stable, be anticoagulated for 4–6 weeks prior to attempts at DC cardioversion or chemical (antiarrhythmic drugs) cardioversion, owing to the risks of thromboembolism and stroke.

Sinus tachycardia

Sinus tachycardia can be a difficult SVT to diagnose, especially when the rate is more rapid as the P waves

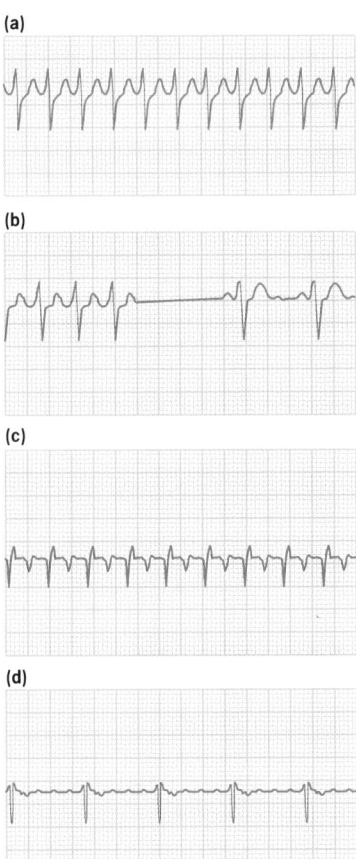

Fig. 13.38 **Two examples of the slowing of tachycardia following the administration of antiarrhythmic drugs.**
(a) A supraventricular tachycardia (rate 205 b.p.m.) before treatment with verapamil.
(b) The result 60 s later. The tachycardia slows to 130 b.p.m. before terminating abruptly and revealing sinus rhythm.
(c) Atrial tachycardia at a rate of 170 b.p.m. It is difficult to discern the atrial tachycardia waves. Verapamil is administered and the result is shown in (d).
(d) Now the atrial tachycardia is easily seen. The proportion of atrial tachycardia beats transmitted to the ventricles has been reduced following the administration of verapamil.

may be superimposed and hidden by the preceding T wave. Sinus tachycardia due to intrinsic sinus node abnormalities is extremely rare. In general sinus tachycardia is a secondary phenomenon and the underlying causes need to be actively investigated. Depending on the clinical setting, acute causes include exercise, emotion, pain, fever, infection, acute heart failure, acute pulmonary embolism and hypovolaemia. Chronic causes include pregnancy, anaemia, hyperthyroidism and cathecholamine excess. The list of possible causes is myriad but the underlying cause should be found and treated rather than treating what in effect is a compensatory physiological response. If necessary, beta-blockers may be used to slow the sinus rate, e.g. in hyperthyroidism (p. 1041).

Junctional tachycardia

In these tachycardias the AV node is an essential component of the re-entry circuit.

Atrioventricular nodal re-entry tachycardia (AVNRT)

This tachycardia is paroxysmal in nature. AVNRT is the commonest cause of SVT in patients with structurally normal hearts. Clinically, the tachycardia often strikes suddenly without obvious provocation, but exertion, coffee, tea and alcohol may aggravate or induce the arrhythmia. The rhythm is rapid (140–280 per minute) and regular. An attack may stop spontaneously or may continue indefinitely until medical intervention. The predominant symptom is palpitations, but chest pain, dyspnoea, presyncope and polyuria may develop. The polyuria occurs because tachycardia leads to an elevated atrial pressure and the release of atrial natriuretic peptide and other hormones.

The rhythm is recognized on ECG by normal regular QRS complexes usually at a rate of 140–240 per minute. Sometimes the QRS complexes will show typical bundle branch block (aberration). P waves are either not visible or are seen immediately before or after the QRS complex because of simultaneous atrial and ventricular activation. Patients with AVNRT are taught how to self-terminate an acute attack using vagal manoeuvres. AV nodal blocking agents such as beta-blockers or calcium channel blockers may suppress recurrent attacks. AVNRT is effectively cured by catheter ablation and this procedure should be offered to patients in whom drug therapy is ineffective, poorly tolerated or unwanted over the long term (p. 753).

Atrioventricular reciprocating tachycardia (AVRT)

This tachycardia usually results in paroxysmal tachycardia and its presentation is very similar to AVNRT. In AVRT there is a large circuit comprising the AV node, the His bundle, the ventricle and an abnormal connection from the ventricle back to the atrium. This abnormal connection consists of myocardial fibres that span the atrioventricular groove and is called an accessory pathway or bypass tract. In contrast to AVNRT, this tachycardia is due to a macro-reentry circuit and each part of the circuit is activated sequentially. As a result atrial activation occurs after ventricular activation and the P wave is usually clearly seen between the QRS and T complexes.

Accessory pathways are most commonly situated on the left atrial free wall but may occur anywhere around the AV groove. Accessory pathways that conduct from the ventricles to the atria only are not visible on the surface ECG during sinus rhythm and are therefore called concealed. Accessory pathways that conduct bidirectionally usually are manifest on the surface ECG. If the accessory pathway conducts from the atrium to the ventricle, then during sinus rhythm the electrical impulse can conduct quickly over this abnormal connection to depolarize part of the ventricles abnormally (pre-excitation). A pre-excited ECG is characterized by a short PR interval and a wide QRS complex that begins as a slurred part known as the δ wave (see Fig. 13.39). Patients with a history of palpitations and a pre-excited ECG have a syndrome known as Wolff–Parkinson–White (WPW) syndrome.

In AVRT in patients with a concealed bypass tract the AV node and ventricles are activated normally (orthodromically) resulting usually in a narrow QRS complex. In patients with accessory pathways that conduct bi-directionally, orthodromic AVRT is the commonest SVT but other forms of tachycardia are possible. Less commonly the tachycardia circuit can be reversed, with activation of the ventricles via the accessory pathway and atrial activation via retrograde conduction through the AV node (antidromic AVRT). This results in a broad complex tachycardia. These patients are also prone to atrial fibrillation. During atrial fibrillation the ventricles may be depolarized by impulses travelling over both the abnormal and the normal pathways. This results in pre-excited atrial fibrillation, a characteristic tachycardia that is both broad complex and irregularly irregular. The conduction ability of the abnormal pathway is depressed by drugs that affect the atrium (e.g. classes I and III, see Table 13.16) but not by verapamil and digoxin, which may allow a higher rate of conduction over the abnormal pathway and precipitate ventricular fibrillation. Therefore, neither verapamil nor digoxin should be used to treat atrial fibrillation associated with the WPW syndrome.

Symptomatic patients with a concealed accessory pathway are initially treated in a similar manner to patients with AVNRT, i.e. AV nodal slowing agents proceeding to radiofrequency ablation. Patients with WPW syndrome are almost always treated with radiofrequency ablation.

Drugs such as classes Ia, Ic and III may be used if ablation is (rarely) unsuccessful or not wanted.

Atrial tachyarrhythmias

Atrial tachyarrhythmias including atrial fibrillation, atrial flutter, atrial tachycardia and atrial ectopic beats all arise from the atrial myocardium. They share common aetiologies, which are listed in Table 13.12.

Atrial fibrillation

This is a common arrhythmia, occurring in 5–10% of patients over 65 years of age. It also occurs, particularly in a paroxysmal form, in younger patients. Any condition resulting in raised atrial pressure, increased atrial muscle mass, atrial fibrosis, or inflammation and infiltration of the atrium may cause atrial fibrillation. There are also many systemic causes of atrial fibrillation (Table 13.12). Hyperthyroidism may provoke atrial fibrillation, sometimes as virtually the only feature of the disease, and thyroid function tests are mandatory in any patient with unaccounted atrial fibrillation. In some patients no cause can be found and this group are labelled as 'lone' atrial fibrillation.

Atrial fibrillation is maintained by continuous, rapid (300–600 per minute) activation of the atria by multiple meandering re-entry wavelets. The atria respond electrically at this rate but there is no coordinated mechanical action and only a proportion of the impulses are conducted to the ventricles.

Symptoms and signs

Symptoms attributable to atrial fibrillation are highly variable. In some patients it is an incidental finding, whilst others attend hospital as an emergency following the onset of atrial fibrillation. Most patients experience some deterioration of exercise capacity or well-being, but this may only be appreciated once sinus rhythm is

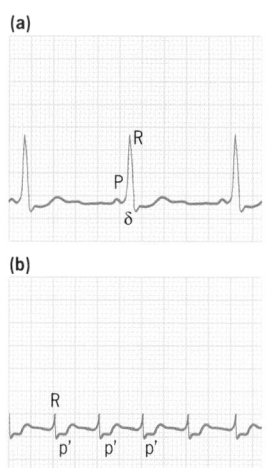

Fig. 13.39 **An ECG showing Wolff–Parkinson–White syndrome.**
(a) A trace taken during sinus rhythm, demonstrating a short PR interval (0.09 s) and broad QRS complex (0.12 s).
(b) Atrioventricular reciprocating tachycardia (AVRT) associated with this syndrome. Note the tachycardia p wave visible between QRS and T wave complexes.

Table 13.12
Causes of atrial arrhythmias

Ischaemic heart disease
Mitral valve disease
Rheumatic heart disease
Hypertension
Cardiomyopathy
Thyrotoxicosis
Atrial septal defect
Acute and chronic alcohol abuse
Cardiac surgery
Pericarditis
Pulmonary embolus
Lone atrial fibrillation (i.e. no cause discovered)
Tachy–brady syndrome

restored. When caused by rheumatic mitral stenosis, the onset of atrial fibrillation results in considerable worsening of cardiac failure.

The patient has a very irregular pulse, as opposed to a basically regular pulse with an occasional irregularity (e.g. extrasystoles) or recurring irregular patterns (e.g. Wenckebach block). The irregular nature of the pulse in atrial fibrillation is maintained during exercise.

The ECG shows fine oscillations of the baseline (so-called fibrillation or φ waves) and no clear P waves. The QRS rhythm is rapid and irregular. Untreated, the ventricular rate is usually 120–180 per minute, but it slows with treatment (Fig. 13.40d, e and f).

Management

When atrial fibrillation is due to an acute precipitating event such as alcohol toxicity, chest infection or hyperthyroidism, the provoking cause should be treated. Strategies for the acute management of AF are ventricular rate control or cardioversion (± anticoagulation). Ventricular rate control is achieved by drugs which block the AV node (see below), while the cardioversion is achieved electrically by DC shock (see p. 733) or medically either by intravenous infusion of an anti-arrhythmic

drug such as a class Ic or a class III agent or by taking an oral agent previously tested in hospital and found to be safe in a particular patient ('pill-in-pocket' approach).

The choice depends upon:

- How well the arrhythmia is tolerated (is cardioversion urgent?).
- Whether anticoagulation is required before considering elective cardioversion (anticoagulants are used to minimize the excess risk of thromboembolism associated with cardioversion unless AF is of less than 1–2 days' duration). Transoesophageal echocardiography is being used to document the presence or not of atrial thrombus as a guide to the necessity of anticoagulation.
- Whether spontaneous cardioversion is likely (previous history? reversible cause?).

In general, each patient deserves at least one cardioversion attempt.

Conversion to sinus rhythm can be achieved by electrical DC cardioversion 200 J, then 2 × 360 J (see p. 733) in about 80% of patients. Biphasic waveform defibrillation is more effective than conventional (monophasic) defibrillation and in future biphasic defibrillators should

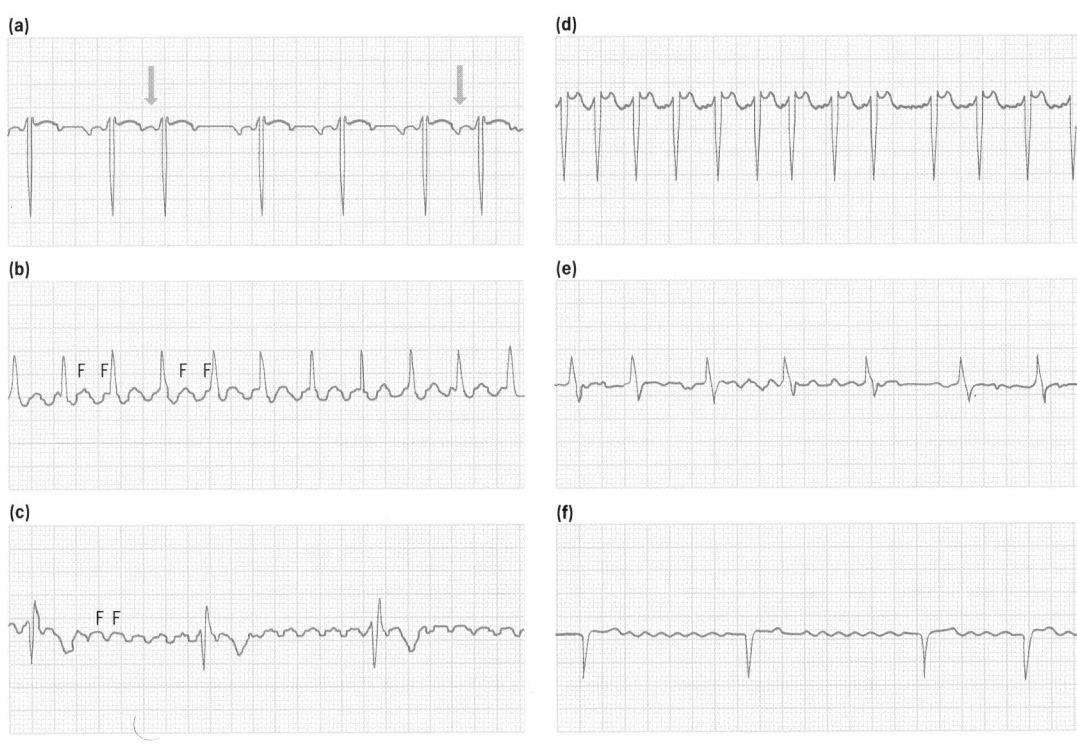

Fig. 13.40 **ECGs of a variety of atrial arrhythmias. (a) Atrial premature beats** (arrows). The premature P wave is different from the sinus P wave and conducts to the ventricle with a slightly prolonged PR interval.
(b) Atrial flutter. Some flutter waves are marked with an F. In this case the flutter frequency is 270 per minute. Every second flutter wave is transmitted to the ventricles, and the ventricular rate is therefore 135 per minute.
(c) Atrial flutter at a frequency of 305 per minute. The ventricular rate is approximately 38 per minute. Therefore, only one in eight flutter waves is transmitted to the ventricles.
(d) Irregular ventricular response. This is typical of rapidly conducted atrial fibrillation.
(e) Moderate conduction of atrial fibrillation. The underlying baseline undulations can now be appreciated.
(f) So-called 'slow' atrial fibrillation. The ventricular response rate is slow and the underlying atrial fibrillation is seen as minor fluctuations of the baseline.

become commonplace. Patients are anticoagulated for 4 weeks before cardioversion.

Two strategies are available for the long-term management of atrial fibrillation:

- 'maintenance of sinus rhythm' (antiarrhythmic drugs plus DC cardioversion)
- 'rate control plus anticoagulation' (AV nodal slowing agents plus warfarin).

Which strategy to adopt needs to be assessed for each individual patient. Factors to consider include the likelihood of maintaining sinus rhythm and the safety/ tolerability of antiarrhythmic drugs in a particular patient. Recurrent paroxysms may be prevented by oral medication. In general, class Ic agents are employed in patients with no significant heart disease and class III agents are preferred in patients with significant structural heart disease. Younger patients with lone paroxysmal atrial fibrillation should be carefully assessed to rule out a single atrial ectopic focus triggering atrial fibrillation. This form of atrial fibrillation can be effectively cured by catheter ablation.

If the arrhythmia is persistent and cannot be converted to sinus rhythm or if sinus rhythm cannot be maintained, AV nodal blocking drugs should be used to control the ventricular response rate. This should generally be below 90 b.p.m. at rest and patients should be able to perform reasonable levels of exercise without excessive tachycardia. This is usually achieved by a combination of beta-blockers, calcium-channel blockers and digoxin. However, beta-blockers and verapamil are commonly required to control the ventricular response rate during activity. Patients with poor rate control despite optimal medical therapy should be considered for AV node ablation and pacemaker implantation ('ablate and pace' strategy). These patients usually experience a marked symptomatic improvement but because of the ongoing risk of thromboembolism require life-long anticoagulation.

Anticoagulation (target INR 2.0–3.0)

This is indicated in patients with atrial fibrillation and one of the following major or two of the moderate risk factors:

Major risk factors
- Prosthetic heart valve
- Rheumatic mitral valve disease
- Prior history of CVA/TIA
- Age >75 years
- Hypertension
- Coronary artery disease with poor LV function.

Moderate risk factors
- Age 65–75 years
- Coronary artery disease but normal LV function
- Diabetes mellitus.

In addition, other features, e.g. left atrial enlargement, LV dysfunction of any cause, evidence of atrial thrombus or a reduced atrial appendage emptying velocity, also encourage anticoagulation with warfarin.

In most other patients aspirin is prescribed. Young patients (< 65 years) with no heart disease (lone AF) usually require no thromboembolic prophylaxis.

Atrial flutter

This is a rhythm disturbance that is usually associated with structural heart disease. The atrial rate is usually around 300 per minute. Symptoms are largely related to the degree of AV block. Most often, every second flutter beat conducts, giving a ventricular rate of 150 per minute. Occasionally, every beat conducts, producing a heart rate of 300 b.p.m. More often, especially when patients are receiving treatment, AV conduction block reduces the heart rate to approximately 75 b.p.m.

The ECG shows regular sawtooth-like atrial flutter waves (F waves) between QRST complexes (Fig. 13.40b and c). If F waves are not clearly visible, it is worth accentuating them by slowing AV conduction by carotid sinus massage or by the administration of AV nodal blocking drugs such as adenosine or verapamil.

Treatment of a symptomatic acute paroxysm is electrical cardioversion Patient who have been in atrial flutter more than 1–2 days should be treated in a similar manner to patients with atrial fibrillation and anticoagulated for 4 weeks prior to cardioversion. Recurrent paroxysms may be prevented by oral medication. In general, class Ic agents are employed in patients with no significant heart disease and class III agents are preferred in patients with significant structural heart disease. AV nodal blocking may be used to control the ventricular rate if the arrhythmia persists. However, the treatment of choice for patients with recurrent atrial flutter is radiofrequency catheter ablation (see p. 753). This technique offers patients whose only arrhythmia is typical atrial flutter an almost certain chance of a cure.

Atrial tachycardia

This is an uncommon arrhythmia. It may present as paroxysmal tachycardia, incessant tachycardia or as atrial tachycardia with AV block. Most are associated with heart disease, but incessant atrial tachycardia may occur in young children with no obvious heart disease. Atrial tachycardia with block is often a result of digitalis poisoning.

Figure 13.41 demonstrates an atrial tachycardia at an atrial rate of 150 per minute. The P waves are abnormally shaped and occur in front of the QRS complexes. Carotid sinus massage may increase AV block during tachycardia thereby facilitating the diagnosis but does not usually terminate the arrhythmia. Treatment options include cardioversion, antiarrhythmic drug therapy to maintain sinus rhythm, AV nodal

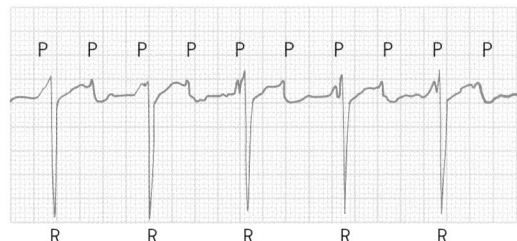

Fig. 13.41 **Atrial tachycardia with second-degree atrioventricular block.** Note the fast atrial (P wave) rate of 150 per minute and the slower ventricular (R wave) rate of 75 per minute. This arrhythmia is most commonly due to digoxin toxicity.

Table 13.13

ECG distinction between supraventricular tachycardia (SVT) with bundle branch block and ventricular tachycardia (VT)

VT is more likely than SVT with bundle branch block when there is:

- a very broad QRS (> 0.14 s)
- atrioventricular dissociation
- a bifid, upright QRS with a taller first peak in V_1
- a deep S wave in V_6
- a concordant (same polarity) QRS direction in all chest leads (V_1–V_6)

slowing agents to control rate and in selected cases radiofrequency catheter ablation.

Atrial ectopic beats

These often cause no symptoms although they may be sensed as an irregularity or heaviness of the heartbeat. On the ECG they appear as early and abnormal P waves, and are usually, but not always, followed by normal QRS complexes (see Fig. 13.40a). Treatment is not normally required unless the ectopic beats provoke more significant arrhythmias, when beta-blockade may be effective.

Ventricular tachyarrhythmias

Ventricular tachyarrhythmias can be considered under the following headings:

- life-threatening ventricular tachyarrhythmias
- torsades de pointes
- normal heart ventricular tachycardias
- non-sustained ventricular tachycardia
- ventricular premature beats.

Life-threatening ventricular tachyarrhythmias

Sustained ventricular tachycardia and ventricular fibrillation with haemodynamic instability (e.g. syncope, hypotension) are life-threatening ventricular tachyarrhythmias.

Sustained ventricular tachycardia

Sustained ventricular tachycardia (> 30 s) often results in presyncope (dizziness), syncope, hypotension and cardiac arrest, although it may be remarkably well tolerated in some patients. Examination reveals a pulse rate typically between 120–220 b.p.m. Usually there are clinical signs of atrioventricular dissociation (i.e. intermittent cannon *a* waves in the neck (p. 712) and variable intensity of the first heart sound).

The ECG shows a rapid ventricular rhythm with broad (often 0.14 s or more), abnormal QRS complexes. AV dissociation may result in visible P waves which appear to march through the tachycardia, capture beats (intermittent narrow QRS complex owing to normal ventricular activation via the AV node and conducting system) and fusion beats (intermediate between ventricular tachycardia beat and capture beat). Supraventricular tachycardia with bundle branch block may resemble ventricular tachycardia on the ECG. However, if a broad complex tachycardia is due to SVT with either right or left bundle branch block, then the QRS morphology should resemble a typical LBBB or RBBB pattern (Figs 13.37 and 13.87). Other ECG criteria to differentiate VT from SVT with aberrancy are indicated in Table 13.13. Eighty per cent of all broad complex tachycardias are due to ventricular tachycardia and the proportion is even higher in patients with structural heart disease. Therefore, in all cases of doubt, ventricular tachycardia should be diagnosed.

Treatment may be urgent depending on the haemodynamic situation. If the patient is haemodynamically compromised (e.g. hypotensive or pulmonary oedema) emergency DC cardioversion may be required. On the other hand, if the blood pressure and cardiac output are well maintained, intravenous therapy with class I drugs or amiodarone is usually advised. First-line drug treatment consists of lidocaine (lignocaine) (50–100 mg i.v. over 5 minutes) followed by a lidocaine infusion (2–4 mg i.v. per minute). DC cardioversion may be necessary if medical therapy is unsuccessful.

Ventricular fibrillation

This is very rapid and irregular ventricular activation with no mechanical effect. The patient is pulseless and becomes rapidly unconscious, and respiration ceases (cardiac arrest). The ECG shows shapeless, rapid oscillations and there is no hint of organized complexes (Fig. 13.42). It is usually provoked by a ventricular ectopic beat. Ventricular fibrillation rarely reverses spontaneously. The only effective treatment is electrical defibrillation. Basic and advanced cardiac life support is needed (see p. 730).

If the attack of ventricular fibrillation occurs during the first day or two of an acute myocardial infarction, it is probable that prophylactic therapy will be unnecessary. If the ventricular fibrillation was not related to an acute infarction the long-term risk of recurrent cardiac arrest and sudden death is high.

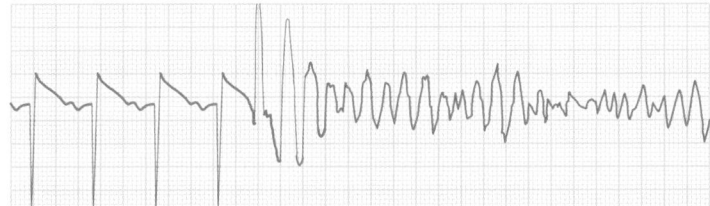

Fig. 13.42 **Four beats of sinus rhythm followed by a ventricular ectopic beat that initiates ventricular fibrillation.** The ST segment during sinus rhythm is elevated owing to acute myocardial infarction in this case.

Long-term management. Survivors of these tachycardias are, in the absence of an identifiable reversible cause (e.g. acute myocardial infarction, severe metabolic disturbance), at high risk of sudden death. Implantable cardioverter–defibrillators are now accepted as first-line therapy in the management of these patients (see p. 753).

Torsades de pointes

Torsades de pointes arises when ventricular repolarization (QT interval) is greatly prolonged (long QT syndrome). The causes of long QT syndrome and torsades de pointes are listed in Table 13.14.

Congenital long QT syndrome may (Jervell–Lange–Nielsen syndrome) or may not (Romano–Ward syndrome) be associated with congenital deafness. QT prolongation and torsades de pointes is usually precipitated by increased adrenergic drive. In contrast, in acquired long QT syndrome, QT prolongation and torsades de pointes is usually provoked by bradycardia.

Torsades de pointes causes palpitations and syncope but usually terminates spontaneously. It may, however, degenerate to ventricular fibrillation resulting in sudden death. It is characterized on the ECG by rapid, irregular, sharp complexes that continuously change from an upright to an inverted position (Fig. 13.43a). Between spells of tachycardia or immediately preceding the onset of tachycardia the ECG shows a prolonged QT

Table 13.14

Causes of long QT syndrome and torsades de pointes tachycardia

Congenital syndromes
Jervell–Lange–Nielsen (autosomal recessive)
Romano–Ward (autosomal dominant)

Electrolyte abnormalities
Hypokalaemia
Hypomagnesaemia
Hypocalcaemia

Drugs
Quinidine (and other class Ia antiarrhythmic drugs)
Sotalol (and other class III antiarrhythmic drugs)
Amitriptyline (and other tricyclic antidepressants)
Chlorpromazine (and other phenothiazine drugs)
Terfenadine and astemizole
Erythromycin and the macrolides
Cisapride (withdrawn in the UK)

Poisons
Organophosphate insecticides

Miscellaneous
Bradycardia
Mitral valve prolapse
Acute myocardial infarction
Prolonged fasting and liquid protein diets (long term)
Central nervous system diseases e.g. dystrophia myotonica

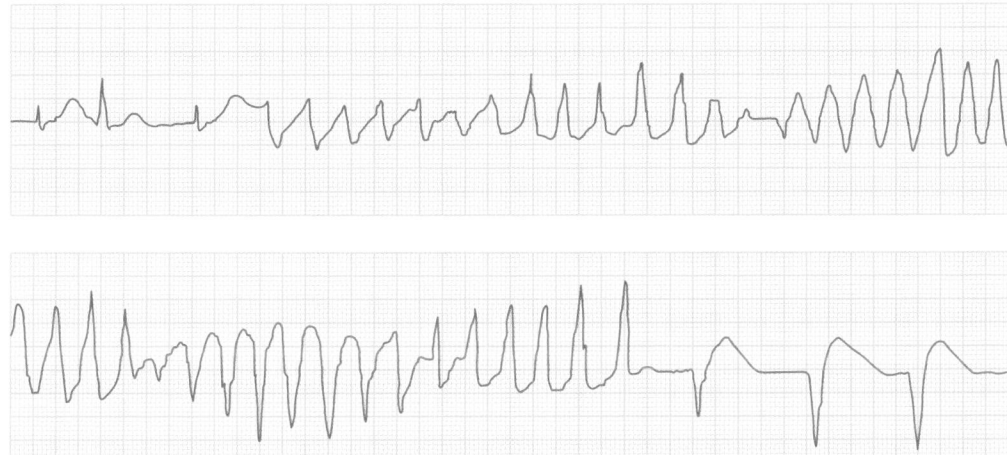

Fig. 13.43 **(a) An ECG demonstrating a supraventricular rhythm** with a long QT interval giving way to atypical ventricular tachycardia (torsades de pointes). The tachycardia is short-lived and is followed by a brief period of idioventricular rhythm.

interval; the corrected QT (see Table 13.6) is equal to or greater than 0.44 s. Figure 13.43b shows a further example of a prolonged QT interval. Acute management is as follows:

- Any electrolyte disturbance is corrected.
- Causative drugs are stopped.
- The heart rate is maintained with atrial or ventricular pacing.
- Intravenous isoprenaline may be effective when QT prolongation is acquired. (Isoprenaline is contraindicated for congenital long QT syndrome.)

Long-term management of acquired long QT syndrome involves avoidance of all drugs known to prolong the QT interval. Congenital long QT syndrome is generally treated by beta-blockade, left cardiac sympathetic denervation, and pacemaker therapy. Patients who remain symptomatic despite conventional therapy and those with a strong family history of sudden death should be considered for implantable defibrillator therapy. The molecular biology of the congenital long QT syndromes has been shown to be heterogenous; a number of mutations in genes coding for potassium or sodium channels have been identified and linked to several chromosomes. The different mutations appear to correlate with different phenotypes and it is likely to be possible to improve therapy for the congenital long QT syndrome on the basis of identification of the mutation involved.

Normal heart ventricular tachycardia

Monomorphic ventricular tachycardia in patients with structurally normal hearts (idiopathic VT) is usually a benign condition with an excellent long-term prognosis.

Normal heart VT either arises from the right ventricular outflow tract or from the left ventricular septum. In symptomatic patients radiofrequency catheter ablation is highly effective, resulting in a cure in >90% cases.

Non-sustained ventricular tachycardia

Non-sustained ventricular tachycardia (NSVT) is defined as ventricular tachycardia, which is ≥3 consecutive beats but lasts <30 s. NSVT in patients with normal hearts usually does not require treatment. In patients with structural heart disease it is an independent risk factor for cardiac mortality. However, NSVT is documented in up to 60% of patients with more advanced heart failure and is associated more with an overall risk of death than with a risk of sudden cardiac death. Beta-blocker therapy is a safe initial drug choice for symptom relief in most patients. In a select group of patients with prior myocardial infarction, ejection fraction ≤35%, non-sustained ventricular tachycardia and inducible, sustained VT/VF on invasive electrophysiological testing, therapy with an implantable defibrillator has been shown to improve survival compared to conventional medical therapy. Whether more NSVT patients should have prophylactic antiarrhythmic therapy to prevent sudden death awaits the results of ongoing clinical trials.

Ventricular premature beats

These may be uncomfortable, especially when frequent. The patient complains of extra beats, missed beats or heavy beats because it may be the premature beat, the post-ectopic pause or the next sinus beat that is noticed by the patient. The pulse is irregular owing to the premature beats. Some early beats may not be felt at

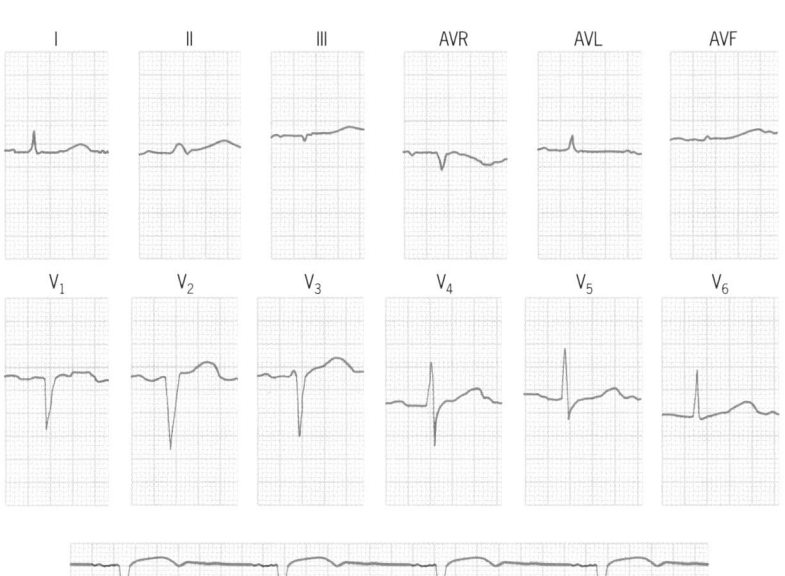

Fig. 13.43 **(b) A 12-lead ECG from an 11-year-old child with a history of syncope,** demonstrating sinus bradycardia with a long QT interval (560 ms). The ECG is typical of a form of hereditary long-QT syndrome.

the wrist. When a premature beat occurs regularly after every normal beat, 'pulsus bigeminus' may occur.

These premature beats (Fig. 13.44) have a broad (>0.12 s) and bizarre QRS complex because they arise from an abnormal (ectopic) site in the ventricular myocardium. Following a premature beat there is usually a complete compensatory pause because the AV node or ventricle is refractory to the next sinus impulse. Early 'R-on-T' ventricular premature beats (occurring simultaneously with the upstroke or peak of the T wave of the previous beat) may induce ventricular fibrillation, particularly in patients following myocardial infarction.

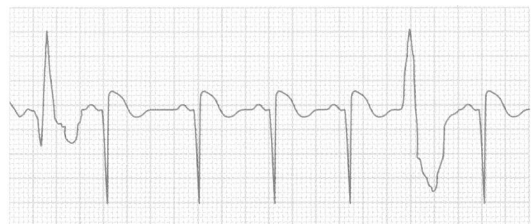

(a) Two ventricular ectopic beats of different morphology (multimorphological).

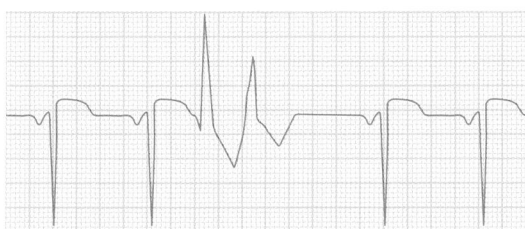

(b) Two ventricular premature beats (VPBs) occurring one after the other (a pair or couplet of VPBs).

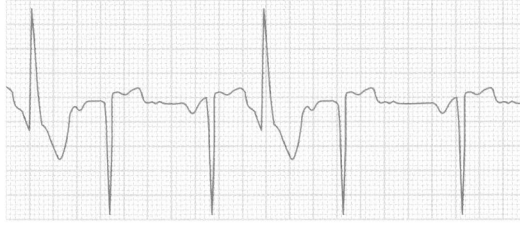

(c) Frequently repetitive ventricular ectopic activity of a single morphology.

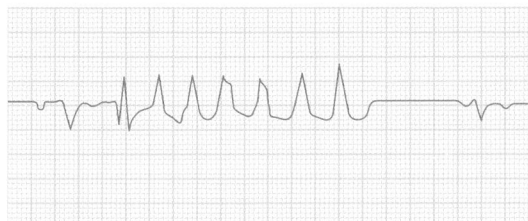

(d) Brief run of ventricular tachycardia (non-sustained ventricular tachycardia) that follows previous ectopic activity.

Fig. 13.44 Varieties of ventricular ectopic activity.

Ventricular premature beats are usually only treated if symptomatic. Usually simple measures such as beta-blocker therapy are all that is required.

Long-term management of cardiac tachyarrhythmias

Options for the long-term management of cardiac tachyarrhythmias include:

- antiarrhythmic drug therapy
- ablation therapy
- device therapy.

To determine the optimal strategy for a given patient the following questions must be addressed:

- Is the principal aim of treatment symptom relief or prevention of sudden death?
- Is maintaining sinus rhythm or controlling ventricular rates the treatment goal?

Commonly employed treatment strategies for the management of specific tachyarrhythmias are outlined in Table 13.15.

Antiarrhythmic drugs

Drugs that modify the rhythm and conduction of the heart are used to treat cardiac arrhythmias. Antiarrhythmic drugs may aggravate or produce arrhythmias (proarrhythmia) and they may also depress ventricular contractility and must therefore be used with caution. They are classified according to their effect on the action potential (Vaughan Williams' classification; Fig. 13.45

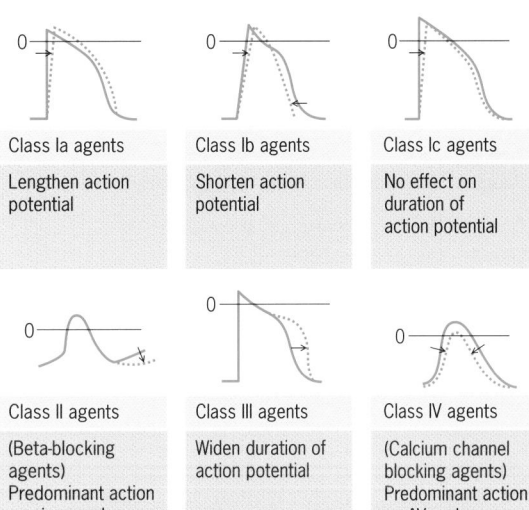

Fig. 13.45 Vaughan Williams' classification of antiarrhythmic drugs based on their effect on cardiac action potentials. 0, 0 mV. The dotted curves indicate the effects of the drugs.

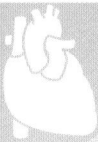

Table 13.15
Long-term management of tachyarrhythmias

Tachycardia	Management aims	Management strategies
AV node re-entry tachycardia (AVNRT)	Relieve symptoms	AV-node-blocking agents Catheter ablation Class Ic or class III
AV reciprocating tachycardia (AVRT)	Relieve symptoms	AV-node-blocking agents Catheter ablation Class Ic or class III
Wolff–Parkinson–White (WPW) syndrome	Relieve symptoms Prevent sudden death (esp. if documented pre-excited atrial fibrillation)	Catheter ablation Class Ic or class III

Atrial fibrillation	Relieve symptoms
	Prevent thromboembolic complications
	Prevent worsening heart failure due to poor rate control
		Maintenance of sinus rhythm:
		    Class Ic or class III ± cardioversion
		    Catheter ablation of ectopic focus (select cases only)
		Rate control plus anticoagulation:
		    AV-node-slowing agents
		    AV node ablation plus pacemaker

Atrial flutter	Relieve symptoms Prevent thromboembolic complications Prevent worsening heart failure due to poor rate control	Class Ic or class III Catheter ablation AV-node-blocking agents
Atrial tachycardia	Relieve symptoms Prevent thromboembolic complications Prevent worsening heart failure due to poor rate control	Class Ic or class III Catheter ablation (select cases only) AV-node-blocking agents
Life-threatening ventricular tachyarrhythmias	Prevent sudden death	Implantable cardioverter defibrillator (ICD) Amiodarone
Congenital long QT	Prevent sudden death	Beta-blockers ± pacemaker ICD Left cardiac sympathetic denervation
Acquired long QT	Prevent sudden death	Avoidance of all QT-prolonging drugs
Normal heart ventricular tachycardias	Relieve symptoms	Beta-blockers, calcium-channel blockers Catheter ablation
Non-sustained VT (NSVT)	Relieve symptoms Prevent sudden death in certain situations	Beta-blockers Class Ic or class III ICD in clearly defined subgroups Catheter ablation if NSVT is a form of ablatable normal heart VT

Table 13.16
Vaughan Williams' classification of antiarrhythmic drugs

Class Ia	Quinidine, procainamide, disopyramide
Class Ib	Lidocaine, mexiletine
Class Ic	Flecainide, propafenone
Class II	β-Adrenergic blocking drugs
Class III	Amiodarone, sotalol, bretylium, ibutilide, dofetilide
Class IV	Verapamil, diltiazem
(Other	Adenosine, digoxin)

and Table 13.16). Another clinical classification is based on the part of the heart that is affected by the anti-arrhythmic drug (Fig. 13.46).

The features of the major antiarrhythmic drugs are given in Table 13.17.

Class I drugs

These are membrane-depressant drugs that reduce the rate of entry of sodium into the cell (sodium-channel blockers). They may slow conduction, delay recovery or reduce the spontaneous discharge rate of myocardial cells. Class Ia drugs (e.g. disopyramide) lengthen the action potential, Class Ib drugs (e.g. lidocaine (ligno-caine)) shorten the action potential, and Class Ic (flecainide, propafenone) do not affect the duration of the action potential. Class I agents have been found to increase mortality compared to placebo in post-myocardial infarction patients with ventricular ectopy (CAST trials – Class Ic agents) and in patients treated for atrial fibrillation (Class Ia agent, quinidine). In view of this, class Ic agents such as flecainide and indeed all other class I drugs should be reserved for patients who do not have significant coronary artery disease, left

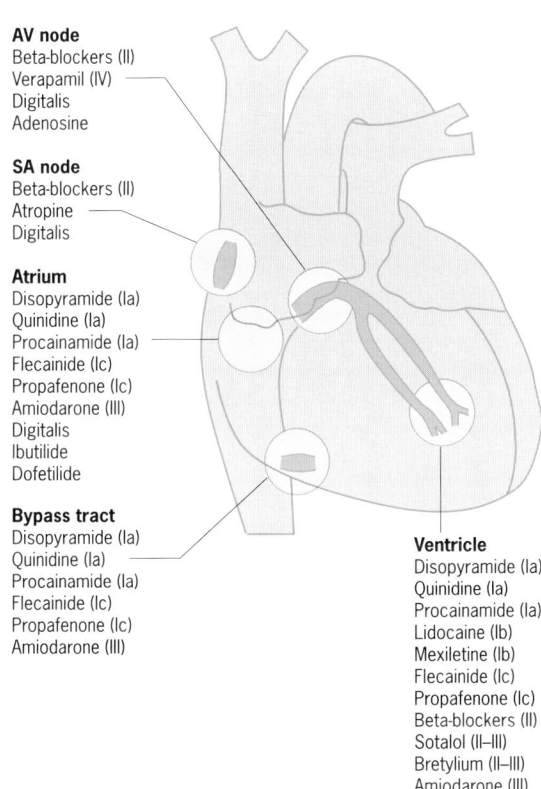

AV node
Beta-blockers (II)
Verapamil (IV)
Digitalis
Adenosine

SA node
Beta-blockers (II)
Atropine
Digitalis

Atrium
Disopyramide (Ia)
Quinidine (Ia)
Procainamide (Ia)
Flecainide (Ic)
Propafenone (Ic)
Amiodarone (III)
Digitalis
Ibutilide
Dofetilide

Bypass tract
Disopyramide (Ia)
Quinidine (Ia)
Procainamide (Ia)
Flecainide (Ic)
Propafenone (Ic)
Amiodarone (III)

Ventricle
Disopyramide (Ia)
Quinidine (Ia)
Procainamide (Ia)
Lidocaine (Ib)
Mexiletine (Ib)
Flecainide (Ic)
Propafenone (Ic)
Beta-blockers (II)
Sotalol (II–III)
Bretylium (II–III)
Amiodarone (III)

Fig. 13.46 **Drugs that affect various parts of the heart.**
The Vaughan Williams' class is given in parentheses.

ventricular dysfunction, or other forms of significant structural hearts disease.

Class II drugs

These antisympathetic drugs prevent the effects of catecholamines on the action potential. Most are β-adrenergic antagonists. Cardioselective beta-blockers (β$_1$) include metoprolol, atenolol and acebutalol. Beta-blockers suppress AV node conduction, which may be effective in preventing attacks of junctional tachycardia, and may help to control ventricular rates during paroxysms of other forms of SVT (e.g. atrial fibrillation). In general beta-blockers are anti-ischaemic, and anti-adrenergic and have proven beneficial effects in patients post-myocardial infarction (by preventing ventricular fibrillation) and in patients with congestive heart failure. It is therefore advisable to consider beta-blocker therapy either alone or in combination with other antiarrhythmic drugs in patients with symptomatic tachyarrhythmias, particularly in patients with coronary artery disease.

Class III drugs

These prolong the action potential and do not affect sodium transport through the membrane. The drugs in this class are amiodarone and sotalol. Sotalol is also a beta-blocker.

Some drugs, such as ibutilide and dofetilide, are only available in some countries. Sotalol may result in acquired long QT syndrome and torsades de pointes. The risk of torsades is increased in the setting of hypokalaemia and particular care should be taken in patients taking diuretic therapy. Amiodarone therapy in contrast to most other antiarrhythmic drugs carries a low risk of proarrhythmia in patients with significant structural heart disease. Because it has many toxic and potentially serious side-effects, patients need to be counselled prior to commencing amiodarone and monitored carefully at regular follow-up intervals. Dofetilide has been used to treat atrial fibrillation and flutter in patients with recent myocardial infarction and poor LV function.

Class IV drugs (see also Table 13.27)

The non-dihydropyridine calcium antagonists that reduce the plateau phase of the action potential are particularly effective at slowing conduction in nodal tissue. Verapamil and diltiazem are two drugs in this group. These drugs can prevent attacks of junctional tachycardia (AVNRT and AVRT) and may help to control ventricular rates during paroxysms of other forms of SVT (e.g. atrial fibrillation).

Drug therapy is commonly used for symptomatic relief in patients who do not have life-threatening tachyarrhythmias. Patient safety is the main factor determining the choice of antiarrhythmic therapy and proarrhythmic risks need to be carefully assessed prior to initiating therapy. As a generalization, class Ic agents are employed in patients with structurally normal hearts and class III agents are used in patients with structural heart disease. In order to administer antiarrhythmic agents as safely as possible it is helpful to be familiar with the different proarrhythmia mechanisms and their main predisposing risk factors (Table 13.18). Consideration of the proarrhythmic risk will help to determine which agent is safest and most appropriate, the level of monitoring required at the time of drug initiation, and whether a non-pharmacological option would carry less risk to the patient. Patients with structurally normal hearts and normal QT intervals, or with implantable defibrillators, are either at very low risk of proarrhythmia or are protected from the life-threatening consequences of proarrhythmic events, and in these patients it is possible to persevere with drug therapy until an efficacious, well-tolerated agent is identified.

Drug therapy in clinical practice

Drug therapy in many individuals does not result in complete abolition of the arrhythmia but is nevertheless successful if it results in substantially fewer and better-tolerated events. Antiarrhythmic drug therapy is usually efficacious in 70–90% of SVT patients. However, up to 50% of these patients have unwanted side-effects.

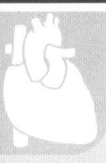

Table 13.17
Details of antiarrhythmic drugs. For class II drugs (beta-blockers) see Table 13.45. Adenosine 0.05–0.25 mg/kg (see p. 741) is given only intravenously

	Quinidine	Disopyramide	Lidocaine (lignocaine)	Mexiletine	Flecainide	Propafenone	Amiodarone	Sotalol	Verapamil	Diltiazem	Digoxin
Class	Ia	Ia	Ib	Ib	Ic	Ic	III	II/III	IV	IV	N/A
Daily dose	250–500 mg orally	100–250 mg × 3 orally	1–4 mg/min (50–150 mg i.v. loading dose)	400–800 mg orally loading, 150–300 mg maintenance	100 mg × 2 orally	150 mg × 3 300 mg × 2 or 300 mg × 3	200 mg × 1–2 orally	80–160 mg × 2–3 orally	0.1 mg/kg i.v. 40–160 mg × 3–4 orally	60–120 mg × 3–4 orally	0.25 mg × 1 orally
Protein binding	75%	40–90%	50–80%	70%	50%	85%	98%	<10%	90%	80%	25%
Half-life	6 hours	5 hours	1.5–2 hours	15 hours	18 hours	6 hours	50 days +	24 hours	6 hours	2–8 hours	36 hours
Plasma therapeutic range	2–5 µg/mL	3–6 µg/mL	2–6 µg/mL	0.5–2.0 µg/mL	0.2–0.8 µg/mL	0.2–1.5 µg/mL	0.2–5.0 µg/mL	0.3–1.5 µg/mL	0.1–0.3 µg/mL	0.02–0.16 µg/mL	1.3–2.6 nmol/L
Indication	AF PSVT VT VPBs WPW	AF PSVT VT VPBs WPW	VT/VF associated with myocardial infarction VPBs	VT especially after myocardial infarction	VT PSVT WPW	VT/VF PSVT WPW	VT/VF WPW PSVT AF	VT WPW PSVT	PSVT	PSVT	AF/AFL PSVT
Side-effects	Nausea Diarrhoea Rash Fever Cinchonism Syncope Blood dyscrasia	Hypotension Anticholinergic effects Dry mouth Urinary hesitancy Blurred vision Heart failure	Confusion Convulsions	Confusion Tremor Bradycardia Hypotension	Dizziness Visual disturbance Arrhythmogenesis	Light-headedness Unusual taste Headache Constipation Arrhythmogenesis	Corneal deposits Photosensitivity Skin pigmentation Thyroid disturbance Pulmonary alveolitis Nightmares Liver disease Neurological	Ventricular arrhythmias Bradycardia Heart failure Bronchospasm Hypotension	Nausea Vomiting Constipation Flushing Headache Bradycardia Fluid retention Hypotension	Nausea Vomiting Constipation Flushing Headache Bradycardia Fluid retention Hypotension	Nausea Anorexia Vomiting Visual disturbance Bradycardia Gynaecomastia

AF, atrial fibrillation; AFL, atrial flutter; N/A, not applicable; PSVT, paroxysmal supraventricular tachycardia; VF, ventricular fibrillation; VPBs, ventricular premature beats; VT, ventricular tachycardia; WPW, Wolff-Parkinson-White syndrome

Table 13.18
Proarrhythmia mechanisms and the predisposing risk factors

Proarrhythmia mechanism	Drug	Predisposing risk factors
Torsades de pointes	Class Ia (quinidine, procainamide, disopyramide) Sotalol 'Pure' class III (ibutilide, dofetilide)	Baseline QT prolongation Female gender Hypokalaemia/diuretic use Clinical heart failure Advanced structural heart disease Conversion of AF to sinus rhythm
Atrial flutter with 1 : 1 AV conduction and wide QRS complexes	Class I_a (quinidine, disopyramide) Class I_c (flecainide, propafenone)	Risk reduced by adding an AV-nodal-slowing agent
'Late' sudden death (arrhythmic mechanism not clearly defined)	Class I_c (flecainide) Quinidine	Myocardial ischaemia

Therefore in only one-third to one-half of all patients will a chosen agent be both effective and well tolerated and hence a satisfactory long-term option for the patient. In the remaining group of patients decisions regarding further therapy need to consider not only alternative drug options but also non-pharmacological options such as catheter ablation.

Catheter ablation

Radiofrequency catheter ablation is frequently employed in the management of symptomatic tachyarrhythmias. Ablations are performed by placing three or four electrode catheters into the heart chambers in order to record and pace from various sites. Pacing the atria or the ventricles is used to trigger the tachycardia and to study the tachycardia mechanism. Successful ablation depends on accurate identification of either the site of origin of a focal tachycardia or of a critical component of a macro-reentry tachycardia. The following tachyarrhythmias can be readily ablated:

- AV node re-entry tachycardia (AVNRT)
- accessory-pathway-mediated tachycardias
- AV reciprocating tachycardia (AVRT)
- WPW syndrome
- normal heart VT
- atrial flutter
- atrial tachycardia.

Symptomatic patients with a pre-excited ECG because of accessory pathway conduction (WPW syndrome) are advised to undergo catheter ablation as first-line therapy owing to the risk of sudden death associated with this condition. This is especially the case in patients with pre-excited atrial fibrillation. Patients with accessory pathways that only conduct retrogradely from the ventricles to the atrium are not at increased risk of sudden death but experience symptoms due to AVRT. These patients are commonly offered an ablation procedure if simple measures such as AV nodal slowing agents fail to suppress tachycardia. The main risk associated with accessory pathway ablation is thromboembolism

in patients with left-sided accessory pathways. Similarly patients with AVNRT are routinely offered an ablation if AV nodal slowing agents are ineffective. Because of the proximity of the ablation site to the compact AV node, the risk of heart block associated with ablation of AVNRT is approximately 1%. The success rate for catheter ablation of AVNRT and accessory pathways is greater than 95%. Patients with normal hearts and documented ventricular tachycardia should be referred for specialist evaluation. Unlike VT in patients with structural heart disease, normal heart VT is not associated with increased risk of sudden death and is easily cured by catheter ablation. Catheter ablation is recommended in patients with atrial flutter that is not easily managed medically. Atrial tachycardia, especially in patients with structurally normal hearts, may also be cured by catheter ablation.

In atrial fibrillation, adequate control of ventricular rates is sometimes not possible despite optimal medical therapy. These patients experience a marked symptomatic improvement following AV node ablation and pacemaker implantation. Unlike other forms of catheter ablation this does not cure the arrhythmia; atrial fibrillation continues and anticoagulation is still required following ablation. In younger patients with structurally normal hearts atrial ectopic beats, which commonly arise from a focus situated in the pulmonary veins, may trigger atrial fibrillation. Catheter ablation of this ectopic focus may cure atrial fibrillation.

Implantable cardioverter–defibrillator (ICD)

Life-threatening ventricular arrhythmias (ventricular fibrillation or rapid ventricular tachycardia with hypotension) carry a mortality within 1 year of up to 40% The implantable cardioverter–defibrillator (ICD) recognizes ventricular tachycardia or fibrillation and automatically delivers pacing or a shock to the heart to cause cardioversion to sinus rhythm.

Modern ICDs are only a little larger than a pacemaker and may be implanted in a pectoral position (Fig. 13.47). The device may have leads to sense and pace both the

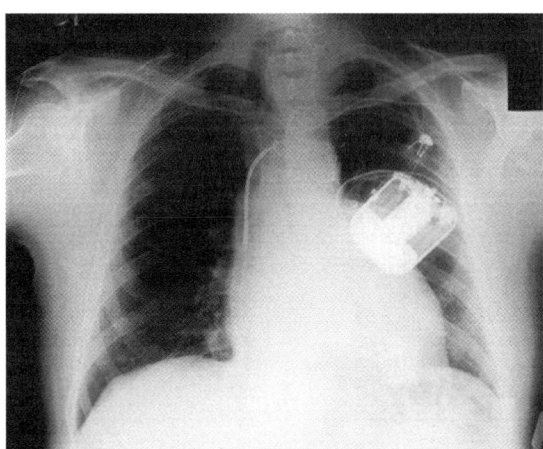

Fig. 13.47 PA X-ray of an 'ICD' in a left pectoral position with a single lead on which are mounted defibrillation electrodes in the superior vena cava and in the right ventricle.

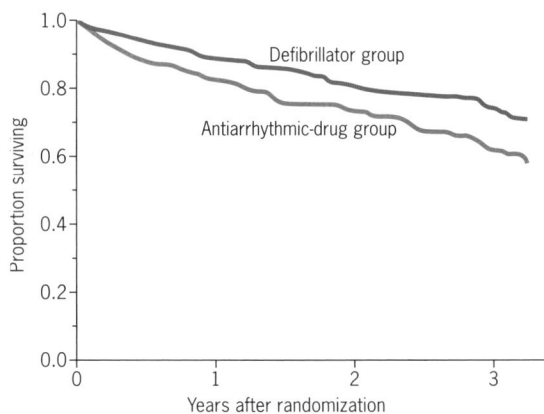

Fig. 13.48 Survival curves of the Multicentre Automatic Defibrillator Implantation Trial (MADIT) following myocardial infarction. Patients with left ventricular ejection fractions of ≤0.35 and documented asymptomatic non-sustained ventricular tachycardia and inducible ventricular tachycardia were randomized to receive an ICD or conventional therapy.

right atrium and ventricle, and the lithium batteries employed are able to provide energy for over 100 shocks each of around 30 J. When an arrhythmia develops that requires treatment by a shock, the device takes up to 15 s to recognize the arrhythmia and charge its capacitors. It then delivers the defibrillating discharge that may be painful if the patient is conscious. However, ventricular tachycardia may often be terminated by overdrive pacing the heart, which is painless.

The ICD is superior to all other treatment options at preventing sudden cardiac death. The use of this device has cut the sudden death rate in patients with a history of serious ventricular arrhythmias to approximately 2% per year. However, the majority of these patients have significant structural heart disease and overall cardiac mortality due to progressive heart failure remains high. Large multicentred prospective trials such as the Antiarrhythmics (amiodarone) Versus Implantable Defibrillator (AVID) trial have proven that implantable defibrillators improve overall survival in patients who have experienced an episode of life-threatening ventricular tachyarrhythmia (Fig. 13.48). As a result ICDs are now first-line therapy in the secondary prevention of sudden death. In patients with cardiomyopathy (dilated or ischaemic) and relatively well-preserved left ventricular function (EF >35%) antiarrhythmic drugs such as amiodarone may be as effective as an ICD.

Implantable cardioverter–defibrillators are also employed in the primary prevention of sudden cardiac death. The chances of surviving an out of hospital cardiac arrest are as low as 10%. Therefore selected patients who have never experienced a spontaneous episode of life-threatening ventricular tachyarrhythmia but who are assessed to be at high risk of sudden death are advised to undergo ICD implantation. One such group is patients with coronary artery disease; significant impairment of left ventricular function, spontaneous

non-sustained ventricular tachycardia in whom sustained ventricular tachycardia was induced by pacing the heart during an electrophysiological study.

FURTHER READING

Ackerman MS, Clapham DE (1997) Ion channels: basic science and chemical disease. *New England Journal of Medicine* **336**: 1575–1580.

Antiarrhythmics Versus Implantable Defibrillators (AVID) Investigators (1997) A comparison of antiarrhythmic-drug therapy with implantable defibrillators in patients resuscitated from near-fatal ventricular arrhythmias. *New England Journal of Medicine* **337**: 1576–1583.

Falk RH (2001) Atrial fibrillation. *New England Journal of Medicine* **344**: 1067–1078.

Huikuri HV, Castellanos A, Myerburg RJ (2001) Sudden death due to cardiac arrhythmias. *New England Journal of Medicine* **345**: 1473–1482.

Mangrum JM, DiMarco JP (2000) The evaluation and management of bradycardia. *New England Journal of Medicine* **342**: 703–709.

Cardiac failure

Cardiac failure occurs when, despite normal venous pressures, the heart is unable to maintain sufficient cardiac output to meet the demands of the body.

The incidence of heart failure increases with advancing age. The average annual incidence is 2–4% between 35 and 64 years, and 10% in patients over 65 years. The prognosis of heart failure has improved over the past 10 years, but the mortality rate is still high with approximately 50% of patients dead at 5 years. Heart failure accounts for 5% of admissions to hospital medical wards with over 100 000 each year in the UK. The cost of managing heart failure in the UK exceeds £600 million. Coronary artery disease is the commonest cause of heart failure in western countries.

The causes of heart failure include:

- *myocardial dysfunction* (e.g. ischaemic heart disease, hypertension, alcohol, cardiomyopathy)
- *volume overload* (e.g. valvular regurgitation – aortic or mitral)
- *obstruction to outflow* (e.g. aortic stenosis)
- *obligatory high output* (e.g. anaemia, thyrotoxicosis, Paget's disease, beriberi, systemic-to-pulmonary shunts)
- *compromised ventricular filling* (e.g. constrictive pericarditis, pericardial tamponade, restrictive cardiomyopathy)
- *altered rhythm* (e.g. atrial fibrillation).

Factors aggravating or precipitating heart failure
Any factor that increases myocardial work may aggravate existing heart failure or initiate failure. These factors must be carefully considered in patients who present with heart failure. The most common are arrhythmias, anaemia, thyrotoxicosis, pregnancy, infective endocarditis, pulmonary infection, change of heart failure therapy including poor compliance. Readmission rates range from 29–47% within 3–6 months of hospital discharge.

Pathophysiology

When the heart fails, considerable changes occur to the heart and peripheral vascular system in response to the haemodynamic changes associated with heart failure (Table 13.19). These physiological changes are compensatory and maintain cardiac output and peripheral perfusion. However, as heart failure progresses, these mechanisms are overwhelmed and become pathophysiological. The development of pathological peripheral vasoconstriction and sodium retention in heart failure by activation of the renin–angiotensin–aldosterone system, is a loss of beneficial compensatory mechanisms and represents cardiac decompensation. Factors involved are venous return, outflow resistance, contractility of the myocardium, and salt and water retention.

Table 13.19
Pathophysiological changes in heart failure

Ventricular dilatation
Myocyte hypertrophy
Increased collagen synthesis
Altered myosin gene expression
Altered sarcoplasmic Ca^{2+}-ATPase density
Increased ANP secretion
Salt and water retention
Sympathetic stimulation
Peripheral vasoconstriction

Venous return (preload)
In the intact heart, myocardial failure leads to a reduction of the volume of blood ejected with each heartbeat and an increase in the volume of blood remaining after systole. This increased diastolic volume stretches the myocardial fibres and, as Starling's law of the heart would suggest, myocardial contraction is restored. However, the failing myocardium results in depression of the ventricular function curve (cardiac output plotted against the ventricular diastolic volume) (see Fig. 13.3, p. 702).

Mild myocardial depression is not associated with a reduction in cardiac output because it is maintained by an increase in venous pressure (and hence diastolic volume). However, the proportion of blood ejected with each heartbeat (ejection fraction) is reduced early in heart failure. Sinus tachycardia also ensures that any reduction of stroke volume is compensated for by the increase in heart rate; cardiac output (stroke volume × heart rate) is therefore maintained.

When there is more severe myocardial dysfunction, cardiac output can be maintained only by a large increase in venous pressure and/or marked sinus tachycardia. The increased venous pressure contributes to the development of dyspnoea, owing to the accumulation of interstitial and alveolar fluid, and to the occurrence of hepatic enlargement, ascites and dependent oedema, due to increased systemic venous pressure. However, the cardiac output at rest may not be much depressed, but myocardial and haemodynamic reserve is so compromised that a normal increase in cardiac output cannot be produced by exercise.

In very severe heart failure the cardiac output at rest is depressed, despite high venous pressures. The inadequate cardiac output is redistributed to maintain perfusion of vital organs, such as the heart, brain and kidneys, at the expense of the skin and muscle.

Outflow resistance (afterload) (see Figs 15.3 and 15.4)
This is the load or resistance against which the ventricle contracts. It is formed by:

- pulmonary and systemic resistance
- physical characteristics of the vessel walls
- the volume of blood that is ejected.

An increase in afterload decreases the cardiac output. This results in a further increase of end-diastolic volume and dilatation of the ventricle itself, which further exacerbates the problem of afterload. This is expressed by Laplace's law: the tension of the myocardium (T) is proportional to the intraventricular pressure (P) multiplied by the radius of the ventricular chamber (R): i.e. $T \propto PR$.

Myocardial contractility (inotropic state)
The state of the myocardium also influences performance. The sympathetic nervous system is activated in heart failure via baroreceptors as an early compensatory mechanism, which provides inotropic support and

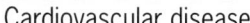
maintains cardiac output. Chronic sympathetic activation, however, has deleterious effects by further increasing neurohormonal activation and myocyte apoptosis. This is compensated by a downregulation of β-receptors. Increased contractility (positive inotropism) can result from increased sympathetic drive, and this is a normal part of the Frank–Starling relationship (see Fig. 13.3, p. 702). Conversely, myocardial depressants (e.g. hypoxia) decrease myocardial contractility (negative inotropism).

Salt and water retention

The increase in venous pressure that occurs when the ventricles fail leads to retention of salt and water and their accumulation in the interstitium, producing many of the physical signs of heart failure. Reduced cardiac output also leads to diminished renal perfusion, activating the renin–angiotensin system and enhancing salt and water retention (see p. 670, Fig. 12.3), which further increases venous pressure (Fig. 13.49). The retention of sodium is in part compensated by the action of circulating atrial natriuretic peptides (p. 592). These are short-chain peptides secreted by the atria in response to distension. These atrial peptides are potent vasodilators with natriuretic properties, and levels rise considerably in heart failure. The effect of their action may represent a beneficial, albeit inadequate, compensatory response tending to reduce cardiac load (preload and afterload) by vasodilatation and by enhancing sodium and water excretion. However, antidiuretic (vasopressin) is also increased in severe chronic heart failure contributing to hyponatraemia that is an ominous prognostic indicator in these patients.

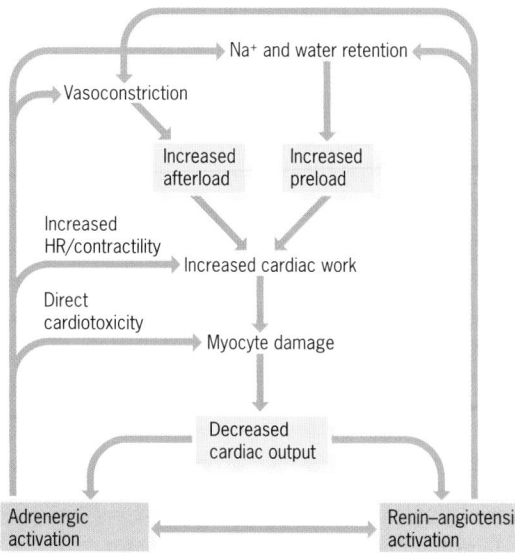

Fig. 13.49 **The compensatory physiological response to heart failure.** Chronic activation of the renin–angiotensin and adrenergic systems results in a 'vicious cycle' of cardiac deterioration that further exacerbates the physiological response.

The interaction of haemodynamic and neurohumoral factors in the progression of heart failure remains unclear. Increased ventricular wall stress promotes ventricular dilatation and further worsens contractile efficiency. In addition, prolonged activation of the sympathetic nervous and renin–angiotensin–aldosterone systems exert direct toxic effects on myocardial cells.

Myocardial remodelling in heart failure

Myocardial hypertrophy is one of the major adaptations to haemodynamic overload of the left ventricle. As cardiac myocytes are terminally differentiated, this occurs by an increase in myocyte size and the growth of non-myocyte components such as vascular smooth muscle cells and fibroblasts. Collagen synthesis may also be increased. These structural changes result in an increase in myocardial volume and mass, impaired systolic and diastolic function, and impaired coronary blood flow.

Changes in myocardial gene expression

Haemodynamic overload of the ventricle stimulates changes in cardiac contractile protein gene expression. The overall effect is to increase protein synthesis, but many proteins also switch to fetal and neonatal isoforms. Human myosin is composed of a pair of heavy chains and two pairs of light chains. Myosin heavy chains (MHC) exist in two isoforms, α and β, that have different contractile properties and ATPase activity. αα-MHC predominates in the atria and ββ-MHC in the ventricles. In animal models, pressure overload results in a shift from αα- to ββ-MHC in the atria, in parallel with atrial size. This results in reduction in atrial contractility but reduced energy demands. This shift is less significant in the human ventricle as the ββ-MHC isoform already predominates. Other genes affected in heart failure include those encoding Na^+–K^+-ATPase, Ca^{2+}-ATPase and $β_1$-adrenoceptors.

Abnormal calcium homeostasis

Calcium ion flux within myocytes plays a pivotal role in the regulation of contractile function. Excitation of the myocyte cell membrane causes the rapid entry of calcium into myocytes from the extracellular space via calcium channels. This triggers the release of intracellular calcium from the sarcoplasmic reticulum and initiates contraction (see Fig. 13.2). Relaxation results from the uptake and storage of calcium by the sarcoplasmic reticulum. In heart failure, there is a prolongation of the calcium current in association with prolongation of contraction and relaxation.

Apoptosis (see also p. 184)

Apoptosis (or 'programmed cell death') is the process by which cells self-destruct following the induction of endonucleases that degrade DNA. It is a normal feature in the developing fetus and in some adult tissues (e.g. thymus). Apoptosis has been demonstrated in animal models of ischaemic reperfusion, rapid ventricular pacing, mechanical stretch, and pressure overload. Apoptosis is associated with irreversible congestive heart failure, and the spiral of ventricular dysfunction, characteristic of heart failure, results from the initiation of apoptosis by cytokines, free radicals and other triggers.

Cardiac hormones

Atrial natriuretic peptide (ANP) is released from atrial myocytes in response to stretch. ANP induces diuresis, natriuresis, vasodilatation and suppression of the renin–angiotensin system. Levels of circulating ANP are increased in congestive cardiac failure and correlate with functional class, prognosis and haemodynamic state. The renal response to ANP is attenuated in heart failure, probably secondary to reduced renal perfusion, receptor downregulation, increased peptide breakdown, renal sympathetic activation, and excessive renin–angiotensin activity. *Brain natriuretic peptide* (so called because it was first discovered in brain) is predominantly secreted by the ventricles and has an action similar to ANP but it has greater diagnostic and prognostic value (p. 592). The therapeutic benefits of the natriuretic peptides have been investigated by administration of ANP and by the inhibition of the enzyme responsible for breakdown of the peptides (neutral endopeptidase – NEP). Initial results suggest that these drugs have a useful therapeutic role.

Endothelial function in heart failure

The endothelium has a central role in the regulation of vasomotor tone. In patients with heart failure, endothelium-dependent vasodilatation in peripheral blood vessels is impaired and may be one mechanism of exercise limitation. The cause of abnormal endothelial responsiveness relates to abnormal release of both nitric oxide and vasoconstrictor substances, such as endothelin (ET). The activity of nitric oxide, a potent vasodilator, is blunted in heart failure. ET secretion from a variety of tissues is stimulated by many factors, including hypoxia, catecholamines, angiotensin II and shear stress. The plasma concentration of ET is elevated in patients with heart failure, and levels correlate with the severity of haemodynamic disturbance. The major source of circulating ET in heart failure is the pulmonary vascular bed.

ET has many actions that potentially contribute to the pathophysiology of heart failure: vasoconstriction, sympathetic stimulation, renin–angiotensin system activation and left ventricular hypertrophy. Acute intravenous administration of endothelin antagonists improves haemodynamic abnormalities in patients with congestive cardiac failure, and oral endothelin antagonists are now being developed. Plasma concentrations of some cytokines, in particular TNF, are increased in patients with heart failure.

Clinical syndromes of heart failure

The terms 'biventricular' or 'congestive' heart failure are used variously but are best restricted to cases where right heart failure results from pre-existing left heart failure.

Biventricular cardiac failure is the most common manifestation of heart failure although it is clinically useful to divide heart failure into the syndromes of left and right cardiac failure, but it is rare for any part of the heart to fail in isolation. Chronic heart failure can be 'compensated' or 'decompensated'. In compensated heart failure symptoms are stable and overt features of fluid retention are absent. Decompensated heart failure refers to an acute or continuing deterioration. Causes, such as ischaemia, arrhythmia, infection and electrolyte disturbance, should be identified and reversed. The natural history of moderate heart failure involves increasingly frequent hospital admissions due to symptom exacerbation.

Left heart failure

Causes include:

- ischaemic heart disease (the most common cause)
- systemic hypertension (chronic or 'malignant')
- mitral and aortic valve disease
- cardiomyopathies.

Mitral stenosis causes left atrial hypertension and signs of left heart failure but does not itself cause failure of the left ventricle.

Symptoms and signs

Symptoms are predominantly fatigue, exertional dyspnoea, orthopnoea and paroxysmal nocturnal dyspnoea.

Physical signs are few and not prominent until a late stage or if ventricular failure is acute. Cardiomegaly is demonstrable with a displaced and often sustained apical impulse. Auscultation reveals a left ventricular third or fourth heart sound that, with tachycardia, is described as a gallop rhythm. Dilatation of the mitral annulus results in functional mitral regurgitation. Crackles are heard at the lung bases. In severe left heart failure the patient has pulmonary oedema (p. 765).

Right heart failure

This syndrome occurs in association with:

- left heart failure
- chronic lung disease (cor pulmonale)
- pulmonary embolism or pulmonary hypertension
- tricuspid valve disease
- pulmonary valve disease
- left-to-right shunts (e.g. atrial or ventricular septal defects)
- isolated right ventricular cardiomyopathy
- mitral valve disease with pulmonary hypertension.

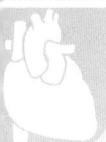

Symptoms and signs

Symptoms include fatigue, breathlessness, anorexia and nausea. They relate to distension and fluid accumulation in areas drained by the systemic veins. Physical signs are usually more prominent than the symptoms, with:

- jugular venous distension (± *v* waves of tricuspid regurgitation)
- tender smooth hepatic enlargement
- dependent pitting oedema
- development of free abdominal fluid (ascites)
- pleural transudates (commonly right-sided).

Dilatation of the right ventricle produces cardiomegaly and may give rise to functional tricuspid regurgitation. Tachycardia and a right ventricular third heart sound are usual.

Systolic versus diastolic heart failure

Systolic and diastolic dysfunction usually coexist.

Systolic ventricular dysfunction is most commonly due to coronary artery disease, usually following myocardial infarction. The left ventricle is usually dilated and fails to contract normally.

Diastolic ventricular dysfunction results from impaired myocardial relaxation, with increased stiffness in the ventricular wall and decreased left ventricular compliance leading to impairment of diastolic ventricular filling and hence decreased cardiac output. Coronary artery disease, hypertension and hypertrophic cardiomyopathy are common causes although infiltrative disease such as amyloid may lead to pure diastolic dysfunction. The incidence remains unclear, although up to 30% of patients with heart failure may have normal systolic contraction. Management is similar to systolic heart failure but there may be an additional place for calcium-channel blockers. Diastolic dysfunction appears to carry a better prognosis.

Cardiac cachexia

The term cardiac cachexia describes the loss of lean (non-oedematous) body mass that occurs in some patients with moderate or severe heart failure. Most patients with cachexia are over 40 years of age, have had heart failure for at least 5 years and are in NYHA (p. 707) functional class 3/4. Its presence is associated with increased morbidity and mortality.

Several mechanisms are thought to contribute to wasting in heart failure, including malabsorption, anorexia caused by intestinal oedema and drugs, and loss of nutrients through the gastrointestinal and renal tracts. Patients with heart failure also have an increased metabolic rate secondary to increased sympathetic activity in association with reduced anabolic metabolism. Tumour necrosis factor alpha (TNF-α) is increased in patients with cardiac cachexia and contributes to the phenomenon. Possible stimuli to TNF-α release include reduced peripheral blood flow, failing myocardium and prostaglandin release. Natriuretic peptide C (CNP) is also elevated in cachectic patients.

Acute heart failure

Acute failure of the heart most commonly occurs in the setting of acute myocardial infarction when there is extensive loss of ventricular muscle. The condition may also occur with rupture of the interventricular septum producing a ventricular septal defect, or be due to acute valvular regurgitation. Common examples of valvular regurgitation are papillary or chordal rupture producing mitral regurgitation, or sudden aortic valve regurgitation in infective endocarditis. Other causes of acute heart failure include obstruction of the circulation by acute pulmonary embolus and cardiac tamponade. In each case severe cardiac failure can occur with a relatively normal heart size.

High-output heart failure

The heart may not be able to meet the demands placed on it in conditions such as anaemia, thyrotoxicosis, beriberi and Gram-negative septicaemia. This form of heart failure presents in much the same manner as low-output states but is associated with tachycardia and a gallop rhythm. Patients are often warm with distended superficial veins. Unlike low-output failure, the oxygen content of systemic venous blood is high owing to the delivery of large amounts of arterial blood to non-metabolizing tissues.

Investigations

A clinical diagnosis of heart failure should always be confirmed using objective measures of left ventricular structure and function (usually echocardiography). Similarly, the underlying cause of heart failure should be established in all patients.

General/diagnostic investigations

- **Chest X-ray** – cardiac size and evidence of pulmonary congestion (initially upper lobe diversion; then fluid in fissures and Kerley B lines – pulmonary venous pressure > 20 mmHg; then frank pulmonary oedema – pulmonary venous pressure > 25 mmHg).
- **Electrocardiogram** – evidence of ischaemia, hypertension or arrhythmia.
- **Echocardiography.** Two-dimensional and Doppler echocardiography establishes the presence of systolic and/or diastolic impairment of the left or right ventricle. They may also reveal the aetiology (valve disease, regional wall motion abnormalities in ischaemic heart disease, cardiomyopathy, amyloid), and may detect intracardiac thrombus. An ejection fraction of < 0.45 is generally accepted as evidence for systolic dysfunction.

- **Blood tests:**
  - Full blood count, liver biochemistry, urea and electrolytes
  - Cardiac enzymes in acute heart failure to diagnose myocardial infarction
  - Thyroid function.
- **Cardiac catheterization.** See page 728.

Functional/prognostic investigations

- **Cardiopulmonary exercise testing.** Peak oxygen consumption (Vo_2) is a strong independent predictor of hospital admission and death in patients with heart failure but is not widely available. A 6-minute exercise walk may be used instead.
- **Ambulatory (24–48 hours) ECG monitoring** – if arrhythmia is suspected.
- **Resting and stress radionuclide angiography (MUGA)** – for estimation of ejection fraction, regional wall motion abnormality.
- **Serum BNP levels** (raised) are over 70% sensitive and specific for detecting left ventricular systolic dysfunction.
- **Plasma endothelin-1 concentration** – raised level independent marker of outcome.

Treatment of heart failure

Measures to prevent heart failure include cessation of smoking, alcohol and illicit drugs, effective treatment of hypertension and hypercholesterolaemia, and pharmacological therapy following myocardial infarction.

Treatment of chronic heart failure is aimed at relieving symptoms, retarding disease progression and improving survival. The management of heart failure requires that any factor aggravating the failure should be identified and treated. Similarly the cause of heart failure must be elucidated and where possible corrected. Community nursing programmes to help with drug compliance and to detect early deterioration may prevent acute hospitalization.

General treatment
Physical activity

For patients with exacerbations of congestive cardiac failure, bed rest reduces the demands of the heart and is useful for a few days. Migration of fluid from the interstitium promotes a diuresis, reducing heart failure. Prolonged bed rest may lead to development of deep vein thrombosis; this can be avoided by daily leg exercises, low-dose subcutaneous heparin and elastic support stockings. Low-level endurance exercise (e.g. 20–30 minutes walking three or five times per week, or 20 minutes cycling at 70–80% of peak heart rate five times per week) is actively encouraged in patients with compensated heart failure in order to reverse 'deconditioning' of peripheral muscle metabolism. Strenuous isometric activity should be avoided.

Dietary modifications

Large meals should be avoided and if necessary weight reduction instituted. Salt restriction is necessary and foods rich in salt or added salt in cooking and at the table should be avoided. A low-sodium diet is unpalatable and of questionable value. In severe heart failure fluid restriction is necessary. Alcohol has a negatively inotropic effect and patients should abstain.

Vaccination

While prospective clinical trials are lacking, it is recommended that patients with heart failure be vaccinated against pneumococcal disease and influenza.

Education

Effective counselling of patients emphasizing weight monitoring and dose adjustment of diuretics may prevent hospitalization.

Drug management (Table 13.20)
Diuretics (see Table 12.3)

These act by promoting the renal excretion of salt and water by blocking tubular reabsorption of sodium and chloride. The resulting loss of fluid reduces ventricular filling pressures (preload), produces consistent haemodynamic and symptomatic benefits in patients with

---

Table 13.20

Treatment of heart failure and non-pharmacological options

Drugs with proven prognostic benefit
Angiotensin-converting enzyme inhibitors/angiotensin II receptor antagonists
Beta-blockers
Spironolactone
Hydralazine plus nitrate

Drugs useful for symptom relief and may improve outcome
Loop diuretics
Digoxin
Antiarrhythmics
Anticoagulants

Research drugs at present
Neuroendopeptidase inhibitors (omapatrillat)
Endothelin A antagonists (bosantan)
Vasopressin antagonists
Anti-TNF antibodies
Natriuretic peptides

Drugs with no prognostic benefit or worsen outcome
Positive inotropic agents
Calcium-channel blockers

Devices and surgery
Coronary artery bypass grafting
Pacemaker/implantable cardioverter–defibrillator
Heart transplantation
Cardiomyoplasty

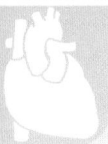

heart failure, and rapidly improves dyspnoea and peripheral oedema. The intravenous administration of loop diuretics such as furosemide (frusemide) relieves pulmonary oedema rapidly by means of arteriolar vasodilatation reducing afterload, an action that is independent of its diuretic effect.

Diuretics act in various ways.

Loop diuretics (p. 675)

Loop diuretics such as furosemide (frusemide) and bumetanide have a rapid onset of action (i.v. – 5 min; oral – 1–2 h) and generally short-lived (4–6 h) diuresis as the concentrating power of the kidney is reduced. These agents also produce marked potassium loss and promote hyperuricaemia, and renal function should be monitored.

Thiazide diuretics (p. 676)

Thiazide diuretics such as bendroflumethazide (bendrofluazide) have a mild diuretic effect. Potassium excretion is enhanced. Thiazides are less effective in patients with reduced glomerular filtration rates. In some patients with severe congestive heart failure oedema may persist despite high dose of loop diuretic. Thiazide diuretics in combination with loop diuretics have a synergistic action and greater diuretic effect. Associated metabolic abnormalities are more likely and close supervision is needed. Metolazone is a powerful thiazide producing profound diuresis acting synergistically with loop diuretics. This combination is only used for the treatment of severe and resistant heart failure.

Although heart failure symptoms are improved by loop diuretic treatment, loop diuretics are not proven to have any survival benefit. In addition, their use may be complicated by overdiuresis and electrolyte depletion (potassium and magnesium), which may predispose to the development of lethal ventricular arrhythmias, hyperkalaemia (potassium-sparing diuretics) and other metabolic disturbances (hyperuricaemia and dyslipidaemia).

Potassium-sparing diuretics (Table 12.3)

Spironolactone is a specific competitive antagonist to aldosterone, producing a weak diuresis but with a potassium-sparing action. A randomized placebo-controlled study, the Randomized Aldactone Evaluation Study (RALES) showed a 30% reduction in all cause mortality when spironolactone (up to 25 mg) was added to conventional treatment in patients with moderate to severe heart failure. The risk of hyperkalaemia was low. Risk factors for developing hyperkalaemia include spironolactone dose > 50 mg/day, high-dose angiotensin-converting enzyme inhibitor (ACEI) and renal impairment. Potassium should be measured 5 days after the initiation of spironolactone until levels are stable and then every 1–3 months.

Table 13.21
Effects of vasodilator drugs used in heart failure

	Reduction in:	
	Preload	Afterload
Nitroprusside	+	+++
Glyceryl trinitrate	+++	+
Isosorbide di/mono nitrate	+++	+
β-Adrenoceptor blockers	+	++
Prazosin	+	++
ACE inhibitors/antagonists	++	++
Hydralazine	0	+++
Calcium-channel blockers	+	++

ACE, angiotensin-converting enzyme

Amiloride and triamterene act at the distal tubule preventing potassium secretion in exchange for sodium. These drugs are weak diuretics but are useful in combination with more powerful loop diuretics. They should be avoided in the presence of renal failure and in patients taking ACE inhibitors unless there is persistent hypokalaemia. There is no evidence as yet that these two potassium-sparing diuretics have any prognostic effect.

Vasodilator therapy (see Table 13.21)

Diuretics and sodium restriction serve to activate the renin–angiotensin system, promoting formation of angiotensin (a potent vasoconstrictor) and an increase in afterload. A variety of other neural and hormonal reactions also serve to increase preload and afterload. These compensatory mechanisms are initially beneficial in maintaining blood pressure and redistributing blood flow, but in the later stages of heart failure they are deleterious and reduce cardiac output. The high venous pressures found in heart failure are also related to the activation of the sympathetic nervous system and the presence of circulating vasoconstrictors, thus shifting the Starling curve to the right.

Angiotensin-converting enzyme inhibitors
(Fig. 18.27, p. 1064)

Several large controlled trials (e.g. CONSENSUS and SOLVD), have established the benefit of ACEI in heart failure (Fig. 13.50). The trials have shown that in addition to producing considerable symptomatic improvement in patients with symptomatic heart failure, prognosis is markedly improved and development of heart failure is slowed. The SAVE study confirmed the benefit of ACEI in patients with asymptomatic heart failure following myocardial infarction, in whom the development of overt heart failure was reduced.

ACEI lower systemic vascular resistance and venous pressure, and reduce levels of circulating catecholamines, thus improving myocardial performance. The beneficial haemodynamic effect of these drugs appears to be

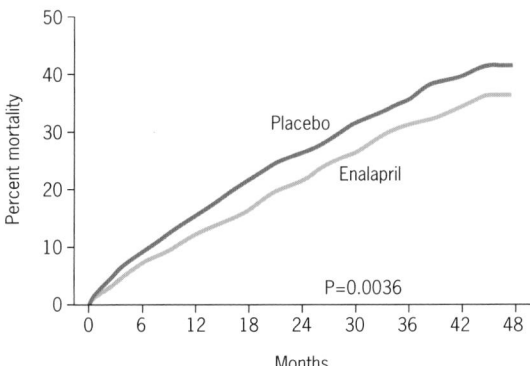

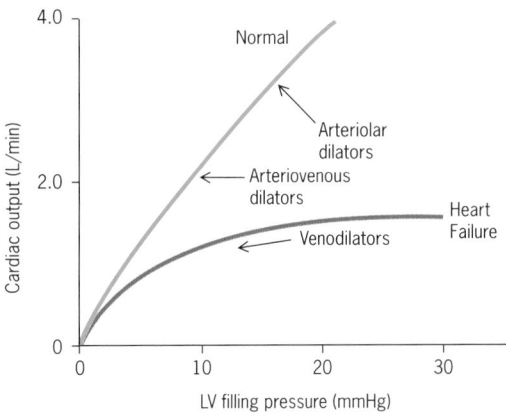

Fig. 13.51 **Effect of vasodilators on cardiac output and left ventricular filling pressure.** Agents with arteriolar and arteriovenous dilating properties reduce the afterload and increase cardiac output. Venodilators reduce the left ventricular filling pressure (and pulmonary oedema) but do not increase cardiac output.

independent of their inhibition of ACE as they are equally effective when plasma renin activity is normal.

These drugs should be carefully introduced to patients with heart failure because of the risk of first-dose hypotension. This is a particular risk in patients who are receiving large doses of diuretics and in the presence of hyponatraemia (<130 mmol/L). In such cases a test dose of ACEI should be commenced and the preceding diuretic doses omitted. Some of these agents are pro-drugs (e.g. enalapril) and require conversion to the active metabolite (enalaprilat) by liver enzymes; these drugs have a delayed onset of action and first-dose hypotension may not occur for several hours. Pro-drugs are best avoided if heart failure results in significantly altered hepatic function. Serious hypotension may result in acute renal failure. Concomitant potassium-sparing diuretics should be discontinued, as ACEI tend to promote potassium retention. Creatinine levels rise by approximately 10–15% during ACE therapy. ACEI are contraindicated in patients with bilateral renal artery stenosis. Between 10 and 15% of patients develop a cough, owing to the inhibition of bradykinin metabolism. A prospective trial looking at dose and survival (ATLAS study) showed no significant mortality difference although high-dose treatment was associated with a significant reduction in all cause mortality and hospitalization.

Arteriolar vasolidators (Fig. 13.51)

Drugs such as α-adrenergic blockers (e.g. prazosin) and direct smooth-muscle relaxants (e.g. hydralazine) are potent arteriolar vasodilators but are not very effective in heart failure. Calcium-channel blockers also reduce afterload, but first-generation calcium antagonists (diltiazem, nifedipine) may have a detrimental effect on left ventricular function in patients with heart failure. The PRAISE 2 trial showed that the second-generation calcium antagonist amlodipine showed no prognostic benefit in patients with heart failure.

Venodilators (Fig. 13.51)

Short- and long-acting nitrates (e.g. glyceryl trinitrate and isosorbide mononitrate) act by reducing preload and lowering venous pressure with resulting reduction in pulmonary and dependent oedema. Reduction of filling pressure does not significantly enhance cardiac output because the heart is operating on the flat portion of the ventricular filling curve. With chronic use, tolerance develops with loss of efficacy and consequent worsening of heart failure. Only combination therapy of nitrate with hydralazine (Veterans Heart Failure Trials, VHeFT) has been shown to improve mortality and exercise performance, and may be useful when ACEI are contraindicated. The benefit of vasodilators is not as great as with ACEI (VHeFT 2).

Angiotensin II receptor antagonist

Angiotensin II (AII) receptor antagonists (e.g. losartan, ibersartan and valsartan) have similar haemodynamic effects to ACEI, but as they do not affect bradykinin metabolism, they do not produce a cough. A recent trial comparing losartan with the ACEI enalapril in patients with heart failure (ELITE 2) showed no benefit of the AII receptor blocker over the ACEI. AII receptor antagonists should be used when ACE inhibitors are contraindicated.

The combination of ACEI and AII receptor antagonists may confer additional benefit compared to ACEI therapy. Recently the Val HeFT study of valsartan and captopril in combination showed that the use of valsartan resulted a significant reduction in hospitalization but no difference in mortality. However, in a small number of patients (7%) valsartan alone resulted in significant reduction in mortality.

β-Adrenoceptor blocking agents

There is now considerable evidence to support the use of beta-blockers in patients with chronic stable heart

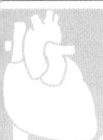

failure. The studies MERIT and CIBIS 2 using the beta-blockers metoprolol and bisoprolol respectively have shown improved symptomatic class, exercise tolerance left ventricular function and mortality in patients with heart failure of any cause. The US Carvedilol Studies using carvedilol, a non-selective vasodilator beta-blocker with additional vasodilator and antioxidant properties, has also demonstrated a significant improvement in mortality. Beta-blocker use should be restricted to those with stable heart failure and their introduction should be cautious because of the potential to cause heart failure decompensation. Following the administration of beta-blockers, the ejection fraction may decline, but usually returns to baseline within a month and then increases after 3 months. Thus, initial doses should be low, and should be titrated slowly over a period of months rather than days.

Inotropic agents

Intravenous inotropes are frequently used to support myocardial function in patients with acute left ventricular failure and following cardiac surgery.

Epinephrine (adrenaline), dobutamine, dopexamine and dopamine are intravenous adrenergic agonists. Dobutamine is predominantly a β_1-adrenoceptor, increasing intracellular cyclic AMP, which in turn increases calcium availability for myocardial contraction. Dobutamine also causes peripheral vasodilatation by an anti-α-adrenergic effect. Dopexamine is a selective β_2 agonist with an additional action on peripheral dopamine receptors that theoretically results in improved renal perfusion. Dopamine is a less selective inotrope that is often used in a low dose to improve renal perfusion (via dopaminergic receptors) although this renal effect has been questioned (p. 940).

β-Adrenergic agonists are used in patients with acute left ventricular failure and in patients with end-stage heart failure as a bridge to transplantation. Intermittent intravenous infusions of dobutamine may produce long-lasting improvements in symptoms and exercise performance at the cost of increased mortality.

Several orally active agents have been tested in patients with chronic congestive cardiac failure, but all apart from digoxin have been associated with increased mortality and are not generally used.

Digitalis glycosides

Digitalis glycosides have been used for many years in patients with heart failure and atrial fibrillation. A large prospective trial (Digoxin Investigation Group (DIG) trial) showed that digoxin combined with ACE inhibitors and diuretics, reduced death and hospitalization resulting from progressive heart failure in patients in sinus rhythm. A small significant increase in deaths presumed to be secondary to myocardial infarction and/or arrhythmia meant that the effect on overall mortality was neutral. Therefore patients who are hospitalized or present with severe heart failure in spite of therapy with vasodilators, beta-blockers, diuretics and also rapid AF, should have digoxin added to their therapeutic regimen.

The half-life of digoxin is approximately 36 hours. It is partly protein-bound, making it liable to drug interaction. As 90% is excreted unchanged in urine, accumulation can occur in renal failure. Digoxin acts as a positive inotrope by competitive inhibition of Na^+–K^+-ATPase, producing high levels of intracellular sodium. This is then exchanged for extracellular calcium. High levels of intracellular calcium result in enhanced actin–myosin interaction and increased contractility (see Fig. 13.2). Digoxin also improves baroreceptor responsiveness, and reduces sympathetic activity and circulating renin.

Digoxin is administered orally (1 mg loading and 0.125–0.25 mg daily according to body mass and renal function). Trough serum levels should be monitored (1.3–2.6 nmol/L) and hypokalaemia should be avoided. The elderly and patients with hyperthyroidism are more prone to digoxin toxicity. In patients with fluctuating renal function, digitoxin, which is metabolized by the liver, is preferable.

With improvement in formulation, digoxin toxicity has become less problematic. The most common features of digoxin toxicity are:

- anorexia, nausea, altered vision
- arrhythmia (e.g. ventricular premature beats especially bigeminy, ventricular tachycardia and AV block)
- digoxin levels >2.5 nmol/L.

Digoxin toxicity is treated by stopping the drug, restoration of serum potassium and management of arrhythmias. Digoxin antibody (Fab fragments) is a specific antidote that is useful for life-threatening toxicity.

β-Adrenergic agonists

Based on the demonstration that the inotropic state of the failing myocardium is impaired and that the myocardial response to adrenergic stimulation is reduced, several adrenergic agonists have been tested in heart failure. All of these agents consistently increase mortality in the longer term and are therefore restricted in use.

Xamoterol, the only oral β-adrenoceptor agonist to be extensively tested, improves exercise tolerance and symptoms in patients with mild heart failure, but increases mortality in patients with moderate to severe heart failure.

Milrinone and enoximone are known as 'inodilator' drugs; they act by inhibiting phosphodiesterase, thus preventing breakdown of cyclic AMP. Accumulation of cAMP produces an increase in contractility and peripheral vasodilatation. The Starling curve is shifted upwards. Although these agents are effective in improving myocardial performance acutely, there is evidence that they increase mortality in the long term.

Anticoagulants

Heart failure is associated with a fourfold increase in the risk of a stroke. Oral anticoagulants are recommended in patients with atrial fibrillation, a previous history of thromboembolism or endocardial thrombus, but their role in patients in sinus rhythm is less certain. Large-scale prospective randomized controlled trials of antithrombotic treatment in heart failure are in progress.

Antiarrhythmic agents

Precipitating factors should be addressed, in particular electrolyte disturbance. Atrial fibrillation is commonly associated with heart failure and leads to a deterioration in symptoms. Restoration of sinus rhythm, either by electrical cardioversion or drugs, is desirable but less successful in the presence of structural heart disease and decompensated heart failure. Rate control with digoxin may be appropriate.

Arrhythmias are frequent in heart failure and are implicated in sudden death. Although treatment of complex ventricular arrhythmias might be expected to improve survival, there is conflicting evidence that this is so. This may be related to the diverse mechanisms of death in patients with heart failure, death commonly being associated with bradyarrhythmias, particularly in patients with non-ischaemic heart failure. Patients with sustained episodes of ventricular tachycardia should receive empirical treatment, usually with an implantable cardioverter–defibrillator (ICD).

The ICD is likely to improve the survival prospects of patients who have not yet developed serious ventricular arrhythmias and is being evaluated in the SCD-HeFT and MADIT II trials. However, it is already clear that when a life-threatening arrhythmia has already been suffered an ICD is the best therapy to prevent mortality due to ventricular arrhythmias.

Beta-blockers, ACEI, some statins and spironolactone may reduce sudden cardiac death in patients with coronary heart disease and heart failure. It should be noted that ACEI probably exert an indirect antiarrhythmic effect by reducing high circulating levels of norepinephrine (noradrenaline) and improving cardiac function

Summary of treatment (see Table 13.22)

All patients with clinical heart failure should receive treatment with diuretics and an ACEI. Patients in atrial fibrillation should be digitalized but patients in sinus rhythm may also be improved by the addition of digoxin or a beta-blocker. Patients with asymptomatic left ventricular dysfunction are at risk of progressive deterioration and should be treated with prophylactic ACEI therapy. Patients with ischaemic heart failure and ongoing ischaemia, and patients intolerant of ACEI or in whom they are contraindicated (hypotension, renal

Table 13.22
Summary of drug treatment for heart failure

Medication	Symptoms	Mortality	SCD	Hospitalization
ACEI	↓↓	↓↓	?(↓)	↓↓
AIIRA	↓↓	↔	↔	?(↓)
Beta-blocker	↓↓	↓↓↓	↓↓↓	↓↓
Glycosides	↓	↔	↔	↓
Diuretics	↓↓↓	↔	↔	?
Spironolactone	↓	↓↓↓	↓↓↓	↓↓

ACEI, angiotensin-converting enzyme inhibitor; AIIRA, angiotensin-II receptor antagonists; SCD, sudden cardiac death; ↓, reduce; ↔, no change

insufficiency or hyperkalaemia), may benefit from nitrate/hydralazine therapy. Spironolactone should also be added to the above treatment regimens.

Non-pharmacological treatment of heart failure

Revascularization

While coronary artery disease is the most common cause of heart failure, the role of revascularization in patients with heart failure is unclear. Patients with angina and left ventricular dysfunction have a higher mortality from surgery (10–20%), but have the most to gain in terms of improved symptoms and prognosis. Factors that must be considered before recommending surgery include age, symptoms and evidence for reversible myocardial ischaemia.

Hibernating myocardium

'Hibernating' myocardium can be defined as reversible left ventricular dysfunction due to chronic coronary artery disease that responds positively to inotropic stress and indicates the presence of viable heart muscle that may recover after revascularization. It is due to reduced myocardial perfusion, which is just sufficient to maintain viability of the heart muscle. Myocardial hibernation results from repetitive episodes of cardiac stunning that occur, for example, with repeated exercise in a patient with coronary artery disease. *Myocardial stunning* is reversible ventricular dysfunction that persists following an episode of ischaemia when the blood flow has returned to normal, i.e. there is a mismatch between flow and function. The prevalence of hibernating myocardium in patients with coronary artery disease can be estimated from the frequency of improvement in regional abnormalities in wall motion after revascularization and is estimated to be 33% of such patients. Techniques to try to identify hibernating myocardium include stress echocardiography, nuclear imaging techniques and positron emission tomography.

The clinical relevance of the hibernating and stunned myocardium is that ventricular dysfunction due to these mechanisms may be wrongly ascribed to myocardial

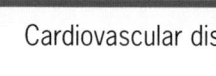

necrosis and scarring which seems untreatable, but will respond to coronary revascularization.

Pacemaker or implantable cardioverter–defibrillator (p. 753)

Pacemakers are indicated in patients with sinoatrial disease and atrioventricular conduction block. Pacemakers are also valuable in patients without AV block but with prolonged PR intervals, left bundle branch block and severe mitral regurgitation. In patients with heart failure and left bundle branch block and NYHA 3 heart failure (MUSTIC study) biventricular pacing is more beneficial than conventional right ventricular pacing. The results showed an improvement in symptoms and exercise tolerance. The effect on prognosis is addressed by an ongoing trial (CARE HF).

Cardiac transplantation

Cardiac transplantation has become the treatment of choice for younger patients with severe intractable heart failure, whose life expectancy is less than 6 months. With careful recipient selection, the expected 1-year survival for patients following transplantation is over 90%, and is 75% at 5 years. Irrespective of survival, quality of life is dramatically improved for the majority of patients. The availability of heart transplantation is limited.

Heart allografts do not function normally. Cardiac denervation results in a high resting heart rate, loss of diurnal blood pressure variation and impaired renin–angiotensin–aldosterone regulation. Some patients develop 'stiff heart' syndrome, caused by rejection, denervation and ischaemic injury during organ harvest and implantation. Transplantation of an inappropriately small donor heart can also result in elevated right and left heart pressure.

The complications of heart transplantation are summarized in Table 13.23. Many (infection, malignancy, hypertension and hyperlipidaemia) are related to immunosuppression. Allograft coronary atherosclerosis is the major cause of long-term graft failure and is present in 30–50% of patients at 5 years. It is due to a 'vascular' rejection process in conjunction with hypertension and hyperlipidaemia.

There are specific contraindications to cardiac transplantation (Table 13.24); notably, high pulmonary vascular resistance is an absolute contraindication. Several alternatives to transplantation are available: cardiomyoplasty (augmentation of left ventricular contraction by wrapping a latissimus dorsi muscle flap around the ventricle), and the Batista procedure (surgical ventricular size reduction and remodelling the geometry of the left ventricle). Both procedures have a high mortality and limited evidence of substantial benefit in the medium term.

Artificial hearts and left ventricular assist devices are used as bridges to transplantation or corrective

surgery. Mechanical devices are also indicated if there is a possibility of spontaneous recovery; for example, acute myocarditis.

The available ventricular assist devices include extracorporeal membrane oxygenation, univentricular and biventricular extracorporeal non-pulsatile devices, extracorporeal and implantable pulsatile devices, and the total artificial heart. Although most of these devices require the patient to be connected to cumbersome extracorporeal drive systems, miniaturization of control and power-supply components has resulted in the development of wearable left ventricular assist devices.

Table 13.23	
Complications of cardiac transplantation	
Allograft rejection	**Allograft vascular disease**
'Humoral'	
'Vascular'	**Hypertension**
'Cell-mediated'	
	Hypercholesterolaemia
Infections	
Early: nosocomial organisms,	**Malignancy**
– staphylococci, Gram-negatives	
Late (2–6 months): opportunistic	
(toxoplasmosis, cytomegalovirus,	
fungi, *Pneumocystis*)	

Table 13.24
Contraindications for cardiac transplantation
Age > 60 years (some variations between centres)
Alcohol/drug abuse
Uncontrolled psychiatric illness
Uncontrolled infection
Severe renal/liver failure
High pulmonary vascular resistance
Systemic disease with multiorgan involvement
Treated cancer in remission but with < 5 years' follow-up
Recent thromboembolism
Other disease with a poor prognosis

Pulmonary oedema

This is a very frightening, life-threatening emergency characterized by extreme breathlessness. The dyspnoea may first occur at night in the form of paroxysmal dyspnoea due to pulmonary congestion. This occurs because of reabsorption of dependent oedema when lying flat, and the relative insensitivity of the respiratory centre at night allows pulmonary congestion to develop.

Pathophysiology

A pressure above 20 mmHg causes increased filtration of fluid out of the capillaries into the interstitial space (interstitial oedema). Further accumulation of fluid disrupts intercellular membranes, leading to the collection of fluid in the alveolar spaces (alveolar oedema). Alveolar oedema occurs when the capillary pressure exceeds the total oncotic pressures (approximately 30 mmHg).

Clinical features

Patients with alveolar oedema are acutely breathless, wheezing, anxious and perspiring profusely. In addition, they have a cough productive of frothy, blood-tinged (pink) sputum, which can be copious. The patient is tachypnoeic with peripheral circulatory shutdown. There is a tachycardia, a raised venous pressure and a gallop rhythm. Crackles and wheezes are heard throughout the chest. The arterial P_{O_2} falls and initially the P_aCO_2 also falls, owing to overbreathing. Later, however, the P_aCO_2 increases because of impaired gas exchange. The chest X-ray shows diffuse haziness, owing to alveolar fluid, and the Kerley B lines of interstitial oedema (see Fig. 13.15). The abnormality can be unilateral, giving the appearance of a tumour that disappears on treatment (a pseudotumour).

Treatment

The patient must be placed in a sitting position. High-concentration oxygen (60% via a variable performance mask) is given. In severe cases it may be necessary to ventilate the patient (see p. 947).

Intravenous diuretic treatment with furosemide (frusemide) or bumetanide is given. These diuretics produce immediate vasodilatation in addition to the more delayed diuretic response.

Morphine (10–20 mg i.v. depending on the size of the patient) together with an antiemetic such as metoclopramide (10 mg i.v.) is given. Morphine sedates the patient and causes systemic vasodilatation; it must be avoided if the systemic arterial pressure is less than 90 mmHg. Respiratory depression occurs with large doses of morphine.

Venous vasodilators, such as glyceryl trinitrate, may produce prompt relief by reducing the preload. Cardiac output may be increased by using arterial vasodilatation, such as occurs with hydralazine (see Table 13.21 and Fig. 13.51).

Aminophylline (250–500 mg or 5 mg/kg i.v.) is infused over 10 minutes. Aminophylline is a phosphodiesterase inhibitor that causes bronchodilatation, vasodilatation and increased cardiac contractility. It must be given slowly because of the risk of precipitating ventricular arrhythmias. It is usually used when bronchospasm is present.

Venesection and mechanical methods of reducing venous return (e.g. sphygmomanometer cuffs inflated to 10 mmHg below diastolic blood pressure and placed around the thighs) are inefficient and rarely used.

In a severe case, after the acute emergency is controlled, a pulmonary artery balloon catheter may be inserted to monitor progress and treatment. Any factor that precipitated the heart failure, such as cardiac arrhythmias or chest infection, should be corrected. The underlying cardiac problem should be diagnosed and treated.

Cardiogenic shock

Shock is a severe failure of tissue perfusion, characterized by hypotension, a low cardiac output and signs of poor tissue perfusion such as oliguria, cold extremities and poor cerebral function. Cardiogenic shock (pump failure) is an extreme type of cardiac failure with a high mortality of approximately 90%. Its most common cause is myocardial infarction and it complicates up to 10% of MI. Other causes are acute massive pulmonary embolus, pericardial tamponade and sudden-onset valvular regurgitation.

Cardiogenic shock is diagnosed when critical impairment of tissue perfusion occurs despite an adequate or elevated pulmonary capillary wedge pressure and in the absence of mechanical circulatory obstruction. An essential element in this diagnosis is the measurement of the pulmonary capillary wedge pressure (see p. 935). In situations where the vascular capacity has expanded or the circulatory fluid volume has decreased, the wedge pressure will be low. In cardiogenic shock the wedge pressure is normal or elevated.

The mortality rate in cardiogenic shock is high, estimated at 80%, because of the vicious downward spiral that occurs: hypotension due to pump failure results in a reduction of coronary flow, which results in further impairment of pump function, and so on.

Treatment

Patients require intensive care, as described in Chapter 15. General measures such as complete rest, continuous 60% oxygen administration and pain and anxiety relief are essential.

The infusion of fluid is necessary if the pulmonary capillary wedge pressure is below 18 mmHg, which is probably the optimal 'filling pressure' with which to prime a failing heart.

Short-acting venous dilators such as glyceryl trinitrate or sodium nitroprusside should be administered intravenously if the wedge pressure is 25 mmHg or more.

Cardiac inotropes such as epinephrine (adrenaline), dobutamine and dopamine may be used to increase aortic diastolic pressure (coronary perfusion pressure). Emergency revascularization of occluded arteries for cardiogenic shock adds benefit compared with medical therapy (including intra-aortic balloon counterpulsation and thrombolytic therapy).

These lead to a temporary improvement; long-term prognosis is not improved unless there is a surgically correctable cause, such as a ruptured interventricular septum or acute mitral regurgitation.

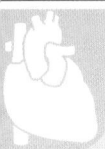

FURTHER READING

Cohn JN (1996) The management of chronic heart failure. *New England Journal of Medicine* **335**: 490–498.

Colucci WS et al. (2000) Intravenous nesiritide a natriuretic peptide in the treatment of decompensated congestive heart failure. *New England Journal of Medicine* **343**: 246–253.

Dries DL (2000) Brain natriuretic peptide as bridge to therapy for heart failure. *Lancet* **355**: 1112–1113.

Gheorghiade M, Bonow RO (2001) Beta blocker therapy for mild to moderate chronic heart failure. *American Journal of Medicine* **III** (Suppl 7A): 1S–94S.

Hunt S (2001) Reinnervation of the transplanted heart. *New England Journal of Medicine* **345**: 762–764.

Marwick TH (1998) The viable myocardium. *Lancet* **341**: 815–816.

Task Force of the Working Group on Heart Failure of the European Society of Cardiology (1997) Treatment of heart failure. *European Heart Journal* **18**: 736–753.

Troughton RW et al. (2000) Treatment of heart failure guided by plasma aminoterminal brain natriuretic peptide (N-BNP) concentrations. *Lancet* **355**: 1126–1130.

Vasan RS, Benjamin EJ (2001) Diastolic heart failure – no time to relax. *New England Journal of Medicine* **344**: 56–59.

Willenheimer R et al. (2000) Value of 6-min-walk test for assessment of severity and prognosis of heart failure. *Lancet* **355**: 515–516.

Ischaemic heart disease

Myocardial ischaemia occurs when there is an imbalance between the supply of oxygen (and other essential myocardial nutrients) and the myocardial demand for these substances. The causes are as follows:

1. Coronary blood flow to a region of the myocardium may be reduced by a mechanical obstruction that is due to:
   - atheroma
   - thrombosis
   - spasm
   - embolus
   - coronary ostial stenosis
   - coronary arteritis (e.g. in SLE).
2. There can be a decrease in the flow of oxygenated blood to the myocardium that is due to:
   - anaemia
   - carboxyhaemoglobulinaemia
   - hypotension causing decreased coronary perfusion pressure.
3. An increased demand for oxygen may occur owing to an increase in cardiac output (e.g. thyrotoxicosis) or myocardial hypertrophy (e.g. from aortic stenosis or hypertension).

In the UK, myocardial ischaemia most commonly occurs as a result of obstructive coronary artery disease (CAD) in the form of coronary atherosclerosis. In addition to this fixed obstruction, variations in the tone of smooth muscle in the wall of a coronary artery may add another element of dynamic or variable obstruction.

CAD is the largest single cause of death in the UK. Each year there are approximately 60 deaths per 100 000 (giving a standardized mortality rate of about 200 per 100 000).

The process of coronary atherosclerosis

Coronary atherosclerosis is a complex inflammatory process characterized by the accumulation of lipid, macrophages and smooth muscle cells in intimal plaques in the large and medium-sized epicardial coronary arteries. The vascular endothelium plays a critical role in maintaining vascular integrity and homeostasis. Mechanical shear stresses (e.g. from morbid hypertension), biochemical abnormalities (e.g. elevated and modified LDL, diabetes mellitus, elevated plasma homocysteine), immunological factors (e.g. free radicals from smoking), inflammation (e.g. infection such as *Chlamydia pneumoniae* and *Helicobactor pylori*) and genetic alteration may contribute to the initial endothelial 'injury' or dysfunction, which is believed to trigger atherogenesis. The development of atherosclerosis follows the endothelial dysfunction, with increased permeability to and accumulation of oxidized lipoproteins, which are taken up by macrophages at focal sites within the endothelium to produce lipid-laden foam cells. Macroscopically, these lesions are seen as flat yellow dots or lines on the endothelium of the artery and are known as 'fatty streaks'. The 'fatty streak' progresses with the appearance of extracellular lipid within the endothelium ('transitional plaque'). Release of cytokines such as platelet-derived growth factor and transforming growth factor-β (TGF-β) by monocytes, macrophages or the damaged endothelium promotes further accumulation of macrophages as well as smooth muscle cell migration and proliferation. The proliferation of smooth muscle with the formation of a layer of cells covering the extracellular lipid, separates it from the adaptive smooth muscle thickening in the endothelium. Collagen is produced in larger and larger quantities by the smooth muscle and the whole sequence of events cumulates as an 'advanced or raised fibrolipid plaque'. The 'advanced plaque' may grow slowly and encroach on the lumen or become unstable, undergo thrombosis and produce an obstruction ('complicated plaque').

Two different mechanisms are responsible for thrombosis on the plaques (Fig. 13.52). The first process is superficial endothelial injury, which involves denudation of the endothelial covering over the plaque. Subendocardial connective tissue matrix is then exposed and platelet adhesion occurs because of reaction with collagen. The thrombus is adherent to the surface of the plaque. The second process is deep endothelial fissuring, which involves an advanced plaque with a lipid core. The plaque cap tears (ulcerates, fissures or ruptures), allowing blood from the lumen to enter the inside of the plaque itself. The core with lamellar lipid surfaces, tissue factor (which triggers platelet adhesion and activation) produced by macrophages and exposed collagen, is highly thrombogenic. Thrombus forms within the plaque, expanding its volume and distorting its shape. Thrombosis may then extend into the lumen.

A 50% reduction in luminal diameter (producing a reduction in luminal cross-sectional area of approximately 70%) causes a haemodynamically significant stenosis. At this point the smaller distal intramyocardial arteries and arterioles are maximally dilated (coronary flow reserve is near zero), and any increase in myocardial oxygen demand provokes ischaemia.

CAD gives rise to a wide variety of clinical presentations. These range from relatively stable angina through to the acute coronary syndromes of unstable angina and myocardial infarction (Fig. 13.53; Fig. 13.54 shows an actual plaque rupture). These will be discussed in detail below.

Risk factors for coronary artery disease

The aetiology of CAD is multifactorial, and a number of 'risk' factors are known to predispose to the condition (Table 13.25). Some of these – such as age, gender, race and family history – cannot be changed, whereas other major risk factors, such as serum cholesterol, smoking habits, diabetes and hypertension, can be modified.

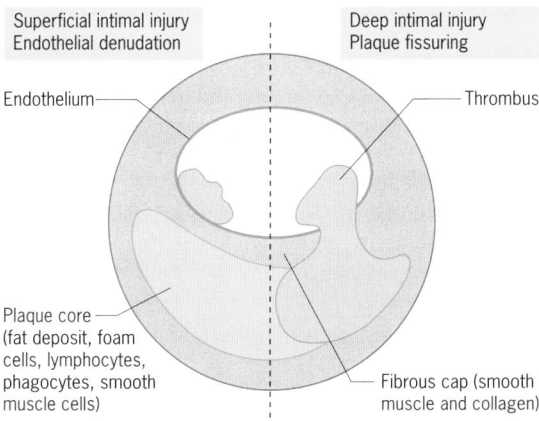

Fig. 13.52 **The mechanisms for the development of thrombosis on plaques.**

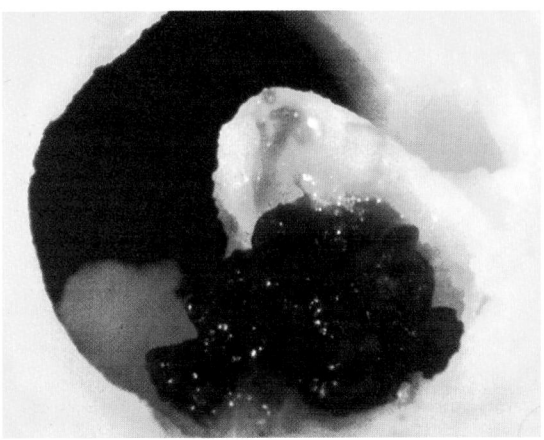

Fig. 13.54 **Acute coronary thrombus.** Cross-section (×30) of the epicardial coronary artery, demonstrating a rupture of the shoulder region of the plaque with a luminal thrombus.

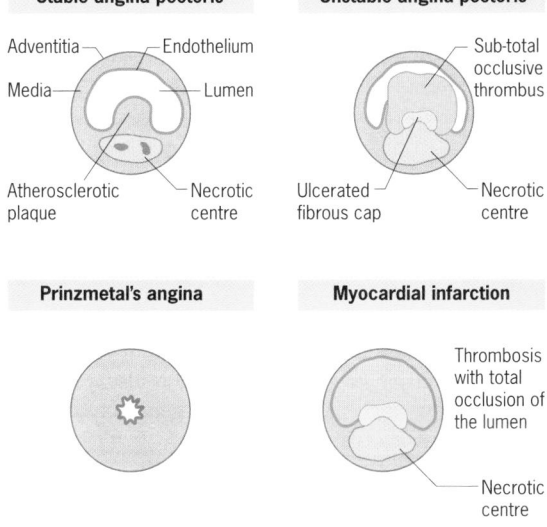

Fig. 13.53 **Relationship between the state of coronary artery vessel wall and clinical syndrome.**

Table 13.25
Risk factors for coronary disease

Fixed
Age
Male sex
Positive family history
Deletion polymorphism in the ACE gene (DD)

Potentially changeable with treatment
Hyperlipidaemia
Cigarette smoking
Hypertension
Diabetes mellitus
Lack of exercise
Blood coagulation factors – high fibrinogen, factor VII
C-reactive protein
Homocysteinaemia
Personality
Obesity
Gout
Soft water
Contraceptive pill
Heavy alcohol consumption

ACE, angiotensin-converting enzyme

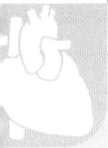
However, not all patients with myocardial infarction are identified by these risk factors.

Traditional risk factors

Age

CAD rates increase with age. Atherosclerosis is rare in childhood, except in familial hyperlipidaemia, but is often detectable in young men between 20 and 30 years of age. It is almost universal in the elderly in the West.

Gender

Men have a higher incidence of coronary artery disease than premenopausal women. However, after the menopause, the incidence of atheroma in women approaches that in men. The reasons for this gender difference are not clearly understood, but probably relate to the loss of the protective effect of oestrogen.

Family history

CAD is often found in several members of the same family. Because the disease is so prevalent and because other risk factors are familial, it is uncertain whether family history, per se, is an independent risk factor. A positive family history is generally accepted to refer to those in whom a first-degree relative has developed ischaemic heart disease before the age of 50 years.

Smoking

In men, the risk of developing CAD is directly related to the number of cigarettes smoked. This relationship is less certain (but still important) in women and cigar and pipe smokers. The risk from smoking declines to almost normal after 10 years of abstention.

Diet

Diets high in fats are associated with ischaemic heart disease, as are those with low intakes of antioxidants. Supplementation with antioxidants has been shown to be unhelpful.

Hypertension

Both systolic and diastolic hypertension are associated with an increased risk of CAD. The risk is the same for men and women. Whilst reduction of blood pressure reduces the risk of a cerebrovascular event, it does not appear to affect the risk of cardiac events such as myocardial infarction.

Hyperlipidaemia (see p. 1107)

High serum cholesterol, especially when associated with a low value of high-density lipoproteins (HDL), is strongly associated with coronary atheroma. There is increasing evidence that high serum triglyceride is also independently linked with coronary atheroma.

Familial hypercholesterolaemia, familial hypercholesterolaemia combined with hypertriglyceridaemia and remnant hyperlipidaemia are also associated with increased risk of coronary atherosclerosis.

Measurement of the fasting lipid profile (total cholesterol, low- and high-density lipoproteins and triglycerides) should be performed on all patients.

Angiographic studies have shown that lowering the serum cholesterol can slow the progression of coronary atherosclerosis, and can cause regression of disease. Large clinical trials have shown that lipid lowering usually with a statin, can decrease total mortality and new coronary events, and reduce the need for revascularization. Management is described on page 1109.

Other risk factors

Diabetes mellitus

Diabetes, or an abnormal glucose tolerance test, is strongly associated with vascular disease. Obesity, particularly central obesity, is associated with CAD, but it is not certain whether obesity itself is independently linked to the condition.

CAD rates also vary among different ethnic groups, by socio-economic status and geographical region.

Sedentary lifestyle

Lack of exercise is an independent risk factor for CAD equal to hypertension, hyperlipidaemia and smoking. Regular exercise probably protects against its development.

Genetic factors

A number of genetic factors have been linked with coronary artery disease. The angiotensin-converting enzyme (ACE) gene contains an insertion/deletion (I/D) polymorphism, the DD genotype of which has been associated with a predisposition to coronary artery disease and myocardial infarction.

Lipoprotein (a)

High plasma Lp(a) concentrations are associated with CAD and, although probably not an independent risk factor, elevated plasma Lp(a) increases the CAD risk associated with more traditional risk factors.

Coagulation factors

Serum fibrinogen is strongly, consistently, and independently related to CAD risk. The pathophysiological mechanism by which fibrinogen levels mediate coronary disease risk is related to its effect on the coagulation cascade, platelet aggregation, endothelial function and smooth muscle cell proliferation and migration.

High levels of *coagulation factor VII* is also a risk factor. Polymorphisms of the factor VII gene may increase the risk of myocardial infarction.

Homocysteine

Homocysteinaemia has emerged as a potential major risk factor in the pathogenesis of CAD and a strong predictor of mortality in this group. Plasma levels of homocysteine are influenced by a variety of genetic and non-genetic factors. The mechanism associating hyper-homocysteinaemia with atherosclerosis is its adverse effect on vascular endothelium. Folic acid in low doses may ameliorate this process.

C-reactive protein (CRP)

CRP is linked with future risk of coronary events independent of the traditional risk factors. This suggests that CRP may be used as a marker for subclinical atherosclerosis and cardiovascular risk. CRP has been positively associated with future cardiovascular events in healthy women, healthy men, elderly patients, and high-risk individuals. In addition, there are associations between CRP and peripheral vascular disease and stroke.

It is clear that many factors influence the development of coronary atheroma. Modification of some of these can help reduce both the development of the coronary artery disease (primary prevention) and slow the progression of established disease (secondary prevention). In addition, for primary prevention for men with high risk factors, aspirin 75 mg per day should be given.

Angina (see also p. 707)

The diagnosis of angina is largely based on the clinical history. The chest pain is generally described as 'heavy', 'tight' or 'gripping'. Typically, the pain is central/retrosternal and may radiate to the jaw and/or arms. Angina can range from a mild ache to a most severe pain that provokes sweating and fear. There may be associated breathlessness. CAD is common, fatal and largely preventable. More than 1.4 million people in the UK suffer from angina. CAD accounts for about 3% of all hospital admissions in England. The prevalence of angina is approximately 2% with an incidence of new cases each year approximately 1 per 1000.

Classical or exertional angina pectoris is provoked by physical exertion, especially after meals and in cold, windy weather, and is commonly aggravated by anger or excitement. The pain fades quickly (usually within minutes) with rest. Occasionally it disappears with continued exertion ('walking through the pain'). Whilst in some patients the pain occurs predictably at a certain level of exertion, in most patients the threshold for developing pain is variable.

Decubitus angina is that occurring on lying down. It usually occurs in association with impaired left ventricular function, as a result of severe coronary artery disease.

Nocturnal angina occurs at night and may wake the patient from sleep. It can be provoked by vivid dreams. It tends to occur in patients with critical coronary artery disease and may be the result of vasospasm.

Variant (Prinzmetal's) angina refers to an angina that occurs without provocation, usually at rest, as a result of coronary artery spasm. It occurs more frequently in women. Characteristically, there is ST segment elevation on the ECG during the pain. Specialist investigation using provocation tests (e.g. hyperventilation, cold-pressor testing or ergometrine challenge) may be required to establish the diagnosis. Arrhythmias, both ventricular tachyarrhythmias and heart block, can occur during the ischaemic episode.

Cardiac syndrome X refers to those patients with a good history of angina, a positive exercise test and angiographically normal coronary arteries. They form a heterogeneous group and the syndrome is much more common in women than in men. Whilst they have a good prognosis, they are often highly symptomatic and can be difficult to treat. A recent study using phosphorus-31 nuclear magnetic resonance spectroscopy of the anterior left ventricular myocardium in women with this syndrome showed an abnormal metabolic response to stress consistent with the suggestion of myocardial ischaemia probably resulting from abnormal dilator responses of the coronary microvasculature to stress. The prognostic and therapeutic implications are not known.

Unstable angina refers to angina of recent onset (less than 1 month), worsening angina or angina at rest, and will be described in more detail on page 773.

Examination and diagnosis

There are usually no abnormal findings in angina, although occasionally a fourth heart sound may be heard. Signs to suggest anaemia, thyrotoxicosis or hyperlipidaemia (e.g. lipid arcus, xanthelasma, tendon xanthoma) should be sought. It is essential to exclude aortic stenosis (i.e. slow-rising carotid impulse and ejection systolic murmur radiating to the neck) as a possible cause for the angina. The blood pressure should be taken to identify coexistent hypertension.

Investigations for angina
Resting ECG

This is usually normal between attacks. Evidence of old myocardial infarction (e.g. pathological Q waves), left ventricular hypertrophy or left bundle branch block may be present. During an attack, transient ST depression, T-wave inversion or other changes of the shape of the T wave may appear.

Exercise ECG

Exercise testing can be very useful both in confirming the diagnosis of angina and in giving some indication as to the severity of the CAD. ST segment depression of ≥1 mm suggests myocardial ischaemia, particularly if typical chest pain occurs at the same time (Fig. 13.20).

The test has a specificity of 80% and a sensitivity of about 70% for CAD. A strongly positive test (within 6 minutes of starting the Bruce protocol) suggests 'prognostic' disease (see surgical management below) and helps to identify patients who should be offered

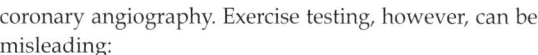

coronary angiography. Exercise testing, however, can be misleading:

- A normal test does not exclude CAD (so-called false-negative test) although these patients, as a group, have a good prognosis.
- Up to 20% of patients with positive exercise tests are subsequently found to have no evidence of coronary artery disease (so-called false-positive test).

Cardiac scintigraphy

Myocardial perfusion scans (see p. 728) both at rest and after stress (i.e. exercise or dobutamine) can be obtained using various contrast agents (e.g. [201]thallium or [99]technetium MIBI – methoxyisobutylisonitrile). Redistribution of the contrast agent is a sensitive indicator of ischaemia and can be particularly useful in deciding if a stenosis seen at angiography is giving rise to ischaemia. A normal perfusion scan makes significant CAD unlikely.

Echocardiography

This can be used to assess ventricular wall involvement and ventricular function. Regional wall motion abnormalities at rest reflect previous ventricular damage. Stress echocardiography, although technically difficult, is useful especially in women with coronary artery disease.

Coronary angiography

This is occasionally useful in patients with chest pain where the diagnosis is unclear. More often, the test is performed to delineate the exact coronary anatomy (Fig. 13.55) in patients being considered for revascularization

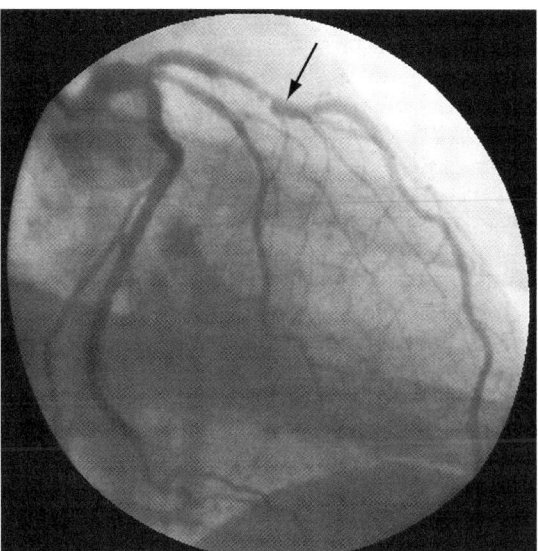

Fig. 13.55 Left coronary angiogram. X-ray contrast material is injected into the ostium of the left main coronary artery. In this example, the left main artery divides into three vessels: left anterior descending (top), diagonal and circumflex (bottom) vessels. In the proximal part of the left anterior descending artery is a severe narrowing due to an atherosclerotic plaque (arrow).

(i.e. coronary artery bypass grafting or coronary angioplasty). Coronary angiography should be performed only when the benefit in terms of diagnosis and potential treatment outweighs the small risk of the procedure (a mortality rate of less than 1 in 1000 cases). The indications for coronary angiography are outlined in Table 13.26.

Lesions with complex morphology (irregular borders, overhanging edges, thrombus or ulceration) appear to identify a subgroup of stenoses associated with disease progression and adverse clinical outcomes.

Treatment of angina
General management

Patients should be informed as to the nature of their condition and reassured that the prognosis is good (annual mortality less than 2%). Underlying problems, such as anaemia or hyperthyroidism, should be treated. Management of coexistent conditions, such as diabetes and hypertension, should be optimized. Risk factors should be evaluated and steps made to correct them where possible; for example, smoking must be stopped, hypercholesterolaemia should be identified and treated (see below), weight loss where appropriate and regular exercise should be encouraged.

Choosing between medical therapy and revascularization (coronary artery bypass grafting and angioplasty) can be difficult and will depend on a number of factors including symptoms, angiographic anatomy and patient/physician preference. The various treatment options are not mutually exclusive and should be considered as complementary.

Medical treatment
Prognostic therapies

Aspirin reduces the risk of coronary events in patients with coronary artery disease. All patients with angina, therefore, should take aspirin (75 mg daily is probably adequate) unless contraindicated.

Lipid-lowering therapy (p. 1109) should be used in patients with total cholesterol above 4.8 mmol/L (particularly if the LDL is >3.3 mmol/L and the HDL is <1.0 mmol/L), despite a low fat diet. If the triglycerides (TGs) are under 3.5 mmol/L, then one of the statins (HMG-CoA reductase inhibitors) should be used. If the TGs are above 3.5 mmol/L, a fibrate is indicated.

Table 13.26
Indications for coronary angiography

Angina refractory to medical therapy
Strongly positive exercise test
Unstable angina
Angina occurring after myocardial infarction
Patients under 50 years with angina or myocardial infarction
Where the diagnosis of angina is uncertain
Severe left ventricular dysfunction after myocardial infarction
Non-Q-wave myocardial infarction

If simple therapy fails to reduce the LDL adequately, then the patient should be referred to a lipidologist. Lipid-lowering therapy can be expected to prevent 20–30 deaths or myocardial infarcts per 1000 patient-years.

Hormone replacement therapy (HRT) appears to be cardioprotective. Exogenous oestrogen increases HDL, decreases oxidation of LDL and has beneficial effects on vasomotion. However, side-effects such as vaginal bleeding, and adverse effects such as the possible increase in risk of breast cancer, have limited its use. HRT is likely to benefit women who have a high risk of developing ischaemic heart disease, and should be considered for all women with established CAD who are not at high risk of breast carcinoma. The Heart and Estrogen/Progestin Replacement Study (HERS) is the first large clinical trial designed to test the efficacy of postmenopausal HRT for secondary prevention of CAD. The result showed that oral conjugated oestrogen plus medoxyprogesterone did not reduce the overall rate of events in postmenopausal women with CAD over an average follow-up of 4.1 years. However, patients receiving HRT had a significant 11% lower LDL cholesterol and 10% higher HDL cholesterol.

Symptomatic treatment

Glyceryl trinitrate (GTN) used sublingually, either as a tablet or as a spray, gives prompt relief (in a few minutes) and can also be used prior to performing activities that the patient knows will provoke angina.

All but the most mildly affected patients will probably require regular prophylactic therapy. The choice of drugs is between beta-blockers, nitrates and calcium-channel blockers. There is no commonly accepted algorithm and treatment needs to be tailored to the individual patient. Some patients will require combination therapy, but there is little evidence that adding a third drug is of benefit. Patients not controlled adequately on medical therapy should be considered for revascularization (see below).

Beta-blockers reduce the heart rate (negative chronotropic effect) and the force of ventricular contraction (negative inotropic effect), both of which reduce myocardial oxygen demand, especially on exertion. They are the drugs of choice in patients with previous myocardial infarction because of their proven benefit in secondary prevention. Atenolol, 50–100 mg daily, is the most commonly prescribed. Metoprolol, 25–50 mg twice daily, is often used if renal function is impaired. Beta-blockers may aggravate coronary artery spasm.

Long-acting nitrates (e.g. isosorbide mononitrate) are particularly useful in patients who gain relief from sublingual GTN. They reduce venous return and hence intracardiac diastolic pressures, reduce the impedance to the emptying of the left ventricle and relax the tone of the coronary arteries. Once-daily preparations are available which have a smooth pharmacokinetic profile and avoid the problem of tolerance. Nitrates should be given with care to patients on other hypotensive agents. Sildenafil should not be given to patients taking nitrates.

Calcium-channel blockers block calcium flux into the cell and the utilization of calcium within the cell (Table 13.27). They relax coronary arteries, cause peripheral vasodilatation and reduce the force of left ventricular contraction, thereby reducing the oxygen demand of the myocardium. The non-dihydropyridine calcium antagonists (e.g. diltiazem and verapamil) also reduce the heart rate and are particularly useful anti-anginal agents, but should be used with caution in combination with beta-blockers. Short-acting dihydropyridines (e.g. nifedipine) can cause reflex tachycardia when used alone. Case-control studies have suggested that high-dose nifedipine is associated with adverse outcome. Slow-release formulations and the third-generation agents (e.g. amlodipine) can be used once daily and have a smooth profile of action with no significant effect on the heart rate and no significant negative inotropic effect.

Nicorandil is a potassium-channel activator with a nitrate component; it has both arterial and venous

Table 13.27
Calcium-channel blockers

	Class 1 (non-dihydropyridine) (e.g. verapamil, diltiazem)	Class 2 (dihydropyridine) (e.g. nifedipine, nicardipine, amlodipine, felodopine, risoldipine)
Effects		
Sinus node suppression	+++	+
AV node suppression	+++	+
Myocardial depression	++	++
Arteriolar vasodilatation	+	+++
Side-effects		
Flushing, ankle oedema, palpitations	+	++
Bradycardia, impaired AV conduction	++	+
Aggravation of heart failure	++	+
Combination with beta-blockers	No	Yes

AV, atrioventricular

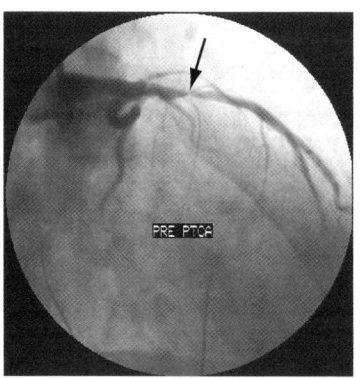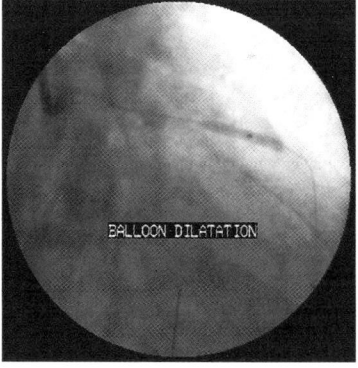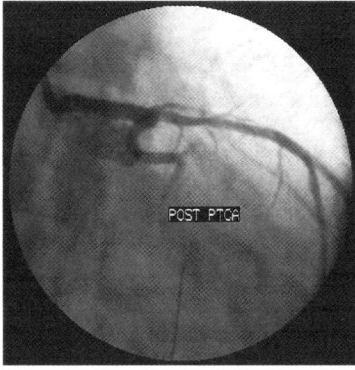

Fig. 13.56 **Percutaneous transluminal coronary angioplasty (PTCA)** demonstrated in a sequence of three films in a patient with a 90% stenosis in the proximal left anterior descending coronary artery (left film taken during coronary angiogram). The middle X-ray shows the inflated angioplasty balloon across the arterial lesion. The right film is taken from the post-PTCA coronary angiogram. It shows virtually complete alleviation of the stenosis.

vasodilating properties. Whilst not used as a first-line drug, it is used when there are contraindications to the above agents and in refractory unstable angina.

Coronary angioplasty

Percutaneous transluminal coronary angioplasty (PTCA) refers to the technique of dilating coronary atheromatous obstructions by inflating a balloon within the obstruction (Fig. 13.56). The balloon, which is mounted on the tip of a very thin catheter, is inserted through the obstruction using X-ray fluoroscopy and is then inflated with dilute contrast material. Multiple inflations of the balloon using a pressure of several atmospheres usually relieve the obstruction.

A number of different mechanisms have been postulated, including fracturing and compression of the plaque, and stretching of the artery. Endothelial denudation, local dissection and distal embolization also occur and may account for some of the complications of the procedure. Whilst PTCA is ideally suited to single, discrete stenoses, multiple lesions may be treated and repeat procedures can be undertaken.

Acute coronary occlusion occurs in a small proportion of cases (2–4%), and local dissection of the coronary artery is frequently observed. PTCAs improve symptoms of angina, but confer no significant prognostic benefit. The risks associated with PTCA are often understated and comprise mortality (1%), acute myocardial infarction (2%), and the need for urgent coronary artery bypass grafting (CABG) (2%).

A number of trials have compared PTCA with medical therapy for stable angina. PTCA may provide more complete relief from angina, but is associated with higher rates of myocardial infarction or bypass surgery (as a result of this procedure).

An increasing number of intracoronary stents (Fig. 13.57) are being used both to 'bale out' in cases of dissection and for the primary treatment of stenoses in large vessels (>3 mm; for example, proximal lesions in big left anterior descending arteries and dominant right

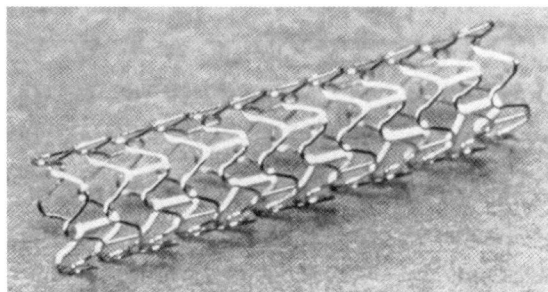

Fig. 13.57 **An intracoronary stent.**

coronary arteries), in coronary vein grafts, and in restenotic lesions following PTCA. The BENESTENT study demonstrated that PTCA plus stent implantation is significantly better than PTCA alone in terms of death, myocardial infarction, occurrence of cerebrovascular accident, the need for CABG or a repeat percutaneous intervention. Stents have a lower incidence of restenosis, which still complicates up to 30% of PTCAs (usually within the first 6 months post-procedure), but are more expensive. Aspirin plus other antiplatelet agents (e.g. clopidogrel) are routinely prescribed following stent insertion. The use of monoclonal antibodies to the glycoprotein IIb/IIIa platelet receptor (the final common pathway of platelet aggregation) in selected high-risk cases may reduce peri-procedural complications. Ongoing studies of new stents and optimal antithrombotic therapies are being carried out, recently intracoronary radiation therapy has been used to prevent restenosis.

Surgical management (Fig. 13.58)

There are two principal indications for coronary artery bypass grafting (CABG):

- *Symptom control* in patients who remain symptomatic despite optimal medical therapy and whose disease is not suitable for PTCA. Surgery provides dramatic relief from angina in about 90% of cases.

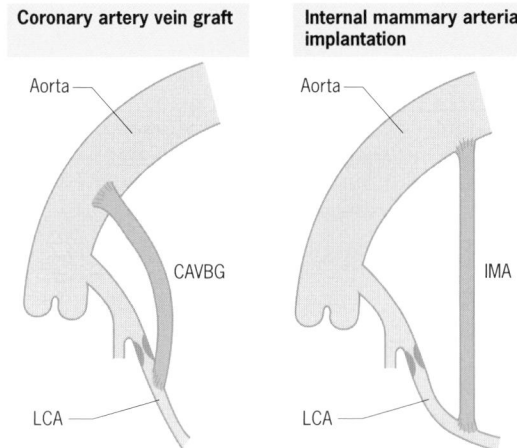

Fig. 13.58 Relief of coronary obstruction by surgical techniques: coronary artery vein bypass grafting (CAVBG) or internal mammary arterial implantation (IMA). In both of these examples, the graft bypasses a coronary obstruction in the left coronary artery (LCA).

- Improved survival in patients with severe three-vessel CAD (significant proximal stenoses in all three main coronary vessels), particularly those with impaired left ventricular function, and in those with left main stem artery disease. These patients obtain *prognostic benefit* from CABG, irrespective of symptoms.

Where possible, the left internal mammary artery (LIMA) is used to bypass proximal stenoses in the left anterior descending artery. Similarly, the right internal mammary artery is increasingly being used to bypass stenoses in the right coronary artery. Reverse saphenous vein grafts are still commonly used in addition to arterial grafts, although the long-term patency is less good with atheromatous occlusion occurring in up to 10% of cases per year. Operative mortality is well below 1% in patients with normal left ventricular function. Perioperative strokes occur in up to 2% of cases, and more subtle neurological deficits are common.

Minimally invasive operative procedures for bypass grafting ('MIDCAB') are being developed which do not require the use of extracorporeal circulatory support. These include laparoscopic approaches and may be of use in certain subgroups of patients (e.g. previous CABG and those with coexistent medical conditions which would increase the operative risks of 'full' CABG).

Aggressive lowering of LDL (to less than 2.5 mmol/L) has shown to be beneficial in patients who have had coronary artery bypass surgery.

PTCA versus bypass surgery

Several studies have compared PTCA with bypass surgery. Both techniques provide excellent symptomatic relief with a similar incidence of major ischaemic complications. The major short-term advantage of PTCA is the avoidance of major open-heart surgery (and a shorter hospital stay). However, up to 50% of patients will require a repeat revascularization procedure within the next 2 years. There is some evidence that diabetic patients have a better 5-year survival after treatment with bypass surgery than with PTCA.

Patients with intractable angina

Some patients remain symptomatic despite medication and are not suitable for (further) revascularization. Transmyocardial laser revascularization (TMR), whereby a laser is used to form channels in the myocardium to allow direct perfusion of the myocardium from blood within the ventricular cavity has been used in some centres but in controlled trials it has not been beneficial.

Spinal cord stimulation (SCS) is accomplished using a flexible electrode in the epidural space at the mid-thoracic level. Stimulation via a pacemaker-like generator reduces angina and has been shown to reduce indices of ischaemia. Similarly, transcutaneous electrical nerve stimulation has been shown to reduce angina and increase exercise capacity in selected patients.

Acute coronary syndrome (ACS)

ACS (also called *unstable angina*) and *myocardial infarction without ST segment elevation* are clinical features of coronary artery disease which lie between stable angina and myocardial infaction with ST elevation or sudden death. ACS is a medical emergency which, untreated, will progress to myocardial infarction in over 10% of cases. Therapy (see below) reduces this rate to less than 5%. However, death within 1 year still occurs in 5–15%.

ACS is a common reason for hospital admission and patients are at increased risk of myocardial infarction, death and other cardiovascular events. Defining high-risk patients is necessary to allow appropriate targeting of treatment strategies and resources. The **P**rospective **R**egistry of **A**cute **I**schaemic **S**yndromes in the **UK** (PRAIS-UK) demonstrated the magnitude of the problem. For all patients, the risk of death, new myocardial infarction, refractory angina or readmission with ACS is 30% at 6 months. Age, diabetes mellitus, troponin level and baseline ECG are good aids to risk stratification (Table 13.28).

Patients require admission for bed rest, oxygen and morphine, plus aspirin and heparin as well as standard medical anti-anginal therapy (i.e. nitrates and beta-blockers). Aspirin decreases the incidence of both death and myocardial infarction. Oral clopidogrel, which inhibits the platelet ADP receptor, should also be given (CURE study – **C**lopidogrel in **U**nstable angina to prevent **R**ecurrent **E**vents trial). Heparin, traditionally given intravenously, should be given for at least 3 days. There is increasing evidence that low-molecular-weight heparins (LMWH), such as dalteparin or enoxaparin, are at least as effective as standard unfractionated heparin and have the advantage of being able to be given subcutaneously and of not require monitoring. Recent trials have shown that infusion of glycoprotein

Table 13.28
Risk stratification in patients with acute coronary syndrome (ACS)

High risk	Intermediate risk	Low risk
Prolonged, ongoing (> 20 min) rest pain	Rest angina (< 20 min or relieved with GTN)	Increased angina severity frequency or duration
Pulmonary oedema or angina with hypotension	New-onset angina (< 4 weeks) Nocturnal angina	Angina provoked at a lower threshold, but no rest pain
Rest angina with dynamic ST changes > 1 mm	Angina with dynamic T wave changes	Normal/unchanged ECG
Raised troponin (I/T)		Normal troponin I/T
Age > 70 years		
Diabetes mellitus		

IIb/IIIa receptor inhibitors (e.g. tirofiban, eptifibatide) may have an additional advantage over heparin plus aspirin in reducing the mortality in high-risk patients. These receptors are activated in the final common pathway of platelet aggregation.

In terms of the short-term risk of death or myocardial infarction, it is possible to risk-stratify patients with ACS into high risk, intermediate risk and low risk (Table 13.28). Those at high risk should proceed promptly to angiography, with a view to proceeding to revascularization, where appropriate, during that admission. Those at low risk can be discharged and then assessed electively as outpatients. In between, there is much controversy regarding the optimal management of patients at intermediate risk, and in particular those who settle on initial medical therapy. Early intervention does not convincingly appear to influence the medium- and long-term outcomes. Attention is increasingly being directed at therapies that can favourably influence the procoagulant/thrombogenic state that seems to persist for several months following presentation. In particular, the prolonged use (weeks to months) of subcutaneous low-molecular-weight heparin and intravenous glycoprotein IIb/IIIa antagonists has been clearly shown to be of benefit (FRISC II and PRISM-PLUS trials).

Irrespective of the immediate success of treatment, early coronary angiography and, depending on the results, referral for revascularization are usually advised.

Thrombolytic therapy has not been shown to be of benefit in patients with ACS. Occasionally, intra-aortic balloon pumping (see p. 734) can be helpful in stabilizing the patient, and to enable angiography (± PTCA) to be undertaken.

Myocardial infarction

Myocardial infarction (MI) is the most common cause of death in the UK. There are approximately 300 000 new myocardial infarctions per year. Only half of those who suffer an MI survive the acute event. A further 10% die in hospital and up to 10% more die in the following 2 years. Fifty per cent of initial survivors are alive at 10 years.

MI almost always occurs in patients with coronary atheroma as a result of plaque rupture with superadded thrombus. This occlusive thrombus consists of a platelet-rich core ('white clot') and a bulkier surrounding fibrin-rich ('red') clot. About 6 hours after the onset of infarction, the myocardium is swollen and pale, and at 24 hours the necrotic tissue appears deep red owing to haemorrhage. In the next few weeks, an inflammatory reaction develops and the infarcted tissue turns grey and gradually forms a thin, fibrous scar.

Remodelling refers to the alteration in size, shape and thickness of both the infarcted myocardium (which thins and expands) and the compensatory hypertrophy that occurs in other areas of the myocardium. The resultant global ventricular dilatation may help maintain the stroke volume of the heart.

The use of thrombolysis (see below) has transformed the acute management of patients with MI. Thrombolysis recanalizes the thrombotic occlusion by lysing the fibrin-rich elements, resulting in restoration of coronary blood flow. Many large trials have established benefits in reducing infarct size, improving myocardial function and improving survival. Paramedic and hospital services should be organized to ensure prompt thrombolysis.

Clinical features

The algorithm for assessing patients with suspected MI is shown in Figure 13.59. MI typically presents with severe chest pain, similar in character to exertional angina. The onset is usually sudden, often occurring at rest, and persists fairly constantly for some hours (often until diamorphine is given). Whilst the pain may be so severe that the patient fears imminent death, it can be less severe, and as many as 20% of patients with MI have no pain. So-called 'silent' myocardial infarctions are more common in diabetics and the elderly. MI is often accompanied by sweating, breathlessness, nausea, vomiting and restlessness.

Patients with acute MI appear pale, sweaty and grey. There may be no specific physical signs unless complications develop (see below). A sinus tachycardia, fourth heart sound and a raised JVP are common. A modest fever (up to 38°C) due to myocardial necrosis often occurs over the course of the first 5 days.

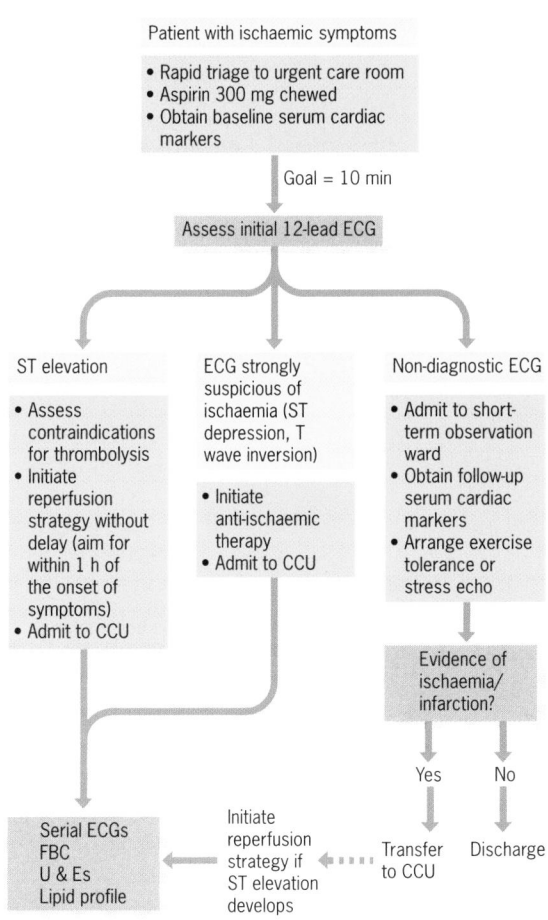

Fig. 13.59 Management of acute myocardial infarction.

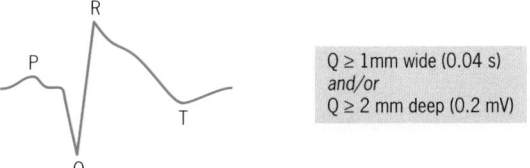

Fig. 13.60 **Electrocardiographic features of myocardial infarction,** showing a Q wave, ST elevation and T wave inversion.

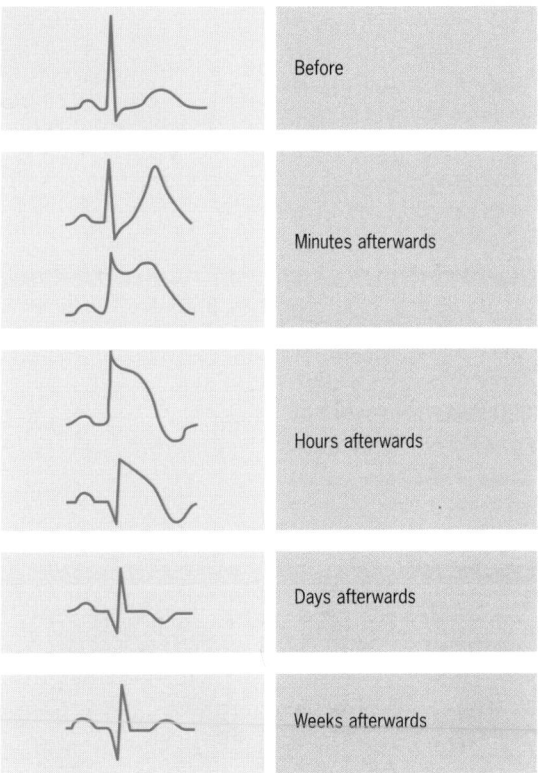

Fig. 13.61 **Electrocardiographic evolution of myocardial infarction.** After the first few minutes the T waves become tall, pointed and upright and there is ST segment elevation. After the first few hours the T waves invert, the R wave voltage is decreased and Q waves develop. After a few days the ST segment returns to normal. After weeks or months the T wave may return to upright but the Q wave remains.

Diagnosis requires at least two of the following:

- a history of ischaemic-type chest pain
- evolving ECG changes
- a rise in cardiac enzymes or troponins.

Investigations

The electrocardiogram

A Q wave is a broad (>1 mm) and deep (>2 mm or more than 25% of the amplitude of the following R wave) negative deflection that starts the QRS complex (Fig. 13.60). It may occur normally in leads AVR and V_1 (and sometimes in lead III) but, in other leads, it is abnormal. Abnormal Q waves are produced by several abnormalities such as left bundle branch block, ventricular tachycardia and the Wolff–Parkinson–White syndrome. The gradual development of Q waves over minutes or hours suggests the occurrence of a full-thickness (as opposed to a subendocardial) MI. They develop because the electrical silence of infarcted cardiac tissue results in a so-called 'window' through which the normal endocardial-to-epicardial activation of the opposite non-infarcted ventricular wall is 'seen', resulting in an unopposed depolarization front moving away from an electrode situated over the epicardial surface of the infarct. Q waves are usually permanent electrocardiographic features following full-thickness MI.

T wave and ST segment changes result from ischaemia and injury. They are therefore often transient, occurring only during the acute attack. The progressive changes or evolution of the ECG during the course of a full-thickness MI are illustrated in Figure 13.61.

With subendocardial infarction (Fig. 13.62), only the endocardial surface is infarcted and Q waves do not develop (so-called 'non-Q-wave MI'). ST segment and T wave changes are therefore the only ECG features of a

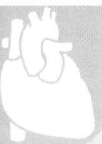

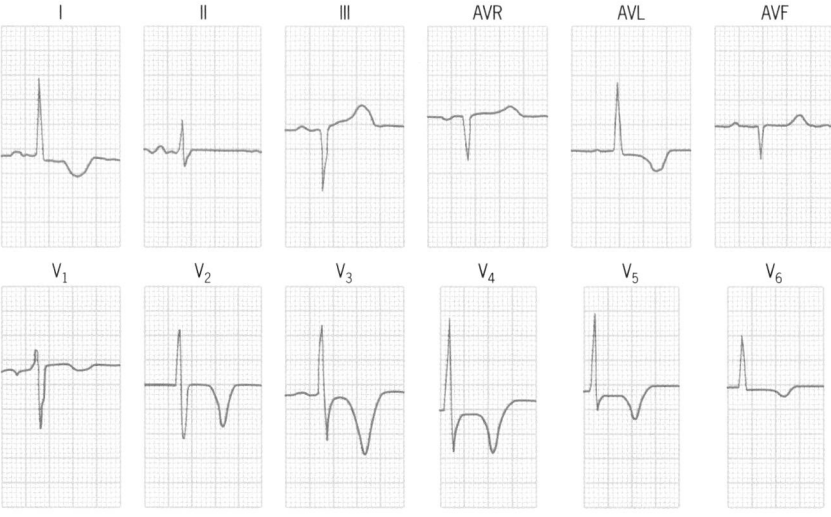

Fig. 13.62 **A widespread (anterolateral) subendocardial myocardial infarction** shown by a 12-lead ECG. Note the deeply inverted, symmetrical T waves in addition to ST depression.

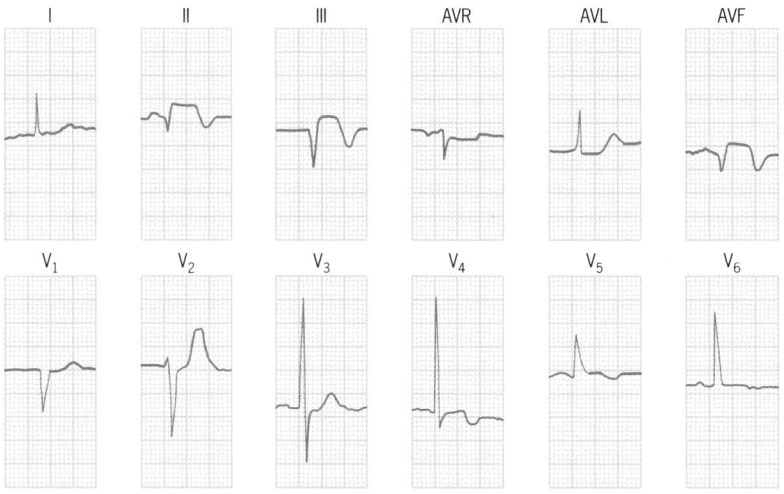

Fig. 13.63 **An acute inferior wall myocardial infarction** shown by a 12-lead ECG. Note the raised ST segment and Q waves in the inferior leads (II, III and AVF). The additional T wave inversion in V_4 and V_5 probably represents anterior wall ischaemia.

Table 13.29
Typical ECG changes in myocardial infarction

Infarct site	Leads showing main changes
Anterior	
Small	V_3–V_4
Extensive	V_2–V_5
Anteroseptal	V_1–V_3
Anterolateral	V_4–V_6, I, AVL
Lateral	I, II, AVL
Inferior	II, III, AVF
Posterior	V_1, V_2 (reciprocal)
Subendocardial	Any lead
Right ventricle	VR_4

subendocardial infarction. Because the injury is endocardial rather than predominantly epicardial, ST segment depression rather than elevation is usual.

ECG changes (Table 13.29) are usually confined to the ECG leads that 'face' the infarction. Therefore, an inferior wall MI is diagnosed when the ECG findings are seen in leads II, III and AVF (Fig. 13.63). Lateral infarction produces changes in leads I, AVL and $V_{5/6}$. In anterior infarction, leads V_2–V_5 may be affected. Changes seen in an anterolateral infarction are demonstrated in Figure 13.64. Because there are no posterior leads, a true posterior wall infarct is usually diagnosed by the appearance of a mirror image or reciprocal changes in leads V_1 and V_2 (i.e. the development of a tall initial R wave, ST segment depression and tall, upright T waves). These reciprocal changes can also be seen in association with other infarctions. For example, in an inferior wall myocardial infarction, anterior ST segment depression may be seen. In right ventricular infarction the ST segment is raised in lead VR_4.

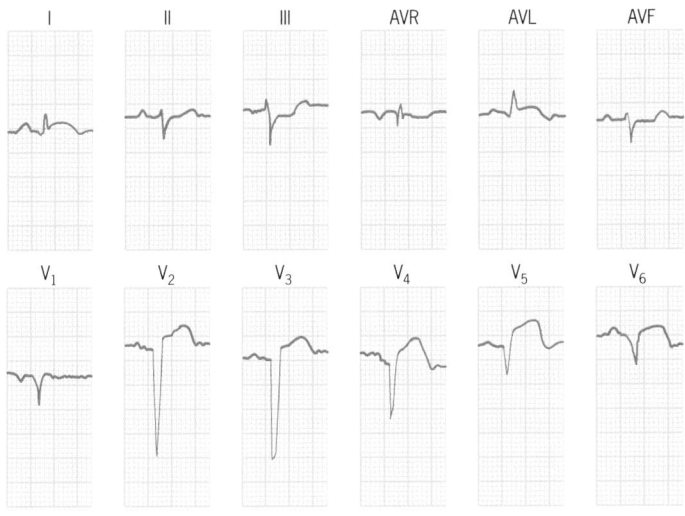

Fig. 13.64 An acute anterolateral myocardial infarction shown by a 12-lead ECG. Note the ST segment elevation in leads I, AVL, and V_2–V_6. The T wave is inverted in leads I, AVL and V_3–V_6. Pathological Q waves are seen in leads V_2–V_6.

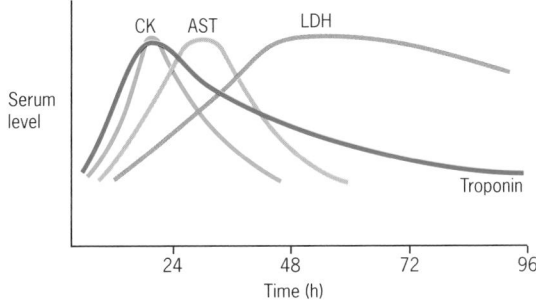

Fig. 13.65 Cardiac markers in acute myocardial infarction. CK, creatine kinase; AST, aspartate aminotransferase; LDH, lactate dehydrogenase.

Cardiac markers (Fig. 13.65)

Necrotic cardiac tissue releases several enzymes and proteins into the serum:

- *Creatine kinase* (CK). This peaks within 24 hours and is usually back to normal by 48 hours. It is also produced by damaged skeletal muscle and brain. Cardiac-specific isoforms can be measured (CK-MB) allowing greater diagnostic accuracy. The size of the enzyme rise is broadly proportional to the infarct size.
- *Cardiac-specific troponins*. Troponin T and troponin I are regulatory proteins with a very high specificity for cardiac injury. They are released early (2–4 hours) and can persist for up to 7 days. Immunoassays specific for these proteins can be performed in the laboratory and at the bedside in as little as 15 minutes using modern automated equipment. They are more sensitive and cardiac specific than CK-MB.
- *Aspartate aminotransferase* (AST) and *lactate dehydrogenase* (LDH). These non-specific enzymes are rarely used now for the diagnosis of MI. LDH peaks at 3–4 days and remains elevated for up to

10 days and can be useful in confirming myocardial infarction in patients presenting several days after an episode of chest pain.
- *Serial cardiac markers*. These should be measured in all patients presenting with suspected MI. Levels greater than twice the upper limit of normal are confirmatory in patients with a good history and/or ECG changes. With successful reperfusion, the enzyme rise should be curtailed.

Management of myocardial infarction

Acute management

The treatment of acute MI is summarized in Figure 13.59. If the diagnosis of MI is suspected, an ECG should be obtained immediately. If diagnostic ST elevation is present (see below), thrombolysis should be commenced without delay (unless contraindicated) and aspirin given (150 mg, chewed). The beneficial effects of aspirin and thrombolysis are synergistic. Adequate analgesia (diamorphine 5–10 mg i.v. combined with antiemetics such as cyclizine 50 mg i.v. or metoclopramide 10 mg i.v.) should be given if required. Thrombolysis should also be started if there is typical chest pain and high serum cardiac markers (troponins can be measured in 15 min).

Thrombolytic treatment can achieve reperfusion in 50–70% of patients (compared with a spontaneous rate of 20–30%). Many large trials have shown that thrombolysis within 12 hours reduces the extent of ventricular damage and mortality rate. The criteria for thrombolysis are outlined in Table 13.30.

Streptokinase (1.5 million units over 1 hour) is the agent used most commonly. Front-loaded tissue-type plasminogen activator (t-PA) achieves higher reperfusion rates but is more expensive than streptokinase and is associated with a higher risk of stroke. t-PA tends to be given in preference to streptokinase in patients under 50 years of age with anterior MIs, where the blood pressure is low (systolic below 100 mmHg), and in those

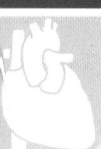

Table 13.30
Criteria for thrombolysis in acute myocardial infarction

Indications	Chest pain consistent with myocardial infarction, within 12 hours AND ST segement elevation (> 1 mm in two or more contiguous leads) or new left bundle branch block or high-serum cardiac markers
Contraindications	Stroke or active bleeding in last 2 months Systolic blood pressure > 200 mmHg Proliferative diabetic retinopathy Pregnancy
Relative contraindications	Prolonged or traumatic resuscitation Recent (< 2 weeks) surgery or trauma Known bleeding diathesis or current use of anticoagulants

patients who have previously received streptokinase. t-PA must be followed by intravenous heparin. t-PA is considerably more effective than streptokinase if it can be given within 4 hours of the onset of chest pain.

There is an approximate 1% risk of stroke and a 0.7% risk of major haemorrhage associated with the use of thrombolysis. Allergic reactions occur in under 2% of patients receiving streptokinase, and hypotension in 10%.

Following initiation of thrombolysis, the patient should be transferred to the coronary care unit. An i.v. beta-blocker such as metoprolol 5–10 mg should be given, particularly if the heart rate is above 100 b.p.m. with persistent pain. Intravenous nitrates are also given for persistent pain or pulmonary oedema (only if the systolic blood pressure is above 100 mmHg). Oxygen 60% is given routinely, by facemask or nasal cannula.

If the ECG is normal or shows only minor or non-specific changes, then take a careful history, examine the patient, and repeat the ECG after 1 hour. With a typical history and no ST elevation, acute coronary syndrome is likely (see p. 773). Alternative diagnoses should also be considered during this period (e.g. aortic dissection, see p. 830).

Whilst thrombolytic therapy is effective in restoring antegrade flow, improving left ventricular function and reducing mortality, reperfusion is unsuccessful in approximately 25% of patients, and early re-occlusion occurs in a further 10%. An increasing number of interventional centres are performing 'primary PTCA' – immediate cardiac catheterization and PTCA – in patients with evolving myocardial infarction. Primary PTCA can be attempted when thrombolysis is contra-indicated (see below), when initial ECG changes are equivocal, and when thrombolysis has failed. However, it requires experienced operators and, ideally, cardio-thoracic surgical backup, a scenario that is not widely available in the UK.

Subsequent management in hospital

The patient should be monitored in the coronary care unit for 48 hours (this is the at-risk time for cardiac arrests secondary to ventricular arrhythmias) to enable prompt resuscitation by specially trained staff as necessary.

Aspirin 75–150 mg daily is given unless contra-indicated. Beta-blockers have been shown to reduce the incidence of sudden death following MI by 20–25% (about 10 lives saved per 1000 patients yearly). All patients – except those with ongoing clinical heart failure – should be treated with beta-blockers for at least 1 year unless contraindicated (e.g. COPD). Patients with ongoing heart failure can be considered for beta-blocker treatment after they have recovered from heart failure, but it is crucial to commence them on a low dose of beta-blocker and titrate upwards. Left ventricular function has prognostic relevance after an MI, with a progressive increase in 1-year mortality following MI as the left ventricular ejection fraction (LVEF) falls below 0.4. With survival benefit from ACE inhibitor treatment, all patients after MI should have their LVEF measured with an echocardiogram prior to discharge and patients with clinical evidence of pulmonary oedema, reduced left ventricular ejection fraction < 0.4, or extensive Q-wave infarct should be commenced on an angiotensin-converting enzyme (ACE) inhibitor. The treatment with an ACE inhibitor should be reviewed after 4–6 weeks as an outpatient. Patients with large anterior Q-wave infarcts should also be anticoagulated with warfarin, usually for 3 months.

Gradual mobilization is commenced on the second day and the patient should be pain-free and fully ambulant before discharge – 5 or 6 days in uncomplicated cases. Prior to discharge, patients should undergo submaximal exercise-tolerance testing. An exercise-tolerance test is used to identify the presence of residual ischaemia and has short- and long-term prognostic value. It is useful for the prescription of rehabilitation programmes. It normally entails submaximal treadmill testing (70% of age-predicted maximal heart rate) at 4–6 days post-MI or symptom-limited treadmill testing at 10–14 days post-MI. Patients with test results suggesting ischaemia should be referred for coronary angiography. Patients with non-Q-wave MI should also be evaluated with coronary angiography.

All patients should be seen by a rehabilitation nurse and dietitian to arrange systematic individualized reha-bilitation. Cardiac rehabilitation should start as soon as possible within the hospital environment beginning with education on MI, advice on risk factor modifica-tion, work prospect, prognosis and the benefit of early mobilization. Risk factors on smoking cessation, physi-cal activity, diet, weight and diabetes should be given. Patients need to be advised that they cannot drive for 1 month, and heavy goods and public service driving licences are withdrawn prior to special assessment.

Follow-up

Structured psychological and physical rehabilitation should be available to all patients after myocardial infarction. Most patients are ready to join the outpatient exercise-training programme 4–8 weeks after MI and attend for 4–12 weeks with 1–6 sessions a week. The majority will be fully recovered at 2 months and able to return to work.

Most patients should be reviewed as outpatients at 6–8 weeks and risk factors should be reviewed and modified if necessary:

- *Give advice and treatment* to maintain blood pressure below 140/85 mmHg.
- *Diabetic patients* must control glucose level meticulously.
- *Lipid-lowering therapy* if the fasting lipid profile is unfavourable (total serum cholesterol > 5 mmol/L or LDL-C > 3 mmol/L), despite a low-fat diet.
- *Aspirin* should be continued indefinitely.

Consideration can be given to withdrawing beta-blockers after 3 years in low-risk, normotensive patients. ACE inhibitors should be continued indefinitely in patients with persistent impairment of left ventricular function (i.e. an ejection fraction < 0.4).

Complications

In the acute phase – the first 2 or 3 days following MI – cardiac arrhythmias, cardiac failure and pericarditis are the most common complications. Later, recurrent infarction, angina, thromboembolism, mitral valve regurgitation and ventricular septal or free wall rupture may occur. Late complications include the post-MI syndrome (Dressler's syndrome), ventricular aneurysm, and recurrent cardiac arrhythmias. Cardiac arrhythmias are described in detail on page 735.

Ventricular extrasystoles

These commonly occur after MI. Their occurrence may precede the development of ventricular fibrillation, particularly if they are frequent (more than five per minute), multiform (different shapes) or R-on-T (falling on the upstroke or peak of the preceding T wave). Treatment has not been shown to reduce the likelihood of subsequent ventricular tachycardia or fibrillation.

Sustained ventricular tachycardia

This may degenerate into ventricular fibrillation or may itself produce serious haemodynamic consequences. It can be treated with intravenous lidocaine (lignocaine) or, if haemodynamic deterioration occurs, synchronized cardioversion (initially 200 J).

Ventricular fibrillation

This may occur in the first few hours or days following an MI in the absence of severe cardiac failure or cardiogenic shock. It is treated with prompt defibrillation (200–360 J). Recurrences of ventricular fibrillation can be treated with lidocaine (lignocaine) infusion or, in cases of poor left ventricular function, amiodarone. When ventricular fibrillation occurs in the setting of heart failure, shock or aneurysm (so-called 'secondary ventricular fibrillation'), the prognosis is very poor unless the underlying haemodynamic or mechanical cause can be corrected. The serum potassium should be above 4.5 mmol/L.

Atrial fibrillation

This occurs in about 10% of patients with MI. It is due to atrial irritation caused by heart failure, pericarditis and atrial ischaemia or infarction. It may be managed with intravenous digoxin (to reduce ventricular rate in 1–2 h) or intravenous amiodarone and by treatment of the underlying pathology. It is not usually a long-standing problem, but it is a risk factor for subsequent mortality.

Sinus bradycardia

This is especially associated with acute inferior wall MI. Symptoms emerge only when the bradycardia is severe. When symptomatic, the treatment consists of elevating the foot of the bed and giving intravenous atropine, 600 μg if no improvement. When sinus bradycardia occurs, an escape rhythm such as idioventricular rhythm (wide QRS complexes with a regular rhythm at 50–100 b.p.m.) or idiojunctional rhythm (narrow QRS complexes) may occur. Usually no specific treatment is required. It has been suggested that sinus bradycardia following MI may predispose to the emergence of ventricular fibrillation. Severe sinus bradycardia associated with unresponsive symptoms or the emergence of unstable rhythms may need treatment with temporary pacing.

Sinus tachycardia

This is produced by heart failure, fever and anxiety. Usually, no specific treatment is required.

Conduction disturbances

These are common following MI. AV nodal delay (first-degree AV block) or higher degrees of block may occur during acute MI, especially of the inferior wall (the right coronary artery usually supplies the SA and AV nodes). Complete heart block, when associated with haemodynamic compromise, may need treatment with atropine or a temporary pacemaker. Such blocks may last for only a few minutes, but frequently continue for several days. Permanent pacing may need to be considered if complete heart block persists for over 2 weeks.

Acute anterior wall MI may also produce damage to the distal conduction system (the His bundle or bundle branches). The development of complete heart block usually implies a large MI and a poor prognosis. The ventricular escape rhythm is slow and unreliable, and a temporary pacemaker is necessary. This form of block is often permanent.

The development of complete AV block (Table 13.31) can be expected in 20–30% of cases where progressive

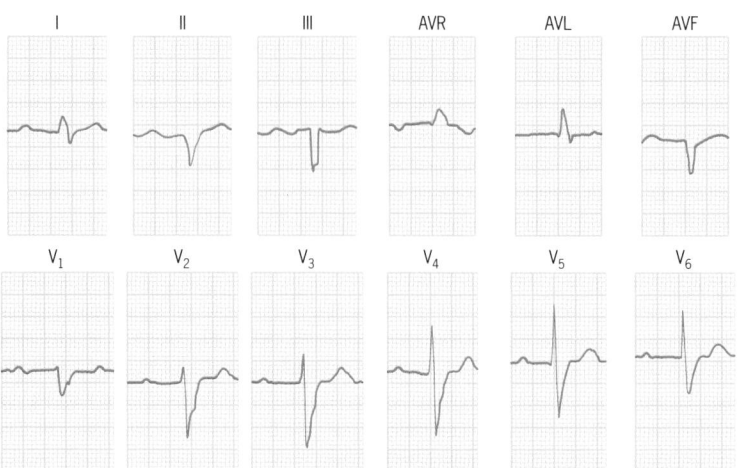

I   II   III   AVR   AVL   AVF

V₁   V₂   V₃   V₄   V₅   V₆

Fig. 13.66 Electrocardiographic picture consistent with bifascicular block with delay in the AV node on the third fascicle. There is a prolonged PR interval (0.32 s), a broad QRS complex with a deep S wave in leads I and V6 (right bundle branch block) and left axis deviation (−75°).

Table 13.31
Progression from different types of fascicular block to complete heart block in patients with acute myocardial infarction

Type of fascicular block	Percentage progressing to complete heart block
LAH	4
LPH	8
Long PR interval	10
LBBB	10
RBBB	20
RBBB + LAH	30
RBBB + LPH	40
RBBB + (LPH or LAH) + Long PR interval	40

LAH, left anterior hemiblock; LPH, left posterior hemiblock; RBBB, right bundle branch block; LBBB, left bundle branch block

---

Table 13.32
Killip (clinical) classification of heart failure in patients with acute myocardial infarction

Class	Description	Incidence (%)	Mortality (%)
I	No heart failure	40	5
II	Mild left ventricular failure	40	20
III	Pulmonary oedema	10	40
IV	Cardiogenic shock	10	90

---

bundle branch block (right bundle branch block and then right bundle branch block with a QRS axis shift) has already occurred (Fig. 13.66).

Cardiac failure and cardiogenic shock.

Heart failure after acute MI is graded according to a clinical classification (Table 13.32). Mild left heart failure (a few basal crackles that persist after coughing, an extra heart sound and upper lobe blood diversion on chest X-ray) occurs in about 40% of patients with acute MI.

Treatment for a few days with low-dose diuretics is usually all that is needed for symptomatic relief, but an ACE inhibitor should be given for prognostic benefit (see p. 760).

A large MI may lead to severe heart failure and pulmonary oedema. In such cases more prolonged and powerful diuretics and vasodilator treatment is necessary. In very severe cases a pulmonary artery balloon catheter is used to measure the pulmonary artery and, indirectly, the left atrial pressures and the cardiac output. Treatment is with loop diuretics, vasodilators (see p. 760) and, occasionally, digoxin.

The Amiodarone Trials meta-analysis showed that amiodarone therapy reduces both arrhythmic deaths (29%) and all-cause mortality (13%) in high-risk patients (i.e. left ventricular dysfunction after MI) (see also p. 751).

Hypotension and raised right-heart filling pressures are characteristically seen in right ventricular infarction that may accompany inferior infarcts. ST segment elevation is seen in V₄R leads on ECG. Echocardiography should be performed to exclude pericardial effusion. Initial treatment is with volume expansion (p. 937).

Severe heart failure may also follow ventricular septal rupture or mitral valve papillary muscle rupture. Both of these conditions present with worsening heart failure, a systolic thrill and a loud pansystolic murmur, widely heard over the precordium. Often, echocardiography and right heart catheterization with a balloon catheter is needed to differentiate between these two conditions. Both are associated with a poor prognosis, but vigorous treatment, including early surgical correction, can be successful in selected cases.

Cardiogenic shock is an extreme form of *cardiac failure* or *circulatory collapse*. Its features and management are described on page 765. The mortality from this condition is about 90%. The majority of those rescued (usually with the help of intra-aortic balloon counterpulsation) have a complication that can be treated surgically, such as left ventricular aneurysm, torrential mitral regurgitation or ventricular septal perforation.

Cardiac rupture results in almost immediate cardiac tamponade and is usually fatal within a few minutes. Electromechanical dissociation – no pulse or cardiac output, but a persistently normal rhythm on ECG – is the classical presentation. Treatment is rarely successful.

Ventricular asynergy and papillary muscle dysfunction (not rupture) may produce mild mitral regurgitation in association with heart failure. This causes a transient, soft, pansystolic murmur in up to half of those with acute MI. In these cases, no specific treatment is necessary for the mitral regurgitation.

Thromboembolism

Bed rest and cardiac failure contribute to the common occurrence of thrombosis and embolism after MI. Only 10% of patients have clinical features of thromboembolism, but in almost 50% of patients who die, there is evidence of emboli. Deep venous thrombosis (p. 832) is the most common manifestation and pulmonary embolism may result from this.

Left ventricular mural thrombus may form on the endocardial surface of the infarcted region. Systemic embolization may occur in over 10% of patients. A review of over 2000 patients with left ventricular dysfunction following MI found a 5-year stroke rate of 8.1%. A decreased ejection systolic fraction and older age were both independent predictors of an increased risk of stroke. Anticoagulant therapy appears to protect against stroke and should be considered in a patient with documented mural thrombus and in those patients with significant left ventricular dysfunction.

Other complications
Pericarditis

This is characterized by sharp chest pain, aggravated by movement and respiration. It is characteristically worse on lying down. There may be a pericardial rub. It is common in the first few days, particularly in anterior wall infarction. ECG shows generalized ST segment elevation (concave upward) with upright, peaked T waves. Asprin, paracetamol, but not NSAIDS are usually effective. Anticoagulation should be avoided.

Post-myocardial infarction syndrome (Dressler's syndrome)

This occurs weeks or months after an acute MI and presents with chest pain, pericardial friction rub, pleurisy with occasional pulmonary infiltrates, fever, malaise, and leucocytosis. Pericardial effusion is common and is usually fibrinous. Autoimmune reaction to myocardial damage is the main aetiology, and antimyocardial antibodies can often be found. Recurrences are common. Differential diagnosis should be made with a new MI or unstable angina. Treatment includes high doses of aspirin (600–900 mg every 4–6 hours), although corticosteroids are often required for recurrent forms. Anticoagulants should be discontinued unless there is a strong evidence for high risk of thromboembolic complications.

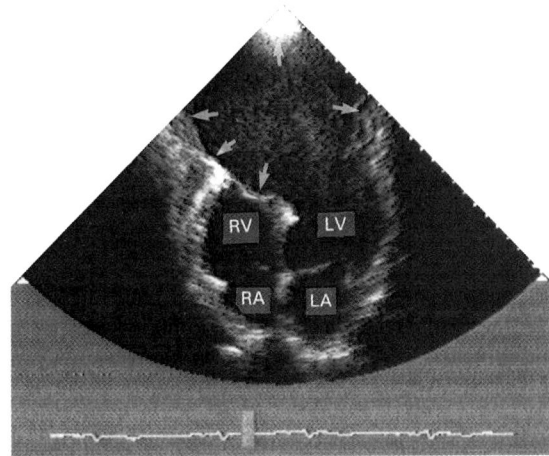

Fig. 13.67 Two-dimensional echocardiogram (apical four-chamber view) showing a very large apical left ventricular aneurysm (arrowed). The relatively static blood in the aneurysm produces a swirling 'smoke' effect. This aneurysm was successfully resected surgically. LV, left ventricle; LA, left atrium; RV, right ventricle; RA, right atrium.

Left ventricular aneurysm

This is a late complication. Patients may present with heart failure, arrhythmias or systemic emboli. It is characterized by ventricular asynergy (often palpable as a double impulse) and ECG shows persistent ST segment elevation. Diagnosis is confirmed by echocardiography (Fig. 13.67). Treatment comprises anticoagulation, ACE inhibitors and antiarrhythmic drugs as necessary. Surgical removal (aneurysectomy) may be helpful in selected cases.

Prognosis

Prognosis following MI is variable. The main prognostic indicators are advanced age and large infarcts (e.g. reduced left ventricular function, large heart on chest X-ray, heart failure). Left ventricular dysfunction, residual myocardial ischaemia and a susceptibility to ventricular arrhythmias are the three main determinants of survival. Patency of the infarct-related artery is associated with a significantly lower long-term mortality.

Overall, approximately 10% of patients surviving the initial heart attack die in the first 2 years, with the 5-year mortality approaching 20%. In young patients (< 50 years) the absolute risk of death is below 3% per year, compared with over 15% in those over 70 years old.

Sudden cardiac death

(see also Box 13.1, p. 731)

Sudden cardiac death is generally defined as death due to cardiac causes which occurs within 6 hours of the onset of symptoms. The causes of sudden cardiac death tend to mirror, in risk factors and prevalence, the predominant cardiac causes of death in a given population.

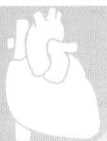

Table 13.33
Causes of sudden cardiac death

Coronary
Acute myocardial infarction
Chronic ischaemic heart disease
Post-coronary-artery bypass surgery
Post-successful resuscitation for cardiac arrest
Congenital anomaly of coronary arteries
Coronary artery embolism
Coronary arteritis

Non-coronary
Hypertrophic cardiomyopathy
Dilated cardiomyopathy (ischaemic or idiopathic)
Arrhythmogenic right ventricular cardiomyopathy
Congenital long QT syndrome
Brugada's syndrome
Valvular heart disease (aortic stenosis, mitral valve prolapse)
Cyanotic heart disease (tetralogy of Fallot, transposition)
Acyanotic heart disease (ventricular septal defect, patent ductus arteriosus)

In developed countries, the majority (80%) is estimated to be due to coronary artery disease, a further 10–15% to cardiomyopathies and 5% to valvular heart disease. Post-mortem studies have revealed that coronary atheroma is present in 80–90% of cases. Forty per cent of all deaths due to coronary atherosclerosis occur suddenly in this way, although up to 50% of patients dying suddenly because of coronary atheroma have no preceding history of coronary disease. The majority of cases of sudden death due to atheroma appear to be due to fatal ventricular arrhythmia, sometimes triggered by acute myocardial ischaemia. Other less common causes of sudden cardiac death are listed in Table 13.33. Patients presenting with a cardiac arrest require immediate cardiopulmonary resuscitation as outlined in Figure 13.30. In those patients that survive a cardiac arrest, an implantable cardiodefibrillator should be considered to prevent further cardiac arrest. Antiarrhythmic drugs such as amiodarone may be used as an alternative to an implantable cardiodefibrillator but are less effective.

Coronary artery disease in women

Until the age of 65, the prevalence of CAD is much less in women than in men and the incidence of MI in women aged 60–70 increases dramatically, corresponding to that in men. Women have a generally poorer survival post-MI than men and have 2-3% higher in-hospital mortality independent of age and other risk factors.

Boersma E et al (2002) Platelet glycoprotein 11b/11a inhibitors in acute coronary syndromes – a meta-analysis. *Lancet* **359**: 189–198.
Buchthal SD et al. (2000) Abnormal myocardial phosporus-31 nuclear magnetic resonance spectroscopy in women with chest pain but normal coronary angiograms. *New England Journal of Medicine* **342**: 829–835.
Cannon RO, Balaban RS (2000) Chest pain in women with normal coronary angiograms. *New England Journal of Medicine* 342: 885–887.
Collins R, Peto R, Baigent C, Sleight P (1997) Aspirin, heparin and fibrinolytic therapy in suspected myocardial infarction. *New England Journal of Medicine* **336**: 847–866.
Davies MJ (1997) The composition of coronary artery plaques. *New England Journal of Medicine* **336**: 1312–1314.
Hamm CW (2001) Acute coronary syndrome without ST elevation: implementation of new guidelines. *Lancet* **358**: 1533–1538.
Kanagasaby RR, Parker DJ (1996) Long term results of coronary bypass grafting. *Current Opinion in Cardiology* **11**: 568–573.
Kolesnik V, Bishop A (2000) Long term inhibition of platelet aggregation. *Lancet* **356**: 768.
Lee TH, Goldman L (2000) Primary care: evaluation of patient with acute chest pain. *New England Journal of Medicine* **342**: 1187–1195.
Pope JH et al. (2000) Missed diagnoses of acute cardiac ischaemia in the emergency department. *New England Journal of Medicine* **342**: 1163–1170.
Speed CA, Shapiro LM (2000) Exercise prescription in cardiac disease. *Lancet* **356**: 1208–1210.

National Service Framework (NSF) for Coronary Heart Disease (CHD)

Plans to reduce CHD-related death in the under-75-years age group by 40% by the year 2010 by the implementation of set standards (Table 13.34) have been published by the Department of Health. The NSF includes a nurse-led audited approach to reduce CHD by lowering saturated fat intake, increasing exercise and, most important, decreasing smoking. The hypertension treatment targets are 140/85 mmHg in patients at risk of or with established coronary artery disease and 130/80 mmHg in diabetics. The cholesterol target is either total cholesterol of <5.0 mmol/L (LDL-cholesterol <3 mmol/L) or a reduction of 30% (whichever is greater).

FURTHER READING

Anderson WD, King SB (1996) A review of randomized trials comparing coronary angioplasty and bypass grafting. *Current Opinion in Cardiology* **11**: 583–590.

FURTHER READING

National Service Framework for Coronary Heart Disease (2000) Department of Health
//www.doh.gov.uk/nsf/chd.htm.

Table 13.34
Standards for the National Service Framework for coronary heart disease

(for further information, see
http://www.doh.gov.uk/nsf/coronarych4.htm)

1. Reduction of risk factors in the population and health inequalities
2. Reduction of the prevalence of smoking
3. Primary care teams to identify and treat all patients with established atherosclerotic disease
4. Primary care teams to identify and treat all patients with cardiovascular risk > 3%/year
5. In acute infarction, access to a defibrillator in 8 min
6. In acute infarction, assessment and treatment (with aspirin) within 60 min
7. In acute infarcts, acute cardiac units should assess and manage all patients appropriately
8. Patients with angina should be professionally assessed and treated
9. Patients with increasing angina should be referred to a cardiologist in 2 weeks
10. Patients with established disease should be investigated and treated appropriately
11. Patients with heart failure should be investigated by echocardiography and managed appropriately

All patients after a cardiac event should receive rehabilitation and secondary prevention lifestyle advice

Valvular heart disease and infective endocarditis

Mitral stenosis

Almost all mitral stenosis is due to rheumatic heart disease.

At least 50% of sufferers have a history of rheumatic fever or chorea. The single most common valve lesion due to rheumatic fever is pure mitral stenosis (50%) (Table 13.35). The mitral valve is affected in over 90% of those with rheumatic valvular heart disease. Rheumatic mitral stenosis is much more common in women. The pathological process results after some years in valve thickening, cusp fusion, calcium deposition, a narrowed (stenotic) valve orifice and progressive immobility of the valve cusps.

Table 13.35
Rheumatic valvular lesions

Valves involved	Percentage of cases
Mitral valve alone	50
Mitral and aortic valves	40
Mitral, aortic and tricuspid	5
Aortic valve alone	2
All other combinations	3

Other causes include:

- Lutembacher's syndrome, which is the combination of acquired mitral stenosis and an atrial septal defect
- a rare form of congenital mitral stenosis
- in the elderly, a syndrome similar to mitral stenosis, which develops because of calcification and fibrosis of the valve, valve ring and subvalvular apparatus (chordae tendineae)
- carcinoid tumours metastasizing to the lung or primary bronchial carcinoid.

Pathophysiology
When the normal valve orifice area of 5 cm^2 is reduced to approximately 1 cm^2, severe mitral stenosis is present. In order that sufficient cardiac output will be maintained, the left atrial pressure increases and left atrial hypertrophy and dilatation occur. Consequently, pulmonary venous, pulmonary arterial and right heart pressures also increase. The increase in pulmonary capillary pressure is followed by the development of pulmonary oedema. This is partially prevented by alveolar and capillary thickening and pulmonary arterial vasoconstriction (reactive pulmonary hypertension). Pulmonary hypertension leads to right ventricular hypertrophy, dilatation and failure. Right ventricular dilatation results in tricuspid regurgitation. Mitral stenosis is frequently associated with complications (Table 13.36).

Symptoms
Usually there are no symptoms until the valve orifice is moderately stenosed (i.e. has an area of 2 cm^2). In Europe this does not usually occur until several decades after the first attack of rheumatic fever, but children of 10–20 years of age in the Middle or Far East may have severe calcific mitral stenosis.

Because of pulmonary venous hypertension and recurrent bronchitis, progressively severe dyspnoea develops. A cough productive of blood-tinged, frothy sputum is quite common, and occasionally frank haemoptysis may occur. The development of pulmonary hypertension eventually leads to right heart failure and its symptoms of weakness, fatigue and abdominal or lower limb swelling.

Table 13.36
Complications of mitral stenosis

Atrial fibrillation
Systemic embolization
Pulmonary hypertension
Pulmonary infarction
Chest infections
Infective endocarditis (rare)
Tricuspid regurgitation
Right ventricular failure

Cardiovascular disease

The large left atrium favours atrial fibrillation, giving rise to symptoms such as palpitations. Atrial fibrillation may result in systemic emboli, most commonly to the cerebral vessels resulting in neurological sequelae, but mesenteric, renal and peripheral emboli are also seen. Clinical pulmonary embolism as a result of mitral stenosis associated with atrial fibrillation is less commonly seen, but it is likely that subclinical pulmonary emboli occur.

Signs (see Clinical memo in Fig. 13.68)

Face

Severe mitral stenosis with pulmonary hypertension is associated with the so-called mitral facies or malar flush. This is a bilateral, cyanotic or dusky pink discoloration over the upper cheeks that is due to arteriovenous anastomoses and vascular stasis.

Pulse

Mitral stenosis may be associated with a small-volume pulse which is usually regular early on in the disease process when most patients are in sinus rhythm. However, as the severity of the disease progresses, many patients develop atrial fibrillation resulting in an irregularly irregular pulse. The development of atrial fibrillation in these patients often causes a dramatic clinical deterioration.

Jugular veins

If right heart failure develops, there is obvious distension of the jugular veins. If pulmonary hypertension or tricuspid stenosis is present, the *a* wave will be prominent provided that atrial fibrillation has not supervened.

Palpation

There is a tapping impulse felt parasternally on the left side which is not localized. This is the result of a palpable first heart sound combined with left ventricular backward displacement produced by an enlarging right ventricle. A sustained parasternal impulse due to right ventricular hypertrophy may also be felt.

Auscultation

Auscultation (Fig. 13.68) reveals a loud first heart sound if the mitral valve is pliable, but it will not occur in calcific mitral stenosis. As the valve suddenly opens with the force of the increased left atrial pressure, an 'opening snap' will be heard. This is followed by a low-pitched 'rumbling' mid-diastolic murmur best heard with the bell of the stethoscope held lightly at the apex with the patient lying on the left side. If the patient is in sinus rhythm, the murmur becomes louder at the end of diastole as a result of atrial contraction (presystolic accentuation).

The severity of mitral stenosis is judged clinically on the basis of several criteria:

- The presence of pulmonary hypertension implies that mitral stenosis is severe. Pulmonary hypertension is recognized by a right ventricular heave, a loud pulmonary component of the second heart sound, with eventually signs of right-sided heart failure, such as oedema and hepatomegaly. Pulmonary hypertension results in pulmonary valvular regurgitation that causes an early diastolic murmur in the pulmonary area known as a Graham–Steell murmur.
- The closeness of the opening snap to the second heart sound is proportional to the severity of mitral stenosis.

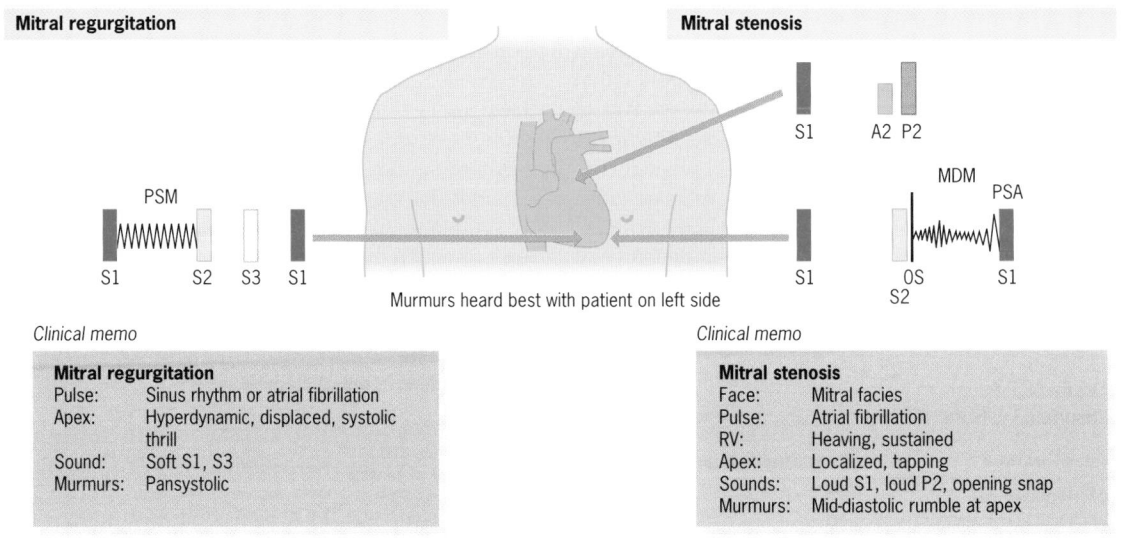

Fig. 13.68 **Auscultatory features associated with mitral regurgitation and mitral stenosis.** A2, aortic component of the second heart sound; MDM, mid-diastolic murmur; OS, opening snap; P2, pulmonary component of the second heart sound; PSA, presystolic accentuation; PSM, pansystolic murmur; S1, first heart sound; S2, second heart sound; S3, third heart sound.

- The length of the mid-diastolic murmur is proportional to the severity.
- As the valve cusps become immobile, the loud first heart sound softens and the opening snap disappears. When pulmonary hypertension occurs, the pulmonary component of the second sound is increased in intensity and the mitral diastolic murmur may become quieter because of the reduction of cardiac output.

Investigations

Chest X-ray

The chest X-ray usually shows a generally small heart with an enlarged left atrium (see Fig. 13.13, p. 717). Pulmonary venous hypertension is usually also present. Late in the course of the disease a calcified mitral valve may be seen on a penetrated or lateral view. The signs of pulmonary oedema or pulmonary hypertension may also be apparent when the disease is severe.

Electrocardiogram

In sinus rhythm the ECG shows a bifid P wave owing to delayed left atrial activation (Fig. 13.69). However, atrial fibrillation is frequently present. As the disease progresses, the ECG features of right ventricular hypertrophy (right axis deviation and perhaps tall R waves in lead V_1) may develop (Fig. 13.70).

Echocardiogram (Fig. 13.24)

Two-dimensional echocardiography is invaluable in assessing the mitral valve apparatus and calculating mitral valve area. The information provides a useful guide in determining whether balloon valvotomy or valve replacement is the treatment of choice in patients symptomatic on medical therapy. Two-dimensional echocardiography also determines left atrial size and right ventricular size and function. Continuous wave (CW) Doppler may also be used to measure mitral valve area and provides an estimate of pulmonary artery pressure through measurement of the degree of tricuspid regurgitation. In many cases, echocardiography alone is sufficient to judge the severity of mitral stenosis such that decisions regarding surgery can be made.

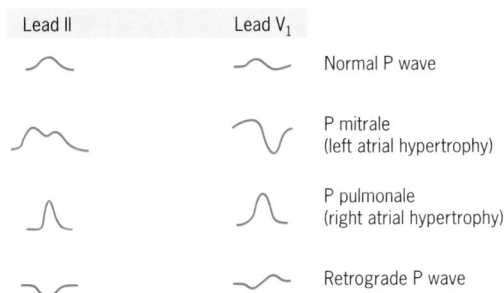

Fig. 13.69 A bifid P wave as seen on the ECG in mitral stenosis (P mitrale). Also shown for comparison are other P wave abnormalities.

Cardiac catheterization

This is required only if an adequate echocardiogram (transthoracic or transoesophageal) is impossible to obtain or if coexisting cardiac problems (e.g. mitral regurgitation or coronary artery disease) are suspected. The typical findings in mitral stenosis are a diastolic pressure that is higher in the left atrium than in the left ventricle (Fig. 13.71). This gradient of pressure is usually proportional to the degree of the stenosis.

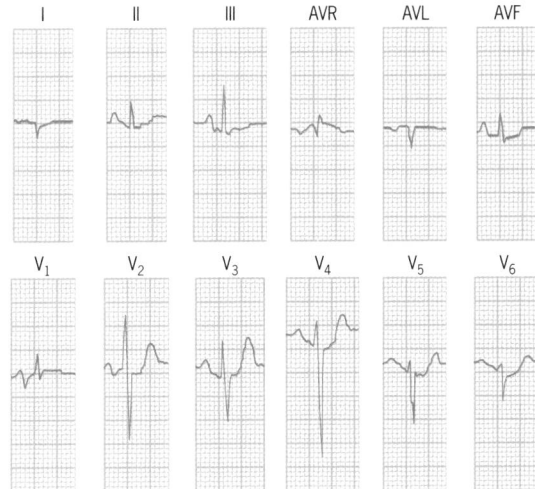

Fig. 13.70 **Severe mitral stenosis** shown by a 12-lead ECG. Note the right axis deviation (frontal plane axis = +120°), the left atrial conduction abnormality (large terminal negative component of the P wave in V_1) and the right ventricular hypertrophy (R wave in V_1 and right axis deviation).

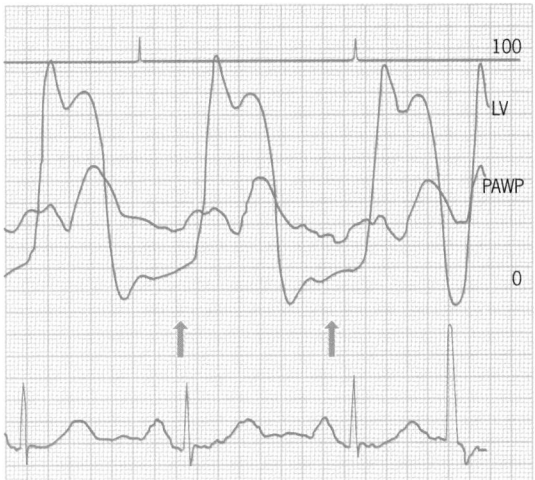

Fig. 13.71 Simultaneous recordings of the ECG, the left ventricular (LV) and the pulmonary arterial wedge pressure (PAWP). The PAWP is almost equivalent to the left atrial pressure. Thus at end-diastole (the onset of the QRS complex) the PAWP is significantly higher than the LV pressure (arrows). The pressure gradient is due to mitral valve stenosis. PAWP is also known as PAOP (occlusion pressure).

Treatment

Mild mitral stenosis may need no treatment other than prompt therapy of attacks of bronchitis. Although infective endocarditis in pure mitral stenosis is uncommon, antibiotic prophylaxis is advised (see p. 35). Early symptoms of mitral stenosis such as mild dyspnoea can usually be treated with low doses of diuretics. The onset of atrial fibrillation requires treatment with digoxin and anticoagulation to prevent atrial thrombus and systemic embolization. If pulmonary hypertension develops or the symptoms of pulmonary congestion persist despite therapy, surgical relief of the mitral stenosis is advised. There are four operative measures.

Trans-septal balloon valvotomy

A catheter is introduced into the right atrium via the femoral vein. The interatrial septum is then punctured and the catheter advanced into the left atrium and across the mitral valve. A balloon is passed over the catheter to lie across the valve, and then inflated briefly to split the valve commissures. The procedure is performed under local anaesthesia in the cardiac catheter laboratory. As with other valvotomy techniques, significant regurgitation may result, necessitating valve replacement (see below). This procedure is ideal for patients with pliable valves in whom there is little involvement of the subvalvular apparatus and in whom there is minimal mitral regurgitation. The procedure cannot be performed when there is heavy calcification or more than mild mitral regurgitation. The presence of thrombus in the left atrium is a contraindication to balloon valvotomy; therefore, transoesophageal echocardiography must be performed prior to this technique in order that left atrial thrombus can be excluded.

Closed valvotomy

This operation is advised for patients with mobile, non-calcified and non-regurgitant mitral valves. The fused cusps are forced apart by a dilator introduced through the apex of the left ventricle and guided into position by the surgeon's finger inserted via the left atrial appendage. Cardiopulmonary bypass is not needed for this operation. Closed valvotomy may produce a good result for 10 years or more. The valve cusps often re-fuse and eventually another operation may be necessary.

Open valvotomy

This operation is often preferred to closed valvotomy. The cusps are carefully dissected apart under direct vision. Cardiopulmonary bypass is required. Open dissection reduces the likelihood of causing traumatic mitral regurgitation.

Mitral valve replacement

Replacement of the mitral valve is necessary if:

- mitral regurgitation is also present

- there is a badly diseased or badly calcified stenotic valve that cannot be reopened without producing significant regurgitation
- there is moderate or severe mitral stenosis and thrombus in the left atrium despite anticoagulation.

Artificial valves (see p. 793) may work successfully for more than 20 years. Anticoagulants are generally necessary to prevent the formation of thrombus, which might obstruct the valve or embolize.

Mitral regurgitation

Of the many causes of mitral valve regurgitation, rheumatic heart disease (50%) and a prolapsing mitral valve are the most common. There are many other causes, which include:

- aortic valve disease
- acute rheumatic fever
- myocarditis
- dilated cardiomyopathy
- hypertensive heart disease
- ischaemic heart disease
- infective endocarditis – mitral regurgitation may result from destruction of the mitral valve leaflets
- hypertrophic cardiomyopathy – left ventricular contraction is disorganized and mitral regurgitation often results
- connective tissue disorders – systemic lupus erythematosus (SLE) may cause mitral regurgitation
- collagen abnormalities – Marfan's syndrome and Ehlers–Danlos syndrome cause mitral regurgitation
- degeneration of the valve cusps or mitral annular calcification – results in mitral regurgitation
- rupture of the chordae tendineae (due to myocardial infarction, infective endocarditis or trauma) – results in acute and very severe mitral regurgitation
- drugs, e.g. fenfluramine is associated with mitral regurgitation.

Pathophysiology

Regurgitation into the left atrium produces left atrial dilatation but little increase in left atrial pressure if the regurgitation is long-standing, as the regurgitant flow is accommodated by the large left atrium. With acute mitral regurgitation the normal compliance of the left atrium does not allow much dilatation and the left atrial pressure rises. Thus, in acute mitral regurgitation the left atrial v wave is greatly increased and pulmonary venous pressure rises to produce pulmonary oedema. Since a proportion of the stroke volume is regurgitated, the stroke volume increases to maintain the forward cardiac output and the left ventricle therefore enlarges.

Symptoms

Mitral regurgitation can be present for many years and the cardiac dimensions greatly increased before any symptoms occur. The increased stroke volume is sensed as a 'palpitation'. Dyspnoea and orthopnoea develop owing to pulmonary venous hypertension occurring as a direct result of the mitral regurgitation and secondarily to left ventricular failure. Fatigue and lethargy develop because of the reduced cardiac output. In the late stages of the disease the symptoms of right heart failure also occur and eventually lead to congestive cardiac failure. Cardiac cachexia may develop. Thromboembolism is less common than in mitral stenosis, but subacute infective endocarditis is much more common.

Signs (see Clinical memo in Fig. 13.68)

The physical signs of uncomplicated mitral regurgitation are:

- laterally displaced, thrusting (hyperdynamic), diffuse apex beat and a systolic thrill
- soft first heart sound, owing to the incomplete apposition of the valve cusps and their partial closure by the time ventricular systole begins
- pansystolic murmur, owing to the occurrence of regurgitation throughout the whole of systole, being loudest at the apex but radiating widely over the precordium and into the axilla
- prominent third heart sound, owing to the sudden rush of blood back into the dilated left ventricle in early diastole (sometimes a short mid-diastolic flow murmur may follow the third heart sound).

The signs related to atrial fibrillation, pulmonary hypertension, and left and right heart failure develop later in the disease. The onset of atrial fibrillation has a much less dramatic effect on symptoms than in mitral stenosis.

Investigations

Chest X-ray

The chest X-ray may show left atrial and left ventricular enlargement. There is an increase in the CTR, and valve calcification is seen.

Electrocardiogram

The ECG shows the features of left atrial delay (bifid P waves) and left ventricular hypertrophy (Fig. 13.72) as manifested by tall R waves in the left lateral leads (e.g. leads I and V_6) and deep S waves in the right-sided precordial leads, (e.g. leads V_1 and V_2). (Note that SV_1 plus RV_5 or RV_6 >35 mm indicates left ventricular hypertrophy.) Left ventricular hypertrophy occurs in about 50% of patients with mitral regurgitation. Atrial fibrillation may be present.

Echocardiogram

The echocardiogram shows a dilated left atrium and left ventricle. There may be specific features of chordal or papillary muscle rupture. CW Doppler can determine the velocity of the regurgitant jet.

The echocardiogram is not as definitive in mitral regurgitation as in mitral stenosis. However, useful information regarding the severity of the condition can be obtained indirectly by observing the dynamics of ventricular function. Transoesophageal echocardiography (TOE) has become an integral part in the assessment of patients at the time of surgery of mitral regurgitation. TOE helps to identify structural valve abnormalities before surgery. Intraoperative TOE can also aid assessment of the efficacy of valve repair.

Cardiac catheterization

This demonstrates a prominent left atrial systolic pressure wave, and when contrast is injected into the left ventricle it is seen regurgitating into an enlarged left atrium during systole.

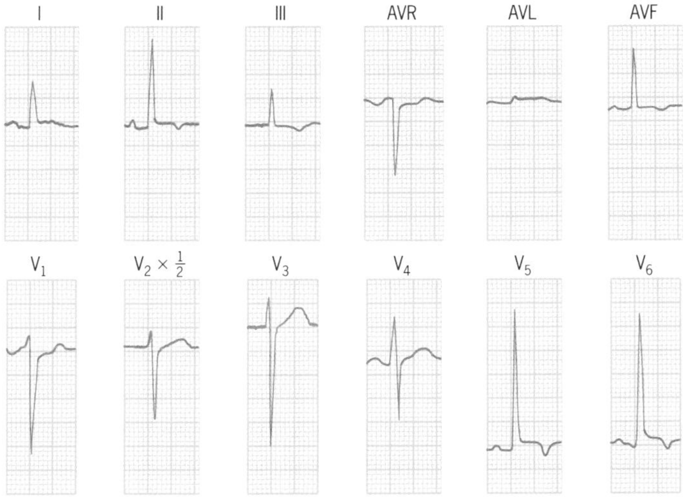

Fig. 13.72 Left ventricular hypertrophy shown in a 12-lead ECG. Note the size of the S wave seen in V_1 (21 mm); S in V_1 + R in V_6 = >35 mm.

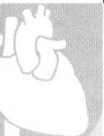

Treatment

Mild mitral regurgitation in the absence of symptoms can be managed conservatively by following the patient with serial echocardiograms. Prophylaxis against endocarditis is required (see p. 35). Any evidence of progressive cardiac enlargement generally warrants early surgical intervention by either mitral valve repair or replacement. The advantages of surgical intervention are diminished in more advanced disease. In patients who are not considered appropriate for surgical intervention, or in whom surgery will be considered at a later date, management usually involves treatment with ACE inhibitors, diuretics and possibly anticoagulants. Sudden torrential mitral regurgitation, as seen with chordal or papillary muscle rupture or infective endocarditis, necessitates emergency mitral valve replacement.

Prolapsing (billowing) mitral valve

This is also known as Barlow's syndrome or floppy mitral valve. It is due to excessively large mitral valve leaflets, an enlarged mitral annulus, abnormally long chordae or disordered papillary muscle contraction. Histology may demonstrate myxomatous degeneration of the mitral valve leaflets. It is more commonly seen in young women than in men or older women and it has a familial incidence. Its cause is unknown but it is associated with Marfan's syndrome, thyrotoxicosis, rheumatic or ischaemic heart disease. It also occurs in association with atrial septal defect and as part of hypertrophic cardiomyopathy. Mild mitral valve prolapse is so common that it should be regarded as a normal variant.

Pathophysiology

During ventricular systole, a mitral valve leaflet (most commonly the posterior leaflet) prolapses into the left atrium. This may result in abnormal ventricular contraction, papillary muscle strain and some mitral regurgitation. Usually the syndrome is not haemodynamically serious. Thromboembolism occurs.

Symptoms

Atypical chest pain is the most common symptom. Usually the pain is left submammary and stabbing in quality. Sometimes it is substernal, aching and severe. Rarely it is similar to typical angina pectoris. Palpitations may be experienced because of the abnormal ventricular contraction or because of the atrial and ventricular arrhythmias that are commonly associated with mitral valve prolapse. Sudden cardiac death due to fatal ventricular arrhythmias is a very rare but recognized complication.

Signs

The most common sign is a mid-systolic click, which is produced by the sudden prolapse of the valve and the tensing of the chordae tendineae that occurs during systole. This may be followed by a late systolic murmur owing to some regurgitation. With more regurgitation, the murmur becomes pansystolic mitral regurgitation.

Investigations

Chest X-ray

The chest X-ray is usually normal unless significant mitral regurgitation is present.

Electrocardiogram

Non-specific ST/T wave changes have been described in 15–30% of cases, but there is no evidence that this is more than in the general population.

Echocardiogram

The diagnosis is confirmed on two-dimensional echocardiography, which typically shows posterior movement of one or both mitral valve cusps into the left atrium during systole.

Cardiac catheterization

Contrast angiograms performed during cardiac catheterization reveal the systolic prolapse of the mitral valve into the left atrium, and mitral regurgitation, if present, is seen. This investigation is not normally required.

Treatment

Usually, beta-blockade is effective for the treatment of the atypical chest pain and palpitations. Sometimes more specific antiarrhythmic drug treatment is necessary. When a prolapsing mitral valve is associated with significant mitral regurgitation and atrial fibrillation, anticoagulation is advised to prevent thromboembolism. Mitral valve prolapse associated with severe mitral regurgitation has a risk of sudden cardiac death. Mitral valve repair is indicated in all such cases. Very occasionally, mitral valve replacement rather than repair may be necessary for severe regurgitation when there is severe prolapse of both leaflets. Prophylaxis against endocarditis (see p. 35) is advised if there is significant mitral valve regurgitation.

Aortic stenosis

There are three causes of aortic valve stenosis:

- Congenital aortic valve stenosis develops progressively because of turbulent blood flow through a congenitally abnormal (usually bicuspid) aortic valve. Most congenitally abnormal aortic valves occur in men.
- Rheumatic fever results in progressive fusion, thickening and calcification of a previously normal three-cusped aortic valve. In rheumatic heart disease the aortic valve is affected in about 40% of cases and there is usually associated mitral valve disease.
- Calcific valvular disease is the commonest cause of aortic stenosis. This is an inflammatory process with

initially thickening of the subendothelium with adjacent fibrosis. The lesions contain lipoproteins which calcify, increasing leaflet stiffness and reducing systolic opening.

Valvular aortic stenosis should be distinguished from other causes of obstruction to left ventricular emptying (Fig. 13.73), which include:

- *supravalvular obstruction* – a congenital fibrous diaphragm above the aortic valve often associated with mental retardation and hypercalcaemia (William's syndrome)

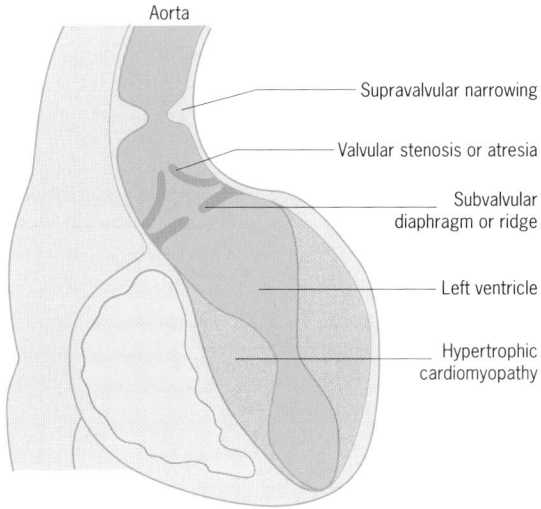

Fig. 13.73 **Several forms of left ventricular outflow tract obstruction.**

- *hypertrophic cardiomyopathy* – septal muscle hypertrophy obstructing left ventricular outflow
- *subvalvular aortic stenosis* – a congenital condition in which a fibrous ridge or diaphragm is situated immediately below the aortic valve.

Pathophysiology

Obstructed left ventricular emptying leads to increased left ventricular pressure and compensatory left ventricular hypertrophy. In turn, this results in relative ischaemia of the left ventricular myocardium, and consequent angina, arrhythmias and left ventricular failure. The obstruction to left ventricular emptying is relatively more severe on exercise. Normally, exercise causes a many-fold increase in cardiac output, but when there is severe narrowing of the aortic valve orifice the cardiac output can hardly increase. Thus, the blood pressure falls, coronary ischaemia worsens, the myocardium fails and cardiac arrhythmias develop. Left ventricular systolic function is typically preserved in patients with aortic stenosis (cf aortic regurgitation).

Symptoms

There are usually no symptoms until aortic stenosis is moderately severe (when the aortic orifice is reduced to one-third of its normal size). At this stage, exercise-induced syncope, angina and dyspnoea develop. When symptoms occur, the prognosis is poor – on average, death occurs within 2–3 years if there has been no surgical intervention.

Signs (see Clinical memo in Fig. 13.74)
Pulse

The carotid pulse is of small volume and is slow-rising or plateau in nature (see p. 710).

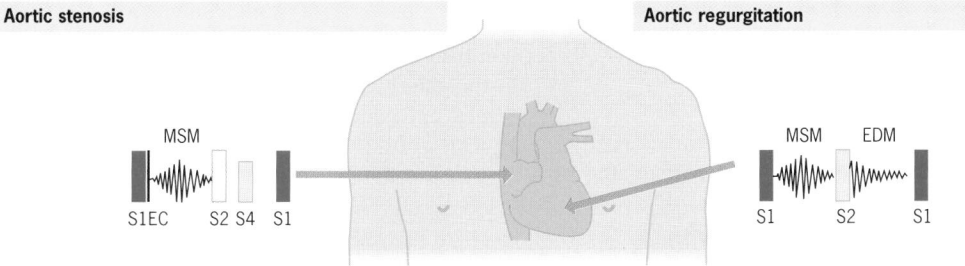

Murmurs heard best with patient leaning forwards and breath held in expiration

Clinical memo

Aortic stenosis	
Pulse:	Sinus rhythm, low volume, slow rising
Aortic area:	Systolic thrill
Apex:	Not displaced, sustained
Sounds:	Ejection click, soft A2, S4
Murmurs:	Systolic, low pitched, ejection, radiating to carotids

Clinical memo

Aortic regurgitation	
Pulse:	Sinus rhythm, large volume, collapsing
Blood pressure:	Wide pulse pressure
Apex:	Displaced, diffuse, hyperdynamic
Murmurs:	(1) High pitched, early diastolic at LSE
	(2) Ejection systolic at base and into neck
	(3) Mid-diastolic rumble at apex (Austin-Flint)

Fig. 13.74 **Auscultatory features of aortic stenosis and aortic regurgitation.** EC, ejection click; EDM, early diastolic murmur; MSM, mid-systolic murmur; S1, first heart sound.

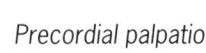

Precordial palpation

The apex beat is not usually displaced because hypertrophy (as opposed to dilatation) does not produce noticeable cardiomegaly. However, the pulsation is sustained and obvious. A double impulse is sometimes felt because the fourth heart sound or atrial contraction ('kick') may be palpable. A systolic thrill may be felt in the aortic area.

Auscultation

The most obvious auscultatory finding in aortic stenosis is an ejection systolic murmur that is usually 'diamond-shaped' (crescendo–decrescendo). The murmur is usually longer when the disease is more severe as a longer ejection time is needed. The murmur is usually rough in quality and best heard in the aortic area. It radiates into the carotid arteries and also the precordium. The intensity of the murmur is not a good guide to the severity of the condition because it is lessened by a reduced cardiac output. In severe cases, the murmur may be inaudible.

Other findings

- There is a systolic ejection click (see p. 714), unless the valve has become immobile and calcified.
- There is a soft or inaudible aortic second heart sound when the aortic valve becomes immobile.
- There is reversed splitting of the second heart sound (splitting on expiration) (see p. 713).
- There is a prominent fourth heart sound (see p. 714), unless coexisting mitral stenosis prevents this.

Investigations

Chest X-ray

The chest X-ray usually reveals a relatively small heart with a prominent, dilated, ascending aorta. This occurs because turbulent blood flow above the stenosed aortic valve produces so-called 'post-stenotic dilatation'. The aortic valve may be calcified. When heart failure occurs, the CTR increases.

Electrocardiogram

The ECG shows left ventricular hypertrophy and left atrial delay. A left ventricular 'strain' pattern due to

'pressure overload' (depressed ST segments and T wave inversion in leads orientated towards the left ventricle, i.e. leads I, AVL, V_5 and V_6) is common when the disease is severe. Usually, sinus rhythm is present, but ventricular arrhythmias may be recorded.

Echocardiogram

The echocardiogram readily demonstrates the thickened, calcified and immobile aortic valve cusps. Left ventricular hypertrophy may also be seen. The gradient across the valve can be estimated by CW Doppler, provided the left ventricular function is reasonable (see Fig. 13.23, p. 724).

Cardiac catheterization

Cardiac catheterization can be used to document the systolic pressure difference (gradient) between the aorta and the left ventricle (Fig. 13.75) and assess left ventricular function. This is rarely necessary since all of this information can be gained non-invasively with echocardiography. Coronary angiography is necessary before recommending surgery.

Treatment

In patients with aortic stenosis, symptoms are a good index of severity and all symptomatic patients should have aortic valve replacement. Asymptomatic patients should be under regular review for assessment of symptoms and echocardiography. Antibiotic prophylaxis against infective endocarditis is essential (see p. 35).

Provided that the valve is not severely deformed or heavily calcified, critical aortic stenosis in childhood or adolescence can be treated by valvotomy (performed under direct vision by the surgeon or by balloon dilatation using X-ray visualization). This produces temporary relief from the obstruction. Aortic valve replacement will usually be needed a few years later. Balloon dilatation (valvuloplasty) has been tried in adults, especially in the elderly, as an alternative to surgery. Generally results are poor and such treatment is reserved for patients unfit for surgery or as a 'bridge' to surgery (as systolic function will often improve).

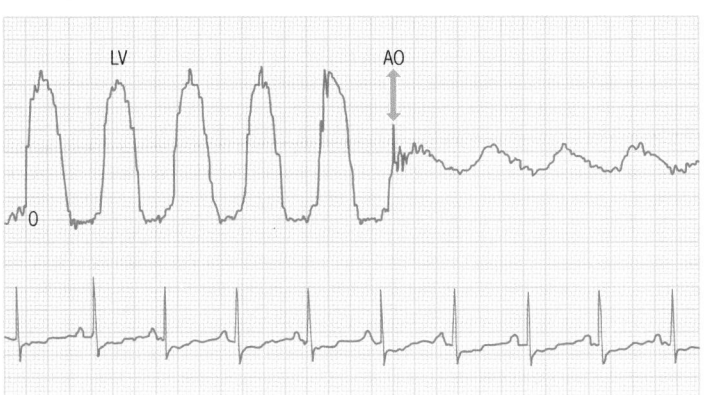

Fig. 13.75 ECG and pressure trace as a cardiac catheter is withdrawn from the left ventricle (LV) to the aorta (AO). Note that the peak systolic pressure changes from 250 to 130 mmHg (arrow). The 120 mmHg peak-to-peak systolic gradient indicates severe aortic valvular stenosis.

Aortic regurgitation

The most common causes of aortic regurgitation are rheumatic fever and infective endocarditis complicating a previously damaged valve. This can be a congenitally abnormal valve (e.g. a bicuspid valve) or one damaged by rheumatic fever. There are numerous other causes and associations (Table 13.37). The majority of patients with aortic regurgitation are men (75%), but rheumatic aortic regurgitation occurs more commonly in women.

Pathophysiology

Aortic regurgitation is reflux of blood from the aorta through the aortic valve into the left ventricle during diastole. If net cardiac output is to be maintained, the total volume of blood pumped into the aorta must increase, and consequently the left ventricular size must enlarge. Because of the aortic run-off during diastole, diastolic blood pressure falls and coronary perfusion is decreased. In addition, the larger left ventricular size is mechanically less efficient so that the demand for oxygen is greater and cardiac ischaemia develops.

Symptoms

In aortic regurgitation, significant symptoms occur late and do not develop until left ventricular failure occurs. As with mitral regurgitation, a common symptom is 'pounding of the heart' because of the increased left ventricular size and its vigorous pulsation. Angina pectoris is a frequent complaint. Varying grades of dyspnoea occur depending on the extent of left ventricular dilatation and dysfunction. Arrhythmias are relatively uncommon.

Signs (see Clinical memo in Fig. 13.74)

The signs of aortic regurgitation are many and are due to the hyperdynamic circulation, reflux of blood into the left ventricle and the increased left ventricular size.

The pulse is bounding or collapsing (see p. 709). The following signs, which are rare, also indicate a hyperdynamic circulation:

- Quincke's sign – capillary pulsation in the nail beds
- De Musset's sign – head nodding with each heart beat
- Duroziez's sign – a to-and-fro murmur heard when the femoral artery is auscultated with pressure applied distally (if found, it is a sign of severe aortic regurgitation)
- pistol shot femorals – a sharp bang heard on auscultation over the femoral arteries in time with each heart beat.

The apex beat is displaced laterally and downwards and is thrusting (hyperdynamic) in quality. On auscultation, there is a high-pitched early diastolic murmur best heard at the left sternal edge in the fourth intercostal space with the patient leaning forward and the breath held in expiration.

Table 13.37
Causes and associations of aortic regurgitation

Acute aortic regurgitation	Chronic aortic regurgitation
Acute rheumatic fever	Rheumatic heart disease
Infective endocarditis	Syphilis
Dissection of the aorta	Arthritides
Ruptured sinus of Valsalva aneurysm	Reiter's syndrome
Failure of prosthetic heart value	Ankylosing spondylitis
	Rheumatoid arthritis
	Hypertension (severe)
	Bicuspid aortic valve
	Aortic endocarditis
	Marfan's syndrome
	Osteogenesis imperfecta

Because of the volume overload there is commonly an ejection systolic flow murmur. The regurgitant jet can impinge on the anterior mitral valve cusp, causing a mid-diastolic murmur (Austin Flint).

Investigations

Chest X-ray

The chest X-ray features are those of left ventricular enlargement and possibly of dilatation of the ascending aorta. The ascending aortic wall may be calcified in syphilis, and the aortic valve may be calcified if valvular disease is responsible for the regurgitation.

Electrocardiogram

The ECG appearances are those of left ventricular hypertrophy due to 'volume overload' – tall R waves and deeply inverted T waves in the left-sided chest leads, and deep S waves in the right-sided leads. Normally, sinus rhythm is present.

Echocardiogram

The echocardiogram demonstrates vigorous cardiac contraction and a dilated left ventricle. The aortic root may also be enlarged. Diastolic fluttering of the mitral leaflets or septum occurs in severe aortic regurgitation (producing the Austin Flint murmur, see p. 716). The regurgitant jet can be detected by CW Doppler.

Cardiac catheterization

During cardiac catheterization, injection of contrast medium into the aorta (aortography) will outline aortic valvular abnormalities and allow assessment of the degree of regurgitation.

Treatment

The underlying cause of aortic regurgitation (e.g. syphilitic aortitis or infective endocarditis) may require specific treatment. The treatment of aortic regurgitation usually requires aortic valve replacement but the timing of surgery is critical.

Because symptoms do not develop until the myocardium fails and because the myocardium does not recover fully after surgery, operation is performed before significant symptoms occur. The timing of the operation is best determined according to haemodynamic, echocardiographic or angiographic criteria.

Both mechanical prostheses and tissue valves are used. Tissue valves are preferred in the elderly and when anticoagulants must be avoided, but are contraindicated in children and young adults because of the rapid calcification and degeneration of the valves.

Antibiotic prophylaxis against infective endocarditis (see p. 35) is necessary even if a prosthetic valve replacement has been performed.

Tricuspid stenosis

This uncommon valve lesion, which is seen much more often in women than in men, is usually due to rheumatic heart disease and is frequently associated with mitral and/or aortic valve disease. Tricuspid stenosis is also seen in the carcinoid syndrome.

Pathophysiology
Tricuspid valve stenosis results in a reduced cardiac output, which is restored towards normal when the right atrial pressure increases. The resulting systemic venous congestion produces hepatomegaly, ascites and dependent oedema.

Symptoms
Usually, patients with tricuspid stenosis complain of symptoms due to associated left-sided rheumatic valve lesions. The abdominal pain (due to hepatomegaly) and swelling (due to ascites) and peripheral oedema that occur are relatively severe when compared with the degree of dyspnoea.

Signs
If the patient remains in sinus rhythm, which is unusual, there is a prominent jugular venous *a* wave. This pre-systolic pulsation may also be felt over the liver. There is usually a rumbling mid-diastolic murmur, which is heard best at the lower left sternal edge and is louder on inspiration. It may be missed because of the murmur of coexisting mitral stenosis. A tricuspid opening snap may occasionally be heard.

Hepatomegaly, abdominal ascites and dependent oedema may be present.

Investigations
Chest X-ray
On the chest X-ray there may be a prominent right atrial bulge.

Electrocardiogram
The enlarged right atrium may be manifested on the ECG by peaked, tall P waves (>3 mm) in lead II.

Echocardiogram
The echocardiogram may show a thickened and immobile tricuspid valve, but this is not so clearly seen as an abnormal mitral valve.

Cardiac catheterization
This demonstrates a diastolic pressure gradient between the right atrium and the right ventricle. Contrast injection will demonstrate a large right atrium.

Treatment
Medical management consists of diuretic therapy and salt restriction. Tricuspid valvotomy is occasionally possible, but tricuspid valve replacement is often necessary. Other valves usually also need replacement because tricuspid valve stenosis is rarely an isolated lesion.

Tricuspid regurgitation

Functional tricuspid regurgitation may occur whenever the right ventricle dilates, e.g. in cor pulmonale, myocardial infarction or pulmonary hypertension.

Organic tricuspid regurgitation may occur with rheumatic heart disease, infective endocarditis, carcinoid syndrome, Ebstein's anomaly (a congenitally malpositioned tricuspid valve) and other congenital abnormalities of the atrioventricular valves.

Symptoms and signs
The valvular regurgitation gives rise to high right atrial and systemic venous pressure. Patients may complain of the symptoms of right heart failure (see p. 758).

Physical signs include a large jugular venous *cv* wave and a palpable liver that pulsates in systole. Usually a right ventricular impulse may be felt at the left sternal edge, and there is a blowing pansystolic murmur, best heard on inspiration at the lower left sternal edge. Atrial fibrillation is common.

Treatment
Functional tricuspid regurgitation usually disappears with medical management. Severe organic tricuspid regurgitation may require operative repair of the tricuspid valve (annuloplasty or plication). Very occasionally, tricuspid valve replacement may be necessary. In drug addicts with infective endocarditis of the tricuspid valve, surgical removal of the valve is recommended to eradicate the infection. This is usually well tolerated in the short term. The insertion of a prosthetic valve for this condition is considered on page 793.

Pulmonary stenosis

This is usually a congenital lesion, but it may rarely result from rheumatic fever or from the carcinoid syndrome.

Congenital pulmonary stenosis may be associated with an intact ventricular septum or with a ventricular septal defect (Fallot's tetralogy).

Pulmonary stenosis may be valvular, subvalvular or supravalvular. Multiple congenital pulmonary arterial stenoses are usually due to infection with rubella during pregnancy.

Symptoms and signs
The obstruction to right ventricular emptying results in right ventricular hypertrophy which in turn leads to right atrial hypertrophy. Severe pulmonary obstruction may be incompatible with life, but lesser degrees of obstruction give rise to fatigue, syncope and the symptoms of right heart failure. Mild pulmonary stenosis may be asymptomatic.

The physical signs are characterized by a harsh mid-systolic ejection murmur, best heard on inspiration, to the left of the sternum in the second intercostal space. This murmur is often associated with a thrill. The pulmonary closure sound is usually delayed and soft. There may be a pulmonary ejection sound if the obstruction is valvular. A right ventricular fourth sound and a prominent jugular venous *a* wave are present when the stenosis is moderately severe. A right ventricular heave (sustained impulse) may be felt.

Investigations
Chest X-ray
The chest X-ray usually shows a prominent pulmonary artery owing to poststenotic dilatation.

Electrocardiogram
The ECG demonstrates both right atrial and right ventricular hypertrophy, although it may sometimes be normal even in severe pulmonary stenosis.

Cardiac catheterization
The passage of a catheter through the right heart allows the level and degree of the stenosis to be established by measuring the systolic pressure gradient.

Treatment
Treatment of severe pulmonary stenosis requires pulmonary valvotomy (balloon valvotomy or direct surgery).

Pulmonary regurgitation

This is the most common acquired lesion of the pulmonary valve. It results from dilatation of the pulmonary valve ring, which occurs with pulmonary hypertension. It is characterized by a decrescendo diastolic murmur beginning with the pulmonary component of the second sound that is difficult to distinguish from the murmur of aortic regurgitation. Pulmonary regurgitation usually causes no symptoms and treatment is rarely necessary.

Prosthetic heart valves

There are two types of prosthetic heart valve: tissue and mechanical. Tissue valves are usually fashioned from a porcine or bovine aortic valve (xenograft); occasionally a human aortic valve is used (homograft). Mechanical valves are of various types, the most common being a ball-and-cage design (Starr–Edwards valve), a tilting disc (Björk–Shiley valve), or a double tilting disc (St Jude valve). The disadvantage of the mechanical valve over the tissue valve is that formal anticoagulation is required. However, mechanical valves are much harder wearing; a tissue valve tends to degenerate after about 10 years. Unlike a tilting disc valve, the ball of a ball-and-cage valve presents some obstruction to flow through the valve. Although ball-and-cage valves have always been mechanically satisfactory, some tilting disc valves have been mechanically insecure. Prosthetic valves may become detached from the valve ring, thrombose, stick, degenerate or become infected. Echocardiography is often helpful, but echoes are scattered from the mechanical valve making assessment of the structure of the valve rather difficult. Transoesophageal echocardiography has largely overcome this problem and is the investigation of choice when prosthetic valve endocarditis is suspected.

FURTHER READING

Carabello BA, Crawford FA (1997) Medical progress: valvular heart disease. *New England Journal of Medicine* **337**: 32–41.
Otto CM (2001) Evaluation and management of chronic mitral regurgitation. *New England Journal of Medicine* **345**: 740–746.

Infective endocarditis

Infective endocarditis is an infection (usually bacterial, occasionally fungal) of the endocardium . It is a serious disease with significant morbidity and mortality, and prompt diagnosis and treatment are essential to minimize sequelae. Mortality without treatment approaches 100%. The disease may occur either as an acute, fulminating infection but more commonly runs an insidious course and is known as subacute (bacterial) endocarditis (SBE). The term 'infective endocarditis' (IE) is preferred because not all the infecting organisms are bacteria. The annual incidence in the UK is 6–7 per 100 000, but it is much more common in developing countries.

Aetiology and pathogenesis
Endocarditis is usually the consequence of two factors: (1) abnormal cardiac endothelium, facilitating bacterial

adherence and growth and (2) the presence of organisms in the bloodstream. Most bacteria (with the exception of some highly virulent species such as *Staphylococcus aureus* and pneumococci) cannot adhere to normal endothelium.

Abnormal vascular endothelium is usually the result of valvular lesions, which create areas of non-laminar blood flow, promoting fibrin and platelet deposition. It is these small thrombi that allow organisms to adhere and grow. As they grow, more fibrin and platelets are deposited, leading to the characteristic infected vegetation.

Local cardiac factors

Common valve lesions associated with endocarditis include those due to rheumatic heart disease, congenital valve disease, mitral valve prolapse and calcification of the aortic valve. Other congenital cardiac lesions, such as ventricular septal defect or persistent ductus arteriosus, are also associated with endocarditis. Prosthetic valves and prosthetic vascular material promote localized fibrin deposition and are thus a risk for endocarditis or endovascular disease.

Factors causing bacteraemia

Organisms causing endocarditis usually arise from the mouth (the majority of cases) or the skin. In some cases the cause of the bacteraemia is unknown; more often, there is an obvious factor that facilitated entry of organisms into the bloodstream. Such risk factors include poor oral hygiene and dental sepsis, dental procedures, cellulitis and soft-tissue infections, intravenous drug abuse (IVDA) and increasingly, medical procedures or devices such as intravascular cannulae (especially central), cardiac surgery, or permanent pacemakers.

Organisms implicated

An extremely large number of organisms have been reported to cause endocarditis, but most cases are due to streptococci or staphylococci.

The oral streptococci account for between a third and a half of cases, and more in undeveloped countries, where iatrogenic endocarditis is rare. This group of α haemolytic streptococci includes species such as *Streptococcus mutans* and *Strep. sanguis*; they are often collectively but somewhat inaccurately known as 'Strep. viridans'. They are obviously often associated with dental disease or procedures.

Enterococci, e.g. *E. faecalis* now cause up to one-fifth of cases. They normally inhabit the gut and perineum, and may cause urinary sepsis; they may be selected by the use of broad-spectrum antibiotics; therefore enterococcal endocarditis is often associated with underlying genitourinary disease or procedures, or prolonged hospitalization.

Staphylococci cause up to a third of cases of native valve endocarditis, and about a half of prosthetic valve infections. Most cases are due to *Staph. aureus*, and this often leads to a dramatic fulminant infection. Methicillin-resistant *Staph. aureus* (MRSA) accounts for an increasing proportion of these cases, especially (but not only) those which are hospital-acquired, and have an equally poor outcome. Coagulase-negative staphylococci ('Staph. epidermidis') infections tend to be more indolent.

Some cases of staphylococcal endocarditis are related to a minor area of soft-tissue infection, and diabetics seem to be at increased risk, but increasingly cases are seen in IVDAs and patients with intravenous catheters, especially if these are long-standing and poorly cared for. Some patients with prosthetic valve endocarditis are directly infected during their surgery, and present within a few weeks or months; infections after this time are usually the consequence of a later bacteraemia.

Candida endocarditis is rare: it is seen in patients who have had prolonged indwelling vascular catheters (especially for total parenteral nutrition) and antibiotic use, and also in IVDAs who dissolve heroin in (infected) lemon juice.

Strep. bovis endocarditis is even rarer, but as there is a well-documented association with bowel malignancy, it should prompt consideration of this diagnosis.

Culture-negative endocarditis accounts for 5–10% of cases. The usual cause is prior antibiotic therapy, but some cases are due to a variety of fastidious organisms that fail to grow in normal blood cultures. These include *Coxiella burnetii*, the cause of Q fever (p. 93), *Chlamydia* spp., *Bartonella* spp. (organisms that cause trench fever and cat-scratch-disease) and *Legionella*.

Pathology

Infection of native valves usually occurs along the edges of the heart valves. The left side is more commonly involved, with mitral and aortic regurgitation being the most common predisposing valve lesions. In IVDAs the valves in the right heart are usually affected. Infection of prosthetic valves tends to involve the valve insertion ring, rather than valve leaflets.

In endocarditis due to congenital lesions such as ventricular septal defects or patent ductus arteriosus, the infection occurs at the site of the 'jet lesion' on the wall opposite the shunt. The characteristic lesion of infective endocarditis is a mass of fibrin, platelets and infecting organisms known as vegetations. The chance of an organism sticking to a vegetation is increased because of the clumping together of bacteria caused by agglutinating antibodies. In acute endocarditis, vegetations may be very large and may embolize. Virulent microorganisms may rapidly destroy the valve cusp, producing ulceration and regurgitation.

The extracardiac manifestations result either from embolization or from the deposition of immune complexes. The latter is thought to be responsible for arthralgia, Roth spots and Janeway lesions, focal glomerulonephritis and acute vasculitis (see below); infarcts and abscesses are produced by emboli.

Clinical presentation

Cardinal features of endocarditis are a heart murmur and fever, and the diagnosis must always be suspected when these features are present. However, the clinical manifestations of IE are often very varied and non-specific; thus there is frequently a considerable delay between presentation and diagnosis.

Clinical syndromes arise from four processes: systemic features of infection, valvular damage, embolization and immune vasculitis. In addition, examination of the patient must include consideration of possible causes/risks of endocarditis, such as dental sepsis, infected lines or other foci of infection. Table 13.38 lists the clinical features of infective endocarditis.

Systemic symptoms

Patients may present with insidious symptoms such as fever, night sweats, weight loss, fatigue, myalgia and arthralgia. More rarely, patients present acutely, either with a severe septicaemic illness, or with a stroke or other embolic event.

Cardiac symptoms and signs

There are three categories of cardiac signs. Features of any predisposing heart disease may be found; a new or changing heart murmur is often (but not always) heard, and patients may present with cardiac failure due to valvular destruction or conduction abnormalities.

Embolic phenomena

Systemic embolization occurs in about one-third of cases, and is a major contributor to the mortality from endocarditis. Pulmonary abscesses or infarction suggest right-sided endocarditis. Endocarditis should be considered in the differential diagnosis of all patients presenting with arterial, pulmonary, coronary or cerebral infarction. Mycotic (infected) aneurysms are occasionally seen and may present after the endocarditis has been treated.

Vascular and inflammatory lesions

Vascular lesions may arise from immune complex deposition or from microembolism. Subungual splinter haemorrhages are the most frequently sought lesions indicative of endocarditis, although they are not specific, occurring in other vasculitides. Many of the lesions described are late phenomena, and are rarely seen with earlier diagnosis and treatment.

Clubbing of the fingers and toes may be seen, as may slight splenomegaly. If a splenic infarct has occurred, the spleen may be painful and tender and a friction rub may be heard over it. Arthritis of the major joints is occasionally seen.

Haematuria is common, owing to glomerulonephritis, or to infarction as a result of emboli. Renal abscesses may also occur.

Petechial haemorrhages are common, and occur on the skin or mucosal surfaces. Rarely they are seen on the retina (Roth spots). Other rare vascular lesions include small, flat, erythematous, non-tender macules, mainly on the thenar and hypothenar eminences (Janeway lesions); and hard, painful, tender, subcutaneous swellings on the fingers, toes, palms and soles, known as Osler's nodes.

Investigations

Blood cultures are a key diagnostic test in IE. They are positive in about three-quarters of cases. At least three sets of samples (i.e. six bottles) should be taken. Special culture techniques may be necessary for unusual microorganisms such as *Brucella*, but modern automated blood culture systems are increasingly good at detecting such pathogens.

Echocardiography

Echocardiography is extremely useful in allowing vegetations to be seen (Fig. 13.76), and should be requested urgently where the diagnosis is suspected. Echocardiography is also useful in documenting valvular dysfunction and other local complications, such as aortic root abscesses; thus it may help to identify patients in need of urgent surgery.

Table 13.38
Clinical features of infective endocarditis

	Approximate %
General systems	
Malaise	95
Clubbing	10
Cardiac	
Murmurs	90
Cardiac failure	50
Arthralgia	25
Pyrexia	90
Skin lesions	
Osler's nodes	15
Splinter haemorrhages	10
Janeway lesions	5
Petechiae	50
Eyes	
Roth spots	5
Conjunctival splinter haemorrhages	Rare
Splenomegaly	40
Neurological	
Cerebral emboli	20
Mycotic aneurysm	10
Renal	
Haematuria	70

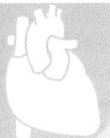

(a)

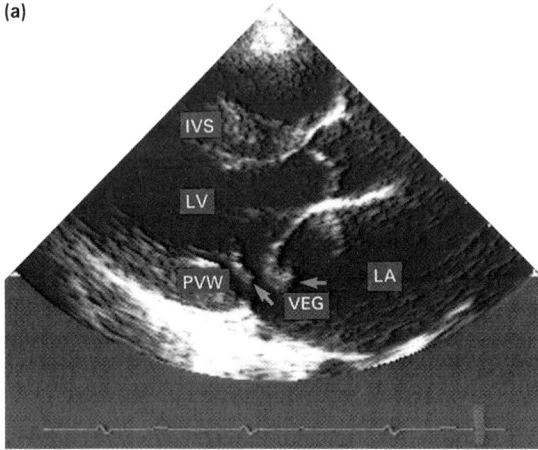

(b)

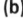

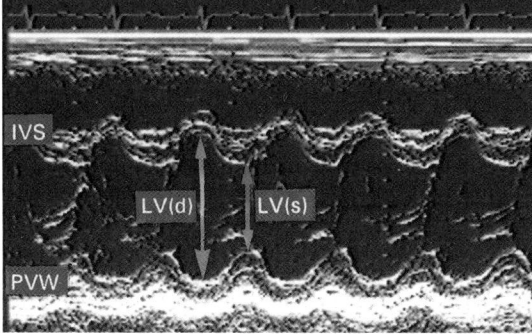

Fig. 13.76 **(a) Two-dimensional echocardiogram (long-axis view) showing vegetations** (arrowed) attached to both the anterior and posterior leaflets of the mitral valve in a patient with infective endocarditis. **(b) M-mode echocardiogram of the left ventricle** in the same patient, showing hyperdynamic contraction associated with volume overloading from the associated severe mitral regurgitation. Compare with Figure 13.22c. IVS, interventricular septum; LV, left ventricle; LV(d) and LV(s), diastolic and systolic left ventricular dimensions; PVW, posterior ventricular wall; LA, left atrium; VEG, vegetation.

Transoesophageal echocardiography is better than transthoracic, especially for visualizing the left heart, small vegetations and prosthetic valves; however, the sensitivity quoted for both techniques varies considerably and a negative echocardiogram does not necessarily exclude the diagnosis.

Serology

Serological tests should be sent when the diagnosis is suspected and blood cultures are negative. They can help diagnose *Coxiella*, *Bartonella*, *Legionella*, and *Chlamydia*, where the organisms will not grow in blood cultures, and may be helpful for *Candida* and *Brucella*. However, negative cultures usually arise because patients have recently received antibiotic therapy.

Other laboratory tests

These are useful to confirm sepsis, though they are non-specific.

- *Blood tests.* A normochromic normocytic anaemia is usual and C-reactive protein and the ESR are increased. A polymorphonuclear leucocytosis is common and thrombocytopenia can occasionally occur.
- *Liver biochemistry* is often mildly disturbed with, in particular, an increased serum alkaline phosphatase.
- *Immunoglobulins and complement.* Serum immunoglobulins are increased, but total complement and C3 complement are decreased owing to immune complex formation. Circulating immune complexes are present in more than 70% of cases but are not routinely measured.
- *Urine.* Proteinuria may occur and microscopic haematuria is nearly always present.

Chest X-ray

This may show evidence of heart failure, or emboli in right-sided endocarditis.

Electrocardiogram

This may show evidence of myocardial infarction (emboli) or conduction defects. The latter should suggest the possibility of valve ring infection or myocardial abscesses.

Management

Therapy of endocarditis is difficult because bacteria reside within a protected site within the vegetation. High concentrations of antibiotic are therefore required for prolonged periods to achieve successful treatment. Where possible, synergistic combinations of antibiotic are used, in order to maximize the microbicidal effect. Given the complex nature of the infection, and the catastrophic consequences of ineffective treatment, optimum management needs close liaison between cardiologists, clinical microbiologists/infectious disease physicians, and possibly cardiac surgeons.

Drug therapy

Endocarditis is treated with bactericidal antibiotics chosen on the basis of the results of the blood culture and antibiotic sensitivity, where possible. The treatment should continue for 4–6 weeks, although recent studies of 2-week short-course therapy have shown that it is highly effective in uncomplicated penicillin-sensitive *Strep. viridans* endocarditis. Typical therapeutic regimens are shown in Table 13.39. Response should be monitored clinically, cardiologically and by change in white cell count and C-reactive protein; failure of response should prompt review of therapy.

The recurrence of fever may suggest inadequate antibiotic therapy or valve ring infection. Emergence of bacterial resistance is uncommon. Recrudescence of fever may also signal a drug reaction, especially if penicillins are being used. The antibiotics may be omitted for 24–72 hours to test this.

Table 13.39
Antibiotics in endocarditis (adapted from BSAC guidelines)

Clinical situation	Suggested antibiotic regimen to start
Clinical endocarditis, culture results awaited, no suspicion of staphylococci	Penicillin 1.2 g 4-hourly, Gentamicin 80 mg 12-hourly
Suspected staphylococcal endocarditis (IVDA, recent intravascular devices or cardiac surgery, acute infection)	Vancomycin 1 g 12-hourly, Gentamicin 80–120 mg 8-hourly
Streptococcal endocarditis (penicillin sensitive)	Penicillin 1.2 g 4-hourly, Gentamicin 80 mg 12-hourly
Enterococcal endocarditis (no high-level gentamicin resistance)	Ampicillin/amoxicillin 2 g 4-hourly, Gentamicin 80 mg 12-hourly
Staphylococcal endocarditis	Vancomycin 1 g 12-hourly, OR Flucloxacillin 2 g 4-hourly, OR Benzylpenicillin 1.2 g 4-hourly, PLUS Gentamicin 80–120 mg 8-hourly

Note:
1. Monitor vancomicin and gentamicin levels, and adjust if necessary
2. Choice of antibiotic for staphylococci depends on sensitivities
3. Optimum choice of therapy needs close liaison with Microbiology/Infectious Diseases

All antibiotics given i.v.

BSAC, British Society for Antimicrobial Chemotherapy

Surgery

There are several situations in which surgery is necessary:

- extensive damage to a valve
- prosthetic valve endocarditis – valve replacement is usually required
- persistent infection despite therapy
- serious embolization
- large vegetations
- myocardial abscesses
- fungal endocarditis – this is often refractory to antimicrobial therapy
- progressive cardiac failure.

The timing of surgery is important. On the one hand the infection should, if possible, be eradicated before surgery is undertaken, but if antibiotic therapy is failing, with progressive cardiac failure or uncontrollable sepsis, or severe emboli, it will not be possible to wait. In general, early surgery is preferable.

Prognosis

The prognosis is worse with acute or *Staph. aureus* endocarditis when cardiac failure is present, when infection occurs on a prosthetic valve, and when the micro-organisms found are resistant to therapy. Overall, the mortality is about 20–30%.

Prophylaxis and prevention (see also p. 80)

Where rheumatic fever is common, control and prevention will prevent rheumatic heart disease, and thus associated endocarditis.

In developed countries, most attention is focused on the role of antibiotic prophylaxis. People with valvular lesions should receive antibiotic therapy before undergoing a procedure likely to result in a bacteraemia such as dental treatment or surgical instrumentation. Current UK recommendations (detailed in the British National Formulary) for dental treatment suggest a single dose of 3 g of amoxicillin 1 hour before the procedure; other antibiotics are advised for different procedures.

Meticulous oral and skin hygiene is probably more significant than antibiotic prophylaxis in preventing endocarditis.

Many cases of hospital-acquired endocarditis can be prevented by better care during insertion and handling of intravascular catheters, and prompt removal if they become infected.

FURTHER READING

Adnan S et al. (1997) Prevention of bacterial endocarditis: recommendation by the American Heart Association. *Circulation* **96**: 358–366.

Mylonakis E, Calderwood SB (2001) Infective endocarditis in adults. *New England Journal of Medicine* **345**: 1318–1330.

Working Party for the British Society for Antimicrobial Chemotherapy (1998) Antimicrobial treatment of streptococcal, enterococcal and staphylococcal endocarditis. *Heart* **79**: 207–210.

Also refer to Websites, e.g.:
http://www.americanheart.org/Scientific/statements.

Congenital heart disease

A congenital cardiac malformation occurs in about 1% of live births. There is an overall male predominance, although some individual lesions (e.g. atrial septal defect and persistent ductus arteriosus) occur more commonly in females. As a result of improved medical and surgical management, more children with congenital cardiac disease are surviving into adolescence and adulthood. In the USA the number of adults with corrected or uncorrected congenital cardiac disorders is increasing by 5% per annum. It is estimated that there are up to one million affected adults in the American population at present. In the UK and Ireland, 3000–4000 operations per annum are performed on children with congenital heart disease, resulting in mortality rates less than 10%. Eighty-five per cent of children born with congenital heart disease survive into adulthood, resulting in 60 000 patients over 16 in the UK who require further medical and surgical management. Thus there is

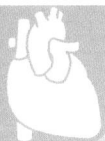
a need for an increased awareness amongst general physicians and cardiologists of the problems posed by these individuals.

The aetiology of congenital cardiac disease is often unknown, but recognized associations include:

- *maternal perinatal rubella infection* (persistent ductus arteriosus, and pulmonary valvular and arterial stenosis)
- *maternal alcohol abuse* (septal defects)
- *maternal drug treatment and radiation*
- *genetic abnormalities* (e.g. the familial form of atrial septal defect and congenital heart block)
- *chromosomal abnormalities* (e.g. septal defects and mitral and tricuspid valve defects are associated with Down's syndrome (trisomy 21) or coarctation of the aorta in Turner's syndrome (45, XO)).

Congenital heart disease should be recognized as early as possible, as the response is usually better the earlier treatment is initiated. Some symptoms, signs and clinical problems are common in congenital heart disease:

- *Central cyanosis* occurs because of right-to-left shunting of blood or because of complete mixing of systemic and pulmonary blood flow. In the latter case, e.g. Fallot's tetralogy, the abnormality is described as *cyanotic* congenital heart disease.
- *Pulmonary hypertension* results from large left-to-right shunts. The persistently raised pulmonary flow leads to the development of increased pulmonary artery vascular resistance and consequent pulmonary hypertension. This is known as the Eisenmenger reaction (or the Eisenmenger complex when due specifically to a ventricular septal defect). The development of pulmonary hypertension significantly worsens the prognosis.
- *Clubbing of the fingers* occurs in congenital cardiac conditions associated with prolonged cyanosis.
- *Paradoxical embolism* of thrombus from the systemic veins to the systemic arterial system may occur when a communication exists between the right and left heart. There is therefore an increased risk of cerebrovascular accidents and also abscesses (as with endocarditis).
- *Polycythaemia* can develop secondary to chronic hypoxaemia leading to a hyperviscosity syndrome and an increased thrombotic risk, e.g. strokes.
- *Growth retardation* is common in children with cyanotic heart disease.
- *Syncope* is common when severe right or left ventricular outflow tract obstruction is present. Exertional syncope, associated with deepening central cyanosis, may occur in Fallot's tetralogy. Exercise increases resistance to pulmonary blood flow but reduces systemic vascular resistance. Thus, the right-to-left shunt increases and cerebral oxygenation falls.
- *Squatting* is the posture adopted by children with Fallot's tetralogy. It results in obstruction of venous return of desaturated blood and an increase in the peripheral systemic vascular resistance. This leads to a reduced right-to-left shunt and improved cerebral oxygenation.

Adolescents and adults with congenital heart disease present with specific common problems related to the long-standing structural nature of these conditions and any surgical treatment:

- endocarditis (particularly in association with otherwise innocuous lesions such as small VSDs or bicuspid aortic valve that can give up to 10% lifetime risk)
- progression of valvular lesions (calcification and stenosis of congenitally deformed valves, e.g. bicuspid aortic valve)
- atrial and ventricular arrhythmias (often quite resistant to treatment)
- sudden cardiac death
- right heart failure (especially when surgical palliation results in the right ventricle providing the systemic supply)
- end-stage heart failure (rarely managed by heart or heart–lung transplantation).

These conditions necessitate active follow-up of adult patients. Pregnancy is normally safe except if pulmonary hypertension or vascular disease is present when the prognosis for both mother and fetus is poor.

Table 13.40 lists the most common congenital lesions and their occurrence in first-degree relatives.

Genetic factors should be considered in all patients presenting with congenital heart disease. For example, parents with a child suffering from Fallot's tetralogy stand a 4% chance of conceiving another child with the disease, and so fetal ultrasound screening of the mother during pregnancy is essential. Parents with congenital heart disease are also more likely to have affected offspring. Fathers have a 2% risk while mothers have a higher risk (around 5%). Individual families can exhibit even higher risks of recurrence.

Table 13.40
Common congenital lesions

	Percentage of congenital lesions	Occurrence in first-degree relatives (%)
Ventricular septal defect	39	4
Atrial septal defect	10	2
Persistent ductus arteriosus	10	4
Pulmonary stenosis	7	
Coarctation of the aorta	7	2
Aortic stenosis	6	4
Fallot's tetralogy	6	4
Others	15	

Ventricular septal defect (VSD)

VSD is the most common congenital cardiac malformation (1 in 500 live births). It may occur as an isolated abnormality or in association with other anomalies. Left ventricular pressure is higher than right ventricular pressure; blood therefore moves from left to right and pulmonary blood flow increases. When pulmonary blood flow is very large, progressive obliteration of the pulmonary vasculature changes eventually causes the pulmonary arterial pressure to equal the systemic pressure (Eisenmenger's complex). Consequently, the shunt is reduced or reversed (becoming right-to-left) and central cyanosis may develop.

Clinical features

A small VSD ('maladie de Roger') presents with a loud and sometimes long systolic murmur in an asymptomatic patient. Such VSDs usually close spontaneously, with 90% no longer patent by 10 years of age. Unfortunately there is a future risk of the development of aortic regurgitation or endocarditis even after spontaneous closure.

Moderate VSDs produce some fatigue and dyspnoea. Physical signs include cardiac enlargement and a prominent apex beat. There is often a palpable systolic thrill at the lower left sternal edge. A loud 'tearing' pansystolic murmur is heard at the same position.

Large VSDs eventually cause pulmonary hypertension (right ventricular parasternal heave and a loud, pulmonary component of the second heart sound). The murmur may be soft as the increased right ventricular pressure may be nearly equal to the left ventricular pressure, so that flow across the VSD is small.

Investigations

A small VSD produces no abnormal X-ray or ECG findings. On the chest X-ray, larger defects show a prominent pulmonary artery owing to increased pulmonary blood flow. In Eisenmenger's complex the radiological signs of pulmonary hypertension (i.e. 'pruned' pulmonary arteries) can be seen. Cardiomegaly occurs when a moderate or a large VSD is present. The ECG shows features of both left and right ventricular hypertrophy. 2-D echocardiography and CW Doppler (Fig. 13.77) can assess the size and location of the VSD, and its haemodynamic consequences.

Treatment

Moderate and large VSDs should be surgically repaired before the development of severe pulmonary hypertension. Infective endocarditis prophylaxis should be advised in all cases.

Atrial septal defect (ASD)

This condition is often first diagnosed in adults and represents one-third of all adult congenital heart disease. It is two to three times more common in women than in men. There are two main types of ASD, ostium

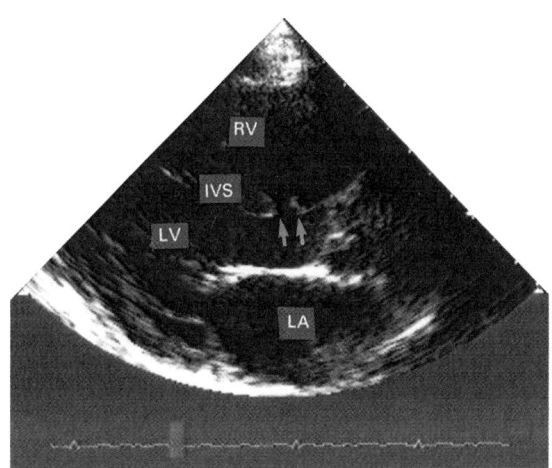

Fig. 13.77 Two-dimensional echocardiogram (long-axis view) showing a ventricular septal defect (arrowed). Colour Doppler would provide graphic demonstration of the left-to-right shunt. RV, right ventricle; IVS, interventricular septum; LV, left ventricle; LA, left atrium.

secundum and ostium primum. The common form is the ostium secundum defect, which involves the fossa ovalis in the atrial mid-septum. This should not be confused with the patent foramen ovale (PFO) which is a normal variant and not a true septal defect. PFOs are usually asymptomatic but are associated with paradoxical emboli and an increased incidence of embolic stroke. Communication at the level of the atria allows left-to-right shunting of blood. Because the pulmonary vascular resistance is low and the right ventricle is easily distended (i.e. it is compliant), there is a considerable increase in right heart output. Above the age of 30 years there may be an increase in pulmonary vascular resistance, which gives rise to pulmonary hypertension. Atrial arrhythmias, particularly atrial fibrillation, are common at this stage.

Clinical features (Box 13.2)

Most children with ASDs are asymptomatic, although they are prone to pulmonary infection. Some complain of dyspnoea and weakness. Palpitations due to atrial arrhythmias are not uncommon. Right heart failure and atrial fibrillation may develop to become the initial presentation in adult life.

Box 13.2

Atrial septal defect

Sternal impulse	Right ventricular heave
Sounds:	Loud P2 Fixed split S2 (A2–P2)
Murmurs	Mid-systolic ejection in pulmonary area Occasional diastolic tricuspid flow murmur

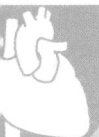
The physical signs of ASD reflect the volume overloading of the right ventricle. Therefore, the splitting of the second sound is wide and fixed (see p. 713). The increased flow through the right heart produces a loud ejection systolic pulmonary flow murmur, and sometimes a diastolic tricuspid flow murmur may be heard. A right ventricular heave can usually be felt.

Investigations
Chest X-ray
This reveals a prominent pulmonary artery and pulmonary plethora. Figure 13.78 shows a more severe case with pulmonary hypertension. There may be noticeable right ventricular enlargement.

Electrocardiogram
This usually shows some degree of right bundle branch block (because of dilatation of the right ventricle) and right axis deviation. Sometimes the ASD is part of a major developmental abnormality involving the ventricular septum and the mitral and tricuspid valves. In this case there is left axis deviation on the ECG.

Echocardiogram
This is usually abnormal if a significant defect is present. Indirect evidence includes right ventricular hypertrophy and pulmonary arterial dilatation, and abnormal motion of the interventricular septum. Subcostal views may demonstrate the ASD (Fig. 13.79). Flow disturbance can be assessed by colour Doppler.

Treatment
A significant ASD (i.e. a pulmonary flow that is more than 50% increased when compared with systemic flow) should be repaired before the age of 10 years or as soon as possible if first diagnosed in adulthood. There is a dilemma with regard to whether less severe shunts should be closed when diagnosed in adulthood. Anecdotal evidence suggests that the shunt might be progressive and that low-risk closure would be appropriate.

There is a good result from surgery unless pulmonary hypertension has developed. Angiographic closure is now possible with significantly lower risk using a transcatheter clamshell device (see Fig. 13.80). A PFO discovered in a patient with an otherwise unexplained

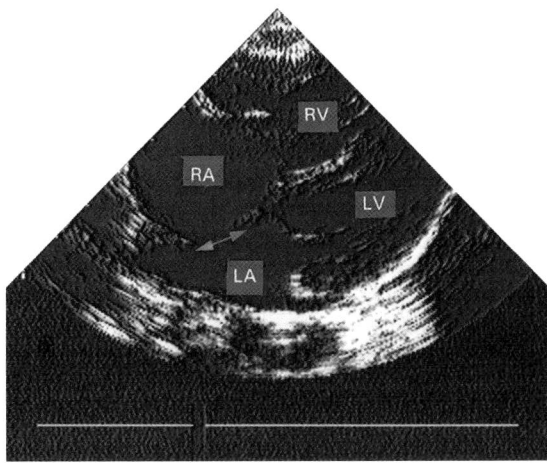

Fig. 13.79 Ostium secundum atrial septal defect (arrowed) in a young girl, shown by a two-dimensional echocardiogram subcostal four-chamber view (similar to Fig. 13.77, but rotated clockwise). Colour Doppler can demonstrate the left-to-right shunt. LA, left atrium; RA, right atrium; LV, left ventricle; RV, right ventricle.

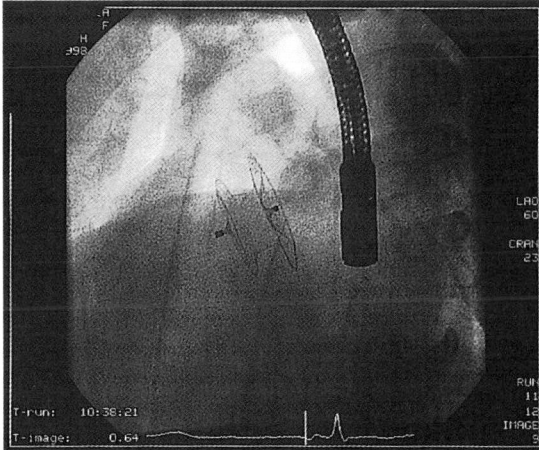

Fig. 13.80 The angiographic appearance of a fully deployed ASD closure device. The device bridges the ASD and wedges against the surfaces of the right and left atrial septa, occluding flow. The metal object in frame is the distal end of a transoesophageal echocardiography probe. Courtesy of Dr D Ward.

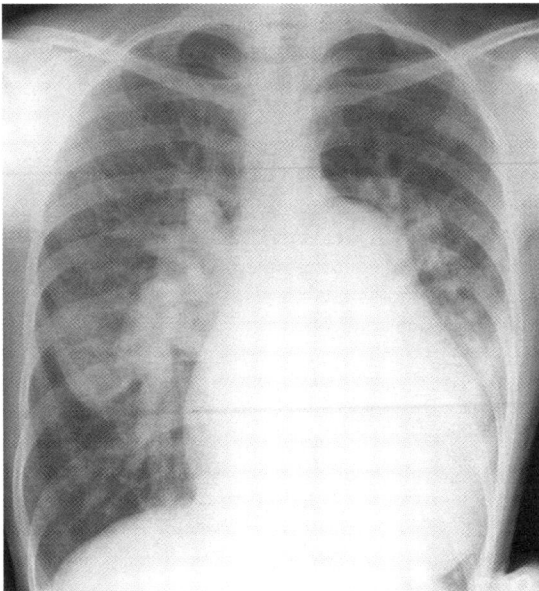

Fig. 13.78 Atrial septal defect shown by a PA chest X-ray from a young woman. The film shows a prominent main pulmonary artery and pulmonary arterial plethora. The heart is increased in size.

thrombotic stroke is now closed in this way to prevent paradoxical thromboembolism. In high-risk groups, for example deep-sea divers, such closures may be undertaken even though the patients are asymptomatic. Uncorrected ASDs do not usually require antibiotic prophylaxis for endocarditis. If there is an accompanying valvular lesion, however, prophylaxis is indicated.

Persistent ductus arteriosus (PDA)

The ductus arteriosus connects the pulmonary artery at its bifurcation to the descending aorta immediately distal to the subclavian artery. In fetal life the ductus diverts blood away from the unexpanded, and hence high-resistance, pulmonary circulation into the systemic circulation, where the blood is reoxygenated as it passes through the placenta. At birth, the high oxygen in the lungs and the reduced pulmonary vascular resistance trigger closure of the duct. If the duct is malformed (i.e. it does not contain sufficient elastic tissue) it will not close. This is more common in females and is sometimes associated with maternal rubella. Premature babies are often born with persistent ducts that are anatomically normal but are immature in that they lack the mechanism to close. Other associations include continual perinatal hypoxaemia and high-altitude environments.

Because aortic pressure exceeds pulmonary artery pressure throughout the cardiac cycle, a persistent duct produces continuous aorta-to-pulmonary artery shunting. This leads to an increased pulmonary venous return to the left heart and an increased left ventricular volume load. If the shunt is large, this results in severe left heart failure and pulmonary hypertension. One-third of individuals with an unrepaired ductus die from heart failure, pulmonary hypertension or endocarditis by the age of 40; two-thirds by the age of 60.

Clinical features

There are often no symptoms until later in life when heart failure or infective endocarditis develops.

The characteristic physical sign is a continuous 'machinery' murmur (due to turbulent aortic-to-pulmonary artery shunting in both systole and diastole), best heard below the left clavicle in the first interspace or over the first rib. A thrill may often be felt. This lessens or disappears as pulmonary hypertension develops leading to shunt reversal. The peripheral pulse is large in volume ('bounding') because of the increased left heart blood flow and the decompression of the aorta into the pulmonary artery.

Investigations

The aorta and pulmonary arterial system are usually prominent on X-ray, although a small ductus shows no abnormality. There is both a left atrial abnormality and left ventricular hypertrophy on the ECG. With the development of Eisenmenger's syndrome, right ventricular hypertrophy may be seen. The echocardiogram shows a dilated left atrium and left ventricle. Right heart changes are apparent in late disease.

Treatment

Premature infants with a persistent duct are treated medically with indometacin, which inhibits prostaglandin production and stimulates duct closure. In other cases the duct can be ligated surgically or angiographically with very little risk. Surgery should be performed as soon as possible and not later than the age of 5 years. Closure is inappropriate if pulmonary hypertension is severe.

Coarctation of the aorta

A coarctation of the aorta is a narrowing of the aorta at, or just distal to, the insertion of the ductus arteriosus, i.e. distal to the left subclavian artery (Fig. 13.81). Rarely it can occur proximal to the left subclavian. It occurs twice as commonly in men as in women. It is also associated with Turner's syndrome (p. 1030). In 80% of cases the aortic valve is bicuspid (and potentially stenotic or endocarditic). Other associations include patent ductus arteriosus, ventricular septal defect, mitral stenosis or regurgitation and circle of Willis aneurysms.

Severe narrowing of the aorta encourages the formation of a collateral arterial circulation involving the periscapular and intercostal arteries. Decreased renal perfusion can lead to the development of systemic hypertension that persists even after surgical correction.

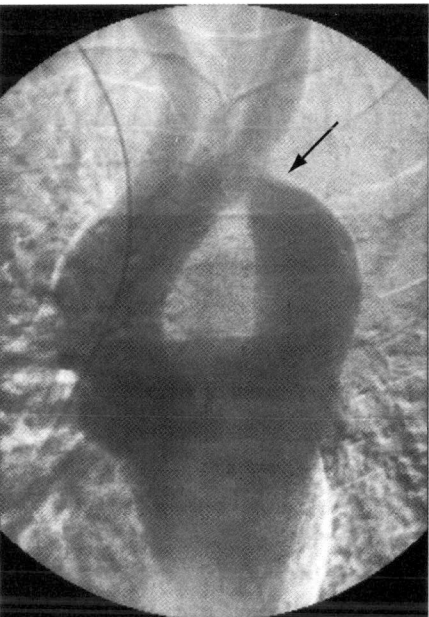

Fig. 13.81 **This aortogram demonstrates a coarctation of the aorta.** Contrast outlines the left ventricle, aorta (ascending, arch and descending) and three major arteries arising from the aorta (innominate, left carotid and left subclavian). Immediately after the left subclavian artery the aorta is very markedly narrowed owing to a coarctation of the aorta.

Clinical features

Coarctation of the aorta is often asymptomatic for many years. Headaches and nosebleeds (due to hypertension) and claudication and cold legs (due to poor blood flow in the lower limbs) may be present.

Physical examination reveals hypertension in the upper limbs, and weak, delayed (radiofemoral delay) pulses in the legs.

A mid-to-late systolic murmur due to turbulent flow through the coarctation may be heard over the upper precordium or the back. Vascular bruits from the collateral circulation may also be heard.

Investigations

The chest X-ray may reveal a dilated aorta indented at the site of the coarctation. This is manifested by an aorta (seen in the upper right mediastinum) shaped like a figure '3'. In adults, tortuous and dilated collateral intercostal arteries may erode the undersurfaces of the ribs ('rib notching').

The ECG demonstrates left ventricular hypertrophy. Echocardiography sometimes shows the coarctation and other associated anomalies. Aortography will show the defect, and digital vascular imaging allows the coarctation to be visualized after the intravenous injection of contrast. CT and MRI scanning can accurately demonstrate the coarctation and quantify flow.

Treatment

Treatment is usually indicated if the pressure gradient across the coarctation is greater than 30 mmHg. This involves surgical excision of the coarctation and end-to-end anastomosis of the aorta. If the coarctation is extensive, prosthetic vascular grafts may be needed. When surgery is performed in early childhood, hypertension usually resolves completely. However, when the operation is performed on adolescents or adults the hypertension persists in 70% because of previous renal damage. There is also an increased risk of accelerated atherosclerosis and strokes in these individuals. Balloon dilatation is used in some centres either for primary disease or post-surgical recurrence although there is a higher incidence of aneurysm formation and post-dilatation recurrence.

Surgical correction in childhood gives a good 25-year survival rate of 83%. If this is delayed until adulthood (20–40), the 25-year survival rate drops to 75%. If coarctation is left uncorrected, however, only 25% of patients are alive at 50 while cardiac failure ensues in two-thirds of surviving patients over 40.

Cyanotic congenital heart disease: Fallot's tetralogy

Most children with cyanotic congenital heart disease do not survive the neonatal period. Fallot's is the most common cyanotic anomaly in those who do survive and is commonest amongst adults. Transposition of the

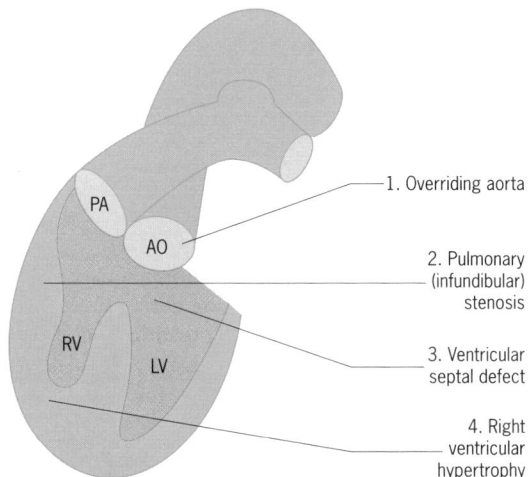

1. Overriding aorta

2. Pulmonary (infundibular) stenosis

3. Ventricular septal defect

4. Right ventricular hypertrophy

Fig. 13.82 **The four features of Fallot's tetralogy.**

great vessels is more common in the neonatal period but more likely to be fatal. Other cyanotic congenital heart disease includes tricuspid atresia, pulmonary atresia and Ebstein's anomaly (dysplastic tricuspid valve).

Fallot's consists of the four features shown in Figure 13.82.

The level of the right ventricular outflow obstruction may be subvalvular, valvular or supravalvular. The most common obstruction is subvalvular, either alone (50%) or in combination with valvular stenosis (25%).

This combination of lesions leads to a high right ventricular pressure and right-to-left shunting of blood through the VSD. Thus the patient is centrally cyanosed.

Clinical features

Children with this condition may present with dyspnoea or fatigue, or with hypoxic episodes on exertion (Fallot's spells) – deep cyanosis and possible syncope. These can even result in seizures, cerebrovascular events or sudden death. Squatting is common.

Adults tend not to suffer 'spells' but fatigue easily with dyspnoea on exertion. Erythrocytosis (polycythaemia) secondary to chronic hypoxaemia commonly results in thrombotic strokes. Endocarditis is common.

Physical signs include a parasternal sustained heave and a systolic ejection murmur, often associated with a thrill in the second left interspace close to the sternum. The second heart sound is usually single because the pulmonary component is too soft to be heard. Central cyanosis is commonly present from birth, and finger clubbing and polycythaemia are obvious after about 12 months. Growth is usually retarded.

Investigations

The chest X-ray shows a large right ventricle and a small pulmonary artery (classically described as 'boot-shaped'). The ECG reveals right ventricular hypertrophy, and the echocardiogram demonstrates discontinuity between the aorta and the anterior wall of the ventricular septum. Cardiac catheterization is performed to evaluate the size and degree of the right ventricular outflow obstruction.

Treatment

Complete surgical correction of this combination of lesions is possible even in infancy. As adults, however, these individuals are at increased risk of right ventricular failure and ventricular arrhythmias due to the trauma from past corrective surgery. Less-damaging procedures are used presently, the long-term results of which are unknown as yet.

Occasionally a palliative procedure – an anastomosis between a subclavian artery and a pulmonary artery (Blalock shunt) – is performed on very young infants or the premature in order to increase blood supply to the lungs. Without intervention, 66% survive to 1 year while only 11% survive to 20 years.

Fallot's spells may need treatment with beta-blockade or, when severe, with diamorphine to relax the right ventricular outflow obstruction. Antibiotic prophylaxis for endocarditis is indicated.

FURTHER READING

Brickner EM et al. (2000) Congenital heart disease in adults. *New England Journal of Medicine* **342**(4): 256–263.
Hunter S (2000) Congenital heart disease in adolescence. *Journal of the Royal College of Physicians of London* **34**(2): 150–152.
Perloff JK (1994) *Congenital Heart Disease*, 4th edn. Philadelphia: WB Saunders.

Marfan's syndrome

Clinical features

Marfan's syndrome (MFS) is one of the most common autosomal dominant inherited disorders of connective tissue, affecting the heart (aortic aneurysm and dissection, mitral valve prolapse) eye (dislocated lenses, retinal detachment) and skeleton (tall, thin body build with long arms, legs and fingers; scoliosis and pectus deformity) (Fig. 13.83).

Clinically, two out of three major systems must be affected, to avoid overdiagnosing the condition. Diagnosis may be confirmed by studying family linkage to the causative gene, or by demonstrating a mutation in the Marfan's syndrome gene (*MFS1*) for fibrillin (FBN-1) on chromosome 15q21.

MFS affects approximately 1 in 5000 population worldwide, and 25% of patients are affected as a result of a new mutation. This group includes many of the more severely affected patients, with high cardiovascular risk. Other known associations with early death due to aortic aneurysm and dissection are: family history of early cardiac involvement; family history of dissection with

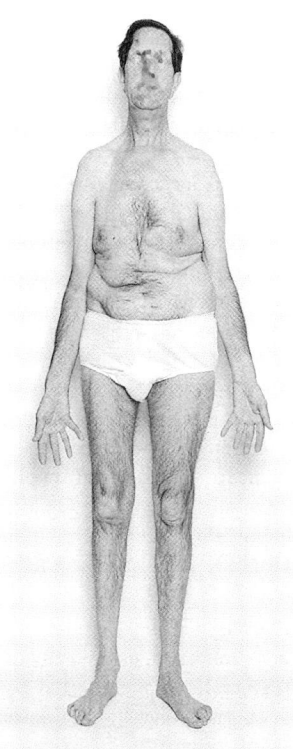

Fig. 13.83 Marfan's syndrome – photograph of 63-year-old man.

an aortic root diameter of < 5 cm; male sex; and extreme physical characteristics, including markedly excessive stature and widespread striae. Histological examination of aortas often shows widespread medial degeneration, described as 'cystic medial necrosis'.

Investigations

- **Chest X-ray.** Often normal but may show signs of aortic aneurysm and unfolding, or of widened mediastinum. Pneumothorax affects 11% and scoliosis is present in 70% of patients.
- **ECG.** May be misleadingly normal with an acute dissection. Usually, in conjunction with mitral valve prolapse 40% of patients have arrhythmia, with premature ventricular and atrial arrhythmias.
- **Echocardiography.** Mitral valve prolapse and mitral regurgitation are seen in the majority of patients. High-quality serial echocardiogram measurements of aortic root diameter in the sinuses of Valsalva, at 90 degrees to the direction of flow are the basis for medical and surgical management (Fig. 13.103).

Management

Beta-blocker therapy slows the rate of dilatation of the aortic root. Lifestyle alterations, involving sports and career choice, may be indicated, because of ocular, cardiac or skeletal involvement. Sports that necessitate prolonged exertion at maximum cardiac output, such as cross-country running, are to be avoided. Sedentary occupations are usually best, as patients tend to suffer from easy fatigability and hypermobile painful joints.

The patient should be monitored with yearly echo-cardiograms up to aortic root diameter 4.5 cm, 6-monthly from 4.5–5 cm, and then referred directly to a surgeon who is experienced in aortic root replacement in Marfan's syndrome for elective surgery.

Pregnancy is generally well tolerated if no serious cardiac problems are present, but is preferably avoided if the aortic root diameter is over 4 cm, with aortic regurgitation. Caesarean section at 39 weeks' gestation is the recommended method of delivery when the aortic root is over 4.5 cm. Beta-blocker therapy may be safely instituted or continued throughout pregnancy, to help prevent aortic dissection.

Careful medical and surgical management have increased the overall survival rate. On average, 13 years of life is added, when surgical survival is compared to that reported in the natural history of MFS.

Genetic counselling

The condition is inherited in an autosomal dominant mode, with each child of one affected parent having a 50–50 chance of inheriting the condition. Males and females are equally often affected. In 25% of all cases, the condition arises as the result of a spontaneous mutation in the sperm or ovum of one of the parents. Fibrillin-1 gene mutations can be identified in 80% of those affected, confirming diagnosis and aiding prognosis.

FURTHER READING

Devereux RB, Roman MJ (1999) Aortic disease in Marfan's syndrome. *New England Journal of Medicine* **340**: 1358–1359.

Pulmonary heart disease (cor pulmonale)

The term 'cor pulmonale' means right heart disease arising secondary to pulmonary hypertension. In some ways it is an unsatisfactory term, in that the causes of cor pulmonale are very diverse and mostly represent very different disease processes. The approach to treatment varies according to the aetiology, as well as specific therapy often being required for the causative disease. The reason for continued use of the term is that most clinically relevant right heart diseases arise secondary to a problem downstream in the circulation from it, and the term 'right heart failure' is therefore also unsatisfactory in this context. Equally, the diseases in question do not inevitably lead to cor pulmonale.

As long as it is remembered that cor pulmonale is not a disease but a final common pathway, then it is still a useful term. Where possible, the two diagnoses should be given together; for example, cystic fibrosis complicated by cor pulmonale, cor pulmonale secondary to multiple pulmonary emboli.

Pure right heart failure does occur, but is rare. Examples include right ventricular myocardial infarction and isolated right-sided heart valve disease.

The causes of acute and chronic cor pulmonale are numerous but, in clinical practice, one disorder of each type predominates. These are pulmonary embolism in acute, and chronic obstructive pulmonary disease (COPD) in chronic cor pulmonale. The causes of cor pulmonale are shown in (Table 13.41).

Acute cor pulmonale (pulmonary embolism)

Thrombus, usually formed in the systemic veins or rarely in the right heart (less than 10% of cases), may dislodge and embolize into the pulmonary arterial system. Post-mortem studies indicate that this is a very common condition (microemboli are found in up to 60% of autopsies) but it is not usually diagnosed this frequently in life. Ten per cent of clinical pulmonary emboli are fatal.

Most clots which cause clinically relevant pulmonary emboli actually come from the pelvic and abdominal veins, but femoral deep venous thrombosis, and even occasionally axillary thrombosis, can be the origin of the clot. Clot forms as a result of a combination of sluggish blood flow, local injury or compression of the vein and

---

Table 13.41
The causes of cor pulmonale

Pulmonary vascular disorders
Acute pulmonary thromboembolism (rarely tumour emboli)
Primary pulmonary hypertension
Multiple pulmonary artery stenoses
Pulmonary veno-occlusive disease
Recurrent pulmonary emboli

Disease of the lung and parenchyma
COPD
All other chronic lung disorders (Ch. 14)

Musculoskeletal disorders (causing chronic underventilation)
Kyphoscoliosis
Poliomyelitis
Myasthenia gravis

Disturbance of respiratory control
Morbid obesity (Pickwickian syndrome)
Obstructive sleep apnoea
Cerebrovascular disease

Left heart disorders
Mitral stenosis
Left atrial myxoma
Left ventricular failure

Miscellaneous
Appetite suppressant drugs (e.g. dexfenfluramine)

a hypercoagulable state. Risk factors are shown in Table 8.26 and discussed on page 465.

After pulmonary embolism, lung tissue is ventilated but not perfused – producing an intrapulmonary dead space and resulting in impaired gas exchange. After some hours the non-perfused lung no longer produces surfactant. Alveolar collapse occurs and exacerbates hypoxaemia. The primary haemodynamic consequence of pulmonary embolism is a reduction in the cross-sectional area of the pulmonary arterial bed which results in an elevation of pulmonary arterial pressure and a reduction in cardiac output. The zone of lung that is no longer perfused by the pulmonary artery may infarct, but often does not do so because oxygen continues to be supplied by the bronchial circulation and the airways.

Clinical features

Sudden onset of unexplained dyspnoea is the most common, and often the only symptom of pulmonary embolism. Pleuritic chest pain and haemoptysis are present only when infarction has occurred. Many pulmonary emboli occur silently, but there are three typical clinical presentations. A clinical deep venous thrombosis is not commonly observed, although detailed investigation of the lower limb and pelvic veins will reveal thrombosis in more than half of the cases.

Small/medium pulmonary embolism

In this situation an embolus has impacted in a terminal pulmonary vessel. Symptoms are pleuritic chest pain and breathlessness. Haemoptysis occurs in 30%, often 3 or more days after the initial event. On examination, the patient may be tachypnoeic with a localized pleural rub and often coarse crackles over the area involved. A pleural effusion (occasionally blood-stained) can develop. The patient may have a fever and cardiovascular examination is normal.

Massive pulmonary embolism

This is a much more rare condition where sudden collapse occurs because of an acute obstruction of the right ventricular outflow tract. The patient has severe central chest pain (cardiac ischaemia due to lack of coronary blood flow) and becomes shocked, pale and sweaty. Syncope may result if the cardiac output is transiently but dramatically reduced, and death may occur. On examination, the patient is tachypnoeic, has a tachycardia with hypotension and peripheral shutdown. The jugular venous pressure (JVP) is raised with a prominent 'a' wave. There is a right ventricular heave, a gallop rhythm and a widely split second heart sound. There are usually no abnormal chest signs.

Multiple recurrent pulmonary emboli

This leads to increased breathlessness, often over weeks or months. It is accompanied by weakness, syncope on exertion and occasionally angina. The physical signs are due to the pulmonary hypertension that has developed from multiple occlusions of the pulmonary vasculature. On examination, there are signs of right ventricular overload with a right ventricular heave and loud pulmonary second sound.

Diagnosis

The symptoms and signs of small and medium-sized pulmonary emboli are often subtle and non-specific, so the diagnosis is often delayed or even completely missed. Pulmonary embolism should be considered if patients present with symptoms of new-onset atrial fibrillation (or other tachycardia), unexplained breathlessness or cough, if no other obvious cause is present.

Investigations

Small/medium pulmonary emboli

- **Chest X-ray** is often normal, but linear atelectasis or blunting of a costophrenic angle (due to a small effusion) is not uncommon. These features develop only after some time. A raised hemidiaphragm is present in some patients. More rarely, a wedge-shaped pulmonary infarct, the abrupt cut-off of a pulmonary artery or a translucency of an underperfused distal zone is seen. Previous infarcts may be seen as opaque linear scars.
- **ECG** is usually normal, except for sinus tachycardia, but sometimes atrial fibrillation or another tachyarrhythmia occurs. There may be evidence of right ventricular strain.
- **Blood tests.** If pulmonary infarction has occurred, there will be a polymorphonuclear leucocytosis, an elevated ESR and increased lactate dehydrogenase levels in the serum.
- **Plasma D-dimer** (see p. 456). If this is undetectable, it excludes a diagnosis of pulmonary embolism.
- **Radionuclide ventilation/perfusion scan ($\dot{V}/\dot{Q}$ scan)** is a good and widely available diagnostic investigation. The pulmonary ^{99m}Tc scintigram demonstrates underperfused areas (Fig. 13.84) which, if not accompanied by a ventilation defect on a ventilation scintigram performed after inhalation of radioactive xenon gas (see p. 849), is highly suggestive of a pulmonary embolus. There are limitations to the test, however. For example, a matched defect may arise with a pulmonary embolus which causes an infarct or from emphysematous bullae. This test is therefore conventionally reported as a probability of pulmonary embolus and should be interpreted in the context of the history, examination and other investigations.
- **Ultrasound scanning** can be performed for the detection of clots in pelvic or ileofemoral veins (see p. 832).

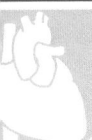

- **Spiral CT scans** with intravenous contrast show good sensitivity and specificity for medium-sized pulmonary emboli. They do not exclude pulmonary emboli in small arteries.
- **MR imaging** gives similar results and is used if CT angiography is contraindicated.

Massive pulmonary emboli

- **Chest X-ray** may show pulmonary oligaemia, sometimes with dilatation of the pulmonary artery in the hila. Often there are no changes.
- **ECG** shows right atrial dilatation with tall peaked T waves in lead II. Right ventricular strain and dilatation give rise to right axis deviation, some degree of right bundle branch block, and T wave inversion in the right precordial leads (Fig. 13.85). The 'classic' ECG pattern with an S wave in lead I,

and a Q wave and inverted T waves in lead III (S^1, Q^{iii}, T^{iii}), is rare.
- **Blood gases** show hypoxia and hypocapnia.
- **Echocardiogram** shows a vigorously contracting left ventricle and occasionally a clot in the right ventricular outflow tract.
- **Pulmonary angiography** is sometimes undertaken if surgery is considered in acute massive embolism. The test is performed by injecting contrast material through a catheter inserted into the main pulmonary artery. Filling defects or obstructed vessels can be delineated (Fig. 13.86). Angiography is hazardous but the risk may be reduced if contrast is injected into each pulmonary artery separately. If the patient is in extremis and the diagnosis is obvious, surgery should proceed without prior angiography.

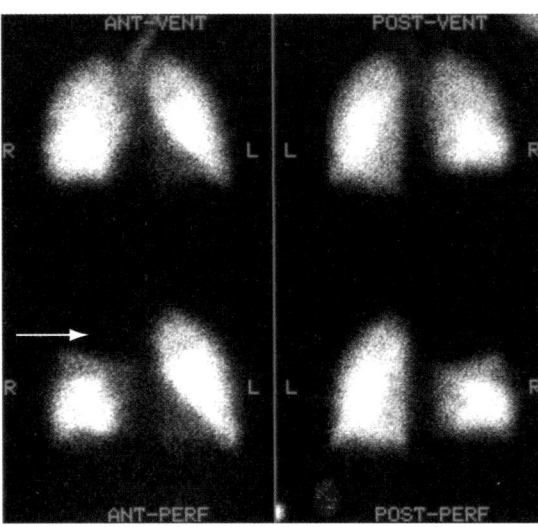

Fig. 13.84 Ventilation (top) **and perfusion** (bottom) **lung scans** which demonstrate absence of perfusion but normal ventilation in the right upper lobe, i.e. probably pulmonary embolism.

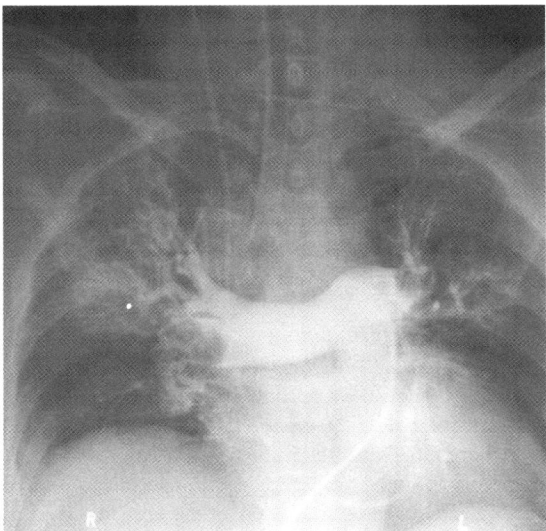

Fig. 13.86 Contrast injected directly into the main pulmonary artery (pulmonary angiogram) demonstrates a large filling defect in the interlobar segment of the right pulmonary artery and extensive occlusion in the proximal left pulmonary artery.

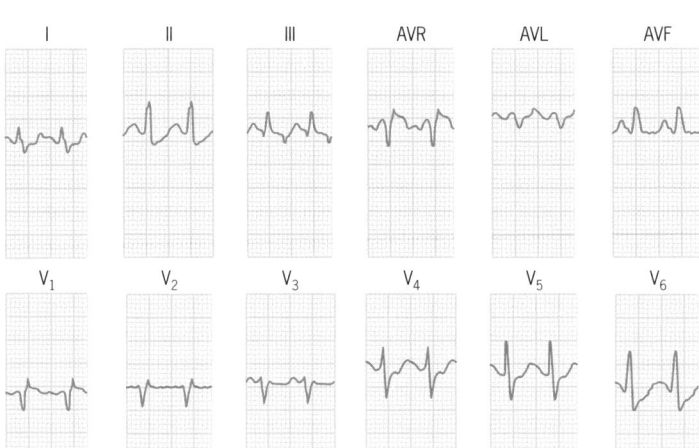

Fig. 13.85 Acute pulmonary embolism shown by a 12-lead ECG. There is an S wave in lead I, a Q wave in lead III and an inverted T wave in lead III (the S1, Q3, T3 pattern). There is sinus tachycardia (160 b.p.m.) and an incomplete right bundle branch block pattern (an R wave in AVR and V_1 and an S wave in V_6).

Multiple recurrent pulmonary emboli

- **Chest X-ray** may be normal. Enlarged pulmonary arterioles with oligaemic lung fields indicate advanced disease.
- **ECG** can be normal or show signs of pulmonary hypertension (Fig. 13.87).
- **Leg imaging** with **ultrasound** and **venography** may show thrombi.
- $\dot{V}/\dot{Q}$ **scan** may show evidence of pulmonary infarcts.
- **Further tests** looking for exercise-induced hypoxaemia and catheter studies to estimate pulmonary artery pressures are often required.

Treatment

Acute management

All patient should receive high-flow oxygen (60–100%) unless they have significant chronic lung disease. Patients with pulmonary infarcts require bed rest and analgesia. In severe cases, intravenous fluids and even inotropic agents to improve the pumping of the right heart are sometimes required and very ill patients will require care on the intensive therapy unit (p. 922).

Prevention of further emboli

The basis of therapy is intravenous heparin. This can be with a bolus of 10 000 units of unfractionated heparin followed by the continuous infusion of 1000–2000 units per hour. A comparison of low-molecular-weight heparin (LMWH) with unfractionated heparin has shown no difference. As LMWHs simplify treatment (p. 468) they are being increasingly used, although they are more expensive. Oral anticoagulants are usually begun after 48 hours and the heparin is tapered off as the oral anticoagulant becomes effective. Oral anticoagulants are continued for 6 weeks to 6 months, depending on the likelihood of recurrence of venous thrombosis or embolism. In some situations, such as after recurrent embolism, lifelong treatment is indicated.

Occasionally, physical methods are required to prevent further emboli. This is usually because recurrent emboli occur despite adequate anticoagulation, but is also indicated in high-risk patients in whom anticoagulation is absolutely contraindicated. The most common method by which pulmonary embolism is treated in this situation is by insertion of a filter in the inferior vena cava above the level of the renal veins.

Dissolution of the thrombus

Fibrinolytic therapy such as streptokinase (250 000 units by i.v. infusion over 30 minutes, followed by streptokinase 100 000 units i.v. hourly for up to 12–72 hours according to manufacturer's instructions) is often used following a major embolism.

Surgery

Surgical embolectomy is rarely necessary, but there may be no alternative when the haemodynamic circumstances are very severe.

Chronic cor pulmonale

Cor pulmonale is enlargement of the right ventricle because of increase in afterload that is due to diseases of the thorax, lung and pulmonary circulation; the presence of right ventricular failure is not necessary for the diagnosis of cor pulmonale.

Pathophysiology

The precise mechanism varies according to the cause of cor pulmonale, but chronic obstructive pulmonary disease (COPD), which is discussed here, is illustrative. Pulmonary vascular resistance is increased because of loss of pulmonary vascular tissue and because of pulmonary vasoconstriction caused by hypoxia and acidosis. The increased pulmonary vascular resistance leads to pulmonary hypertension, which initially occurs only during an acute respiratory infection. Eventually, the pulmonary hypertension becomes persistent and progressively more severe. The pulmonary vascular bed is gradually obliterated by muscular hypertrophy of the arterioles and thrombus formation. Right ventricular function is progressively compromised because of the increased pressure load. Hypoxia further impairs right ventricular function and, as it develops, left ventricular function is also depressed.

Clinical features

Chest pain, exertional dyspnoea, syncope and fatigue are common symptoms, and sudden death occurs. Other symptoms are due to the cause of the pulmonary hypertension.

On physical examination, there is a prominent *a* wave in the jugular venous pulse, a right ventricular (parasternal) heave, and a loud pulmonary component

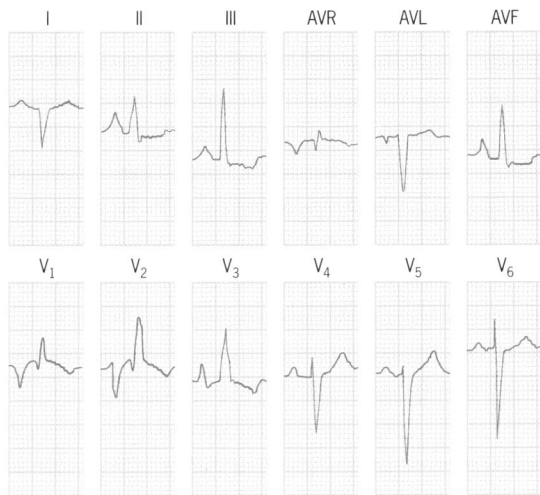

I	II	III	AVR	AVL	AVF

V₁	V₂	V₃	V₄	V₅	V₆

Fig. 13.87 **Pulmonary hypertension** shown by a 12-lead ECG. There is right axis deviation (+120°), right ventricular hypertrophy (dominant secondary R wave [R'] in V_1) and a combination of left and right atrial conduction abnormalities.

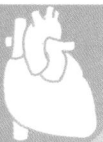
to the second heart sound. Other findings include a right ventricular fourth heart sound, a systolic pulmonary ejection click, a mid-systolic ejection murmur, and an early diastolic murmur due to pulmonary regurgitation (Graham Steell murmur). If tricuspid regurgitation develops, there is a pansystolic murmur and a large jugular *cv* venous wave (p. 711).

Investigations

- **Chest X-ray** may show right ventricular enlargement and right atrial dilatation. The pulmonary artery is usually prominent and the enlarged proximal pulmonary arteries taper rapidly. Peripheral lung fields are oligaemic.
- **ECG** demonstrates right ventricular hypertrophy (right axis deviation, possibly a dominant R wave in lead V_1, and inverted T waves in right precordial leads) and a right atrial abnormality (tall peaked P waves in lead II) (Fig. 13.87).
- **Echocardiography** will usually demonstrate right ventricular dilatation and/or hypertrophy. It is often possible to measure the peak pulmonary artery pressure indirectly with Doppler echocardiography. The echocardiogram may also reveal the cause of pulmonary hypertension, such as an intracardiac shunt.

Other investigations may also be required to evaluate the cause of pulmonary hypertension and to look for treatable conditions, such as left-to-right shunts, mitral stenosis or left atrial tumours. Direct measurement of pulmonary artery pressure and pulmonary wedge pressure by cardiac catheterization is necessary in some patients with severe pulmonary hypertension of unknown cause. Pulmonary angiography may be indicated if multiple pulmonary emboli are suspected, but is dangerous.

If no other cause is found, then a diagnosis of primary pulmonary hypertension is made (p. 808).

Treatment

Treatment is determined by the condition underlying pulmonary hypertension. Diuretic treatment is used for right ventricular failure, but care should be taken to avoid excessive fluid depletion as this will result in reduced output from the impaired right ventricle. Hypoxia is avoided by the use of oxygen therapy when safe and necessary. In those with COPD and some others, long-term oxygen therapy (LTOT) improves symptoms and prognosis. In contrast to their enormous value in those with left ventricular impairment, angiotensin-converting enzyme inhibitors are seldom useful and may make matters worse.

Primary pulmonary hypertension

Primary pulmonary hypertension (PPH) is an uncommon disease characterized by increased pulmonary artery pressure and increased pulmonary vascular resistance without an obvious cause. The normal pulmonary artery pressure in a person living at sea level has a peak systolic value of 18–25 mmHg, an end-diastolic value of 6–10 mmHg and a mean value ranging from 12–16 mmHg. Definite pulmonary hypertension is present when pulmonary artery systolic and mean pressures exceed 30 and 20 mmHg, respectively. There is a female-to-male preponderance (1.7:1), with patients most commonly presenting in the third and fourth decades.

Pathophysiology

Three histological patterns have been described.

- *Plexogenic pulmonary arteriopathy* is found in 30–60% of patients and is more prevalent in younger women. The histology is characterized by medial hypertrophy, concentric laminar intimal fibrosis, and plexiform lesions.
- *Thrombotic pulmonary arteriopathy* affects men and women equally and accounts for 40–50% of the cases. Histologically it is characterized by eccentric intimal fibrosis with medial hypertrophy, fibroelastic intimal pads, and scattered evidence of old recanalized thrombus appearing as fibrous webs.
- *Pulmonary veno-occlusive disease* occurs in less than 10% of cases and is histologically characterized by widespread intimal proliferation and fibrosis of the intrapulmonary veins and venules.

It is difficult to distinguish these three subsets on clinical grounds. A chest radiograph and perfusion lung scan is helpful.

The underlying haemodynamic derangement is an increased resistance to pulmonary blood flow, and marked increase in pulmonary arterial pressure possibly due to endothelin-1; the pulmonary capillary wedge pressure remains normal. Pulmonary function is usually normal in PPH, although a mild restrictive pattern is sometimes seen. Hypoxia is common.

Specific risk factors in the development of pulmonary hypertension. Obesity, portal hypertension, anorexigens, human immunodeficiency virus, systemic hypertension and chronically increased blood flow have all been implicated in the development of primary pulmonary hypertension. The gene for PPH (*PPP1*) has been mapped to chromosome 2q 31–33 and mutations in the *BMPR 2* gene (bone morphogenetic protein receptor, a member of the TGF-β-receptor family) has been found in some patients.

Diagnosis

The *history* usually reveals the gradual onset of shortness of breath on exertion, progressing until the patient is dyspnoeic with minimal activity. The average duration from symptom onset until diagnosis is 2.5 years. Other common *symptoms* are fatigue, angina pectoris which represents right ventricular ischaemia, syncope, near syncope and peripheral oedema. The physical examination is characteristic. Increased JVP, a reduced carotid pulse, and an easily palpable right ventricular lift are typical. Most patients have increased pulmonic component of second heart sound and right-sided third and fourth heart sounds. Tricuspid and pulmonary regurgitation and peripheral cyanosis and oedema may be noted. Clubbing is not a feature.

Chest X-ray generally shows enlarged central pulmonary arteries and clear lung fields. *ECG* shows right axis deviation and right ventricular hypertrophy. The *echocardiogram* demonstrates right ventricular enlargement, a reduction in left ventricular cavity size, and abnormal septal configuration consistent with right ventricular pressure overload. Ventricular filling is markedly dependent on atrial systole. *Lung function studies* show hypoxia, hypocapnia and an abnormal diffusing capacity for carbon monoxide. A *perfusion lung scan* may be normal or abnormal with multiple diffuse patchy filling defects of a non-segmental nature and not suggestive of pulmonary thromboembolism. *Pulmonary angiography* and *cardiac catheterization* should be performed.

Prognosis

Several studies have reported a mean survival of 2–3 years from the time of diagnosis. The cause of death is usually right ventricular failure or sudden death. Increased right atrial pressure above 15 mmHg and cardiac index below 2 L/min/m^2 are haemodynamic predictors of poor prognosis.

Management

Lifestyle changes, digoxin, diuretics, oral anticoagulants, supplemental oxygen therapy and vasodilators are mainstays in treatment of PPH. Continuous infusion of prostacyclin has now been shown in prospective randomized trials to improve quality of life and symptoms related to PPH, exercise tolerance, haemodynamics and survival. It has been reported recently that the long-term treatment with aerosolized iloprost (a stable prostacyclin analogue) was safe and has sustained effects on exercise capacity and pulmonary haemodynamics in patients with primary pulmonary hypertension. Endothelin-receptor antagonists are also being used. Heart and lung transplantation is used for younger patients.

FURTHER READING

Fedullo PF et al (2001) Chronic thromboembolic pulmonary hypertension. *New England Journal of Medicine* **345**: 1465–1472.

Hoeper MM et al. (2000) Long-term treatment of primary pulmonary hypertension with aerosolized iloprost, a prostacycline analogue. *New England Journal of Medicine* **342**: 1866–1870.

Loscalzo J (2001) Genetic clues to the cause of primary pulmonary hypertension. *New England Journal of Medicine* **345**: 367–371.

Pulmonary hypertensive diseases – review (1999) *European Respiratory Journal* **14**(6): 1246–1250.

Myocardial and endocardial disease

Atrial myxoma

This is the most common primary cardiac tumour. It occurs at all ages and show no sex preference. Although most myxomas are sporadic, some are familial or are part of a multiple system syndrome. Histologically they are benign. The majority of myxomas are solitary, usually develop in the left atrium and are polypoid, gelatinous structures attached by a pedicle to the atrial septum. The tumour may obstruct the mitral valve or may be a site of thrombi that then embolize. It is also associated with constitutional symptoms: the patient may present with dyspnoea, syncope or a mild fever. The physical signs are a loud first heart sound, a tumour 'plop' (a loud third heart sound produced as the pedunculated tumour comes to an abrupt halt), a mid-diastolic murmur, and signs due to embolization. A raised ESR is usually present.

The diagnosis is easily made by echocardiography because the tumour is demonstrated as a dense space-occupying lesion (Fig. 13.88). Surgical removal usually results in a complete cure.

Myxomas may also occur in the right atrium or in the ventricles. Other primary cardiac tumours include rhabdomyomas and sarcomas.

Myocardial disease

Myocardial disease that is not due to ischaemic, valvular or hypertensive heart disease or a known infiltrative,

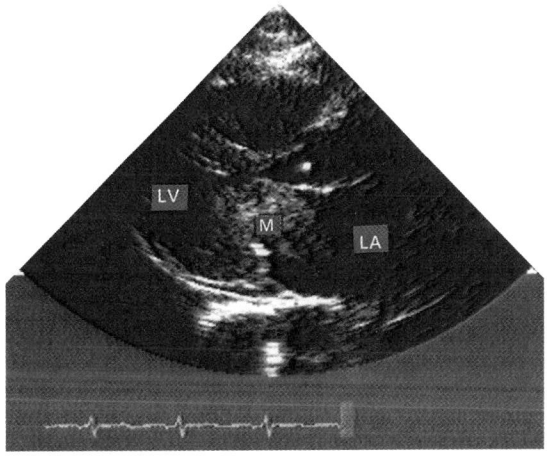

Fig. 13.88 Atrial myxoma shown by a two-dimensional echocardiogram (long-axis view). The myxoma is an echo-dense mass obstructing the mitral valve orifice. It was removed surgically. LV, left ventricle; LA, left atrium; M, mass.

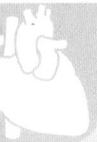

metabolic/toxic or neuromuscular disorder may be caused by:

- an acute or chronic inflammatory pathology (myocarditis)
- idiopathic myocardial disease (cardiomyopathy).

Myocarditis

Acute inflammation of the myocardium has many causes (Table 13.42). Establishment of a definitive aetiology with isolation of viruses or bacteria is difficult in routine clinical practice.

In western societies, the commonest causes of infective myocarditis are Coxsackie or adenoviral infection. Myocarditis in association with HIV infection is seen at post-mortem in up to 20% of cases but causes clinical problems in <10% of cases. Chagas' disease, due to *Trypanosoma cruzi*, which is endemic in South America is one of the commonest causes of myocarditis world-wide.

Clinical features

Patients present with an acute illness, often characterized by fever and cardiac failure. There may be a history of previous respiratory or febrile illness. Physical examination reveals soft heart sounds, a prominent third sound and tachycardia (gallop rhythm). Often a pericardial friction rub may be heard. Presentation may occasionally mimic that of acute myocardial infarction, or be with syncope or sudden cardiac death due to conduction system involvement or ventricular arrhythmia.

Investigations

- **Chest X-ray** may show some cardiac enlargement, depending on the stage and virulence of the disease.
- **ECG** demonstrates ST and T wave abnormalities and arrhythmias. Heart block may be seen with diphtheritic myocarditis, Lyme disease and Chagas' disease (see below).
- **Cardiac enzymes** are elevated.
- **Viral antibody titres** may be increased. However, since enteroviral infection is common in the general population, specific diagnosis requires the demonstration of acutely rising titres or, preferably, demonstration of active viral replication within myocardial tissue.
- **Endomyocardial biopsy** may show acute inflammation but false negatives are common by conventional criteria. Biopsy is of limited value outside specialized units.

Treatment

General management includes bed rest and the eradication of any acute infection. Therapy is aimed towards the management of cardiac failure and the treatment of cardiac arrhythmias. Immunosuppression has not been shown to be beneficial, although in the future more accurate diagnosis may lead to selective use of immunosuppressive or antiviral therapy, depending on the underlying aetiology. The prognosis depends on aetiology and is usually good, although a chronic cardiomyopathy may ensue.

Giant cell myocarditis

This is a severe form of myocarditis characterized by the presence of multinucleated giant cells within the myocardium. The cause is unknown but it may be associated with thymoma and autoimmune disease. It has a rapidly progressive course and a poor prognosis. Immunosuppression is recommended.

Chagas' disease

Chagas' disease is caused by the protozoan *Trypanosoma cruzi* and is endemic in South America where upwards of 20 million people are infected. Acutely, features of myocarditis are present with fever and congestive heart failure. Chronically, there is progression to a dilated cardiomyopathy with a propensity towards heart block and ventricular arrhythmias. Treatment is aimed at preventing further infection and the management of heart failure. Amiodarone is helpful for the control of ventricular arrhythmias.

Cardiomyopathy

Cardiomyopathy is a general term indicating disease of the cardiac muscle. Diseases are classified on predominant clinical presentations:

- *dilated cardiomyopathy* – ventricular dilatation
- *hypertrophic cardiomyopathy* – myocardial hypertrophy
- *restrictive cardiomyopathy* – impaired ventricular filling.

Table 13.42
Causes of myocarditis

Idiopathic

Infective
Viral: Coxsackievirus, adenovirus, CMV, echovirus, influenza, polio, hepatitis, HIV
Parasitic: Trypanosoma cruzi, Toxoplasma gondii (a cause of myocarditis in the newborn or immunocompromised)
Bacterial: Streptococcus (most commonly rheumatic carditis), diphtheria (toxin-mediated heart block common)
Spirochaetal: Lyme disease (heart block common), leptospirosis
Fungal
Rickettsial

Toxic

Drugs causing hypersensitivity reactions, e.g. methyldopa, penicillin, sulphonamides, antituberculous

Radiation may cause myocarditis but pericarditis more common

Autoimmune – an autoimmune form with autoactivated T cells and organ-specific antibodies may occur

arrhythmogenic right ventricular cardiomyopathy – prominent right ventricular involvement with a high frequency of ventricular arrhythmias

Dilated cardiomyopathy (DCM)

DCM is characterized by dilatation and impaired systolic function of the left ventricle and/or right ventricle, in the absence of abnormal loading conditions (e.g. hypertension, valve disease).

A large number of cardiac and systemic diseases can cause cardiac dilatation and systolic impairment (Table 13.43) but in the majority of patients no cause is found and the condition is termed 'idiopathic'.

At least 25% of 'idiopathic' cases are now known to be familial (Fig. 13.89). In the majority of familial cases inheritance is autosomal dominant, but X-linked and recessive cases occur. In a limited number of cases the responsible genes have been identified. Many of these are genes encoding cytoskeletal or associated myocyte proteins (dystrophin in X-linked cardiomyopathy, actin, desmin and lamin a/c in autosomal dominant DCM) (Fig. 13.90). Many of these have prominent associated features such as skeletal myopathy or conduction system disease and therefore differ from the majority of cases of DCM. The aetiology in the majority of cases remains unknown. Other potential causes of DCM include persistent viral infection and autoimmune disease. Evidence for the latter includes associations with specific HLA subtypes and the frequent finding of circulating cardiac-specific autoantibodies.

Clinical features

Presentation is generally with congestive heart failure and therefore symptoms and signs are those of left and/or right heart failure. Additionally patients may present with syncope due to ventricular arrhythmia or conduction disease or with pulmonary or systemic embolism. Occasionally, initial presentation is with sudden cardiac death. Increasingly, evaluation of relatives of DCM patients is allowing identification of early asymptomatic disease, prior to the onset of these complications. Clinical evaluation should include careful family history and construction of a pedigree where appropriate.

Investigations

- **Chest X-ray** demonstrates generalized cardiac enlargement.
- **ECG** shows diffuse non-specific ST segment and T wave changes. Sinus tachycardia, conduction abnormalities and arrhythmias (i.e. atrial fibrillation, ventricular premature contractions or ventricular tachycardia) are also seen.
- **Echocardiogram** reveals dilatation of the left and/or right ventricle with poor global contraction function (Fig. 13.91).
- **Angiography** should be performed to exclude coronary artery disease in all individuals at risk (generally patients > 40 years or younger if symptoms or risk factors are present).
- **Biopsy** is generally not indicated outside specialist care.

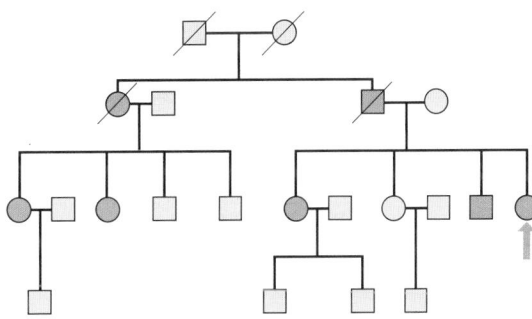

Fig. 13.89 **Pedigree of a family with dilated cardiomyopathy.** Blue symbols are affected family members. The arrow indicates the index case.

Table 13.43
Causes of dilated cardiomyopathy (DCM)

Genetic	e.g. autosomal dominant DCM, X-linked cardiomyopathy
Inflammatory	Post-infective, autoimmune, connective tissue diseases (systemic lupus erythematosus, systemic sclerosis)
Metabolic	e.g. glycogen storage disease
Nutritional	Thiamin, selenium deficiency
Endocrine	Acromegaly, thyrotoxicosis, myxoedema, diabetes mellitus
Infiltrative	Hereditary haemochromatosis
Neuromuscular	e.g. muscular dystrophy, Friedreich's ataxia, mitochondrial myopathies
Toxic	Alcohol, cocaine, doxorubicin, cyclophosphamide, cobalt
Haematological	Sickle cell anaemia, thrombotic thrombocytopenic purpura

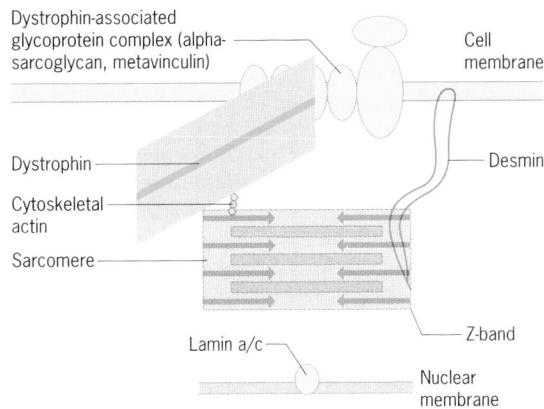

Fig. 13.90 **Schematic representation of myocyte proteins implicated in dilated cardiomyopathy (DCM).** See also Fig. 13.1.

(a)

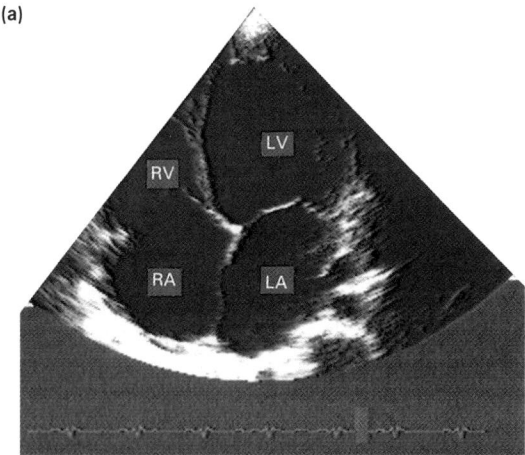

(b)

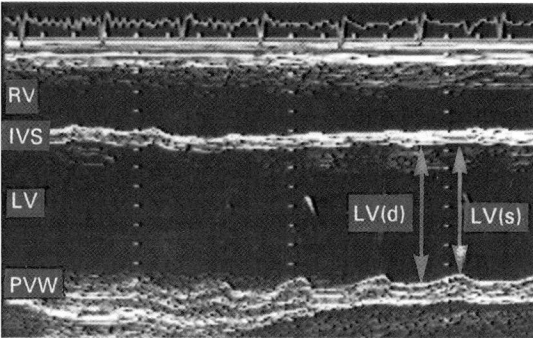

Fig. 13.91 **Dilated cardiomyopathy** shown in two-dimensional (apical four-chamber view) and M-mode echocardiograms. The heart has a 'globular' appearance with all four chambers dilated. The extremely impaired left ventricular function can be appreciated from the M-mode recording. Compare the systolic shortening fraction with that of Figures 13.22 and 13.74. LA, left atrium; RA, right atrium; LV, left ventricle; LV(d) and LV(s), diastolic and systolic left ventricular dimensions; IVS, interventricular septum; PVW, posterior ventricular wall.

Treatment

The goals of management are to relieve symptoms, retard disease progression and prevent complications. Treatment involves conventional management of heart failure (p. 759). Diuretics are highly effective for the relief of congestive symptoms but should not be used in isolation since they exacerbate activation of neurohormones that may contribute to disease progression. ACE-inhibitors and beta-blockers, by antagonizing activation of the renin–angiotensin–aldosterone (RAAS) and sympathetic nervous systems respectively, retard disease progression and are indicated in most cases. Beta-blockers may also help prevent arrhythmias. In specific cases, permanent pacing, anti-arrhythmic therapy or implantable cardioverter–defibrillators may be indicated. Severe ventricular dilatation and dysfunction, documented atrial fibrillation or a history of embolization are indications for anticoagulant treatment. Cardiac transplantation remains the principal option for advanced disease refractory to medical therapy. Potential

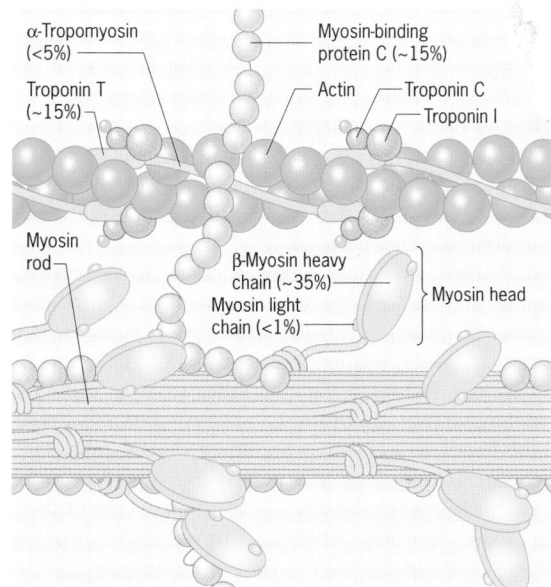

Fig. 13.92 **Sarcomeric proteins implicated in hypertrophic cardiomyopathy.** Reproduced with permission from Spirito P et al. (1997) The management of hypertrophic cardiomyopathy. *New England Journal of Medicine* **336**: 775–785. © Massachusetts Medical Society.

alternatives to transplantation are discussed in the section on heart failure (p. 764). There is currently no specific treatment for idiopathic DCM although preliminary studies have investigated the role of growth hormone, immunoadsorption and anti-cytokine therapy.

Hypertrophic cardiomyopathy (HCM)

Hypertrophic cardiomyopathy is characterized by variable myocardial hypertrophy, most commonly involving the interventricular septum, and disorganization ('disarray') of cardiac myocytes and myofibrils (Fig. 13.92). Twenty-five percent of patients have dynamic left ventricular outflow tract obstruction due to the combined effects of hypertrophy, systolic anterior motion (SAM) of the anterior mitral valve leaflet and rapid ventricular ejection.

The majority of cases are familial, autosomal dominant, and due to mutations in the genes encoding sarcomeric proteins.

The salient clinical and morphological features of the disease vary according to the underlying genetic mutation. For example, marked hypertrophy is common with beta-myosin heavy chain mutations whereas mutations in troponin T may be associated with mild hypertrophy but a high risk of sudden death. Modifying genetic factors may also influence the phenotype in HCM. These include polymorphisms of components of the renin–angiotensin–aldosterone system which influence myocyte growth.

The hypertrophy may not manifest before completion of the adolescent growth spurt, making the diagnosis in en difficult. HCM due to myosin-binding protein C ~~~ot manifest until the sixth decade of life or Sporadic cases of HCM occur, but the aetiology is ~wn. HCM may also be associated with Noonan's ~rome, Friedreich's ataxia, glycogen storage disease, ~ mitochondrial myopathies.

Clinical features

Patients with HCM present with chest pain, dyspnoea, syncope or presyncope (typically with exertion), cardiac arrhythmias and sudden death. Sudden death may occur at any age but the highest rates (up to 6% per annum) occur in adolescents or young adults. Risk factors for sudden death are discussed below. Dyspnoea is common and is due to impaired relaxation of the heart muscle. Left ventricular filling – and therefore left ventricular emptying – is impaired, compounded by outflow obstruction in about one-third of cases. Systolic ventricular function remains good until the very late stages of disease when progressive dilatation may occur. Atrial fibrillation occurs (the prevalence increasing with increasing duration of disease) and is associated with worsening symptoms due to reduction in ventricular filling.

The classical physical findings are:

- double apical pulsation (forceful atrial contraction producing a fourth heart sound).
- jerky carotid pulse because of rapid ejection and sudden obstruction to left ventricular outflow during systole
- ejection systolic murmur due to left ventricular outflow obstruction late in systole – it can be increased by manoeuvres that decrease afterload, e.g. standing or Valsalva, and decreased by manoeuvres that increase afterload and venous return, e.g. squatting
- pansystolic murmur due to mitral regurgitation (secondary to SAM)
- fourth heart sound (if not in AF).

Investigations

- **Chest X-ray** is usually unremarkable.
- **ECG** demonstrates left ventricular hypertrophy (see Fig. 13.72) and ST and T wave changes. Abnormal Q waves, most commonly in the inferolateral leads occur in 25–50% of patients.
- **Echocardiogram** is usually diagnostic and in the most typical cases shows asymmetric left ventricular hypertrophy (involving septum more than posterior wall), systolic anterior motion of the mitral valve, and a vigorously contracting ventricle (Fig. 13.93). However any pattern of hypertrophy may be seen, including concentric and apical hypertrophy. Certain mutations, e.g. involving the troponin gene, are associated with minimal or even no hypertrophy.

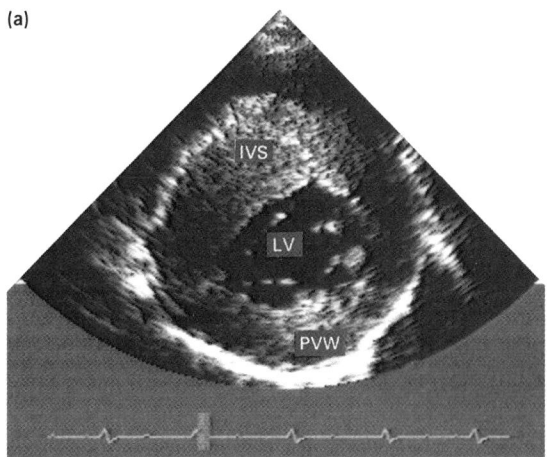

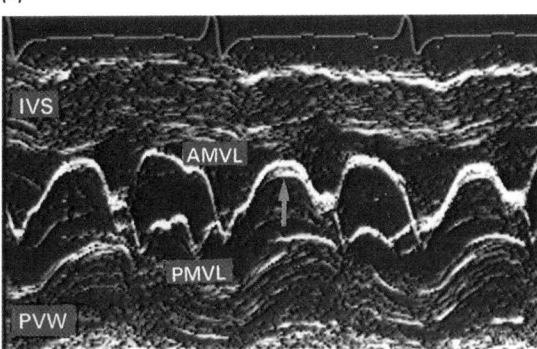

Fig. 13.93 Hypertrophic cardiomyopathy shown by a **(a)** two-dimensional echocardiogram (short-axis view) and **(b)** M-mode recording. The grossly thickened interventricular septum is shown, resulting in a small left ventricular cavity. This condition is associated with an abnormal anterior motion of the mitral valve during systole (arrowed). IVS, interventricular septum; LV, left ventricle; PVW, posterior ventricular wall; AMVL, PMVL, anterior and posterior mitral valve leaflets.

- **Pedigree analysis** generally reveals autosomal dominant inheritance and may provide prognostic information (e.g. history of sudden death). Genetic analysis where available confirms the diagnosis, may provide prognostic information and facilitates evaluation of relatives.
- **Exercise test and ECG ambulatory recording** also provide prognostic information.

Treatment

The overriding concern in the management of HCM is the prevention of sudden death. Several risk factors for sudden death have been identified. Massive left ventricular hypertrophy (>30 mm) is a recognized risk factor but the majority of sudden deaths do not occur in individuals with massive hypertrophy, and other risk factors must be considered. These include genotype, family history of sudden cardiac death, abnormal blood pressure response during exercise, non-sustained ventricular tachycardia on Holter monitoring and recurrent syncope. The presence of two or more of these risk factors is associated with a substantial risk of sudden death. Implantable defibrillators effectively prevent sudden death in high-risk cases. In patients in whom the risk is less high, amiodarone is an appropriate alternative.

Chest pain and dyspnoea are treated with beta-blockers and verapamil, either alone or in combination. If these are ineffective, disopyramide is a useful second-line therapy for patients with obstruction. In selected cases only (e.g. elderly patients) with significant left outflow obstruction and recalcitrant symptoms, dual-chamber pacing may be of use. Alcohol (non-surgical) ablation of the septum may also be useful and its long-term effects are under investigation. Occasionally, resection of septal myocardium may be indicated. Vasodilators should be avoided because they may aggravate left ventricular outflow obstruction or cause refractory hypotension.

Restrictive cardiomyopathy

Some cardiomyopathies do not present with muscular hypertrophy or ventricular dilatation. Instead, the ventricular filling is restricted (as with constrictive pericarditis), resulting in symptoms and signs of heart failure. Dilatation of the atria and thrombus formation commonly occur.

Conditions associated with this form of cardiomyopathy include amyloidosis, sarcoidosis, Loeffler's endocarditis and endomyocardial fibrosis; in the latter two conditions there is myocardial and endocardial fibrosis associated with eosinophilia. Amyloidosis is the most common form of restrictive cardiomyopathy. The idiopathic form of restrictive cardiomyopathy may be familial.

Clinical features

Dyspnoea, fatigue and embolic symptoms are the presenting features. Restriction to ventricular filling (especially right) results in persistently elevated venous pressures, consequent hepatic enlargement, ascites, and dependent oedema.

Physical signs are similar to those of constrictive pericarditis – a high jugular venous pressure with diastolic collapse (Friedreich's sign) and elevation of venous pressure with inspiration (Kussmaul's sign). A fourth heart sound is common in early disease and cardiac enlargement and a third heart sound may be present in advanced disease. In idiopathic restrictive cardiomyopathy, however, cardiac size may remain normal.

Investigations

- **Chest X-ray** may show pulmonary venous congestion. The cardiac silhouette can be normal or show cardiomegaly and/or atrial enlargement.
- **ECG** usually has low-voltage and ST segment T wave abnormalities.
- **Echocardiogram** shows symmetrical myocardial thickening and often a normal systolic ejection fraction, but impaired ventricular filling.
- **Cardiac catheterization** and haemodynamic study help distinction from constrictive pericarditis.
- **Endomyocardial biopsy** in contrast with other cardiomyopathies is often useful in this condition and may permit a specific diagnosis such as amyloidosis to be made.

Treatment

There is no specific treatment. Cardiac failure and embolic manifestations should be treated. Cardiac transplantation should be considered in some severe cases, especially the idiopathic variety. In primary amyloidosis, combination therapy with melphalan plus prednisolone with or without colchicine may improve survival. However, patients with cardiac amyloidosis have a worse prognosis than those with other forms of the disease, and the disease often recurs after transplantation. Liver transplantation may be effective in familial amyloidosis (due to production of mutant prealbumin) and may lead to reversal of the cardiac abnormalities.

Arrhythmogenic right ventricular cardiomyopathy

Arrhythmogenic right ventricular cardiomyopathy (ARVC) is characterized by progressive fibrofatty replacement of the right ventricular myocardium (Fig. 13.94). This leads to ventricular arrhythmia and risk of sudden death in its early stages and right ventricular or biventricular failure in its later stages. It is familial in at least 50% of cases, most commonly with an autosomal dominant pattern of inheritance. A rare form of ARVC

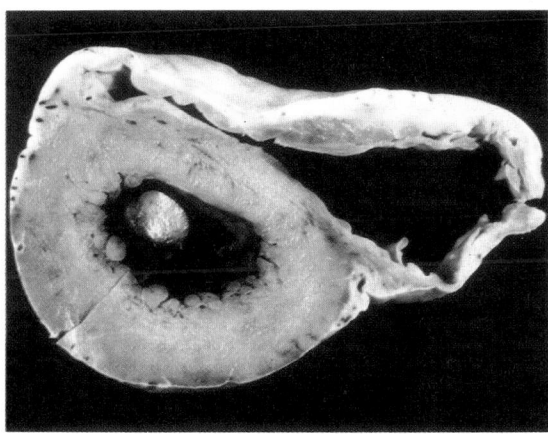

Fig. 13.94 Gross pathological specimen demonstrating thinning and fibrofatty replacement of RV free wall. From Basso et al. (1996) *Circulation* **94**: 983–991 with permission.

which is associated with dermatological abnormalities (Naxos disease) is caused by a mutation in a gene encoding a myocyte structural protein (plakoglobin) found in desmosomes and gap junctions.

Clinical features

Presentation is most commonly with severe symptomatic ventricular arrhythmias or syncope. Occasionally presentation is with right heart failure. Heart failure, however, is more commonly associated with a later stage of disease, in which left ventricular dilatation may also occur, and severity of arrhythmia may paradoxically diminish. The condition is often asymptomatic and the first presentation may be with sudden death or alternatively it may be diagnosed as a result of routine medical evaluation or family screening.

Investigations

- **Chest X-ray** is usually unremarkable except in advanced disease.
- **ECG** most commonly demonstrates T wave inversion in precordial leads related to the right ventricle (V_1–V_3). Small-amplitude potentials occurring at the end of the QRS complex (epsilon waves) may be present (Fig. 13.95). Incomplete or complete RBBB is seen.
- **Echocardiogram.** In early cases is often normal and in more advanced cases may demonstrate right ventricular dilatation and aneurysm formation, associated in some cases with concomitant left ventricular dilatation.
- **MRI** demonstrates morphological abnormalities of the RV and is capable of demonstrating fatty infiltration.
- **RV angiography** demonstrates enlargement and abnormal motion of right ventricular myocardium.
- **RV biopsy** may demonstrate fibro-fatty replacement but is often falsely negative.
- **Holter monitoring** often demonstrates frequent extrasystoles of right ventricular origin and runs of non-sustained or sustained ventricular tachycardia.

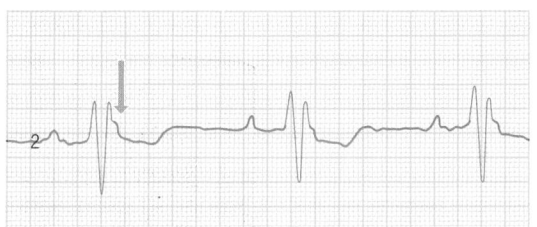

Fig. 13.95 **Electrocardiogram from an adult with arrhythmogenic right ventricular cardiomyopathy** (ARVC) demonstrating RBBB and precordial T wave insertion with epsilon waves visible at the terminal of the QRS complex (arrow).

Treatment

Beta-blockers are first-line treatment for patients with non-life-threatening arrhythmias. Amiodarone or sotalol may be used for symptomatic arrhythmias, and for refractory or life-threatening arrhythmias an ICD may be required. Occasionally cardiac transplantation is indicated, either for intractable arrhythmia or cardiac failure.

FURTHER READING

Corrado D, Basso C, Thiene G (2000) Arrhythmogenic right ventricular cardiomyopathy: diagnosis, prognosis and treatment. *Heart* **83**: 588–585.

Elliott PM, Poloniecki J, Dickie S, Sharma S, Monserrat L, Varnava A, Mahon NG, McKenna WJ (2000) Sudden death in hypertrophic cardiomyopathy: identification of high risk patients. *Journal of the American College of Cardiology* **36**: 2212–2218.

Elliott PM et al. (2001) Relation between severity of left ventricular hypertrophy and prognosis in patients with HCM. *Lancet* **357**: 420–424.

Franz W-M, Müller OJ, Katus HA (2001) Cardiomyopathies: from genetics to the prospect of treatment. *Lancet* **358**: 1627–1637.

Pericardial disease

The normal pericardium lubricates the surface of the heart, prevents sudden deformation or dislocation of the heart, and acts as a barrier to the spread of infection. It normally contains up to 50 ml of serous fluid. There are three common presentations of pericardial disease:

- acute pericarditis
- pericardial effusion
- constrictive pericarditis.

Acute pericarditis (< 6 weeks)

Acute pericarditis has numerous aetiologies, but Coxsackie and echovirus infections and myocardial infarction are the most common causes in the UK.

Acute pericarditis is initially dry and fibrinous. However, almost all aetiologies of this condition also induce the formation of a pericardial effusion.

Viral

This is often sudden in onset and tends to affect young adults. Usually, the illness lasts only a few weeks and the prognosis is good. However, recurrences as well as sudden death do occur. Serial serological tests are helpful in diagnosing a viral aetiology of acute pericarditis. A fourfold or greater increase in viral antibody titres

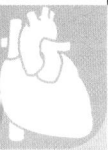
is indicative of viral infection. HIV should be excluded in young patients with large pericardial effusions, co-existent pulmonary infiltrates and fever.

Post-myocardial infarction

This occurs in about 20% of patients within the first few days following MI. The likelihood of post-MI pericarditis is higher in patients with anterior MI, Q-wave MI, and high serum cardiac enzymes. A pericardial friction rub, recurrence of chest pain and fever are typical. Persistence of positive T waves or reversal of negative T waves may be seen in the ECG. Post-MI pericarditis is usually fibrinous and rarely causes haemodynamic compromise. Thrombolytic treatment may reduce the prevalence of post-MI pericarditis. Non-steroidal anti-inflammatory drugs, other than aspirin, as well as corticosteroids, should be used cautiously as they may increase risk of myocardial rupture. *Dressler's syndrome* occurs a month to one year later (p. 781).

Uraemic/dialysis-related

This is seen usually in the terminal stages of uraemia and is often asymptomatic; intensive dialysis is required. Uraemic pericarditis should be distinguished from pericarditis that occasionally occurs in patients on chronic haemodialysis possibly caused by infection or an immune reaction to haemodialysis equipment.

Bacterial

Purulent pericarditis may rarely occur with septicaemia or pneumonia. It may stem from an early postoperative infection after thoracic surgery or trauma or may complicate endocarditis. A swinging fever, dyspnoea, and substantial leucocytosis with a marked leftward shift are common. *Staphylococcus* and *Haemophilus influenzae* account for two-thirds of such cases. *Staphylococcus aureus* is a frequent cause of purulent pericarditis in HIV patients. Antibiotics are the mainstay of treatment and surgical drainage may be indicated. This form of pericarditis, especially staphylococcal, is fulminant and often fatal.

Other endemic infectious pericarditis includes myco-plasmosis, Lyme pericarditis, borreliosis and *Chlamydia* which are often effusive and require pericardial drainage. The diagnosis is based on serological tests of pericardial fluid and identification of organisms in pericardial or myocardial biopsies.

Tuberculous

Typical presentation is with chronic low-grade fever, particularly in the evening, associated with features of acute pericarditis, dyspnoea, malaise, night sweats, and weight loss. Pericardial aspiration is often required to make the diagnosis. The effusion may be blood-stained, but is usually serous. Antituberculous chemotherapy is needed. Constrictive pericarditis is a frequent outcome of acute tuberculous pericarditis.

Fungal

Fungal pericarditis is a common complication of endemic fungal infections, such as histoplasmosis and coccidioidomycosis but may be also caused by *Candida albicans*, especially in immunocompromised patients, drug addicts or after cardiac surgery. Treatment includes antifungal therapy with amphotericin B and pericardial drainage.

Malignant

Carcinoma of the bronchus, carcinoma of the breast and Hodgkin's disease are the most common causes. Leukaemia and malignant melanoma are also associated with pericarditis. Chest pain is usually atypical. Pericardial friction rub is often absent. A substantial pericardial effusion is very typical and is due to the obstruction of the lymphatic drainage from the heart. The effusion is often haemorrhagic. Pericardiocentesis is useful in establishing the diagnosis in the majority of cases. Pleural effusion and abdominal distress due to congestion of the liver are common. ST segment elevation is not typical but QRS alternans caused by an increased mobility of the heart within the pericardium space is characteristic.

Radiation and therapy for thoracic tumours may cause radiation injury to the pericardium resulting in serous or haemorrhagic pericardial effusion and pericardial fibrosis. Cancer chemotherapy with doxorubicin and cyclophosphamide may also cause pericarditis. Absence of neoplastic cells in the pericardial fluid often helps with these diagnoses.

Automimmune

Collagen vascular disorders of rheumatoid arthritis, e.g. rheumatic fever, SLE, scleroderma, can cause a pericarditis.

Other causes

These include familial, idiopathic, and post-surgical (post-pericardotomy) syndrome of hypothyroidism. Drugs, e.g. procainamide, hydralazine, isoniazid, doxorubicin, and cyclophosphamide, can also cause pericarditis.

Clinical features

Pericardial inflammation gives rise to chest pain that is substernal and sharp. It is relieved by sitting forward and made worse by lying down and, like pleurisy, is aggravated by movement and respiration. It may be referred to the neck or shoulders.

The cardinal clinical sign is a pericardial friction rub. It is characteristically a leathery triphasic sound heard best at the lower left sternum with the patient leaning forward. It also may be heard as a biphasic 'to-and-fro' rub. Large pericardial effusion may compress adjacent bronchi and lung tissue and may cause dyspnoea. There is usually a fever when pericarditis is due to viral or bacterial infection, rheumatic fever or myocardial infarction.

Investigations

The ECG is diagnostic. During the first week there is ST segment elevation, concave upwards, in all leads facing the epicardial surface – i.e. the anterior, lateral and inferior leads (Fig. 13.96). Only 'cavity' leads AVR, V_1 and rarely V_2 show ST depression. Later ST segment normalizes and T wave inversion may be seen without a decrease in R wave amplitude or the appearance of pathological Q waves. As the illness improves the T waves become normal but occasionally may persist in patients with chronic pericarditis. Sinus tachycardia is a common finding in acute pericarditis and may by due to fever or haemodynamic embarrassment. Rhythm and conduction abnormalities are not typical unless the myocardium is involved. Leucocytosis is common at early stages but later may be replaced by lymphocytosis.

Cardiac enzymes may be elevated if there is associated myocarditis.

Treatment

The cause of the pericarditis must be treated if possible. Treatment consists of anti-inflammatory drugs and rest. Aspirin is given at high doses (600–900 mg every 6 hours). Indometacin at a dose of 25–100 mg every 4 hours or ibuprofen 400 mg every 6 hours can be used for symptom relief (not post-MI, p. 779). Occasionally, if pericarditis is severe or recurrent, systemic corticosteroids may be needed. Prednisone is started at a dose of 20–80 mg daily followed by a gradual decrease in dose in 5–7 days after clinical signs are resolved. If pericarditis is resistant to corticosteroids, azathioprine 50–100 mg daily or colchicine 1–2 mg/dL may be effective. Pericardiotomy may be indicated for cure of recurrent forms refractory to medical treatment.

Pericardial effusion

The effusion collects in the closed pericardium, and when the pericardium can distend no further this produces mechanical embarrassment to the circulation by preventing ventricular filling. This is called cardiac tamponade.

Clinical features

The effusion obscures the apex beat and the heart sounds are soft and distant. Although a friction rub may be heard in the early stages, it may be quieter once the fluid accumulates, as this separates the visceral and parietal pericardia. Features of cardiac tamponade include a raised jugular venous pressure with sharp diastolic collapse, *y* descent (Friedreich's sign), a paradoxical pulse, increased neck vein distension during inspiration (Kussmaul's sign) and reduced cardiac output. Pericardial effusion may compress the base of the left lung, and an area of dullness can be detected by percussion below the angle of the left scapula (Ewart's sign).

Investigations

ECG shows low voltages and the chest X-ray may demonstrate a large globular or pear-shaped heart with sharp outlines. Typically, the pulmonary veins are not distended. Echocardiography is the most useful technique for demonstrating the effusion and right ventricular collapse during late diastole (see Fig. 13.25, p. 726). Doppler may show an increased flow through tricuspid and pulmonary valves and a decreased mitral flow during inspiration. Magnetic resonance imaging may also help to detect haemopericardium or loculated pericardial effusions.

Treatment

Cardiac tamponade is a medical emergency and the effusion must be tapped. Pericardiocentesis is also indicated when a malignant, tuberculous or a purulent pericarditis is suspected. In the UK, malignancy is the most common cause of reaccumulation of pericardial effusion. Reaccumulation may require pericardial fenestration (i.e. the creation of a pericardial window), either transcutaneously via a balloon pericardiotomy under local anaesthesia, or by using a conventional surgical approach.

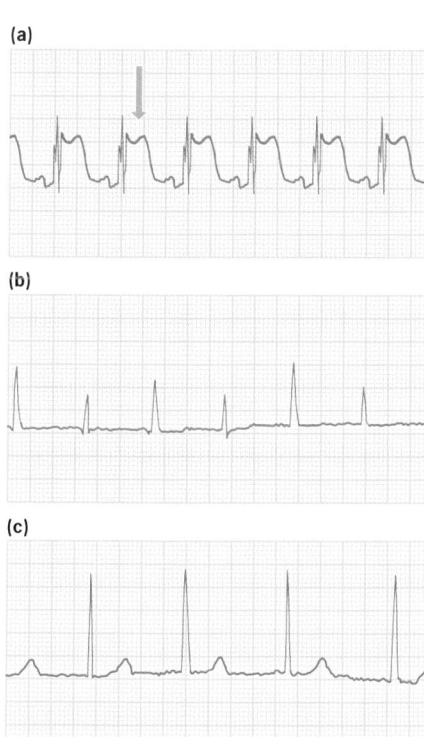

(a)

(b)

(c)

Fig. 13.96 ECGs associated with pericarditis. (a) Acute pericarditis. Note the raised ST segment, concave upwards (arrow). **(b) Chronic phase of pericarditis** associated with a pericardial effusion. Note the T wave flattening and inversion and the alternation of the QRS amplitude (QRS alternans). **(c)** The same patient after evacuation of the pericardial fluid. Note that the QRS voltage has increased and the T waves have returned to normal.

Constrictive pericarditis

Following certain forms of pericarditis (tuberculous effusion, haemopericardium, bacterial infection or rheumatic heart disease), the pericardium may become thick, fibrous and calcified. The heart is then encased in a solid shell and cannot fill properly. Myocardial contractility is usually preserved but is impaired at late stages owing to fibrosis, atrophy, and calcification of subepicardial layers of myocardium. Constrictive pericarditis also develops late after open-heart surgery.

Clinical features

Typical signs are of systemic venous congestion – ascites, dependent oedema, hepatomegaly and jugular venous distension, without much breathlessness or pulmonary venous distension. There are signs of impaired ventricular filling (Kussmaul's sign), Friedreich's sign and pulse paradoxus. Fatigue and exercise intolerance are common symptoms. Sinus tachycardia often occurs to compensate low cardiac output.

Atrial fibrillation is common (30%), and a loud third heart sound (a pericardial knock) due to rapid ventricular filling may be heard. This is an early third heart sound.

Other causes of ascites must be excluded. Restrictive cardiomyopathy is a close mimic.

Investigations

- **Chest X-ray** shows a relatively small heart with obvious calcification seen on a lateral film or by using fluoroscopy (see Fig. 13.97). The ECG may show low QRS voltages and T wave inversion.

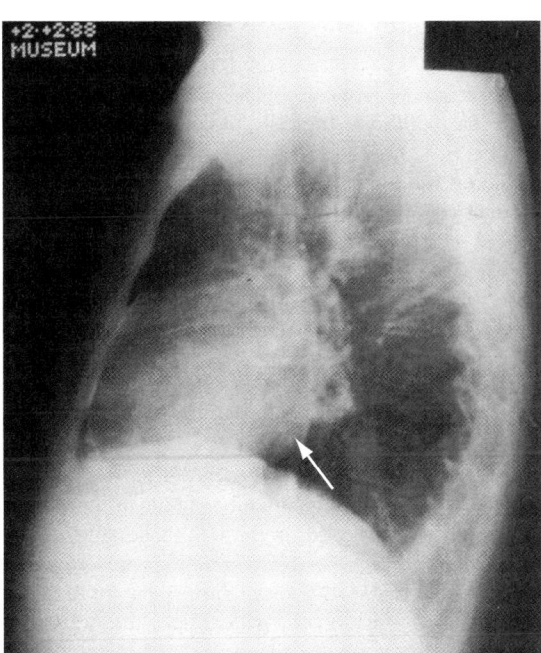

Fig. 13.97 Chest X-ray showing pericardial calcification (arrow).

- **Echocardiography** may demonstrate the thickened pericardium with calcification predominantly over the right heart and relative immobility of the heart. Typically, the ventricular cavities are small with normal wall thickness and dilated atria. An abnormal septal motion is often present. The pericardial effusion is usually absent. CT is also good for detecting the thickness and the calcification of the pericardium.
- **Cardiac catheterization and MRI scan** may be useful in difficult cases. Typically, the diastolic pressures are equal in all four chambers; the left and right ventricular end-diastolic pressures, the left and right atrial pressures are all equal or differ by less than 5 mmHg.

Treatment

Surgical removal of a substantial portion of the thickened pericardium provides a cure in about half the cases. In others, persistent constriction, atrial fibrillation and myocardial fibrosis prevent full recovery.

FURTHER READING

Hancock EW (1990) Neoplastic pericardial disease. Review. *Cardiology Clinics* **8**(4): 673–682.

Karliner JS (2000) Fulminating myocarditis. *New England Journal of Medicine* **342**: 734–735.

McCarthy RE et al. (2000) Long-term outcome of fulminant myocarditis as compared with acute (nonfulminant). *New England Journal of Medicine* **342**: 690–695.

Maisch B (1994) Pericardial diseases, with a focus on etiology, pathogenesis, pathophysiology, new diagnostic imaging methods, and treatment. Review. *Current Opinion in Cardiology* **9**(3): 379–388.

Zales VR, Wright KL (1997) Endocarditis, pericarditis and myocarditis. *Paediatric Annals* **26**: 116–121.

Systemic hypertension

Definitions of normotension and hypertension

Epidemiological studies have clearly demonstrated that elevated arterial blood pressure is a major cause of premature vascular disease leading to cerebrovascular events, ischaemic heart disease and peripheral vascular disease. Blood pressure is a characteristic of each individual, like height and weight, with marked interindividual variation, and has a continuous (bell-shaped) distribution. The levels of blood pressure observed depend on the characteristics of the population studied – in particular, the age and ethnic background. Blood pressure in industrialized countries rises with age, certainly up to the seventh decade. This rise is more marked for systolic pressure and is more pronounced in men. Diastolic pressure may level off or even gradually start to decline after age of 70 years Hypertension remains one of the commonest chronic conditions in the developed world. Depending on the criteria used for the diagnosis, hypertension can be said to be present in 20–30% of the adult population. Hypertension rates are much higher in black Africans with up to 40–45% of adults being affected.

The definition of an abnormal blood pressure remains a controversial issue, but that best accepted is: that level of blood pressure above which investigation and treatment do more good than harm. In a recent study in Framingham USA, 'normal' blood pressure in women was 122 ± 5 systolic and 77 ± 6 diastolic. Corresponding figures in men were 122 ± 5 and 78 ± 5. The WHO International Society of Hypertension classifies non-hypertensive subjects with a systolic pressure of 130–139 mmHg or a diastolic pressure of 85–89 mmHg as having a 'high' normal blood pressure.

It is well recognized that the risk of mortality or morbidity rises progressively with increasing systolic and diastolic pressures, with each measure having independent prognostic value; for example, isolated systolic hypertension is associated with a two- to threefold increase in cardiac mortality.

All adults should have blood pressure measured routinely at least every 5 years until the age of 80 years. Seated blood pressure when measured after 5 minutes resting is usually sufficient, but standing blood pressure should be measured in diabetic and elderly subjects to exclude orthostatic hypotension. Patients should be seated, and the cuff deflated at 2 mm/s and the blood pressure measured to the nearest 2 mmHg. A single reading of blood pressure may be misleading; as blood pressure will fall with repeated measurements in a large number of patients. Indeed, when assessing the cardiovascular risk, the average blood pressure at separate visits is more accurate than measurements taken at a single visit.

Causes

The great majority of patients with hypertension have primary elevation of blood pressure (i.e. cause not known – essential hypertension) which can be ameliorated only by life-long pharmacological therapy.

Essential hypertension

Essential hypertension has a multifactorial aetiology.

Genetic factors

Blood pressure tends to run in families and children of hypertensive parents tend to have higher blood pressure than age-matched children of people with normal blood pressure. Clearly this familial concordance of blood pressure may be explained, at least in part by shared environmental influences. However, there still remains a large, still unidentified genetic component.

Fetal factors

Studies have consistently shown a relationship between lower birth weight and subsequent higher blood pressure. This relationship may be due to fetal adaptation to intrauterine undernutrition with long-term changes in blood vessel structure or in the function of crucial hormonal systems.

Environmental factors

Amongst the several environmental factors that have been proposed, the following seem to be the most significant:

Obesity. Fat people have higher blood pressures than thin people. There is a risk, however, of overestimation if the blood pressure is measured with a small cuff. Adjust the bladder size to the arm circumference. Sleep disorders (p. 869) often seen with obesity may be an additional risk factor.

Alcohol intake. Most studies have shown a close relationship between the consumption of alcohol and blood pressure level. However, subjects who consume small amounts of alcohol seem to have lower blood pressure level than those who consume no alcohol.

Sodium intake. A high sodium intake has been suggested to be an important determinant of blood pressure differences between and within populations around the world. Populations with higher sodium intake have higher average blood pressures than those with lower sodium intake. Migration from a rural to an urban environment is associated with an increase in blood pressure that is in part related to the amount of salt in the diet. Finally, studies of the restriction of salt intake have shown a beneficial effect on blood pressure in hypertensives. There is some evidence that a high potassium diet can protect against the effects of a high sodium intake.

Stress. Whilst acute pain or stress can raise blood pressure, it has been difficult to study the relationship between chronic stress and blood pressure and, therefore, it remains uncertain whether chronic 'job strain' can be implicated in the pathophysiology of essential hypertension.

Humoral mechanisms

The autonomic nervous system, as well as the renin–angiotensin, natriuretic peptide and kallikrein–kinin system, plays a role in the physiological regulation of short-term changes in blood pressure and has been implicated in the pathogenesis of essential hypertension. However, there is no convincing evidence that any of these systems is directly involved in the maintenance of hypertension.

Insulin resistance

An association between diabetes and hypertension has long been recognized and a syndrome has been described of hyperinsulinaemia, glucose intolerance, reduced levels of HDL cholesterol, hypertriglyceridaemia

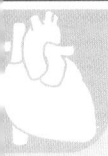

and central obesity (all of which are related to insulin resistance) in association with hypertension. This association (also called the 'metabolic syndrome' or 'syndrome X') is a major risk factor for cardiovascular disease. However, it has been difficult to define the mechanism linking the insulin resistance with hypertension. A new adipocyte hormone, resistin, may be the link between increased fat mass and insulin resistance.

Secondary hypertension

Secondary hypertension is where blood pressure elevation is the result of a specific and potentially treatable cause. These patients may be amenable to curative treatment, thereby sparing them from life-long medical therapy that is frequently unpleasant, sometimes ineffective, and always expensive. Secondary forms of hypertension include the following:

Renal diseases

These account for over 80% of the cases of secondary hypertension. The common causes are diabetic nephropathy, chronic glomerulonephritis, adult polycystic disease, chronic tubulointerstitial nephritis, and reno-vascular disease. Hypertension can itself cause or worsen renal disease. The mechanism of this blood pressure elevation is primarily due to sodium and water retention, although there can be inappropriate elevation of plasma renin levels.

Endocrine causes

These include:

- Conn's syndrome
- adrenal hyperplasia
- phaeochromocytoma
- Cushing's syndrome
- acromegaly.

Cardiovascular causes

The major cause is coarctation of the aorta.

Drugs

There are many drugs that have been shown to cause or aggravate hypertension, or interfere with the response to some antihypertensive agents. The oral contraceptive pill, steroids, carbenoxolone and vasopressin may all cause hypertension. Patients taking monoamine oxidase inhibitors, who consume tyramine-containing foods, may develop paroxysms of severe hypertension.

Pregnancy

Cardiac output rises in pregnancy but, owing to a relatively greater fall in peripheral resistance, blood pressure in pregnant women is usually lower than in those not pregnant. Hypertension detected in the first half of pregnancy or persisting after delivery is usually due to pre-existing essential hypertension. Hypertension presenting in the second half of pregnancy – or 'pregnancy-induced hypertension' – usually resolves after delivery. Pre-eclampsia is a syndrome consisting of pregnancy-induced hypertension with proteinuria. The primary pathology is unknown, but is likely to involve a disturbance of the uteroplacental circulation. Hypertension in pregnancy, together with pulmonary embolus, are the commonest causes of maternal death, with a rate of 10 per million pregnancies. Furthermore, the critical condition of eclampsia which is associated with severe hypertension, may ultimately lead to convulsions, cerebral and pulmonary oedema, jaundice, clotting abnormalities and fetal death.

Pathophysiology

The pathogenesis of *essential hypertension* remains unclear. In some young hypertensive patients, there is an early increase in cardiac output, in association with increased pulse rate and circulating catecholamines. This could result in changes in baroreceptor sensitivity, which would then operate at a higher blood pressure level.

In *chronic hypertension*, the cardiac output is normal and it is an increased peripheral resistance that maintains the elevated blood pressure. The resistance vessels (the small arteries and arterioles) show structural changes in hypertension. These are an increase in wall thickness with a reduction in the vessel lumen diameter. There is also some evidence for rarefaction (decreased density) of these vessels. These mechanisms would result in an increased overall peripheral vascular resistance.

Hypertension also causes changes in the large arteries. There is thickening of the media, an increase in collagen and the secondary deposition of calcium. These changes result in a loss of arterial compliance, which in turn leads to a more pronounced arterial pressure wave. Atheroma develops in the large arteries owing to the interaction of these mechanical stresses and low growth factors (see p. 766). Endothelial dysfunction with alternations in agents such as nitric oxide and endothelins appear to be involved.

Left ventricular hypertrophy develops as a result of the increased peripheral vascular resistance, and the increased left ventricular load, and is a significant prognostic indicator of future cardiovascular events.

Changes in the *renal vasculature* eventually lead to a reduced renal perfusion, reduced glomerular filtration rate and, finally, a reduction in sodium and water excretion. The decreased renal perfusion may lead to activation of the renin–angiotensin system (renin converts angiotensinogen to angiotensin I, which is in turn converted to angiotensin II by the angiotensin-converting enzyme) with increased secretion of aldosterone and further sodium and water retention.

Complications

Cerebrovascular disease and coronary artery disease are the most common causes of death in hypertension, although hypertensive patients are also prone to renal failure and peripheral vascular disease.

In the Framingham studies, hypertensives had a six-fold increase in stroke (both haemorrhagic and athero-thrombotic) compared with normotensives. There was also a threefold increase in cardiac death (due either to coronary events or to cardiac failure). Furthermore, peripheral arterial disease was as twice as common in hypertensives. High normal blood pressure is also associated with an increased risk of cardiovascular events.

Malignant hypertension

Malignant or accelerated hypertension is said to occur when blood pressure rises rapidly and is considered with severe hypertension (diastolic blood pressure >140 mmHg) (p. 826). The characteristic histological change is fibrinoid necrosis of the vessel wall and, unless treated, it may lead to death from progressive renal failure, heart failure or stroke. The changes in the renal circulation result in rapidly progressive renal failure, proteinuria and haematuria. There is also a high risk of cerebral oedema and haemorrhage with resultant encephalopathy, and in the retina there may be flame-shaped haemorrhages, cotton wool spots, hard exudates and papilloedema. Without effective treatment there is a 1-year survival of less than 20%.

Assessment

The management of patients should be considered in three stages: assessment, non-pharmacological treatment, and drug treatment. During the assessment period, secondary causes of hypertension should be excluded, the target-organ effect of the blood pressure should be evaluated, and any concomitant conditions (e.g. dyslipi-daemia or diabetes) identified.

History

The patient with mild hypertension is usually asympto-matic. Features in the history such as attacks of sweating, headaches and palpitations may point towards the diagnosis of phaeochromocytoma. Higher levels of blood pressure may be associated with headaches, epistaxis or nocturia. Breathlessness may be present owing to left ventricular hypertrophy or cardiac failure, whilst angina or symptoms of peripheral arterial occlusive disease suggests the diagnosis of atheromatous renal artery stenosis This is usually a local manifestation of more generalized atherosclerosis and as such, the patients are often elderly with coexistent vascular disease (Fig. 13.98). Fibromuscular disease of the renal arteries is a term that encompasses a group of conditions in which fibrous or muscular proliferation results in a variety of morpholog-ically simple or complex stenoses (Fig. 13.99) and tend to occur in younger patients than those with athero-sclerosis. Malignant hypertension may present with severe headaches, visual disturbances, fits, transient loss of consciousness or symptoms of heart failure.

Examination

The elevated blood pressure is usually the only abnormal sign. Signs of an underlying cause should be sought, such as renal artery bruits in renovascular hypertension, or radiofemoral delay in coarctation of the aorta. The cardiac examination may also reveal features of left ven-tricular hypertrophy and a loud aortic second sound. If cardiac failure develops, there may be a sinus tachy-cardia and a third heart sound.

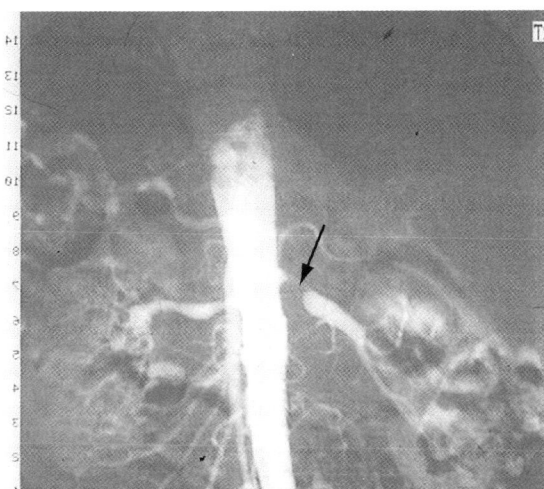

Fig. 13.98 Digital subtraction angiography, showing typical unilateral atheromatous renal artery stenosis with post-stenotic dilatation.

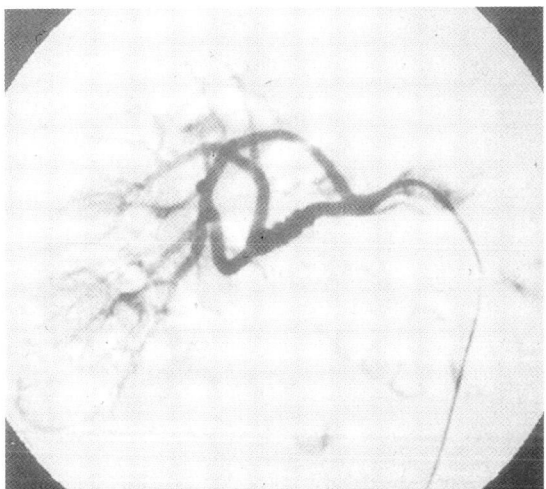

Fig. 13.99 Digital subtraction angiography showing typical fibromuscular dysplasia which involves the distal part of the right renal artery and also one of its branches.

Cardiovascular disease

Fundoscopy is an essential part of the examination of any hypertensive patient (Fig. 13.100). The abnormalities are graded according to the Keith–Wagener classification:

Grade 1 – tortuosity of the retinal arteries with increased reflectiveness (silver wiring)

Grade 2 – grade 1 plus the appearance of arteriovenous nipping produced when thickened retinal arteries pass over the retinal veins

Grade 3 – grade 2 plus flame-shaped haemorrhages and soft ('cotton wool') exudates actually due to small infarcts

Grade 4 – grade 3 plus papilloedema (blurring of the margins of the optic disc).

Grades 3 and 4 are diagnostic of malignant hypertension.

Ambulatory blood pressure monitoring

Indirect automatic blood pressure measurements can be made usually over a 24-hour period using a measuring device worn by the patient. The clinical role of such devices remains uncertain, although they are used to confirm the diagnosis in those patients with 'white-coat' hypertension – i.e., in those subjects whose blood pressure is completely normal at all stages except during a clinical consultation (Fig. 13.101a). These patients do not have any evidence of target-organ damage and unnecessary treatment can be avoided. These devices may also be used to monitor the response of patients to drug treatment and, in particular, can be used to determine the adequacy of 24-hour control with once-daily medication (Fig. 13.101b, c).

Ambulatory blood pressure recordings seem to be better predictors of cardiovascular risk than clinic measurements. Analysis of the diurnal variation in blood pressure suggests that those hypertensives with loss of the usual nocturnal fall in blood pressure ('non-dippers') have a worse prognosis than those who retain this pattern.

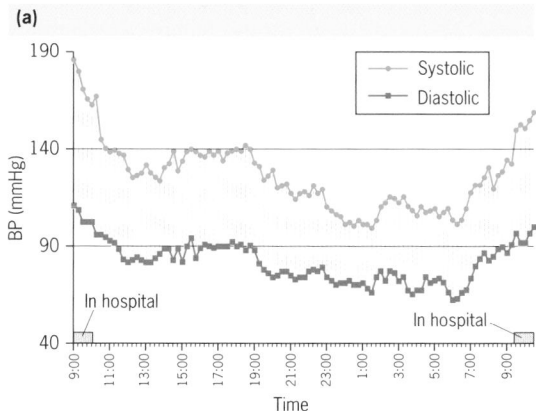

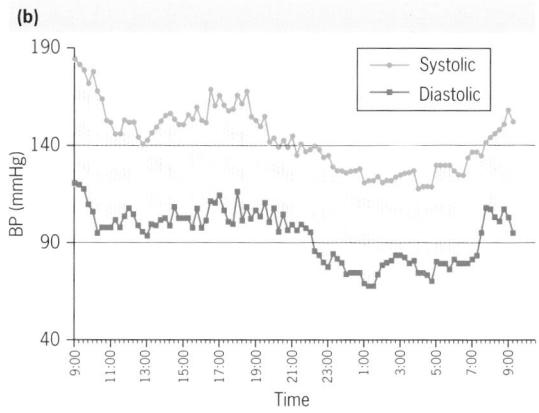

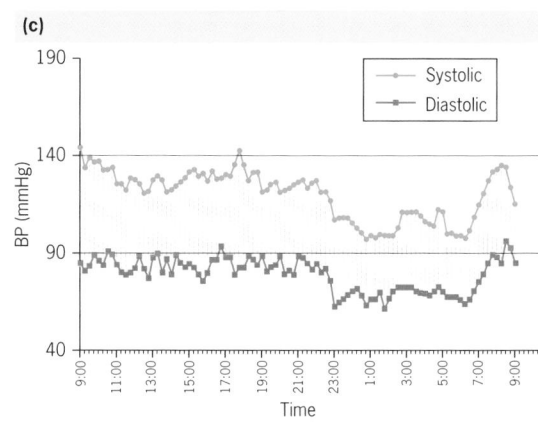

Fig. 13.101 **24-hour ambulatory blood pressure monitoring, showing: (a)** white-coat hypertension; **(b)** pre-treatment; **(c)** after 3 months' treatment.

Fig. 13.100 **Fundus showing hypertensive changes:** Grade 4 retinopathy with papilloedema, haemorrhages and exudates.

Investigations

Routine investigation of the hypertensive patient should include:

- chest X-ray
- ECG
- echocardiogram
- urinalysis
- fasting blood for lipids and glucose
- serum urea, creatinine and electrolytes.

If the urea or creatinine is elevated, more specific renal investigations are indicated – creatinine clearance, renal ultrasound (in case of polycystic kidney disease, or parenchymal renal artery disease) and a renal isotope scan or renal angiography if renovascular disease (either atheromatous or fibromuscular dysplasia) is suspected. A low serum potassium may indicate an endocrine disorder (either primary hyperaldosteronism or gluco-corticoid excess), and aldosterone, cortisol and renin measurements must then be made, preferably prior to initiating pharmacological therapy. Clinical suspicion of phaeochromocytoma should be investigated further with measurement of urinary metanephrines and plasma or urinary catecholamines.

The ECG may show evidence of coronary artery disease or left ventricular hypertrophy, although echo-cardiography is a far more sensitive method for detection of left ventricular hypertrophy. The chest X-ray may show cardiomegaly or pulmonary congestion if heart failure is developing. Rib notching on the X-ray may be a sign of coarctation of the aorta and should be investigated further with an MRI scan.

Treatment

Unless the patient has severe or malignant hypertension, there should be a period of assessment with repeated blood pressure measurements, combined with advice and non-pharmacological measures prior to the initiation of drug therapy. The guidelines of the third working party of the British Hypertension Society (BHS) suggest the following (Fig. 13.102):

- Use of non-pharmacological therapy (weight reduction, low-fat and -sodium diet, limited alcohol consumption, dynamic exercise, and increased fruit and vegetable consumption) in all hypertensive and borderline hypertensive people.
- The initiation of antihypertensive therapy in subjects with sustained systolic blood pressure (BP) >160 mmHg, or sustained diastolic BP >100 mmHg.
- Decide on treatment in subjects with sustained systolic blood pressure between 140–159 mmHg, or sustained diastolic BP between 90–99 mmHg, according to the presence or absence of target organ damage or a 10-year coronary heart disease risk >15%.

- In patients with diabetes mellitus, the initiation of antihypertensive drug therapy if systolic BP is sustained >140 mmHg, or diastolic BP is sustained >90 mmHg.
- In non-diabetic hypertensive subjects, the recommended optimal BP is <140/85 mmHg. The BHS acknowledges, however, that in some hypertensive subjects these levels may be difficult to achieve.
- In the absence of contraindications or compelling indications for other antihypertensive agents, low-dose thiazide diuretics or beta-blockers are preferred as first-line therapy for the majority of hypertensive subjects. In the absence of compelling indications for beta-blockade, diuretics or long-acting dihydropyridine calcium antagonists are preferred to beta-blockers in older subjects
- For most hypertensives, a combination of antihypertensive drugs will be required to achieve the recommended targets for blood pressure control.

Drug treatment (Table 13.44)

The decision to commence specific drug therapy should usually be made only after a careful period of assessment, of up to 6 months, with repeated measurements of blood pressure. The aim of drug treatment to reduce the risk of complications of hypertension should be carefully explained to the patient. All of the drugs used to treat hypertension can be associated with side-effects and, since the benefits of drug treatment are not immediately apparent to the patient, compliance is a major problem. Several classes of drugs are available to treat hypertension. The most appropriate 'first-line' treatment depends on the individual patient characteristics.

Diuretics

Thiazide diuretics such as bendroflumethazide (bendro-fluazide) (2.5–5 mg daily) and cyclopenthiazide (0.25–0.5 mg daily) are well-established agents which have been shown to reduce the risk of stroke in patients with hypertension. The lower doses seems to be equally effective as higher doses in the reduction of blood pressure and most have a duration of up to 24 hours. The major concern with these agents is their adverse metabolic effects, particularly increased serum cholesterol, impaired glucose tolerance, hyperuricaemia (which may precipitate gout) and hypokalaemia. These tend to occur with higher doses of thiazide diuretics.

Loop diuretics such as furosemide (frusemide) (40 mg daily) do have a hypotensive effect, but are not routinely used in the treatment of essential hypertension. Potassium-sparing diuretics such as amiloride (5–10 mg daily) or spironolactone (50–200 mg daily) are not effective agents when used alone, with the exception of spironolactone in the treatment of hypertension and hypokalaemia associated with primary hyper-aldosteronism.

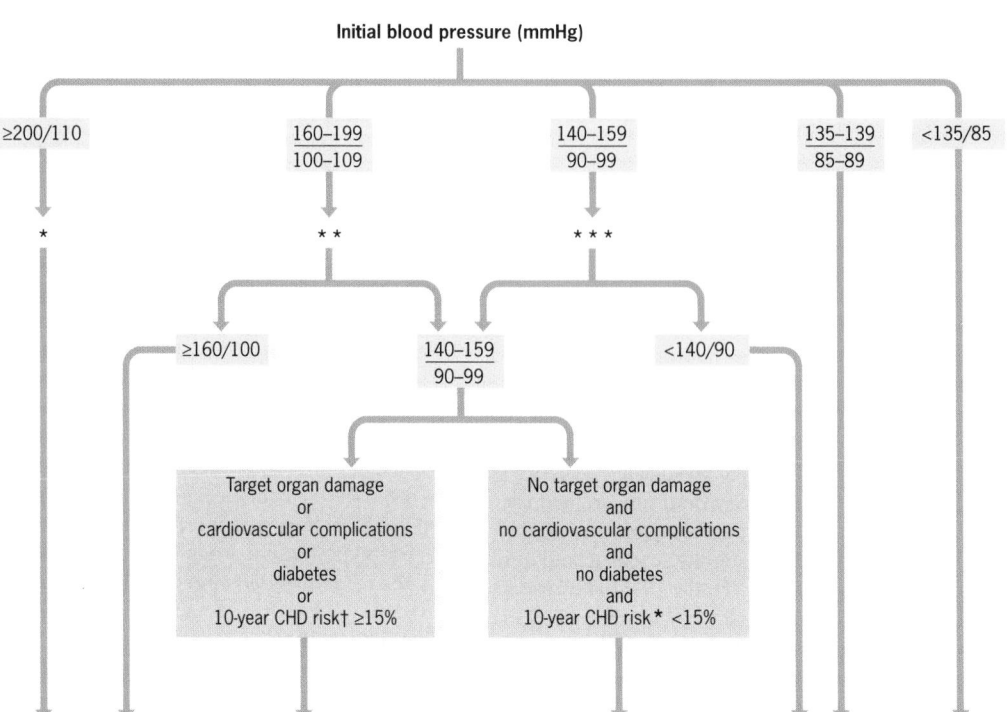

Fig. 13.102 **Blood pressure thresholds and drug treatment in hypertension.** From Ramsay LE et al. (1999) *British Medical Journal* **309**: 630.

Table 13.44
Advantages and disadvantages of drugs used in hypertension with respect to associated conditions

	Diuretic	Beta-blocker	ACE inhibitor/Angiotensin II receptor antagonist	Calcium channel blockers	Alpha-blocker
Diabetes	Care*	Care*	Yes	Yes	Yes
Gout	No	Yes	Yes	Yes	Yes
Dyslipidaemia	Care[†]	Care[†]	Yes	Yes	Yes
Ischaemic heart disease	Yes	Yes	Yes	Yes	Yes
Heart failure	Yes	Care[‡]	Yes	Care[§]	Yes
Asthma	Yes	No	Yes	Yes	Yes
Peripheral vascular disease	Yes	Care	Care[¶]	Yes	Yes
Renal artery stenosis	Yes	Care	No	Yes	Yes
Pregnancy	Caution	Not in late pregnancy	No	No	Caution

* Diuretics may aggravate diabetes: beta-blockers worsen glucose intolerance and mask symptoms of hypoglycaemia
[†] Both diuretics and beta-blockers disturb the lipid profile
[‡] There is evidence for beneficial effects of some beta-blockers when used cautiously in heart failure
[§] Verapamil and diltiazem may exacerbate heart failure, although amlodipine appears to be safe
[¶] Patients with peripheral vascular disease may also have renal artery stenosis; therefore ACE inhibitors should be used cautiously

Beta-blockers

The beta-blockers have also been shown to improve the prognosis of hypertensives. They have been suggested to exert their effects by attenuating the effects of the sympathetic nervous and the renin–angiotensin systems. They reduce the force of cardiac contraction, as well as resting and exercise-induced increase in heart rate. But, there are differences between these antihypertensive drugs (Table 13.45):

- *Cardioselectivity.* Some have less effect on the β_2 (non-cardiac) receptors and are therefore said to be relatively cardioselective. These include atenolol and bisoprolol.
- *Intrinsic sympathomimetic activity.* Some agents have partial agonist activity and cause less bradycardia. These include oxprenolol and pindolol.
- *Lipid solubility.* The agents that are less lipid-soluble are less likely to cause central nervous system side-effects. These include atenolol.

The major side-effects of this class of agents are bradycardia, bronchospasm, cold extremities, fatigue, bad dreams and hallucinations. These agents are especially useful in the treatment of patients with both hypertension and angina.

Angiotensin-converting enzyme (ACE) inhibitors

These drugs block the conversion of angiotensin I to angiotensin II, which is a potent vasoconstrictor. They also block the degradation of bradykinin, a potent vasodilator. There is evidence, however, that black African patients respond less well to ACE inhibitors unless combined with diuretics. They are particularly useful in diabetics with nephropathy, where they have been shown to slow disease progression, and in those patients with symptomatic or asymptomatic left ventricular dysfunction, where they have been shown to improve survival.

The major potential side-effects are profound hypotension following the first dose, which is usually seen in sodium-depleted patients or in those on treatment with large doses of diuretics, and deterioration of renal function in those with severe bilateral renovascular disease (in whom the production of angiotensin II is playing a major role in maintaining renal perfusion by causing efferent arteriolar constriction at the glomerulus). They also cause mild dry cough in a number of antihypertensive patients, especially if prescribed at high doses.

These are several ACE inhibitors available and there are no significant differences between them in terms of blood pressure effect other than the half-life and therefore the frequency at which they have to be prescribed for 24-h blood pressure control; those with the longest duration of action may be taken once-daily, which is clearly a benefit in terms of compliance. The drugs include captopril (50–150 mg daily in divided doses), enalapril or lisinopril (10–20 mg daily), and trandolapril (1–4 mg daily).

Angiotensin II receptor antagonists

This group of agents selectively block the receptors for angiotensin II. They share many of the actions of ACE inhibitors but, since they do not have any effect on bradykinin, do not cause a cough. They are currently used for patients who cannot tolerate ACE inhibitors because of persistent cough. The agents include losartan (50–100 mg daily), candesartan (16 mg daily) valsartan (80–160 mg daily), irbesartan (75–300 mg daily).

Calcium-channel blockers

These agents effectively reduce blood pressure by causing arteriolar dilatation, and some also reduce the force of cardiac contraction. Like the beta-blockers, they are especially useful in patients with concomitant ischaemic heart disease. The major side-effects are particularly seen with the short-acting agents and include headache, sweating, swelling of the ankles, palpitations and flushing. Many of these side-effects can be lessened by the co-administration of a beta-blocker. The short-acting agents, such as nifedipine (10–20 mg three times daily) are being replaced by once-daily agents that are very well tolerated and include amlodipine (5–10 mg daily) and nifedipine LA (20–90 mg daily).

Alpha-blockers

These agents cause postsynaptic α_1-receptor blockade with resulting vasodilatation and blood pressure reduction. Earlier short-acting agents caused serious first-dose hypotension, but the newer longer-acting agents

Table 13.45
Main properties of the beta-blockers commonly used for hypertension

	Cardiac selectivity	Intrinsic sympathomimetic activity	Lipid solubility	Plasma half-life (hours)	Usual dosage
Acebutalol	+	+	0	5	400 mg once or twice daily
Atenolol	+	0	0	6	50 mg once daily
Bisoprolol	++	0	0	10–12	10–20 mg once daily
Oxprenolol	0	++	+	1.5	20–80 mg three times daily
Propranolol	0	0	+++	5	80–160 mg twice daily
Timolol	0	0	+	5	5–20 mg twice daily

are far better tolerated. These include doxazosin (1–4 mg daily). Labetalol is an agent that has combined alpha- and beta-blocking properties, but is not commonly used, except in pregnancy-induced hypertension.

Other vasodilators

These include hydralazine (up to 100 mg daily) and minoxidil (up to 50 mg daily). Both are extremely potent vasodilators that are reserved for patients resistant to other forms of treatment. Hydralazine can be associated with tachycardia, fluid retention and a systemic lupus erythematosus-like syndrome. Minoxidil can cause severe oedema and excessive hair growth. If these agents are used, it is usually in combination with a beta-blocker.

Sodium nitroprusside is a potent arterial and venous dilator. It is now only used intravenously, in hypertensive crises when prompt blood pressure reduction is required (e.g. dissecting aortic aneurysm).

Centrally acting drugs

Reserpine is used in a low dose of 0.05 mg per day, which provides almost all its antihypertensive action with fewer side-effect than higher doses. It has a slow onset of action (measured in weeks). Methyldopa is still widely used despite central and potentially serious hepatic and blood side-effects. It acts on central α_2-receptors, usually without slowing the heart. Clonidine and moxonidine provide all the benefits of methyldopa with none of the rare (but serious) autoimmune reactions.

Other agents

Adrenergic neurone-blocking drugs, such as guanethidine, are hardly ever used.

Drug selection

Treatment is normally commenced with a single agent (monotherapy). The target of therapy should be to maintain diastolic blood pressure in the range of 80–90 mmHg with systolic blood pressure below 160 mmHg, or even lower in diabetic patients (see above).

The most appropriate first-line agent will depend on the patient's age, ethnic background, sex and any concomitant illnesses. Conventionally, thiazide diuretics and beta-blockers have been used as first-line agents with the other agents reserved for those in whom these prove ineffective. However, as our understanding of the adverse metabolic actions of these traditional agents increases, more patients are being prescribed calcium antagonists and ACE inhibitors as first-line treatment. There is some evidence that the drugs differ in their ability to reverse left ventricular hypertrophy (with the ACE inhibitors, A II blockers being the most effective) although larger long-term studies are required to confirm these findings. If monotherapy is unsuccessful, it is appropriate to move to combination therapy and certain combinations have been found to be particularly effective. These include the combination of an ACE inhibitor or beta-blocker with a diuretic, and the combination of a calcium antagonist with a beta-blocker. Resistant hypertension is most commonly due to non-compliance with medication, although it may reflect an unrecognized underlying cause (e.g. secondary hypertension or unrecognized coarctation of the aorta), or may genuinely be due to refractory hypertension requiring multiple combination therapy

Management of severe or malignant hypertension

Patients with severe hypertension (diastolic pressure >140 mmHg), malignant hypertension (grades 3 or 4 retinopathy), hypertensive encephalopathy or with severe hypertensive complications, such as cardiac failure, should be admitted to hospital for immediate initiation of treatment. However, it is unwise to reduce the blood pressure too rapidly since this may lead to cerebral, renal, retinal or myocardial infarction, and the blood pressure response to therapy must be carefully monitored, preferably in a high-dependency unit. In most cases, the aim is to reduce the diastolic blood pressure to 100–110 mmHg over 24–48 hours. This is usually achieved with oral medication e.g. atenolol or amlodipine. The blood pressure can then be normalized over the next 2–3 days.

When rapid control of blood pressure is required (e.g. in an aortic dissection), the agent of choice is intravenous sodium nitroprusside. Alternatively, an infusion of labetalol can be used. The infusion dosage must be titrated against the blood pressure response. Fenoldopam, a selective peripheral dopamine receptor agonist, has recently been introduced and is effective as nitroprusside.

Management of hypertension in pregnancy

Many antihypertensive agents are contraindicated in pregnancy. Mild hypertension can be treated with methyldopa, which has been established as being safe in pregnancy, or labetalol. Pre-eclamptic hypertension can be treated with the same agents, or nifedipine, although the only method for reversal of overt pre-eclampsia is delivery. More severe hypertension or eclampsia requires treatment with intravenous hydralazine and may even require termination of the pregnancy.

Prognosis

The prognosis from hypertension depends on a number of features:

- the level of blood pressure
- the presence of target-organ changes (retinal, renal, cardiac or vascular)
- coexisting risk factors for cardiovascular disease, such as hyperlipidaemia, diabetes, smoking, obesity, male sex
- age at presentation.

Several studies have confirmed that the treatment of hypertension, even mild hypertension, will reduce the risk not only of stroke but of coronary artery disease as well.

FURTHER READING

British Hypertension Society Working Party (1999) Guidelines for the management of hypertension: report of the third working party. *Journal of Human Hypertension* **13**: 569–592.

Hansson L et al. (1998) Hypertension Optimal Treatment (HOT) randomised trial. *Lancet* **351**: 1755–1762.

Medical Research Council Working Party (1985) MRC trial of treatment of mild hypertension: principal results. *British Medical Journal* **291**: 97–104.

Swales JD (1994) *Textbook of Hypertension*. Oxford: Blackwell Scientific.

Vasan RS et al (2001) Impact of high-normal blood pressure on the risk of cardiovascular disease. *New England Journal of Medicine* **345**: 1291–1297.

Heart disease in the elderly

As the average age of the population increases, and as patients with cardiac disease survive for longer periods of time, the number of elderly patients with heart disease has increased markedly and is likely to continue to escalate in years to come. The elderly are vulnerable to hypertension, coronary artery disease, heart failure, arrhythmias and degenerative pathologies.

Normal findings

Diagnosis of mild forms of heart disease may be difficult in the elderly. The wear and tear of age results in some features that would be regarded as abnormal in the young. For example, a fourth heart sound and a systolic aortic ejection murmur are common findings on examining normal elderly adults. Basal crackles in the elderly are common and may not necessarily imply left-sided heart failure. The ECG often shows slight PR interval prolongation (up to 0.22 s), left axis deviation and T wave flattening. On the chest X-ray there is frequently a degree of tissue calcification. This is seen in the valvular annuli, the aortic arch, and the coronary and pulmonary vasculature, but the cardiac silhouette is usually normal although changes in the shape of the chest wall may distort normal anatomy. The echocardiogram may show mild myocardial hypertrophy and buckling of the ventricular septum mimicking hypertrophic cardiomyopathy.

It is sometimes difficult to diagnose and define hypertension in the elderly. Cuff blood pressure usually overestimates intravascular pressure since the arterial wall is stiff (pseudohypertension). Normally, blood pressure steadily increases with age, at least up to the age of 70 years, furthermore blood pressure is particularly labile in the elderly. In the very old (>80 years) there is only a weak association between 'hypertension' and diseases such as stroke, myocardial infarction and heart failure.

Disease presentation

Cardiac disease often presents in unexpected ways in an old person. It is not unusual for significant bradycardia to present as a fractured hip owing to a fall resulting from transient asystole. Left heart failure may present as an acute confusional state due to poor cerebral perfusion, rather than with the classical symptom of breathlessness, and frequently accompanies pneumonia. Myocardial infarction may not cause any chest pain ('silent' myocardial infarction) in up to 20% of patients but presents as weakness, abdominal pain, confusion, or a more general deterioration in well-being. Infective endocarditis can cause much diagnostic confusion particularly in the elderly who may not display fever, and present with symptoms from almost any organ system. Elderly patients may present with heart failure despite a normal-sized heart on X-ray and normal systolic myocardial function on echocardiogram (diastolic heart failure).

Treatment

Age is no bar to effective treatment of heart disease and the principles of treatment of heart disease in the elderly are usually no different from those governing treatment in the young. Drug pharmacokinetics are changed in the elderly: absorption is reduced, renal and hepatic clearance are delayed, body fat increases and lean body mass decreases. Elderly patients frequently have coexistent disease and are taking other medication which interacts with both their cardiac medication and their heart disease. For example, non-steroidal anti-inflammatory drugs for arthritis may cause fluid retention and worsen heart failure. Old people may forget to take their medication or be confused about the correct dose and timing.

In general, therapy in elderly patients (who have a limited life span) is more likely to be focused on effective relief of symptoms rather than substantial prolongation of life. Recent studies strongly suggest that systolic hypertension results in a marked increase in cardiac and cerebrovascular complications, and that this risk can be effectively reduced with adequate blood pressure control. Coronary angioplasty, mitral and, less commonly, aortic valvuloplasty can be undertaken in patients too frail for cardiac surgery, which carries a much greater (approximately two to five times) risk in the elderly. As with younger patients, the absolute risk of cardiac surgery is dependent upon the state of the myocardium, the extent of cardiac disease and the condition of other organ systems.

Specific heart problems in the elderly

There are a few cardiac conditions that are largely confined to the elderly.

Aortic sclerosis

Aortic sclerosis results from fibrosis and calcification on the aortic side of an otherwise normal trileaflet aortic valve. The resultant obstruction to left ventricular outflow is often trivial; however, true aortic stenosis requiring aortic valve replacement may be necessary if the obstruction is severe.

Mitral annulus calcification

Mitral annulus calcification occurs predominantly in elderly women. It is diagnosed from the chest X-ray and it is not usually responsible for any symptoms.

Endocarditis

A non-bacterial thrombotic form of endocarditis (marantic endocarditis) may occur in the elderly. It is sometimes associated with malignancy and presents with cachexia, thrombosis and embolization. Anticoagulation may be needed.

Lev's disease

Disruption of His–Purkinje conduction by fibrosis and calcification is most common in the old when it is known as Lev's disease. It presents with Stokes–Adams attacks and must be treated by pacemaker insertion. Age is not a contraindication to pacing, even when the most sophisticated physiological devices are used. Pacemakers should be prescribed on similar criteria in the young and the old.

Carotid sinus hypersensitivity

This is a common cause of syncope in the elderly and is responsible for many admissions for falls, fractures, and dizzy spells. The syndrome is frequently not diagnosed. It is thought to be due to abnormal sensitivity of the carotid baroreceptors resulting in a fall in heart rate, a drop in blood pressure, or both. Diagnosis is made by carotid sinus massage (after excluding carotid stenosis by auscultation). Treatment with a pacemaker may significantly help some patients with the syndrome (see p. 737).

Atrial fibrillation

Atrial fibrillation is much more common in the elderly and is a common cause of stroke in this group of patients. It is often well tolerated and may not need any active treatment for control of heart rate. Anticoagulation is usually advised (see p. 744), except in the very elderly, those prone to falls and those who cannot be relied upon to take their medication regularly.

FURTHER READING

Martin A, Camm AJ (1994) *Heart Disease in the Elderly.*
   Chichester: John Wiley.

Peripheral vascular disease

Peripheral arterial disease

This is due to atherosclerosis involving the aorta, iliac and/or any other peripheral vessel (Table 13.46). It occurs over the age of 40 years in patients who are smokers with other risk factors for atherosclerosis (Table 13.25, p. 767). The age affected prevalence of peripheral arterial disease is 12% affecting men and women equally.

Symptoms

Often both limbs are affected, but usually one is more severely affected than the other. There is cramp-like pain, usually in the calves during exercise and relieved by rest (intermittent claudication). The thighs and buttocks are sometimes involved. The Leriche syndrome is due to severe atheromatous disease of the distal aorta leading to thigh claudication and male impotence.

Rest pain, which is often worse at night, is sometimes relieved by dangling the legs over the edge of the bed. The feet are cold, sometimes with discoloration due to peripheral cyanosis.

Five to ten per cent of patients have critical leg ischaemia with pain in the foot, ulceration or gangrene. These patients with severe disease have an annual mortality from cardiovascular causes of 25%.

Signs

- A cold limb with dry skin and lack of hair.
- Diminished or absent pulses to diseased areas.
- Ulceration.
- Gangrene; dark discoloration, usually starting at the toes.

Investigations
Doppler ultrasound

Measurement of the cuff pressure at which blood flow is detectable by Doppler in the peripheral arteries is a good guide to the severity of arterial disease. It is expressed as a ratio of ankle/brachial pressure index (ABPI). With intermittent claudication, the ratio is from 0.4–0.9. With critical leg ischaemia the values are 0.04–0.4. After exercise there is a further fall in the pressure ratio in patients with arterial disease and this is a highly sensitive test.

Table 13.46

Common sites of clinically significant atherosclerosis, in order of frequency

Abdominal aorta and iliac arteries
Proximal coronary arteries
Femoral and popliteal arteries, and thoracic aorta
Internal carotid arteries
Vertebrobasilar system

ABPI > 1.30 indicates non-compressible calcified vessels and the test is invalid.

B-mode ultrasonography and Doppler combined (duplex imaging) gives a detailed image of the lower limb arteries from the aorta to the pedal vessels with detection of any stenotic areas and also the direction of blood flow.

MRI and spiral CT angiography

MRI avoids exposure to X-rays and is accurate in detecting arterial stenosis.

Angiography

This is performed via a percutaneous catheter inserted into the brachial or other artery. With digital subtraction imaging, an intravenous injection has been used with good definition using only small doses of contrast. These investigations are now less often required because of good Doppler images.

Intravascular ultrasonography and angioscopy are invasive techniques that are being used for intraluminal visualization, particularly after angioplasty and stenting.

Management
General

Risk factors should be reduced. In particular, smoking should be stopped as this slows progression of the disease. Both diabetes mellitus and hypertension should be treated aggressively but whether this prevents progression of the disease is debatable. A weight-reduction programme should be introduced. Hypercholesterolaemia should be treated (see p. 1109) as this reduces disease progression judged angiographically and by reduction in symptoms.

The limbs should be kept warm but local heat should not be applied. Foot care should be introduced to avoid infection and trauma of the feet. Elderly patients often need regular visits to a chiropodist. Supervised exercise programmes significantly increase walking distances and quality of life.

Low-dose aspirin should be given to reduce the risk of myocardial infarction and stroke, with a possible reduction in the rate of re-occlusion following angioplasty. Vasodilators should not be used for claudication. Anticoagulants are of no benefit. Pentoxifylline and naftidrofuryl have limited effects on symptoms.

Surgery

Surgery should not be considered for 3 months after intermittent claudication has developed, to allow time for collaterals to develop. In 75% of patients the disease remains static.

Aorto-iliac bypass grafts give good results, but reconstructive surgery for blockages below the inguinal ligament is less successful. In the short term, percutaneous transluminal angioplasty via a catheter inserted into the artery is useful for local iliac or femoral stenoses; over

2–5 years, the results are similar to those of medical therapy. Insertion of a stent may improve on these results.

Amputation is necessary for severely ischaemic limbs, usually those with gangrene. Rehabilitation may take months in the elderly and is often unsuccessful.

Prognosis

The severity of peripheral arterial disease is closely associated with the risk of myocardial infarction, cerebrovascular disease and death from vascular causes; the reduction in risk factors is the most useful therapy.

Acute ischaemia of the legs

This is due to atherosclerosis with an acute thrombosis or from an embolism from the heart (e.g. in atrial fibrillation) or from an atheromatous central vessel.

The clinical picture is of an acutely painful, pale, paralysed, pulseless limb.

Treatment is surgical, with removal of the clot. Anticoagulants with heparin can help some patients. Intra-arterial thrombolysis, usually with streptokinase, provides successful recannalization in about 50% of patients. Further revascularization surgery is usually required later. If gangrene develops, amputation is necessary.

Aortic aneurysms

An aortic aneurysm refers to a permanent localized dilatation of the aorta with a diameter of at least 1.5 times that of the expected diameter.

Abdominal aneurysms

The most common aortic aneurysms are abdominal between the renal and iliac arteries. They are usually due to atherosclerosis. The incidence increases with age, with men being affected four to five times more frequently.

Asymptomatic aneurysms may be found as a pulsatile mass on examination or as calcification on an X-ray. A CT scan or ultrasound of the abdomen will demonstrate the size of the aneurysm, the thickness of the aortic wall and whether any leak has occurred. An expanding aneurysm may cause epigastric or back pain. Rupture presents with epigastric pain radiating through to the back. A pulsatile mass is felt and the patient is shocked. Treatment of symptomatic aneurysms is surgical. A ruptured aneurysm requires emergency surgery, but even then the mortality is high.

Large, asymptomatic aneurysms should also be treated surgically (except in the very old) because those larger than 5 cm diameter have a high risk of rupture. Follow-up with ultrasound is required with small aneurysms and surgery offered when the aneurysm reaches 5 cm.

Some atherosclerotic aneurysms are associated with a severe periadventitial inflammatory and fibrotic response. Patients present with severe abdominal and sometimes back pain. Inflammatory markers are raised. Steroids relieve symptoms; surgical repair is difficult.

Thoracic aneurysms

These can be divided into ascending, arch or descending aortic aneurysms (the most common).

Ascending thoracic aortic aneurysms most often result from cystic medial degeneration/necrosis. This describes mucosal degeneration of the collagen and elastic tissue of the media, often with cystic changes. It occurs in patients with hypertension and in diseases of collagen, e.g. Marfan's (p. 803). Descending thoracic aortic and arch aneurysms are usually due to atherosclerosis. Syphilis as a cause of aneurysms is now rare.

Forty per cent are asymptomatic at diagnosis, but when large they can give rise to chest pain or to evidence of pressure on other organs, such as the superior vena cava or the oesophagus. They can rupture. Transoesophageal echocardiography is accurate in diagnosis. Asymptomatic aneurysms should probably be resected when they reach 6–7 cm, possibly smaller if the patient has Marfan's syndrome (p. 803). Arch aneurysms are technically the most difficult to deal with and carry a higher mortality.

Dissecting aortic aneurysms

Aortic dissection usually begins with a tear in the intima. Blood penetrates the diseased medial layer and then cleaves the lamina plain of the intima in two, leading to a dissection of variable length. In a small number of cases no tear is found and it is proposed that a haemorrhage within the media is the first step.

Aortic dissections are of three types:

- DeBakey I – originates in the ascending aorta, propagates at least to the aortic arch and often beyond
- DeBakey II – originates in, and is confined to, the ascending aorta
- DeBakey III – originates in the distal aorta and extends distally down the aorta.

The major symptom is severe and central chest pain, often radiating to the back. The pain radiates down the arms and into the neck and can be difficult to distinguish from myocardial infarction.

On examination, the patient is usually shocked and there may be neurological signs owing to the involvement of the spinal vessels. The peripheral pulses may be absent, but this is not invariable. Half of the patients are hypertensive and this should be controlled immediately.

The diagnosis is suggested by the presence of back pain in addition to chest pain and no ECG or enzyme changes of myocardial infarction. The chest X-ray may show a wide mediastinum, and CT scanning and ultrasonography with transoesophageal echocardiography are diagnostic (Fig. 13.103). MRI is highly accurate and is the gold standard. Aortography is now rarely necessary to confirm the diagnosis.

Emergency surgery is necessary for acute proximal dissections. Acute distal aortic dissections are best treated medically to control pain and hypertension. Five-year survival in both groups is in the region of 70–80%.

Thromboangiitis obliterans (Buerger's disease)

This disease, involving the small vessels of the lower limbs, occurs in young men who smoke. It is thought by some workers to be indistinguishable from atheromatous disease. However, pathologically there is inflammation of the arteries and sometimes veins that may indicate a separate disease entity. Clinically it presents with severe claudication and rest pain leading to gangrene. A thrombophlebitis is sometimes present.

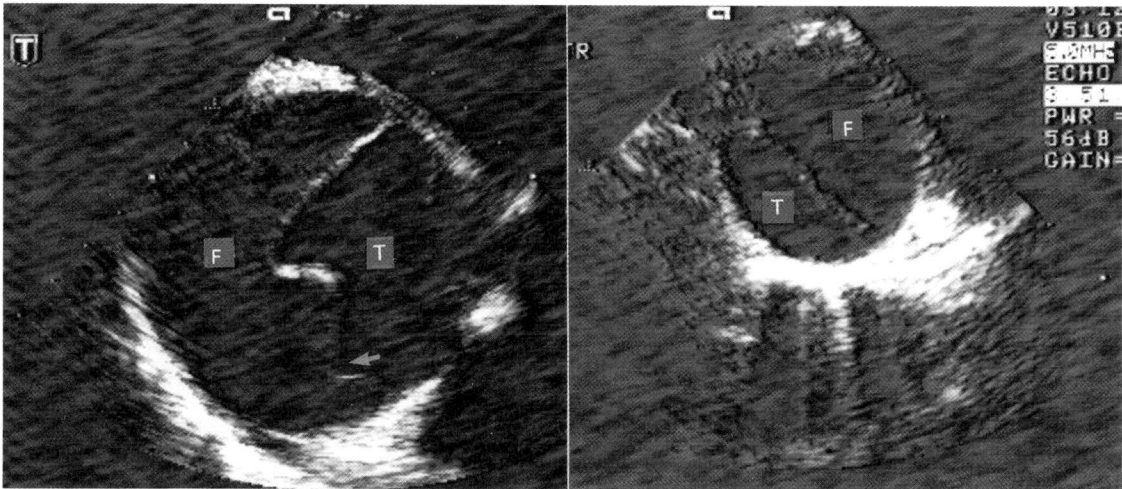

Fig. 13.103 **Two-dimensional transoesophageal echocardiograms from a patient with Marfan's syndrome** resulting in dissection of the aorta. From its position in the oesophagus, the transducer can be aimed forward to visualize the greatly enlarged ascending aorta (left), or backwards to show the descending thoracic aorta (right). In both views the dissected intima is seen within the aortic lumen. The main entry point to the false lumen is seen in the ascending aorta (arrowed), just above the aortic valve. T, true lumen; F, false lumen.

Treatment is as for all peripheral vascular disease, but patients must stop smoking.

Takayasu's syndrome

This is rare, except in Japan. It is known as 'pulseless disease' or the aortic arch syndrome. It is of unknown aetiology and occurs in young females. There is a vasculitis involving the aortic arch as well as other major arteries. There is also a systemic illness, with pain and tenderness over the affected arteries. Absent peripheral pulses and hypertension are usually found. Corticosteroids help the constitutional symptoms. Heart failure and cerebrovascular events eventually occur, but most patients survive for at least 5 years.

Cardiovascular syphilis

This gives rise to:

- uncomplicated aortitis
- aortic aneurysms, usually in the ascending part
- aortic valvulitis with regurgitation
- stenosis of the coronary ostia.

The diagnosis is confirmed by serology. Treatment is with penicillin. Aneurysms and valvular disease are treated as necessary by the usual methods.

Connective tissue disorders

These cause vasculitis and can give rise to peripheral vascular disease. They are discussed on page 565.

Raynaud's disease and phenomenon

Raynaud's phenomenon consists of spasm of the arteries supplying the fingers or toes and is usually precipitated by cold and relieved by heat. When Raynaud's phenomenon occurs without any underlying disorder, it is then known as Raynaud's disease. This is a common disease affecting 5% of the population and occurring predominantly in young women.

The disorder is usually bilateral and fingers are affected more commonly than toes. There is an initial pallor of the skin resulting from vasoconstriction and this is followed by cyanosis due to sluggish blood flow. Redness finally occurs owing to hyperaemia. The duration of the attacks can be variable and can sometimes last for hours. Numbness and burning of the fingers usually occurs and pain can be severe, particularly in the rewarming phase.

Between the attacks the pulses and the digits appear normal, but trophic changes with small areas of gangrene can occur in severe and persistent cases.

Diagnosis

Primary Raynaud's disease must be differentiated from secondary causes of Raynaud's phenomenon, which are chiefly disorders of connective tissue, particularly systemic sclerosis. It can also occur in cryoglobulinaemia

and as a side-effect of drug treatment, especially with beta-blocking agents.

Treatment (see also p. 562)

No treatment is usually required for the attacks but any underlying disease must be looked for. The hands and feet should be kept warm, and smoking should be stopped.

Beta-blockers should be stopped. Nifedipine 10 mg three times daily may be helpful. Lumbar sympathectomy may help lower limb symptoms.

Peripheral venous disease

Varicose veins

Varicose veins are a common problem, sometimes giving rise to pain. They are treated by injection or surgery.

Venous thrombosis

Thrombosis can occur in any vein, but the veins of the leg and the pelvis are the most common sites.

Superficial thrombophlebitis

This commonly involves the saphenous veins and is often associated with varicosities. Occasionally the axillary vein is involved, usually as a result of trauma. There is local superficial inflammation of the vein wall, with secondary thrombosis.

The clinical picture is of a painful, tender, cord-like structure with associated redness and swelling.

The condition usually responds to symptomatic treatment with rest, elevation of the limb and analgesics (e.g. non-steroidal anti-inflammatory drugs). Anticoagulants are not necessary, as embolism does not occur from superficial thrombophlebitis.

Deep-vein thrombosis

A thrombus forms in the vein, and any inflammation of the vein wall is secondary to this.

Thrombosis commonly occurs after periods of immobilization, but it can occur in normal individuals for no obvious reasons. The precipitating factors are discussed on page 465.

A deep-vein thrombosis in the legs occurs in 50% of patients after prostatectomy (without prophylactic heparin) or following a cerebral vascular event. In addition, 10% of patients with a myocardial infarct have a clinically detected deep-vein thrombosis.

Thrombosis can occur in any vein of the leg, but is particularly found in veins of the calf. It is often undetected; autopsy figures give an incidence of over 60% in hospitalized patients.

Axillary vein thrombosis occasionally occurs, sometimes related to trauma, but usually for no obvious reason.

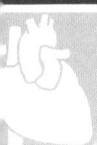
Clinical features

The individual may be asymptomatic, presenting with clinical features of pulmonary embolism (see p. 804).

A major presenting feature is pain in the calf, often with swelling, redness and engorged superficial veins. The affected calf is often warmer and there may be ankle oedema. Homan's sign (pain in the calf on dorsiflexion of the foot) is often present, but is not diagnostic and occurs with all lesions of the calf.

Thrombosis in the iliofemoral region can present with severe pain, but there are often few physical signs apart from occasional swelling of the thigh and/or ankle oedema.

Complete occlusion, particularly of a large vein, can lead to a cyanotic discoloration of the limb and severe oedema, which can very rarely lead to venous gangrene.

Pulmonary embolism can occur with any deep-vein thrombosis but is more frequent from an iliofemoral thrombosis and is rare with thrombosis confined to veins below the knee. In 20–30% of patients, spread of thrombosis can occur proximally without clinical evidence, so careful monitoring of the leg, usually by ultrasound, is required.

Investigations

Clinical diagnosis is unreliable and confirmation of an iliofemoral thrombosis can usually be made with ultrasound or Doppler ultrasound. Below-knee thromboses can be detected reliably only by venography. A venogram is performed by injecting a vein in the foot with contrast which will detect virtually all thrombi that are present.

Treatment

The main aim of therapy is to prevent pulmonary embolism, and all patients with thrombi above the knee must be anticoagulated. Anticoagulation of below-knee thrombi is controversial, but as it reduces proximal extension it is usually recommended for 6 weeks. Bed rest is advised until the patient is fully anticoagulated. The patient should then be mobilized, with an elastic stocking giving graduated pressure over the leg.

Unfractionated heparin is given normally for at least 2–3 days, whilst warfarin, which is started immediately, becomes effective. Laboratory monitoring is essential with daily activated partial thromboplastin time (APTT, p. 457). Low-molecular-weight heparins (see p. 468) are replacing unfractionated heparin as they are more effective, they do not require monitoring and there is less risk of bleeding. DVTs are now being treated at home with low-molecular-weight heparin. The duration of warfarin treatment is debatable – 3 months is the period usually recommended, but 4 weeks is long enough if a definite risk factor (e.g. bed rest) has been present. The target INR should be at 2.5. Anticoagulants do not lyse the thrombus that is already present.

Thrombolytic therapy (see p. 467) is occasionally used for patients with a large iliofemoral thrombosis.

Prognosis

Destruction of the deep-vein valves produces a clinically painful, swollen limb that is made worse by standing and is accompanied by oedema and sometimes venous eczema. It occurs in approximately half of the patients with a clinically symptomatic deep-vein thrombosis, and it means that elastic support stockings are then required for life.

Prevention

Subcutaneous low-molecular weight heparin (see p. 468) should be given to patients with cardiac failure, a myocardial infarct or surgery to the leg or pelvis.

Early ambulation is indicated as most thromboses occur within the first 72 hours following surgery. Leg exercises should be encouraged and patients should not sit in a chair with their legs immobilized on a stool. An elastic support stocking should be given to patients at high risk (e.g. those with a history of thrombosis or with obesity).

FURTHER READING

Adam J, van der Vliet, Boll APM (1997) Abdominal aortic aneurysm. *Lancet* **349**: 863–866.

Dinguid DL (2001) Choosing a parenteral anticoagulant agent. *New England Journal of Medicine* **345**: 1340–1341.

Dormandy JA, Rutherford RB (2000) Management of peripheral arterial disease. *Journal of Vascular Surgery* **31**: S1–S296.

Hiatt WR (2001) Medical treatment of peripheral arterial disease and claudication. *New England Journal of Medicine* **344**: 1608–1621.

Kelly J et al (2001) Screening for subclinical deep vein thrombosis. *Quarterly Journal of Medicine* **94**: 511–519.

Kouchoukos NT, Dougenis D (1997) Surgery of the thoracic aorta. *New England Journal of Medicine* **336**: 1876–1888.

Rosendaal FR (1997) Risk factors for venous thrombosis. *Seminars in Haematology* **34**: 171–187.

Respiratory disease

14

The main role of the respiratory system is to work closely with the heart and blood to extract oxygen from the external environment and dispose of waste gases, principally carbon dioxide. This requires the lungs to function as an efficient bellows, expelling used air, bringing fresh air in and mixing it efficiently with the air remaining in the lungs. The lungs have to provide a large surface area for gas exchange and the alveoli walls have to present minimal resistance to gas diffusion. This means the lungs have to present a large area to the environment and this can be damaged by dusts, gases and infective agents. Host defence is therefore a key priority for the lung and is achieved by a combination of structural and immunological defences.

Structure of the respiratory system

The nose

The anterior one-third of the nasal cavity is divided into right and left halves by the nasal septum (Fig. 14.1). The nasal vestibule leads to the internal ostium (a) which is the narrowest part of the nasal cavity. This causes a 50% increased resistance to airflow when breathing through the nose rather than through the mouth. The respiratory

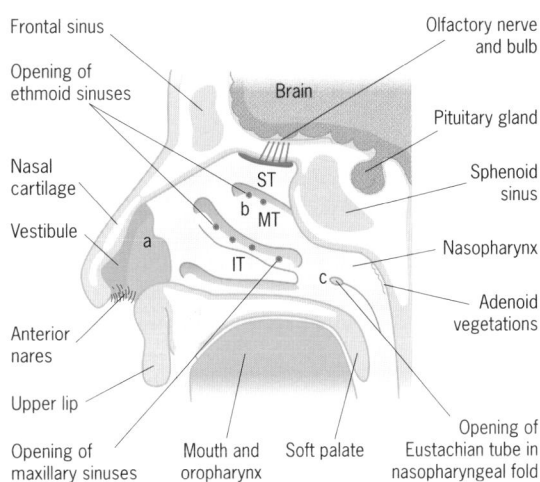

Fig. 14.1 **The anatomy of the nose in longitudinal section.**
IT, inferior turbinate; MT, middle turbinate; ST, superior turbinate;
a, internal ostium; b, respiratory region; c, choanae.

region (b) is divided by three folds arising from the lateral wall, termed the superior, middle and inferior turbinates. Behind these turbinates are situated the openings of the nasolacrimal duct and the frontal, ethmoidal and maxillary sinuses. The olfactory region for smell is found above the superior turbinate. The nasal cavities communicate with the nasopharynx via the posterior nasal apertures (the choanae (c)), and the Eustachian tube opens into this area just above the soft palate.

The pharynx and larynx

The pharynx is divided by the soft palate into an upper nasopharyngeal and lower oropharyngeal region. There are numerous collections of lymphoid tissue arranged in a circular fashion around the nasopharynx; these include the adenoids. The tonsils lie between the anterior and posterior fauces, separating the mouth from the oropharynx.

The larynx consists of a number of articulated cartilages, vocal cords, muscles and ligaments, all of which serve to keep the airway open during breathing and occlude it during swallowing.

The main motor nerve to the larynx is the recurrent laryngeal nerve. The left recurrent laryngeal nerve leaves the vagus at the level of the aortic arch, hooking round it to run upwards through the mediastinum between the trachea and the oesophagus; it can be affected by disease in these areas. The principal tensor of the vocal cords is the external branch of the superior laryngeal nerve, which can be injured during thyroidectomy.

The trachea, bronchi and bronchioles

The trachea is 10–12 cm in length. It lies slightly to the right of the midline and divides at the carina into right and left main bronchi. The carina lies under the junction of the manubrium sternum and the second right costal cartilage. The right main bronchus is more vertical than the left and, hence, inhaled material is more likely to pass into it.

The right main bronchus divides into the upper lobe bronchus and the intermediate bronchus, which further subdivides into the middle and lower lobe bronchi. On the left the main bronchus divides into upper and lower lobe bronchi only. Each lobar bronchus further divides into segmental and subsegmental bronchi. There are about 25 divisions in all between the trachea and the alveoli.

Of the first seven divisions, the bronchi have:

- walls consisting of cartilage and smooth muscle
- epithelial lining with cilia and goblet cells
- submucosal mucus-secreting glands
- endocrine cells – Kulchitsky or APUD (amine precursor and uptake decarboxylation) containing 5-hydroxytryptamine.

In the next 16–18 divisions the bronchioles have:

- no cartilage and a muscular layer that progressively becomes thinner
- a single layer of ciliated cells but very few goblet cells
- granulated Clara cells that produce a surfactant-like substance.

The ciliated epithelium is an important defence mechanism. Each cell contains approximately 200 cilia beating at 1000 beats per minute in organized waves of contraction. Each cilium consists of nine peripheral parts and two inner longitudinal fibrils in a cytoplasmic matrix (Fig. 14.2). Nexin links join the peripheral pairs. Dynein arms consisting of ATPase protein project towards the adjacent pairs. Bending of the cilia results from a sliding movement between adjacent fibrils powered by an ATP-dependent shearing force developed by the dynein arms. Absence of dynein arms leads to immotile cilia. Mucus, which contains macrophages, cell debris, inhaled particles and bacteria, is moved by the cilia towards the larynx at about 1.5 cm/min (the 'mucociliary escalator', see below).

The bronchioles finally divide within the acinus into smaller respiratory bronchioles that have alveoli arising from the surface (Fig. 14.3). Each respiratory bronchiole supplies approximately 200 alveoli via alveolar ducts. The term 'small airways' refers to bronchioles of less than 2 mm; there are 30 000 of these in the average lung.

The alveoli

There are approximately 300 million alveoli in each lung. Their total surface area is 40–80 m². The epithelial lining consists largely of *type I pneumocytes* (Fig. 14.4). These cells have an extremely attenuated cytoplasm, and thus provide only a thin barrier to gas exchange. They are derived from type II pneumocytes. *Type I cells* are connected to each other by tight junctions that limit the fluid movements in and out of the alveoli. *Type II*

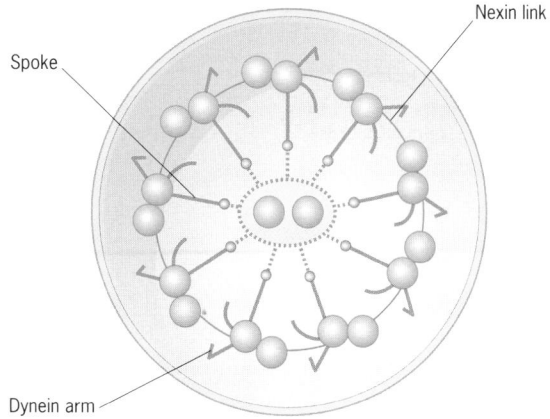

Fig. 14.2 Cross-section of a cilium. Nine outer microtubular doublets and two central single microtubules are linked by spokes, nexin links and dynein arms.

pneumocytes are slightly more numerous than type I cells but cover less of the epithelial lining. They are found generally in the borders of the alveolus and contain distinctive lamellar vacuoles, which are the source of surfactant. Macrophages are also present in the alveoli and are involved in the defence mechanisms of the lung.

The pores of Kohn are holes in the alveolar wall allowing communication between alveoli of adjoining lobules.

The lungs

The lungs are separated into lobes by invaginations of the pleura, which are often incomplete. The right lung has three lobes, whereas the left lung has two. The position of the oblique fissures and the right horizontal fissure are shown in Figure 14.5. The upper lobe lies mainly in front of the lower lobe and therefore signs on the right side in the front of the chest found on physical examination are due to lesions mainly of the upper lobe or part of the middle lobe.

Each lobe is further subdivided into bronchopulmonary segments by fibrous septa that extend inwards from the pleural surface. Each segment receives its own segmental bronchus.

The bronchopulmonary segment is further divided into individual lobules approximately 1 cm in diameter and generally pyramidal in shape, the apex lying towards the bronchioles supplying them. Within each lobule a terminal bronchus supplies an acinus and within this structure further divisions of the bronchioles eventually give rise to the alveoli.

A chest X-ray (Fig. 14.6) illustrates the above features.

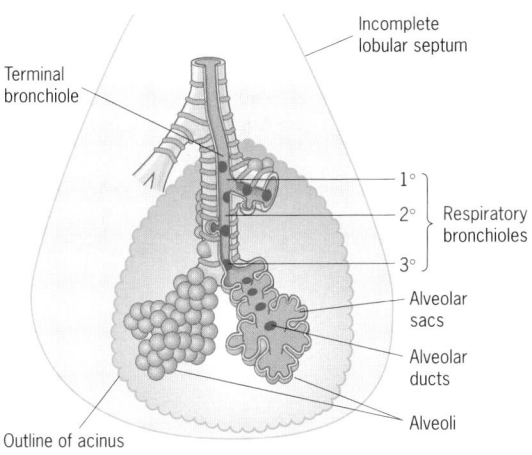

Fig. 14.3 Branches of a terminal bronchiole ending in the alveolar sacs.

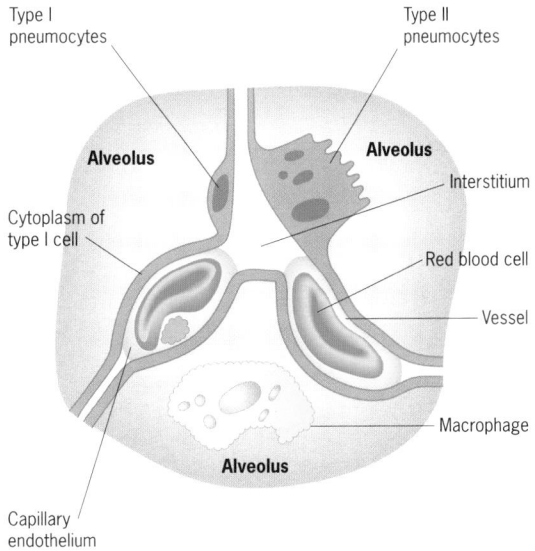

Fig. 14.4 The structure of alveoli, showing the pneumocytes and capillaries.

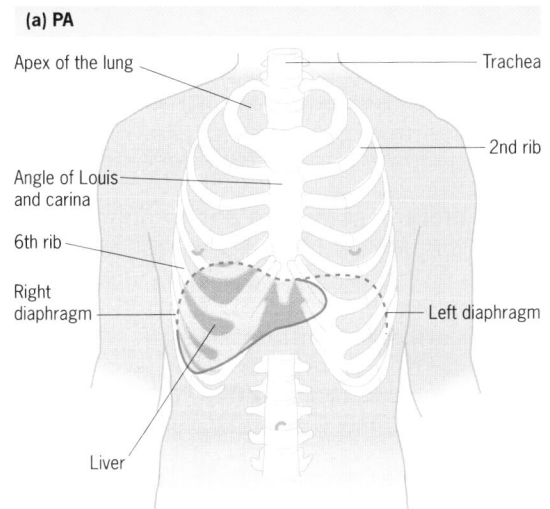

Fig. 14.5 Surface anatomy of the chest. (a) PA; (b) lateral.

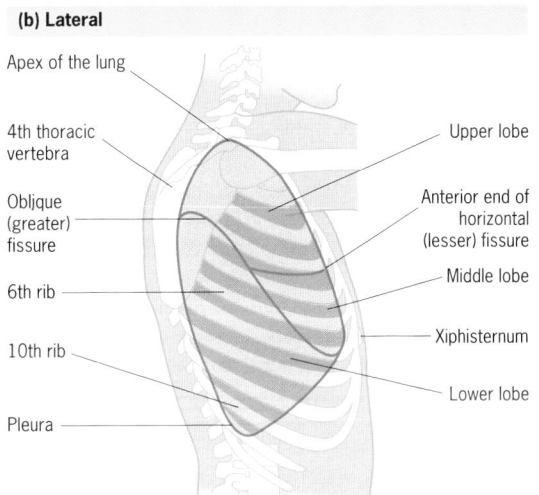

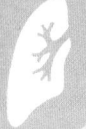

(a)

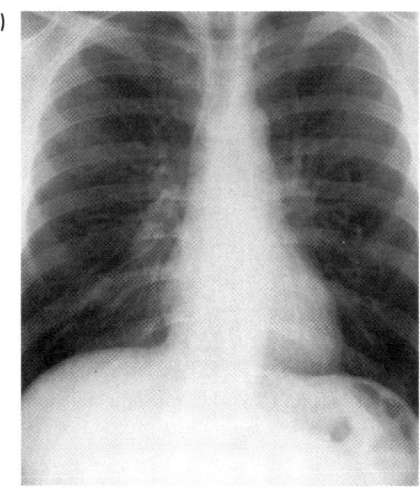

(b)

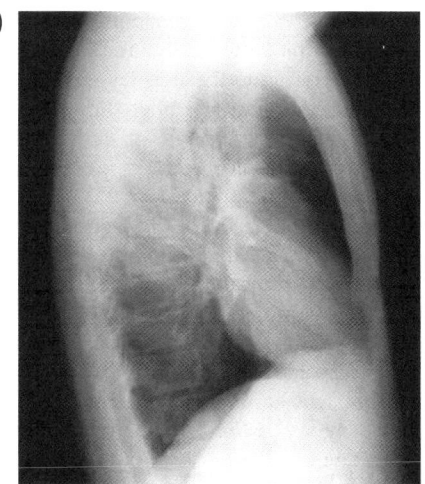

(a) PA

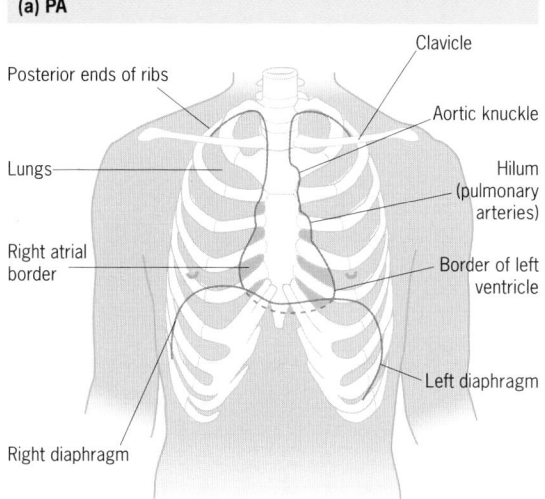

Posterior ends of ribs

Clavicle

Aortic knuckle

Lungs

Hilum (pulmonary arteries)

Right atrial border

Border of left ventricle

Left diaphragm

Right diaphragm

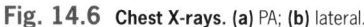

(b) Lateral

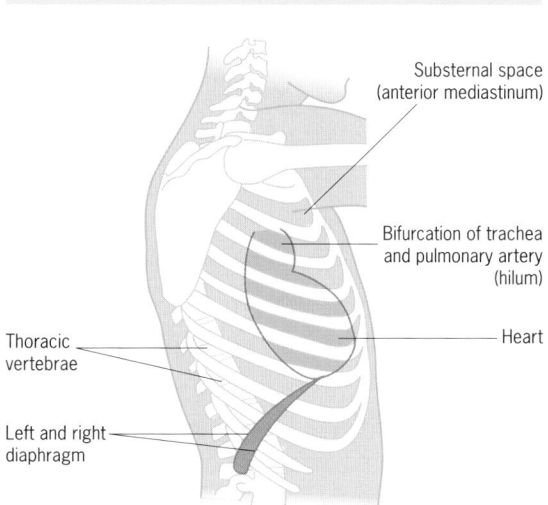

Substernal space (anterior mediastinum)

Bifurcation of trachea and pulmonary artery (hilum)

Heart

Thoracic vertebrae

Left and right diaphragm

Fig. 14.6 **Chest X-rays. (a)** PA; **(b)** lateral.

The pleura

The pleura is a layer of connective tissue covered by a simple squamous epithelium. The visceral pleura covers the surface of the lung, lines the interlobar fissures, and is continuous at the hilum with the parietal pleura, which lines the inside of the hemithorax. At the hilum the visceral pleura continues alongside the branching bronchial tree for some distance before reflecting back to join the parietal pleura. In health, the pleurae are in apposition apart from a small quantity of lubricating fluid, so the pleural cavity is only a potential space.

The diaphragm

The diaphragm is lined by parietal pleura and peritoneum. Its muscle fibres arise from the lower ribs and insert into the central tendon. Motor and sensory nerve fibres go separately to each half of the diaphragm via the phrenic nerves. Fifty per cent of the muscle fibres are of the slow-twitch type with a low glycolytic capacity; they are relatively resistant to fatigue.

Pulmonary vasculature and lymphatics

The lung is unusual in having a dual blood supply. It receives deoxygenated blood from the right ventricle via the pulmonary artery and also has a systemic supply throughout the bronchial circulation.

The pulmonary artery divides to accompany the bronchi. The arterioles accompanying the respiratory bronchioles are thin-walled and contain little smooth muscle. The pulmonary venules drain laterally to the periphery of the lobules, pass centrally in the interlobular and intersegmental septa, and eventually join to form the four main pulmonary veins.

The bronchial circulation arises from the descending aorta. These bronchial arteries supply tissues down to the level of the respiratory bronchiole. The bronchial veins drain into the pulmonary vein, forming part of the physiological shunt observed in normal individuals.

Lymphatic channels lie in the potential interstitial space between the alveolar cells and the capillary endothelium of the pulmonary arterioles.

The tracheobronchial lymph nodes are arranged in five main groups: paratracheal, superior tracheobronchial, subcarinal, bronchopulmonary and pulmonary. In practical terms these form a continuous network of nodes from the lung substance up to the trachea.

Nerve supply to the lung

The innervation of the lung remains incompletely understood. Parasympathetic (from the vagus) and sympathetic (from the adjacent sympathetic chain) nerve supplies entwine in a plexus at the nerve root and branches accompany the pulmonary arteries and the airways. Airway smooth muscle is innervated by vagal afferents, postganglionic cholinergic vagal efferents and vagally derived non-adrenergic non-cholinergic (NANC) fibres. Neurotransmitters (peptides and purines) may be involved. Three muscarinic receptor subtypes have been identified: M_1 receptors on parasympathetic ganglia, a smaller number of M_2 receptors on cholinergic nerve terminals, and M_3 receptors on airway smooth muscle. The parietal pleura is innervated from intercostal and phrenic nerves but the visceral pleura has no innervation.

FURTHER READING

Brewis RAL, Corrin B, Gibson GJ, Geddes DM (1995) *Respiratory Medicine*, 2nd edn, vols 1 and 2. London: WB Saunders.

Physiology of the respiratory system

The nose

The major functions of nasal breathing are:

- to heat and moisten the air
- to remove particulate matter.

About 10 000 L of particle-laden air are inhaled daily. Deposited particles are removed from the nasal mucosa within 15 minutes, compared with 60–120 days from the alveolus. The relatively low flow rates and turbulence of inspired air are ideal for particle deposition, and few particles greater than 10 microns pass through the nose. Nasal secretion contains many protective proteins in the form of antibodies, lysozyme and interferon. In addition, the cilia of the nasal epithelium move the mucous gel layer rapidly back to the oropharynx where it is swallowed. Bacteria have little chance of settling in the nose. Mucociliary protection against viral infections is more difficult because viruses bind to receptors on epithelial cells. The majority of rhinoviruses bind to an adhesion molecule, intercellular adhesion molecule 1 (ICAM-1), shared by neutrophils and eosinophils. Many noxious gases, such as SO_2, are almost completely removed by nasal breathing.

Breathing

Lung ventilation can be considered in two parts:

- the mechanical process of inspiration and expiration
- the control of respiration to a level appropriate for the metabolic needs.

Mechanical process

Inspiration is an active process and results from the descent of the diaphragm and movement of the ribs upwards and outwards under the influence of the intercostal muscles. In resting healthy individuals, contraction of the diaphragm is responsible for most inspiration. Respiratory muscles are similar to other skeletal muscles but are less prone to fatigue. However, weakness may play a part in respiratory failure resulting from neurological and muscle disorders and possibly with severe chronic airflow limitation.

Expiration follows passively as a result of gradual lessening of contraction of the intercostal muscles, allowing the lungs to collapse under the influence of their own elastic forces.

Inspiration against increased resistance may require the use of the accessory muscles of ventilation, such as the sternomastoid and scalene muscles. Forced expiration is also accomplished with the aid of accessory muscles, chiefly those of the abdominal wall, which help to push up the diaphragm.

The lungs have an inherent elastic property that causes them to tend to collapse away from the thoracic wall, generating a negative pressure within the pleural space. The strength of this retractive force relates to the volume of the lung; for example, at higher lung volumes the lung is stretched more, and a greater negative intrapleural pressure is generated.

Lung compliance is a measure of the relationship between this retractive force and lung volume. It is defined as the change in lung volume brought about by unit change in transpulmonary (intrapleural) pressure and is measured in litres per kilopascal (L/kPa). At the end of a quiet expiration, the retractive force exerted by the lungs is balanced by the tendency of the thoracic wall to spring outwards. At this point, respiratory muscles are resting and the volume of the lung is known as the *functional residual capacity* (FRC).

Diseases that affect the movement of the thoracic cage and diaphragm can have a profound effect on ventilation. These include diseases of the thoracic spine such as ankylosing spondylitis and kyphoscoliosis, neuropathies (e.g. the Guillain–Barré syndrome), injury to the phrenic nerves, and myasthenia gravis.

The control of respiration

Coordinated respiratory movements result from rhythmical discharges arising in an anatomically ill-defined group of interconnected neurones in the reticular substance of the brainstem, known as the respiratory centre. Motor discharges from the respiratory centre travel via the phrenic and intercostal nerves to the respiratory musculature.

The pressures of oxygen and carbon dioxide in arterial blood are closely controlled. In a typical normal adult at rest:

- The pulmonary blood flow of 5 L/min carries 11 mmol/min (250 mL/min) of oxygen from the lungs to the tissues.
- Ventilation at about 6 L/min carries 9 mmol/min (200 mL/min) of carbon dioxide out of the body.
- The normal pressure of oxygen in arterial blood (P_aO_2) is between 11 and 13 kPa (83 and 98 mmHg).
- The normal pressure of carbon dioxide in arterial blood (P_aCO_2) is 4.8–6.0 kPa (36–45 mmHg).

Ventilation is controlled by a combination of neurogenic and chemical factors (Fig. 14.7).

Breathlessness on physical exertion is normal and not considered a symptom unless the level of exertion is very light, such as when walking slowly. Recent surveys of healthy Western populations reveal that over 20% of the general population report themselves as breathless on relatively minor exertion Although breathlessness is a very common symptom, the sensory and neural mechanisms underlying it remain obscure. The sensation of breathlessness is derived from at least three sources:

- *Changes in lung volume.* These are sensed by receptors in thoracic wall muscles signalling changes in their length.
- *The tension developed by contracting muscles.* This can be sensed by Golgi tendon organs. The tension developed in normal muscle can be differentiated from that developed in muscles weakened by fatigue or disease.
- *Central perception of the sense of effort.*

The airways of the lungs

From the trachea to the periphery, the airways become smaller in size (although greater in number). The cross-sectional area available for airflow increases as the

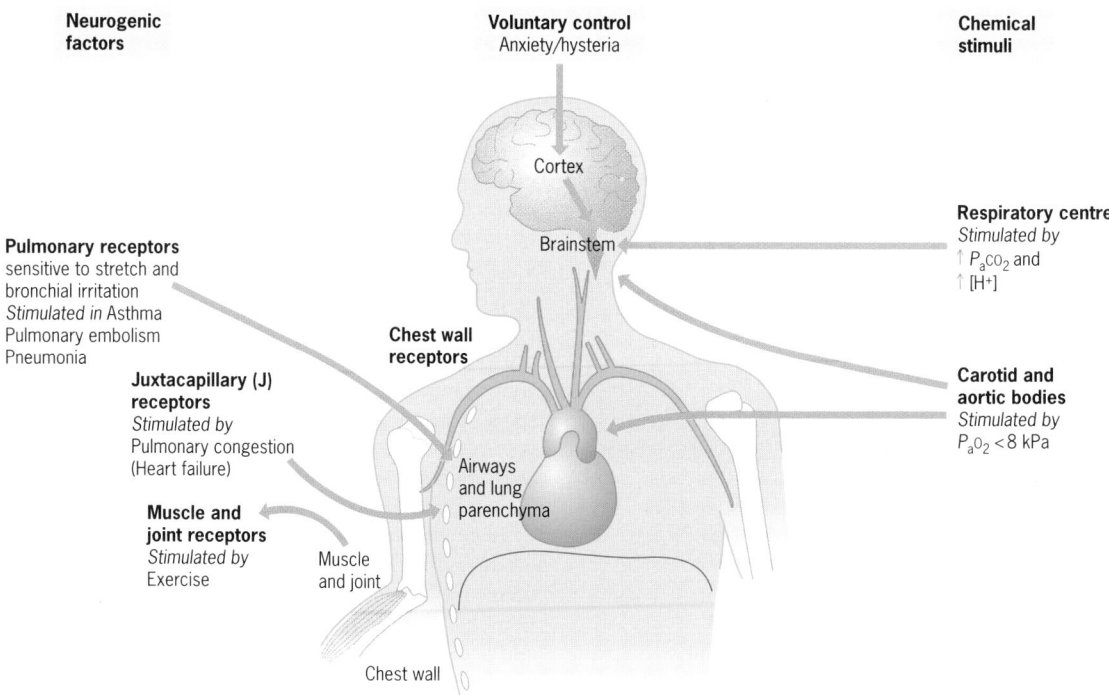

Fig. 14.7 Chemical and neurogenic factors in the control of ventilation. The strongest stimulant to ventilation is a rise in P_aCO_2 which increases [H⁺] in CSF. Sensitivity to this may be lost in COPD. In these patients hypoxaemia is the chief stimulus to respiratory drive; oxygen treatment may therefore reduce respiratory drive and lead to a further rise in P_aCO_2. An increase in [H⁺] due to metabolic acidosis as in diabetic ketoacidosis will increase ventilation with a fall in P_aCO_2 causing deep sighing (Kussmaul) respiration. The respiratory centre is depressed by severe hypoxaemia and sedatives (e.g. opiates) and stimulated by doxapram, large doses of aspirin and pyrexia. COPD, chronic obstructive pulmonary disease. Derived from Manning HL, Schwartzstein RM (1995) *New England Journal of Medicine* **333**: 1547–1553.

total number of airways increases. The flow of air is greatest in the trachea and slows progressively towards the periphery (as the velocity of airflow depends on the ratio of flow to cross-sectional area). In the terminal airways, gas flow occurs solely by diffusion. The resistance to airflow is very low (0.1–0.2 kPa/L in a normal tracheobronchial tree), steadily increasing from the small to the large airways.

Airways expand as lung volume is increased, and at full inspiration (*total lung capacity*, TLC) they are 30–40% larger in calibre than at full expiration (*residual volume*, RV). In chronic obstructive pulmonary disease (COPD) the small airways are narrowed and this can be partially compensated by breathing at a larger lung volume.

Control of airway tone

This is under the control of the autonomic nervous system. Bronchomotor tone is maintained by vagal efferent nerves and, even in a normal subject, is reduced by atropine or β-adrenoceptor agonists. The many adrenoceptors on the surface of bronchial muscles respond to circulating catecholamines; sympathetic nerves do not directly innervate them. Airway tone shows a *circadian rhythm*, which is greatest at 04.00 and lowest in the mid-afternoon. Tone can be increased briefly by inhaled stimuli acting on epithelial nerve endings, which trigger reflex bronchoconstriction via the vagus.

These stimuli include cigarette smoke, inert dust and cold air; airway responsiveness to these increases following respiratory tract infections even in healthy subjects. In asthma, the airways are very irritable and as the circadian rhythm remains the same, asthmatic symptoms are usually worst in the early morning.

Airflow

Movement of air through the airways results from a difference between the pressure in the alveoli and the atmospheric pressure; a positive alveolar pressure occurs in expiration and a negative pressure occurs in inspiration. During quiet breathing the sub-atmospheric pleural pressure throughout the breathing cycle slightly distends the airways. With vigorous expiratory efforts (e.g. cough), although the central airways are compressed by positive pleural pressures exceeding 10 kPa, the airways do not close completely because the driving pressure for expiratory flow (alveolar pressure) is also increased.

Alveolar pressure P_{ALV} is equal to the elastic recoil pressure (P_{EL}) of the lung plus the pleural pressure (P_{PL}).

When there is no airflow (i.e. during a pause in breathing) the tendency of the lungs to collapse (the positive recoil pressure) is exactly balanced by an equivalent negative pleural pressure.

As air flows from the alveoli towards the mouth there is a gradual loss of pressure owing to flow resistance. In forced expiration, as mentioned above, the driving

pressure raises both the alveolar pressure and the intrapleural pressure. Between the alveolus and the mouth, a point will occur (C in Fig. 14.8) where the airway pressure will equal the intrapleural pressure, and airway compression will occur. However, this compression of the airway is temporary, as the transient occlusion of the airway results in an increase in pressure behind it (i.e. upstream) and this raises the intra-airway pressure so that the airways open and flow is restored. The airways thus tend to vibrate at this point of 'dynamic compression'.

The elastic recoil pressure of the lungs decreases with decreasing lung volume and the 'collapse point' moves upstream (i.e. towards the smaller airways – see Fig. 14.8(c)). Where there is pathological loss of recoil pressure (as in chronic obstructive pulmonary disease, COPD), the 'collapse point' starts even further upstream and these patients are often seen to 'purse their lips' in

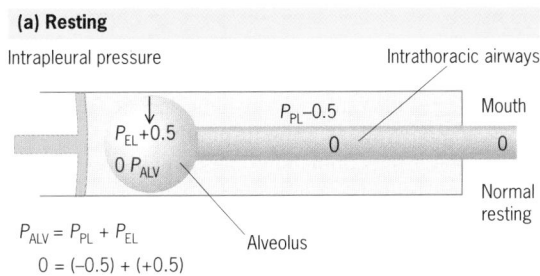

(a) Resting

$$P_{ALV} = P_{PL} + P_{EL}$$
$$0 = (-0.5) + (+0.5)$$

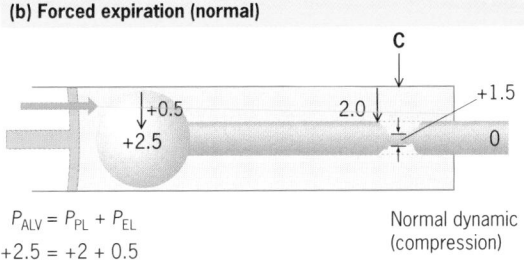

(b) Forced expiration (normal)

$$P_{ALV} = P_{PL} + P_{EL}$$
$$+2.5 = +2 + 0.5$$

Normal dynamic (compression)

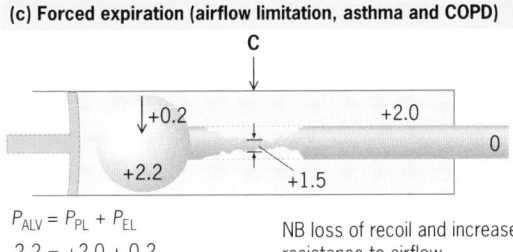

(c) Forced expiration (airflow limitation, asthma and COPD)

$$P_{ALV} = P_{PL} + P_{EL}$$
$$2.2 = +2.0 + 0.2$$

NB loss of recoil and increased resistance to airflow

Fig. 14.8 Diagrams showing ventilatory forces. (a) During resting at functional residual capacity. **(b)** During forced expiration in normal subjects. **(c)** During forced expiration in a patient with COPD. The respiratory system is represented as a piston with a single alveolus and the collapsible part of the airways within the piston (see text). C, compression point; P_{ALV}, alveolar pressure; P_{EL}, elastic recoil pressure; P_{PL}, pleural pressure.

order to increase airway pressure so that their peripheral airways do not collapse. The expiratory airflow limitation is the disordered physiology that underlies chronic airflow limitation. The measurement of the forced expiratory volume in 1 second (FEV_1) is a useful clinical index of this phenomenon.

On inspiration, the intrapleural pressure is always less than the intraluminal pressure within the intrathoracic airways, so there is no limitation to airflow with increasing effort. Inspiratory flow is limited only by the power of the inspiratory muscles.

Flow–volume loops

The relationship between maximal flow rates on expiration and inspiration is demonstrated by the maximal flow–volume (MFV) loops. Figure 14.9(a) shows this in a normal subject.

In subjects with healthy lungs the clinical importance of flow limitation will not be apparent, since maximal flow rates are rarely achieved even during vigorous exercise. However, in patients with severe COPD, limitation of expiratory flow occurs even during tidal breathing at rest (see Fig. 14.9(b)). To increase ventilation these patients have to breathe at higher lung volumes and also allow more time for expiration by increasing flow rates during inspiration, where there is relatively less flow limitation. Thus patients with severe airflow limitation have a prolonged expiratory phase to their respiration.

The measure of the volume that can be forced in from RV in 1 second (FIV_1) will always be greater than that which can be forced out from TLC in 1 second (FEV_1). Thus, the ratio of FEV_1 to FIV_1 is below 1. The only exception to this occurs when there is significant obstruction to the airways outside the thorax, such as with a tumour mass in the upper part of the trachea. Under these circumstances expiratory airway narrowing is prevented by the tracheal resistance (a situation similar to pursing the lips) and expiratory airflow becomes more effort-dependent. During forced inspiration this same resistance causes such negative intraluminal pressure that the trachea is compressed by the surrounding atmospheric pressure. Inspiratory flow thus becomes less effort-dependent, and the ratio of FEV_1 to FIV_1 becomes greater than 1. This phenomenon, and the characteristic flow–volume loop, is used to diagnose extrathoracic airways obstruction (Fig. 14.9(c)).

When obstruction occurs in large airways within the thorax (lower end of trachea and main bronchi), expiratory flow is impaired more than inspiratory flow but a characteristic plateau to expiratory flow is seen (Fig. 14.9(d)).

Ventilation and perfusion relationships

For efficient gas exchange it is important that there is a match between ventilation of the alveoli ($\dot{V}_A$) and their perfusion ($\dot{Q}$). There is a wide variation in the $\dot{V}_A/\dot{Q}$

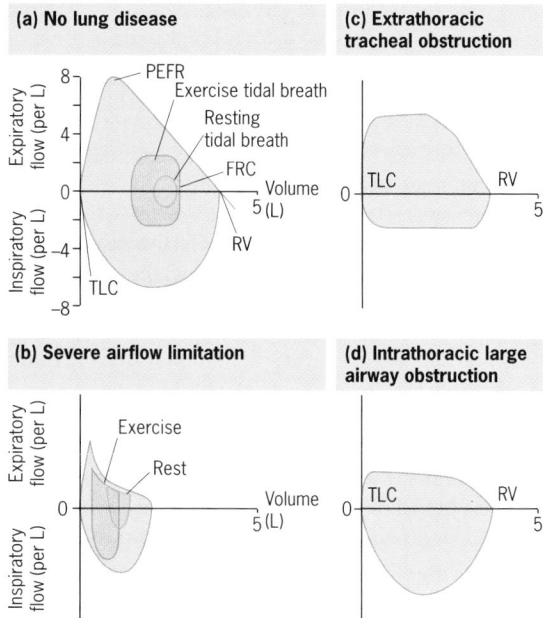

Fig. 14.9 **(a and b) Maximal flow–volume loops, showing the relationship between maximal flow rates on expiration and inspiration. (a)** In a normal subject. **(b)** In a patient with severe airflow limitation. Flow–volume loops during tidal breathing at rest (starting from the functional residual capacity (FRC)) and during exercise are also shown. The highest flow rates are achieved when forced expiration begins at total lung capacity (TLC) and represent the peak expiratory flow rate (PEFR). As air is blown out of the lung, so the flow rate decreases until no more air can be forced out, a point known as the residual volume (RV). Because inspiratory airflow is only dependent on effort, the shape of the maximal inspiratory flow–volume loop is quite different, and inspiratory flow remains at a high rate throughout the manoeuvre. **(c and d) Flow–volume loops of patients with large airway (tracheal) obstruction, showing plateauing of maximal expiratory flow high in the lung volume. (c)** Extrathoracic tracheal obstruction with a proportionally greater reduction of maximal inspiratory (as opposed to expiratory) flow rate. **(d)** Intrathoracic large airway obstruction; the expiratory plateau is more pronounced and inspiratory flow rate is less reduced than in (c). In severe airflow limitation the ventilatory demands of exercise cannot be met (cf. a and b), greatly reducing effort tolerance.

ratio throughout both normal and diseased lung. In the normal lung the extreme relationships between alveolar ventilation and perfusion are:

- ventilation with reduced perfusion (physiological deadspace)
- perfusion with reduced ventilation (physiological shunting).

These and the 'ideal' match are illustrated in Figure 14.10. In normal lungs there is a tendency for ventilation not to be matched by perfusion towards the apices, with the reverse occurring at the bases.

An increased physiological shunt results in arterial hypoxaemia. The effects of an increased physiological deadspace can usually be overcome by a compensatory

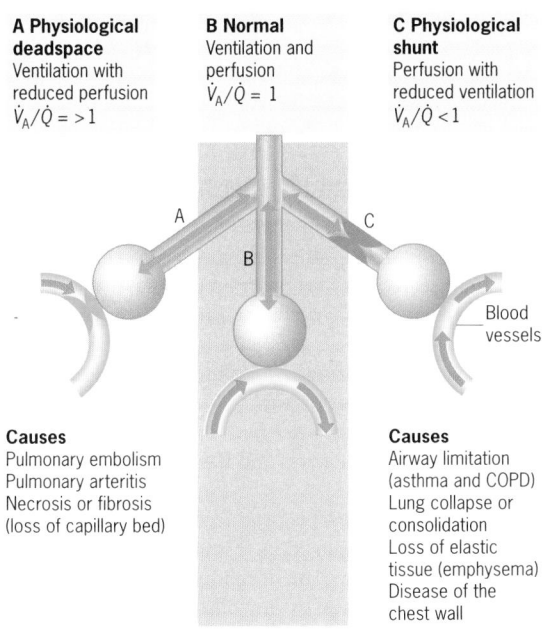

A Physiological deadspace
Ventilation with reduced perfusion
$\dot{V}_A/\dot{Q} = >1$

B Normal
Ventilation and perfusion
$\dot{V}_A/\dot{Q} = 1$

C Physiological shunt
Perfusion with reduced ventilation
$\dot{V}_A/\dot{Q} <1$

Blood vessels

Causes
Pulmonary embolism
Pulmonary arteritis
Necrosis or fibrosis
(loss of capillary bed)

Causes
Airway limitation (asthma and COPD)
Lung collapse or consolidation
Loss of elastic tissue (emphysema)
Disease of the chest wall

Fig. 14.10 **Relationships between ventilation and perfusion: a schematic diagram showing the alveolar–capillary interface.** The centre (B) shows normal ventilation and perfusion. On the left (A) there is a block in perfusion (physiological deadspace), while on the right (C) there is reduced ventilation (physiological shunting).

increase in the ventilation of normally perfused alveoli. In advanced disease this compensation cannot occur, leading to increased alveolar and arterial P_{CO_2}, together with hypoxaemia which cannot be compensated by increasing ventilation.

Hypoxaemia occurs more readily than hypercapnia because of the different ways in which oxygen and carbon dioxide are carried in the blood. Carbon dioxide can be considered to be in simple solution in the plasma, the volume carried being proportional to the partial pressure. Oxygen is carried in chemical combination with haemoglobin in the red blood cells, and the relationship between the volume carried and the partial pressure is not linear (see Fig. 15.5). Alveolar hyperventilation reduces the alveolar P_{CO_2} and diffusion leads to a proportional fall in the carbon dioxide content of the blood. However, as the haemoglobin is already saturated with oxygen, there is no significant increase in the blood oxygen content as a result of increasing the alveolar P_{O_2} through hyperventilation. The hypoxaemia of even a small amount of physiological shunting cannot therefore be compensated for by hyperventilation.

The P_aO_2 and P_aCO_2 of some individuals who have mild disease of the lung causing slight $\dot{V}_A/\dot{Q}$ mismatch may still be normal. Increasing the requirements for gas exchange by exercise will widen the $\dot{V}_A/\dot{Q}$ mismatch and the P_aO_2 will fall. $\dot{V}_A/\dot{Q}$ mismatch is by far the most common cause of arterial hypoxaemia.

Alveolar stability

The alveoli of the lung are essentially hollow spheres. Surface tension acting at the curved internal surface tends to cause the sphere to decrease in size. The surface tension within the alveoli would make the lungs extremely difficult to distend were it not for the presence of surfactant. The type II cells within the alveolus secrete an insoluble lipoprotein largely consisting of dipalmitoyl lecithin, which forms a thin monomolecular layer at the air–fluid interface. Surfactant reduces surface tension so that alveoli remain stable.

Fluid surfaces covered with surfactant exhibit a phenomenon known as hysteresis; that is, the surface-tension-lowering effect of the surfactant can be improved by a transient increase in the size of the surface area of the alveoli. During quiet breathing, small areas of the lung undergo collapse, but it is possible to re-expand these rapidly by a deep breath; hence the importance of sighs or deep breaths as a feature of normal breathing. Failure of such a mechanism – which can occur, for example, in patients with fractured ribs – gives rise to patchy basal lung collapse. Surfactant levels may be reduced in a number of diseases that cause damage to the lung (e.g. pneumonia). Lack of surfactant plays a central role in the respiratory distress syndrome of the new-born. Severe reduction in perfusion of the lung causes impairment of surfactant activity and may well account for the characteristic areas of collapse associated with pulmonary embolism.

FURTHER READING

Manning HL, Schwartzstein RM (1995) Pathology of dyspnoea. *New England Journal of Medicine* **333**: 1547–1553.

Defence mechanisms of the respiratory tract

Pulmonary disease often results from a failure of the many defence mechanisms that usually protect the lung in a healthy individual (Fig. 14.11). These can be divided into physical and physiological mechanisms and humoral and cellular mechanisms.

Physical and physiological mechanisms
Humidification
This prevents dehydration of the epithelium.

Particle removal
Over 90% of particles greater than 10 μm diameter are removed in the nostril or nasopharynx. This includes most pollen grains which are typically > 20 microns in diameter. Particles between 5–10 microns become

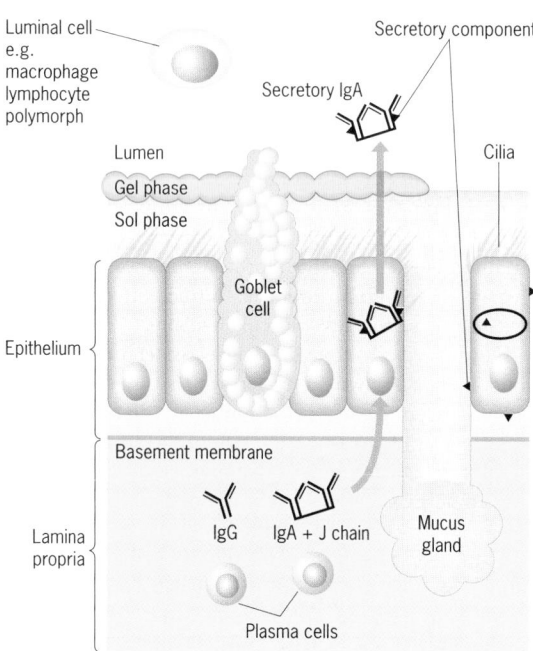

Fig. 14.11 Defence mechanisms present at the epithelial surface.

impacted in the carina. Particles smaller than 1 micron tend to remain airborne, thus the particles capable of reaching the deep lung are confined to the 1–5 micron range.

Particle expulsion
This is effected by coughing, sneezing or gagging.

Respiratory tract secretions
The mucus of the respiratory tract is a gelatinous substance consisting chiefly of acid and neutral polysaccharides. The mucus consists of a 5 mm thick gel that is relatively impermeable to water. This floats on a liquid or sol layer that is present around the cilia of the epithelial cells. The gel layer is secreted from goblet cells and mucous glands as distinct globules that coalesce increasingly in the central airways to form a more or less continuous mucus blanket. Under normal conditions the tips of the cilia are in contact with the under surface of the gel phase and coordinate their movement to push the mucus blanket upwards. Whilst it may only take 30–60 minutes for mucus to be cleared from the large bronchi, there may be a delay of several days before clearance is achieved from respiratory bronchioles. One of the major long-term effects of cigarette smoking is a reduction in mucociliary transport. This contributes to recurrent infection and in the larger airways it prolongs contact with carcinogens. Air pollutants, local and general anaesthetics and bacterial and viral infections also reduce mucociliary clearance.

Congenital defects in mucociliary transport occur. In the *'immotile cilia'* syndrome there is an absence of the

dynein arms in the cilia themselves, and in *cystic fibrosis* an abnormal mucus is associated with ciliary dyskinesia. Both diseases are characterized by recurrent infections and eventually with the development of bronchiectasis.

Humoral and cellular mechanisms

Non-specific soluble factors
- *α₁-Antitrypsin* ($α_1$-antiprotease, see p. 864) is present in lung secretions derived from plasma. It inhibits chymotrypsin and trypsin and neutralizes proteases and elastase.
- *Lysozyme* is an enzyme found in granulocytes that has bactericidal properties.
- *Lactoferrin* is synthesized from epithelial cells and neutrophil granulocytes and has bactericidal properties.
- *Interferon* (see p. 197) is produced by most cells in response to viral infection. It is a potent modulator of lymphocyte function. It renders other cells resistant to infection by any other virus.
- *Complement* is present in secretions and is derived by diffusion from plasma. In association with antibodies, it plays an important cytotoxic role.
- *Surfactant protein* A (SP$_A$) is one of four species of surfactant proteins which opsonizes bacteria/particles, enhancing phagocytosis by macrophages.
- *Defensins* are bactericidal peptides present in the azurophil granules of neutrophils.

Pulmonary alveolar macrophages
These are derived from precursors in the bone marrow and migrate to the lungs via the bloodstream. They phagocytose particles, including bacteria, and are removed by the mucociliary escalator, lymphatics and bloodstream. They are the dominant cell in the airways at the level of the alveoli and comprise 90% of all cells obtained by bronchoalveolar lavage.

Alveolar macrophages work principally as scavengers and are not particularly good at presenting antigens to the immune system. Dendritic cells form a network throughout the airways and are thought to be the key antigen-presenting cell in the airway.

Lymphoid tissue (see also p. 199)
The lung contains large numbers of lymphocytes which are scattered throughout the airways. In animals, aggregates of bronchus-associated lymphoid tissue (BALT) can be identified but these are not normally found in humans. Sensitized lymphocytes contribute to local immunity through differentiation into IgA-secreting plasma cells. IgG and IgE are found in low concentrations in airway secretions from a combination of local and systemic production.

In addition to these resident cells, the lung has the usual range of acute inflammatory responses and can mobilize neutrophils promptly in response to injury or infection (see p. 192) and play a major part in inflammatory conditions such as asthma (p. 878).

FURTHER READING

Stockley RA (1998) Role of bacteria in the pathogenesis and progression of acute and chronic lung infection. *Thorax* **53**: 58–62.

Wanner A, Salathé M, O'Riordan TG (1996) Mucociliary clearance in the airways. *American Journal of Respiratory and Critical Care Medicine* **154**: 1868–1882.

Symptoms

Runny, blocked nose and sneezing

Nasal symptoms are extremely common. The differentiation between the common cold or allergic rhinitis as a cause of 'runny nose' (rhinorrhoea), nasal blockage and attacks of sneezing is difficult. In allergic rhinitis, symptoms may be seasonal, following contact with grass pollen, or perennial, when the house-dust mite is the important allergen. Colds are frequent during the winter but, if more than three occur, the patient is probably suffering from perennial rhinitis rather than from infection due to a virus. Patients may be able to identify the cause of their symptoms if, for example, they sneeze whilst walking in the park in summer or after making beds.

Nasal secretions are usually thin and runny in rhinitis but thicker and yellowish green in the common cold. Nose bleeds and blood-stained nasal discharge are common occurrences and are not as serious as haemoptysis. Nevertheless, a blood-stained nasal discharge associated with nasal obstruction and pain may be the presenting feature of a nasal tumour. Total nasal blockage with loss of smell is often a feature of nasal polyps.

Cough

Cough is the most common manifestation of lower respiratory tract disease. Smokers often have a morning cough with little sputum. Cough is the cardinal feature of chronic bronchitis, while sputum production and coughing, particularly at night, can be symptoms of asthma. Cough also occurs in asthmatics after mild exertion or following a forced expiration. A cough can also occur for psychological reasons.

A worsening cough is the most common presenting symptom of a bronchial carcinoma. The explosive character of a normal cough is lost when laryngeal paralysis is present – a bovine cough – usually resulting from carcinoma of the bronchus infiltrating the left recurrent laryngeal nerve. Cough may be accompanied by stridor in whooping cough and in the presence of laryngeal or tracheal obstruction.

Cough may persist in some individuals for many weeks following a respiratory tract infection, perhaps as the result of persisting bronchial inflammation and increased airway responsiveness, a process that may settle with inhaled corticosteroid treatment.

Sputum

Approximately 100 mL of mucus is produced daily in a healthy, non-smoking individual. This flows at a regular pace up the airways, through the larynx, and is swallowed. Excess mucus is expectorated as sputum. The most common cause of excess mucus production is cigarette smoking.

Mucoid sputum is clear and white but can contain black specks resulting from the inhalation of carbon. Yellow or green sputum is due to the presence of cellular material, including bronchial epithelial cells, or neutrophil or eosinophil granulocytes. Yellow sputum is not necessarily due to infection, as eosinophils in the sputum, as seen in asthma, can give the same appearance. The production of large quantities of yellow or green sputum is characteristic of bronchiectasis.

Haemoptysis (blood-stained sputum) varies from small streaks of blood to massive bleeding. The following should be borne in mind.

- The most common cause of haemoptysis is acute infection, particularly in exacerbations of chronic obstructive pulmonary disease (COPD) but it should not be attributed to this without investigation.
- Other common causes are pulmonary infarction, bronchial carcinoma and tuberculosis.
- In lobar pneumonia, the sputum is rusty in appearance when blood is present.
- Pink, frothy sputum is seen in pulmonary oedema.
- In bronchiectasis, the blood is often mixed with purulent sputum.
- Massive haemoptyses (> 200 mL of blood in 24 hours) are usually due to bronchiectasis or tuberculosis.
- Uncommon causes of haemoptyses are idiopathic pulmonary haemosiderosis, Goodpasture's syndrome, microscopic polyangiitis, trauma, blood disorders and benign tumours.

Haemoptysis should always be investigated. Often, the diagnosis can be made from a chest X-ray.

Firm plugs of sputum may be coughed up by patients suffering from an exacerbation of allergic bronchopulmonary aspergillosis. Sometimes such sputum may appear as firm threads representing casts from inflamed bronchi.

Breathlessness (Table 14.1)

Breathlessness should be assessed in relation to the patient's lifestyle. For example, a moderate degree of breathlessness may be totally disabling if the patient has to climb many flights of stairs to reach home. A grading for breathlessness is given on page 707.

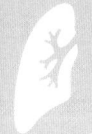

Table 14.1
Respiratory sensations described by patients with different chest diseases

Sensation	Asthma	Chronic obstructive pulmonary disease (COPD)	Pulmonary fibrosis	Chest wall disease	Congestive heart failure	Pulmonary vascular disease
Rapid breathing					√	√
Shallow breathing	√					
Incomplete exhalation	√					
Increased effort	√	√	√	√		
Feeling of suffocation (heavy breathing)	√	√				
Chest tightness	√					

Dyspnoea should be used to describe a sense of awareness of increased respiratory effort that is unpleasant and that is recognized by the patient as being inappropriate. It is highly unlikely that this term will be used by the patient. Patients may complain of tightness in the chest; this must be differentiated from angina. Respiratory sensations described by patients with different chest diseases are shown in Table 14.1.

Orthopnoea (see p. 707) is breathlessness on lying down and is partly due to the weight of the abdominal contents pushing the diaphragm further into the thorax. Such patients are also made uncomfortable by bending over.

Tachypnoea and hyperpnoea refer, respectively, to an increased rate of breathing and an increased level of ventilation, which may be appropriate to the situation (e.g. during exercise).

Hyperventilation is inappropriate overbreathing. This may occur at rest or on exertion and results in a lowering of the alveolar and arterial $P\text{CO}_2$ (see p. 1251).

Paroxysmal nocturnal dyspnoea is described on page 707.

Wheezing

Wheezing is a common complaint and is the result of airflow limitation due to any cause. The symptom of wheezing is not diagnostic of asthma; it may be absent in the early stages of this disease, and may also occur in patients with bronchiolitis or chronic obstructive pulmonary disease.

Chest pain

The most common type of chest pain encountered in respiratory disease is a localized sharp pain, often referred to as pleuritic. It is made worse by deep breathing or coughing and can be precisely localized by the patient. Localized anterior chest pain may be accompanied by tenderness of a costochondral junction as a symptom of costochondritis. Pain in the shoulder tips suggests irritation of the diaphragmatic pleura, whereas central chest pain radiating to the neck and arms is typically of cardiac origin. Retrosternal soreness may occur in patients with tracheitis, and a constant, severe, dull pain may be the result of invasion of the thoracic wall by carcinoma.

FURTHER READING

Irwin RS, Madison JM (2000) The diagnosis and treatment of cough. *New England Journal of Medicine* **343**: 1715–1721.

Pasterkamp H, Kraman SS, Wodicka GR (1997) Respiratory sounds. Advances beyond the stethoscope. *American Journal of Respiratory and Critical Care Medicine* **156**: 974–987.

Examination of the respiratory system

The nose

The anterior part of the nose can be examined using a nasal speculum and light source. In allergic rhinitis the mucosa lining the nasal septum and inferior turbinate appear swollen and a dark red or plum colour. Nasal polyps can also be identified, as can a frequent site of nasal haemorrhage (Little's area).

The chest (Table 14.2)

Examination of the chest

Inspection

Look for mental alertness, cyanosis, breathlessness at rest, use of accessory muscles and any deformity or scars on the chest. A coarse tremor or flap of the outstretched hands indicates CO_2 intoxication. Prominent veins on the chest may imply obstruction of the superior vena cava. The jugular venous pressure should be assessed and the respiratory rate counted in selected cases. Reduced movement of one side of the chest, over-expansion of the chest and intercostal indrawing with large changes in respiratory pressure are additional features.

Table 14.2
Physical signs of respiratory disease

Pathological process	Chest wall movement	Mediastinal displacement	Percussion note	Breath sounds	Vocal resonance	Added sounds
Consolidation (i.e. lobar pneumonia)	Reduced on affected side	None	Dull	Bronchial	Increased	Fine crackles
Collapse Major bronchus	Reduced on affected side	Towards lesion	Dull	Diminished or absent	Reduced or absent	None
Peripheral bronchus	Reduced on affected side	Towards lesion	Dull	Bronchial	Increased	Fine crackles
Fibrosis Localized	Reduced on affected side	Towards lesion	Dull	Bronchial	Increased	Coarse crackles
Generalized (e.g. cryptogenic fibrosing alveolitis)	Reduced on both sides	None	Normal	Vesicular	Increased	Fine crackles
Pleural effusion (> 500 mL)	Reduced on affected side	Away from lesion (in massive effusion)	Stony dull	Vesicular reduced or absent	Reduced or absent	None
Large pneumothorax	Reduced on affected side	Away from lesion	Normal or hyperresonant	Reduced or absent	Reduced or absent	None
Asthma	Reduced on both sides	None	Normal	Vesicular Prolonged expiration	Normal	Expiratory polyphonic wheeze
Chronic obstructive pulmonary disease	Reduced on both sides	None	Normal	Vesicular Prolonged expiration	Normal	Expiratory polyphonic wheeze and coarse crackles

Cyanosis (see p. 709) is a dusky colour of the skin and mucous membranes, owing to the presence of more than 5 g/dL of desaturated haemoglobin. When due to central causes, cyanosis is visible on the tongue (especially the underside) and lips, and indicates a P_aO_2 below 6 kPa. Patients with central cyanosis will also be cyanosed peripherally. Peripheral cyanosis without central cyanosis is caused by a reduced peripheral circulation and is noted on the fingernails and skin of the extremities with associated coolness of the skin.

Finger clubbing is present when the normal angle between the base of the nail and the nail fold is lost. The base of the nail is fluctuant owing to increased vascularity, and there is an increased curvature of the nail in all directions, with expansion of the end of the digit. Some causes of clubbing are given in Table 14.3. Clubbing is not seen in COPD.

Palpation and percussion

The position of the trachea is assessed by placing a finger in the suprasternal notch. The position of the apex beat is noted and the supraclavicular fossa is examined for enlarged lymph nodes. The distance between the sternal notch and the cricoid cartilage (three to four finger breadths in full expiration) is reduced in patients with severe airflow limitation. Chest expansion should be assessed by palpation. A tape measure may be used if

Table 14.3
Some causes of finger clubbing

Respiratory
Bronchial carcinoma, especially epidermoid (squamous cell) type (major cause)
Chronic suppurative lung disease
  Bronchiectasis
  Lung abscess
  Empyema
Pulmonary fibrosis (e.g. cryptogenic fibrosing alveolitis)
Pleural and mediastinal tumours (e.g. mesothelioma)
Cryptogenic organizing pneumonia

Cardiovascular
Cyanotic heart disease
Subacute infective endocarditis

Miscellaneous
Congenital – no disease
Cirrhosis
Inflammatory bowel disease

precise measurements are needed, e.g. in ankylosing spondylitis. Local discomfort over the sternochondral joints may suggest costochondritis. Compression of the chest laterally and anteroposteriorly may produce localized pain suggestive of a rib fracture. *Percussion* should be performed symmetrically on both sides for comparison. The clavicle should be percussed routinely. Liver dullness is usually detected anteriorly at the level of the sixth rib. Liver and cardiac dullness are lost with over-inflated lungs. The percussion note is dull over consolidation and stony dull over a pleural effusion.

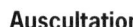

Auscultation

The diaphragm of the stethoscope should be used, although the bell may be useful for hairy chests. The patient is asked to take deep breaths through the mouth. Inspiration sounds more prolonged than expiration. Healthy lungs filter off most of the high-frequency component, which is mainly due to turbulent flow in the larynx. Normal breath sounds are harsher anteriorly over the upper lobes (particularly on the right) and described as vesicular. Vesicular sounds may be loud in a thin healthy subject or soft in patients with emphysema. Breath sounds are reduced or absent in a pneumothorax, over a pleural effusion, or when the bronchus to a lobe is obstructed by a carcinoma.

Bronchial breathing

These abnormal breath sounds are heard best over consolidated or collapsed lung and sometimes over areas of localized fibrosis or bronchiectasis. Such areas conduct the high-frequency hissing component of breath sounds well. Characteristically, the noise heard during inspiration and expiration is equally long but separated by a short silent phase. Bronchial breathing can be imitated by listening over the larynx, particularly if the subject breathes with the vocal cords in a position to sound a whispered 'eee'. Whispering pectoriloquy (whispered, higher-pitched, sounds heard distinctly through a stethoscope) invariably accompanies bronchial breathing.

Added sounds

The terms 'rhonchi', 'rales' and 'crepitations' have been replaced with the simple terms wheezes and crackles.

Wheeze. Wheeze is usually heard during expiration and results from vibrations in the collapsible part of the airways when apposition occurs as a result of the flow-limiting mechanisms. Wheezes are heard in asthma and in chronic obstructive pulmonary disease, but are not invariably present. In the most severe cases of asthma a wheeze may not be heard, as the airflow may be insufficient to generate the sound. Wheezes may be monophonic (single large airway obstruction) or polyphonic (narrowing of many small airways). An end-inspiratory (as opposed to expiratory) 'squeak' may be heard in obliterative bronchiolitis.

Crackles. These brief crackling sounds are probably produced by opening of previously closed bronchioles, and their timing during breathing is of significance – early inspiratory crackles are associated with diffuse airflow limitation, whereas late inspiratory crackles are characteristically heard in pulmonary oedema, fibrosis of the lung and bronchiectasis. They may be described as fine or coarse.

Pleural rub. This is a creaking or groaning sound that is usually well localized. It is indicative of inflammation and roughening of the pleural surfaces, which normally glide silently over one another.

Vocal resonance. Healthy lung attenuates high-frequency notes, leaving the booming low-pitched components of speech. Consolidated lung has the reverse effect, transmitting the high frequencies; the spoken word then takes on a bleating quality. Whispered (and therefore high-pitched) speech can barely be heard over healthy lung, whereas consolidation allows its clear transmission. Sonorous sounds such as 'ninety-nine' are well transmitted across healthy lung to produce vibration that can be felt over the chest wall. Consolidated lung transmits these low-frequency noises less well, and pleural fluid severely dampens or obliterates the vibrations altogether. Tactile vocal fremitus is the palpation of this vibration, usually by placing the edge of the hand on the chest wall. For all practical purposes this duplicates the assessment of vocal resonance and is no longer considered a routine part of the chest examination.

Additional bedside tests

Since so many patients with respiratory disease have airflow limitation, airflow should be routinely measured at the bedside using a peak flow meter or spirometer. This will provide a much more accurate assessment of airflow limitation than any physical sign.

Investigation of respiratory disease

Haematological and biochemical tests

It is useful to measure:

- haemoglobin, to detect the presence of anaemia or polycythaemia
- packed cell volume (secondary polycythaemia occurs with chronic hypoxia)
- routine biochemistry (often disturbed in carcinoma and infection).

Other blood investigations sometimes required include α_1-antitrypsin levels, *Aspergillus* antibodies, viral and mycoplasma cytology, autoantibody profiles and specific IgE measurements.

Sputum

Sputum should be inspected for colour:

- yellowish green indicates inflammation (infection or allergy)
- the presence of blood suggests neoplasm or pulmonary infarct.

Microbiological studies (Gram stain and culture) are not helpful in upper respiratory tract infections or in acute or chronic bronchitis. They are of value in:

- pneumonia
- the diagnosis of tuberculosis (Ziehl–Nielsen stain)
- unusual clinical problems
- *Aspergillus* lung disease.

Cytology

This is extremely useful in the diagnosis of bronchial carcinoma. Advantages are:

- a quick result
- cheapness
- it is non-invasive.

However, its value depends on the production of sputum and the presence of a reliable cytologist. Sputum can be induced following the inhalation of nebulized hypertonic saline (5%). This is unpleasant and for important samples it is better to proceed to transtracheal aspiration or more usually bronchoscopy and bronchial washings (see p. 853).

Transtracheal aspiration

This technique involves pushing a needle through the cricothyroid membrane, through which a catheter is threaded to a position just above the carina. This procedure induces coughing, and specimens are collected by aspiration or by the introduction and subsequent aspiration of sterile saline. It is an excellent technique (although not often required) for assessing infection in the lower respiratory tract because it avoids contamination of the specimen with bacteria from the pharynx and mouth.

Imaging

Radiology is an essential part of examination of the chest. Diseases such as tuberculosis or lung cancer may not be detectable on clinical examination but are obvious on the chest X-ray. Conversely, the abnormal physical signs in asthma or chronic bronchitis may be associated with a normal chest X-ray.

Chest X-ray

The following must be taken into account when viewing films:

- *Centring of the film.* The distance between each clavicular head and the spinal processes should be equal.
- *Penetration.*
- *The view.* Routine films are taken P–A, i.e. the film is placed in front of the patient with the X-ray source behind. Anteroposterior (AP) films are taken only in very ill patients who are unable to stand up and be taken to the radiology department; the cardiac outline appears bigger and the scapulae cannot be moved out of the way.

The following should be noted:

- the shape and bony structure of the chest wall
- whether the trachea is central
- whether the diaphragm is elevated or flat
- the shape, size and position of the heart
- the shape and size of the hilar shadows
- the vascular shadowing and the size and shape of any abnormalities of the lungs.

X-ray abnormalities

Collapse and consolidation

A chest X-ray showing collapse of a whole lung is shown in Figure 14.12 and causes are shown in Table 14.4. Loss of volume in the relevant hemithorax should raise the possibility of lobar collapse. The lung lobes collapse in characteristic directions. The lower lobes collapse downward and towards the mediastinum, the left upper lobe collapses forwards against the anterior chest wall, while the right upper lobe collapses upwards and outwards, forming the appearance of an arch over the remaining lung. The right middle lobe collapses anteriorly and inward, obscuring the right heart border. If a whole lung collapses, the mediastinum will shift towards the side of the collapse. Consolidated lobes remain the same size, and uncomplicated consolidation should not cause mediastinal shift or loss of lung volume.

Pleural effusion (see Fig. 14.44)

Pleural effusions need to be more than 500 mL to cause much more than blunting of the costophrenic angle. On an erect film they produce a characteristic shadow with

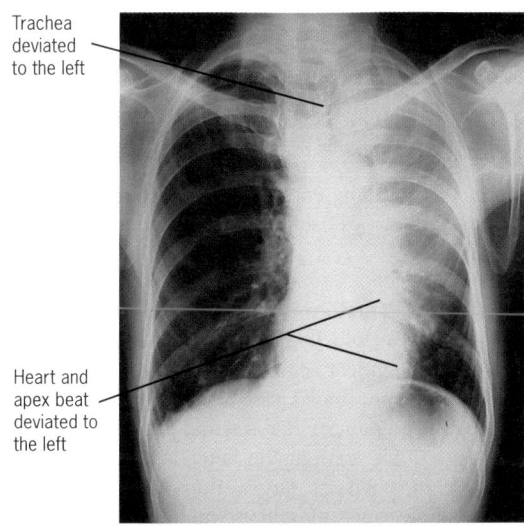

Trachea deviated to the left

Heart and apex beat deviated to the left

Fig. 14.12 Collapse of the left lung. Chest X-ray showing a raised left diaphragm and compensatory emphysema of the right lung.

Table 14.4
Causes of collapse of the lung

Enlarged tracheobronchial lymph nodes due to: Malignant disease Tuberculosis	Bronchial casts or plugs (e.g. allergic bronchopulmonary aspergillosis)
Inhaled foreign bodies (e.g. peanuts) in children, usually in the right main bronchus	Retained secretions – postoperatively and in debilitated patients

Table 14.5
Causes of round shadows (> 3 cm) in the lung

Carcinoma	Aspergilloma
Metastatic tumours (usually multiple shadows)	Rheumatoid nodules
	Tuberculoma (may be calcification within the lesion)
Lung abscess (usually with fluid level)	
	Rare causes:
Encysted interlobar effusion (usually in horizontal fissure)	Bronchial carcinoid
	Cylindroma
	Chondroma
Hydatid cysts (rare and often with a fluid level)	Lipoma
Arteriovenous malformations (usually adjacent to a vascular shadow)	Other shadows related to mediastinum:
	Pericardium ⎫ Seen on
	Oesophagus ⎬ lateral
	Spinal cord ⎭ chest X-ray

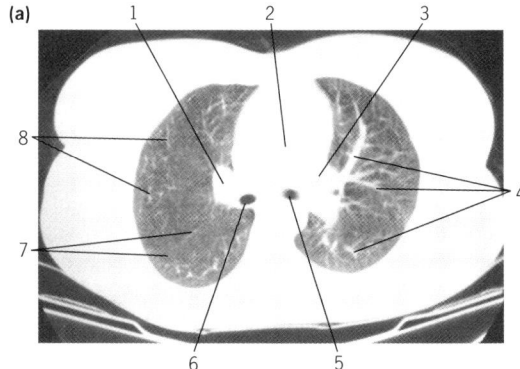

a curved upper edge rising into the axilla. If very large, the whole of one side of the thorax may be opaque, with shift of the mediastinum to the opposite side.

Fibrosis
Localized fibrosis causes streaky shadowing, and the accompanying loss of lung volume causes mediastinal structures to move to the same side. More generalized fibrosis in the lung can lead to a honeycomb appearance (see p. 904), seen as diffuse shadows containing multiple circular translucencies a few millimetres in diameter.

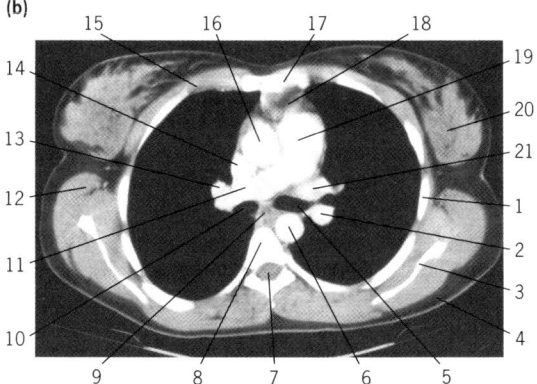

Round shadows
Lung cancer is the commonest cause of large round shadows but many other causes are recognized (Table 14.5).

Miliary mottling
This term describes numerous minute opacities, 1–3 mm in size, which are caused by many pathological processes. The most common causes are miliary tuberculosis, pneumoconiosis, sarcoidosis, fibrosing alveolitis (idiopathic pulmonary fibrosis) and pulmonary oedema (see Fig. 13.15), though the latter is usually perihilar and accompanied by larger, fluffy shadows. A rare but striking cause of miliary mottling is pulmonary microlithiasis.

Computed tomography

Modern CT scanners provide excellent images of the lungs and mediastinal structures. Different settings are required to show the parenchymal tissue and the central structures (Fig. 14.13). Mediastinal structures may be shown more clearly by injecting intravenous contrast medium to enhance the vascular structures.

The advent of rapid *volumetric* or *'spiral' scanning* means that scans can be obtained rapidly (within seconds) during contrast injection. This is a useful technique for directly demonstrating pulmonary emboli within pulmonary vessels. *Conventional CT* is valuable

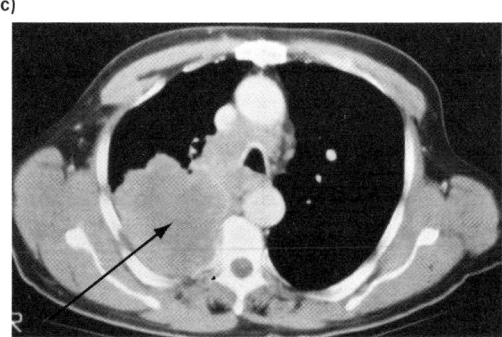

Fig. 14.13 **CT scan of the lung.**
(a) Lung setting – showing normal lung markings. 1, right hilum; 2, mediastinum; 3, left hilum; 4, lung vessels; 5, L. main bronchus; 6, R. main bronchus; 7, position of oblique fissure; 8, peripheral lung vessels.
(b) Mediastinal (soft tissue) setting – showing normal mediastinal structures following intravenous contrast enhancement. 1, rib; 2, descending L. pulmonary artery; 3, scapula; 4, subcutaneous fat; 5, L. main bronchus; 6, descending aorta; 7, spinal canal; 8, vertebral body; 9, oesophagus; 10, R. main bronchus; 11, R. pulmonary artery; 12, muscle; 13, R. superior pulmonary vein; 14, superior vena cava; 15, costal cartilage; 16, ascending aorta; 17, sternum; 18, thymic remnant; 19, pulmonary trunk; 20, breast tissue; 21, L. superior pulmonary vein.
(c) Post-contrast scan showing large right upper zone carcinoma with enlarged lymph nodes in the mediastinum surrounding the trachea.

in bronchial carcinoma staging to demonstrate mediastinal, pleural or chest wall invasion and to determine operability.

Enlarged mediastinal nodes (> 1 cm) may be either malignant or reactive and may require biopsy. Scanning should include assessment of liver, adrenals and brain, which are likely sites for metastatic disease.

High-resolution CT scanning (sampling lung parenchyma with 1–2 mm thickness scans at 10–20 mm intervals) allows assessment of diffuse lung parenchymal processes, particularly interstitial disease. It is valuable in the following situations:

- Detection of diffuse interstitial pulmonary involvement in any type of interstitial lung disease, including sarcoidosis, cryptogenic and extrinsic allergic alveolitis, occupational lung disease, and any other form of interstitial pulmonary fibrosis.
- Bronchiectasis. High-resolution CT has a sensitivity and specificity of greater than 90%. Inspiratory and expiratory scans may allow demonstration of air trapping in small airway disease. This technique has replaced bronchography.
- Distinguishing emphysema from interstitial lung disease or pulmonary vascular disease as a cause of a low gas transfer factor with otherwise normal lung function
- Diagnosis of lymphangitis carcinomatosa.

Magnetic resonance imaging

Problems with motion artefact, both respiratory and cardiac, make magnetic resonance imaging (MRI) less valuable than CT in assessment of lung parenchyma. In the mediastinum, MRI is becoming the investigation of choice for assessing vascular and solid masses. The use of ECG-gating allows accurate images of the heart and aortic aneurysms to be obtained. The main strength of MRI in staging lung cancer is for assessing tumour invasion in the mediastinum, chest wall and particularly at the lung apex, by virtue of its ability to produce good images in the sagittal and coronal planes. Vascular structures can be clearly differentiated as flowing blood produces a signal void on MR.

Scintigraphic imaging

This technique is used widely for the detection of pulmonary emboli.

Perfusion scan

Macro-aggregated human albumin labelled with technetium-99m is injected intravenously. The particles are of such a size that they impact in pulmonary capillaries, where they remain for a few hours. A gamma camera is then used to detect the position of the macro-aggregated human albumin. The resultant pattern indicates the distribution of pulmonary blood flow; cold areas occur where there is defective blood flow (e.g. in pulmonary emboli).

Ventilation–perfusion scan (see p. 805)

Xenon-133 gas is inhaled into the lung and its distribution is detected at the same time as the perfusion scan. Using the two scans, a pulmonary embolus can be seen to cause a striking diminution of perfusion relative to ventilation. Other lung diseases (e.g. asthma or pneumonia) impair both ventilation and perfusion. Unfortunately, however, a pulmonary embolus often produces substantial changes in the lung substance (e.g. atelectasis) so that such a clear distinction is not always obvious. Nevertheless, this is a better technique than perfusion scan alone.

Respiratory function tests (Table 14.6)

In clinical practice, airflow limitation can be assessed by relatively simple tests that have good intra-subject repeatability. Normal values are required for their interpretation since these tests vary considerably, not only with sex, age and height, but also within individuals of the same age, sex and height. The standard deviation about the mean for a group of individuals is therefore very high; for example, the standard deviation for the peak expiratory flow rate is approximately 50 L/min, and for the FEV_1 it is approximately 0.4 L. Repeated measurements of lung function are useful for assessing the progression of disease in an individual patient.

Tests of ventilatory function

These tests are used mainly to assess the degree of airflow limitation present during expiration.

Peak expiratory flow rate (PEFR)

This is an extremely simple and cheap test. Subjects are asked to take a full inspiration to total lung capacity and then blow out forcefully into the peak flow meter (Fig. 14.14), which is held horizontally. The lips must be placed tightly around the mouthpiece. The best of three tests is recorded.

Although reproducible, PEFR is not a good measure of airflow limitation since it measures the expiratory flow rate only in the first 2 ms of expiration and overestimates lung function in patients with moderate airflow limitation. PEFR is best used to monitor progression of disease and its treatment. Regular measurements of peak flow rates on waking, during the afternoon, and before bed demonstrate the wide diurnal variations in airflow limitation that characterize asthma and allow an objective assessment of treatment to be made (Fig. 14.15).

Spirometry

The spirometer measures the FEV_1 and the forced vital capacity (FVC). Both the FEV_1 and FVC are related to height, age and sex. The technique involves a maximum inspiration followed by a forced expiration (for as long as possible) into the spirometer. The act of expiration triggers the moving record chart, which measures volume against time. The record chart moves for a total

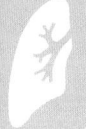

Table 14.6
Respiratory function tests and exercise tests

Test	Use	Advantages	Disadvantages
PEFR	Monitoring changes in airflow limitation in asthma	Portable Can be used at the bedside	Effort-dependent Poor measure of chronic airflow limitation
FEV, FVC, FEV$_1$/FVC	Assessment of airflow limitation The best single test	Reproducible Relatively effort-independent	Bulky equipment but smaller portable machines available
Flow–volume curves	Assessment of flow at lower lung volumes Detection of large airway obstruction both intra- and extrathoracic (e.g. tracheal stenosis, tumour)	Recognition of patterns of flow–volume curves for different diseases	Sophisticated equipment needed for full test but expiratory loop now possible with compact spirometry
Airways resistance	Assessment of airflow limitation	Sensitive	Technique difficult to perform
Lung volumes	Differentiation between restrictive and obstructive lung disease	Effort independent, complements FEV$_1$	Sophisticated equipment needed
Gas transfer	Assessment and monitoring of extent of interstitial lung disease and emphysema	Non-invasive (compared with lung biopsy or radiation from repeated chest X-rays and CT)	Sophisticated equipment needed
Blood gases	Assessment of respiratory failure	Can detect early lung disease when measured during exercise	Invasive
Pulse oximetry	Postoperative, sleep studies and respiratory failure	Continuous monitoring Non-invasive	Measures saturation only
Exercise tests (6 min walk)	Practical assessment for disability and effects of therapy	No equipment required	Time-consuming Learning effect At least two walks required
Cardiorespiratory assessment	Early detection of lung/heart disease Fitness assessment	Differentiates breathlessness due to lung or heart disease	Expensive and complicated equipment required

(a) Peak flow meter

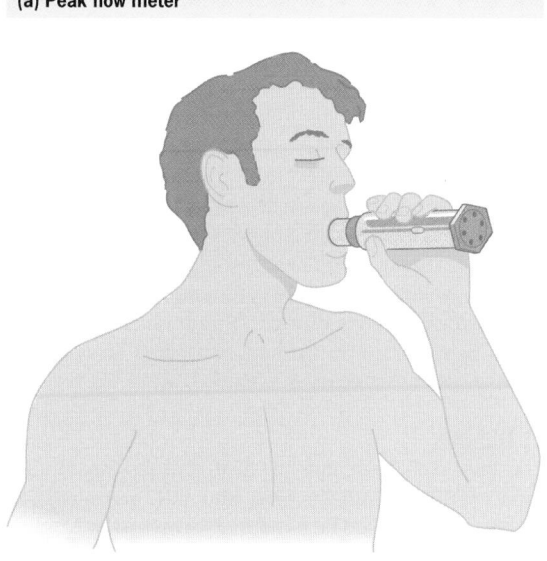

(b) Graph of normal readings

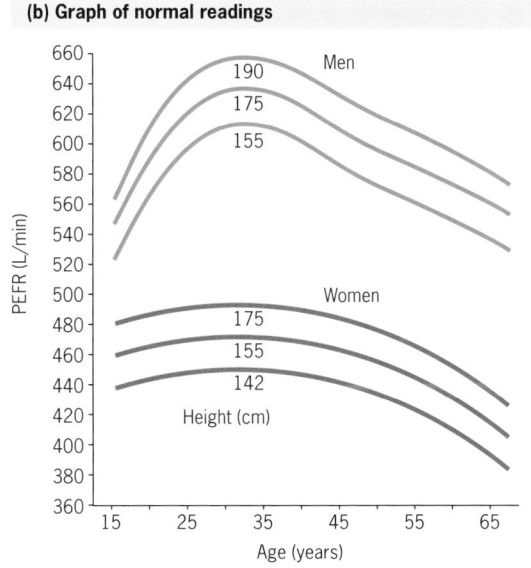

Fig. 14.14 Peak flow measurements. (a) Peak flow meter: the lips should be tight around the mouthpiece. **(b)** Graph of normal readings for men and women.

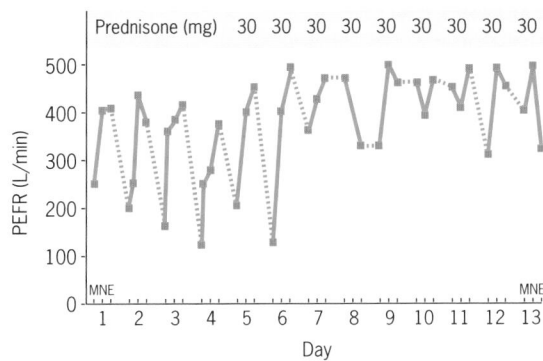

Fig. 14.15 Diurnal variability in airflow limitation, showing the effect of steroids. M, morning; N, noon; E, evening.

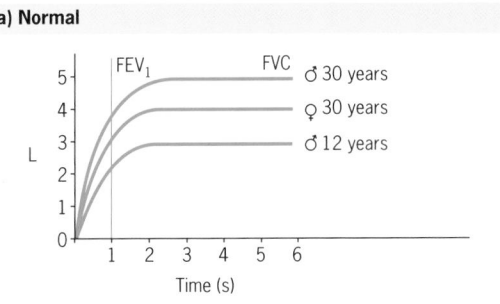

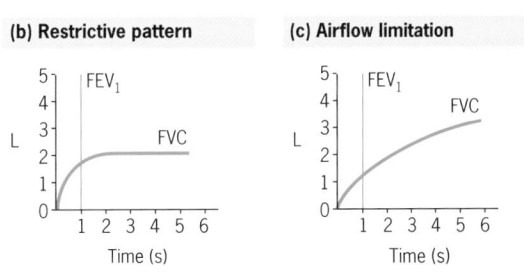

Fig. 14.16 Spirometry. Graphs showing **(a)** normal patterns for age and sex, **(b)** restrictive pattern (FEV_1 and FVC reduced), **(c)** airflow limitation (FEV_1 only reduced).

of 5 s, but expiration should continue until all the air has been expelled from the lungs, as patients with severe airflow limitation may have a very prolonged forced expiratory time. This is demonstrated on the record chart in Figure 14.16.

The FEV_1 expressed as a percentage of the FVC is an excellent measure of airflow limitation. In normal subjects it is around 75%. With *increasing airflow limitation* the FEV_1 falls proportionately more than the FVC, so that the FEV_1/FVC ratio is reduced. With *restrictive lung disease* the FEV_1 and the FVC are reduced in the same proportion and the FEV_1/FVC ratio remains normal or may even increase because of the enhanced elastic recoil.

In chronic airflow limitation (particularly in emphysema and asthma) the total lung capacity (TLC) is usually increased, yet there is nearly always some reduction in the FVC. This is the result of disease in the small airways causing obstruction to airflow before the normal RV is reached. This trapping of air within the lung (giving an increased RV) is a characteristic feature of these diseases.

Other tests

Tests such as the measurement of airways resistance in a body plethysmograph are more sensitive but the equipment is expensive and the necessary manoeuvres are too exhausting for many patients with chronic airflow limitation.

Flow–volume loops

The ability to measure flow rates against volume (flow–volume loops, see Fig. 14.9) enables a more sophisticated analysis to be made of the site of airflow limitation within the lung. At the start of expiration from TLC, the site of maximum resistance is the large airways, and this accounts for the flow reduction in the first 25% of the curve. As the lung volume reduces further, so the elastic pressures within the lung holding open the smaller airways reduce, and disease of the lung parenchyma or the small airways themselves becomes apparent. For example, in diseases such as chronic obstructive pulmonary disease (COPD), where the brunt of the disease falls upon the smaller airways, expiratory flow rates at 50% or 25% of the vital capacity may be disproportionately reduced when compared with flow rates at larger lung volumes.

Lung volume

The subdivisions of the lung volume are shown in Figure 14.17. Tidal volume and vital capacity can be measured using a simple spirometer, but the TLC and RV need to be measured by an alternative technique. TLC is measured by connecting the lungs to a reservoir containing a known amount of non-absorbable gas (helium) that can readily be measured. If the concentration of the gas in the reservoir is known at the start of the test and is measured after equilibration of the gas has occurred (when the patient has breathed in and out of the reservoir), the dilution of the gas will reflect the TLC. This technique is known as *helium dilution*. RV can be calculated by subtracting the vital capacity from the TLC.

The TLC measured using this technique is inaccurate if large cystic spaces are present in the lung, because the helium cannot diffuse into them. Under these circumstances the thoracic gas volume can be measured more accurately using a body plethysmograph. The difference between the two measurements can be used to define the extent of non-communicating air space within the lungs.

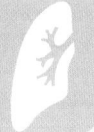

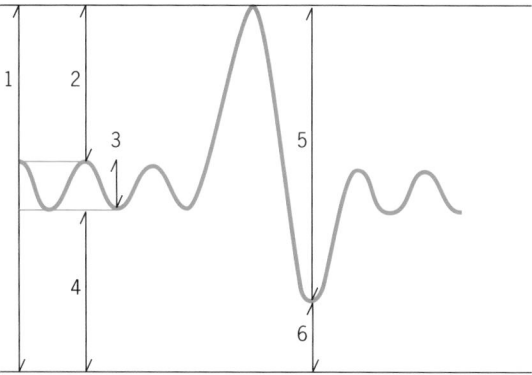

1 Total lung capacity   4 Functional residual capacity
2 Inspiratory reserve volume   5 Vital capacity
3 Tidal volume   6 Residual volume

Fig. 14.17 **The subdivisions of the lung volume.**

Transfer factor

This measures the transfer of gas across the alveolar–capillary membrane and reflects the uptake of oxygen from the alveoli into the red cells. A low concentration of carbon monoxide is inhaled and is avidly taken up in a linear fashion by circulating haemoglobin, the amount of which must be known when the test is performed. In normal lungs the transfer factor is a true measure of the diffusing capacity of the lungs for oxygen and depends on the thickness of the alveolar–capillary membrane. In lung disease the diffusing capacity (D_{CO}) also depends on the $\dot{V}_A/\dot{Q}$ relationship as well as on the area and thickness of the alveolar membrane. To control for differences in lung volume, the uptake of carbon monoxide is related to the lung volume; this is known as the transfer coefficient (K_{CO}).

Gas transfer is usually reduced in patients with severe degrees of emphysema and fibrosis. Overall gas transfer can be thought of as a relatively non-specific test of lung function but one that can be particularly used in the early detection and assessment of progress of diseases affecting the lung parenchyma (e.g. cryptogenic pulmonary fibrosis, sarcoidosis, asbestosis).

Measurement of blood gases

This technique is described on page 945.

Measurement of the partial pressures of oxygen and carbon dioxide within arterial blood is an extremely useful test in diseases of the respiratory and circulatory systems. It is essential in the management of cases of respiratory failure and severe asthma, when repeated measurements are often the best guide to therapy.

Arterial oxygen saturation (S_aO_2) can be continuously measured using an oximeter with either ear or finger probes. The oximeter measures the differential absorption of light by oxy- and deoxyhaemoglobin and measures saturation to within 5% of that obtained by blood gas analysis.

Exercise tests

The predominant symptom in respiratory medicine is that of breathlessness. The degree of disability produced by breathlessness can be assessed before and after treatment by asking the patient to walk for 6 minutes along a measured track. This has been shown to be a reproducible and useful test once the patient has undergone an initial training walk to overcome the learning effect.

Exercise tests incorporating assessment of both lung and heart function are of particular value in the investigation of breathlessness. Such tests involve the use of sophisticated equipment enabling measurement of uptake of oxygen ($\dot{V}O_2$), work performed, heart rate and blood pressure together with serial ECGs. Correlation of these variables allows:

- the early detection of lung disease
- the detection of myocardial ischaemia
- the distinction between lung and heart disease
- assessment of fitness.

Pleural aspiration

Diagnostic aspiration is necessary for all but very small effusions. A needle attached to a 20 mL syringe is inserted through an intercostal space over an area of dullness. Fluid is withdrawn and the presence of any blood is noted. Samples are sent for protein estimation, cytology and bacteriological examination, including culture and Ziehl–Nielsen stain for tuberculosis. Large amounts of fluid can be aspirated through a large needle to help relieve extreme breathlessness. Because of the risk of introducing infection into the pleural space, with the subsequent development of an empyema, this technique must be performed using full aseptic precautions.

Pleural aspiration and drainage are now often performed using ultrasound to localize the fluid.

Pleural biopsy

Experienced operators obtain tissue in nearly all patients and, provided multiple specimens are taken, positive results may be expected in up to 80% of cases of tuberculosis and in 60% of cases of malignancy. The technique is illustrated in Figure 14.18. If tissue is not obtained by blind pleural biopsy, the pleura can be examined by fibreoptic thoracoscopy and any lesions biopsied, yielding results in a further 80% (see Practical box 14.1).

Intercostal drainage

This is carried out when large effusions are present producing severe breathlessness or for drainage of an empyema (see Practical box 14.2). Pleurodesis is performed for recurrent/malignant effusion.

Mediastinoscopy and scalene node biopsy

This technique can be used in the management of carcinoma of the bronchus. It involves inspection of the mediastinal structures using a mediastinoscope inserted

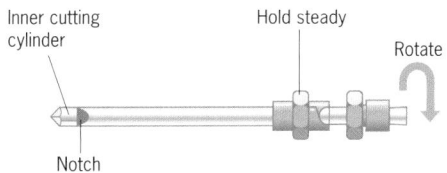

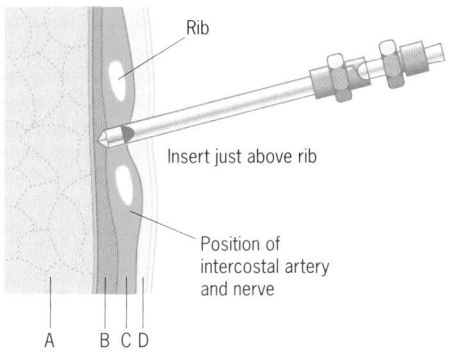

Fig. 14.18 Technique of pleural biopsy. The biopsy needle is shown penetrating the chest wall. A, lung parenchyma; B, pleural space; C, muscle; D, skin and subcutaneous tissue.

by blunt dissection downwards from behind the proximal end of the clavicle. Subsequent biopsy of tissue will reveal the presence or absence of malignant cells in enlarged lymph nodes previously detected by CT, allowing accurate staging of the disease.

Fibreoptic bronchoscopy (Practical box 14.3)

Central bronchial lesions can be biopsied readily.

Washings can be taken from lobes containing more peripheral lesions for cytological examination for malignant cells, and appropriate staining and culture for *Pneumocystis carinii, Mycobacterium,* etc.

Diffuse parenchymal lung disease can be investigated using transbronchial biopsy. The biopsy forceps are pushed as far as possible to the periphery of the lung, the patient is asked to breathe in and the forceps are opened. The patient then breathes out and the jaws of the forceps are closed, removing a small piece of peripheral airway and surrounding lung parenchyma.

Large peripheral lesions can be biopsied under biplanar screening but most peripheral lesions are better sampled by percutaneous aspiration or biopsy using X-ray or CT control.

Bronchoalveolar lavage

This technique can be used both in patients who have disease confined to one lobe and in those with more diffuse lung disease. The tip of the fibreoptic bronchoscope is lodged in the segmental orifice and 20 mL of 0.9% sterile saline is squirted down the suction port of the bronchoscope and immediately aspirated. This is repeated five times; about 40–60% of the total volume is

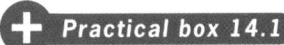

Practical box 14.1

Pleural biopsy

1. Pleural biopsy is best performed after the aspiration of diagnostic fluid samples but before draining large volumes of fluid.
2. A small skin incision is made, as the end of the Abrams' pleural biopsy needle is blunt.
3. Once in place through the pleura, the back part of the needle is rotated to open the notch; this is kept pointing forward.
4. With lateral pressure the needle is withdrawn so that the notch will snag against the pleura.
5. The needle is held firmly and the hexagonal grip is twisted clockwise to cut the biopsy. To avoid damage to the intercostal vessel or nerve, the notch should never be directed upwards when the biopsy is taken.
6. Several biopsies should be taken at different angles by repeated insertion of the needle.
7. Specimens should be put in sterile saline for culture for tuberculosis and into 10% formol saline for histological examination.

Practical box 14.2

Intercostal drainage

1. Carefully sterilize the skin over the aspiration site. Sterile gloves, cap, gown and mask must be worn.
2. Anaesthetize the skin, muscle and pleura with 2% lidocaine (lignocaine).
3. Make a small incision, then push a 28 French gauge Argyle catheter into the pleural space.
4. Attach to three-way tap and 50 mL syringe.
5. Aspirate up to 1000 mL. Stop aspiration if patient becomes uncomfortable – shock may ensue if too much fluid is withdrawn too quickly.
6. A Silastic pigtail catheter can be inserted under X-ray/ultrasound control and attached to tubing and bag for slower aspiration. For drainage and effusions, an 8–12 French gauge pigtail is inserted using the Seldinger technique in which the needle used to enter the pleural space is withdrawn over a control wire along which the catheter is then passed. A 14–16 French gauge pigtail catheter is used for drainage of empyema.

For pleurodesis

Tetracycline 500 mg or bleomycin 15 units in 30–50 mL sodium chloride 0.9% solution is instilled into the pleural cavity to achieve pleurodesis in recurrent/malignant effusion.

recovered. Fluid is strained through two layers of surgical gauze and the volume is noted. The cells are then spun down and resuspended at a concentration of 1×10^7 cells/mL for differential counting. Since there is a considerable overlap in the distribution of cells seen in bronchoalveolar wash specimens in different diseases, this technique has no value in diagnosis. However, it can be used to monitor progression of disease, since

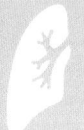

 Practical box 14.3

Fibreoptic bronchoscopy

This enables the direct visualization of the bronchial tree as far as the subsegmental bronchi under a local anaesthetic. Informed consent should be obtained.

Indications

- Lesions requiring biopsy seen on chest X-ray.
- Haemoptysis.
- Stridor.
- Positive sputum cytology for malignant cells with no chest X-ray abnormality.
- Collection of bronchial secretions for bacteriology, especially tuberculosis.
- Recurrent laryngeal nerve paralysis of unknown aetiology.
- Infiltrative lung disease (to obtain a transbronchial biopsy).
- Investigation of collapsed lobes or segments and aspiration of mucus plugs.

Procedure

1. The patient is starved overnight.
2. Atropine 0.6 mg i.m. is given 30 min before the procedure.
3. Topical anaesthesia (lidocaine (lignocaine) 2% gel) is applied to the nose, nasopharynx and pharynx.
4. Intravenous sedation (e.g. diazepam 10 mg or midazolam 2.5–10 mg) is given.
5. The bronchoscope is passed through the nose, nasopharynx and pharynx under direct vision to minimize trauma.
6. Lidocaine (2 mL of 4%) is dropped through the instrument on to the vocal cords.
7. The bronchoscope is passed through the cords into the trachea.
8. All segmental and subsegmental orifices should be identified.
9. Biopsies and brushings should be taken of macroscopic abnormalities or occasionally from peripheral lesions under radiographic control.

Disadvantages

- All patients require sedation to tolerate the procedure.
- Minor and transient cardiac dysrhythmias occur in up to 40% of patients on passage of the bronchoscope through the larynx.
- Oxygen supplementation is required in patients with P_aO_2 below 8 kPa.
- Fibreoptic bronchoscopy should be performed with care in the very sick, and transbronchial biopsies avoided in ventilated patients owing to the increased risk of pneumothorax.
- Massive bleeding may occur on accidental biopsy of vascular lesions or carcinoid tumours. Rigid bronchoscopy may be required to allow adequate access to the bleeding point for haemostasis.

---

improvement is characterized by a reduction in the number of cells and a return towards the normal proportions of different cell types.

Skin-prick tests

Allergen solutions are placed on the skin (usually the volar surface of the forearm) and the epidermis is broken using a 1 mm tipped lancet. A separate lancet should be used for each allergen. If the patient is sensitive to the allergen a weal develops and the diameter of the induration should be measured after 10 minutes. A weal of at least 3 mm diameter is regarded as positive provided that the negative control test is truly negative. The results should be interpreted in the light of the history. Skin tests are not affected by bronchodilators or corticosteroids but antihistamines should be discontinued at least 48 hours before testing.

FURTHER READING

Armstrong P, Wilson AG, Dee P, Hansell DM (1994) *Imaging of Diseases of the Chest*, 2nd edn. Chicago, Mosby Year Book.

Smoking and air pollution

Smoking

Prevalence

General household surveys in the UK have shown a continuing decline in the prevalence of cigarette smoking in men but not in women. Recent data suggest that this may have levelled off and further efforts to reduce the prevalence of smoking are undoubtedly required. At present, 44% of men and 34% of women aged 16 years and over have smoked tobacco in some form. Manufactured cigarettes were smoked by an equal proportion of both sexes (34%). Cigarette smoking is most common between the ages of 16 and 24 years (42% in both sexes). At the age of 15 more girls (27%) than boys (18%) smoke cigarettes. A greater proportion of professional workers than manual workers have given up smoking. In the USA the proportion of adult males and females who smoke is less than 30%. However, cigarette consumption is rising in Central and Eastern Europe and China.

Toxic effects

Cigarette smoke contains polycyclic aromatic hydrocarbons and nitrosamines, which are potent carcinogens and mutagens in animals. It causes release of enzymes from neutrophil granulocytes and macrophages that are capable of destroying elastin and leading to lung damage. Pulmonary epithelial permeability increases even in symptomless cigarette smokers, and correlates with the concentration of carboxyhaemoglobin in blood. This altered permeability possibly allows easier access to carcinogens.

The dangers

Cigarette smoking is addictive. People usually start smoking in adolescence for psychosocial reasons and, once it is a regular habit, the pharmacological properties of nicotine play an important part in persistence, conferring some advantage to the smoker's mood. Very few cigarette smokers (less than 2%) can limit themselves to occasional or intermittent smoking. The dangers are listed in Table 14.7.

There is a significant dose–response relationship between the smoking of 0–40 cigarettes daily and lung cancer mortality (Table 14.8). Sputum production and airflow limitation increase with daily cigarette consumption, and effort tolerance decreases, partly owing to high levels of carboxyhaemoglobin in bronchitis patients. Smoking and asbestos exposure are synergistic in producing bronchial carcinoma, increasing the risk in asbestos workers by up to five to eight times that of nonsmokers exposed to asbestos.

Cigarette smokers who change to other forms of tobacco can reduce the risk, even if they continue to inhale, and are better off changing to cigars or pipes. However all pipe and cigar smokers also have a greater risk of lung cancer than lifelong non-smokers or former smokers.

Environmental tobacco smoke ('passive smoking') has been shown to cause more frequent and more severe attacks of asthma in children and possibly increases the number of cases of asthma. It is also associated with a small but definite increase in lung cancer.

Stopping smoking

If the entire population could be persuaded to stop smoking, the effect on healthcare use would be enormous. National campaigns, bans on advertising and a substantial increase in the cost of cigarettes are the most certain ways of achieving this. Only one in five general practitioners actively encourage their patients to give up smoking, yet simple advice and follow-up can motivate some 50% of their patients to stop. In smoking withdrawal clinics, success rates of 80% can be achieved in the first month, though only 15–20% of patients remain abstinent in the long term. Nicotine chewing gum has been advocated but is probably no better than verbal advice. Nicotine patches are available over the counter and are better than placebo in helping smokers to stop, though they must not be used by those suffering from heart disease. Chest symptoms usually have to be severe to stop patients from smoking. The introduction of amfebutamone/buproprion (a norepinephrine (noradrenaline) and dopamine reuptake inhibitor) may prove a significant step forward in providing pharmacological support to those who wish to give up their habit.

Air pollution

Atmospheric air pollution, due to the burning of coal for energy and heat, has been a characteristic of urban living in developed countries for at least two centuries. It consists of black smoke and sulphur dioxide (SO_2). Air pollution of this type peaked in the 1950s in the UK, until legislation led to restrictions on coal burning. Such pollution continues to increase in newly industrialized countries (India, China) and continues in Eastern

Table 14.7
The dangers of cigarette smoking

General	Passive smoking
Lung cancer	Risk of asthma, pneumonia
COPD	and bronchitis in infants of
Carcinoma of the oesophagus	smoking parents
Ischaemic heart disease	An increase in cough and
Peripheral vascular disease	breathlessness in smokers
Bladder cancer	and non-smokers with
An increase in abnormal	COPD and asthma
spermatozoa	Increased cancer risk
Memory problems	

Maternal smoking
A decrease in birthweight of
  the infant
An increase in fetal and
  neonatal mortality
An increase in asthma

Table 14.8
Effects of smoking on the lung

Large airways	Small airways
Increase in submucosal	Increase in number and
gland volume	distribution of goblet cells
Increase in number of	Airway inflammation and fibrosis
goblet cells	Epithelial metaplasia/dysplasia
Chronic inflammation	Carcinoma
Metaplasia and dysplasia	
of the surface epithelium	**Parenchyma**
	Proximal acinar scarring
	Increase in alveolar
	macrophage numbers
	Emphysema (centri-acinar,
	pan-acinar)

Europe and Russia. The combustion of petroleum and diesel oil in motor vehicles has led to new air pollution, consisting of primary pollutants such as the oxides of nitrogen (NO and NO_2), diesel particulates, poly-aromatic hydrocarbons and the secondary pollutant ozone (O_3) generated by photochemical reactions in the atmosphere. Levels of NO_2 can be higher in poorly ventilated kitchens and living rooms where gas is used for cooking and in fires. In Europe 70% of the particulates present in urban air result from the combustion of diesel fuel. Very small particles (< 2.5 μm, Particulate matter $PM_{2.5}$) remain airborne for long periods and are carried into rural areas. In the UK, ozone concentrations are highest in sunny rural areas.

Epidemiology

Classical studies in the 1950s showed that winter-time episodes of severe air pollution (smog) were associated with substantial numbers of deaths from respiratory disease, particularly when temperature inversion trapped black smoke and SO_2 over urban areas. Air pollution of this type continues to cause excess deaths from respiratory and cardiovascular disease in older populations, and symptoms of bronchitis in children. Pollution resulting primarily from motor vehicles has been shown to cause:

- Increased deaths from respiratory and cardiovascular causes in the elderly – particulates less than 10 μm in diameter (PM_{10}).
- Increased respiratory symptoms, hospital admissions and reduced lung function in children and younger adults – SO_2, NO_2, O_3, PM_{10}. Frequently there is a lag of 1–2 days between peaks in air pollution and disease effects.
- Increase in lung cancer – polyaromatic hydrocarbons.

It has been proposed at various times that air pollutants are one of the causes of the dramatic increase in asthma and other allergic diseases (Table 14.9).

However, there is no current evidence that this is true. On the other hand, both NO_2 and ozone have been shown to enhance the nasal and lung airway responses to inhaled allergen, in those with established allergic disease.

Management

Asthmatics are advised not to exercise outdoors during periods of poor air quality and to increase their anti-inflammatory medication (i.e. inhaled sodium cromoglicate/nedocromil or inhaled corticosteroids).

Short- and long-term measures are required to reduce air pollution, particularly diesel particulates (which are predicted to increase as more diesel engines are used). Such measures include increased motor engine efficiency, catalytic converters, diesel particulate traps and decreased reliance on cars and trucks.

FURTHER READING

Koenig JQ (1999) Air pollution and asthma. *Journal of Allergy and Clinical Immunology* **104**: 717–722.

Kunzil N et al. (2000) Public health impact of outdoor and traffic-related air pollution: a European assessment. *Lancet* **356**: 795–801.

Salvi S et al. (1999) Is diesel exhaust a cause for increasing allergies? *Clinical and Experimental Allergy* **29**: 4–8.

Ware JH (2000) Particulate air pollution and mortality. *New England Journal of Medicine* **343**: 1798–1799.

Diseases of the upper respiratory tract

The common cold (acute coryza)

This highly infectious illness causes a mild systemic upset and prominent nasal symptoms. It is due to infection by rhinoviruses, the majority of which belong to the picornavirus group and exist in at least 100 different

Table 14.9
Air pollutants and their health effects

	Average concentration	Poor air quality	Susceptible individuals	Mechanism of health effects
Sulphur dioxide (SO_2)	5–15 ppb	> 125 ppb	Asthmatics	Bronchoconstriction through neurogenic mechanism
Ozone (O_3)	10–30 ppb	> 90 ppb	All affected, particularly during exercise	Restrictive lung defect Airway inflammation Enhanced response to allergen
Nitrogen dioxide (NO_2)	25–40 ppb	> 100 ppb	Allergic individuals	Airway inflammation Enhanced response to allergen
Particulate matter (PM_{10})	25–30 μg/m³	> 70 μg/m³	Elderly Allergic individuals	Airway and alveolar inflammation Enhanced production selectively of the allergy antibody (IgE)

ppb, parts per billion

antigenic strains. Infectivity from close personal contact (nasal mucus on hands) or droplets is high in the early stages of the infection, and spread is facilitated by overcrowding and poor ventilation. On average, individuals suffer two to three colds per year; but the incidence lessens with age, presumably as a result of accumulating immunity to the causative virus strains. The incubation is from 12 hours to an upper limit of 5 days.

The clinical features are tiredness, slight pyrexia, malaise and a sore nose and pharynx. Profuse, watery nasal discharge, eventually becoming thick and mucopurulent, persists for up to a week. Sneezing is present in the early stage. Secondary bacterial infection occurs only in a minority.

Sinusitis

Sinusitis is an infection of the paranasal sinuses that often complicates upper respiratory tract infections (e.g. coryza and allergic rhinitis). Acute infections are usually caused by *Streptococcus pneumoniae* and *Haemophilus influenzae*. Symptoms include frontal headache and facial pain and tenderness, usually with nasal discharge, but are often difficult to differentiate from symptoms of the common cold. Sinusitis is a frequent finding in aspirin intolerant subjects and in those with severe asthma.

Treatment is with antibiotics. Many strains of *H. influenzae* are now resistant to amoxicillin, so co-amoxiclav or cefaclor are preferred. In addition, nasal treatment with decongestants such as xylometazoline or anti-inflammatory therapy with topical corticosteroids such as fluticasone propionate nasal spray should be given to reduce swelling of the mucosa and unblock the sinus openings. Rare complications include local and cerebral abscesses. Chronic sinusitis can be a cause of headaches, but more often headaches are due to tension.

Rhinitis

Rhinitis is present if sneezing attacks, nasal discharge or blockage occur for more than an hour on most days for:

- a limited period of the year (seasonal rhinitis)
- throughout the whole year (perennial rhinitis).

Seasonal rhinitis

This is often called 'hayfever' and is the most common of all allergic diseases. It is better described as seasonal allergic rhinitis. World-wide prevalence rates vary from 2% to 20%. Prevalence is maximum in the second decade, and up to 30% of young British people suffer symptoms in June and July.

Nasal irritation, sneezing and watery rhinorrhoea are the most troublesome symptoms, but many also suffer from itching of the eyes and soft palate and occasionally even itching of the ears because of the common innervation of the pharyngeal mucosa and the ear. In addition, approximately 20% suffer from seasonal attacks of

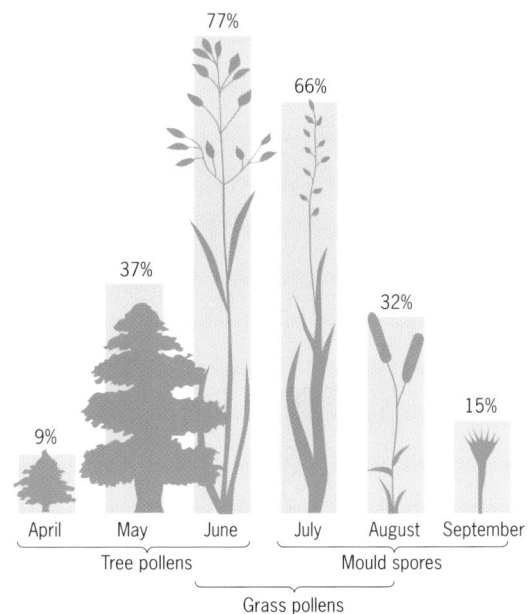

Fig. 14.19 Seasonal allergic rhinitis. Bar graph showing the proportion of patients whose symptoms are worst in the month or months indicated. The causative agents are also shown.

asthma. The common seasonal allergens are shown in Figure 14.19. Since pollination of plants that give rise to high pollen counts varies from country to country, seasonal rhinitis and accompanying conjunctivitis and asthma may occur at different times of the year.

Perennial rhinitis

Patients with perennial rhinitis rarely have symptoms that affect the eyes or throat. Half have symptoms predominantly of sneezing and watery rhinorrhoea, whilst the other half complain mostly of nasal blockage. The patient may lose the sense of smell and taste. A swollen mucosa can obstruct drainage from the sinuses, causing sinusitis in half of the patients. Perennial rhinitis is most frequent in the second and third decades, decreasing with age, and can be divided into four main types.

Perennial allergic rhinitis

The major cause of this in allergic patients is the faecal particles of the house-dust mite *Dermatophagoides pteronyssinus* or *D. farinae*; these particles are approximately 20 μm in diameter (Fig. 14.20), not dissimilar in size to pollen grains. The house-dust mite itself is under 0.5 mm in size, invisible to the naked eye (Fig. 14.20), and is found in dust throughout the house, particularly in older, damp dwellings. It depends for nourishment on desquamated human skin scales and is found in abundance (4000 mites per gram of surface dust) in human bedding.

The next most common allergens come from domestic pets (especially cats) and are proteins derived from

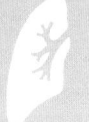

House-dust mite and faeces (80%)

500 μm

20 μm

Pollen grains (70%)

30 μm

Domestic pets (40%)

Moulds (20%)

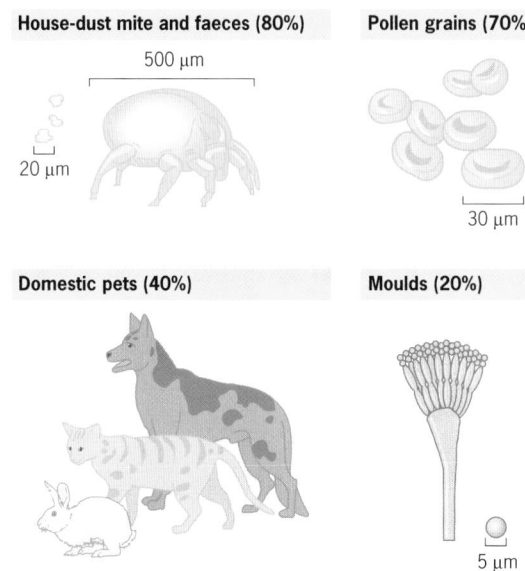

5 μm

Fig. 14.20 **Common allergens causing allergic rhinitis and asthma:** the house-dust mite, faeces of house-dust mites, pollen grains, domestic pets and moulds. Percentages are those of positive skin-prick tests to these allergens in patients with allergic rhinitis.

urine or saliva spread over the surface of the animal as well as skin protein. Allergy to urinary protein from small mammals is a major cause of morbidity amongst laboratory workers.

Industrial dust, vapours and fumes cause occupationally related perennial rhinitis more often than asthma.

The presence of perennial rhinitis makes the nose more reactive to non-specific stimuli such as cigarette smoke, washing powders, household detergents, strong perfumes and traffic fumes. Although patients often think they are allergic to these stimuli, these are irritant responses and do not involve allergic immune reactions.

Perennial non-allergic rhinitis with eosinophilia

No extrinsic allergic cause can be identified in these patients, either from the history or on skin testing; but, as in patients with perennial allergic rhinitis, eosinophilic granulocytes are present in nasal secretions. Aspirin and NSAID intolerance is found in this group.

Vasomotor rhinitis

These patients with perennial rhinitis have no demonstrable allergy or eosinophilia in nasal secretions. They may be suffering from non-specific nasal hyperreactivity that is due to an imbalance of the autonomic nervous system innervating the erectile tissue (sinusoids) in the nasal mucosa.

Nasal polyps

These are round, smooth, soft, semi-translucent, pale or yellow, glistening structures attached to the sinus mucosa by a relatively narrow stalk or pedicle, occurring in patients with both allergic and vasomotor rhinitis. They contain mast cells, eosinophils and mononuclear cells in large numbers and cause nasal obstruction, loss of smell and taste, and mouth breathing, but rarely sneezing, since the mucosa of the polyp is largely denervated. The mechanism(s) of their formation is not known.

Pathogenesis

Sneezing, increased secretion and changes in mucosal blood flow are mediated both by efferent nerve fibres and by released mediators (see p. 878). Mucus production results largely from parasympathetic stimulation, whilst blood vessels are under both sympathetic and parasympathetic control. Sympathetic fibres maintain tonic contraction of blood vessels, keeping the sinusoids of the nose partially constricted with good nasal patency. Stimulation of the parasympathetic system dilates these blood vessels. This stimulation varies spontaneously in a cyclical fashion so that air intake alternates slowly over several hours from one nostril to the other. The erectile cavernous nasal sinusoids can be influenced by emotion, which, in turn, can affect nasal patency.

Allergic rhinitis develops as a result of interaction between the inhaled allergen and adjacent molecules of IgE antibody present on the surface of mast cells found in increased numbers in nasal secretions and within the nasal epithelium. Release of preformed mediators, in particular histamine, causes an increase in permeability of the epithelium, allowing allergen to reach IgE-primed mast cells in the lamina propria. Sneezing, largely caused by histamine, results from stimulation of afferent nerve endings and begins within minutes of the allergen entering the nose. This is followed by nasal exudation and secretion and eventually nasal blockage at a maximum of 15–20 minutes after contact with the allergen. The cysteinyl leukotrienes and vasodilator prostaglandins (PGD_2, PGE_2 and PGI_2) released from mast cells, eosinophils and macrophages are especially potent in causing nasal blockage.

Although the mast cell contains or can generate many other potent vasomotor and chemotactic factors (see Fig. 14.34), the exact role for each of these has still to be evaluated. It is likely that histamine plays a more significant role in the development of allergic rhinitis than of asthma, since the antihistamines are effective treatment for allergic rhinitis but are of little value in the everyday management of asthma. The increase in nasal response observed as the pollen season progresses is in part explained by a progressive increase in mast cells colonizing the mucosa. The mechanisms for recruitment of mast cells under these circumstances probably involve the release of stem cell factor (c-kit) and interleukin-3 from epithelial cells and interleukins -3, -4 and -9 from T cells.

Investigations and diagnosis

A detailed history is mandatory for the diagnosis of allergic factors in rhinitis.

Skin-prick testing indicates that the mechanisms leading to allergic rhinitis (or asthma) are present in human skin. A positive test does not necessarily mean that the particular allergen producing the weal causes the respiratory disease. However, if there is a positive clinical history for that allergen, a causative role is likely. Specific serum IgE antibody against the particular allergen (RAST test) provides the same information as the skin-prick test. Blood tests are much more expensive and should be reserved for use in patients who cannot be skin tested for some reason (e.g. dermatographism, active eczema or using antihistamines and unable to stop for 3 days before skin tests).

Treatment

Allergen avoidance

Removal of a household pet or total enclosure of industrial processes releasing sensitizing agents can lead to cure of rhinitis and, indeed, asthma.

Pollen avoidance is impossible. Contact may be diminished by wearing sunglasses, driving with the car windows shut, avoiding walks in the countryside (particularly in the late afternoon when the number of pollen grains is highest at ground level), and keeping the bedroom window shut at night. These measures are rarely sufficient in themselves to control symptoms. Exposure to pollen is generally lower at the seaside, where sea breezes keep pollen grains inland.

The house-dust mite infests most areas of the house, but particularly the bedroom. Mite counts are extremely low in hospitals where carpets are absent, floors are cleaned frequently and mattresses and pillows are covered in plastic sheeting that can be wiped down. Mite allergen exposure can be reduced by enclosing bedding in fabric specifically designed to prevent the passage of mite allergen, while allowing water vapour through. This is both comfortable and reduces symptoms. Acaricides are less effective and cannot be recommended. Increased room ventilation and reduced soft furnishings including carpets, curtains and soft toys are all helpful in reducing the mite load.

Antihistamines

Antihistamines remain the most common therapy for rhinitis, and many can be purchased directly over the counter in the UK. They are particularly effective against sneezing, but are less effective against rhinorrhoea and have little influence on nasal blockage. The first-generation antihistamines cause sedation. Second-generation drugs such as cetirizine (10 mg once daily), loratadine (10 mg once daily) and fexofenadine 120 mg or 160 mg twice daily are highly specific for H_1 receptors; they do not cross the blood–brain barrier and are therefore not associated with sedation. Fatal cardiac arrhythmias (torsades de pointes) have been described with terfenadine and astemizole and these drugs should be replaced with those that do not influence the ECG QT interval. Antihistamines also control itching in the eyes and palate.

Decongestants

Drugs with sympathomimetic activity (α-adrenergic agents) are widely used for the treatment of nasal obstruction. They may be taken orally or more commonly as nasal drops or sprays (e.g. ephedrine nasal drops). Xylometazoline and oxymetazoline are widely used because they have a prolonged action and tachyphylaxis does not develop. Secondary nasal hyperaemia can occur some hours later as a rebound effect and rhinitis medicamentosa can develop if patients go on taking increasing quantities of the local decongestant to overcome this phenomenon. Local decongestants may be the only effective treatment for vasomotor rhinitis, but patients must be warned about rebound nasal obstruction and must use the drug carefully. Usually, such preparations should be prescribed for only a limited period to open the nasal airways for administration of other therapy, particularly topical corticosteroids.

Anti-inflammatory drugs

Sodium cromoglicate and nedocromil sodium influence a number of aspects of inflammation, including mast cell and eosinophil activation and nerve function. They act by blocking an intracellular chloride channel and preventing cell activation. Sodium cromoglicate applied topically in spray or powder form is of limited value in the treatment of allergic rhinitis, though along with nedocromil sodium, it is very effective in the management of allergic conjunctivitis.

Corticosteroids

The most effective treatment for rhinitis is to use small doses of topically administered corticosteroid preparations (e.g. beclometasone spray twice daily or fluticasone propionate spray once daily). The amount used is insufficient to cause systemic effects and the effect is primarily anti-inflammatory. Preparations should be started prior to the beginning of seasonal symptoms. The combination of a topical corticosteroid with a nonsedative antihistamine taken regularly is particularly effective. Special attention needs to be given to teaching patients how to use the aqueous dispensers or metered-dose inhalers to produce optimal drug deposition. It may be necessary to use an α-adrenergic agonist to decongest the nose prior to taking the topical corticosteroid.

If other therapy has failed, seasonal and perennial rhinitis respond readily to a short course (2 weeks) of treatment with oral prednisolone 5–10 mg daily. Nasal polyps respond well to such oral doses of corticosteroids and their recurrence may be prevented by continuous application of topical corticosteroids.

Pharyngitis

The most common viruses causing pharyngitis belong to the adenovirus group, which consists of about 32 serotypes. Endemic adenovirus infection causes the common sore throat, in which the oropharynx and soft palate are reddened and the tonsils are inflamed and swollen. Within 1–2 days the tonsillar lymph nodes enlarge. Occasionally, localized epidemics occur, particularly in schools in the summer-time, with episodes of fever, conjunctivitis, pharyngitis and lymphadenitis of the neck glands; these are due to adenovirus serotype 8. These diseases are self-limiting, and symptomatic treatment is all that is required.

In the past about one-third of sore throats were due to bacterial infections, e.g. haemolytic streptococcus, but this proportion appears to be falling. Persistent and severe tonsillitis requires antibiotic therapy. Phenoxymethylpenicillin (500 mg four times a day) or cefaclor (250 mg three times daily) can be used. Avoid amoxicillin and ampicillin if there is a possibility of infectious mononucleosis (p. 49).

Acute laryngotracheobronchitis

Acute laryngitis is an occasional but striking complication of upper respiratory tract infections, particularly those caused by viruses of the parainfluenza group and the measles virus. Inflammatory oedema extends to the vocal cords and the epiglottis, causing considerable narrowing of the airway; in addition, there may be associated tracheitis or tracheobronchitis. Children under the age of 3 years are most severely affected. The voice becomes hoarse, the cough assumes a barking quality (croup) and there is audible laryngeal stridor. Progressive airways obstruction may occur, with recession of the soft tissue of the neck and abdomen during inspiration, and in severe cases central cyanosis may occur. Inhalation of steam may be helpful; in severe cases endotracheal intubation may be necessary. Oxygen and adequate fluids should be given. Rarely, a tracheostomy may be required.

Acute epiglottitis

This is caused by *H. influenzae* type b. Since the advent of the Hib immunization there has been an 88% reduction in notification in England and Wales (Fig. 14.21). However, where the vaccine is not available, *H. influenzae* type b can cause life-threatening infection of the epiglottis, a condition that is rare over the age of 5 years. The young child becomes extremely ill with a high fever, and severe airflow obstruction may rapidly occur. This is a life-threatening emergency and requires urgent endotracheal intubation and intravenous ceftazidime (25–150 mg/kg in children). Chloramphenicol (50–100 mg/kg in children) can also be used. The epiglottis, which is red and swollen, should not be inspected until facilities to maintain the airways are available.

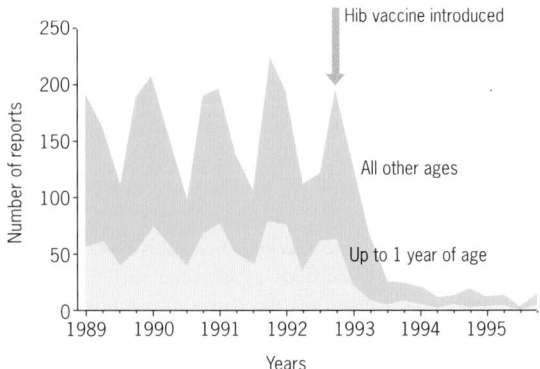

Fig. 14.21 **Laboratory reports of *Haemophilus influenzae* type b by age, England and Wales 1989–95.** From Salisbury DM, Begg NT (1996), with permission. © HMSO.

Other manifestations of *H. influenzae* type b (Hib) are meningitis, septic arthritis and osteomyelitis. Immunization is achieved with a purified polyribosylribitol phosphate from the capsule of Hib linked to a non-toxic diphtheria toxin PRP-T to increase immunogenicity. It is highly effective when given to infants at 2, 3 and 4 months with primary immunization against diphtheria, tetanus and pertussis (DTP), reducing death rates from Hib infections virtually to zero.

Influenza (see also p. 58)

The influenza virus belongs to the orthomyxovirus group and exists in two main forms, A and B. Influenza B is associated with localized outbreaks of milder nature, whereas influenza A is the cause of world-wide pandemics. Influenza A has a capacity to develop new antigenic variants at irregular intervals. Human immunity develops against the haemagglutinin (H) antigen and the neuraminidase (N) antigen on the viral surface. Major shifts in the antigenic make-up of influenza A viruses provide the necessary conditions for major pandemics, whereas minor antigenic drifts give rise to less severe epidemics because immunity in the population is less blunted.

The most serious pandemic of influenza occurred in 1918, and was associated with more than 20 million deaths world-wide. In 1957, a major shift in the antigenic make-up of the virus led to the appearance of influenza A2 type H2-N2, which caused a world-wide pandemic. A further pandemic occurred in 1968 owing to the emergence of Hong Kong influenza type H3-N2, and minor antigenic drifts have caused outbreaks around the world ever since. In 1997, avian H5N1 strain of influenza A was found in humans and represented a major change in viral surface antigens.

Clinical features

The incubation period of influenza is usually 1–3 days. The illness starts abruptly with a fever, shivering and generalized aching in the limbs. This is associated with severe headache, soreness of the throat and a persistent dry cough that can last for several weeks. Influenza viruses can cause a prolonged period of debility and depression that may take weeks or months to clear; this is known as the postviral syndrome.

Complications

Secondary bacterial infection, particularly with *Strep. pneumoniae* and *H. influenzae*, is common following influenza virus infection. Rarer, but more serious, is the development of pneumonia caused by *Staph. aureus*, which has a mortality of up to 20%. Postinfectious encephalomyelitis rarely occurs after infection with influenza virus.

Diagnosis and treatment

Laboratory diagnosis is not usually necessary, but a definitive diagnosis can be established by demonstrating a fourfold increase in the complement-fixing antibody or the haemagglutinin antibody when measured before and after an interval of 1–2 weeks or demonstration of the virus in throat or nasal secretion.

Treatment is by bed rest and paracetamol, together with antibiotics for individuals who have chronic bronchitis, heart or renal disease.

The recent introduction of neuraminidase inhibitors may prove helpful in shortening the duration of symptoms in patients with influenza. The cost–benefit of zanamivir and oseltamivir remains unproven but these are currently recommended in the UK for patients with suspected influenza over the age of 65 and 'at-risk' adults, as part of a strategy to reduce admissions to hospital when influenza is circulating in the community.

Prophylaxis

Protection by influenza vaccines is only effective in up to 70% of people and is of short duration, usually lasting for only a year. Influenza vaccine should not be given to individuals who are allergic to egg protein as some are manufactured in chick embryos. New vaccines have to be prepared to cover each change in viral antigenicity and are therefore in limited supply at the start of an epidemic. Routine vaccination is now recommended for all individuals over 65 years of age and also for younger people with chronic heart disease, chronic lung disease (including asthma), chronic renal failure, diabetes mellitus and those who are immunosuppressed. During pandemics key hospital and health service personnel should also be vaccinated.

Inhalation of foreign bodies

Children inhale foreign bodies, e.g. peanuts, more commonly than adults. In the adult, inhalation often occurs after an excess of alcohol or under general anaesthesia (loose teeth or dentures).

When the foreign body is large it may impact in the trachea. The person chokes and then becomes silent; death occurs unless the material is quickly removed (see Emergency box 14.1).

Impaction usually occurs in the right main bronchus and produces:

- choking
- persistent monophonic wheeze
- later, persistent suppurative pneumonia
- lung abscess (common).

 Emergency box 14.1

Treatment of inhaled foreign bodies (Heimlich manoeuvre)

Emergency

The Heimlich manoeuvre is used to expel the obstructing object:

1. Stand behind the patient.
2. Encircle your arms around the upper part of the abdomen just below the patient's rib cage.
3. Give a sharp, forceful squeeze, forcing the diaphragm sharply into the thorax. This should expel sufficient air from the lungs to force the foreign body out of the trachea.

Non-emergency

Rigid bronchoscopy should be performed.

FURTHER READING

Couch RB (2000) Drug therapy: prevention and treatment of influenza. *New England Journal of Medicine* **343**: 1778–1787.

Dunn CJ, Goa KL (1999) Zanamivir: a review of its use in influenza. *Drugs* **58**: 761–764.

Gubareva LV, Hayden FG (2000) Influenza neuraminidase inhibitors. *Lancet* **355**: 827–835.

Rusznak C, Davies RJ (1998) ABC of allergies. Diagnosing allergy. *British Medical Journal* **316**: 686–689.

Salisbury DM, Begg NT (1996) *Immunisation Against Infectious Disease: Haemophilus influenzae type B*. London: HMSO, pp. 77–83.

Diseases of the lower respiratory tract

Acute bronchitis

Acute bronchitis in previously healthy subjects is often viral. Bacterial infection with organisms such as *Strep. pneumoniae* and *H. influenzae* is a common sequel to viral infections, and is more likely to occur in individuals who are cigarette smokers and in those with chronic obstructive pulmonary disease (COPD).

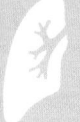

The illness begins with an irritating, unproductive cough, together with discomfort behind the sternum. This may be associated with tightness in the chest, wheezing and shortness of breath. The cough becomes productive, the sputum being yellow or green. There is a mild fever and a neutrophil leucocytosis; wheeze with occasional crackles can be heard on auscultation. In otherwise healthy adults the disease improves spontaneously in 4–8 days without the patient becoming seriously ill.

Treatment with antibiotics may be given (e.g. amoxicillin 250 mg three times daily), though it is not known whether this hastens recovery in otherwise healthy individuals.

Chronic obstructive pulmonary disease (COPD)

The term 'chronic obstructive pulmonary disease' (COPD) was introduced to bring together a variety of clinical syndromes associated with destruction of the lung and airflow obstruction. The terms 'chronic obstructive airways disease' (COAD) and 'chronic obstructive lung disease' (COLD) are used as synonyms in different parts of the world. Prior to 1979, patients with these conditions were often classified in terms of symptoms (chronic bronchitis, chronic asthma), by pathological changes (emphysema) or physiological correlates (pink puffers, blue bloaters). It was the recognition that these entities overlapped and often coexisted which led to the recognition of the need for the new term COPD.

Definitions in COPD

Chronic bronchitis is a symptom definition which has a morphological correlate. Patients with chronic bronchitis produce increased amounts of mucoid sputum for all or part of the year. The symptoms are usually worse in the winter and the patient experiences infective exacerbations when the sputum goes green or brown. For epidemiological purposes, chronic bronchitis is defined as a patient who produces sputum on most days for at least 3 months of each year in more than one consecutive year. This definition is useful for surveys and for clinical trials since it excludes patients with one bad year of sputum production after a bout of pneumonia, but patients with COPD may have symptoms of chronic bronchitis without necessarily meeting the epidemiological definition. Patients with chronic bronchitis will show mucus gland hyperplasia in their large airways (the morphological correlate).

Emphysema is defined pathologically as dilatation and destruction of the lung tissue distal to the terminal bronchiole. There are several varieties (distinguished on the basis of the area of the lung which is destroyed). Emphysema has a radiological correlate in that patients who have lost more than 40% of their lung tissue will show hyperlucency of their lungs and in addition,

the lung fields will be increased in area, because of air trapping. Destruction of the lung tissue leads to loss of elastic recoil and collapse of small airways during expiration. This in turn causes air trapping and an increase in residual volume. In addition, the disturbance of ventilation leads to $\dot{V}/\dot{Q}$ mismatching and consequent hypoxaemia.

Some patients with COPD show significant reversibility to bronchodilators. There is continuing controversy as to whether these patients have a form of asthma. The 'Dutch hypothesis' suggests that patients develop mild asthma which progresses to COAD, whereas the 'British hypothesis' is that these patients have a distinct condition caused by exposure to smoke and pollution with destruction of the lung substance, rather than inflammation of the airways mucosa, as the principal cause of the physiological abnormalities. Given that asthma is defined by airways physiology, emphysema by pathology and bronchitis by history, it is clear that these conditions are not mutually exclusive, hence the need for the term COPD.

Clinical observations led to the suggestion that there were two distinct types of patient, types A and B:

- The *type A* fighter is *pink and puffing*. Although the person is very breathless, arterial tensions of oxygen and carbon dioxide are relatively normal and there is no cor pulmonale. These individuals were thought to be suffering predominantly from emphysema with little bronchitis.
- The *type B* non-fighter, on the other hand, is *blue and bloated*. The person does not appear to be breathless, but has marked arterial hypoxaemia, carbon dioxide retention, secondary polycythaemia and cor pulmonale. These patients were thought to be suffering predominantly from chronic bronchitis.

Although this was an attractive concept with some clinical usefulness, the existence of two separate disorders is not supported by CT or post-mortem studies that have shown no difference in the degree of mucous gland hyperplasia or in the amount of emphysema in patients with type A compared with type B disease. It thus appears that the distinction between type A and type B patients simply reflects the development of type 1 and type 2 respiratory failure (p. 944).

Epidemiology and aetiology

In the UK, COPD, diagnosed on the basis of a reduction in FEV_1 of two standard deviations below predicted, occurs in 18% of male and 14% of female smokers and in 7% and 6% of those who have never smoked. In the USA similar prevalence figures have been obtained and many developing countries are showing an increased prevalence. There is no doubt that cigarette smoking is a major factor in the development of COPD. COPD is much more common in cigarette smokers, it is also related to the number of cigarettes smoked per day. The

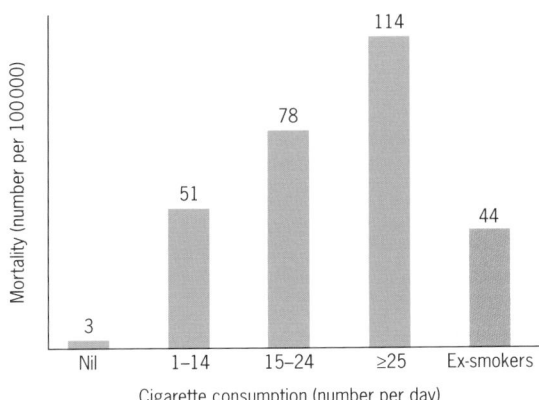

Fig. 14.22 Bronchitis death rates per 100 000 British male doctors according to their smoking habits. From Doll R, Peto R (1976) *British Medical Journal* **2**: 1525.

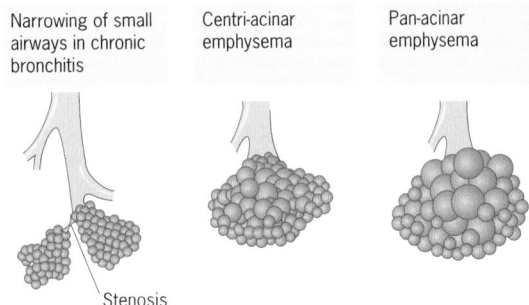

Fig. 14.23 Pathological features of chronic bronchitis and emphysema.

risk of death from COPD in patients smoking 30 cigarettes daily is 20 times that of a non-smoker. The bronchitis mortality amongst male doctors in relation to the number of cigarettes smoked is shown in Figure 14.22. Autopsy studies have also shown that substantial numbers of centri-acinar emphysematous spaces are found in the lungs of 50% of British smokers over the age of 60 years and are unrelated to the diagnosis of significant respiratory disease before death.

Climate and air pollution are of less importance, but there is a great increase in mortality from COPD during periods of heavy atmospheric pollution (p. 856). The effect of urbanization, social class and occupation may also play a part in aetiology, but these effects are difficult to separate from that of smoking. Some animal studies suggest that diet could be a risk factor for COPD; but this has not been proven in humans. The socio-economic burden of COPD is considerable. In the UK, COPD causes approximately 18 million lost working days for men and 2.1 million lost working days for women per year, accounting for some 7% of all days of sickness absence from work. Nevertheless, the number of patients discharged from hospitals in the UK with this diagnosis has been steadily falling; the death rate has also fallen in the last 25 years from 200 to 70 per 100 000.

Pathophysiology

In COPD the pathological changes of bronchitis and emphysema typically coexist. In this section we have separated them for clarity.

Chronic bronchitis

The most consistent pathological finding in chronic bronchitis is hypertrophy of the mucus-secreting glands of the bronchial tree. The hypertrophy of these mucous glands is evenly distributed throughout the lung, and is mainly seen in the larger bronchi. In addition, the number of the mucus-secreting goblet cells increases. This leads to increased mucus production and the regular expectoration of sputum. In more advanced cases, the bronchi themselves are obviously inflamed and pus is seen in the lumen. Microscopically there is infiltration of the walls of the bronchi and bronchioles with acute and chronic inflammatory cells. In contrast to asthma, the lymphocytic infiltrate is predominantly $CD8^+$. The epithelial layer may become ulcerated and, when the ulcers heal, squamous epithelium may replace the columnar cells. The inflammation leads to widespread narrowing in the small airways.

The small airways are particularly affected early in the disease, initially without the development of any significant breathlessness. This initial inflammation of the small airways is reversible and accounts for the improvement in airway function if smoking is stopped early.

Further progression of the disease leads to progressive squamous cell metaplasia, and fibrosis of the bronchial walls. The physiological consequences of these changes is the development of airflow limitation. If the airway narrowing is combined with emphysema (causing loss of the elastic recoil of the lung) the resulting airflow limitation is even more severe.

Emphysema (Fig. 14.23)

Emphysema is classified according to the site of damage:

- *Centri-acinar emphysema*. Distension and damage of lung tissue is concentrated around the respiratory bronchioles, whilst the more distal alveolar ducts and alveoli tend to be well preserved. This form of emphysema is extremely common; when of modest extent, it is not necessarily associated with disability. Severe centri-acinar emphysema is associated with substantial airflow limitation.
- *Pan-acinar emphysema*. This is less common. Here, distension and destruction appear to involve the whole of the acinus, and in the extreme form the lung becomes a mass of bullae. Severe airflow limitation and $\dot{V}_A/\dot{Q}$ mismatch occur. This type of emphysema occurs in α_1-antitrypsin deficiency (see p. 377).
- *Irregular emphysema*. There is scarring and damage affecting the lung parenchyma patchily without particular regard for acinar structure.

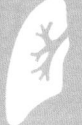
Emphysema leads to expiratory airflow limitation and air trapping. The loss of lung elastic recoil results in an increase in TLC while the loss of alveoli with emphysema results in decreased gas transfer.

$\dot{V}_A/\dot{Q}$ mismatch occurs partly because of damage and mucus plugging of smaller airways from chronic bronchitis, and partly because of the rapid expiratory closure of the smaller airways owing to loss of elastic recoil from emphysema. This leads to a fall in P_aO_2 and an increase in the work of respiration.

CO_2 excretion is not impaired to the same extent and indeed many patients will show low normal P_aCO_2 values. These patients are the 'pink puffers' who seek to maintain normal blood gases by increasing their respiratory effort. Other patients fail to maintain their respiratory effort and as a consequence their carbon dioxide levels increase. In the short term, the rise in CO_2 leads to stimulation of respiration but in the long term, these patients often become insensitive to CO_2 and come to depend on hypoxaemia to drive their ventilation. These patients appear less breathless and because they run low P_aO_2 values, they start to retain fluid and stimulate the growth of erythrocytes. In consequence they become bloated, plethoric and cyanosed, the typical appearance of the 'blue bloater'. Attempts to abolish hypoxaemia by administering oxygen can make the situation much worse by decreasing respiratory drive in these patients who rely on hypoxia to drive their ventilation.

Carbon dioxide is normally the major stimulant of the respiratory centre. In the face of a prolonged high P_aCO_2 this sensitivity is diminished and hypoxaemia becomes the chief drive to respiration. In this situation an attempt to abolish hypoxaemia by administration of oxygen can result in an increase in P_aCO_2 by decreasing the respiratory drive, worsening respiratory failure.

Pathogenesis

Cigarette smoking

Bronchoalveolar washes have shown that smokers have neutrophil granulocytes present within the lumen of the lung that are absent in non-smokers. Additionally, the small airways of smokers are infiltrated by granulocytes. These granulocytes are capable of releasing elastases and proteases, which possibly help to produce emphysema. It is suggested that an imbalance between protease and antiprotease activity may produce the damage. α_1-Antitrypsin is a major serum antiprotease which can be inactivated by cigarette smoke (see below).

The hypertrophy of mucous glands in the larger airways is thought to be a direct response to persistent irritation resulting from the inhalation of cigarette smoke. The smoke has an adverse effect on surfactant, favouring overdistension of the lungs.

Infections

Patients with COPD cope badly with respiratory infections, which are often the precipitating cause of acute exacerbations of the disease. However, the role of infection in the development of the progressive airflow limitation that characterizes disabling COPD is far less clear. Prompt use of antibiotics and routine influenza vaccinations are appropriate.

α_1-Antitrypsin deficiency (see also p. 377)

α_1-Antitrypsin inhibitor is an antiproteinase inhibitor produced in the liver, secreted into the blood and which diffuses into the lung. Here it functions as an antiprotease that inhibits neutrophil elastase, a proteolytic enzyme capable of destroying alveolar wall connective tissue.

More than 75 alleles of the α_1-antitrypsin inhibitor gene have been described. The three main phenotypes are MM (normal), MZ (heterozygous deficiency) and ZZ (homozygous deficiency). About 1 child in 5000 in Britain is born with the homozygous deficiency, but not all develop chest disease. Those who do develop breathlessness under the age of 40 years have radiographic evidence of basal emphysema and are usually, but not always, cigarette smokers. Hereditary deficiency of α_1-antitrypsin inhibitor accounts for about 2% of emphysema cases. A small minority develop liver disease (see p. 377).

Clinical features

Symptoms

The characteristic symptoms of COPD are cough with the production of sputum, wheeze and breathlessness following many years of a smoker's cough. Colds seem to 'go down to the chest' and frequent infective exacerbations occur, giving purulent sputum. Symptoms can be worsened by factors such as cold, foggy weather and atmospheric pollution. With advanced disease, breathlessness becomes severe even after mild exercise such as dressing.

Signs

In mild disease there are no signs apart from 'wheeze' throughout the chest. In severe disease, the patient is tachypnoeic, with prolonged expiration. The accessory muscles of respiration are used and there may be intercostal indrawing on inspiration and pursing of the lips on expiration (see p. 839). Chest expansion is poor, the lungs are hyperinflated, and there is loss of the normal cardiac and liver dullness.

Patients who remain responsive to CO_2 are usually breathless and rarely cyanosed. Heart failure and oedema are rare features except as terminal events. Patients who become insensitive to CO_2 are often oedematous and cyanosed but not particularly breathless. Those with hypercapnia may have peripheral vasodilatation, a bounding pulse and when the P_aCO_2 is above about 10 kPa, a coarse flapping tremor of the outstretched hands. Severe hypercapnia will lead to confusion and progressive drowsiness. At this stage papilloedema may be present but is neither specific nor sensitive as a diagnostic feature.

Complications

Respiratory failure

The later stages of COPD are characterized by the development of respiratory failure. For practical purposes this is said to occur when there is either a P_aO_2 of less than 8 kPa (60 mmHg) or a P_aCO_2 of more than 7 kPa (55 mmHg) (see Ch. 15).

The persistence of chronic alveolar hypoxia and hypercapnia leads to constriction of the pulmonary arterioles and subsequent pulmonary arterial hypertension. Cardiac output is normal or increased but salt and fluid retention occurs as a result of renal hypoxia.

Cor pulmonale

Patients with advanced COPD may develop cor pulmonale (see p. 807), which is defined as heart disease secondary to disease of the lung. It is characterized by pulmonary hypertension, right ventricular hypertrophy, and eventually right heart failure. On examination, the patient is centrally cyanosed (owing to the lung disease) and, when heart failure develops, the patient becomes more breathless and ankle oedema occurs. Initially a prominent parasternal heave may be felt that is due to right ventricular hypertrophy and a loud pulmonary second sound may be heard. In very severe pulmonary hypertension there is incompetence of the pulmonary valve. With right heart failure, tricuspid incompetence may develop with a greatly elevated jugular venous pressure (JVP), ascites and upper abdominal discomfort owing to swelling of the liver.

Diagnosis

This is usually clinical. There is a history of breathlessness and sputum production in a lifetime smoker. In the absence of a history of cigarette smoking one should consider a working diagnosis of asthma unless there is a family history of lung disease suggestive of a deficiency of α_1-antitrypsin inhibitor.

The patient may have signs of hyperinflation and typical pursed lip respiration. No individual clinical feature is diagnostic. Emphysema is often incorrectly diagnosed on signs of over-inflation of the lungs (e.g. loss of liver dullness on percussion), but this may occur with other diseases such as asthma. Furthermore, centri-acinar emphysema may be present without signs of over-inflation. Some elderly men develop a barrel-shaped chest as a result of osteoporosis of the spine, and a consequent decrease in height.

Investigations

- **Lung function tests** show evidence of airflow limitation (see Figs 14.9 and 14.16). The ratio of the FEV_1 to the FVC is reduced and the PEFR is low. In many patients the airflow limitation is reversible to some extent (usually a change in FEV_1 of <15%), and the distinction between asthma and COPD can be difficult. Lung volumes may be normal or increased, and the gas transfer coefficient of carbon monoxide is low when significant emphysema is present.
- **Chest X-ray** is often normal, even when the disease is advanced. The classic features are the presence of bullae, severe over-inflation of the lungs with low, flattened diaphragms, and a large retrosternal air space on the lateral film. There may also be a deficiency of blood vessels in the peripheral half of the lung fields compared with relatively easily visible proximal vessels.
- **Haemoglobin level and PCV** can be elevated as a result of persistent hypoxaemia (secondary polycythaemia, see p. 441).
- **Blood gases** are often normal. In the advanced case there is evidence of hypoxaemia and hypercapnia.
- **Sputum examination** is unnecessary in the ordinary case as *Strep. pneumoniae* or *H. influenzae* are the only common organisms to produce acute exacerbations. Occasionally *Moraxella catarrhalis* may be the causative bacterium for the infection.
- **Electrocardiogram**. In advanced cor pulmonale the P wave is taller (P pulmonale) and there may be right bundle branch block (RSR′ complex) and the changes of right ventricular hypertrophy (see p. 807).
- **Echocardiogram** is performed to assess cardiac function.
- α_1-**Antitrypsin levels.** The normal range is 2–4 g/L.

Treatment

Persuading the patient to stop smoking is vital. Even at a late stage of the disease this may slow down the rate of deterioration and prolong the time before disability and death occur (Fig. 14.24). Accompanying heart failure should be treated (see p. 759).

Drug therapy

This is used both for the short-term management of exacerbations and for the long-term relief of symptoms. In many cases the therapy is similar to that used in asthma (see p. 881).

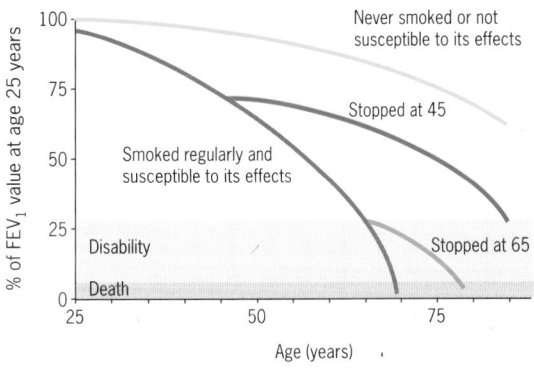

Fig. 14.24 Influence of smoking on airflow limitation.
From Fletcher CM, Peto R (1977) *British Medical Journal* **1**: 1645.

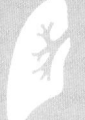

Bronchodilators

Many patients feel less breathless following the inhalation of a β-adrenergic agonist such as salbutamol (200 μg every 4–6 hours). More prolonged and greater broncho-dilatation results from the use of anti-muscarinic agents: ipratropium bromide 40 μg four times daily or oxi-tropium bromide 200 μg twice daily. Objective evidence of improvement in the peak flow or FEV_1 may be small and decisions to continue or stop therapy should be based on the patient's reported symptoms. Long-acting preparations of theophylline are of little benefit.

Corticosteroids

In symptomatic patients with COPD, a trial of cortico-steroids is always indicated, since a proportion of patients have a large, unsuspected, reversible element to their disease and airway function may improve considerably. Prednisolone 30 mg daily should be given for 2 weeks, with measurements of lung function before and after the treatment period. If there is objective evidence of a substantial degree of improvement in airflow limitation (FEV_1 increase > 15%), prednisolone should be discontinued and replaced by inhaled corticosteroids (beclometasone 400 μg twice daily in the first instance, adjusted according to response). The long-term value of regular inhaled corticosteroids in all patients with COPD has not been proven.

Antibiotics

Prompt antibiotic treatment shortens exacerbations and should always be given in acute episodes as it may prevent hospital admission and further lung damage. Patients can be given a supply of antibiotics to keep at home to start as soon as their sputum turns yellow or green. Amoxicillin-resistant *H. influenzae* is an increasing problem, occurring in 10–20% of isolates from sputum and likely to become more common over the next decade. Resistance to cefaclor 500 mg 8-hourly or cefixime 400 mg once daily is significantly less frequent while co-amoxiclav is a useful alternative.

Long-term treatment with antibiotics remains controversial. They were once thought to be of no value, but eradication of infection and keeping the lower respiratory tract free of bacteria may help to prevent deterioration in lung function.

Diuretic therapy (see p. 679)

This is necessary for all oedematous patients. Daily weights should be recorded during acute inpatient episodes.

α₁-Antitrypsin replacement

Weekly or monthly infusions of α₁-antitrypsin have been recommended for patients with serum levels of this compound below 310 mg/L and abnormal lung function. Whether this modifies the long-term progression of the disease has still to be determined.

Mucolytics and vaccines

Although mucus production is increased, mucolytics are not beneficial. It is vital that patients be encouraged to cough up sputum, and a physiotherapist can provide valuable training and advice. Symptomatic treatment with steam inhalations may help to liquefy the sputum so that it can be more easily coughed up. Patients with COPD should receive yearly influenza vaccine. These patients should also receive one dose of the polyvalent pneumococcal polysaccharide vaccine (a single dose usually provides lifelong immunity).

Treatment of respiratory failure

There are many causes of respiratory failure (Fig. 14.25) but COPD is by far the most common. The primary aim of the management of respiratory failure is to improve the P_aO_2 by continuous oxygen therapy. In type I respiratory failure (low P_aO_2, normal P_aCO_2) it is safe to administer as much oxygen as is required to return the P_aO_2 to normal. In type II respiratory failure the P_aCO_2 is elevated and giving additional oxygen will nearly always lead to a rise in the P_aCO_2 (see p. 944). Small increases in P_aCO_2 can be tolerated but not if the pH falls dramatically. The pH should not be allowed to fall below 7.25; under such circumstances, increased ventilation must be achieved either by the use of a respiratory stimulant or by artificial ventilation.

Figure 14.26 shows a fixed-performance mask (Venturi mask) for the administration of oxygen. This style of mask is used to deliver low concentrations of oxygen. It should be compared with the variable-performance face mask (see Fig. 15.21).

Initially, 24% oxygen is given, which is only slightly greater than the concentration of oxygen in air. However, because of the shape of the oxygen–haemoglobin dissociation curve (see Fig. 15.5), this small increase in oxygen is valuable. The concentration of inspired oxygen can be gradually increased if the P_aCO_2 does not rise unacceptably.

Additional measures

- *Removal of retained secretions*. The patient should be encouraged to cough to remove secretions. Physiotherapy is helpful. If this fails, bronchoscopy and/or aspiration via an endotracheal tube may be necessary. A tracheostomy is only rarely required.
- *Secondary polycythaemia*. Venesection is recommended if the packed cell volume is greater than 55%.
- *Respiratory support* (see p. 946). Non-invasive ventilatory techniques can be very helpful in avoiding the need for endotracheal intubation. The best current technique uses tight-fitting facial masks to deliver bilevel positive airway pressure ventilatory support (BiPAP). Assisted ventilation with an endotracheal tube is occasionally used for patients with COPD with severe respiratory failure when there is a definite precipitating factor and the

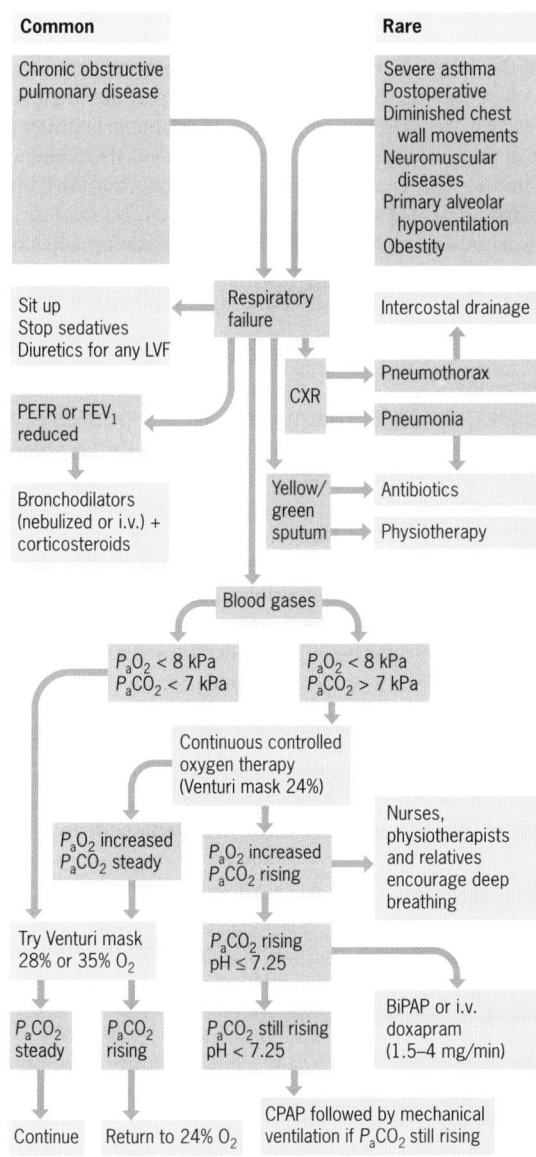

Fig. 14.25 Algorithm for the treatment of respiratory failure. LVF, left ventricular failure; CPAP, continuous positive airway pressure; BiPAP, bilevel positive airway pressure.

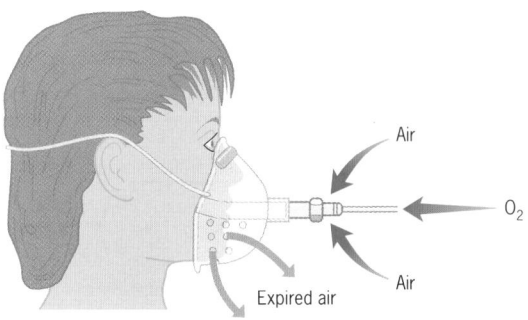

Fig. 14.26 'Fixed-performance' device for administration of oxygen to spontaneously breathing patients (Venturi mask). Oxygen is delivered through the injector of the Venturi mask at a given flow rate. A fixed amount of air is entrapped and the inspired oxygen can be predicted accurately. Masks are available to deliver 24%, 28% and 35% oxygen.

- *Corticosteroids, antibiotics and bronchodilators* should be administered in the acute phase and then reassessed once the patient has recovered (see above).

Further management at home

Oxygen

Two controlled trials (chiefly in males) have indicated that life can be prolonged by the continuous administration of oxygen at 2 L/min via nasal prongs to achieve an oxygen saturation of greater than 90% for large proportions of the day and night. Survival curves from these two studies are shown in Figure 14.27.

Only 30% of those not receiving long-term oxygen therapy survived for more than 5 years. A fall in pulmonary artery pressure was achieved if oxygen was given for 15 hours daily, but substantial improvement in mortality was only achieved by the administration of oxygen for 19 hours daily. These results suggest that long-term continuous domiciliary oxygen therapy will benefit patients who have:

- COPD with an FEV_1 of less than 1.5 L.
- A P_aO_2 on air of less than 7.3 kPa (55 mmHg) with or without hypercapnia. Measurements should be taken on two occasions at least 3 weeks apart after appropriate bronchodilator therapy.
- Carboxyhaemoglobin of less than 3% (i.e. patients who have stopped smoking).

The provision of 19 hours of oxygen daily at a flow rate of 1–3 L/min using a 28% oxygen mask is best achieved using an oxygen concentrator. To achieve this with oxygen cylinders would require 20 standard cylinders per week, which is unacceptably expensive. Oxygen concentrators are available through the UK national health service for patients who fulfil the above criteria.

overall prognosis is reasonable. Assessing the relative reversibility in an acute setting can present a difficult ethical problem.

- *Respiratory stimulants.* The use of respiratory stimulants has declined in recent years, largely because of the increasing availability of respiratory support services. Doxapram, 1.5–4.0 mg/min by slow i.v. infusion, may help in the short term to arouse the patient and to stimulate coughing, with clearance of some secretions.

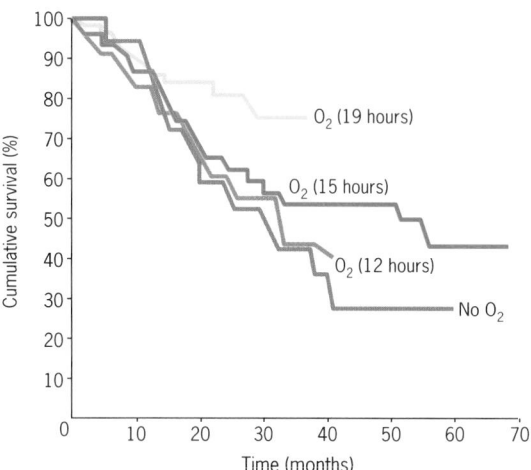

Fig. 14.27 Cumulative survival curves for patients receiving oxygen. Oxygen doses are in hours per day.

Drugs

Pulmonary hypertension can be partially relieved by the use of oral β-adrenergic stimulants such as salbutamol (4 mg three times daily), but whether this is useful in the long term is unknown.

The sensation of breathlessness can be reduced by the use of either promethazine 125 mg daily or dihydrocodeine 1 mg/kg by mouth. Reduced breathlessness and increased exercise tolerance also result from the combined administration of dihydrocodeine and oxygen delivered from a portable cylinder. Although opiates are the most effective treatment for intractable breathlessness they depress ventilation and carry risk of increasing respiratory failure.

Surgery

Some patients with large emphysematous bullae (which reduce lung capacity) can benefit from bullectomy, enabling adjacent areas of collapsed lung to re-expand and function again. In addition, carefully selected patients with severe COPD (FEV$_1$ < 1 L), can benefit from *lung volume reduction surgery*. This increases elastic recoil, reducing the expiratory collapse of the airway and also reducing expiratory airflow limitation. It also enables the diaphragm to work at a better advantage. Overall, ventilation is improved and patients are less breathless.

Single lung transplantation (see p. 873) is used for end-stage emphysema, with 3-year survival rates of 75%. The principal benefit is to improve quality of life but it does not statistically improve survival. Lung volume reduction surgery offers an intermediate option for patients who have severe emphysema. A recent control trial in severe emphysema, however, showed an increased mortality and no improvement in their condition.

Exercise training

A modest increase in exercise capacity with diminution in the sense of breathlessness and improved general well-being can result from exercise training. Regular training periods can be instituted at home; climbing stairs or walking fixed distances combined with regular clinic visits for encouragement. Breathing exercises are probably of less value. Quality of life can be improved by a multidisciplinary approach emphasizing physiotherapy, exercise, education and smoking cessation, although this does not alter life expectancy or the rate of decline in lung function.

Prognosis

In general, 50% of patients with severe breathlessness die within 5 years (Fig. 14.27), but even in the severe group, stopping smoking will improve the prognosis.

Nocturnal hypoxia

It has been shown that patients with COPD who show severe arterial hypoxaemia also suffer from profound nocturnal hypoxaemia which may drop the P_aO_2 as low as 2.5 kPa (19 mmHg), particularly during the rapid eye movement (REM) phase of sleep.

Because patients with COPD are already hypoxic, the fall in P_aO_2 produces a much larger fall in oxygen saturation (owing to the steepness of the oxygen–haemoglobin dissociation curve) and desaturation of up to 50% occurs. The mechanism is alveolar hypoventilation due to:

- inhibition of intercostal and accessory muscles in REM sleep
- shallow breathing in REM sleep, which reduces ventilation, particularly in severe COPD
- an increase in upper airway resistance because of a reduction in muscle tone.

These nocturnal hypoxaemic episodes are associated with a further rise in pulmonary arterial pressure owing to vasoconstriction, and the majority of deaths in patients with COPD occur during the night, possibly from cardiac arrhythmias. These patients additionally show severe secondary polycythaemia, partly as a result of the severe nocturnal hypoxaemia.

Each episode of desaturation is usually terminated by arousal from sleep, so that normal sleep is reduced and the patient suffers from daytime sleepiness.

Treatment

Patients with arterial hypoxaemia should not be given sleeping tablets, which will further depress respiratory drive. Treatment is with nocturnal administration of oxygen and ventilatory support.

Positive-pressure ventilation can be administered non-invasively through a tightly fitting nasal mask with bilevel positive airway pressure – inspiratory to provide inspiratory assistance and expiratory to prevent alveolar closure, each adjusted independently. The use of these devices to maintain adequate ventilation during sleep and to allow respiratory muscles to rest at night are effective in chronic chest wall disease (e.g. kyphoscoliosis) or neuromuscular disease (e.g. previous poliomyelitis). These devices, however, have not led to improvement in respiratory function, respiratory muscle strength, exercise tolerance or breathlessness in patients with COPD.

Obstructive sleep apnoea

This condition occurs most often in overweight middle-aged men and affects 1–2% of the population. It can occur in children, particularly those with enlarged tonsils. The major symptoms and their frequency are listed in Table 14.10. During sleep, activity of the respiratory muscles is reduced, especially during REM sleep when the diaphragm is virtually the only active muscle. Apnoeas occur when the airway at the back of the throat is sucked closed when breathing in during sleep. When awake this tendency is overcome by the action of opening muscles of the upper airway – the genioglossus and palatal muscles, which become hypotonic during sleep (Fig. 14.28). Partial narrowing results in snoring, occlusion in apnoea and critical narrowing in hypopnoeas. Apnoea leads to hypoxia and increasingly strenuous respiratory efforts until the patient overcomes the resistance. The combination of the effort and the central hypoxic stimulation wakes the patient from sleep. These awakenings are so brief that the patient remains unaware of them but may be woken hundreds of times per night leading to sleep deprivation, especially a reduction in REM sleep, with consequent daytime sleepiness and impaired intellectual performance. Important contributory factors are obesity, a small pharyngeal opening and coexistent COPD.

Correctable factors occur in about one-third of cases and include:

- encroachment on pharynx – obesity, acromegaly, enlarged tonsils
- nasal obstruction – nasal deformities, rhinitis, polyps, adenoids
- respiratory depressant drugs – alcohol, sedatives, strong analgesics.

Table 14.10
Signs of obstructive sleep apnoea

Loud snoring (95%)	Nocturnal choking (30%)
Daytime sleepiness (90%)	Reduced libido (20%)
Unrefreshed sleep (40%)	Morning drunkenness (5%)
Restless sleep (40%)	Ankle swelling (5%)
Morning headache (30%)	

Diagnosis

In many cases this can be made on the combination of a good history of the snore–silence–snore cycle reported by the patient's relatives, supported by non-invasive ear or finger oximetry performed at home. Characteristically, arterial oxygen saturation will fall significantly in a cyclical manner. If the oximetry is negative or equivocal, inpatient assessment is indicated, preferably in a room specifically adapted for sleep studies rather than a normal ward side room. Oximetry is supplemented by video recording. Full polysomnographic studies are rarely necessary for clinical diagnosis but are useful in research labs. These involve oximetry, direct measurements of thoracic and abdominal movement to assess breathing, and electroencephalography to record patterns of sleep and arousal. Some centres also measure oronasal airflow.

The diagnosis of sleep apnoea/hypopnoea is confirmed if there are more than 15 apnoeas or hypopnoeas in any 1 hour of sleep.

Management

Management consists of correction of treatable factors (see above) with, if necessary, nasal continuous positive airway pressure (CPAP) delivered by a nasal mask during sleep. Such systems raise the pressure in the pharynx by about 1 kPa, keeping the walls apart.

Bronchiectasis

The term 'bronchiectasis' is used to describe abnormal and permanently dilated airways. Bronchial walls become inflamed, thickened and irreversibly damaged. The mucociliary transport mechanism is impaired and frequent bacterial infections ensue. Clinically, the disease is characterized by cough production of large amounts of sputum and dilated and thickened bronchi, detected on CT scanning of the thorax.

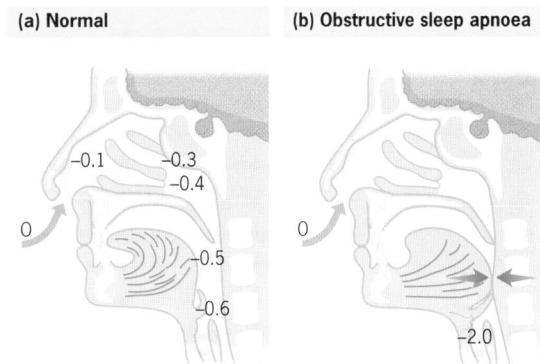

Fig. 14.28 **Section through head, showing pressure changes (in kPa) in (a) the normal situation and (b) obstructive sleep apnoea.** There is a pressure drop during inspiration as air is sucked through the turbinates. In patients with obstructive sleep apnoea this is sufficient to collapse the pharynx, obstructing inspiration.

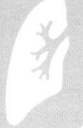

Respiratory disease

Aetiology

The causes are shown in Table 14.11. Cystic fibrosis is the most common cause in developed countries.

Clinical features

Patients with mild bronchiectasis only produce yellow or green sputum after an infection. Localized areas of the lung may be particularly affected, when sputum production will depend on position. As the condition worsens, the patient suffers from persistent halitosis, recurrent febrile episodes with malaise, and episodes of pneumonia. Clubbing occurs, and coarse crackles can be heard over the infected areas, usually the bases of the lungs. When the condition is severe there is continuous production of foul-smelling, thick, khaki-coloured sputum. Haemoptysis, either as blood-stained sputum or as a massive haemorrhage, can occur. Breathlessness may result from airflow limitation.

Investigations

- **Chest X-ray** may be normal or may show dilated bronchi with thickened bronchial walls and sometimes multiple cysts containing fluid.
- **High-resolution CT scanning** (see p. 849) shows bronchial dilatation and wall thickening and is the investigation of choice (Fig. 14.29).
- **Bronchography** is rarely required except if the diagnosis is in doubt or where there is reason to believe that the disease may be localized and

therefore amenable to surgical treatment. The left lower lobe and lingula are the most common sites for localized disease. The investigation is performed during fibreoptic bronchoscopy.

- **Sputum** examination with culture and sensitivity of the organisms is essential for adequate treatment. The major pathogens are *Staph. aureus, Pseudomonas aeruginosa, H. influenzae* and anaerobes. Other pathogens include *Strep. pneumoniae* and *Klebsiella pneumoniae*. *Aspergillus fumigatus* can be isolated from 10% of sputum specimens in cystic fibrosis, but the role of this organism is uncertain.
- **Sinus X-rays.** Thirty per cent have concomitant purulent rhinosinusitis.
- **Serum immunoglobulins.** Ten per cent of adults have immune deficiency.
- **Sweat electrolytes** – if appropriate (see p. 872).
- **Mucociliary clearance** (nasal clearance of saccharin). A 1 mm cube of saccharin is placed on the inferior turbinate and the time to taste measured (normally less than 30 minutes).

Treatment

Postural drainage

Postural drainage is of vital importance and patients must be trained by physiotherapists to tip themselves into a position in which the lobe to be drained is uppermost at least three times daily for 10–20 minutes. Most patients find that lying over the side of the bed with head and thorax down is the most effective position.

Antibiotics

Experience from the treatment of cystic fibrosis suggests that bronchopulmonary infections need to be eradicated if progression of the disease is to be halted. In mild cases, intermittent chemotherapy with cefaclor 500 mg three times daily or ciprofloxacin 500 mg twice daily may be the only therapy needed. Flucloxacillin 500 mg 6-hourly is the best treatment if *Staph. aureus* is isolated.

Table 14.11
Causes of bronchiectasis

Congenital	Immunological over-response
Deficiency of bronchial wall elements	Allergic bronchopulmonary aspergillosis
Pulmonary sequestration	Post-lung transplant
Mechanical bronchial obstruction	**Immune deficiency**
Intrinsic	*Primary*
Foreign body	Panhypogammaglobulinaemia
Inspissated mucus	Selective immunoglobulin
Post-tuberculous stenosis	deficiencies (IgA and IgG$_2$)
Tumour	
	Secondary
Extrinsic	HIV and malignancy
Lymph node	
Tumour	**Mucociliary clearance defects**
	Genetic
Postinfective bronchial damage	Primary ciliary dyskinesia (Kartagener's syndrome with dextrocardia and situs inversus)
Bacterial and viral pneumonia, including pertussis, measles and aspiration pneumonia	Cystic fibrosis
	Acquired
Granuloma and fibrosis	Young's syndrome – azoospermia, sinusitis
Tuberculosis, sarcoidosis and fibrosing alveolitis	

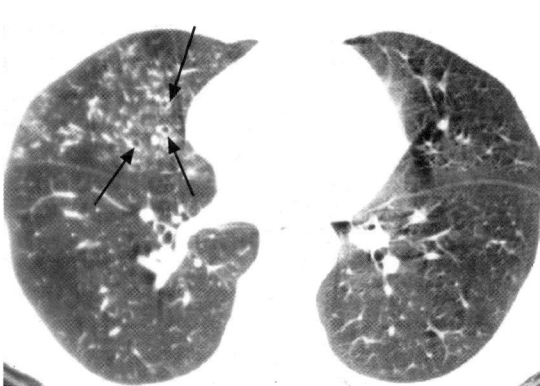

Fig. 14.29 CT scan showing bronchiectasis in the right middle lobe. Note dilated bronchi with thickened wall and adjacent artery giving a signet ring appearance.

If the sputum remains yellow or green despite regular physiotherapy and intermittent chemotherapy, or if lung function deteriorates despite treatment with bronchodilators, it is likely that there is infection with *P. aeruginosa*. Treatment requires parenteral or aerosol chemotherapy at regular 3-month intervals. Ceftazidime 2 g intravenously 8-hourly or by inhalation (1 g twice daily) has been shown to be effective. Ciprofloxacin 750 mg twice daily orally may be equally effective in the short term, but rapid development of resistance is a problem. High sputum levels of some antibiotics, e.g. tobramycin, can be achieved by inhalation.

Bronchodilators

Bronchodilators are useful in patients with demonstrable airflow limitation.

Anti-inflammatory agents

Inhaled or oral steroids can decrease the rate of progression.

Surgery

Unfortunately, it is rare for bronchiectasis to be sufficiently localized for surgery to be of any value. Heart or heart–lung transplantation is sometimes required.

Complications

The incidence of complications has fallen with antibiotic therapy. Pneumonia, pneumothorax, empyema and metastatic cerebral abscess can occur. Severe, life-threatening haemoptysis can also occur, particularly in patients with cystic fibrosis.

Massive haemoptysis originates from the high-pressure systemic bronchial arteries and has a mortality of 25%. Other causes that should be considered apart from bronchiectasis, include pulmonary tuberculosis (most common), aspergilloma, lung abscess and infection, and primary and secondary malignant tumours.

Treatment of the haemoptysis consists of bed rest and antibiotics, when most stop bleeding. Blood transfusion is given if required. Urgent fibreoptic bronchoscopy is occasionally necessary to detect the source of bleeding. If the haemoptysis does not settle rapidly the treatment of choice is bronchial artery embolization. Surgical resection may be required if embolization fails.

Prognosis

The advent of effective antibiotic therapy has greatly improved the prognosis. Ultimately, most patients with severe bronchiectasis will develop respiratory failure because of chronic deterioration of the lung tissue. Cor pulmonale is also a well-recognized complication.

Cystic fibrosis

In cystic fibrosis (CF) there is an alteration in the viscosity and tenacity of mucus production at epithelial surfaces. The classical form of the syndrome includes bronchopulmonary infection and pancreatic insufficiency, with a high sweat sodium and chloride concentration. It is an autosomal recessive inherited disorder with a carrier frequency in Caucasians of 1 in 22 (see p. 185). There is a gene mutation on the long arm of chromosome 7 (7q21.3 → 7q22.1). The commonest abnormality is a specific deletion at position 508 in the amino acid sequence [ΔF_{508}] – which results in a defect in a transmembrane regulator protein (see p. 188). This is the cystic fibrosis transmembrane conductance regulator (CFTR) which represents a critical chloride channel (Fig. 14.30). The

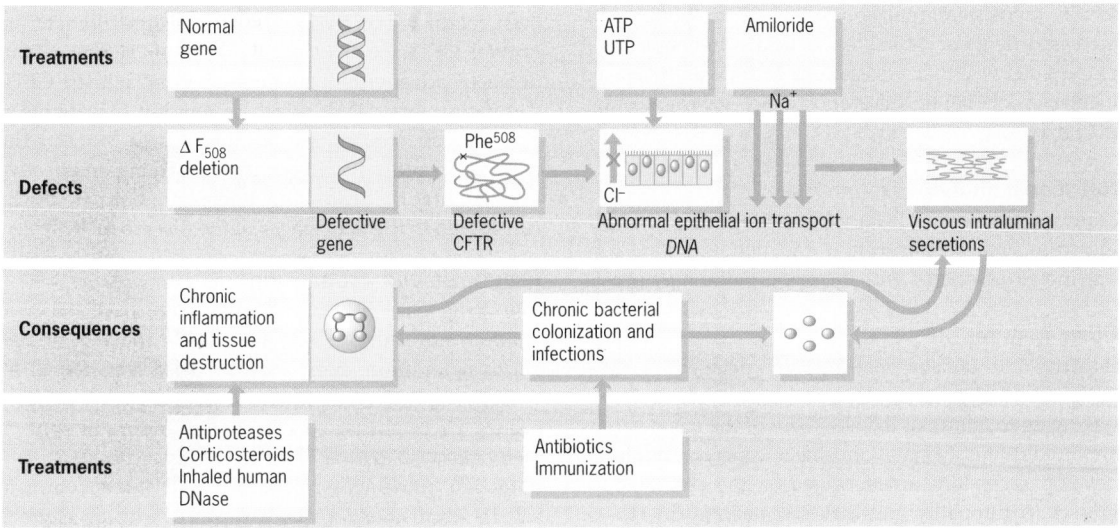

Fig. 14.30 **Cystic fibrosis:** abnormalities and therapeutic advances (see text). CFTR, cystic fibrosis transmembrane conductance regulator.

mutation alters the secondary and tertiary structure of the protein, leading to a failure of opening of the chloride channel in response to elevated cyclic AMP in epithelial cells. This results in a decreased excretion of chloride into the airway lumen and a threefold increase in the reabsorption of sodium into the epithelial cells. With less excretion of salt there is less excretion of water and increased viscosity and tenacity of airway secretions. A possible reason for the high salt content of sweat is that there is a CFTR-independent mechanism of chloride secretion in the sweat gland with an impaired reabsorption of sodium chloride in the distal end of the duct. Many genetic variants are known. The frequency of ΔF_{508} mutation in CF is 70% in the USA and UK, under 50% in southern Europe and 30% in Ashkenazi families.

Clinical features
Respiratory effects
Although the lungs of babies born with CF are structurally normal at birth, respiratory symptoms are usually the presenting feature. CF is now the most common cause of recurrent bronchopulmonary infection in childhood, and is an important cause in early adult life. Sinusitis is almost inevitable and finger clubbing eventually occurs. Breathlessness and haemoptysis occur in the later stages as airflow limitation develops. Older children may also develop nasal polyps. Spontaneous pneumothorax may occur. Respiratory failure and cor pulmonale eventually develop.

Gastrointestinal effects
About 85% of patients have symptomatic steatorrhoea owing to pancreatic dysfunction (see p. 402). Children may be born with meconium ileus owing to the viscid consistency of meconium in CF, and later in life develop the meconium ileus equivalent (MIE) syndrome, an important cause of small intestinal obstruction unique to CF. Cholesterol gallstones appear to occur with increased frequency. Cirrhosis develops in about 5% of older patients. Other associations include an increased incidence of peptic ulceration and gastrointestinal malignancy.

Nutritional effects
Many patients suffer from malnutrition mainly resulting from both malabsorption and maldigestion. Poor nutrition is associated with increased pulmonary sepsis.

Other features
Puberty and skeletal maturity are delayed in most patients with the disease. Males are almost always infertile owing to failure of development of the vas deferens and epididymis. Females are able to conceive, but often develop secondary amenorrhoea as the disease progresses. Arthropathy and diabetes mellitus (in 11% of adults with CF) also occur.

Diagnosis
The diagnosis of CF in older children and adults may be difficult. It depends on the clinical history together with:

- a family history of the disease
- a high sweat sodium concentration over 60 mmol/L (meticulous technique by laboratories performing regular sweat analysis is essential, but the test is still difficult to interpret in adults)
- blood DNA analysis of gene defect
- radiology showing features seen in bronchiectasis (see p. 870)
- absent vas deferens and epididymis
- blood immunoreactive trypsin levels are not useful diagnostically but may be useful in screening.

Treatment
Antibiotic treatment for the respiratory disease is as described under bronchiectasis on page 870; treatment of pancreatic insufficiency and malnutrition is described on page 402.

Better understanding of the basic abnormality in CF has led to dramatic changes in treatment. Potential treatments to improve hydration of secretions include blocking of sodium reabsorption with amiloride or stimulating chloride secretion with a triphosphate nucleotide (adenosine or uridine triphosphates, ATP and UTP) which stimulate nucleotide receptors by a pathway independent of cAMP. DNA from dead inflammatory cells is an important contributor to the viscosity of sputum. Human DNase capable of degrading DNA has been cloned, sequenced and expressed by recombinant techniques. Inhalation of this material has been shown to improve FEV_1 by 20% in some individuals. Similarly, inhaled antibiotics and corticosteroids are used in the hope of reducing inflammation and improving lung function. Human experimental studies have been conducted on the delivery to the epithelium of the normal CFTR gene using, as a vector, a replication-deficient adenovirus containing normal human CFTR complementary DNA which is trophic for epithelial cells. These studies are in their early stages. The recent difficulties have been in establishing an effective vector. Lung or heart–lung transplantation should be considered in the later stages of the disease (p. 823).

Prognosis and counselling
The prognosis has consistently improved; 90% of children now survive into their teens and the median survival for those born after 1990 is estimated at 40 years. Progressive respiratory failure almost inevitably occurs. Of particular concern is the finding in sputum of *Burkholderia cepacia* (formerly *Pseudomonas*), a plant pathogen, previously considered a harmless commensal. Its acquisition can be associated with accelerated disease and rapid death. Multiple antibiotic resistance is

common and spread is from person to person. Drastic strategies to limit transmission include rigid segregation of both inpatients and outpatients and the instruction to CF sufferers not to socialize together. Groups formed for mutual support and education have been disrupted, leading to considerable distress.

Genetic screening is available for the four most common mutations and this identifies 85–95% of carriers. Screening for the carrier state should be offered to persons or couples with a family history of CF, together with counselling (see p. 186).

Chronic cough

Pathological coughing results from two mechanisms:

- stimulation of sensory nerves in the epithelium by secretions, foreign bodies, cigarette smoke and tumours
- sensitization of the cough reflex in which there is an abnormal increase in the sensitivity of the cough receptors demonstrable by inhalation of the tussive agents capsaicin or hypotonic chloride solutions.

Sensitization of the cough reflex presents clinically as a persistent tickling sensation in the throat with paroxysms of coughing induced by changes in air temperature, aerosol sprays, perfumes and cigarette smoke. It is found in association with viral infections, oesophageal reflux, postnasal drip, cough variant asthma, idiopathic cough, and in 15% of patients taking angiotensin-converting enzyme (ACE) inhibitors. The association with the latter implicates neuroactive peptides – prostaglandins E_2 and $F_{2\alpha}$ and bradykinin as a cause of the cough. In the absence of chest X-ray abnormalities, possible investigations include:

- ENT examination and sinus CT for postnasal drip
- lung function tests and histamine bronchial provocation testing (p. 880) for cough variant asthma
- ambulatory oesophageal pH monitoring for oesophageal reflux
- CT scan of thorax for interstitial lung disease
- $\dot{V}_A/\dot{Q}$ scans for recurrent pulmonary embolism
- fibreoptic bronchoscopy for inhaled foreign body or tumour
- ECG, echocardiography and exercise testing for cardiac causes
- hyperventilation testing and psychiatric appraisal.

The absence of any pathology makes the management of unexplained cough difficult. Morphine will depress the sensitized cough reflex but its unwanted effects limit its use in the long term. Dihydrocodeine linctus may be of value in some patients. Demulcent preparations and cough sweets provide temporary relief only.

Patients taking ACE inhibitors should be changed to an angiotensin-II receptor antagonist, e.g. losartan (see p. 761).

Lung and heart–lung transplantation
Indications and donor selection
Indications for this treatment are patients under 60 years with a life expectancy of less than 18 months, no underlying cancer and no serious systemic disease. The main diseases treated by transplantation are:

- pulmonary fibrosis
- primary pulmonary hypertension
- cystic fibrosis
- bronchiectasis
- emphysema – particularly α_1-antitrypsin inhibitor deficiency
- Eisenmenger's syndrome.

Donor selection includes age under 40 years, good cardiac and lung function, and chest measurements slightly smaller than those of the recipient. Matching for ABO blood group is essential, but rhesus blood group compatibility is not essential. Since donor material is limited, single lung transplantation is preferred to double lung or heart–lung transplantation and can be successfully undertaken in pulmonary fibrosis, pulmonary hypertension and emphysema. Bilateral lung transplantation is required in infective conditions to prevent spillover of bacteria from the diseased lung to a single lung transplant. Eisenmenger's syndrome requires heart–lung transplant.

Complications and their treatment
- *Early* – post-transplant pulmonary oedema requires diuretics and respiratory support by ventilation.
- *Infections*, particularly within first 3 months:
  Bacterial pneumonia – antibiotics
  Cytomegalovirus – ganciclovir
  Herpes simplex – aciclovir
  P. carinii – prophylactic co-trimoxazole.
- *Immunosuppression* is with ciclosporin or tacrolimus, azathioprine or mycophenolate mofetil and prednisolone.
- *Rejection*:
  Early (first few weeks) – high-dose i.v. corticosteroids
  Late (after 3 months) – in obliterative bronchiolitis, high-dose i.v. corticosteroids are sometimes effective. Post-transplant lymphoproliferative disease may respond to rituximab, a monoclonal antibody which causes lysis of B lymphocytes.

Prognosis. There is a 2-year survival of 75% and 5-year survival of almost 50%.

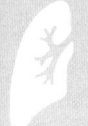

FURTHER READING

Barnes PJ (2000) Chronic obstructive pulmonary disease. *New England Journal of Medicine* **343**: 269–280.

British Thoracic Society (1998) Smoking cessation guidelines and their cost-effectiveness. *Thorax* **53** (Suppl 5): S1–S38.

Geddes D et al. (2000) Effect of lung volume reduction surgery in patients with severe emphysema. *New England Journal of Medicine* **343**: 239–245.

Griffiths TL et al. (2000) Pulmonary rehabilitation. *Lancet* **355**: 362–368.

Jones NL, Killian KJ (2000) Exercise limitation in health and disease. *New England Journal of Medicine* **343**: 632–641.

McNicholas WT (1998) Respiratory disorders during sleep. *European Respiratory Monographs* 3(10).

Plant PK et al. (2000) Early use of non-invasive ventilation for acute exacerbations of COPD. *Lancet* **355**: 1931–1935.

Super M (2000) CFTR and disease: implications for drug development. *Lancet* **355**: 1840–1842.

Wood AJJ (1996) Management of pulmonary disease in cystic fibrosis. *New England Journal of Medicine* **335**: 179–188.

Wright J, Johns R, Watts I, Melville A, Sheldon T (1997) Health effects of obstructive sleep apnoea and the effectiveness of continuous positive airways pressure: a systemic review of the research evidence. *British Medical Journal* **314**: 851–860.

Asthma

Asthma is a common chronic inflammatory condition of the lung airways whose cause is incompletely understood. Symptoms are cough, wheeze, chest tightness and shortness of breath, often worse at night. It has three characteristics:

- *airflow limitation* which is usually reversible spontaneously or with treatment
- *airway hyperresponsiveness* to a wide range of stimuli (see below)
- *inflammation of the bronchi* with eosinophils, T lymphocytes and mast cells with associated plasma exudation, oedema, smooth muscle hypertrophy, mucus plugging and epithelial damage.

In chronic asthma, inflammation may be accompanied by irreversible airflow limitation.

The underlying pathology in pre-school children may be different, in that they may not exhibit appreciable bronchial hyperreactivity. There is no evidence that chronic inflammation is the basis for the episodic wheezing associated with viral infections.

Prevalence

In many countries the prevalence of asthma is increasing, particularly in the second decade of life where this disease affects 10–15% of the population. There is also a geographical variation, with asthma being common in more developed countries, some of the highest rates being in New Zealand, but being much rarer in Far Eastern countries such as China and Malaysia, and in Africa and Central and Eastern Europe. Long-term follow-up in developing countries suggests that the disease may become more frequent as individuals become more 'westernized'. Studies of occupational asthma suggest that a high percentage of the workforce, perhaps up to 20%, may become asthmatic if exposed to potent sensitizers.

Classification

Asthma can be divided into:

- *extrinsic* – implying a definite external cause
- *intrinsic or cryptogenic* – when no causative agent can be identified.

Extrinsic asthma occurs most frequently in atopic individuals who show positive skin-prick reactions to common inhalant allergens. Positive skin-prick tests to inhalant allergens are shown in 90% of children with persistent asthma, whereas only 50% of adults show this phenomenon. Childhood asthma is often accompanied by eczema (see p. 1282). An important and often overlooked cause of late-onset asthma in adults is sensitization to chemicals or biological products in the workplace. A proportion of these cases are atopic, e.g. laboratory animal workers, but many are not accompanied by IgE sensitization.

Intrinsic asthma often starts in middle age ('late onset'). Nevertheless, many patients with adult-onset asthma show positive skin tests and on close questioning give a history of respiratory symptoms compatible with childhood asthma.

Although this classification is useful in thinking about asthma, it is of little value in clinical practice. Non-atopic individuals may develop asthma in middle age from extrinsic causes such as sensitization to occupational agents or aspirin intolerance, or because they were given β-adrenoceptor-blocking agents for concurrent hypertension or angina. Extrinsic causes must be considered in all cases of asthma and, where possible, avoided.

Aetiology and pathogenesis

There are two major factors involved in the development of asthma and many other stimuli that can precipitate attacks (Fig. 14.31).

Atopy and allergy

The term 'atopy' was used by clinicians at the beginning of the century to describe a group of disorders, including asthma and hayfever, that appeared:

- to run in families
- to have characteristic wealing skin reactions to common allergens in the environment
- to have circulating antibody in their serum that could be transferred to the skin of non-sensitized individuals.

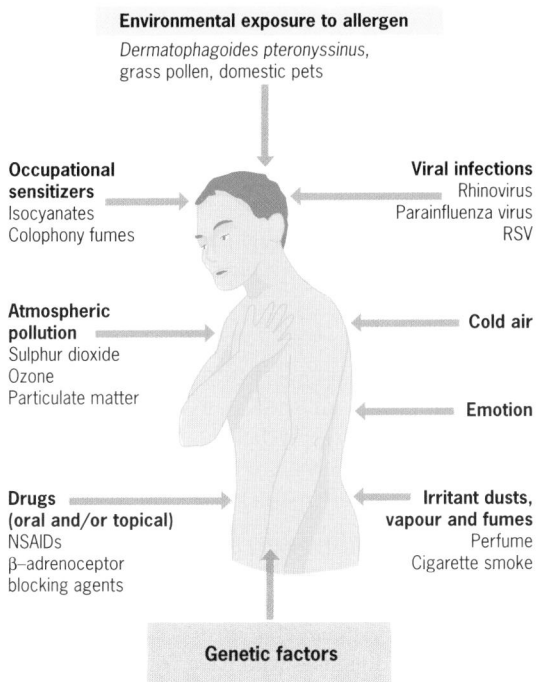

Fig. 14.31 Causes and triggers of asthma. RSV, respiratory syncytial virus; NSAIDs, non-steroidal anti-inflammatory drugs.

The term is best used to describe those individuals who readily develop antibodies of IgE class against common materials present in the environment. Such antibodies are present in 30–40% of the UK population, and there is a link between serum IgE levels and both the prevalence of asthma and airway responsiveness to histamine or methacholine. Genetic and environmental factors affect serum IgE levels. The use of candidate groups for linkage and DNA microsatellite markers to scan the entire genome has uncovered 5 or 6 chromosomal regions of interest containing candidate genes. Some of these, in combination with environmental factors, may turn out to play a key role in the development of asthma. The genes controlling the production of the cytokines IL-3, IL-4, IL-5, IL-9, IL-13 and GM-CSF – which in turn affect mast and eosinophil cell development and longevity as well as IgE production – are present in a cluster on chromosome 5q31–33 (the IL-4 gene cluster).

Early childhood exposure to allergens and maternal smoking have a major influence on IgE production. Much current interest focuses on the role of intestinal bacteria and childhood infections in shaping the immune system in early life. It has been suggested that growing up in a relatively clean environment may predispose towards an IgE response to allergens. Conversely, growing up in a dirtier environment may allow the immune system to avoid developing allergic responses. The allergens involved in asthma are similar to those in rhinitis, though the particle size of pollens (> 20 microns) means that they are much more likely to cause conjunctivitis, rhinitis and pharyngitis than asthma. Allergens from the faecal particles of the house-dust mite are the most important extrinsic cause of asthma world-wide. Cockroach allergy has been implicated in asthma in US inner-city children. The fungal spores from *Aspergillus fumigatus* give rise to a complex series of lung disorders, including asthma (see p. 902).

Increased responsiveness of the airways of the lung (airway hyperresponsiveness)

Bronchial hyperresponsiveness can be demonstrated by asking the patient to inhale gradually increasing concentrations either of histamine or methacholine (*bronchial provocation tests*). This induces a transient episode of airflow limitation in susceptible individuals (approximately 20% of the population); the dose of the agonist (provocation dose) necessary to produce a 20% fall in FEV_1 is known as the $PD_{20}FEV_1$. Patients with clinical symptoms of asthma respond to very low doses of methacholine; i.e. they have a low $PD_{20}FEV_1$ (< 11 µmol). In general, the greater the degree of hyperreactivity, the more persistent the symptoms and the greater the need for treatment.

Some patients also react to methacholine but at *higher doses* and include those with:

- attacks of asthma only on extreme exertion
- wheezing or prolonged periods of coughing following a viral infection
- cough variant asthma
- problems with asthma only during the pollen season
- allergic rhinitis, but not complaining of any lower respiratory symptoms until specifically questioned
- some subjects with no respiratory symptoms.

Although the degree of hyperresponsiveness can itself be influenced by allergic mechanisms (see p. 876 and Fig. 14.34), its pathogenesis and mode of inheritance probably involve a combination of airway inflammation and tissue remodelling.

Precipitating factors
Occupational sensitizers

Over 200 materials encountered at the workplace are known to give rise to occupational asthma. The important causes are recognized occupational diseases in the UK, and patients in insurable employment are therefore eligible for statutory compensation provided they apply within 10 years of leaving the occupation in which the asthma developed (Table 14.12). The development of asthma following exposure to some of these materials is linked to the development of specific IgE antibodies in some cases, whilst in others the cause has yet to be determined. Reactive chemicals such as isocyanates and acid anhydrides bond chemically to epithelial cells to activate them as well as provide haptens against which T cells can be directed. The risk of developing occupational asthma increases in smokers (especially for acid anhydrides).

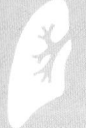

Table 14.12
Occupational asthma in the UK

Cause	Source
Non-IgE related	
Isocyanates	Polyurethane varnishes
	Industrial coatings
	Spray painting
Colophony fumes	Soldering/welders
	Electronics industry
IgE related	
Allergens from animals and insects	Laboratories
Allergens from flour and grain	Farmers
	Millers/bakers
	Grain handlers
Proteolytic enzymes	Manufacture (but not use) of 'biological' washing powders
Complex salts of platinum	Metal refining
Acid anhydrides and polyamine hardening agents	Industrial coatings

The proportion of employees developing occupational asthma depends primarily upon the level of exposure. Proper enclosure of industrial processes or appropriate ventilation can greatly reduce the risk. Atopic individuals develop occupational asthma more rapidly when exposed to agents causing the development of specific IgE antibody. Non-atopic individuals can also develop asthma when exposed to such agents, but usually after a longer period.

Non-specific factors

The characteristic feature of bronchial hyperreactivity in asthmatics means that as well as reacting to specific antigens their airways will also respond to a wide variety of non-specific stimuli.

Cold air and exercise

Most asthmatics experience an attack of wheezing after prolonged and continuous exercise. Typically, the attack does not occur during the exercise period but at its conclusion. The inhalation of cold, dry air will also precipitate an attack. It has been shown that exercise-induced wheeze is driven by histamine and leukotrienes which are released from mast cells when the epithelial lining fluid of the bronchi becomes hyperosmolar owing to drying and cooling during exercise. Exercise and cold air provocation tests can be performed to demonstrate the phenomenon.

Atmospheric pollution and irritant dusts, vapours and fumes

Many patients with asthma experience worsening of symptoms on contact with cigarette smoke, car exhaust fumes, strong perfumes or high concentrations of dust in the atmosphere. Major epidemics have been recorded when large amounts of allergens are released into the air, e.g. soy bean epidemic in Barcelona. Further minor epidemics of the disease have occurred during periods of heavy atmospheric pollution in industrial areas, caused by the presence of high concentrations of sulphur dioxide, ozone and nitrogen dioxide in the air.

Diet

Increased intakes of fresh fruit and vegetables has been shown to be protective, possibly owing to the increased intake of antioxidants.

Emotion

It is well known that emotional factors may influence asthma, but there is no evidence that patients with the disease are any more psychologically disturbed than their non-asthmatic peers.

Drugs

Non-steroid anti-inflammatory drugs (NSAIDs). NSAIDs, particularly aspirin, have a major role in the development and precipitation of attacks in approximately 5% of patients with asthma. This effect is especially prevalent in those individuals who have both nasal polyps and asthma. The precise mechanism involved is unknown, but it is thought that treatment with these drugs leads to an imbalance in the metabolism of arachidonic acid. NSAIDs inhibit arachidonic acid metabolism via the cyclo-oxygenase (COX) pathway, preventing the synthesis of prostaglandins. It is suggested that under these circumstances there is a reduced production of prostaglandin E_2 which, in a sub-proportion of genetically susceptible subjects, induces the overproduction of cysteinyl leukotrienes by eosinophils, mast cells and macrophages. In such patients there is evidence for polymorphisms involving the promoter region of the LTC_4 synthase gene that controls the level of activity of this terminal enzyme of the leukotriene-generating pathway (Fig. 14.32).

Beta-blockers. The airways of the lung have a direct parasympathetic innervation that tends to produce bronchoconstriction. There is no direct sympathetic innervation of the smooth muscle of the bronchi, and antagonism of parasympathetically induced bronchoconstriction is critically dependent upon circulating epinephrine (adrenaline) acting through β_2-receptors on the surface of smooth muscle cells. Inhibition of this effect by β-adrenoceptor-blocking drugs such as propranolol leads to bronchoconstriction and airflow limitation, but only in asthmatic subjects. The so-called selective β_1-adrenergic-blocking drugs such as atenolol may still induce attacks of asthma; their use in asthmatic patients for hypertension or angina should be questioned.

Allergen-induced asthma

The experimental inhalation of allergen by atopic asthmatic individuals leads to the development of four types of reaction, as illustrated in Figure 14.33.

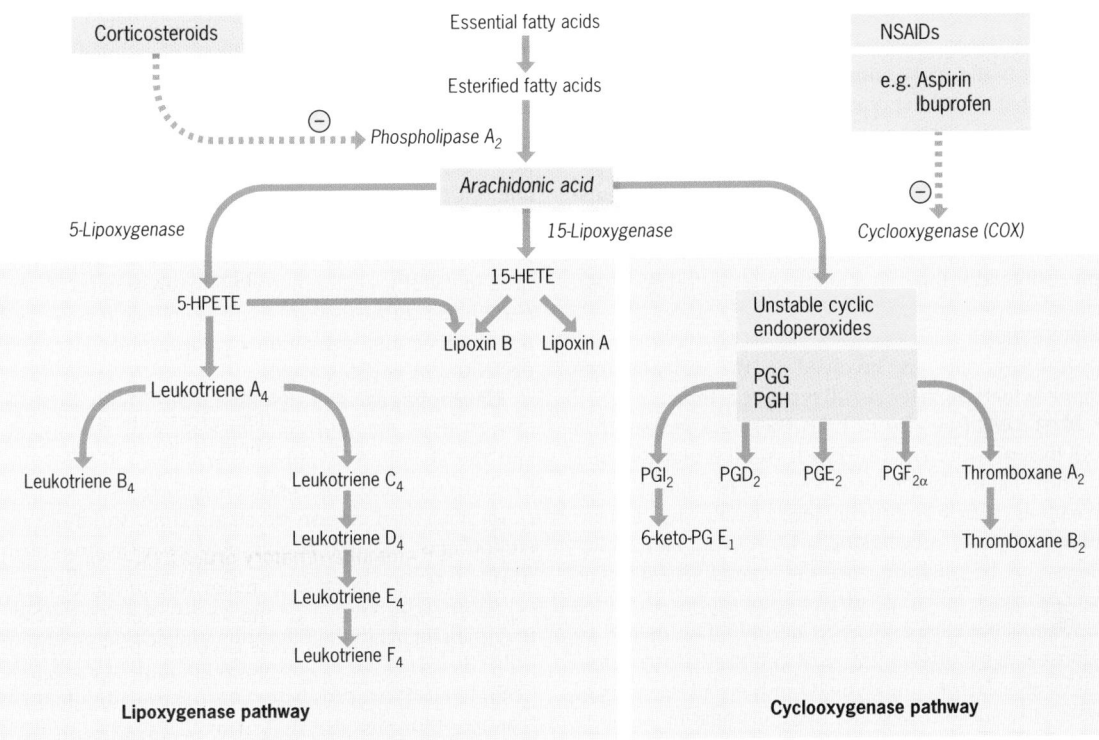

Fig. 14.32 Arachidonic acid metabolism and the effect of drugs. The enzyme cyclo-oxygenase occurs in two isoforms, COX-1 (constitutive) and COX-2 (inducible).

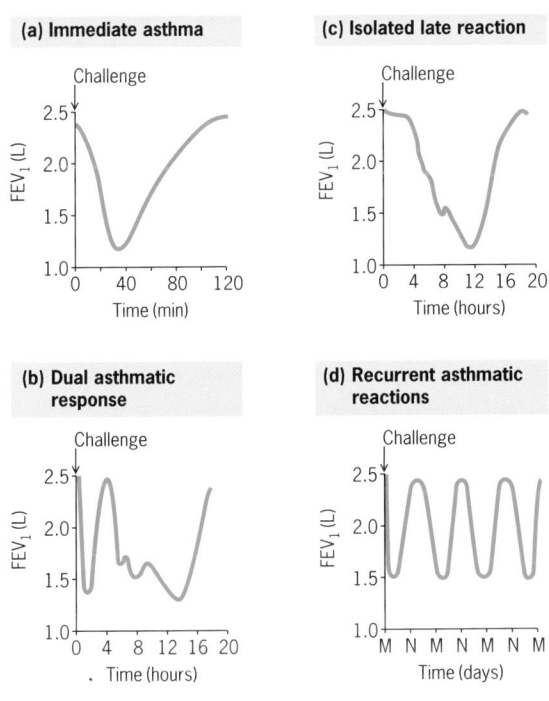

Fig. 14.33 Different types of asthmatic reactions following challenge with allergen. (a) Immediate asthma. **(b)** Dual asthmatic response. **(c)** Isolated late reaction. **(d)** Recurrent asthmatic reactions. M, midnight; N, noon.

Immediate asthma (early reaction)

This is the most common reaction, in which airflow limitation begins within minutes of contact with the allergen, reaches its maximum in 15–20 minutes and subsides by 1 hour.

Late-phase reactions

Following an immediate reaction many asthmatics subsequently develop a more prolonged and sustained attack of airflow limitation that responds poorly to inhalation of bronchodilator drugs such as salbutamol. Alternatively, the inhalation of some materials, particularly occupational sensitizers such as the isocyanates, may cause the development of an isolated late reaction with no preceding immediate response.

Dual asthmatic response

This is a combination of an early reaction followed by a late reaction.

Recurrent asthmatic reactions

The development of the late-phase reaction is associated with an increase in the underlying level of airway hyperreactivity such that individuals may show continuing episodes of asthma on subsequent days.

Pathogenesis

The pathogenesis of asthma is complex and not fully understood. It involves a number of cells, mediators,

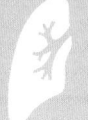
nerves and vascular leakage that can be activated by several different mechanisms, of which exposure to allergens is the most important (Fig. 14.34). It is now appreciated that the varying clinical severity and chronicity of asthma is dependent on an interplay between a special type of airway inflammation and airway wall remodelling. It is a chronic inflammatory disease of the airways driven by Th2-type T lymphocytes which leads to IgE synthesis through production of IL-4 and eosinophilic inflammation through IL-5 (Fig. 14.34).

Inflammation

Several key cells are involved in the inflammatory response that characterizes all types of asthma.

Mast cells (see also p. 195). These are increased in both the epithelium and surface secretions of asthmatics and can generate and release powerful mediators acting on smooth muscle and small blood vessels, such as histamine, tryptase, prostaglandin D_2 (PGD_2) and leukotriene C_4 (LTC_4), which cause the immediate asthmatic reaction. Since potent β_2-adrenoceptor agonists such as salbutamol have little effect on airway inflammation or hyperreactivity but inhibit mast cell mediator release, many other factors are involved in the pathogenesis of late and recurrent asthmatic reactions leading to more severe disease.

Eosinophils. These cells are found in large numbers in the bronchial wall and secretions of asthmatics. They are attracted to the airways by the eosinophilopoietic cytokines IL-3, IL-5 and GM-CSF as well as by chemokines which act on type 3 C-C chemokine receptors (CCR-3) (i.e. eotaxin, RANTES, MCP-1, MCP-3 and MCP-4). These mediators also prime eosinophils for enhanced mediator secretion. When activated, they release LTC_4, and basic proteins such as major basic protein (MBP), eosinophil cationic protein (ECP) and peroxidase (EPX) that are toxic to epithelial cells. Both the number and activation of eosinophils is rapidly decreased by corticosteroids.

Macrophages and lymphocytes. These cells are abundant in the mucous membranes of the airways and the alveoli. Macrophages may have a role in the initial uptake and presentation of allergens to lymphocytes. They can release prostaglandins, thromboxane, leukotrienes C_4 and B_4 and platelet activating factor (PAF). T helper lymphocytes (CD4) show evidence of activation (Fig. 14.34) and the release of their cytokines may play a part in the migration and activation of mast cells (IL-3, IL-4, IL-9) and eosinophils (IL-3, IL-5, GM-CSF). In addition, production of IL-4 leads to the maintenance of the allergic (Th2) T cell phenotype, favouring switching of antibody production by B lymphocytes to

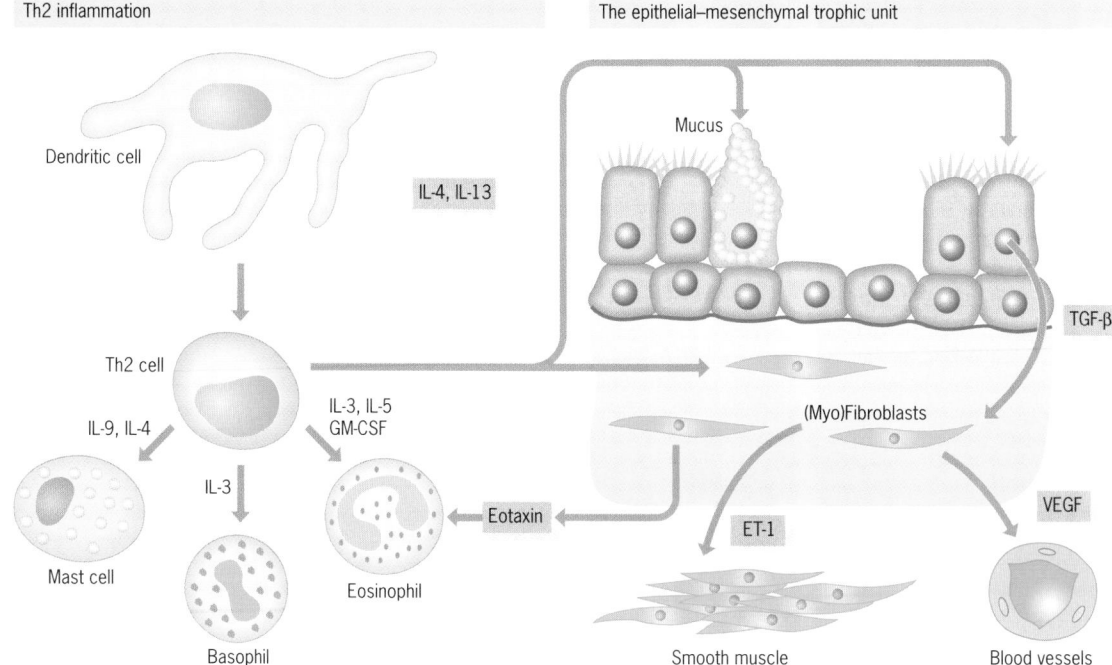

Fig. 14.34 Pathogenesis of asthma. Antigen-presenting cells (dendritic cell) activate Th2 T cells causing them to release cytokines which attract mast cells and eosinophils. IL-9 and IL-4 activate mast cells to release LTC_4, PGD_2 and histamine which act on smooth muscle and blood vessels. IL-3, IL-5 and GM-CSF attract eosinophils; these are also attracted by chemokines which act on type 3 C-C chemokine receptors (CCR-3, e.g. eotaxin, RANTES, MCP-1, -3 and -4). Activated eosinophils release LTC_4, MBP, ECP and peroxidase (EPX) which are toxic to epithelial cells. IL-4 and IL-13 produced by activated T cells maintain the allergic reaction and cause mucus secretion and smooth muscle contraction.
IL, interleukin; GM-CSF, granulocyte and macrophage colony-stimulating factor; RANTES, regulated upon activation, normal T cell expressed and secreted; MBP, major basic protein; ECP, eosinophilic cationic protein; LTC_4, leukotriene C_4; MCP, monocytic chemoattractant protein; PGD_2, prostaglandin D_2; TGF-β, transforming growth factor-β; VEGF; vascular endothelial growth factor; ET-1, endothelin-1.

IgE. In asthma there occurs a selective upregulation of Th2 T cells with reduced evidence of the Th1 phenotype (producing interferon-γ and IL-2). This polarization is thought to be mediated by dendritic cells and involves a combination of antigen presentation, costimulation and exposure to polarizing cytokines. The activity of both macrophages and lymphocytes is influenced by corticosteroids but not β_2-adrenoceptor agonists.

Remodelling

A characteristic feature of chronic asthma is an alteration of structure and functions of the formed elements of the airways. Together, these structural changes interact with inflammatory cells and mediators to cause the characteristic features of the disease. Deposition of matrix proteins, swelling and cellular infiltration cause an expansion of the submucosa beneath the epithelium so that for a given degree of smooth muscle shortening there is excess airway narrowing. Swelling outside the smooth muscle layer (in the adventitia) spreads the retractile forces exerted by the surrounding alveoli over a greater surface area so that the airways close more easily. These factors as well as an alteration of smooth muscle contractility cause the bronchial hyperresponsiveness characteristic of asthma. Several factors contribute to these changes.

The epithelium. In asthma the epithelium of the conducting airways is damaged with loss of ciliated columnar cells onto the lumen. The epithelium also undergoes metaplasia with a resultant increase in the number and activity of mucus-secreting goblet cells. The epithelium is a major source of mediators, cytokines and growth factors that serve to enhance inflammation and promote tissue remodelling. Damage and activation of the epithelium make it more vulnerable to infection by common respiratory viruses, e.g. rhinovirus, coronavirus, and to the effects of air pollutants.

Epithelial basement membrane. A pathognomonic feature of asthma is the deposition of repair collagens (types I, III and V) on the lamina reticularis beneath the basement membrane. This, along with the deposition of other matrix proteins such as laminin, tenascin and fibronectin, causes the appearance of a thickened basement membrane observed by light microscopy in asthma. This collagen reflects activation of an underlying sheath of fibroblasts that transform into contractile myofibroblasts. Aberrant signalling between the epithelium and underlying myofibroblasts is thought to be the principal cause of airway wall remodelling, since the cells are prolific producers of a range of tissue growth factors such as epidermal growth factors (EGF), transforming growth factor-β (TGF-β), connective tissue-derived growth factor, platelet-derived growth factor (PDGF), endothelin (ET), insulin-like growth factors (IGF), nerve growth factors and vascular endothelial growth factors (Fig. 14.34). The same interaction between epithelium and mesenchymal tissues is central to branching morphogenesis in the developing fetal lung. It has been suggested that these mechanisms are reactivated in asthma (but not in other airways disease), but instead of causing airway growth and branching, they lead to thickening of the airway wall (remodelling). Increased deposition of collagens, proteoglycans and matrix proteins creates a microenvironment conducive to ongoing inflammation since these complex molecules possess important cell-signalling functions which prolong inflammatory cell survival and prime them for mediator secretion.

Smooth muscle. A prominent feature of asthma is hyperplasia of the helical bands of airways smooth muscle. In addition to increasing in amount, the smooth muscle alters in function to contract more easily and stay contracted because of a change in actin–myosin cross-link cycling. These changes allow the asthmatic airways to contract too much and too easily at the least provocation.

Nerves. Neural reflexes, both central and peripheral, contribute to the irritability of asthmatic airways. Central reflexes involve stimulation of nerve endings in the epithelium and submucosa with transmission of impulses via the spinal cord and brain back down to the airways where release of acetylcholine from nerve endings stimulates M_2 receptors on smooth muscle causing contraction. Local neural reflexes involve antidromic neurotransmission and the release of a variety of neuropeptides. Some of these are smooth muscle contractants (substance P, neurokinin A), some are vasoconstrictors (e.g. calcitonin gene related peptide, CGRP) and some vasodilators (e.g. neuropeptide Y, vasoactive intestinal polypeptide). Bradykinin generated by tissue and serum proteolytic enzymes (including most or all tryptase activity) is also a potent stimulus of local neural reflexes involving (non-myelinated) nerve fibres.

Clinical features

Patients experiencing asthma exhibit symptoms that are virtually identical to those suffering from airflow limitation caused by COPD (see p. 864). Wheezing attacks and episodic shortness of breath are almost universal. Symptoms are usually worst during the night. Cough is a frequent symptom that sometimes predominates and is often misdiagnosed as being due to bronchitis. Nocturnal cough can be a presenting feature.

There is a tremendous variation in the frequency and duration of the attacks. Some patients have only one or two attacks a year that last for a few hours, whilst others have attacks lasting for weeks. Some patients can have chronic symptoms. Attacks may be precipitated by all the factors illustrated in Figure 14.31. Asthma is a major cause for impaired quality of life with impact on work, recreational, as well as physical activities and emotions.

Investigations

There is no single satisfactory diagnostic test for all asthmatic patients.

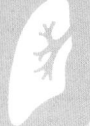

Peak expiratory flow charts

Measurements of PEFR on waking, prior to taking a bronchodilator and before bed after a bronchodilator, are particularly useful in demonstrating the variable airflow limitation that characterizes the disease. An example is shown in Figure 14.15 on page 851. The diurnal variation in PEF is a good measure of asthma activity.

This measure is also of help in the longer-term assessment of the patient's disease and its response to treatment. Peak flows need to be measured over several days and preferably over a weekend or short holiday if the effect of work exposure is also being studied.

Reversibility

Asthma can be diagnosed on the basis of demonstrating a greater than 15% improvement in FEV_1 or PEFR following the inhalation of a bronchodilator. However, this degree of response may often not be present if the asthma is in remission or in very severe chronic disease, when little reversibility can be demonstrated, or if the patient is already being treated with long-acting bronchodilators.

Exercise tests

These have been widely used in the diagnosis of asthma in children. Ideally, the child should run for 6 minutes on a treadmill at a workload sufficient to increase the heart rate above 160 beats per minute. Alternative methods use cold air challenge or isocapnoeic hyperventilation (forced overbreathing with artificially maintained P_aCO_2). A negative test does not automatically rule out asthma.

Histamine or methacholine bronchial provocation test (see p. 875)

This test indicates the presence of airway hyperresponsiveness, a feature found in most asthmatics, and can be particularly useful in investigating those patients whose main symptom is cough. The test should not be performed on individuals who have poor lung function ($FEV_1 < 1.5$ L) or a history of 'brittle' asthma.

Trial of corticosteroids

All patients who present with severe airflow limitation should undergo a formal trial of steroids. Prednisolone 30 mg orally should be given daily for 2 weeks with lung function measured before and immediately after the course. A substantial improvement in FEV_1 (>15%) confirms the presence of a reversible element and indicates that the administration of inhaled steroids will prove beneficial to the patient. If the trial is for 2 weeks or less, the oral steroids can be withdrawn without tailing off the dose, and should be replaced by inhaled corticosteroids in those who have responded and are thought will benefit.

Blood and sputum tests

Patients with asthma may have an increase in the number of eosinophils in peripheral blood ($>0.4 \times 10^9$/L).

The presence of large numbers of eosinophils in the sputum is a more useful diagnostic tool.

Chest X-ray

There are no diagnostic features of asthma on the chest X-ray, although during an acute episode or in chronic severe disease overinflation is characteristic. A chest X-ray may be helpful in excluding a pneumothorax, which can occur as a complication, or in detecting the pulmonary shadows associated with allergic bronchopulmonary aspergillosis.

Skin tests

Skin-prick tests should be performed in all cases of asthma to help identify extrinsic causes.

Allergen provocation tests

Allergen challenge is not required in the clinical investigation of patients, except in cases of suspected occupational asthma. Another controversial exception is the investigation of food allergy causing asthma. This diagnosis is difficult, although many patients are concerned about the possibility. If the patient has asthma without any other systemic features, then food allergy is most unlikely to be the cause. Open food challenges are unreliable and if the diagnosis is seriously entertained, blind oral challenges with the food disguised in opaque gelatine capsules are necessary to confirm or refute a causative link (see p. 249).

Management

Asthma is extremely common and causes considerable morbidity. The aims of treatment are:

- to abolish symptoms
- to restore normal or best possible long-term airway function
- to reduce the risk of severe attacks
- to enable normal growth to occur in children
- to minimize absence from school or employment.

This involves:

- patient and family education about asthma
- patient and family participation in treatment
- avoidance of identified causes where possible
- use of the lowest effective doses of convenient medications to minimize short-term and long-term side-effects.

Many asthmatics belong to self-help groups whose aim is to further their understanding of the disease and to foster self-confidence and fitness.

Control of extrinsic factors

Measures must be taken to avoid causative allergens such as the house-dust mite, pets, moulds and certain foodstuffs (see allergic rhinitis), particularly in childhood.

Avoidance of the house-dust mite is now possible with effective and comfortable covers for bedding and changes to living accommodation. Active and passive smoking should be avoided, as should beta-blockers in either tablet or eyedrop form.

Individuals intolerant to aspirin may benefit, though are rarely cured, by avoiding salicylates. Other agents (e.g. preservatives and colouring materials such as tartrazine) should be avoided if shown to be a causative factor. Fifty per cent of individuals sensitized to occupational agents may be cured if they are kept permanently away from exposure. The remaining 50% continue to have symptoms that may be as severe as when exposed to materials at work. This is particularly so if they had been symptomatic for a long time before the diagnosis was made.

This emphasises:

- the importance of the rapid identification of extrinsic causes of asthma and their removal wherever possible (e.g. occupational agents, family pets)
- once extrinsic asthma is initiated, it may become self-perpetuating.

Drug treatment

The mainstay of asthma therapy is the use of therapeutic agents delivered as aerosols or powders directly into the lungs (Practical box 14.4). The advantages of this method of administration are that drugs are delivered direct to the lung and the first-pass metabolism in the liver is avoided; both these factors mean that much lower doses are necessary and unwanted effects are minimized or absent.

Both national and international guidelines have been published on the stepwise treatment of asthma (Box 14.1) based on three important factors:

- Asthma self-management with regular asthma monitoring using peak flow meters and individual treatment plans discussed with each patient and written down.
- The appreciation that asthma is an inflammatory disease and that anti-inflammatory (controller) therapy should be started even in mild cases.
- Use of short-acting inhaled bronchodilators (e.g. salbutamol and terbutaline) only to relieve breakthrough symptoms. Increased use of bronchodilator treatment to relieve increasing symptoms is an important index of deteriorating disease.

A list of drugs used in asthma is shown in Box 14.2.

 Practical box 14.4

Inhaled therapy

Use of an inhaler
1. The canister is shaken.
2. The patient exhales to functional residual capacity (not residual volume), i.e. normal expiration.
3. The aerosol nozzle is placed to the open mouth.
4. The patient simultaneously inhales rapidly and activates the aerosol.
5. Inhalation is completed.
6. The breath is held for 10 seconds if possible.

Even with good technique only 15% of the contents is inhaled and 85% is deposited on the wall of the pharynx and ultimately swallowed.

Spacers
These are plastic conical spheres inserted between the patient's mouth and the inhaler. They are designed to reduce particle velocity so that less drug is deposited in the mouth. Spacers also diminish the need for coordination between aerosol activation and inhalation. They are useful in children and in the elderly.

Box 14.1

The stepwise management of asthma

Step	PEFR	Treatment
1 Occasional symptoms, less frequent than daily	100% predicted	As-required bronchodilators If used more than once daily, move to step 2
2 Daily symptoms	≤ 80% predicted	Anti-inflammatory drugs Sodium cromoglicate or low-dose inhaled corticosteroids up to 800 µg If not controlled, move to step 3
3 Severe symptoms	50–80% predicted	High-dose inhaled corticosteroids up to 2000 µg daily
4 Severe symptoms uncontrolled with high-dose inhaled corticosteroids	50–80% predicted	Add regular long-acting β_2 agonists (e.g. salmeterol)
5 Severe symptoms deteriorating	≤ 50% predicted	Add prednisolone 40 mg daily
6 Severe symptoms deteriorating in spite of prednisolone	≤ 30% predicted	Hospital admission

Short-acting bronchodilator treatment taken at any step on as-required basis

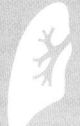

Box 14.2

Drugs used in asthma

Inhaled steroids

Short-acting relievers (salbutamol, terbutaline)

Long-acting relief/disease controllers

Long-acting β₂ agonists – salmeterol, formoterol
Leukotriene modifiers – montelukast, zafirlukast, pranlukast, zileuton

Other agents with bronchodilator activity

Anticholinergic agents (ipratropium, oxitropium)
Theophylline preparations

Steroid-sparing agents

Methotrexate
Ciclosporin
Gold
Intravenous immunoglobulin
Anti-IgE monoclonal antibody

β₂-adrenergic agonists

The most widely used bronchodilator preparations contain β_2-adrenergic agonists that are selective for the respiratory tract and do not stimulate the β_1-adrenoceptors of the myocardium. These drugs are potent bronchodilators because they cause relaxation of bronchial smooth muscle. Such treatment is very effective in relieving symptoms but does little for the underlying inflammatory nature of the disease. Only the mildest asthmatics with intermittent attacks should rely on bronchodilator treatment alone. Inhalants such as salbutamol (100 µg) or terbutaline (250 µg) should be prescribed as two puffs as required. Some patients use nebulizers at home for self-administration of salbutamol or terbutaline. Such treatment is very effective but patients must not rely on repeated home administration of nebulized β_2-adrenoceptor agonists for worsening asthma, and must be encouraged to seek medical advice urgently if their condition does not improve. The excessive use of β_2 agonists has been linked to the two epidemics of asthma mortality in the 1960s and 1980s although the link has not been conclusively proven.

Salmeterol and formoterol (eformoterol) are highly selective and potent long-acting β_2-adrenoceptor agonists effective by inhalation for up to 12 hours, thereby reducing the need for administration to once or twice daily. Long-acting β_2-adrenoceptor agonists are now used routinely for maintenance therapy in patients who are not controlled on standard doses of inhaled steroids. Tablets of β_2-adrenoceptor agonists are less effective than when the drug is inhaled. To help those who cannot coordinate activation of the aerosol and inhalation, several breath-activated or dry powder devices have been developed.

Anticholinergic bronchodilators

Muscarinic receptors are found in the respiratory tract; large airways contain mainly M_3 receptors whereas the peripheral lung tissue contains M_3 and M_1 receptors (see p. 837). Non-selective muscarinic antagonists – ipratropium bromide (20–40 mg three or four times daily) or oxitropium bromide (200 mg twice daily) – by aerosol inhalation are useful bronchodilators, particularly in COPD, and may be additive to β_2-adrenoceptor stimulants.

Anti-inflammatory drugs

Sodium cromoglicate and nedocromil sodium prevent activation of many inflammatory cells, particularly mast cells, eosinophils and epithelial cells, but not lymphocytes, by blocking a specific chloride channel which in turn prevents calcium influx. These drugs are effective in patients with milder asthma. Sodium cromoglicate is taken regularly either in the form of a Spincap containing 20 mg or in aerosol form from a metered-dose inhaler delivering 5 mg per puff. The dose should be two puffs four times daily from an inhaler, or one Spincap three or four times daily. Nedocromil sodium is taken as an aerosol at a dose of 4 mg (two puffs) two to four times daily.

Inhaled corticosteroids

All patients who have regular persisting symptoms need regular treatment with inhaled corticosteroids delivered in a stepwise fashion or as a high dose followed by a reduction to maintenance levels. Beclometasone dipropionate is the most widely used inhaled steroid and is available in doses of 50, 100, 200 and 250 µg per puff. Other inhaled steroids include budesonide, fluticasone, mometasone and triamcinolone.

Much of the inhaled dose does not reach the lung but is either swallowed or exhaled. Deposition in the lung varies between 10–25% depending on inhaler technique and the technical characteristics of the aerosol device. Drug which is deposited in the airways reaches the systemic circulation directly, through the bronchial circulation, while any drug that is swallowed has to pass through the liver before it can reach the systemic circulation. Gram for gram, fluticasone and mometasone are more potent than beclometasone with considerably less systemic bioavailability, owing to their greater sensitivity to hepatic metabolism. The newer hydrofluoroalkane (HFA) aerosols of beclometasone deliver a higher proportion of useable drug than the old CFC-based aerosols, and the effective dosage of HFA-beclometasone is equivalent to the same dose of HFA-fluticasone, whereas previously the effective dose ratio was 2 : 1. Absorption of beclometasone and budesonide does not seem to present a risk at doses up to 800 µg/day, but when using high-dose inhaled steroids in patients who have not responded to standard doses, fluticasone or mometasone may be preferred because of their lower bioavailability. Recent studies indicate that in patients with moderate asthma, addition of an inhaled long-acting β₂ agonist such as salmeterol or formoterol (eformoterol) is more effective than doubling the dose of inhaled corticosteroid, when patients are taking beclometasone 800 μg/day or equivalent.

The unwanted effects of inhaled corticosteroids are oral candidiasis, which may develop in 5% of patients, and hoarseness due to the effect of corticosteroids on the laryngeal muscles. Subcapsular cataract formation is rare but can occur. Abnormalities of bone metabolism can be detected when inhaled steroids are taken in high doses (beclometasone or budesonide > 800 μg daily). In children, inhaled steroids at doses greater than 400 μg daily have been shown to retard short-term growth. Inhaled corticosteroid use should be stepped down once asthma comes under control.

Oral corticosteroids

Oral corticosteroids may be necessary for those individuals not controlled on inhaled corticosteroids. The dose should be kept as low as possible to minimize side-effects. The effect of short-term treatment with prednisolone 30 mg daily is shown in Figure 14.15 on page 851. Some patients require continuing treatment with oral corticosteroids. Several studies suggest that treatment with low doses of methotrexate (15 mg weekly) can significantly reduce the dose of prednisolone needed to control the disease in some patients, and ciclosporin also improves lung function in some steroid-dependent asthmatics. Several other steroid-sparing strategies have also been tried with varying degrees of success.

Cysteinyl leukotriene receptor antagonists (LTRAs)

This new class of anti-asthma therapy targets one of the principal asthma mediators by inhibiting the cysteinyl LT receptor. Montelukast and zafirlukast are given orally and are effective in a subpopulation of patients. However, at present it is not possible to predict which individuals will benefit: a 4-week trial of LTRA therapy is recommended before a decision is made to continue or stop. LTRAs should be considered in any patient who is not controlled on low to medium doses of inhaled steroids. Their action is additive to that of long-acting β₂ agonists. LTRAs are particularly useful in patients with aspirin-intolerant asthma and on those patients requiring high-dose inhaled or oral corticosteroids.

Newer agents that modulate IgE-associated inflammation are being developed. These have their effects on IL-4 (a soluble recombinant of IL-4 receptor can be delivered in nebulized form) or on free IgE (a recombinant humanized monoclonal antibody that complexes with free IgE – rhuMAB-E25 or omalizumab – blocking its interaction with mast cells and basophils).

Antibiotics

There is no evidence that antibiotics are helpful in the management of patients who suffer from properly diagnosed asthma. However, wheezing frequently occurs in exacerbations of COPD associated with infected sputum. Yellow or green sputum containing eosinophils and bronchial epithelial cells may be coughed up in acute exacerbations of asthma. This is not normally due to bacterial infection and antibiotics are not required. Occasionally, mycoplasma and chlamydia infections can cause chronic relapsing asthma. The use of appropriate antimicrobials is worthwhile only if a bacterial diagnosis has been established.

Management of asthma exacerbations

(Emergency box 14.2)

The term 'status asthmaticus' was defined as asthma that had failed to resolve with therapy in 24 hours.

 Emergency box 14.2

Treatment of severe asthma

At home

1. The patient is assessed. Tachycardia, a high respiratory rate and inability to speak in sentences indicate a severe attack.
2. If the PEFR is less than 150 L/min (in adults), an ambulance should be called. (All doctors should carry peak flow meters.)
3. Nebulized salbutamol 5 mg or terbutaline 10 mg is administered.
4. Hydrocortisone sodium succinate 200 mg i.v. is given.
5. Oxygen 40–60% is given if available.
6. Prednisolone 60 mg is given orally.

At hospital

1. The patient is reassessed.
2. Oxygen 40–60% is given.
3. The PEFR is measured using a low-reading peak flow meter, as an ordinary meter measures only from 60 L/min upwards. Measure O₂ saturation with a pulse oximeter.

4. Nebulized salbutamol 5 mg or terbutaline 10 mg is repeated and administered 4-hourly.
5. Add nebulized ipratropium bromide 0.5 mg to nebulized salbutamol/terbutaline.
6. Hydrocortisone 200 mg i.v. is given 4-hourly for 24 hours.
7. Prednisolone is continued at 60 mg orally daily for 2 weeks.
8. Arterial blood gases are measured; if the P_aCO_2 is greater than 7 kPa, ventilation should be considered.
9. A chest X-ray is performed to exclude pneumothorax.
10. One of the following intravenous infusions is given if no improvement is seen:

    salbutamol 3–20 μg/min, or
    terbutaline 1.5–5.0 μg/min.

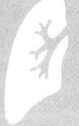

Although this term is still used occasionally, it has now been discarded and replaced by 'acute severe asthma', i.e. severe asthma that has not been controlled by the patient's use of medication. Patients with severe asthma exacerbations typically have:

- inability to complete a sentence in one breath
- respiratory rate ≥ 25 breaths per minute
- tachycardia ≥ 110 beats/min (pulsus paradoxus, p. 710, is not useful as it is only present in 45% of cases)
- PEFR < 50% of predicted normal or best.

Features of life-threatening attacks are:

- a silent chest, cyanosis or feeble respiratory effort
- exhaustion, confusion or coma
- bradycardia or hypotension
- PEFR < 30% of predicted normal or best (approximately 150 L/min in adults).

Arterial blood gases should always be measured in asthmatic patients requiring admission to hospital. Pulse oximetry is useful in monitoring oxygen saturation during the admission and reduces the need for repeat arterial puncture. Features suggesting very severe life-threatening attacks are:

- a high $P_aCO_2 > 6$ kPa
- severe hypoxaemia $P_aO_2 < 8$ kPa irrespective of treatment with oxygen
- a low and falling arterial pH.

Treatment is commenced with 5 mg of nebulized salbutamol or 10 mg terbutaline with oxygen as the driving gas. A chest X-ray is taken to exclude a pneumothorax. If no improvement occurs with nebulized therapy, 250 µg of salbutamol or terbutaline should be administered by intravenous infusion over 10 minutes. Intravenous aminophylline is sometimes used for severe asthma but has a narrow therapeutic index. Hydrocortisone 200 mg i.v. should be administered 4-hourly for 24 hours, and 60 mg of prednisolone should be given orally daily. Patients who do not respond to this regimen may require ventilation.

Ideally patients should be kept in hospital for at least 5 days, since the majority of sudden deaths occur 2–5 days after admission. During this time oxygen saturation should be monitored by oximetry. Oral corticosteroids can be reduced from 60 mg to 30 mg once improvement occurs. Further reduction should be gradual on an outpatient basis until an appropriate maintenance dose or substitution by inhaled corticosteroid aerosols can be achieved.

If the PEFR is greater than 150 L/min, patients may improve dramatically on nebulized therapy and may not require hospital admission. Their regular treatment should be increased, to include treatment for 2 weeks with 30 mg of prednisolone followed by a gradual reduction in the oral dose and substitution by an inhaled corticosteroid preparation.

Management of catastrophic sudden severe (brittle) asthma

This is an unusual variant of asthma in which patients are at risk from sudden death in spite of the fact that their asthma may be well controlled between attacks. Severe life-threatening attacks may occur within hours or even minutes. Such patients require a carefully worked out management plan agreed by respiratory physician, primary care physician and patient, and require:

- emergency supplies of medications at home, in the car and at work
- oxygen and resuscitation equipment at home and at work
- nebulized β_2 agonists at home and at work
- self-injectable epinephrine (adrenaline): two Epipens of 0.3 mg epinephrine at home, at work and to be carried by patient at all times
- prednisolone 60 mg
- Medic Alert bracelet.

The patient should attend the nearest hospital immediately. Admission to intensive care may be required.

Prognosis of asthma

Although asthma often improves in children as they reach their teens, it is now realized that the disease frequently returns in the second, third and fourth decades. In the past the data indicating a natural decrease in asthma through teenage years have led to childhood asthma being treated as an episodic disorder. However, it is now increasingly considered that airway inflammation is present continuously from an early age and usually persists even if the symptoms resolve. Moreover, airways remodelling accelerates the process of decline in lung function over time. This has led to a reappraisal of the treatment strategy for asthma, mandating the early use of effective controller drugs and environmental measures from the time asthma is first diagnosed.

FURTHER READING

Barnes PJ (2000) New directions in allergic diseases: mechanism-based anti-inflammatory therapies. *Journal of Allergy and Clinical Immunology* **106**: 5–16.

Bousquet J et al (2000) Asthma: from bronchoconstriction to airways inflammation and remodelling. *American Journal of Respiratory and Critical Care Medicine* **161**: 1720–1745.

British Thoracic Society (1997) The British guidelines on asthma management. *Thorax* **52** (Suppl 1): S1–S21.

British Thoracic Society (2000) Aspirin intolerance and related syndromes. *Thorax* **55** (Suppl 2): S1–S90.

Christiansen SC (2000) Day care siblings and asthma – please sneeze on my child. *New England Journal of Medicine* **343**: 574–575.

Chung KF, Godard P (2000) Difficult therapy-resistant asthma. *European Respiratory Reviews* 10(69).

Holgate ST (1998) Asthma and allergy. *Quarterly Journal of Medicine* **91**: 171–184.

Venables KM, Chan-Yeung M (1997) Occupational asthma. *Lancet* **349**: 1465–1469.

Pneumonia

Pneumonia may be defined as an inflammation of the substance of the lungs. It is usually caused by bacteria. Clinically it presents as an acute illness characterized in the majority of cases by the presence of cough, purulent sputum and fever together with physical signs or radiological changes compatible with consolidation of the lung. The advent of antibiotics has decreased dramatically the mortality from pneumonia among young people but it remains a dangerous condition. Pneumonia is a major cause of death in individuals over the age of 70 years. Bacterial pneumonia is more frequent in HIV-infected individuals than in the general population, particularly in HIV-infected intravenous drug users. The causative agents are the same as found in non-HIV community-acquired pneumonia.

Classification

Pneumonia can be classified both anatomically and on the basis of the aetiology.

Classification by site

Pneumonias are either localized, with the whole of one or more lobes affected, or diffuse, when they primarily affect the lobules of the lung, often in association with the bronchi and bronchioles – a condition referred to as 'bronchopneumonia'.

Classification by aetiology

An aetiological factor can be discovered in approximately 75% of patients. The term 'atypical pneumonia' has been used to describe pneumonia caused by agents such as *Mycoplasma*, *Legionella*, *Chlamydia* and *Coxiella burnetii*. While these pneumonias can differ from pneumococcal disease, there is a considerable overlap in clinical presentation and as these agents account for almost one-fifth of the cases of pneumonia (Table 14.13), the term 'atypical' has been dropped. Pneumonias may also result from:

- chemical causes, such as in the aspiration of vomit (see p. 890)
- radiotherapy (see p. 907)
- allergic mechanisms (see p. 902).

Mycobacterium tuberculosis is a cause of pneumonia; it is considered separately, since both its mode of presentation and its treatment are very different from the other infective agents.

Precipitating factors

- *Strep. pneumoniae* – often follows viral infection with influenza or parainfluenza.
- Hospitalized 'ill' patients – often infected with Gram-negative organisms.
- Cigarette smoking (the strongest independent risk factor for invasive pneumococcal disease).
- Alcohol excess.
- Bronchiectasis (e.g. in cystic fibrosis).
- Bronchial obstruction (e.g. carcinoma) – occasionally associated with infection with 'non-pathogenic' organisms.
- Immunosuppression (e.g. AIDS or treatment with cytotoxic agents) – organisms include *Pneumocystis*

Table 14.13
The aetiology of pneumonia in the UK

Infecting agent	Frequency as a cause of pneumonia (%)	Clinical circumstances
Streptococcus pneumoniae	50	Community pneumonia patients usually previously fit
Mycoplasma pneumoniae	6	As above
Influenza A virus (usually with a bacterial component)	5	As above
Haemophilus influenzae	5	Pre-existing lung disease: COPD
Chlamydia pneumoniae	5	Community-acquired pneumonia
Chlamydia psittaci	3	Contact with birds (though not inevitable)
Staphylococcus aureus	2	Children, intravenous drug abusers, associated with influenza virus infections
Legionella pneumophila	2	Institutional outbreaks (hospitals and hotels), sporadic, endemic
Coxiella burnetii	1	Abattoir and animal-hide workers
Pseudomonas aeruginosa	< 1	Cystic fibrosis
Pneumocystis carinii *Actinomyces israelii* *Nocardia asteroides* *Cytomegalovirus* *Aspergillus fumigatus*	< 1	AIDS, lymphomas, leukaemias, use of cytotoxic drugs and corticosteroids
Anaerobic organisms	< 1	Inhalation pneumonia, alcohol abuse, postoperative
None isolated	20	–

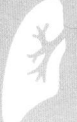

carinii, Mycobacterium avium-intracellulare, cytomegalovirus.

- Intravenous drug abuse – frequently associated with *Staph. aureus* infection.
- Inhalation from oesophageal obstruction – often associated with infection with anaerobes.

Clinical features

The clinical presentation varies according to the immune state of the patient and the infecting agent. In the most common type of pneumonia – caused by *Strep. pneumoniae* – there is often a preceding history of a viral infection.

With *Strep. pneumoniae* infection the patient rapidly becomes more ill with a high temperature (up to 39.5°C), pleuritic pain and a dry cough. A day or two later, rusty-coloured sputum is produced and at about the same time the patient may develop labial herpes simplex. The patient breathes rapidly and shallowly, the affected side of the chest moves less, and signs of consolidation may be present together with a pleural rub. See Box 14.3 for severe community-acquired pneumonia.

Investigations

Chest X-ray confirms the area of consolidation (Fig. 14.35), but radiological changes lag behind the clinical course so that X-ray changes may be minimal at the start of the illness. Conversely, consolidation may remain on the chest X-ray for several weeks after the patient is clinically cured. The chest X-ray always returns to normal by 6 weeks, except in patients with severe airflow limitation. Persistent changes on the chest X-ray after this time suggest a bronchial abnormality, usually a carcinoma, with persisting secondary pneumonia. Chest X-rays should rarely be repeated more frequently than

at weekly intervals during the acute illness and then at 6 weeks after discharge from hospital.

In *Strep. pneumoniae* pneumonia, there is often a white blood cell count that is greater than $15 \times 10^9/L$ (90% polymorphonuclear leucocytosis) and an erythrocyte sedimentation rate (ESR) greater than 100 mm/h.

Types of pneumonia

The individual features of various pneumonias are given below. The overall investigation and management is shown in Figure 14.36 and discussed on page 890.

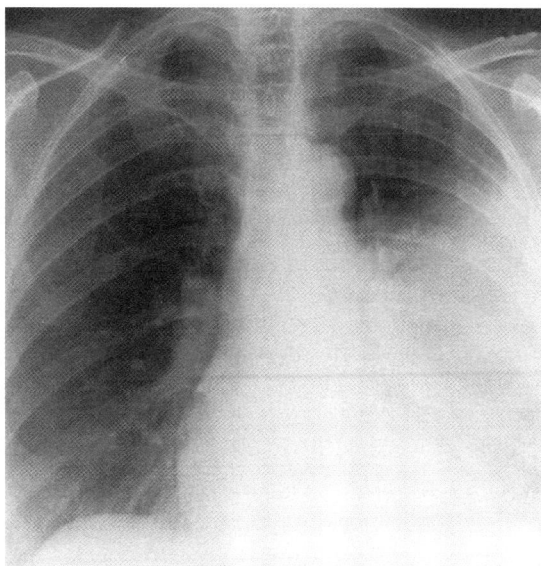

Fig. 14.35 Chest X-ray to show lobar pneumonia.

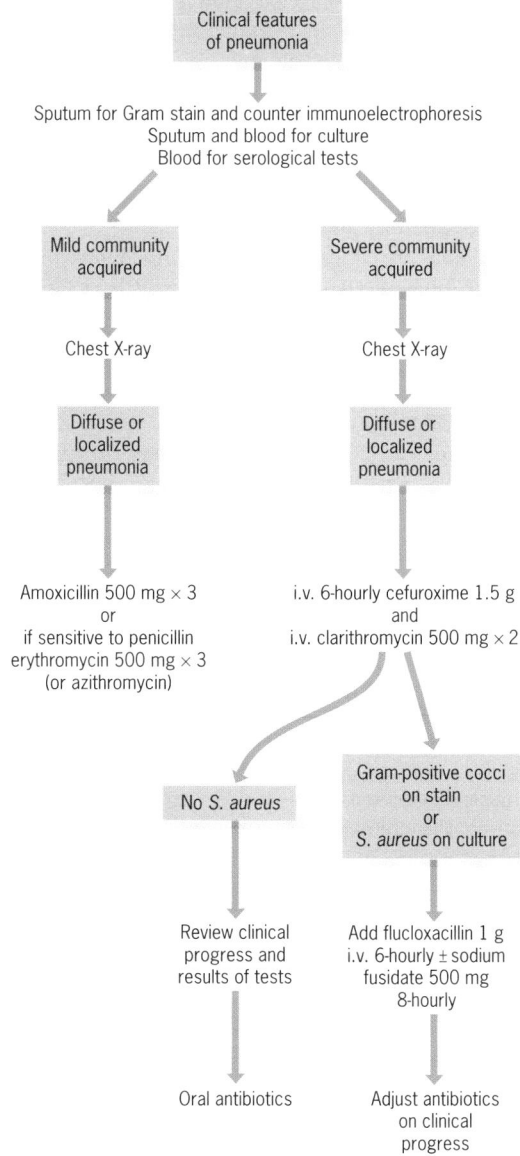

Fig. 14.36 Algorithm for the management of pneumonia (see also p. 890).

Mycoplasma pneumonia

Mycoplasma pneumonia is relatively common and occurs in cycles of 3–4 years. It often occurs in patients in their teens and twenties, frequently amongst those living in boarding institutions. Generalized features such as headaches and malaise often precede the chest symptoms by 1–5 days. Cough may not be obvious initially and physical signs in the chest may be scanty.

On chest X-ray, usually only one lobe is involved but sometimes there may be dramatic shadowing in both lungs. There is frequently no correlation between the X-ray appearances and the clinical state of the patient.

The white blood cell count is not raised. Cold agglutinins occur in half of the cases. The diagnosis is confirmed by a rising antibody titre. Treatment is with erythromycin 500 mg four times daily for 7–10 days. Tetracycline is also effective.

Although most patients recover in 10–14 days, the disease can be protracted, with cough and X-ray appearance lasting for weeks and relapses occurring. Lung abscesses and pleural effusions are rare.

Extrapulmonary complications can occur at any time during the illness and occasionally dominate the clinical picture. Most are rare but they include:

- myocarditis and pericarditis
- rashes and erythema multiforme
- haemolytic anaemia and thrombocytopenia
- myalgia and arthralgia
- meningoencephalitis and other neurological abnormalities
- gastrointestinal symptoms (e.g. vomiting, diarrhoea).

Viral pneumonia

Viral pneumonia is uncommon in adults, bacteria being the usual cause of the pneumonia per se. Influenza A virus or adenovirus infection can occasionally produce pneumonia.

Other pneumonias

Haemophilus influenzae

H. influenzae is frequently identified in the yellow-green sputum produced during exacerbation of chronic bronchitis. It is therefore not surprising that this organism may be the cause of pneumonia in people suffering from COPD. The pneumonia can be diffuse or confined to one lobe. There are no special features to separate it from other bacterial causes of pneumonia. It responds well to treatment with oral cefaclor 500 mg 8-hourly.

Chlamydia psittaci (see also p. 69)

Typically the individual has been exposed to infected birds, especially parrots, but cases may occur without a history of contact. The incubation period is 1–2 weeks and the disease may pursue a very low-grade course over several months. Symptoms include malaise, high fever, cough and muscular pains. The liver and spleen are occasionally enlarged, and scanty 'rose spots' may be seen on the abdomen. The chest X-ray shows segmental or a diffuse pneumonia. Occasionally the illness presents with a high, swinging fever and dramatic prostration with photophobia and neck stiffness that can be confused with meningitis. The diagnosis is confirmed by the demonstration of a rising titre of complement-fixing antibody. Macrolides or tetracycline are the antibiotics of choice.

Chlamydia pneumoniae

Outbreaks of *Chlamydia pneumoniae* have been reported in institutions and within families, suggesting person-to-person spread without any avian or animal reservoir. Serological tests on patients admitted to hospital with community-acquired pneumonia suggest that 5–10% may be the result of *C. pneumoniae* infection. In general, disease is mild with 50% of *C. pneumoniae* infections presenting as pneumonia, 28% as acute bronchitis, 10% with a 'flu-like illness and 12% with upper respiratory illnesses. Type-specific microimmunofluorescence tests are required to distinguish *C. pneumoniae* from *C. psittaci* and *C. trachomatis*. Treatment is with erythromycin or tetracycline.

Staphylococcus aureus

In general *Staph. aureus* causes a pneumonia only after a preceding influenzal viral illness. The infection starts in the bronchi, leading to patchy areas of consolidation in one or more lobes, which break down to form abscesses. These may appear as cysts on the chest X-ray.

Pneumothorax, effusion and empyemas are frequent. Septicaemia develops with metastatic abscesses in other organs.

Fulminating staphylococcal pneumonia can lead to death in hours. All patients with this type of pneumonia are very ill; intravenous antibiotics must be administered promptly, but are not always effective.

Areas of pneumonia (septic infarcts) are also seen in staphylococcal septicaemia. This is frequently seen in intravenous drug abusers, and in patients with central catheters being used for parenteral nutrition. The infected puncture site is the source of the *Staphylococcus*. Pulmonary symptoms are often few but breathlessness and cough occur and the chest X-ray reveals areas of consolidation. Abscess formation is frequent.

Diagnosis and treatment are shown in Figure 14.36.

Coxiella burnetii (Q-fever) (see also p. 93)

The patient develops systemic symptoms of fever, malaise and headache, often associated with multiple lesions on the chest X-ray. The illness may run a chronic course and is occasionally associated with endocarditis. Diagnosis is made by an increase in the titre of complement-fixing antibody. Treatment is usually with macrolides or tetracycline. Severe cases may require rifampicin.

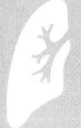
Legionella pneumophila

Three epidemiological patterns of this disease are recognized:

- outbreaks among previously fit individuals staying in hotels, institutions or hospitals where the shower facilities or cooling systems have been contaminated with the organism
- sporadic cases occurring in many parts of the world where the source of the infection is unknown; most cases involve middle-aged and elderly men who are smokers, but it is also being seen in children
- outbreaks occurring in immunocompromised patients, e.g. on corticosteroid therapy.

Legionella grows well in water up to 40°C in temperature, and the infection is almost certainly spread by the aerosol route. Adequate chlorination and temperature control of the water supply are important factors in the prevention of the disease.

The incubation period is 2–10 days. Males are affected twice as commonly as females. The infection may be mild, but the characteristic picture is of malaise, myalgia, headache and a fever with rigors and a pyrexia of up to 40°C. Half of the patients have gastrointestinal symptoms, with nausea, vomiting, diarrhoea and abdominal pain. Patients may be acutely ill, with mental confusion and other neurological signs. Haematuria occurs and occasionally renal failure.

The patient is tachypnoeic with initially a dry cough that later may become productive and purulent. The chest X-ray usually shows lobar and then multilobar shadowing, sometimes with a small pleural effusion. Cavitation is rare.

A strong presumptive diagnosis of *L. pneumophila* infection is possible in the majority of patients if they have three of the four following features:

- a prodromal virus-like illness
- a dry cough, confusion or diarrhoea
- lymphopenia without marked leucocytosis
- hyponatraemia.

Hypoalbuminaemia and high serum levels of liver aminotransferases are also common in this disease.

Diagnosis is confirmed by a fourfold increase in antibody titre in the blood, but the quickest way is by the direct immunofluorescent staining of the organism in the pleural fluid, sputum or bronchial washings. The organism is not seen on Gram staining. Culture on special media is possible but takes up to 3 weeks. A urinary antigen test is commercially available and is highly specific.

Treatment is usually with one of the macrolides, clarithromycin now being the drug of choice. Ciprofloxacin is also effective and rifampicin can be used in addition in ill patients. Mortality can be up to 30% in elderly patients but most patients recover fully.

Prevention is with chlorination and sealing of water supplies.

Gram-negative bacteria

These are the cause of many hospital-acquired pneumonias but they are occasionally responsible for cases in the community.

Klebsiella pneumoniae

Pneumonia due to *Klebsiella* usually occurs in elderly people with a history of heart or lung disease, diabetes, alcohol excess or malignancy. The onset is often sudden, with severe systemic upset. The sputum is purulent, gelatinous or blood-stained. The upper lobes are more commonly affected and the consolidation is often extensive. There is often swelling of the infected lobe so that on the lateral chest X-ray there is bulging of the fissures. The organism can be found in the sputum or in the blood.

Treatment is dependent on the sensitivity of the organism, but a cephalosporin is usually required. The mortality is high, partly owing to the presence of the predisposing condition.

Pseudomonas aeruginosa

Pneumonia due to *Pseudomonas* is of considerable significance in patients with cystic fibrosis, since it correlates with a worsening clinical condition and mortality. It is also seen in patients with neutropenia following cytotoxic chemotherapy. The isolation of *P. aeruginosa* from sputum must be interpreted with care because the organism grows well on bacterial culture medium and may simply represent contamination from the upper airways.

Treatment. *Pseudomonas* and other Gram-negative infections respond well to treatment with the 4-quinolone antibiotic ciprofloxacin (200–400 mg i.v. over 30–60 minutes twice daily) or ceftazidime (2 g bolus i.v. 8-hourly). Ticarcillin (15–20 g daily i.v. infusion) and piperacillin are active against these bacilli. These penicillins are usually given in combination with an aminoglycoside, e.g. gentamicin or netilmicin, for maximum benefit.

Treatment regimens may have to be modified in the light of sensitivity testing. Aminoglycosides are nephrotoxic and ototoxic, so blood levels should be monitored.

Moraxella catarrhalis

This organism has been found to be associated with exacerbations of COPD and occasionally with fatal pneumonia. Some strains produce a β-lactamase capable of destroying amoxicillin. The exact role of this organism in bronchopulmonary infection remains to be determined.

Anaerobic bacteria

Infections with these organisms usually occur in patients with an underlying condition, such as diabetes, and are often associated with aspiration. Bacteroides is the most common organism and is sensitive to metronidazole. The prognosis depends largely on the precipitating cause.

Pneumonias due to opportunistic infections

Immunocompromised patients develop pneumonia with all the usual organisms and with a number of organisms which do not normally cause illness in healthy hosts. However, with HAART therapy (p. 146) the incidence of these infections has fallen dramatically.

Pneumocystis carinii

This is by far the most common opportunistic infection, accounting for 50% of the cases of pneumonia in patients with acquired immunodeficiency syndrome (AIDS) (see p. 139) particularly when the CD4 lymphocyte count is $\leq 200/mm^3$. It is also seen in patients receiving immunosuppressive therapy. In the developing world, however, *Pneumocystis carinii* pneumonia (PCP) is not infrequently found in malnourished children. *P. carinii* is found in the air, and pneumonia arises from reinfection rather than reactivation of persisting organisms acquired in childhood. Clinically the pneumonia is associated with a high fever, breathlessness and dry cough. In patients with AIDS, the clinical features are described on page 139. The typical radiographic appearance of PCP is of a diffuse bilateral alveolar and interstitial shadowing beginning in the perihilar regions and spreading out in a butterfly pattern. Other chest X-ray appearances include localized infiltration, nodules, cavitation or a pneumothorax. In patients receiving aerosolized pentamidine for prophylaxis, infiltrates may be localized to the upper zones. (For CT appearances see p. 139.) Investigation includes induction of sputum with hypertonic saline or fibreoptic bronchoscopy with bronchoalveolar lavage; the diagnosis can be made in 90% of cases by staining sputum using indirect immunofluorescence with monoclonal antibodies.

Other causes of shadowing on the chest X-ray in AIDS patients include:

- cytomegalovirus
- *M. avium-intracellulare*
- *M. tuberculosis*
- *L. pneumophila*
- *Cryptococcus*
- pyogenic bacteria
- Kaposi's sarcoma
- lymphoid interstitial pneumonia
- non-specific interstitial pneumonitis.

Treatment of PCP is with high-dose co-trimoxazole (see p. 139).

Actinomyces israeli (see also p. 92)

The clinical picture is that of severe pneumonia, lung abscess or empyema. Treatment is surgical drainage when appropriate, with high-dose intravenous penicillin for 4–6 weeks.

Nocardia asteroides

This produces a similar picture to *Actinomyces*, though of greater severity. The chest X-ray often shows irregular opacities in one or both lungs, particularly in the mid-zones. Treatment is with sulfadiazine in doses up to 9 g daily.

Cytomegalovirus (see also p. 141)

Bronchitis and pneumonia may occur but these are usually a more minor part of the generalized systemic illness.

Aspergillus fumigatus (see also p. 140)

This fungus gives rise to a widespread invasion of lung tissue in patients who are immunocompromised. It is a serious pneumonia that is usually rapidly fatal. Treatment is with amphotericin and flucytosine.

Mycobacterium avium-intracellulare (MAI)

This bacterium causes lung disease in patients with AIDS primarily as part of disseminated disease when CD4 lymphocyte counts are $\leq 100/mm^3$ with the pulmonary complications being of less significance than the extrapulmonary involvement. Therapeutic regimens include combinations of rifabutin or rifampicin, ethambutol and clofazimine. Clarithromycin and azithromycin may prove to be particularly efficacious.

Cryptococcus

Infection with this fungus is usually disseminated but pulmonary involvement includes intrathoracic lymph node enlargement and effusions.

Kaposi's sarcoma (see also pp. 144 and 1308)

This malignancy affecting HIV-infected homosexual men is now seen less often since the introduction of HAART (see p. 146). Intrathoracic involvement usually follows cutaneous manifestations and includes nodules or infiltrates in the lungs with lymph node enlargement and endobronchial lesions. Symptoms are those of progressive dyspnoea and cough. Chest X-ray appearances are non-specific. Bronchoscopy reveals multiple red or purple flat lesions which are not biopsied because of difficulty with histological diagnosis in crushed fragments and risk of haemorrhage. Treatment is with chemotherapy, vincristine 2 mg and bleomycin 10 mg/m² every 3 weeks.

Lymphoid interstitial pneumonia

This condition is more common in children than in adults and is characterized by infiltration with lymphocytes, plasma cells and immunoblasts. It is thought to be a viral pneumonia and causes diffuse reticulonodular infiltrates on the chest X-ray. Corticosteroid therapy appears to be of benefit, as is zidovudine.

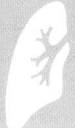

Rare causes of pneumonia

Pneumonia may be seen as a minor feature in the course of infection by *Bordetella pertussis,* typhoid and paratyphoid bacillus, brucellosis, leptospirosis and a number of viral infections including measles, chickenpox and glandular fever. Details of these infections are described in Chapter 2.

Aspiration pneumonia

The acute aspiration of gastric contents into the lungs can produce an extremely severe and sometimes fatal illness owing to the intense destructiveness of gastric acid. This has been termed Mendelson's syndrome and can complicate anaesthesia, particularly during pregnancy.

In the absence of a tracheo-oesophageal fistula, aspiration occurs only during periods of impaired consciousness (e.g. during sleep), in reflux oesophagitis with an oesophageal stricture, or in bulbar palsy. Because of the bronchial anatomy, the most usual sites for spillage are the apical and posterior segments of the right lower lobe. The persistent pneumonia is often due to anaerobes and it may progress to lung abscess or even bronchiectasis. It is vital to identify any underlying problem, since appropriate corrective measures can lead to resolution of the pulmonary problems.

Treatment is discussed on page 891.

Cryptogenic organizing pneumonia (COP)

This condition, also called bronchiolitis obliterans organizing pneumonia (BOOP) is an organizing pneumonia of unknown aetiology. No infective agent has been described. Typically, patients present with single or recurrent episodes of malaise associated with cough, breathlessness and fever. Pleuritic chest pain is sometimes present but finger clubbing is very rare. Chest X-rays show confluent bilateral parenchymal shadowing. Lung function tests may show a restrictive defect. The white blood count is normal, but the ESR may be raised. Open lung biopsy will reveal characteristic buds of connective tissue in respiratory bronchioles and in alveolar ducts. These are diagnostic, but the diagnosis is usually made on history and X-ray appearances. The disease responds rapidly to corticosteroid treatment but may recur episodically especially in older women.

Diffuse pneumonia (bronchopneumonia)

Diffuse pneumonia is very common. It is differentiated from severe bronchitis by signs of bronchial breathing or patchy shadows on the chest X-ray. Widespread diffuse pneumonia is a common terminal event, resulting from an inability of patients dying from other conditions (e.g. cancer) to cough up retained secretions, allowing infection to develop throughout the lungs. Decisions on therapy will vary according to the particular clinical circumstances but aggressive antibacterial treatment is rarely appropriate.

General management of pneumonia

Refer to the algorithm given in Figure 14.36. Sputum and blood should always be sent for culture but antibiotic treatment should not be delayed. Severe cases need to be admitted to hospital and a chest X-ray performed. Other investigations, e.g. blood gases, are useful to detect respiratory failure and provide a baseline for comparison if the patient deteriorates.

Further investigations may be necessary for the diagnosis of certain types of pneumonia:

- *Pneumococcal antigen* – counterimmunoelectrophoresis (CIE) of sputum, urine and serum (three to four times more sensitive than sputum or blood cultures)
- *Mycoplasma antibodies* (IgM and IgG) – in acute and convalescent samples – cold agglutinins present in 50%
- *Legionella and Chlamydia antibodies* – immunofluorescent tests
- *Legionella antigen* – in urine.

The choice of antibiotics is inevitably empirical, especially in those patients treated in the community. Empirical therapy is largely directed at *Strep. pneumoniae* infections. Apart from mycoplasma, the other pathogens are responsible for a small minority of infections. Acquired antibiotic resistance of common respiratory bacterial pathogens is recognized as a concern, but is currently rare in the UK and rarely causes clinical failure. There is at present no convincing evidence that newer antibiotics provide any significant therapeutic advantage over established therapies. For treatment of mild community-acquired pneumonia, oral amoxicillin remains the preferred agent, but should be given at a dose of 500 mg 8-hourly. Oral erythromycin (or azithromycin, which is better tolerated) is an alternative choice for those sensitive to penicillin. For more severe cases treated in hospital, combined therapy with amoxicillin and a macrolide (erythromycin or azithromycin) is recommended. When oral therapy is contraindicated, parenteral ampicillin or benzylpenicillin should be combined with clarithromycin. If *Staph. aureus* infection is suspected or is proven on culture, intravenous flucloxacillin ± sodium fusidate should be added. Fluoroquinolones are recommended for those intolerant of penicillins or macrolides. For severe cases requiring intensive care, parenteral antibiotics should be given with the combination of a broad-spectrum lactamase-stable beta-lactam antibiotic combined with clarithromycin. Parenteral therapy is only required in a minority of patients with non-severe pneumonia. Parenteral antibiotics should be switched to oral once the temperature has settled for a period of 24 hours and provided there is no contraindication to oral therapy. The choice of antibiotics may be narrowed

Criteria for the diagnosis of *severe community-acquired pneumonia*

Clinical features

- Respiratory rate ≥30/min
- Diastolic blood pressure ≤60 mmHg
- Confusion
- High mortality particularly in those > 65 years old
- Co-morbidity

Investigations

- Chest X-ray – more than one lobe involved
- $P_aO_2 < 8$ kPa
- Low albumin (< 35 g/L)
- White cell count (low < 10^9/L or high > 20×10^9/L)
- Raised serum urea (> 7 mmol/L)
- Blood culture – positive

once microbiological results are available but up to 10% of pneumonias may have mixed infection, which may reduce the opportunity to narrow down the antibiotic coverage.

The overall mortality for patients admitted to hospital with community-acquired pneumonia is currently 5%, except for pneumonia due to *Staph. aureus* where it exceeds 25%. Patients who die from pneumonia usually have not received the appropriate antibiotics in sufficient doses before or during the early stages of hospital admission.

Box 14.3 shows features of *severe community-acquired pneumonia* which indicate a poorer prognosis. In spite of treatment in the intensive care unit, approximately 50% of such patients will die.

General measures

These include care of the mouth and skin. Fluids should be encouraged, to avoid dehydration. The patient is normally nursed sitting up or in the most comfortable position. Cough should normally be encouraged, but if it is unproductive and distressing, suppressants such as codeine linctus can be given. Physiotherapy is needed to help and encourage the patient to cough. Pleuritic pain may require analgesia, but powerful analgesia (e.g. opiates) should be used with care because they cause respiratory depression. In severe hypoxia, oxygen therapy should be given. However, since the hypoxia is often due to a physiological shunt, it may make little difference to the hypoxaemia.

Hospital-acquired (nosocomial) pneumonias

Patients with mild forms of hospital-acquired pneumonias need to be reviewed carefully to make sure that there is nothing else responsible for their deterioration (e.g. heart failure, pulmonary embolism). Although very mild forms of hospital-acquired pneumonia may be treated with co-amoxiclav 500 mg three times daily, most cases will have co-morbidities which will dictate more aggressive antibiotic therapy. These should be managed in the same way as severe community-acquired pneumonias once appropriate samples for culture and sensitivities have been taken. Gram-negative bacteria are common and treatment should normally include a third-generation cephalosporin (e.g. cefuroxime) and aminoglycosides (e.g. gentamicin). Patients with chronic chest infection and others in whom *Pseudomonas* infection is suspected should receive i.v. ciprofloxacin or ceftazidime. Immunosuppressed patients may require very high-dose broad-spectrum antibiotics as well as antifungal and antiviral agents. Aspiration pneumonia (p. 890) is relatively common in hospital and usually involves infection with multiple bacteria, including anaerobes. The oral route is usually inappropriate in these patients. A combination of metronidazole (intravenous or rectal) and either co-amoxiclav or cefuroxime i.v. is recommended.

Complications of pneumonia

Lung abscess

This term is used to describe severe localized suppuration in the lung associated with cavity formation on the chest X-ray, often with the presence of a fluid level, and not due to tuberculosis.

There are many causes of lung abscesses, but the most common is aspiration, particularly amongst alcohol abusers following aspiration pneumonia. Lung abscesses also frequently follow the inhalation of a foreign body into a bronchus and occasionally occur when the bronchus is obstructed by a bronchial carcinoma. Chronic or subacute lung abscesses follow an inadequately treated pneumonia.

Abscesses may develop during the course of specific pneumonias, particularly when the infecting agent is *Staph. aureus* or *Klebsiella pneumoniae*. Septic emboli, usually staphylococci, result in multiple lung abscesses. Infarcted areas of lung may occasionally cavitate and rarely become infected. Amoebic abscesses may occasionally develop in the right lower lobe following transdiaphragmatic spread from an amoebic liver abscess.

The clinical features are those of persisting and worsening pneumonia associated with the production of large quantities of sputum, which is often foul-smelling owing to the growth of anaerobic organisms. There is usually a swinging fever; malaise and weight loss occur. The chest signs may be few but clubbing often develops if the condition is not rapidly cured. The patient is often anaemic with a high ESR.

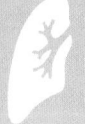

Empyema

Empyema means the presence of pus within the pleural cavity. This usually arises from bacterial spread from a severe pneumonia or after the rupture of a lung abscess into the pleural space. Typically an empyema cavity becomes infected with anaerobic organisms and the patient is severely ill with a high fever and a neutrophil granulocytosis.

Investigations

Bacteriological investigation of lung abscess and empyema is best conducted on specimens obtained by transtracheal aspiration, bronchoscopy or percutaneous transthoracic aspiration with ultrasound or CT guidance. Bronchoscopy is helpful to exclude carcinomas and foreign bodies.

Treatment

Although anaerobic organisms are found in up to 70% of lung abscesses and empyemas, there is usually a mixed flora, often with aerobes, particularly *Strep. milleri*. Anaerobic cocci, black-pigmented bacteroids and fusobacteria are the anaerobes found most commonly.

Empyemas should be treated by prompt tube drainage or by rib resection and drainage of the empyema cavity under ultrasound control. Appropriate antibiotic treatment is given for up to 6 weeks. Antibiotics should be given to cover both aerobic and anaerobic organisms. An appropriate initial choice is cefuroxime 1 g i.v. 6-hourly and metronidazole 500 mg i.v. 8-hourly for 5 days, followed by oral cefaclor and metronidazole for a prolonged period depending on bacterial sensitivities. Abscesses occasionally require surgery.

FURTHER READING

Bartlett JG, Mundy LM (1995) Community-acquired pneumonia. *New England Journal of Medicine* **333**: 1618–1624.
Lim WS et al. (2000) Predicting severity in community acquired pneumonia. *Thorax* **55**: 219–223.
Miller R (1996) HIV-associated respiratory disease. *Lancet* **348**: 307–312.
Nuorte JP et al. (2000) Smoking and pneumococcal disease. *New England Journal of Medicine* **342**: 681–689.
Stout JE, Yu VL (1997) Legionellosis. *New England Journal of Medicine* **337**: 682–687.

Tuberculosis (see also p. 89)

Following many decades of decline, tuberculosis is on the increase in developed countries, because of AIDS and the use of immunosuppressive drugs which depress the host defence mechanisms, decreased socioeconomic conditions, as well as increased immigration of persons from areas of high endemicity. In developing countries it is 20–50 times more common.

Epidemiology

Tuberculosis is the world's leading cause of death from a single infectious disease, with two million deaths (without HIV infection) in 1990. This is the result of:

- inadequate programmes for disease control
- multiple drug resistance (MDR)
- co-infection with HIV
- a rapid rise in the world's population of young adults – the age group with the highest mortality from tuberculosis.

In the UK the number of cases is stable, with 7000 new cases per year. The incidence of tuberculosis in immigrants from the Asian subcontinent and from the West Indies are respectively forty and four times as common as in the native white population. This has led to great variation in the frequency of the disease in different areas of the UK. Tuberculosis is a notifiable disease.

The high frequency of *Mycobacterium tuberculosis* in India (two million new cases per year) and Africa is the result of poor nutrition, overcrowding, lack of control measures, inadeqately supervised treatment and the cost of drugs.

Pathology

The first infection with *M. tuberculosis* is known as primary tuberculosis. It is usually subpleural, often in the mid to upper zones. Within an hour of reaching the lung, tubercle bacilli reach the draining lymph nodes at the hilum of the lung and a few escape into the bloodstream.

The initial reaction comprises exudation and infiltration with neutrophil granulocytes. These are rapidly replaced by macrophages that ingest the bacilli. These interact with T lymphocytes, with the development of cellular immunity that can be demonstrated 3–8 weeks after the initial infection by a positive reaction in the skin to an intradermal injection of protein from tubercle bacilli (tuberculin/PPD).

At this stage the classical pathology of tuberculosis can be seen. Granulomatous lesions consist of a central area of necrotic material of a cheesy nature, called caseation, surrounded by epithelioid cells and Langerhans' giant cells with multiple nuclei, both cells being derived from the macrophage. Lymphocytes are present and there is a varying degree of fibrosis. Subsequently the caseated areas heal completely and many become calcified. It is known that at least 20% of these calcified primary lesions contain tubercle bacilli, initially lying dormant but capable of being activated by depression of the host defence system. Reactivation leads to typical post-primary pulmonary tuberculosis with cavitation, usually in the apex or upper zone of the lung. 'Post-primary tuberculosis' refers to all forms of tuberculosis that occur after the first few weeks of the primary infection when immunity to the mycobacterium has developed.

Clinical features and investigations

Primary tuberculosis is symptomless in the great majority of individuals. Occasionally there may be a vague illness, sometimes associated with cough and wheeze. A small transient pleural effusion or erythema nodosum may occur occasionally, both representing hypersensitivity manifestations of the infective process.

Enlargement of lymph nodes compressing the bronchi can give rise to collapse of segments or lobes of the lung. Apart from cough and a monophonic wheeze, the individual remains remarkably well and the collapse disappears as the primary complex heals. Occasionally, persistent collapse can give rise to subsequent bronchiectasis, often in the middle lobe (Brock's syndrome).

The manifestations of primary and post-primary tuberculosis are shown in Figure 14.37, together with the times when they usually occur. Extrapulmonary manifestations are summarized on page 89. Miliary tuberculosis can occur within a year of the primary infection, or can occasionally occur much later as a manifestation of reactivation or, rarely, reinfection with tubercle bacillus.

Reactivation in the lung, or indeed in any extrapulmonary location, can occur as immunity wanes, usually with age or chronic ill-health. All manifestations are shown in Figure 14.37.

Miliary tuberculosis

This disease is the result of acute diffuse dissemination of tubercle bacilli via the bloodstream. It can be a difficult diagnosis to make, especially in older people, where it is particularly covert. This form of disseminated tuberculosis is universally fatal without treatment.

It may present in an entirely non-specific manner with the gradual onset of vague ill-health, loss of weight and then fever. Occasionally the disease presents as tuberculous meningitis. Usually there are no abnormal physical signs in the early stages, although eventually the spleen and liver become enlarged. Choroidal tubercles are seen in the eyes. These lesions are about one-quarter of the diameter of the optic disc and are yellowish and slightly shiny and raised in nature, later becoming white in the centre. There may be one or many in each eye.

The chest X-ray may be entirely normal in miliary tuberculosis as the tubercles are not visible until uniform miliary shadows 1–2 mm in diameter are seen throughout the lung; they have a hard outline. The lesions can increase in size up to 5–10 mm. Sarcoidosis and staphylococcal or *Mycoplasma* pneumonia can mimic the chest X-ray appearance of miliary tuberculosis. CT scanning may reveal lung parenchymal abnormalities at an earlier stage.

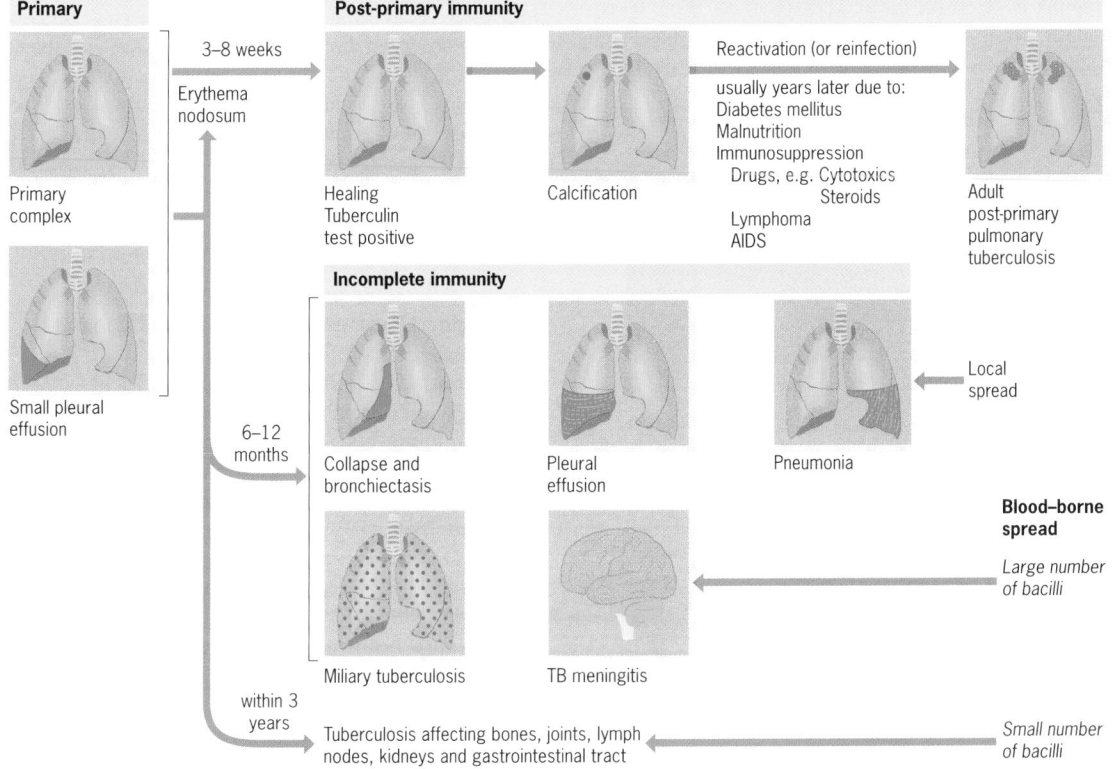

Fig. 14.37 Manifestations of primary and post-primary tuberculosis.

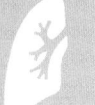

The Mantoux test is positive but may be negative in 30–50% of people with very severe disease. Transbronchial biopsies are frequently positive before any abnormality is visible on the chest X-ray.

Biopsy and culture of liver and bone marrow may be necessary in patients presenting with a pyrexia of unknown origin (PUO). A trial of antituberculous therapy can be used in individuals with a PUO. The fever should settle within 2 weeks of starting chemotherapy if it is due to tuberculosis. This approach is used in susceptible individuals when a diagnosis cannot be confirmed.

Adult post-primary pulmonary tuberculosis

Typically there is gradual onset of symptoms over weeks or months. Tiredness, malaise, anorexia and loss of weight together with a fever and cough remain the outstanding features of pulmonary tuberculosis. Drenching night sweats are now rather uncommon and are more usually due to anxiety. Sputum in tuberculosis may be mucoid, purulent or blood-stained. Many patients suffer a dull ache in the chest and it is not uncommon for patients to complain of recurrent colds. A pleural effusion or pneumonia can be the presenting feature of tuberculosis.

Physical examination reveals little. Finger clubbing is only present if the disease is advanced and associated with considerable production of purulent sputum. There are often no physical signs in the chest even in the presence of extensive radiological changes, though occasionally persistent crackles may be heard. Physical signs of an associated effusion, pneumonia or fibrosis may be present.

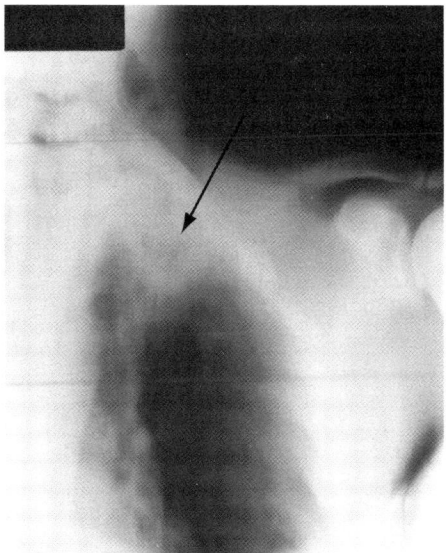

Fig. 14.38 Chest X-ray showing tuberculosis of left upper lobe with cavitation.

Chest X-ray

An abnormal chest X-ray is often found with no symptoms, but the reverse is extremely rare – pulmonary tuberculosis is unlikely in the absence of any radiographic abnormality.

The chest X-ray (Fig. 14.38) typically shows patchy or nodular shadows in the upper zones, loss of volume, and fibrosis with or without cavitation. Calcification may be present. The X-ray appearances alone may strongly suggest tuberculosis, but every effort must be made to obtain microbiological evidence. A single X-ray does not give an indication of the activity of the disease. Very similar chest X-ray appearances occur in histoplasmosis and other fungal infections of the lung, including cryptococcosis, coccidioidomycosis, blastomycosis and aspergillosis as well as in bronchial carcinoma.

Lymph node presentation of tuberculosis

The patient presents with a tender lump or fluctuant mass, usually supraclavicular or in the anterior triangle of the neck.

This form of tuberculosis is discussed on page 89.

Tuberculosis in HIV-infected persons (see also p. 143)

Tuberculosis in an HIV-infected person is an AIDS-defining illness. Disease may arise from rapid progression of primary infection, by reactivation and by reinfection. The clinical pattern of disease is described on page 143. Treatment is with conventional therapy but four rather than three drugs and it should be supervised (directly observed therapy short course, DOTS). Adverse reactions are common and the prognosis may be poor, especially if treatment is not supervised. Multiple drug resistance (MDR) occurs in about 6% of cases of tuberculosis in HIV-positive individuals.

Diagnosis

The diagnosis of tuberculosis is made on the basis of the following investigations:

- **Imaging.** Chest X-ray (see above), and CT scan if necessary.
- **Staining.** The sputum is stained with Ziehl–Nielsen (ZN) stain for acid and alcohol-fast bacilli (AAFB) or an auramine–phenol fluorescent test performed.
- **Culture.** The sputum is cultured on Ogana or Lowenstein–Jensen medium for 4–8 weeks. Liquid culture (Baltec (Becton-Dickinson)) is now used in many laboratories and has the advantage of shorter culture times. Cultures to determine the sensitivity of the bacillus to antibiotics take a further 3–4 weeks.
- **Fibreoptic bronchoscopy** with washings from the affected lobes is useful if no sputum is available. This has replaced former techniques such as gastric washings. Transbronchial biopsies can also be obtained for histology and microbiological assessment.

- **Biopsies** of the pleura, lymph nodes and solid lesions within the lung (tuberculomas) may be required to confirm the diagnosis.

The slow growth of *M. tuberculosis* in culture has hindered the ability to make a rapid definitive diagnosis. Radiolabelled DNA and RNA probes specific for various mycobacterial species can identify organisms in culture. The sensitivity of these methods has been enhanced by amplifying target DNA using the polymerase chain reaction. This allows direct testing of sputum and other fluids to provide a laboratory diagnosis within 48 hours. This is still not entirely reliable and should not be accepted as a final diagnosis, particularly in the difficult case when it is most likely to be used. ELISA techniques have been developed which have high specificities, but unfortunately low sensitivity.

Treatment

Bed rest does not affect the outcome of the disease. Some patients will require hospitalization for a brief period; these include ill patients, smear-positive, highly infectious patients (particularly multidrug-resistant TB), those in whom the diagnosis is uncertain and those individuals from whom it is essential to gain cooperation. The most important factor in the successful treatment of tuberculosis is the continuous self-administration of drugs for 6 months; lack of patient compliance is a major reason why 5% of patients do not respond to treatment. In vitro resistance to one or more of the antituberculous drugs used to occur in fewer than 1% of patients in the UK, but the rate of resistance is gradually increasing.

Directly observed therapy short course (DOTS)

In order to improve compliance, special clinics are used to supervise treatment regimens directly. Incentives to attend (e.g. free meals) may be helpful. The effectiveness of DOTS is, however, variable in different countries and compliance is still a problem. Long-stay hospital treatment is required only for persistently uncooperative patients, many of whom are homeless and abuse alcohol.

Six-month regimen

Six-months' treatment with once-daily rifampicin 600 mg and isoniazid 300 mg is standard practice for patients with pulmonary and lymph node disease. (For those whose bodyweight is below 55 kg, rifampicin is reduced to 450 mg daily.) These are given as combination tablets and are taken 30 minutes before breakfast, since the absorption of rifampicin is influenced by food. This is supplemented for the first 2 months by pyrazinamide at a dose of 1.5 g (bodyweight < 50 kg) or 2.0 g daily. Pyrazinamide is of particular value in treating mycobacteria present within macrophages, and for this reason it may have a very valuable effect on preventing subsequent relapse. Pyridoxine 10 mg daily is given to reduce the risk of isoniazid-induced neuropathy.

Longer regimens

Treatment of bone tuberculosis should be continued for a total of 9 months and of tuberculous meningitis for 1 year. The drugs used are the same as for pulmonary tuberculosis, with pyrazinamide prescribed for the first 2 months only and for drug-resistant disease.

Drug-resistant organisms

The development of resistance after initial drug sensitivity (*secondary drug resistance*) occurs in patients who do not comply with the treatment regimens. *Primary drug resistance* is seen in immigrants to the UK and those exposed to others infected with resistant organisms. Multidrug resistance is a major therapeutic problem with a high mortality and occurs mainly in HIV-infected patients. Nosocomial transmission of multidrug-resistant tuberculosis to healthcare workers and to other patients is recognized and poses a major public health problem. The drug treatment of suspected drug resistance in HIV-positive and HIV-negative patients is as follows:

- with multiple drug resistance use at least three drugs to which the organism is sensitive
- with resistance to one of the four main drugs, use the other three.

Therapy should be continued for up to 2 years and in HIV-positive patients for at least 12 months after negative cultures. Second-line drugs available for treatment of resistant *M. tuberculosis* are capreomycin, cycloserine, clarithromycin, azithromycin, ciprofloxacin, ofloxacin, ethionamide, kanamycin and amikacin.

Unwanted effects of drug treatment

Rifampicin induces liver enzymes, which may be transiently elevated in the serum of many patients. The drug should be stopped only if the serum bilirubin becomes elevated or if transferases are >3× elevated, which is extremely rare. Thrombocytopenia has been reported. Rifampicin stains body secretions pink and the patients should be warned of the change in colour of their urine, tears and sweat. Induction of liver enzymes means that concomitant drug treatment may be made less effective (see Ch. 16). Oral contraception will not be effective, so alternative birth-control methods should be used.

Isoniazid has very few unwanted effects. At high doses it may produce a polyneuropathy but this is extremely rare when the normal dose of 200–300 mg is given daily. Nevertheless, it is customary to prescribe pyridoxine 10 mg daily to prevent this effect (see Fig. 5.7). Occasionally, isoniazid gives rise to allergic reactions in the form of a skin rash and fever, with hepatitis occurring in fewer than 1% of cases. The latter, however, may be fatal if the drug is continued.

Pyrazinamide may cause hepatic toxicity, though recent experience suggests that this is much rarer with present dosage schedules. Pyrazinamide reduces the renal excretion of urate and may precipitate hyperuricaemic gout.

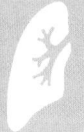

Ethambutol can cause a dose-related optic retro-bulbar neuritis that presents with colour blindness for green, reduction in visual acuity and a central scotoma (commoner at doses of 25 mg/kg). This usually reverses provided the drug is stopped when symptoms develop; patients should therefore be warned of its effects. All patients prescribed the drug should be seen by an ophthalmologist prior to treatment and doses of 15 mg/kg should be used.

Streptomycin can cause irreversible damage to the vestibular nerve. It is more likely to occur in the elderly and in those with renal impairment. Allergic reactions to streptomycin are more common than to rifampicin, isoniazid and pyrazinamide. This drug is used only if patients are very ill, have multidrug-resistant TB and are not responding adequately to therapy.

Follow-up

Patients should be seen regularly for the duration of chemotherapy and once more after 3 months, since relapse, though very unlikely, usually occurs within this period of time. Patients with multidrug-resistant TB should be followed up for at least 1 year after treatment is completed.

Chemoprophylaxis

Patients who have any chest X-ray changes compatible with previous tuberculosis and who are about to undergo long-term treatment that has an immuno-suppressive effect, such as renal dialysis or treatment with corticosteroids, should receive chemoprophylaxis with isoniazid 200–300 mg daily.

Prevention
BCG vaccination

Vaccination with BCG (bacille Calmette–Guérin) has been given to schoolchildren in the UK since 1954. BCG is live attenuated vaccine derived from *M. bovis* (a bovine strain of *M. tuberculosis*) that lost its virulence after growth in the laboratory for many passages. Early trials showed that it decreases the risk of developing tuberculosis by about 70%. With the continuing decrease in the incidence of tuberculosis in most parts of the UK it is becoming less cost-effective to administer this vaccine, and the procedure is being stopped in many areas of the UK. However, in other areas of the UK with a high immigrant population, the vaccine is being administered at birth rather than at the traditional age of 13 years. This is to prevent the disease from developing in young children, where it can progress extremely rapidly and in whom any delay in diagnosis can be fatal. BCG has been shown to be particularly effective in preventing miliary tuberculosis and tuberculous meningitis. In meta-analysis the protective efficacy is around 50%. However, the efficacy of BCG vaccination varies throughout the world from zero to 94% protection and appears to depend on latitude, being most beneficial in Norway, Sweden and Denmark (80–94%) and least so in the southern states of the USA and in India (0–20%). This lack of efficacy is thought to be related to a number of local factors including the frequency of infection with environmental mycobacteria (e.g. *M. fortuitum, M. kansasii*), which may induce a degree of protection similar to but not enhanced by BCG.

BCG is given only to individuals who are tuberculin-negative; those with positive tests are further screened by a chest X-ray. BCG should be given at a dose of 0.1 mL intradermally to children and adults, but at a dose of 0.05 mL to infants percutaneously. The practice of BCG vaccination in the UK, thereby producing cellular immunity and a positive tuberculin test, means that the Mantoux test is of no value in clinical practice for diagnosis of active disease, although it is in the USA where BCG is not used.

Contact tracing

Tuberculosis is spread from person to person and effective tracing of close contacts has helped to limit spread of the disease as well as to identify diseased individuals at an early stage. Screening procedures involve screening all close family members or other individuals who share the same kitchen and bathroom facilities. Occasionally, close contacts at work or school may also be screened. Contacts who are ill should be thoroughly investigated for tuberculosis. If they are well, a chest X-ray is taken and a tuberculin test is performed (Practical box 14.5).

In adults, even if the tuberculin test is positive, provided the chest X-ray is negative nothing more need be done. In patients with HIV infection, who have not had BCG, chemoprophylaxis with isoniazid is given, reducing the relative risk of developing active TB by 40% in highly endemic areas.

In children, a positive tuberculin test is usually taken as evidence of infection, and treatment is instituted. If the tuberculin test is negative in children and young adults (< 35 years), it is repeated at 6 weeks, and if it remains negative then BCG is administered. If it has become positive (without BCG), this is again taken as an indication of active disease and the individual is treated.

Children under the age of 1 year who have a family member with tuberculosis are given chemoprophylaxis with a daily dose of isoniazid 5–10 mg/kg for 6 months together with immunization with a strain of BCG that is resistant to isoniazid.

In general, in the UK much greater emphasis is placed on contact tracing and investigation of those under the age of 35 years and in some immigrant groups (African, Asian and Eastern European) in whom the disease is more prevalent.

Practical box 14.5

Tuberculin testing

Mainly used for:

- Contact tracing
- BCG vaccination programmes.

It is rarely of any value in the diagnosis of tuberculosis.

Patients are tested with:

- Purified protein derivative (PPD) of *Mycobacterium tuberculosis*.

The test is based on cell-mediated immunity with the development of induration and inflammation at the site of infection due to infiltration with mainly T lymphocytes. In patients with AIDS the test may be falsely negative owing to impairment of delayed hypersensitivity.

The Mantoux test

This is used for individual patients.

1. 0.1 mL of a 1:1000 strength PPD (equivalent to 10 tuberculin units) is injected intradermally.
2. The induration (not the erythema) is measured after 72 hours. The test is positive if the induration is 10 mm or more in diameter.

The Heaf test

This is a simple test used for large-scale screening.

1. A small amount of PPD (100 000 IU/mL) is placed on the flexor surface of the left forearm.
2. The 6-point disposable apparatus is actuated through the solution.
3. The Heaf reaction is graded 0–4 depending on the degree of induration: 0 and 1 (where there is only discrete induration at the puncture site) is a negative result after 3–10 days.

Other mycobacteria

M. kansasii occurs in water and milk, though not in soil. Disease caused by this mycobacterium has mainly been described in Europe and the USA. It rarely causes a relatively benign type of human pulmonary disease, more common in HIV+ individuals, usually in middle-aged males. Men working in dusty jobs (e.g. miners) appear to be especially at risk, as are those who have underlying COPD. *M. avium-intracellulare* is a cause of pulmonary infection in AIDS patients (see p. 143).

FURTHER READING

British Thoracic Society (2000) Management of opportunist mycobacterial infections. *Thorax* **55**: 210–218.

British Thoracic Society (2000) Control and prevention of tuberculosis in the UK. *Thorax* **55**: 887–901.

Fine PEM (1995) Variation in protection by BCG: implications of and for heterologous immunity. *Lancet* **346**: 1339–1345.

Small PM, Fujiwara PI (2001) Management of tuberculosis in the United States. *New England Journal of Medicine* **345**: 189–200.

Walley et al. (2001) Effectiveness of DOTS for tuberculosis in Pakistan. *Lancet* **357**: 664–669.

Diffuse diseases of the lung parenchyma

A wide variety of disorders can affect the parenchyma of the lungs. Many different terms have been used to describe these, but the term diffuse parenchymal lung disease (DPLD) is increasingly favoured across the world. The commonest forms of DPLD are sarcoidosis and cryptogenic fibrosing alveolitis. Taken together, DPLD accounts for about 15% of respiratory clinical practice. Pathological features typically include granuloma formation and fibrosis, often with progressive destruction of the lung parenchyma. However, the presentation and outcomes of DPLD vary widely. There is a serious lack of hard evidence regarding the management of DPLD, but the morbidity of the diseases themselves and their therapies can be high. Accurate diagnosis and appropriate specialist management are essential if an optimum outcome is to be achieved.

Granulomatous lung disease

A granuloma is a mass or nodule composed of chronically inflamed tissue formed by the response of the mononuclear phagocyte system (macrophage/histiocyte) to a slowly soluble antigen or irritant. If the foreign substance is inert (e.g. an inhaled dust), the phagocytes turn over slowly; if the substance is toxic or reproducing, the cells turn over faster, producing a granuloma. A granuloma is characterized by epithelioid multinucleate giant cells, as seen in tuberculosis. Granulomas are also seen in other infections, including fungal and helminthic, in sarcoidosis, and in extrinsic allergic alveolitis, and can also be due to foreign bodies (e.g. talc). Granulomatosis with pulmonary vasculitis is discussed on page 900.

Sarcoidosis

Sarcoidosis is a multisystem granulomatous disorder, commonly affecting young adults and usually presenting with bilateral hilar lymphadenopathy, pulmonary infiltration and skin or eye lesions. The diagnosis is confirmed on the histological evidence of widespread, non-caseating, epithelioid granulomas in more than one organ. Beryllium poisoning can rarely produce a clinical and histological picture identical to sarcoidosis, though contact with this element is now strictly controlled.

Epidemiology and aetiology

Sarcoidosis is a common disease of unknown aetiology that is often detected by routine chest X-ray. There is great geographical variation. The prevalence in the UK is approximately 19 in 100 000 of the population. It is common in the USA but is uncommon in Japan. The course of the disease is much more severe in American blacks than in whites. There is no relation with any histocompatibility antigen, but cases of sarcoidosis are seen within families, possibly suggesting an environmental factor. Other aetiological factors suggested are an atypical mycobacterium or fungus, the Epstein–Barr virus, and occupational, genetic, social or other environmental factors (a higher incidence occurs in rural than in urban populations). None of these has been substantiated.

Immunopathology

- Typical sarcoid granulomas consist of focal accumulations of epithelioid cells, macrophages and lymphocytes, mainly T cells.
- There is depressed cell-mediated reactivity to tuberculin and other antigens such as *Candida albicans*.
- There is overall lymphopenia: circulating T lymphocytes are low but B cells are slightly increased.
- Bronchoalveolar lavage shows a great increase in the number of cells; lymphocytes are greatly increased (particularly CD4 helper cells).
- The number of alveolar macrophages is increased but they represent a reduced percentage of the total number of cells.
- Transbronchial biopsies show infiltration of the alveolar walls and interstitial spaces with leucocytes, mainly T cells, prior to granuloma formation.

It seems likely that the decrease in circulating T lymphocytes and changes in delayed hypersensitivity responses are the result of sequestration of lymphocytes within the lung. There is no evidence to suggest that patients with sarcoidosis suffer from an overall defect in cellular immunity, since the frequency of fungal, viral and bacterial infections is not increased and there is no substantiated evidence of a greater risk of developing malignant neoplasms.

Clinical features

The peak incidence is in the third and fourth decades, with a female preponderance. Sarcoidosis can affect many different organs of the body. The most common presentation is with respiratory symptoms or abnormalities found on chest X-ray (50%). Fatigue or weight loss occurs in 5%, peripheral lymphadenopathy in 5% and a fever in 4%. A chest X-ray may be negative in up to 20% of non-respiratory cases, though lesions may be detected later.

Bilateral hilar lymphadenopathy

This is a characteristic feature of sarcoidosis. It is often symptomless and simply detected on a routine chest X-ray. Occasionally, the bilateral hilar lymphadenopathy is associated with a dull ache in the chest, malaise and a mild fever.

Although the chest X-ray may not show any evidence of infiltration in the lung fields, evidence from CT scanning (Fig. 14.39), transbronchial biopsies and

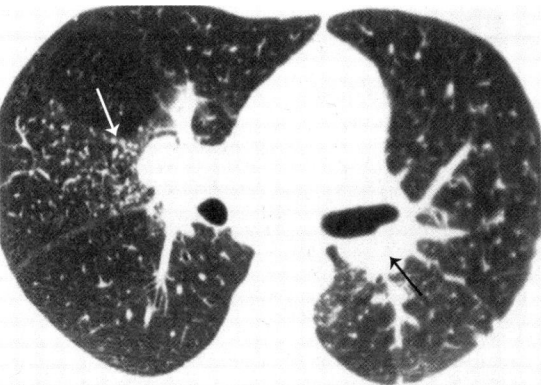

Fig. 14.39 CT scan in sarcoidosis. Note enlarged glands at the hilum (black arrow) and nodular shadowing, particularly in right middle lobe (white arrow).

bronchoalveolar lavage indicates that the lung parenchyma is nearly always involved.

The differential diagnosis of the bilateral hilar lymphadenopathy includes:

- lymphoma – though it is rare for this to affect only the hilar lymph nodes
- pulmonary tuberculosis – though it is rare for the hilar lymph nodes to be symmetrically enlarged
- carcinoma of the bronchus with malignant spread to the contralateral hilar lymph nodes – again it is rare for this to give rise to a typical symmetrical picture.

In the early stages it may be difficult to distinguish enlarged lymph nodes on the chest X-ray from the pulmonary arteries, and lymph node enlargement is not always symmetrical. It is for these reasons that, in the absence of erythema nodosum (see below), further confirmation of the disease process is advisable.

Pulmonary infiltration

This type of sarcoidosis may be progressive and may lead to increasing effort dyspnoea and eventually cor pulmonale and death. The chest X-ray shows a mottling in the mid-zones proceeding to generalized fine nodular shadows. Eventually, widespread pulmonary line shadows develop, reflecting the underlying fibrosis. A honeycomb appearance can occasionally occur. Pulmonary function tests show a typical restrictive lung defect (see below).

The combination of pulmonary infiltration and normal lung function tests is highly suggestive of sarcoidosis. The principal differential diagnoses are tuberculosis, pneumoconiosis, cryptogenic fibrosing alveolitis and alveolar cell carcinoma. However, these other conditions do have their own X-ray appearances and usually cause both symptoms and abnormal lung function tests.

Extrapulmonary manifestations

Skin and ocular sarcoidosis are the most common extrapulmonary presentations.

Skin lesions occur in 10% of cases. Sarcoidosis is the most common cause of erythema nodosum (see p. 1297). The association of bilateral symmetrical hilar lymphadenopathy with erythema nodosum occurs only in sarcoidosis. A chilblain-like lesion known as lupus pernio is also seen, as are nodules (see p. 1300).

Ocular and associated effects. Anterior uveitis is common and may present with misting of vision, pain and a red eye, but posterior uveitis may present simply as progressive loss of vision. Although ocular sarcoidosis accounts for about 5% of uveitis presenting to ophthalmologists, evidence of asymptomatic uveitis may be found in up to 25% of patients with sarcoidosis. Conjunctivitis may occur and retinal lesions have also been reported.

Keratoconjunctivitis sicca and lacrimal gland enlargement may also occur. *Uveoparotid fever* is a syndrome of bilateral uveitis and parotid gland enlargement together with occasional development of facial nerve palsy and is sometimes seen with sarcoidosis.

Metabolic manifestations. It is rare for sarcoidosis to present with problems of calcium metabolism, though hypercalcaemia is found in 10% of established cases. Hypercalcaemia and hypercalciuria can lead to the development of renal calculi and nephrocalcinosis. The cause of the hypercalcaemia is due to an increase in circulating 1,25-dihydroxyvitamin D_3, with the 1α-hydroxylation occurring in sarcoid macrophages in the lung in addition to that taking place in the kidney.

The central nervous system. Involvement of the central nervous system (CNS) is rare (2%) but can lead to severe neurological disease (see p. 1197).

Bone and joint involvement. Arthralgia without erythema nodosum is seen in 5% of cases. Bone cysts are found, particularly in the digits, with associated swelling. In the absence of swelling, routine X-rays of the hands are unnecessary.

Hepatosplenomegaly. Sarcoidosis is a cause of hepatosplenomegaly, though it is rarely of any clinical consequence.

Cardiac involvement. Cardiac involvement is rare (3%). Ventricular dysrhythmias, conduction defects and cardiomyopathy with congestive cardiac failure may be seen.

Investigations

- **Imaging.** Chest X-ray (see above). CT is useful for assessment of diffuse lung involvement.
- **Full blood count.** There is mild normochromic, normocytic anaemia with raised ESR.
- **Serum biochemistry.** There is raised serum calcium and hypergammaglobulinaemia.
- **Transbronchial biopsy** is the most useful investigation. Positive results are seen in 90% of cases of pulmonary sarcoidosis with or without X-ray evidence of lung involvement. The test provides positive histological evidence of a

granuloma in approximately one-half of patients with clinically extrapulmonary sarcoidosis in whom the chest X-ray is normal.

- **Serum level of angiotensin-converting enzyme** (ACE) is two standard deviations above the normal mean value in over 75% of patients with untreated sarcoidosis. Raised (but lower) levels are also seen in patients with lymphoma, pulmonary tuberculosis, asbestosis and silicosis, limiting the diagnostic value of the test. However, the test is useful in assessing the activity of the disease and therefore as a guide to treatment with corticosteroids. Reduction of serum ACE during treatment with corticosteroids has not, however, been proved to reflect resolution of the disease.
- **Lung function tests** show a restrictive lung defect with pulmonary infiltration. There is a decrease in TLC, a decrease in both FEV_1 and FVC, and a decrease in gas transfer.
- **The tuberculin skin test** is negative in 80% of patients with sarcoidosis; this is of interest but has no diagnostic value.

Treatment

Both the need to treat and the value of corticosteroid therapy are contested in many aspects of this disease. Hilar lymphadenopathy on its own with no evidence of chest X-ray involvement of the lungs or decrease in lung function tests does not require treatment. Persisting infiltration on the chest X-ray or abnormal lung function tests are unlikely to improve without corticosteroid treatment. If the disease is not improving spontaneously 6 months after diagnosis, treatment should be started with prednisolone 30 mg for 6 weeks, reducing to alternate-day treatment with prednisolone 15 mg for 6–12 months. Although there have been no controlled trials that have proved the efficacy of such treatment, it is difficult to withhold corticosteroids when there is continuing deterioration of the disease. Systemic prednisolone should be given for patients suffering from involvement of the eyes or persistent hypercalcaemia. If the erythema nodosum of sarcoidosis is severe or persistent it will respond rapidly to a 2-week course of prednisolone 5–15 mg daily, as will patients with uveoparotid fever. Myocardial sarcoidosis and neurological manifestations are also treated with prednisolone.

Prognosis

Sarcoidosis is a much more severe disease in certain racial groups, particularly American blacks, where death rates of up to 10% have been recorded. It is probable that the disease is fatal in fewer than 5% of cases in the UK, most often as a result of respiratory failure and cor pulmonale but, rarely, from myocardial sarcoidosis and renal damage. The chest X-ray provides a guide to prognosis. The disease remits within 2 years in over two-thirds of patients with hilar lymphadenopathy alone, in approximately one-half with hilar lymph-adenopathy plus chest X-ray evidence of pulmonary infiltration, but in only one-third of patients with X-ray evidence of infiltration without any demonstrable lymphadenopathy. Lung function tests are the most useful tests in monitoring progression.

Langerhans' cell histiocytosis (LCH)

This rare disease (a prevalence of 1 per 50 000) is characterized histologically by proliferation of LCH cells identified by the presence of Birbeck granules on electron-microscopy or the CD_{1a} antigen on the surface of the cells. There is a wide variation in clinical presentation, from unifocal bone lesions in older children (which may regress spontaneously), to more disseminated disease in younger children (with a high mortality). Chest X-rays show multiple small cysts (honeycomb lung), fibrosis or widespread nodular shadows. Etoposide treatment is justified for advanced progressive disease.

Pulmonary vasculitis and granulomatosis

The classification of pulmonary vasculitis and granulomatous disorders is unsatisfactory. In broad terms it is reasonable to consider two main groups: the respiratory manifestations of systemic connective tissue diseases and disorders associated with the presence of anti-neutrophil cytoplasmic antibodies (ANCAs).

Pulmonary vasculitis with connective tissue disease

Rheumatoid disease (see also p. 542)
The features of respiratory involvement in rheumatoid disease are illustrated in Figure 14.40.

Pleural adhesions, thickening and effusion are the most common lesions. The effusion is often unilateral and tends to be chronic. It has a low glucose content but this can occur in any chronic pleural effusion. Several forms of parenchymal disease can occur in patients with rheumatoid arthritis. These include fibrosing alveolitis, rheumatoid nodules, cryptogenic organizing pneumonia, and lymphoid interstitial pneumonia. Moreover, some patients will have modified presentations because they are already on disease-modifying drugs such as prednisolone or methotrexate for their arthritis.

Fibrosing alveolitis occurring in rheumatoid arthritis can be considered as a variant of the cryptogenic form of the disease (see p. 904). The clinical features and gross appearance are the same but the disease is often more chronic. Rheumatoid nodules appear on the chest X-ray as single or multiple nodules ranging in size from a few millimetres to a few centimetres. The nodules frequently cavitate. They usually produce no symptoms but can give rise to a pneumothorax or pleural effusion.

Obliterative disease of the small bronchioles is rare. It is characterized by progressive breathlessness and irreversible airflow limitation. Corticosteroids may prevent progression.

Involvement by rheumatoid arthritis of the cricoarytenoid joints gives rise to dyspnoea, stridor, hoarseness and occasionally severe obstruction necessitating tracheostomy. *Caplan's syndrome* is due to a combination of dust inhalation and the disturbed immunity of rheumatoid arthritis. It occurs particularly in coal-worker's pneumoconiosis but it can occur in individuals exposed to other dusts, such as silica and asbestos. Typically the lesions appear as rounded nodules 0.5–5.0 cm in diameter, though sometimes they become incorporated into large areas of fibrosis that are indistinguishable radiologically from progressive massive fibrosis. There may not be much evidence of simple pneumoconiosis prior to the development of the nodule. These lesions may precede the development of the arthritis. Rheumatoid factor is always present in the serum.

Systemic lupus erythematosus (see also p. 558)
Pleurisy is the most common respiratory manifestation of this disease, occurring in up to two-thirds of cases, with or without an effusion. Effusions are usually small and bilateral. Basal pneumonitis is often present, perhaps as a result of poor movement of the diaphragm, or restriction of chest movements because of pleural pain. Pneumonia also occurs, because of either infection or the disease process itself. In contrast to rheumatoid arthritis, diffuse pulmonary fibrosis is rare.

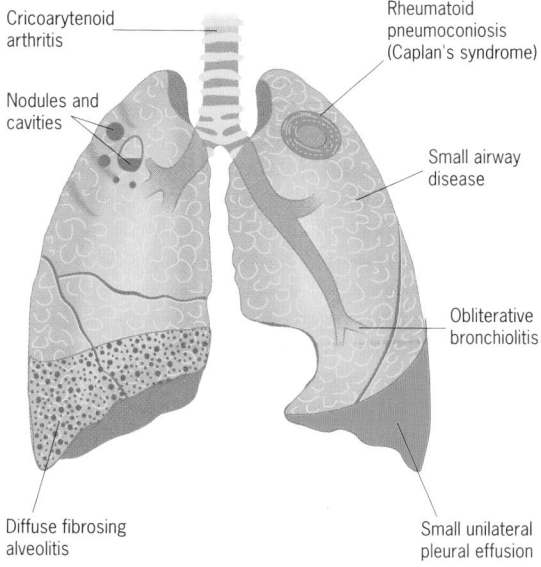

Fig. 14.40 **Respiratory manifestations of rheumatoid disease.**

Systemic sclerosis (see pp. 561 and 1298)

Autopsy studies have indicated that there is almost always some diffuse fibrosis of alveolar walls and obliteration of capillaries and the alveolar space. Severe changes result in nodular then streaky shadowing on the chest X-ray, followed by cystic changes, ending up with a honeycomb lung. Lung function tests indicate a restrictive defect and poor gas transfer. Pneumonia may occur owing to aspiration from the dilated oesophagus (see p. 267). Breathlessness may be worsened by restriction of chest wall movement owing to thickening and contraction of the skin and trunk.

Granulomatous vasculitides

Antineutrophil cytoplasmic antibodies
(see also pp. 516 and 608)

Antineutrophil cytoplasmic antibodies (ANCAs) are found in the acute phase of vasculitides, particularly Wegener's granulomatosis, Churg–Strauss syndrome and microscopic polyangiitis (polyarteritis) associated with neutrophil infiltration of the vessel wall.

Two major ANCA reactivities are recognized: proteinase-3 (PR3) ANCA and myeloperoxidase (MPO) ANCA.

About 10% of all vasculitis patients are ANCA-negative: this is more common in Wegener's granulomatosis limited to the upper respiratory tract. Ten to fifteen per cent of cases of progressive glomerulonephritis with anti-glomerular basement membrane (GBM) antibodies are MPO ANCA-positive and these are the most likely to suffer pulmonary haemorrhage.

Wegener's granulomatosis

This granulomatous disease of unknown aetiology is one of the primary systemic vasculitides in which the small arteries are predominantly affected (the other is the Churg–Strauss syndrome, see below). It is characterized by lesions involving the upper respiratory tract, the lungs and the kidneys. Often the disease starts with severe rhinorrhoea with subsequent nasal mucosal ulceration followed by cough, haemoptysis and pleuritic pain. Occasionally there may be involvement of the skin and nervous system. A chest X-ray usually shows single or multiple nodular masses or pneumonic infiltrates with cavitation. The most remarkable radiographic feature is the migratory pattern, with large lesions clearing in one area and new lesions appearing in another. The typical histological changes are usually best seen in the kidneys, where there is a necrotizing microvascular glomerulonephritis. This disease responds well to treatment with cyclophosphamide 150–200 mg daily. A variant of Wegener's granulomatosis called 'midline granuloma' affects the nose and paranasal sinuses and is particularly mutilating; it has a poor prognosis.

The Churg–Strauss syndrome

This condition occurs in patients, usually male, in their fourth decade who have a triad of rhinitis and asthma, eosinophilia and systemic vasculitis. The aetiology is uncertain, with some believing that it represents an unusual progression of allergic disease in a subset of predisposed individuals. Others believe it is a primary vasculitis which presents like asthma because of the involvement of eosinophils.

The pathology of this condition is dominated by an eosinophilic infiltration with a characteristic high blood eosinophil count, vasculitis of small arteries and veins, and extravascular granulomas. Typically it involves the lungs, peripheral nerves and skin but kidney involvement is uncommon. Transient patchy pneumonia-like shadows may occur, but sometimes these can be massive and bilateral. Skin lesions include tender subcutaneous nodules as well as petechial or purpuric lesions. ANCA is usually positive. The disease responds well to corticosteroids. Occasionally Churg–Strauss syndrome may be revealed when oral steroids are withdrawn in patients being treated for asthma. There is no reason to think that other anti-asthma drugs precipitate the condition.

Microscopic vasculitis (polyangiitis)

This involves the kidneys and the lungs where it results in recurrent haemoptysis. ANCA is usually positive. In the early literature there was confusion between this condition, the Churg–Strauss syndrome and polyarteritis nodosa. The latter, however, is ANCA-negative and rarely involves the lungs.

Pulmonary infiltration with eosinophilia

The common types and characteristics of these diseases are shown in Table 14.14. They range from very mild, simple, pulmonary eosinophilias to the often fatal hypereosinophilic syndrome.

Simple and prolonged pulmonary eosinophilia

Simple pulmonary eosinophilia is a relatively mild illness with a slight fever and cough and usually lasting for less than 2 weeks. Occasionally, the disease becomes more prolonged, with a high fever lasting for over a month. There is usually an eosinophilia in the blood and this condition is then called prolonged pulmonary eosinophilia. In both conditions the chest X-ray shows either localized or diffuse opacities. The simple form is probably due to a transient allergic reaction in the alveoli. Many allergens have been implicated, including *Ascaris lumbricoides*, *Ankylostoma*, *Trichuris*, *Trichinella*,

Table 14.14
Common types and characteristics of pulmonary infiltration with eosinophilia

Disease	Symptoms	Blood eosinophils (%)	Multisystem involvement	Duration	Outcome
Simple pulmonary eosinophilia	Mild	10	None	<1 month	Good
Prolonged pulmonary eosinophilia	Mild/moderate	>20	None	>1 month	Good
Asthmatic bronchopulmonary eosinophilia	Moderate/severe	5–20	None	Years	Fair
Tropical pulmonary eosinophilia	Moderate/severe	>20	None	Years	Fair
Hypereosinophilic syndrome	Severe	>20	Always	Months/years	Poor

Taenia and *Strongyloides*. Drugs such as aspirin, penicillin, nitrofurantoin and sulphonamides have been implicated. Often, no allergen is identified. No treatment is required and the disease is self-limiting. In the more chronic form all unnecessary treatment should be withdrawn and where appropriate, worms are treated. Corticosteroid therapy is indicated, with resolution of the disease over the ensuing weeks.

Asthmatic bronchopulmonary eosinophilia

This is characterized by the presence of asthma, transient fleeting shadows on the chest X-ray, and blood or sputum eosinophilia. By far the most common cause worldwide is allergy to *A. fumigatus* (see below), although *Candida albicans* and other mycoses may be the allergen in a small number of patients. In many, no allergen can be identified. Whether these cases are intrinsic or driven by an unidentified extrinsic factor is uncertain.

Diseases caused by *Aspergillus fumigatus*

The various types of lung disease caused by *A. fumigatus* are illustrated in Figure 14.41.

The spores of *A. fumigatus* (diameter 5 mm) are readily inhaled and are present in the atmosphere throughout the year, though they are at their highest concentration in the late autumn. They can be grown from the sputum in up to 15% of patients with chronic lung disease in whom they do not produce disease. They are an important cause of extrinsic asthma in atopic individuals.

Allergic bronchopulmonary aspergillosis

In this rare disease, *Aspergillus* actually grows in the walls of the bronchi and eventually produces proximal bronchiectasis. There are episodes of eosinophilic pneumonia throughout the year, particularly in late autumn and winter. The episodes present with a wheeze, cough, fever and malaise. They are associated with expectoration of firm sputum plugs containing the fungal mycelium, which results in the clearing of the pulmonary infiltrates on the chest X-ray. Occasionally the large mucus plugs obliterate the bronchial lumen, causing collapse of the lung.

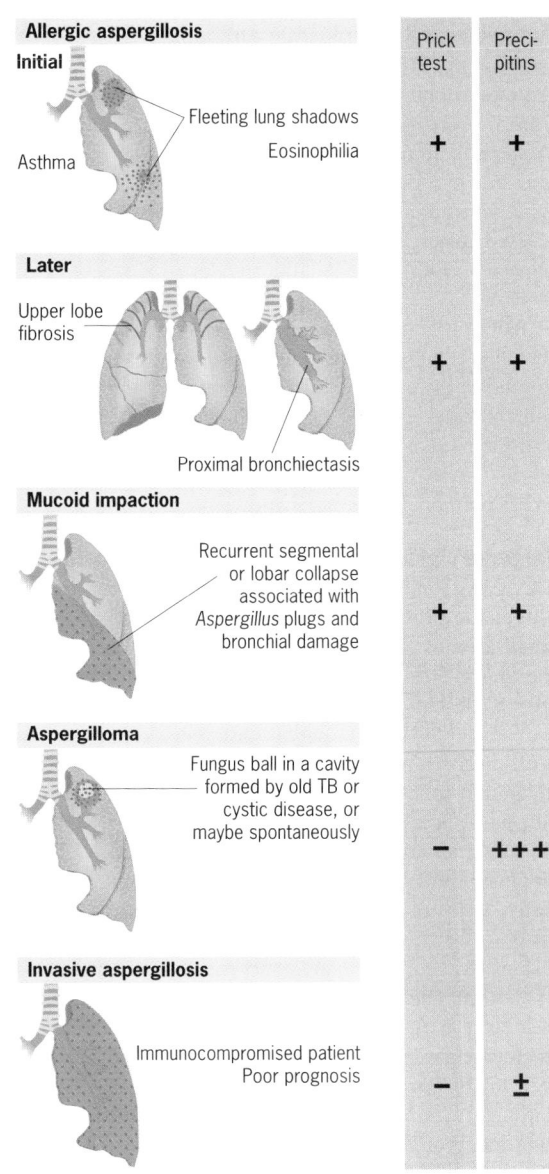

Fig. 14.41 Diseases caused by *Aspergillus fumigatus*.

Left untreated, repeated episodes of eosinophilic pneumonia can result in progressive pulmonary fibrosis that usually affects the upper zones and can give rise to a chest X-ray appearance similar to that produced by tuberculosis.

The peripheral blood eosinophil count is usually raised, and total levels of IgE are usually extremely high (both that specific to *Aspergillus* and non-specific). Skin-prick testing to protein allergens from *A. fumigatus* gives rise to positive immediate skin tests. Sputum may show eosinophils and mycelia, and precipitating antibodies are usually, but not always, found in the serum.

Treatment is with prednisolone 30 mg daily, which readily causes clearing of the pulmonary infiltrates. Frequent episodes of the disease can be prevented by long-term treatment with prednisolone, but doses as high as 10–15 mg daily are usually required. Several anti-fungal agents have been tried in the past without success, but there is now evidence that concurrent treatment with itraconazole helps. The asthma component responds to inhaled corticosteroids although they do not influence the occurrence of pulmonary infiltrates. Lung function tests show a decrease in lung volumes and gas transfer in more chronic cases, but in all cases evidence of reversible airflow limitation can be demonstrated.

Aspergilloma and invasive aspergillosis

Aspergilloma is the growth of *A. fumigatus* within previously damaged lung tissue where it forms a ball of mycelium within lung cavities. Typically the chest X-ray shows a round lesion with an air 'halo' above it. Continuing antigenic stimulation gives rise to large quantities of precipitating antibody in the serum. The aspergilloma itself causes little trouble, though occasionally massive haemoptysis may occur, requiring resection of the area of damaged lung containing the aspergilloma. Although treatment with antifungal agents, such as amphotericin, has been tested in both allergic bronchopulmonary aspergillosis and aspergilloma, this has had little success. Invasive aspergillosis is a well-recognized complication of immunosuppression and requires aggressive antifungal therapy usually with amphotericin (250 µg/kg) combined with flucytosine (200 mg/kg i.v. daily in four doses).

Tropical pulmonary eosinophilia

This term is reserved for an allergic reaction to micro-filaria from *Wuchereria bancrofti*. The condition is seen in the Asian subcontinent and presents with cough and wheeze together with fever, lassitude and weight loss. The typical appearance of the chest X-ray is of bilateral hazy mottling that is frequently uniformly distributed in both lung fields. Individual shadows may be as large as 5 mm or may become more confluent, giving the appearance of pneumonia.

The disease is characterized by a very high eosinophil count in peripheral blood. The filarial complement fixation test is positive in almost every case, although the microfilaria are seldom found. The treatment of choice is diethylcarbamazine at a dose of 5 mg/kg body-weight for 10–14 days; this usually produces a good response.

The hypereosinophilic syndrome

This disease is characterized by eosinophilic infiltration in various organs, sometimes associated with an eosinophilic arteritis. The heart muscle is particularly involved, but pulmonary involvement in the form of a pleural effusion or interstitial lung disease occurs in about 40% of cases. Typical features are fever, weight loss, recurrent abdominal pain, persistent non-productive cough and congestive cardiac failure. Corticosteroid treatment may be of value in some cases.

Goodpasture's syndrome and idiopathic pulmonary haemosiderosis

Goodpasture's syndrome (see also p. 605)

The disease often starts with an upper respiratory tract infection followed by cough and intermittent haemo-ptysis, tiredness and eventually anaemia, though massive bleeding may occur. The chest X-ray shows transient blotchy shadows that are due to intrapulmonary haemorrhage. These features usually precede the development of an acute glomerulonephritis by several weeks or months. The course of the disease is variable: some spontaneously improve while others proceed to renal failure.

The disease usually occurs in individuals over 16 years of age. It is due to a type II cytotoxic reaction driven by antibodies directed against the basement membrane of both kidney and lung. It has been proposed that there may be a shared antigen. ANCA may be positive. An association with influenza A2 virus has been reported.

Treatment is with corticosteroids, but in some cases dramatic improvement has been seen with plasma-pheresis to remove the antibodies.

Idiopathic pulmonary haemosiderosis

This is clinically similar to Goodpasture's syndrome, but there are no anti-basement-membrane antibodies and the kidneys are less frequently involved. Most cases occur in children under 7 years of age. The child develops a chronic cough and anaemia and the chest X-ray shows diffuse shadows that are due to intrapulmonary bleeding, and eventually miliary nodulation. Characteristically, haemosiderin-containing macrophages are found in the sputum. There is an association with a sensitivity to cows' milk, and an appropriate diet is usually tried.

The prognosis in general is poor and treatment with corticosteroids or azathioprine is usually given.

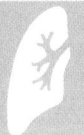

Pulmonary fibrosis and honeycomb lung

Pulmonary fibrosis is the end result of many diseases of the respiratory tract. It may be:

- localized (e.g. following unresolved pneumonia)
- bilateral (e.g. in tuberculosis)
- widespread (e.g. in cryptogenic fibrosing alveolitis, in industrial lung disease, or due to drugs such as busulfan, bleomycin and cyclophosphamide).

Sometimes a typical radiological appearance is seen that is known as 'honeycomb lung'. This reflects the presence diffusely in both lungs of thick-walled cysts 0.5–2.0 cm diameter. These cystic air spaces probably represent dilated and thickened terminal and respiratory bronchioles. The main causes are shown in Table 14.15.

Cryptogenic fibrosing alveolitis (CFA)

This relatively rare disorder, known in the USA as *idiopathic pulmonary fibrosis*, causes diffuse fibrosis throughout the lung fields, usually in late middle age. The cause is unknown, but in a few cases it may be the

Table 14.15
The main causes of honeycomb lung

Localized	Diffuse
Systemic sclerosis	Cryptogenic fibrosing alveolitis
Sarcoidosis	Rheumatoid lung
Tuberculosis	Langerhans' cell histiocytosis
Asbestosis	Tuberous sclerosis
Berylliosis	Neurofibromatosis

result of occupational exposure to metal or wood dust, while many patients show features of autoimmunity.

Pathogenesis

The pathogenesis of damage and fibrosis is complex and several factors are thought to be involved (Fig. 14.42). Macrophages and alveolar epithelial cells are activated by several mechanisms (see p. 194) and produce growth factors including fibronectin, platelet-derived growth factor, transforming growth factor-β, and insulin-like growth factor-1. These stimulate the deposition of type I and III collagens. Histologically there are two main features:

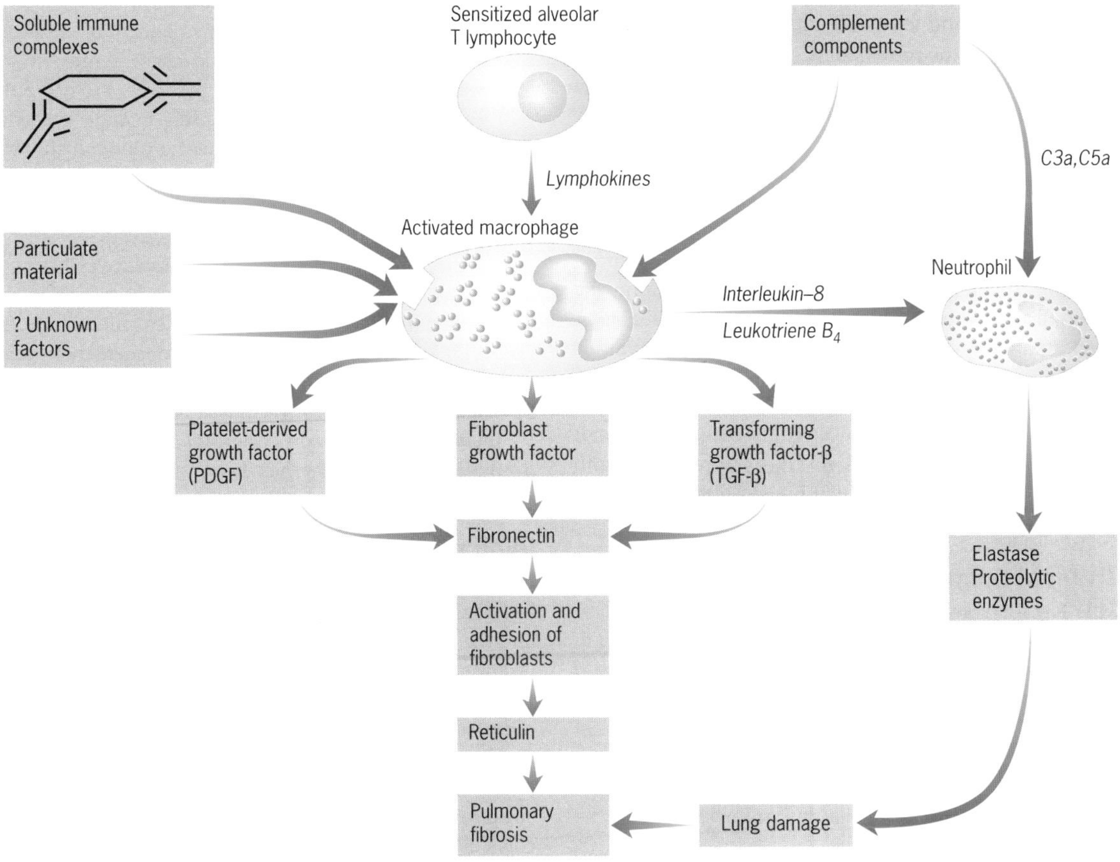

Fig. 14.42 Pathogenesis of pulmonary fibrosis. Macrophages can be activated by several factors, such as soluble immune complexes and sensitized T lymphocytes, resulting in the release of various cytokines leading to fibrosis.

- cellular infiltration with T lymphocytes and plasma cells and thickening and fibrosis of the alveolar walls
- alveolitis – increased cells within the alveolar space (mainly macrophages and type II pneumocytes shed from the alveolar walls).

Clinical features

The main features are progressive breathlessness and cyanosis, which eventually lead to respiratory failure, pulmonary hypertension and cor pulmonale. Gross finger clubbing occurs in two-thirds of cases and fine bilateral end-inspiratory crackles are heard on auscultation. An acute form known as the *Hamman–Rich syndrome* occurs in a small proportion of cases. The chest X-ray appearance initially is of ground-glass appearance, progressing to obvious small nodular shadows with streaky fibrosis and finally a honeycomb lung. A number of autoimmune diseases are seen in association with this condition. For example, autoimmune hepatitis occurs in 5–10% of cases. Similar lung changes are also seen in rheumatoid arthritis, systemic lupus erythematosus, dermatomyositis, systemic sclerosis and Sjögren's syndrome, often associated with Raynaud's phenomenon. CFA has also been reported in association with coeliac disease, ulcerative colitis and renal tubular acidosis.

Investigations

- **Chest X-ray** shows irregular reticulonodular shadowing, often maximal in the lower zones.
- **High-resolution CT scan** shows characteristic changes of peripheral reticular and ground-glass opacification, seen best in the basal regions but extending all over the lungs (Fig. 14.43).
- **Respiratory function tests** show a restrictive ventilatory defect – the lung volumes are reduced, the FEV_1 and FVC ratio is normal to high (with both values being reduced), and carbon monoxide expiratory gas transfer is reduced. Peak flow rates may be normal.

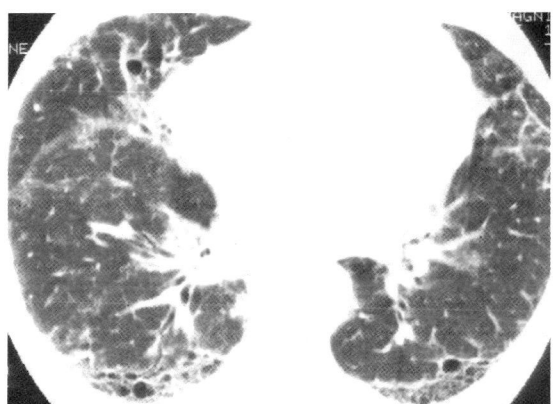

Fig. 14.43 CT scan showing cryptogenic fibrosing alveolitis.

- **Blood gases** show an arterial hypoxaemia caused by a combination of alveolar–capillary block and ventilation–perfusion mismatch with normal or low P_aCO_2 owing to hyperventilation.
- **Blood tests.** Antinuclear antibodies and rheumatoid factors are present in one-third of patients. The ESR and immunoglobulins are mildly elevated.
- **Bronchoalveolar lavage** shows increased numbers of cells, particularly neutrophils and macrophages.
- **Histological confirmation** is necessary in some patients. Transbronchial lung biopsy is rarely diagnostic, but can exclude other conditions such as sarcoidosis or lymphangitis carcinomatosa. An open or thoracoscopic lung biopsy to obtain a larger specimen is usually needed to make a clear histological diagnosis.

Differential diagnosis

The diagnosis of CFA is usually made in a patient presenting with the above signs and characteristic CT changes. The differential diagnosis of the chest X-ray appearance includes extrinsic allergic alveolitis, bronchiectasis, chronic left heart failure, sarcoidosis, industrial lung disease and lymphangitis carcinomatosa.

Prognosis and treatment

The median survival time for patients with CFA is approximately 5 years, although with the acute form mortality is very high. Treatment with prednisolone (30 mg daily) is usually prescribed for disabling disease, though its benefit has still to be proved by appropriate controlled trials. Azathioprine or cyclophosphamide may be added if there is no response. Supportive treatment includes domiciliary oxygen therapy. In severe disease, single lung transplantation can be offered.

Extrinsic allergic alveolitis

In this disease there is a widespread diffuse inflammatory reaction in both the small airways of the lung and alveoli. It is due to the inhalation of a number of different antigens, the most common being microbial spores contaminating vegetable matter (e.g. straw, hay, mushroom compost). Some examples are illustrated in Table 14.16. By far the most common of these diseases world-wide is farmer's lung, which affects up to 1 in 10 of the farming community in disadvantaged, wet communities around the world. In the West the incidence is declining as more mechanized farming procedures and informed animal husbandry are introduced.

Pathogenesis

Histologically there is an initial infiltration of the small airways and alveolar walls with neutrophils followed by T lymphocytes and macrophages, leading to the development of small non-caseating granulomas. These comprise multinucleated giant cells, occasionally containing

Table 14.16
Extrinsic allergic (bronchiolar) alveolitis – some causes

Disease	Situation	Antigens
Farmer's lung	Forking mouldy hay or any other mouldy vegetable material	Thermophilic actinomycetes and *Micropolyspora faeni*
Bird fancier's lung	Handling pigeons, cleaning lofts or budgerigar cages	Proteins present in the 'bloom' on the feathers and in excreta
Maltworker's lung	Turning germinating barley	*Aspergillus clavatus*
Humidifier fever	Contaminated humidifying systems in air conditioners or humidifiers in factories (especially in printing works)	Possibly a variety of bacteria or amoeba (e.g. *Naegleria gruberi*)
Mushroom workers	Turning mushroom compost	Thermophilic actinomycetes

the inhaled antigenic material. The allergic response to the inhaled antigens involves both cellular immunity and the deposition of immune complexes causing foci of inflammation through the activation of complement via the classical pathway. Some of the inhalant materials may also lead to inflammation by directly activating the alternative complement pathway. These mechanisms attract and activate alveolar and interstitial macrophages, so that continued antigenic exposure results in the progressive development of pulmonary fibrosis.

Clinical features

Typically fever, malaise, cough and shortness of breath come on several hours after exposure to the causative antigen. For example, a farmer forking hay in the morning may notice symptoms during the late afternoon and evening with resolution by the following morning. On examination the patient may have a fever, tachypnoea and coarse end-inspiratory crackles and wheezes throughout the chest. Cyanosis caused by ventilation–perfusion mismatch may be severe even at rest. Continued exposure leads to a chronic illness characterized by severe weight loss, effort dyspnoea and cough as well as the features of fibrosing alveolitis (see p. 905).

Investigations

- **Chest X-ray** shows fluffy nodular shadowing with the subsequent development of streaky shadows, particularly in the upper zones. In very advanced cases, honeycomb lung occurs.
- **Lung function tests** show a restrictive ventilatory defect with a decrease in carbon monoxide gas transfer.
- **Polymorphonuclear leucocyte count** is raised in acute cases. Eosinophilia is not a feature.

- **Precipitating antibodies** are present in the serum. One-quarter of pigeon fanciers have precipitating IgG-antibodies against pigeon protein and droppings in their serum, but only a small proportion have lung disease. Precipitating antibodies are evidence of exposure, not disease.
- **Bronchoalveolar lavage** shows increased T lymphocytes and granulocytes.

Differential diagnosis

Although extrinsic allergic alveolitis due to inhalation of the spores of *Micropolyspora faeni* is common among farmers, it is probably more common for these individuals to suffer from asthma related to inhalation of antigens from a variety of mites that infest stored grain and other vegetable material. These include *Lepidoglyphus domesticus, L. destructor* and *Acarus siro*. Symptoms of asthma resulting from inhalation of these allergens are often mistaken for farmer's lung. Lung function tests will effectively discriminate between the disorders. Pigeon fancier's lung is quite common, but alveolitis from budgerigars, parrots and parakeets is very rare.

Management

Prevention is the aim. This can be achieved by changes in work practice, with the use of silage for animal fodder and the drier storage of hay and grain. Pigeon fancier's lung is more difficult to control since affected individuals remain strongly attached to their hobby. Prednisolone, initially in large doses of 30–60 mg daily, may achieve regression during the early stages of the disease. Established fibrosis will not resolve and in some patients the disease may progress inexorably to respiratory failure in spite of intensive therapy. Farmer's lung is a recognized occupational disease in the UK and sufferers are entitled to compensation, depending upon their degree of disability.

Humidifier fever

Humidifier fever, one cause of building-related illnesses (p. 998), may present with the typical features of extrinsic allergic alveolitis without any radiographic changes. This disease has occurred in outbreaks in factories in the UK, particularly in printing works. In North America it is more commonly found in office blocks with contaminated air-conditioning systems. The cause remains unknown but probably involves several bacteria or even amoebae and their constituent products.

Humidifier fever may be effectively prevented by sterilization of the re-circulating water used in large humidifying plants.

Drug-induced lung disease

Drugs may produce a wide variety of disorders of the respiratory tract. The mechanisms are varied and include direct toxicity (e.g. bleomycin), immune complex formation with arteritis, hypersensitivity (involving both T cell and IgE mechanisms) and autoimmunity.

Pulmonary infiltrates with fibrosis may result from the use of a number of cytotoxic drugs used in the treatment of cancer. The most common cause of these reactions is bleomycin. The pulmonary damage is dose-related, occurring when the total dosage is greater than 450 mg, but will regress in some cases if the drug is stopped. The most sensitive test is a decrease in carbon monoxide gas transfer, and therefore gas transfer should be measured repeatedly during treatment with the drug. The use of corticosteroids may help resolution. Drugs affecting the respiratory tract are shown in Table 14.17, together with the types of reaction they

produce. The list is not exhaustive; for example, over 20 different drugs are known to produce a systemic lupus erythematosus-like syndrome, sometimes complicated by pulmonary infiltrates and fibrosis. Paraquat ingestion (see p. 987) causes severe pulmonary oedema and death, and pulmonary fibrosis develops in many of those who survive.

Radiation damage

Irradiation of the lung during radiotherapy can cause a radiation pneumonitis. Patients complain of breathlessness and a dry cough. Radiation pneumonitis results in a restrictive lung defect. Corticosteroids should be given in the acute stage.

Table 14.17
Drug-induced respiratory disease

Disease	Drugs
Asthma ± rhinitis	Penicillins
	Sulphonamides
	Cephalosporins
	Aspirin
	NSAIDs
	Tartrazine
	Iodine-containing contrast media
	Non-selective β-adrenoceptor-blocking drugs (e.g. propranolol)
	Suxamethonium
	Thiopental
Diffuse lung injury infiltrate and/or fibrosis	Amiodarone
	Hexamethonium
	Nitrofurantoin
	Paraquat
	Continuous oxygen
	Cytotoxic agent (many, particularly busulfan, CCNU, bleomycin, methotrexate)
Pulmonary eosinophilia	Antibiotics
	Penicillin
	Tetracycline
	Sulphonamides
	NSAIDs
	Antidepressants
	Antiepileptic
	Phenytoin
	Carbamazepine
	Others
	Chlorpropamide
	Cytotoxic agents
Opportunistic pulmonary infections	Corticosteroids
	Azathioprine
	Other cytotoxic drugs
Respiratory depression	Sedatives
	Opiates
SLE-like syndrome including pulmonary infiltrates, effusions and fibrosis	Hydralazine
	Procainamide
	Isoniazid
	Phenytoin
	ACE inhibitors

CCNU, chloroethyl-cyclohexyl-nitrosourea (lomustine); NSAIDs, non-steroidal anti-inflammatory drugs; SLE, systemic lupus erythematosus

FURTHER READING

British Thoracic Society (1999) The diagnosis, assessment and treatment of diffuse parenchymal lung disease in adults. *Thorax* **54** (S2): S1–S30.
Gross TJ, Hunninghake GW (2001) Idiopathic pulmonary fibrosis. *New England Journal of Medicine* **345**: 517–525.
Newman LS, Rose CS, Maier LA (1997) Sarcoidosis. *New England Journal of Medicine* **336**: 1224–1234.
Savage COS, Harper L, Adu D (1997) Primary systemic vasculitis. *Lancet* **349**: 558–562.
Vassallo R et al. (2000) Pulmonary Langerhans cell histiocytosis. *New England Journal of Medicine* **342**: 1969–1978.

Occupational lung disease

Exposure to dusts, gases, vapours and fumes at work can lead to the development of the following types of lung disease:

- acute bronchitis and even pulmonary oedema from irritants such as sulphur dioxide, chlorine, ammonia or the oxides of nitrogen
- pulmonary fibrosis due to mineral dust
- occupational asthma (see Table 14.12) – this is now the commonest industrial lung disease in the developed world
- extrinsic allergic alveolitis (see Table 14.16)
- bronchial carcinoma due to industrial agents (e.g. asbestos, polycyclic hydrocarbons, radon in mines).

The degree of fibrosis that follows inhalation of mineral dust varies. While iron (siderosis), barium (baritosis) and tin (stannosis) lead to dramatic dense nodular shadowing on the chest X-ray, their effect on lung function and symptoms is minimal. Exposure to silica or asbestos, on the other hand, leads to extensive fibrosis and disability. Coal dust has an intermediate fibrogenic effect and accounts for 90% of all compensated industrial lung diseases in the UK. The term 'pneumoconiosis' means the accumulation of dust in the lungs and the reaction of the tissue to its presence. The term is not

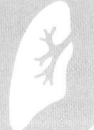

wide enough to encompass all occupational lung disease and is now generally used only in relation to coal dust and its effects on the lung.

Coal-worker's pneumoconiosis

Improved conditions and the progressive contraction of the coal industry in the UK have led to a considerable reduction in the number of cases of pneumoconiosis. The disease is caused by dust particles approximately 2–5 μm in diameter that are retained in the small airways and alveoli of the lung. The incidence of the disease is related to total dust exposure, which is highest at the coal face, particularly if ventilation and dust suppression are poor. Two very different syndromes result from the inhalation of coal.

Simple pneumoconiosis

This simply reflects the deposition of coal dust in the lung. It produces fine micronodular shadowing on the chest X-ray and is by far the most common type of pneumoconiosis. It is graded on the chest X-ray appearance according to standard categories set by the International Labour Office (see below). Considerable dispute remains about the effects of simple pneumoconiosis on respiratory function and symptoms. In many cases the symptoms are due to COPD related to cigarette smoking, but this is not always the case. Recent changes to UK workers compensation legislation means that coal miners who develop COPD may be compensated for their disability regardless of their chest X-ray appearance.

Categories of simple pneumoconiosis are as follows:

1. small round opacities definitely present but few in number
2. small round opacities numerous but normal lung markings still visible
3. small round opacities very numerous and normal lung markings partly or totally obscured.

The importance of simple pneumoconiosis is that it may lead to the development of progressive massive fibrosis (PMF) (see below). PMF virtually never occurs on a background of category 1 simple pneumoconiosis but occurs in about 7% of those with category 2 simple pneumoconiosis and in 30% of those with category 3. Miners with category 1 pneumoconiosis are unlikely to receive compensation unless they also have evidence of COPD. Those with more extensive radiographic changes may be compensated solely on the basis of their X-ray appearances.

Progressive massive fibrosis

In PMF, patients develop round fibrotic masses several centimetres in diameter, almost invariably in the upper lobes and sometimes having necrotic central cavities. The pathogenesis of PMF is still not understood, though it seems clear that some fibrogenic promoting factor is present in individuals developing the disease. At one time this was thought to be *M. tuberculosis*, but it is more probably due to immune complexes, analogous to the development of large fibrotic nodules in coal miners with rheumatoid arthritis (Caplan's syndrome). Both rheumatoid factor and antinuclear antibodies are often present in the serum of patients with PMF, as is also seen in those suffering from asbestosis and silicosis. Pathologically there is apical destruction and disruption of the lung, resulting in emphysema and airway damage. Lung function tests show a mixed restrictive and obstructive ventilatory defect with loss of lung volume, irreversible airflow limitation and reduced gas transfer.

The patient with PMF suffers considerable effort dyspnoea, usually with a cough. The sputum can be black. The disease can progress (or even develop) after exposure to coal dust has ceased and may lead to respiratory failure.

Silicosis

This disease is uncommon though it may still be encountered in workers in foundries where sand used in moulds has to be removed from the metal casts (fettling), in sand blasting, and amongst stonemasons, pottery and ceramic workers. Silicosis is caused by the inhalation of silica (silicon dioxide). This dust is highly fibrogenic. For example, a coal miner can remain healthy with 30 g of coal dust in his lungs but 3 g of silica is sufficient to kill. Silica seems particularly toxic to alveolar macrophages and readily initiates fibrogenesis (see Fig. 14.42). The chest X-ray appearances and clinical features of silicosis are similar to those of PMF, but distinctive thin streaks of calcification may be seen around the hilar lymph nodes ('eggshell' calcification).

Asbestosis

Asbestos is a mixture of silicates of iron, magnesium, nickel, cadmium and aluminium, and has the unique property of occurring naturally as a fibre. It is remarkably resistant to heat, acid and alkali, and has been widely used for roofing, insulation and fireproofing. Asbestos has been mined in southern Africa, Canada and eastern Europe. Several different types of asbestos are recognized: about 90% of asbestos is chrysotile, 6% crocidolite and 4% amosite. Chrysotile or white asbestos is the softest asbestos fibre. Each fibre is often as long as 2 cm but only a few microns thick. It is less fibrogenic than crocidolite. Crocidolite (blue asbestos) is particularly resistant to chemical destruction and exists in straight fibres up to 50 mm in length and 1–2 μm in width. Crocidolite is the most likely type of asbestos to produce asbestosis and mesothelioma. This may be due to the fact that it is readily trapped in the lung. Its long, thin shape means that it can be inhaled, but subsequent rotation against the long axis of the smaller airways, particularly in turbulent airflow during expiration, causes the fibres to impact. Crocidolite is also particularly resistant to macrophage and neutrophil enzymatic destruction.

Exposure to asbestos occurred particularly in ship-building yards and in power stations, but its ubiquitous use meant that low levels of exposure were common. Up to 50% of urban dwellers have been found to have evidence of asbestos bodies (asbestos fibre covered in protein secretions) in their lungs at post-mortem. Regulations in the UK prevent the use of crocidolite and severely restrict the use of chrysotile. Careful dust control measures are enforced, which should eventually abolish the problem. Workers continue to be exposed to blue asbestos in the course of demolition or in the replacement of insulation, and it should be remembered that there is a considerable time lag between exposure and development of the disease, particularly mesothelioma (20–40 years).

A synergistic relationship between asbestosis and cigarette smoking and the development of bronchial carcinoma, usually adenocarcinoma, exists; the risk is multiplied fivefold above the risk attributable to smoking. The risk of lung cancer is also increased in non-smokers, especially in those who have parenchymal asbestosis but also in those with pleural plaques without parenchymal fibrosis.

The diseases caused by asbestos are summarized in Table 14.18. Bilateral diffuse pleural thickening, asbestosis, mesothelioma and asbestos-related carcinoma of the bronchus are all eligible for industrial injuries benefit in the UK, but account for only one-quarter of the number of cases of compensation compared with coal-worker's pneumoconiosis.

Asbestosis is defined as fibrosis of the lungs caused by asbestos dust, which may or may not be associated with fibrosis of the parietal or visceral layers of the pleura. It is a progressive disease characterized by breathlessness and accompanied by finger clubbing and bilateral basal end-inspiratory crackles. Fibrosis, not detectable on chest X-ray, may be revealed on CT scan. No treatment is known to alter the progress of the disease, though corticosteroids are often prescribed.

The number of cases of mesothelioma has increased progressively since the mid-1980s and has now reached over 1000 cases per year. Pleural effusions are the most common presentation of mesothelioma, typically with persistent chest wall pain, which should raise the index of suspicion even if the initial pleural fluid or biopsy samples are non-diagnostic. Often thoracoscopic biopsy is needed to obtain sufficient tissue for diagnosis. In the event of a positive pleural biopsy diagnosis, local radiotherapy should be given to prevent the seeding of mesothelioma cells down the needle track. No treatment influences the universally fatal outcome.

Table 14.18

The effects of asbestos on the lung

	Exposure	Chest X-ray	Lung function	Symptoms	Outcome
Asbestos bodies	Light	Normal	Normal	None	Evidence of asbestos exposure only
Pleural plaques	Light	Pleural thickening (parietal pleura) and calcification (also in diaphragmatic pleura)	Mild restrictive ventilatory defect	Rare, occasional mild effort dyspnoea	No other sequelae
Effusion	First two decades following exposure	Effusion	Restrictive	Pleuritic pain, dyspnoea	Often recurrent
Bilateral diffuse pleural thickening	Light/moderate	Bilateral diffuse thickening (of both parietal and visceral pleura) more than 5 mm thick and extending over more than one-quarter of the chest wall	Restrictive ventilatory defect	Effort dyspnoea	May progress in absence of further exposure
Mesothelioma	Light (interval of 20–40 years from exposure to disease)	Pleural effusion, usually unilateral	Restrictive ventilatory defect	Pleuritic pain, increasing dyspnoea	Median survival 2 years
Asbestosis	Heavy (interval of 5–10 years from exposure to disease)	Diffuse bilateral streaky shadows, honeycomb lung	Severe restrictive ventilatory defect and reduced gas transfer	Progressive dyspnoea	Poor, progression in some cases after exposure ceases
Asbestos-related carcinoma of the bronchus		The features of asbestosis, bilateral diffuse pleural thickening or bilateral pleural plaques plus those of bronchial carcinoma			Fatal

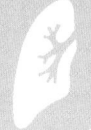

Byssinosis

This disease occurs world-wide but is declining rapidly in areas where the numbers of people employed in cotton mills are falling. In the UK the disease used to occur in areas of Lancashire and Northern Ireland but is now a historical footnote. The symptoms start on the first day back at work after a break (Monday sickness) with improvement as the week progresses. Tightness in the chest, cough and breathlessness occur within the first hour in dusty areas of the mill, particularly in the blowing and carding rooms where raw cotton is cleaned and the fibres are straightened.

The exact nature of the disease and its aetiology remain disputed. Two important features are that pure cotton does not cause the disease, and that cotton dust has some effect on airflow limitation in all those exposed. Individuals with asthma are particularly badly affected by exposure to cotton dust. The most likely aetiology is endotoxins from bacteria present in the raw cotton causing constriction of the airways of the lung. There are no changes on the chest X-ray and there is considerable dispute as to whether the progressive airflow limitation seen in some patients with the disease is due to the cotton dust or to other factors such as cigarette smoking or coexistent asthma.

Berylliosis

Beryllium–copper alloy has a high tensile strength and is resistant to metal fatigue, high temperature and corrosion. It is used in the aerospace industry, in atomic reactors and in many electrical devices.

Although beryllium is inhaled into the lungs, it causes a systemic illness with a clinical picture similar to sarcoidosis. The major chronic problem is that of progressive dyspnoea with pulmonary fibrosis. However, strict control of levels in the working atmosphere have made the disease a rarity.

FURTHER READING

Beckett WS (2000) Occupational respiratory disorders. *New England Journal of Medicine* **342**: 406–413.
Wagner GR (1997) Asbestosis and silicosis. *Lancet* **349**: 1311–1315.

Lung cysts

These may be congenital, bronchogenic cysts or may result from a sequestrated pulmonary segment. Hydatid disease causes fluid-filled cysts. Thin-walled cysts are due to lung abscesses, which are particularly found in staphylococcal pneumonia, tuberculous cavities, septic pulmonary infarction, primary bronchogenic carcinoma, cavitating metastatic neoplasm, or paragonimiasis caused by the lung fluke *Paragonimus westermani*.

Tumours of the respiratory tract

Bronchial carcinoma accounts for 95% of all primary tumours of the lung. Alveolar cell carcinoma accounts for 2% of lung tumours and other less malignant or benign tumours account for the remaining 3%.

Benign tumours

Pulmonary hamartoma

This is the most common benign tumour of the lung and is usually seen on the X-ray as a very well-defined round lesion 1–2 cm in diameter in the periphery of the lung. Growth is extremely slow, but the tumour may reach several centimetres in diameter. Rarely it arises from a major bronchus and causes obstruction.

Bronchial carcinoid

This rare tumour resembles intestinal carcinoid tumour and is locally invasive, eventually spreading to mediastinal lymph nodes and finally to distant organs. It is a highly vascular tumour that projects into the lumen of a major bronchus causing recurrent haemoptysis. It grows slowly and eventually blocks the bronchus, leading to lobar collapse. As foregut derivatives, bronchial carcinoids may produce ACTH but do not usually produce the 5-hydroxytryptamine that is seen in midgut or hindgut carcinoid tumours.

Cylindroma, chondroma and lipoma

These are extremely rare tumours that may grow in the bronchus or trachea, causing obstruction.

Tracheal tumours

Benign tumours include squamous papilloma, leiomyoma, haemangiomas and tumours of neurogenic origin.

Malignant tumours

Tracheal carcinoma

Primary tumours of the trachea are rare – their incidence relative to laryngeal and bronchial tumours is 1 : 75 and 1 : 180 respectively. The majority are malignant and cause severe and rapidly progressive dyspnoea and stridor. Flow–volume curves show typical and dramatic reductions in inspiratory flow (extrathoracic tracheal tumours) (see p. 840). Diagnosis is confirmed by sputum examination and bronchoscopy. Rapid and effective destruction of tumour (p. 914) provides temporary relief of symptoms. Radiotherapy is often given and occasionally surgery may be possible but the prognosis is very poor.

Bronchial carcinoma

This is the most common malignant tumour in the West and is the third most common cause of death in the UK after heart disease and pneumonia. Mortality rates world-wide are highest in Scotland, closely followed by England and Wales. In the UK, 32 000 people die each year from bronchial carcinoma, with a male-to-female ratio of 3 : 1. Although the mortality rate from this disease has levelled off in men, it continues to rise in women, accounting for 1 in 8 of all deaths from malignant disease in women, second only to carcinoma of the breast.

The strength of the association between cigarette smoking and bronchial carcinoma overshadows any other aetiological factors (Table 14.19), but there is a higher incidence of bronchial carcinoma in urban compared with rural areas, even when allowance is made for cigarette smoking. Passive smoking (the frequent inhalation of other people's smoke by non-smokers) increases the risk of bronchial carcinoma by a factor of 1.5. Occupational factors include exposure to asbestos, and an association is also claimed for workers in contact with arsenic, chromium, iron oxide, petroleum products and oils, coal tar, products of coal combustion, and radiation. Tumours associated with occupational factors are mostly adenocarcinomas and appear to be less related to cigarette smoking.

Cell types

Bronchial carcinoma is divided into small-cell carcinoma and non-small-cell carcinoma, a division based on the characteristics of the disease and its response to treatment. Studies of mean doubling times of carcinomas indicate that development from the initial malignant change to presentation takes many years; for adenocarcinoma it takes approximately 15 years, for squamous carcinoma 8 years and for small-cell carcinoma 3 years.

Non-small-cell carcinoma

Squamous or *epidermoid carcinoma* is the most common carcinoma in this group, accounting for approximately 40% of all carcinomas. Most present as obstructive lesions of the bronchus leading to infection. It occasionally

cavitates (10%) at presentation but widespread metastases occur relatively late. The cells are usually well differentiated but occasionally anaplastic. Local spread is common.

Large-cell carcinoma is a less well-differentiated tumour that metastasizes early. It accounts for 25% of all tumours.

Adenocarcinoma arises peripherally from mucous glands in the small bronchi and often produces a subpleural mass. Invasion of the pleura and the mediastinal lymph nodes is common, as are metastases to the brain and bones. Adenocarcinoma accounts for approximately 10% of all bronchial carcinomas and frequently arises in or around scar tissue. It is the most common bronchial carcinoma associated with asbestos and is proportionally more common in non-smokers, in women, in the elderly, and in the Far East.

Alveolar cell carcinoma (also termed bronchiolar carcinoma) accounts for only 1–2% of lung tumours and occurs either as a peripheral solitary nodule or as diffuse nodular lesions of multicentric origin. Occasionally this tumour is associated with expectoration of very large volumes of mucoid sputum.

Small-cell carcinoma

This tumour, often called oat-cell carcinoma, accounts for 20–30% of all lung cancers. It arises from endocrine cells (Kulchitsky cells). These cells are members of the APUD system, which explains why many polypeptide hormones are secreted by these tumours. Some of these polypeptides act in an autocrine fashion: they feed back on the cells and cause cell growth. Small-cell carcinoma is considered to be a systemic disease. Although the tumour is rapidly growing and highly malignant, it is the only one of the bronchial carcinomas that responds to chemotherapy.

Clinical features

The frequencies of the common symptoms of lung cancer on presentation are shown in Table 14.20. Chest pain and discomfort are often described as fullness and pressure in

Table 14.19
Death rates from lung cancer (age standardized) per 100 000 according to smoking habits in male British doctors

Death rate		Number of cigarettes per day	Death rate
Non-smokers	10	1–14	78
Ex-smokers	43	15–24	127
Continuing smokers		25 or more	251
Any tobacco	104		
Pipe/cigar	58		
Cigarettes	140		

Table 14.20
The frequency of the common presenting symptoms of bronchial carcinoma

Symptom	Frequency (%)
Cough	41
Chest pain	22
Cough and pain	15
Coughing blood	7
Chest infection	< 5
Malaise	< 5
Weight loss	< 5
Shortness of breath	< 5
Hoarseness	< 5
Distant spread	< 5
No symptoms	< 5

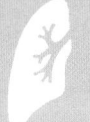

the chest. Sometimes the pain may be pleuritic owing to invasion of the pleura or ribs.

Often there are no abnormal physical signs. Enlarged supraclavicular lymph nodes can be found with small-cell carcinoma. There may be signs of a pleural effusion or of lobar collapse. Signs of an unresolved pneumonia or of associated underlying disease (e.g. diffuse pulmonary fibrosis in asbestosis) may be present.

Direct spread

The tumour may directly involve the pleura and ribs. Carcinoma in the apex of the lung can erode the ribs and involve the lower part of the brachial plexus (C8, T1 and T2), causing severe pain in the shoulder and down the inner surface of the arm (Pancoast's tumour). The sympathetic ganglion can also be involved, producing Horner's syndrome. Further extension may involve the recurrent laryngeal nerve as it passes down the aortic arch, causing unilateral vocal cord paresis with hoarseness and a bovine cough, and rarely the tumour causes spinal cord compression.

Bronchial carcinoma can also directly invade the phrenic nerve, causing paralysis of the ipsilateral hemidiaphragm. It can involve the oesophagus, producing progressive dysphagia, and the pericardium, producing pericardial effusion and malignant dysrhythmias. Superior vena caval obstruction causes early morning headache, facial congestion and oedema involving the upper limbs; the jugular veins are distended, as are the veins on the chest that form a collateral circulation with veins arising from the abdomen.

Metastatic complications

Bony metastases are common, giving rise to severe pain and pathological fractures. There is frequent involvement of the liver. Secondary deposits in the brain present as a change in personality, epilepsy or as a focal neurological lesion. Secondary deposits in the adrenal gland are a very frequent post-mortem finding but may often be asymptomatic.

Non-metastatic extrapulmonary manifestations

Although approximately 10% of small-cell tumours are thought to produce ectopic hormones at some stage, clinically important extrapulmonary manifestations are relatively rare apart from finger clubbing (Table 14.21).

Hypertrophic pulmonary osteoarthropathy (HPOA) (see p. 572) occurs in approximately 3% of all bronchial carcinomas, particularly squamous-cell carcinomas and adenocarcinomas. Symptoms include joint stiffness and severe pain in the wrists and ankles, sometimes associated with gynaecomastia. X-rays show a characteristic proliferative periostitis at the distal ends of long bones, which have an onion-skin appearance. HPOA is invariably associated with clubbing of the fingers. It may regress after resection of the lung tumour or as a result of vagotomy at thoracotomy.

Table 14.21

Non-metastatic extrapulmonary manifestations of bronchial carcinoma (percentage of all cases)

Metabolic (universal at some stage) Loss of weight Lassitude Anorexia	**Vascular and haematological** (rare) Thrombophlebitis migrans Non-bacterial thrombotic endocarditis Microcytic and normocytic anaemia Disseminated intravascular coagulopathy Thrombotic thrombocytopenic purpura Haemolytic anaemia
Endocrine (10%) (usually small-cell carcinoma) Ectopic adrenocorticotrophin syndrome Syndrome of inappropriate secretion of antidiuretic hormone (SIADH) Hypercalcaemia (usually squamous cell carcinoma) Rarer: hypoglycaemia, thyrotoxicosis, gynaecomastia	**Skeletal** Clubbing (30%) Hypertrophic osteoarthropathy (± gynaecomastia) (3%)
Neurological (2–16%) Encephalopathies – including subacute cerebellar degeneration Myelopathies – motor neurone disease Neuropathies – peripheral sensorimotor neuropathy Muscular disorders – polymyopathy, myasthenic syndrome (Eaton–Lambert syndrome)	**Cutaneous** (rare) Dermatomyositis Acanthosis nigricans Herpes zoster

Investigations

Chest X-ray

By the time the lung cancer is causing symptoms, it will almost always be visible on chest X-rays. Asymptomatic tumours may be seen on chest X-ray if they are more than 1 cm in diameter. CT scanning will detect smaller masses but is not suitable for screening purposes. A minority of tumours are confined to the central airways and mediastinum without obvious change on the plain chest X-ray. These will be readily seen at bronchoscopy or on CT scanning. In general, investigation of isolated haemoptysis with a normal chest X-ray is unrewarding but a normal chest X-ray should not deter from further investigation if there are other symptoms suggestive of bronchial carcinoma. About 70% of all primary lung cancers arise in the hilar region including virtually all small-cell lung cancers and most squamous cell carcinomas. Adenocarcinoma occurs more often in the periphery than the other cell types.

Carcinomas causing partial obstruction of a bronchus interrupt the mucociliary escalator, and bacteria are retained within the affected lobe. This gives rise to the so-called secondary pneumonia that is commonly seen on a chest X-ray of a patient presenting with bronchial carcinoma.

Bronchial carcinoma can also appear as round shadows on a chest X-ray (see p. 848). Characteristically the edge of the tumour has a fluffy or spiked appearance, though sometimes it may be entirely smooth with cavitation, particularly when the tumour is epidermoid in type.

The hilar lymph nodes on the side of the tumour are frequently involved in carcinoma of the lung. Bronchial carcinoma is also a common cause of large pleural effusions. Carcinoma can spread through the lymphatic channels of the lung to give rise to lymphangitis carcinomatosa; in bronchial carcinoma this is usually unilateral and associated with striking dyspnoea. The chest X-ray shows streaky shadowing throughout the lung. Bilateral lymphangitis carcinomatosa is more often due to metastatic spread, usually from tumours below the diaphragm (the stomach and colon) or from breast cancers.

Computed tomography

CT is particularly useful for identifying disease in the mediastinum, such as enlarged lymph nodes (see Fig. 14.13, p. 848) or local spread of the tumour, and for identifying secondary spread of carcinoma to the opposite lung by detecting masses too small to be seen on the chest X-ray. Lymph nodes larger than 1 cm are considered pathological, although whether they are due to metastatic tumour, reactive hyperplasia or previous lung disease (e.g. tuberculosis) can only be determined by biopsy. A normal CT scan prior to surgery excludes the need for mediastinoscopy and node biopsy. CT scanning should be extended to include the liver, adrenal glands and the brain since there are common sites for metastases.

Magnetic resonance imaging

MRI is not useful for the diagnosis of primary lung tumours but is very useful for staging as it provides better images of the mediastinum than CT (see p. 849).

Fibreoptic bronchoscopy (see also p. 853)

This technique is used to define the bronchial anatomy and to obtain biopsy and cytological specimens. If the carcinoma involves the first 2 cm of either main bronchus, the tumour is inoperable as there would be insufficient resection margins for pneumonectomy. Widening and loss of the sharp angle of the carina indicates the presence of enlarged mediastinal lymph nodes, either malignant or reactive. These can be biopsied by passage of a needle through the bronchial wall. Vocal cord paresis on the left indicates involvement of the recurrent laryngeal nerve and inoperability.

Transthoracic fine-needle aspiration (FNA) biopsy

Peripheral lung lesions cannot be seen by fibreoptic bronchoscopy and samples may be obtained by direct aspiration through the chest wall under appropriate X-ray or CT screening. Specimens can be obtained from 75% of peripheral lesions that could not be biopsied transbronchially. Pneumothorax is common (25% of patients), occasionally requiring drainage. Mild haemoptysis occurs in 5%. Implantation metastases do not occur. Although useful if positive, negative FNA is not very helpful. For this reason some physicians prefer to refer direct for thoracotomy.

Other investigations

These include a full blood count for the detection of anaemia, biochemistry for liver involvement, hypercalcaemia and hyponatraemia. Other complications are addressed as and when they arise.

Treatment (see also p. 503)

Unlike cancers at some other sites, there has been no improvement in survival from carcinoma of the bronchus apart from small-cell cancer (see below). Only 20% of patients are alive 1 year after diagnosis and only 6–8% after 5 years (cf. 50% for breast or cervix).

Surgery

The only treatment of any curative value for non-small-cell cancer of the lung is surgery. Only 20–25% of all cases are suitable for resection and only 25–30% of these survive for 5 years. Exploratory thoracotomy should be avoided in patients over 65 years as the operative mortality rate exceeds the expected 5-year survival rate.

Preoperative assessment. This requires blood tests and imaging as described above. Because of their common aetiology, COPD is frequently present. An FEV_1 of less than 1.5 L is not compatible with an active life following pneumonectomy, although the surgery itself can be successfully accomplished. This also applies when the gas-transfer test is reduced by 50%.

Radiation therapy for cure

High-dose radiotherapy (65 Gy or 6500 rads) can produce results that are as good as those of surgery in patients who are fit and who have slowly growing squamous carcinoma. It is the treatment of choice if the tumour is inoperable for reasons such as poor lung function. Radiation pneumonitis (defined as an acute infiltrate precisely confined to the radiation area and occurring within 3 months of radiotherapy) develops in 10–15% of cases. Radiation fibrosis, a fibrotic change occurring within a year or so of radiotherapy and not precisely confined to the radiation area, occurs to some degree in all cases. These complications are usually of little importance.

Symptomatic radiation treatment

Bone pain, haemoptysis and the superior vena cava syndrome respond favourably to irradiation in the short term.

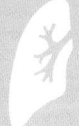

Chemotherapy

Small-cell cancer. Single or combination chemotherapy has resulted in a fivefold increase in median survival from 2 to 10 months. A small number of patients enjoy several years of remission. Good results have been achieved with the combination of etoposide and cisplatin (see p. 503). The unwanted effects are greater than with single-agent chemotherapy with etoposide alone, which should be reserved for elderly patients and those with additional medical or physical disabilities.

Non-small-cell lung cancer (NSCLC). Treatment regimens change frequently and such treatment is best supervised by a specialized oncologist. Response rates with single-agent treatment with newly introduced drugs exceed 20%. Gemcitabine, a pyrimidine antimetabolite, has less toxicity but equivalent antitumour effect to ifosfamide, vindesine and mitomycin C. Combination chemotherapy including cisplatin leads to a better response rate in non-operable NSCLC with median survivals of 6 months and 10–12 months in responding patients. Most patients achieve their best response after two or three courses of treatment. Adjuvant chemotherapy with radiotherapy improves response rate and extends median survival. Preoperative (neoadjuvant) chemotherapy increases by half the number of previously inoperable NSCLC patients who can undergo surgical resection with 30% survival at 3 years.

Laser therapy, endobronchial irradiation and tracheobronchial stents

These techniques are used in the palliation of inoperable lung cancer in selected patients with tracheobronchial narrowing from intraluminal tumour or extrinsic compression causing disabling breathlessness, intractable cough and complications, including infection, haemoptysis and respiratory failure.

A neodymium-Yag (Nd-Yag) laser passed through a fibreoptic bronchoscope can be used to vaporize inoperable fungating intraluminal carcinoma involving short segments of trachea or main bronchus. Benign tumours, strictures and vascular lesions can also be treated effectively with immediate relief of symptoms.

Endobronchial irradiation (*brachytherapy*) is useful for the treatment of both intraluminal tumour and malignant extrinsic compression. A radioactive source is afterloaded into a catheter placed adjacent to the carcinoma under fibreoptic bronchoscope control. Radiation dose falls rapidly with distance from the source, minimizing damage to adjacent normal tissue. Reduction in endoscopically assessed tumour size occurs in 70–95% of cases.

Tracheobronchial stents made of silicone or as expandable metal springs are available for insertion into strictures caused by tumour or from external compression or when there is weakening and collapse of the tracheobronchial wall.

Terminal care (see p. 507)

Patients dying of cancer of the lung need attention to their overall well-being. Palliative care must not be ignored simply because they cannot be cured. Much can be done to make the patient's remaining life symptom-free and as active as possible. As compared to patients with fatal cancers at other sites, patients with lung cancer tend to remain relatively independent and pain-free, but die more rapidly once they reach the terminal phase.

Daily treatment with prednisolone (up to 15 mg daily) may improve appetite. Morphine or diamorphine must be given regularly for pain, either in the form of a sustained-release morphine sulphate tablet twice daily or else as regular elixirs or injections. Many patients benefit from a continuous subcutaneous injection of opiates given by a pump. Candidiasis and other infections in the mouth are common and must be looked for and treated. Patients taking opiates are frequently constipated, so regular laxatives should be prescribed. Short courses of palliative radiotherapy are helpful for bone pain, severe cough or haemoptysis.

Both the patient and the relatives may require counselling, a task that should be shared between the respiratory teams, the primary care team and the nurses, social workers, hospital chaplains and doctors, who make up the palliative care team.

Secondary tumours

Metastases in the lung are very common and usually present as round shadows (1.5–3.0 cm diameter). They may be detected on chest X-ray in patients already diagnosed as having carcinoma. *Typical sites for the primary tumour include the kidney, prostate, breast, bone, gastrointestinal tract, cervix or ovary.*

Metastases nearly always develop in the parenchyma and are often relatively asymptomatic even when the chest X-ray shows extensive pulmonary metastases. Rarely metastases may develop in the bronchi, when they may present with haemoptysis.

Carcinoma, particularly of the stomach, pancreas and breast, can involve mediastinal glands and spread along the lymphatics of both lungs (lymphangitis carcinomatosa), leading to progressive and severe breathlessness. On the chest X-ray, bilateral lymphadenopathy is seen together with streaky basal shadowing fanning out over both lung fields.

Occasionally a pulmonary metastasis may be detected as a *solitary round shadow* on chest X-ray in an asymptomatic patient. The most common primary tumour to do this is a renal cell carcinoma.

The differential diagnosis includes:

- primary bronchial carcinoma
- tuberculoma
- benign tumour of the lung
- hydatid cyst.

Single pulmonary metastases can be removed surgically but, as CT scans usually show the presence of small metastases undetected on chest X-ray, surgery is seldom performed.

Screening for lung cancer

Screening programmes (yearly chest X-ray, 4-monthly sputum cytology) have been tried in high-risk groups but the success rate is minimal, underlining the need for prevention.

FURTHER READING

American Society of Clinical Oncology (1997) Clinical practice guidelines for the treatment of unresectable non-small-cell lung cancer. *Journal of Clinical Oncology* **15**: 2996–3018.
Hoffman RS (2000) Lung cancer: clinical/pathological features, staging and treatment. *Lancet* **355**: 479–485.
Mulshine JL (2000) Prospects for lung cancer screening. *Lancet* **355**: 592–593.
Seijo LM, Sternman DH (2001) Interventional pulmonology. *New England Journal of Medicine* **344**: 740–749.

Disorders of the chest wall and pleura

Trauma
Trauma to the thoracic wall can cause penetrating wounds and lead to pneumothorax or haemothorax.

Rib fractures
Rib fractures are caused by trauma or coughing (particularly in the elderly), and can occur in patients with osteoporosis. Pathological rib fractures are due to metastatic spread from carcinoma of the bronchus, breast, kidney, prostate or thyroid. Ribs can also become involved by a mesothelioma. Fractures may not be readily visible on a PA chest X-ray, so lateral X-rays and oblique views may be necessary.

Pain prevents adequate chest expansion and coughing and this can lead to pneumonia.

Treatment is with adequate oral analgesia, by local infiltration or an intercostal nerve block.

Two fractures in one rib can lead to a flail segment with paradoxical movement, i.e. part of the chest wall moves inwards during inspiration. This can produce inefficient ventilation and may require intermittent positive-pressure ventilation, especially if several ribs are similarly affected.

Rupture of the trachea or a major bronchus
Rupture of the trachea or even a major bronchus can occur during deceleration injuries, leading to pneumothorax, surgical emphysema, pneumomediastinum and haemoptysis. Surgical emphysema is caused by air leaking into the subcutaneous connective tissue; this can also occur after the insertion of an intercostal drainage tube. A pneumomediastinum occurs when air leaks from the lung inside the parietal pleura and extends along the bronchial walls.

Rupture of the oesophagus (p. 268)
Rupture of the oesophagus leads to mediastinitis usually with mixed bacterial infections. This is a serious complication of external injury, endoscopic procedures, bougienage or necrotic carcinoma, and requires vigorous antibacterial chemotherapy.

Lung contusion
This causes widespread fluffy shadows on the chest X-ray owing to intrapulmonary haemorrhage. This may give rise to acute respiratory distress syndrome (see p. 951).

Kyphoscoliosis
Kyphoscoliosis may be congenital, owing to disease of the vertebrae such as tuberculosis or osteomalacia, or due to neuromuscular disease such as Friedreich's ataxia or poliomyelitis. The respiratory effects of severe kyphoscoliosis are often more pronounced than might be expected and respiratory failure and death often occur in the fourth or fifth decade. The abnormality should be corrected at an early stage if possible. Positive airway pressure ventilation delivered through a tightly fitting nasal mask is the treatment of choice for respiratory failure (see p. 950).

Ankylosing spondylitis (see also p. 548)
Limitation of chest wall movement is often well compensated by diaphragmatic movement, and so the respiratory effects of this disease are relatively mild. It is occasionally associated with upper lobe fibrosis.

Pectus excavatum and carinatum
Pectus excavatum causes few problems other than embarrassment about the deep vertical furrow in the chest, which can be corrected surgically. The heart is seen to lie well to the left on the chest X-ray. Pectus carinatum (pigeon chest) is often the result of rickets but is rarely seen in the West now. No treatment is required.

Pleurisy
This is the term used to describe pain arising from any disease of the pleura. The localized inflammation produces sharp localized pain, made worse on deep inspiration, coughing and occasionally on twisting and bending movements. Pleurisy occurs with pneumonia, pulmonary infarct and carcinoma. Rarer causes include rheumatoid arthritis and systemic lupus erythematosus.

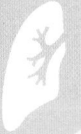

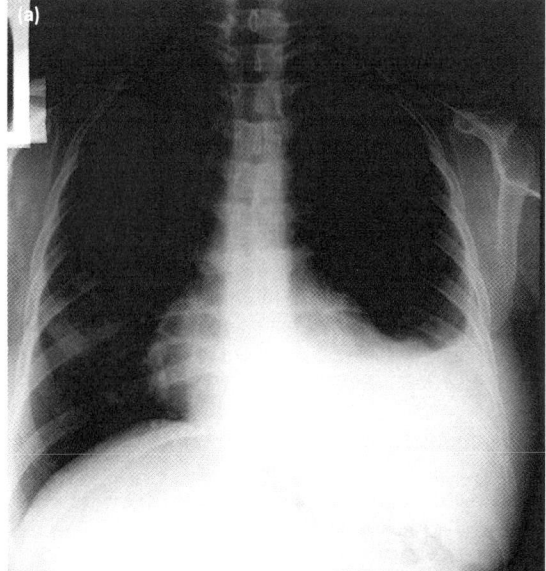 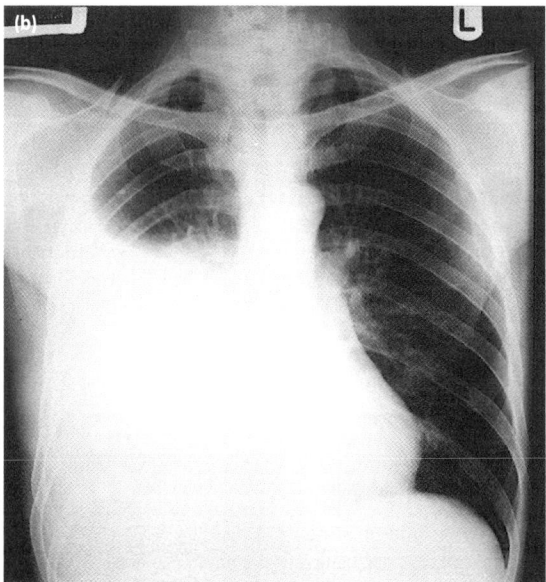

Fig. 14.44 Radiographs showing (a) small and (b) large pleural effusions.

Epidemic myalgia (Bornholm disease) is due to infection by Coxsackie B virus. This illness is common in young adults in the late summer and autumn and is characterized by an upper respiratory tract illness followed by pleuritic pain in the chest and upper abdomen with tender muscles. The chest X-ray remains normal and the illness clears within a week.

Pleural effusion

A pleural effusion is an excessive accumulation of fluid in the pleural space. It can be detected on X-ray when 300 mL or more of fluid is present and clinically when 500 mL or more is present. The chest X-ray appearances (Fig. 14.44) range from the obliteration of the costophrenic angle to dense homogeneous shadows occupying part or all of the hemithorax. Fluid below the lung (a subpulmonary effusion) can simulate a raised hemidiaphragm. Fluid in the fissures may resemble an intrapulmonary mass. The physical signs are shown in Table 14.2 on page 845.

Diagnosis

This is by pleural aspiration (see p. 852). The fluid that accumulates may be a transudate or an exudate.

Transudates

Effusions that are transudates can be bilateral, but are often larger on the right side. The protein content is less than 30 g/L and the lactic dehydrogenase is less than 200 IU/L. Causes include:

- heart failure
- hypoproteinaemia (e.g. nephrotic syndrome)
- constrictive pericarditis

- hypothyroidism
- ovarian tumours producing right-sided pleural effusion – Meigs' syndrome.

Exudates

The protein content of exudates is > 30 g/L and the lactic dehydrogenase is > 200 IU/L. Causes include:

- bacterial pneumonia (common)
- carcinoma of the bronchus and pulmonary infarction – fluid may be blood-stained (common)
- tuberculosis
- connective-tissue disease
- post-myocardial infarction syndrome (rare)
- acute pancreatitis (high amylase content) (rare)
- mesothelioma (rare)
- sarcoidosis (very rare)
- yellow-nail syndrome (effusion due to lymphoedema) (very rare)
- familial Mediterranean fever (rare).

Pleural biopsy (see p. 852) may be necessary if the diagnosis has not been established by simple aspiration.

Treatment is of the underlying condition unless there is an empyema which requires drainage in its own right.

Management of malignant pleural effusions

Malignant pleural effusions that reaccumulate and are symptomatic can be aspirated to dryness followed by the instillation of a sclerosing agent such as tetracycline or bleomycin. Effusions should be drained slowly since rapid shift of the mediastinum causes severe pain and occasionally shock. This treatment produces only temporary relief.

Chylothorax

This is due to the accumulation of lymph in the pleural space, usually resulting from leakage from the thoracic duct following trauma or infiltration by carcinoma.

Empyema

This is the presence of pus in the pleural space and can be a complication of pneumonia (see p. 892).

Pneumothorax

'Pneumothorax' means air in the pleural space. It may be spontaneous or occur as a result of trauma to the chest. Spontaneous pneumothorax usually occurs in young males, the male-to-female ratio being 6 : 1. It is caused by the rupture of a pleural bleb, usually apical, and is thought to be due to congenital defects in the connective tissue of the alveolar walls. Both lungs are affected with equal frequency. Often these patients are tall and thin.

In patients over 40 years of age, the usual cause is underlying COPD. Rarer causes include bronchial asthma, carcinoma, a lung abscess breaking down and leading to bronchopleural fistula, and severe pulmonary fibrosis with cyst formation.

Pneumothorax is localized if the visceral pleura has previously undergone adhesion to the parietal pleura, or generalized if the whole hemithorax contains air. It may be spontaneous or occur as a result of trauma to the chest. Normally the pressure in the pleural space is negative but this is lost once a communication is made with atmospheric pressure; the elastic recoil pressure of the lung then causes it to partially deflate. If the communication between the airways and the pleural space remains (an open pneumothorax), a bronchopleural fistula is created. Once the communication between the lung and the pleural space is obliterated, air will be reabsorbed at a rate of 1.25% of the total radiographic volume of the hemithorax per day. Thus, a 50% collapse of the lung will take about 40 days to reabsorb completely once the pneumothorax is closed.

It has been postulated that a valvular mechanism may develop through which air can be sucked into the pleural space during inspiration but not expelled during expiration. The intrapleural pressure remains positive throughout breathing, the lung deflates further, the mediastinum shifts, and venous return to the heart decreases, with increasing respiratory and cardiac embarrassment. This is called tension pneumothorax and is very rare unless the patient is on positive ventilation.

The usual presenting features are sudden onset of unilateral pleuritic pain or progressively increasing breathlessness. If the pneumothorax enlarges, the patient becomes more breathless and may develop pallor and tachycardia. There may be few physical signs if the pneumothorax is small.

The characteristic features and management are shown in Figure 14.45. The main aim is to get the patient back to active life as soon as possible.

The procedure for simple aspiration is shown in Practical box 14.6.

 Practical box 14.6

Simple aspiration

1. Infiltrate 2% lidocaine (lignocaine) down to the pleura in the second intercostal space in the mid-clavicular line.
2. Push a 3–4 cm 16 French gauge cannula through the pleura.
3. Connect the cannula to a three-way tap and 50 mL syringe.
4. Aspirate up to 2.5 L of air. Stop if resistance to suction is felt or the patient coughs excessively.
5. Repeat chest X-ray (in expiration) in the X-ray department.

FURTHER READING

Miller AC, Harvey JE (1993) Guidelines for the management of spontaneous pneumothorax. *British Medical Journal* **307**: 114–116.
Sahn SA, Heffner JE (2000) Spontaneous pneumothorax. *New England Journal of Medicine* **342**: 868–874.

Disorders of the diaphragm

Diaphragmatic fatigue

The diaphragm can become fatigued if the force of contraction during inspiration exceeds 40% of the force it can develop in a maximal static effort. When this occurs acutely in patients with exacerbations of COPD or cystic fibrosis or in quadriplegics, positive-pressure ventilation is required. Further rehabilitation requires exercises to increase the strength and endurance of the diaphragm by breathing against a resistance for 30 minutes a day.

Unilateral diaphragmatic paralysis

This is common and symptomless. The affected diaphragm is usually elevated and moves paradoxically on inspiration. It can be diagnosed thoroughly when a sniff causes the paralysed diaphragm to rise, the unaffected diaphragm to descend. Causes include:

- surgery
- carcinoma of the bronchus with involvement of the phrenic nerve
- neurological, including poliomyelitis, herpes zoster
- trauma to cervical spine, birth injury, subclavian vein puncture
- infection: tuberculosis, syphilis, pneumonia.

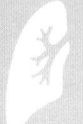
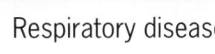

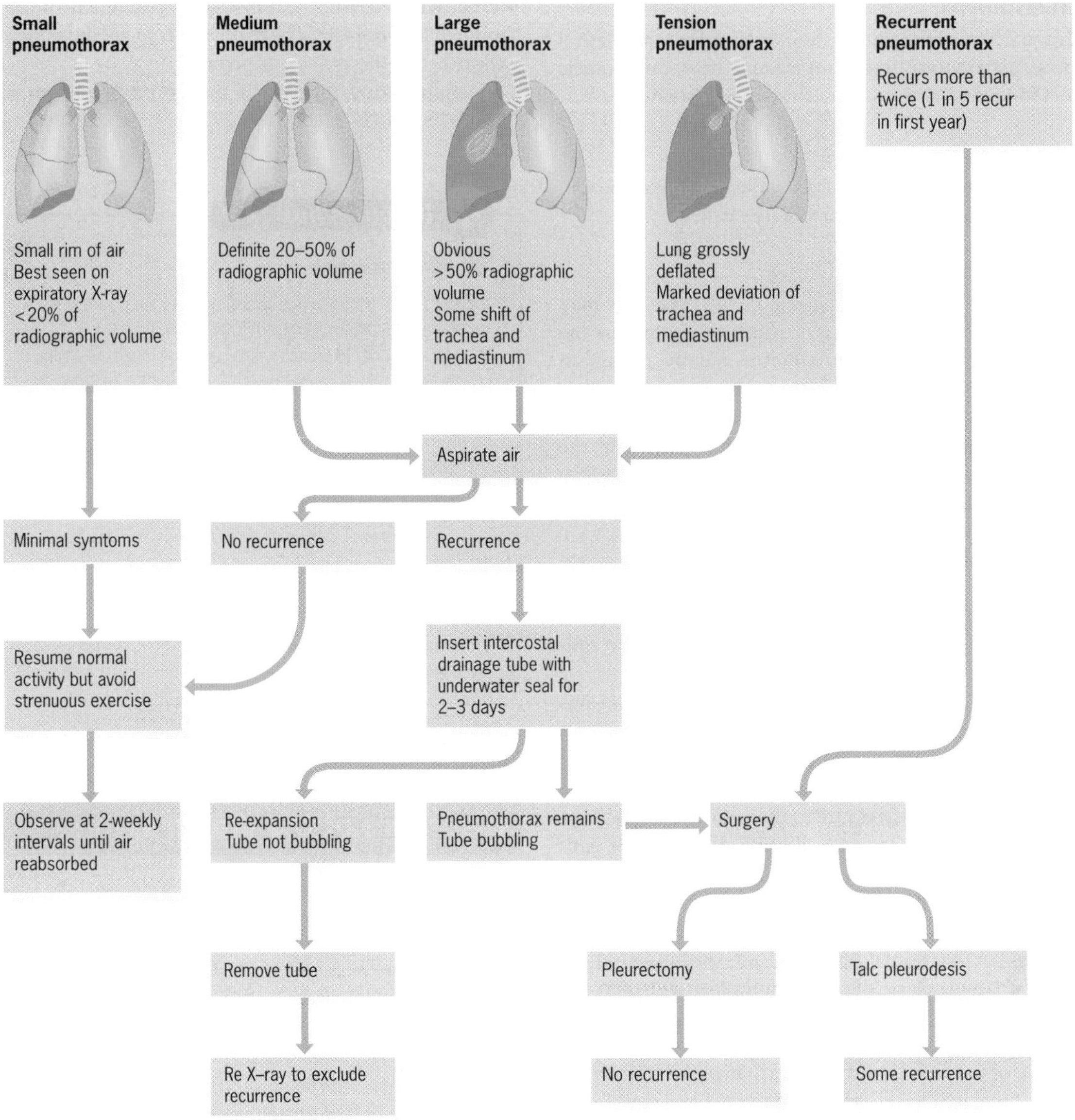

Small pneumothorax

Small rim of air
Best seen on expiratory X-ray
<20% of radiographic volume

Medium pneumothorax

Definite 20–50% of radiographic volume

Large pneumothorax

Obvious >50% radiographic volume
Some shift of trachea and mediastinum

Tension pneumothorax

Lung grossly deflated
Marked deviation of trachea and mediastinum

Recurrent pneumothorax

Recurs more than twice (1 in 5 recur in first year)

Aspirate air

Minimal symtoms

No recurrence

Recurrence

Resume normal activity but avoid strenuous exercise

Insert intercostal drainage tube with underwater seal for 2–3 days

Observe at 2-weekly intervals until air reabsorbed

Re-expansion
Tube not bubbling

Pneumothorax remains
Tube bubbling

Surgery

Remove tube

Pleurectomy

Talc pleurodesis

Re X–ray to exclude recurrence

No recurrence

Some recurrence

Fig. 14.45 Pneumothorax: an algorithm for management.

Bilateral diaphragmatic weakness or paralysis

This causes breathlessness in the supine position and is a cause of sleep apnoea leading to daytime headaches and somnolence. Tidal volume is decreased and respiratory rate increased. Vital capacity is substantially reduced when lying down, and sniffing causes a paradoxical inward movement of the abdominal wall best seen in the supine position. Causes include viral infections, multiple sclerosis, motor neurone disease, poliomyelitis, Guillain–Barré syndrome, quadriplegia after trauma, and rare muscle diseases. Treatment is either diaphragmatic pacing or night-time assisted ventilation.

Complete eventration of the diaphragm

This is a congenital condition (invariably left-sided) in which muscle is replaced by fibrous tissue. It presents as marked elevation of the left hemidiaphragm, sometimes associated with gastrointestinal symptoms. Partial eventration, usually on the right, causes a hump (often anteriorly) on the diaphragmatic shadow on X-ray.

Diaphragmatic hernias

These are most commonly through the oesophageal hiatus, but occasionally occur anteriorly, through the foramen of Morgagni, posterolaterally through the foramen of Bochdalek, or at any site following traumatic tears.

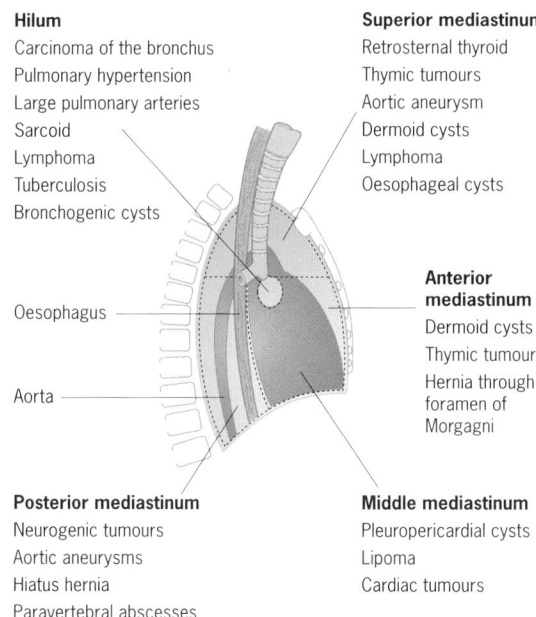

Hilum	Superior mediastinum
Carcinoma of the bronchus	Retrosternal thyroid
Pulmonary hypertension	Thymic tumours
Large pulmonary arteries	Aortic aneurysm
Sarcoid	Dermoid cysts
Lymphoma	Lymphoma
Tuberculosis	Oesophageal cysts
Bronchogenic cysts	

Oesophagus

Anterior mediastinum
Dermoid cysts
Thymic tumours
Hernia through foramen of Morgagni

Aorta

Posterior mediastinum	Middle mediastinum
Neurogenic tumours	Pleuropericardial cysts
Aortic aneurysms	Lipoma
Hiatus hernia	Cardiac tumours
Paravertebral abscesses	

Fig. 14.46 Subdivisions of the mediastinum and mass lesions.

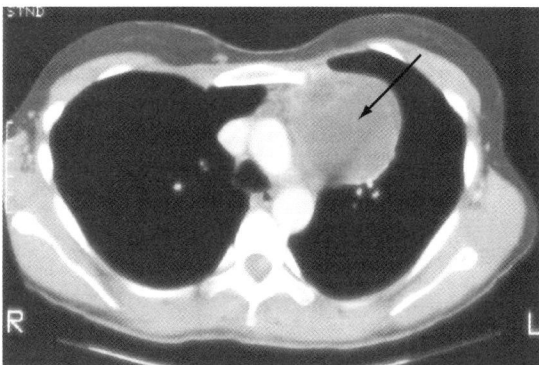

Fig. 14.47 CT scan of a dermoid cyst in the mediastinum.

Hiccups

Hiccups are due to involuntary diaphragmatic contractions with closure of the glottis and are extremely common. Occasionally patients present with persistent hiccups. This can be as a result of diaphragmatic irritation (e.g. subphrenic abscess) or a metabolic cause (e.g. uraemia). Treatment for persistent hiccups is with chlorpromazine 50 mg three times daily, or diazepam 5 mg three times daily. The cause should be treated, if known.

Mediastinal lesions

The mediastinum is defined as the region between the pleural sacs. It is additionally divided as shown in Figure 14.46. Tumours affecting the mediastinum are rare. Masses are detected very accurately on CT scan (Fig. 14.47).

Retrosternal or intrathoracic thyroid

The most common mediastinal tumour is a retrosternal or intrathoracic thyroid, which is nearly always an extension of the thyroid present in the neck. Enlargement of the thyroid by a colloid goitre or malignant disease and, rarely, in thyrotoxicosis causes displacement of the trachea and oesophagus to the opposite side. Symptoms of compression develop insidiously before producing the cardinal feature of dyspnoea. Very occasionally an intrathoracic thyroid may be the cause of dysphagia and, rarely, of hoarseness of the voice and vocal cord paralysis from stretching of the recurrent laryngeal nerve. The treatment is surgical removal.

Thymic tumours

The thymus is large in childhood and occupies the superior and anterior mediastinum. It involutes with age but may be enlarged by cysts, which are rarely symptomatic, or by tumours, which may cause myasthenia gravis or may lead to compression of the trachea or, rarely, the oesophagus. Surgery is the treatment of choice. Approximately half of the patients presenting with a thymic tumour have myasthenia gravis.

Pleuropericardial cysts

These cysts, which may be up to 10 cm in diameter, are filled with clear fluid and are usually situated anteriorly in the cardiophrenic angle on the right in 70% of cases. Infection only rarely occurs; malignant change does not occur. The diagnosis is usually made by needle aspiration. No treatment is required, but these patients should be followed up as an increase in cyst size suggests an alternative pathology; surgical excision is then advisable.

FURTHER READING

Cibella F et al. (1997) Evaluation of diaphragmatic fatigue in obstructive sleep apnoea during non-REM sleep. *Thorax* **52**: 731–735.

Karamanoukian HL et al. (1997) Congenital diaphragmatic hernia. *Thorax* **52**: 209–212.

Intensive care medicine

Intensive care medicine (or 'critical care medicine') is concerned predominantly with the management of patients with acute life-threatening conditions ('the critically ill') in specialized units. As well as emergency cases, such units admit high-risk patients electively after major surgery (Table 15.1). Intensive care medicine also encompasses the resuscitation and transport of those who become acutely ill, or are injured, either elsewhere in the hospital (e.g. in coronary care units, acute admissions wards, postoperative recovery areas, or accident and emergency units) or in the community. The value of extending the responsibilities of the intensive care team to encompass the management of seriously ill patients throughout the hospital, including critically ill patients who have been discharged to the ward ('outreach care') is now widely accepted. Teamwork and a multidisciplinary approach are central to the provision of intensive care and are most effective when directed and coordinated by committed specialists. Guidance for involving the critical care team is shown in Box 15.1.

Intensive care units (ICUs) are usually reserved for patients with established or potential organ failure and must therefore provide facilities for the diagnosis, prevention and treatment of multiple organ failure. They

Table 15.1
Some common indications for admission to intensive care

Surgical emergencies	Medical emergencies
Acute intra-abdominal catastrophe	*Respiratory failure*
Ruptured/leaking abdominal aortic aneurysm	Exacerbation of chronic obstructive pulmonary disease (COPD)
Perforated viscus, especially with faecal soiling of peritoneum (often complicated by septic shock)	Acute severe asthma
	Severe pneumonia (may be complicated by septic shock)
Trauma (often complicated by hypovolaemic and later septic shock)	Meningococcal infection
Multiple injuries	Status epilepticus
Massive blood loss	Severe diabetic ketoacidosis
Severe head injury	Coma
Obstetric emergencies	**Elective surgical**
Severe pre-eclampsia/eclampsia	Extensive/prolonged procedure, e.g. oesophagogastrectomy
Amniotic fluid embolism	Cardiothoracic surgery
	Major head and neck surgery
	Coexisting cardiovascular or respiratory disease

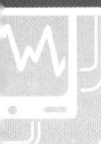

Box 15.1

Guidance for involving a Medical Emergency or 'Patient at Risk' team

(Modified from Lee A et al. (1995) The medical emergency team. *Anaesthesia and Intensive Care* 23: 188–186)

This system should be activated if the following criteria are fulfilled and the patient is being actively treated:

- Heart rate below 40 b.p.m.
- Heart rate above 120 b.p.m.
- Systolic blood pressure above 200 mmHg
- Systolic blood pressure below 80 mmHg
- Urine output less than 0.5 mL/kg/h for 2 consecutive hours
- Respiratory rate above 30 breaths per minute
- Respiratory rate below 8 breaths per minute
- Oxygen saturation less than 90% whilst receiving supplemental oxygen
- Glasgow coma score less than 8
- Core temperature greater than 39°C
- Core temperature less than 35°C.

FURTHER READING

Lyons RA, Wareham K, Hutchings HA, Major E, Ferguson B (2000) Population requirement for adult critical care beds: a prospective quantitative and qualitative study. *Lancet* 355: 595–598.

McQuillan P, Pilkington S, Allan A, Taylor B, Short A, Morgan G, Nielsen M, Bennett D, Smith C (1998) Confidential inquiry into quality of care before admission to intensive care. *British Journal of Medicine* 316: 1853–1858.

Vincent JL, Burchardi H (1999) Do we need intermediate care units? *Intensive Care Medicine* 25: 1345–1349.

General aspects of intensive care management

Critically ill patients require multidisciplinary care with:

- Intensive skilled nursing care (usually 1:1 nurse/patient ratio).
- Regular physiotherapy.
- Careful management of pain and distress with analgesics and sedation as necessary.
- Constant reassurance and support (critically ill patients easily become disorientated and psychologically disturbed).
- Nutritional support (enteral nutrition should always be used if possible). Recent laboratory studies have shown various nutrients to have positive immunomodulatory effects (immunonutrition) including glutamine, polyunsaturated fatty acids and arginine. Confirmatory randomized studies are awaited. Growth hormone should not be used.
- H_2-receptor antagonists in selected cases to prevent stress-induced ulceration.
- TED stockings and subcutaneous heparin to prevent venous thrombosis.
- Care of the mouth, prevention of constipation and of pressure sores.

are fully equipped with monitoring and technical facilities, including an adjacent laboratory (or 'near patient testing' devices) for the rapid determination of blood gases and simple biochemical data such as serum potassium, blood glucose and blood lactate levels. Patients can receive continuous expert nursing care and the constant attention of appropriately trained medical staff. High dependency units (HDUs) offer a level of care intermediate between that available on the general ward and that provided in an ICU. They provide monitoring and support for patients at risk of developing organ failure, including facilities for short-term ventilatory support and immediate resuscitation. They can also provide a 'step-down' facility for patients being discharged from intensive care (sometimes called a 'progressive care unit').

The provision of staff and the level of technical support must match the needs of the individual patient and resources are used more efficiently when they are combined in a single critical care facility rather than being divided between physically and managerially separate units.

In the UK about 1–2% of the acute beds in a hospital are usually allocated to intensive care, but elsewhere in the developed world the proportion is often much higher. Recent estimates in the UK suggest that to meet the needs of a population of 500 000 requires 30 intensive care and 55 high dependency beds in a single critical care area. These numbers increase to 48 and 81 respectively if resources are divided among three separate critical care areas.

In many critically ill patients the underlying diagnosis is initially unclear, but in all cases the immediate objective is to preserve life and prevent, reverse or minimize damage to vital organs such as the liver and kidneys. This involves a rapid assessment of the physiological derangement followed by prompt institution of measures to support cardiovascular and respiratory function in order to restore perfusion of vital organs, improve delivery of oxygen to the tissues and encourage the removal of carbon dioxide and other waste products of metabolism. The patient's condition and response to treatment should be closely monitored throughout. The underlying diagnosis can then be established later as the results of investigations become available, a more detailed history is obtained and a more thorough physical examination is performed.

Discharge of patients from intensive care should normally be planned in advance and should ideally take place during normal working hours. Planned discharge may involve a period in a 'step-down' area. Premature or unplanned discharge, especially during the night, has been associated with higher hospital mortality rates. A summary including 'points to review' should be included in the clinical notes and there should be a detailed handover to the receiving team (medical and nursing). The intensive care team should continue to review the patient, who may deteriorate following discharge, on the ward and should be available at all times for advice on further management (e.g. tracheostomy care, nutritional support). In this way deterioration and re-admission to intensive care (which is associated with a particularly poor outcome) or even cardiorespiratory arrest may be avoided.

This chapter concentrates on cardiovascular and respiratory problems. Many patients also have failure of other organs such as the kidney and liver; treatment of these is dealt with in more detail in the appropriate chapters.

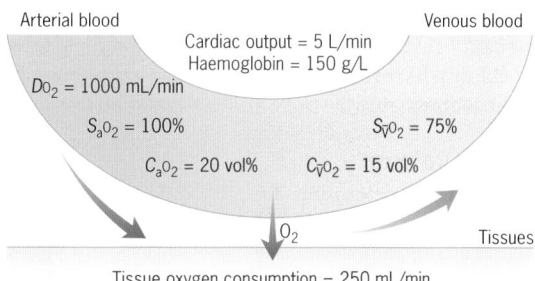

Fig. 15.1 **Tissue oxygen delivery and consumption.** Oxygen delivery (Do_2) = cardiac output × (haemoglobin concentration × oxygen saturation (S_aO_2) × 1.34). In normal adults it is roughly 1000 mL/min, of which 250 mL is taken up by tissues. Mixed venous blood is thus 75% saturated with oxygen. $C_{\bar{v}}O_2$, mixed venous oxygen content; $S_{\bar{v}}O_2$, mixed venous oxygen saturation. From Singer M, Grant I (eds) (1999) *ABC of Intensive Care*. London: BMJ Books, with permission.

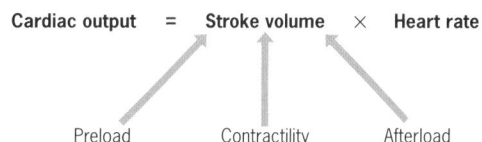

Fig. 15.2 **The determinants of cardiac output.**

FURTHER READING

Cook D, Guyatt G, Marshall J et al. (1998) A comparison of sucralfate and ranitidine for the prevention of upper gastrointestinal bleeding in patients requiring mechanical ventilation. *New England Journal of Medicine* **338**: 791–797.

Goldfrad C, Rowan K (2000) Consequences of discharges from intensive care at night. *Lancet* **335**: 1138–1142.

Jolliet P, Pichard C (1999) Immunonutrition in the critically ill. *Intensive Care Medicine* **25**: 631–633.

Applied cardiorespiratory physiology

Oxygen delivery and consumption (Fig. 15.1)

Oxygen delivery (oxygen dispatch) is defined as the total amount of oxygen delivered to the tissues per unit time. It is dependent on the volume of blood flowing through the microcirculation per minute (i.e. the total cardiac output, $\dot{Q}_t$) and the amount of oxygen contained in that blood (i.e. the arterial oxygen content, C_aO_2). Oxygen is transported both in combination with haemoglobin and dissolved in plasma. The amount combined with haemoglobin is determined by the oxygen capacity of the haemoglobin (usually taken as 1.34 mL of oxygen per gram of haemoglobin) and its percentage saturation with oxygen (So_2), while the volume dissolved in plasma depends on the partial pressure of oxygen (Po_2). Except when hyperbaric oxygen is administered, the amount of dissolved oxygen in plasma is insignificant.

Clinically, however, the utility of this global concept of oxygen dispatch is limited because it fails to account for changes in the relative flow to individual organs and its distribution through the microcirculation (i.e. the efficiency with which oxygen delivery is matched to the metabolic requirements of individual tissues or cells). Furthermore, some organs (such as the heart) have high oxygen requirements relative to their blood flow and may become hypoxic even if the overall oxygen delivery is apparently adequate.

Cardiac output

Cardiac output is the product of heart rate and stroke volume, and is affected by changes in either (Fig. 15.2).

Heart rate

When heart rate increases, the duration of systole remains essentially unchanged, whereas diastole, and thus the time available for ventricular filling, becomes progressively shorter, and the stroke volume eventually falls. In the normal heart this occurs at rates greater than about 160 beats per minute, but in those with cardiac pathology, especially when this restricts ventricular filling (e.g. mitral stenosis), stroke volume may fall at much lower heart rates. Furthermore, tachycardias cause a marked increase in myocardial oxygen consumption ($\dot{V}_mO_2$) and this may precipitate ischaemia in areas of the myocardium that have reduced coronary perfusion. When the heart rate falls, a point is reached at which the increase in stroke volume is insufficient to compensate for bradycardia and again cardiac output falls.

Alterations in heart rate are often caused by disturbances of rhythm (e.g. atrial fibrillation, complete heart block) in which ventricular filling is not augmented by atrial contraction and stroke volume therefore falls.

Stroke volume

Three factors determine the stroke volume: preload, myocardial contractility and afterload (see p. 702).

Preload

This is defined as the tension of the myocardial fibres at the end of diastole, just before the onset of ventricular contraction, and is therefore related to the degree of stretch of the fibres. As the end-diastolic volume of the ventricle increases, tension in the myocardial fibres is increased and stroke volume rises (Fig. 15.3). $\dot{V}_mO_2$ increases only slightly with an increase in preload and this is therefore the most efficient way of improving cardiac output.

Myocardial contractility

This refers to the ability of the heart to perform work, independent of changes in preload and afterload. The state of myocardial contractility determines the response of the ventricles to changes in preload and afterload. Contractility is often reduced in intensive care patients, as a result of either pre-existing myocardial damage (e.g. ischaemic heart disease), or the acute disease process itself (e.g. sepsis). Changes in myocardial contractility alter the slope and position of the Starling curve; the resulting worsening ventricular performance is manifested as a depressed, flattened curve (Fig. 15.3).

Afterload

This is defined as the myocardial wall tension developed during systolic ejection. In the case of the left ventricle, the resistance imposed by the aortic valve, the peripheral vascular resistance and the elasticity of the major blood vessels are important determinants of afterload. Ventricular wall tension will also be increased by ventricular dilatation, an increase in intraventricular pressure or a reduction in ventricular wall thickness.

Decreasing the afterload can increase the stroke volume achieved at a given preload (Fig. 15.4), whilst reducing $\dot{V}_mO_2$. The reduction in wall tension may also lead to an increase in coronary blood flow, thereby improving the myocardial oxygen supply/demand ratio. Excessive reductions in afterload will cause hypotension.

Increasing the afterload, on the other hand, can cause a fall in stroke volume and is a potent cause of increased $\dot{V}_mO_2$. Right ventricular afterload is normally negligible because the resistance of the pulmonary circulation is very low.

Oxygenation of the blood

Oxyhaemoglobin dissociation curve

The saturation of haemoglobin with oxygen is determined by the partial pressure of oxygen (PO_2) in the blood, the relationship between the two being described by the oxyhaemoglobin dissociation curve (Fig. 15.5). The sigmoid shape of this curve is important clinically for a number of reasons:

- Modest falls in the partial pressure of oxygen in the arterial blood (P_aO_2) may be tolerated (since oxygen content is relatively unaffected) provided that the percentage saturation remains above 90%.
- Increasing the P_aO_2 to above normal has only a minimal effect on oxygen content unless hyberbaric oxygen is administered (when the amount of oxygen in solution in plasma becomes significant).
- Once on the steep 'slippery slope' of the curve (percentage saturation below about 90%), a small decrease in P_aO_2 can cause large falls in oxygen content, while increasing P_aO_2 only slightly, e.g. by administering 28% oxygen to a patient with chronic obstructive pulmonary disease (COPD), can lead to a useful increase in oxygen saturation and content.

The P_aO_2 is in turn influenced by the alveolar oxygen tension (P_AO_2), the efficiency of pulmonary gas exchange, and the partial pressure of oxygen in mixed venous blood ($P_{\bar{v}}O_2$).

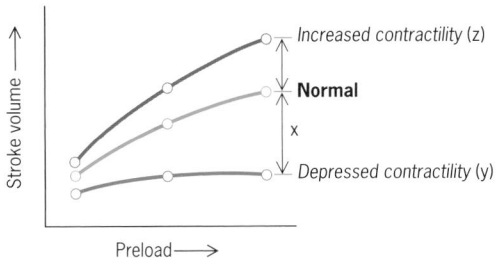

Fig. 15.3 Ventricular function (Starling curve). As the preload is increased, the stroke volume rises. If the ventricle is overstretched, the stroke volume will fall (x). In myocardial failure, the curve is depressed and flattened (y). Increasing contractility shifts the curve upwards and to the left (z).

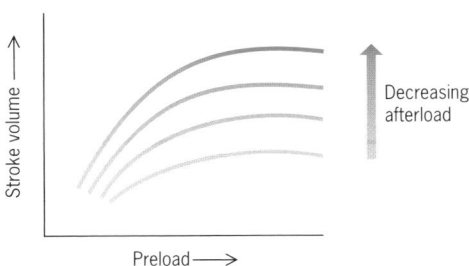

Fig. 15.4 The effect of changes in afterload on the ventricular function curve. At any given preload, decreasing afterload increases the stroke volume.

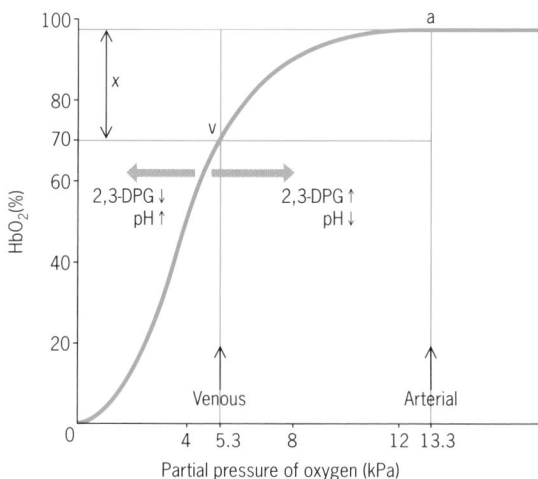

Fig. 15.5 The oxyhaemoglobin dissociation curve: a, arterial point; v, venous point; x, arteriovenous oxygen content difference. HbO_2 is the oxygen saturation of haemoglobin. The curve will move to the right in the presence of acidosis (metabolic or respiratory), pyrexia or an increased red cell 2,3-DPG concentration. For a given arteriovenous oxygen content difference, the mixed venous Po_2 will then be higher. Furthermore, if the mixed venous Po_2 is unchanged, the arteriovenous oxygen content difference increases and more oxygen is offloaded to the tissues (see p. 409).

Alveolar oxygen tension (P_AO_2)

The partial pressures of inspired gases are shown in Figure 15.6. By the time the inspired gases reach the alveoli they are fully saturated with water vapour at body temperature (37°C), which has a partial pressure of 6.3 kPa (47 mmHg), and contain CO_2 at a partial pressure of approximately 5.3 kPa (40 mmHg). The P_AO_2 is thereby reduced to approximately 13.4 kPa (100 mmHg).

The clinician can influence P_AO_2 by administering oxygen or by increasing the barometric pressure. Because of the reciprocal relationship between the partial pressures of oxygen and carbon dioxide in the alveoli, a small increase in P_aO_2 can be produced by lowering the P_ACO_2 (e.g. by using mechanical ventilation).

Pulmonary gas exchange

In *normal* subjects there is a small alveolar–arterial oxygen difference ($P_{A–a}O_2$). This is due to:

- a small (0.133 kPa, 1 mmHg) pressure gradient across the alveolar membrane
- a small amount of blood (2% of total cardiac output) bypassing the lungs via the bronchial and thebesian veins
- a small ventilation/perfusion mismatch.

Pathologically there are three causes of an increased $P_{A–a}O_2$ difference, as follows:

Diffusion defect

This is not a major cause of hypoxaemia even in conditions such as fibrosing alveolitis, in which the

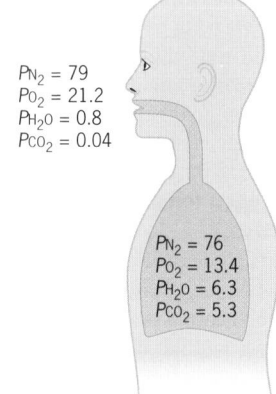

Fig. 15.6 The partial pressures of inspired and alveolar gas: values given in kiloPascals.

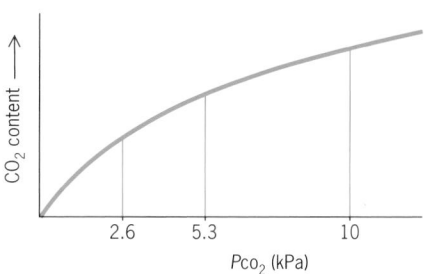

Fig. 15.7 The carbon dioxide dissociation curve. Note that in the physiological range the curve is essentially linear.

alveolar–capillary membrane is considerably thickened. Certainly carbon dioxide is not affected, as it is more soluble than oxygen.

Right-to-left shunts

In certain congenital cardiac lesions, such as Fallot's tetralogy and when a segment of lung is completely unventilated, a considerable amount of blood bypasses the lungs and causes arterial hypoxaemia. This hypoxaemia cannot be corrected by administering oxygen to increase the P_AO_2, because blood leaving normal alveoli is already fully saturated and further increases in Po_2 will not significantly affect its oxygen content. On the other hand, because of the shape of the carbon dioxide dissociation curve (Fig. 15.7), the high Pco_2 of the shunted blood can be compensated for by overventilating patent alveoli, thus lowering the CO_2 content of the effluent blood. Indeed, many patients with acute right-to-left shunts hyperventilate in response to the hypoxia or stimulation of mechanoreceptors in the lung, so that the P_aCO_2 is normal or low.

Ventilation/perfusion mismatch (see Ch. 14)

Diseases of the lung parenchyma result in $\dot{V}/\dot{Q}$ mismatch, producing an increase in alveolar deadspace and hypoxaemia. The increased deadspace can be compensated by increasing overall ventilation. In contrast to the hypoxia resulting from a true right-to-left shunt, that due to areas of low $\dot{V}/\dot{Q}$ can be partially corrected by administering oxygen and thereby increasing the $P_{A}O_2$ even in poorly ventilated areas of lung.

Mixed venous oxygen tension ($P_{\bar{v}}O_2$) and saturation ($S_{\bar{v}}O_2$)

The $P_{\bar{v}}O_2$ is the partial pressure of oxygen in pulmonary arterial blood that has been thoroughly mixed during its passage through the heart. Assuming $P_{a}O_2$ remains constant, $P_{\bar{v}}O_2$ and $S_{\bar{v}}O_2$ will fall if more oxygen has to be extracted from each unit volume of blood arriving at the tissues. A low $P_{\bar{v}}O_2$ therefore indicates either that oxygen delivery has fallen or that tissue oxygen requirements have increased without a compensatory rise in cardiac output. If $P_{\bar{v}}O_2$ falls, the effect of a given degree of pulmonary shunting on arterial oxygenation will be exacerbated. Thus, worsening arterial hypoxaemia does not necessarily indicate a deterioration in pulmonary function but may instead reflect a fall in cardiac output and/or a rise in oxygen consumption.

Conversely a rise in $P_{\bar{v}}O_2$ and $S_{\bar{v}}O_2$ may reflect impaired tissue oxygen extraction (due to microcirculatory dysfunction) and/or a reduced oxygen uptake/consumption (due, for example, to a mitochondrial defect) as is seen in severe sepsis (see below).

Disturbances of acid–base balance

The physiology of acid–base control is discussed on page 689. Acid–base disturbances can be described in relation to the diagram illustrated in Figure 12.13 which shows $P_{a}CO_2$ plotted against arterial [H$^+$].

Both acidosis and alkalosis can occur, each of which may be either metabolic (primarily affecting the bicarbonate component of the system) or respiratory (primarily affecting $P_{a}CO_2$). Compensatory changes may also be apparent. In clinical practice, arterial [H$^+$] values outside the range 18–126 nmol/L (pH 6.9–7.7) are very rarely encountered.

Blood gas and acid–base values (normal ranges) are shown in Table 15.2. Blood gas analysis see p. 945.

Table 15.2
Arterial blood gas and acid–base values (normal ranges)

H$^+$	35–45 nmol/L	pH 7.35–7.45
P_{O_2}	10–13.3 kPa	(75–100 mmHg)
P_{CO_2}	4.8–6.1 kPa	(36–46 mmHg)
Base deficit	± 2.5	
Plasma HCO$_3^-$	22–26 mmol/L	
O$_2$ saturation	95–100%	

Respiratory acidosis. This is caused by retention of carbon dioxide. The $P_{a}CO_2$ and [H$^+$] rise. A chronically raised $P_{a}CO_2$ is compensated by renal retention of bicarbonate and the [H$^+$] returns towards normal. A constant arterial bicarbonate concentration is then usually established within 5 days. This represents a primary respiratory acidosis with a compensatory metabolic alkalosis (see p. 696). Common causes of respiratory acidosis include ventilatory failure and COPD (type II respiratory failure where there is a high $P_{a}CO_2$ and a low $P_{a}O_2$ – see Ch. 14).

Respiratory alkalosis. In this case the reverse occurs and there is a fall in $P_{a}CO_2$ and [H$^+$], often with a small reduction in bicarbonate concentration. If hypocarbia persists, some degree of renal compensation may occur, producing a metabolic acidosis, although in practice this is unusual. A respiratory alkalosis is often produced, intentionally or unintentionally, when patients are mechanically ventilated; it may also be seen with hypoxaemic (type I) respiratory failure (see Ch. 14), spontaneous hyperventilation and in those living at high altitudes.

Metabolic acidosis (p. 693). This may be due to excessive acid production, most commonly lactate and H$^+$ (lactic acidosis) as a consequence of anaerobic metabolism during an episode of shock or following cardiac arrest. A metabolic acidosis may also develop in chronic renal failure or in diabetic ketoacidosis. It can also follow the loss of bicarbonate from the gut, for example, or from the kidney in renal tubular acidosis. Respiratory compensation for a metabolic acidosis is usually slightly delayed because the blood–brain barrier initially prevents the respiratory centre from sensing the increased blood [H$^+$]. Following this short delay, however, the patient hyperventilates and 'blows off' carbon dioxide to produce a compensatory respiratory alkalosis. There is a limit to this respiratory compensation, since in practice values for $P_{a}CO_2$ less than about 1.4 kPa (11 mmHg) are never achieved. It should also be noted that respiratory compensation cannot occur if the patient's ventilation is controlled or if the respiratory centre is depressed, for example by drugs or head injury.

Metabolic alkalosis. This can be caused by loss of acid, for example from the stomach with nasogastric suction, or in high intestinal obstruction, or excessive administration of absorbable alkali. Overzealous treatment with intravenous sodium bicarbonate is implicated. Respiratory compensation for a metabolic alkalosis is often slight, and it is rare to encounter a $P_{a}CO_2$ above 6.5 kPa (50 mmHg), even with severe alkalosis.

Shock and acute disturbances of haemodynamic function

Shock is difficult to define. The term is used to describe acute circulatory failure with inadequate or

Table 15.3
Causes of shock

Hypovolaemic	Obstructive
Exogenous losses (e.g. haemorrhage, burns)	Obstruction to outflow (e.g. pulmonary embolus)
Endogenous losses	Restricted cardiac filling (e.g. cardiac tamponade, tension pneumothorax)
Cardiogenic (e.g. ischaemic cardiac damage)	
	Distributive (e.g. sepsis, anaphylaxis)
	Vascular dilatation
	Sequestration
	Arteriovenous shunting
	Maldistribution of flow
	Myocardial depression

inappropriately distributed tissue perfusion resulting in generalized cellular hypoxia.

Causes of shock

The causes of shock are shown in Table 15.3. Often shock can result from a combination of these factors (e.g. in sepsis, distributive shock is frequently complicated by hypovolaemia and myocardial depression).

Pathophysiology

The sympatho-adrenal response to shock

(Fig. 15.8)
Hypotension stimulates the baroreceptors, and to a lesser extent the chemoreceptors, causing increased sympathetic nervous activity. Later this is augmented by the release of catecholamines from the adrenal medulla. The resulting vasoconstriction, together with increased myocardial contractility and heart rate, help to restore blood pressure and cardiac output. Reduction in perfusion of the renal cortex stimulates the juxtaglomerular apparatus to release renin. This converts angiotensinogen to angiotensin I, which is in turn converted in the lungs and by the vascular endothelium to the potent vasoconstrictor angiotensin II. Angiotensin II then stimulates secretion of aldosterone by the adrenal cortex, causing sodium and water retention (p. 1064). This helps to restore the circulating volume (see p. 669).

Neuroendocrine response

- There is *release of pituitary hormones* such as adrenocorticotrophic hormone (ACTH), vasopressin (antidiuretic hormone, ADH) and endogenous opioid peptides.
- There is *release of cortisol* which causes fluid retention and antagonizes insulin.
- There is *release of glucagon* which raises the blood sugar level.

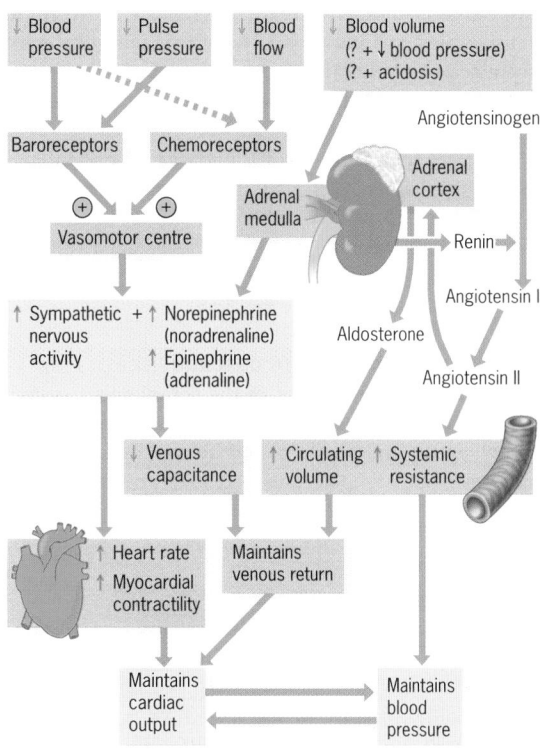

Fig. 15.8 The sympatho-adrenal response to shock.

Release of pro- and anti-inflammatory mediators (see also Ch. 4)

The presence of severe infection (often with bacteraemia or endotoxaemia) or of large areas of damaged tissue (e.g. following trauma or major surgery) can trigger a massive inflammatory response with systemic activation of leucocytes and release of a variety of potentially damaging 'mediators'. Although beneficial when targeted against local areas of infection or necrotic tissue, dissemination of this response can produce shock and widespread tissue damage.

Microorganisms and their toxic products

In sepsis/septic shock the inflammatory cascade is triggered by the presence in the bloodstream of microorganisms, their cell wall components (e.g. endotoxin) and/or exotoxins (antigenic proteins produced by bacteria such as staphylococci, streptococci and pseudomonas). Endotoxin is a lipopolysaccharide (LPS) derived from the cell wall of Gram-negative bacteria which is a potent trigger of the inflammatory response. The lipid A portion of LPS can be bound by a protein normally present in human serum known as lipopolysaccharide binding protein (LBP). The LBP/LPS complex attaches to the cell surface marker CD14, this complex then binds to toll-like receptors (TLRs) which transduce the signal

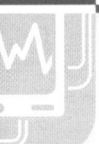

into the cell. Another recently described mechanism in this complex area involves TREM-I (triggering receptor expressed in myeloid cells) (see p. 198). Specific kinases then phosphorylate IκB, releasing the nuclear transcription factor NFκB which passes into the nucleus where it promotes the synthesis of a wide variety of inflammatory mediators. Cell wall components from Gram-positive bacteria, some of which are similar in structure to LPS (e.g. lipoteichoic acid), can also trigger a systemic inflammatory response, probably through similar, but not identical pathways (see Fig. 15.9).

Activation of complement cascade (see p. 195)
One of the many functions of the complement system is to attract and activate leucocytes, which then marginate on to endothelium and release inflammatory mediators such as proteases and toxic free radicals of oxygen and other reactive oxygen and nitrogen species (see below).

Cytokines (see also p. 197)
Proinflammatory cytokines such as the interleukins (ILs) and tumour necrosis factor (TNF) are important mediators of the systemic inflammatory response. TNF-α release initiates many of the responses to endotoxin, for example, and acts synergistically with IL-1, in part through induction of cyclo-oxygenase, platelet-activating factor (PAF) and nitric oxide synthase (see below). The cytokine network is extremely complex, with many endogenous self-regulating mechanisms. For example, naturally occurring soluble TNF receptors are shed from cell surfaces during the inflammatory response, binding to TNF and thereby reducing its biological activity. An endogenous inhibitory protein that binds competitively to the IL-1 receptor has also been identified.

In addition to pro-inflammatory mediators such as TNF, anti-inflammatory cytokines, e.g. IL-10, are released. The ratio of IL-10 to TNF, and of TNF to TNF receptors, has been shown to be related to mortality in severe sepsis/septic shock. When excessive, this compensatory anti-inflammatory response syndrome (CARS) may be associated with an inappropriate immune hyporesponsiveness.

Platelet-activating factor
This vasoactive lipid is released from various cell populations, such as leucocytes and macrophages, in shock. Its effects, which are caused both directly and through the secondary release of other mediators, include hypotension, increased vascular permeability and platelet aggregation.

Products of arachidonic acid metabolism
(see Fig. 14.32)
Arachidonic acid, derived from the breakdown of membrane phospholipid, is metabolized to form prostaglandins and leukotrienes, which are important inflammatory mediators (see p. 192).

Lysosomal enzymes
These can cause myocardial depression and coronary vasoconstriction. Furthermore, lysosomal enzymes can convert inactive kininogens to vasoactive kinins such as bradykinins. These substances cause vasodilatation and increased capillary permeability, as well as myocardial depression. They can also activate clotting mechanisms.

Adhesion molecules (see also p. 192)
Adhesion of activated leucocytes to the vessel wall and their subsequent extravascular migration is a key component of the sequence of events leading to endothelial injury, tissue damage and organ dysfunction. This process is mediated by inducible intercellular adhesion molecules (ICAMs) found on the surface of leucocytes and endothelial cells. Expression of these molecules can be induced by endotoxin and pro-inflammatory cytokines such as IL-1 and TNF-α. Several families of molecules are involved in promoting leucocyte–endothelial interaction. The selectins are 'capture' molecules and initiate the process of leucocyte rolling on vascular endothelium, whilst members of the immunoglobulin superfamily (ICAM-1 and vascular cell adhesion molecule-1) are involved in the formation of a more secure bond which leads to leucocyte migration into the tissues.

Endothelium-derived vasoactive mediators
Endothelial cells synthesize a number of mediators which contribute to the regulation of blood vessel tone and the fluidity of the blood; these include nitric oxide

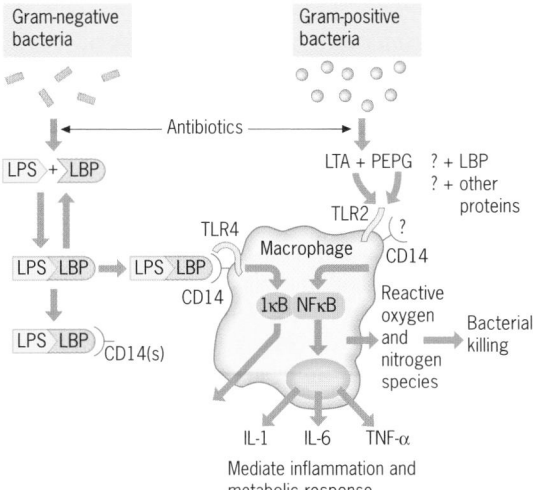

Fig. 15.9 Induction of synthesis of cytokines, free radicals and nitric oxide by bacterial cell wall components. LPS, lipopolysaccharide; LPB, lipopolysaccharide binding protein; LTA, lipoteichoic acid; NFκB, nuclear factor kappa B; IκB inhibitory factor kappa B; PEPG, peptidoglycan-G; TLR, toll-like receptors.

prostacyclin and endothelin-1 (a potent vasoconstrictor). Nitric oxide (NO) is synthesized from the terminal guanidino-nitrogen atoms of the amino acid L-arginine under the influence of nitric oxide synthase (NOS). NO inhibits platelet aggregation and adhesion and produces vasodilatation by activating guanylate cyclase in the underlying vascular smooth muscle to form cyclic guanosine monophosphate (cGMP) from guanosine triphosphate (GTP) (Fig. 15.10). There is evidence for the existence of several distinct NOS enzymes, as listed below.

- **Constitutive or endothelial NOS** (cNOS or eNOS) present in endothelial cells is responsible for the basal release of NO and is involved in the physiological regulation of vascular tone, blood pressure and tissue perfusion.
- **Neuronal NOS** (nNOS). The role of nerves containing nNOS is uncertain but they probably provide neurogenic vasodilator tone. In the central nervous system nNOS may be a regulator of local cerebral blood flow as well as fulfilling a number of other physiological functions, such as the acute modulation of neuronal firing behaviour.
- **Inducible NOS** (iNOS) is induced in vascular endothelial smooth muscle cells and monocytes within 4–18 hours of stimulation with certain cytokines, such as TNF-α, and endotoxin. The resulting prolonged increase in NO formation is believed to be an important cause of the sustained vasodilatation, hypotension and reduced reactivity to adrenergic agonists ('vasoplegia') that characterizes septic shock. This mechanism may also be involved in severe prolonged haemorrhage/traumatic shock. The NO generated by macrophages contributes to their role as highly effective killers of intracellular and extracellular pathogens, in part as a consequence of its ability to bind to cytochrome oxidase and inhibit electron transport, but also via the production of the highly reactive radical peroxynitrite.

Redox imbalance

In health the balance between reducing and oxidizing conditions (redox) is controlled by antioxidants which may either prevent radical formation (e.g. transferrin and lactoferrin which bind iron, a catalyst for radical formation) or remove/inactivate reactive oxygen and nitrogen species (e.g. enzymes such as superoxide dismutases, vitamins C and E, and sulphydryl group donors such as glutathione). There are also mechanisms to remove and repair oxidatively damaged molecules and in particular to preserve DNA integrity. In severe systemic inflammation the uncontrolled production of oxygen-derived free radicals and reactive nitrogen species e.g. superoxide ($O_2^{\cdot-}$), hydroxylradicals ($^{\cdot}OH$), hydrogen peroxide (H_2O_2) and peroxynitrite ($ONOO^-$) particularly by activated polymorphonuclear leucocytes can overwhelm these defensive mechanisms and cause:

- lipid and protein peroxidation
- damage to cell membranes
- increased capillary permeability
- impaired mitochondrial respiration
- DNA strand breakage
- apoptosis (p. 162).

Haemodynamic and microcirculatory changes

In septic shock there is:

- vasodilatation
- maldistribution of regional blood flow
- abnormalities in the microcirculation
  - — arteriovenous shunting
  - — 'stop-flow' capillaries (flow is intermittent)
  - — 'no-flow' capillaries (capillaries are obstructed)
  - — failure of capillary recruitment
  - — increased capillary permeability with interstitial oedema.

Although these *microvascular abnormalities* may partly account for the reduced oxygen extraction often seen in septic shock, there is probably also a *primary defect of cellular oxygen utilization* owing to mitochondrial dysfunction (see above). Initially, before hypovolaemia supervenes, or when therapeutic replacement of circulating volume has been adequate, *cardiac output is usually high and peripheral resistance is low*. These changes are associated with impaired oxygen consumption, a reduced arteriovenous oxygen content difference, an increased $S_{\bar{v}}O_2$ and a lactic acidosis (so-called 'tissue dysoxia'). Vasodilatation and increased permeability also occur in anaphylactic shock.

In the initial stages of other forms of shock, and sometimes when hypovolaemia and myocardial depression

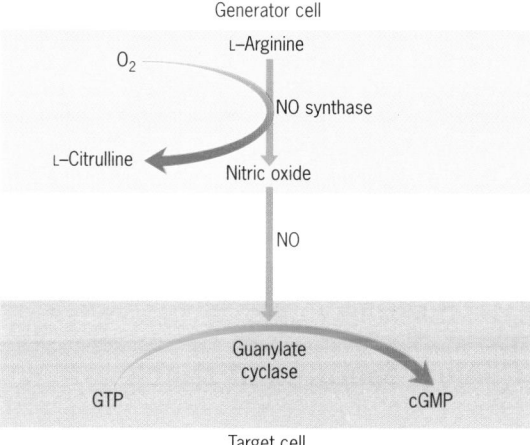

Fig. 15.10 **Synthesis and biochemical action of nitric oxide.**

supervene in sepsis and anaphylaxis, cardiac output is low and increased sympathetic activity causes constriction of both precapillary arterioles and, to a lesser extent, the postcapillary venules. This helps to maintain the systemic blood pressure. In addition, the hydrostatic pressure within the capillaries falls and fluid is mobilized from the extravascular space into the intravascular compartment.

Disseminated intravascular coagulation (DIC)

The inflammatory response to shock, tissue injury and infection is frequently associated with systemic activation of the clotting cascade, leading to platelet aggregation and widespread thrombosis. Plasminogen is converted to plasmin, which breaks down thrombus, liberating fibrin/fibrinogen degradation products (FDPs). Circulating levels of FDPs are therefore increased, the thrombin time, PTT and PT are prolonged and platelet and fibrinogen levels fall. Activation of the coagulation cascade can be confirmed by demonstrating increased plasma levels of 'D' dimers. The development of DIC often heralds the onset of multiple organ failure. Because clotting factors and platelets are consumed in DIC, they are unavailable for haemostasis elsewhere and a coagulation defect results – hence the alternative name for DIC is 'consumption coagulopathy'. In some cases a microangiopathic haemolytic anaemia develops. DIC is particularly associated with septic shock, especially when due to meningococcal infection (see p. 98). Treatment is supportive with infusions of fresh frozen plasma, platelets and occasionally factor VIII concentrates.

Reperfusion injury

Restoration of flow to previously hypoxic tissues can exacerbate cell damage through the generation of large quantities of reactive oxygen species (see above) (Fig. 15.11). The gut mucosa seems to be especially vulnerable to this 'ischaemia-reperfusion injury'.

Metabolic response to trauma, major surgery and severe infection

This is initiated and controlled by the neuroendocrine system and various cytokines (e.g. IL-6) acting in concert, and is characterized by an increase in energy expenditure ('hypermetabolism'). Gluconeogenesis is stimulated by increased glucagon and catecholamine levels, whilst hepatic mobilization of glucose from glycogen is increased. Catecholamines inhibit insulin release and reduce peripheral glucose uptake. Combined with elevated circulating levels of other insulin antagonists such as cortisol, these changes ensure that the majority of patients are hyperglycaemic ('insulin resistance'). Later hypoglycaemia may be precipitated by depletion of hepatic glycogen stores and inhibition of gluconeogenesis. Free fatty acid synthesis is also increased, leading to hypertriglyceridaemia.

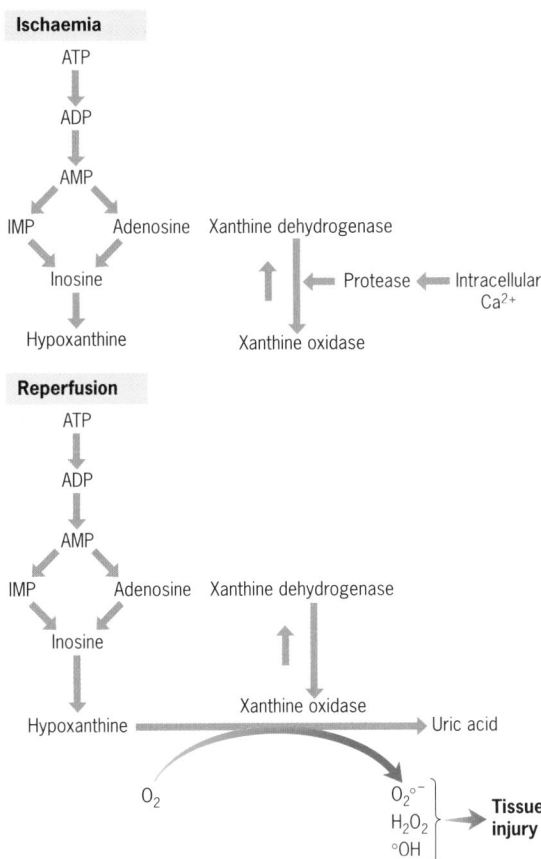

Fig. 15.11 Generation of reactive oxygen species following ischaemia and reperfusion.

Protein breakdown is initiated to provide energy from amino acids, and hepatic protein synthesis is preferentially augmented to produce the 'acute phase reactants' (see p. 194). The amino acid glutamine (which is indispensable in this situation) is mobilized from muscle for use as a metabolic fuel in rapidly dividing cells such as leucocytes and enterocytes. Glutamine is also required for hepatic production of the free radical scavenger glutathione. When severe and prolonged, this catabolic response can lead to considerable weight loss. Protein breakdown is associated with wasting and weakness of skeletal and respiratory muscle, prolonging the need for mechanical ventilation and delaying mobilization. Tissue repair, wound healing and immune function may also be compromised.

Clinical features of shock

Although many clinical features are common to all types of shock, there are certain important respects in which they differ (Box 15.2).

Box 15.2

Haemodynamic changes in shock

Hypovolaemic shock
Low central venous pressure (CVP) and pulmonary artery
   occlusion pressure (PAOP)
Low cardiac output
Increased systemic vascular resistance

Cardiogenic shock
Signs of myocardial failure
Increased systemic vascular resistance
CVP and PAOP high (except when hypovolaemic)

Cardiac tamponade
Parallel increases in CVP and PAOP
Low cardiac output
Increased systemic vascular resistance

Pulmonary embolism
Low cardiac output
High CVP, high pulmonary artery pressure but low PAOP
Increased systemic vascular resistance

Anaphylaxis
Low systemic vascular resistance
Low CVP and PAOP
High cardiac output

Septic shock
Low systemic vascular resistance
Low CVP and PAOP
Cardiac output usually high
Myocardial depression – low ejection fraction
Stroke volume maintained by ventricular dilatation
Cardiac output increased by tachycardia

Hypovolaemic shock
- Inadequate tissue perfusion:
    - (a) Skin – cold, pale, blue, slow capillary refill, 'clammy'
    - (b) Kidneys – oliguria, anuria
    - (c) Brain – drowsiness, confusion and irritability
- Increased sympathetic tone:
    - (a) Tachycardia, narrowed pulse pressure, 'weak pulse'
    - (b) Sweating
    - (c) Blood pressure – may be maintained initially (despite up to a 25% reduction in circulating volume if the patient is young and fit), but later hypotension supervenes
- Metabolic acidosis – compensatory tachypnoea.

Additional clinical features may occur in the following types of shock.

Cardiogenic shock (see p. 765)
Signs of myocardial failure, e.g. raised jugular venous pressure (JVP), pulsus alternans, 'gallop' rhythm, basal crackles, pulmonary oedema.

Obstructive shock
- Elevated JVP
- Pulsus paradoxus and muffled heart sounds in cardiac tamponade
- Signs of pulmonary embolism (see p. 805).

Anaphylactic shock (see p. 961)
- Signs of profound vasodilatation:
    - (a) Warm peripheries
    - (b) Low blood pressure
- Erythema, urticaria, angio-oedema, pallor, cyanosis

- Bronchospasm, rhinitis
- Oedema of the face, pharynx and larynx
- Pulmonary oedema
- Hypovolaemia due to capillary leak
- Nausea, vomiting, abdominal cramps, diarrhoea.

Sepsis, severe sepsis and septic shock
- Pyrexia and rigors, or hypothermia (unusual)
- Nausea, vomiting
- Vasodilatation, warm peripheries
- Bounding pulse
- Rapid capillary refill
- Hypotension (septic shock)
- Occasionally signs of cutaneous vasoconstriction
- Other signs:
    - (a) Jaundice
    - (b) Coma (rare)
    - (c) Bleeding due to coagulopathy (e.g. from vascular puncture sites, GI tract and surgical wounds)
    - (d) Rash and meningism.

The diagnosis of sepsis is easily missed, particularly in the elderly when the classical signs may not be present. Mild confusion, tachycardia and tachypnoea may be the only clues, sometimes associated with unexplained hypotension, a reduction in urine output, a rising plasma creatinine and glucose intolerance.

The clinical signs of sepsis are not always associated with bacteraemia and can occur with non-infectious processes such as pancreatitis or severe trauma. The term 'systemic inflammatory response syndrome' (SIRS) has been suggested to describe the disseminated inflammation that can complicate this diverse range of disorders (Box 15.3). The usefulness of this terminology has, however, been questioned.

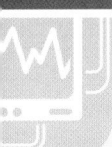

Box 15.3

Terminology used in systemic inflammation and sepsis

Infection

Invasion of normally sterile host tissue by microorganisms

Bacteraemia

Viable bacteria in blood

Systemic inflammatory response syndrome (SIRS)

The systemic inflammatory response to a variety of severe clinical insults. The response is manifested by two or more of the following:

- Temperature $> 38°C$ or $< 36°C$
- Heart rate > 90 beats/min
- Respiratory rate > 20 breaths/min or $P_a co_2 < 4.3$ kPa
- White cell count $> 12 \times 10^9$/L, $< 4 \times 10^9$/L or $> 10\%$ immature forms

Compensatory anti-inflammatory response syndrome (CARS)

Release of anti-inflammatory mediators which downregulate the inflammatory response. If excessive, may lead to inappropriate immune hyperresponsiveness

Sepsis

SIRS resulting from documented infection

Severe sepsis

Sepsis associated with organ dysfunction, hypoperfusion or hypotension. Hypoperfusion and perfusion abnormalities may include, but are not limited to, lactic acidosis, oliguria or an acute alteration in mental state

Septic shock

Severe sepsis with hypotension (systolic BP < 90 mmHg or a reduction of > 40 mmHg from baseline) in the absence of other causes for hypotension and despite adequate fluid resuscitation

(Patients receiving inotropic or vasopressor agents may not be hypotensive when perfusion abnormalities are documented)

Refractory shock

Shock unresponsive to conventional therapy (intravenous fluids and inotropic/vasoactive agents) within 1 hour

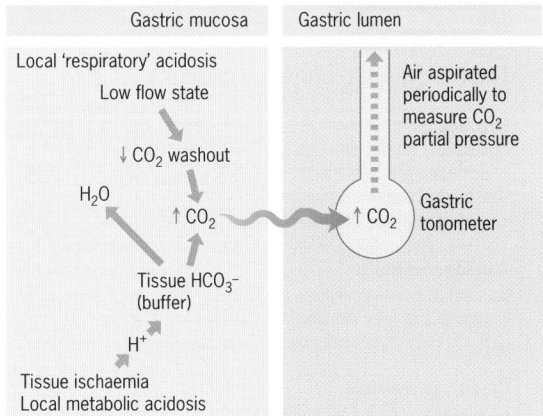

Fig. 15.12 Gastric tonometry. A silastic balloon is passed into the stomach. Equilibration of carbon dioxide partial pressure between mucosa and balloon takes up to 30 minutes. Low flow states and tissue ischaemia are associated with a rise in carbon dioxide partial pressure. From Singer M, Grant I (eds) (1999) *ABC of Intensive Care*. London: BMJ Books, with permission.

Monitoring critically ill patients

Invasive monitoring is associated with a small, but significant, risk of complications and should therefore only be used when the potential benefits outweigh the dangers. Likewise invasive devices should be removed as soon as possible. In general invasive monitoring will be required in the more seriously ill patients and in those who fail to respond to initial treatment. Clinical assessment must never be neglected.

Assessment of tissue perfusion

- *Pale, cold skin*, delayed capillary refill and the absence of visible veins in the hands and feet indicate poor perfusion. (Peripheral skin temperature measurements can help clinical evaluation as vasoconstriction is an early compensatory response.)
- *Urinary flow* is a sensitive indicator of renal perfusion and haemodynamic performance.
- *Metabolic acidosis with raised lactate concentration* may suggest that tissue perfusion is sufficiently compromised to cause cellular hypoxia and anaerobic glycolysis. Persistent, severe lactic acidosis is associated with a very poor prognosis. In many critically ill patients, especially those with sepsis, however, lactic acidosis can also be caused by metabolic disorders unrelated to tissue hypoxia and may be exacerbated by reduced clearance owing to hepatic or renal dysfunction.
- *Gastric tonometry* (Fig. 15.12). The earliest compensatory response to hypovolaemia or a low cardiac output, and the last to resolve after resuscitation is splanchnic vasoconstriction. In sepsis, gut mucosal ischaemia may be precipitated by disturbed microcirculatory flow combined with increased oxygen requirements. Mucosal acidosis is therefore an early sign of shock. Changes in intramucosal pH or $P co_2$ have been suggested as a guide to the adequacy of resuscitation, although the clinical value of this technique is questionable.

Blood pressure

Alterations in blood pressure are often interpreted as reflecting changes in cardiac output. However, if there is vasoconstriction with a high peripheral resistance, the blood pressure may be normal, even when the cardiac output is reduced. Conversely, the vasodilated patient may be hypotensive despite a very high cardiac output.

Radial artery cannulation

Technique

1 The procedure is explained to the patient.

2 The arm is supported, with the wrist extended, by an assistant. (Gloves should be worn)

3 The radial artery is palpated where it arches over the head of the radius.

4 In conscious patients, local anaesthetic is injected to raise a weal over the artery, taking care not to puncture the vessel or obscure its pulsation.

5 A small skin incision is made over the proposed puncture site.

6 A small parallel-sided cannula (20 gauge for adults, 22 gauge for children) is used in order to allow blood flow to continue past the cannula.

7 The cannula is inserted over the point of maximal pulsation and advanced in line with the direction of the vessel at an angle of approximately 30°.

8 'Flashback' of blood into the cannula indicates that the radial artery has been punctured.

9 To ensure that the shoulder of the cannula enters the vessel the needle and cannula are lowered and advanced a few millimetres into the vessel.

10 The cannula is threaded off the needle into the vessel and the needle withdrawn.

11 The cannula is connected to a non-compliant manometer line filled with heparinized saline. This is then connected via a transducer and continuous flush device to a monitor, which records the arterial pressure.

Complications

- Thrombosis
- Loss of arterial pulsation
- Distal ischaemia, e.g. digital necrosis (rare)
- Accidental injection of drugs – can produce vascular occlusion
- Disconnection – rapid blood loss.

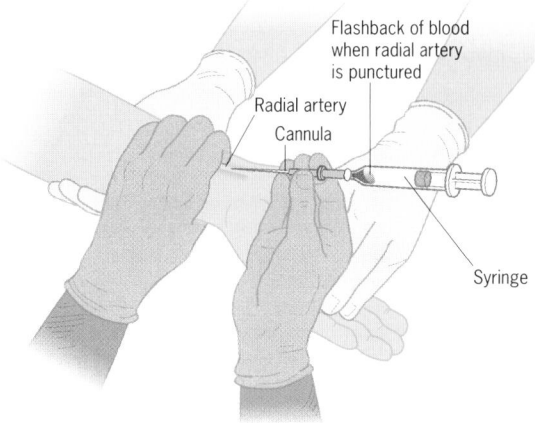

Fig. 15.13 **Cannulation of the radial artery.**

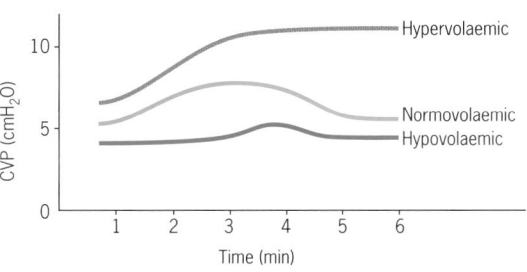

Fig. 15.14 **The effects of rapid administration of a 'fluid challenge' to patients with a central venous pressure within the normal range.** From Sykes MK (1963) Venous pressure as a clinical indication of adequacy of transfusion. *Annals of the Royal College of Surgeons of England* **33**: 185–197.

The absolute level of blood pressure is also important, since hypotension may jeopardize perfusion of vital organs. The adequacy of blood pressure in an individual patient must always be assessed in relation to the premorbid value. Blood pressure is traditionally measured using a sphygmomanometer but if rapid alterations are anticipated, continuous monitoring using an intra-arterial cannula is indicated (Practical box 15.1, Fig. 15.13).

Central venous pressure (CVP)

This provides a fairly simple method of assessing the adequacy of a patient's circulating volume and the contractile state of the myocardium. The absolute value of the CVP is not as important as its response to a fluid challenge (the infusion of 100–200 mL of fluid over a few minutes) (Fig. 15.14). The hypovolaemic patient will initially respond to transfusion with little or no change in CVP, together with some improvement in cardiovascular function (falling heart rate, rising blood pressure and increased peripheral temperature). As the normovolaemic state is approached, the CVP usually rises slightly and stabilizes, while other cardiovascular values normalize. At this stage, volume replacement should be slowed, or even stopped, in order to avoid overtransfusion (indicated by an abrupt and sustained rise in CVP, often accompanied by some deterioration in the patient's condition). In cardiac failure the venous pressure is usually high; the patient will not improve in response to volume replacement, which will cause a further, sometimes dramatic, rise in CVP.

The central venous catheter is usually inserted via a percutaneous puncture of a subclavian or internal jugular vein (Practical box 15.2, Fig. 15.15). Techniques using a guidewire are generally safer and more reliable than the catheter over needle devices (Fig. 15.16). They can also be used in conjunction with a vein dilator for

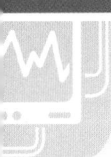

 Intensive care medicine

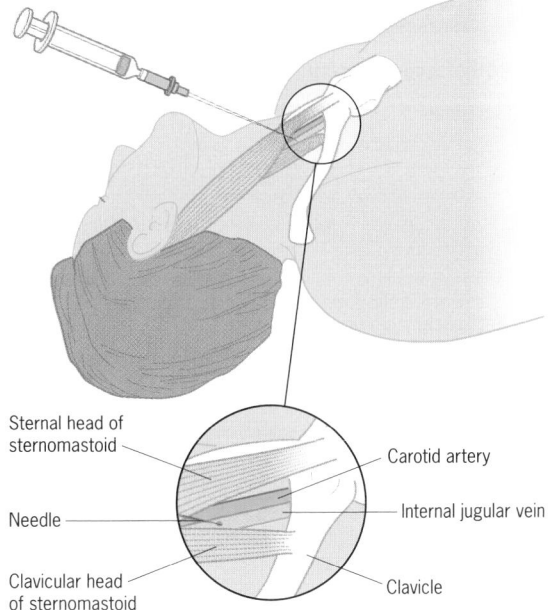

➕ Practical box 15.2

Internal jugular vein cannulation

Technique

1. The procedure is explained to the patient.
2. The patient is placed head-down to distend the central veins (this facilitates cannulation and minimizes the risk of air embolism but may exacerbate respiratory distress and is dangerous in those with raised intracranial pressure).
3. The skin is cleaned. Sterile precautions are taken throughout the procedure.
4. Local anaesthetic (1% plain lidocaine (lignocaine)) is injected intradermally to raise a weal at the apex of a triangle formed by the two heads of sternomastoid with the clavicle at its base.
5. A small incision is made through the weal.
6. The cannula or needle is inserted through the incision and directed laterally downwards and backwards in the direction of the nipple until the vein is punctured just beneath the skin and deep to the lateral head of sternomastoid.
7. Check that venous blood is easily aspirated.
8. The cannula is threaded off the needle into the vein.
9. The CVP manometer line is connected.
10. If the catheter is in a large vein, venous blood will flow back when the giving-set tap is open and the infusion bottle is on the floor.
11. The CVP is measured. The fluid level in the manometer should then fall rapidly and fluctuate with respiration.
12. A chest X-ray should be taken to verify that the tip of the catheter is in the superior vena cava and to exclude pneumothorax.

Possible complications

- Haemorrhage
- Accidental arterial puncture (carotid or subclavian)
- Pneumothorax
- Damage to thoracic duct on left
- Air embolism
- Thrombosis
- Catheter-related sepsis

Fig. 15.15 **Cannulation of right internal jugular vein with a catheter over the needle device.**

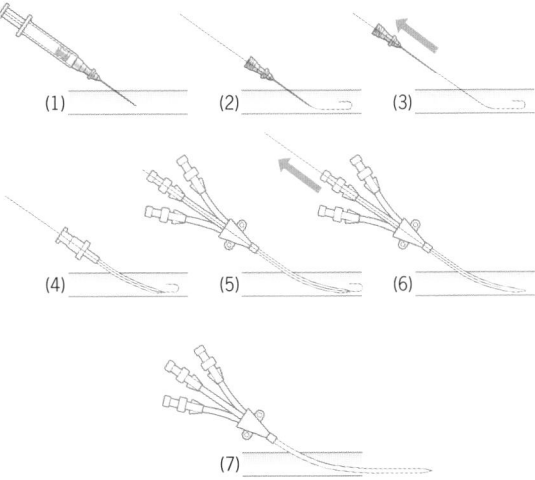

Fig. 15.16 **Seldinger technique – insertion of a catheter over guidewire.** (1) Puncture vessel; (2) advance guidewire; (3) remove needle; (4) dilate vessel; (5) advance catheter over guidewire; (6) remove guidewire; (7) catheter in situ. From Hinds CJ, Watson JD (1994) *Intensive Care: A Concise Textbook*. London: Baillière Tindall, with permission.

inserting introducers of pulmonary artery catheters, multilumen catheters and double lumen cannulae for haemofiltration.

The CVP may be read intermittently using a manometer system (Fig. 15.17) or continuously using a transducer and bedside monitor. It is essential that the pressure recorded always be related to the level of the right atrium. Various landmarks are advocated (e.g. sternal notch with the patient supine, sternal angle or mid-axilla when patient at 45 degrees), but it is largely immaterial which is chosen provided it is used consistently in an individual patient. Pressure measurements should be obtained at end-expiration.

The following are common pitfalls in interpreting central venous pressure readings:

Blocked catheter. This results in a sustained high reading, with a damped or absent waveform which often does not correlate with clinical assessment.

Manometer or transducer wrongly positioned. Failure to level the system is a common cause of erroneous readings.

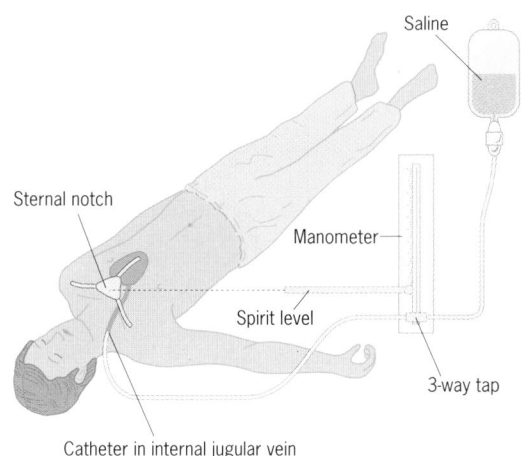

Fig. 15.17 **Central venous pressure measurement using a manometer system.** The reading must be referred to the level of the right atrium (indicated by the axillary fold or, provided the patient is supine, the sternal notch) using a spirit level.

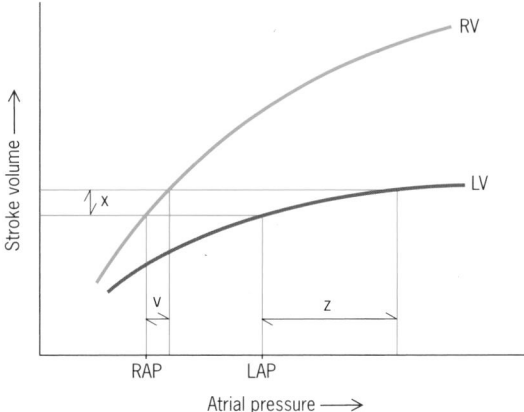

Fig. 15.18 **Left ventricular (LV) and right ventricular (RV) function curves in a patient with left ventricular dysfunction.** Since the stroke volume of the two ventricles must be the same (except perhaps for a few beats during a period of circulatory adjustment), left atrial pressure (LAP) must be higher than right atrial pressure (RAP). Moreover, an increase in stroke volume (x) produced by a small rise in RAP (v) will be associated with a marked increase in LAP (z).

Catheter tip in right ventricle. If the catheter is advanced too far, an unexpectedly high pressure with pronounced oscillations is recorded. This is easily recognized when the waveform is displayed.

Left atrial pressure

In uncomplicated cases, careful interpretation of the CVP is an adequate guide to the filling pressures of both sides of the heart. In many critically ill patients, however, this is not the case and there is a disparity in function between the two ventricles. Most commonly, left ventricular performance is worst, so that the left ventricular function curve is displaced downward and to the right (Fig. 15.18). High right ventricular filling pressures, with normal or low left atrial pressures, are less common but may occur in right ventricular ischaemia and in situations where the pulmonary vascular resistance (i.e. right ventricular afterload) is raised, such as in acute respiratory failure and pulmonary embolism.

If there is a disparity in ventricular function after cardiac surgery, then the left atrium can be cannulated directly. If the chest is not open, however, some other means of determining left ventricular filling pressure must be devised.

Pulmonary artery pressure

A 'balloon flotation catheter' enables prompt and reliable catheterization of the pulmonary artery. These 'Swan–Ganz' catheters can be inserted centrally (see Fig. 15.16) or through the femoral vein, or via a vein in the antecubital fossa. Passage of the catheter from the major veins, through the chambers of the heart, into the pulmonary artery and into the wedged position is monitored and guided by the pressure waveforms recorded from the distal lumen (Fig. 15.19 and Practical box 15.3).

A chest X-ray should always be obtained to check the final position of the catheter. In difficult cases screening with an image intensifier may be required.

Once in place, the balloon is deflated and the pulmonary artery mean, systolic and end-diastolic pressures (PAEDP) can be recorded. The pulmonary artery occlusion pressure (PAOP, otherwise known as pulmonary artery wedge pressure – PAWP) is measured by reinflating the balloon, thereby propelling the catheter distally until it impacts in a medium-sized pulmonary artery. In this position there is a continuous column of fluid between the distal lumen of the catheter and the left atrium, so that PAOP is usually a reflection of left atrial pressure.

The technique is generally safe – the majority of complications are related to user inexperience. Pulmonary artery catheters should preferably be removed within 72 hours, since the incidence of complications, especially infection, then increases progressively (Table 15.4).

Cardiac output

The only quantitatively accurate methods for measuring cardiac output are invasive. Of these, the thermodilution technique is most commonly used clinically. This uses a modified pulmonary artery catheter with a lumen opening in the right atrium and a thermistor located a few centimetres from its tip. A known volume (usually 10 mL) of cold 5% dextrose is injected as a bolus into the right atrium. This mixes with, and cools, the blood passing through the heart and the transient fall in temperature is continuously recorded by the thermistor in the pulmonary artery. The cardiac output is computed from the total amount of indicator (i.e. cold) injected, divided by the average concentration, i.e. the amount of cooling, and the time taken to pass the thermistor. It is now

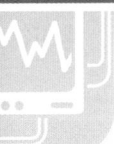

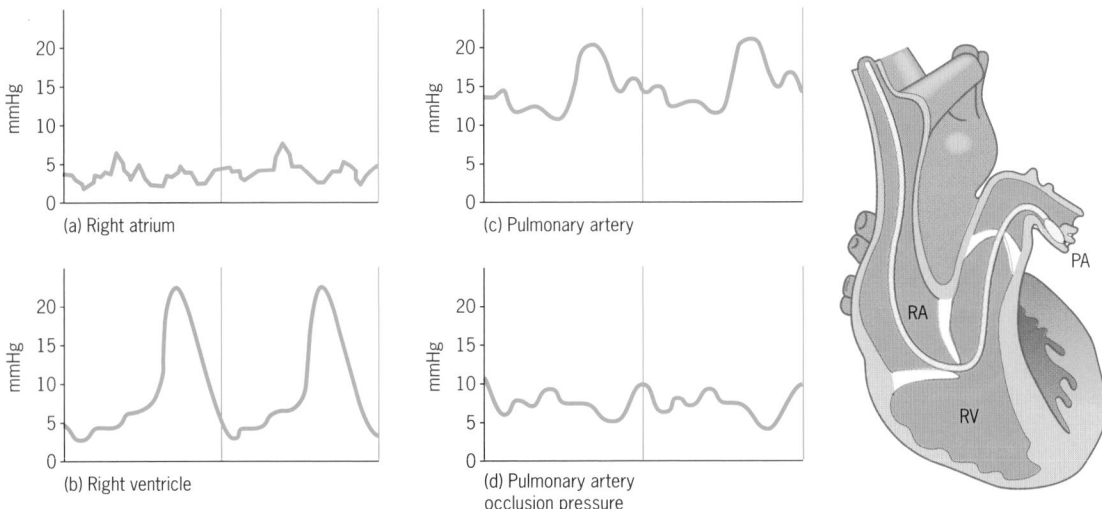

Fig. 15.19 **Passage of pulmonary artery balloon flotation catheter through the chambers of the heart into the 'wedged' position.** See Practical box 15.3.

✚ Practical box 15.3

Passage of a pulmonary artery balloon flotation catheter through the chambers of the heart into the 'wedged' position

(a) Once in the thorax, marked respiratory oscillations are seen. The catheter should be advanced further towards the lower superior vena cava/right atrium, where oscillations become more pronounced. The balloon should then be inflated and the catheter advanced.

(b) When the catheter is in the right ventricle, there is no dicrotic notch and the diastolic pressure is close to zero. The patient should be returned to the horizontal, or slightly head-up, position before advancing the catheter further.

(c) When the catheter reaches the pulmonary artery a dicrotic notch appears and there is elevation of the diastolic pressure. The catheter should be advanced further with the balloon inflated.

(d) Reappearance of a venous waveform indicates that the catheter is 'wedged'. The balloon is deflated to obtain the pulmonary artery pressure. The balloon is inflated intermittently to obtain the pulmonary artery occlusion (also known as pulmonary artery, or capillary, 'wedge') pressure.

Table 15.4

Balloon flotation pulmonary artery catheters: some complications in addition to those associated with central venous cannulation

Complication	Comments
Arrhythmias	Occur during passage of catheter through right ventricle Usually benign Can often be prevented with lidocaine (lignocaine)
Sepsis	Occurs at insertion site Bacteraemia or endocarditis may develop
Knotting	Occurs when catheter coils in right ventricle and is then withdrawn
Valve trauma	Occurs if catheter is withdrawn with balloon inflated, also tricuspid and pulmonary valves repeatedly open and close on the catheter
Thrombosis/embolism	
Pulmonary infarction	Occurs if catheter remains in 'wedged' position
Pulmonary artery rupture	Usually fatal May occur if balloon is inflated when catheter already 'wedged'
Balloon rupture/leak/embolism	Rare

possible to measure cardiac output continuously using a modified pulmonary artery catheter which transmits low heat energy into the surrounding blood and constructs a 'thermodilution curve'. These catheters also optically measure and continuously display $S_{\bar{v}}O_2$.

In general, pulmonary artery catheters enable the clinician to optimize cardiac output and oxygen delivery, while minimizing the risk of pulmonary oedema. They also allow the rational use of inotropes and vasoactive agents. However, their clinical value, and in particular their influence on outcome, is still a matter of controversy.

Non-invasive techniques for assessing cardiac function

The most useful technique for determining cardiac output and myocardial function non-invasively is Doppler ultrasonography. A probe is passed into the oesophagus to continuously monitor velocity waveforms from the descending aorta (Fig. 15.20). Although reasonable

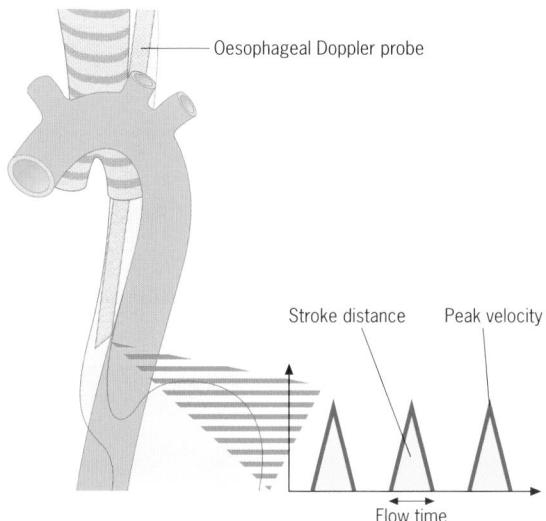

Oesophageal Doppler probe

Stroke distance   Peak velocity

Flow time

Fig. 15.20 Doppler ultrasonography. An oesophageal Doppler probe continuously measures velocity waveforms from the descending thoracic aorta. With a nomogram, stroke distance (area under waveform) provides an estimate of stroke volume. Acceleration and peak velocity indicate myocardial performance, while flow time is related to circulating volume and peripheral resistance. From Singer M, Grant I (eds) (1999) *ABC of Intensive Care*. London: BMJ Books, with permission.

estimates of stroke volume and cardiac output can be obtained, the technique is best used for trend analysis rather than for making absolute measurements. It is particularly valuable for perioperative optimization of the circulating volume and cardiac performance.

If there is disagreement between clinical signs and a monitored variable it should be assumed that the monitor is incorrect until all sources of potential error have been checked and eliminated. Changes and trends in monitored variables are always more informative than a single reading.

Management of shock (see Fig. 15.21)

Delays in making the diagnosis and in initiating treatment, as well as inadequate resuscitation, contribute to the development of multiple organ failure (MOF) and must be avoided (see p. 943).

A *patent airway* must be maintained and oxygen must be given. If necessary, an oropharyngeal airway or an endotracheal tube is inserted. The latter has the advantage of preventing aspiration of gastric contents. Very rarely emergency tracheostomy is indicated (see below). Some patients may require mechanical ventilation.

The *underlying cause of shock should be corrected* – for example, haemorrhage should be controlled or infection eradicated. In patients with septic shock, every effort must be made to identify the source of infection and isolate the causative organism. As well as a thorough history and clinical examination, X-rays, ultrasonography and

CT scanning may be required to locate the origin of the infection. Appropriate samples (urine, sputum, cerebrospinal fluid, pus drained from abscesses) should be sent to the laboratory for microscopy, culture and sensitivities. Several blood cultures should be performed and 'blind', broad-spectrum antibiotic therapy (p. 34) should be commenced. If an organism is isolated, therapy can be adjusted appropriately. The choice of antibiotic depends on the likely source of infection, previous antibiotic therapy and known local resistance patterns, as well as on whether it was acquired in hospital or in the community. Abscesses must be drained and infected indwelling catheters removed.

Whatever the aetiology of the haemodynamic abnormality, *tissue blood flow must be restored* by achieving and maintaining an adequate cardiac output, as well as ensuring that arterial blood pressure is sufficient to maintain perfusion of vital organs. Traditionally a mean arterial pressure (MAP) ≥60 mmHg has been considered to be adequate, but there is some evidence to suggest that 80 mmHg may be a more appropriate target and some now believe that in most cases the aim should be to achieve the patient's premorbid blood pressure.

Preload and volume replacement

Optimizing preload is the most efficient way of increasing cardiac output. Volume replacement is obviously essential in hypovolaemic shock but is also required in anaphylactic and septic shock because of vasodilatation, sequestration of blood and loss of circulating volume because of capillary leak.

In obstructive shock, high filling pressures may be required to maintain an adequate stroke volume. Even in cardiogenic shock, careful volume expansion may, on occasions, lead to a useful increase in cardiac output. On the other hand, patients with severe cardiac failure, in whom ventricular filling pressures may be markedly elevated, often benefit from measures to reduce preload (and afterload) – such as the administration of diuretics and vasodilators (see below).

The circulating volume must be replaced quickly (in minutes not hours) to reduce tissue damage and prevent acute renal failure. Fluid is administered via wide-bore intravenous cannulae to allow large volumes to be given quickly, and the effect is continuously monitored.

Care must be taken to prevent volume overload, which leads to cardiac dilatation, a reduction in stroke volume, and a rise in left atrial pressure with a risk of pulmonary oedema. Pulmonary oedema is more likely in very ill patients because of a low colloid osmotic pressure (usually due to a low serum albumin) and disruption of the alveolar–capillary membrane (e.g. in acute lung injury). Left ventricular filling pressures should therefore not be allowed to rise to more than 15–18 mmHg in most critically ill patients. In general, however, many more patients are undertransfused rather than overtransfused.

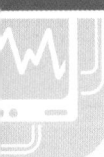
Restore delivery of oxygen to the tissues rapidly
and completely to prevent organ damage

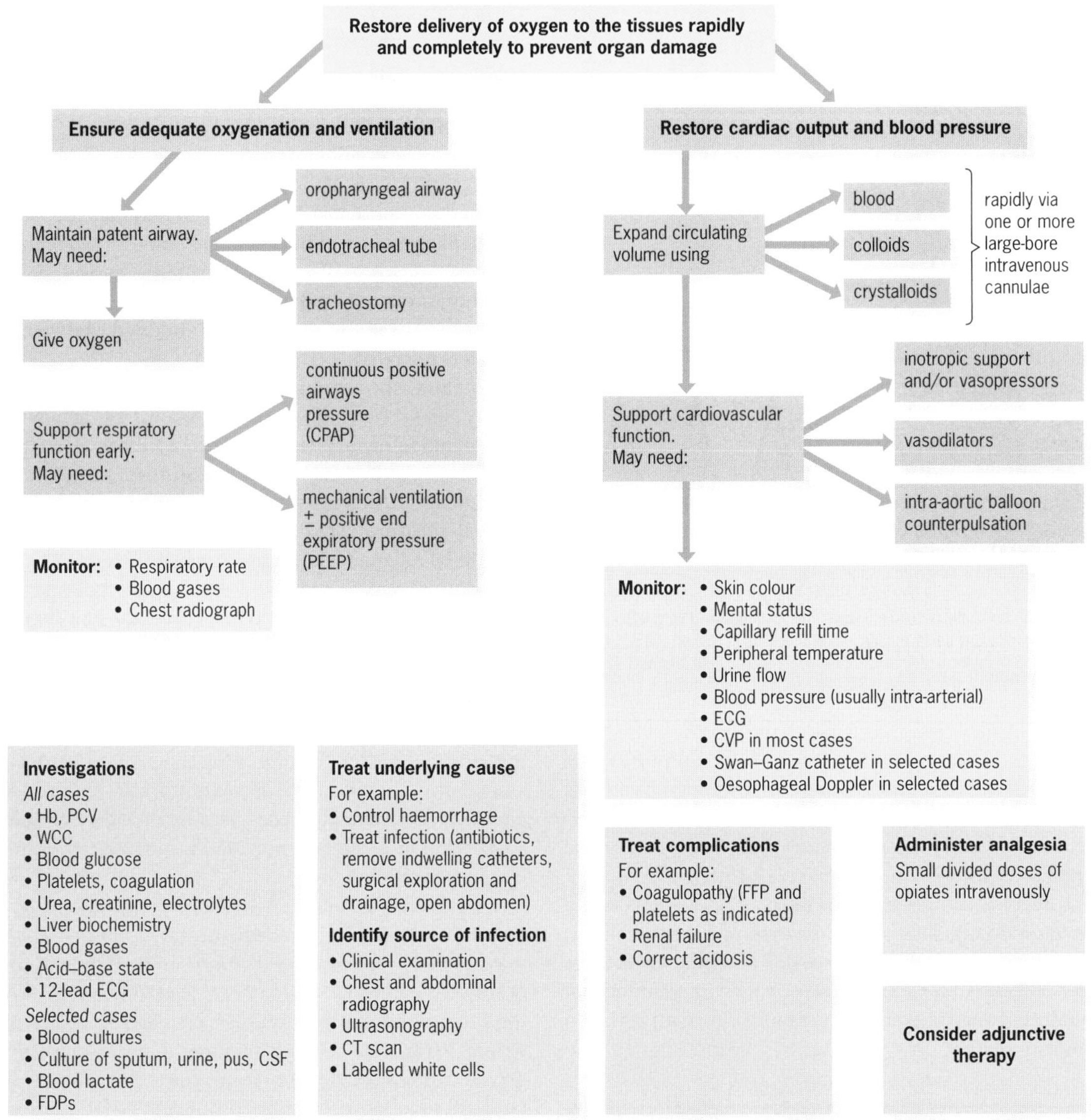

Ensure adequate oxygenation and ventilation

Maintain patent airway.
May need:
- oropharyngeal airway
- endotracheal tube
- tracheostomy

Give oxygen

Support respiratory
function early.
May need:
- continuous positive airways pressure (CPAP)
- mechanical ventilation ± positive end expiratory pressure (PEEP)

Monitor:
- Respiratory rate
- Blood gases
- Chest radiograph

Restore cardiac output and blood pressure

Expand circulating
volume using
- blood
- colloids
- crystalloids
} rapidly via one or more large-bore intravenous cannulae

Support cardiovascular
function.
May need:
- inotropic support and/or vasopressors
- vasodilators
- intra-aortic balloon counterpulsation

Monitor:
- Skin colour
- Mental status
- Capillary refill time
- Peripheral temperature
- Urine flow
- Blood pressure (usually intra-arterial)
- ECG
- CVP in most cases
- Swan–Ganz catheter in selected cases
- Oesophageal Doppler in selected cases

Investigations

All cases
- Hb, PCV
- WCC
- Blood glucose
- Platelets, coagulation
- Urea, creatinine, electrolytes
- Liver biochemistry
- Blood gases
- Acid–base state
- 12-lead ECG

Selected cases
- Blood cultures
- Culture of sputum, urine, pus, CSF
- Blood lactate
- FDPs

Treat underlying cause
For example:
- Control haemorrhage
- Treat infection (antibiotics, remove indwelling catheters, surgical exploration and drainage, open abdomen)

Identify source of infection
- Clinical examination
- Chest and abdominal radiography
- Ultrasonography
- CT scan
- Labelled white cells

Treat complications
For example:
- Coagulopathy (FFP and platelets as indicated)
- Renal failure
- Correct acidosis

Administer analgesia
Small divided doses of opiates intravenously

Consider adjunctive therapy

Fig. 15.21 Management of shock. Patients require intensive nursing care.

Choice of fluid for volume replacement

Blood

This is conventionally given for haemorrhagic shock as soon as it is available. In extreme emergencies, cross-match can be performed in about 30 minutes and is as safe as the standard procedure (see p. 446).

Although red cell transfusion will augment oxygen-carrying capacity, and hence global oxygen delivery, tissue oxygenation is also dependent on microcirculatory flow. This is influenced by the viscosity of the blood and hence the packed cell volume (PCV). Conventionally a PCV of 30–35% has been considered to provide the optimal balance between oxygen-carrying capacity and tissue flow, although it is well recognized that previously

fit patients with haemorrhagic shock can tolerate extremely low Hb concentrations provided their circulating volume and cardiac output are maintained. Transfusion of old stored red cells, which are poorly deformable, may be associated with microvascular occlusion and worsening tissue hypoxia.

Complications of blood transfusion are discussed on page 447. Special problems arise when large volumes of stored blood are transfused rapidly. These include:

Temperature changes. Bank blood is stored at 4°C and transfusion may result in hypothermia, peripheral veno-constriction (which slows the rate of the infusion) and arrhythmias. If possible blood should therefore be warmed during massive transfusion and in those at risk of hypothermia (e.g. during prolonged major surgery with open body cavity).

Coagulopathy. Stored blood has virtually no effective platelets and is deficient in clotting factors. Large transfusions can therefore produce a coagulation defect. This may need to be treated by replacing clotting factors with fresh frozen plasma and administering platelet concentrates.

Metabolic acidosis/alkalosis. Stored blood is preserved in citrate/phosphate/dextrose (CPD) solution, and metabolic acidosis attributable solely to blood transfusion is rare and in any case seldom requires correction. A metabolic alkalosis often develops 24–48 hours after a large blood transfusion, probably mainly owing to metabolism of the citrate. This will be exacerbated if any preceding acidosis has been corrected with intravenous sodium bicarbonate.

Hypocalcaemia. Stored blood is anticoagulated with citrate, which binds calcium ions. This can reduce total body ionized calcium levels and cause myocardial depression. This is uncommon in practice, but can be corrected by administering 10 mL of 10% calcium chloride intravenously. Routine treatment with calcium is not recommended.

Increased oxygen affinity. In stored blood, the red cell 2,3-DPG content is reduced, so that the oxyhaemoglobin dissociation curve is shifted to the left. The oxygen affinity of haemoglobin is therefore increased and oxygen unloading is impaired. This effect is less marked with CPD blood. Red cell levels of 2,3-DPG are substantially restored within 12 hours of transfusion.

Hyperkalaemia. Plasma potassium levels rise progressively as blood is stored. However, hyperkalaemia is rarely a problem as rewarming of the blood increases red cell metabolism – the sodium pump becomes active and potassium levels fall.

Microembolism. Microaggregates in stored blood may be filtered out by the pulmonary capillaries. This process is thought by some to contribute to acute lung injury (ALI) (see p. 952).

Red cell concentrates

Nutrient additive solutions – saline, adenine, glucose and mannitol (SAGM) – are available which allow red cell storage in the absence of plasma (see p. 450).

Concern about the supply, cost and safety of blood, including the risk of disease transmission and immune suppression, has encouraged a conservative approach to transfusion. Recent evidence suggests that in normovolaemic critically ill patients a restrictive strategy of red cell transfusion (Hb maintained at 7.0–9.0 g/dL) is at least as effective, and may be safer than a liberal transfusion strategy (Hb maintained at 10–12 g/dL). However, in some groups of patient (e.g. the elderly and those with significant cardiac or respiratory disease) it may be beneficial to maintain Hb at the higher level.

Blood substitutes

Attempts to develop an effective and safe oxygen-carrying blood substitute have so far been unsuccessful.

Crystalloid solutions

Crystalloid solutions such as saline are cheap, convenient to use and free of side-effects, but the administration of large volumes of these fluids to critically ill patients should, in general, be avoided. They are rapidly lost from the circulation into the extravascular spaces, and volumes of crystalloid several times that of colloid are required to achieve an equivalent haemodynamic response.

Colloidal solutions

These produce a greater and more sustained increase in circulating volume, with associated improvements in cardiovascular function and oxygen transport. They also increase colloid osmotic pressure. Despite these theoretical advantages, one systematic review has suggested that resuscitation with colloids rather than crystalloids may be associated with an increased risk of death. Many remain unconvinced by this controversial review, however, and would consider it reasonable to use crystalloids initially but to use colloids in addition if there is continued need for volume replacement in excess of about 1 L.

Polygelatin solutions (Haemaccel, Gelofusin) have an average molecular weight of 35 000, which is iso-osmotic with plasma. They are cheap and do not interfere with crossmatching. Large volumes can be administered, as clinically significant coagulation defects are unusual and renal function is not impaired. However, because they readily cross the glomerular basement membrane, their half-life in the circulation is only approximately 4 hours and they can promote an osmotic diuresis, although allergic reactions can occur. These solutions are particularly useful during the acute phase of resuscitation, especially when volume losses are continuing; but in many patients, colloids with a longer half-life will be required later to achieve haemodynamic stability.

Hydroxyethyl starch (HES) has a mean molecular weight of approximately 450 000 and a half-life of about 12 hours. Volume expansion is equivalent to, or slightly greater than, the volume infused. The incidence of allergic reactions is approximately 0.1%. Although more expensive than gelatins, HES is a useful volume expander.

Dextrans are polymolecular polysaccharides which have a powerful osmotic effect. They interfere with crossmatching and have a small rate of allergic reactions (0.1–1%) which may be life-threatening. Normally a dose of 1.5 g dextran per kilogram of bodyweight should not be exceeded because of the risk of renal damage. In practice, dextrans are rarely used in the UK because of the availability of other agents.

Human albumin solution (HAS) is a natural colloid which has been used for volume replacement in shock and burns, and for the treatment of hypoproteinaemia. HAS is not generally recommended for routine volume replacement, because supplies are limited and other cheaper solutions are equally effective. Controversially a recent systematic review suggested that the administration of human albumin to patients with hypovolaema, burns or hypoalbuminaemia might increase mortality. Nevertheless many remain sceptical of these findings and some clinicians continue to administer albumin especially to patients with burns and children with septic shock.

Myocardial contractility and inotropic agents

Myocardial contractility can be impaired by many factors such as hypoxaemia and hypocalcaemia, as well as by some drugs (e.g. beta-blockers, antiarrhythmics and sedatives).

Severe lactic acidosis can depress myocardial contractility and may limit the response to inotropes. Attempted correction of acidosis with intravenous sodium bicarbonate, however, generates additional carbon dioxide which diffuses across cell membranes, producing or exacerbating intracellular acidosis. Other disadvantages of bicarbonate therapy include sodium overload and a left shift of the oxyhaemoglobin dissociation curve. Ionized calcium levels may be reduced and, combined with the fall in intracellular pH, this may impair myocardial performance. Treatment of lactic acidosis should therefore concentrate on correcting the cause. Bicarbonate should only be administered to correct *extreme persistent metabolic acidosis* (see p. 696).

If the signs of shock persist despite adequate volume replacement, and perfusion of vital organs is jeopardized, pressor agents should be administered to improve cardiac output and blood pressure. In some cases inotropic agents are given in an attempt to redistribute blood flow (e.g. dopamine has been used to increase renal perfusion, dopexamine to improve splanchnic perfusion – see below). All inotropes increase myocardial oxygen consumption, particularly if a tachycardia develops, and this can lead to an imbalance between myocardial oxygen supply and demand, with the development or extension of ischaemic areas. For this reason inotropes should be used with caution, particularly in cardiogenic shock following myocardial infarction and in those known to have ischaemic heart disease.

Many of the most seriously ill patients become increasingly resistant to the effects of pressor agents, an observation attributed to 'downregulation' of adrenergic receptors and NO-induced 'vasoplegia' (p. 929).

All inotropic agents should be administered via a large central vein, and their effects carefully monitored. Some of the currently available inotropes are considered here (see also p. 762 and Table 15.5).

Epinephrine (adrenaline)

Epinephrine stimulates both α- and β-adrenergic receptors, but at low doses β effects seem to predominate. This produces a tachycardia, with an increase in cardiac index and a fall in peripheral resistance. At higher doses, α-mediated vasoconstriction develops. If this produces a useful increase in perfusion pressure and an increase in urine output, renal failure can be avoided. However, epinephrine can cause excessive vasoconstriction, with worrying reductions in splanchnic flow, particularly at higher doses. Cardiac output may fall, prolonged high-dose administration can cause peripheral gangrene and metabolic acidosis is common. For these reasons the minimum effective dose should be used for as short a time as possible.

Norepinephrine (noradrenaline)

This is predominantly an α-adrenergic agonist. It is particularly useful in those with severe hypotension associated with a low systemic vascular resistance, for example in septic shock. There is a risk of producing excessive vasoconstriction with impaired organ perfusion and increased afterload. Norepinephrine administration should normally therefore be accompanied by full haemodynamic monitoring, including invasive or non-invasive determination of cardiac output (see p. 935) and calculation of the peripheral resistance.

Dopamine

Dopamine is a natural precursor of epinephrine which acts on β receptors and α receptors, as well as dopaminergic D_1 and D_2 receptors.

In low doses (e.g. 1–3 µg/kg/min), dopaminergic vasodilatory receptors in the renal, mesenteric, cerebral and coronary circulations are activated. D_1 receptors are located on postsynaptic membranes and mediate vasodilatation, whilst D_2 receptors are presynaptic and potentiate these vasodilatory effects by preventing the release of epinephrine (adrenaline). Renal and hepatic flow increase, urine output is improved and it is possible that failure of these vital organs can be prevented (but see below). The importance of the renal vasodilator effect of dopamine has, however, been questioned and it has been suggested that the increased urine output is largely attributable to the rise in cardiac output, combined with a decrease in aldosterone concentration and inhibition of tubular sodium reabsorption mediated via D_1 stimulation.

In moderate doses (e.g. 3–10 µg/kg/min), dopamine increases heart rate, myocardial contractility and cardiac output. In some patients the dose of dopamine is limited by β-receptor effects such as tachycardia and arrhythmias.

In higher doses (e.g. > 10 mg/kg/min) the increased epinephrine (adrenaline) produced is associated with vasoconstriction. This increases afterload and raises ventricular filling pressures.

Table 15.5
Receptor actions of sympathomimetic and dopaminergic agents

	β_1	β_2	α_1	α_2	D_1	D_2	Dose dependence
Epinephrine (adrenaline)							++++
Low dose	++	+	+	±	−	−	
Moderate dose	++	+	++	+	−	−	
High dose	++(+)	+(+)	++++	+++	−	−	
Norepinephrine (noradrenaline)	++	0	+++	+++	−	−	+++
Isoprenaline	+++	+++	0	0	−	−	
Dopamine							+++++
Low dose	±	0	±	+	++	+	
Moderate dose	++	+	++	+	++(+)	+	
High dose	+++	++	+++	+	++(+)	+	
Dopexamine	+	+++	0	0	++	+	++
Dobutamine	++	+	±	?	0	0	++

Receptor	Action
β_1 – postsynaptic	Positive inotropism and chronotropism Renin release
β_2 – presynaptic	Stimulates norepinephrine (noradrenaline) release
β_2 – postsynaptic	Positive inotropism and chronotropism Vascular dilatation Relaxes bronchial smooth muscle
α_1 – postsynaptic	Constriction of peripheral, renal and coronary vascular smooth muscle Positive inotropism Antidiuresis
α_2 – presynaptic	Inhibition of norepinephrine (noradrenaline) release, vasodilatation
α_2 – postsynaptic	Constriction of coronary arteries Promotes salt and water excretion
D_1 – postsynaptic	Dilates renal, mesenteric and coronary vessels Renal tubular effect (natriuresis, diuresis)
D_2 – presynaptic	Inhibits norepinephrine (noradrenaline) release Inhibits adrenaline release

Dopexamine

Dopexamine is an analogue of dopamine which activates β_2 receptors as well as D_1 and D_2 receptors. Dopexamine is a very weak positive inotrope, but is a powerful splanchnic vasodilator, reducing afterload and improving blood flow to vital organs, including the kidneys. In septic shock, dopexamine can increase cardiac index and heart rate, but causes further reductions in peripheral resistance. It is most useful in those with low cardiac output and peripheral vasoconstriction and has been used as an adjunct to the perioperative management of high-risk patients (see below).

Dobutamine

Dobutamine is closely related to dopamine and has predominantly β_1 activity. Dobutamine has no specific effect on the renal vasculature but urine output often increases as cardiac output and blood pressure improve. It reduces systemic resistance, as well as improving cardiac performance, thereby decreasing afterload and ventricular filling pressures. Dobutamine is therefore useful in patients with cardiogenic shock and cardiac failure. In septic shock, dobutamine increases cardiac output and oxygen delivery.

Phosphodiesterase inhibitors (e.g. amrinone, milrinone, enoximone)

These agents have both inotropic and vasodilator properties. Because the phosphodiesterase type III inhibitors bypass the β-adrenergic receptor they do not cause tachycardia and are less arrhythmogenic than β agonists. They may be useful in patients with receptor 'downregulation', those receiving beta-blockers, for weaning patients from cardiopulmonary bypass and for patients with cardiac failure. In vasodilated septic patients, however, they may precipitate or worsen hypotension.

Guidelines for use of inotropic and vasopressor agents

Many still consider dopamine in low to moderate doses to be the first-line agent for restoring blood pressure, although others favour dopexamine as a means of increasing cardiac output and organ blood flow. High-dose dopamine is usually best avoided. Dobutamine is particularly indicated in patients in whom the vasoconstriction caused by dopamine could be dangerous (i.e. patients with cardiac disease and septic patients with fluid overload or myocardial failure). The combination of dobutamine and norepinephrine (noradrenaline) is

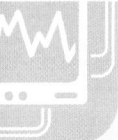

currently popular for the management of patients who are *shocked with a low systemic resistance* (e.g. septic shock). Dobutamine is given to achieve an optimal cardiac output, while norepinephrine is used to restore an adequate blood pressure by reducing vasodilatation. In some *vasodilated septic patients* with a high cardiac output, norepinephrine is used alone.

Epinephrine (adrenaline), because of its potency, remains a useful agent in patients with *refractory hypotension,* although adverse effects are common. This agent is still preferred by some as a cheap, effective agent for the management of septic shock, especially when haemodynamic monitoring is not available.

The value of inhibiting nitric oxide synthesis (e.g. with *N*-monomethyl-L-arginine) and of alternative vasoconstrictors such as vasopressin and angiotensin in septic shock remains uncertain.

High-risk surgical patients (Box 15.4)

These patients benefit from intensive perioperative circulatory support, in particular maintenance of an adequate circulating volume, and postoperative admission to ICU/HDU. Morbidity and mortality have been reduced by preoperative admission to intensive care for optimization of cardiovascular function. In such cases volume replacement and administration of inotropes or vasopressors should be guided by pulmonary artery catheterization or an oesophageal Doppler probe.

Targeting 'supranormal' values for oxygen delivery (Do_2) and oxygen consumption (Vo_2)

Although resuscitation has conventionally aimed at achieving normal haemodynamics, survival of many critically ill patients is associated with raised values for cardiac output, Do_2 and Vo_2. Aggressive fluid resuscitation and inotropic support aimed at achieving these 'supranormal values' has been associated with improved outcome when instituted early in major trauma and high-risk surgical patients. In such cases benefit may be largely related to optimal expansion of the circulating

---

Box 15.4

Patients at risk of developing perioperative multi-organ failure

(Modified from Shoemaker WC et al. (1988) *Chest* 94: 1176–1178)

- Patients with jeopardized cardiorespiratory function
- Patients with trauma to two body cavities requiring multiple blood transfusions
- Patients undergoing surgery involving extensive tissue dissection, e.g. oesophagectomy, pancreatectomy, aortic aneurysm surgery
- Patients undergoing emergency surgery for intra-abdominal or intrathoracic catastrophic states, e.g. faecal peritonitis, oesophageal perforation.

---

volume with consequent improvements in oxygen delivery and regional flow. Targeting 'supranormal values' is of no benefit when started after admission to intensive care.

Vasodilator therapy (see p. 760)

In selected cases, afterload reduction may be used to increase stroke volume and decrease myocardial oxygen requirements by reducing the systolic ventricular wall tension. Vasodilatation also decreases heart size and the diastolic ventricular wall tension so that coronary blood flow is improved. The relative magnitude of the falls in preload and afterload depends on the pre-existing haemodynamic disturbance, concurrent volume replacement and the agent selected (see below).

Vasodilator therapy is most beneficial in patients with cardiac failure in whom the ventricular function curve is flat (see Fig. 15.3) and falls in preload have only a limited effect on stroke volume.

This form of treatment, often combined with inotropic support, may therefore be useful in cardiogenic shock and in the management of patients with pulmonary oedema associated with low cardiac output. Vasodilators may also be valuable in shocked patients who remain vasoconstricted and oliguric despite restoration of an adequate blood pressure.

Such therapy is potentially dangerous and should be guided by continuous haemodynamic monitoring.

The agents used most commonly to achieve vasodilatation in the critically ill are those which act directly on the vessel wall.

Hydralazine predominantly affects arterial resistance vessels. It therefore reduces afterload and blood pressure, while cardiac output and heart rate usually increase. Hydralazine is usually given as an intravenous bolus to control acute increases in blood pressure.

Sodium nitroprusside (SNP) dilates arterioles and venous capacitance vessels, as well as the pulmonary vasculature by donating nitric oxide. SNP therefore reduces the afterload and preload of both ventricles and can improve cardiac output and the myocardial oxygen supply/demand ratio. On the other hand, it has been suggested that SNP can exacerbate myocardial ischaemia by producing a 'steal' phenomenon in the coronary circulation. The effects of SNP are rapid in onset and spontaneously reversible within a few minutes of discontinuing the infusion. A large overdose of SNP can cause cyanide poisoning, with intracellular hypoxia caused by inhibition of cytochrome oxidase, the terminal enzyme of the respiratory chain. This is manifested as a metabolic acidosis and a fall in the arteriovenous oxygen content difference.

Nitroglycerine (NTG) and *isosorbide dinitrate* (ISDN) are both predominantly venodilators. They are of most value in those with cardiac failure in whom preload reduction may reduce ventricular wall tension and improve coronary perfusion without adversely affecting cardiac performance. Furthermore, these agents may reverse myocardial ischaemia by increasing and redistributing coronary blood flow. They are therefore often used in preference to SNP in patients with cardiac failure and/or myocardial ischaemia. Both NTG and ISDN reduce pulmonary vascular resistance, an effect that can occasionally be exploited in patients with a low cardiac output secondary to pulmonary hypertension.

Mechanical support of the myocardium

Intra-aortic balloon counterpulsation (IABCP) is the technique used most widely for mechanical support of the failing myocardium. It is discussed on page 734.

Sepsis and multiple organ failure (MOF)

(also known as multiple organ dysfunction syndrome – MODS)

Sepsis is being diagnosed with increasing frequency and is now the commonest cause of death in non-coronary adult intensive care units. The in-hospital incidence of severe sepsis is conservatively in the order of two cases per 100 admissions and length of stay is dramatically longer than for those without sepsis. Mortality rates are high (between 20 and 70%) and are closely related to the number of organs which fail and the duration of organ dysfunction. Those who die are overwhelmed by persistent or recurrent sepsis, with fever, intractable hypotension and failure of several organs.

Sequential failure of vital organs occurs progressively over weeks, although the pattern of organ dysfunction is variable. In most cases the lungs are the first to be affected (acute lung injury – ALI; acute respiratory distress syndrome – ARDS; see p. 951) in association with cardiovascular instability and deteriorating renal function. Damage to the mucosal lining of the gastrointestinal tract as a result of reduced splanchnic flow followed by reperfusion, allows bacteria within the gut lumen, or their cell wall components, to gain access to the circulation. The liver defences, which are often compromised by poor perfusion, are overwhelmed and the lungs and other organs are exposed to bacterial toxins and inflammatory mediators released by liver macrophages. Some have therefore called the gut the 'motor of multiple organ failure'. Secondary pulmonary infection, complicating ALI/ARDS also frequently acts as a further stimulus to the inflammatory response. Later, renal failure and liver dysfunction develop (see p. 944). Gastrointestinal failure, with an inability to tolerate enteral feeding and paralytic ileus, is common. Ischaemic colitis, acalculous cholecystitis, pancreatitis and gastrointestinal haemorrhage may also occur. Features of central nervous system dysfunction include impaired consciousness and disorientation, progressing to coma. Characteristically, these patients initially have a hyperdynamic circulation with vasodilatation and a high cardiac output, associated with an increased metabolic rate. Eventually, however, cardiovascular collapse supervenes and is the usual terminal event.

Table 15.6
Some of the therapeutic strategies tested in randomized, controlled phase II or III trials in human sepsis

High-dose steroids
Endotoxin antibodies
Bactericidal permeability-increasing protein
TNF antibodies
Soluble TNF receptors
Interleukin-1 receptor antagonists
Platelet-activating factor antagonists
N-acetyl cysteine
Nitric oxide synthase inhibition
Antithrombin ⎫
Activated protein C ⎭ recent trials suggest some possible benefit

Treatment

Initial attempts to combat the high mortality associated with sepsis concentrated on cardiovascular and respiratory support in the hope that survival could be prolonged until surgery, antibiotics and the patient's own defences had eradicated the infection and injured tissues were repaired. Despite some success, mortality rates remained unacceptably high. Aggressive fluid resuscitation and inotropic support have met with only limited success, and controlled trials have demonstrated that, when instituted following admission to intensive care have shown no benefit in controlled trials.

So far, attempts to improve outcome by modulating the inflammatory response or neutralizing endotoxin (Table 15.6) have also proved disappointing and in some cases may even have been harmful.

Despite this apparent lack of progress many clinicians believe that advances have been made and that some individuals who would in the past have died now survive. Prevention of organ damage in those at risk is crucial. Aggressive early resuscitation is essential. Advances in nursing care and in the organization of hospital-wide critical care provision may all contribute to better outcomes.

FURTHER READING

Astiz MA, Rackow EC (1998) Septic shock. *Lancet* **251**: 1501–1505.

Bone RC (1996) Sir Isaac Newton, sepsis, SIRS and CARS. *Critical Care Medicine* **24**: 1125–1128.

Gan TJ, Arrowsmith JE (1997) The oesophageal Doppler monitor. *British Medical Journal* **315**: 893–894.

Hayes MA, Timmins AC, Yau EHS, Palazzo M, Watson D, Hinds CJ (1996) Oxygen transport patterns in patients with sepsis syndrome or septic shock: influence of treatment and relationship to outcome. *Critical Care Medicine* **25**: 926–936.

Hébert PC, Wells G, Blajchman MA et al. (1999) A multicenter, randomised, controlled clinical trial of transfusion requirements in critical care. *New England Journal of Medicine* **340**: 409–417.

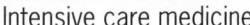

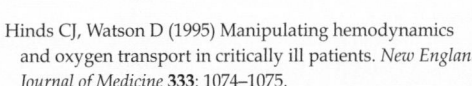

Hinds CJ, Watson D (1995) Manipulating hemodynamics
and oxygen transport in critically ill patients. *New England
Journal of Medicine* **333**: 1074–1075.

Landry DW, Oliver JA (2001) The pathogenesis of
vasodilatory shock. *New England Journal of Medicine* **345**:
588–595.

Sands KE, Bates DW, Lanken PN et al. (1997) Epidemiology
of sepsis syndrome in 8 academic medical centres. *JAMA*
278: 234–240.

Soni N (1996) Swan song for the Swan–Ganz catheter?
British Medical Journal **313**: 763–764.

Task Force of the American College of Critical Care
Medicine, Society of Critical Care Medicine (1999)
Practice parameters for haemodynamic support of sepsis
in adult patients with sepsis. *Critical Care Medicine* **27**:
639–660.

Renal failure

Acute renal failure is a common and serious complication of critical illness which adversely affects the prognosis. The importance of preventing renal failure by rapid and effective resuscitation, as well as the avoidance of nephrotoxic drugs (especially NSAIDs), and control of infection cannot be overemphasized. Shock and sepsis are the most common causes of acute renal failure in the critically ill, but diagnosis of the cause of renal dysfunction is necessary to exclude reversible pathology, especially obstruction (see Ch. 11).

Oliguria is usually the first indication of renal impairment and immediate attempts should be made to optimize cardiovascular function, particularly by expanding the circulating volume and restoring blood pressure to premorbid levels. Restoration of the urine output is a good indicator of successful resuscitation. Low-dose dopamine may be used to enhance renal blood flow and improve urine output, although recent evidence suggests that this agent is not an effective means of preventing or reversing renal impairment (p. 762). Some believe that dobutamine is at least as effective. If these measures fail to reverse oliguria, administration of diuretics such as furosemide (frusemide), or less often mannitol, is recommended. Currently furosemide infusions are most frequently employed (see Ch. 11), but mannitol is specifically indicated in rhabdomyolysis and may be useful in the prevention of renal failure due to radio contrast media. If oliguria persists, it is important to reduce crystalloid intake and review drug doses.

Intermittent haemodialysis has a number of disadvantages in the critically ill. In particular it is frequently complicated by hypotension and it may be difficult to remove sufficient volumes of fluid. Peritoneal dialysis is also frequently unsatisfactory in these patients and is contraindicated in those who have undergone intra-abdominal surgery. The use of continuous veno-venous

haemofiltration, usually with dialysis (CVVHD), is therefore preferred (see Ch. 11) and is indicated for fluid overload, electrolyte disturbances (especially hyperkalaemia), severe acidosis and, to a lesser extent, uraemia.

If the underlying problems resolve, renal function almost invariably recovers within a few days to several weeks later.

FURTHER READING

Australian and New Zealand Care Society (ANZICS)
Clinical Trials Group (2000) Low-dose dopamine in
patients with early renal dysfunction: a placebo-
controlled randomised trial. *Lancet* **356**: 2139–2143.

Respiratory failure

Types and causes

The respiratory system consists of a gas exchanging organ (the lungs) and a ventilatory pump (respiratory muscles/thorax), either or both of which can fail and precipitate respiratory failure. Respiratory failure occurs when pulmonary gas exchange is sufficiently impaired to cause hypoxaemia with or without hypercarbia. In practical terms, respiratory failure is present when the P_aO_2 is < 8 kPa (60 mmHg) or the P_aCO_2 is > 7 kPa (55 mmHg). It can be divided into:

- type I respiratory failure, in which the P_aO_2 is low and the P_aCO_2 is normal or low
- type II respiratory failure, in which the P_aO_2 is low and the P_aCO_2 is high.

Type I or '*acute hypoxaemic*' respiratory failure occurs with diseases that damage lung tissue. Hypoxaemia is due to right-to-left shunts or $\dot{V}/\dot{Q}$ mismatch. Common causes include pulmonary oedema, pneumonia, acute lung injury and, in the chronic situation, fibrosing alveolitis.

Type II or '*ventilatory failure*' occurs when alveolar ventilation is insufficient to excrete the volume of carbon dioxide being produced by tissue metabolism. Inadequate alveolar ventilation is due to reduced ventilatory effort, inability to overcome an increased resistance to ventilation, failure to compensate for an increase in deadspace and/or carbon dioxide production, or a combination of these factors. The most common cause is chronic obstructive pulmonary disease (COPD). Other causes include chest-wall deformities, respiratory muscle weakness (e.g. Guillain–Barré syndrome) and depression of the respiratory centre (e.g. overdose).

Deterioration in the mechanical properties of the lungs and/or chest wall increases the work of breathing and the oxygen consumption/carbon dioxide production of the respiratory muscles. The concept that respiratory muscle fatigue (either acute or chronic) is a major factor in the pathogenesis of respiratory failure is controversial.

Monitoring of respiratory failure

A clinical assessment of respiratory distress should be made on the following criteria (those marked with an asterisk may be indicative of respiratory muscle fatigue):

- the use of accessory muscles of respiration, intercostal recession
- tachypnoea*
- tachycardia
- sweating
- pulsus paradoxus (rarely present)
- inability to speak, unwillingness to lie flat
- agitation, restlessness, diminished conscious level
- asynchronous respiration (a discrepancy in the timing of movement of the abdominal and thoracic compartments)*
- paradoxical respiration (abdominal and thoracic compartments move in opposite directions)*
- respiratory alternans (breath-to-breath alteration in the relative contribution of intercostal/accessory muscles and the diaphragm).*

Blood gas analysis should be performed to guide oxygen therapy and to provide an objective assessment of the severity of the respiratory failure. The *most sensitive clinical* indicator of increasing respiratory difficulty is a rising respiratory rate. *Measurement of tidal volume* is a less sensitive indicator.

Vital capacity is often a better guide to deterioration and is particularly useful in patients with respiratory inadequacy that is due to neuromuscular problems – such as the Guillain–Barré syndrome, in which the vital capacity decreases as weakness increases.

Pulse oximetry

Lightweight oximeters which measure the changing amount of light transmitted through pulsating arterial blood and provide a continuous, non-invasive assessment of S_aO_2 can be applied to an ear lobe or finger. These devices are reliable, easy to use and do not require calibration, although remember that pulse oximetry is not a very sensitive guide to *changes* in oxygenation. An S_aO_2 within normal limits in a patient receiving supplemental oxygen in no way excludes the possibility of hypoventilation. Readings may be inaccurate in those with poor peripheral perfusion.

Blood gas analysis

Errors can result from malfunctioning of the analyser or incorrect sampling of arterial blood.

- The sample should be analysed immediately or the syringe should be immersed in iced water (the end having first been sealed with a cap) to prevent the continuing metabolism of white cells causing a reduction in Po_2 and a rise in Pco_2.
- The sample must be adequately anticoagulated to prevent clot formation within the analyser. However, excessive dilution of the blood with heparin, which is acidic, will significantly reduce its pH. Heparin (1000 i.u./mL) should just fill the deadspace of the syringe, i.e. approximately 0.1 mL. This will adequately anticoagulate a 2 mL sample.
- Air almost inevitably enters the sample. The gas tensions within these air bubbles will equilibrate with those in the blood, thereby lowering the Pco_2 and usually raising the Po_2 of the sample. However, provided the bubbles are ejected immediately by inverting the syringe and expelling the air that rises to the top of the sample, their effect is insignificant.

Disposable pre-heparinized syringes are available for blood gas analysis.

Normal values of blood gas analysis are shown in Table 15.2. Interpretation of the results of blood gas analysis can be considered in two separate parts:

- disturbances of acid–base balance (see pp. 689 and 926)
- alterations in oxygenation.

Correct interpretation requires a knowledge of the history, the age of the patient, the inspired oxygen concentration, any other relevant treatment (e.g. the administration of sodium bicarbonate, and the ventilator settings for those on mechanical ventilation). It is the oxygen content of the arterial blood that is most important and this is determined by the percentage saturation of haemoglobin with oxygen. The relationship between the latter and the P_aO_2 is determined by the oxyhaemoglobin dissociation curve (Fig. 15.5).

Capnography

Continuous breath-by-breath analysis of expired carbon dioxide concentration can be used to:

- confirm tracheal intubation
- continuously monitor end tidal Pco_2, which approximates to P_aco_2 in normal subjects (may be useful when transporting critically ill patients, for example)
- detect apparatus malfunction
- detect alterations in lung function.

Management of respiratory failure

Standard management of patients with respiratory failure includes:

- administration of supplemental oxygen
- treatment for airways obstruction

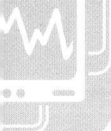

- measures to limit pulmonary oedema
- control of secretions
- treatment of pulmonary infection.

The load on the respiratory muscles should be reduced by improving lung mechanics. Correction of abnormalities which may lead to respiratory muscle weakness, such as hypophosphataemia and malnutrition, is also necessary.

Oxygen therapy

Methods of oxygen administration

Oxygen is initially given via a face mask. In the majority of patients (except patients with COPD and chronically elevated P_aCO_2) the concentration of oxygen given is not vital and oxygen can therefore be given by a 'variable performance' device such as a simple face mask or nasal cannulae (Fig. 15.22).

With these devices the inspired oxygen concentration varies from about 35% to 55%, with oxygen flow rates of between 6 and 10 L/min. Nasal cannulae are often preferred because they are less claustrophobic and do not interfere with feeding or speaking, but they can cause ulceration of the nasal or pharyngeal mucosa. Higher concentrations of oxygen can be administered by using a mask with a reservoir bag attached (Fig. 15.22(c)). Figure 15.22 should be compared with the fixed performance mask shown in Fig. 14.26, with which the oxygen concentration can be controlled. This latter type of mask is used in patients with COPD and chronic type II failure, although the dangers of reducing hypoxic drive have been overemphasized – hypoxaemia is more dangerous than hypercapnia.

Oxygen toxicity

Experimentally, mammalian lungs have been shown to be damaged by continuous exposure to high concentrations of oxygen, but oxygen toxicity in humans is less well proven. Nevertheless, it is reasonable to assume that high concentrations of oxygen might damage the lungs, and so the lowest inspired oxygen concentration compatible with adequate arterial oxygenation should be used. Dangerous hypoxia should never be tolerated through a fear of pulmonary oxygen toxicity.

Respiratory support

If, despite the above measures, the patient continues to deteriorate or fails to improve, the institution of some form of respiratory support should be considered (Table 15.7).

Intermittent positive-pressure ventilation (IPPV) is achieved by intermittently inflating the lungs with a positive pressure delivered by a ventilator via an endotracheal tube or a tracheostomy. A number of refinements and modifications of IPPV have been introduced over the years (Table 15.7). *Controlled mechanical ventilation* (CMV) with the abolition of spontaneous breathing rapidly leads to atrophy of respiratory muscles so that assisted modes that are triggered by the patient's inspiratory efforts (see below) are preferred.

The rational use of mechanical ventilation depends on a clear understanding of its potential beneficial effects, as well as its dangers.

Beneficial effects of mechanical ventilation

- *Improved carbon dioxide elimination.* By adjusting the volume of ventilation, the P_aCO_2 can be controlled.
- *Relief from exhaustion.* Mechanical ventilation removes the work of breathing, 'rests' the respiratory muscles and relieves the extreme exhaustion that may be present in patients with respiratory failure. In some cases, if ventilation is not instituted, this exhaustion may culminate in respiratory arrest.

Effects on oxygenation. Application of positive pressure can prevent or reverse atelectasis. In those with severe pulmonary parenchymal disease, the lungs may be very stiff and the work of breathing is therefore greatly increased. Under these circumstances the institution of

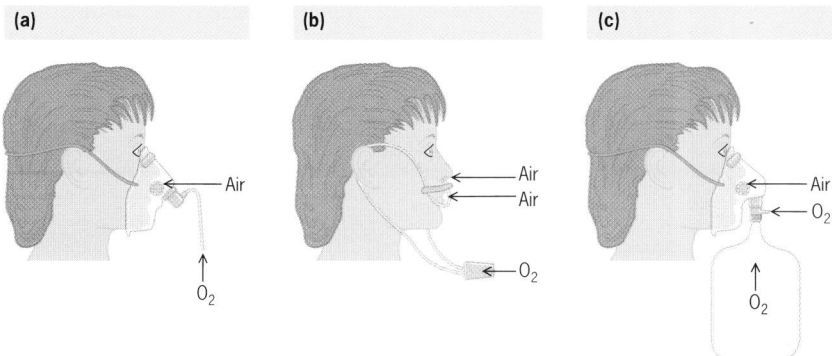

Fig. 15.22 Methods of administering supplemental oxygen to the unintubated patient. **(a)** Simple face mask. **(b)** Nasal cannulae. **(c)** Mask with reservoir bag.

Table 15.7
Techniques for respiratory support

Technique	Comment
Invasive respiratory support	
Intermittent positive-pressure ventilation (IPPV)	May be given with positive end-expiratory pressure (PEEP)
Continuous positive airway pressure (CPAP)	Given via endotracheal tube
Synchronized intermittent mandatory ventilation (SIMV) (volume or pressure controlled)	May be given with pressure support and CPAP
Pressure support ventilation (PSV)	Usually given with CPAP
'Lung-protective' ventilatory strategies to minimize ventilator-induced lung injury	Low tidal volume, reduced airway pressures. Can use with SIMV, PEEP and prolonged inspiratory phase
High-frequency jet ventilation (HFJV)	May be useful in those with lung leak (e.g. bronchopleural fistula)
Extracorporeal techniques	May be useful in severe acute respiratory failure
Non-invasive respiratory support	
Continuous positive airway pressure (CPAP)	Given by mask
Non-invasive IPPV and SIMV	Given via nasal or face mask
Bilevel positive airway pressure (BiPAP)	Inspiratory or expiratory

respiratory support may significantly reduce total body oxygen consumption; consequently $P_{\bar{v}}O_2$ – and thus P_aO_2 – may improve. Because ventilated patients are connected to a leak-free circuit, it is possible to administer high concentrations of oxygen (up to 100%) accurately and to apply a positive end-expiratory pressure (PEEP). In selected cases the latter may reduce shunting and increase P_aO_2 (see below).

Indications for mechanical ventilation

Acute respiratory failure, with signs of severe respiratory distress (e.g. respiratory rate > 40/min, inability to speak, patient exhausted) persisting despite maximal therapy. Confusion, restlessness, agitation, a decreased conscious level, a rising P_aCO_2 (> 8 kPa) and extreme hypoxaemia (< 8 kPa), despite oxygen therapy, are further indications.

Acute ventilatory failure due, for example, to myasthenia gravis or Guillain–Barré syndrome. Mechanical ventilation should usually be instituted when the vital capacity has fallen to 10 mL/kg or less. This will avoid complications such as atelectasis and infection as well as preventing respiratory arrest. The tidal volume and respiratory rate are relatively insensitive in the above conditions and change late in the course of the disease. A high P_aCO_2 (particularly if rising) is an indication for urgent artificial ventilation.

Other indications include:

- prophylactic postoperative ventilation in high-risk patients
- head injury – to avoid hypoxia and hypercarbia which increase cerebral blood flow and intracranial pressure, hyperventilation to reduce intracranial pressure
- trauma – chest injury and lung contusion
- severe left ventricular failure with pulmonary oedema
- coma with breathing difficulties, e.g. following drug overdose.

Institution of invasive respiratory support

This requires tracheal intubation. If the patient is conscious the procedure must be fully explained before anaesthesia is induced. The complications of tracheal intubation are given in Table 15.8.

Intubating patients in severe respiratory failure is an extremely hazardous undertaking and should only be performed by experienced staff. In extreme emergencies it may be preferable to ventilate the patient by hand using an oropharyngeal airway, a face mask and a self-inflating bag with added oxygen until experienced help arrives.

The patient is usually hypoxic and hypercarbic, with increased sympathetic activity; the stimulus of laryngoscopy and intubation can precipitate dangerous arrhythmias and even cardiac arrest. Except in an extreme emergency, therefore, the ECG and oxygen saturation should be monitored, and the patient pre-oxygenated with 100% oxygen before intubation. Resuscitation drugs should be immediately available. If time allows, the circulating volume should be optimized and, if necessary, inotropes commenced before attempting intubation. In some cases it may be appropriate to establish intra-arterial and central venous pressure monitoring before instituting mechanical ventilation, although many patients will not tolerate the supine or head-down position. In some deeply comatose patients, no sedation may be required, but in the majority of patients a short-acting intravenous anaesthetic agent followed by muscle relaxation will be necessary.

Tracheostomy

Tracheostomy may be required for the long-term control of excessive bronchial secretions, particularly in those with a reduced conscious level, and/or to maintain an airway and protect the lungs in those with impaired pharyngeal and laryngeal reflexes. Tracheostomy is also performed when intubation is likely to be prolonged

Table 15.8
Complications of endotracheal intubation

Complication	Comments
Immediate	
Tube in one or other (usually the right) bronchus	Avoid by checking both lungs are being inflated; i.e. both sides of the chest move and air entry is heard on auscultation
	Obtain chest X-ray to check position of tube and to exclude lung collapse
Tube is in oesophagus	Gives rise to hypoxia and abdominal distension
	Detected by capnography
Early	
Migration of the tube out of the trachea	
Leaks around the tube	
Obstruction of tube because of kinking or secretions	*A dangerous complication*
	The patient becomes distressed, cyanosed and has poor chest expansion
	The following should be performed immediately:
	• Manual inflation with 100% oxygen
	• Endotracheal suction
	• Check position of tube
	• Deflate cuff
	• Check tube for 'kinks'
	If no improvement, ventilate with face mask and then insert new endotracheal tube
Late	
Sinusitis	
Mucosal oedema and ulceration	
Laryngeal injury	
Tracheal narrowing and fibrosis	
Tracheomalacia	

Table 15.9
Complications of tracheostomy

As for endotracheal intubation (Table 15.8), plus:

Early
Death
Surgical complications
  Pneumothorax
  Haemorrhage
Tube misplaced in pretracheal subcutaneous tissues
Subcutaneous emphysema

Intermediate
Erosion of tracheal cartilages
  (may cause tracheo-oesophageal fistula)
Erosion of innominate artery (may lead to fatal haemorrhage)
Stomal infection
Pneumonia

Late
Failure of stoma to heal
Tracheal stenosis at level of stoma, cuff or tube tip
Collapse of tracheal rings at level of stoma
Cosmetic

(> 14 days for example), for patient comfort and to facilitate weaning from mechanical ventilation.

Tracheostomy can be performed at the bedside in an ICU. A percutaneous dilatational technique, which is quick and economical, is increasingly considered to be the technique of choice in critically ill patients and can be used in an emergency. Alternatively, the trachea can be opened through the second, third and fourth tracheal rings via a transverse skin incision in theatre.

A life-threatening obstruction of the upper respiratory tract that cannot be bypassed with an endotracheal tube should have a *cricothyroidotomy*, which is safer, quicker and easier to perform than a formal tracheostomy.

Surgical tracheostomy has a mortality rate of up to 5%. Complications of tracheostomy are shown in Table 15.9. With any tracheostomy, care should be taken to ensure that the tube is not blocked by secretions.

Minitracheostomy involves inserting a small-diameter uncuffed tube percutaneously into the trachea via the cricothyroid membrane using a guidewire. It can be performed under local anaesthesia. This technique facilitates the clearance of copious secretions in those who are unable to cough effectively, although, because these tubes have no cuff, patients must be able to protect their airway.

Dangers of mechanical ventilation

Airway complications. There may be complications with endotracheal intubation with additional local complications of a tracheostomy (see above) (Tables 15.8 and 15.9).

Disconnection, failure of gas or power supply, mechanical faults. These are unusual but dangerous. A method of manual ventilation, such as a self-inflating bag, and oxygen must always be available by the bedside.

Cardiovascular complications. The intermittent application of positive pressure to the lungs and thoracic wall impedes venous return and distends alveoli, thereby 'stretching' the pulmonary capillaries and causing a rise in pulmonary vascular resistance. Both these mechanisms can produce a fall in cardiac output.

Respiratory complications. Mechanical ventilation can be complicated by a deterioration in gas exchange because of $\dot{V}/\dot{Q}$ mismatch and collapse of peripheral alveoli. Traditionally the latter was prevented by using high tidal volumes (10–15 mL/kg) but there is increasing evidence to suggest that high inflation pressures, with overdistension of compliant alveoli, perhaps exacerbated by the repeated opening and closure of distal airways, can disrupt the alveolar–capillary membrane, increase microvascular permeability and release inflammatory mediators leading to *'ventilator-induced lung* *injury'*. Extreme overdistension of the lungs during mechanical ventilation with high tidal volumes and PEEP can rupture alveoli and cause air to dissect centrally along the perivascular sheaths. This *'barotrauma'* may be complicated by pneumomediastinum, subcutaneous emphysema, pneumoperitoneum, pneumothorax, and intra-abdominal air. The risk of pneumothorax is increased in those with destructive lung disease (e.g. necrotizing pneumonia, emphysema), asthma or fractured ribs.

A *tension pneumothorax* can be rapidly fatal in ventilated patients. Suggestive signs include the development or worsening of hypoxia, hypercarbia, fighting the ventilator, an unexplained increase in airway pressure, as well as hypotension and tachycardia, sometimes accompanied by a rising CVP. Examination may reveal unequal chest expansion, mediastinal shift (deviated trachea, displaced apex beat) and a hyperresonant hemithorax. Although, traditionally, breath sounds are diminished over the pneumothorax, this sign can be extremely misleading in ventilated patients. If there is time, the diagnosis can be confirmed by chest X-ray.

Ventilator-associated pneumonia. Nosocomial pneumonia occurs in as many as one-third of patients receiving mechanical ventilation and is associated with a significant increase in mortality. It can be difficult to diagnose. There is now good evidence that leakage of infected oropharyngeal secretions past the tracheal cuff is largely responsible. Bacterial colonization of the oropharynx may be promoted by regurgitation of colonized gastric fluid and the risk of nosocomial pneumonia can be reduced by nursing patients in the semi-recumbent, rather than the supine, position.

Gastrointestinal complications. Initially, many ventilated patients will develop abdominal distension associated with an ileus. The cause is unknown, although the use of non-depolarizing neuromuscular blocking agents and opiates may in part be responsible.

Salt and water retention. Mechanical ventilation, particularly with PEEP, causes increased ADH secretion and possibly a reduction in circulating levels of atrial natriuretic peptide. Combined with a fall in cardiac output and a reduction in renal blood flow, these can cause salt and water retention. This fluid retention is often particularly noticeable in the lungs.

Positive end-expiratory pressure (PEEP)

A positive airway pressure can be maintained at a chosen level throughout expiration by attaching a threshold resistor valve to the expiratory limb of the circuit. PEEP re-expands underventilated lung units, and redistributes lung water from the alveoli to the perivascular interstitial space, thereby reducing shunt and increasing the P_aO_2. Unfortunately, however, the inevitable rise in mean intrathoracic pressure that follows the application of PEEP may further impede venous return, increase pulmonary vascular resistance and thus reduce cardiac output. This effect is probably least when the lungs are stiff. The fall in cardiac output can be ameliorated by expanding the circulating volume, although in some cases inotropic support may be required. Thus, although arterial oxygenation is often improved by the application of PEEP, a simultaneous fall in cardiac output can lead to a reduction in total oxygen delivery.

PEEP should be considered if it proves difficult to achieve adequate oxygenation of arterial blood (more than 90% saturation) without raising the inspired oxygen concentration to potentially dangerous levels (conventionally 50%). Most recommend that end-expiratory pressures of 15 cmH_2O should not be exceeded. Many use lower levels of PEEP (5–7 cmH_2O) in the majority of mechanically ventilated patients in order to maintain lung volume.

Other techniques for respiratory support
Continuous positive airway pressure (CPAP)

The application of CPAP achieves for the spontaneously breathing patient what PEEP does for the ventilated patient. Oxygen and air are delivered under pressure via an endotracheal tube, a tracheostomy or a tightly fitting face mask. Not only can this improve oxygenation, but the lungs become less stiff, and the work of breathing is reduced.

Pressure support ventilation (PSV)

Spontaneous breaths are augmented by a pre-set level of positive pressure (usually between 5 and 20 cmH_2O) triggered by the patient's spontaneous respiratory effort and applied until inspiratory flow falls below a certain level. Tidal volume is determined by the set pressure, the patient's effort and pulmonary mechanics. The level of pressure support can be reduced progressively as the patient improves.

Intermittent mandatory ventilation (IMV)

This technique allows the patient to breathe spontaneously between the 'mandatory' tidal volumes delivered by the ventilator. These mandatory breaths are timed to coincide with the patient's own inspiratory effort (synchronized IMV, or SIMV). SIMV can be used with or without CPAP and spontaneous breaths may be assisted with pressure support. SIMV is used extensively as an alternative to CMV.

'Lung-protective' ventilatory strategies

These are designed to avoid exacerbating or perpetuating lung injury by avoiding overdistension of alveoli, minimizing airway pressures and preventing the repeated opening and closure of distal airways. Alveolar volume is maintained with PEEP, and sometimes by prolonging the inspiratory phase, while tidal volumes are limited to 4–8 mL/kg in order to achieve a plateau airway pressure of 30 cmH$_2$O or less. Peak airway pressures should not exceed 35–40 cmH$_2$O. An alternative is to deliver a constant pre-set inspiratory pressure for a prescribed time in order to generate a low tidal volume at reduced airway pressures ('pressure-limited' mechanical ventilation). Respiratory rate can be increased to improve CO$_2$ removal and avoid severe acidosis (pH < 7.2), but hypercarbia is frequent and should be accepted ('permissive hypercarbia'). Both techniques can be used with SIMV. Ventilation with low tidal volumes has been shown to improve outcome in patients with acute lung injury (ALI) or the acute respiratory distress syndrome (ARDS) (see p. 951).

Extracorporeal gas exchange (ECGE)

In patients with severe refractory respiratory failure veno-venous bypass through a membrane lung (extracorporeal membrane oxygenation – ECMO, or extracorporeal carbon dioxide removal – ECCO$_2$R) can be used to reduce ventilation requirements, thereby minimizing further ventilation-induced lung damage and encouraging resolution of the lung injury. Although randomized controlled trials have indicated that this technique does not improve outcome in adults, some authorities remain convinced that, when used by experienced teams in specialist centres, extracorporeal gas exchange can significantly reduce the high mortality associated with severe ARDS.

Non-invasive ventilation (NIV)

Non-invasive respiratory support is only suitable for patients who are conscious, cooperative and able to protect their airway; they must also be able to expectorate effectively. Positive pressure is applied to the airways using a tight-fitting face or nasal mask so that tracheal intubation is avoided. Techniques include mask CPAP, pressure support ventilation, positive-pressure ventilation or bilevel positive airway pressure (BiPAP). With the latter technique, inspiratory and expiratory pressure levels and times are set independently and unrestricted spontaneous respiration is possible throughout the respiratory cycle. BiPAP can also be patient triggered. There is a reduced risk of ventilator-associated pneumonia and improved patient comfort, with preservation of airway defence mechanisms, speech and swallowing. Spontaneous coughing and expectoration are not hampered and sedation may be avoided. Institution of non-invasive respiratory support can rest the respiratory muscles, reduce respiratory acidosis and breathlessness, improve clearance of secretions and re-expand collapsed lung segments. The intubation rate, length of ICU and hospital stay and, in some categories of patient, mortality may all be reduced. NIV is useful in acute hypercapnic respiratory failure associated with COPD, provided the patient is not profoundly hypoxic, and in patients with acute hypoxaemic respiratory failure due, for example, to community-acquired pneumonia. NIV may also be useful as a means of avoiding tracheal intubation in immunocompromised patients with acute respiratory failure and as an aid to weaning. Non-invasive techniques can be used for the long-term support of patients with chronic respiratory failure.

Weaning

Weakness and wasting of respiratory muscles is an inevitable consequence of the catabolic response to critical illness and may be exacerbated by the reduction in respiratory work during mechanical ventilation. Often abnormalities of gas exchange and lung mechanics persist. Not surprisingly, therefore, many patients experience difficulty in resuming spontaneous ventilation. In a significant proportion of patients who have undergone a prolonged period of respiratory support the situation is further complicated by the development of a neuropathy, a myopathy or both.

Critical illness polyneuropathy/myopathy

This acquired polyneuropathy has most often been described in association with persistent sepsis and multiple organ failure (see below). It is characterized by a primary axonal neuropathy involving both motor and, to a lesser extent, sensory nerves. Clinically the initial manifestation is often difficulty in weaning the patient from respiratory support. There is muscle wasting, the limbs are weak and flaccid, and deep tendon reflexes are reduced or absent. Cranial nerves are relatively spared. Nerve conduction studies confirm axonal damage. The cerebrospinal fluid (CSF) protein concentration is normal or minimally elevated. These findings differentiate critical illness neuropathy from Guillain–Barré syndrome, in which nerve conduction studies show evidence of demyelination and CSF protein is usually high.

The cause of critical illness polyneuropathy is not known and there is no specific treatment. With resolution of the underlying critical illness, recovery can be expected after 1–6 months, although weaning from respiratory support and rehabilitation are likely to be prolonged.

Critical illness can also be complicated by various myopathies, including a severe quadriplegic myopathy, which have been particularly associated with the administration of steroids and muscle relaxants to mechanically ventilated patients with acute, severe asthma. Often the most severely ill patients will have a combined neuropathy and myopathy.

Criteria for weaning patients from mechanical ventilation

Clinical assessment is of paramount importance when deciding whether a patient can be weaned from the ventilator. The patient's conscious level, psychological state, metabolic function, the effects of drugs and cardiovascular performance must all be taken into account. Objective criteria are based on an assessment of pulmonary gas exchange (blood gas analysis), lung mechanics and muscular strength.

Techniques for weaning

Patients who have received mechanical ventilation for less than 24 hours – for example, after elective major surgery – can usually resume spontaneous respiration immediately and no weaning process is required. This procedure can also be adopted for those who have been ventilated for longer periods but who clearly fulfil objective criteria for weaning. Methods of weaning include:

- The traditional method is to allow the patient to breathe entirely spontaneously for a short time, following which respiratory support is reinstituted. The periods of spontaneous breathing are gradually increased and the periods of respiratory support are reduced. Initially it is usually advisable to ventilate the patient throughout the night. This method can be stressful and tiring for both patients and staff, although some patients do not tolerate SIMV and the traditional method of weaning may then be necessary.
- SIMV provides a smooth, controlled method of weaning and can be commenced at an earlier stage than is possible using the traditional method. The application of inspiratory pressure support and CPAP is often used in combination with SIMV (see above).
- CPAP can prevent the alveolar collapse, hypoxaemia and fall in compliance that might otherwise occur when patients start to breathe spontaneously. It is therefore often used during weaning with SIMV/pressure support and in spontaneously breathing patients prior to extubation.
- Non-invasive ventilation via facial or nasal mask.
- BiPAP, CPAP. Tracheostomy is used frequently in critically ill patients to facilitate weaning from mechanical ventilation (see above).

Extubation

This should not be considered until patients can cough, swallow, protect their own airway and are sufficiently alert to be cooperative. Patients are assessed on their ability to breathe spontaneously via the endotracheal tube over a period of time. In those who have undergone prolonged mechanical ventilation, this period may need to be 24–48 hours, or even longer, while patients ventilated for less than 12–24 hours can often be extubated within 10–15 minutes. During this 'trial of spontaneous respiration' the patient should be observed closely for any signs of respiratory distress.

FURTHER READING

The Acute Respiratory Distress Syndrome Network (2000) Ventilation with lower tidal volumes as compared with traditional tidal volumes for acute lung injury and the acute respiratory distress syndrome. *New England Journal of Medicine* **342**: 1301–1308.

Brochard L, Rauss A, Benito S et al. (1994) Comparison of three methods of gradual withdrawal from ventilatory support during weaning from mechanical ventilation. *American Journal of Respiratory Critical Care Medicine* **150**: 896–903.

Confalorieri M, Potena A, Carbone G, Della Porta R, Tolley EA, Meduri GU (1999) Acute respiratory failure in patients with severe community-acquired pneumonia: a prospective evaluation of non-invasive ventilation. *American Journal of Respiratory Critical Care Medicine* **160**: 1585–1591.

Drakulovic MB, Torres A, Bauer TT, Nicolas JM, Moguè S, Ferrer M (1999) Supine body position as a risk factor for nosocomial pneumonia in mechanically ventilated patients: a randomised trial. *Lancet* **354**: 1851–1858.

Hillberg RE, Johnson DC (1997) Noninvasive ventilation. *New England Journal of Medicine* **337**: 1746–1752.

Plant PK, Owen JL, Elliott MW (2000) Early use of non-invasive ventilation for acute exacerbations of chronic obstructive pulmonary disease on general respiratory wards: a multicentre randomised controlled trial. *Lancet* **355**: 1931–1935.

Young PJ, Ridley SA (1999) Ventilator-associated pneumonia. *Anaesthesia* **54**: 1183–1197.

Acute lung injury/acute respiratory distress syndrome

Definition and causes (see Table 15.10)

Acute lung injury (ALI) and acute respiratory distress syndrome (ARDS) are diagnosed in an appropriate clinical setting with one or more recognized risk factors. ALI/ARDS can be defined as follows:

- Respiratory distress.
- Stiff lungs (reduced pulmonary compliance resulting in high inflation pressures).
- Chest radiograph: new bilateral, diffuse, patchy or homogeneous pulmonary infiltrates.
- Cardiac: no apparent cardiogenic cause of pulmonary oedema (pulmonary artery occlusion pressure < 18 mmHg if measured or no clinical evidence of left atrial hypertension).
- Gas exchange abnormalities: ALI – arterial oxygen tension/fractional inspired oxygen (P_aO_2/F_1O_2) ratio < 40 kPa (< 300 mmHg); ARDS P_aO_2/F_1O_2 (< 26.6 kPa) (< 200 mmHg) (in both cases despite normal arterial carbon dioxide tension and regardless of positive end-expiratory pressure). The criterion for arterial oxygen tension/fractional inspired oxygen is arbitrary and the value of differentiating ALI from ARDS has been questioned.

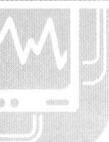

Table 15.10
Disorders associated with acute lung injury/acute respiratory distress syndrome

Indirect
Sepsis/septic shock
Systemic inflammatory response
    (e.g. pancreatitis, cardiopulmonary bypass),
    severe non-thoracic trauma, severe burns
Haematological
    Massive blood transfusion
    Transfusion reaction
    Disseminated intravascular coagulation
Obstetric
    Amniotic fluid embolism
    Eclampsia
Drug overdose
    Heroin
    Barbiturates
Miscellaneous
    High altitude

Direct
Lung contusion
Blast injury
Pneumonia
Pulmonary aspiration
    Gastric contents
    Near drowning
Inhalation injury
    Smoke
    Corrosive gases

ALI/ARDS can occur as a non-specific reaction of the lungs to a wide variety of direct and indirect pulmonary insults. By far the commonest predisposing factor is sepsis, and 20–40% of patients with severe sepsis will develop ALI/ARDS (Table 15.10).

Pathogenesis and pathophysiology of ALI/ARDS

Acute lung injury can be considered as the earliest manifestation of a generalized inflammatory response with endothelial dysfunction and is therefore frequently associated with the development of MODS.

Non-cardiogenic pulmonary oedema
This is the cardinal feature of ALI and is the first and clinically most evident sign of a generalized increase in vascular permeability caused by the microcirculatory changes and release of inflammatory mediators described previously (see p. 927), with activated neutrophils playing a particularly important role. The pulmonary epithelium is also damaged in the early stages, reducing surfactant production and lowering the threshold for alveolar flooding.

Pulmonary hypertension
This is a common feature. Initially, mechanical obstruction of the pulmonary circulation may occur as a result of

vascular compression by interstitial oedema whilst local activation of the coagulation cascade leads to thrombosis and obstruction in the pulmonary microvasculature. Later, pulmonary vasoconstriction may develop in response to increased autonomic nervous activity and circulating substances such as catecholamines, serotonin, thromboxane and complement. Those vessels supplying alveoli with low oxygen tensions constrict (the 'hypoxic vasoconstrictor response'), diverting pulmonary blood flow to better oxygenated areas of lung, thus limiting the degree of shunt.

Haemorrhagic intra-alveolar exudate
This exudate is rich in platelets, fibrin, fibrinogen and clotting factors and may inactivate surfactant and stimulate inflammation, as well as promoting hyaline membrane formation.

Fibrosis
Within days of the onset of lung injury, formation of a new epithelial lining is underway and activated fibroblasts accumulate in the interstitial spaces. Subsequently, interstitial fibrosis progresses, with loss of elastic tissue and obliteration of the lung vasculature, together with lung destruction and emphysema. In those who recover, the lungs are substantially remodelled.

Physiological changes
Shunt and deadspace increase, compliance falls, and there is evidence of airflow limitation. Although the lungs in ALI and ARDS are diffusely injured, the pulmonary lesions, when identified as densities on a CT scan, are predominantly located in dependent regions. This is partly explained by the effects of gravity on the distribution of extravascular lung water and areas of lung collapse.

Clinical presentation of ALI/ARDS

The first sign of the development of ALI/ARDS is often an unexplained tachypnoea, followed by increasing hypoxaemia, with central cyanosis, and breathlessness. Fine crackles are heard throughout both lung fields. Later, the chest X-ray shows bilateral diffuse shadowing, interstitial at first, but subsequently with an alveolar pattern and air bronchograms that may then progress to the picture of complete 'white-out' (Fig. 15.23). The differential diagnosis includes cardiac failure and pneumonia.

Management of ALI/ARDS

This is based on treatment of the underlying condition (e.g. eradication of sepsis), avoidance of complications such as ventilator-associated pneumonia, and supportive measures.

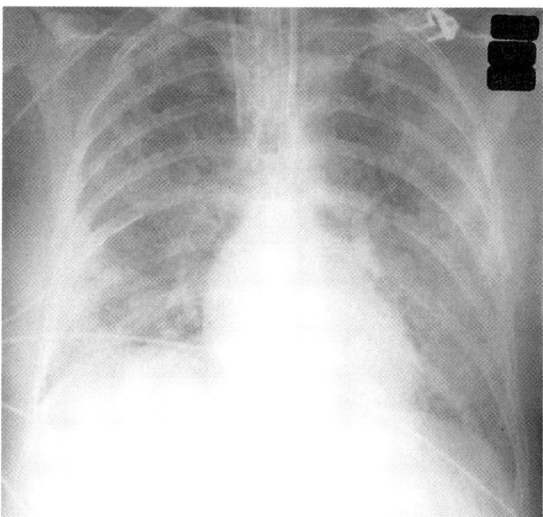

Fig. 15.23 Chest radiograph appearances in adult respiratory distress syndrome. Bilateral diffuse alveolar shadowing with air bronchograms and no cardiac enlargement.

Mechanical ventilation

Strategies designed to minimize ventilator-induced lung injury and encourage lung healing should be used (see p. 949).

Pulmonary oedema limitation. Pulmonary oedema formation should be limited by minimizing left ventricular filling pressure with fluid restriction, the use of diuretics and, if these measures fail, preventing fluid overload by haemofiltration. The aim should be to achieve a consistently negative fluid balance. If possible, plasma oncotic pressure should be maintained by using colloidal solutions to expand the intravascular volume. In patients with ALI/ARDS, however, colloids are unlikely to be retained within the vascular compartment; once they enter the interstitial space, the transvascular oncotic gradient is lost and the main determinants of interstitial oedema formation become the microvascular hydrostatic pressure and lymphatic drainage. There is therefore some controversy concerning the relative merits of colloids or crystalloids for volume replacement in patients likely to develop ALI/ARDS, or in whom the condition is established. Cardiovascular support and the reduction of oxygen requirements are also important.

Prone position. When the patient is changed from the supine to the prone position lung densities in the dependent region are redistributed and shunt fraction is reduced. A reduced pleural pressure gradient, more uniform alveolar ventilation, caudal movement of the diaphragm, redistribution of perfusion and recruitment of collapsed alveoli may all contribute to the improvement in gas exchange. Body position changes can be achieved with minimal complications despite the presence of multiple indwelling vascular lines. Repeated position changes between prone and supine may allow reductions in airway pressures and the inspired oxygen fraction. The response to prone positioning is, however, variable and it seems that this strategy does not improve overall outcome.

Inhaled nitric oxide. This vasodilator, when inhaled, can improve $\dot{V}/\dot{Q}$ matching by increasing perfusion of ventilated lung units, as well as reducing pulmonary hypertension. It has been shown to improve oxygenation in so-called responders with ALI/ARDS but so far has not been shown to increase survival. Its administration requires specialized monitoring equipment, as products of its combination with oxygen include toxic nitrogen dioxide.

Aerosolized prostacyclin. This appears to have similar effects to inhaled NO. As with inhaled NO, the response to aerosolized prostacyclin is, however, variable and although it has been shown to improve oxygenation its effect on outcome has yet to be established.

Aerosolized surfactant. Surfactant replacement therapy reduces morbidity and mortality in neonatal respiratory distress syndrome and is beneficial in animal models of ALI/ARDS. In adults with ARDS, however, the value of surfactant administration remains uncertain.

High-dose steroids. Administration of high-dose steroids to patients with established ALI/ARDS does not appear to improve outcome, and current evidence suggests that prophylactic administration to those at risk is of no value. There is, however, some anecdotal evidence that the administration of corticosteroids to patients in the fibroproliferative stage of the disease (e.g. 10–14 days after the onset) may reduce mortality, provided there is no evidence of infection.

Prognosis

There is increasing evidence that mortality from ALI/ARDS has fallen over the last decade, from around 60% to between 30 and 40%, perhaps as a consequence of improved general care, the increasing use of management protocols, and attention to infection control and nutrition, as well as the introduction of novel treatments and lung-protective strategies for respiratory support. Prognosis is, however, still very dependent on aetiology. When ARDS occurs in association with intra-abdominal sepsis, mortality rates remain very high, whereas much lower mortality rates are to be expected in those with 'primary' ARDS (pneumonia, aspiration, lung contusion). Mortality rises with increasing age and failure of other organs. Most of those dying with ARDS now do so as a result of MODS and haemodynamic instability rather than impaired gas exchange.

FURTHER READING

Ware LB, Matthay MA (2000) The acute respiratory distress syndrome. *New England Journal of Medicine* **342**: 1334–1349.

Wyncoll DLA, Evans TW (1999) Acute respiratory distress syndrome. *Lancet* **354**: 497–501.

Patient selection – denying, limiting and withdrawing treatment

For many critically ill patients, intensive care is undoubtedly life-saving and resumption of a normal lifestyle is to be expected. In the most seriously ill patients, however, immediate mortality rates are high, a significant number die soon after discharge from the intensive care unit, and the quality of life for some of those who do survive may be poor. Moreover, intensive care is expensive, particularly for those with the worst prognosis, and resources are limited.

Inappropriate use of intensive care facilities has other implications. The patient may experience unnecessary suffering and loss of dignity, while relatives may also have to endure considerable emotional pressures. In some cases treatment may simply prolong the process of dying, or sustain life of dubious quality, and in others the risk of interventions may outweigh the potential benefits.

Both for a humane approach to the management of critically ill patients and to ensure that limited resources are used appropriately, it is therefore important to avoid admitting patients who cannot benefit from intensive care and to limit further aggressive therapy when the prognosis is clearly hopeless. Needless to say such decisions can be extremely difficult and every case must be assessed individually, taking into account the patient's previous health and quality of life, the primary diagnosis, the medium- and long-term prognosis of the underlying condition (both in terms of survival and quality of life) and the survivability of the acute illness. Age alone should not be a consideration. When in doubt, active measures should continue but should be reviewed regularly in the light of response to treatment and any further information which may become available. Decisions to limit therapy, not to resuscitate in the event of cardiorespiratory arrest, or to withdraw treatment should be made jointly by the medical staff of the unit, the primary physician or surgeon, the nurses and if possible the patient, normally in consultation with the patient's family. Withdrawal or limitation of active treatment should not be viewed negatively as the cessation of all medical or nursing care. Rather a positive approach should be adopted to ensuring that the patient dies with dignity, free of pain and distress, and that family and friends receive support and comfort.

Scoring systems

A variety of scoring systems have been developed that can be used to evaluate the severity of a patient's illness. Some have included an assessment of the patient's previous state of health and the severity of the acute disturbance of physiological function (acute physiology, age, chronic health evaluation – APACHE, and simplified acute physiology score – SAPS). Other systems have been designed for particular categories of patient (e.g. the injury severity score for trauma victims).

The APACHE and SAPS scores are widely applicable and have been extensively validated. They can quantify accurately the severity of illness and predict the overall mortality for large groups of critically ill patients, and are therefore useful for defining the 'casemix' of patients when auditing a unit's clinical activity, for comparing results nationally or internationally, and as a means of characterizing groups of patients in clinical studies. Although the APACHE and SAPS methodologies can also be used to estimate risks of mortality, no scoring system has yet been devised that can predict with certainty the outcome in an individual patient. They must not, therefore, be used in isolation as a basis for limiting or discontinuing treatment.

The Therapeutic Intervention Scoring System (TISS) scores interventions and nursing activities for each day of admission. Such information may provide estimates of resource consumption and indices of nursing dependency. This may not only be related to prognosis but can also be used to estimate costs. Current estimates of daily costs of intensive care in the UK vary from £800–1600; high dependency and ward care costs are approximately 50% and 20% of intensive care budgets respectively.

FURTHER READING

Bion J (1995) Rationing intensive care. *British Medical Journal* **310**: 682–683.

Knaus WA, Wagner DP, Draper EA et al. (1991) The APACHE III prognostic system: risk prediction of hospital mortality for critically ill hospitalized adults. *Chest* **100**: 1619–1636.

Brain death

Brain death means 'the irreversible loss of the capacity for consciousness combined with the irreversible loss of the capacity to breathe'. Both these are essentially functions of the brainstem. Death, if thought of in this way, can arise either from causes outside the brain (i.e. respiratory and cardiac arrest) or from causes within the cranial cavity. With the advent of artificial ventilation it became possible to support such a dead patient temporarily, although in all cases cardiovascular failure eventually supervenes and progresses to asystole.

Before considering a diagnosis of brainstem death it is essential that certain preconditions and exclusions be fulfilled.

Preconditions

- The patient must be in apnoeic coma (i.e. unresponsive and on a ventilator, with no spontaneous respiratory efforts).

- Irremediable structural brain damage due to a disorder that can cause brainstem death must have been diagnosed with certainty (e.g. head injury, intracranial haemorrhage).

Exclusions

- The possibility that unresponsive apnoea is the result of poisoning, sedative drugs or neuromuscular blocking agents must be excluded.
- Hypothermia must be excluded as a cause of coma. The central body temperature should be more than 35°C.
- There must be no significant metabolic or endocrine disturbance that could produce or contribute to coma or cause it to persist.
- There should be no profound abnormality of the plasma electrolytes, acid–base balance, or blood glucose levels.

Diagnostic tests for the confirmation of brain death

All brainstem reflexes are absent in brain death.

Tests

The following tests should not be performed in the presence of seizures or abnormal postures.

- Oculocephalic reflexes should be absent: when the head is rotated from side to side, the eyes move with the head and therefore remain stationary relative to the orbit. In a comatose patient whose brainstem is intact, the eyes will rotate relative to the orbit (i.e. doll's eye movements will be present).
- The pupils are fixed and unresponsive to bright light. Both direct and consensual light reflexes are absent. The size of the pupils is irrelevant, although most often they will be dilated.
- Corneal reflexes are absent.
- There are no vestibulo-ocular reflexes on caloric testing (see p. 1140).
- There is no motor response within the cranial nerve territory to painful stimuli applied centrally or peripherally. Spinal reflexes may be present.

- There is no gag or cough reflex in response to pharyngeal, laryngeal or tracheal stimulation.
- Spontaneous respiration is absent. The patient should be ventilated with 5% CO_2 in 95% O_2 for 10 minutes and then temporarily disconnected from the ventilator for up to 10 minutes. Oxygenation is maintained by insufflation with 100% oxygen via a catheter placed in the endotracheal tube. The patient is observed for any signs of spontaneous respiratory efforts. A blood gas sample should be obtained during this period to ensure that the $P_a CO_2$ is sufficiently high to stimulate spontaneous respiration (> 6.7 kPa (50 mmHg)).

The examination should be performed and repeated by two senior doctors.

In the UK it is not considered necessary to perform confirmatory tests such as EEG and carotid angiography.

The primary purpose of establishing a diagnosis of brainstem death is to demonstrate beyond doubt that it is futile to continue mechanical ventilation and other life-supporting measures.

In suitable cases, and provided the assent of relatives has been obtained (easier if the patient was carrying an organ donor card), the organs of those in whom brainstem death has been established may be used for transplantation. In the UK each region has a transplant coordinator who can help with the process, as well as providing information, training and advice about organ donation. They should be informed of all potential donors. In all cases in the UK the coroner's consent must be obtained.

FURTHER READING

Pallis C, Harley DH (1996) *ABC of Brain Death*, 2nd edn. London: BMJ Publishing Group.
Wijdicks EF (2001) The diagnosis of brain death. *New England Journal of Medicine* **344**: 1215–1221.

GENERAL FURTHER READING

Hinds CJ, Watson JD (1994) *Intensive Care: A Concise Textbook*. London: Baillière Tindall.

Drug therapy and poisoning 16

Drug therapy

The principles of drug therapy

Introduction

In order to use drugs safely and effectively, the clinician needs to have an understanding of the best way to administer drugs to patients, and how to get the right amount of drug at the target tissue. To achieve this it is necessary to have some knowledge of how the body handles drugs, (*pharmacokinetics*). Knowledge of how drugs work at a cellular and molecular level (*pharmacodynamics*) is also useful in predicting drug interactions, drug adverse effects and the consequences of overdose.

How the body handles drugs

Understanding of pharmacokinetic principles is essential in determining the dosage interval of drugs, and how to modify the dose of oral and intravenous drugs to obtain optimum therapeutic plasma concentrations and avoid drug toxicity (see Fig. 16.1).

Pharmacokinetics is divided into four main processes: absorption, distribution, metabolism and elimination.

Absorption

This depends on a number of factors including formulation, route of administration, lipid solubility, and gastric acidity.

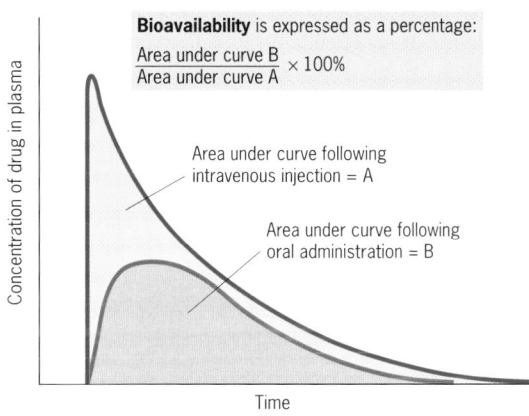

Bioavailability is expressed as a percentage:
$$\frac{\text{Area under curve B}}{\text{Area under curve A}} \times 100\%$$

Area under curve following intravenous injection = A

Area under curve following oral administration = B

Fig. 16.1 Bioavailability of drugs. Graph showing the concentration of a drug in the plasma following intravenous (A) and oral (B) administration.

Formulation is the way that a drug is packaged. In most drugs the active agent represents only a small proportion of the total weight of the tablet or capsule, which may also contain diluents, lubricating or disintegrating agents which may affect absorption. With some drugs, such as digoxin and ciclosporin, and sustained-release products absorption is affected by the formulation used, and in this case the exact manufacturer should be specified to ensure similar effects.

Route of administration. Drugs are usually given orally but can also be given by many other routes, e.g. intravenous, intramuscular, transdermal, buccal, rectal, intrapulmonary. These routes can bypass the 'first-pass metabolism' in the liver, leading to enhanced bioavailability. Bioavailability is the term used to describe how much of an orally administered drug gets into the general circulation and is calculated as shown in Figure 16.1.

Lipid solubility. Drugs are absorbed across membranes more easily if they are lipid-soluble. Most drugs are weak acids or weak bases and exist in two forms: ions and undissociated molecules. Absorption depends on the dissociation constant (pK) of the drug and the surrounding pH. Weak acids such as aspirin will be better absorbed from the stomach as the acid environment ensures that most of the drug is unionized and therefore lipid-soluble. Basic drugs are largely ionized at the pH of the stomach and therefore less well absorbed. Nevertheless many drugs are absorbed well in the small bowel where they are present for a longer duration.

Distribution

Distribution of a drug refers to its movement to tissues other than the blood plasma, principally into extravascular fluid and into cells. V_d is the apparent volume into which the drug has been dissolved and is equal to the total amount of drugs in the body divided by the drug concentration in the plasma. Highly lipid-soluble drugs such as glyceryl trinitrate and anaesthetic gases rapidly diffuse into fatty tissue resulting in a low plasma concentration and hence a high V_d. Many drugs bind strongly to plasma proteins (Box 16.1), which inhibits diffusion of drugs outside the vascular compartments.

Metabolism

Metabolism of drugs occurs principally in the liver. This means that impaired liver function will impair metabolism and increase the potential toxicity of many drugs. As all of the portal circulation passes through the liver, some drugs (see Box 16.2) are extensively metabolized before they reach the systemic circulation, and their oral dose needs to be higher than the parenteral dose to achieve similar plasma concentrations. This phenomenon is known as presystemic or 'first-pass' metabolism.

Liver drug metabolism occurs in two stages:

- *Phase I* is the modification of the drug, by oxidation, reduction or hydrolysis, by a family of enzymes known as cytochrome p450 enzymes (see p. 964).
- *Phase II* is the conjugation of the resulting molecule with glucuronic acid, sulphate, acetate or other substances to render it more soluble and therefore able to be excreted in the urine. The amount of cytochrome p450 enzymes can be affected by certain drugs. Anticonvulsants such as barbiturates and phenytoin have the property of increasing the amount of these enzymes, whereas other drugs such as erythromycin and cimetidine reduce them. Cytochrome p450 enzyme induction and inhibition is a major cause of drug interactions (see Table 16.3).

Some drugs are inactive in the form in which they are normally administered, but are activated by hepatic or cellular metabolism. These are known as pro-drugs and some examples are given in Box 16.3.

Box 16.2

Drugs which have extensive pre-systemic (first-pass) metabolism

- Verapamil
- Propranolol
- Lidocaine (lignocaine)
- Glyceryl trinitrate
- Isosorbide dinitrate
- Morphine
- Pethidine
- Clomethiazole

There is a risk of overdose with these drugs in patients with hepatic failure.

Box 16.1

Protein binding

Most drugs are bound to plasma proteins, particularly albumin. This inhibits the passage of drugs outside the circulation and prevents glomerular filtration and excretion in urine. Drugs can be displaced from their protein binding site by another drug, but this normally has little clinical effect on plasma concentration because the free drug is rapidly redistributed in the interstitial fluid and excreted in the urine.

Box 16.3

Examples of pro-drugs

Form administered	Metabolized to
Enalapril	Enalaprilat
Minoxidil	Minoxidil sulphate
Glyceryl trinitrate	Nitric oxide
Ganciclovir	Ganciclovir phosphate
Azathioprine	6-Mercaptopurine

Other drugs, such as benzodiazepines are metabolized to pharmacologically active molecules, which may greatly increase their effective duration of action. Diazepam (half-life 43 hours) is converted to desmethyldiazepam which has a half-life of over 70 hours.

Elimination

Elimination of most drugs is principally via the kidney, either the parent drug if it is water-soluble, or the conjugated drug if it is lipid-soluble. Extreme care should be taken in prescribing for patients with renal impairment; serious toxicity may occur with drugs such as digoxin and gentamicin. Most drugs are secreted in small amounts in other body fluids such as sweat and breast milk (see p. 955).

Kinetics of drug metabolism and elimination

First order kinetics. The rate at which a drug is metabolized and eliminated is generally proportional to the dose given. Elimination itself depends both on clearance and the volume of distribution. With most drugs there is an exponential reduction in plasma concentration with time and these drugs obey 'first-order kinetics'. The time required to decrease the plasma concentration of the drug by half is the plasma half-life ($t_{1/2}$) (Fig. 16.2). Thus for any drug that has 'first-order' elimination, by the end of the first half-life the drug will be reduced by 50%, by the end of the second half-life by 25%, and so on. Drugs can thus be considered to be eliminated after 3–5 half lives.

Zero-order kinetics. With drugs obeying zero-order kinetics, e.g. ethanol, phenytoin, the body can only eliminate a certain amount of a drug over a period of time as their enzyme metabolism is saturable. Thus the rate of metabolism is independent of the drug concentration, i.e. a small increase in the administered drug produces a large increase in plasma concentration which could lead to toxicity.

Mechanisms of drug action (pharmacodynamics)

Most drugs affect the normal functioning of mammalian cells or disrupt the normal function of pathogens. There are a limited number of ways which drugs can interact with mammalian cells, the most common are:

- binding to specialized receptors (Fig. 16.3; see also p. 156)
- inhibition of enzyme function (see p. 964)
- blocking or opening of membrane ion channels (see p. 155).

Some commonly used drugs, such as insulin, thyroxine and vitamins are essentially replacement therapies.

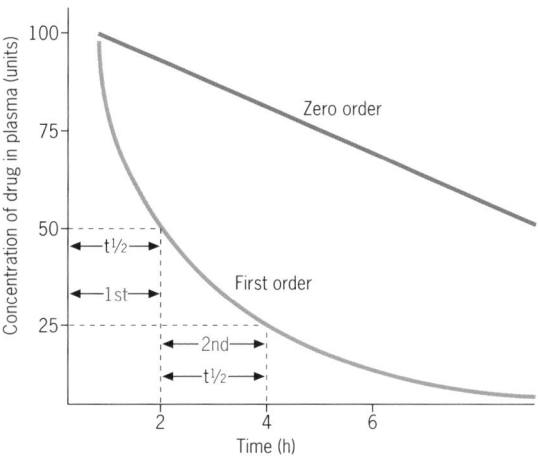

Fig. 16.2 **Kinetics of drug metabolism and elimination.** Most drugs are eliminated by a first-order process, with some exponential reduction in plasma concentration with time. Some substances, such as ethanol, are eliminated by a zero-order process, which means that the rate of metabolism is independent of drug concentration.

Increasingly, drugs are being developed with novel modes of action, such as monoclonal antibodies which bind to specific endogenous proteins (such as abciximab which inactivates glycoprotein IIa/IIIb on the surface of platelets) or the currently experimental gene therapies designed to replace defective or missing genes (see p. 467).

Anticancer (cytotoxic) drugs are effective because malignant cells lack some of the protective mechanisms which prevent healthy cells dividing when they are damaged. Most of these drugs damage or alter DNA. Healthy cells respond to this damage by stopping dividing, or undergoing apoptosis (programmed cell death, p. 162). Cancer cells have several defective genes (such as that which produces p53 protein) which allow cells to continue to divide in the face of drugs which cause DNA damage. Dividing cells are much more vulnerable to these damaging agents, which explains the selectivity of cytotoxic drugs towards cancer cells.

Antibiotics and antiviral drugs

Drugs which are effective in killing or preventing replication of pathogens must have a selective toxicity towards that organism. In the case of bacteria, there are several structural and biochemical differences between prokaryotic and eukaryotic cells which have been exploited as drug targets (see Fig. 16.4). In the case of antiviral agents, it has been much more difficult to find such targets, as viruses use mammalian cell biochemical pathways to replicate their genetic material and synthesize protein. Attack on these pathways is likely to cause damage to the host cell machinery.

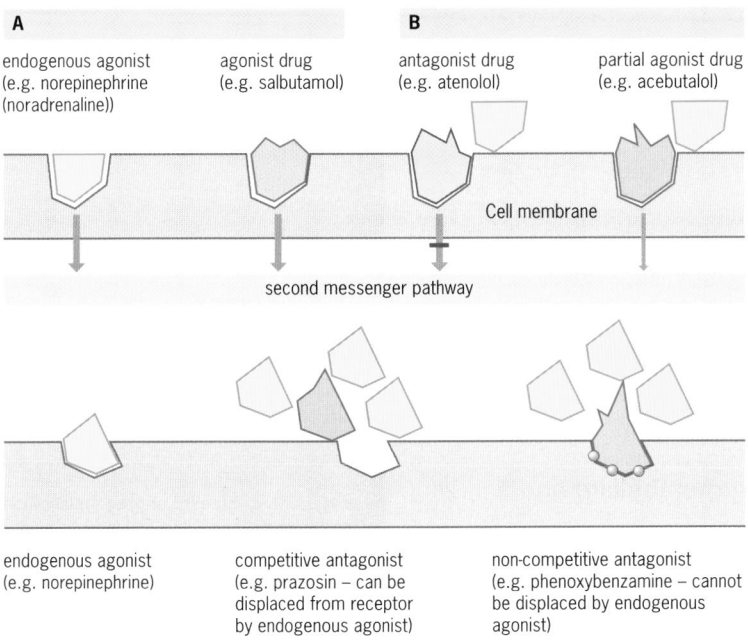

Fig. 16.3 **Drug–receptor interaction. (A)** An **agonist** (either endogenous or drug) binds to a receptor, activating a second-messenger pathway. **(B)** An **antagonist** binds to a receptor but does not activate the second-messenger pathway and also prevents any other ligand binding to the receptor (competitively or non-competitively). A **partial agonist** binds to a receptor but only partially stimulates the second-messenger pathway and also prevents an endogenous agonist binding to this receptor.

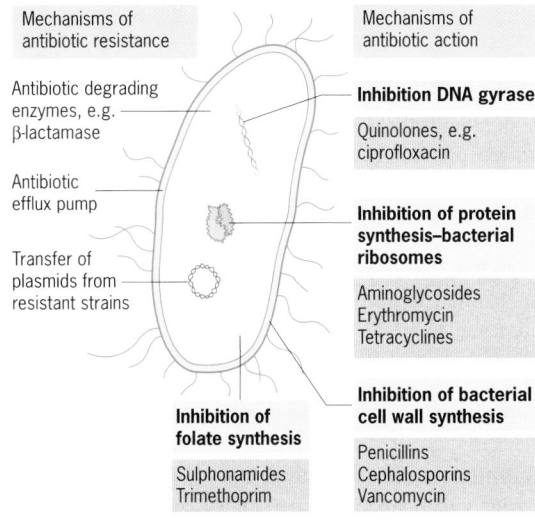

Fig. 16.4 **Mechanisms of antibiotic action and resistance** (see also Fig. 2.4).

Adverse effects of drugs

All drugs which have a proven therapeutic benefit may cause adverse effects. Despite this, a large number of effective drugs produce no adverse effects in the vast majority of patients who take them. This is in part due to the pressures on pharmaceutical companies to produce safe and effective medicines, but also due to increasingly stringent governmental regulations which regulate the use of new drugs, and organizations which monitor the safety of existing compounds. New drugs are now subjected to a rigorous programme of preclinical and clinical testing (see p. 961) before they are licensed for general use (Table 16.1) and are also monitored for safety following licensing.

The size of the problem

Overall, approximately 10–20% of hospital inpatients suffer an adverse drug reaction. Up to 5% of hospital admissions are directly due to adverse drug reactions and about 0.25–0.5% of deaths are attributable to treatment rather than the disease for which the drugs were being used. Unwanted effects of drugs are more common in elderly patients, rising from 3% in 10- to 20-year-olds to 20% in patients over 80 years. The likelihood of adverse reactions increases sharply with the number of drugs administered (Fig. 16.5), partly because such patients are likely to be more unwell, provoking a drug–host reaction, and partly because the potential for drug–drug interaction increases in a factorial manner with each new drug which is added to the regimen.

Types of adverse drug reactions

There are two main types of adverse drug reactions:

- dose-dependent (also called type A, augmented, predictable)
- dose-independent (type B, bizarre, unpredictable, idosyncratic).

Table 16.1
Evaluation of new drugs

Phase 1
Healthy human subjects (usually men)
First use in man
Evaluation of safety and toxicity
Pharmacokinetic assessment
Sometimes pharmacodynamic assessment
Approximately 100 subjects

Phase II
First assessment in patients
Safety and toxicity evaluated
Dose range identified
Pharmacokinetic and pharmacodynamic monitoring
Approximately 500 subjects

Phase III
Use in wider patient population
Efficacy main objective
Safety and toxicity also carefully monitored
Often multicentre trials
Approximately 2000 patients involved

Phase IV
Postmarketing surveillance
All patients prescribed drug monitored
Efficacy, safety and toxicity measured
Quantification of unusual drug adverse effects
Yellow card and Prescription Event Monitoring
Often very large numbers of patients observed

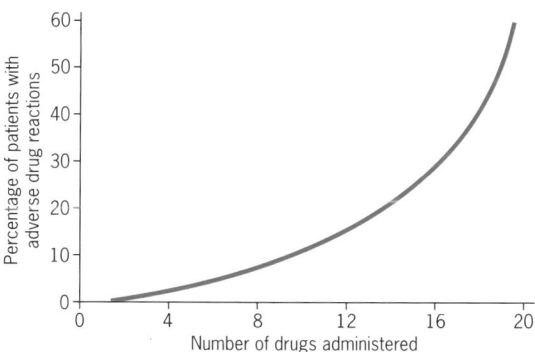

Fig. 16.5 Adverse drug reactions. The number of adverse drug reactions increases with the number of drugs administered. After Smith JW et al. (1966) *Annals of Internal Medicine* **65**: 631.

Dose-dependent reactions

These often result from the known pharmacological effect of the drug and are increasingly likely as the dose is increased. Good examples of such a reaction is gout resulting from treatment with a thiazide diuretic or bone marrow suppression following therapy with methotrexate. As a general rule, dose-dependent reactions are less serious and rapidly resolve on stopping the drug. However, some dose-dependent reactions such as eighth nerve damage with aminoglycoside antibiotics or myocardial damage following doxorubicin therapy are serious, largely irreversible and are due to mechanisms which are not completely understood.

Dose-independent reactions

In these reactions there is a large variability between individuals in their susceptibility to an adverse effect; many different mechanisms operate, most of which are not understood. The adverse reactions are often serious and life-threatening; patients should be warned about particular symptoms suggestive of such an adverse reaction.

Anaphylactic reactions (type I hypersensitivity)

These are more common in patients with a history of anaphylaxis with drugs, foods (such as nuts) or insect stings and in atopic individuals with a history of asthma and eczema.

Typically anaphylaxis occurs on the second or third exposure to the drug, and may occur following administration of only very small amounts. The mechanism involves recognition of the drug (or a drug–protein complex) by IgE molecules on the surface of mast cells and subsequent degranulation with release of histamine and other inflammatory mediators.

The onset of the clinical syndrome of anaphylaxis is often dramatic and rapid. Prompt recognition and treatment can be life-saving (Emergency box 16.1).

! Emergency box 16.1

Anaphylactic shock

Usually follows injections or occasionally insect bites or nut ingestion.

Clinical features (rapid and dramatic)
- Bronchospasm causing breathlessness
- Facial and laryngeal oedema
- Hypotension causing dizziness and collapse
- Nausea, vomiting and diarrhoea

Treatment
Lay patient down with feet raised.
Ensure airway free.
Monitor blood pressure.
Establish venous access.
Give oxygen.
Give (in following order):

1. 0.5 mL of 1 in 1000 epinephrine (adrenaline) intramuscularly (0.5 mg) – repeat after 5 minutes if shock persists
2. Antihistamine (such as chlorphenamine (chlorpheniramine) 10 mg) by slow intravenous injection continuing for 48 h
3. Hydrocortisone 100 mg intravenously.

If hypotension persists, give rapid intravenous infusion (colloid is better than crystalloid fluids) 1–2 litres.

If hypoxia is severe, assisted ventilation may be necessary.

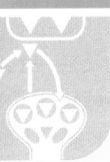

Penicillin antibiotics are notorious for causing ana-phylaxis, even though the incidence of severe reactions is very low. Other likely causes are radio-opaque contrast media, local anaesthetics and streptomycin.

Type II reactions (p. 216)

These reactions occur because of interaction of the drug and a circulating or membrane-bound protein (see drug-induced haemolytic anaemia, p. 437) to cause production of a circulating antibody of the IgG or IgM class with subsequent complement activation. The most common target for this type of immune-mediated damage is the haematological system resulting in Coombs-positive haemolytic anaemia (e.g. with methyldopa and penicillin) or thrombocytopenia (e.g. with quinine). It is likely that some examples of agranulocytosis or marrow aplasia are due to this mechanism of adverse reaction.

Type III (Arthus, serum sickness or immune complex) reaction (p. 218)

This type of reaction used to occur most commonly following injection of foreign serum to treat infectious diseases (e.g. antitetanus serum). It also occurs with antibiotics such as penicillins, streptomycin and sulphonamides as well as with the antithyroid drugs propylthiouracil and carbimazole. It is thought to be caused by the formation of antibody–antigen complexes which lodge in the small blood vessels of the skin, kidney and joints, and may mimic systemic lupus erythematosus, in which such complexes are also found (see p. 558).

The classic clinical presentation occurs several days after starting therapy and includes fever, urticaria, arthropathy, lymphadenopathy and proteinuria. Eosinophilia is a common and diagnostically useful feature. Other skin rashes, particularly maculopapular in type are also characteristic.

Type IV reactions (cell-mediated hypersensitivity) (p. 214)

The typical example of a type IV reaction is the contact dermatitis which is sometimes produced following application of antibiotic or other topical therapy on the skin. It is thought to be due to the formation of hapten–protein complexes which trigger a lymphocytic cellular immune reaction.

Pseudoallergic reactions

These reactions mimic those detailed above, but are not thought to involve immune recognition. They are due to release of immunological mediators by other mechanisms. They typically occur on first-time exposure to the drug rather than after previous sensitization. Examples of this type of reaction include:

- itching, bronchospasm and vasodilatation following treatment with intravenous morphine
- flushing, urticaria, bronchospasm and even circulatory shock caused by aspirin
- bronchospasm and hypotension caused by N-acetylcysteine used in the treatment of paracetamol poisoning. This occurs in approximately 5% of patients and responds to intravenous antihistamines.

Long-term adverse effects of drugs

Adverse effects which occur months or years after institution of a particular drug therapy may not obviously be connected with the agent responsible and will only be discovered by taking a careful drug history. Some of these long-term effects are dose-dependent and can be anticipated (such as movement disorders with neuroleptic agents) whereas others are idiosyncratic (such as pulmonary fibrosis with amiodarone). Table 16.2 details some of the more common long-term effects of drugs.

Carcinogenesis

Certain drugs which damage DNA predispose towards cancer. Many cancers are due to acquired defects in tumour suppressor genes which limit cellular division (such as the p53 gene, p. 184) and oncogenes, which promote cellular growth. Most cytotoxic chemotherapy relies on its ability to damage DNA. The antitumour effect is achieved by stimulating the transcription of

Table 16.2
Delayed and long-term adverse effects of drugs

Drug	Effect	Mechanism
Corticosteroids	Osteoporosis	Protein catabolism
Anticonvulsants	Megaloblastic anaemia	Folate antagonism
Amiodarone	Pulmonary fibrosis	Unknown
Neuroleptics	Movement disorders	Probably dopamine antagonism
Thiazide diuretics	Gout	Impaired urate excretion
Methysergide	Retroperitoneal fibrosis (peri-aortitis)	Unknown
Cytotoxic drugs	Malignancy	DNA damage
Analgesics	Tubulointerstitial nephritis	Unknown
Methyldopa	Haemolytic anaemia	Immune stimulation
Hydralazine	SLE	Unknown

tumour suppressor genes in normal cells, resulting in arrested cellular division, leaving tumour cells vulnerable to the effects of DNA damage. Whereas DNA damage is often repairable, cumulative damage due to cytotoxic drugs, environmental factors and genetic predisposition may allow disabling of sufficient regulatory systems to cause uncontrolled proliferation and cancer. Examples include the increase in risk of bladder cancer in patients taking cyclophosphamide and of leukaemias in patients taking all types of alkylating agents.

Recognition of abnormal cells is one of the important functions of the immune system and powerful immunosuppressant drugs such as ciclosporin have been linked with an increase in lymphoma (although this does not seem to be as large a problem as once feared).

Cancers of the breast and endometrium are known to be hormone-dependent and there is evidence of a link between oestrogen and breast cancer, in addition to the established association between unopposed oestrogen therapy and endometrial cancer.

Factors predisposing to adverse drug effects

Prescribing factors

Serious and avoidable toxicity to patients is, and will continue to be, due to lack of care in prescribing and dispensing medication. Common causes include:

- *errors in prescribing* (poor handwriting or doctor inattention), e.g. chlorpromazine instead of chlorpropamide or milligrams instead of micrograms
- *errors in dispensing*
- *errors in administration*, e.g. extravasation or intra-arterial injection of cytotoxic drugs
- *wrong or insufficient advice given to patient* – written information such as steroid cards or anticoagulant cards are very useful to prevent problems.

Drug interactions

Most patients in hospital are prescribed more than one drug and a large number of adverse drug reactions are due to drug interactions. There are a very large number of potential drug interactions, only a handful of which are commonly encountered which cause serious problems (Table 16.3). Drugs can interact to cause both inhibition and potentiation of the effect of either or both components of the interaction. Interactions causing adverse effects are due to potentiation, and are conveniently grouped according to pharmaceutic, pharmacokinetic and pharmacodynamic mechanisms.

Pharmaceutic interactions

These are due to interaction between drugs outside the body, which normally leads to inactivation of one or

Table 16.3
Some potentially serious drug interactions

Drug	Interacting drug	Problem caused
Warfarin	Cimetidine Erythromycin Ciprofloxacin Imidazoles Sulphonamides	Uncontrolled bleeding
Theophylline	Cimetidine Erythromycin Ciprofloxacin	Convulsions Arrhythmias
Digoxin	Amiodarone Verapamil Quinidine Diuretics	Arrhythmias Heart block
Beta-blockers	Verapamil Diltiazem	Bradycardia, asystole
Lithium	Thiazide diuretics	Ataxia, convulsions
Azathioprine Mercaptopurine	Allopurinol	Bone marrow failure
Phenytoin	Cimetidine Isoniazid Sulphonamides Imidazoles	Ataxia
	Oral contraceptive pill	Reduced effect

both components, for instance as a result of incompatibility of infusion solutions which leads to precipitation or inactivation of one component. An example is the co-infusion of heparin and hydrocortisone leading to the inactivation of heparin.

Pharmacokinetic interactions

These interactions can be subdivided into the familiar categories which describe the pharmacokinetic process – absorption, distribution, metabolism and elimination.

Absorption

Absorption of tetracyclines and iron supplements can be impaired by concurrent administration of calcium, aluminium and magnesium salts. Similarly, the bile salt binding resin colestyramine will also bind with other drugs such as digoxin and warfarin and inhibit their absorption. Broad-spectrum antibiotics such as amoxicillin interfere with the normal gut bacterial flora which is involved in both synthesizing vitamin K (thus causing a potentiation of the effect of warfarin) and the enterohepatic recycling of oestrogen, reducing the contraceptive effectiveness of this hormone.

Distribution

Displacement of one drug from its binding to a plasma protein or tissue by another can often be demonstrated in a test-tube, but only rarely does this mechanism lead to a clinically significant drug interaction. This is because the increased amount of free (unbound) drug is

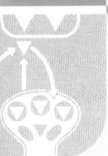

Table 16.4
Cytochrome p450 enzyme-inducing drugs

Alcohol
Carbamazepine
Griseofulvin
Phenobarbital
Phenytoin
Prednisolone
Rifampicin

now available for metabolism or excretion and there is rapid re-establishment of previous unbound concentration of drug.

The situations where clinically relevant interactions occur are when there is concomitant inhibition of metabolism or excretion alongside displacement from the binding sites. This appears to be the mechanism explaining the potentially serious interaction between quinidine and digoxin, where quinidine both displaces digoxin from its tissue binding site and impairs renal excretion.

Metabolism

Enzyme induction. Interference with liver metabolism is one of the most common causes of serious drug interaction. Drugs (Table 16.4) such as rifampicin and phenytoin cause induction of the mixed function cytochrome p450 enzymes, which are responsible for liver metabolism of most drugs, leading to more rapid destruction, reduced plasma concentrations and lack of effect of drugs which are metabolized by these enzymes, and consequent therapeutic failure. The three major drug-metabolizing enzymes of the p450 superfamily of haem protein enzyme isoforms are CYP1A2, CYP2D6 and CYP3A4, although many others are involved.

Enzyme inhibition. Serious drug interactions are often due to drugs which inhibit liver p450 enzymes. There are a limited number of such drugs, which include cimetidine, erythromycin, ciprofloxacin and sodium valproate. Not all these drugs will inhibit all p450 isoenzymes, and therefore such interactions are not entirely predictable. Some interactions in this category are given in Table 16.3 and involve drugs with a low therapeutic ratio, particularly warfarin, theophylline and phenytoin. Theophylline toxicity is commonly caused by co-administration of erythromycin or ciprofloxacin to patients with airflow obstruction and chest infection who are also prescribed theophylline or aminophylline.

Other enzymes responsible for drug metabolism can also be inhibited and result in drug interactions. The administration of the xanthine oxidase inhibitor allopurinol in patients treated with 6-mercaptopurine (6MP) or azathioprine (which is metabolized to 6MP) constitutes a potentially fatal combination as 6MP is itself metabolized by xanthine oxidase.

Elimination (p. 637)

The inhibition of renal tubular excretion of benzylpencillin by probenecid has been used as a useful drug interaction, to increase the plasma concentration of penicillin when it was first discovered and in short supply. Harmful interactions can also be caused by inhibition of renal tubular transport, as is the case with aspirin and other non-steroidal analgesics reducing methotrexate and lithium excretion. Lithium excretion is also impaired by thiazide and (to a lesser extent) loop diuretics, as a result of increased proximal resorption of monovalent cations in response to enhanced distal tubular excretion.

Pharmacodynamic interactions

The body's normal homeostatic mechanisms will often come into play to prevent a potential undesirable effect of a drug. When another drug is added which predisposes to the same unwanted effect by a different mechanism, it is much more likely that the undesired effect will happen. An example of this is the reduction in cardiac output resulting from treatment with verapamil for angina. Heart rate and contractility is maintained by upregulation of the sympathetic supply to the heart. If a β-adrenoceptor blocker is added then heart failure or symptomatic bradycardia may result.

A similar example is the profound hypotension that may follow the first dose of an ACE inhibitor in patients with heart failure who are treated with high doses of loop diuretics. Blood pressure is normally maintained in patients on loop diuretics by activation of the renin–angiotensin system which is suddenly withdrawn when ACE inhibitors are given.

Although the precise mechanisms are less clear, drugs which cause sedation or confusion will often have a synergistic effect. Well-known examples are the combination of alcohol and benzodiazepines and combination of opiates and antipsychotics leading to enhanced sedation.

Toxicity with digoxin is greatly enhanced by reduction in plasma potassium concentration, which is caused most commonly by treatment with loop and thiazide diuretics. Conversely, treatment with potassium-sparing diuretics such as amiloride or triamterene can cause serious toxicity due to hyperkalaemia when co-prescribed with ACE inhibitors.

Use of drugs in pregnancy

Pregnancy poses particular problems in the use of drugs. Most drugs will passively diffuse across the placenta and some are actively transported. The potential benefit of the drug to the mother has to be considered in relation to the potential risk to the fetus. As a general rule, all drugs should be avoided in pregnancy unless there is a compelling reason for their use. Some drugs

Table 16.5
Common adverse effects of drugs in pregnancy
All drugs should be avoided in pregnancy unless benefit clearly outweighs risk

Drug	Effect
ACE inhibitors/α-receptor antagonists	Renal damage and oligohydramnios
Retinoic acid derivatives	Multiple gross abnormalities (up to 2 years after stopping)
Alcohol	Fetal alcohol syndrome and growth retardation
	Withdrawal syndrome in newborn
Aminoglycosides	Vestibular damage (esp. streptomycin)
Amiodarone	Neonatal goitre
Warfarin	Bone abnormalities and neonatal haemorrhage
Sedatives, tranquillizers and hypnotics	Sedation or apnoea in neonate
Beta-blockers	May cause growth retardation
Carbamazepine	Neural tube defects (may be reduced with folate supplementation)
Carbimazole	Neonatal hypothyroidism
Chloramphenicol	Grey baby syndrome
Glucocorticoids	Neonatal adrenal suppression in high doses
Cytotoxic drugs	Most are potently teratogenic
NSAIDs	Delayed closure of ductus arteriosus
Opiate analgesics	Neonatal depression and withdrawal syndrome
Phenytoin	Hare lip, cleft palate and cardiac abnormalities
Antimalarial drugs	Methaemoglobinaemia and haemolysis in neonate
Stilbestrol	Vaginal carcinoma in offspring
Tetracyclines	Damage to bones and teeth
Valproate	Neural tube defects

NSAIDs, non-steroidal anti-inflammatory drugs

have been definitely linked to fetal abnormalities (Table 16.5). The safety of most drugs has not been firmly established, as the effects may not be apparent for many years after birth. The past use of stilbestrol in pregnant women with threatened abortion has resulted in adenocarcinoma of the vagina in female children developing in their teens and early twenties. This devastating adverse effect was only recognized because this is normally an extremely rare tumour. There is the possibility that use of other drugs in pregnancy predisposes to more common conditions such as diabetes or hypertension. Such an association would not be easily recognized.

Effects on fertilization and implantation

The principal mode of contraceptive action of progestogens is to prevent implantation which normally occurs between 2 and 3 weeks after fertilization. Intrauterine contraceptive devices have a similar effect. Damage to the embryo before implantation results in failure of implantation and is therefore unlikely to cause fetal abnormalities.

Effects on fetal development

The intrauterine period between 2 weeks and 3 months is when the most serious abnormalities of fetal development can be caused by drugs. It is during this period that the major organs are being formed. Even one dose of a drug administered at the critical time has been shown to have a major effect in animal studies. The mechanisms of damage are not yet known, but the molecular basis of differentiation of embryonic cells is an intense area of basic research.

Toxicity to the formed fetus

During the second and third trimester of pregnancy the fetal adverse effects of drugs administered to the mother are generally an exaggeration of effects seen in the adult. Exceptions to this rule are the damage to tissues which are still developing such as teeth and bones by tetracycline antibiotics and impairment of brain development by coumarin anticoagulants. Particular care must be taken with drugs given shortly before delivery. Analgesics such as pethidine and tranquillizers such as benzodiazepines may severely impair neonatal respiration. In addition the newborn lacks many enzymes necessary for the efficient metabolism of drugs.

Breast-feeding

Although most drugs can be detected in breast milk, the dose administered to the infant is generally low. This is because, unless there is concentration of drug by breast tissue, the concentration in milk tends to be similar to that of maternal plasma. Clearly in this case the final concentration in infant's plasma is likely to be much less than that in the mother's. Despite this, it is known that some drugs do cause problems via breast-feeding. Examples are carbimazole, which may affect infant thyroid function and tetracyclines which are also excreted in milk. As with pregnancy, avoid all drugs in nursing mothers unless there is a compelling need. If drug therapy in a nursing mother is necessary, the risk to the baby must be balanced against the benefits of breast-feeding before advising whether breast-feeding should continue. A list of drugs excreted in breast milk and known to cause problems is given in an appendix to the *British National Formulary*.

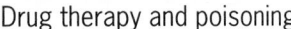

Use of drugs in children and the elderly

Initial evaluation of the safety and efficacy of drugs is normally carried out in healthy volunteers and patients aged between 18 and 65. For new drugs in particular, the likelihood of adverse effects are not known in children or the elderly, and information only slowly becomes available through published case reports and monitoring systems (see Table 16.1).

Children

There are several reasons why drugs may have different effects in the young compared with adults.

- Dosage is more difficult to calculate and formulations are often different to make oral medicines acceptable to the young. Administration of a precise oral dose is often impossible in babies who spit out unpleasant-tasting syrup.
- Absorption of oral drugs may be affected in infants because of reduced gastric acidity.
- Skin absorption of topical drugs and disinfecting agents is enhanced in premature babies, sometimes leading to serious toxicity from steroids, iodine and aminoglycoside antibiotics.
- Adults typically have 20% of their bodyweight as fat; the premature baby may have as little as 1%. This will have a very marked effect to increase plasma concentration of fat-soluble drugs when given on a dose/kg basis.
- The metabolism of certain drugs such as chloramphenicol and theophylline is markedly less rapid in the newborn compared with children and adults. Use of the former has been associated with cardiovascular collapse and 'the grey baby syndrome'.
- Renal excretion of drugs rapidly improves during the first few days of life, making the safe and effective use of aminoglycoside antibiotics, in particular, very difficult.

Adverse effects and the elderly

As the proportion of elderly patients increases in industrialized countries, it is becoming more apparent that this group are more likely to suffer adverse effects of drugs. Reasons for this include:

- Confused patients have difficulty in remembering the correct dose, especially if many different medicines are prescribed.
- Interactions between different drugs – polypharmacy is more common in the elderly.
- Altered drug absorption, distribution, metabolism and excretion owing to concomitant disease processes.
- Pharmacodynamic adverse effects, particularly exaggerated CNS and cardiovascular effects of

Table 16.6
Pharmacodynamic adverse effects of drugs in the elderly

Effect	Drugs
Bradycardia	β-Adrenoceptor blockers Verapamil and diltiazem Digoxin
Postural hypotension	Nitrates Diuretics Tricyclic antidepressants α-Adrenoceptor blockers
Glucose intolerance	Diuretics
Bladder function	Diuretics
Bowel function constipation diarrhoea	e.g. verapamil e.g. metformin
Temperature regulation	Phenothiazines
Confusion	Tranquillizers Anticonvulsants Antimuscarinics Hypnotics Opiates Anaesthesia

certain drugs (Table 16.6). Elderly patients are also much more prone to complain of constipation with drugs which have this adverse effect.

- Non-steroidal anti-inflammatory drugs (NSAIDs) are very commonly prescribed in the elderly and cause a disproportionate number of serious adverse effects in this group of patients.

Drugs and coexistent diseases

Diseases can predispose towards adverse drug reactions by two main mechanisms.

Pharmacokinetic mechanisms

Alteration in absorption may result from previous gastric surgery or intestinal malabsorption due to conditions such as coeliac disease. Infective diarrhoea may increase transit time sufficiently to impair the absorption of many drugs, including oral contraceptives. Oedema of the gut in patients with severe heart failure has been suggested as a reason for reduced efficacy of oral furosemide (frusemide) in this condition.

Reduced plasma albumin concentration because of poor nutrition or renal or hepatic disease will cause little change in the active unbound fraction of protein-bound drugs but will cause a reduction in total plasma concentration. This would have little effect were it not for the fact that total, rather than unbound drug is usually measured when therapeutic drug monitoring is employed, leading to a tendency to overdosing.

Metabolism of many drugs is largely dependent on normal hepatic function and extreme caution must be taken in prescribing to patients with liver failure. In particular reduced metabolism of opiate analgesics, anticoagulants, anticonvulsant drugs and theophylline may cause serious toxicity. If it is necessary to administer a drug which is metabolized by the liver in a patient with hepatic impairment then close monitoring of the effect and/or frequent measurements of plasma concentrations should be done (if such assays are appropriate and available). Reduced metabolism of one drug does not always predict that other drugs which are metabolized by the liver will be similarly affected. Patients with cardiac failure generally have reduced hepatic blood flow and consequently reduced hepatic metabolism of many drugs.

The major route of excretion for most drugs is via the kidneys. In drugs which are not subject to hepatic metabolism, renal excretion is the main factor which determines the concentration of active drug circulating in the plasma. Particular care must be taken with drugs with a low therapeutic ratio which are principally excreted by the kidneys, such as digoxin, lithium and aminoglycoside antibiotics.

Pharmacodynamic mechanisms

It is not surprising that a certain disease will often be exacerbated by a drug that is known to cause this disease as a side-effect. For instance, asthmatics are very sensitive to β-adrenoceptor blocking drugs (see p. 876) and will almost invariably become more wheezy if such agents are inadvertently taken; those with acne will often encounter a worsening of their skin problem when glucocorticoids are prescribed. This is not always the case; patients with liver disease will not necessarily encounter further hepatic damage when antituberculous drugs are given, although, of course, particular caution must be taken in such situations.

Genetic factors and response to drugs

Our genetic make-up can profoundly influence the way in which we react to drugs owing to both pharmacokinetic and pharmacodynamic mechanisms. Susceptibility may be due to a single gene variation or due to several genes having an additive effect. With the sequencing of the human genome, many more common adverse drug reactions will be found to have a genetic basis.

Genetic causes of altered pharmacokinetics
The best-known genetic cause of altered drug handling is acetylator phenotype. Certain drugs are metabolized by acetylation in the liver and individuals can be classified as slow acetylators or fast acetylators. Most populations show a distinct bimodal distribution in their

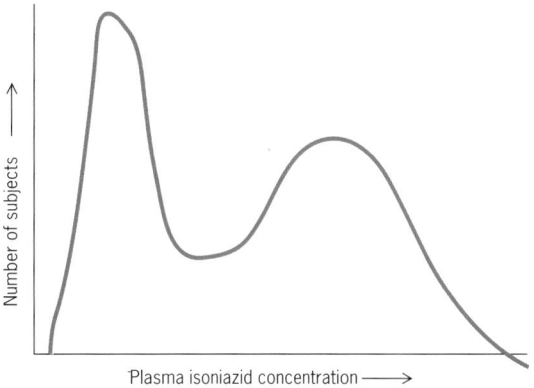

Fig. 16.6 **Bimodal distribution of acetylator status.** Plasma isoniazid concentration shows two distinct groups. Modified from Evans DAP et al. (1960) *British Medical Journal* **2**: 485.

acetylator status (see Fig. 16.6), which is likely to be due to a single gene variation. Those who acetylate slowly will have higher plasma concentrations of drug for any given dose and will tend to develop adverse effects more readily. The antituberculous drug isoniazid will cause a polyneuropathy more commonly in patients with slow acetylator status; inhibition of metabolism of the anticonvulsant phenytoin when prescribed concurrently with isoniazid is also more common in slow acetylators. Rapid acetylators may, conversely, be more likely to relapse because of inadequate plasma concentrations of isoniazid. SLE is more likely to develop with procainamide and hydralazine in slow acetylators.

Debrisoquine hydroxylation is also markedly deficient is certain individuals (about 8% of the British population), and such deficiency shows autosomal dominant inheritance. Debrisoquine is rarely used in the treatment of hypertension, not least because almost 1 in 10 patients will have defective metabolism resulting in enhanced adrenergic blockade with the risk of severe hypotension. The same hydroxylase enzyme is involved in metabolism of several beta-blockers and the antidepressant nortriptyline, although it is not clear whether hydroxylation status predicts adverse effects with these drugs.

The rare failure to metabolize suxamethonium resulting in prolonged muscular paralysis is due to a genetic defect in the production of plasma pseudocholinesterase. The condition is autosomal recessive and affects about 1 in 2500 patients.

Genetic causes of altered pharmacodynamic response
Glucose-6-phosphate-dehydrogenase (G6PD) (p. 433) deficiency is a fairly common X-linked recessive disorder. Individuals with this trait are less able to synthesize NADPH in response to oxidative stress and are susceptible to red cell haemolysis and methaemoglobinaemia when challenged with certain oxidizing drugs as well as broad beans. Drugs that are likely to be a problem in

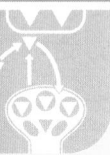

Table 16.7
Commonly used drugs which may precipitate acute porphyria – *a complete list is given in the British National Formulary*

ACE inhibitors
Anticonvulsants
Antihistamines
Barbiturates
Benzodiazepines
Calcium-channel blockers
Cephalosporins
Diuretics
Erythromycin
Flucloxacillin
Methyldopa
Metoclopramide
Oral hypoglycaemics
Sex steroids
Sulphonamides
Theophylline
Tricyclic antidepressants

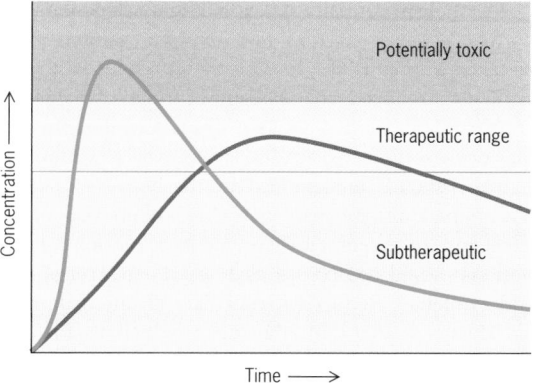

Fig. 16.7 Relationships between blood drug concentration, its effect and time after oral administration.

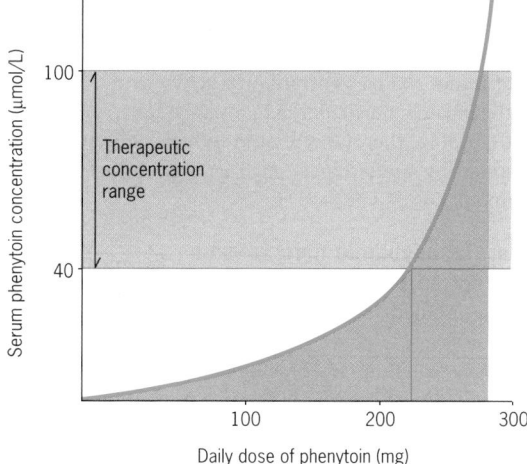

Fig. 16.8 Saturation kinetics as exhibited by phenytoin. The measurements were obtained from one patient on several maintenance doses of phenytoin and show a curvilinear relationship between dose and serum concentration. Note the relatively small dose range compatible with a therapeutic concentration.

G6PD deficiency are given in Table 8.14. Antimalarial drugs, particularly primaquine, can produce severe haemolysis resulting in renal failure.

Acute porphyrias (see p. 1119) can be precipitated by a large number of drugs (Table 16.7).

Malignant hyperthermia (see p. 1224) is a rare but potentially fatal condition, where autosomal dominant inheritance can often be shown. General anaesthesia (particularly when volatile anaesthetics and suxamethonium are given) provokes muscular rigidity, hyperpyrexia, sweating, cyanosis, and rapid respiration. Intravenous dantrolene has been advocated as a useful therapy.

Gilbert's syndrome (p. 347) is exacerbated by oestrogens and improved by low doses of barbiturates, which induce the defective enzyme UDP glucuronosyl transferase.

Monitoring the effect of drugs

As a result of genetic or environmental factors (including other drug therapy), the effect of the same dose of drug in different individuals will differ.

The *therapeutic ratio* of a drug is the ratio between the dose required to produce a toxic effect and the dose required to produce the desired effect (Fig. 16.7). For drugs with a low therapeutic ratio, that is drugs in which toxicity occurs at a dose only marginally higher than the therapeutic dose, monitoring the effect to establish a safe dose is necessary.

Therapeutic drug monitoring

This procedure involves measuring the plasma concentration of a potentially toxic drug and is only useful if:

- there is a reliable and available plasma drug assay

- plasma concentrations correlate well with therapeutic efficacy and toxicity (i.e. the therapeutic range is well documented).

Monitoring of the plasma concentration of phenytoin is essential because of saturation kinetics. When the concentration in plasma reaches a certain level, the metabolizing enzymes are saturated and the drug is eliminated by zero-order kinetics (Fig. 16.8.)

Table 16.8 details those drugs in which therapeutic drug monitoring is routinely employed.

Monitoring of drug effect in individuals

Dosage of other drugs may be adjusted according to their pharmacodynamic effect. A familiar example of this is the use of the International Normalized Ratio (INR) for adjusting the dose of warfarin and other coumarin anticoagulants. Other examples are the estimation of circulating thyroid hormone concentrations (or TSH) in

Table 16.8
Drugs for which therapeutic drug monitoring is used

Drug	Therapeutic plasma concentration range	Toxic levels	Optimum time for sampling after dose (hours)
Carbamazepine	20–50 μmol/L	> 50 μmol/L	> 8
Digoxin	1.3–2.6 nmol/L	> 2.6 nmol/L	> 8
Gentamicin	Trough < 2 mg/L	> 12 mg/L	6–8 (immediately pre-dose)
	Peak 5–10 mg/L	> 12 mg/L	> 1
Lithium	0.6–1.0 mmol/L	> 1.5 mmol/L	> 10
Phenytoin	40–80 μmol/L	> 80 μmol/L	> 10
Theophylline	55–110 μmol/L	> 110 μmol/L	> 4
Ciclosporin	50–200 μg/L	> 200 μg/L	Pre-dose

patients treated with carbimazole, and routine measurement of white cell and platelet count in patients receiving cytotoxic chemotherapy. For many drugs, e.g. penicillins, the therapeutic ratio is so high that there is little chance of toxicity with standard doses so monitoring of plasma concentrations is unnecessary.

Monitoring of adverse drug effects in populations

In order to identify less common adverse effects of new drugs or rare adverse effects of established drugs, pharmacoepidemiologists have developed a variety of approaches. In the UK the *yellow card system* has been useful. This system invites clinicians and pharmacists to report all definite or suspected adverse reactions to the Committee on Safety of Medicines. This should be done for newly introduced products as well as for serious or unusual reactions to established products. Clearly the efficacy of such a system inevitably is reduced by the low reporting rate, but the yellow card system has uncovered a number of adverse effects and drug interactions, including thromboembolism in oral contraceptive users and jaundice with halothane. Complementary to this system is *prescription event monitoring*, in which prescriptions for a certain drug are identified at the Prescription Pricing Authority office. A sample of patients or their doctors are then sent a questionnaire to determine if certain adverse effects are occurring at a greater incidence than that found for a comparable drug prescribed for the same clinical indication.

FURTHER READING

Birkett DJ (1998) *Pharmacokinetics made easy.* Sydney: McGraw-Hill.

Edwards IR, Aronson JK (2000) Adverse drug reactions, definitions, diagnosis and management. *Lancet* **356**: 1255–1259. First of six articles.

Ito S (2000) Drug therapy for breast-feeding women. *New England Journal of Medicine* **343**: 118–126.

Meyer UA (2000) Pharmacogenetics and adverse drug reactions. *Lancet* **356**: 1667–1671.

Rang HP, Dale M, Ritter JM (1999) *Pharmacology*, 4th edn. Edinburgh: Churchill Livingstone.

Ritter JM, Lewis LD, Mant TGKA (1998) *Textbook of Clinical Pharmacology*, 4th edn. London: Edward Arnold.

Clinical trials

There is now general acceptance that treatments should be introduced into, and used in, routine clinical care, only if they have been demonstrated to be effective in formal clinical trials. There are two types of controlled clinical trial:

- the prospective controlled trial
- the historical controlled trial.

Although clinical trials were originally introduced to investigate the efficacy of drugs (Tables 16.9 and 16.10), the methodology now encompasses surgical procedures, and devices.

Prospective controlled trials

In this type of trial, patients with a particular condition are given, prospectively, one of two (or more) treatments. Treatments are usually allocated randomly (a 'randomized' controlled trial, RCT). In order to reduce patient bias, the patients themselves are often unaware of their treatment allocations (a 'single-blind' trial); and in order to reduce doctor bias the treatment allocation may also be withheld from the investigators (a 'double-blind' controlled trial). In order to recruit sufficient numbers of patients in a clinical trial it is often necessary to conduct it at a number of locations (a 'multicentre' trial). The gold standard for demonstrating the efficacy of a treatment is thus the *prospective, randomized, double-blind, multicentre, controlled trial.*

Prospective randomized controlled trials are generally designed either to show that one treatment is better than another (a 'superiority' trial), or that one treatment is similar to another (an 'equivalence' trial). In a *superiority trial* the study treatment is usually compared to placebo, to no treatment, or to current standard practice. With drugs, the comparators may include different doses of the study ('active') drug in order to define the optimum treatment regimen. In an *equivalence trial* the study treatment is usually compared to another treatment (e.g. another drug for the same condition).

Historical controlled trials

Despite the pre-eminence of the prospective, randomized controlled trial there are many treatments that have never been subjected to this technique yet their efficacy is unquestioned. Examples include insulin in the treatment of diabetic ketoacidosis, thyroxine for hypothyroidism, vitamin B_{12} in pernicious anaemia, and defibrillation for ventricular fibrillation.

In a historical controlled trial the outcome in patients treated with the study drug is compared to that of previous patients with the particular disease. The circumstances when it is legitimate for a treatment to be accepted into routine use on the basis of favourable comparisons with historical controls are generally limited to circumstances when all the following conditions are satisfied:

- There should be a biologically plausible reason why the treatment might be effective. From a knowledge of the underlying nature of the condition, and the properties of the treatment, it should be reasonable to be able to infer likely benefit.
- There should be no other effective form of treatment. If there is, then the study treatment should be compared with alternatives in a prospective, randomized controlled trial.
- The disease, if untreated, should result in death or permanent disability.
- The condition should have a known, and predictable, natural history.

New treatments that fulfil these stringent requirements are uncommon. Historical controlled trials are most frequently (though often inappropriately) used in the assessment of, for example, new anticancer treatments: in most instances prospective, comparative, randomized, controlled trials would be more informative.

Assessing clinical trials

In assessing the relevance and reliability of a clinical trial, a number of features need to be taken into account:

- *Was ethical approval obtained?* All clinical trials should have received approval, before the start of the study, from a properly constituted research ethics committee. In particular, patients taking part in the study should have given their full, and informed, consent to participate.
- *Randomization.* In any randomized controlled trial the method of randomization should be robust. In particular, the investigator should be unaware of which treatment a patient about to enter a trial will receive. This avoids selection bias.
- *Maintaining 'blindness'.* Although, ideally, in prospective randomized controlled trials neither investigator nor patient is aware of the treatment allocation until the end of the study, this is not always possible. Side-effects, for example, may make it obvious which treatment a patient has been given. Nevertheless, maintaining blindness is necessary

where the outcome is subjective (e.g. relief of pain, alleviation of depression) if bias is to be avoided.

- *Are the results generalizable?* (Box 16.4). Were the patients enrolled into the study a reasonable reflection of those likely to be treated in routine clinical practice (a so-called 'pragmatic' trial)? Or were they a selected population that excluded significant patient groups (e.g. the elderly). If the latter, view the conclusions with caution.
- *Were the treated and control groups comparable?* Were the treated and control groups broadly similar in their 'baseline' characteristics? Were they, for example, of similar age, severity and duration of illness? If not, are they likely to bias the results? Or has the statistical analysis (most often using Cox's proportional hazards model) tried to adjust for them? Table 16.9 shows an RCT where the baseline characteristics were comparable.
- *Outcomes.* There are two ways to look at the outcome(s) of a clinical trial. One is to include only those patients who completed the study ('per protocol' analysis) and the other is to include all patients from the time of randomization ('intention-to-treat' analysis). Ideally there should be no difference, but in reality the results of a per protocol analysis are usually more advantageous to a treatment than an intention-to-treat analysis. The reason is that the intention-to-treat analysis will take account of patients who have withdrawn from the trial because of intolerance to the treatment or adverse reactions. It is therefore a much more robust approach. Table 16.10 shows the results of an 'intention to treat' trial, with fewer fits with $MgSO_4$ than with diazepam.

Box 16.4

Criteria for assessing the 'generalizability' of a clinical trial in routine clinical care

1. Were the patients typical of those you would expect to see in your own practice?
2. Was there only a small difference in the numbers of patients considered for entry and those ultimately randomized?
3. Were patients treated in circumstances similar to your own practice?
4. Was the dose and duration of treatment the same as that normally recommended (e.g. in the *British National Formulary*)?
5. Was (were) the outcome(s) a direct measure of actual clinical benefit?
6. Were the results analysed by intention-to-treat?
7. Are the results comparable to those of other RCTs with the same drug and for the same condition?

Positive answers (out of 7)
6–7 – probably generalizable
3–5 – possibly generalizable
1–2 – not generalizable (at least at the present time)

Table 16.9

Randomized comparative trial of parenteral magnesium sulphate and diazepam in the treatment of eclamptic fits: baseline characteristics

	MgSO$_4$ (n = 452)	Diazepam (n = 453)
Mean age (years)	22.1	22.3
Primiparous	293	302
Twins/triplets	14	16
Previous history of epilepsy	9	8
Blood pressure (mmHg) at start of treatment		
Diastolic > 110	238	228
Systolic > 170	161	166
Gestational age (weeks)		
< 34	119	103
34–37	110	107
> 37	168	180
Not known	56	62

Collaborative Eclampsia Trialists (1995) Which anticonvulsant for women with eclampsia? *Lancet* **345**: 1455–1462

Table 16.10

Randomized comparative trial of parenteral magnesium sulphate and diazepam in the treatment of eclamptic fits: results

	MgSO$_4$ (n = 453)	Diazepam (n = 452)	Relative risk (95% CI)
Further fits	60	126	0.48 (0.36–0.63)
Death	17	23	0.74 (0.40–1.36)
Respiratory depression	35	33	
Pneumonia	9	14	
Renal failure	28	29	
Stroke	13	17	

Collaborative Eclampsia Trialists (1995) Which anticonvulsant for women with eclampsia? *Lancet* **345**: 1455–1462

- *Analysis of a superiority trial.* The aim of a superiority trial is to determine whether one treatment (or dose) is better (more effective) than another. It is usual to estimate the probability of any difference being due to chance, and if this is less than 1 in 20 ($p < 0.05$) it is regarded as 'statistically significant'. There are, though, two caveats. First, any difference may still be due to the play of chance and consequently it is wise to await the results of at least two independent studies before adopting a new treatment. Secondly, a trial may show no 'statistically significant' difference, when one in fact exists, because too few patients have been included. The 'power' of a study (the number of patients needed in each treatment group in order to detect a predefined difference) should have been defined at the outset. If not, the results of the study should be extremely carefully interpreted.
- *Effect size.* The size of the difference in a superiority trial (the 'effect' size) may or may not be clinically relevant even if statistically significant. For example, if a trial of a new analgesic for mild pain showed that a new treatment relieved pain in 94% of patients compared to 92% of patients given an older treatment, few clinicians would be impressed even if the effect size (2%) were statistically significant. On the other hand, a reduction in the 30-day mortality after acute myocardial infarction from 8% to 6%, by giving streptokinase, is of real clinical advantage even though the effect size is 2%.
- *Analysis of an equivalence trial.* Here, the aim is to determine whether two (or possibly more) treatments produce similar benefits. It is necessary, during the design of such trials, to decide what difference is unimportant and then to calculate the number of patients needed in order to have an 80% or 90%

chance of showing this. In equivalence trials such power calculations show that the number of patients required is invariably greater than that needed for superiority trials. The results of equivalence trials are usually reported as a 'hazard ratio' (the ratio of the response rate to the study treatment to that of the comparator) with its 95% confidence intervals. A hazard ratio of around 1.0 (with a confidence interval of, say, 0.9 to 1.2) would indicate that the two treatments were indeed likely to be equivalent. A hazard ratio of 0.5 (confidence interval 0.3 to 0.7) would suggest inequivalence, and superiority of the study treatment. By contrast, a hazard ratio of 2.0 (confidence interval 1.7 to 2.3) would suggest that the new treatment is inferior. In equivalence trials, it should be obvious that the comparator itself must have been shown to be effective.

The development of formal approaches to the evaluation of the effectiveness of both new and established therapeutic measures has been a major advance. It allows practitioners to be confident that the treatments they offer to patients are likely to be beneficial, and it provides patients themselves with reassurance about the treatments they receive.

Evidence-based medicine (EBM) is regarded by many as the hallmark of good practice and relies heavily on the results of randomized controlled trials (RCTs) particularly by meta-analysis.

Meta-analysis, an analysis of all controlled trials that have been performed in a particular area, will help minimize random errors in the assessment of treatment effects, as more patients and treatments are included than in an individual trial. Meta-analysis should be performed carefully because of the heterogeneity of trials.

There is an enormous economic pressure on pharmaceutical companies to market their drugs. Therefore all trials should be scrupulously monitored with the financial benefits to individuals and organizations clearly stated and declared.

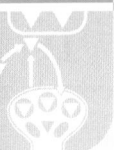

FURTHER READING

Benson K, Hartz AJ (2000) A comparison of observational studies and randomized controlled trials. *New England Journal of Medicine* **342**: 1878–1886.

Collins R, MacMahon S (2001) Reliable assessment of the effects of treatment on mortality and major morbidity. I Clinical trials, II Observational studies. *Lancet* **357**: 373–380, 455–462.

Concato J, Shah N, Horwitz RI (2000) Randomised controlled trials, observational studies, and hierarchy of research designs. *New England Journal of Medicine* **342**: 1887–1892.

Statistical analyses

Statistics has become of immense importance in clinical science. Its relevance is not confined to those who undertake research but also to everyone who wants to understand the relevance of research studies to their clinical practice. This brief account of some of the concepts and terms, used by statisticians, does not replace the more detailed accounts to be found in some of the excellent books that are now available.

The average

Clinical studies may describe, quantitatively, the value of a particular variable (e.g. height, weight, blood pressure, haemoglobin) in a sample of a defined population. The 'average' value (or 'central tendency' in statistical parlance) may be expressed as the mean, median or mode depending on the circumstances:

- The *mean* is the average of a distribution of values that are grouped symmetrically around a central tendency.
- The *median* is the middle value in a sample. It is used, particularly, where the values in a sample are asymmetrically distributed around a central tendency.
- The *mode* is the interval, in a distribution of values, that contains more values than any other.

In a symmetrically distributed population the mean, median and mode are the same.

The average value of a sample, on its own, is of only modest interest. Of equal (and often greater) relevance is the confidence we can place on this sample average truly reflecting the average value of the population from which it has been drawn. This is most often expressed as a *confidence interval* which expresses the probability of a sample mean being a certain distance from the population mean. If, for example, the mean systolic blood pressure sample of 100 undergraduates is 124 mm mercury, with a 95% confidence interval of ± 15 mm mercury, we can be confident that if we replicated the study 100 times the value of the mean would be within the range 109–139 mm mercury on 95 occasions. It is intuitively

obvious that the larger the sample the less will be the size of the confidence interval and vice versa.

Correlation

In clinical studies two, or more, variables may be measured in the same individuals in a sample population (e.g. weight and blood pressure). The degree of correlation, between the two, can be investigated by estimating the *correlation coefficient*. This coefficient (often abbreviated to 'r') measures the degree of association between the variables and may range from 1 to –1. If $r = 1$ then there is complete and direct concordance between the two variables; if $r = -1$ there is complete but inverse concordance; and where $r = 0$ there is no concordance. Standard statistical tables enable the investigator to determine the probability that r is due to chance. As in other areas of statistics, if the probability is less than 1 in 20 ($p < 0.05$) then by custom and practice it is regarded as 'statistically significant'. There are, however, two caveats. First, the 1 in 20 rule is a convention and does not exclude the possibility that a presumed association is due to chance. Second, the fact that there is an association between two variables does not necessarily mean that it is causal. A correlation between blood pressure and weight, with $r = 0.75$ and $p < 0.05$, does not necessarily mean that weight has a direct effect on blood pressure.

Correlation analyses can become very complicated. The simplest (least squares linear regression analysis) presumes a straight-line relationship between two normally distributed variables. More complicated techniques can be used to estimate r where a non-linear relationship is presumed (or assumed); where the distributions deviate from normal; where the scales of one or both the variables are intervals or ranks; or where a correlation between three or more variables is sought.

Hypothesis testing

Much of statistics is concerned with testing hypotheses. The basic assumption – known as the '*null hypothesis*' – is that there is no difference between two variables in one (or more) groups. The reason for this confusing terminology is that statistical techniques are designed to assess the extent by which a zero difference might be due to the play of chance (or to sampling error). In the analysis of a prospective, randomized, placebo-controlled trial the null hypothesis asserts that there is no difference between the results in patients treated with placebo and those on the active treatment. Statistical tests are used to determine the probability that the observed difference is due to chance. Where this is less than 1 in 20 ($p < 0.05$) it is described as 'statistically significant'. Again, as with correlations, the 1 in 20 rule is arbitrary and is a convention that has been widely adopted.

The choice of statistical test to examine the null hypothesis is a complicated one. It is dependent on the type of data collected; whether it is ordinal, cardinal or categorical; and whether it conforms to a normal (parametric), or other (non-parametric), distribution. Those most commonly used include Student's t test (parametric) and the χ^2 test, analysis of variance and various tests for non-parametric data. In some circumstances it is possible to use the confidence intervals of the means of two (or more) groups to test the null hypothesis.

When the results of a statistical test indicate rejection of the null hypothesis, and that the probability of the results being due to chance are less than 1 in 20 ($p < 0.05$) it means that 95 times out of 100 we are correct in our decision; but that 5 times out of 100 we will be wrong. Statisticians call erroneous rejection of the null hypothesis a *type 1 error*. In this situation the null hypothesis is actually true, although we believe it to have been false. Erroneous acceptance of the null hypothesis when there is, indeed, a difference is known as a *type 2 error*. Type 1 errors can be reduced by requiring a higher level of probability (e.g. $p < 0.01$) but can never be absolutely excluded. Type 2 errors are usually the result of too few participants in the study and can be avoided by estimating the number of subjects needed to examine specific levels of difference. Such estimates are known as 'power calculations'.

Ratios

Statisticians have developed a range of techniques to address various problems raised by the analysis of ratios. The most important relates to the analysis of case-control studies.

A case-control study is almost the reverse of a randomized controlled trial. Instead of following, prospectively, two or more cohorts and comparing a specific outcome the case-control technique examines patients with a specific outcome and retrospectively studies possible causal factors. For example, an investigator may wish to discover whether there is an association between upper gastrointestinal bleeding and exposure to non-steroidal anti-inflammatory drugs (NSAIDs). The cases are all patients in a particular population with upper gastrointestinal bleeding, and the controls are a random sample of people drawn from the same population without upper gastrointestinal bleeding. The use of NSAIDs is then compared between the two groups giving rise to a '2 × 2' table:

NSAID exposure	Cases	Controls
Yes	a	c
No	b	d

From this the odds ratio can calculated:

Odds ratio $= a/c \div b/d$

It is also possible to derive, reasonably simply, the confidence intervals around this ratio. The odds ratio expresses the extent to which the use of an NSAID is associated with an increase in the risk of upper gastrointestinal bleeding. An odds ratio of two would suggest a twofold increase in the risk of upper gastrointestinal bleeding, above that in the normal population; and an odds ratio of 10 a 10-fold increase.

Other statistical techniques

Statisticians have developed a range of sophisticated methods to handle a wide variety of biomedical problems. Unless a clinical investigator is supremely (and, probably, unreasonably) confident its is wise to seek professional statistical advise in the analysis of numerical data that look complicated. In doing so it is invariably wiser to do so at the time the study is being designed rather than after the results have been generated.

FURTHER READING

Bland M (2000) *An Introduction to Medical Statistics*, 3rd edn. Oxford: Oxford University Press.

Daly LE, Bourke GJ (2000) *Interpretation and Uses of Medical Statistics*, 5th edn. Oxford: Blackwell Science.

Shakespeare TP, Gebski VJ, Veness MJ, Simes J (2001) Improving interpretation of clinical studies by use of confidence levels, clinical significance curves, and risk–benefit contours. *Lancet* **357**: 1349–1353.

Poisoning

The nature of the problem

In many hospitals in the developed world, acute poisoning is one of the most common reasons for acute admission to a medical ward. In such cases poisoning is usually by self-administration of prescribed and over-the-counter medicines, or illicit drugs. Poisoning in children aged less than 6 months is most commonly iatrogenic and involves overtreatment with, for example, paracetamol. Children between 8 months and 5 years of age also ingest poisons accidentally. Drugs may be administered deliberately to cause harm, as in Münchausen's syndrome by proxy, or for financial or sexual gain. Occupational poisoning as a result of dermal or inhalational exposure to chemicals is a common occurrence in the developing world and still occurs in the developed world. Sometimes inappropriate treatment of a patient by a doctor is responsible for the development of poisoning, for example digoxin toxicity.

In adults, self-poisoning is commonly a 'cry for help'. Those involved are most often females under the age of 35 who are in good physical health. They take an overdose in circumstances where they are likely to be found, or in the presence of others. In those older than 55 years of age, men predominate and the overdose is usually

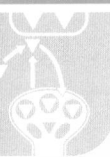

taken in the course of a depressive illness or because of poor physical health.

A third of patients admitted with an overdose state that they are unaware of the toxic effects of the substance involved; the majority take whatever drug is easily available at their home (Box 16.5). Studies of the agents involved reveal that:

- Acute overdoses usually involve more than one agent.
- Alcohol is the most commonly implicated second agent in mixed self-poisonings – 60% of men and 45% of women consume some alcohol at the same time as the drug.
- There is often a poor correlation between the drug history and the toxicological analytical findings. Therefore, a patient's statement about the type and amount of drug ingested cannot always be relied upon.

In England and Wales there are some 100 000 hospital admissions each year for self-poisoning. The most common agents involved are paracetamol, benzodiazepines, antidepressants and NSAIDs. A similar pattern exists in other developed countries. In contrast, in the developing world, pesticide poisoning is far commoner with some 1 million cases of serious unintentional pesticide poisonings annually and 2 million hospitalized deliberate pesticide ingestions. In addition, ingestion of heating fuels (e.g. petroleum distillates), antimalarials, antituberculous drugs and traditional medicine is reported frequently.

The majority of cases of self-poisoning do not require intensive medical management, but all patients require a sympathetic and caring approach, a psychiatric and social assessment and, sometimes, psychiatric treatment. However, as the majority of patients ingest relatively non-toxic agents, all that is required is good supportive care and, when appropriate, the administration of specific antidotes such as N-acetylcysteine. The in-hospital mortality in most developed countries is now approximately 0.5%. Most 'poison' deaths (80% of some 4500 in the UK) occur outside hospital; the commonest causes are poisoning due to carbon monoxide, tricyclic antidepressants, paracetamol, and analgesic combinations containing paracetamol and an opioid.

The approach to the patient

History

Eighty per cent of adults are conscious on arrival at hospital and the diagnosis of self-poisoning can usually be made from the history (Box 16.6). It should be emphasized that in any patient with an altered level of consciousness, drug overdose must always be considered in the differential diagnosis.

Examination

On arrival at hospital the patient must be assessed urgently in the accident and emergency department. The following should be evaluated:

- *Level of consciousness* – the Glasgow Coma Scale should be used (see p. 1159).
- *Ventilation* – pulse oximetry can be used to measure oxygen saturation. The displayed reading may be inaccurate when the saturation is below 70%, there is poor peripheral perfusion and in the presence of carboxyhaemoglobin and methaemoglobin. Only measurement of arterial blood gases will indicate the presence both of hypercapnia and hypoxia.
- *Blood pressure and pulse rate*.
- *Pupil size* and reaction to light.
- Evidence of intravenous drug abuse.
- *A head injury* complicating poisoning.

If the patient is unconscious the following should also be checked:

- *Cough and gag reflex* – present or absent
- *Temperature* – measured with a low-reading rectal thermometer.

Some of the physical signs that may aid identification of the agents responsible for poisoning are shown in Table 16.11.

Box 16.5

Prevention of self-poisoning

Patients usually take what is readily available at home.

- Small amounts only of drugs should be bought.
- Foil-wrapped drugs are less likely to be taken.
- Keep drugs in a safe place.
- Keep drugs and liquids in their original containers.
- Child-proof drug containers should be used.
- Doctors should be careful in prescribing all drugs.
- Prescriptions for any susceptible patient (e.g. depressed) must be monitored carefully.
- Household products should be kept safely, away from children.

SELF-POISONING CAN KILL
All people must be aware of the dangers.

Box 16.6

Diagnostic process in acute poisoning

- Obtain history if possible from the patient or a relative/friend/paramedic.
- Is there circumstantial evidence of an overdose?
- Are the circumstances in which the patient has been found suggestive of an overdose?
- Was a suicide note left?
- Are the symptoms suggestive of an overdose?
- Do the physical signs suggest an overdose? (Table 16.11)

Table 16.11
Some physical signs of poisoning

Features	Likely poisons
Constricted pupils	Opioids Organophosphorus insecticides Nerve agents
Dilated pupils	Tricyclic antidepressants Amfetamines Cocaine Anticholinergic drugs
Convulsions	Tricyclic antidepressants Theophylline Opioids Mefenamic acid Isoniazid Amfetamines
Dystonic reactions	Metoclopramide Phenothiazines
Delirium and hallucinations	Anticholinergic drugs Amfetamines Cannabis Recovery from tricyclic antidepressant overdose
Loss of vision	Methanol Quinine
Divergent strabismus	Tricyclic antidepressants
Papilloedema	Carbon monoxide Methanol
Nystagmus	Phenytoin Carbamazepine
Hypertonia and hyperreflexia	Tricyclic antidepressants Anticholinergic drugs
Tinnitus and deafness	Salicylates Quinine
Hyperventilation	Salicylates Phenoxyacetate herbicides Theophylline Hyperthermia MDMA (Ecstasy)
Blisters	Usually occur in comatose patients

Box 16.7

Management strategy in acute poisoning

- Provide supportive treatment.
- Is the use of an antidote appropriate? (Table 16.15)
- Is it appropriate to attempt to reduce poison absorption?
- Is it appropriate to perform toxicological investigations? (Table 16.12)
- Will non-toxicological investigations assist? (Table 16.13)
- Should urine alkalinization, multiple-dose activated charcoal, and haemodialysis be employed to increase poison elimination?

Table 16.12
Poisons for which emergency measurement of blood concentrations is appropriate

Aspirin
Digoxin
Ethanol (in monitoring treatment of ethylene glycol and methanol poisoning)
Ethylene glycol
Iron
Lithium (NB Do **not** use a lithium heparin tube!)
Methanol
Paracetamol
Paraquat
Quinine
Theophylline

Non-toxicological investigations (Table 16.13)

Some routine investigations are of value in the differential diagnosis of coma or the detection of poison-induced hypokalaemia, hyperkalaemia, hypoglycaemia, hyperglycaemia and hepatic renal failure or of acid–base disturbances (Table 16.14). Measurement of carboxyhaemoglobin, methaemoglobin and cholinesterase activities are of assistance in the diagnosis and management respectively of cases of poisoning due to carbon monoxide, methaemoglobin-inducing agents such as nitrites, and organophosphorus insecticides.

Principles of management (Box 16.7)

Most patients with self-poisoning require only general care and support of the vital systems. However, for a few drugs additional therapy is required.

Toxicological investigations

On admission, or at an appropriate time post-overdose, a timed blood sample should be taken if the drugs shown in Table 16.12 have been ingested. The determination of the concentrations of these drugs will be valuable in management. Drug screens on blood and urine are occasionally indicated in severely poisoned patients in whom the cause of coma is unknown. Poison Information Services will advise.

Care of the unconscious patient

(see also p. 1161)

In all cases the patient should be nursed in the lateral position with the lower leg straight and the upper leg flexed; in this position the risk of aspiration is reduced. A clear passage for air should be ensured by the removal of any obstructing object, vomit or dentures, and by backward pressure on the mandible. Nursing care of the mouth and pressure areas should be instituted. Immediate catheterization of the bladder in unconscious patients is usually unnecessary as it can be emptied by gentle suprapubic pressure. Insertion of a venous cannula is usual, but administration of intravenous fluids is

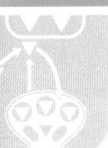

Table 16.13
Relevant non-toxicological investigations

Serum sodium (e.g. hyponatraemia in MDMA poisoning) and potassium (e.g. hypokalaemia in theophylline poisoning and hyperkalaemia in digoxin poisoning) concentrations

Plasma creatinine concentration (e.g. renal failure in ethylene glycol poisoning)

Acid–base disturbances, including metabolic acidosis (Table 16.14)

Blood sugar concentration (e.g. hypoglycaemia in insulin poisoning or hyperglycaemia in salicylate poisoning)

Serum calcium concentration (e.g. hypocalcaemia in ethylene glycol poisoning)

Liver function (e.g. in paracetamol poisoning)

Serum creatine kinase (rhabdomyolysis)

Carboxyhaemoglobin concentration (in carbon monoxide poisoning)

Methaemoglobinaemia (e.g. in nitrite poisoning)

Cholinesterase activities (e.g. organophosphorus insecticide poisoning)

ECG (e.g. wide QRS in tricyclic antidepressant poisoning)

X-ray for ingestion/injection of radiopaque substances

MDMA, 3,4-methylenedioxy-methamfetamine

Table 16.14
Some poisons inducing metabolic acidosis

Carbon monoxide
Cocaine
Cyanide
Ethanol
Ethylene glycol
Iron
Methanol
Paracetamol
Salicylates
Tricyclic antidepressants

unnecessary unless the patient has been unconscious for more than 12 hours or is hypotensive.

Respiratory support

If respiratory depression is present, as determined by pulse oximetry or preferably by arterial blood gas analysis, an oropharyngeal airway should be inserted, and supplemental oxygen should be administered. Pulse oximetry alone will not detect hypercapnia. Loss of the cough or gag reflex is the prime indication for intubation. The gag reflex can be assessed by positioning the patient on one side and making him or her gag using a suction tube. In many severely poisoned patients the reflexes are depressed sufficiently to allow intubation without the use of sedatives or relaxants. The complications of endotracheal tubes are discussed on page 948.

If ventilation remains inadequate after intubation, as shown by hypoxaemia and hypercapnia, intermittent positive-pressure ventilation (IPPV) should be instituted.

Cardiovascular support

Although hypotension (systolic blood pressure below 80 mmHg) is a recognized feature of acute poisoning, the classic features of shock – tachycardia and pale cold skin – are observed only rarely. In patients with marked hypotension, volume expansion with gelatins or etherified starches (e.g. hetastarch, hexastarch) should be used, guided by monitoring of central venous pressure (CVP). Urine output (aiming for 35–50 mL/h) is also a useful guide to the adequacy of the circulation.

If a patient fails to respond to the above measures, more intensive therapy is required (see p. 936).

Arrhythmias are observed occasionally in poisoned patients, for example after the ingestion of a tricyclic antidepressant or theophylline. All patients with shock should have ECG monitoring. Known arrhythmogenic factors such as hypoxia, acidosis and hypokalaemia should be corrected.

Other problems
Body temperature
Hypothermia – a rectal temperature below 35°C – is a recognized complication of poisoning, especially in older patients or those who are comatose. The patient should be covered with a 'space blanket' and, if necessary, given intravenous and intragastric fluids at normal body temperature. Inspired gases should also be warmed to 37°C. *Hyperthermia* can develop with CNS stimulant ingestion. Removal of clothing and sponging with tepid water will promote evaporation.

Rhabdomyolysis
Rhabdomyolysis can occur from pressure necrosis in drug-induced coma, or it may complicate, for example, MDMA (Ecstasy, p. 1259) abuse in the absence of coma. Patients with rhabdomyolysis are at risk of developing firstly, renal failure from myoglobinaemia, particularly if they are hypovolaemic and have an acidosis, and, secondly, wrist or ankle drop from the development of a compartment syndrome (see p. 530).

Convulsions
These may occur, for example, in poisoning due to tricyclic antidepressants, mefenamic acid or opioids. Usually the fits are short-lived but, if they are prolonged, diazepam 10–20 mg i.v. should be administered. Persistent fits must be controlled rapidly to prevent severe hypoxia, brain damage and laryngeal trauma. If diazepam in repeated doses is ineffective, the patient should also receive a loading dose of phenytoin (15 mg/kg) administered intravenously at a rate of not more than 50 mg per minute, with blood pressure and ECG monitoring.

Stress ulceration and bleeding
Medication to prevent stress ulceration of the stomach should be started on admission in all patients who are

unconscious and require intensive care. An H_2-receptor antagonist or a proton pump inhibitor should be administered intravenously.

Specific management

Antidotes

Specific antidotes are available for only a small number of poisons (Table 16.15).

Antidotes may exert a beneficial effect by:

- forming an inert complex with the poison (e.g. desferrioxamine, dicobalt edetate, dimercaprol, DMSA, DMPS, digoxin-specific antibody fragments, hydroxocobalamin, penicillamine, pralidoxime,

protamine, Berlin (Prussian) blue, sodium calcium edetate)
- accelerating the detoxification of the poison (e.g. methionine, *N*-acetylcysteine, sodium thiosulphate)
- reducing the rate of conversion of the poison to a more toxic compound (e.g. ethanol, fomepizole)
- competing with toxic substances for essential receptor sites (e.g. oxygen, naloxone, vitamin K_1)
- blocking essential receptors through which the toxic effects are mediated (e.g. atropine)
- bypassing the effect of the poison (e.g. oxygen).

Reduction of poison absorption

Inhaled

To reduce poison absorption through the lungs, the casualty should be removed from the toxic atmosphere, without the rescuers themselves being put at risk.

Skin

If clothing is contaminated this should be removed to reduce dermal absorption. In addition, contaminated skin should be washed thoroughly with soap and water.

Gut decontamination

The efficacy of current methods to remove unabsorbed drug from the gastrointestinal tract remains unproven. The two major international societies of clinical toxicology (*American Academy of Clinical Toxicology* (AACT) and the *European Association of Poisons Centres and Clinical Toxicologists* (EAPCCT)) have produced **Position Statements** on each method and are quoted (in italics) below.

Gastric lavage

Gastric lavage involves the insertion of a large-bore orogastric tube into the stomach. Small amounts (200–300 mL in an adult) of warm (38°C) fluid (water or 0.9% saline) are introduced and removed by suction. Lavage is continued until the recovered solution is clear of particulate matter.

Gastric lavage *should not be employed routinely in the management of poisoned patients*. The amount of marker removed by gastric lavage is highly variable and diminishes with time. There is no certain evidence that its use improves clinical outcome and it may cause significant morbidity. Gastric lavage should only be *considered*, therefore, if a patient has ingested a potentially life-threatening amount of a poison and the procedure can be undertaken within 1 hour of ingestion. Gastric lavage is contraindicated if airway-protective reflexes are lost (unless the patient is intubated) and also if a hydrocarbon with high aspiration potential or a corrosive substance has been ingested.

Syrup of ipecacuanha

Syrup of ipecacuanha contains two alkaloids, emetine and cephaeline, which induce vomiting by a central action and by a local action (emetine).

Table 16.15
Antidotes of value in poisoning

Poison	Antidote
Anticoagulants (oral)	Vitamin K_1
Arsenic	DMSA Dimercaprol (BAL)
Benzodiazepines	Flumazenil
β-Adrenoceptor blocking drugs	Atropine Glucagon
Carbon monoxide	Oxygen
Cyanide	Oxygen Dicobalt edetate Hydroxocobalamin Sodium nitrite Sodium thiosulphate
Digoxin	Digoxin-specific antibody fragments
Ethylene glycol	Ethanol Fomepizole
Iron salts	Desferrioxamine
Lead (inorganic)	Sodium calcium edetate DMSA
Methaemoglobinaemia	Methylthioninium chloride (methylene blue)
Methanol	Ethanol Fomepizole
Mercury (inorganic)	DMPS Dimercaprol (BAL) Penicillamine
Opioids	Naloxone
Organophosphorus insecticides	Atropine Pralidoxime
Paracetamol	*N*-acetylcysteine or methionine
Thallium	Berlin (Prussian) blue

DMSA, dimercaptosuccinic acid (succimer); DMPS, dimercaptopropanesulphonate (unithiol)

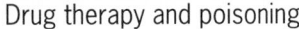
Syrup of ipecacuanha *should not be administered in the management of poisoned patients.* The amount of marker removed in studies was highly variable and diminished with time. There is no evidence that it improves the clinical outcome and therefore its administration, even in children, should be abandoned.

Single-dose activated charcoal

Activated charcoal has a highly developed internal pore structure which is able to adsorb a wide variety of compounds and drugs, e.g. aspirin, carbamazepine, aminophylline, digoxin, barbiturates, phenytoin, paracetamol. It does not absorb strong acids and alkalis, ethanol, ethylene glycol, iron, lithium, mercury and methanol.

Single-dose activated charcoal *should not be administered routinely in the management of poisoned patients.* Based on volunteer studies, the effectiveness of activated charcoal decreases with time; the greatest benefit is within 1 hour of ingestion. The administration of activated charcoal should only be *considered* if a patient (with an intact or protected airway) has ingested a potentially toxic amount of a poison (which is known to be adsorbed to charcoal) up to 1 hour previously. Again, there is no evidence that this improves the clinical outcome. For multiple-dose active charcoal use, see below.

Cathartics

The administration of a cathartic alone has *no role in the management of the poisoned patient* and is not recommended as a method of gut decontamination. Experimental data are conflicting regarding the use of cathartics in combination with activated charcoal. No clinical studies have been published to investigate the ability of a cathartic, with or without activated charcoal, to reduce the bioavailability of drugs or to improve the outcome of poisoned patients. Based on available data, the routine use of a cathartic in combination with activated charcoal is not recommended.

Whole bowel irrigation

Whole bowel irrigation (WBI) requires the insertion of a nasogastric tube into the stomach and the introduction of polyethylene glycol electrolyte solution 1500–2000 mL/h in an adult. WBI is continued until the rectal effluent is clear.

WBI should not be used routinely in the management of the poisoned patient. Although some volunteer studies have shown substantial decreases in the bioavailability of ingested drugs, no controlled clinical trials have been performed and there is no conclusive evidence that WBI improves the outcome of the poisoned patient. Based on volunteer studies, WBI should be *considered* for potentially toxic ingestions of sustained-release or enteric-coated drugs. There are insufficient data to support or exclude the use of WBI for potentially toxic ingestions of iron, lead, zinc, or packets of illicit drugs; WBI remains a theoretical option for these ingestions. WBI is contraindicated in patients with bowel obstruction, perforation, ileus, and in patients with haemodynamic instability or compromised unprotected airways. WBI should be used cautiously in debilitated patients, or in patients with medical conditions that may be further compromised by its use.

Increasing poison elimination

Treatments that might speed poison elimination are forced diuresis, urine alkalinization, acid diuresis, multiple-dose activated charcoal, dialysis and haemoperfusion.

Forced diuresis

The efficacy of forced diuresis depends on the poison being excreted unchanged by the kidney or as an active metabolite. Most drugs are either degraded by the liver to non-toxic metabolites or have such large volumes of distribution that there is insufficient active drug elimination in urine for forced diuresis to be of any clinical value. The amount removed in this way is insignificant compared to that removed by hepatic metabolism and *forced diuresis should not be used.*

Urine alkalinization

Most drugs, particularly unionized, lipid-soluble molecules, are largely reabsorbed by the renal tubules. Increasing the concentration of ionized drug in the urine should reduce reabsorption and further enhance elimination. This is achieved by manipulating urine pH which enhances ionization and hence elimination of weakly acidic compounds such as salicylates, phenobarbital, and chlorophenoxy herbicides. In practice, urine alkalinization is only employed commonly in salicylate intoxication. Methodology is described under aspirin poisoning (p. 979).

Urine acidification

Although, theoretically, induction of urine acidification increases the elimination of basic drugs such as amfetamines, there is no evidence that it is of clinical value in cases of poisoning.

Multiple-dose activated charcoal

Multiple doses of activated charcoal aid the elimination of some drugs from the circulation by interrupting their enterohepatic circulation and also by adsorbing the drug that has diffused into the intestinal juices. The rate of transfer of the latter is dependent upon the blood supply to the gut, the area of mucosa available for transfer, and the concentration gradient of the drug across the mucosa. The adsorptive capacity of charcoal is such that as zero concentrations of free drug are present in luminal fluid, the diffusion gradient still remains as high as possible. The process has been termed 'gut dialysis' since, in effect, the intestinal mucosa is being used as a semipermeable membrane.

Although many studies have demonstrated that multiple-dose activated charcoal increases drug elimination significantly, this therapy has not yet been shown to reduce morbidity and mortality. Multiple-dose activated charcoal should be *considered* only if a patient has ingested a life-threatening amount of carbamazepine, dapsone, phenobarbital, quinine or theophylline. In all of these cases there are data to confirm enhanced elimination, though no controlled studies have demonstrated clinical benefit. Adults should receive 50–100 g initially, followed by 50 g 4-hourly or 25 g 2-hourly until charcoal appears in the faeces or recovery occurs.

Dialysis

Haemodialysis in acute poisoning is most commonly indicated for the treatment of acute renal failure and only infrequently to increase the elimination of poisons. The rate of elimination across the dialysis membrane depends upon a number of variables including the molecular weight of the poison, the extent to which it is protein-bound, the concentration gradient, and pH of blood and dialysate. Haemodialysis is of little value in patients who ingest poisons with large volumes of distribution, e.g. tricyclic antidepressants, because the plasma contains only a small proportion of the total amount of drug in the body. *Haemodialysis is indicated* in patients with severe clinical features and high plasma concentrations of ethanol, ethylene glycol, isopropanol, lithium, methanol or salicylate.

Peritoneal dialysis increases the elimination of poisons such as ethylene glycol and methanol but is much less efficient than haemodialysis.

Haemoperfusion

This technique is *not available routinely*. It involves the passage of blood through an adsorbent material, e.g. activated charcoal, but is no better than oral multidose activated charcoal (p. 978) for the removal of phenobarbital, carbamazepine and theophylline. Other barbiturate and non-barbiturate hypnotics can be removed effectively but are now only rarely prescribed.

FURTHER READING

AACT/EAPCCT (1997) Position Statement: Gastric lavage. *Journal of Toxicology–Clinical Toxicology* **35**: 711–719.

AACT/EAPCCT (1997) Position Statement: Ipecac syrup. *Journal of Toxicology–Clinical Toxicology* **35**: 699–709.

AACT/EAPCCT (1997) Position Statement: Single-dose activated charcoal. *Journal of Toxicology–Clinical Toxicology* **35**: 721–741.

AACT/EAPCCT (1997) Position Statement: Cathartics. *Journal of Toxicology–Clinical Toxicology* **35**: 743–752.

AACT/EAPCCT (1997) Position Statement: Whole bowel irrigation. *Journal of Toxicology–Clinical Toxicology* **35**: 753–762.

AACT/EAPCCT (1999) Position Statement and Practice Guidelines on the use of multi-dose activated charcoal in the treatment of acute poisoning. *Journal of Toxicology–Clinical Toxicology* **37**: 731–751.

Specific poisons

Drugs and chemicals

In this section only specific treatment regimens will be discussed and are in alphabetical order. The general principles of management of self-poisoning will always be required. All drug doses relate to adults.

Amfetamines

Amfetamines are CNS and cardiovascular stimulants. These effects are mediated by increasing synaptic concentrations of epinephrine (adrenaline) and dopamine. Poisoning is usually the result of their use for pleasurable purposes.

Clinical features

These drugs cause euphoria, extrovert behaviour, a lack of desire to eat or sleep, tremor, dilated pupils, tachycardia and hypertension. More severe intoxication is associated with agitation, paranoid delusions, hallucinations and violent behaviour. Convulsions, rhabdomyolysis, hyperthermia and cardiac arrhythmias may develop in severe intoxication. Rarely, intracerebral and subarachnoid haemorrhage may occur and be fatal.

Treatment

Agitation is controlled by diazepam 10–20 mg i.v. or chlorpromazine 50–100 mg i.m. The peripheral sympathomimetic actions of amfetamines may be antagonized by β-adrenoceptor blocking drugs.

Aspirin

Aspirin is metabolized to salicylic acid (salicylate) by hydrolases present in many tissues, especially the liver, and subsequently to salicyluric acid and salicyl phenolic glucuronide (Fig. 16.9); these two pathways become saturated in overdose, with the following consequences:

- The plasma salicylate concentration increases more than proportionately with increasing dose.
- The time needed to eliminate a given fraction of a dose increases with increasing dose.
- Renal excretion of salicylic acid becomes increasingly significant after overdose; this excretion pathway is extremely sensitive to changes in urinary pH, e.g. increasing urinary pH from 7 to 8 increases the renal excretion of salicylates by a factor of 10.

Salicylates stimulate the respiratory centre, increase the depth and rate of respiration, and induce a respiratory alkalosis. Compensatory mechanisms, including renal excretion of bicarbonate and potassium, result in a metabolic acidosis. Salicylates also interfere with carbohydrate, fat and protein metabolism, disrupt oxidative phosphorylation, producing increased concentrations of lactate, pyruvate and ketone bodies, all of which contribute to the acidosis.

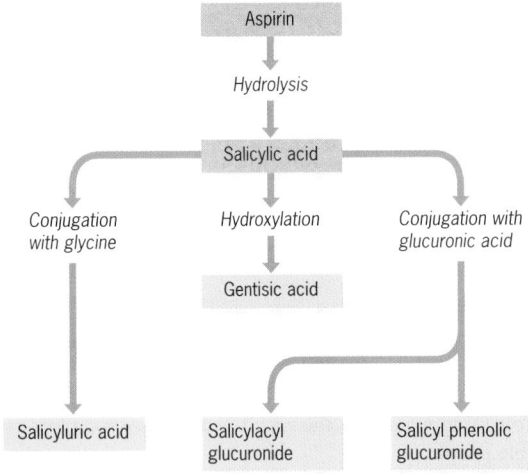

Fig. 16.9 The metabolism of aspirin.

Clinical features

After an overdose, symptoms include hyperventilation, sweating, nausea, vomiting, epigastric pain, tinnitus, and deafness can develop. Respiratory alkalosis and metabolic acidosis supervene and a mixed acid–base disturbance is commonly observed. Rarely, in severe cases non-cardiogenic pulmonary oedema, renal failure, tetany, coma and convulsions may ensue.

Management

For all cases (patients must be assessed in hospital):

- Plasma salicylate concentration. The severity of salicylate poisoning can only be assessed by blood concentration. Initial and repeat levels after 2–4 hours should be performed.
- Serum urea and electrolytes.
- Arterial blood gases.
- Intravenous fluids and electrolytes to correct any dehydration or electrolyte imbalance.
- Gastric lavage or activated charcoal (50–100 g) may be considered in a patient who has taken a large amount of aspirin less than 1 hour previously, though there is little evidence of benefit.

Moderate cases – plasma salicylate concentration 500–700 mg/L (3.62–5.07 mmol/L) – should receive *urine alkalinization*. Approximately 225 ml of an 8.4% (1 mmol bicarbonate/mL) solution of sodium bicarbonate is infused intravenously over 1 hour to ensure a urinary pH (measured by narrow-range indicator paper or pH meter) of more than 7.5 and preferably close to 8.5.

Urine alkalinization is a metabolically invasive procedure requiring frequent biochemical monitoring and medical and nursing expertise.

NB:
- Forced alkaline diuresis with large fluid volumes should not be used.
- Administration of sodium bicarbonate will exacerbate pre-existing hypokalaemia (this should have been corrected).

Severe cases – plasma salicylate concentration > 700 mg/L (5.07 mmol/L) – particularly those with coma and metabolic acidosis, require haemodialysis.

β-Adrenoceptor blocking drugs
Clinical features

In mild poisoning sinus bradycardia is the only feature but, if a substantial amount has been ingested, coma, convulsions and hypotension develop. Less commonly delirium, hallucinations and cardiac arrest supervene.

Treatment

Atropine 0.6–1.2 mg i.v. may be given but it is usually less effective than glucagon 50–150 µg/kg (typically 5–10 mg in an adult) followed by an infusion of 1–5 mg/h. Glucagon acts by bypassing the blocked β-receptor thus activating adenyl cyclase and promoting formation of cyclic AMP from ATP; cyclic AMP in turn exerts a direct β-stimulant effect on the heart.

Batteries (disc)

Children occasionally ingest disc button batteries, less commonly larger batteries. In the past there was concern that disc batteries might leak and release mercuric oxide but this metal has now been removed in Europe as a result of legislation. Most disc batteries will pass through the gut in 2 or 3 days. If they lodge in the oesophagus, removal by endoscopy is performed.

Benzodiazepines

Benzodiazepines are commonly taken in overdose but rarely produce severe poisoning except in the elderly or those with chronic respiratory disease.

Clinical features

Benzodiazepines produce drowsiness, ataxia and dysarthria. Coma and respiratory depression develop in severe intoxication.

Treatment

If respiratory depression is present, flumazenil 0.5 mg i.v. should be administered in an adult and this dose may be repeated, if necessary.

Cannabis (marijuana)

Cannabis is usually smoked but may be ingested as a 'cake', made into a tea or injected intravenously. It is the drug most widely abused in most developed countries. The major psychoactive constituent is delta-9-tetrahydrocannabinol (THC). THC possesses activity at the benzodiazepine, opioid and cannabinoid receptors.

Clinical features

Initially there is euphoria followed by drowsiness. A tachycardia is often present. High doses (and chronic use) may lead to psychosis. Intravenous injection leads to watery diarrhoea, tachycardia, hypotension and arthralgia.

Treatment

Reassurance is usually the only treatment required, though sedation with intravenous diazepam 10–20 mg i.v. or chlorpromazine 50–100 mg i.m. in adults may be required.

Carbamate insecticides

Carbamate insecticides inhibit acetylcholinesterase but the duration of this effect is comparatively short-lived since the carbamate–enzyme complex tends to dissociate spontaneously.

Clinical features

The features are similar to those of organophosphorus insecticide poisoning (see p. 985).

Treatment

Occasionally atropine 0.6–2 mg i.v. is required and recovery invariably occurs within 24 hours.

Carbon monoxide

The commonest source of carbon monoxide is an improperly maintained and ventilated heating system. In addition, inhalation of methylene chloride (found in paint strippers) may also lead to carbon monoxide poisoning as methylene chloride is metabolized in vivo to carbon monoxide. The affinity of haemoglobin for carbon monoxide is some 240 times greater than that for oxygen. Carbon monoxide combines with haemoglobin to form carboxyhaemoglobin, thereby reducing the total oxygen-carrying capacity of the blood and increasing the affinity of the remaining haem groups for oxygen. This results in tissue hypoxia. In addition, carbon monoxide also inhibits cytochrome oxidase a_3.

Clinical features

Symptoms of mild to moderate exposure to carbon monoxide may be mistaken for a viral illness. A peak carboxyhaemoglobin (COHb) concentration of less than 10% is not normally associated with symptoms, and peak COHb concentrations of 10–30% may result only in headache and mild exertional dyspnoea. Higher concentrations of COHb are associated with coma, convulsions and cardiorespiratory arrest. Neuropsychiatric features occur after apparent recovery from carbon monoxide intoxication.

Treatment

In addition to removing the patient from carbon monoxide exposure, high-flow oxygen should be administered using a tightly fitting face mask. Endotracheal intubation and mechanical ventilation may be required in those who are unconscious. Several controlled studies of hyperbaric oxygen have not shown long-term clinical benefit.

Chloroquine

Chloroquine poisoning is common in Africa, the Far East and West Pacific.

Clinical features

Hypotension is often the first clinical manifestation of poisoning. It may progress to cardiogenic shock, pulmonary oedema and cardiac arrest. Agitation and acute psychosis, convulsions and coma may ensue. Hypokalaemia is common and is due to chloroquine-induced potassium channel blockade.

Treatment

Hypokalaemia should be corrected. There is some evidence that mechanical ventilation, the administration of epinephrine (adrenaline) and high doses of diazepam reduce morbidity and mortality. Multiple-dose activated charcoal may enhance chloroquine elimination.

Cocaine (p. 1259)

Cocaine may be abused by smoking, ingestion, injection or snorting it intranasally. Cocaine blocks the reuptake of biogenic amines. Inhibition of dopamine reuptake is responsible for the psychomotor agitation which commonly accompanies cocaine use. Blockade of norepinephrine (noradrenaline) reuptake produces tachycardia, and inhibition of serotonin reuptake may induce hallucinations. Cocaine also enhances CNS arousal by potentiating the effects of excitatory amino acids.

Clinical features

After initial euphoria, cocaine produces agitation, tachycardia, hypertension, sweating, hallucinations, convulsions, metabolic acidosis, hyperthermia, rhabdomyolysis, and ventricular arrhythmias. Dissection of the aorta, myocarditis, myocardial infarction, dilated cardiomyopathy, subarachnoid haemorrhage, and cerebral haemorrhage also occur.

Treatment

Diazepam 10–20 mg i.v. is used to control agitation and convulsions. Active external cooling should be used for hyperthermia. β-Adrenoceptor blockers are contra-indicated for treatment of hypertension and severe tachycardia as propranolol particularly can cause paradoxical hypertension.

Cyanide

Cyanide and its derivatives are used widely in industry. Hydrogen cyanide is also released during the thermal decomposition of polyurethane foams. Cyanide reversibly inhibits cytochrome oxidase a_3 so that cellular respiration ceases.

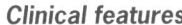

Clinical features

Inhalation of hydrogen cyanide gas may produce symptoms within seconds and death within minutes. In contrast, the ingestion of a cyanide salt may not produce features for 1 hour. After exposure initial symptoms are non-specific and include a feeling of constriction in the chest and dyspnoea. Coma, convulsions and metabolic acidosis may then supervene.

Treatment

Oxygen should be administered and, if available, dicobalt edetate 300 mg should be administered i.v.; the dose may be repeated in severe cases. An alternative antidote is hydroxocobalamin 5 g i.v. (although this is not available in all countries at this dosage) which may be repeated as necessary. If these two preferred antidotes are not available sodium nitrite 300 mg i.v. and sodium thiosulphate 12.5 g i.v. should be administered. Sodium nitrite produces methaemoglobinaemia; methaemoglobin combines with cyanide to form cyanmethaemoglobin. Sodium thiosulphate and hydroxocobalamin enhance endogenous cyanide detoxification mechanisms. Dicobalt edetate (and the free cobalt contained in the preparation) complexes free cyanide.

Digoxin

Toxicity occurring during chronic administration is common, though acute poisoning is infrequent.

Clinical features

These include nausea, vomiting, dizziness, anorexia and drowsiness. Rarely, confusion, visual disturbances and hallucinations occur. Sinus bradycardia is often marked and may be followed by supraventricular arrhythmias with or without heart block, ventricular premature beats and ventricular tachycardia. Hyperkalaemia occurs owing to the inhibition of the sodium–potassium-activated ATPase pump.

Treatment

Sinus bradycardia, atrioventricular block and sinoatrial standstill are often reduced or even abolished by atropine 0.6–2.4 mg i.v. If cardiac output is compromised, however, digoxin-specific antibody fragments 6–8 mg/kg bodyweight should be administered.

Ecstasy (3,4-methylenedioxy-methamfetamine, MDMA) (p. 1259)

Ecstasy is often taken in the setting of a rave where dancing is fast and prolonged. It is likely that the pharmacological effects of the drug (which are similar to those of the closely related amfetamines) are compounded by physical exertion and dehydration.

Clinical features

Mild abuse is characterized by agitation, tachycardia, hypertension, widely dilated pupils, trismus and sweating. In more severe cases, hyperthermia, disseminated intravascular coagulation, rhabdomyolysis, acute renal failure and hyponatraemia (secondary to inappropriate antidiuretic hormone secretion) predominate.

Treatment

Reassurance and rehydration. If necessary, diazepam 5–10 mg i.v. should be given for severe agitation or convulsions. If hyperthermia is present, dantrolene 1 mg/kg bodyweight i.v. should be administered. Deaths occur from hyperpyrexia, dehydration and renal and liver failure. Self-induced water intoxication occurs.

Ethanol (see p. 250)

Ethanol is commonly ingested in beverages and deliberately with other substances in overdose. It is also present in many cosmetic and antiseptic preparations. Following absorption, ethanol is oxidized to acetaldehyde and then to acetate. Ethanol is a CNS depressant and the features of ethanol intoxication are generally related to blood concentrations and are shown in Table 21.15.

Clinical features

In children in particular, severe hypoglycaemia may accompany alcohol intoxication owing to inhibition of gluconeogenesis. Hypoglycaemia is also observed in adults who are malnourished or who have fasted in the previous 24 hours. In severe cases of intoxication, coma and hypothermia are often present and lactic acidosis, ketoacidosis and acute renal failure have been reported.

Treatment

As ethanol-induced hypoglycaemia is not responsive to glucagon, intravenous glucose 25 g (50 ml of 50% dextrose should be given). Haemodialysis should be considered if the blood ethanol concentration exceeds 5000 mg/L (32.5 mmol/L) and, particularly, if severe metabolic acidosis is present.

Ethylene glycol

Ethylene glycol is a common constituent of antifreeze fluid used in car radiators. Ethylene glycol itself is non-toxic but is metabolized to toxic products (Fig. 16.10).

Clinical features

Initially the features of ethylene glycol poisoning are similar to ethanol intoxication (though there is no ethanol on the breath). Coma and convulsions follow and a variety of neurological abnormalities including nystagmus and ophthalmoplegias may be observed. Severe metabolic acidosis, hypocalcaemia and the presence of calcium oxalate crystalluria are well-recognized complications.

Treatment

Supportive measures to combat shock, hypocalcaemia, and metabolic acidosis should be instituted. Inhibitors

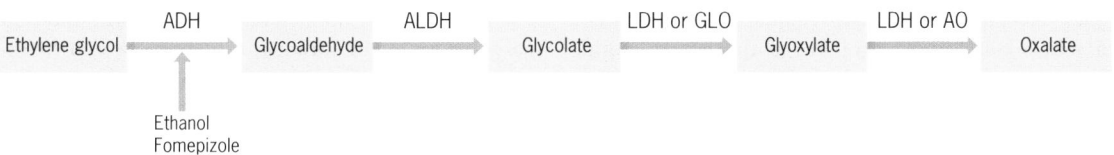

Fig. 16.10 **The metabolism of ethylene glycol.** ADH, alcohol dehydrogenase; ALDH, aldehyde dehydrogenase; LDH, lactate dehydrogenase; GLO, glycolic acid oxidase; AO, aldehyde oxidase.

of alcohol dehydrogenase (either ethanol or fomepizole) should be given to inhibit ethylene glycol metabolism (Fig. 16.10) and, secondly, haemodialysis should be employed to remove ethylene glycol, its aldehyde metabolites and glycolate. A loading dose of ethanol 50 g (conveniently given orally as 125 ml of gin, whisky or vodka) should be administered followed by an intravenous infusion of ethanol 10–12 g/h to produce blood ethanol concentrations of 500–1000 mg/L (11–22 mmol/L). The infusion is continued until ethylene glycol is no longer detectable in the blood. If haemodialysis is employed, the rate of ethanol administration will need to be increased to 17–22 g/h as ethanol is dialysable. Alternatively, fomepizole 15 mg/kg bodyweight (available on a named-patient basis) can be administered over 30 minutes followed by four 12-hourly doses of 10 mg/kg, then 15 mg/kg every 12 hours until ethylene glycol concentrations are less than 200 mg/L. If dialysis is employed the frequency of fomepizole dosing should be increased to 4-hourly during dialysis because fomepizole is dialysable.

Household products

The agents most commonly involved are bleach, cosmetics, toiletries, detergents, disinfectants and petroleum distillates such as paraffin and white spirit. Ingestion of household products is usually accidental and is most common among children less than 5 years of age. If the ingestion is accidental, adverse features very rarely occur except in the case of petroleum distillates where aspiration is a recognized complication because of their low surface tension.

Powder detergents, sterilizing tablets, denture-cleaning tablets and industrial bleaches (which contain high concentrations of sodium hypochlorite) are corrosive to the mouth and pharynx if ingested. Endotracheal intubation or tracheostomy may be required for life-threatening pharyngeal or laryngeal oedema. Gastric aspiration and lavage and dilution or neutralization of the alkali is contraindicated as it causes further damage and a risk of aspiration. Careful upper GI endoscopy is required to estimate the extent of injury. Oesophageal strictures occur.

Nail polish and nail polish remover contain acetone, which may produce coma if ingested in substantial quantities. Inhalation by small children of substantial quantities of talcum powder has occasionally given rise to severe pulmonary oedema and death.

Iron

Unless more than 60 mg of elemental iron per kg body-weight is ingested, adverse features are unlikely to develop. As a result poisoning is seldom severe but deaths still occur. Iron salts have a direct corrosive effect on the upper gastrointestinal tract.

Clinical features

The initial features are characterized by nausea, vomiting (the vomit may be grey or black in colour), abdominal pain and diarrhoea. Severely poisoned patients develop haematemesis, hypotension, coma and shock at an early stage. Most patients only suffer mild gastrointestinal symptoms. A small minority deteriorate 12–48 hours after ingestion and develop shock, metabolic acidosis, acute renal tubular necrosis and hepatocellular necrosis. Rarely, up to 6 weeks after ingestion, intestinal strictures due to corrosive damage may occur.

Treatment

Serum iron should be measured approximately 4 hours after ingestion. Desferrioxamine therapy is not required unless the concentration exceeds the predicted normal iron-binding capacity (> 5 mg/L, 90 µmol/L). If a patient develops coma or shock, desferrioxamine should be given without delay in a dose of 15 mg/kg/h i.v. (total amount of infusion not to exceed 80 mg/kg in 24 hours). If the recommended rate of administration is exceeded, or the therapy is continued for several days, adverse effects including pulmonary oedema have been reported.

Lead

Exposure to lead occurs occupationally and the current practice in many countries is to recommend that workers over 18 years of age should cease working with lead when their blood lead concentration is above 600 µg/L (2.9 µmol/L), or 300 µg/L (1.45 µmol/L) for a woman of reproductive capacity, or 500 µg/L (2.4 µmol/L) for all employees aged under 18 years. Children who chew on lead-painted items in their homes (pica) may develop lead poisoning. The use of lead-containing cosmetics or 'drugs' has also resulted in lead poisoning.

Clinical features

Mild intoxication may result in no more than lethargy and occasional abdominal discomfort, though abdominal pain, vomiting, constipation and encephalopathy (seizures, delirium, coma) may develop in more severe cases. Encephalopathy is more common in children than in adults but is now rare in the developed world. Typically, though very rarely, lead poisoning results in foot drop attributable to peripheral motor neuropathy. A bluish discoloration of the gum margins owing to the deposition of lead sulphide is observed occasionally.

Treatment

The social and occupational dimensions of lead poisoning must be recognized. Simply giving children chelation therapy and then returning them to a contaminated home environment is of no value. Similarly, returning a worker to an environment where he was exposed previously and excessively to lead is inappropriate.

The decision to use chelation therapy is based not only on the blood lead concentration but on the presence of symptoms. Although sodium calcium edetate 75 mg/kg bodyweight per day for 5 days is some four times more efficient in increasing lead excretion than oral dimercaptosuccinic acid (DMSA) 30 mg/kg bodyweight for 5 days, it has to be given intravenously and may result in increased uptake of lead into the brain. Oral DMSA, if available, is preferred.

Lithium (see p. 1248)

Lithium toxicity is usually the result of therapeutic overdosage (chronic toxicity) rather than deliberate self-poisoning (acute toxicity).

Chronic toxicity is usually associated with serum concentrations above 1.5 mmol/L (10.4 mg/L). Acute massive overdose may produce concentrations of 5 mmol/L (34.7 mg/L) without causing toxic features (see p. 1248).

Treatment

Forced diuresis with sodium chloride 0.9% is effective in increasing elimination of lithium, though haemodialysis is far superior and should be undertaken particularly if neurological features are present, if renal function is impaired and if chronic toxicity or acute on chronic toxicity are the modes of presentation.

Mercury

Metallic mercury is very volatile and when spilled has a large surface area so that high atmospheric concentrations may be produced in enclosed spaces, particularly when environmental temperatures are high. Thus, great care should be taken in clearing up a spillage of mercury if a thermometer or sphygmomanometer is broken. If ingested, metallic mercury will usually be eliminated per rectum, though small amounts may be found in the appendix. Mercury salts are well absorbed following ingestion as are organometallic compounds where mercury is covalently bound to carbon.

Clinical features

Inhalation of acute mercury vapour causes headache, nausea, cough, chest pain, bronchitis and occasionally pneumonia. Proteinuria and nephrotic syndrome are observed rarely. In addition, a fine tremor and neuro-behavioural impairment occurs and peripheral nerve involvement has also been observed. Ingestion of inorganic and organic mercury compounds causes an irritant gastroenteritis with corrosive ulceration, bloody diarrhoea and abdominal cramps and may lead to circulatory collapse and shock.

Mercurous compounds are less corrosive and toxic than mercuric salts.

Treatment

DMPS (dimercaptopropanesulphonate) is probably the antidote of choice and is given orally in a dose of 30 mg/kg per day. At least 5 days' treatment is usually required. Alternatives are dimercaprol (BAL), which must be administered intramuscularly, and penicillamine.

Methanol

Methanol is used widely as a solvent and is found in antifreeze solutions. Methanol is metabolized to formaldehyde and formate (Fig. 16.11). The concentration of formate increases greatly and is accompanied by accumulation of hydrogen ions causing metabolic acidosis.

Clinical features

Methanol causes inebriation and drowsiness. After a latent period coma supervenes. Blurred vision and diminished visual acuity occur. The presence of dilated pupils that are unreactive to light suggests that permanent blindness is likely to ensue. A severe metabolic acidosis may develop and be accompanied by hyperglycaemia and a raised serum amylase activity. A blood methanol concentration of 500 mg/L (15.63 mmol/L) confirms serious poisoning. The mortality correlates well with the severity and duration of metabolic acidosis. Survivors may show permanent neurological sequelae including parkinsonian-like signs as well as blindness.

Treatment

Treatment is similar to that of ethylene glycol poisoning (see p. 983). Metabolic acidosis should be corrected, methanol metabolism should be inhibited by the administration of ethanol or fomepizole (if available), and haemodialysis should be considered to remove high

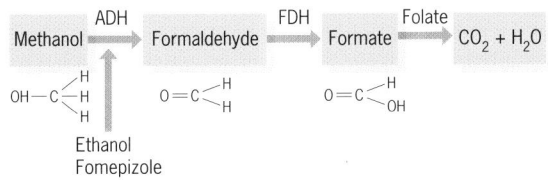

Fig. 16.11 The metabolism of methanol. ADH, alcohol dehydrogenase; FDH, formaldehyde dehydrogenase.

circulating methanol concentrations. Folinic acid 30 mg i.v. 6-hourly may protect against ocular toxicity by accelerating formate metabolism.

Monoamine oxidase inhibitors

These are now used less frequently in the treatment of depression because of the dangers of dietary and drug interactions. Hence, poisoning with them is correspondingly uncommon. A reversible type A MOAI inhibitor, moclobemide, is now marketed.

Clinical features

Features after overdose may be delayed for 12–24 hours. They include excitement, restlessness, hyperpyrexia, hyperreflexia, convulsions, opisthotonos, rhabdomyolysis and coma. Sinus tachycardia and either hypo- or hypertension are also observed.

Treatment

Treatment is supportive with control of convulsions and marked excitement; diazepam 10–20 mg i.v. in an adult should be given as necessary and repeated. Dantrolene 1 mg/kg i.v. should be administered if hyperpyrexia develops. Hypotension should be treated with plasma expansion and hypertension by the administration of an α-adrenoceptor blocker such as chlorpromazine.

Non-steroidal anti-inflammatory agents (NSAIDs)

Self-poisoning with NSAIDs has increased, particularly now that ibuprofen is available without prescription. In most cases minor gastrointestinal disturbance is the only feature but, in more severe cases, coma, convulsions, metabolic acidosis and renal failure have occurred. Poisoning with mefenamic acid commonly results in convulsions though these are usually short-lived.

Treatment is symptomatic and supportive.

Opiates and opioids

Clinical features

Cardinal signs of opiate poisoning are pinpoint pupils, reduced respiratory rate and coma. Hypothermia, hypoglycaemia and convulsions are occasionally observed in severe cases. In severe heroin overdose, non-cardiogenic pulmonary oedema has been reported.

Treatment

Naloxone 1.2 mg i.v. in an adult (5–10 μg per kg bodyweight in a child) will reverse severe respiratory depression and coma at least partially. In severe poisoning larger initial doses or repeat doses will be required. It should be remembered that the duration of action of naloxone is often less than the drug taken in overdose; e.g. methadone, which has a very long half-life. For this reason an infusion of naloxone may be required. Non-cardiogenic pulmonary oedema should be treated with mechanical ventilation.

Organophosphorus insecticides

Organophosphorus (OP) insecticides are used widely throughout the world. Intoxication may follow ingestion, inhalation or dermal absorption. Organophosphorus insecticides inhibit acetyl cholinesterase causing accumulation of acetylcholine at central and peripheral cholinergic nerve endings, including neuromuscular junctions. Many OP insecticides require biotransformation before becoming active and so the features of intoxication are delayed.

Clinical features

Poisoning is characterized by anxiety, restlessness, tiredness, headache, and muscarinic features such as nausea, vomiting, abdominal colic, diarrhoea, tenesmus, sweating, hypersalivation, and chest tightness. Miosis may be present. Nicotinic effects include muscle fasciculation and flaccid paresis of limb, respiratory, and, occasionally, extraocular muscles. Respiratory failure will ensue in severe cases and is exacerbated by the development of bronchial secretions and pulmonary oedema. Coma and convulsions occur in severe poisoning. Diagnosis is confirmed by measuring the erythrocyte cholinesterase activity; plasma cholinesterase activity is less specific but may also be depressed.

Treatment

Mild cases require no specific treatment other then the removal of soiled clothing; contaminated skin should be washed with soap and water to prevent further absorption. Atropine 0.6–2 mg i.v. should be given to reduce bronchial secretions. In addition, pralidoxime, which reactivates phosphorylated acetylcholinesterase, should be given in symptomatic patients where the diagnosis has been confirmed. The dose is 30 mg/kg by slow i.v. injection which should be repeated 4- to 6-hourly; in severe cases an infusion of pralidoxime 8–10 mg/kg/h is used.

Paracetamol (acetaminophen)

Paracetamol is the most common form of poisoning encountered in the UK. In therapeutic dose, paracetamol is conjugated with glucuronide and sulphate. A small amount of paracetamol is metabolized by mixed function oxidase enzymes to form a highly reactive compound (N-acetyl-p-benzoquinoneimine, NAPQI), which is then immediately conjugated with glutathione and subsequently excreted as cysteine and mercapturic conjugates. In overdose, large amounts of paracetamol are metabolized by oxidation because of saturation of the sulphate conjugation pathway. Liver glutathione stores become depleted so that the liver is unable to deactivate the toxic metabolite (NAPQI). Paracetamol-induced renal damage probably results from a mechanism similar to that which is responsible for hepatotoxicity.

The severity of paracetamol poisoning is dose-related. There is, however, some variation in individual susceptibility to paracetamol-induced hepatotoxicity. Patients with pre-existing liver disease, those with a high alcohol intake and poor nutrition, those receiving enzyme-inducing drugs, those suffering from anorexia nervosa and other eating disorders and HIV infection should be considered to be at greater risk and given treatment at plasma paracetamol concentrations lower than those normally used for interpretation (Fig. 16.12).

Clinical features

Following the ingestion of an overdose of paracetamol, patients usually remain asymptomatic for the first 24 hours or at the most develop anorexia, nausea and vomiting. Liver damage is not usually detectable by routine liver function tests until at least 18 hours after ingestion of the drug. Liver damage usually reaches a peak, as assessed by measurement of aminotransferase (ALT/AST) activity and prothrombin time (INR), at 72–96 hours after ingestion. Without treatment, a small percentage of patients will develop fulminant hepatic failure. Renal failure due to acute tubular necrosis occurs in 25% of patients with severe hepatic damage and in a few without evidence of serious disturbance of liver function.

Management

- Admit the patient.
- Take blood for urgent estimation of the plasma paracetamol concentration as soon as 4 hours or more have elapsed since ingestion. Check INR, plasma creatinine and ALT.
- Assess whether the patient is at increased risk of liver damage.
- Give treatment (below) if needed (Fig 16.12).

The treatment protocol is dependent on the time of presentation.

< 8 hours after ingestion

- If the plasma paracetamol concentration is not available within 8 hours of the overdose and, if 10–15 g (20–30 tablets) or > 150 mg/kg paracetamol has been ingested, treatment should be started at once and stopped if the plasma paracetamol concentration subsequently indicates that treatment is not required.
- Check INR, plasma creatinine and ALT on the completion of treatment and before discharge.

8–15 hours after ingestion

- Urgent action is required because the efficacy of treatment declines progressively from 8 hours after overdose. If > 150 mg/kg paracetamol has been ingested, start treatment immediately.
- In patients already receiving treatment, only discontinue if the plasma paracetamol concentration is below the relevant treatment line (Fig. 16.12) and there is no abnormality of the INR, plasma creatinine or ALT and the patient is asymptomatic. Do not discontinue the infusion if there is any doubt as to the timing of the overdose.
- At the end of treatment, measure INR, plasma creatinine and ALT. If any test is abnormal or the patient is symptomatic, further monitoring is required and expert advice should be sought.
- Patients with normal INR, plasma creatinine and ALT and who are asymptomatic may be discharged.

15–24 hours after ingestion

- Urgent action is required because the efficacy of treatment is limited more than 15 hours after overdose. Start treatment immediately if > 150 mg/kg paracetamol has been ingested.
- The prognostic accuracy of the '200 mg/L line' after 15 hours is uncertain but a plasma paracetamol concentration above the extended treatment line should be regarded as carrying serious risk of severe liver damage.
- At the end of treatment, check INR, plasma creatinine and ALT. If any test is abnormal or the patient is symptomatic, further monitoring is required and expert advice should be sought.

Methionine and *N*-acetylcysteine (NAC) have emerged as effective protective agents provided that they are administered within 8–10 hours of ingestion of the overdose. Both substances act by replenishing cellular glutathione stores, though NAC may also repair oxidation damage caused by NAPQI. Methionine appears more

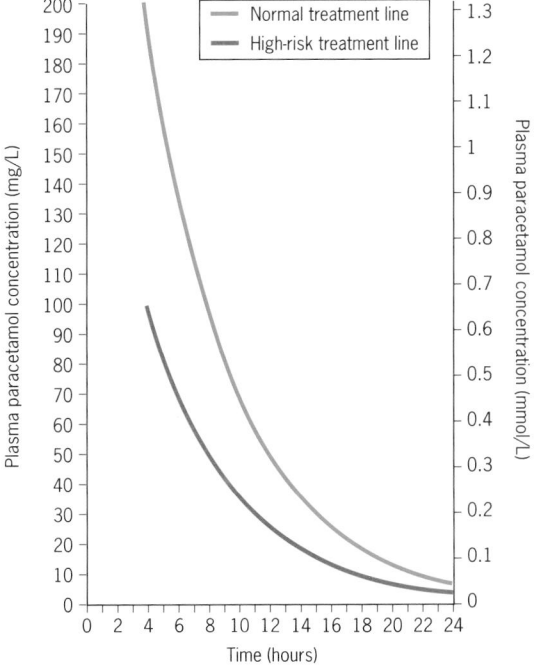

Fig. 16.12 Nomogram for paracetamol. From *British National Formulary* (1998) with permission. For definition of 'high-risk patients' see text.

> **Box 16.8**
>
> **Antidote regimens for paracetamol poisoning**
>
> **_N_-acetylcysteine (intravenously)**
> 150 mg/kg over 15 min, then 50 mg/kg in 500 mL of 5% dextrose in the next 4 hours and 100 mg/kg in 1000 mL of 5% dextrose over the ensuing 16 hours.
>
> Total dose: 300 mg/kg over 20–25 hours.
>
> **Methionine (orally)**
> 2.5 g initially, then 2.5 g 4-hourly for a further three doses.
>
> Total dose: 10 g methionine over 12 hours.
>
> **_N_-acetylcysteine (orally)**
> 140 mg/kg initially, then 60 mg/kg every 4 hours for 17 additional doses.
>
> Total dose: 1330 mg/kg over 72 hours.

effective when given orally than when administered intravenously. As oral NAC induces vomiting (as does paracetamol ingestion), the intravenous route is preferred. The main treatment regimens used internationally are shown in Box 16.8.

Some 5% of patients treated with intravenous NAC develop rash, angio-oedema, hypotension and bronchospasm. These reactions, which are related to the initial bolus, are seldom serious and discontinuing the infusion is usually all that is required. In more severe cases chlorphenamine (chlorpheniramine) 10–20 mg i.v. in an adult may be given.

If liver or renal failure ensues, this should be treated conventionally though there is evidence that a continuing infusion of NAC (continue 16-h infusion until recovery) will improve the morbidity and mortality. Liver transplantation has been performed successfully in patients with paracetamol-induced fulminant hepatic failure (p. 357).

Paraquat

Poisoning with paraquat is very uncommon in the UK but is a common cause of morbidity and mortality in the developing world.

Following ingestion, ulcers in the mouth and oesophagus develop, accompanied by vomiting and diarrhoea, which are induced by paraquat and partly by the co-formulants. In severe cases of poisoning multiple organ failure develops. The prognosis may be determined by measurement of the plasma paraquat concentration.

Treatment is supportive.

Phenothiazines

Phenothiazines have varying antimuscarinic, extra-pyramidal and sedative effects.

In overdose, impairment of consciousness, hypotension and respiratory depression develop. These effects are less likely to be observed in those who are taking the drug therapeutically.

Benzatropine 2 mg i.v. in an adult is occasionally required for the treatment of dyskinesia and oculogyric crisis.

Quinine

Quinine poisoning is relatively common in Western Europe, probably because of its use for the treatment of leg cramps. It is also ingested in overdose in the developing world where it is employed as an antimalarial.

In addition to the development of tinnitus and deafness, a substantial number of patients develop oculotoxicity including blindness which may be irreversible. Ventricular arrhythmias, convulsions and coma are observed in severe cases.

Treatment is supportive. There is evidence that multiple-dose activated charcoal increases quinine elimination (but see p. 978).

Selective serotonin reuptake inhibitors (SSRIs)

Citalopram, fluoxetine, fluvoxamine, paroxetine and sertraline are antidepressants that inhibit serotonin reuptake. They lack the anticholinergic actions of tricyclic antidepressants.

Even large overdoses appear to be relatively safe unless potentiated by ethanol. Most patients will show no signs of toxicity but drowsiness, nausea, diarrhoea, and sinus tachycardia have been reported. Rarely, junctional bradycardia, seizures, and hypertension have been encountered and influenza-like symptoms may develop.

Supportive measures are all that are required.

Theophylline

Poisoning may complicate therapeutic use as well as being the result of deliberate self-poisoning. If a slow-release preparation is involved, peak plasma concentrations may not be attained until 6–12 hours after overdosage and the onset of toxic features is correspondingly delayed.

Clinical features

Nausea, vomiting, hyperventilation, haematemesis, abdominal pain, diarrhoea, sinus tachycardia, supraventricular and ventricular arrhythmias, hypotension, restlessness, irritability, headache, hyperreflexia, tremors, and convulsions have been observed. Hypokalaemia probably results from activation of Na^+/K^+-ATPase. A mixed acid–base disturbance is common. Most symptomatic patients have plasma theophylline concentrations in excess of 25 mg/L (430 μmol/L). Convulsions are seen more commonly when concentrations are > 50 mg/L (> 860 μmol/L). Plasma potassium concentrations of < 2.6 mmol/L, acidaemia, hypotension, seizures and arrhythmias are indicators of severe poisoning.

Treatment

There is good evidence that multiple-dose activated charcoal enhances the elimination of theophylline

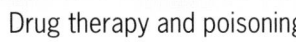
(p. 978). However, protracted theophylline-induced vomiting may mitigate the benefit of this therapy, unless vomiting is suppressed by ondansetron 8 mg i.v. in an adult. Correction of hypokalaemia to prevent or treat tachyarrhythmias is of great importance. A non-selective β-adrenoceptor blocking drug, such as propranolol, is also useful in the treatment of tachyarrhythmias secondary to hypokalaemia but should only be given to those without a history of respiratory disease. Convulsions should be treated with diazepam 10–20 mg i.v. in an adult.

Tricyclic antidepressants

Tricyclic antidepressants block the reuptake of norepinephrine (noradrenaline) into peripheral and intracerebral neurones, thereby increasing the concentration of monoamines in these areas. These drugs also have anticholinergic actions and class 1 antiarrhythmic (quinidine-like) activity.

Clinical features

Features of poisoning usually appear within 1 hour after ingestion. Drowsiness, sinus tachycardia, dry mouth, dilated pupils, urinary retention, increased reflexes, and extensor plantar responses are the most common features of mild poisoning. Severe intoxication leads to coma, often with divergent strabismus and convulsions. Plantar, oculocephalic, and oculovestibular reflexes may be temporarily abolished. An ECG will often show a wide QRS interval and there is a reasonable correlation between the width of the QRS complex and the severity of poisoning. Metabolic acidosis and cardiorespiratory depression are observed in severe cases.

Treatment

The majority of patients recover with supportive therapy alone though a small percentage of patients will require mechanical ventilation for 24–48 hours. The onset of supraventricular tachycardia and ventricular tachycardia should be treated with sodium bicarbonate (8.4%) 50 mmol (50 mL) intravenously over 20 minutes, even if there is no acidosis present. In addition, adequate oxygenation, control of convulsions and correction of acidosis should be undertaken. If ventricular tachycardia is compromising cardiac output, lidocaine (lignocaine) 50–100 mg i.v. should be administered in an adult.

Volatile substance abuse (p. 1259)

Volatile substances are either 'bagged' (sprayed into a plastic bag and then inhaled until the subject passes out) or 'huffed' (sprayed on to a cloth held to the mouth). Volatile substances abused in this way include organic solvents, hydrocarbon mixtures such as petrol, and aerosol propellants. Glues (containing toluene) are most often sniffed from a plastic bag and repeated abuse in this manner leads to the development of erythematous spots around the mouth and nose ('glue-sniffer's rash').

Clinical features

The clinical features are similar to those of alcohol intoxication with initial CNS stimulation followed by depression. Thus, euphoria, blurring of vision, tinnitus, slurring of speech, ataxia, feelings of omnipotence, impaired judgement, irritability and excitement are observed commonly. Convulsions and coma, which is usually short-lived, may occur. Some chronic abusers report psychotic symptoms, listlessness and anorexia. Chronic abuse of toluene-containing glues has also resulted in muscle weakness, gastrointestinal complaints (abdominal pain and haematemesis) and neuropsychiatric disorders (altered mental status, cerebellar abnormalities, peripheral neuropathy). In addition, hypokalaemia, hypophosphataemia and hyperchloraemia have been reported. Rhabdomyolysis occurs in a substantial minority of these patients.

Marine animals

Ciguatera fish poisoning

Over 400 fish species have been reported as ciguatoxic (*Cigua* is Spanish for poisonous snail), though barracuda, red snapper, amberjack and grouper are most commonly implicated. Ciguatera fish contain ciguatoxin, maitotoxin and scaritoxin, which are lipid-soluble, heat-stable compounds that are derived from dinoflagellates such as *Gambierdiscus toxicus*. The mechanisms of toxicity in man appear to involve more than just inhibition of acetylcholinesterase activity, which has been found in vitro.

Clinical features

The onset of symptoms may occur from a few minutes to 30 hours after ingestion of toxic fish. Typically, features appear between 1 and 6 hours and include abdominal cramps, nausea, vomiting and watery diarrhoea. In some cases, numbness and paraesthesiae of the lips, tongue and throat occur. Other features described include malaise, dry mouth, metallic taste, myalgia, arthralgia, blurred vision, photophobia and transient blindness. In more severe cases, hypotension, cranial nerve palsies and respiratory paralysis have been reported. The mortality in severe cases may be as high as 12%. Recovery takes from 48 hours to 1 week in the mild form and from 1 to several weeks in the severe form.

Treatment is symptomatic, although in a few patients atropine has lessened some of the cardiovascular and gastrointestinal manifestations.

Jelly fish

Most of the jelly fish found in North European coastal waters are non-toxic as their stings cannot penetrate human skin. A notable exception is the 'Portuguese man-o'-war' (*Physalia physalis*), whose sting contains a toxic peptide, phospholipase A, and a histamine-liberating factor.

Local pain occurs followed by myalgia, nausea, griping abdominal pain, dyspnoea and even death.

Adhesive tape may be used to remove any tentacles still adherent to the bather. Local analgesia and antihistamine creams provide symptomatic relief.

Paralytic shell fish poisoning

This is uncommon and is caused by bivalve molluscs being contaminated with neurotoxins, including saxitoxin, produced by the toxic dinoflagellates, *Gonyaulax catenella* and *Gonyaulax tamarensis*.

Symptoms develop within 30 minutes of ingestion. The illness is characterized by paraesthesiae of the mouth, lips, face and extremities and is often accompanied by nausea, vomiting and diarrhoea. In more severe cases, dysphonia, dysphagia, muscle weakness, paralysis, ataxia and respiratory depression occur.

Treatment is symptomatic and supportive.

Scrombrotoxic fish poisoning

This is due to the action of bacteria such as *Proteus morgani* and *Klebsiella pneumoniae* in decomposing the flesh of fish such as tuna, mackerel, bonito and skipjack if the fish are stored at insufficiently low temperatures. The spoiled fish can contain excessively high concentrations of histamine (muscle histidine is broken down by the bacteria to histamine), though the precise role of histamine in the pathogenesis of the clinical syndrome is uncertain.

The mean incubation period is 30 minutes. The illness is characterized by flushing, headache, sweating, dizziness, burning of the mouth and throat, abdominal cramps, nausea, vomiting and diarrhoea and is usually short-lived; the mean duration is 4 hours.

Treatment is symptomatic and supportive. Antihistamines may alleviate the symptoms.

Stings from marine animals

Several species of fish have venomous spines in their fins. These include the weaver fish, short-spine cottus, spiny dogfish and the stingray. Bathers and fishermen may be stung if they tread on or handle these species.

The immediate result of a sting is intense local pain, swelling, bruising, blistering, necrosis and, if the poisoned spine is not removed, chronic sepsis (though this is uncommon). Occasionally, systemic symptoms including vomiting, diarrhoea, hypotension and tachycardia occur.

Immersing the affected part in hot water may relieve local symptoms as this denatures the thermolabile toxin.

Venomous animals

Insect stings and bites

Insect stings from wasps and bees and bites from ants produce pain and swelling at the puncture site. Following the sting or bite, patients should be observed for 2 hours for any signs of evolving urticaria, pruritus, bronchospasm or oropharyngeal oedema. The onset of anaphylaxis requires urgent treatment (see p. 961).

Scorpions

Scorpion stings are a serious problem in North Africa, the Middle East and the Americas. Scorpion venoms stimulate the release of acetylcholine and catecholamines causing both cholinergic and adrenergic symptoms.

Severe pain occurs immediately at the site of puncture, followed by swelling. Signs of systemic involvement, which may be delayed for 24 hours, include vomiting, sweating, piloerection, abdominal colic, diarrhoea. In some cases, depending on the species, shock, respiratory depression and pulmonary oedema may develop.

Local infiltration with anaesthetic or a ring block will usually alleviate local pain, though systemic analgesia may be required. Specific antivenom, if available, should be administered as soon possible.

Venomous snakes

Snake bite is common in some tropical countries. For example, in Sri Lanka there are some 6 bites per 100 000 population and 900 deaths per year. In Nigeria there are some 500 bites per 100 000 population with a 12% mortality. In Myanmar there are 15 deaths per 100 000 population from snake bites. In the US (population 250 million) there are some 45 000 bites per year (7000 by venomous species) with 9–14 deaths annually. In the UK (population 50 million) approximately 100 people are admitted to hospital annually but no deaths have occurred since 1970. In Australia there are 2–3 deaths annually.

There are three main groups of venomous snakes, representing some 200 species, which have in their upper jaws a pair of enlarged teeth (fangs) that inject venom into the tissues of their victim. These are Viperidae (Old World adders and vipers, American rattlesnakes, moccasins, lanceheaded vipers and Asian pit vipers), Elapidae (cobras, kraits, mambas, coral snakes, Australian venomous snakes) and Hydrophiidae (sea snakes).

Clinical features

Viperidae

Russell's viper is the most important cause of snake-bite mortality in India, Pakistan and Burma. There is local swelling at the site of the bite, which may become massive. Local tissue necrosis may occur, particularly with cobra bites. Evidence of systemic involvement occurs within 30 minutes, including vomiting, evidence of shock and hypotension. Haemorrhage due to incoagulable blood can be fatal.

Elapidae

There is not usually any swelling at the site of the bite, except with Asian cobras and African spitting cobras – here the bite is painful and is followed by local tissue necrosis. Vomiting occurs first followed by shock and then neurological symptoms and muscle weakness,

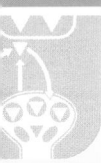

with paralysis of the respiratory muscles in severe cases. Cardiac muscle can be involved.

Hydrophiidae

Systemic features are muscle involvement, myalgia and myoglobinuria, which can lead to acute renal failure. Cardiac and respiratory paralysis may occur.

Management

A firm pressure bandage should be placed over the bite and the limb immobilized. This greatly delays the spread of the venom.

Arterial tourniquets should not be used, and incision or excision of the bite area should not be performed. The type of snake should be identified if possible.

In about 50% of cases no venom has been injected by the bite and antivenoms are not generally indicated (unless systemic effects are present), as they can cause severe allergic reactions. Nevertheless, careful observation for 12–24 hours is necessary and antivenom must always be given when indicated, as the mortality of snake bite is 10–15% with certain snakes.

General supportive measures should be given as necessary, as for all poisoning. These include diazepam for anxiety and intravenous fluids with volume expanders for hypotension. Treatment of acute respiratory, cardiac and renal failure is instituted as necessary.

Specific measures (i.e. antivenoms) can rapidly neutralize venom, but only if an amount in excess of the amount of venom is given. Antivenoms cannot reverse the effects of the venom so they must be given early. They do minimize some of the local effects and may prevent necrosis at the site of the bite. Antivenoms should be administered intravenously by slow infusion, the same dose being given to children and adults.

Allergic reactions are frequent, and epinephrine (adrenaline) (1 in 1000 solution) should be available. Antivenoms are usually rapidly effective. In severe cases the antivenom infusion should be continued even with allergic reactions, with subcutaneous injections of epinephrine being given as necessary. Large quantities of antivenom may be required. Some forms of neurotoxicity, such as those induced by the death adder, respond to anticholinesterase therapy with neostigmine and atropine.

Local wounds often require little treatment. If necrosis is present, antibiotics should be given together with initially minimal surgical treatment. Skin grafting may be required later. Antitetanus prophylaxis must be given.

Antivenoms must be kept readily available in all snake-infested areas.

Spiders

The black widow spider (*Latrodectus mactans*) is found in North America and the tropics and occasionally in Mediterranean countries.

The bite quickly becomes painful and generalized muscle pain, sweating, headache and shock may occur.

No systemic treatment is required except in cases of severe systemic toxicity, when specific antivenom should be given, if this is available.

Plants

Many plants are known to be poisonous, but it is unusual for severe poisoning to occur in practice. Poisonous plants commonly ingested include hemlock, laburnum, deadly nightshade and green potatoes. Deadly nightshade (*Atropa belladonna*) contains oscyamine and hyoscine and causes anticholinergic effects – a dry mouth, nausea and vomiting – leading to blurred vision, hallucinations, confusion and hyperpyrexia.

Mushrooms

Most mushrooms and edible fungi are not poisonous, but transient nausea, vomiting and diarrhoea can occur occasionally after ingestion of some varieties. There are a few species which are toxic:

- *Amanita phalloides* (death cap mushroom), which contains phallotoxins and amatoxins, both of which interfere with cell metabolism (inhibition of RNA polymerase II). Amatoxins are not inactivated by cooking. Hepatocellular necrosis follows 72 hours after ingestion and some varieties cause renal failure. Treatment is with gastric aspiration and general support; haemodialysis and liver/renal transplantation may be necessary.
- Other poisonous mushrooms include *Amanita muscaria* (fly agaric), which contains muscarine and other hallucinogenic substances, *Coprinus atramentarius* (ink cap) which contains a dehydrogenase inhibitor with a disulfiram-like effect (flushing, rash); and *Amanita pantherina* (false blusher) which has atropine-like effects.

Overdose of magic mushrooms (which contain the hallucinogen psilocybin) produces severe gastroenteritis as well as psychiatric symptoms.

FURTHER READING

Theakston RDG, Warrell DA (1991) Antivenoms: a list of hyperimmune sera currently available for the treatment of envenoming by bites and stings. *Toxicon* **29**: 1419–1470.

Warrell DA (ed) (1999) WHO/SEARO Guidelines for the clinical management of snake bites in the South-East Asian Region. *South East Asian Journal of Tropical Medicine and Public Health* **30** (Suppl 1): 1–86.

POISONING INFORMATION SERVICES (UK)

UK National Poisons Information Service (0870) 600 6266.

Environmental medicine   17

Heat

In health, the body core temperature is maintained at 37°C by the hypothalamic thermoregulatory centre.

Heat is produced by cellular metabolism, and lost through the skin by both vasodilatation and sweating and through the lungs in expired air. Profuse sweating occurs when the ambient temperature is greater than 32.5°C and during exercise. Evaporation of sweat is the vital mechanism cooling the body.

Heat acclimatization

Acclimatization to hot climates takes several weeks. Sweat volume increases and its salt content falls. Increased evaporation cools down the body.

Heat cramps

Painful muscle (usually leg) cramps often occur in well-acclimatized fit young people when they exercise in hot weather. Cramps are probably the result of low extracellular sodium caused by replenishment of water but not salt during prolonged sweating. They can be prevented by increasing dietary salt and respond to combined salt and water replacement.

Heat illness (heat exhaustion)

In high environmental temperatures, particularly with high humidity, vigorous exercise in clothing which inhibits heat loss can provoke a sudden elevation in core temperature. Weakness/exhaustion, dizziness and syncope, with a core temperature > 37°C define *heat illness* (*exertional heat illness* after exercise). Temperature elevation is more important than water and sodium loss. Heat *illness* may progress to heat *injury*, a serious medical emergency.

Management

Remove the patient from any heat source. Cool with cold sponging and fans. Give oxygen by mask. Other causes of hyperpyrexia, e.g. malaria, should be considered.

Oral rehydration with both salt and water (25 g of sodium chloride per 5 L of water) is given in the first 24 hours, with adequate replacement thereafter. In severe heat illness, intravenous fluids are needed. Isotonic saline is usually given, depending on serum sodium. Careful monitoring is required. Secondary potassium loss must be corrected.

Heat injury (heat stroke)

Heat *injury* is an acute life-threatening situation when core temperature rises above 41°C. There is headache, nausea, vomiting and weakness. The skin is hot. Sweating is often absent, but this is not invariable, even in severe heat injury. Brain involvement leads to confusion, delirium and coma.

Heat injury develops in unacclimatized people in hot, humid windless climates, even without exercise. Sweating may be limited by prickly heat. Excessive exercise in inappropriate clothing, e.g. exercising on land in a wetsuit, can lead to heat injury in temperate climates. Old age, diabetes, drugs (e.g. alcohol, anticholinergics, diuretics and phenothiazines) are all further precipitating factors. The pathogenesis of heat injury is a fall in cardiac output, lactic acidosis and intravascular coagulation. *Diagnosis* is clinical.

- Remove the patient from the hot area immediately.
- Cool with sponging and icepacks.
- Manage in intensive care (monitor biochemistry, clotting and muscle enzymes).
- Give fluids with caution: hypovolaemia is often absent.

Prompt treatment is essential and can lead to rapid and complete recovery. Delay may be fatal. Prevention is by acclimatization, fluids and common sense.

Complications

These are hypovolaemia (shock), intravascular coagulation, cerebral oedema, rhabdomyolysis, and renal and hepatic failure. Their management is described in appropriate chapters.

Malignant hyperpyrexia (see p. 1224)

> **FURTHER READING**
>
> Simon H (1993) Hyperthermia. *New England Journal of Medicine* **329**: 483–487.

Cold

Hypothermia is defined as a core (i.e. rectal) temperature below 35°C. It is frequently lethal when core temperature falls below 32°C.

Frostbite is local cold injury when tissue freezes.

Hypothermia

Hypothermia occurs in many settings.

At home

Hypothermia occurs in cold climates when there is poor heating, inadequate clothing and poor nutrition. Depressant drugs (e.g. hypnotics), alcohol, hypothyroidism or intercurrent illness also contribute. Hypothermia is commonly seen in the poor and elderly, the latter having a diminished ability to sense cold and often loss of insulating fat. Infants and neonates become hypothermic rapidly at room temperature because of their relatively large surface area and lack of subcutaneous fat.

During exposure to extremes of temperature

Hypothermia is a prominent cause of death in climbers, skiers, polar travellers and in wartime. Wet, cold conditions with windchill, physical exhaustion, injuries and inadequate clothing are contributory.

Following immersion in cold water

Dangerous hypothermia can develop after 1 hour's immersion at water temperatures of 15–20°C. Below 12°C limbs rapidly become numb and paralysed. Recovery takes some hours after rescue.

Clinical features

Mild hypothermia (core 32–35°C) causes shivering and initially quite intense cold. Though alert the subject may not act appropriately to rewarm (e.g. huddling, extra clothing or exercise). As core temperature falls below 32°C, severe hypothermia causes impaired judgement (including awareness of cold), drowsiness and coma. Death follows, usually from ventricular fibrillation.

Diagnosis

If a thermometer (low-reading) is available diagnosis is straightforward. If not, a rapid clinical assessment is reliable. A person who *feels* icy to touch – the abdomen, groin and axillae – is hypothermic. If clammy and uncooperative, sleepy or in a coma, core temperature is almost certainly below 32°C – a medical emergency.

Sequelae

Pulse rate and volume fall; respiration becomes shallow and slow. Muscle stiffness develops and tendon reflexes become sluggish. Systemic blood pressure falls. As coma ensues, pupillary and other brainstem reflexes are lost (pupils are fixed and may be dilated in severe hypothermia).

Metabolic changes are variable, either metabolic acidosis or alkalosis developing. Arterial oxygen tension may appear normal since it is measured at room temperature, but the measurement is falsely high as arterial Po_2 falls 7% for each degree Celcius (C) fall in temperature.

Ventricular arrhythmias (tachycardia/fibrillation) or asystole is the usual cause of death. 'J' waves – rounded waves above the isoelectric line immediately after the QRS complex – are pathognomonic of hypothermia. Prolongation of PR and QT intervals and QRS complex occurs.

Principles of management

- Rewarm gradually.
- Correct metabolic abnormalities
- Anticipate and treat dysrhythmias.
- Check for hypothyroidism (see p. 1037).

If the patient is awake, with core temperature above 32°C, place them in a warm room, use a 'space blanket', and give warm fluids orally. Outdoors, add extra dry clothing, huddle together and use a warmed sleeping bag. Rewarming may take several hours. Avoid alcohol: it may add to confusion, boost confidence factitiously, cause peripheral vasodilatation (and further heat loss), or precipitate hypoglycaemia.

Severe hypothermia

In severe hypothermia, people look dead. Always exclude hypothermia before diagnosing brain death (p. 954). Warm gradually, aiming at a 1°C per hour increase in core temperature. Cover with a 'space blanket' and place in a warm room. Direct surface heat from an electric blanket is also helpful. Treat any underlying condition promptly, e.g. sepsis. Monitor all vital functions. Correct dysrhythmias. Drug screening is essential.

Give warm i.v. fluids slowly. Correct metabolic abnormalities. Hypothyroidism, if present, should be treated with triiodothyronine 10 micrograms i.v. 8-hourly. Various methods of artificial rewarming exist – inhaled humidified air, gastric or peritoneal lavage, and haemodialysis. These are rarely used.

Prevention

Hypothermia prevention is especially necessary in the elderly. Improved home heating and insulation, central heating in bedrooms and electric blankets are helpful. Finance is often needed. Supervision should be given during cold spells; warm food and extra blankets must be provided.

Frostbite

Ice crystals form within skin and superficial tissues when the tissue temperature falls to –3°C: ambient temperatures generally must be below –6°C.

Recognition

Frostbitten tissue is pale, greyish and initially doughy to touch. Later it freezes hard, when it looks and feels like meat taken from a deep freeze. Frostbite can easily occur when working or exercising in low temperatures. Typically it develops without the patient's knowledge. Below –5°C, hands or feet that have lost their feeling are at risk of frostbite.

Management

The frostbitten patient should, if possible, be transported (or walk, even on frostbitten feet) to a place of safety before treatment commences. Warm with a companion's body or by immersion in water at 39–42°C (hand hot). Continue until obvious thawing occurs. This may be painful. Blisters form within several days and, depending on the degree of frostbite, a blackened carapace or shell develops as the blisters regress or burst. Dry, non-adherent dressings and strict aseptic precautions are essential. Frostbitten tissues are anaesthetic and at risk from infection and further trauma. Recovery takes place over many weeks. Surgery may be required, but should be avoided in the early stages.

FURTHER READING

Lazar HL (1997) Editorial: The treatment of hypothermia. *New England Journal of Medicine* **337**: 1545–1547.

High altitudes

The partial pressure of ambient (and hence alveolar and arterial) oxygen falls in a near-linear relationship to altitude (Fig. 17.1).

Below 3000 m there are few clinical effects. Commercial aircraft are pressurized to 2750 m. The resulting hypoxia causes breathlessness only in those with severe cardiorespiratory disease. The incidence of thromboembolism is slightly greater in (sedentary) travellers on long flights than in a similar population at sea level. Above 3000–3500 m hypoxia causes a spectrum of related clinical syndromes that affect visitors to high altitudes, principally climbers, trekkers, skiers and troops (Table 17.1). These occur largely during acclimatization. Acclimatization takes several weeks and enables humans to live (permanently if necessary) up to

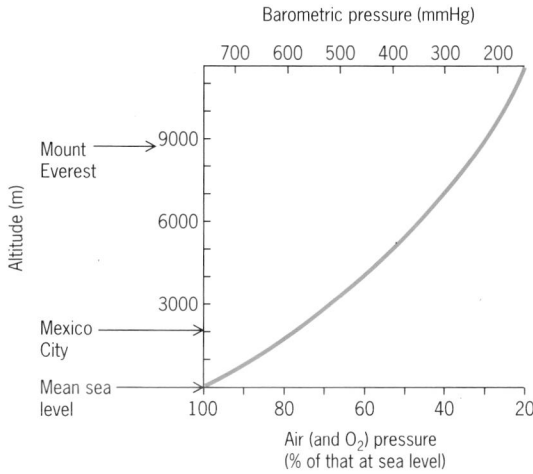

Fig. 17.1 The decrease in oxygen and barometric pressure with increasing altitude.

Table 17.1
Conditions caused by sustained hypoxia

Condition	Incidence (%)	Usual altitude (m)
Acute mountain sickness	70	3500–4000
Acute pulmonary oedema	2	4000
Acute cerebral oedema	1	4500
Retinal haemorrhage	50	5000
Deterioration	100	5600
Chronic mountain sickness	Rare	4500

about 5600 m. At greater heights, although people can survive for days or weeks, deterioration due to chronic hypoxia is inevitable.

Ascent of the world's highest summits is possible without the use of supplementary oxygen. At the summit of Everest (nearly 9000 m) the barometric pressure is 34 kPa (253 mmHg). An acclimatized mountaineer has an alveolar Po_2 of 4.0–4.7 kPa (30–35 mmHg) – near man's absolute physiological limit.

Acute mountain sickness (AMS)
This describes malaise, nausea, headache and lassitude common for a few days above 3500 m. Following arrival at this altitude there is usually a latent interval of 6–36 hours before symptoms begin. Treatment is rest, with analgesics if necessary. Recovery is usually spontaneous.

Prophylactic treatment with acetazolamide, a carbonic anhydrase inhibitor and a respiratory stimulant is of some value in preventing AMS. Acclimatizing, i.e. ascending gradually, is the best prophylaxis.

In the minority, more serious sequelae of high-altitude pulmonary oedema and high-altitude cerebral oedema develop.

High-altitude pulmonary oedema
Predisposing factors include youth, rapidity of ascent, heavy exertion and severe AMS. Breathlessness, with frothy blood-stained sputum indicates established oedema. Unless treated rapidly this leads to cardio-respiratory failure and death. Milder forms are common, presenting with less severe breathlessness.

High-altitude cerebral oedema
Cerebral oedema is another sequel of hypoxia. It is the result of abrupt increase in cerebral blood flow that occurs even at modest altitudes of 3500–4000 m. Headache is usual, and is accompanied by drowsiness, ataxia, and papilloedema. Coma and death follow if the condition progresses.

Treatment
Any but the milder forms of AMS require urgent treatment. Oxygen should be given if available, and descent to a lower altitude should take place as quickly as possible. Nifedipine reduces pulmonary hypertension and is used in the treatment of pulmonary oedema. Dexamethasone is effective in reducing brain oedema. Portable pressure bags, in which the patient is inserted, are helpful in increasing barometric pressure; these have become widely used.

Retinal haemorrhages
Small 'flame' haemorrhages in the retinal nerve fibre layer are common above 5000 m. They are usually symptomless. Rarely they cover the macula, causing painless loss of central vision. Recovery is usual.

Deterioration
Prolonged residence between 5600 and 7000 m leads to weight loss, anorexia and listlessness after several weeks. Above 7500 m, deterioration develops more quickly, although it is possible to survive for a week or more at altitudes over 8000 m.

Chronic mountain sickness
This rare syndrome occurs in long-term residents at high altitudes after several decades. It has been described in the Andes and in central Asia.

Polycythaemia, drowsiness, cyanosis, finger clubbing, congested cheeks and ear lobes, and right ventricular enlargement occur. It is gradually progressive.

By way of contrast, coronary artery disease and hypertension are rare in high-altitude native populations.

FURTHER READING

Clarke C (2001) High altitude and mountaineering expeditions. In: Warrell D, Anderson S (eds) *Expedition Medicine*. London: Royal Geographical Society.

Hackett PH, Roach RC (2001) High-altitude illness. *New England Journal of Medicine* 345: **107**–114.

UIAA Mountain Medicine Data Centre leaflets available from British Mountaineering Council, 177–179 Burton Road, Manchester M20 2BB. Tel: 0161-445-4747; Fax: 0161-445-4500. www.thebmc.co.uk.

Information: Wilderness Medical Society, PO Box 2463, Indianapolis, Indiana 462206, USA. www.wms.org.

Diving

Ambient pressures at various depths are shown in Table 17.2.

Various methods are used to supply air to a diver. With the simplest (e.g. a snorkel), the limiting factor which occurs below 0.5 m, is respiratory effort sucking air into the lungs. At greater depths this 'forced negative-pressure ventilation' causes pulmonary capillary damage and haemorrhagic oedema. Scuba divers – the usual sports diving down to 50 m – carry bottled compressed air.

Table 17.2
Pressure in relation to sea depth

Sea depth (m)	Absolute pressure (atmospheres)	mmHg
0	1	760
10	2	1520
50	6	4560
90	10	7600

Divers who work at great depths for commercial purposes or exploration breathe helium–oxygen or nitrogen–oxygen mixtures delivered by hose from the surface.

Complex problems can affect divers at all depths.

Compression problems (descent)

Middle ear barotrauma ('squeeze') is common and caused by inability to equalize pressure in the middle ear – usually the result of Eustachian tube blockage. Deafness occurs and eventual tympanic membrane rupture, with acute vertigo.

Sinus barotrauma ('squeeze') – is due to blockage of the nasal and paranasal sinus ostia with intense local pain.

Treatment and prevention. Treatment is with decongestants. Avoid diving with any respiratory infection.

Nitrogen narcosis

When compressed air is breathed below 30 m, narcotic effects of nitrogen impair brain function. Changes of mood and performance may be hazardous. These reverse rapidly on ascent.

Nitrogen narcosis is avoided by replacing air with helium–oxygen mixtures, enabling descent to 700 m.

At these great depths direct effect of pressure on neurones can cause tremor, hemiparesis and cognitive impairment.

Oxygen narcosis

Pure oxygen is not used for diving because oxygen is toxic. Lung damage (atelectasis, endothelial cell damage and pulmonary oedema) occurs when the alveolar oxygen pressure exceeds 1.5 atmospheres (5 m of water). At around 10 m of water the nervous system is affected. Apprehension, nausea and sweating is followed by muscle twitching and generalized convulsions with possible underwater fatalities.

Decompression problems (i.e. ascent)
Breath-hold (shallow-water) diving

Shallow-water swimmers and free divers deliberately hyperventilate prior to a dive to drive off CO_2 – reducing the stimulus to breathe. The subsequent breath-hold causes a rise in P_aCO_2 and a fall of P_aO_2. However, on surfacing, decompression further lowers P_aO_2. This may cause syncope.

Decompression sickness

Decompression sickness ('the bends') occurs in divers on returning to the surface and is caused by the release of bubbles of inert gases (nitrogen or helium). Bubbles develop only if ascent is too rapid. Decompression tables indicate the time needed for safe return from given depths.

The bends can be mild (type 1 non-neurological bends), with skin irritation, mottling or joint pain only. Type 2 (neurological) bends are more serious – cortical blindness, hemiparesis, sensory disturbances or cord lesions develop. If nitrogen bubbles form in pulmonary vessels, divers experience retrosternal discomfort, dyspnoea and cough ('the chokes'). These develop within minutes or hours of a dive.

Treatment is with oxygen. All but the mildest forms of decompression sickness (i.e. skin mottling alone) require recompression in a pressure chamber.

A long-term problem is aseptic necrosis (e.g. of the hip) due to nitrogen bubbles causing infarction of nutrient arteries of bone. Neurological damage may also persist.

Lung rupture, pneumothorax and surgical emphysema

These emergencies occur principally when divers 'breath-hold' while making emergency ascents after losing their gas supply. There is severe dyspnoea, cough and haemoptysis. Pneumothorax and emphysema usually respond to 100% oxygen. Air embolism may occur and should be treated with recompression and hyperbaric oxygen.

FURTHER READING

Bennett P, Elliot D (1993) *The Physiology and Medicine of Diving*, 4th edn. London: WB Saunders.
Melamed Y, Shupak A, Bitterman H (1992) Medical problems associated with underwater diving. *New England Journal of Medicine* **326**: 30–36.

DIVING INFORMATION

Institute of Naval Medicine, Undersea Medicine Division, Alverstoke, Gosport, Hampshire PO12 2DL. Tel: 01705 768026.
UK Diving emergencies: Ministry of Defence, Duty Diving Medical Officer. Tel: 07831 151523.

Ionizing radiation

Ionizing radiation is either penetrating (X-rays, gamma rays or neutrons) or non-penetrating (alpha or beta particles). Penetrating radiation affects the whole body, while non-penetrating radiation affects only the skin.

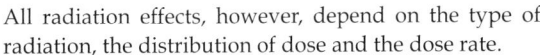

All radiation effects, however, depend on the type of radiation, the distribution of dose and the dose rate.

Radiation dosage is measured in joules per kilogram (J/kg); 1 J/kg is also known as 1 gray (1 Gy). This is equivalent to 100 rads. Radioactivity is measured in becquerels (Bq); 1 Bq is equal to the amount of radioactive material in which there is one disintegration per second. One curie (Ci) is equal to 3.7×10^{10} Bq.

Radiation differs in the density of ionization it causes. Therefore a dose-equivalent called a sievert (Sv) is used. This is the absorbed dose weighted for the damaging effect of the radiation. The annual background radiation is approximately 2.5 mSv. A chest X-ray gives 0.02 mSv, while a CT scan of the abdomen/pelvis is 10 mSv.

Excessive exposure to ionizing radiation occurs following accidents in hospitals, industry, nuclear power plants and strategic nuclear explosions.

Mild acute radiation sickness

Nausea, vomiting and malaise follow doses of approximately 1 Gy. Lymphopenia occurs within several days, followed 2–3 weeks later by a fall in all white cells and platelets. There is a late risk of leukaemia and solid tumours.

Severe acute radiation sickness

Many systems are affected; the extent of the damage depends on the dose of radiation received. The effects of radiation are summarized in Table 17.3.

Haemopoietic syndrome

Absorption of doses between 2 and 10 Gy is followed by early and transient vomiting in some individuals, followed by a period of relative well-being. Lymphocytes are particularly sensitive to radiation damage and severe lymphopenia develops over several days. A decrease in granulocytes and platelets occurs 2–3 weeks later as no new cells are being formed by the damaged marrow. Thrombocytopenia with bleeding develops and frequent overwhelming infections occur, with a very high mortality.

Gastrointestinal syndrome

Absorption of doses greater than 6 Gy causes vomiting several hours after exposure. This then stops, only to recur some 4 days later accompanied by severe diarrhoea. Owing to radiation inhibition of cell division, the villous lining of the intestine becomes denuded. Intractable bloody diarrhoea follows, with dehydration, secondary infection and death.

CNS syndrome

Exposures above 30 Gy are followed rapidly by nausea, vomiting, disorientation and coma. Death due to severe cerebral oedema follows within 36 hours.

Radiation dermatitis

Skin erythema, purpura, blistering and secondary infection occur. Total loss of body hair is a bad prognostic sign and usually follows an exposure of at least 5 Gy.

Late effects of radiation exposure

Survivors of the nuclear bombing of Hiroshima and Nagasaki have provided information on the long-term effects of radiation. The risk of developing acute myeloid leukaemia or cancer, particularly of the skin, thyroid and salivary glands, increases. Infertility, teratogenesis and cataract are also late sequelae of radiation exposure.

Treatment

Acute radiation sickness is a medical emergency. Hospitals should be informed immediately of the type and length of exposure so that suitable arrangements can be made to receive the patient. The initial radiation dose absorbed can be reduced by removing clothing contaminated by radioactive materials.

Treatment of radiation sickness is largely supportive and consists of prevention and treatment of infection, haemorrhage and fluid loss. Storage of the patient's white cells and platelets for future use should be considered, if feasible.

Accidental ingestion of, or exposure to, bone-seeking radioisotopes (e.g. strontium-90 and caesium-137) should be treated with chelating agents (e.g. EDTA) and massive doses of oral calcium. Radioiodine contamination should be treated immediately with potassium iodide 133 mg per day. This will block 90% of radioiodine absorption by the thyroid if given immediately before exposure.

Table 17.3
The effects of radiation

Acute effects	Delayed effects
Haemopoietic syndrome	Infertility
Gastrointestinal syndrome	Teratogenesis
CNS syndrome	Cataract
Radiation dermatitis	Neoplasia
	Acute myeloid leukaemia
	Thyroid
	Salivary glands
	Skin
	Others

Electric shock

Electric shock may produce clinical effects in several ways:

- *Pain and psychological sequelae.* The common 'electric shock' is usually a painful, but harmless, stimulus but an unpleasant and frightening experience. It produces no lasting neurological damage or skin damage.

- *Cardiac, neurological and muscle damage.* Ventricular fibrillation, muscular contraction and spinal cord damage follow a major shock. These are seen typically following a lightning strike which is a very high voltage and amperage current.
- *Electrical burns.* These commonly only involve the skin (lightning may cause a fern-shaped burn), but subcutaneous or deep injuries can occur.

Smoke

Air pollution is discussed on page 855.

Smoke consists of particles of carbon in hot air and gases. These particles are coated with organic acids and aldehydes and synthetic materials. On combustion, other toxins such as carbon monoxide, sulphur dioxide, sulphuric and hydrochloric acids are released. Polyvinyl chloride is no longer used in household goods.

Respiratory symptoms may be immediate or delayed. Patients are dyspnoeic and tachypnoeic. Laryngeal stridor may require intubation. Hypoxia and pulmonary oedema can be fatal.

Patients should breathe through an aspirator or wet towel. Remove the patient from the smoke. Give O_2 and ITU support. Smoke alarms should be used in households.

Noise

Sound intensity is expressed as the square of sound pressure. The bel is a ratio and is equivalent to a 10-fold increase in sound intensity; a decibel (dB) is one-tenth of a bel. Sound is made up of a number of frequencies ranging from 30 Hz to 20 kHz, with most being between 1 and 4 kHz. When measuring sound, these different frequencies must be taken into account. In practice a scale known as A-weighted sound is used; sound levels are then reported as dB(A). A hazardous sound source is defined as one with an overall sound pressure greater than 90 dB(A).

Repeated prolonged exposure to loud noise, particularly between 2–6 kHz, causes first temporary and later permanent hearing loss by physically destroying hair cells in the organ of Corti and, eventually, auditory neurones. This is a common occupational problem, not only in industry and the armed forces, but also in the home (electric drills and sanders), in sport (motor racing), and in entertainment (pop stars, disc jockeys and their audiences).

Serious noise-induced hearing loss is almost wholly preventable by personal protection (ear muffs, ear plugs). Little help can be offered once deafness becomes established.

Other effects of noise

Noise is undoubtedly irritative and increases or produces anxiety. It has been suggested that excess noise affects child development and reading skills.

Drowning and near-drowning

Drowning is the third commonest cause of accidental death in the UK; it caused over 500 000 deaths worldwide in 2000. Approximately 40% of drownings occur in children under five. People also drown after an epileptic seizure or a myocardial infarct whilst in water. Exhaustion, alcohol, drugs and hypothermia all contribute to drowning.

'Dry' drowning

Between 10% and 15% of drownings occur without water aspiration into the lungs. Laryngeal spasm occurs, apnoea, anoxia and cardiac arrest.

'Wet' drowning

Aspiration of fresh water affects pulmonary surfactant, with alveolar collapse and ventilation/perfusion mismatch and hypoxaemia. Aspiration of hypertonic seawater (5% NaCl) pulls additional fluid into the lungs with further ventilation/perfusion mismatch. In practice, however, there is little difference between saltwater and freshwater drowning. In both, severe hypoxaemia develops rapidly after water aspiration. Severe metabolic acidosis develops in the majority of survivors.

Emergency treatment of near-drowning

Patients can survive for up to 30 minutes under water without suffering brain damage – and for longer if the water temperature is near 0°C. This is probably related to the protective role of the diving reflex – submersion causes reflex slowing of the pulse and vasoconstriction. In addition, hypothermia decreases oxygen consumption. CPR should be started immediately (see p. 1730).

Resuscitation should always be attempted, even in the absence of a pulse and the presence of fixed dilated pupils. Patients frequently make a dramatic recovery. All patients should be subsequently admitted to hospital for intensive monitoring. Survivors are liable to develop acute respiratory distress syndrome (ARDS).

Prognosis

This is good if the patient regains consciousness promptly but poor if they remain in coma 30 minutes after resuscitation.

FURTHER READING

Modell JH (1993) Drowning. *New England Journal of Medicine* **328**: 253–256.

Travel

Motion sickness

This common problem, particularly in children, is caused by repetitive stimulation of the labyrinth. It occurs frequently at sea and in cars, but may occur on horseback or on less usual forms of transport such as camels or elephants. It is a major issue in space travel. Nausea, sweating, dizziness, vertigo and profuse vomiting occur, accompanied by an irresistible desire to stop moving.

Prophylactic antihistamines or vestibular sedatives (hyoscine or cinnarizine) are of some value.

Jet-lag

Jet-lag, or circadian dyschronism, is a well-known phenomenon after changing time-zones, particularly from West to East. Fatigue, intense insomnia, headache, irritability, poor concentration and loss of appetite are common. Symptoms last several days.

Mechanisms are poorly understood but relate to the hypothalamic body clock, sited within the suprachiasmatic nuclei. The clock is regulated by various zeitgebers ('time-givers'), e.g. light and melatonin.

Management of jet-lag includes its acceptance as a phenomenon causing poor performance and waiting for 3–5 days to recover. Various hypnotics can help insomnia, but their place is disputed. Oral melatonin is widely used to reduce jet-lag. This increases sleepiness and hastens resetting of the body clock. Melatonin is not available on prescription.

FURTHER READING

Waterhouse J, Reilly T, Atkinson G (1997) Jet-lag. *Lancet* **350**: 1611–1616.

Building-related illnesses

Modern office buildings have a controlled environment with automated heating, ventilation and air-conditioning systems, often without outdoor air. More than half the adult workforce in developed countries work in offices.

Non-specific building-related illness

Headache, fatigue and difficulty in concentrating sometimes in apparent epidemics, are common complaints of office-workers. Psychological factors may have a role. Temperature, humidity, dust, volatile organic compounds (e.g. paints, solvents) have all been implicated. Maintenance of continuous outdoor air supply is recommended. However, changes in ventilation sometimes fail to improve matters.

Specific building-related illness

Legionnaires' disease (see p. 888) is frequently due to contamination of air-conditioned systems. Humidifier fever (p. 906) is also due to contaminated systems, probably by fungi, bacteria and protozoa. Many common viruses are easily transmitted in the enclosed environment (e.g. the common cold, influenza and rarely pulmonary tuberculosis). Allergic disorders (e.g. rhinitis, asthma and dermatitis) also occur owing to exposure to indoor allergens such as dust mites and plants. Office equipment (e.g. fumes from photocopiers) has also been implicated. Passive smoking (p. 855) is also a problem.

FURTHER READING

Menzies J, Bourbeau T (1997) Building-related illnesses. *New England Journal of Medicine* **337**: 1524–1531.

Endocrine disease

Hormonal activity

Hormones are chemical messengers produced by a variety of specialized secretory cells. They may be transported in the blood to a distant site of action (the classic 'endocrine' effect) or act directly upon nearby cells ('paracrine' activity). In the hypothalamus, elsewhere in the brain and in the gastrointestinal tract there are many such cells secreting hormones, some of which have true endocrine or paracrine activity, while others behave more like neurotransmitters or neuromodulators. At the molecular level there is little difference in the way cellular activity is regulated between classical neurotransmitters that act across synaptic clefts, intercellular factors acting across gap junctions, classic endocrine and paracrine activity and a variety of other chemical messengers involved in cell regulation – such as cytokines, growth factors and interleukins; progress in basic cell biology has revealed the biochemical similarities in the messengers, receptors and intracellular post-receptor mechanisms underlying all these aspects of cell function.

Synthesis, storage and release of hormones

Hormones may be of several chemical structures: polypeptide, glycoprotein, steroid or amine. Hormone release is the end-product of a long cascade of intracellular events. In the case of polypeptide hormones, neural or endocrine stimulation of the cell leads to increased transcription from DNA to a specific mRNA, which is in turn translated to the peptide product. This is often in the form of a precursor molecule that may itself be biologically inactive. This 'prohormone' may be further processed before being packaged into granules, in the Golgi apparatus. These granules are then transported to the plasma membrane before release, which is itself regulated by a complex combination of intracellular regulators. Hormone release may be in a brief spurt caused by the sudden stimulation of granules, often induced by an intracellular Ca^{2+}-dependent process, or it may be 'constitutive' (immediate and continuous secretion).

Plasma transport

Most classical hormones are secreted into the systemic circulation where they travel to have effects elsewhere in the body. In contrast, hypothalamic releasing hormones are released into the pituitary portal system so that much higher concentrations of the releasing hormones reach the pituitary than occur in the systemic circulation.

Table 18.1
Plasma hormones with important binding proteins

Hormone	Binding protein(s)
Thyroxine (T_4)	Thyroxine-binding globulin (TBG)
	Thyroxine-binding prealbumin (TBPA)
	Albumin
Triiodothyronine (T_3) (less bound than T_4)	Thyroxine-binding globulin (TBG)
	Albumin
Cortisol	Cortisol-binding globulin (CBG)
Testosterone, oestradiol	Sex hormone-binding globulin (SHBG)
Insulin-like growth factor-I (IGF-I)	IGF-binding proteins (mainly IGF–BP3)

Many hormones are bound to proteins within the circulation. In most cases, only the free (unbound) hormone is available to the tissues and thus biologically active. This binding serves to buffer against very rapid changes in plasma levels of the hormone, and some binding protein interactions may also be involved in the active regulation of hormone action. This principle is important in interpreting many tests of endocrine function, which often measure total rather than free hormone, since binding proteins are frequently altered in disease states. Binding proteins comprise both specific, high-affinity proteins of limited capacity, such as thyroxine-binding globulin (TBG) and other less-specific low-affinity ones, such as prealbumin and albumin. The clinically relevant binding proteins are shown in Table 18.1.

Hormone action and receptors

Hormones act by binding to specific receptors in the target cell, which may be at the cell surface and/or within the cell. Most hormone receptors are proteins with complex tertiary structures, parts of which complement the tertiary structure of the hormone to allow highly specific interactions, while other parts are responsible for the effects of the activated receptor within the cell. Many hormones bind to specific cell-surface receptors where they trigger internal messengers, while others bind to nuclear receptors which interact directly with DNA. Cell-surface receptors usually contain hydrophobic sections which span the lipid-rich plasma membrane, while nuclear receptors contain characteristic amino-acid sequences to bind nuclear DNA (e.g. so-called 'zinc fingers', see p. 166) as in the glucocorticoid receptor.

In order to achieve these intracellular effects, hormone receptors interact with a variety of other regulatory factors within the cell membrane, in the cytosol or within the nucleus of the cell. In each case, binding of the hormone to its receptor results in a conformational change in the structure of the receptor which may result in a number of possible outcomes, which are illustrated in Fig. 3.4 (p. 158):

- activation of, or modified binding to, other regulatory factors within the cell membrane or cytosol (e.g. binding of transmembrane receptors to the cell-membrane G-proteins, thereby activating the stimulatory or inhibitory effects of the latter on other intracellular mediators)
- activation of enzyme activity in the receptor or its regulatory factors (e.g. receptor adenylate cyclase, other protein kinases, phospholipase C) to generate a variety of intracellular 'second messengers' (e.g. cAMP, cGMP, phosphatidylinositol metabolites, calmodulin) which usually form a complex, branching and interacting intracellular cascade of enzyme activation and inhibition and/or mobilization of intracellular stores of ions (primarily calcium)
- opening or closing of cell membrane ion channels or other membrane transporters
- altered binding of the receptor to DNA or to nuclear transcription factors in order to stimulate or inhibit transcription of one or more genes
- altered activity of cell membrane channels or transporters (e.g. for glucose, potassium or for other ions)
- dimerization of the receptor, or internalization of some cell-surface receptors.

These immediate effects of hormone binding may then cause rapid alterations in cell-membrane ion transport or intracellular calcium concentrations, or slower responses such as DNA, RNA and protein synthesis.

In each case, binding of the hormone to its receptor is the first step in a complex cascade of interrelated intracellular events which eventually lead to the overall effects of that hormone on cellular function.

Common 'second messengers' involved in these cascades include *cyclic AMP* (for adrenocorticotrophic hormone (ACTH), luteinizing hormone (LH), follicle-stimulating hormone (FSH) and parathyroid hormone (PTH)), *a calcium-phospholipid system* (for thyrotrophin-releasing hormone (TRH), vasopressin and angiotensin II), *tyrosine kinase* and *other intracellular kinases* (for insulin and insulin-like growth factor-1 (IGF-1)) and *membrane-bound phosphoinositide pathways*.

Some general characteristics of selected hormone systems are shown in Table 18.2.

The sensitivity and/or number of receptors for a hormone are often decreased after prolonged exposure to a high hormone concentration, the receptors thus becoming less sensitive ('downregulation', e.g. angiotensin II receptors, β-adrenoceptors). The reverse is true when stimulation is absent or minimal, the receptors showing increased numbers or sensitivity ('upregulation').

Abnormal receptors are an occasional, though rare, cause of endocrine disease (see p. 1006), but are being recognized and characterized more frequently owing to advances in molecular endocrinology.

Control and feedback

Most hormone systems are controlled by some form of feedback; an example is the hypothalamic–pituitary–thyroid axis (Fig. 18.1).

Table 18.2
Characteristics of some different hormone systems

	Peptides and catecholamines	Steroids and thyroid hormones
Protein binding	Sometimes for growth hormone and insulin-like growth factor	Yes
Changes in plasma concentrations	Rapid changes	Slow fluctuations
Plasma half-life	Short (seconds to minutes)	Long (minutes to days)
Type of receptors	Cell membrane	Intracellular
Mechanism	Activate preformed enzymes	Stimulate protein synthesis
Secretion	Secretory granules	Direct passage rapidly
	Constitutive + bursts	Related to secretion rate
Speed of effect	Rapid (seconds to minutes)	Slow (hours to days)

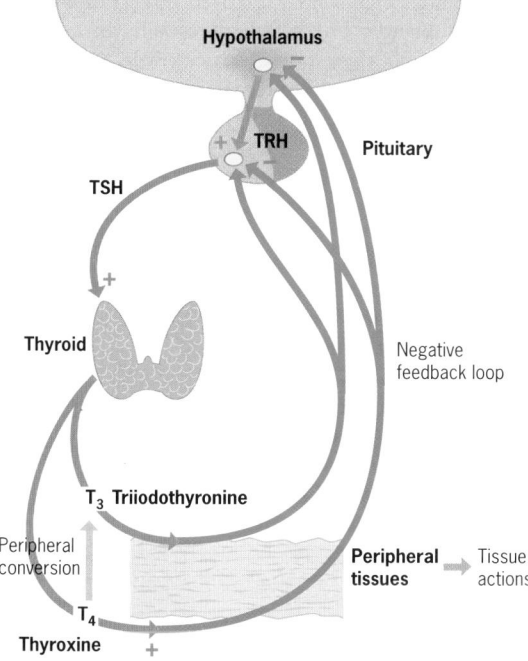

Fig. 18.1 The hypothalamic–pituitary–thyroid axis. The green line indicates negative feedback at the hypothalamic and pituitary level.

- TRH (thyrotrophin-releasing hormone) is secreted in the hypothalamus and travels via the portal system to the pituitary where it stimulates the thyrotrophs to produce thyroid-stimulating hormone (TSH).
- TSH is secreted into the systemic circulation where it stimulates increased thyroidal iodine uptake and thyroxine (T_4) and triiodothyronine (T_3) synthesis and release.
- Serum levels of T_3 and T_4 are thus increased by TSH; in addition, the conversion of T_4 to T_3 (the more active hormone) in peripheral tissues is stimulated by TSH.
- T_3 and T_4 then enter cells where they bind to nuclear receptors and promote increased metabolic and cellular activity.
- Levels of T_3 (from the blood and from local conversion of T_4) are sensed by receptors in the pituitary and possibly the hypothalamus. If they rise above normal, TRH and TSH production is suppressed, leading to reduced T_3 and T_4 secretion.
- Peripheral T_3 and T_4 levels thus fall to normal.
- If, however, T_3 and T_4 levels are low (e.g. after thyroidectomy), increased amounts of TRH and thus TSH are secreted, stimulating the remaining thyroid to produce more T_3 and T_4; blood levels of T_3 and T_4 may be restored to normal, although at the expense of increased TSH drive, reflected by a high TSH level ('compensated euthyroidism'). Conversely, in thyrotoxicosis when factors other than TSH itself are maintaining high T_3 and T_4 levels, the same mechanisms lead to suppression of TSH secretion.

This is known as a 'negative feedback' system, referring to the effect of T_3 and T_4 on the pituitary and hypothalamus, which represents the most common mechanism for regulation of circulating hormone levels. There are also 'positive feedback' systems, classically seen in the regulation of the normal menstrual cycle (p. 1015).

Patterns of secretion

Hormone secretion may be continuous or intermittent. The former is shown by the thyroid hormones, where T_4 has a half-life of 7–10 days and T_3 of about 6–10 hours. Levels over the day, month and year show little variation.

In contrast, secretion of the gonadotrophins, LH and FSH, is normally pulsatile, with major pulses released every 1–2 hours depending on the phase of the menstrual cycle. Continuous infusion of LH to produce a steady equivalent level does not produce the same result (e.g. ovulation in the female) as the intermittent pulsatility, and may indeed produce downregulation. Thus a long-acting superactive gonadotrophin-releasing hormone (GnRH) analogue, such as buserelin, produces downregulation of the GnRH receptors and subsequent very low androgen or oestrogen levels, which are clinically valuable both in carcinoma of the prostate in men and in ovulation-induction regimens in infertile women. In contrast, pulsatile GnRH administration can produce normal menstrual cyclicity, ovulation and fertility in women with hypothalamic amenorrhoea but intact pituitary LH and FSH stores.

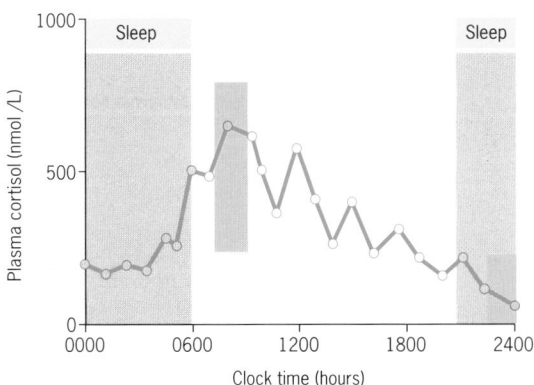

Fig. 18.2 Plasma cortisol levels during a 24-hour period.
Note both the pulsatility and the shifting baseline. Normal ranges for 0900h (180–700 nmol/L) and 2400h (less than 100 nmol/L; must be taken when asleep) are shown in the orange boxes. Purple shading shows sleep.

Biological rhythms

Circadian means changes over the 24 hours of the day–night cycle and is best shown for the pituitary–adrenal axis. Figure 18.2 shows plasma cortisol levels measured over 24 hours – levels are highest in the early morning and lowest overnight. Additionally, cortisol release is pulsatile, following the pulsatility of pituitary ACTH. Thus 'normal' cortisol levels vary during the day and great variations can be seen in samples taken only 30 minutes apart (Fig. 18.2). The circadian (light–dark) rhythm is seen in reverse with the pineal hormone, melatonin, which shows high levels during dark. Melatonin may be involved in entraining other hormonal rhythms and systems to the current light–dark cycle, but there is no known clinical syndrome related to abnormalities of this hormone, though a synthetic preparation is widely used for 'jet-lag' (p. 998).

The *menstrual cycle* is the best example of a longer and more complex (28-day) biological rhythm (see p. 1015).

Other regulatory factors

- *Stress.* Physiological 'stress' and acute illness produce rapid increases in ACTH and cortisol, growth hormone (GH), prolactin, epinephrine (adrenaline) and norepinephrine (noradrenaline). These can occur within seconds or minutes.
- *Sleep.* Secretion of GH and prolactin is increased during sleep, especially the rapid eye movement (REM) phase.
- *Feeding and fasting.* Many hormones regulate the body's control of energy intake and expenditure and are therefore profoundly influenced by feeding and fasting. Thus, secretion of insulin is increased and growth hormone decreased after ingestion of food, and secretion of a number of hormones is altered during prolonged food deprivation.

All these factors must be considered when attempting to measure hormone levels in normal individuals and in patients with disease. For example, cortisol levels will often be high and fail to suppress during standard tests in a patient who is severely stressed by serious illness, and growth hormone will usually be low in postprandial individuals during the daytime.

Testing endocrine function

Ideally, the *activity* of hormones would be measured at the cellular level, but this is usually impossible. Measurement of hormone *levels* in body fluids is the normal substitute but, although usually an excellent approximation, does not always reflect the current tissue action of the relevant hormone. Most commonly, hormone levels in the blood (or, more technically, levels in plasma or serum) are measured and all references to hormone levels in this chapter refer to blood/plasma levels unless stated otherwise.

Basal blood levels

Assays for all clinically relevant hormones are available. Obviously the time, day and condition of measurement may make great differences to hormone levels and the method and timing of samples will depend upon the characteristics of the endocrine system involved. There may also be sex, developmental and age differences.

Basal levels are especially useful for systems with long half-lives (e.g. T_4 and T_3). These vary little over the short term and random samples are therefore satisfactory.

Basal samples for other hormones may also be satisfactory if interpreted with respect to normal ranges for the time of day/month, diet or posture concerned. Examples are FSH, oestrogen and progesterone (varying with time of cycle) and renin/aldosterone (varying with sodium intake, posture and age). For these hormones, all relevant details must be recorded or the results may prove uninterpretable.

Stress-related hormones

Stress-related hormones (e.g. catecholamines, prolactin, GH, ACTH and cortisol) may require samples to be taken via an indwelling needle some time after initial venepuncture; otherwise, high levels may be artefactual.

Urine collections

Collections over 24 hours have the advantage of providing an 'integrated mean' of a day's secretion but in practice are often incomplete or wrongly timed. They also vary with sex and body size or age. Written instructions should be provided for the patient to ensure accurate collection.

Saliva

Saliva is sometimes used for steroid estimations, especially in children.

Stimulation and suppression tests

Stimulation and suppression tests are used when basal levels give equivocal information. In general, stimulation tests are used to confirm suspected deficiency and suppression tests to confirm suspected excess of hormone secretion. These tests are valuable in many instances.

For example, where the secretory capacity of a gland is damaged, maximal stimulation by the trophic hormone will give a diminished output. Thus, in the synacthen (SYNthetic-ACTH-en) test for adrenal reserve (Fig. 18.3(a) and Box 18.1), the healthy subject shows a normal response while the subject with primary hypoadrenalism (Addison's disease) demonstrates an impaired cortisol response to ACTH.

A patient with a hormone-producing tumour usually fails to show normal negative feedback. A patient with Cushing's disease (excess pituitary ACTH) will thus fail to suppress ACTH and cortisol production when given a dose of synthetic steroid, in contrast to normal subjects. Figure 18.3(b) shows the response of a normal

---

Box 18.1

Short tetracosactide (synacthen) test

Indication
Diagnosis of Addison's disease
Screening test for ACTH deficiency

Procedure
Intravenous cannula for sampling
Any time of day, but best at 0900h; non-fasting
Tetracosactide 250 µg, i.v. or i.m. at time 0
Measure serum cortisol at time 0 and time +30 min

Normal response
30 min cortisol > 600 nmol/L*
(400–600 nmol/L borderline and may indicate deficiency)

---

* Precise cortisol normal ranges are variable between laboratories and assays – appropriate local reference ranges must be used

---

subject given dexamethasone 1 mg at midnight; cortisol is suppressed the following morning. The subject with Cushing's disease shows inadequate suppression.

The detailed protocol for each test must be followed exactly, since even slight differences in technique will produce variations in results.

Measurement of hormone concentrations

Circulating levels of most hormones are very low (10^{-9}–10^{-12} mol/L) and cannot be measured by simple chemical techniques. Hormones are therefore usually measured by immunoassays which rely on highly specific antibodies (polyclonal or now usually monoclonal) which bind specifically to the hormone being measured during the assay incubation. This hormone–antibody interaction is measured by use of labelled hormone after separation of bound and free fractions (Fig. 18.4).

Immunoassay is sensitive but has limitations. In particular, the immunological activity of a hormone, as used in developing the antibody, may not necessarily correspond to biological activity. Other measurement techniques include high-pressure liquid chromatography (HPLC).

Endocrine disease: an introduction

See Figure 18.5.

Epidemiology

The most common endocrine disorders, excluding diabetes mellitus (Ch. 19), are:

- thyroid disorders, affecting 4–8 new patients per primary care physician each year (the most

---

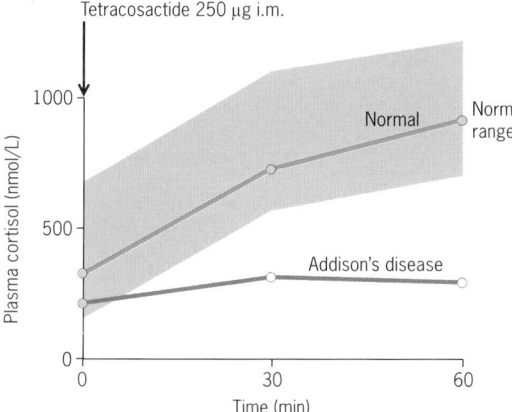

(a) Short ACTH stimulation test

Tetracosactide 250 µg i.m.

Plasma cortisol (nmol/L) — Time (min)

Normal
Normal range
Addison's disease

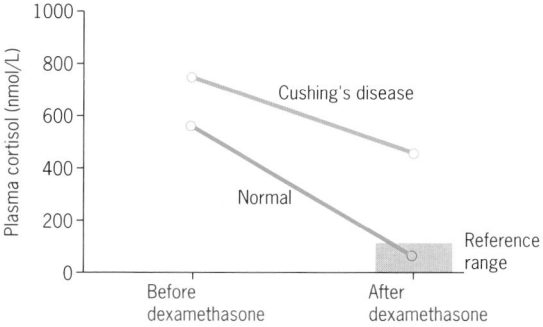

(b) Dexamethasone suppression test

Plasma cortisol (nmol/L)

Cushing's disease
Normal
Reference range

Before dexamethasone — After dexamethasone

Fig. 18.3 Synacthen and dexamethasone tests. (a) Short ACTH stimulation test showing a normal response in a healthy subject and a decreased response in a patient with Addison's disease. **(b)** Dexamethasone suppression tests in a normal subject and in a patient with Cushing's disease showing inadequate suppression.

(a)   **(b)**

Solid phase

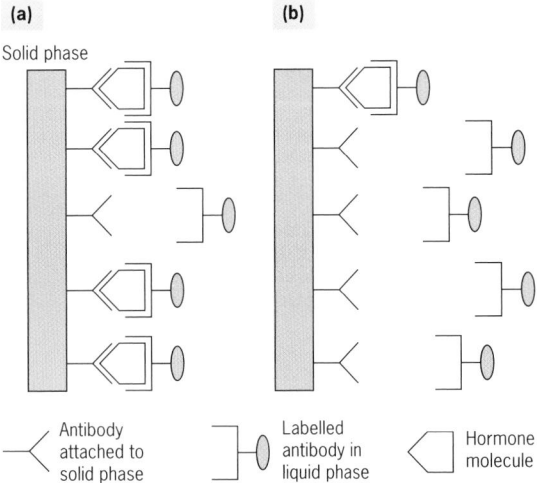

⊏─< Antibody
attached to
solid phase

⊏─⊐ Labelled
antibody in
liquid phase

<─ Hormone
molecule

Fig. 18.4 Principles of measurement of hormone levels in plasma by immunoassay (precise details vary with different assays and manufacturers). Immunoassays use two antibodies specific to the hormone being measured – one typically attached to a solid phase and one labelled antibody in the liquid phase.

(a) High hormone levels in plasma: large amount of hormone binds to antibody on solid phase – large amount of labelled antibody linked to solid phase via molecules of the hormone.

(b) Low hormone levels in plasma: less hormone, and therefore less labelled antibody, is linked to the solid phase. Label (radioactive, chemiluminescent, enzymatic or fluorescent) can be measured in either solid or liquid phase after separation of phases; levels of label will be proportional to the amount of hormone in the sample.

common problems are thyrotoxicosis, primary hypothyroidism and goitre)

- subfertility, affecting 5–10% of all couples, often with an endocrine component
- menstrual disorders and excessive hair growth in young women, most commonly polycystic ovary syndrome (PCOS)
- osteoporosis, especially in postmenopausal women largely owing to gonadal steroid deficiency
- primary hyperparathyroidism, affecting about 0.1% of the population
- disorders of growth or puberty.

While most other endocrine conditions are very uncommon, they often affect young people and are usually curable or completely controllable with appropriate therapy.

Hormones as therapy

Hormones are also widely used therapeutically:

- The oral contraceptive pill is the choice of perhaps 20–30% of women aged 18–35 years using contraception.
- Hormone replacement therapy (HRT; oestrogens ± progestogens) is increasingly used for postmenopausal women (see p. 1017).
- Corticosteroid therapy is widely used in non-endocrine disease such as asthma (see p. 881).

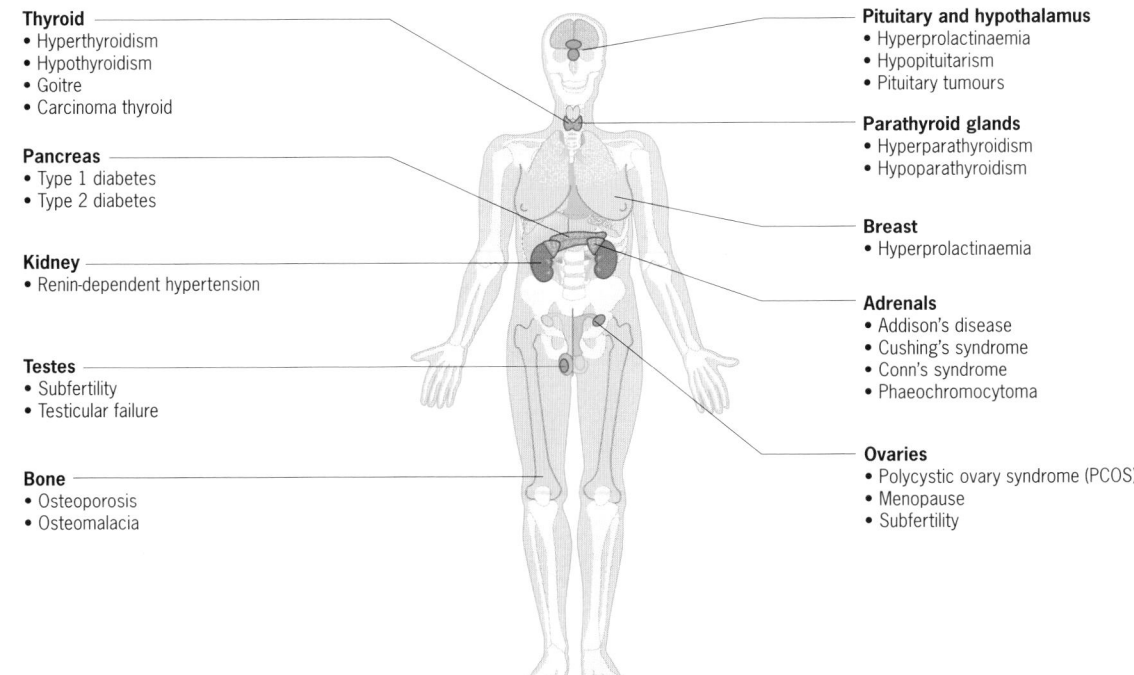

Thyroid
- Hyperthyroidism
- Hypothyroidism
- Goitre
- Carcinoma thyroid

Pancreas
- Type 1 diabetes
- Type 2 diabetes

Kidney
- Renin-dependent hypertension

Testes
- Subfertility
- Testicular failure

Bone
- Osteoporosis
- Osteomalacia

Pituitary and hypothalamus
- Hyperprolactinaemia
- Hypopituitarism
- Pituitary tumours

Parathyroid glands
- Hyperparathyroidism
- Hypoparathyroidism

Breast
- Hyperprolactinaemia

Adrenals
- Addison's disease
- Cushing's syndrome
- Conn's syndrome
- Phaeochromocytoma

Ovaries
- Polycystic ovary syndrome (PCOS)
- Menopause
- Subfertility

Fig. 18.5 The major endocrine organs and common endocrine problems.

Box 18.2

Common presenting complaints in endocrine disease

Body size and shape
Short stature
Tall stature
Excessive weight or
   weight gain
Loss of weight

'Metabolic' effects
Tiredness
Weakness
Increased appetite
Decreased appetite
Polydipsia/thirst
Polyuria/nocturia
Tremor
Palpitation
Anxiety
Heat or cold intolerance

Local effects
Swelling in the neck
Carpal tunnel syndrome
Bone or muscle pain
Protrusion of eyes
Visual loss (acuity and/or fields)
Headache

Reproduction/sex
Loss or absence of libido
Impotence
Oligomenorrhoea/
   amenorrhoea
Subfertility
Galactorrhoea
Gynaecomastia
Delayed puberty
Precocious puberty

Skin
Hirsutism
Hair thinning
Pigmentation
Dry skin
Greasy skin
Acne
Flushing
Excess sweating

Box 18.3

Endocrine disease: past, family and social histories

Past history
Necessary details may include:
● previous pregnancies (ease of conception, postpartum haemorrhage)
● relevant surgery (e.g. thyroidectomy, orchidopexy)
● radiation (e.g. to neck, gonads, thyroid)
● drug exposure (e.g. chemotherapy, sex hormones, oral contraceptives)
● in childhood, developmental milestones and growth.

Family history
Family history of:
● autoimmune disease
● endocrine disease, including tumours
● essential hypertension
● diabetes.

Family details of:
● height
● weight
● body habitus
● hair growth
● age of sexual development.

Social history
● Detailed records of alcohol intake (e.g. in subfertility, obesity)
● Drug abuse (e.g. cannabis and subfertility)
● Full details of occupation, access to drugs or chemicals
● Diet (e.g. salt, liquorice, iodine).

Symptoms

Common endocrine presenting symptoms are shown in Box 18.2, which demonstrates the many effects that hormonal abnormalities can produce.

Hormones produce widespread effects upon the body; focal symptoms are less common than with other systems. Many endocrine symptoms are diffuse and vague, and the differential diagnosis is often wide.

History and examination

A detailed history including the past, family and social history should be taken (Box 18.3).

A full drug history is mandatory as endocrine problems are quite often iatrogenic (Table 18.3).

Physical signs are listed under the relevant systems.

Specific points about endocrine disease

Autoimmune disease

Organ-specific autoimmune diseases can affect every major endocrine organ (Table 18.4). They are characterized by the presence of specific antibodies in the serum, often present years before clinical symptoms are evident. The conditions are usually more common in women and have a strong genetic component, often with an identical-twin concordance rate of 50% and with HLA associations (see individual diseases). Several of the autoantigens have been identified.

Endocrine tumours

Hormone-secreting tumours occur in all endocrine organs, most commonly pituitary, thyroid and parathyroid. Fortunately, they are more commonly benign than malignant. While often considered to be 'autonomous' – that is, independent of the physiological control mechanisms – many do show evidence of feedback occurring at a higher 'set-point' than normal (e.g. ACTH secretion from a pituitary basophil adenoma).

The molecular basis of some of these tumours is sometimes a very specific mutation of a single gene, such as the mutations of the *Ret*-proto-oncogene in MEN 2 (see p. 1067), but more commonly a wide variety of different lesions in tumour suppressor genes, growth factor receptors and other intracellular mediators have been identified.

Enzymatic defects

The biosynthesis of most hormones involves many stages. Deficient or abnormal enzymes can lead to absent or reduced production of the secreted hormone.

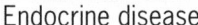
Table 18.3
Drugs and endocrine disease

Drug*	Effect
Drugs inducing endocrine disease	

Chlorpromazine
Metoclopramide
  (dopamine agonists)
Oestrogens
	Increase prolactin,
	  causing galactorrhoea

Iodine Amiodarone	Hyperthyroidism
Lithium Amiodarone	Hypothyroidism
Chlorpropamide	Inappropriate ADH secretion
Ketoconazole Metyrapone, aminoglutethimide	Hypoadrenalism
Drugs simulating endocrine disease	
Sympathomimetics Amfetamines	Mimic thyrotoxicosis or phaeochromocytoma
Liquorice Carbenoxolone	Increase mineralocorticoid activity; mimic aldosteronism
Purgatives	Hypokalaemia
Diuretics	Secondary aldosteronism
ACE inhibitors	Hypoaldosteronism
Drugs affecting hormone binding proteins	
Anticonvulsants	Bind to TBG – decrease total T_4
Oestrogens	Raise TBG and CBG – increase total T_4/cortisol
Exogenous hormones or stimulating agents	
Use, abuse or misuse, by patient or doctor, of the following:	
Steroids	Cushing's syndrome Diabetes
Thyroxine	Thyrotoxicosis factitia
Vitamin D preparations Milk and alkali preparations	Hypercalcaemia
Insulin Sulphonylureas	Hypoglycaemia

*Drugs causing gynaecomastia are listed in Table 18.15
Amiodarone may cause both hypo- or hyperthyroidism

In general, severe deficiencies present early in life with obvious signs; partial deficiencies usually present later with mild signs or are only evident under stress. An example of an enzyme deficiency is congenital adrenal hyperplasia (CAH). Again the molecular basis has usually been identified as mutations or deletions of the gene encoding the relevant enzymes.

Receptor abnormalities (see p. 156)
Hormones work by activating cellular receptors. There are rare conditions in which hormone secretion and control are normal but the receptors are defective; thus, if androgen receptors are defective, normal levels of androgen will not produce masculinization (e.g. testicular feminization). There are also a number of rare syndromes of diabetes and insulin resistance from receptor abnormalities (p. 1071); other examples include nephrogenic diabetes insipidus, thyroid hormone resistance and pseudohypoparathyroidism.

FURTHER READING

Davis JR et al. (1996) Molecular biology techniques in endocrinology. *Clinical Endocrinology* **45**: 125–133.
Diagnostic evaluation update (1997) *Endocrinology and Metabolism Clinics of North America* **26**: 4.
Epidemiology and clinical decision-making (1997) *Endocrinology and Metabolism Clinics of North America* **26**: 1–3.
Funder JW et al. (1996) Mineralocorticoid receptors and glucocorticoid receptors. *Clinical Endocrinology* **45**: 651–656.
Harris PE et al. (1996) Gs protein mutations and the pathogenesis and function of pituitary tumors. *Metabolism* **45** (Suppl 1): 120–122.
Spiegel AM et al. (1996) Mutations in G proteins and G-protein-coupled receptors in endocrine disease. *Journal of Clinical Endocrinology and Metabolism* **81**: 2434–2442.

Central control of endocrine function

Anatomy
Many peripheral hormone systems are controlled by the hypothalamus and pituitary. The hypothalamus is sited at the base of the brain around the third ventricle and above the pituitary stalk, which leads down to the pituitary itself, carrying the hypophyseal–pituitary portal blood supply.

The anatomical relationships of the hypothalamus and pituitary (Fig. 18.6) include the optic chiasm just above the pituitary fossa; any expanding lesion from the pituitary or hypothalamus can thus produce visual field defects by pressure on the chiasm. Such upward expansion of the gland through the diaphragma sellae is termed 'suprasellar extension'. Lateral extension of pituitary lesions may involve the vascular and nervous structures in the cavernous sinus and may rarely reach the temporal lobe of the brain. The pituitary is itself encased in a bony box; any lateral, anterior or posterior expansion must cause bony erosion.

Embryologically, the anterior pituitary is formed from Rathke's pouch (ectodermal) which meets an outpouching of the third ventricular floor which becomes the posterior pituitary.

Physiology
Hypothalamus
This contains many vital centres for such functions as appetite, thirst, thermal regulation and sleeping/waking.

Table 18.4
Types of autoimmune disease

Organ and frequency if known	Antibody	Antigen if known	Clinical syndrome
Stimulating			
Thyroid (1 in 100)	Thyroid-stimulating immunoglobulin (TSI, TSAb) Thyroid growth immunoglobulin	TSH receptor	Graves' disease, neonatal thyrotoxicosis Goitre
Destructive			
Thyroid (1 in 100)	Thyroid microsomal antibody Thyroglobulin	Thyroid peroxidase enzyme (TPO)	Primary hypothyroidism (myxoedema)
Adrenal (1 in 20 000)	Adrenal cortex	21-Hydroxylase enzyme	Primary hypoadrenalism (Addison's disease)
Pancreas (1 in 500)	Islet cell	GAD (see p. 1074)	Type 1 (insulin-dependent) diabetes
Stomach	Gastric parietal cell Intrinsic factor		Pernicious anaemia
Skin	Melanocyte		Vitiligo
Ovary (1 in 500)	Ovary		Primary ovarian failure
Testis	Testis		Primary testicular failure
Parathyroid	Parathyroid chief cell		Primary hypoparathyroidism
Pituitary	Pituitary-specific cells		Selective hypopituitarism (e.g. GH deficiency, diabetes insipidus)

Frequencies are approximate and refer to the population in Northern Europe
GAD, glutamic acid dehydrogenase
NB: Other related diseases include myasthenia gravis and autoimmune liver diseases

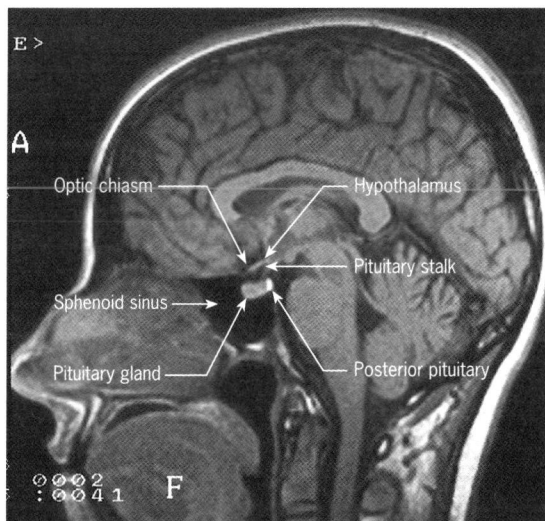

Fig. 18.6 **MR image of a sagittal section of the brain, showing the pituitary fossa and adjacent structures.** By kind permission of Dr Martin Jeffree.

It acts as an integrator of many neural and endocrine inputs to control the release of pituitary hormone-releasing factors. It plays a role in the circadian rhythm, menstrual cyclicity, and responses to stress, exercise and mood.

Hypothalamic neurones secrete pituitary hormone-releasing and -inhibiting factors and hormones into the portal system which runs down the stalk to the pituitary. As well as the classical hormones described in Table 18.5, the hypothalamus also contains large amounts of other neuropeptides and neurotransmitters such as neuropeptide Y, vasoactive intestinal peptide (VIP) and nitric oxide that can also alter pituitary hormone secretion but whose role is less well defined.

Synthetic hypothalamic hormones and their antagonists are available for the testing of many aspects of endocrine function and for treatment.

Anterior pituitary

Hormone secretion is controlled by hypothalamic releasing or inhibitory hormones (Table 18.5 and Fig. 18.7). Many hormones are under dual control by both stimulatory and inhibitory hypothalamic factors. Examples are:

- Growth hormone release is stimulated by growth hormone-releasing hormone (GHRH) but inhibited by somatostatin (growth hormone release inhibitory hormone, GHRIH).
- TSH release is stimulated by TRH but partially inhibited by somatostatin.

Some hormones have a dual stimulatory control. For example, corticotropin-releasing hormone (CRH) and vasopressin are both endogenous stimulators of ACTH release. Uniquely, prolactin is under predominant inhibitory dopaminergic control with some stimulatory TRH control.

Table 18.5
Nomenclature and biochemistry of hypothalamic, pituitary and peripheral hormones

Hypothalamic hormones	Pituitary hormones	Peripheral hormones
Gonadotrophin-releasing hormone (GnRH, LHRH) (*Decapeptide*)	Luteinizing hormone (LH) Follicle-stimulating hormone (FSH) (*Two-chain α, β peptides*)	Oestrogens/androgens (*Steroid ring*)
Prolactin inhibiting factor (PIF – dopamine) (*Amine*)	Prolactin (PRL) (*Single chain peptide*)	–
Growth hormone-releasing hormone (GHRH) (*Peptide*) Somatostatin (GHRIH) (*Cyclic peptide*)	Growth hormone (GH) (*Peptide*)	Insulin-like growth factor-I (IGF-1) (*Peptide*)
Thyrotrophin-releasing hormone (TRH) (*Tripeptide*)	Thyroid-stimulating hormone (TSH) (*Two-chain α, β peptide*)	Thyroxine (T$_4$), triiodothyronine (T$_3$) (*Thyronines*)
Corticotropin-releasing hormone (CRH) (*Single-chain peptide*)	Adrenocorticotrophic hormone (ACTH) (*Single-chain peptide*)	Cortisol (*Steroid ring*)
Vasopressin (antidiuretic hormone; ADH) (*Nonapeptide*)	–	–
Oxytocin (*Nonapeptide*)	–	–

NB: The α chains of LH, FSH and TSH are identical
GHRIH, growth hormone release inhibitory hormone

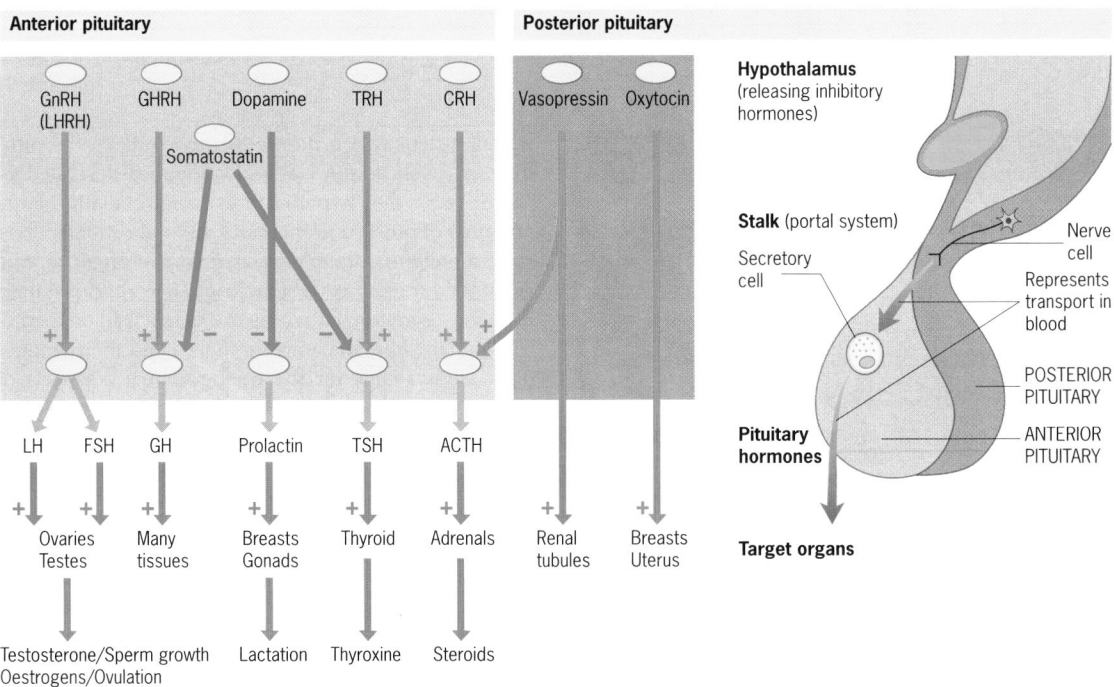

Fig. 18.7 Hypothalamic releasing hormones and the pituitary trophic hormones. See the text for abbreviations and an explanation.

Posterior pituitary

This, in contrast, acts merely as a storage organ. Antidiuretic hormone (ADH, vasopressin) and oxytocin, both nonapeptides, are synthesized in the supraoptic and paraventricular nuclei in the anterior hypothalamus. They are then transported along the axon and stored in the posterior pituitary. This means that damage to the stalk or pituitary alone does not prevent synthesis and release of ADH and oxytocin. ADH is discussed on page 1057; oxytocin produces milk ejection and uterine myometrial contraction.

Presentations of hypothalamic and pituitary disease

Pituitary space-occupying lesions and tumours

Pituitary tumours (Table 18.6) are the most common cause of pituitary disease, and most of these are benign pituitary adenomas, usually monoclonal in origin. Problems may be caused by excess hormone secretion, by local effects of a tumour, or as the result of inadequate production of hormone by the remaining normal pituitary – hypopituitarism. The great majority of pituitary tumours are benign pituitary adenomas.

Investigations

The investigation of a possible or proven tumour follows three lines.

Is there a tumour?

If there is, how big is it and what local anatomical effects is it exerting? Pituitary and hypothalamic space-occupying lesions, hormonally active or not, can cause symptoms by pressure on, or infiltration of:

- the visual pathways, with field defects and visual loss

and more rarely:

- the cavernous sinus, with III, IV and VI cranial nerve lesions
- bony structures and the meninges surrounding the fossa, causing headache
- hypothalamic centres: altered appetite, obesity, thirst, somnolence/wakefulness or precocious puberty
- the ventricles, causing interruption of cerebrospinal fluid (CSF) flow leading to hydrocephalus
- the sphenoid sinus with invasion causing CSF rhinorrhoea.

Investigations:

- **Lateral skull X-ray.** This may show enlargement of the fossa. Although an X-ray is rarely requested as a definitive investigation, this remains a common incidental finding.
- **Visual fields.** These should be plotted formally by automated computer perimetry or Goldmann perimetry, but clinical assessment by confrontation at the bedside using a small red pin as target is also sensitive and valuable. Common defects are upper-temporal quadrantanopia and bitemporal hemianopia (see p. 1130). Subtle defects may also be revealed by delay or attenuation of visual evoked potentials (VEPs).
- **MRI of the pituitary.** MRI is superior to CT scanning (Fig. 18.8) and will readily show any significant pituitary mass. However, small lesions within the pituitary fossa on MRI consistent with small pituitary microadenomas are very common, reported in as many as 10% of normal individuals in some studies. Such small lesions are sometimes detected during MRI scanning of the head for other reasons – so-called 'pituitary incidentalomas'.

Is there a hormonal excess?

There are three major conditions usually caused by secretion from pituitary adenomas which will show positive immunostaining for the relevant hormone:

- prolactin excess (prolactinoma or hyperprolactinaemia) – histologically, prolactinomas are 'chromophobe' adenomas (a description of their appearance on classical histological staining)
- GH excess, leading to acromegaly or gigantism – somatotroph adenomas, usually 'acidophil', and sometimes due to specific G-protein mutations (see p. 156)

Table 18.6
Characteristics of common pituitary and related tumours

Tumour or condition	Usual size	Most common clinical presentation
Prolactinoma	Most < 10 mm (microprolactinoma)	Galactorrhoea, amenorrhoea, hypogonadism, impotence
	Some > 10 mm (macroprolactinoma)	As above plus headaches, visual field defects and hypopituitarism
Acromegaly	Few mm to several cm	Change in appearance, visual field defects and hypopituitarism
Cushing's disease	Most small – few mm (some cases are hyperplasia)	Central obesity, Cushingoid appearance (local symptoms rare)
Nelson's syndrome	Often large – > 10 mm	Post-adrenalectomy, pigmentation, sometimes local symptoms
Non-functioning tumours	Usually large – > 10 mm	Visual field defects; hypopituitarism (microadenomas may be incidental finding)
Craniopharyngioma	Often very large and cystic (skull X-ray abnormal in > 50%; calcification common)	Headaches, visual field defects, growth failure (50% occur below age 20; about 15% arise from within sella)

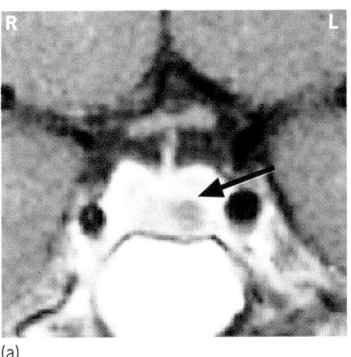
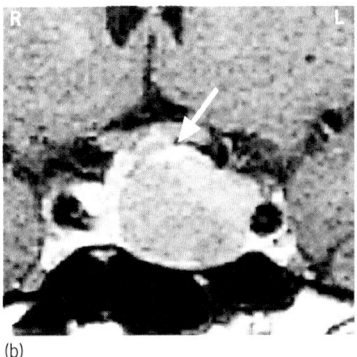
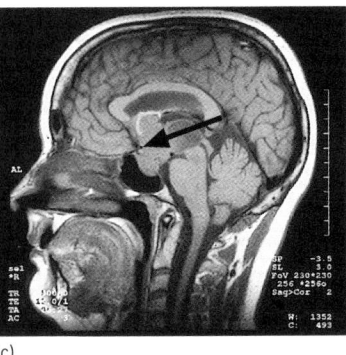

(a) (b) (c)

Fig. 18.8 **(a) Coronal MRI of pituitary**, showing a left-sided lucent intrasellar microadenoma (arrowed). The pituitary stalk is deviated slightly to the right. **(b) Coronal MRI of pituitary**, showing macroadenoma with moderate suprasellar extension, and lateral extension compressing left cavernous sinus. The top of the adenoma is compressing the optic chiasm (arrowed). **(c) Sagittal MRI of head**, showing a pituitary macroadenoma with massive suprasellar extension (arrow).

- Cushing's disease and Nelson's syndrome (excess ACTH secretion) – corticotroph adenomas, usually 'basophil'.

Many tumours are able to synthesize several pituitary hormones, and occasionally more than one hormone is secreted in clinically-significant excess (e.g. both GH and prolactin).

The clinical features of acromegaly and Cushing's disease or hyperprolactinaemia are usually (but not always) obvious, and are discussed on pages 1033, 1027, and 1052. Hyperprolactinaemia may be clinically 'silent'. Tumours producing LH, FSH or TSH are well described but very rare.

Some pituitary tumours cause no clinically apparent hormone excess and are referred to as 'non-functioning' tumours, which are common and usually 'chromophobe' adenomas. Laboratory studies such as immunocyto-chemistry show that these tumours may often produce LH and FSH or the α subunit of LH, FSH and TSH (see Table 18.5), and occasionally ACTH.

Is there a deficiency of any hormone?

Clinical examination may give clues; thus, short stature in a child with a pituitary tumour is likely to be due to GH deficiency. A slow, lethargic adult with pale skin is likely to be deficient in TSH and/or ACTH. Milder deficiencies may not be obvious, and require specific testing (see Table 18.9).

Treatment

Treatment depends on the type and size of tumour (Table 18.7) and is discussed in more detail in the relevant sections (acromegaly, see p. 1034; prolactinoma, see p. 1028). In general, therapy has three aims:

Removal/control of tumour

Surgery via the trans-sphenoidal route is usually the treatment of choice. Very large tumours are occasionally removed via the open transfrontal route.

Radiotherapy may be by an external three-beam technique, stereotactic or rarely via implant of yttrium needles. It is usually employed when surgery is impracticable or incomplete as it controls but rarely abolishes tumour mass. The standard regimen involves a dose of about 45 Gy, given as 20–25 fractions via three fields.

Octreotide or dopamine agonists sometimes cause shrinkage of specific types of tumour (see p. 1034).

Reduction of excess hormone secretion

Reduction is usually obtained by surgical removal but sometimes by medical treatment. Useful control can be achieved with dopamine agonists for prolactinomas or somatostatin analogues for acromegaly, but ACTH secretion usually cannot be controlled by medical means. Growth hormone antagonists are being trialled for acromegaly (p. 1035).

Replacement of hormone deficiencies

Replacement of hormone deficiencies is detailed in Table 18.10.

Small tumours producing no significant symptoms, pressure or endocrine effects may be observed with appropriate clinical, visual field, imaging and endocrine assessments.

Differential diagnosis of pituitary or hypothalamic masses

Although pituitary adenomas are the most common mass lesion of the pituitary, a variety of other conditions may also present as a pituitary or hypothalamic mass and form part of the differential diagnosis.

Other tumours

Craniopharyngioma, a usually cystic hypothalamic tumour, which is often calcified, arising from Rathke's pouch often mimics an intrinsic pituitary lesion. It is the most common pituitary tumour in children but may present at any age.

Table 18.7
Comparisons of primary treatments for pituitary tumours

Treatment method	Advantages	Disadvantages
Surgical		
Trans-sphenoidal adenomectomy or hypophysectomy	Relatively minor procedure Potentially curative for microadenomas and smaller macroadenomas	Some extrasellar extensions may not be accessible Risk of CSF leakage and meningitis
Transfrontal	Good access to suprasellar region	Major procedure; danger of frontal lobe damage High chance of subsequent hypopituitarism
Radiotherapy		
External (40–50 Gy)	Non-invasive Reduces recurrence rate after surgery	Slow action, often over many years Not always effective Possible late risk of tumour induction
Stereotactic	Precise administration of high dose to lesion	Long-term follow-up data limited
Yttrium implantation	High local dose	Only ever used in a few centres
Medical		
Dopamine agonist therapy (e.g. bromocriptine)	Non-invasive; reversible	Usually not curative Significant side-effects in minority
Somatostatin analogue therapy (octreotide, lanreotide)	Non-invasive; reversible	Usually not curative; expensive; side-effects

Uncommon tumours include meningiomas, gliomas, chondromas, germinomas and pinealomas. Secondary deposits occasionally present as apparent pituitary tumours, often presenting with headache and diabetes insipidus.

Hypophysitis and other inflammatory masses
A variety of inflammatory masses may occur in the pituitary or hypothalamus. These include rare pituitary-specific conditions (e.g. postpartum hypophysitis, lymphocytic hypophysitis, giant cell hypophysitis), or pituitary manifestations of more generalized disease processes (sarcoidosis, Langerhans' cell histiocytosis, Wegener's granulomatosis).

Other lesions
Carotid artery aneurysms may masquerade as pituitary tumours. Cystic lesions may also present as a pituitary mass, including arachnoid and Rathke cleft cysts.

Hypopituitarism
Pathophysiology
Deficiency of hypothalamic releasing hormones or of pituitary trophic hormones is either selective or multiple. There are, for example, rare isolated deficiencies of LH/FSH and ACTH, some of which may be congenital, autoimmune or idiopathic in nature.

Multiple deficiencies usually result from tumour growth or other destructive lesions. There is generally a progressive loss of anterior pituitary function, usually in the order shown from left to right in Figure 18.7. GH and gonadotrophins are usually first affected. Hyperprolactinaemia, rather than prolactin deficiency, occurs relatively early because of loss of tonic inhibitory control by dopamine. TSH and ACTH are usually last to

be affected. *Panhypopituitarism* refers to deficiency of all anterior pituitary hormones; it is most commonly caused by pituitary tumours, surgery or radiotherapy. Multiple deficiencies can also rarely result from congenital defects, e.g. mutation of the gene for the pituitary-specific transcription factor 'Pit-1' causes deficiency in GH, prolactin and TSH.

Vasopressin and oxytocin secretion will be significantly affected only if the hypothalamus is involved, either by a hypothalamic tumour or by major suprasellar extension of a pituitary lesion. Posterior pituitary deficiency is rare in an uncomplicated pituitary adenoma.

Causes
Disorders causing hypopituitarism are listed in Table 18.8. Pituitary and hypothalamic tumours, and surgical or radiotherapy treatment, are the most common.

Clinical features
Symptoms and signs depend upon the extent of hypothalamic and/or pituitary deficiencies, and mild deficiencies may not lead to any complaint by the patient. In general, symptoms of deficiency of a pituitary-stimulating hormone are the same as primary deficiency of the peripheral endocrine gland (e.g. TSH deficiency and primary hypothyroidism cause similar symptoms due to lack of thyroid hormone secretion). Thus, secondary hypothyroidism and adrenal failure both lead to tiredness and general malaise; hypothyroidism may cause slowness of thought and action, dry skin and cold intolerance, while hypoadrenalism may cause mild hypotension, hyponatraemia and ultimately cardiovascular collapse during severe intercurrent stressful illness. Loss of libido, loss of secondary sexual hair, amenorrhoea and impotence are symptoms of gonadotrophin and thus

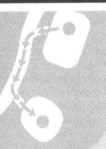

Table 18.8
Causes of hypopituitarism

Congenital
Isolated deficiency of
   pituitary hormones
   (e.g. Kallmann's syndrome)
Pit-1 deficiency

Infective
Basal meningitis
   (e.g. tuberculosis)
Encephalitis
Syphilis

Vascular
Pituitary apoplexy
Sheehan's syndrome
   (postpartum necrosis)
Carotid artery aneurysms

Immunological
Pituitary antibodies

Neoplastic
Pituitary or hypothalamic
   tumours
Craniopharyngioma
Meningiomas
Gliomas
Pinealoma
Secondary deposits,
   especially breast
Lymphoma

Traumatic
Skull fracture through base
Surgery, especially transfrontal
Perinatal trauma

Infiltrations
Sarcoidosis
Langerhans' cell histiocytosis
Hereditary haemochromatosis
Hypophysitis
   Postpartum
   Lymphocytic
   Giant cell

Others
Radiation damage
Fibrosis
Chemotherapy
Empty sella syndrome

'Functional'
Anorexia nervosa
Starvation
Emotional deprivation

gonadal deficiencies, while hyperprolactinaemia may cause galactorrhoea and hypogonadism. GH deficiency is relatively clinically 'silent' except in children, though recent evidence suggests that it may cause markedly impaired well-being in some adults. Weight may increase (due to hypothyroidism) or decrease in severe combined deficiency (pituitary cachexia). Long-standing panhypopituitarism may give the classic picture of pallor with hairlessness ('alabaster skin').

Particular syndromes related to hypopituitarism are:

Kallmann's syndrome
This syndrome is isolated gonadotrophin (GnRH) deficiency (p. 1020).

Sheehan's syndrome
This situation, now rare, is pituitary infarction following postpartum haemorrhage.

Pituitary apoplexy
A pituitary tumour may occasionally infarct or haemorrhage into itself. This may produce severe headache sometimes followed by acute life-threatening hypopituitarism.

The 'empty sella' syndrome
An 'empty sella' is sometimes reported on pituitary imaging. This is sometimes due to a defect in the diaphragma and extension of the subarachnoid space (cisternal herniation) or may follow spontaneous

Table 18.9
Tests for hypothalamic-pituitary (HP) function

- All hormone levels are measured in plasma unless otherwise stated.
- Tests **shown in bold** are those normally measured on a single basal 0900h sample in the initial assessment of pituitary function.

Axis	Pituitary hormone	End-organ product/function	Common dynamic tests	Other tests
Anterior pituitary				
HP-ovarian	**LH** **FSH**	**Oestradiol** Progesterone (day 21 of cycle)		Ovarian ultrasound LHRH test*
HP-testicular	**LH** **FSH**	**Testosterone**		Sperm count LHRH test*
Growth	GH	IGF-1 IGF-BP3	Insulin tolerance test	GH response to sleep, exercise or arginine infusion GHRH test*
Prolactin	**Prolactin**			
HP-thyroid	**TSH**	**Free T$_4$**, T$_3$		TRH test*
HP-adrenal	ACTH	**Cortisol**	Insulin tolerance test Short synacthen (tetracosactide) test	Glucagon test CRH test* Metyrapone test
Posterior pituitary				
Thirst and osmoregulation		**Plasma/urine osmolality**	Water deprivation test	Hypertonic saline infusion

*Releasing hormone tests were a traditional part of pituitary function testing, but have been largely replaced by the advent of more reliable assays for basal hormones. They test only the 'readily releasable pool' of pituitary hormones and normal responses may be seen in hypopituitarism

infarction of a tumour. All or most of the sella turcica is devoid of apparent pituitary tissue, but, despite this, pituitary function is usually normal, the pituitary being eccentrically placed and flattened against the floor or roof of the fossa.

Investigations

Each axis of the hypothalamic–pituitary system requires separate investigation. However, the presence of normal gonadal function (ovulatory/menstruation or normal libido/erections) suggests that multiple defects of anterior pituitary function are unlikely.

Tests range from the simple basal levels (e.g. T_4 or free T_4 for the thyroid axis), to stimulatory tests for the pituitary, and tests of feedback for the hypothalamus (Table 18.9). Assessment of the hypothalamo-pituitary–adrenal axis remains critical but controversial: basal 0900h cortisol levels above 500 nmol/L, and probably above 400 nmol/L, indicate an adequate reserve, while levels below 100 nmol/L predict an inadequate stress response. In many cases basal levels are equivocal and a dynamic test is essential: the insulin tolerance test (Box 18.4) is widely regarded as the 'gold standard' but the synacthen test (see Box 18.1), though an indirect measure, is used by many as a routine test of hypothalamic–pituitary–adrenal status. Overall the assessment of adrenal reserve is best left in the hands of a specialist endocrinologist.

Treatment

Steroid and thyroid hormones are essential for life. Both are given as oral replacement drugs, as in primary thyroid and adrenal deficiency, aiming to restore the patient to clinical and biochemical normality (Table 18.10) and levels may be monitored by routine hormone assays. Sex hormone production is replaced with androgens and oestrogens, both for symptomatic control and to prevent long-term problems related to deficiency

---

Box 18.4

Insulin tolerance test

Indication
Diagnosis or exclusion of ACTH and growth hormone deficiency

Procedure
Should only be performed in experienced, specialist units
Exclude cardiovascular disease (ECG), epilepsy or unexplained blackouts; exclude severe untreated hypopituitarism (basal cortisol must be > 100 nmol/L; normal free T_4)
Intravenous hydrocortisone and glucose available for emergency
Overnight fast, begin at 0800–0900h
Soluble insulin, 0.15 Units/kg, i.v. at time 0
Glucose, cortisol and GH at 0, 30, 45, 60, 90, 120 min

Normal response
Cortisol rises above 550 nmol/L*
GH rises above 20 mU/L (severe deficiency = < 9 mU/L (3 ng/L))
Glucose must be < 2.2 mmol/L to achieve adequate stress response

* Precise cortisol normal ranges are variable between laboratories and assays – appropriate local reference ranges must be used

---

(e.g. osteoporosis). When fertility is desired, gonadal function may be stimulated directly by human chorionic gonadotrophin (HCG, mainly acting as LH), purified or biosynthetic gonadotrophins, or indirectly by pulsatile gonadotrophin-releasing hormone (GnRH – also known as luteinizing hormone-releasing hormone, LHRH); all are expensive and time-consuming and should be restricted to specialist units.

GH therapy is given in the growing child, under the care of a paediatric endocrinologist. In adult GH deficiency, GH therapy also produces improvements in body composition, work capacity and psychological well-being, together with reversal of lipid abnormalities

---

Table 18.10
Replacement therapy for hypopituitarism

Axis	Usual replacement therapies
Adrenal	Hydrocortisone 15–40 mg daily (starting dose 10 mg on rising/5 mg lunchtime/5 mg evening) (Normally no need for mineralocorticoid replacement)
Thyroid	Thyroxine 100–150 µg daily
Gonadal	
Male	Testosterone intramuscularly, orally, as patch or implant
Female	Cyclical oestrogen/progestogen orally or as patch
Fertility	HCG plus FSH (purified or recombinant) or pulsatile GnRH to produce testicular development, spermatogenesis or ovulation
Growth	Recombinant human GH used routinely to achieve normal growth in children Also advocated for replacement therapy in adults where GH has effects on muscle mass and well-being
Thirst	Desmopressin (DDAVP) 10–20 µg one to three times daily by nasal spray or orally 100–200 µg three times daily Carbamazepine and thiazides are rarely used in mild diabetes insipidus
Breast (Prolactin inhibition)	Dopamine agonist as replacement inhibition (e.g. bromocriptine 2.5–15 mg daily)

associated with a high cardiovascular risk, and this may result in significant symptomatic benefit in some cases. Although now licensed for such use in most countries, the long-term safety and efficacy of GH therapy in adults is not yet fully established, and its cost is £2500–6000 per annum.

Two points should be noted:

- Thyroid replacement should not commence until normal glucocorticoid function has been demonstrated or replacement steroid therapy initiated, as an adrenal 'crisis' may otherwise be precipitated.
- Glucocorticoid deficiency may mask impaired urine concentrating ability, diabetes insipidus only becoming apparent after steroid replacement.

FURTHER READING

Ho KKY (2000) Diagnosis of adult GH deficiency. *Lancet* **356**: 1125–1126.

Lamberts SWJ, de Herder WW, van der Lely AJ (1998) Pituitary insufficiency. *Lancet* **352**: 127–134.

Plowman PN (1999) Pituitary adenoma radiotherapy – when and how? *Clinical Endocrinology* **51**: 265–272.

Vance ML, Mauras N (1999) Drug therapy: growth hormone therapy in adults and children. *New England Journal of Medicine* **341**: 1206–1216.

Reproduction and sex

The normal physiology of the female and male reproductive systems will be considered first, followed by their common disorders. Some relevant terminology is set out in Box 18.5.

Embryology

Up to 8 weeks of gestation the sexes share a common development, with a primitive genital tract including the Wolffian and Müllerian ducts. There are additionally a primitive perineum and primitive gonads.

- In the presence of a Y chromosome the potential testis develops while the ovary regresses.
- In the absence of a Y chromosome, the potential ovary develops and related ducts form a uterus and the upper vagina.

Production of Müllerian inhibitory factor from the early 'testis' produces atrophy of the Müllerian duct, while, under the influence of testosterone and dihydrotestosterone, the Wolffian duct differentiates into an epididymis, vas deferens, seminal vesicles and prostate. Androgens induce transformation of the perineum to include a penis, penile urethra and scrotum containing the testes, which descend in response to androgenic stimulation. At birth, testicular volume is 0.5–1 mL.

Physiology

The male

An outline of the hypothalamic–pituitary–testicular axis is shown in Figure 18.9.

1. Pulses of GnRH (LHRH) are released from the hypothalamus and stimulate LH and FSH release from the pituitary.
2. LH stimulates testosterone production from Leydig cells of the testis.
3. Testosterone acts systemically to produce male secondary sexual characteristics, anabolism and the maintenance of libido. It also acts locally within

---

Box 18.5

Definitions in reproductive medicine

Menarche	Age at first period
Primary amenorrhoea	Failure to begin spontaneous menstruation by age 16
Secondary amenorrhoea	Absence of menstruation for 3 months in a woman who has previously had cycles
Oligomenorrhoea	Irregular long cycles; often used for any length of cycle above 32 days
Dyspareunia	Pain or discomfort in the female during intercourse
Libido	Sexual interest or desire; often difficult to assess and is greatly affected by stress, tiredness and psychological factors
Menstruation	Onset of spontaneous (usually regular) uterine bleeding in the female
Impotence	Inability of the male to achieve or sustain an erection adequate for satisfactory intercourse
Azoospermia	Absence of sperm in the ejaculate
Oligospermia	Reduced numbers of sperm in the ejaculate; normal values are disputed
Virilization	Occurrence of male secondary sexual characteristics in the female

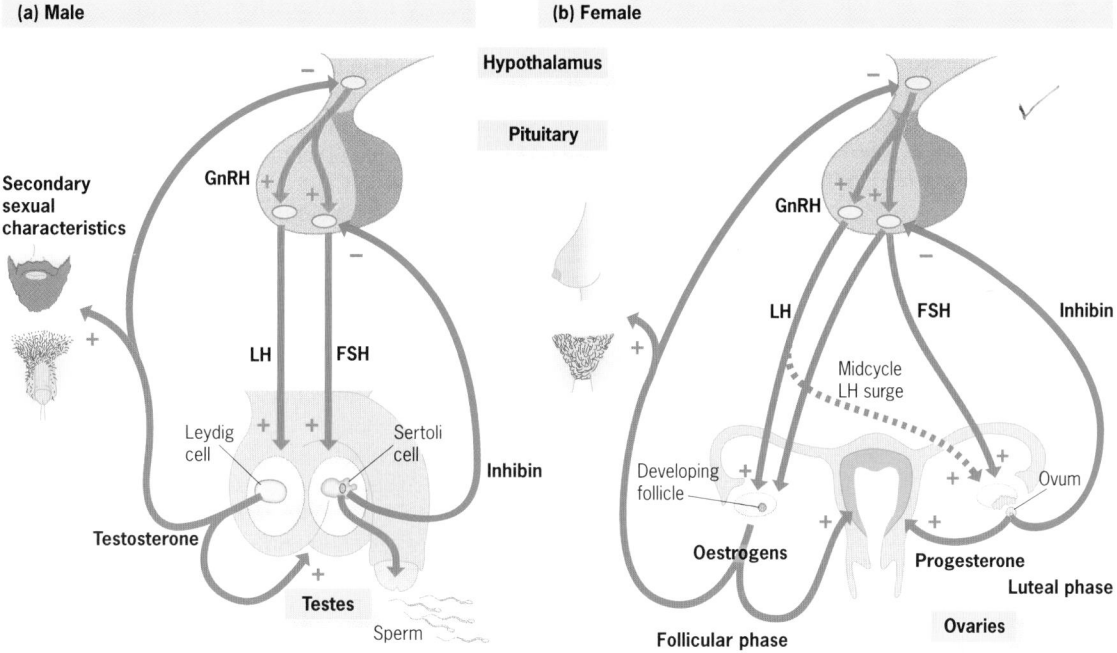

Fig. 18.9 **Male and female hypothalamic–pituitary–gonadal axes.** Note the close parallels. The green lines indicate negative feedback.

the testis to aid spermatogenesis. Testosterone circulates largely bound to sex hormone-binding globulin (SHBG) (see p. 1000). Testosterone feeds back on the hypothalamus/pituitary to inhibit GnRH secretion.

4. FSH stimulates the Sertoli cells in the seminiferous tubules to produce mature sperm and the inhibins A and B.
5. Inhibin causes feedback on the pituitary to decrease FSH secretion.

The secondary sexual characteristics of the male for which testosterone is necessary are the growth of pubic, axillary and facial hair, enlargement of the external genitalia, deepening of the voice, sebum secretion, muscle growth and frontal balding.

The female
The female situation is more complex (Figs 18.9 and 18.10).

1. In the adult female, higher brain centres impose a menstrual cycle of 28 days upon the activity of hypothalamic GnRH.
2. Pulses of GnRH, at about 2-hour intervals, stimulate release of pituitary LH and FSH.
3. LH stimulates ovarian androgen production by the ovarian theca cells.
4. FSH stimulates follicular development and aromatase activity (an enzyme required to convert ovarian androgens to oestrogens) in the ovarian

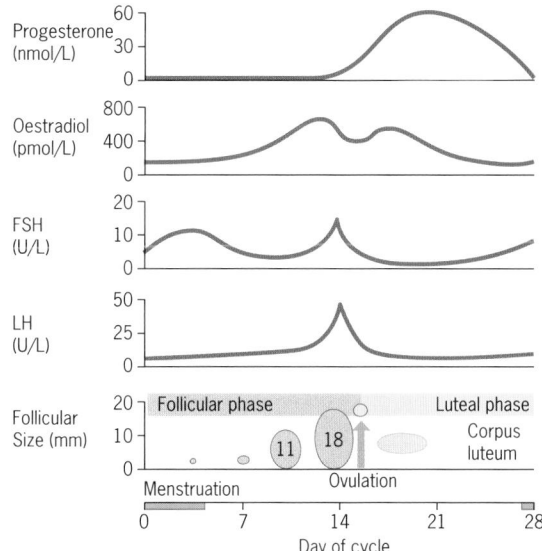

Fig. 18.10 **Hormonal and follicular changes during the normal menstrual cycle.**

granulosa cells. FSH also stimulates release of inhibin from ovarian stromal cells which inhibits FSH release.
5. Although many follicles are 'recruited' for development in early folliculogenesis, by day 8–10 a 'leading' (or 'dominant') follicle is selected for development into a mature Graafian follicle.

6. Oestrogens show a double feedback action on the pituitary (Fig. 18.9), initially inhibiting gonadotrophin secretion (negative feedback), but later high-level exposure results in increased GnRH secretion and increased LH sensitivity to GnRH (positive feedback), which leads to the mid-cycle LH surge inducing ovulation from the leading follicle (Fig. 18.10).

7. The follicle then differentiates into a corpus luteum, which secretes both progesterone and estradiol during the second half of the cycle (luteal phase).

8. Oestrogen initially and then progesterone cause uterine endometrial proliferation in preparation for possible implantation; if implantation does not occur, the corpus luteum regresses and progesterone secretion and inhibin levels fall so that the endometrium is shed (menstruation) allowing increased GnRH and FSH secretion.

9. If implantation and pregnancy follow, human chorionic gonadotrophin (HCG) production from the corpus luteum maintains corpus luteum function until 10–12 weeks of gestation, by which time the placenta will be making sufficient oestrogen and progesterone to support itself.

Oestrogens also induce secondary sexual characteristics, especially development of the breast and nipples, vaginal and vulval growth and pubic hair development. They also induce growth and maturation of the uterus and Fallopian tubes. They circulate largely bound to SHBG.

Physiology of prolactin secretion

The hypothalamic–pituitary control of prolactin secretion is illustrated in Figure 18.11.

Prolactin is under tonic dopamine inhibition, while other factors known to increase prolactin secretion (e.g. TRH) are probably of less importance. Prolactin stimulates milk secretion but also reduces gonadal activity. It decreases GnRH pulsatility at the hypothalamic level and, to a lesser extent, blocks the action of LH on the ovary or testis, producing hypogonadism. These actions may be clinically relevant.

Puberty

The mechanisms initiating puberty are poorly understood but are thought to result from withdrawal of central inhibition of GnRH release.

LH and FSH are both low in the prepubertal child. In early puberty, FSH begins to rise first, initially in nocturnal pulses; this is followed by a rise in LH with a subsequent increase in testosterone/oestrogen levels. The milestones of puberty in the two sexes are shown in Figure 18.12.

In boys, pubertal changes begin at between 10 and 14 years and are complete at between 15 and 17 years. The genitalia develop, testes enlarge and the area of pubic hair increases. Peak height velocity is reached between ages 12 and 17 years during stage 4 of testicular development. Full spermatogenesis occurs comparatively late.

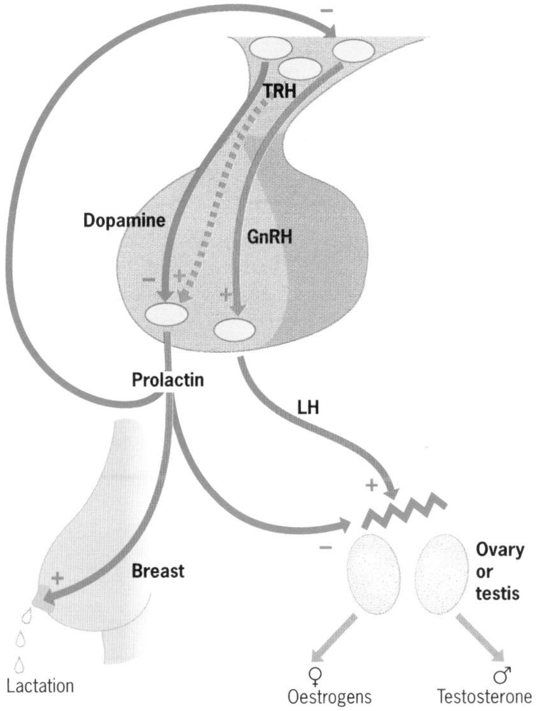

Fig. 18.11 **The control of prolactin secretion.**

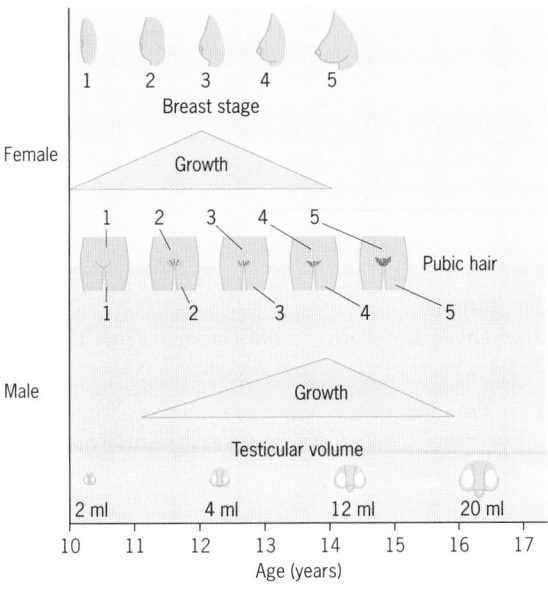

Fig. 18.12 The age of development of features of puberty. Stages and testicular size show mean ages, and all vary considerably between individuals. The same is true of height spurt, shown here in relation to other data. Numbers 2 to 5 indicate stages of development (see the text).

In girls, events start a year earlier. Breast bud enlargement begins at ages 9–13 years and continues to 12–18 years. Pubic hair growth commences at ages 9–14 years and is completed at 12–16 years. Menarche occurs relatively late (age 11–15 years) but peak height velocity is reached earlier (at age 10–13 years), and growth is completed much earlier than in boys.

Precocious puberty

Development of secondary sexual characteristics, or menarche in girls, at or before the age of 9 years is premature. All cases require specialist assessment by a paediatric endocrinologist.

Idiopathic (true) precocity is most common in girls and very rare in boys. This is a diagnosis of exclusion. With no apparent cause for premature breast or pubic hair development, and an early growth spurt, it may be normal and may run in families. Treatment with long-acting GnRH analogues (given by nasal spray, by subcutaneous injection or by implant) causes suppression of gonadotrophin release via downregulation of the receptor – and therefore reduced sex hormone production – and is moderately effective; cyproterone acetate, an antiandrogen with progestational activity, may also be used.

The following are other forms of precocity:

- *Cerebral precocity*. Many causes of hypothalamic disease, especially tumours, may present in this way. In boys this must be rigorously excluded.
- *McCune–Albright syndrome*. This is usually in girls, with precocity, polyostotic fibrous dysplasia and skin pigmentation (café-au-lait).
- *Premature thelarche*. This is early breast development alone, usually transient, at age 2–4 years. It may regress or persist until puberty. There is no evidence of follicular development.
- *Premature adrenarche*. This is early development of pubic hair without significant other changes, usually after age 5 years and more commonly in girls.

Delayed puberty

Over 95% of children show signs of pubertal development by age 14 years. In its absence, investigation should begin by age 15 years. Causes of hypogonadism (see below) are clearly relevant but most cases represent constitutional delay.

In constitutional delay, pubertal development, bone age and stature are in parallel. A family history may confirm that other family members experienced the same delayed development, which is common in boys but very rare in girls.

In boys, a testicular volume > 5 mL indicates the onset of puberty. A rising serum testosterone is an earlier clue.

In girls, the breast bud is the first sign. Ultrasound allows accurate assessment of ovarian and uterine development.

Basal LH/FSH levels may identify the site of a defect, and GnRH (LHRH) tests can indicate the stage of early puberty.

If any progression into puberty is evident clinically, investigations are not required. When delay is great and problems are serious (e.g. severe teasing at school), low-dose short-term sex hormone therapy is used. Specialist assessment is advisable.

The menopause

The menopause, or cessation of periods, naturally occurs about the age of 45–55 years. During the late forties, FSH initially, and then LH concentrations begin to rise, probably as follicle supply diminishes. Oestrogen levels fall and the cycle becomes disrupted. Most women notice irregular scanty periods coming on over a variable period, though in some sudden amenorrhoea or menorrhagia occur. Eventually the menopausal pattern of low estradiol levels with grossly elevated LH and FSH levels (usually > 50 and > 25 U/L, respectively) is established. Menopause may also occur surgically, with radiotherapy to the ovaries and with ovarian disease (e.g. premature menopause).

Clinical features and treatment

Features of oestrogen deficiency are hot flushes (which occur in most women and can be disabling), vaginal dryness and atrophy of the breasts. There may also be vague symptoms of loss of libido, loss of self-esteem, non-specific aches and pains, irritability, depression, loss of concentration and weight gain. Women show a rapid loss of bone density in the 10 years following the menopause (osteoporosis, see p. 579) and the premenopausal protection from ischaemic heart disease disappears.

Symptomatic patients should be treated and many physicians also recommend the widespread, near universal, use of hormone replacement therapy (HRT), though uptake remains less frequent in the UK than in the USA. In treatment, some of the usual hazards of oestrogens apply (see below). However, current evidence suggests that, when given with a progestogen, the benefits of HRT far outweigh the small risks, unless there are clear contraindications. The overall benefits may be summarized as follows, though randomized trial data are still awaited (studies are in progress) for some of these conclusions:

- *Symptomatic improvement in most menopausal symptoms* for the majority of women. Oestrogen-deficient symptoms respond well to oestrogen replacement, the vaguer symptoms generally, but not always, less well. Vaginal symptoms respond to local oestrogen preparations.
- *Protection against fractures of wrist, spine and hip, secondary to osteoporosis* (see Ch. 10), at least where HRT is used before the age of 60 years when loss of

bone mass is maximal. This is due to predominant protection of trabecular bone (p. 574).

- *Other effects* include possible reductions in the incidence of Alzheimer's disease and large bowel cancer in women taking HRT.

Apart from individual risks from oestrogen therapy (e.g. migraine, thrombosis) – and even here the effect of HRT may not parallel those of the 'pill' since the oestrogen dose is smaller – the main concerns have been induction of cancer of the uterus or breast. In HRT, oestrogen should be given cyclically with a progestogen (if the uterus is present) to prevent endometrial carcinoma from unopposed oestrogen action. Given with a progestogen, the risk of uterine cancer is not significantly increased, while the data on breast carcinoma are conflicting (current best evidence appears to indicate a slightly increased *incidence* of breast carcinoma, but slightly lower breast cancer *mortality* and a clear reduction in overall mortality on HRT). There is of course the inconvenience of withdrawal bleeds, unless a hysterectomy has been performed. Bleeding can now often be avoided by regimens which include continuous oestrogen and progesterone, but individual patient response is variable. The preferred route of administration has been oral, but oestrogen implants and skin patches are also widely used. The optimal length of treatment with HRT remains to be clearly proven, but most physicians who favour the use of HRT would recommend at least 10 years' treatment from the menopause, and some advocate indefinite therapy.

Selective oestrogen receptor modulators, SERMs (e.g. raloxifene), have been introduced and offer a potentially attractive combination of positive oestrogen effects on bone and cardiovascular system with no effects on oestrogen receptors of uterus and breast; long-term outcome studies, however, are still awaited.

Premature menopause

The most common cause of premature menopause in women (before age 40) is ovarian failure, which may be autoimmune or of unknown aetiology. HRT should be given, as the risk of osteoporosis and premature ischaemic heart disease far outweigh the risks.

The ageing male

In the male there is no sudden 'change of life'. However, there is a progressive loss in sexual function with reduction in morning erections and frequency of intercourse.

The age of onset varies widely, but overall testicular volume diminishes and sex hormone-binding globulin (SHBG) and gonadotrophin levels gradually rise. If premature hypogonadism is present for any reason, replacement testosterone therapy should be given to prevent osteoporosis (see p. 578). More widespread androgen replacement of the ageing male is under evaluation,

primarily in the USA, with promising early results but no long-term follow-up data are available.

Conversely, lowering of androgens forms part of the therapy of prostate hypertrophy and prostate cancer. Finasteride, an inhibitor of 5α-reductase, is used in benign prostatic hypertrophy. It prevents the conversion of testosterone to dihydrotestosterone, which causes prostatic hypertrophy, and is effective, though somewhat delayed in action (see p. 664). GnRH analogues are used to lower testosterone levels and induce disease remission in patients with prostate cancer.

Clinical features of disorders of sex and reproduction

A detailed history and examination of all systems is required (Box 18.6).

Tests of gonadal function

The patient and partner are their own best assay for gonadal endocrine function. A man having regular satisfactory intercourse or a woman with regular ovulatory periods is most unlikely to have significant endocrine disease, assuming the history is accurate (check with the partner!). When symptoms are present, much can be deduced by basal measurements of the gonadotrophins, oestrogens/testosterone and prolactin:

- *Low testosterone or estradiol with high gonadotrophins* indicates primary gonadal disease.
- *Low levels of LH/FSH and of testosterone/estradiol* imply hypothalamic–pituitary disease.
- *Confirmation of normal female reproductive endocrinology* requires the demonstration of ovulation. This is achieved by measurement of luteal phase serum progesterone and/or by serial ovarian ultrasound in the follicular phase.

Box 18.6

Sexual and menstrual disorders

History
Libido
Potency
Frequency of intercourse
Menstruation – relationship of symptoms to cycle
Breasts (? galactorrhoea)
Hirsutism

Physical signs
Evidence of systemic disease
Secondary sexual characteristics
Genital size (testes, ovaries, uterus)
Clitoromegaly
Breast development, gynaecomastia
Galactorrhoea
Extent/distribution of hair

Table 18.11
Tests of gonadal function

Test	Uses/comments
Male	
Basal testosterone	Normal levels exclude hypogonadism
Sperm count	Normal count excludes deficiency Motility and abnormal sperm forms should be noted
Female	
Basal estradiol	Normal levels exclude hypogonadism
Luteal phase progesterone (days 18–24 of cycle)	If >30 nmol/L, suggests ovulation
Ultrasound of ovaries	To confirm ovulation
Both sexes	
Basal LH/FSH	Demonstrates state of feedback system for hormone production (LH) and germ cell production (FSH)
HCG test (testosterone or estradiol measured)	Response shows potential of ovary or testis; failure demonstrates primary gonadal problem
Clomifene test (LH and FSH measured)	Tests hypothalamic negative feedback system; clomifene is oestrogen antagonist
Post-coital test	Demonstrates state of sperm and sperm–mucus interaction
LHRH test (now rarely used)	Shows adequacy (or otherwise) of LH and FSH stores in pituitary

- *Complete demonstration of normal male and female function* requires a pregnancy. In the male, in the first instance there should be a healthy sperm count ($20–200 \times 10^6$/mL), good motility (> 60% grade I) and few abnormal forms (< 20%).
- *Hyperprolactinaemia* can be confirmed or excluded by direct measurement. Levels may increase with stress; ideally, a cannula should be inserted and samples taken through it 30 minutes later.
- *The clomifene test* examines hypothalamic negative feedback. Clomifene is a competitive oestrogen antagonist that binds to, but does not activate, oestrogen receptors, thus inducing a rise in gonadotrophin secretion in the normal subject.

More detailed tests are indicated in Table 18.11.

Disorders in the male

Hypogonadism
Clinical features
Male hypogonadism may be a presenting complaint or an incidental finding, such as during investigation for

Table 18.12
Effects of androgens and consequences of androgen deficiency in the male

Physiological effect	Consequences of deficiency
General	
Maintenance of libido	Loss of libido
Deepening of voice	High-pitched voice (if prepubertal)
Frontotemporal balding	Smooth skin
Facial, axillary and limb hair	Decreased hair
Maintenance of erectile and ejaculatory function	Loss of erections/ejaculation
Pubic hair	
Maintenance of male pattern	Thinning and loss of pubic hair
Testes and scrotum	
Maintenance of testicular size/ consistency (needs gonadotrophins as well)	Small soft testes
Rugosity of scrotum	Poorly developed penis/scrotum
Stimulation of spermatogenesis	Subfertility
Musculoskeletal	
Epiphyseal fusion	Eunuchoidism (if prepubertal)
Maintenance of muscle bulk	Decreased muscle bulk and power
Maintenance of bone mass	Osteoporosis

subfertility. The testes may be small and soft. Except with subfertility, the symptoms are usually of androgen deficiency, primarily poor libido, impotence and loss of secondary sexual hair (Table 18.12) rather than deficiency of semen production. Sperm makes up only a very small proportion of seminal fluid volume.

Causes of male hypogonadism are shown in Table 18.13.

Investigations
Testicular disease may be immediately apparent but basal levels of testosterone, LH and FSH should be measured. These will allow the distinction between primary gonadal (testicular) failure and hypothalamic–pituitary disease to be made. Depending on the causes, semen analysis, chromosomal analysis (e.g. to exclude Klinefelter's syndrome) and bone age estimation are required.

In clear-cut gonadotrophin deficiency, pituitary MRI scan, prolactin levels and other pituitary function tests are needed. However, equivocal lowering of serum testosterone (7–10 nmol/L) without elevation of gonadotrophins is a relatively common biochemical finding, and is a frequent cause of referral in men with poor libido or erectile dysfunction. Such tests are compatible with mild gonadotrophin deficiency, but may also be seen in acute illness of any cause and often simply represent the lower end of the normal range or the normal circadian rhythm of testosterone when bloods

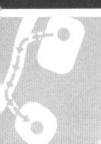

Table 18.13
Causes of male hypogonadism

Reduced gonadotrophins (hypothalamic–pituitary disease)
Hypopituitarism
Selective gonadotrophic deficiency (Kallmann's syndrome)
Severe systemic illness
Severe underweight

Hyperprolactinaemia

Primary gonadal disease (congenital)
Anorchia/Leydig cell agenesis
Chromosome abnormality (e.g. Klinefelter's syndrome)
Enzyme defects
5α-Reductase deficiency

Primary gonadal disease (acquired)
Testicular torsion
Castration
Local testicular disease
Chemotherapy/radiation toxicity
Renal failure
Cirrhosis/alcohol
Sickle cell disease

Androgen receptor deficiency/abnormality

are checked in afternoon or evening surgeries. A therapeutic trial of testosterone replacement is often justified and forms part of the investigation in many patients; full pituitary evaluation may be required in such cases to exclude other pituitary disease. 'Anabolic' steroid (i.e. androgen) abuse causes similar biochemical findings, and an index of suspicion is required if the patient appears well virilized.

Treatment

The cause can rarely be reversed. Replacement therapy should be commenced (Table 18.14). Primary gonadal failure should be treated with androgens. Patients with hypothalamic–pituitary disease are given LH and FSH (purified or synthetic) or pulsatile GnRH if fertility is required; otherwise they should receive androgen replacement.

Special instances of hypogonadism

Cryptorchidism

By the age of 5 years both testes should be in the scrotum. After that age the germinal epithelium is increasingly at risk, and lack of descent by puberty is associated with subfertility. Surgical exploration and orchidopexy are usually undertaken but a short trial of HCG occasionally induces descent: an HCG test with a testosterone response 72 hours later excludes anorchia. Intra-abdominal testes have an increased risk of developing malignancy; if presentation is after puberty, orchidectomy is advised.

Klinefelter's syndrome

Klinefelter's syndrome (seminiferous tubule dysgenesis), a chromosomal disorder (47XXY) affecting 1 in 1000 males, involves both loss of Leydig cells and seminiferous tubular dysgenesis. Patients usually present with poor sexual development, small or undescended testes, gynaecomastia or infertility. They are occasionally mentally retarded. Clinical examination shows small pea-size but firm testes, usually gynaecomastia and often signs of androgen deficiency. Confirmation is by chromosomal analysis. Treatment is androgen replacement therapy unless testosterone levels are normal. No treatment is possible for the abnormal seminiferous tubules and infertility.

Kallmann's syndrome

This is due to isolated GnRH deficiency. It is often associated with decreased or absent sense of smell (anosmia), and sometimes with other bony (cleft-palate), renal and cerebral abnormalities (e.g. colour blindness). It is often familial and is usually X-linked; one sex-linked form is due to an abnormality of a cell adhesion molecule. Management is that of secondary hypogonadism (see p. 1020). Fertility is possible.

Oligospermia or azoospermia

These may be secondary to androgen deficiency and can be corrected by androgen replacement. More often they result from primary testicular diseases, in which case they are rarely treatable.

Table 18.14
Androgen replacement therapy

Preparation	Dose	Remarks
Testosterone mixed esters	250 mg i.m. every 3 weeks	Usual first-line maintenance therapy
Testosterone enanthate		Injection can be painful
Testosterone propionate	50–100 mg i.m. every 1–2 weeks	Frequent injections needed as half-life is short
		Good initial therapy
Testosterone undecanoate	80–240 mg daily, orally in divided doses	Variable dose, irregular absorption
		Expensive
Testosterone transdermal		Convenient but expensive

Mesterolone and methyltestosterone are no longer advised; they are weakly active and can cause cholestasis

Azoospermia with normal testicular size and low FSH levels suggests a vas deferens block, which is sometimes reversible by surgical intervention.

Lack of libido and erectile dysfunction ('impotence')

Impotence is common in hypogonadism, but most patients with impotence have normal hormones and many have no definable organic cause. A careful history of physical disease, related symptoms, stress and psychological factors, together with drug and alcohol abuse, must be taken. The presence of nocturnal emissions and frequent satisfactory morning erections largely excludes endocrine disease as a cause.

True erectile difficulty may be psychological, neurogenic, vascular, endocrine or related to drugs and often includes contributions from several causes. *Vascular disease* may be more common than realized and is often associated with vascular problems elsewhere. The *endocrine* causes are those of hypogonadism (see above) and can be excluded by normal testosterone, gonadotrophin and prolactin levels. *Autonomic neuropathy*, most commonly from diabetes mellitus, is a common partial, if not total, identifiable cause (see p. 1098). Many drugs produce impotence (see Table 21.28).

Psychogenic impotence is frequently a diagnosis of exclusion, though complex tests of penile vasculature and function are available in some centres.

Offending drugs should be stopped. Sildenafil a phosphodiesterase inhibitor which increases penile blood flow (see p. 1098) is first choice for therapy. Other methods of treatment include intracavernosal injections of alprostadil, papaverine or phentolamine, vacuum expanders and penile implants. New agents are under development.

If no organic disease is found, or if there is clear evidence of psychological problems, the couple should receive psychosexual counselling.

Gynaecomastia

Gynaecomastia is development of breast tissue in the male. Causes are shown in Table 18.15.

Pubertal gynaecomastia occurs in perhaps 50% of normal boys, often asymmetrically. It usually resolves spontaneously within 6–18 months, but after this duration may require surgical removal, as fibrous tissue will have been laid down. The cause is thought to be relative oestrogen excess.

In the older male, gynaecomastia requires a full assessment to exclude potentially serious underlying disease, such as bronchial carcinoma and testicular tumours (e.g. Leydig cell tumour). Drug effects are common (especially digoxin and spironolactone), and once these and significant liver disease are excluded most cases have no definable cause. Surgical removal is occasionally necessary.

Table 18.15
Causes of gynaecomastia

Physiological	**Drugs**
Neonatal	Oestrogenic
Pubertal	oestrogens
Old age	digitalis
	cannabis
Hyperthyroidism	diamorphine
	Anti-androgens
Liver disease	spironolactone
Oestrogen-producing	cimetidine
tumours (testis, adrenal)	cyproterone
	Others
HCG-producing tumours	gonadotrophins
(testis, lung)	cytotoxics
Starvation/refeeding	
Carcinoma of breast	

Disorders in the female

Hypogonadism

Impaired ovarian function, whether primary or secondary, will lead both to oestrogen deficiency and abnormalities of the menstrual cycle. The latter is very sensitive to disruption, cycles becoming anovulatory and irregular before disappearing altogether. Symptoms will depend on the age at which the failure develops. Thus, before puberty, primary amenorrhoea will occur, possibly with delayed puberty; if after puberty, secondary amenorrhoea and hypogonadism will result.

Oestrogen deficiency

The physiological effects of oestrogens and symptoms/signs of deficiency are shown in Table 18.16.

Amenorrhoea

Absence of periods or markedly irregular infrequent periods (oligomenorrhoea) are the commonest presentation of female gonadal disease. The clinical assessment of such patients is shown in Box 18.7, and common causes listed in Table 18.17.

Polycystic ovary syndrome

Polycystic ovary syndrome is the most common cause of oligomenorrhoea and amenorrhoea in clinical practice and should always be considered in the context of menstrual dysfunction.

Weight-related amenorrhoea

A minimum bodyweight is necessary for regular menstruation. While anorexia nervosa is the extreme form (see p. 1266), this condition is common and may be seen at weights within the 'normal' range. The biochemistry is indistinguishable from gonadotrophin deficiency and some patients have additional mild endocrine disease (e.g. polycystic ovarian disease). Restoration of

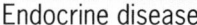

Table 18.16
Effects of oestrogens and consequences of oestrogen deficiency

Physiological effect	Consequence of deficiency
Breast	
Development of connective and duct tissue	Small, atrophic breast
Nipple enlargement and areolar pigmentation	
Pubic hair	
Maintenance of female pattern	Thinning and loss of pubic hair
Vulva and vagina	
Vulval growth	Atrophic vulva
Vaginal glandular and epithelial proliferation	Atrophic vagina
Vaginal lubrication	Dry vagina and dyspareunia
Uterus and tubes	
Myometrial and tubal hypertrophy	Small, atrophic uterus and tubes
Endometrial proliferation	Amenorrhoea
Skeletal	
Epiphyseal fusion	Eunuchoidism (if prepubertal)
Maintenance of bone mass	Osteoporosis

bodyweight to above the 50th centile for height is usually effective in restoring menstruation, but in the many cases where this cannot be achieved then oestrogen replacement must be considered. Similar problems occur with intensive physical training in athletes and dancers.

Hypothalamic amenorrhoea
Amenorrhoea with low oestrogen and gonadotrophins in the absence of organic pituitary disease, weight loss or excessive exercise is described as hypothalamic amenorrhoea. This may be related to 'stress', to previous weight loss or stopping the contraceptive pill, but some patients appear to have defective cycling mechanisms without apparent explanation.

Hypothyroidism
Oligomenorrhoea and amenorrhoea are frequent findings in severe hypothyroidism in young women.

Other
Pregnancy must always be considered as a possible cause. The possibility of genital tract abnormalities, such as an imperforate hymen, should also be remembered, especially in primary amenorrhoea. Severe illness, even in the absence of weight loss, can lead to amenorrhoea, as can stopping the contraceptive pill.

Investigations
Basal levels of FSH, LH, oestrogen and prolactin allow initial distinction between primary gonadal and

---

Box 18.7

Clinical assessment of amenorrhoea

History	Examination
? Pregnant	General health
Date of onset	Body shape and skeletal abnormalities
Age of menarche, if any	
Sudden or gradual onset	Weight and height
General health	Hirsutism and acne
Weight, absolute and changes in recent past	Evidence of virilization
	Maturity of secondary sexual characteristics
Stress (job, lifestyle, exams, relationships)	Galactorrhoea
Excessive exercise	Normality of vagina, cervix and uterus
Drugs	
Hirsutism, acne, virilization	
Headaches/visual symptoms	
Sense of smell	
Past history of pregnancies	
Past history of gynaecological surgery	

hypothalamic–pituitary causes (Table 18.17). Ovarian biopsy may occasionally be necessary to confirm the diagnosis of primary ovarian failure, although elevation of LH and FSH to menopausal levels is usually adequate. Subsequent investigations are shown in Table 18.17.

Treatment
Treatment is that of the cause wherever possible (e.g. hypothyroidism, low weight, stress, excessive exercise).

Primary ovarian disease is rarely treatable except in the rare condition of 'resistant' ovary, where high-dose gonadotrophin therapy can occasionally lead to folliculogenesis. Hyperprolactinaemia should be corrected (see below). Polycystic ovarian syndrome is discussed in detail below. In all other cases oestrogen replacement is usually indicated to prevent the long-term consequences of deficiency.

Hirsutism and polycystic ovary syndrome
Pathophysiology
The extent of normal hair growth varies between individuals, families and races, being more extensive in the Mediterranean and some Asian subcontinent populations. These variations in body hair in the normal population, and the more extensive hair growth seen in patients complaining of hirsutism, represent a continuum from no visible hair to extensive cover with thick dark hair. It is therefore impossible to draw an absolute dividing line between 'normal' and 'abnormal' degrees of facial and body hair in the female. Soft vellous hair is normally present all over the body and this type of hair on the face and elsewhere is 'normal' and is not sex-hormone dependent, nor is normal hair on the forearm or lower leg. Hair in the beard, moustache, breast, chest, axilla, abdominal midline, pubic and thigh areas is sex-hormone dependent. Any excess in the latter regions is thus usually a marker of increased ovarian or adrenal androgen production.

Table 18.17
Amenorrhoea – differential diagnosis and investigation

Diagnosis	Biochemical markers	Secondary tests
Polycystic ovarian syndrome*		
	Normal/slightly high testosterone	Serum androgens
	Normal/high LH	SHBG
	Normal FSH	Ultrasound of ovary
	Normal/high prolactin	Progesterone challenge
	Variable estradiol	
Ovarian failure		
Ovarian dysgenesis*	High FSH	Repeat FSH
Premature ovarian failure*	High LH	Karyotype
Steroid biosynthetic defect*	Low estradiol	Ultrasound of ovary/uterus
(Oophorectomy)	Normal prolactin	Laparoscopy/biopsy of ovary
(Chemotherapy)		HCG stimulation
Resistant ovary syndrome		
Gonadotrophin failure (see also hypothalamic causes below)		
Hypothalamic–pituitary disease*	Low LH	Pituitary MRI if diagnosis unclear
Kallmann's syndrome*	Low FSH	Clomifene test
Anorexia*	Low estradiol	Possibly LHRH test
Weight loss*	Normal/low prolactin	Serum thyroxine
General illness*		
Possible hypothalamic causes		
Hypothalamic amenorrhoea*	Variable LH	Serum thyroxine
Weight gain/loss*	Variable FSH	Serum testosterone, SHBG
Exercise-induced amenorrhoea	Normal prolactin	
Post-pill amenorrhoea	Low/normal estradiol	Pituitary MRI unless diagnosis clear
Hyperprolactinaemia		
Prolactinoma*	High prolactin	Repeat prolactin (if > 2000 mU/L then pituitary tumour likely)
Idiopathic hyperprolactinaemia*	Normal/low LH	
Hypothyroidism*	Normal/low FSH	Serum thyroxine
Polycystic ovarian disease*	Normal/low estradiol	Pituitary MRI
Other endocrine disease		
Hypothyroidism	Variable LH/FSH/estradiol	Serum thyroxine/TSH
Cushing's syndrome	Variable prolactin	Clinically appropriate endocrine and imaging techniques
Androgen excess		
Gonadal or adrenal tumour	Testosterone > 5 nmol/L	Imaging ovary/adrenal
Uterine/vaginal abnormality		
Imperforate hymen*	Normal hormones	Examination under anaesthetic
Absent uterus*		Ultrasound of pelvis
Lack of endometrium		Progesterone challenge
Physiological		
Pregnancy	High estradiol/prolactin	Pregnancy test
Lactation	High prolactin	

*These conditions may present as primary amenorrhoea
SHBG, sex hormone binding globulin

Some authorities divide patients with hirsutism into those with no elevation of serum androgen levels and no other clinical features (usually labelled 'idiopathic hirsutism') and those with an identifiable endocrine imbalance (most commonly polycystic ovary syndrome (PCOS), or rarely other causes). However, studies suggest that most patients with 'idiopathic hirsutism' have some radiological or biochemical evidence of PCOS on more detailed investigation, and indeed several studies have demonstrated evidence of mild PCOS in up to 20%

of the normal female population. Therefore, in routine clinical practice, the majority of patients with objective signs of androgen-dependent hirsutism will have PCOS, and investigation is mainly required to exclude rarer and more serious causes of virilization.

PCOS, originally known in its severe form as the *Stein–Leventhal syndrome*, is characterized by multiple small cysts within the ovary and by excess androgen production from the ovaries and to a lesser extent from the adrenals, although whether the basic defect is in the ovary, adrenal or pituitary remains unknown. The precise levels of androgens in blood vary widely from patient to patient. In addition, oestrogens are converted to androgens in adipose tissue, which represents a further source of androgen excess in obese patients. The response of the hair follicle to circulating androgens also seems to vary between individuals with otherwise identical clinical and biochemical features, and the reason for this variation in end-organ response remains poorly understood.

The ovarian 'cysts' represent arrested follicular development. Studies have shown an association of polycystic ovarian syndrome with anovulation and insulin resistance, which may also be associated with hypertension, hyperlipidaemia and increased cardiovascular disease. The precise mechanisms which link the aetiology of polycystic ovaries, hyperandrogenism, anovulation and insulin resistance remain to be elucidated.

Familial or idiopathic hirsutism does occur, but usually involves a distribution of hair growth which is not typically androgenic. Similarly, non-androgen-dependent hair growth occurs with drugs such as phenytoin, diazoxide, minoxidil and ciclosporin. Iatrogenic hirsutism also occurs after treatment with androgens, or more weakly androgenic drugs such as progestagens or danazol.

Rarer, and more serious, endocrine causes of hirsutism and virilization include congenital adrenal hyperplasia (CAH, see p. 1054), Cushing's syndrome (p. 1052) and virilizing tumours of the ovary and adrenal. All these conditions should be considered in any patient with hirsutism – as this may be their only presenting complaint.

Clinical features

The complaint of hirsutism is common and often accompanied by severe anxiety and social stress.

The extent and severity of hirsutism

This should be recorded objectively, ideally using a scoring system, to document the problem and to monitor treatment. The method and frequency of physical removal (e.g. shaving, plucking) should also be recorded. Most patients who complain of hirsutism will have an objective excess of hair on examination, but occasionally very little will be found (and appropriate counselling is then indicated).

Age and speed of onset

Hirsutism related to PCOS usually begins around the time of the menarche and increases slowly and steadily in the teens and twenties. Rapid progression and prepubertal or late onset suggest a more serious cause.

Accompanying virilization

Hirsutism due to PCOS may be severe and affect all androgen-dependent areas on the face and body. However, more severe virilization (clitoromegaly, frontal balding, male phenotype) implies substantial androgen excess, and usually indicates a rarer cause rather than PCOS.

Menstruation

Most patients with hirsutism will have some disturbance of menstruation. The greater the disruption the more likely it is that there is a serious cause.

Weight

Many patients with hirsutism are also overweight or obese. This worsens the underlying androgen excess and insulin resistance and inhibits the response to treatment, and is an indication for appropriate advice on diet and exercise. In severe cases the insulin resistance may have a visible manifestation as acanthosis nigricans on the neck and in the axillae (see Fig. 22.23).

Presentation

Typically, PCOS presents with amenorrhoea/oligomenorrhoea, hirsutism and acne, usually beginning shortly after menarche. It is sometimes associated with marked obesity, but weight may be normal. Mild virilization may occur in severe cases. Clinical, biochemical and radiological features of PCOS merge imperceptibly into those of the normal populations, and the incidence of the syndrome will therefore depend on the diagnostic criteria used by the clinician, and indeed by the patient when deciding whether or not to seek medical advice. In practice, patients may present with any of the clinical features (menstrual disturbance, hirsutism or acne) alone or in various combinations.

Investigations

A variety of investigations may aid the diagnosis of patients with hirsutism:

- **Serum testosterone** may be elevated in PCOS and is invariably substantially raised in virilizing tumours (usually > 5 nmol/L). Patients with hirsutism and normal testosterone level frequently have low levels of sex hormone-binding globulin (SHBG), leading to high free androgen levels.
- **Other androgens.** Androstenedione and dehydroepiandrosterone sulphate are frequently elevated in PCOS, and even more elevated in congenital adrenal hyperplasia and virilizing tumours.
- **17-α-Hydroxyprogesterone** is elevated in classical CAH (congenital adrenal hyperplasia), but may be apparent in late-onset CAH only after stimulation tests.
- **Gonadotrophin levels.** LH hypersecretion is a consistent feature of PCOS, but the pulsatile nature of secretion of this hormone means that a 'classic' increased LH/FSH ratio is not always observed on a random sample.

- **Oestrogen levels.** Estradiol is usually normal in PCOS, but estrone levels (which are rarely measured) are elevated because of peripheral conversion. Levels are variable in other causes.
- **Ovarian ultrasound.** The most useful investigation in PCOS is ovarian ultrasound (Fig. 18.13), although a skilled observer is necessary. The typical ultrasonic features are those of a thickened capsule, multiple 3–5 mm cysts and a hyperechogenic stroma. It should also be noted that prolonged hyperandrogenization from any cause may lead to polycystic changes in the ovary. Ultrasound may also reveal virilizing ovarian tumours, although these are often small.
- **Serum prolactin.** Mild hyperprolactinaemia is common in PCOS but rarely exceeds 1500 mU/L.

If a virilizing tumour is suspected clinically or after investigation, then more complex tests may include dexamethasone suppression tests, CT or MRI of adrenals, and selective venous sampling.

Differential diagnosis

Most patients presenting with a combination of hirsutism and menstrual disturbance will be shown to have polycystic ovary syndrome, but the rarer alternative diagnoses should be excluded, e.g. late-onset congenital adrenal hyperplasia (early-onset, raised serum 17-α-OH-progesterone), Cushing's syndrome (look for other clinical features) and virilizing tumours of the ovary or adrenals (severe virilization, markedly elevated serum testosterone).

Treatments

The underlying cause should be removed in the rare instances where this is possible (e.g. drugs, adrenal or ovarian tumours). Treatment of CAH and Cushing's are discussed on page 1055 and page 1053, respectively. Other therapy depends upon whether the aim is to reduce hirsutism, regularize periods or produce fertility.

Local therapy for hirsutism

Plucking, bleaching, depilatory cream or wax and shaving may all help and are often underused. Electrolysis is effective but expensive and often requires long-term treatment. Laser hair removal shows promise, but has not been evaluated in long-term studies and is very expensive.

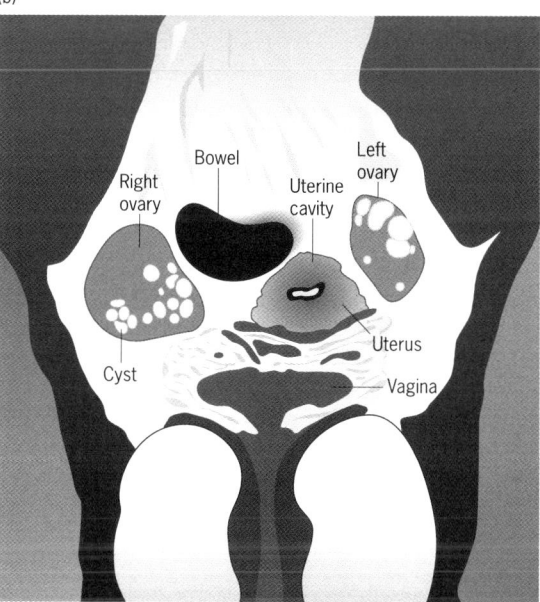
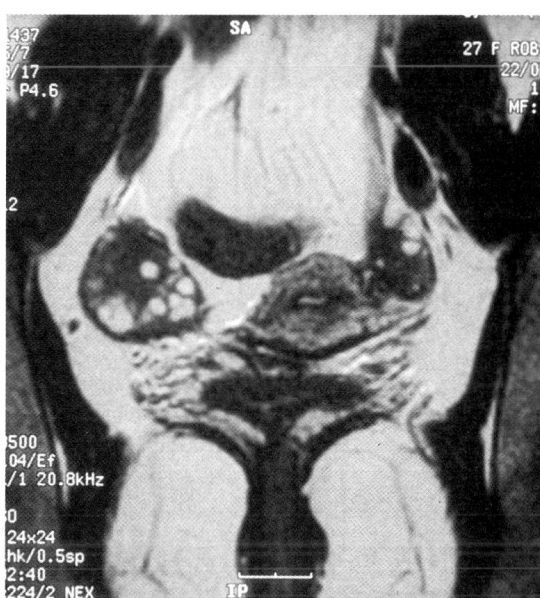

Fig. 18.13 **Polycystic ovarian syndrome. (a) Longitudinal transvaginal ultrasound of ovary**, revealing multiple cysts with central ovarian stroma showing increased echo texture. **(b) MR image (coronal) of polycystic ovaries**, also showing pelvic anatomy. Reproduced by kind permission of Barbara Hochstein and Geoffrey Cox, Auckland Radiology Group.

Systemic therapy for hirsutism

This always requires a year or more of treatment for maximal benefit, and long-term treatment is frequently required as the problem tends to recur when treatment is stopped. The patient must therefore always be an active participant in the decision to use systemic therapy and must understand the rare risks as well as the benefits.

- *Oestrogens* (e.g. oral contraceptives) suppress ovarian androgen production and reduce free androgens by increasing SHBG levels. Combined pills, which contain a non-androgenic progestogen (e.g. co-cyprindiol), have an advantage over older combined pills, will result in a slow improvement in hirsutism in a majority of cases and should normally be used first unless there is a contraindication. Long-term follow-up studies of the use of the 'pill' for contraception gives firm reassurance about the safety of the long-term treatment which is very often required. After the menopause, HRT preparations which contain medroxyprogesterone (rather than more androgenic progestagens) may be helpful.
- *Cyproterone acetate* (50–100 mg daily) is an antiandrogen but is also a progestogen, teratogenic and a weak glucocorticoid. Given continuously it produces amenorrhoea, and so is normally given for days 1–14 of each cycle. In women of childbearing age, contraception is essential.
- *Spironolactone* (200 mg daily) also has antiandrogen activity and can cause useful improvements in hirsutism in selected cases.
- *Finasteride* (5 mg daily), a 5α-reductase inhibitor which prevents the formation of dihydrotestosterone in the skin, has also been shown to be effective but long-term experience is still awaited.

It should be noted that none of these drugs is actually licensed in the UK for the treatment of hirsutism; while spironolactone and cyproterone are widely used, both are subject to Committee of Safety of Medicine (CSM) warnings. Flutamide, another antiandrogen, is not used owing to the high incidence of hepatic side-effects.

Treatment of menstrual disturbance

Cyclical oestrogen/progestogen will regulate the menstrual cycle and remove the symptom of oligo- or amenorrhoea. This is most frequently an additional benefit of the treatment of hirsutism, but may also be used when menstrual disturbance is the only symptom.

Recent interest has focused on the use of drugs to improve the hyperinsulinaemia associated with PCOS. Early studies of metformin (500 mg three times daily) are optimistic, reporting improvements in menstrual cyclicity and incidence of ovulation, but long-term evaluation is still awaited. Glitazones are also being tried.

Treatment for fertility

- Clomifene 50–200 mg can be given daily on days 2–6 of the cycle (or tamoxifen 10–40 mg daily), sometimes combined with 5000 U of HCG intramuscularly on day 12/13. This can occasionally cause ovarian hyperstimulation and specialist supervision is essential. The CSM has recommended that clomifene should not normally be used for longer than six cycles (owing to a possible increased risk of ovarian cancer in patients treated for longer than recommended).
- *Reverse circadian rhythm.* Prednisolone (2.5 mg in the morning, 5 mg on retiring) suppresses pituitary production of ACTH upon which adrenal androgens partly depend. Regular ovulatory cycles often ensue. Steroid instruction leaflet and a card must be supplied.

More intensive techniques to stimulate ovulation may also be indicated in specialist hands, including low-dose *gonadotrophin therapy*, and ovarian hyperstimulation techniques associated with in vitro fertilization.

Wedge resection of the ovary was a traditional therapy which is now rarely required, although laparoscopic ovarian electrodiathermy has gained some popularity in recent years.

Oral contraception

The combined oestrogen–progestogen pill is widely used for contraception and has a low failure rate (< 1 per 100 woman-years). 'Pills' contain 20–50 μg of oestrogen, usually ethinylestradiol, together with a variable amount of one of several progestogens. The mechanism of action is twofold:

- suppression by oestrogen of gonadotrophins, thus preventing follicular development, ovulation and luteinization
- progestogen effects on cervical mucus, making it hostile to sperm, and on tubal motility and the endometrium.

Side-effects of these preparations are shown in Box 18.8. Most of the serious ones are rare and are less common on typical modern 20–30 μg oestrogen pills, although evidence suggests that thromboembolism may be slightly more common on 'third-generation pills' containing desogestrel and gestodene (approx. 30/100 000 woman-years compared with 15/100 000 on older pills and 5/100 000 on no treatment). While some problems require immediate cessation of the pill, the importance of other milder side-effects must be judged against the hazards of pregnancy occurring with inadequate contraception, especially if other effective methods are not practicable or acceptable.

It is clear, however, that the hazards of the combined pill are greater in women aged over 35 years, especially

Adverse effects and drug interactions of oral contraceptives (mixed oestrogen-progesterone combinations)

General
Weight gain
Loss of libido
Pigmentation (chloasma)
Breast tenderness
Increased growth rate of some malignancies

Cardiovascular
Increased blood pressure*
Deep vein thrombosis*
Myocardial infarction
Stroke

Gastrointestinal
Nausea and vomiting
Abnormal liver biochemistry*
Gallstones increased
Hepatic tumours

Nervous system
Headache
Migraine*
Depression*

Malignancy
Possible increase in cancer of the breast
    (but reduced risk of ovarian and endometrial cancer)

Gynaecological
Amenorrhoea
'Spotting'
Cervical erosion

Haematological
Increased clotting tendency

Endocrine/metabolic
Mild impairment of glucose tolerance
Worsened lipid profile, though variable

Drug interactions (reduced contraceptive effect owing to
    enzyme induction)
Antibiotics
Barbiturates
Phenytoin
Carbamazepine
Rifampicin
St. John's Wort

*Common reasons for stopping oral contraceptives

in smokers and those with other risk factors for cardio-vascular disease (e.g. hypertension, hyperlipidaemia, smoking). The 'mini-pill' (progestogen only, usually norethisterone) is less effective but is often suitable where oestrogens are contraindicated (Box 18.8). A progesterone antagonist, mifepristone, in combination with a prostaglandin analogue, induces abortion of pregnancy at up to 9 weeks' gestation. It prevents progesterone-induced inhibition of uterine contraction.

Hyperprolactinaemia

Hyperprolactinaemia has many causes. Common pathological causes include prolactinoma, co-secretion of prolactin in acromegaly, stalk compression due to pituitary adenomas and other pituitary masses, polycystic ovary syndrome, hypothyroidism and 'idiopathic' hyperprolactinaemia; rarer causes are oestrogen therapy (e.g. the 'pill'), renal failure, liver failure, postictal and chest wall injury. Dopamine antagonist drugs are a common iatrogenic cause (metoclopramide, domperidone and most other antiemetics except cyclizine, phenothiazines). Physiological hyperprolactinaemia occurs in pregnancy, lactation and severe stress, as well as during sleep and coitus. The range of serum prolactin seen in common causes of hyperprolactinaemia is illustrated in Figure 18.14. Mildly increased prolactin levels (400–600 mU/L) may be physiological and asymptomatic but higher levels require a diagnosis. Levels above 5000 mU/L always imply a prolactin-secreting pituitary tumour.

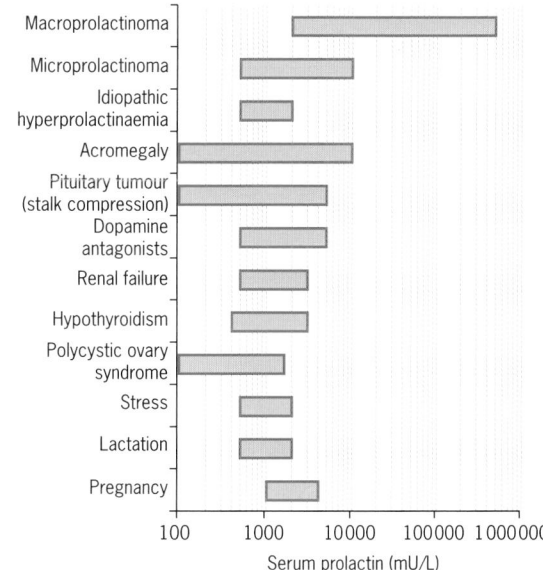

Fig. 18.14 Range of serum prolactin seen in common causes of hyperprolactinaemia.

Clinical features

Hyperprolactinaemia stimulates milk production in the breast and inhibits GnRH and gonadotrophin secretion per se. It usually presents with:

- galactorrhoea, spontaneous or expressible (60% of cases)
- oligomenorrhoea or amenorrhoea
- decreased libido in both sexes
- decreased potency in men
- subfertility
- symptoms or signs of oestrogen or androgen deficiency – in the long term osteoporosis may result, especially in women
- delayed or arrested puberty in the peripubertal patient.

Additionally, headaches and/or visual field defects may be present if there is a pituitary tumour (more common in men). Not all patients with galactorrhoea have hyperprolactinaemia, but the other causes are poorly understood – 'normoprolactinaemic galactorrhoea' and duct ectasia.

Investigations

Hyperprolactinaemia should be confirmed by repeat measurement. Further tests are appropriate after physiological and drug causes have been excluded:

- **Visual fields** should be checked.
- **Hypothyroidism** must be excluded since this is a cause of hyperprolactinaemia.
- **Anterior pituitary function** should be assessed if there is any clinical evidence of hypopituitarism or radiological evidence of a pituitary tumour (Table 18.9; Box 18.1 and Box 18.4).
- **MRI of the pituitary** is necessary if there are any clinical features suggestive of a pituitary tumour, and desirable in all cases when prolactin is significantly elevated (above 1000 mU/L).

In the presence of a pituitary mass on MRI, the level of prolactin helps determine whether the mass is a prolactinoma or a non-functioning pituitary tumour causing stalk-disconnection hyperprolactinaemia: levels of above 5000 mU/L in the presence of a macroadenoma, or above 2000 mU/L in the presence of a microadenoma (or of no radiological abnormality), strongly suggest a prolactinoma (see p. 1009). Macroprolactinoma refers to tumours above 10 mm diameter, microprolactinoma to smaller ones.

Treatment

Hyperprolactinaemia should usually be treated to avoid the long-term effects of oestrogen deficiency (even if the patient would otherwise welcome the lack of periods!) or testosterone deficiency in the male. Exceptions include minor elevations (400–1000 mU/L) with preservation of normal regular menstruation (or normal male testosterone levels) and postmenopausal patients with microprolactinomas who have chosen not to take oestrogen replacement. Hyperprolactinaemia is controlled with a dopamine agonist. Bromocriptine is the longest-established therapy: initial doses should be small (e.g. 1 mg) and taken with food, or at bedtime. The dose should be gradually increased, usually to 2.5 mg two or three times daily, judged on clinical response and prolactin levels. Side-effects, which prevent effective therapy in a minority of cases, include nausea and vomiting, dizziness and syncope, constipation and cold peripheries. Alternative drugs more specific for the D_2 dopamine receptor, which are longer acting and better tolerated, include cabergoline (500 µg once or twice a week) and quinagolide (75–150 µg once daily).

Definitive therapy will depend upon the size of the tumour, the patient's wishes, including desire for fertility, and local expertise and facilities. In most cases a dopamine agonist will be the first, and usually only, therapy. Prolactinomas usually shrink in size on a dopamine agonist; in macroadenomas any pituitary mass effects commonly resolve and in most cases it is simply sufficient to continue successful dopamine agonist therapy in the long term. Prolactin should therefore always be measured before surgery on a pituitary mass. Microprolactinomas may not recur after several years of dopamine agonist therapy in a substantial minority of cases, but in the majority hyperprolactinaemia will recur if treatment is stopped.

Trans-sphenoidal surgery in the most skilled hands may restore normoprolactinaemia in patients with microadenoma, but is rarely completely successful with macroadenomas and risks damage to normal pituitary function. Therefore most patients and physicians elect to continue medical therapy rather than proceed to surgery. Some surgeons believe that long-term bromocriptine increases the hardness of the adenoma and makes resection more difficult – but others dissent from this view.

Radiotherapy usually controls adenoma growth and is slowly effective in lowering prolactin but causes progressive hypopituitarism. It may be advocated after medical tumour shrinkage or after surgery in larger tumours, especially where families are complete, but many workers simply advocate continuation of dopamine agonist therapy in responsive cases.

Rarely, tumours enlarge during pregnancy to produce headaches and visual defects. Dopamine agonists, which are traditionally stopped during pregnancy, should be restarted.

Subfertility

This term, kinder than 'infertility', is defined as the inability of a couple to conceive after 1 year of unprotected intercourse. Investigation requires the combined skills of gynaecologist, endocrinologist and, ideally, andrologist. Both partners must be considered and every aspect of the physiology critically examined.

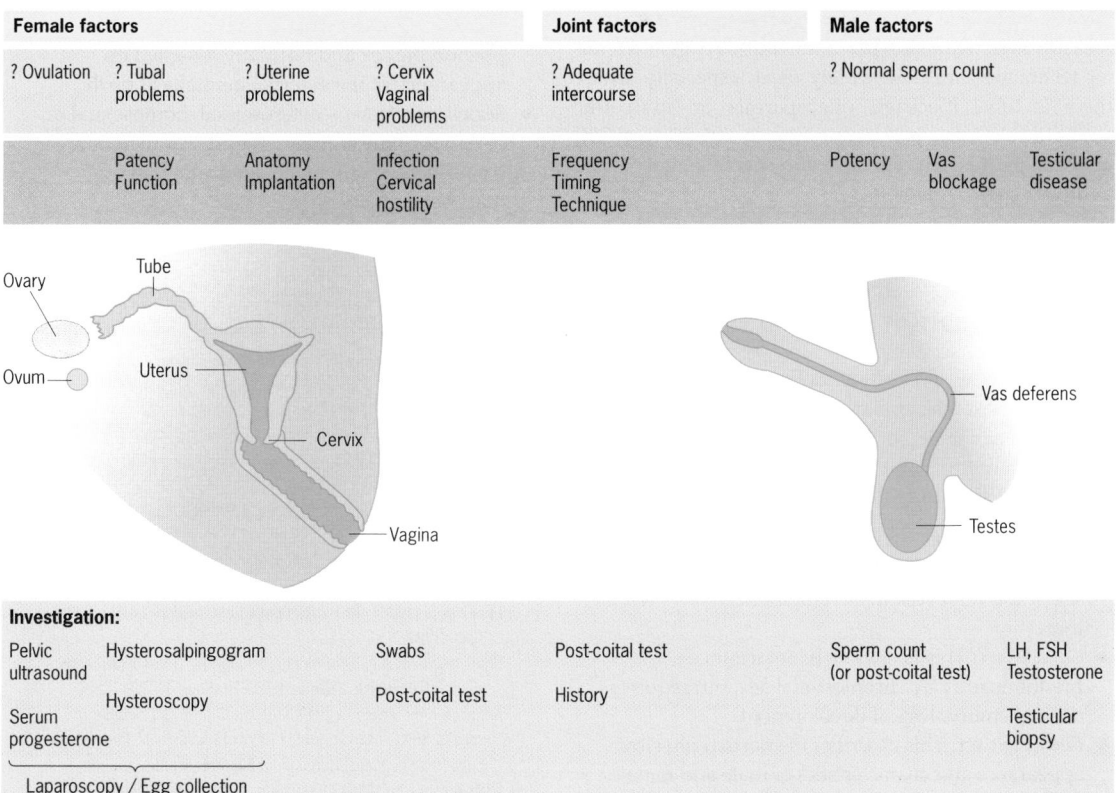

Female factors				Joint factors	Male factors		
? Ovulation	? Tubal problems	? Uterine problems	? Cervix Vaginal problems	? Adequate intercourse	? Normal sperm count		
	Patency Function	Anatomy Implantation	Infection Cervical hostility	Frequency Timing Technique	Potency	Vas blockage	Testicular disease

Investigation:

Pelvic ultrasound	Hysterosalpingogram		Swabs	Post-coital test	Sperm count (or post-coital test)	LH, FSH Testosterone
Serum progesterone	Hysteroscopy		Post-coital test	History		Testicular biopsy

Laparoscopy / Egg collection

Fig. 18.15 **Major factors involved in subfertility and their investigation.** LH, luteinizing hormone; FSH, follicle-stimulating hormone.

Causes (Fig. 18.15)

A significant proportion of couples have both male and female contributing factors.

Inadequate intercourse, hostile cervical mucus and vaginal factors are uncommon (5%). Fifteen per cent of cases appear to be idiopathic, and natural fertility decreases with increasing age.

Male factors

About 30–40% of couples have a major identifiable male factor. There is some evidence that male sperm counts are declining in many populations. Untreated male hypogonadism of any cause (see Table 18.13) is likely to be associated with subfertility.

Female factors

Female tubal problems account for perhaps 20%; a similar proportion have ovulatory disorders. Any cause of oligomenorrhoea or amenorrhoea (see Table 18.17) is likely to be associated with suboptimal ovulation or anovulation.

Clinical assessment

Both partners should be seen and the following factors checked:

- *The man.* Look for previous testicular damage (orchitis, trauma), undescended testes, urethral symptoms and venereal problems, local surgery, and use of alcohol and drugs. A semen analysis early in the investigations is essential.
- *The woman.* Look for previous pelvic infection, regularity of periods, previous surgery, alcohol intake and smoking, and adequacy of bodyweight (see p. 1021).
- *Together.* Check the frequency and adequacy of intercourse, and the use of lubricants.

Examination should include an assessment of secondary sexual characteristics, body habitus and general health. In men, the size and consistency of the testes are important, plus exclusion of a varicocele. In women, a vaginal examination allows a check on the uterus and ovaries.

Investigations

Appropriate tests for particular defects are shown in Figure 18.15.

Treatment

Counselling of both partners is essential. Any defect(s) found should be treated if possible. Ovulation can

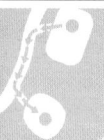

usually be induced by exogenous hormones if simpler measures fail, while in vitro fertilization (IVF) and similar techniques are now widely used, especially where there is tubal blockage, oligospermia or 'idiopathic subfertility'. Intracytoplasmic sperm injection (ICSI) appears particularly effective for severe oligospermia and poor sperm function.

Disorders of sexual differentiation

Disorders of sexual differentiation are rare but may affect chromosomal, gonadal, endocrine and phenotypic development (Table 18.18). Such cases always require extensive, multidisciplinary clinical management. An individual's sex can be defined in several ways:

- *Chromosomal sex.* The normal female is 46XX, the normal male 46XY. The Y chromosome confers male sex; if it is not present, development follows female lines.
- *Gonadal sex.* This is obviously determined predominantly by chromosomal sex, but requires normal embryological development.
- *Phenotypic sex.* This describes the normal physical appearance and characteristics of male and female body shape. This in turn is a manifestation of gonadal sex and subsequent sex hormone production.

- *Social sex (gender).* This is heavily dependent on phenotypic sex and normally assigned on appearance of the external genitalia at birth.
- *Sexual orientation* – heterosexual, homosexual or bisexual. Some studies suggest that there may be some element of genetic determination of homosexuality.

FURTHER READING

Bagatell CJ, Bremner WJ (1996) Drug therapy: androgens in men – uses and abuses. *New England Journal of Medicine* **334**: 707–714.

Baird DT (1997) Amenorrhoea. *Lancet* **350**: 275–279.

Balen A (1999) Pathogenesis of polycystic ovary syndrome – the enigma unravels? *Lancet* **354**: 966–967.

Greendale GA, Lee NP, Arriola ER (1999) The menopause. *Lancet* **353**: 571–580

Gruber CJ et al. (2002) Production and actions of estrogens. *New England Journal of Medicine* **346**: 340–352.

Hughes IA (2001) Sex differentiation. *Endocrinology* **142**: 3281–3287.

Kyel-Mensah AA, Jacobs HS (1995) The investigation of female infertility. *Clinical Endocrinology* **43**: 251–256.

Molitch ME, Thorner MO, Wilson C (1997) Therapeutic controversy: management of prolactinomas. *Journal of Endocrinology and Metabolism* **82**: 996–1000.

Rittmaster RS (1997) Hirsutism. *Lancet* **349**: 191–195.

Table 18.18
Disorders of sexual differentiation

Condition	Chromosomes	Gonads	Phenotype	Remarks
Turner's syndrome	45X	Streak	Female	Often morphological features (e.g. short stature, web neck, coarctation of aorta)
Gonadal dysgenesis	46XY	Streak or minimal testes*	Immature female	
Congenital adrenal hyperplasia	46XX	Ovary	Female with variable virilization	Obvious androgen excess
Virilizing tumour	46XX	Ovary	Female with variable virilization	Obvious androgen excess
True hermaphroditism	46XX/XY or mosaic	Testis and ovary	Male or ambiguous	
Klinefelter's syndrome	47XXY	Small testes	Male, often with gynaecomastia	Many are hypogonadal
Testicular feminization	46XY	Testes*	Ambiguous or infantile female	Androgen receptor defective
Testicular synthetic defects	46XY	Testes*	Cryptorchid, ambiguous	
5α-Reductase deficiency	46XY	Testes	Cryptorchid, ambiguous	Impaired conversion of testosterone to dihydrotestosterone
Anorchia	46XY	Absent	Immature female	

*Gonadectomy advised because of high risk of malignancy

The growth axis

Physiology and control of growth hormone (GH) (Fig. 18.16)

GH is the pituitary factor responsible for stimulation of body growth in humans. Its secretion is stimulated by GHRH, released into the portal system from the hypothalamus; it is also under inhibitory control by GHRIH (somatostatin). GH stimulates the hepatic production of an intermediate insulin-like growth factor-1 (IGF-1, previously known as somatomedin C) that actually stimulates growth. Plasma levels of IGF-1, however, reflect local growth activity poorly, partly as there are multiple IGF-binding proteins (IGF-BP) – IGF-BP3 being most important. The metabolic actions of the system are:

- increasing collagen and protein synthesis
- promoting retention of calcium, phosphorus and nitrogen, necessary substrates for anabolism
- opposing the action of insulin.

GH release is intermittent and mainly nocturnal, especially during REM sleep. The frequency and size of GH pulses increase during the growth spurt of adolescence and decline thereafter. Acute stress and exercise both stimulate GH release while, in the normal subject, hyperglycaemia suppresses it.

IGF-1 may, in addition, play a major role in maintaining neoplastic growth. A relationship has been shown between circulating IGF-1 concentrations and breast cancer in premenopausal women and prostate cancer in men.

Normal growth

There are factors other than GH involved in linear growth in the human.

- *Genetic factors.* Children of two short parents will probably be short and vice versa
- *Nutritional factors.* Adequate nutrients must be available. Impaired growth can result from inadequate dietary intake or small-bowel disease (e.g. coeliac disease).
- *General health.* Any serious systemic disease in childhood is likely to reduce growth (e.g. renal failure).
- *Intrauterine growth retardation.* These infants often grow poorly in the long term, while infants with simple prematurity usually catch up. There is evidence that low birthweight may predispose to hypertension, diabetes and other health problems in later adult life.
- *Emotional deprivation and psychological factors.* These can impair growth by complex, poorly understood mechanisms, probably involving temporarily decreased GH secretion.

The relevant aspects of history and examination in the assessment of problems are shown in Box 18.9.

Assessment of growth

Charts showing ranges of height and weight for normal British children are available (Fig. 18.17), and other national data are available. Height must be measured very carefully, ideally at the same time of day on the same instrument by the same observer.

In general, there are three overlapping phases of growth: infantile (0–2 years), which appears largely substrate (food) dependent; childhood (age 2 years to

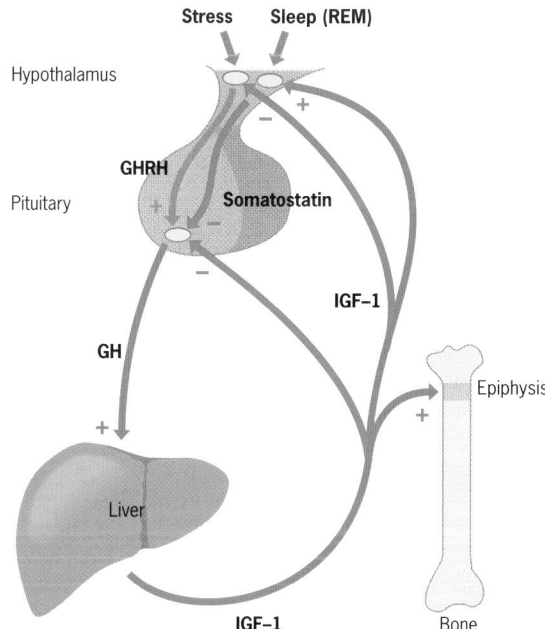

Fig. 18.16 The control of growth hormone (GH) and insulin-like growth factor-1 (IGF-1) secretion and action.

Box 18.9

Assessment of problems of growth and development

History
Pregnancy records
Rate of growth (home/school records, e.g. heights on kitchen door)
Comparison with peers at school and siblings
Change in appearance (old photographs)
Change in shoe/glove/hat size or frequency of 'growing out'
Age of appearance of pubic hair, breasts, menarche

Physical signs
Evidence of systemic disease
Body habitus, size, relative weight, proportions (span versus height)
Skin thickness, interdental separation
Facial features
Spade hands/feet
Grading of secondary sexual characteristics

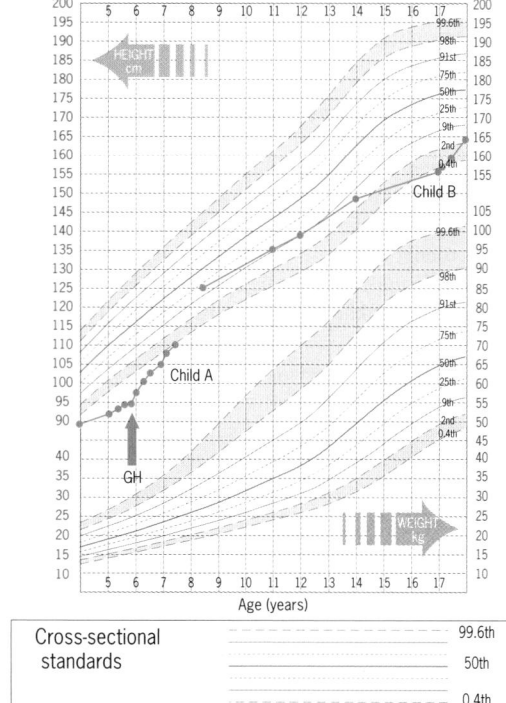

Age (years)

Cross-sectional standards	99.6th
	50th
	0.4th

Fig. 18.17 **A height chart for boys. Child A illustrates the course of a child with hypopituitarism**, initially treated with cortisol and thyroxine, but showing growth only after growth hormone treatment. **Child B shows the course of a child with constitutional growth delay without treatment.** Chart © the Child Growth Foundation.

puberty), which is largely GH dependent; and the adolescent 'growth spurt', dependent on GH and sex hormones.

Height velocity is more helpful than current height. It requires at least two measurements some months apart and, ideally, multiple serial measurements. Height velocity is the rate of current growth (cm per year), while already attained height is largely dependent upon previous growth.

Standard deviation scores (SDS) based on the degree of deviation from age–sex norms are widely used by experts – these and growth velocities are far more sensitive than simple charts in assessing growth. Computer programs also allow calculation of many of these indices.

The approximate future height of a child ('mid-parental height') can be simply predicted from the parental heights. For a boy, this is:

$$[(Maternal\ height + 14\ cm\ (5.5\ inches) + Paternal\ height)/2]$$

and for a girl:

$$[(Paternal\ height - 14\ cm\ (5.5\ inches) + Maternal\ height)/2].$$

Thus, with a father of 180 cm and mother of 154 cm, the predicted heights are 174 cm for a son and 160 cm for a daughter.

Growth failure: short stature

When children or their parents complain of short stature, particular attention should focus on:

- intrauterine growth retardation, weight and gestation at birth
- possible systemic disorders – any system, but especially small-bowel disease
- evidence of skeletal, chromosomal or other congenital abnormalities
- endocrine status – particularly thyroid
- dietary intake and use of drugs, especially steroids for asthma
- emotional, psychological, family and school problems.

School, general practitioner, clinic and home records of height and weight should be obtained if possible to allow growth-velocity calculation. If unavailable, such data must be obtained prospectively.

A child with normal growth velocity is unlikely to have significant endocrine disease. However, low growth velocity without apparent systemic cause requires further investigation. Sudden cessation of growth suggests major physical disease; if no gastrointestinal, respiratory, renal or skeletal abnormality is apparent, then a cerebral tumour or hypothyroidism is likeliest.

Consistently slow-growing children require full endocrine assessment. Features of the more common causes of growth failure are given in Table 18.19.

Around the time of puberty, where constitutional delay is clearly shown and symptoms require intervention, then very-low-dose sex steroids in 3–6-month courses will usually induce acceleration of growth.

Investigations
Systemic disease having been excluded, the following should be undertaken:

- **Thyroid function tests** – serum TSH and T_4 to exclude hypothyroidism.
- **GH status.** Basal levels are of little value, though urinary GH measurements may prove to be of some value in screening. Dynamic tests include the GH response to insulin (the 'gold standard'; Box 18.4), arginine, exercise, clonidine and Bovril. Tests should only be performed in centres experienced in their use and interpretation. Normal responses depend on test and GH assay used.
- **Assessment of bone age.** Non-dominant hand and wrist X-rays allow assessment of bone age by comparison with standard charts.

Table 18.19
Clinical features of common causes of short stature

Cause	Family history	Growth pattern, clinical features and puberty	Bone age	Remarks
Constitutional delay	Often present	Slow from birth, immature but appropriate with late but spontaneous puberty	Moderate delay	Often difficult to differentiate from GH deficiency Growth velocity measurement vital
Familial short stature	Positive	Slow from birth, clinically normal with normal puberty	Normal	Need heights of family members Growth velocity normal
GH insufficiency	Rare	Slow growth, immature, often overweight, delayed puberty	Moderate delay, increasing with time	Early investigation and treatment vital Increased suspicion if child is plump
Primary hypothyroidism	Rare	Slow growth, immature and delayed puberty	Marked delay	Measure TSH, T_4 in all cases of short stature Clear clinical signs not obvious
Small bowel disease	Sometimes	Slow, immature, usually thin for height, delayed puberty	Delayed	Diarrhoea and/or macrocytosis/anaemia Occasionally no GI symptoms

Treatment

Systemic illness should be treated and primary hypothyroidism replaced with thyroxine.

For GH insufficiency, recombinant GH is given as nightly injections in doses of 0.17–0.35 mg/kg per week. Treatment is expensive and should be supervised in expert centres. Human GH (collected from pituitaries) was previously used but was withdrawn as cases of Creutzfeldt–Jakob disease were reported.

GH treatment in so-called 'short normal' children has not been shown to produce any worthwhile increase in final height. In Turner's syndrome (see p. 1030) large doses of GH are effective in increasing final height especially in combination with appropriate very-low-dose oestrogen replacement. Familial cases of resistance to GH owing to an abnormal GH receptor (Laron-type dwarfism) are well described. They are very rare but may respond to therapy with synthetic IGF-1.

Tall stature

The most common causes are hereditary (two tall parents!), idiopathic (constitutional) or early development. It can occasionally be due to hyperthyroidism. Other causes include chromosomal abnormalities (e.g. Klinefelter's syndrome, Marfan's syndrome) or metabolic abnormalities. GH excess is a very rare cause and is usually clinically apparent.

Growth hormone excess: gigantism and acromegaly

GH stimulates skeletal and soft-tissue growth. GH excess therefore produces gigantism in children (if acquired before epiphyseal fusion) and acromegaly in adults.

Acromegaly

This is due to a pituitary tumour in almost all cases. Hyperplasia due to GHRH excess is very rare. Overall incidence is approximately 3–4/million per year and prevalence 50–80/million.

Clinical features

Symptoms and signs of acromegaly are shown in Figure 18.18. One-third of patients present with changes in appearance, one-quarter with visual field defects or headaches; in the remainder the diagnosis is made by an alert observer in another clinic, e.g. GP, diabetic, hypertension, dental, dermatology.

Investigations

- **GH levels** may exclude acromegaly if undetectable but a detectable value is non-diagnostic. Normal adult levels are < 1 mU/L for most of the day except during stress or a 'GH pulse'.
- **The glucose tolerance test** is diagnostic. Acromegalics fail to suppress GH below 1 mU/L and some show a paradoxical rise; about 25% of acromegalics have a diabetic glucose tolerance test.
- **IGF-1 levels** are almost always raised in acromegaly – a single plasma level of IGF-1 reflects mean 24-hour GH levels and is useful in diagnosis.
- **Visual field defects** are common.
- **MRI scan of pituitary** – will almost always reveal the pituitary adenoma.
- **Pituitary function** – partial or complete anterior hypopituitarism is common.
- **Prolactin** – mild to moderate hyperprolactinaemia occurs in 30% of patients (Fig. 18.14). In some, the adenoma secretes both GH and prolactin.

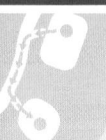

Symptoms		Signs

<table>
<tr><td>

Symptoms

Change in appearance
Increased size of hands/feet
Headaches
Excessive sweating
Visual deterioration
Tiredness
Weight gain
Amenorrhoea
  oligomenorrhoea
  in women
Galactorrhoea
Impotence or poor libido
Deep voice
Goitre
Breathlessness
Pain/tingling in hands
Polyuria/polydipsia
Muscular weakness
Joint pains

Old photographs are
  frequently useful
Symptoms of
  hypopituitarism may also
  be present

</td><td>

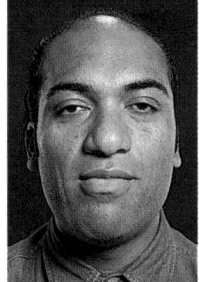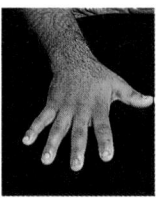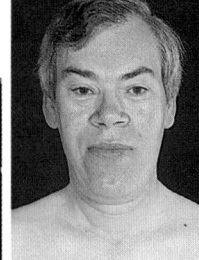

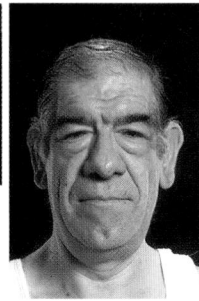

</td><td>

Signs

Prominent supraorbital ridge
Prognathism
Interdental separation
Large tongue
Hirsutism
Thick greasy skin
Spade-like hands and feet
Tight rings
Carpal tunnel syndrome
Visual field defects
Galactorrhoea
Hypertension
Oedema
Heart failure
Arthropathy
Proximal myopathy
Glycosuria
  (plus possible signs of
  hypopituitarism)

</td></tr>
</table>

Fig. 18.18 **The signs of acromegaly.** Bold type indicates signs of greater discriminant value.

Management and treatment

Untreated acromegaly results in markedly reduced survival with most deaths from heart failure, coronary artery disease and hypertension-related causes. In addition, there is an increase in deaths due to neoplasia, particularly large-bowel tumours. Treatment is therefore indicated in all except the elderly or those with minimal abnormalities. There is now consensus agreement that the aim of therapy should be to achieve a mean growth hormone level below 5 mU/L, which has been shown to reduce mortality to normal levels.

Complete cure is often slow, if possible at all. The choice lies between trans-sphenoidal surgery, trans-frontal surgery, external radiotherapy, octreotide, and dopamine agonists. Progress can be assessed by mean GH levels and by serial IGF-1 measurements. The general pros and cons of surgery, radiotherapy and medical treatment are discussed on page 1010.

When present, hypopituitarism should be corrected (see p. 1013) and concurrent diabetes and/or hypertension should be treated conventionally; both usually improve with treatment of the acromegaly.

Surgery

Trans-sphenoidal surgery is generally agreed as the appropriate first-line therapy. It will result in clinical remission in a majority of cases (60–80%) with pituitary microadenoma, but in only 50% of those with macroadenoma. Transfrontal surgery is rarely required except for massive macroadenomas.

External radiotherapy

External radiotherapy is normally used after pituitary surgery fails to normalize GH levels rather than as primary therapy. It is often combined with medium-term treatment with a somatostatin analogue or a dopamine agonist because of the slow biochemical response to radiotherapy, which may take 10 years or more.

Somatostatin analogues

Octreotide and lanreotide are synthetic analogues of somatostatin (GHRIH, p. 1031) which are the treatment of choice in resistant cases, and employed as a short-term treatment while other modalities become effective. Long-acting preparations (monthly for octreotide, every 10–14 days for lanreotide) are now replacing older subcutaneous regimens. Both are generally well tolerated but are associated with an increased incidence of gallstones and are expensive.

Dopamine agonists

Dopamine agonists now play a lesser role. They can be given to shrink tumours prior to definitive therapy or to control symptoms and persisting GH secretion; they are probably most effective in mixed growth-hormone-producing (somatotroph) and prolactin-producing (mammotroph) tumours. The doses are bromocriptine 10–60 mg daily or cabergoline 0.5 mg daily (higher than for prolactinomas) but should be started slowly (see p. 1028). Given alone they rarely reduce GH to 'safe' levels – but may be useful for mild residual disease or in combination with somatostatin analogues.

Growth hormone antagonists

Pegvisomant is a GH receptor antagonist which has its effect by binding to and preventing dimerization of the GH receptor. It has shown considerable promise in clinical trials and has recently been licensed for use. Its main role is likely to be in treatment of patients in whom GH cannot be reduced to safe levels with somatostatin analogues alone.

FURTHER READING

Colao A, Lombardi G (1998) Growth-hormone and prolactin excess. *Lancet* **352**: 1455–1461.

Drake WM, Howell SJ, Monson JP, Shalet SM (2001) Optimising GH therapy in adults and children. *Endocrine Reviews* **22**: 425–450.

Le Roith D (1997) Insulin-like growth factors. *New England Journal of Medicine* **336**: 633–640.

Melmed S (1995) Recent advances in pathogenesis, diagnosis and management of acromegaly. *Journal of Clinical Endocrinology and Metabolism* **80**: 3395–3402.

Orme SM et al. for the UK Acromegaly Study Group (1998) Mortality and cancer incidence in acromegaly: a retrospective cohort study. *Journal of Clinical Endocrinology and Metabolism* **83**: 2730–2734.

Utiger RD (2000) Treatment of acromegaly. *New England Journal of Medicine* **342**: 1210–1211.

The thyroid axis

The metabolic rate of many tissues is controlled by the thyroid hormones, and overactivity and underactivity of the gland pose the most common of all endocrine problems.

Anatomy

The thyroid gland consists of two lateral lobes connected by an isthmus. It is closely attached to the thyroid cartilage and to the upper end of the trachea, and thus moves on swallowing. It is often palpable in normal women.

Embryologically it originates from the base of the tongue and descends to the middle of the neck. Remnants of thyroid tissue can sometimes be found at the base of the tongue (lingual thyroid) and along the line of descent. The gland has a rich blood supply from superior and inferior thyroid arteries.

The thyroid consists of follicles lined by cuboidal epithelioid cells. Inside is the colloid, which is an iodinated glycoprotein, thyroglobulin, synthesized by the follicular cells. Each follicle is surrounded by basement membrane, between which are parafollicular cells containing calcitonin-secreting C cells.

Biochemistry

The thyroid hormones, T_4 and T_3, are synthesized within the gland (Fig. 18.19).

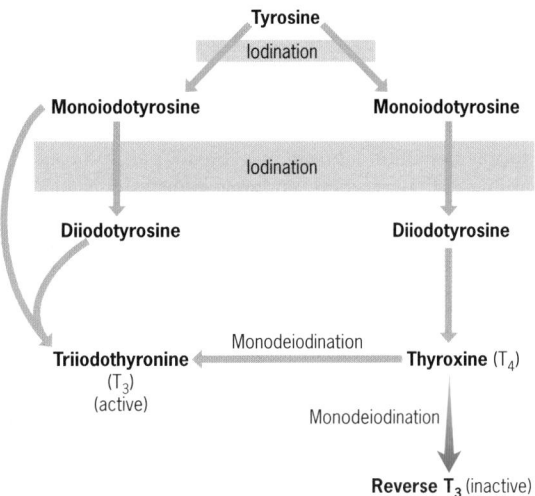

Fig. 18.19 Synthesis and metabolism of the thyroid hormones.

More T_4 than T_3 is produced, but T_4 is converted in some peripheral tissues (liver, kidney and muscle) to the more active T_3 by 5′-monodeiodination; an alternative 3′-monodeiodination yields the inactive reverse T_3 (rT_3). The latter step occurs particularly in severe non-thyroidal illness (see below).

In plasma, more than 99% of all T_4 and T_3 is bound to hormone-binding proteins (thyroxine-binding globulin, TBG; thyroid-binding prealbumin, TBPA; and albumin). Only free hormone is available for tissue action, where T_3 binds to specific nuclear receptors within the cell. Factors affecting TBG are shown in Table 18.20; all may result in confusing thyroid function test results.

Table 18.20
Factors affecting thyroxine-binding globulin (TBG) levels

Increased TBG
Hereditary
Pregnancy
Oestrogen therapy
Oral contraceptive use
Hypothyroidism
Phenothiazines
Acute viral hepatitis

Decreased TBG
Hereditary
Androgens
Corticosteroid excess
Thyrotoxicosis
Nephrotic syndrome
Major illness
Malnutrition
Chronic liver disease

Drug causing altered binding
Non-steroidal anti-inflammatory drugs
Phenytoin

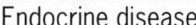
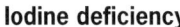

Iodine deficiency

Globally, dietary iodine deficiency is a major cause of thyroid disease as iodine is an essential requirement for thyroid hormone synthesis. The recommended daily intake of iodine should be at least 140 µg, and dietary supplementation of salt and bread has reduced the number of areas where 'endemic goitre' still occurs (see below).

Physiology of the hypothalamic–pituitary–thyroid axis (see Fig. 18.1)

1. TRH is released in the hypothalamus and stimulates release of TSH from the pituitary.
2. TSH stimulates the TSH receptor in the thyroid to increase synthesis of both T_4 and T_3 and also to release stored hormone, producing increased plasma levels of T_4 and T_3.
3. T_3 feeds back on the pituitary and perhaps hypothalamus to reduce TRH and TSH secretion.

Thyroid function tests

Immunoassays for total T_4, free T_4, total T_3, free T_3 and TSH are widely available. There are only minor circadian rhythms, and measurements may be made at any time. Particular uses of the tests are summarized in Table 18.21, with typical findings in common disorders.

TSH measurement

Current assays differentiate between normal and low TSH levels and can thus discriminate between hyperthyroidism, hypothyroidism and euthyroidism. There are pitfalls, however. These are mainly with hypopituitarism, with the 'sick euthyroid' syndrome and with dysthyroid eye disease, all of which may give 'false' (i.e. misleading, not incorrect) low results implying hyperthyroidism. As a single test of thyroid function it is the most sensitive in most circumstances, but many laboratories prefer to perform at least two tests – for example, TSH plus free T_4 or free T_3 where hyperthyroidism is suspected, TSH plus serum free T_4 where hypothyroidism is likely.

'Free' T_4 tests

These attempt to measure only the unbound active hormone. Although not perfect, they are in routine clinical use in most laboratories. TBG is sometimes measured directly.

TRH test

This has been rendered almost obsolete except for investigation of hypothalamic–pituitary dysfunction.

Problems in interpretation of thyroid function tests

There are three major areas of difficulty.

Serious acute or chronic illness

Thyroid function is affected in several ways, with reduced concentration and affinity of binding proteins, decreased peripheral conversion of T_4 to T_3 with more rT_3 and reduced hypothalamic–pituitary TSH production. Systemically ill patients can therefore have an apparently low total and free T_4 and T_3 with a normal or low basal TSH (the 'sick euthyroid' syndrome). Levels are usually only mildly below normal and are thought to be mediated by interleukins IL-1 and IL-6; the tests should be repeated after resolution of the underlying illness.

Pregnancy and oral contraceptives

These lead to greatly increased TBG levels and thus to high or high-normal total T_4. Free T_4 is usually normal. The normal physiological changes during pregnancy are not fully understood but rarely cause clinical problems, although TSH is often slightly suppressed in the first trimester.

Drugs

Many drugs affect thyroid function tests by interfering with protein binding. The most common are listed in Table 18.20. Basal TSH should be measured.

Antithyroid antibodies

Serum antibodies to the thyroid are common and may be either destructive or stimulating; both occasionally coexist in the same patient.

Table 18.21

Characteristics of thyroid function tests in common thyroid disorders (the clinically most informative tests in each situation are shown in bold)

	TSH (0.3–3.5 mU/L)	Total T$_4$ (60–160 mmol/L)	Free T$_4$ (10–25 pmol/L)	T$_3$ (1.2–3.1 nmol/L)
Thyrotoxicosis	**Suppressed (< 0.05 mU/L)**	Increased	**Increased**	**Increased**
Primary hypothyroidism	**Increased (> 10 mU/L)**	Low/low-normal	Low/low-normal	Normal or low
TSH deficiency	Low-normal or subnormal	Low/low-normal	**Low/low-normal**	Normal or low
T$_3$ toxicosis	Suppressed (< 0.05 mU/L)	Normal	Normal	**Increased**
Compensated euthyroidism	Slightly increased (5–10 mU/L)	Normal	**Normal**	Normal

Destructive antibodies may be directed against the microsomes or against thyroglobulin; the antigen for thyroid microsomal antibodies is the thyroid peroxidase (TPO) enzyme. TPO antibodies are found in up to 20% of the normal population, especially older women, but only 10–20% of these develop overt hypothyroidism.

TSH receptor antibodies (TRAb), which are IgG antibodies, can be measured in two ways:

- by the inhibition of binding of TSH to its receptors (TSH-binding inhibitory immunoglobulin, TBII)
- by demonstrating that they stimulate the release of cyclic AMP (thyroid-stimulating immunoglobulin/antibody TSI, TSAb).

Hypothyroidism

Pathophysiology

Underactivity of the thyroid is usually primary, from disease of the thyroid, but may be secondary to hypothalamic–pituitary disease (reduced TSH drive) (Table 18.22). It is one of the most common endocrine conditions with a UK prevalence of 1.4% in women, but under 0.1% in men.

Causes of primary hypothyroidism

Atrophic (autoimmune) hypothyroidism

This is the most common cause of hypothyroidism and is associated with antithyroid autoantibodies leading to lymphoid infiltration of the gland and eventual atrophy and fibrosis. It is six times more common in females and the incidence increases with age. The condition is associated with other autoimmune disease such as pernicious anaemia, vitiligo and other endocrine deficiencies (p. 1009). In some instances intermittent hypothyroidism occurs with recovery; antibodies which block the TSH receptor may sometimes be involved in the aetiology.

Hashimoto's thyroiditis

This form of autoimmune thyroiditis, again more common in women and most common in late middle age, produces atrophic changes with regeneration, leading to goitre formation. The gland is usually firm and rubbery but may range from soft to hard. TPO antibodies are present, often in very high titres (> 1000 IU/L). Patients may be hypothyroid or euthyroid, though they may go through an initial toxic phase, 'Hashi-toxicity'. Thyroxine therapy may shrink the goitre even when the patient is not hypothyroid, though this may take a long time.

Postpartum thyroiditis

This is usually a transient phenomenon observed following pregnancy and may involve hyperthyroidism, hypothyroidism or the two sequentially. It is believed to result from the modifications to the immune system

Table 18.22
Causes of hypothyroidism

PRIMARY	Post-surgery
Congenital	**Post-irradiation**
Agenesis	Radioactive iodine therapy
Ectopic thyroid remnants	External neck irradiation
Defects of hormone synthesis	**Infiltration**
Iodine deficiency	Tumour
Dyshormonogenesis	
Antithyroid drugs	**SECONDARY**
Other drugs (e.g. lithium,	**Hypopituitarism**
amiodarone, interferon)	Isolated TSH deficiency
Autoimmune	**Peripheral resistance to**
Atrophic thyroiditis	**thyroid hormone**
Hashimoto's thyroiditis	
Postpartum thyroiditis	
Infective	
Post-subacute thyroiditis	

necessary in pregnancy, and histologically is a lymphocytic thyroiditis. The process is normally self-limiting, but when conventional antibodies are found there is a high chance of this proceeding to permanent hypothyroidism.

Iodine deficiency

In mountainous areas (the Alps, Himalayas, South America, Central Africa) dietary iodine deficiency still exists, in some areas as 'endemic goitre' where goitre, occasionally massive, is common. The patients may be euthyroid or hypothyroid depending on the severity of iodine deficiency. The mechanism is thought to be borderline hypothyroidism leading to TSH stimulation and thyroid enlargement in the face of continuing iodine deficiency.

Dyshormonogenesis

This rare condition is due to genetic defects in the synthesis of thyroid hormones; patients develop hypothyroidism with a goitre. One particular familial form is associated with sensorineural deafness (Pendred's syndrome).

Clinical features (Fig. 18.20)

Hypothyroidism may produce many symptoms. The alternative term 'myxoedema' refers to the accumulation of mucopolysaccharide in subcutaneous tissues. The classic picture of the slow, dry-haired, thick-skinned, deep-voiced patient with weight gain, cold intolerance, bradycardia and constipation makes the diagnosis easy. Milder symptoms are, however, more common and hard to distinguish from other causes of non-specific tiredness. Many cases are detected on biochemical screening.

Symptoms
Tiredness/malaise
Weight gain
Anorexia
Cold intolerance
Poor memory
Change in appearance
Depression
Poor libido
Goitre
Puffy eyes
Dry, brittle
unmanageable hair
Dry, coarse skin
Arthralgia
Myalgia
Muscle weakness/Stiffness
Constipation
Menorrhagia or
oligomenorrhoea
in women
Psychosis
Coma
Deafness

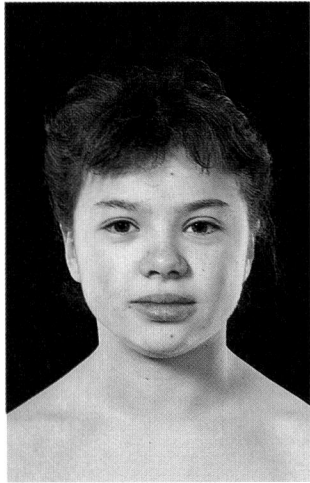

Signs	
Mental slowness	
Ataxia	
Poverty of movement	Periorbital oedema
Deafness	Deep voice
Psychosis/dementia (rare)	Goitre
'Peaches and	**Dry skin**
cream' complexion	Overweight/obesity
Dry thin hair	
Loss of eyebrows	Myotonia
	Muscular hypertrophy
Hypertension	Proximal myopathy
Hypothermia	**Slow-relaxing reflexes**
Heart failure	
Bradycardia	Anaemia
Pericardial effusion	
Cold peripheries	
Carpal tunnel syndrome	
Oedema	

Fig. 18.20 **The symptoms and signs of hypothyroidism.** Bold type indicates signs of greater discriminant value. A history from a relative is often revealing. Symptoms of other autoimmune disease may be present.

Special difficulties in diagnosis may arise in certain circumstances:

- *Children with hypothyroidism* may not show classic features but often have a slow growth velocity, poor school performance and sometimes arrest of pubertal development.
- *Young women with hypothyroidism* may not show obvious signs. Hypothyroidism should be excluded in all patients with oligomenorrhoea/amenorrhoea, menorrhagia, infertility or hyperprolactinaemia.
- *The elderly* show many clinical features that are difficult to differentiate from normal ageing.

Investigation of primary hypothyroidism

Serum TSH is the investigation of choice; a high TSH level confirms primary hypothyroidism. A low total or free serum T_4 level confirms the hypothyroid state and is necessary as, if there is hypothalamic and pituitary disease, the TSH may be low or normal.

Thyroid and other organ-specific antibodies may be present. Other abnormalities include the following:

- *anaemia*, which is usually normochromic and normocytic in type but may be macrocytic (sometimes this is due to associated pernicious anaemia) or microcytic (in women, due to menorrhagia)
- *increased serum aspartate transferase levels*, from muscle and/or liver
- *increased serum creatine kinase levels*, with associated myopathy
- *hypercholesterolaemia*

- *hyponatraemia* due to an increase in ADH and impaired free water clearance.

Treatment

Replacement therapy with thyroxine (i.e. T_4) is given for life. The starting dose will depend upon the severity of the deficiency and on the age and fitness of the patient, especially cardiac performance. In the young and fit, 100 µg daily is suitable, while 50 µg daily (increased to 100 µg after 2–4 weeks) is more appropriate for the small, old or frail. Patients with ischaemic heart disease require even lower initial doses, especially if the hypothyroidism is severe and long-standing. Most physicians would then begin with 25 µg daily and perform serial ECGs, increasing the dose at 3- to 4-week intervals if angina does not occur or worsen and the ECG does not deteriorate. Some, however, would use T_3 beginning with 2.5 µg 8-hourly, doubling the dose every 48 hours up to 10 µg three times daily. If progress is satisfactory, T_4 (100 µg daily) is then started and T_3 is discontinued 5 days later.

Adequacy of replacement should be assessed clinically and by thyroid function tests after at least 6 weeks on a steady dose; the aim is to restore T_4 and TSH to well within the normal range. If serum TSH remains high, the dose of T_4 should be increased in increments of 25–50 µg and the tests repeated 6 weeks later. This stepwise progression should be continued until TSH becomes normal, though some physicians believe that complete well-being is only restored in some patients when the T_4 is high-normal and the TSH is slightly suppressed. The usual maintenance dose is 100–150 μg given as a single daily dose; over-replacement may increase the risk of atrial fibrillation in those aged over 60. An annual thyroid function test is recommended – this is usually performed in the primary care setting, often assisted and prompted by district 'thyroid registers'.

Clinical improvement on T_4 may not begin for 2 weeks or more and full resolution of symptoms may take 6 months. The importance of lifelong therapy must be emphasized and the possibility of other autoimmune endocrine disease developing, especially Addison's disease or pernicious anaemia, should be considered. During pregnancy, an increase in T_4 dosage of about 25–50 μg is often needed to maintain normal TSH levels, and the necessity of optimal replacement during pregnancy is emphasized by the finding of reductions in cognitive function in children of mothers with elevated TSH during pregnancy.

Borderline hypothyroidism or 'compensated euthyroidism'

Patients are frequently seen with low-normal serum T_4 levels and slightly raised TSH levels. Sometimes this follows surgery or radioactive iodine therapy when it can reasonably be seen as 'compensatory'. Treatment with thyroxine is normally recommended where the TSH is consistently above 10 mU/L, or when possible symptoms, high-titre thyroid antibodies or lipid abnormalities are present. Where the TSH is only marginally raised, the tests should be repeated 3–6 months later. Conversion to overt hypothyroidism is more common in men or when TPO antibodies are present. In practice, vague symptoms in patients with marginally elevated TSH (below 10 mU/L) rarely respond to treatment, but a 'therapeutic trial' of replacement may be needed to confirm that symptoms are unrelated to the thyroid.

Myxoedema coma

Severe hypothyroidism, especially in the elderly, may present with confusion or even coma. Myxoedema coma is very rare: hypothermia is often present and the patient may have severe cardiac failure, hypoventilation, hypoglycaemia and hyponatraemia. The mortality was previously at least 50% and patients require full intensive care. Optimal treatment is controversial and data lacking; most physicians would advise T_3 orally or intravenously in doses of 2.5–5 μg every 8 hours, then increasing as above. Large intravenous doses should not be used. Additional measures, though unproven, should include:

- oxygen (by ventilation if necessary)
- monitoring of cardiac output and pressures via a Swan–Ganz catheter
- gradual rewarming
- hydrocortisone 100 mg i.v. 8-hourly
- glucose infusion to prevent hypoglycaemia.

'Myxoedema madness'

Depression is common in hypothyroidism but rarely with severe hypothyroidism in the elderly the patient may become frankly demented or psychotic, sometimes with striking delusions. This may occur shortly after starting T_4 replacement.

Screening for hypothyroidism

The incidence of congenital hypothyroidism is approximately 1 in 3500 births. Untreated, severe hypothyroidism produces permanent neurological and intellectual damage ('cretinism'). Routine screening of the newborn using a blood-spot, as in the Guthrie test, to detect a high TSH level as an indicator of primary hypothyroidism is efficient and cost-effective; cretinism is prevented if T_4 is started within the first few months of life.

Screening of elderly patients for thyroid dysfunction has a low pick-up rate, is controversial and not currently recommended. However, patients who have undergone thyroid surgery or received radioiodine should have regular thyroid function tests, as should those receiving lithium or amiodarone therapy.

Hyperthyroidism

Hyperthyroidism (thyroid overactivity, thyrotoxicosis) is common, affecting perhaps 2–5% of all females at some time and with a sex ratio of 5 : 1, most often between ages 20 and 40 years. Nearly all cases (> 99%) are caused by intrinsic thyroid disease; a pituitary cause is extremely rare (Table 18.23).

Table 18.23
Causes of hyperthyroidism

Common
Graves' disease (autoimmune)
Toxic multinodular goitre
Solitary toxic nodule/adenoma

Uncommon
Acute thyroiditis
    viral (e.g. De Quervain's)
    autoimmune
    post-irradiation
    post-partum
Gestational thyrotoxicosis (hCG stimulated)
Exogenous iodine
Drugs – amiodarone
Thyrotoxicosis factitia (secret T_4 consumption)

Rare
TSH-secreting pituitary tumours
Metastatic differentiated thyroid carcinoma
hCG-producing tumours
Hyperfunctioning ovarian teratoma (struma ovarii)

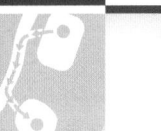

Graves' disease

This is the most common cause of hyperthyroidism and is due to an autoimmune process. Serum IgG antibodies bind to the thyroid TSH receptor stimulating thyroid hormone production, behaving like TSH. These TSH receptor antibodies can be measured in serum. There is an association with HLA-B8, DR3 and DR2 and 50% concordance is seen amongst monozygotic twins with a 5% concordance rate in dizygotic twins.

Yersinia enterocolitica as well as *Escherichia coli* and other Gram-negative organisms contain TSH binding sites. This raises the possibility that the initiating event in the pathogenesis may be an infection with possible 'molecular mimicry' in a genetically susceptible individual, but the precise initiating mechanisms remain unproven in most cases.

Thyroid eye disease accompanies the hyperthyroidism in many cases (see below) but other components of Graves' disease, e.g. Graves' dermopathy, are very rare. Rarely lymphadenopathy and splenomegaly may occur. Graves' disease is also associated with other autoimmune disorders such as pernicious anaemia, vitiligo and myasthenia gravis.

The natural history is one of fluctuation, many patients showing a pattern of alternating relapse and remission; perhaps only 40% of subjects have a single episode. Many patients eventually become hypothyroid.

Other causes of hyperthyroidism/thyrotoxicosis

Toxic solitary adenoma/nodule (Plummer's disease)

This is the cause of about 5% of cases of hyperthyroidism. It does not usually remit after a course of antithyroid drugs.

Toxic multinodular goitre

This commonly occurs in older women. Again, antithyroid drugs are rarely successful in inducing a remission – although they can control the hyperthyroidism.

de Quervain's thyroiditis

This is transient hyperthyroidism from an acute inflammatory process, probably viral in origin. Apart from the toxicosis, there is usually fever, malaise and pain in the neck with tachycardia and local thyroid tenderness. Thyroid function tests show initial hyperthyroidism, the erythrocyte sedimentation rate (ESR) and plasma viscosity are raised, and thyroid uptake scans show suppression of uptake in the acute phase, though hypothyroidism, usually transient, may then follow after a few weeks. Treatment of the acute phase is with aspirin, using short-term prednisolone in severely symptomatic cases.

Postpartum thyroiditis

This is described on page 1043.

Clinical features of hyperthyroidism

The symptoms and signs of hyperthyroidism affect many systems (Fig. 18.21).

Symptomatology and signs vary with age and with the underlying aetiology.

- *The eye signs, pretibial myxoedema and thyroid acropachy* occur only in Graves' disease. Pretibial myxoedema is an infiltration on the shin, essentially occurring only with eye disease (see below). Thyroid acropachy is very rare and consists of clubbing, swollen fingers and periosteal new bone formation.
- *In the elderly*, a frequent presentation is with atrial fibrillation, other tachycardias and/or heart failure, often with few other signs. Thyroid function tests are mandatory in any patient with atrial fibrillation.
- *Children* frequently present with excessive height or excessive growth rate, or with behavioural problems such as hyperactivity. They may also show weight gain rather than loss.
- *So-called 'apathetic thyrotoxicosis'* in some elderly patients presents with a clinical picture more like hypothyroidism. There may be very few signs and a high degree of clinical suspicion is essential.

Differential diagnosis

Hyperthyroidism is often clinically obvious but treatment should never be instituted without biochemical confirmation.

Differentiation of the mild case from anxiety states may be difficult; useful positive clinical markers are eye signs, a diffuse goitre, proximal myopathy and wasting. The hyperdynamic circulation with warm peripheries seen with hyperthyroidism can be contrasted with the clammy hands of anxiety.

Investigations

Serum TSH is suppressed in hyperthyroidism (< 0.05 mU/L), except for the very rare instances of TSH hypersecretion. Diagnosis is confirmed with a raised serum T_4, free T_4 or T_3; T_4 is almost always raised but T_3 is more sensitive as there are occasional cases of isolated 'T_3 toxicosis'. TPO and thyroglobulin antibodies are present in most cases of Graves' disease.

TSH receptor antibodies are not measured routinely, but are commonly present: thyroid stimulating immunoglobin (TSI) 80% positive, TSH-binding inhibitory immunoglobin (TBII) 60–90% in Graves' disease (see p. 1040).

Treatment

Three possibilities are available: antithyroid drugs, radioiodine and surgery. Practices and beliefs differ widely within and between countries.

Symptoms		Signs	
Weight loss		**Tremor**	Proximal myopathy
Increased appetite		**Hyperkinesis**	Proximal muscle wasting
Irritability/behaviour change		Irritability	Onycholysis
Restlessness		Psychosis	Palmar erythema
Malaise			
Stiffness		**Tachycardia or atrial**	Graves' dermopathy*
Muscle weakness		**fibrillation**	Thyroid acropachy
Tremor		**Full pulse**	Pretibial myxoedema
Choreoathetosis		**Warm vasodilated**	
Breathlessness		**peripheries**	
Palpitation		Systolic hypertension	
Heat intolerance		Cardiac failure	
Itching			
Thirst		**Exophthalmos***	
Vomiting		**Lid lag and 'stare'**	
Diarrhoea		Conjunctival oedema	
Eye complaints*		Ophthalmoplegia*	
Goitre		Periorbital oedema	
Oligomenorrhoea		**Goitre, bruit**	
Loss of libido		Weight loss	
Gynaecomastia			
Onycholysis			
Tall stature (in children)			
Sweating			
*Only in Graves' disease		*Only in Graves' disease	

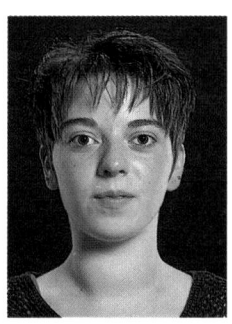
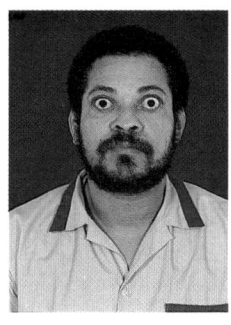

Fig. 18.21 **The symptoms and signs of hyperthyroidism.** Bold type indicates signs of greater discriminant value.

Table 18.24
Drugs used in the treatment of hyperthyroidism

Drug	Usual starting dose	Side-effects	Remarks
Antithyroid drugs			
Carbimazole	20–40 mg 8-hourly, or in single dose	Rash, nausea, vomiting, arthralgia, agranulocytosis (0.1%), jaundice	Active metabolite is methimazole Mild immunosuppressive activity
Propylthiouracil	100–200 mg 8-hourly	Rash, nausea, vomiting agranulocytosis	Additionally blocks conversion of T_4 to T_3
Beta-blocker for symptomatic control			
May need higher doses than normal in hyperthyroidism as metabolism is increased			
Propranolol	40–80 mg every 6–8 hours	Avoid in asthma Use with care in heart failure	Use agents without intrinsic sympathomimetic activity as receptors highly sensitive

Antithyroid drugs

Carbimazole is most often used in the UK, and propylthiouracil is also used. Methimazole, the active metabolite of carbimazole, is used in the USA. These drugs inhibit the formation of thyroid hormones and also have other minor actions; carbimazole/methimazole is also an immunosuppressive agent. Initial doses and side-effects are detailed in Table 18.24.

Although thyroid hormone synthesis is reduced very quickly, the long half-life of T_4 (7 days) means that clinical benefit is not apparent for 10–20 days. As many of the manifestations of hyperthyroidism are mediated via the sympathetic system, beta-blockers may be used to provide rapid partial symptomatic control; they also decrease peripheral conversion of T_4 to T_3. Drugs preferred are those without intrinsic sympathomimetic activity, e.g. propranolol (Table 18.24). They should not be used alone for hyperthyroidism except when the condition is self-limiting, as in subacute thyroiditis.

Subsequent management is either by gradual dose titration or a 'block and replace' regimen. Neither regimen has been shown to be unequivocally superior.

Gradual dose titration

1. Review after 4–6 weeks and reduce dose of carbimazole depending on clinical state and T_4/T_3 levels. TSH levels may remain suppressed for several months and are unhelpful at this stage.
2. When clinically and biochemically euthyroid, stop beta-blockers.
3. Review after 2–3 months and, if controlled, reduce carbimazole.
4. Gradually reduce dose to 5 mg daily over 6–24 months if hyperthyroidism remains controlled.
5. When the patient is euthyroid on 5 mg daily carbimazole, discontinue.

Propylthiouracil is used in similar fashion (Table 18.24).

'Block and replace' regimen

With this policy, full doses of antithyroid drugs, usually carbimazole 40 mg daily, are given to suppress the thyroid completely while replacing thyroid activity with 100 µg of thyroxine daily once euthyroidism has been achieved. This is continued usually for 18 months, the claimed advantages being the avoidance of over- or under-treatment and the better use of the immunosuppressive action of carbimazole. This regimen is contraindicated in pregnancy as T_4 crosses the placenta less well than carbimazole.

Relapse

About 50% of patients will relapse after a course of carbimazole or propylthiouracil, mostly within the following 2 years but occasionally much later. Long-term antithyroid therapy is then used or surgery or radiotherapy is considered (see below). Most patients (90%) with hyperthyroidism have a diffuse goitre but those with large single or multinodular goitres are unlikely to remit after a course of antithyroid drugs. Severe biochemical hyperthyroidism is also less likely to respond.

Toxicity

The major side-effect is agranulocytosis that occurs in approximately 1 in 1000 patients usually within 3 months of treatment. All patients must be warned to seek immediate medical attention if they develop unexplained fever or sore throat – written information is essential. Rashes are more frequent and usually require a change of drug. If toxicity occurs on carbimazole, propylthiouracil may be used and vice versa; side-effects are only occasionally repeated on the other drug.

Radioactive iodine

Radioiodine is now more widely used in the UK, as has previously happened elsewhere, although it is contraindicated in pregnancy and while breast-feeding. Iodine-131 in an empirical dose (usually 200–500 MBq), accumulates in the thyroid and destroys the gland by local radiation – though it takes several months to be fully effective. Strict radiation safety rules apply in the UK and may be inconvenient or disconcerting for some patients. Patients must be rendered euthyroid before treatment though they have to stop antithyroid drugs at least 4 days before radioiodine, and not recommence until 3 days after radioiodine (many patients who are well controlled before radioactive iodine do not need to restart at all).

Early discomfort in the neck and immediate worsening of hyperthyroidism are sometimes seen; if worsening occurs, the patient should receive propranolol (Table 18.24); if necessary carbimazole can be restarted. Euthyroidism normally returns in 2–3 months. Patients with dysthyroid eye disease are more likely to show worsening of eye problems after radioiodine than after antithyroid drugs; this represents a partial contraindication, although worsening can usually be prevented by steroid administration.

Apart from the immediate problems above, a major complication is the progressive incidence of subsequent hypothyroidism affecting the majority of subjects over the following 20 years. Though 75% of patients are rendered euthyroid in the short term, a small proportion remain hyperthyroid; increasing the radioiodine dose improves the speed and rate of response but increases the rate of hypothyroidism. Long-term surveillance of thyroid function is necessary with frequent tests in the first year after therapy, and at least annually thereafter.

Risk of carcinogenesis has been long debated, but it is now clear that overall cancer incidence and mortality are not increased after radioactive iodine (and indeed are significantly reduced in some studies) but the risk of thyroid cancer is significantly increased although the risk remains very low in absolute terms.

Surgery: subtotal thyroidectomy

Thyroidectomy should be performed only in patients who have previously been rendered euthyroid. Conventional practice is to stop the antithyroid drug 10–14 days before operation and to give potassium iodide (60 mg three times daily), which reduces the vascularity of the gland.

The operation should be performed only by experienced surgeons to reduce the chance of complications:

- Early postoperative bleeding causing tracheal compression and asphyxia is a rare emergency requiring immediate removal of all clips/sutures to allow escape of the blood/haematoma.
- Laryngeal nerve palsy occurs in 1%. Vocal chord movement should be checked preoperatively. Mild hoarseness is more common and thyroidectomy is best avoided in professional singers!
- Transient hypocalcaemia occurs in up to 10% but with permanent hypoparathyroidism in fewer than 1%.
- Recurrent hyperthyroidism occurs in 1–3% within 1 year, then 1% per year.

- Hypothyroidism occurs in about 10% of patients within 1 year, and this percentage increases with time. It is likeliest if TPO antibodies are positive. Automated computer thyroid registers with annual TSH screening are used in some regions, and have demonstrated that a high proportion of patients become hypothyroid in the long term.

Choice of therapy

Indications for either surgery or radioiodine are:

- patient choice
- persistent drug side-effects
- poor compliance with drug therapy
- recurrent hyperthyroidism after drugs.

Particular indications for surgery include:

- a large goitre, which is unlikely to remit after antithyroid medication.

Special situations in hyperthyroidism
Thyroid crisis or 'thyroid storm'

This rare condition, with a mortality of 10%, is a rapid deterioration of hyperthyroidism with hyperpyrexia, severe tachycardia and extreme restlessness. It is usually precipitated by stress, infection, surgery in an unprepared patient, or radioiodine therapy. With careful management it should no longer occur and most cases referred as 'crisis' are simply severe but uncomplicated thyrotoxicosis.

Treatment is urgent. Propranolol in full doses is started immediately together with potassium iodide, antithyroid drugs, corticosteroids (which suppress many of the manifestations of hyperthyroidism) and full supportive measures.

Hyperthyroidism in pregnancy and neonatal life

Maternal hyperthyroidism during pregnancy is uncommon and usually mild. Diagnosis can be difficult because of misleading thyroid function tests, although TSH is largely reliable. The pathogenesis is almost always Graves' disease. Thyroid-stimulating immunoglobulin (TSI) crosses the placenta to stimulate the fetal thyroid. Carbimazole also crosses the placenta, but T_4 does so poorly so a 'block-and-replace' regimen is contraindicated. The smallest dose of carbimazole necessary is used and the fetus must be monitored (see below). The paediatrician should be informed and the infant checked immediately after birth – overtreatment with carbimazole can cause fetal goitre. Breast-feeding while on usual doses of carbimazole or propylthiouracil appears to be safe.

If necessary (high doses needed, poor patient compliance or drug side-effects), surgery can be performed, preferably in the second trimester. Radioactive iodine is absolutely contraindicated.

The fetus and maternal Graves' disease

Any mother with a history of Graves' disease may have circulating TSI. Even if she has been treated (e.g. by surgery), the immunoglobulin may still be present to stimulate the fetal thyroid, and the fetus can thus become hyperthyroid, while the mother remains euthyroid.

Any such patient should therefore be monitored during pregnancy. Fetal heart rate provides a direct biological assay of fetal thyroid status, and monitoring should be performed at least monthly. Rates above 160 per minute are strongly suggestive of fetal hyperthyroidism and maternal treatment with carbimazole and/or propranolol may be used. To prevent the mother becoming hypothyroid, T_4 may be given as this does not easily cross the placenta. Sympathomimetics, used to prevent premature labour, are contraindicated as they may provoke fatal tachycardia in the fetus.

Hyperthyroidism may also develop in the neonatal period as TSI has a half-life of approximately 3 weeks. Manifestations in the newborn include irritability, failure to thrive and persisting weight loss, diarrhoea and eye signs. Thyroid function tests are difficult to interpret as neonatal normal ranges vary with age.

Untreated neonatal hyperthyroidism is probably associated with hyperactivity in later childhood.

Thyroid hormone resistance

Thyroid hormone resistance is an inherited condition caused by an abnormality of the thyroid hormone receptor. Mutations to the receptor result in the need for higher levels of thyroid hormones to achieve the same intracellular effect. As a result, the normal feedback control mechanisms (see Fig. 18.1, p. 1001) result in high blood levels of thyroxine with a normal TSH in order to maintain a euthyroid state. This has two consequences:

- First, thyroid function tests appear abnormal even when the patient is euthyroid and requires no treatment; this is not a particular problem as free T_4 and TSH levels are measured.
- Second, different tissues contain different thyroid hormone receptors and, in some families, receptors in certain tissues may have normal activity. In this case the level of thyroid hormones to maintain euthyroidism at pituitary and hypothalamic levels (which controls secretion of TSH) may be higher than that required in other tissues such as heart and bone, so that these tissues may exhibit 'thyrotoxic' effects in spite of a normal serum TSH. This 'partial thyroid hormone resistance' can be very difficult to manage effectively.

Long-term consequences of hyperthyroidism

Long-term follow-up studies of hyperthyroidism show a slight increase in overall mortality, which affects all

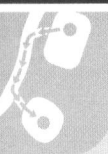

age groups, is not fully explained and tends to occur in the first year after diagnosis. Thereafter, the only long-term risk of adequately treated hyperthyroidism appears to be an increased risk of osteoporosis.

Thyroid eye disease

This is also known as dysthyroid eye disease or ophthalmic Graves' disease.

Pathophysiology

The ophthalmopathy of Graves' disease is due to a specific immune response that causes retro-orbital inflammation. Swelling and oedema of the extraocular muscles lead to limitation of movement and to proptosis which is usually bilateral but can sometimes be unilateral. Ultimately increased pressure on the optic nerve may cause optic atrophy. Histology shows focal oedema and glycosaminoglycan deposition followed by fibrosis. The precise autoantigen which leads to the immune response remains to be identified, but it appears to be an antigen in retro-orbital tissue with similar immunoreactivity to the TSH receptor.

Eye disease is a manifestation of Graves' disease and can occur in patients who may be hyperthyroid, euthyroid or hypothyroid. TSH receptor antibodies are almost invariably found in the serum but their role in the pathogenesis in unclear. Ophthalmopathy is more common in smokers.

Clinical features

The clinical appearances are characteristic (Fig. 18.21) but thyroid eye disease demonstrates a wide range of severity. A high proportion of patients with Graves' disease notice some soreness, painful watering or prominence of the eyes and the 'stare' of lid retraction is relatively common. More severe proptosis occurs in a minority of cases, and limitation and discomfort of eye movement and visual impairment due to optic nerve compression are relatively uncommon. Proptosis and lid retraction may limit the ability to close the eyes completely so that corneal damage may occur. There is periorbital oedema and conjunctural oedema and inflammation.

Eye manifestations do not parallel the degree of biochemical thyrotoxicosis, nor the need for antithyroid therapy, but exacerbation of eye disease is more common after radioiodine treatment (15% vs 3% on antithyroid drugs). Only 5-10% of cases threaten sight, but the discomfort and cosmetic problems cause great patient anxiety.

Investigations

Few investigations are necessary if the appearances are characteristic and bilateral. TSH, T$_3$ and free T$_4$ are measured.

There are a variety of grading systems but none is universally accepted. It is essential to clearly document eye movements and the degree of oedema and inflammation. The exophthalmos should be measured to allow progress to be monitored. If appearances or measurements are markedly discrepant in the two eyes, other retro-orbital space-occupying lesions should be considered: MRI of the orbits will exclude other causes and show enlarged muscles and oedema.

Treatment

If the patient is thyrotoxic this should be treated, but this will not directly result in an improvement of the ophthalmopathy, and hypothyroidism must be avoided as this may exacerbate the eye problem. Smokers should be advised to stop. Treatment of the eyes may be either local or systemic, and always requires close liaison between specialist endocrinologist and ophthalmologist:

- *Methylcellulose or hypromellose eyedrops* are given to aid lubrication and improve comfort.
- *Some patients gain relief by sleeping upright.* The eyelids can be taped to ensure closure at night.
- *Systemic steroids* (prednisolone 30–120 mg daily) usually reduce inflammation if more severe symptoms are present. Pulse intravenous methylprednisolone may be more rapidly effective in severe cases.
- *Irradiation of the orbits* (20 Gy in divided doses) is used in severe instances. This improves inflammation and occular motility but has little effect on proptosis.
- *Lid surgery* will protect the cornea if lids cannot be closed.
- *Surgical decompression of the orbit(s)* is occasionally needed.
- *Corrective eye muscle surgery* may improve diplopia due to muscle changes, but should be deferred until the situation has been stable for 6 months. Plastic surgery around the eyes may also be of value.

Goitre (thyroid enlargement)

Goitre is more common in women than in men and may be either physiological or pathological.

Clinical features

Goitres are present on examination in up to 9% of the population. Most commonly a goitre is noticed as a cosmetic defect by the patient or by friends or relatives. The majority are painless, but pain or discomfort can occur in acute varieties. Large goitres can produce dysphagia and difficulty in breathing, implying oesophageal or tracheal compression.

A small goitre may be more easily visible (on swallowing) than palpable. Clinical examination should record the size, shape, consistency and mobility of the gland as well as whether its lower margin can be demarcated (thus implying the absence of retrosternal extension). A bruit may be present. Associated lymph nodes should be sought and the tracheal position determined if possible. Examination should never omit an assessment of the patient's clinical thyroid status.

Specific enquiry should be made about any medication, especially iodine-containing preparations, and possible exposure to radiation.

Particular points of note are:

- Puberty and pregnancy may produce a diffuse increase in size of the thyroid.
- Pain in a goitre may be caused by thyroiditis, bleeding into a cyst or (rarely) a thyroid tumour.
- Excessive doses of carbimazole or propylthiouracil will induce goitre.
- Iodine deficiency and dyshormonogenesis (see above) can also cause goitre.

Assessment

There are two major aspects of any goitre: its pathological nature and the patient's thyroid status.

The nature can often be judged clinically. Goitres (Table 18.25) are usually separable into diffuse and nodular types, the causes of which differ.

Diffuse goitre

Simple goitre

In this instance no clear cause is found for enlargement of the thyroid, which is usually smooth and soft. It may be associated with thyroid growth-stimulating antibodies.

Autoimmune thyroid disease

Hashimoto's thyroiditis and thyrotoxicosis are both associated with firm diffuse goitre of variable size. A bruit is often present in thyrotoxicosis.

Thyroiditis

Acute tenderness in a diffuse swelling, sometimes with severe pain, is suggestive of an acute viral thyroiditis

(de Quervain's). This is usually associated with a systemic viral illness and may produce transient clinical hyperthyroidism with an increase in serum T_4 (see p. 1040).

Nodular goitres

Multinodular goitre

Most common is the multinodular goitre, especially in older patients. The patient is usually euthyroid but may be hyperthyroid or borderline with suppressed TSH levels but normal T_4 and T_3. Multinodular goitre is the most common cause of tracheal and/or oesophageal compression and can cause laryngeal nerve palsy. It may also extend retrosternally. The classical 'multinodular goitre' is usually readily apparent clinically, but it should be noted that modern, high-resolution ultrasound frequently reports multiple small nodules in glands which are clinically diffusely enlarged and associated with autoimmune thyroid disease. These nodules are also found in up to 40% of the normal population.

Solitary nodular goitre

Such a goitre presents a difficult problem of diagnosis. Malignancy should be considered in any solitary nodule – however, the majority of such nodules are cystic or benign and, indeed, may simply be the largest nodule of a multinodular goitre. The diagnostic challenge is to identify the small minority of malignant nodules, which require surgery, from the majority of benign nodules, which do not. A history of pain, rapid enlargement or associated lymph nodes in such a situation suggests the possibility of thyroid carcinoma, but investigations are paramount. Risk factors for malignancy include previous irradiation, long-standing iodine deficiency and occasional familial cases.

Solitary toxic nodules (Plummer's syndrome) are quite uncommon and may be associated with T_3 toxicosis.

Fibrotic goitre

Fibrotic goitre (Riedel's thyroiditis) is a rare condition, usually producing a 'woody' gland. It is associated with other midline fibrosis and is often difficult to distinguish from carcinoma, being irregular and hard.

Malignancy

In addition to thyroid carcinomas (see below), the thyroid is rarely the site of a metastatic deposit or the site of origin of a lymphoma.

Investigations

Clinical findings will dictate appropriate initial tests:

- **Thyroid function tests** – TSH plus free T_4 or T_3 (see Table 18.21).
- **Ultrasound.** Ultrasound with high resolution is a sensitive method for delineating nodules and can demonstrate whether they are cystic or solid.

Table 18.25
Goitre - causes and types

Diffuse	Nodular
Simple	Multinodular goitre
Physiological (puberty, pregnancy)	Solitary nodular
Autoimmune	Fibrotic (Reidel's
Graves' disease	thyroiditis)
Hashimoto's disease	Cysts
Thyroiditis	
Acute (de Quervain's thyroiditis)	**Tumours**
Iodine deficiency (endemic goitre)	Adenomas
Dyshormonogenesis	Carcinoma
Goitrogens (e.g. sulphonylureas)	Lymphomas
	Miscellaneous
	Sarcoidosis
	Tuberculosis

In addition, a multinodular goitre may be demonstrated when only a single nodule is palpable. Unfortunately, even cystic lesions can be malignant and thyroid tumours may arise within a multinodular goitre; therefore fine needle aspiration (see below) is often required and performed under ultrasound control at the same time as the scan.

- **Chest and thoracic inlet X-rays** to detect tracheal compression and large retrosternal extensions in patients with very large goitre or clinical symptoms.
- **Fine needle aspiration (FNA).** In patients with a solitary nodule or a dominant nodule in a multinodular goitre, there is a 5% chance of malignancy; in view of this, FNA should be performed. This can be done in the outpatient clinic. Cytology in expert hands can usually differentiate the suspicious or definitely malignant nodule.

  FNA has reduced the need for isotope scans and reduces the necessity for surgery, but there is a 5% false-negative rate which must be borne in mind (and the patient appropriately counselled). Continued observation is required when an isolated thyroid nodule is assumed to be benign without excision.

- **Thyroid scan.** FNA has largely replaced isotope scans in the diagnosis of thyroid nodules. Thyroid scan (^{125}I or ^{131}I) can be useful to distinguish between functioning (hot) or non-functioning (cold) nodules. A hot nodule is rarely malignant; however, a cold nodule is malignant in 10% of cases.

Treatment

Many goitres are small, cause no symptoms and can be observed (including self-monitoring by the patient in the long term). In particular, during puberty and pregnancy a goitre associated with euthyroidism rarely requires intervention and the patient can be reassured that spontaneous resolution is likely. When thyroid function is abnormal the patient should be rendered euthyroid. Indications for surgical intervention are:

- *The possibility of malignancy.* A history of rapid growth, pain, cervical lymphadenopathy, change in voice or previous irradiation to the neck are worrying features. A positive or suspicious FNA makes surgery mandatory and surgery may be necessary if doubt persists even in the presence of a negative FNA (especially if the patient is concerned by the false negative rate).
- *Pressure symptoms on the trachea or, more rarely, oesophagus.* The possibility of retrosternal extension should be excluded.
- *Cosmetic reasons.* A large goitre is often a considerable anxiety to the patient even though functionally and anatomically benign.

Thyroid carcinoma

Types of thyroid carcinoma, their characteristics and treatment are listed in Table 18.26. While not common, these tumours are responsible for 400 deaths annually in the UK. In 90% of cases they present as thyroid nodules (see above), but occasionally with cervical lymphadenopathy (about 5%), or with lung, cerebral, hepatic or bone metastases.

Carcinomas derived from thyroid epithelium may be papillary or follicular (differentiated) or anaplastic (undifferentiated), while medullary carcinomas (about 5% of all thyroid cancers) arise from the calcitonin-producing C cells. Lymphomas also arise within the thyroid. The pathogenesis of thyroid epithelial carcinomas is not understood except for occasional familial papillary carcinoma and those cases related to previous head-and-neck irradiation or ingestion of radioactive iodine (e.g. post-Chernobyl). These tumours are minimally active hormonally and are extremely rarely associated with hyperthyroidism; over 90%, however, secrete thyroglobulin, which can therefore act as a tumour marker.

Papillary and follicular carcinomas

The primary treatment is surgical, normally total or near-total thyroidectomy for local disease. Regional, or more extensive, neck dissection is needed where there is local nodal spread or involvement of local structures.

Table 18.26
Types of thyroid malignancy

Cell type	Frequency	Behaviour	Spread	Prognosis
Papillary	70%	Occurs in young people	Local, sometimes lung/bone secondaries	Good, especially in young
Follicular	20%	More common in females	Metastases to lung/bone	Good if resectable
Anaplastic	< 5%	Aggressive	Locally invasive	Very poor
Lymphoma	2%	Variable		Sometimes responsive to radiotherapy
Medullary cell	5%	Often familial	Local and metastases	Poor, but indolent course

Most tumours will take up iodine. If initial disease is extensive (or 'high risk') or if thyroglobulin levels rise during follow-up, patients may be given a therapeutic radioiodine dose (high dose: 5.5–7.5 MBq), which will be taken up by remaining thyroid tissue or metastatic lesions. After ablation of normal thyroid in this way, radioiodine scanning may be used to localize residual disease (using low doses) or to treat it (using high doses). Local invasion and lymph node involvement is most common and lungs and bone are the most common sites of distant metastases.

Where surgical excision is histologically complete and/or radioiodine therapy and scanning completed, patients may be placed on suppressive doses of thyroxine (sufficient to suppress TSH levels below the normal range) and patient progress monitored both clinically and biochemically using serum thyroglobulin levels as a tumour marker (levels are low on thyroxine unless there is residual tumour). Suppression of TSH also minimizes stimulation of any residual differentiated carcinoma.

The prognosis is extremely good when these types of tumour are excised while confined to the thyroid gland, and the specific therapies available lead to a relatively good prognosis even in the presence of metastases at diagnosis. Age below 40 years and papillary tumours do better than those over 40 and with a follicular histology.

Anaplastic carcinomas and lymphoma

These do not respond to radioactive iodine, and external radiotherapy produces only a brief respite.

Medullary carcinoma

Medullary carcinoma, often associated with multiple endocrine neoplasia (MEN 2, see p. 1067), is usually treated by total thyroidectomy. Local invasion or metastasis is frequent, and the tumour responds poorly to treatment, although progression is often slow. The patient's family should be screened for this and other endocrine neoplastic conditions.

FURTHER READING

Dayan CM (2001) Interpretation of thyroid function tests. *Lancet* **357**: 615–624.

Dayan CM, Daniels GH (1996) Medical progress: chronic autoimmune thyroiditis. *New England Journal of Medicine* **335**: 99–107.

Franklyn JA, Maisonnneuve P, Sheppard M, Betteridge J, Boyle P (1999) Cancer incidence and mortality after radioiodine treatment for hyperthyroidism: a population based cohort study. *Lancet* **353**: 2111–2115.

Kendall-Taylor P (2001) Thyroid cancer in the UK: can we do it better? *Clinical Endocrinology* **54**: 705–706.

Lazarus JH (1997) Hyperthyroidism. *Lancet* **349**: 339–343.

Lindsay RS, Toft AD (1997) Hypothyroidism. *Lancet* **349**: 413–417.

Vanderpump MPJ, Ahlqvist JAO, Franklyn JA, Clayton RN (1996) Consensus statement for good practice and audit measures in the management of hypothyroidism and hyperthyroidism. *British Medical Journal* **313**: 539–544.

Weetman AP (2000) Medical progress: Graves' disease. *New England Journal of Medicine* **343**: 1236–1248.

The glucocorticoid axis

Adrenal anatomy and function

The human adrenals weigh 8–10 g together and comprise an outer cortex with three zones (reticularis, fasciculata and glomerulosa) producing steroids, and an inner medulla that synthesizes, stores and secretes catecholamines (see adrenal medulla, p. 1066).

The adrenal steroids are grouped into three classes based on their predominant physiological effects.

Glucocorticoids

These are so named after their effects on carbohydrate metabolism. Major actions are listed in Table 18.27. The relative potency of common steroids is shown in Table 18.28.

Mineralocorticoids

Their predominant effect is on the extracellular balance of sodium and potassium in the distal tubule of the kidney. Aldosterone, produced solely in the zona glomerulosa, is the predominant mineralocorticoid in humans (about 50%); corticosterone makes a small contribution. The weak mineralocorticoid activity of cortisol is also important since it is present in considerable excess, but the mineralocorticoid receptor in the kidney is largely protected from this excess by the intrarenal conversion ('shuttle') of cortisol to the inactive cortisone by the enzyme 11β-hydroxysteroid dehydrogenase.

Table 18.27
The major actions of glucocorticoids

Increased or stimulated	Decreased or inhibited
Gluconeogenesis	Protein synthesis
Glycogen deposition	Host response to infection
Protein catabolism	Lymphocyte transformation
Fat deposition	Delayed hypersensitivity
Sodium retention	Circulating lymphocytes
Potassium loss	Circulating eosinophils
Free water clearance	
Uric acid production	
Circulating neutrophils	

Table 18.28

The relative glucocorticoid and mineralocorticoid potency of equal amounts of common natural and synthetic steroids

Steroid	Glucocorticoid effect	Mineralocorticoid effect
Cortisol (hydrocortisone)*	1	1
Prednisolone	4	0.7
Dexamethasone	40	2
Aldosterone	0.1	400
Fludrocortisone	10	400

*Cortisol is arbitrarily defined as 1

Androgens

Although secreted in considerable quantities, most have only relatively weak intrinsic androgenic activity until metabolized peripherally to testosterone or dihydrotestosterone.

Biochemistry

All steroids have the same basic skeleton (Fig. 18.22(b)) and the chemical differences between them are slight. The major biosynthetic pathways are shown in Figure 18.22(a).

Physiology

Glucocorticoid production by the adrenal is under hypothalamic–pituitary control (Fig. 18.23). Corticotropin-releasing hormone (CRH) is secreted in the hypothalamus in response to circadian rhythm, stress and other stimuli. CRH travels down the portal system to stimulate ACTH release from the anterior pituitary corticotrophs. ACTH is derived from the prohormone pro-opiomelanocortin, which undergoes complex processing within the pituitary to produce ACTH and a number of other peptides including beta-lipotrophin and beta-endorphin. Many of these peptides, including ACTH, contain melanocyte-stimulating hormone (MSH) like sequences which cause pigmentation when levels of ACTH are markedly raised.

Circulating ACTH stimulates cortisol production in the adrenal. The cortisol secreted (or any other synthetic corticosteroid administered to the patient) causes negative feedback on the hypothalamus and pituitary to inhibit further CRH/ACTH release. The set-point of this system clearly varies through the day according to the circadian rhythm, and is usually overridden by severe stress.

Following adrenalectomy or other adrenal damage (e.g. Addison's disease), cortisol secretion will be absent or reduced; ACTH levels will therefore rise.

Mineralocorticoid secretion is mainly controlled by the renin–angiotensin system (see p. 1064).

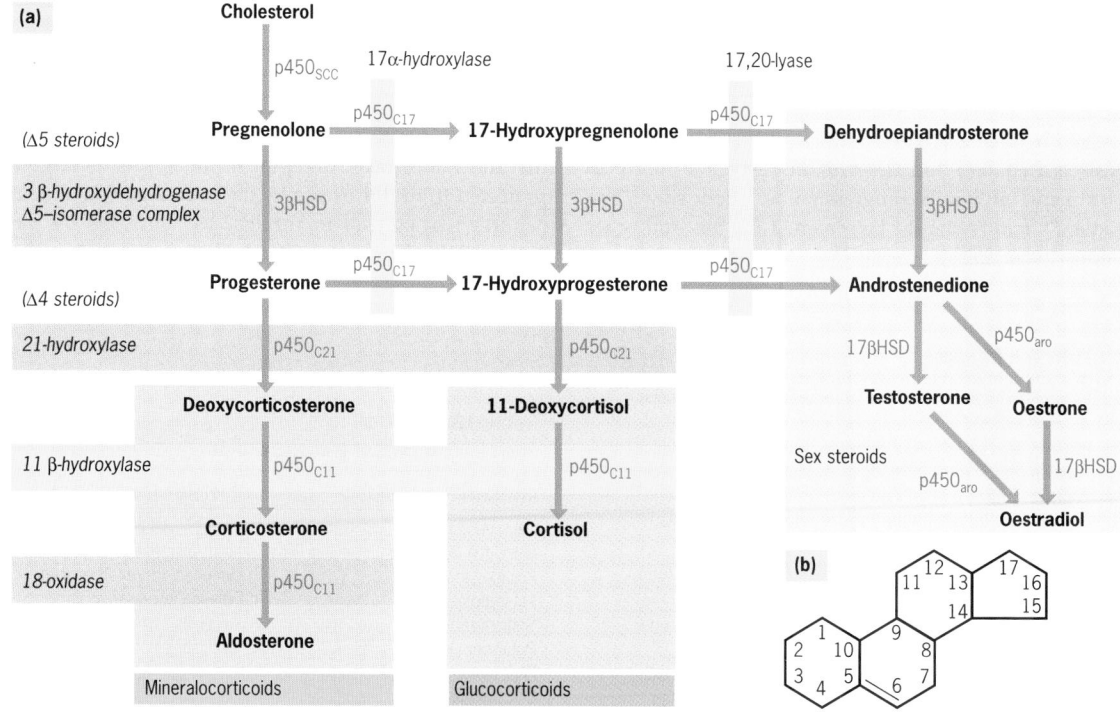

Fig. 18.22 **(a) The major steroid biosynthetic pathways.** Enzymes catalysing reactions are in red: p450 enzymes are in mitochondria and each catalyses several reaction steps; 3βHSD (hydroxysteroid dehydrogenase) is in cytoplasm, bound to endoplasmic reticulum; 17βHSD and p450$_{aro}$ are found mainly in gonads. **(b) The steroid molecule.**

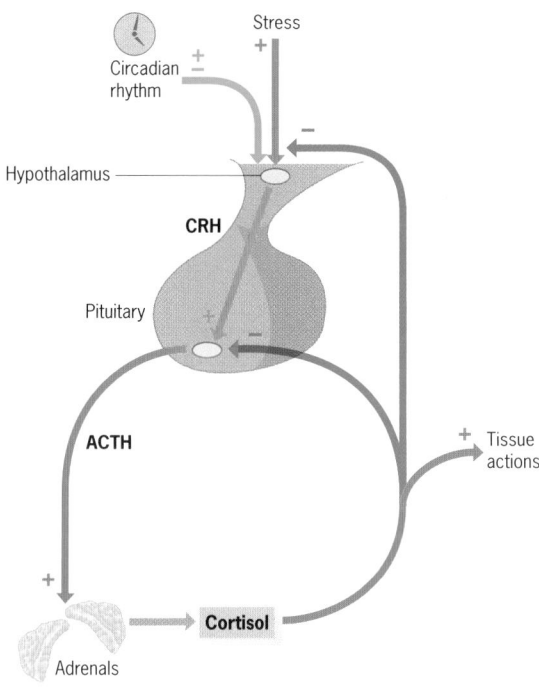

Fig. 18.23 Control of the hypothalamic–pituitary–adrenal axis. CRH, corticotropin-releasing hormone.

In figure labels:
- Circadian rhythm
- Stress
- Hypothalamus
- CRH
- Pituitary
- ACTH
- Tissue actions
- Cortisol
- Adrenals

Investigation of glucocorticoid abnormalities

Basal levels

ACTH and cortisol are released episodically and in response to stress. The following precautions are therefore necessary when taking a blood sample:

- Sampling time should be recorded accurately. Conventionally, basal levels are obtained at between 0800h and 0900h near the peak of the circadian variation.
- Stress should be minimized.
- Sampling should be delayed for 48 hours after admission if Cushing's syndrome is suspected.
- Appropriate reference ranges (for time and assay method) should be used.

Suppression and stimulation tests are used in suspected excess and deficient cortisol production, respectively.

Dexamethasone suppression tests

Administration of a synthetic glucocorticoid to a normal subject produces prompt feedback suppression of CRH and ACTH levels and thus of endogenous cortisol secretion (dexamethasone is not measured by most cortisol assays). Three forms of the test, used in the diagnosis and differential diagnosis of Cushing's syndrome, are available (Table 18.29).

Table 18.29

Details of dexamethasone suppression and ACTH (synacthen) tests in the diagnosis of Cushing's syndrome and Addison's disease

Test and protocol	Measure	Normal test result or positive suppression	Use and explanation
Dexamethasone			
Overnight			
Take 1 mg on going to bed at 2300h	Plasma cortisol at 0900h next morning	Plasma cortisol < 100 nmol/L	Outpatient screening test Some 'false positives'
'Low-dose'			
0.5 mg 6-hourly Eight doses from 0900h on day 0	Plasma cortisol at 0900h on days 0 and +2	Plasma cortisol < 50 nmol/L on second sample	For diagnosis of Cushing's syndrome
'High-dose' used in differential diagnosis			
2 mg 6-hourly Eight doses from 0900h on day 0	Plasma cortisol at 0900h on days 0 and +2	Plasma cortisol on day +2 less than 50% of that on day 0 suggests pituitary-dependent disease	Differential diagnosis of Cushing's syndrome Pituitary-dependent disease suppresses in about 90% of cases
ACTH (synacthen)			
Short			
Tetracosactide 250 μg i.v. or i.m. at time 0	Plasma cortisol at times 0, +30 min	Cortisol at +30 min > 600 nmol/L	To exclude primary adrenal failure
Long			
Depot tetracosactide 1 mg i.m. at time 0	Plasma cortisol at times 0, +1, +2, +3, +4, +5, +8 and +24 h	Maximum > 1000 nmol/L Rise > 550 nmol/L	To demonstrate or exclude adrenal suppression (rather than primary adrenal failure)

Plasma cortisol values are very dependent upon the assay used – local reference ranges must be consulted

ACTH stimulation tests

Synthetic ACTH (tetracosactide, or synacthen, which consists of the first 24 amino acids of human ACTH) is given to stimulate adrenal cortisol production. Details are given in Table 18.29 and Box 18.1 on page 1003.

Addison's disease: primary hypoadrenalism

Pathophysiology and causes

In this condition there is destruction of the entire adrenal cortex. Glucocorticoid, mineralocorticoid and sex steroid production are therefore all reduced. This differs from hypothalamic–pituitary disease, in which mineralocorticoid secretion remains largely intact, being predominantly stimulated by angiotensin II. Adrenal sex steroid production is also largely independent of pituitary action. In Addison's disease reduced cortisol levels lead, through feedback, to increased CRH and ACTH production, the latter being directly responsible for the hyperpigmentation.

Incidence. Addison's disease is rare, with an incidence of 3–4/million/year and prevalence of 40–60/million. Primary hypoadrenalism shows a marked female preponderance and is now most often caused by autoimmune disease (> 90% in UK) rather than tuberculosis (< 10%). All other causes are rare (Table 18.30). Autoimmune adrenalitis results from the destruction of the adrenal cortex by organ-specific autoantibodies, with 21-hydroxylase as the common antigen. There are associations with other autoimmune conditions in the polyglandular autoimmune syndromes Types I and II (e.g. type I diabetes mellitus, pernicious anaemia, thyroiditis, hypoparathyroidism, premature ovarian failure).

Clinical features

These are shown in Figure 18.24. The symptomatology of Addison's disease is often vague and non-specific.

Table 18.30
Causes of primary hypoadrenalism

Autoimmune disease (approx. 90% in UK)	Infiltration
	Malignant destruction
Tuberculosis (< 10% in UK)	Amyloid
Surgical removal	Schilder's disease (adrenal leucodystrophy)
Haemorrhage/infarction	
Meningococcal septicaemia	
Venography	

These symptoms may be the prelude to an Addisonian crisis with severe hypotension and dehydration precipitated by intercurrent illness, accident or operation.

Pigmentation (dull, slaty, grey-brown) is the predominant sign in over 90% of cases.

Postural systolic hypotension, due to hypovolaemia and sodium loss, is present in 80–90% of cases, even if supine blood pressure is normal. Mineralocorticoid deficiency is the cause.

Investigations

Once Addison's disease is suspected, investigation is urgent. If the patient is seriously ill or hypotensive, hydrocortisone 100 mg should be given intramuscularly together with intravenous saline. Ideally this should be done immediately after a blood sample is taken for later measurement of plasma cortisol. Alternatively, an ACTH stimulation test can be performed immediately. Full investigation should be delayed until emergency treatment (see below) has improved the patient's condition. Otherwise, tests are as follows:

- **Single cortisol measurements** are of little value, although a random cortisol below 100 nmol/L during the day is highly suggestive, and a random cortisol > 550 nmol/L makes the diagnosis unlikely (but not impossible).

Symptoms
Weight loss
Anorexia
Malaise
Weakness
Fever
Depression
Impotence/amenorrhoea
Nausea/vomiting
Diarrhoea
Confusion
Syncope from postural hypotension
Abdominal pain
Constipation
Myalgia
Joint or back pain

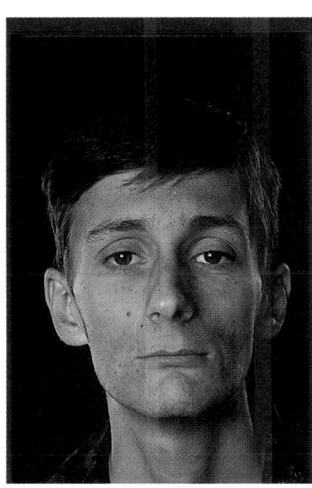

Signs
Pigmentation, especially of new scars and palmar creases
Buccal pigmentation
Postural hypotension
Loss of weight
General wasting
Dehydration
Loss of body hair
(Vitiligo)

Fig. 18.24 **The symptoms and signs of primary hypoadrenalism (Addison's disease).** Bold type indicates signs of greater discriminant value.

- **The short ACTH stimulation test** should be performed (see Table 18.29). An absent or impaired cortisol response is seen, confirmed if necessary by a long ACTH stimulation test to exclude adrenal suppression by steroids or ACTH deficiency.
- **A 0900h plasma ACTH level** – a high level (> 80 ng/L) with low or low-normal cortisol confirms primary hypoadrenalism.
- **Electrolytes and urea** classically show hyponatraemia, hyperkalaemia and a high urea, but they can be normal.
- **Blood glucose** may be low, with symptomatic hypoglycaemia.
- **Adrenal antibodies** are present in many cases of autoimmune adrenalitis.
- **Chest and abdominal X-rays** may show evidence of tuberculosis and/or calcified adrenals.
- **Serum aldosterone** is reduced with high plasma renin activity.
- **Hypercalcaemia and anaemia** (after rehydration) are sometimes seen. They resolve on treatment, but are occasionally the first clue to the diagnosis.

Treatment

Acute hypoadrenalism needs urgent treatment (Emergency box 18.1).

Long-term treatment is with replacement glucocorticoid and mineralocorticoid; tuberculosis must be treated if present or suspected. Replacement dosage details are shown in Table 18.31. Dehydroepiandrosterone (DHEA) replacement has also been advocated, and early studies suggest that this may cause symptomatic improvements, but long-term results are still awaited.

Adequacy of glucocorticoid dose is judged by:

- clinical well-being and restoration of normal, but not excessive, weight
- normal cortisol levels during the day while on replacement hydrocortisone (this cannot be used for synthetic steroids).

Fludrocortisone replacement is assessed by:

- restoration of serum electrolytes to normal
- blood pressure response to posture (it should not fall > 10 mmHg systolic after 2 minutes' standing)
- suppression of plasma renin activity to normal.

Patient advice

All patients requiring replacement steroids should:

- know how to increase steroid replacement dose for intercurrent illness
- carry a 'Steroid Card'
- wear a Medic-Alert bracelet (or similar), which gives details of their condition so that emergency replacement therapy can be given if found unconscious
- keep an (up-to-date) ampoule of hydrocortisone at home in case oral therapy is impossible, and the general practitioner has to be called.

Secondary hypoadrenalism

This may arise from hypothalamic–pituitary disease (inadequate ACTH production) or from long-term steroid therapy leading to hypothalamic–pituitary–adrenal suppression.

Most patients with the former have panhypopituitarism (see p. 1011) and need T_4 replacement as well as cortisol; in this case hydrocortisone must be started before T_4.

Emergency box 18.1

Management of acute hypoadrenalism

- Clinical context: hypotension, hyponatraemia, hyperkalaemia, hypoglycaemia, dehydration, pigmentation often with precipitating infection, infarction, trauma or operation. The major deficiencies are of salt, steroid and glucose.

Assuming normal cardiovascular function, the following are required:

- One litre of normal saline should be given over 30–60 minutes with 100 mg of intravenous bolus hydrocortisone.
- Subsequent requirements are several litres of saline within 24 hours (assessing with central venous pressure line if necessary) plus hydrocortisone, 100 mg i.m., 6-hourly, until the patient is clinically stable.
- Glucose should be infused if there is hypoglycaemia.
- Oral replacement medication is then started, unless unable to take oral medication, initially hydrocortisone 20 mg, 8-hourly, reducing to 20–30 mg in divided doses over a few days (Table 18.31).
- Fludrocortisone is unnecessary acutely as the high cortisol doses provide sufficient mineralocorticoid activity – it should be introduced later.

Table 18.31

Average replacement steroid dosages for adults with primary hypoadrenalism

Drug	Dose
Glucocorticoid	
Hydrocortisone	20–30 mg daily
	e.g. 10 mg on waking, 5 mg at 1200h, 5 mg at 1800h
or	
Prednisolone	7.5 mg daily
	5 mg on waking, 2.5 mg at 1800h
rarely	
Dexamethasone	0.75 mg daily
	0.5 mg on waking, 0.25 mg at 1800h
Mineralocorticoid	
Fludrocortisone	50–300 µg daily

The most common cause of secondary hypoadrenalism is long-term corticosteroid medication for non-endocrine disease. The hypothalamic–pituitary axis and the adrenal may both be suppressed and the patient may have vague symptoms of feeling unwell. The long ACTH stimulation test should demonstrate a delayed cortisol response. Weaning off steroids is often a long and difficult process.

Cushing's syndrome

Cushing's syndrome is the term used to describe the clinical state of increased free circulating glucocorticoid. It occurs most often following the therapeutic administration of synthetic steroids or ACTH (see below). All the spontaneous forms of the syndrome are rare.

Pathophysiology and causes

Spontaneous Cushing's syndrome is rare, with an incidence of < 5/million/year.

Causes of Cushing's syndrome are usually subdivided into two groups (Table 18.32):

- increased circulating ACTH from the pituitary (65% of cases), known as Cushing's disease, or from an 'ectopic', non-pituitary, ACTH-producing tumour elsewhere in the body (10%) with consequential glucocorticoid excess
- a primary excess of endogenous cortisol secretion (25% of spontaneous cases) by an adrenal tumour or nodular hyperplasia, with subsequent (physiological) suppression of ACTH. Rare cases are due to aberrant expression of receptors for other hormones (e.g. GIP, LH or catecholamines) in adrenal cortical cells.

Clinical features

The predominant clinical features of Cushing's syndrome are those of glucocorticoid excess and are illustrated in Figure 18.25.

- *Pigmentation* occurs only with ACTH-dependent causes.
- *A Cushingoid appearance* can be caused by excess alcohol consumption (pseudo-Cushing's syndrome) – the pathophysiology is poorly understood.
- *Impaired glucose tolerance* or frank diabetes are common, especially in the ectopic ACTH syndrome.
- *Hypokalaemia* due to the mineralocorticoid activity of cortisol is common with ectopic ACTH secretion.

Diagnosis

There are two phases to the investigation:

1. confirmation of the presence or absence of Cushing's syndrome
2. differential diagnosis of its cause (e.g. pituitary, adrenal or ectopic).

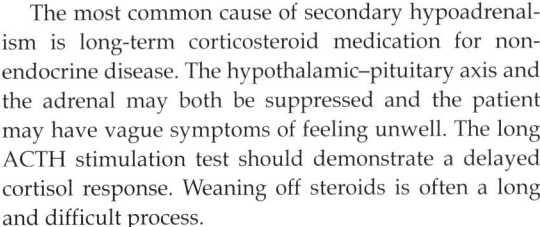

Table 18.32
Causes of Cushing's syndrome

ACTH-dependent disease
Pituitary-dependent (Cushing's disease)
Ectopic ACTH-producing tumours
ACTH administration

Non-ACTH-dependent causes
Adrenal adenomas
Adrenal carcinomas
Glucocorticoid administration

Others
Alcohol-induced pseudo-Cushing's syndrome

Confirmation

Most obese, hirsute, hypertensive patients do not have Cushing's syndrome and some cases of genuine Cushing's have relatively subtle clinical signs. Confirmation rests on demonstrating inappropriate cortisol secretion, not suppressed by exogenous glucocorticoids: difficulties occur with obesity and depression where cortisol dynamics are often abnormal. Random cortisol measurements are of no value. Occasional patients are seen with so-called 'cyclical Cushing's' where the abnormalities come and go.

Investigations to confirm the diagnosis include:

- **48-hour low-dose dexamethasone test** (see Table 18.29). Normal individuals suppress plasma cortisol to < 50 nmol/L. Patients with Cushing's syndrome fail to show complete suppression of plasma cortisol levels (although levels may fall substantially in a few cases). This test is highly sensitive (> 97%). The overnight dexamethasone test is slightly simpler, but has a higher false-positive rate.
- **24-hour urinary free cortisol measurements.** This is simple, but less reliable – repeatedly normal values (corrected for body mass) render the diagnosis most unlikely, but some patients with Cushing's have normal values on some collections (approximately 10%).
- **Circadian rhythm.** After 48 hours in hospital, cortisol samples are taken at 0900h and 2400h (without warning the patient). Normal subjects show a pronounced circadian variation (see Fig. 18.2, p. 1002); those with Cushing's syndrome have high midnight cortisol levels (> 100 nmol/L), though the 0900h value may be normal.
- **Other tests.** There are frequent exceptions to the classic responses to diagnostic tests in Cushing's syndrome. If any clinical suspicion of Cushing's remains after preliminary tests then specialist investigations are still indicated, these may include insulin stress test, desmopressin stimulation test and CRH tests.

Symptoms	Signs	
Weight gain (central)	Moon face	Oedema
Change of appearance	**Plethora**	**Proximal myopathy**
Depression	Depression/psychosis	Proximal muscle
Insomnia	Acne	wasting
Amenorrhoea/	Hirsutism	Glycosuria
oligomenorrhoea	Frontal balding (female)	
Poor libido	**Thin skin**	
Thin skin/easy bruising	**Bruising**	
Hair growth/acne	Poor wound healing	
Muscular weakness	Pigmentation	
Growth arrest in children	Skin infections	
Back pain	**Hypertension**	
Polyuria/polydipsia	Osteoporosis	
Psychosis	**Pathological fractures**	
	(especially vertebrae and ribs)	
Old photographs may	Kyphosis	
be useful	'Buffalo hump'	
	(dorsal fat pad)	
	Central obesity	
	Striae (purple or red)	
	Rib fractures	

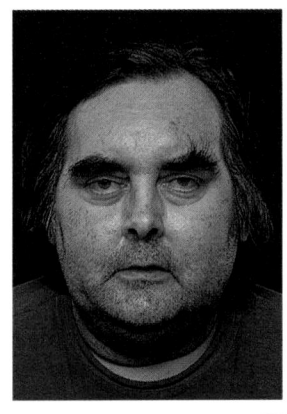
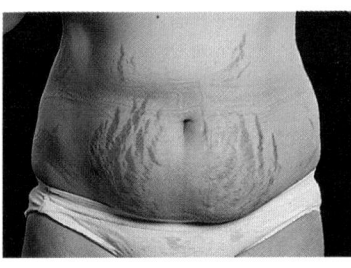

Fig. 18.25 **The symptoms and signs of Cushing's syndrome.** Bold type indicates signs of most value in discriminating Cushing's syndrome from simple obesity and hirsutism.

Differential diagnosis of the cause

This can be extremely difficult since all causes can result in clinically identical Cushing's syndrome. The classical ectopic ACTH syndrome is distinguished by a short history, pigmentation and weight loss, unprovoked hypokalaemia, clinical or chemical diabetes and plasma ACTH levels above 200 ng/L, but many ectopic tumours are benign and mimic pituitary disease closely both clinically and biochemically. Severe hirsutism/virilization suggests an adrenal tumour.

Biochemical and radiological procedures for diagnosis include:

- **Adrenal CT or MRI scan.** Adrenal adenomas and carcinomas causing Cushing's syndrome are relatively large and always detectable by CT scan. Carcinomas are distinguished by large size, irregular outline and signs of infiltration or metastases. Bilateral adrenal hyperplasia may be seen in ACTH-dependent causes or in ACTH-independent nodular hyperplasia.
- **Pituitary MRI.** A pituitary adenoma may be seen but the adenoma is often small and not visible in a significant proportion of cases.
- **Plasma potassium levels.** Hypokalaemia is common with ectopic ACTH secretion. (All diuretics must be stopped.)
- **High-dose dexamethasone test** (Table 18.29). Failure of significant plasma cortisol suppression suggests an ectopic source of ACTH or an adrenal tumour.

- **Plasma ACTH levels.** Low or undetectable ACTH levels (< 10 ng/L) on two or more occasions are a reliable indicator of non-ACTH-dependent disease.
- **CRH test.** An exaggerated ACTH and cortisol response to exogenous CRH suggests pituitary-dependent Cushing's disease, as ectopic sources rarely respond.
- **Chest X-ray** is mandatory to look for a carcinoma of the bronchus or a bronchial carcinoid. Carcinoid lesions may be very small; if ectopic ACTH is suspected, whole-lung and mediastinal CT scanning should be performed.

Further investigations may involve selective catheterization of the inferior petrosal sinus to measure ACTH for pituitary lesions, or blood samples taken throughout the body in a search for ectopic sources. Bronchoscopy, cytology and regional arteriograms are occasionally necessary. Radiolabelled octreotide (^{111}In octreotide) is occasionally helpful in locating ectopic ACTH sites.

Treatment

Untreated Cushing's syndrome has a very bad prognosis, with death from hypertension, myocardial infarction, infection and heart failure. Whatever the underlying cause, cortisol hypersecretion should be controlled prior to surgery or radiotherapy. Considerable morbidity and mortality is otherwise associated with operating on unprepared patients, especially when abdominal surgery is required. The usual drug is metyrapone, an

11β-hydroxylase blocker, which is given in doses of 750 mg to 4 g daily in three to four divided doses. Ketoconazole (200 mg three times daily) is also used and is synergistic with metyrapone. Plasma cortisol should be monitored, aiming to reduce the mean level during the day to 150–300 nmol/L, equivalent to normal production rates. Aminoglutethimide and trilostane (which reversibly inhibits 3β-hydroxysteroid dehydrogenase/δ-5, 4 isomers) are occasionally used.

Choice of further treatment depends upon the cause.

Cushing's disease (pituitary-dependent hyperadrenalism)

- *Trans-sphenoidal removal of the tumour* is the treatment of choice. Selective adenomectomy nearly always leaves the patient ACTH-deficient immediately postoperatively, and this is a good prognostic sign. Overall, pituitary surgery results in remission in 75–80% of cases – but results vary considerably and an experienced surgeon is essential.
- *External pituitary irradiation* alone is slow acting, only effective in 50–60% even after prolonged follow–up and mainly used after failed pituitary surgery. Children, however, respond much better to radiotherapy, 80% being cured.
- *Medical therapy* to reduce ACTH (e.g. bromocriptine, cyproheptadine) is rarely effective.
- *Bilateral adrenalectomy* is an effective last resort if other measures fail to control the disease. Some centres are performing this laparoscopically.

Other causes

Adrenal adenomas should be resected after achievement of clinical remission with metyrapone or ketoconazole. Contralateral adrenal suppression may last for years.

Adrenal carcinomas are highly aggressive and the prognosis is poor. In general, if there are no widespread metastases, tumour bulk should be reduced surgically. The adrenolytic drug op'DDD (Mitotane) may inhibit growth of the tumour and prolong survival, though it can cause nausea and ataxia. Some would also give radiotherapy to the tumour bed after surgery.

Tumours secreting ACTH ectopically should be removed if possible. Otherwise chemotherapy/radiotherapy may be used, depending on the tumour. Control of the Cushing's syndrome with metyrapone, ketoconazole or trilostane (a 3β-hydroxysteroid dehydrogenase) is beneficial for symptoms, and bilateral adrenalectomy may be appropriate to give complete control of the Cushing's syndrome if prognosis from the tumour itself is reasonable.

If the source of ACTH is not clear, cortisol hypersecretion should be controlled with medical therapy until a diagnosis can be made.

Nelson's syndrome

Nelson's syndrome is increased pigmentation (because of high levels of ACTH) associated with an enlarging pituitary tumour, which occurs in about 20% of cases after bilateral adrenalectomy for Cushing's disease. The syndrome is rare now that adrenalectomy is an uncommon primary treatment, and its incidence may be reduced by pituitary radiotherapy soon after adrenalectomy. The Nelson's adenoma may be treated by pituitary surgery and/or radiotherapy (unless given previously).

Incidental adrenal tumours ('incidentalomas')

With the advent of abdominal CT, MRI and high-resolution ultrasound scanning, unsuspected adrenal masses have been discovered in 1% of scans. These obviously include the adrenal tumours described above, but cysts, myelolipomas and metastases are also seen. Functional tests to exclude secretory activity should be performed (adenomas often secrete cortisol at a low level); if none is found then most authorities recommend removal of large (> 4–5 cm) and functional tumours but observation of smaller hormonally inactive lesions.

Congenital adrenal hyperplasia (CAH)
Pathophysiology

This condition results from an autosomal recessive deficiency of an enzyme in the cortisol synthetic pathways. There are six major types, but most common is 21-hydroxylase deficiency which occurs in about 1 in 15 000 births and which has been shown to be due to defects on chromosome 6 near the HLA-region affecting one of the cytochrome p450 enzymes ($p450_{C21}$).

As a result, cortisol secretion is reduced and feedback leads to increased ACTH secretion to maintain adequate cortisol – this in turn leads to diversion of the steroid precursors into the androgenic steroid pathways (see Fig. 18.22(a)). Thus, 17-hydroxyprogesterone, androstenedione and testosterone levels are increased, leading to virilization. Aldosterone synthesis may be impaired with resultant salt wasting.

The other forms affect 11β-hydroxylase, 17α-hydroxylase, 3β-hydroxysteroid dehydrogenase and a cholesterol side-chain cleavage enzyme ($p450_{scc}$) (see Fig. 18.22(a)).

Clinical features

If severe, this presents at birth with sexual ambiguity or adrenal failure (collapse, hypotension, hypoglycaemia), sometimes with a salt-losing state (hypotension, hyponatraemia). In the female, clitoral hypertrophy, urogenital abnormalities and labioscrotal fusion are common, but the syndrome may be unrecognized in the male. Precocious puberty with hirsutism is a later presentation, whereas rare, milder cases only present in adult life, usually accompanied by primary amenorrhoea. Hirsutism developing before puberty is suggestive of CAH.

Investigations

Expert advice is essential in the confirmation and differential diagnosis of 21-hydroxylase deficiency, and with ambiguous genitalia such advice must be sought urgently before any assignment of gender is made.

- 17-Hydroxyprogesterone levels are increased.
- Urinary pregnanetriol excretion is increased.
- Basal ACTH levels are raised.

Treatment

Replacement of glucocorticoid activity, and mineralocorticoid activity if deficient, is as for primary hypoadrenalism (see above). Correct dosage is often difficult to establish in the child but should ensure normal 17-hydroxyprogesterone levels while allowing normal growth; excessive replacement leads to stunting of growth.

Uses and problems of therapeutic steroid therapy

Apart from their use as therapeutic replacement for endocrine deficiency states, synthetic glucocorticoids are widely used for many non-endocrine conditions (Box 18.10). Short-term use (e.g. for acute asthma) carries only small risks of significant side-effects except for the simultaneous suppression of immune responses. The danger lies in their continuance, often through medical oversight or patient default. In general, therapy for 3 weeks or less, or a dose of prednisolone less than 10 mg per day, will not result in significant long-term suppression of the normal adrenal axis.

Long-term therapy with synthetic or natural steroids will, in most respects, mimic endogenous Cushing's syndrome. Exceptions are the relative absence of hirsutism, acne, hypertension and severe sodium retention, as the common synthetic steroids have low androgenic and mineralocorticoid activity.

Excessive doses of steroids may also be absorbed from skin when strong dermatological preparations are used, but inhaled steroids rarely cause Cushing's syndrome, although they commonly cause adrenal suppression.

The major hazards are detailed in Box 18.11. In the long term, many are of such severity that the clinical need for high-dose steroids should be continually and critically assessed. Steroid-sparing agents (e.g. azathioprine) should always be considered and screening and prophylactic therapy for osteoporosis introduced.

Supervision of steroid therapy

All patients receiving steroids should carry a 'Steroid Card'. They should be made aware of the following points:

- Long-term steroid therapy must never be stopped suddenly.
- Doses should be reduced very gradually, with most being given in the morning at the time of withdrawal – this minimizes adrenal suppression. Many authorities believe that 'alternate-day therapy' produces less suppression.

Box 18.10

Common therapeutic uses of glucocorticoids

Respiratory disease
Asthma
Chronic obstructive pulmonary disease
Sarcoidosis
Hayfever (usually topical)
Prevention/treatment of ARDS (see p. 951)

Cardiac disease
Post-myocardial infarction syndrome

Renal disease
Some nephrotic syndromes
Some glomerulonephritides

Gastrointestinal disease
Ulcerative colitis
Crohn's disease
Autoimmune hepatitis

Rheumatological disease
Systemic lupus erythematosus
Polymyalgia rheumatica
Cranial arteritis
Juvenile idiopathic arthritis
Vasculitides
Rheumatoid arthritis

Neurological disease
Cerebral oedema

Skin disease
Pemphigus, eczema

Tumours
Hodgkin's lymphoma
Other lymphomas

Transplantation
Immunosuppression

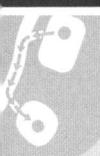

Endocrine disease

- Doses need to be increased in times of serious intercurrent illness (defined as presence of a fever), accident and stress. Double doses should be taken during these times.
- Other physicians, anaesthetists and dentists must be told about steroid therapy.
- Patients should also be informed of potential side-effects and all this information should be documented in the clinical record.

Steroids and surgery

Any patient receiving steroids or who has recently received them (within the last 12 months) and may still have adrenal suppression requires careful control of steroid medication around the time of surgery. Details are shown in Table 18.33.

FURTHER READING

Boscard M et al. (2001) Cushing's syndrome. *Lancet* **357**: 783–791.

Howlett TA (1997) An assessment of optimal hydrocortisone replacement therapy. *Clinical Endocrinology* **46**: 263–268.

Oelkers W (1996) Current concepts: adrenal insufficiency. *New England Journal of Medicine* **335**: 1206–1212.

Oelkers W (1999) Dehydroepiandrosterone for adrenal insufficiency. *New England Journal of Medicine* **341**: 1073–1074.

Box 18.11

Major adverse effects of corticosteroid therapy

Physiological
Adrenal and/or
    pituitary suppression

Pathological
Cardiovascular
Increased blood pressure

Gastrointestinal
Peptic ulceration
    exacerbation (possibly)
Pancreatitis

Renal
Polyuria
Nocturia

Central nervous
Depression
Euphoria
Psychosis
Insomnia

Endocrine
Weight gain
Glycosuria/hyperglycaemia/
    diabetes
Impaired growth
Amenorrhoea

Bone and muscle
Osteoporosis
Proximal myopathy and wasting
Aseptic necrosis of the hip
Pathological fractures

Skin
Thinning
Easy bruising

Eyes
Cataracts (including inhaled
    drug)

**Increased susceptibility to
    infection**
(signs and fever are frequently
    masked)
Septicaemia
Reactivation of TB
Skin (e.g. fungi)

Table 18.33
Steroid cover for operative procedures

Procedure	Premedication	Intra- and postoperative	Resumption of normal maintenance
Simple procedures (e.g. gastroscopy, simple dental extractions)	Hydrocortisone 100 mg i.m.	–	Immediately if no complications and eating normally
Minor surgery (e.g. laparoscopic surgery, veins, hernias)	Hydrocortisone 100 mg i.m.	Hydrocortisone 20 mg orally 6-hourly or 50 mg i.m. every 6 hours for 24 h if not eating	After 24 h if no complications
Major surgery (e.g. hip replacement, vascular surgery)	Hydrocortisone 100 mg i.m.	Hydrocortisone 50–100 mg i.m. every 6 hours for 72 h	After 72 h if normal progress and no complications Perhaps double normal dose for next 2–3 days
GI tract surgery or major thoracic surgery (not eating or ventilated)	Hydrocortisone 100 mg i.m.	Hydrocortisone 100 mg i.m. every 6 hours for 72 h or longer if still unwell	When patient eating normally again Until then, higher doses (to 50 mg 6-hourly) may be needed

The thirst axis

Thirst and water regulation are largely controlled by vasopressin, also known as antidiuretic hormone (ADH), which is synthesized in the hypothalamus, and then migrates in neurosecretory granules along axonal pathways to the posterior pituitary. Pituitary disease alone without hypothalamic involvement therefore does not lead to ADH deficiency as the hormone can still 'leak' from the damaged end of the intact axon.

At normal concentrations the kidney is the predominant site of action of vasopressin. Vasopressin acts via two receptors known as V1 and V2 (p. 672). Stimulation of the V2 receptors allows the collecting tubule to become permeable to water, thus permitting reabsorption of hypotonic luminal fluid. Vasopressin therefore reduces diuresis and results in overall retention of water. At high concentrations vasopressin also causes vasoconstriction via the V1 receptors.

Changes in plasma osmolality are sensed by osmoreceptors in the anterior hypothalamus. Vasopressin secretion is suppressed at levels below 280 mOsm/kg, thus allowing maximal water diuresis. Above this level, plasma vasopressin increases in direct proportion to plasma osmolality. At the upper limit of normal (295 mOsm/kg) maximum antidiuresis is achieved and thirst is experienced at about 298 mOsm/kg (Fig. 18.26).

Other factors affecting vasopressin release are shown in Table 18.34.

Disorders of vasopressin secretion or activity include:

- deficiency as a result of hypothalamic disease ('cranial' diabetes insipidus)
- inappropriate excess of the hormone
- 'nephrogenic' diabetes insipidus – a rare condition in which the renal tubules are insensitive to vasopressin, an example of a receptor abnormality.

While all these are uncommon, they need to be distinguished from the occasional patient with 'primary polydipsia' and those whose renal tubular function has been impaired by electrolyte abnormalities, such as hypokalaemia or hypercalcaemia.

Diabetes insipidus (DI)
Clinical features

Deficiency of vasopressin or insensitivity to its action leads to polyuria, nocturia and compensatory polydipsia. Daily urine output may reach as much as 10–15 L, leading to dehydration that may be very severe if the thirst mechanisms or consciousness are impaired or the patient is denied fluid.

Causes of DI are listed in Table 18.35. The most common is hypothalamic–pituitary surgery, following which transient DI is common, frequently remitting after a few days or weeks. Primary overdrinking (polydipsia) is a common differential diagnosis.

DI may be masked by simultaneous cortisol deficiency – cortisol replacement allows a water diuresis and DI then becomes apparent.

DIDMOAD (Wolfram) syndrome is a rare autosomal recessive disorder comprising Diabetes Insipidus, Diabetes Mellitus, Optic Atrophy and Deafness. MR scanning may show an absent or poorly developed posterior pituitary.

Biochemistry

- High or high-normal plasma osmolality with low urine osmolality (in primary polydipsia plasma osmolality tends to be low)
- Resultant high or high-normal plasma sodium
- High 24-h urine volumes (less than 2 L excludes need for further investigation)
- Failure of urinary concentration with fluid deprivation
- Restoration of urinary concentration with vasopressin or an analogue.

The latter two points may be studied with a formal water-deprivation test (Box 18.12). In normal subjects, plasma osmolality remains normal while urine osmolality rises above 600 mOsm/kg. In DI, plasma osmolality rises while the urine remains dilute, only concentrating after exogenous vasopressin is given (in 'cranial' DI)

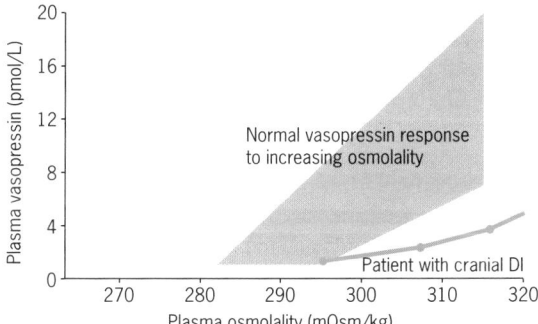

Fig. 18.26 Plasma vasopressin response to increasing osmolality in normal subjects and in a patient with DI.

Table 18.34	
Factors affecting vasopressin release	
Increased by:	**Decreased by:**
Increased osmolality	Decreased osmolality
Hypovolaemia	Hypervolaemia
Hypotension	Hypertension
Nausea	Ethanol
Hypothyroidism	α-Adrenergic stimulation
Angiotensin II	
Epinephrine (adrenaline)	
Cortisol	
Nicotine	
Antidepressants	

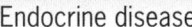
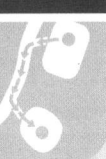

Table 18.35
Causes of diabetes insipidus

Cranial diabetes insipidus	Nephrogenic diabetes insipidus
Familial (e.g. DIDMOAD)	Familial (e.g. vasopressin receptor gene, aquaporin-2 gene defect)
Idiopathic (often autoimmune)	
Tumours	
Craniopharyngioma	Idiopathic
Hypothalamic tumour, e.g. glioma	Renal disease (e.g. renal tubular acidosis)
Metastases, especially breast	Hypokalaemia
Lymphoma/leukaemia	Hypercalcaemia
Pituitary with suprasellar extension (rare)	Drugs (e.g. lithium, demethylchlortetracycline (demeclocycline), glibenclamide)
Infections	
Tuberculosis	
Meningitis	Sickle cell disease
Cerebral abscess	
Infiltrations	
Sarcoidosis	
Langerhans' cell histiocytosis	
Post-surgical	
Transfrontal	
Trans-sphenoidal	
Post-radiotherapy (cranial)	
Vascular	
Haemorrhage/thrombosis	
Sheehan's syndrome	
Aneurysm	
Trauma (e.g. head injury)	

Mild temporary nephrogenic DI can occur after prolonged polyuria due to any cause, including cranial DI and primary polydipsia

---

Box 18.12

Water deprivation test

Indication
Diagnosis or exclusion of diabetes insipidus

Procedure
Fasting and no fluids from wakening (or overnight if only mild DI is expected and polyuria is only modest)
Monitor serum and urine osmolality, urine volume and weight hourly for up to 8 hours
Ideally, monitor osmolalities prospectively during test – proceed to desmopressin administration if serum osmolality > 300 mOsm/kg and/or urine osmolality > 600 mOsm/kg
If osmolalities cannot be monitored, abandon fluid deprivation if weight loss > 3% occurs
Give desmopressin, 2 µg i.m. at end of test. Allow free fluid but measure urine osmolality for 2–4 hours

Normal response
Serum osmolality remains within normal range (275–295 mOsm/kg)
Urine osmolality rises to > 600 mOsm/kg

Diabetes insipidus
Serum osmolality rises above normal without adequate concentration of urine osmolality
Response to desmopressin indicates cranial (pituitary) DI rather than nephrogenic DI

---

or not concentrating after vasopressin if nephrogenic DI is present. This test can give equivocal results and measurement of vasopressin during the test is helpful.

Treatment
The synthetic vasopressin analogue desmopressin (DDAVP) is the treatment of choice. It is given intranasally as a spray 10–20 µg once or twice daily, orally as 200 µg three times daily, or intramuscularly 2–4 µg daily. Response is variable and must be monitored carefully with fluid input/output charts and plasma osmolality measurements. Where there is a reversible underlying cause (e.g. a hypothalamic tumour) this should be treated.

Alternative agents in mild DI, probably working by sensitizing the renal tubules to endogenous vasopressin, include thiazide diuretics, carbamazepine (200–400 mg daily) or chlorpropamide (200–350 mg daily).

Nephrogenic diabetes insipidus
In this condition, renal tubules are resistant to normal or high levels of plasma vasopressin. It may be inherited as a rare sex-linked recessive, with an abnormality in the vasopressin-2 receptor, or as an autosomal post-receptor defect in an ADH-sensitive water channel,

called aquaporin-2. More commonly it can be acquired as a result of renal disease, sickle cell disease, drug ingestion (e.g. lithium), hypercalcaemia or hypokalaemia. Wherever possible the cause should be reversed.

Other causes of polyuria and polydipsia
Diabetes mellitus, hypokalaemia and hypercalcaemia should be excluded. In the case of diabetes mellitus the cause is an osmotic diuresis secondary to glycosuria which leads to dehydration and an increased perception of thirst owing to hypertonicity of the extracellular fluid.

Primary or hysterical polydipsia
This is a relatively common cause of thirst and polyuria. It is a psychiatric disturbance characterized by the excessive intake of water. Plasma sodium and osmolality fall as a result and the urine produced is appropriately dilute. Vasopressin levels become virtually undetectable. Prolonged primary polydipsia may lead to the phenomenon of 'renal medullary washout', with a fall in the concentrating ability of the kidney.

Characteristically the diagnosis is made by a water-deprivation test. A low plasma osmolality is usual at the start of the test, and since vasopressin secretion and action can be stimulated, the patient's urine becomes concentrated (albeit 'maximum' concentrating ability may be impaired); the initially low urine osmolality gradually increases with the duration of the water deprivation.

Syndrome of inappropriate antidiuretic hormone (SIADH)

Clinical features

Inappropriate secretion of ADH leads to retention of water and hyponatraemia. The presentation is usually vague, with confusion, nausea, irritability and, later, fits and coma. There is no oedema. Mild symptoms usually occur with plasma sodium levels below 125 mmol/L and serious manifestations are likely below 115 mmol/L. The elderly may show symptoms with milder abnormalities.

The syndrome must be distinguished from those causing similar dilutional hyponatraemia from excess infusion of dextrose/water solutions or diuretic administration (thiazides or amiloride, see p. 680).

Diagnosis

The usual features are:

- dilutional hyponatraemia due to excessive water retention
- low plasma osmolality with 'inappropriate' urine osmolality which is higher than plasma osmolality
- continued urinary sodium excretion > 30 mmol/L
- absence of hypokalaemia (or hypotension)
- normal renal and adrenal and thyroid function.

The causes are listed in Table 18.36.

Treatment

The underlying cause should be corrected where possible. Symptomatic relief can be obtained by the following measures:

- Fluid intake should be restricted to 500–1000 mL daily. If tolerated, and complied with, this will correct the biochemical abnormalities in almost every case.
- Plasma osmolality and sodium and bodyweight should be measured frequently.
- If water restriction is poorly tolerated or ineffective, demethylchlortetracycline (600–1200 mg daily) may be given; this inhibits the action of vasopressin on the kidney, causing a reversible form of nephrogenic diabetes insipidus. It often, however, causes photosensitive rashes.
- When the syndrome is very severe, rarely hypertonic saline (300 mmol/L slowly i.v.) is given and furosemide (frusemide) may be used. These treatments are potentially dangerous and should only be used with extreme caution.

Disorders of calcium metabolism

Serum calcium levels are mainly controlled by parathyroid hormone (PTH) and vitamin D. Hypercalcaemia is much more common than hypocalcaemia and is frequently detected incidentally with multichannel biochemical analysers. Mild asymptomatic hypercalcaemia occurs in about 1 in 1000 of the population, with an incidence of 25–30 per 100 000 population. It occurs mainly in elderly females, and is usually due to primary hyperparathyroidism (primary HPT).

Parathyroid hormone

There are normally four parathyroid glands which are situated posterior to the thyroid, but occasionally additional glands exist or they may be found elsewhere in the neck or mediastinum. PTH, an 84-amino-acid hormone derived from a 115-residue preprohormone, is secreted from the chief cells of the four parathyroid glands. PTH levels rise as serum ionized calcium falls. The latter is detected by specific calcium-sensing receptors on the plasma membrane of the parathyroid cells. PTH has several major actions, all serving to increase plasma calcium by:

- increasing osteoclastic resorption of bone (occurring rapidly)
- increasing intestinal absorption of calcium (a slow response)
- increasing synthesis of $1,25\text{-}(OH)_2D_3$
- increasing renal tubular reabsorption of calcium
- increasing excretion of phosphate.

PTH effects are mediated at specific membrane receptors on the target cells, resulting in an increase of adenyl cyclase messenger activity.

Table 18.36

Common causes of the syndrome of inappropriate ADH secretion (SIADH)

Tumours	Metabolic causes
Small-cell carcinoma of lung	Alcohol withdrawal
Prostate	Porphyria
Thymus	
Pancreas	**Drugs**
Lymphomas	Chlorpropamide
	Carbamazepine
Pulmonary lesions	Cyclophosphamide
Pneumonia	Vincristine
Tuberculosis	Phenothiazines
Lung abscess	

CNS causes
Meningitis
Tumours
Head injury
Subdural haematoma
Cerebral abscess
SLE vasculitis

PTH measurements

PTH measurements use two-site immunoradiometric assays that measure only the intact PTH molecule; interpretation requires a simultaneous calcium measurement in order to differentiate most causes of hyper- and hypocalcaemia. Urinary cyclic adenosine monophosphate (cyclic AMP) concentration is an index of the bioactivity of PTH. Vitamin D metabolism is discussed on p. 576.

Hypercalcaemia

Pathophysiology and causes

The major causes of hypercalcaemia are listed in Table 18.37; primary hyperparathyroidism and malignancies are by far the most common (> 90% of cases). Hyperparathyroidism itself may be primary, secondary or tertiary. Primary hyperparathyroidism is caused by single (> 80%) parathyroid adenomas or by diffuse hyperplasia of all the glands (15–20%); multiple parathyroid adenomas are rare. Involvement of multiple parathyroid glands may be part of a familial syndrome (e.g. multiple endocrine neoplasia (MEN) syndrome type 1 or 2a). Parathyroid carcinoma is rare (< 1%), though it usually produces severe and intractable hypercalcaemia.

Primary hyperparathyroidism is of unknown cause, though it appears that adenomas are monoclonal. Hyperplasia may also be monoclonal. Chromosomal rearrangements in the 5′ regulatory region of the parathyroid hormone gene have been identified, and inactivation of some tumour suppressor genes at a variety of sites may also be involved.

Secondary hyperparathyroidism (see p. 646) is physiological compensatory hypertrophy of all parathyroids because of hypocalcaemia, such as occurs in renal failure or vitamin D deficiency. PTH levels are raised but calcium levels are low or normal, and PTH falls to normal after correction of the cause of hypocalcaemia where this is possible.

Tertiary hyperparathyroidism is the development of apparently autonomous parathyroid hyperplasia after long-standing secondary hyperparathyroidism, most often in renal failure. Plasma calcium and phosphate are both raised, the latter often grossly so. Parathyroidectomy is necessary at this stage.

Symptoms and signs

Mild hypercalcaemia (e.g. adjusted calcium < 3 mmol/L) is frequently asymptomatic, but more severe hypercalcaemia can produce a number of symptoms:

- *General features.* There may be tiredness, malaise, dehydration and depression.
- *Renal features.* Renal colic from stones, polyuria or nocturia, haematuria and hypertension occur. The polyuria results from the effect of hypercalcaemia on renal tubules, reducing their concentrating ability – a form of mild nephrogenic diabetes insipidus. Primary HPT is present in about 5% of patients who present with renal calculi.
- *Bones.* There may be bone pain. Hyperparathyroidism mainly affects cortical bone, and bone cysts and locally destructive 'brown tumours' occur but only in advanced disease. Only 5–10% of all cases have definite bony lesions even when sought.
- *Abdominal.* There may be abdominal pain, sometimes due to peptic ulceration.
- *Chondrocalcinosis and ectopic calcification.* These are occasional features.
- *Corneal calcification.* This is a marker of long-standing hypercalcaemia but causes no symptoms.

Table 18.37
Causes of hypercalcaemia

Excessive parathormone (PTH) secretion
Primary hyperparathyroidism (commonest by far), adenoma (common), hyperplasia or carcinoma (rare)
Tertiary hyperparathyroidism
Ectopic PTH secretion (very rare indeed)

Malignant disease (second commonest cause)
Myeloma
Secondary deposits in bone
Production of osteoclastic factors by tumours
PTH-related protein secretion

Excess action of vitamin D
Iatrogenic or self-administered excess
Granulomatous diseases, e.g. sarcoidosis, TB
Lymphoma

Excessive calcium intake
'Milk–alkali' syndrome

Other endocrine disease (mild hypercalcaemia only)
Thyrotoxicosis
Addison's disease

Drugs
Thiazide diuretics
Vitamin D analogues
Lithium administration (chronic)
Vitamin A

Miscellaneous
Long-term immobility
Familial hypocalciuric hypercalcaemia

There may also be symptoms from the underlying cause. Malignant disease is usually advanced by the time hypercalcaemia occurs, typically with bony metastases. The common primary tumours are bronchus, breast, myeloma, oesophagus, thyroid, prostate, lymphoma and renal cell carcinoma. True 'ectopic PTH secretion' by the tumour is very rare, and most cases are associated with raised levels of PTH-related protein. This is a 144-amino-acid polypeptide, the initial sequence of which shows an approximate homology with the biologically active part of PTH, which is necessary in fetal development but does not have a clearly defined role in the adult. Local bone resorbing cytokines and prostaglandins may be involved locally where there are metastatic skeletal lesions, leading to local mobilization of calcium by osteolysis with subsequent hypercalcaemia.

Severe hypercalcaemia (> 3 mmol/L) is usually associated with malignant disease, hyperparathyroidism, renal failure or vitamin D therapy.

Investigations and differential diagnosis
Biochemistry

- *Several* fasting serum calcium and phosphate samples should be performed.
- *Serum PTH.* The hallmark of primary hyperparathyroidism is hypercalcaemia and hypophosphataemia with detectable or elevated intact PTH levels during hypercalcaemia. When this combination is present in an asymptomatic patient then further investigation is usually unnecessary.
- There is often a mild *hyperchloraemic acidosis.*
- *Renal function* is usually normal but should be measured as a baseline.

Where PTH is undetectable or equivocal, a number of other tests may lead to the diagnosis

- *Protein electrophoresis:* to exclude myeloma
- *Serum TSH:* to exclude hyperthyroidism
- *0900h cortisol and/or synacthen test:* to exclude Addison's disease
- *Serum ACE:* helpful in the diagnosis of sarcoidosis
- *Hydrocortisone suppression test:* hydrocortisone 40 mg three times daily for 10 days leads to suppression of plasma calcium in sarcoidosis, vitamin D-mediated hypercalcaemia and some malignancies.

Imaging
Abdominal X-rays may show renal calculi or nephrocalcinosis. High-definition hand X-rays can show subperiosteal erosions in the middle or terminal phalanges. DXA bone density scan is useful to detect bone effects in asymptomatic patients with HPT in whom conservative management is planned.

Parathyroid imaging is generally indicated only for patients who have undergone previous parathyroid surgery, as techniques have an overall sensitivity of just 60–70% and a substantial false-positive rate, which is far less accurate than the expert surgical success rate of at least 90%. Methods include:

- ultrasound which, though insensitive for small tumours, is simple and safe
- high-resolution CT scan or MRI (the most sensitive technique)
- radioisotope subtraction scanning – a picture of the parathyroid tissue derived from the difference in uptake between ^{201}Th (taken up by thyroid and parathyroid) and ^{99m}Tc (by thyroid only).

Treatment of hypercalcaemia
Details of emergency treatment for severe hypercalcaemia are given in Emergency box 18.2. Thereafter, treatment is management of the underlying disease.

Treatment of primary hyperparathyroidism
Medical management
There are no effective medical therapies at present for primary hyperparathyroidism, but a high fluid intake should be maintained, a high calcium or vitamin D intake avoided, and exercise encouraged. New therapeutic agents that target the calcium-sensing receptors in the kidney may be of value in the future.

> **Emergency box 18.2**
>
> **Treatment of acute hypercalcaemia**
>
> Acute hypercalcaemia often presents with dehydration, nausea and vomiting, nocturia and polyuria, drowsiness and altered consciousness. The serum Ca^{2+} is over 3 mmol/L and sometimes as high as 5 mmol/L. While investigation of the cause is under way, immediate treatment is mandatory if the patient is seriously ill or if the Ca^{2+} is above 3.5 mmol/L. Specialist help is advised.
>
> - Adequate rehydration is essential – usually at least 4–6 L of saline on day 1, and 3–4 L for several days thereafter. Central venous pressure (CVP) may need to be monitored to control the hydration rate.
> - Intravenous bisphosphonates are now the treatment of choice for hypercalcaemia of malignancy or of undiagnosed cause. Pamidronate is preferred (15–60 mg as an intravenous infusion in 0.9% saline or dextrose over 2–8 hours or, if less urgent, over 2–4 days).
> - Calcitonin (200 units i.v. 6-hourly) has a short-lived action and is now little used.
> - Prednisolone (30–60 mg daily) is effective in some instances (e.g. in myeloma, sarcoidosis and vitamin D excess) but in most cases is ineffective.
> - Oral phosphate (sodium cellulose phosphate 5 g three times daily) produces diarrhoea. Intravenous phosphate rapidly lowers plasma Ca^{2+} but is dangerous and should not be used.

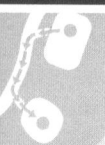
Surgery

Indications for surgery in primary hyperparathyroidism remain controversial. There is agreement that surgery is indicated for:

- patients with renal stones or impaired renal function
- bone involvement or marked reduction in cortical bone density
- unequivocal marked hypercalcaemia (> 3.0 mmol/L)
- the uncommon younger patient, below age 50 years
- a previous episode of severe acute hypercalcaemia.

The situation where plasma calcium is mildly raised (2.65–3.00 mmol/L) is more controversial. Most authorities feel that young patients should be operated on, as should those who have reduced cortical bone density or significant hypercalciuria, as this is associated with stone formation.

In older patients without these problems, or in those unfit for or unwilling to have surgery, conservative management is indicated. Regular measurement of serum calcium and of renal function is necessary. Bone density of cortical bone should be estimated every 3–5 years.

Surgical technique and complications

Parathyroid surgery should be performed only by experienced surgeons, as the minute glands may be very difficult to define, and it is difficult to distinguish between an adenoma and normal parathyroid. In expert centres over 90% of operations are successful, involving removal of the adenoma, or removal of all four hyperplastic parathyroids.

Other than postoperative hypocalcaemia (see below), the other rare complications are those of thyroid surgery – bleeding and recurrent laryngeal nerve palsies (< 1%). Vocal cord function should be checked preoperatively.

If initial exploration is unsuccessful, a full work-up including venous catheterization and scanning is essential, remembering that parathyroid tissue can be ectopic.

Postoperative care

The major danger after operation is hypocalcaemia, which is more common in patients with significant bone disease – the 'hungry bone' syndrome. Some authorities pretreat such patients with alfacalcidol 2 μg daily from 2 days preoperatively for 10–14 days. Chvostek's and Trousseau's signs (see p. 1062) should be checked regularly in all these patients. Plasma calcium measurements are performed daily for at least 2–5 days (more often if low) – a mild transient hypoparathyroidism often continues for 1–2 weeks. Depending on its severity, oral or intravenous calcium (for details see p. 1063) should be given temporarily, as only a few patients (< 1%) will develop long-standing surgical hypoparathyroidism.

Familial hypocalciuric hypercalcaemia

This uncommon autosomal dominant, and usually asymptomatic, condition demonstrates increased renal reabsorption of calcium despite hypercalcaemia. PTH levels are normal or slightly raised and urinary calcium is low. It is caused by mutations in the calcium-ion-sensing G-protein-coupled receptor gene in the kidney and parathyroid gland. In the past it was frequently detected only after operation when removal of hyperplastic glands was unsuccessful in lowering the hypercalcaemia. Family members are often affected and surgery is not indicated as the course appears benign.

Hypocalcaemia and hypoparathyroidism
Pathophysiology

Hypocalcaemia may be due to deficiencies of calcium homeostatic mechanisms, secondary to high phosphate levels or other causes of hypocalcaemia (Table 18.38). All forms of hypoparathyroidism, except transient surgical effects, are uncommon.

Causes

- *Renal failure* is the most common cause of hypocalcaemia.
- *Hypocalcaemia after thyroid or parathyroid surgery* is common but usually transient – fewer than 1% of thyroidectomies leave permanent damage (see above).
- *Idiopathic hypoparathyroidism* is one of the rarer autoimmune disorders, often accompanied by vitiligo, cutaneous moniliasis and other autoimmune disease.

The *DiGeorge syndrome* is a familial condition where the hypoparathyroidism is associated with intellectual impairment, cataracts and calcified basal ganglia, and occasionally with specific autoimmune disease.

Pseudohypoparathyroidism is a syndrome of end-organ resistance to PTH owing to a mutation in the $G_{S\alpha}$-protein which is coupled to the PTH receptor. It is associated with short stature, short metacarpals, subcutaneous calcification and sometimes by intellectual impairment. Variable degrees of resistance involving other G-protein-linked hormone receptors may also be seen (TSH, LH, FSH).

Pseudo-pseudohypoparathyroidism describes the phenotypic defects but without any abnormalities of calcium metabolism. These individuals may share the same gene defect as pseudohypoparathyroidism and occur in the same families.

Clinical features

Hypoparathyroidism presents as neuromuscular irritability and neuropsychiatric manifestations. Paraesthesiae, circumoral numbness, cramps, anxiety and tetany (Box 18.13) are followed by convulsions, laryngeal stridor, dystonia and psychosis. Two signs of hypocalcaemia are Chvostek's sign (gentle tapping over the facial nerve causes twitching of the ipsilateral facial muscles) and Trousseau's sign, where inflation of the sphygmomanometer cuff above systolic pressure for

Table 18.38
Causes of hypocalcaemia

Increased phosphate levels
Chronic renal failure (common)
Phosphate therapy

Hypoparathyroidism
Surgical – after neck exploration (thyroidectomy,
  parathyroidectomy – common)
Congenital deficiency (DiGeorge syndrome)
Idiopathic hypoparathyroidism (rare)
Severe hypomagnesaemia

Vitamin D deficiency
Osteomalacia/rickets
Vitamin D resistance

Resistance to PTH
Pseudohypoparathyroidism

Drugs
Calcitonin
Bisphosphonates

Other
Acute pancreatitis (quite common)
Citrated blood in massive transfusion (not uncommon)
Low plasma albumin, e.g. malnutrition, chronic liver disease
Malabsorption, e.g. coeliac disease

Box 18.13

Causes of tetany

In the presence of alkalosis
Hyperventilation
Excess antacid therapy
Persistent vomiting
Hypochloraemic alkalosis, e.g. primary hyperaldosteronism

In the presence of hypocalcaemia (see Table 18.38)

---

3 minutes induces tetanic spasm of the fingers and wrist. Severe hypocalcaemia may cause papilloedema and frequently a prolonged QT interval on the ECG.

Investigations
The clinical history and picture is usually diagnostic and is confirmed by a low serum calcium (after correction for any albumin abnormality). Additional tests include:

* **serum and urine creatinine** for renal disease
* **PTH levels** in the serum: absent or inappropriately low in hypoparathyroidism, high in other causes of hypocalcaemia
* **parathyroid antibodies** (present in idiopathic hypoparathyroidism)
* **25-hydroxy vitamin D serum level** (low in vitamin D deficiency)
* **X-rays** of metacarpals, showing short fourth metacarpals which occur in pseudo-hypoparathyroidism.

Treatment
Urgency of treatment depends on the severity of the symptoms and the degree of hypocalcaemia. If they are severe with tetany, intravenous calcium is given: 10 mL initially, then 10–40 mL, of 10% calcium gluconate in 1 litre of 150 mmol/L saline over 4–8 hours. Oral calcium supplements 2–10 g daily (40–200 mmol calcium) are rarely sufficient alone.

Alpha-hydroxylated derivatives of vitamin D are preferred for their shorter half-life, and especially in renal disease as the others require renal hydroxylation. Usual daily maintenance doses are 0.25–2 μg for alfacalcidol (1α-OH-D_3). During treatment, plasma calcium must be monitored frequently to detect hypercalcaemia.

FURTHER READING

Al Zahrani A, Levine MA (1997) Primary hyperparathyroidism. *Lancet* **349**: 1233–1238.
Pearce SHS (1998) Calcium homeostasis and disorders of the calcium-sensing receptor. *Journal of the Royal College of Physicians of London* **32**: 10–14.
Strewler GJ (2000) The physiology of parathyroid hormone-related protein. *New England Journal of Medicine* **342**: 177–185.
Thakker RV (2001) Genetic development in hypoparathyroidism. *Lancet* **357**: 974–976.
Toft AD (2000) Surgery for hyperparathyroidism – sooner rather than later. *Lancet* **355**: 1478–1479.

Endocrinology of blood pressure control

The control of blood pressure (BP) is complex, involving neural, cardiac, hormonal and many other mechanisms.

BP is dependent upon cardiac output and peripheral resistance. Although cardiac output can be increased in endocrine disease (e.g. hyperthyroidism), the main role of hormonal mechanisms is control of peripheral resistance and of circulating blood volume. The oral contraceptive pill is a common endocrine cause of mild hypertension.

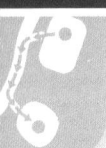

Endocrine disease

When to investigate for secondary hypertension

Endocrine causes account for less than 5% of all hypertension (Table 18.39). It is impracticable and unnecessary to screen all hypertensive patients for secondary causes. The highest chances of detecting such causes are in:

- subjects under 35 years, especially those without a family history of hypertension
- those with accelerated (malignant) hypertension
- those with indications of renal disease (e.g. proteinuria, unequal renal sizes)
- those with hypokalaemia before diuretic therapy
- those resistant to conventional antihypertensive therapy (e.g. more than three drugs)
- those with unusual symptoms (e.g. sweating attacks or weakness).

The renin–angiotensin–aldosterone axis: biochemistry and actions

The renin–angiotensin–aldosterone system is illustrated in Figure 18.27.

Angiotensinogen, an alpha$_2$-globulin of hepatic origin, circulates in plasma. The enzyme, renin, is secreted by the kidney in response to decreased renal perfusion pressure or flow; it cleaves the decapeptide *angiotensin I* from angiotensinogen. Angiotensin I is inactive but is further cleaved by angiotensin-converting enzyme (ACE; present in lung and vascular endothelium) into the active peptide, *angiotensin II*, which has two major actions (mediated by two types of receptor, AT-I and AT-II):

- it causes rapid, powerful vasoconstriction
- it stimulates the adrenal zona glomerulosa to increase aldosterone production.

The vasoconstrictor action of angiotensin II occurs in seconds to minutes, while aldosterone causes sodium retention and urinary potassium loss, leading to increased total body sodium and BP over hours to days.

As BP increases and sodium is retained, the stimuli to renin secretion are reduced. Dietary sodium excess also

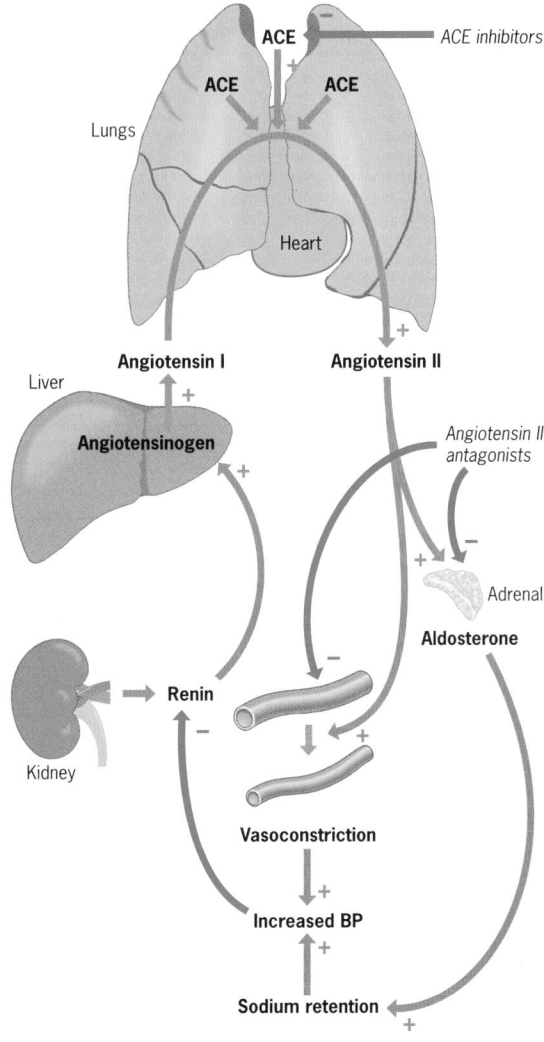

Fig. 18.27 The renin–angiotensin–aldosterone system. ACE, angiotensin-converting enzyme.

Table 18.39
Endocrine causes of hypertension

Excessive renin, and thus angiotensin II, production
Renal artery stenosis
Other local renal disease
Renin-secreting tumours

Excessive production of catecholamines
Phaeochromocytoma

Excessive GH production
Acromegaly

Excessive aldosterone production
Adrenal adenoma (Conn's syndrome)
Idiopathic adrenal hyperplasia
Dexamethasone-suppressible hyperaldosteronism

Excessive production of other mineralocorticoids
Cushing's syndrome (massive excess of cortisol, a weak mineralocorticoid)
Congenital adrenal hyperplasia (in some cases)
Tumours producing other mineralocorticoids, e.g. corticosterone

Exogenous 'mineralocorticoids' or enzyme inhibitors
Liquorice ingestion (inhibits 11β-hydroxylase)
Abuse of mineralocorticoid preparations

suppresses renin secretion, whereas sodium deprivation or urinary sodium loss will increase it.

The renin–angiotensin system can be blocked at several points with renin inhibitors, angiotensin-converting enzyme inhibitors (ACEI) and angiotensin II receptor antagonists (A-IIRA). The latter two are useful agents in treatment of hypertension and heart failure (see pp. 825 and 760) though have differences in action: ACEIs also block kinin production while A-IIRAs are specific for the AT-II receptor.

Atrial and brain natriuretic factors/peptides (ANP and BNP)

Atrial natriuretic peptides, a family of varying length forms, are secreted from atrial granules in response to atrial stretch. They produce marked effects on the kidney, increasing sodium and water excretion and glomerular filtration rate and lowering BP, plasma renin activity and plasma aldosterone (p. 592).

Brain natriuretic peptide is found in the ventricle as well as the brain and has moderate sequence homology with ANP; normally its circulating level is much less than for ANP but may exceed it in congestive cardiac failure.

ANP and BNP appear to play a significant role in cardiovascular and fluid homeostasis, but there is no evidence of primary defects in their secretion causing disease. BNP may accurately reflect the presence and severity of heart failure and appears to be useful in defining prognosis and the need for adjustment of treatment.

It may prove possible to enhance the action of ANP with agents that both inhibit the endopeptidases that break down ANP and inhibit ACE, as the receptors concerned are similar. Long-term clinical studies are awaited.

Renin (and angiotensin) dependent hypertension

Many forms of unilateral and bilateral renal diseases are associated with hypertension. The classic example is renal artery stenosis: the major hypertensive effects of this and other situations such as renin-secreting tumours are directly or indirectly due to angiotensin II.

Angiotensin II receptor antagonists (e.g. losartan, valsartan, candesartan and irbesartan) are effective in hypertension and congestive cardiac failure, though not more so than angiotensin-converting enzyme inhibitors (ACEI), producing much the same clinical effects, though apparently with fewer side-effects (e.g. no cough and less hyperkalaemia).

Renal artery stenosis

This is discussed on page 623.

Disorders of aldosterone secretion

Primary hyperaldosteronism

Pathophysiology

This rare condition (< 1% of all hypertension) is caused by excess aldosterone production leading to sodium retention, potassium loss and the combination of hypokalaemia and hypertension.

Causes (see Table 18.39)

Adrenal adenomas (Conn's syndrome) account for 60% of cases; 30% are due to bilateral adrenal hyperplasia of uncertain aetiology.

Clinical features

The usual presentation is with hypertension and hypokalaemia (< 3.5 mmol/L), although 20–40% of patients have initial potassium levels of 3.5–4.2 mmol/L. The few symptoms are non-specific; rarely muscle weakness, nocturia and tetany are seen. The hypertension may be severe and associated with renal, cardiac and retinal damage.

Adenomas, often very small, are more common in young females, while bilateral hyperplasia rarely occurs before age 40 years and is more common in males.

Investigations

The characteristic features are as follows:

- **Hypokalaemia.** A high-salt diet should be given for several days before testing and diuretics must be stopped 3 weeks before investigation; plasma samples must be separated quickly.
- **Urinary potassium loss.** Levels > 30 mmol daily during hypokalaemia are inappropriate.
- **An elevated plasma aldosterone : renin ratio** is a valuable screening test.
- **Elevated plasma aldosterone levels** that are not suppressed with 0.9% saline infusion (300 mmol over 4 hours) or fludrocortisone administration.
- **Suppressed plasma renin activity.** Beta-blockers and other drugs may interfere with renin activity.

Once a diagnosis of hyperaldosteronism is established, differentiation of adenoma from hyperplasia involves adrenal CT or MRI (not infallible as tumours may be very small), complex biochemical testing including diurnal/postural changes in plasma aldosterone levels (which tend to rise with adenomas between 0900h supine and 1300h erect samples; in contrast they fall with hyperplasia), measurement of 18-OH cortisol levels (raised in adenoma), adrenal scintillation scanning, and venous catheterization for aldosterone levels.

A rare cause is glucocorticoid (or dexamethasone)-suppressible hyperaldosteronism caused by a chimeric gene on chromosome 8. A fusion gene resulting from an unusual cross-over at meiosis between the genes encoding aldosterone synthase and adrenal 11β-hydroxylase produces aldosterone which is under ACTH control. Treatment with glucocorticoid resolves the problem.

Treatment

An adenoma should be removed surgically – often laparoscopically; BP falls in 70% of patients. Those with hyperplasia should be treated with the aldosterone antagonist spironolactone (100–400 mg daily); frequent side-effects include nausea, rashes and gynaecomastia. Amiloride (10–40 mg daily) is a less effective alternative, used especially as spironolactone in long-term use has been linked with tumour development in animals. Calcium-channel blockers are also moderately effective in controlling the hypertension.

Secondary hyperaldosteronism

This situation arises when there is excess renin (and hence angiotensin II) stimulation of the zona glomerulosa. Common causes are accelerated hypertension and renal artery stenosis, when the patient will be hypertensive. Causes associated with normotension include congestive cardiac failure and cirrhosis, where excess aldosterone production contributes to sodium retention.

Angiotensin-converting enzyme inhibitors (e.g. captopril, enalapril or lisinopril), and angiotensin II antagonists (e.g. losartan, irbesartan) are effective in heart failure, both symptomatically and in increasing life expectancy (see p. 760). Spironolactone is of value in both situations, and 25 mg/day has recently been shown to improve survival in heart failure (see p. 760).

Hypoaldosteronism

Except as part of primary hypoadrenalism (Addison's disease, see p. 1050), this is very uncommon. Causes include hyporeninaemic hypoaldosteronism, aldosterone biosynthetic defects, and drugs (e.g. ACE inhibitors, heparin).

The adrenal medulla

The major catecholamines, norepinephrine (noradrenaline) and epinephrine (adrenaline), are produced in the adrenal medulla (Fig. 18.28), although most norepinephrine is derived from sympathetic neuronal release. While norepinephrine and epinephrine undoubtedly produce hypertension when infused, they probably play little part in BP regulation in normal humans.

Phaeochromocytoma

Phaeochromocytomas, tumours of the sympathetic nervous system, are very rare (less than 1 in 1000 cases of

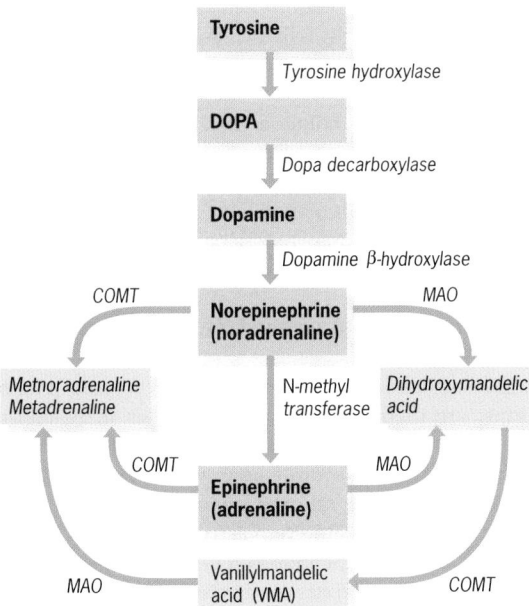

Fig. 18.28 The synthesis and metabolism of catecholamines. COMT, catechol-O-methyl transferase; MAO, monoamine oxidase.

hypertension). Ninety per cent arise in the adrenal, while 10% occur elsewhere in the sympathetic chain. Twenty-five per cent are multiple and 10% are malignant, though this cannot be determined on simple histological examination. Some are associated with MEN 2 syndromes (see below). Most tumours release both norepinephrine (noradrenaline) and epinephrine (adrenaline) but large tumours and extra-adrenal tumours produce almost entirely norepinephrine.

Clinical features

The clinical features are those of catecholamine excess and are frequently, but not necessarily, intermittent (Table 18.40). The diagnosis should particularly be considered when cardiovascular instability has been demonstrated, and in severe hypertension in pregnancy.

Diagnosis

Specific tests are:

- **Measurement of urinary metabolites** (preferably metanephrines rather than vanillylmandelic acid (VMA) – Fig. 18.28) is a useful screening test; normal levels on three 24-hour collections of metanephrines virtually exclude the diagnosis. Many drugs and dietary vanilla interfere with these tests.
- **Plasma and urinary catecholamines** are measured directly.
- **Clonidine suppression and glucagon stimulation** tests may be appropriate, but should only be performed in specialist centres.

Table 18.40
Symptoms and signs of phaeochromocytoma

Symptoms	Signs
Anxiety or panic attacks	Hypertension – intermittent
Palpitations	or constant
Tremor	Tachycardia plus arrhythmias
Sweating	Bradycardia
Headache	Orthostatic hypotension
Flushing	Pallor or flushing
Nausea and/or vomiting	Glycosuria
Weight loss	Fever
Constipation or diarrhoea	(Signs of hypertensive damage)
Raynaud's phenomenon	
Chest pain	
Polyuria/nocturia	

- **CT scans**, initially of the abdomen, are helpful to localize the tumours which are often large.
- **MRI** usually shows the lesion clearly.
- **Scanning with [^{131}I]metaiodobenzylguanidine** (mIBG) produces specific uptake in sites of sympathetic activity with about 90% success. It is particularly useful with extra-adrenal tumours.

Treatment

Tumours should be removed if this is possible; 5-year survival is about 95% where not malignant. Medical preoperative and perioperative treatment is vital and includes complete alpha- and beta-blockade with phenoxybenzamine (20–80 mg daily initially in divided doses), then propranolol (120–240 mg daily), plus transfusion of whole blood to re-expand the contracted plasma volume. The alpha-blockade must precede the beta-blockade, as worsened hypertension may otherwise result. Labetolol is not recommended. Surgery in the unprepared patient is fraught with dangers of both hypertension and hypotension; expert anaesthesia and an experienced surgeon are both vital and sodium nitroprusside should be available in case sudden severe hypertension develops.

When operation is not possible, combined alpha- and beta-blockade can be used long term. Radionucleotide treatment with mIBG has been attempted with limited success.

Patients should be kept under clinical and biochemical review after tumour resection as over 10% recur or develop a further tumour. Catecholamine excretion measurements should be performed at least annually.

FURTHER READING

Bouloux PM, Fakeeh M (1995) Investigation of phaeochromocytoma. *Clinical Endocrinology* **43**: 657–664.
Burnie M, Brunner HR (2000) Angiotensin II receptor antagonists. *Lancet* **355**: 637–645.
Stewart PM (1999) Mineralocorticoid hypertension. *Lancet* **353**: 1341–1347.

Other endocrine disorders

Diseases of many glands

Multiple gland failure (polyglandular autoimmune syndromes)

These are caused by autoimmune disease as detailed in Table 18.4 on page 1007. Most common are the associations of primary hypothyroidism and type 1 diabetes, and either of these with Addison's disease or pernicious anaemia.

Multiple endocrine neoplasia

This is the name given to the simultaneous or metachronous occurrence of tumours involving a number of endocrine glands (Table 18.41). They are inherited in an autosomal dominant manner and arise from the expression of recessive oncogenic mutations, most of which have now been isolated. Affected persons may pass on the mutation to their offspring in the germ cell, but for the disease to become evident a somatic mutation must also occur, such as deletion or loss of a normal homologous chromosome. The defect in MEN 1 is in a novel gene (*menin*) on the long arm of chromosome 11 which encodes for a 610-amino-acid protein. MEN 2a and 2b are caused by mutations of the *Ret*-proto-oncogene on chromosome 10. This gene encodes for a transmembrane glycoprotein receptor. For MEN 2a the mutation is in the extracellular domain, for 2b in the intracellular domain.

Management

Treatment is surgical.

For type 1, all four parathyroid glands are removed (as all may be involved), followed by vitamin D (1,25-dihydrocalciferol) replacement therapy. Pancreatic tumours are often multiple and recurrence after partial pancreatectomy is invariable. Other tumours are treated surgically if necessary.

Type 2 tumours may also be recurrent or bilateral and a careful follow-up is necessary.

Screening

A careful family history should first be taken. If the precise gene mutation has been identified in a particular family, then family members at risk can be screened directly for the presence of the mutation. In affected individuals, biochemical screening is then required. If initial biochemical screening is negative, this does not exclude later involvement and needs repeating at regular (1- to 5-year) intervals.

Screening for type 1

This consists of calcium estimation. If this is elevated, other manifestations of MEN 1 should be sought.

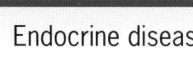

Table 18.41
Multiple endocrine neoplasia (MEN) syndromes

Organ	Frequency	Tumours/manifestations
Type 1		
Parathyroid	95%	Adenomas/hyperplasia
Pituitary	70%	Adenomas – prolactinoma, ACTH or growth hormone secreting (acromegaly)
Pancreas	50%	Islet cell tumours (secreting insulin, glucagon, somatostatin, VIP, pancreatic polypeptide, growth hormone-releasing factor)
		Zollinger–Ellison syndrome (gastrinoma). Non-functional tumour
Adrenal	40%	Non-functional adenoma
Thyroid	20%	Adenomas – multiple or single
Type 2a		
Adrenal	Most	Phaeochromocytoma (70% bilateral)
		Cushing's syndrome
Thyroid	Most	Medullary carcinoma (calcitonin producing)
Parathyroid	60%	Hyperplasia
Type 2b		
Type 2a with Marfanoid phenotype and intestinal and visceral ganglioneuromas but not hyperparathyroidism		

Neuromas also present around lips and tongue

Screening for type 2

- *Medullary carcinoma of thyroid (MCT)* – pentagastrin and calcium infusion test with measurement of calcitonin to pick up 'C' cell hyperplasia. Total thyroidectomy is then indicated to prevent tumour development. With the known presence of the gene defect, total thyroidectomy in childhood is often recommended.
- *Phaeochromocytoma* – metanephrine or catecholamine estimations.

Ectopic hormone secretion

This terminology refers to hormone synthesis, and normally secretion, from a neoplastic non-endocrine cell, most usually seen in tumours that have some degree of embryological resemblance to specialist endocrine cells. The clinical effects may be those of the hormone produced, with or without manifestations of systemic malignancy. The most common situations seen are the following:

- *Hypercalcaemia of malignant disease*, often from squamous cell tumours of lung and breast, often with bone metastases. Where metastases are not present, most cases are mediated by secretion of PTH-related protein (PTHrP), which has considerable sequence homology to PTH; a variety of other factors may sometimes be involved, but very rarely PTH itself (see p. 1061). Treatment is also discussed on page 1061.
- *SIADH* (see p. 1059). Again, this is most common from a primary lung tumour.
- *Ectopic ACTH syndrome* (see p. 1053). Small-cell carcinoma of the lung, carcinoid tumours and medullary thyroid carcinomas are the most common causes, though many other tumours rarely cause it.

- *Production of insulin-like activity* may result in hypoglycaemia (see p. 1103).

Endocrine treatment of other malignancies

Endocrine forms of treatment for malignancy have been used for many years; for example oophorectomy for breast cancer and orchidectomy for prostatic malignancy. More acceptable therapies include the anti-oestrogen tamoxifen for breast carcinoma and the GnRH analogues, buserelin and goserelin, for prostatic cancer.

FURTHER READING

Mulligan LM, Ponder BA (1995) Genetic basis of endocrine disease: MEN type 2. *Journal of Clinical Endocrinology and Metabolism* **80**: 1989–1995.

Shreaves R, Jenkins PJ, Wass JAH (eds) (1997) *Clinical Endocrine Oncology*. Oxford: Blackwell Science.

Trump D et al. (1996) Clinical studies of MEN type 1. *Quarterly Journal of Medicine* **89**: 653–659.

CHAPTER BIBLIOGRAPHY

Besser GM, Thorner MO (1993) *Atlas of Endocrine Imaging*. London: Mosby.

Brook CGD, Hindmarsh PC (2001) *Clinical Paediatric Endocrinology*, 4th edn. Oxford: Blackwell Science.

Conn PM, Melmed S (eds) (1997) *Endocrinology: Basic and Clinical Principles*. New Jersey: Humana Press.

Greenspan FS, Gordon J, Strewler MD (eds) (1997) *Basic and Clinical Endocrinology*, 4th edn. Los Altos: Lange Medical.

Grossman A (ed.) (1997) *Clinical Endocrinology*, 2nd edn. Oxford: Blackwell Science.

Diabetes mellitus and other disorders of metabolism

Hyperglycaemia, insulin and insulin action

Introduction

Diabetes mellitus is a syndrome characterized by chronic hyperglycaemia and relative insulin deficiency, resistance, or both. It affects more than 120 million people world-wide, and it is estimated that it will affect 220 million by the year 2020. Diabetes is usually irreversible and, although patients can have a reasonably normal lifestyle, its late complications result in reduced life expectancy and major health costs. These include macrovascular disease, leading to an increased prevalence of coronary artery disease, peripheral vascular disease and stroke, and microvascular damage causing diabetic retinopathy and nephropathy, and contributing to diabetic neuropathy.

Insulin structure and secretion

Insulin is the key hormone involved in the storage and controlled release within the body of the chemical energy available from food. It is coded for on chromosome 11 and synthesized in the beta-cells of the pancreatic islets. The synthesis, intracellular processing and secretion of insulin by the beta-cell is typical of the way that the body produces and manipulates many peptide hormones. The manufacture and release of insulin from the beta-cell is illustrated in Figure 19.1. Figure 19.2 illustrates the cellular events triggering the release of insulin-containing granules. After secretion, insulin enters the portal circulation and is carried to the liver, its prime target organ. About 50% of secreted insulin is extracted and degraded in the liver; the residue is broken down by the kidneys. C-peptide is only partially extracted by the liver (and hence provides a useful index of the rate of insulin secretion), but is mainly degraded by the kidneys.

An outline of glucose metabolism

Blood glucose levels are closely regulated in health and rarely stray outside the range of 3.5–8.0 mmol/L (63–144 mg/dL), despite the varying demands of food, fasting and exercise. The principal organ of glucose homeostasis is the liver, which absorbs and stores glucose (as glycogen) in the post-absorptive state and releases it into the circulation between meals to match the rate of glucose utilization by peripheral tissues. The liver also combines 3-carbon molecules derived from

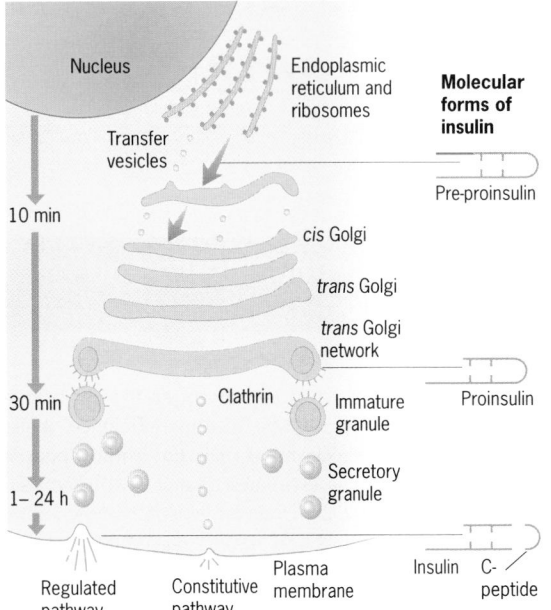

breakdown of fat (glycerol), muscle glycogen (lactate) and protein (e.g. alanine) into the 6-carbon glucose molecule by the process of gluconeogenesis.

Glucose production

About 200 g of glucose is produced and utilized each day. More than 90% is derived from liver glycogen and hepatic gluconeogenesis, and the remainder from renal gluconeogenesis.

Glucose utilization

The brain is the major consumer of glucose. Its requirement is 1 mg/kg bodyweight per minute, or 100 g daily in a 70 kg man. Glucose uptake by the brain is obligatory and is not dependent on insulin, and the glucose used is oxidized to carbon dioxide and water. Other tissues, such as muscle and fat, are facultative glucose consumers. The effect of insulin peaks associated with meals is to lower the threshold for glucose entry into cells; at other times, energy requirements are largely met by fatty-acid oxidation. Glucose taken up by muscle is stored as glycogen or broken down to lactate, which re-enters the circulation and becomes a major substrate for hepatic gluconeogenesis. Glucose is used by fat tissue as a source of energy and as a substrate for triglyceride synthesis; lipolysis releases fatty acids from triglyceride together with glycerol, another substrate for hepatic gluconeogenesis.

Hormonal regulation

Insulin is the major regulator of intermediary metabolism, although its actions are modified in many respects

Fig. 19.1 Part of a beta-cell. The ribosomes manufacture pre-proinsulin from insulin mRNA. The hydrophobic 'pre' portion of pre-proinsulin allows it to transfer to the Golgi apparatus, and is subsequently enzymatically cleaved off. Proinsulin is parcelled into secretory granules in the Golgi apparatus. These mature and pass towards the cell membrane where they are stored before release. The proinsulin molecule folds back on itself and is stabilized by disulphide bonds. The biochemically inert peptide fragment known as connecting (C) peptide splits off from proinsulin in the secretory process, leaving insulin as a complex of two linked peptide chains. Equimolar quantities of insulin and C-peptide are released into the circulation. A small amount of insulin is secreted by the beta-cell directly via the 'constitutive pathway', which bypasses the secretory granules.

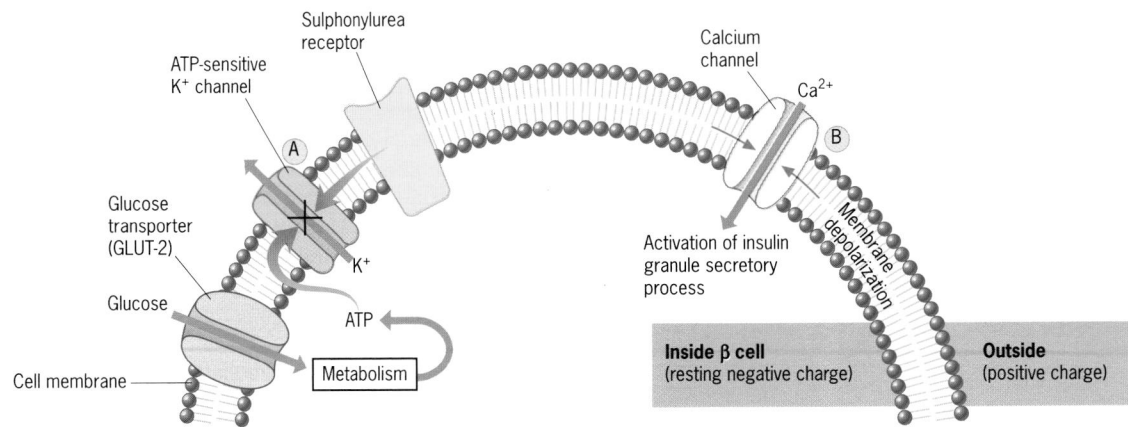

Fig. 19.2 Local forces regulating insulin secretion from beta-cells. Glucose enters the beta-cell via the GLUT-2 transporter protein, which is closely associated with the glycolytic enzyme glucokinase. Metabolism of glucose within the beta-cell generates ATP. ATP closes potassium channels in the cell membrane (A). If a sulphonylurea binds to its receptor, this also closes potassium channels. Closure of potassium channels predisposes to cell membrane depolarization, allowing calcium ions to enter the cell via calcium channels in the cell membrane (B). The rise in intracellular calcium triggers activation of calcium-dependent phospholipid protein kinase which, via intermediary phosphorylation steps, leads to fusion of the insulin-containing granules with the cell membrane and exocytosis of the insulin-rich granule contents. Similar mechanisms operate to cause hormone-granule secretion in many other endocrine cells.

by other hormones. Its actions in the fasting and postprandial states differ (Fig. 19.3). In the fasting state its main action is to regulate glucose release by the liver, and in the postprandial state it additionally facilitates glucose uptake by fat and muscle. The effect of counter-regulatory hormones (glucagon, epinephrine (adrenaline), cortisol and growth hormone) is to cause greater production of glucose from the liver and less utilization of glucose in fat and muscle for a given level of insulin.

Glucose transport

Cell membranes are not inherently permeable to glucose. A family of specialized glucose-transporter (GLUT) proteins carry glucose through the membrane into cells.

- GLUT-1 – enables basal non-insulin-stimulated glucose uptake into many cells.
- GLUT-2 – transports glucose into the beta-cell: a prerequisite for glucose sensing.

- GLUT-3 – enables non-insulin-mediated glucose uptake into brain neurones.
- GLUT-4 – enables much of the peripheral action of insulin. It is the channel through which glucose is taken up into muscle and adipose tissue cells following stimulation of the insulin receptor (Fig. 19.4).

The insulin receptor

This is a glycoprotein (400 kDa), coded for on the short arm of chromosome 19, which straddles the cell membrane of many cells (Fig. 19.4). It consists of a dimer with two alpha-subunits, which include the binding sites for insulin, and two beta-subunits, which traverse the cell membrane. When insulin binds to the alpha-subunits it induces a conformational change in the beta-subunits, resulting in activation of tyrosine kinase and initiation of a cascade response involving a host of other intracellular substrates. One consequence of this is migration of the GLUT-4 glucose transporter to the cell surface and increased transport of glucose into the cell. The insulin–receptor complex is then internalized by the cell, insulin is degraded, and the receptor is recycled to the cell surface.

FURTHER READING

Epstein FH (1999) Glucose transporters and insulin action. *New England Journal of Medicine* **341**: 248–255.

Fasting

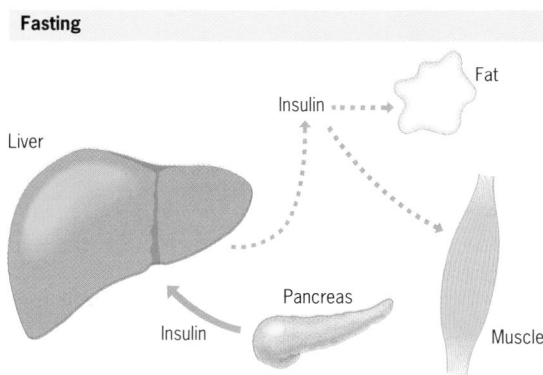

Postprandial

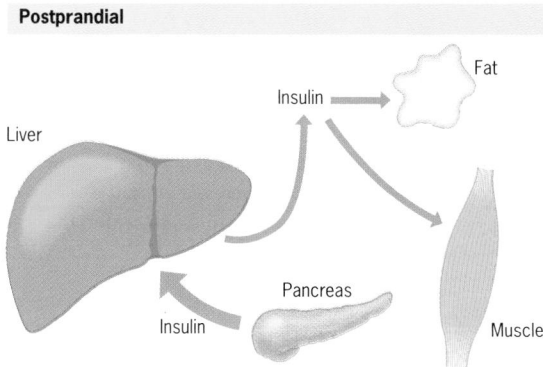

Fig. 19.3 Fasting and postprandial effects of insulin. In the fasting state insulin concentrations are low and it acts mainly as a hepatic hormone, modulating glucose production (via glycogenolysis and gluconeogenesis) from the liver. Hepatic glucose production rises as insulin levels fall. In the postprandial state insulin concentrations are high and it then suppresses glucose production from the liver and promotes the entry of glucose into peripheral tissues (increased glucose utilization).

Types of diabetes

Diabetes may be primary or secondary (Table 19.1). Although secondary diabetes accounts for barely 1–2% of all new cases at presentation, it should not be missed because the cause can often be treated. Type 1 diabetes (insulin-dependent diabetes mellitus) and type 2 diabetes (non-insulin-dependent diabetes mellitus) represent two distinct diseases from the epidemiological point of view, but clinical distinction can sometimes be difficult. The two diseases should, in clinical terms, be seen as a spectrum, distinct at the two ends but overlapping to some extent in the middle (Table 19.2). Varying degrees of insulin secretory failure may be present in both forms of diabetes. This recognizes that some patients with immune-mediated diabetes may not at first require insulin, whereas many with type 2 diabetes will eventually do so.

Type 1 diabetes mellitus
Epidemiology

Type 1 diabetes is a disease resulting in insulin deficiency. In Western countries almost all patients have the immune-mediated form of the disease (type 1A). Type 1

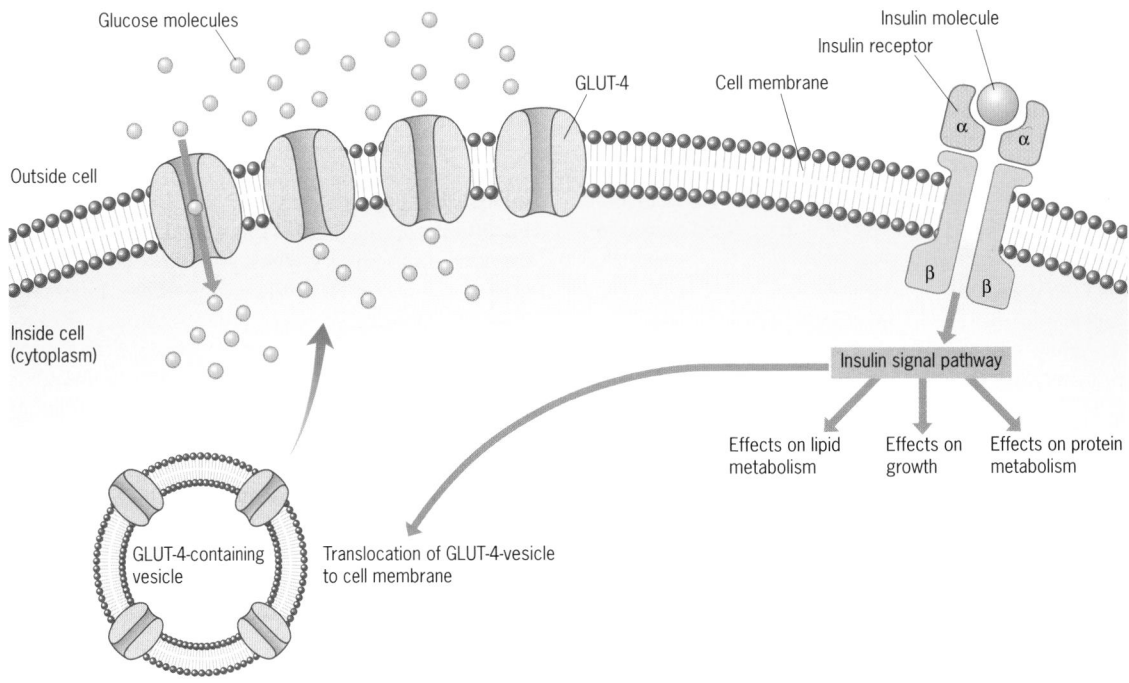

Fig. 19.4 **Insulin signalling in peripheral cells.** The insulin receptor consists of alpha- and beta-subunits linked by disulphide bridges. The beta-subunits straddle the cell membrane. The transporter protein GLUT-4 is stored in intracellular vesicles. The binding of insulin to its receptor initiates many intracellular actions including translocation of these vesicles to the cell membrane, carrying GLUT-4 with them.

Table 19.1
Causes of secondary diabetes

Liver disease	Drug-induced disease
Cirrhosis	Thiazide diuretics
	Corticosteroid therapy
Pancreatic disease	
Cystic fibrosis	**Insulin-receptor**
Chronic pancreatitis	**abnormalities**
Malnutrition-related pancreatic disease	Congenital lipodystrophy
Pancreatectomy	Acanthosis nigricans
Hereditary haemochromatosis	
Carcinoma of the pancreas	**Genetic syndromes**
	Friedreich's ataxia
Endocrine disease	Dystrophia myotonica
Cushing's syndrome	
Acromegaly	
Thyrotoxicosis	
Phaeochromocytoma	
Glucagonoma	

diabetes is prominent as a disease of childhood, reaching a peak incidence around the time of puberty, but can present at any age. A 'slow-burning' variant with slower progression to insulin deficiency occurs in later life and is sometimes called latent autoimmune diabetes of adults (LADA). This may be difficult to distinguish from type 2 diabetes. Clinical clues are considerable weight loss; hyperglycaemia which fails to correct with diet and tablet treatment; the presence of 3+ or more ketonuria at diagnosis, and autoantibody tests indicating autoimmune disease. The highest rates of type 1 diabetes in the world are seen in Finland and other Northern European countries, with the exception of the island of Sardinia, which for unknown reasons has the second highest rate in the world (Fig. 19.5). The incidence of type 1 diabetes appears to be increasing in most populations. In Europe the annual increase is of the order of 3–4%, and is most marked in children under the age of 5 years.

Causes

Type 1 diabetes belongs to a family of HLA-associated immune-mediated organ-specific diseases. Genetic susceptibility is polygenic, with the greatest contribution from the HLA region. Autoantibodies directed against pancreatic islet constituents appear in the circulation within the first few years of life, and predate clinical onset by many years. Autoantibodies are also found in older patients with LADA and predict progression to insulin therapy in this group. A subtype of type 1 diabetes

Table 19.2
The spectrum of diabetes: a comparison of type 1 and type 2 diabetes mellitus

	Type 1 (insulin dependent)	Type 2 (non-insulin dependent)
Epidemiology	Younger (usually < 30 years of age) Usually lean Increased in those of N. European ancestry Seasonal incidence	Older (usually > 30 years of age) Often overweight All racial groups. Increased in peoples of Asian, African, Polynesian and American-Indian ancestry
Heredity	HLA-DR3 or DR4 in > 90% 30–50% concordance in identical twins	No HLA links ~ 50% concordance in identical twins
Pathogenesis	Autoimmune disease: Islet cell antibodies Autoimmunity to glutamic acid decarboxylase (GAD) and IA-2 Insulitis Association with other autoimmune diseases Immunosuppression after diagnosis delays beta-cell destruction	No immune disturbance Insulin resistance
Clinical	Insulin deficiency May develop ketoacidosis Always need insulin	Partial insulin deficiency May develop hyperosmolar state 50% come to need insulin when beta-cells fail after many years
Biochemical	Eventual disappearance of C-peptide	C-peptide persists

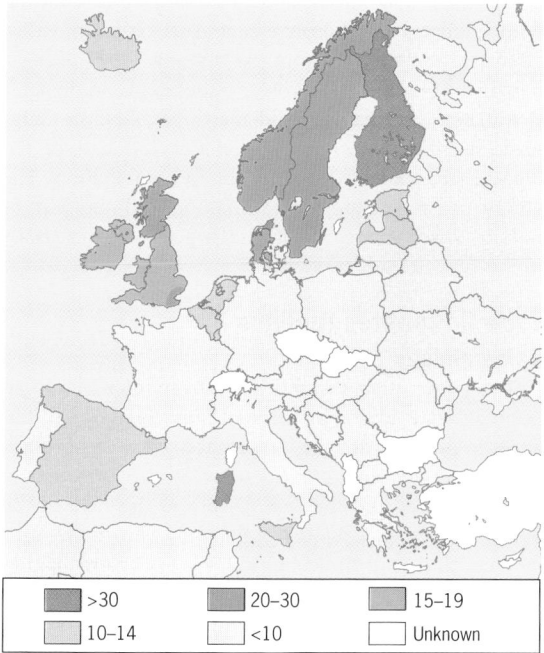

Fig. 19.5 Age-standardized incidence rates of type 1 diabetes (onset 0–14 years) in Europe, per 100 000 per year. From Green A, Gale EAM et al. (1992) *Lancet* **339**: 905–909.

Legend: >30 20–30 15–19 10–14 <10 Unknown

(type 1B) has recently been described in Japanese patients with an abrupt onset, no autoimmune disease and high serum pancreatic enzyme concentrations at diagnosis. This has not been described in other populations.

Genetic susceptibility

Type 1 diabetes is not genetically predetermined, but increased susceptibility to the disease may be inherited.

Inheritance

The identical twin of a patient with type 1 diabetes has a 30–50% chance of developing the disease. Since twins with identical genes may never develop the disease, non-genetic factors must also be involved. The child of an insulin-dependent diabetic patient has an increased chance of developing type 1 diabetes. The risk of developing diabetes by age 20, curiously, is greater with a diabetic father (3–6%) than with a diabetic mother (2–3%). If one child in a family has type 1 diabetes, each sibling has a ~ 6% risk of developing diabetes by age 20. If siblings are HLA-identical (share the same HLA type as the affected child), the risk rises to about 20%. Longer-term follow-up has, however, shown that the lifetime risk of diabetes in first-degree relatives is considerably greater than this.

HLA system. The HLA genes on chromosome 6 are highly polymorphic, and modulate the immune defence system of the body. More than 90% of type 1 diabetes patients carry HLA-DR3 and/or DR4, compared with 35% of the general population. The relative risk conferred by DR3 is about 7, and by DR4 about 9; but DR3/DR4 heterozygotes have a relative risk of 14, showing an additive effect. In contrast, HLA-DR2 is protective. These associations are due to linkage disequilibrium. In other words, the (as yet unknown) genes causing diabetes tend to be transmitted along with these particular HLA types. Even stronger associations have been reported with the DQ region, and substitution of aspartate at position 57 of the HLA-DQ β chain by another amino acid (e.g. in HLA-DQ*0302) considerably increases susceptibility to type 1 diabetes, as do alleles coding for arginine at position 52 on the A chain.

Other gene regions. Genome-wide searches for regions conferring susceptibility to, or protection against, type 1 diabetes have been carried out, and 10–20 regions of interest have been identified. These are designated *IDDM1* (HLA locus), *IDDM2* and so on. It is already clear that individually these make a much smaller contribution to genetic susceptibility than the HLA region. An intensive search to identify these genes and their products is under way.

A DNA region close to the insulin gene on chromosome 11 is designated as *IDDM2*, and short, intermediate and long insertions (see p. 175) have been reported. Homozygosity of the short (class I) allele is found in some 80% of patients with type 1 diabetes as against 40% of controls.

Autoimmunity and insulin-dependent diabetes mellitus

Several pieces of evidence suggest that type 1 diabetes is an immune-mediated disease. These include the HLA associations described above, and associations with other organ-specific autoimmune diseases including autoimmune thyroid disease, Addison's disease and pernicious anaemia. Autopsies of patients who died soon after diagnosis show infiltration of the pancreatic islets by mononuclear cells. This appearance, known as insulitis, resembles that in other autoimmune diseases such as thyroiditis. Autoantibodies directed against islet constituents are also present in some 90% of newly presenting patients. These were first demonstrated by washing serum from newly diagnosed patients across pancreatic sections, and demonstrating the presence of antibodies binding to the islets by immunofluorescence. These were known as islet cell antibodies (ICA), and usually became undetectable within a few years of diagnosis. A number of islet antigens have now been characterized, and include insulin itself, the enzyme glutamic acid decarboxylase (GAD), and the intracellular portion of two islet peptides from the tyrosine phosphatase family (Fig. 19.6). Confirmation of the autoimmune nature of the disease came from the observation that treatment with immunosuppressive agents such as ciclosporin following diagnosis prolongs beta-cell survival.

Environmental factors

The incidence of childhood type 1 diabetes is rising steadily, suggesting that environmental factor(s) are involved in its pathogenesis. Early exposure to enteroviruses such as Coxsackie B4 has often been suspected, but the role of viruses in the causation of the disease has yet to be confirmed.

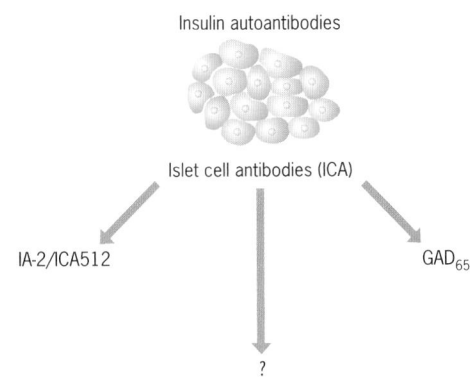

Fig. 19.6 Islet autoantibodies. Islet cell antibodies are detected by a fluorescent antibody technique which detects binding of autoantibodies to islet cells. Much of this staining reaction is due to antibodies specific for glutamic acid decarboxylase (GAD) and protein tyrosine phosphatase – IA-2 (also known as ICA512). Not all the staining seen with ICA is due to these two autoantibodies, so it is assumed that other islet autoantibodies are also involved. Insulin autoantibodies also appear in the circulation but do not contribute to the ICA reaction.

Pre-type 1 diabetes and prevention of type 1 diabetes

Prospective study of first-degree relatives of children with diabetes has shown that islet autoantibodies appear in the circulation in the first few years of life – demonstrating that the process culminating in diabetes is initiated very early – and many years before diagnosis. Further, they can predict development of the disease, especially when present in combination. The ability to predict the disease has opened the way to possible disease prevention, and large multicentre trials of this type are under way.

Type 2 diabetes mellitus
Epidemiology

Unlike type 1 diabetes, this is relatively common in all populations enjoying an affluent lifestyle. Large differences in prevalence exist, presumably because of differences in genetic susceptibility between ethnic groups. In poor countries diabetes is a disease of the rich, but in rich countries it is a disease of the poor. The disease may be present in a subclinical form for years before diagnosis, and the incidence increases markedly with age and degree of obesity. The onset may be accelerated by the stress of pregnancy, drug treatment or intercurrent illness. Estimates of prevalence using the WHO criteria would suggest an overall prevalence of around 2% in the UK. Type 2 diabetes is three to four times as prevalent in people of African and Caribbean ancestry and four to seven times more prevalent in people of Hispanic American origin and in those from South Asia and Arabia living Western lifestyles, than in white Europeans. Indolent well-fed populations are two to twenty times as likely to develop type 2 diabetes as lean populations of the same race. Unfortunately, people in Westernized countries gain on average nearly 1 gram in weight every day of their adult life between the ages of 25–55 years. This gain, due to a tiny excess in energy intake over expenditure – 90 kcal or one chocolate-coated digestive biscuit per day – is the result of reduced exercise in a population rather than of increased food intake. Further, our sedentary lifestyle means that the proportion of obese young adults is rising rapidly, and epidemic obesity will create a huge public health problem for the future. The increasing numbers of obese adolescents presenting with type 2 diabetes is already a matter for concern in the USA and other parts of the world. Diabetes prevalence increases with age and 10% of people of Northern European stock will develop diabetes by the age of 70. This proportion rises towards 30% in those with a family history of diabetes and in those from some ethnic groups.

Causes of type 2 diabetes
Genetics

Early studies in volunteers suggested that identical twins of patients with type 2 diabetes had a greater than 90% chance of developing diabetes, but population-based studies have revised this estimate downwards to 50% or less; the risk to non-identical twins or siblings is of the order of 15–25%. These observations confirm a genetic component to the disease, but suggest that this may have been overestimated in the past. Type 2 diabetes is a polygenic disorder, but the genes responsible for the great majority of cases of type 2 diabetes have yet to be identified. This situation seems set to change,

and as genetic causes are discovered the phenotypic differences between people currently lumped together as having 'type 2 diabetes' will probably be explained.

The genetic causes of some rare forms of type 2 diabetes have, however, emerged over the last 15 years. Dozens of mutations of the insulin receptor have been described but these affect a tiny proportion of all type 2 patients. These usually cause type 2 diabetes with obesity, marked insulin resistance, hyperandrogenism in women and often an area of hyperpigmented skin (acanthosis nigricans). Individuals with some mutations or deletions of mitochondrial DNA develop type 2 diabetes or impaired glucose tolerance, often associated with rare neurological syndromes.

Rare genetic abnormalities affecting the structure of the insulin molecule have been described. These are associated with hyperinsulinaemia and varying degrees of glucose intolerance.

A rare variant of type 2 diabetes is referred to as 'maturity-onset diabetes of the young' (MODY). This is dominantly inherited. Five variants have been described. The different MODY genotypes are associated with different clinical phenotypes (Table 19.3). MODY should be considered in young people presenting with a typical family history (diabetes affecting a parent and 50% expression of the disease in the family) plus a form of early-onset diabetes which appears easy to control.

Environmental factors: early and late

A strong association has been noted between low weight at birth and at 12 months of age and glucose intolerance later in life, particularly in those who gain

Table 19.3
Maturity-onset diabetes of the young (MODY)

	HNF-4a (MODY 1)	Glucokinase (MODY 2)	HNF-1a (MODY 3)	IPF-1 (MODY 4)	HNF-1b (MODY 5)
Chromosomal location	20q	7p	12q	13q	17q
Proportion of all MODY cases	5%	15%	65%	< 1% (MODY)	1%
Clinical features	Onset in teens/twenties	Present from birth	Onset in teens/twenties	?Early adulthood	?Early adulthood
	Progressive hyperglycaemia	Little deterioration with age	Progressive hyperglycaemia	Progression unclear currently	Progression unclear currently
Microvascular complications	Frequent	Rare	Frequent	Few data	Frequent
Non-diabetes-related features	None	Reduced birthweight	Low renal threshold for glucose and aminoaciduria	Pancreatic agenesis in homozygotes	Renal cysts Proteinuria Renal failure

The glucokinase gene is intimately involved in the glucose-sensing mechanism within the pancreatic beta-cell. The hepatic nuclear factor (HNF) genes and the insulin promoter factor-1 (IPF-1) gene control nuclear transcription in the beta-cell where they regulate its development and function. Abnormal nuclear transcription genes may cause pancreatic agenesis or more subtle progressive pancreatic damage

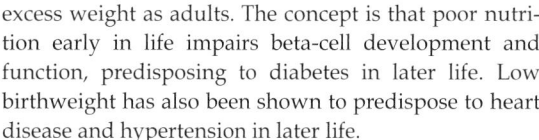

excess weight as adults. The concept is that poor nutrition early in life impairs beta-cell development and function, predisposing to diabetes in later life. Low birthweight has also been shown to predispose to heart disease and hypertension in later life.

Immunology

There is no evidence of immune involvement in the pathogenesis of type 2 diabetes, but as noted earlier a proportion of late-onset patients carry islet autoantibodies – ICA and GAD – at diagnosis, and these are more likely to progress to insulin therapy. Such cases are probably type 1 diabetes masquerading as type 2 diabetes.

Abnormalities of insulin secretion and action

There has been considerable controversy as to the relative importance of secretory failure versus insulin resistance in the pathogenesis of type 2 diabetes, but both factors are involved. Although insulin can bind normally to its receptor on the surface of cells in type 2 diabetes, unknown genetic abnormalities attenuate insulin signalling within the cell, producing 'insulin resistance'. Furthermore, patients with type 2 diabetes cannot secrete enough insulin to overcome this burden of insulin resistance. Depleted numbers of beta-cells are thus in a state of high-output failure. This leads to increased glucose production from the liver (owing to inadequate suppression by insulin) and inadequate uptake of glucose peripherally.

Patients with type 2 diabetes, unlike those with type 1 diabetes, retain about 50% of their beta-cell mass at the time of diagnosis. In addition, almost all show islet amyloid deposition at autopsy, derived from a peptide known as amylin or islet amyloid polypeptide (IAPP) which is co-secreted with insulin. It is not known if this is a cause or consequence of beta-cell secretory failure. Abnormalities of insulin secretion manifest early in the course of type 2 diabetes. Normal subjects have a biphasic insulin response to intravenous glucose, but the first-phase insulin response to it is lost as hyperglycaemia develops, and insulin secretion in response to oral glucose is delayed and exaggerated. The majority of patients manifest reduced insulin secretion relative to the prevailing glucose concentration, and progressive beta-cell loss occurs in many patients, although not to the extent seen in type 1 diabetes. It is not known whether this is due to 'exhaustion' of surviving beta-cells or to some independent process of damage. Obesity is present in 80% of patients with type 2 diabetes, but insulin resistance may also be marked in lean individuals.

Overview and prevention

Whether an individual develops type 2 diabetes or not is largely due to genetic factors. *When* a person develops diabetes is far more important. Diabetes diagnosed between the ages of 40 to 59 can cause a reduction in life expectancy by 5–10 years. In contrast type 2 diabetes diagnosed after the age of 70 has little appreciable effect on life expectancy. Epidemiological studies suggest that keeping slim and taking plenty of exercise has a marked effect in deferring the onset of type 2 diabetes, and may even offer lifelong protection against the disease.

FURTHER READING

EURODIAB ACE Study Group (2000) Variation and trends in incidence of childhood diabetes in Europe. *Lancet* **355**: 873–876.

Gale EAM (2001) The discovery of type 1 diabetes. *Diabetes* **50**: 217–226.

Gerich JE (1998) The genetic basis of type 2 diabetes mellitus: impaired insulin secretion versus impaired insulin sensitivity. *Endocrine Reviews* **19**: 491–503.

Groop LC (1997) Editorial: The molecular genetics of non-insulin-dependent diabetes mellitus. *Journal of Internal Medicine* **241**(2): 95–101.

Hattersley AT (1998) Maturity-onset diabetes of the young: clinical heterogeneity explained by genetic heterogeneity. *Diabetic Medicine* **15**: 15–24.

Hoppener JWM, Ahren B, Lips CJM (2000) Islet amyloid and type 2 diabetes mellitus. *New England Journal of Medicine* **343**: 411–419.

Jung RT (1997) Obesity as a disease. *British Medical Bulletin* **53**: 307–321.

King H, Aubert RE, Herman WH (1998) Global burden of diabetes 1995–2025: prevalence, numerical estimates and projections. *Diabetes Care* **21**: 1414–1431.

Lernmark A (1999) Type 1 diabetes. *Clinical Chemistry* **45**: 1331–1338.

Whitelaw DC, Gilbey SG (1998) Insulin resistance. *Annals of Clinical Biochemistry* **35**: 567–583.

Clinical presentation of diabetes

Acute and subacute presentations often overlap.

Acute presentation

Young people often present with a 2- to 6-week history and report the classic triad of symptoms:

- polyuria – due to the osmotic diuresis that results when blood glucose levels exceed the renal threshold
- thirst – due to the resulting loss of fluid and electrolytes
- weight loss – due to fluid depletion and the accelerated breakdown of fat and muscle secondary to insulin deficiency.

Ketoacidosis may be the presenting feature if these early symptoms are not recognized and treated in a type 1 diabetes patient.

Subacute presentation

The clinical onset may be over several months or years, particularly in older patients. Thirst, polyuria and weight loss are usual features, but medical attention is sought for such symptoms as lack of energy, visual blurring (owing to glucose-induced changes in refraction), or pruritus vulvae or balanitis that is due to *Candida* infection.

Complications as the presenting feature

These include:

- staphylococcal skin infections
- retinopathy noted during a visit to the optician
- a polyneuropathy causing tingling and numbness in the feet
- impotence
- arterial disease, resulting in myocardial infarction or peripheral gangrene.

Asymptomatic diabetes

Glycosuria or a raised blood glucose may be detected on routine examination (e.g. for insurance purposes) in individuals who have no symptoms of ill-health. Glycosuria is not diagnostic of diabetes but indicates the need for further investigations. About 1% of the population have renal glycosuria. This is an inherited low renal threshold for glucose, transmitted either as a Mendelian dominant or recessive trait.

Physical examination at diagnosis

This is often unrewarding in younger patients, but evidence of weight loss and dehydration may be present, and the breath may smell of ketones. Older patients may present with established complications, and the presence of the characteristic retinopathy is diagnostic of diabetes. In occasional patients there will be physical signs of an illness causing secondary diabetes (Table 19.1).

Diagnosis and investigation of diabetes

The diagnosis is usually simple. Blood glucose is so closely controlled by the body that even small deviations become important.

- In *symptomatic* patients, a single elevated plasma glucose ≥ 11 mmol/L, measured by a reliable method, indicates diabetes.
- In *asymptomatic or mildly symptomatic* patients, the diagnosis is made on:
  (a) two, fasting venous plasma glucose levels above 7.0 mmol/L (126 mg/dL); OR
  (b) two, random values ≥ 11.1 mmol/L (200 mg/dL) in venous plasma.
- A glucose tolerance test (Box 19.1) is only needed for borderline cases.

Impaired glucose tolerance

Two per cent of the population will be found to have unsuspected diabetes on an oral glucose tolerance test. Five per cent or more will fall into an intermediate category referred to as 'impaired glucose tolerance' (IGT). This is not a clinical entity but a risk factor for future diabetes and cardiovascular disease. The criteria for this category are given in Box 19.1. On follow-up, only 2–4% yearly will have gone on to develop diabetes. Obesity and lack of regular physical exercise make progression to frank diabetes more likely. The classification is complicated by the poor reproducibility of the oral glucose tolerance test. The group is heterogeneous; some patients are obese, some have liver disease, and others are on medication that impairs glucose tolerance.

Box 19.1

New WHO diagnostic criteria – 1999

New WHO criteria are:

- Fasting plasma glucose > 7.0 mmol/L (126 mg/dL)
- Random plasma glucose > 11.1 mmol/L (200 mg/dL)
- One abnormal laboratory value is diagnostic in symptomatic individuals; two values are needed in asymptomatic people.

The glucose tolerance test is only required for borderline cases and for diagnosis of gestational diabetes.

The glucose tolerance test – WHO criteria

	Normal	Impaired glucose tolerance	Diabetes mellitus
Fasting	Less than 7.0 mmol/L	Less than 7.0 mmol/L	More than 7.0 mmol/L
2 h after glucose	Less than 7.8 mmol/L	Between 7.8 and 11.0 mmol/L	11.1 mmol/L or more

- Adult: 75 g glucose in 300 mL water.
- Child: 1.75 g glucose/kg bodyweight.
- Only a fasting and a 120-min sample are needed.
- Results are for venous plasma – whole blood values are lower.

Note: There is no such thing as mild diabetes. All patients who meet the criteria for diabetes are liable to disabling long-term complications.

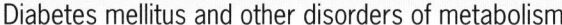
Individuals with IGT have the same increased risk of cardiovascular disease as people with frank diabetes (twice that of people with normal glucose tolerance), but they do not develop the specific microvascular complications of diabetes. A new category of 'impaired fasting glucose' has been delineated on screening by fasting glucose alone. This category only overlaps with IGT to a limited extent, and therefore the associated risk of cardiovascular disease and future diabetes is not directly comparable.

Other investigations

No further tests are needed to diagnose diabetes. Other routine investigations include screening the urine for protein, a full blood count, urea and electrolytes, liver biochemistry and random lipids. The latter test is useful to exclude an associated hyperlipidaemia and, if elevated, should be repeated fasting after diabetes has been brought under control. Diabetes may be secondary to other conditions (see Table 19.1), may be precipitated by underlying illness and be associated with auto-immune disease or hyperlipidaemia. Hypertension is present in one-third of European patients with type 2 diabetes and in 50% of African and Caribbean patients.

Treatment of diabetes

The role of patient education and community care

The care of diabetes is based on self-management by the patient, who is helped and advised by those with specialized knowledge. The quest for improved glycaemic control has made it clear that whatever the technical expertise applied, the outcome depends on willing cooperation by the patient. This in turn depends on an understanding of the risks of diabetes and the potential benefits of glycaemic control and other measures such as maintaining a lean weight, stopping smoking and taking care of the feet. If accurate information is not supplied, misinformation from friends and other patients will take its place. For this reason the best time to educate the patient is at the time of diagnosis. Organized education programmes will involve all healthcare workers, including nurse specialists, dietitians and chiropodists.

Diet

The diet for a diabetic patient is in principle no different from the diet considered healthy for the population as a whole.

Carbohydrate

This should consist of unrefined carbohydrate rather than simple sugars such as sucrose. Carbohydrate is absorbed relatively slowly from fibre-rich foods, preventing the rapid swings in circulating glucose seen when refined sugars are ingested. For example, the glucose peak seen in the blood after eating an apple is much flatter than that seen after drinking the same amount of carbohydrate as apple juice.

The *glycaemic index* is the ratio of the area under the blood glucose curve after eating a particular food divided by the area after taking the same amount of carbohydrate as glucose. Foods with a lower glycaemic index generally aid the metabolic control of diabetes.

Calories

Calories should be tailored to the needs of the diabetic patient. The total amount of carbohydrate in the diet should provide 50–55% of the total calories, with fat approximately 30% and protein 15%.

- An overweight patient is started on a reducing diet of approximately 4–6 MJ (1000–1600 kcal) daily.
- A lean patient is put on an isocaloric diet.
- Patients who are underweight because of untreated diabetes require energy supplementation.

Prescribing a diet

Most people find it extremely difficult to modify their eating habits, and repeated advice and encouragement are needed if this is to be achieved. A diet history is taken, and the diet prescribed should involve the least possible interference with the lifestyle of the patient. Patients on insulin or oral agents should be advised to eat the same amount at the same time each day. Patients on insulin require snacks between meals and at bedtime to buffer the effect of injected insulin. Alcohol is not forbidden, but its energy content should be taken into account. Patients on insulin should be warned to avoid alcoholic binges since these may precipitate severe hypoglycaemia.

Tablet treatment for type 2 diabetes

Diet and lifestyle changes are the key to successful treatment of type 2 diabetes. If satisfactory metabolic control (see 'Measuring control' below) of diabetes is not established by these measures after several weeks, then tablets may be needed in addition. Tablets should only be introduced after the patient has witnessed the improvement obtained by changes in diet and lifestyle – this will establish the concept that controlling diabetes is not just a matter of swallowing tablets.

Sulphonylureas (Table 19.4)

Their principal action is to promote insulin secretion in response to glucose and other secretagogues.

Sulphonylureas close ATP-sensitive potassium channels on the beta-cell membrane, and the resulting depolarization promotes calcium influx, a signal for insulin release (see Fig. 19.2). Sulphonylureas were in addition believed to increase insulin sensitivity in peripheral tissues, but this view is now largely discounted. Sulphonylureas are therefore ineffective in patients without a functional beta-cell mass and should be avoided in young ketotic patients, who require early

Table 19.4
Properties of the most commonly used sulphonylureas

Drug	Features
Tolbutamide	Lower maximal efficacy than other sulphonylureas
	Short half-life – preferable in elderly
	Largely metabolized by liver – can use in renal impairment
Glibenclamide	Long biological half-life
	Active metabolites
	Renal excretion – avoid in renal impairment
Gliclazide	Fairly long biological half-life
	Largely metabolized by liver – can use in renal impairment
	More costly
Chlorpropamide	Very long biological half-life
	Renal excretion – avoid in renal impairment
	1–2% develop inappropriate ADH-like syndrome
	Facial flush with alcohol
	Very inexpensive – important issue for developing countries

insulin therapy, and they are usually avoided in pregnancy (p. 1101). However, recently glibenclamide which does not cross the human placenta, has been used in pregnancy. Insulin should be substituted during major surgery or severe intercurrent illness.

Sulphonylureas should be used with care in patients with liver disease, and only those primarily excreted by the liver should be given to patients with renal impairment. All encourage weight gain and are therefore not drugs of first choice in obese patients. Tolbutamide is the safest drug in the very elderly because of its short duration of action. Glimepiride is a more recently developed sulphonylurea with similar potency to other agents but with the advantage of once-daily administration.

Drug interactions and side-effects. All sulphonylureas bind to circulating albumin and may be displaced by other drugs, such as sulphonamides, that compete for their binding sites. They interact with warfarin.

Hypoglycaemia is the most common and dangerous side-effect. Because the action of many sulphonylureas persists for more than 24 hours, recurrent or prolonged hypoglycaemia is likely, and hospital admission is advisable. Skin rashes and other sensitivity reactions do rarely occur.

Biguanides

The mechanism of action of metformin remains unclear but it reduces gluconeogenesis, thus suppressing hepatic glucose output, and it increases insulin sensitivity. Unlike the sulphonylureas it does not induce hypoglycaemia in normal volunteers. It is usually reserved for patients in middle or old age, particularly for the overweight since it does not promote weight gain. It may be given in combination with sulphonylureas when a single agent has proved to be ineffective.

Its side-effects include anorexia, epigastric discomfort and diarrhoea. A barium enema should never be ordered without testing the effect of stopping metformin! Lactic acidosis has occurred in patients with severe hepatic or renal disease, and metformin is contraindicated when these are present.

Alpha-glucosidase inhibitors

An alternative approach to the treatment of overweight patients with type 2 diabetes is to use drugs which inhibit the enzymes involved in the breakdown of carbohydrates in the intestine. Acarbose is a sham sugar that competitively inhibits alpha-glucosidase enzymes situated on the brush border of the intestine. As a result, dietary carbohydrate is poorly absorbed, and the postprandial rise in blood glucose is reduced. Undigested starch may as a result enter the large intestine where it is broken down by fermentation. Abdominal discomfort, flatulence and diarrhoea can result, and dosage needs careful adjustment to avoid these side-effects. Very little acarbose enters the circulation, since it is mainly inactivated in the gut, but liver dysfunction may rarely occur with high doses.

Thiazolidinediones

The thiazolidinediones (more conveniently known as the 'glitazones') reduce insulin resistance by interaction with peroxisome proliferator-activated receptor-gamma (PPAR-gamma), a nuclear receptor which regulates genes involved in lipid metabolism and insulin action. Two different heterozygous mutations which damage the function of PPAR-gamma have been found in a small number of patients who all have severe insulin resistance, type 2 diabetes mellitus and hypertension at an unusually early age. These loss-of-function mutations provide genetic evidence that this receptor is important in the control of insulin sensitivity and blood pressure in humans. The paradox that glucose metabolism should respond to a drug that binds to nuclear receptors mainly found in fat cells is still not fully understood. One suggestion is that they act indirectly via the glucose–fatty acid cycle, lowering free fatty acid levels and thus promoting glucose consumption by muscle.

The glitazones lower circulating insulin relative to plasma glucose, but do not return glucose levels to normal. This might explain why they appear more useful in combination with other agents than when used alone. The glitazones reduce hepatic glucose production, an effect that is synergistic with that of metformin, and also enhance peripheral glucose uptake. They thus potentiate the effect of endogenous insulin. As monotherapy, their glucose-lowering effect is similar to or less than that of other oral agents.

Troglitazone, the first agent in this class, was withdrawn because of problems with hepatic toxicity. Rosiglitazone and pioglitazone are currently licensed in the UK and USA. Two-monthly liver function tests are recommended for the first year of treatment. In the UK the licence is limited to use as combination therapy with either a sulphonylurea or metformin. They appear to be useful in patients who cannot tolerate metformin. They tend to cause weight gain and to cause a degree of salt and water retention. Anaemia is an occasional side-effect. The place of this group of agents is not yet clear, owing to the paucity of comparative controlled clinical trials.

New drugs for type 2 diabetes

Repaglinide is the first of a new class of insulin secretagogues known as the meglitinides. Meglitinide itself is the non-sulphonylurea moiety of glibenclamide. As with the sulphonylureas, it acts via closure of the K^+-ATP channel in the beta-cells (Fig. 19.2), although its receptor-binding characteristics are different. Repaglinide is a short-acting agent that promotes insulin secretion in response to meals, and which might thus reduce between-meal hypoglycaemia. It is more expensive than standard sulphonylureas. Whether it has advantages over established short-acting sulphonylureas such as tolbutamide has not been addressed by clinical trials.

Orlistat causes fat malabsorption by rendering intestinal lipase enzymes less effective, and therefore reducing the absorption of fat from the diet; it may therefore be regarded as the 'rich man's tapeworm'. It can contribute to weight loss in patients who are already under careful dietary supervision, possibly because it has the effect of inducing unpleasant steatorrhoea in those who do not curtail their fat intake. Its place in diabetes management remains unclear.

Insulin treatment

Insulin is found in every creature with a backbone, and the central part of the molecule shows few species differences. Small differences in the amino acid sequence may alter the antigenicity of the molecule. Beef insulin differs from human insulin by three amino acids and readily induces antibody formation, whereas pork insulin, which differs by only one amino acid, is relatively non-immunogenic.

Soluble insulins

Animal insulins are still used widely in developing countries but have now largely been replaced in most of the West by biosynthetic human insulin. This is produced by adding a DNA sequence coding for proinsulin into cultured yeast or bacterial cells. The proinsulin is subsequently enzymatically cleaved to insulin.

Soluble human or animal insulins have a pharmacodynamic profile which only roughly approximates to the effect of natural insulin in normal people (Fig. 19.7). These are the standard insulins for use in multiple dose regimens and for continuous intravenous infusion in labour and during medical emergencies. Soluble human or animal insulin formulations have a number of

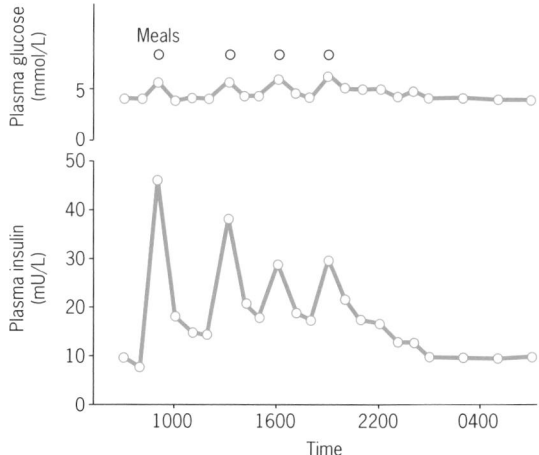

Fig. 19.7 Glucose and insulin profiles in normal subjects.

limitations. The short-acting preparations enter the circulation too slowly, reaching a peak 60–90 minutes after injection, and their effect persists too long after meals predisposing to hypoglycaemia. This delay in absorption is due mainly to the fact that soluble insulin forms hexamers, in which six insulin molecules form around a zinc core. These hexamers are too big to be easily absorbed from subcutaneous tissues and dissociate relatively slowly following injection.

It has been known for many years that insulin can be delivered by other routes, including inhalation, and early clinical trials suggest that this may become a feasible means of maintenance therapy. Various methods are in development, but the principle is to disperse the insulin into particles sufficiently fine to reach the alveoli. The main limitation is that only about 10% of the inhaled dose reaches the circulation, and this is likely to have cost implications.

Rapid-acting insulin analogues

The recombinant DNA technology which allowed the manufacture of human insulin has led to the development of insulin analogues, in which the structure of the insulin molecule is modified in such a way as to change its pharmacokinetics without altering the biological effect. Insulin analogues such as insulin lispro and insulin aspart have a modification of small numbers of the amino acids on the B chain producing insulins which dissociate much more rapidly from hexamers, and thus enter the circulation more rapidly, and equally importantly disappear from the circulation more rapidly, than soluble insulin (Fig. 19.8).

Prolonged-acting insulins

- *Protamine* or zinc can be added to human and animal insulins to aid the formation of insulin crystals. Crystals dissolve slowly; insulin

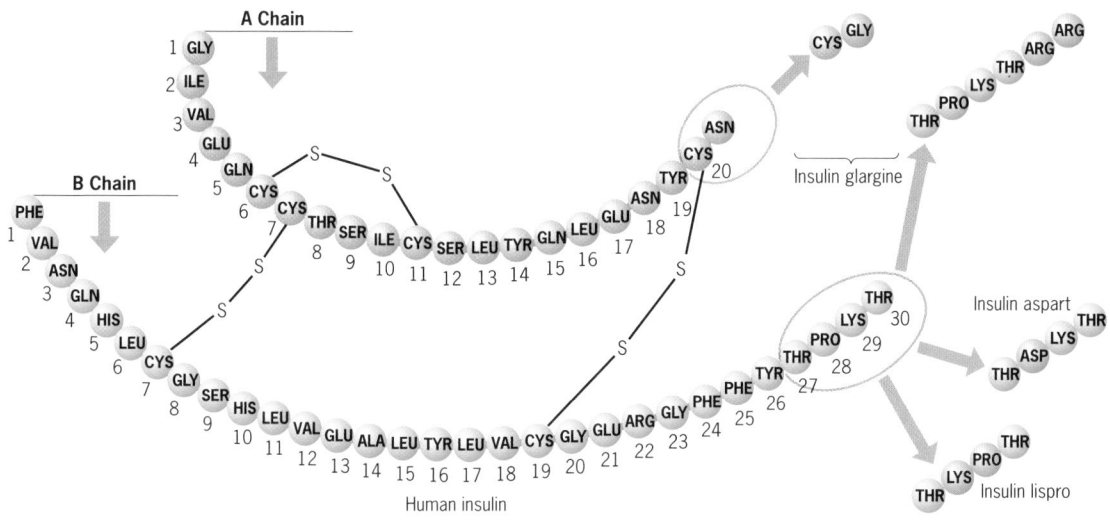

Fig. 19.8 Amino acid structure of human insulin. Lispro is a genetically engineered rapidly acting insulin analogue created by reversing the order of the amino acids proline and lysine in positions 28 and 29 of the B chain. Insulin aspart is a similar analogue created by replacing proline at position 28 of the B chain with an aspartic acid residue. Insulin glargine is a genetically engineered long-acting insulin created by replacing asparagine in position 21 of the A chain with a glycine residue and adding two arginines to the end of the B chain.

prepared in this way is cloudy in appearance. Protamine or NPH (neutral protamine Hagedorn) insulin, also known as isophane insulin, can be premixed with soluble insulin to form stable mixtures. A range of these mixtures is available, but the combination of 30% soluble with 70% NPH is the most widely used.

- *Zinc* insulins are prepared by precipitation of insulin crystals in the presence of excess zinc. The duration of action of the insulin is proportional to the size of the crystals. Since an excess of zinc is present in the vial, these insulins cannot be premixed with soluble insulin, but both zinc and protamine insulins can be mixed in the syringe with soluble insulin immediately prior to injection.

- *Insulin glargine* has its structure modified (Fig. 19.8) to reduce its solubility at physiological pH, thus prolonging its duration of action. It is injected as a slightly acidic (pH 4) solution and then precipitates in the tissues. The precipitates then dissolve slowly from the injection site, giving the preparation a longer duration of action and a less peaked concentration profile in the blood than conventional long-acting insulins.

Practical management of diabetes

All patients with diabetes require diet therapy. Good glycaemic control is unlikely to be achieved with insulin or oral therapy when diet is neglected, especially when the patient is also overweight.

Regular exercise helps to control weight and reduces cardiovascular risk. Walking instead of using transport, gardening regularly, renting an allotment or getting a dog are all more likely to provide prolonged benefit than buying membership to a gym or 'health club'.

Type 2 diabetes

The great majority of patients presenting over the age of 40 will have type 2 diabetes. An approach to their management is illustrated in Figure 19.9. Diet alone should be tried in the first instance, and dietary knowledge and compliance should always be reassessed with care before proceeding to the next step. This is of particular importance in the obese patient who fails to lose weight.

In type 2 diabetes there is a progressive secretory failure of the beta-cells. The diabetes slowly worsens over years and those patients who are initially adequately controlled with diet, or diet and a tablet, will need gradual increases of their treatment over time, even when adhering well to their diet. An annual review is a convenient way of ensuring that a regular review, and increment, of treatment occurs. For most patients tablets will eventually fail to achieve adequate metabolic control and a change to insulin treatment will become necessary. The most widespread error in management at this stage is procrastination; the patient whose control is inadequate on oral therapy should start insulin without undue delay. (Consider insulin in all type 2 patients if $HbA_{1c} > 9\%$ and in selected cases when $HbA_{1c} > 8\%$.)

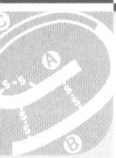

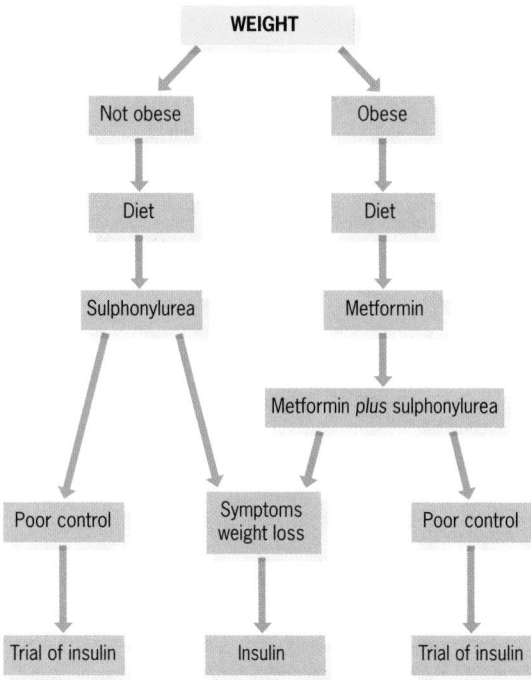

Fig. 19.9 **Conventional treatment pathway for type 2 diabetes.** Diet is the first line of treatment, followed by metformin for the overweight and a sulphonylurea for the lean. Sulphonylureas and insulin should be used with caution in the obese since they predispose to weight gain. (See p. 1079 regarding the use of thiazolidinediones.)

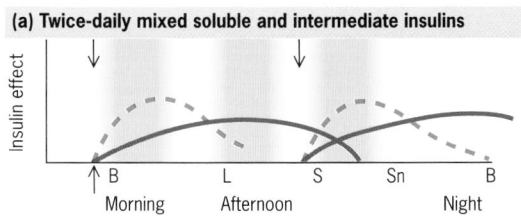

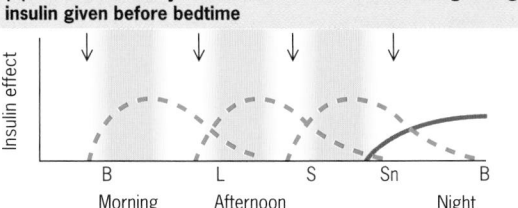

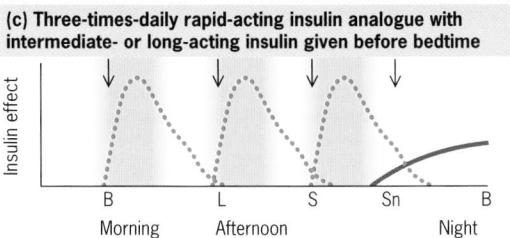

Fig. 19.10 **Insulin regimens.** Profiles of soluble insulins are shown as dashed lines, intermediate- or long-acting insulin as solid lines and rapid-acting insulin analogues as dotted lines. The arrows indicate when the injections are given. B, breakfast; L, lunch; S, supper; Sn, snack (bedtime).

There is little consensus regarding insulin therapy in type 2 diabetes, but an intermediate insulin given at night with metformin during the day is initially as effective as multidose insulin regimens in controlling glucose levels, and is less likely to promote weight gain. A second morning dose of insulin may become necessary to control postprandial hyperglycaemia. Twice-daily injections of premixed soluble and isophane insulins (e.g. Mixtard or Humulin M insulins) are widely used and reasonably effective (Fig. 19.10a). More aggressive treatment, such as with multiple injections or pumps, may be justified in younger patients with type 2 diabetes.

Type 1 diabetes

Insulin is always indicated in a patient who has been in ketoacidosis, and is usually indicated in patients who present under the age of 40 years.

Principles of insulin treatment

Injections

The needles used to inject insulin are very fine and sharp. Even though most injections are virtually painless, patients are understandably apprehensive and treatment begins with a lesson in injection technique.

Insulin is usually administered by a pen injection device but can be drawn up from a vial into special plastic insulin syringes marked in units (100 U in 1 mL). Injections are given into a pinch on the skin on the abdomen, thighs or upper arm, and the needle is usually inserted to its full length. Five types of needle are available for pen injection devices. Adults usually use a 30 gauge 8 mm needle; children a 31 gauge 6 mm needle. Both reusable and disposable pen devices are available.

The injection site used should be changed regularly to prevent areas of lipohypertrophy. The rate of insulin absorption depends on local subcutaneous blood flow, and is accelerated by exercise, local massage or a warm environment. Absorption is more rapid from the abdomen than from the arm, and is slowest from the thigh. All these factors can influence the shape of the insulin profile.

All patients need careful training for a life with insulin. This is best achieved outside hospital whilst living that life, provided that adequate facilities exist for outpatient diabetes education. A scheme for adjusting insulin regimens is given in Table 19.5.

Table 19.5
Guide to adjusting insulin dosage according to blood glucose test results

	Blood glucose persistently too high	Blood glucose persistently too low
Before breakfast	Increase evening long-acting insulin	Reduce evening long-acting insulin
Before lunch	Increase morning short-acting insulin	Reduce morning short-acting insulin or increase mid-morning snack
Before evening meal	Increase morning long-acting insulin or lunch short-acting insulin	Reduce morning long-acting insulin or lunch short-acting insulin or increase mid-afternoon snack
Before bed	Increase evening short-acting insulin	Reduce evening short-acting insulin

Insulin administration

In normal subjects a sharp increase in insulin occurs after meals; this is superimposed on a constant background of secretion (Fig. 19.7). Insulin therapy attempts to reproduce this pattern, but ideal control is usually impossible to achieve for four reasons:

- In normal subjects, insulin is secreted directly into the portal circulation and reaches the liver in high concentration; about 50% of the insulin produced by the pancreas is cleared by the liver. In contrast, insulin injected subcutaneously passes into the systemic circulation before passage to the liver. Insulin-treated patients therefore have lower portal levels of insulin and higher systemic levels relative to the physiological situation.
- Subcutaneous soluble insulin takes 60–90 minutes to achieve peak plasma levels, so the onset and offset of action are too slow.
- The absorption of subcutaneous insulin into the circulation is variable. The longer-acting the preparation, the more erratic the absorption.
- Basal insulin levels are constant in the normal state, but injected insulin invariably peaks and declines, with resulting swings in metabolic control.

Young people with type 1 diabetes can be started on injections of an intermediate-acting insulin at a dose of 8–10 U twice-daily. Some recovery of endogenous insulin secretion may occur over the first few months (the 'honeymoon period') and the insulin dose may need to be reduced or even stopped for a period. Requirements rise thereafter and a multiple injection regimen with soluble insulin and an intermediate-acting insulin at night is then appropriate for most younger patients (Fig. 19.10b). The advantages of multiple injection regimens are that the insulin and the food go in at roughly the same time so that meal times and sizes can vary, without greatly disturbing metabolic control. The flexibility of multiple injection regimens is of great value to patients with busy jobs, shift workers and those who travel regularly. Some type 1 diabetes patients will opt for twice-daily mixed insulin injections (Fig. 19.10a) and put up with the lifestyle restrictions that this

imposes (with twice-daily regimens, the size and timing of meals is fixed more rigidly). Target blood glucose values should normally be 4–7 mmol/L before meals, 4–10 mmol/L after meals. Practical advice on insulin adjustment is given in Table 19.5.

When to use insulin analogues

Hypoglycaemia between meals and particularly at night is the limiting factor for many patients on multiple injection regimens. The more expensive rapid-acting insulin analogues (Fig. 19.10c) are a useful substitute for soluble insulin in some patients. Curiously, they offer particular benefit in reducing the frequency of nocturnal hypoglycaemia owing to reduced carry-over effect from the day-time. High or erratic morning blood sugar readings can prove a problem for about a quarter of all patients on conventional multiple injection regimens, because of waning of the bedtime intermediate-acting insulin and variable absorption. The long-acting insulin analogue insulin glargine and others in development hold promise of improving this problem.

Infusion devices

CSII (continuous subcutaneous insulin infusion) is delivered by a small pump strapped around the waist that infuses a constant trickle of insulin via a needle in the subcutaneous tissues. Meal-time doses are delivered when the patient touches a button on the side of the pump.

This approach is particularly useful in the overnight period, especially since the basal overnight infusion rate can be programmed to fit each patient's needs. Disadvantages include the nuisance of being attached to a gadget, skin infections, and the risk of ketoacidosis if the flow of insulin is broken (since these patients have no protective reservoir of depot insulin). Infusion pumps should only be used by specialized centres able to offer a round-the-clock service to their patients.

Complications of insulin therapy

At the injection site

Shallow injections result in intradermal insulin delivery and painful, reddened lesions or even scarring. Injection site abscesses occur but are extremely rare.

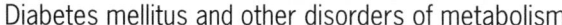
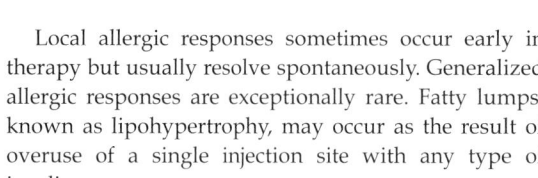

Local allergic responses sometimes occur early in therapy but usually resolve spontaneously. Generalized allergic responses are exceptionally rare. Fatty lumps, known as lipohypertrophy, may occur as the result of overuse of a single injection site with any type of insulin.

Insulin resistance

The most common cause of mild insulin resistance is obesity. Occasional unstable patients require massive insulin doses, often with a fluctuating requirement. There are often associated behavioural problems. Insulin resistance associated with antibodies directed against the insulin receptor has been reported in patients with acanthosis nigricans.

Weight gain

Many patients show weight gain on insulin treatment, especially if the insulin dose is increased inappropriately – insulin makes you feel hungry! Sticking to a careful dietary regimen is particularly important when on insulin. As a general rule the heavier a patient is when starting insulin, and the heavier they have been in the past, the more weight they tend to gain.

Whole pancreas and pancreatic islet transplantation

Transplantation of a whole pancreas at the time of kidney or heart transplantation has been undertaken as a research procedure in small numbers of cases for 20 years. A few patients have been able to become free of insulin injections for a year or two, but the majority have not. The whole pancreas graft adds risk to the transplant procedure: graft pancreatitis, abscess formation, septicaemia. All patients still need daily cytotoxic drug treatment to prevent graft rejection.

A research centre in Edmonton, Canada, has recently had greater success in transplanting pancreatic islets, isolated from cadavers, into the liver bed of small numbers of type 1 diabetic patients. In early 2001, 13 of 15 patients had become free of insulin injections for over 1 year, but still needed daily cytotoxic drug treatment to prevent graft rejection. Much research effort is being expended in seeing if these results can be duplicated in other centres and in larger numbers of patients.

FURTHER READING

Chandalia M, Garg A, Lutjohann D et al. (2000) Beneficial effects of high dietary fibre intake in patients with type 2 diabetes mellitus. *New England Journal of Medicine* **342**: 1392–1398.

DeFronzo RA (1999) Pharmacologic therapy for type 2 diabetes mellitus. *Annals of Internal Medicine* **131**: 281–303.

Frost G, Dornhorst A (2000) The relevance of the glycaemic index to our understanding of dietary carbohydrates. *Diabetic Medicine* **17**: 336–345.

Owens DA, Zinman B, Bolli GB (2001) Insulins today and beyond. *Lancet* **358**: 739–746.

Rendell M (2000) Dietary treatment of diabetes mellitus. *New England Journal of Medicine* **342**: 1440–1441.

Schoonjans K, Auwerx J (2000) Thiazolidinediones: an update. *Lancet* **355**: 1008–1010.

Shapiro AMJ, Lakey JRT, Ryan EA et al. (2000) Islet transplantation in seven patients with type 1 diabetes mellitus using a glucocorticoid-free immunosuppressive regimen. *New England Journal of Medicine* **343**: 230–238.

Hypoglycaemia during insulin treatment

This is the most common complication of insulin therapy, and limits what can be achieved with insulin treatment. It is a major cause of anxiety for patients and relatives. Symptoms develop when the blood glucose level falls below 3 mmol/L and typically develop over a few minutes, with most patients experiencing 'adrenergic' features of sweating, tremor and a pounding heartbeat. Physical signs include pallor and a cold sweat. Many patients with long-standing diabetes report loss of these warning symptoms and are at a greater risk of progressing to more severe hypoglycaemia. Such patients appear pale, drowsy or detached, signs that their relatives quickly learn to recognize. Behaviour is clumsy or inappropriate, and some become irritable or even aggressive. Others slip rapidly into hypoglycaemic coma. Occasionally, patients develop convulsions during hypoglycaemic coma, especially at night. This must not be confused with idiopathic epilepsy, particularly as patients with frequent hypoglycaemia often have abnormalities on the electroencephalogram. Another presentation is with a hemiparesis that resolves within a few minutes when glucose is administered.

Hypoglycaemia is a common problem. Virtually all patients experience intermittent symptoms and one in three will go into a coma at some stage in their lives. A small minority suffer attacks that are so frequent and severe as to be virtually disabling. Hypoglycaemia results from an imbalance between injected insulin and a patient's normal diet, activity and basal insulin requirement. The times of greatest risk are before meals and during the night. Irregular eating habits, unusual exertion and alcohol excess may precipitate episodes; other cases appear to be due simply to variation in insulin absorption.

Hypoglycaemic unawareness. People with diabetes have an impaired ability to counter-regulate glucose levels after hypoglycaemia. The glucagon response is invariably deficient, even though the alpha-cells are preserved and respond normally to other stimuli. The epinephrine (adrenaline) response may also fail in patients with a long duration of diabetes, and this is associated with loss of warning symptoms. Recurrent hypoglycaemia may itself induce a state of hypoglycaemia unawareness, and the ability to recognize the condition may sometimes be restored by relaxing control for a few weeks.

Nocturnal hypoglycaemia. Basal insulin requirements fall during the night but increase again from about 4 a.m. onwards, at a time when levels of injected insulin are falling. As a result many patients awake with high blood glucose levels, but find that injecting more insulin at night increases the risk of hypoglycaemia in the early hours of the morning. The problem may be helped by (a) checking that a bedtime snack is taken regularly, (b) for patients taking twice daily mixed insulin to separate their evening dose and take the intermediate insulin at bedtime rather than before supper, (c) reducing the dose of soluble insulin before supper, since the effects of this persist well into the night, and (d) changing patients on a multiple injection regimen with soluble insulin to a rapid-acting insulin analogue. The new longer-acting insulin analogues with a flatter profile of action overnight may also prove of value.

Urgent treatment of hypoglycaemia

Patients and their families quickly learn to recognize and treat the symptoms of hypoglycaemia.

Mild hypoglycaemia

Any form of rapidly absorbed carbohydrate will relieve the early symptoms, and sufferers should always carry glucose or sweets. Drowsy individuals will be able to take carbohydrate in liquid form (e.g. Lucozade). All patients and their close relatives need careful training about the risks of hypoglycaemia. They should be warned not to take more carbohydrate than necessary, since this causes a rebound to hyperglycaemia. The dangers of alcohol excess and hypoglycaemia while driving need to be emphasized.

Severe hypoglycaemia

The diagnosis of severe hypoglycaemia resulting in confusion or coma is simple and can usually be made on clinical grounds, backed by a bedside blood test. If real doubt exists, blood should be taken for glucose estimation before treatment is given. Patients should carry a card or wear a bracelet or necklace identifying themselves as diabetic, and these should be looked for in unconscious patients.

Unconscious patients should be given either intramuscular glucagon (1 mg) or intravenous glucose (25–50 mL of 50% dextrose solution) followed by a flush of normal saline to preserve the vein (since 50% dextrose scleroses veins). Glucagon acts by mobilizing hepatic glycogen, and works almost as rapidly as glucose. It is simple to administer and can be given at home by relatives. It does not work after a prolonged fast. Oral glucose is given to replenish glycogen reserves once the patient revives.

Measuring the metabolic control of diabetes

The 'artificial pancreas' is a system of blood glucose control that works by continuous blood glucose analysis. This is fed into a computer, which delivers an appropriate amount of insulin into the circulation. Patients on insulin need to devise their own simplified form of this feedback loop.

Urine tests

Some patients will not perform capillary blood glucose monitoring at home. Urine tests give such patients some feedback on whether their diet and treatment are achieving reasonable metabolic control. They are simple to perform using dipsticks, and it can usually be assumed that a patient with consistently negative tests and no symptoms of hypoglycaemia is fairly well controlled. Even so, the correlation between urine tests and simultaneous blood glucose is poor for three reasons:

- Changes in urine glucose lag behind changes in blood glucose.
- The mean renal threshold is around 10 mmol/L but the range is wide (7–13 mmol/L). The threshold also rises with age.
- Urine tests can give no guidance concerning blood glucose levels below the renal threshold.

Blood glucose testing

This provides the best assessment of day-to-day control. The fasting blood glucose concentration is a useful guide to therapy in tablet-treated type 2 diabetes, but random blood glucose test (e.g. in the clinic) is of limited value. Patients may easily be taught to provide their own profiles by testing finger-prick blood samples with reagent strips and reading these with the aid of a meter. Most patients are willing and able to provide reasonably accurate results provided they have been properly taught. Blood is taken from the side of a finger tip (not from the tip, which is densely innervated) using a special lancet usually fitted to a spring-loaded device. There is a huge variety of finger-pricking devices and of blood glucose test meters. Patients will normally be able to talk through the use of various devices with a Diabetes Nurse Specialist to select the most appropriate devices for their own purposes. Patients are asked to take regular profiles (e.g. four daily samples on two days each week) and to note these in a diary or record book. Home blood glucose monitoring is an essential aid to good glycaemic control. Patients on insulin are encouraged to adjust their insulin dose as appropriate (Table 19.5) and should ideally be able to obtain advice over the telephone when needed.

Glycosylated haemoglobin (HbA$_1$ or HbA$_{1c}$) and fructosamine

Glycosylation of haemoglobin occurs as a two-step reaction, resulting in the formation of a covalent bond between

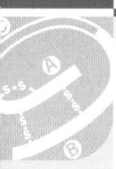
the glucose molecule and the terminal valine of the β chain of the haemoglobin molecule. The rate at which this reaction occurs is related to the prevailing glucose concentration. Glycosylated haemoglobin is expressed as a percentage of the normal haemoglobin (normal range approximately 4–8% depending on the technique of measurement). This test provides an index of the average blood glucose concentration over the life of the haemoglobin molecule (approximately 6 weeks). The figure will be misleading if the life-span of the red cell is reduced or if an abnormal haemoglobin or thalassaemia is present. Although the glycosylated haemoglobin test provides a rapid assessment of the level of glycaemic control in a given patient, blood glucose testing is needed before the clinician can know what to do about it.

Glycosylated plasma proteins ('fructosamine') may also be measured as an index of control. Glycosylated albumin is the major component and fructosamine measurement relates to glycaemic control over the preceding 2–3 weeks. It is useful in patients with a haemoglobinopathy and in pregnancy (when haemoglobin turnover is changeable) and other situations where changes of treatment need a swift means of assessing progress.

Targets

Data from the UK Prospective Diabetic Study (UKPDS) and the Diabetes Control and Complications Trial (DCCT) suggest that under ideal circumstances patients with both type 1 diabetes and type 2 diabetes would be aiming to run their glycosylated haemoglobin readings in the region of 7–7.5% (in assays where the upper limit of the non-diabetic range is 6%), or corrected fructosamine readings of 350 mg/100 g protein, in order to reduce the risk of long-term microvascular complications (Table 19.6). Hypoglycaemia, patterns of eating and lifestyle, weight problems and problems accepting and coping with diabetes limit what can be achieved. Some will, but most will not, be able to reach these target values, particularly as their duration of diabetes increases. Realistic goals should be set for each patient taking into account what is likely to be achievable.

Does good metabolic control of diabetes matter?

Blood glucose is just one measure of the diverse metabolic consequence of diabetes which not only affects carbohydrate metabolism but also the metabolism of lipids and proteins. Studies in experimental animals strongly suggest that improved metabolic control prevents complications and this has been confirmed in humans. The DCCT in the USA compared standard and intensive insulin therapy in a large prospective controlled trial of young patients with type 1 diabetes. Despite intensive therapy, mean blood glucose levels were still 40% above the non-diabetic range, but even at this level of control, the risk of progression to retinopathy was reduced by 60%, nephropathy by 30% and neuropathy by 20% over the 7 years of the study. Near-normoglycaemia should, therefore, be the goal for all young patients with type 1 diabetes. The unwanted effects of this policy include weight gain and a two- to threefold increase in the risk of severe hypoglycaemia. Control should be less strict in those with a history of recurrent severe hypoglycaemia.

The UKPDS compared standard and intensive treatment in a large prospective controlled trial of type 2 diabetes patients. There was a 25% overall reduction in microvascular disease end points, a 33% reduction in albuminuria and a 30% reduction in the need for laser treatment for retinopathy in the more intensively treated patients. There appeared to be little difference in outcome between the tools used to achieve good metabolic control (metformin, sulphonylurea or insulin). A proportion of the total patients in the UKPDS were further randomized into standard and intensive blood pressure control groups. Cardiovascular risk was very considerably reduced in the intensive treatment arm.

Can established complications be halted or reversed by intensive insulin therapy? Insulin infusion devices have made near-normal blood glucose control possible for closely supervised groups of patients. Studies in patients with established retinopathy have shown that patients with early retinopathy benefit from 2–3 years of intensive therapy, but that patients with more advanced retinal changes generally do not.

Table 19.6
Target goals for HbA$_{1c}$, total cholesterol and blood pressure in diabetic patients

Parameter	Ideal	Reasonable but not ideal	Less than satisfactory
HbA$_{1c}$	< 7.5%	< 8.5%	> 8.5%
Total cholesterol	< 5.0 mmol/L	< 6.5 mmol/L	> 6.5 mmol/L*
Blood pressure	< 130/80 mmHg	< 145/90 mmHg	> 145/90 mmHg

* > 5.0 mmol/L over 50 years of age

Box 19.2

Regular checks for patients with diabetes

These items are modified from those set out in 'The European Patients' Charter' (1991) published by the St Vincent Declaration Steering Committee of the WHO. The charter sets out goals for both the healthcare team and the patient.

Checked each visit

- Review of self-monitoring results and current treatment.
- Talk about targets and change where necessary.
- Talk about any general or specific problems.
- Continued education.

Checked at least once a year

- Biochemical assessment of metabolic control (e.g. glycated Hb test).
- Measure bodyweight.
- Measure blood pressure.
- Measure plasma lipids (except in extreme old age).
- Measure visual acuity.
- Examine state of retina (ophthalmoscope or retinal photo).
- Test urine for proteinuria.
- Test blood for renal function (creatinine).
- Check condition of feet, pulses and neurology.
- Review cardiovascular risk factors.
- Review self-monitoring and injection techniques.
- Review eating habits.

Retinopathy may show a transient deterioration when strict control is first established. These observations suggest that microvascular lesions are self-perpetuating once a threshold level of damage has been reached.

Regular checks for patients with diabetes

Box 19.2 is modified from the guidelines set out in *The European Patients' Charter* (1991) published by the St Vincent Declaration Steering Committee of the WHO. The charter sets out goals for both the healthcare team and the patient.

FURTHER READING

DCCT/Epidemiology of Diabetes Interventions and Complications Research Group (2000) Retinopathy and nephropathy in patients with type 1 diabetes four years after a trial of intensive insulin therapy. *New England Journal of Medicine* **342**: 381–389.

Mogensen CE (1998) Combined high blood pressure and glucose in type 2 diabetes: double jeopardy. *British Medical Journal* **317**: 693–694.

St Vincent Declaration Steering Committee of WHO Europe (1991) The European Patients' Charter. *Diabetic Medicine* **8**: 782–783.

Wallace TM, Matthews DR (2000) Poor glycaemic control in type 2 diabetes: a conspiracy of disease, suboptimal therapy and attitude. *Quarterly Journal of Medicine* **93**: 369–374.

Psychosocial implications of diabetes

Patients starting tablet or insulin treatment should be encouraged to live as normal a life as possible, but this is not easy. Tact, empathy, encouragement and practical support are needed from all members of the clinical team. Diabetes, like any chronic disease, has psychological sequelae. Most patients will experience periods of not coping, of helplessness, of denial and of acceptance often fluctuating over time. Other problems include:

- *It is impossible to take a holiday from diabetes* – yet the human psyche is poorly developed to cope with unremitting adversity.
- *Concessions or sympathy are often denied* to the person with diabetes, since its presence is invisible.
- *The treatment is complex and demanding*, and the person with diabetes is expected to make trade-offs between short-term and long-term well-being.
- *Embarrassing loss of control over personal behaviour* or consciousness can occur in insulin-treated patients after only a slight miscalculation.
- *Risk-taking behaviour* is indulged in by all human beings when emotion is in conflict with logical thought, but its effects can be much greater for the person with diabetes (particularly the risks of unplanned pregnancy, alcohol and tobacco).
- *Poor self-image* is a very common problem.
- *Eating disorders* are more common in people with diabetes – 30–40% of young women with diabetes will exhibit a clinically significant eating disorder.
- *Insulin omission* is common since non-adherence to treatment regimens is universal in all illness. Insulin omission is also very common in young women where the pressure to lose weight overcomes concerns about long-term complications.

Adolescence

Adolescence magnifies the internal conflicts that all human beings cope, or intermittently fail to cope, with during life. A period of poor metabolic control, or dropping out of medical care for a time and re-emerging with complications, is very common. Diabetic Holiday Camps (for example run by Diabetes UK) help prevent a feeling of isolation and not knowing anyone else with the same problem. Separate adolescent clinics allow:

- *Treatment without marginalization* in a larger group of older people
- *Meeting peers with similar problems* in the waiting room
- *Gradual separation from parents* and assumption of personal responsibility for the illness
- *Age-appropriate literature* to be available.

Practical aspects

On a practical level patients need to inform the driving and vehicle licensing authority and their insurance companies after diagnosis. They would also be wise to inform their family, friends and employers in case unexpected hypoglycaemia occurs. Insulin treatment can be undertaken by people in most walks of life; a few jobs are unsuitable. These include driving Heavy Goods or Public Service vehicles, working at heights, piloting aircraft or working close to dangerous machinery in motion. Certain professions such as the police and the armed forces are barred to all diabetic patients. There are few other limitations, although a considerable amount of ill-informed prejudice exists. Doctors can sometimes help support patients in the face of misinformed work practices.

Diabetic metabolic emergencies

The main terms used are defined in Table 19.7.

Diabetic ketoacidosis

Diabetic ketoacidosis is the hallmark of type 1 diabetes. It is usually seen in the following circumstances:

- previously undiagnosed diabetes
- interruption of insulin therapy
- the stress of intercurrent illness.

The majority of cases reaching hospital could have been prevented by earlier diagnosis, better communication between patient and doctor, and better patient education. The most common error of management is for patients to reduce or omit insulin because they feel unable to eat owing to nausea or vomiting. This is a factor in at least 25% of all hospital admissions. Insulin should never be stopped.

Pathogenesis

Ketoacidosis is a state of uncontrolled catabolism associated with insulin deficiency. Insulin deficiency is a necessary precondition since only a modest elevation in insulin levels is sufficient to inhibit hepatic ketogenesis, and stable patients do not readily develop ketoacidosis when insulin is withdrawn. Other factors include counter-regulatory hormone excess and fluid depletion. The combination of insulin deficiency with excess of its hormonal antagonists leads to the parallel processes shown in Figure 19.11. In the absence of insulin, hepatic glucose production accelerates, and peripheral uptake by tissues such as muscle is reduced. Rising glucose levels lead to an osmotic diuresis, loss of fluid and electrolytes, and dehydration. Plasma osmolality rises and renal perfusion falls. In parallel, rapid lipolysis occurs, leading to elevated circulating free fatty-acid levels. The free fatty acids are broken down to fatty acyl-CoA within the liver cells, and this in turn is converted to ketone bodies within the mitochondria (Fig. 19.12). Accumulation of ketone bodies produces a metabolic

Table 19.7
Terms used in uncontrolled diabetes

Ketonuria	Detectable ketone levels in the urine; it should be appreciated that ketonuria occurs in fasted non-diabetics and may be found in relatively well-controlled patients with insulin-dependent diabetes mellitus
Ketosis	Elevated plasma ketone levels in the absence of acidosis
Diabetic ketoacidosis	A metabolic emergency in which hyperglycaemia is associated with a metabolic acidosis due to greatly raised (> 5 mmol/L) ketone levels
Non-ketotic hyperosmolar state	A metabolic emergency in which uncontrolled hyperglycaemia induces a hyperosmolar state in the absence of significant ketosis
Lactic acidosis	A metabolic emergency in which elevated lactate levels induce a metabolic acidosis In diabetic patients it is rare and associated with biguanide therapy

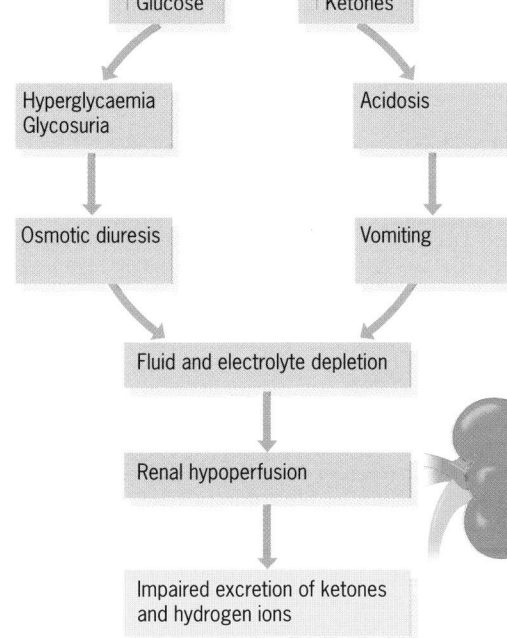

Fig. 19.11 Dehydration occurs during ketoacidosis as a consequence of two parallel processes. Hyperglycaemia results in osmotic diuresis, and hyperketonaemia results in acidosis and vomiting. Renal hypoperfusion then occurs and a vicious circle is established as the kidney becomes less able to compensate for the acidosis.

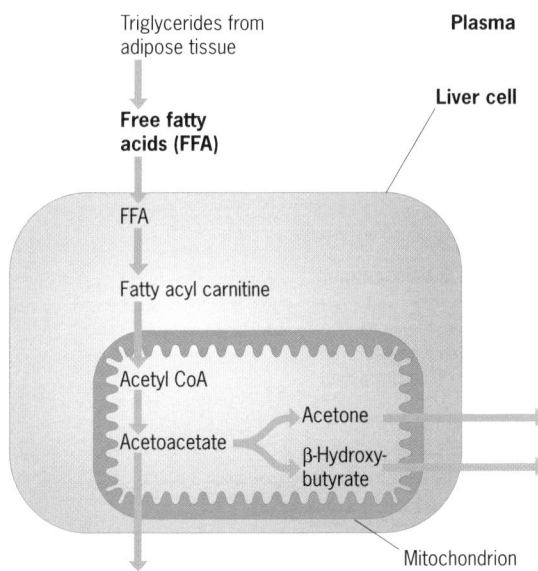

Fig. 19.12 **Ketogenesis.** During insulin deficiency, lipolysis accelerates and free fatty acids taken up by liver cells form the substrate for ketone formation (acetoacetate, acetone and β-hydroxybutyrate) within the mitochondrion. These ketones pass into the blood producing acidosis.

Plasma

Triglycerides from adipose tissue

Free fatty acids (FFA)

Liver cell

FFA

Fatty acyl carnitine

Acetyl CoA

Acetoacetate

Acetone

β-Hydroxy-butyrate

Mitochondrion

acidosis. Vomiting leads to further loss of fluid and electrolytes. The excess ketones are excreted in the urine but also appear in the breath, producing a distinctive smell similar to that of acetone. Respiratory compensation for the acidosis leads to hyperventilation, graphically described as 'air hunger'. Progressive dehydration impairs renal excretion of hydrogen ions and ketones, aggravating the acidosis. As the pH falls below 7.0 ($[H^+] > 100$ nmol/L), pH-dependent enzyme systems in many cells function less effectively. Untreated, severe ketoacidosis is invariably fatal.

Clinical features

The features of ketoacidosis are those of uncontrolled diabetes with acidosis, and include prostration, hyperventilation (Kussmaul respiration), nausea, vomiting and, occasionally, abdominal pain. The latter is sometimes so severe as to cause confusion with a surgical acute abdomen.

Some patients are mentally alert at presentation, but confusion and stupor are common. Up to 5% present in coma. Evidence of marked dehydration is present and the eyeball is lax to pressure in severe cases. Hyperventilation is present but becomes less marked in very severe acidosis owing to respiratory depression. The smell of ketones on the breath allows an instant diagnosis to be made by those able to detect the odour. The skin is dry and the body temperature is often subnormal, even in the presence of infection; in such cases, pyrexia may develop later.

Diagnosis

This is confirmed by demonstrating hyperglycaemia with ketonaemia or heavy ketonuria, and acidosis. No time should be lost and treatment is started as soon as the first blood sample has been taken. Hyperglycaemia is demonstrated by dipstick, while a blood sample is sent to the laboratory for confirmation. Ketonaemia is confirmed by centrifuging a blood sample and testing the plasma with a dipstick that measures ketones. An arterial blood sample is taken for blood gas analysis.

Management

The principles of management are as follows (Emergency box 19.1).

- Replace the *fluid losses* with normal saline.
- Replace the *electrolyte losses*. Potassium levels need to be monitored with great care. Patients have a total body potassium deficit although initial plasma levels may not be low. Insulin therapy leads to uptake of potassium by the cells with a consequent fall in plasma K^+ levels. Potassium is therefore given as soon as insulin is started.
- *Restore the acid–base balance.* A patient with healthy kidneys will rapidly compensate for the metabolic acidosis once the circulating volume is restored. Bicarbonate is seldom necessary and is only considered if the pH is below 7.0 ($[H^+] > 100$ nmol/L), and is best given as an isotonic (1.26%) solution.
- *Replace the deficient insulin.* Modern treatment is with relatively modest doses of insulin, which lower blood glucose by suppressing hepatic glucose output rather than by stimulating peripheral uptake, and are therefore much less likely to produce hypoglycaemia. Soluble insulin is given as an intravenous infusion where facilities for adequate supervision exist, or as hourly intramuscular injections. The subcutaneous route is avoided because subcutaneous blood flow is reduced in shocked patients.
- *Monitor blood glucose closely.* Hourly measurement is needed in the initial phases of treatment.
- *Replace the energy losses.* When plasma glucose falls to near-normal values (12 mmol/L), saline infusion should be replaced with 5% dextrose containing 20 mmol/L of potassium chloride. The insulin infusion rate is reduced and adjusted according to blood glucose.
- *Seek the underlying cause.* Physical examination may reveal a source of infection (e.g. a perianal abscess). Two common markers of infection are misleading: fever is unusual even when infection is present, and polymorpholeucocytosis is present even in the absence of infection. Relevant investigations include a chest X-ray, urine and blood cultures, and an ECG (to exclude myocardial infarction). If infection is suspected, broad-spectrum antibiotics are started once the appropriate cultures have been taken.

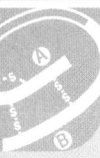

Emergency box 19.1

Guidelines for the diagnosis and management of diabetic ketoacidosis

Diagnosis
- Hyperglycaemia: measure blood glucose.
- Ketonaemia: test plasma with ketostix/Acetest.
- Acidosis: measure blood gases.

Investigations
- Blood glucose
- Urea and electrolytes
- Full blood count
- Blood gases
- Blood and urine culture
- Chest X-ray
- ECG
- Cardiac enzymes.

Phase 1 Management
- Insulin: soluble insulin i.v. 6 units/hour by infusion, or 20 units i.m. stat. followed by 6 units i.m. hourly.
- Fluid replacement: 0.9% sodium chloride with 20 mmol KCl per litre. An average regimen would be 1 L in 30 minutes, then 1 L in 1 hour, then 1 L in 2 hours, then 1 L in 4 hours, then 1 L in 6 hours.
- Adjust KCl concentration depending on results of 2 hours' blood K measurement.

   IF:
- Blood pressure below 80 mmHg, give plasma expander.
- pH below 7.0 give 500 mL of sodium bicarbonate 1.26% plus 10 mmol KCl⁻. Repeat if necessary to bring pH up to 7.0.

Phase 2 Management
- When blood glucose falls to 10–12 mmol/L swap infusion fluid to 1 litre 5% dextrose plus 20 mmol KCl⁻ 6-hourly. Continue insulin with dose adjusted according to hourly blood glucose test results.

Phase 3 Management
- Once stable and able to eat and drink normally, transfer patient to four times daily subcutaneous insulin regimen (based on previous 24 hours' insulin consumption, and trend in consumption).

Special measures
- Broad-spectrum antibiotic if infection likely.
- Bladder catheter if no urine passed in 2 hours.
- Nasogastric tube if drowsy.
- Consider CVP pressure monitoring if shocked or if previous cardiac or renal impairment.
- Consider s.c. prophylactic heparin in comatose, elderly or obese patients.

Subsequent management
- Monitor glucose hourly for 8 hours.
- Monitor electrolytes 2-hourly for 8 hours.
- Adjust K⁺ replacement according to results.

Note: The regimen of fluid replacement set out above is a guide for patients with severe ketoacidosis. Excessive fluid can precipitate pulmonary and cerebral oedema; inadequate replacement may cause renal failure. Fluid replacement must therefore be tailored to the individual and monitored carefully throughout treatment.

Problems of management

- *Hypotension.* This may lead to renal shutdown. Plasma expanders (or whole blood) are therefore given if the systolic blood pressure is below 80 mmHg. A central venous pressure line is useful in this situation. A bladder catheter is inserted if no urine is produced within 2 hours, but routine catheterization is not necessary.
- *Coma.* The usual principles apply (see p. 1161). It is essential to pass a nasogastric tube to prevent aspiration since gastric stasis is common and carries the risk of aspiration pneumonia if a drowsy patient vomits.
- *Cerebral oedema.* This rare, but feared, complication has mostly been reported in children or young adults. Excessive rehydration and use of hypertonic fluids such as 8.4% bicarbonate may sometimes be responsible. The mortality is high.
- *Hypothermia.* Severe hypothermia with a core temperature below 33°C may occur and may be overlooked unless a rectal temperature is taken with a low-reading thermometer.
- *Late complications.* These include stasis pneumonia and deep-vein thrombosis, and occur especially in the comatose or elderly patient.
- *Complications of therapy.* These include hypoglycaemia and hypokalaemia, due to loss of K⁺ in the urine from osmotic diuresis. Overenthusiastic fluid replacement may precipitate pulmonary oedema in the very young or the very old. Hyperchloraemic acidosis may develop in the course of treatment since patients have lost a large variety of negatively charged electrolytes, which are replaced with chloride. The kidneys usually correct this spontaneously within a few days.

Subsequent management

Intravenous dextrose and insulin are continued until the patient feels able to eat and keep food down. The drip is then taken down and a similar amount of insulin is given as three injections of soluble insulin subcutaneously at meal times and a dose of intermediate-acting insulin at night.

Sliding-scale regimens are often unnecessary and may even delay the establishment of stable blood glucose levels. The treatment of diabetic ketoacidosis is incomplete without a careful enquiry into the causes of the episode and advice as to how to avoid its recurrence.

Non-ketotic hyperosmolar state

This condition, in which severe hyperglycaemia develops without significant ketosis, is the metabolic emergency characteristic of uncontrolled type 2 diabetes. Patients present in middle or later life, often with previously undiagnosed diabetes. Common precipitating factors include consumption of glucose-rich fluids (e.g. Lucozade), concurrent medication such as thiazide diuretics or steroids, and intercurrent illness. Non-ketotic coma and ketoacidosis represent two ends of a spectrum rather than two distinct disorders (Box 19.3). The biochemical differences may partly be explained as follows:

- *Age.* The extreme dehydration characteristic of non-ketotic coma may be related to age. Old people experience thirst less acutely, and more readily become dehydrated. In addition, the mild renal impairment associated with age results in increased urinary losses of fluid and electrolytes.
- *The degree of insulin deficiency.* This is less severe in non-ketotic coma. Endogenous insulin levels are sufficient to inhibit hepatic ketogenesis, whereas glucose production is unrestrained.

Clinical features

The characteristic clinical features on presentation are dehydration and stupor or coma. Impairment of consciousness is directly related to the degree of hyperosmolality. Evidence of underlying illness such as pneumonia or pyelonephritis may be present, and the hyperosmolar state may predispose to stroke, myocardial infarction or arterial insufficiency in the lower limbs.

Investigations and treatment

These are, with some exceptions, according to the guidelines for ketoacidosis. The plasma osmolality is usually extremely high. It can be measured directly or calculated as $(2(Na^+ + K^+) + glucose + urea)$ all in mmol/L. Many patients are extremely sensitive to insulin and the glucose concentration may plummet. The resultant change in osmolality may cause cerebral damage. It is sometimes useful to infuse insulin at a rate of 3 U per hour for the first 2–3 h, increasing to 6 U/h if glucose is falling too slowly. Normal saline is the standard fluid for replacement. Avoid half-normal saline (0.45%), since rapid dilution of the blood may cause more cerebral damage than a few hours of exposure to hypernatraemia.

Prognosis

The reported mortality ranges as high as 20–30%, mainly because of the advanced age of the patients and the frequency of intercurrent illness. Unlike ketoacidosis, non-ketotic hyperglycaemia is not an absolute indication for subsequent insulin therapy, and survivors may do well on diet and oral agents.

Lactic acidosis

Lactic acidosis may occur in diabetic patients on biguanide therapy. The risk in patients taking metformin

---

Box 19.3

Electrolyte changes in diabetic ketoacidosis and non-ketotic hyperosmolar state

Examples of blood values

	Severe ketoacidosis	Non-ketotic hyperosmolar coma
Na$^+$ (mmol/L)	140	155
K$^+$ (mmol/L)	5	5
Cl$^-$ (mmol/L)	100	110
HCO$_3^-$ (mmol/L)	5	30
Urea (mmol/L)	8	15
Glucose (mmol/L)	30	50
Arterial pH	7.0	7.35

The normal range of **osmolality** is 285–300 mOsm/kg. It can be measured directly, or can be calculated approximately from the formula:

$$Osmolality = 2(Na^+ + K^+) + glucose + urea.$$

For example, in the example of severe ketoacidosis given above:

$$Osmolality = 2(140 + 5) + 30 + 8 = 328 \text{ mOsm/kg}$$

and in the example of non-ketotic hyperosomolar coma:

$$Osmolality = 2(155 + 5) + 50 + 15 = 385 \text{ mOsm/kg}.$$

The normal **anion gap** is less than 17. It is calculated as $(Na^+ + K^+) - (Cl^- + HCO_3^-)$. In the example of ketoacidosis the anion gap is 40, and in the example of non-ketotic hyperosmolar coma the anion gap is 20. Mild hyperchloraemic acidosis may develop in the course of therapy. This will be shown by a rising plasma chloride and persistence of a low bicarbonate even though the anion gap has returned to normal.

is extremely low provided that the therapeutic dose is not exceeded and the drug is withheld in patients with advanced hepatic or renal dysfunction.

Patients present in severe metabolic acidosis with a large anion gap (calculated as $(Na^+ + K^+) - (Cl^- + HCO_3^-)$, normally less than 17 mmol/L), usually without significant hyperglycaemia or ketosis. Treatment is by rehydration and infusion of isotonic 1.26% bicarbonate. The mortality is in excess of 50%.

Complications of diabetes

When insulin was introduced it was assumed that it would provide complete and adequate replacement therapy, just as thyroxine does in hypothyroidism. Time proved that insulin-treated patients still have a considerably reduced life expectancy. Those diagnosed before the age of 20 years in older studies had only a 50–60% chance of living past the age of 50 years, although there are indications of a steady improvement in survival. The excess deaths in early-onset patients are mainly related to diabetic nephropathy, but there is also a considerable excess cardiovascular mortality. Heart disease, peripheral vascular disease and stroke are the major causes of death in patients over the age of 50 years.

Macrovascular complications (Table 19.8)

Diabetes is a risk factor in the development of *atherosclerosis*. This risk is related to that of the background population. For example, Japanese diabetics are much less likely to develop atherosclerosis than patients in Europe but are much more likely to develop it than non-diabetic Japanese. The excess risk to diabetics compared with the general population increases as one moves down the body:

- Stroke is twice as likely.
- Myocardial infarction is 3–5 times as likely and women with diabetes lose their premenopausal protection from coronary artery disease.
- Amputation of a foot for gangrene is 50 times as likely.

The UKPDS and DCCT studies have shown that intensive treatment of diabetes has only a small effect upon the cardiovascular risk of type 2 diabetes or type 1 diabetes patients.

Table 19.8
Diabetic risk factors for macrovascular complications

Duration
Increasing age
Systolic hypertension
Hyperinsulinaemia due to insulin resistance associated with obesity
and syndrome X
Hyperlipidaemia, particularly hypertriglyceridaemia
Proteinuria (including microalbuminuria)
Other factors are the same as for the general population

Type 2 diabetes tends to cluster with other cardiovascular risk factors such as hypertension, central obesity and lipid abnormalities. This is sometimes called '*syndrome X*' or '*the metabolic syndrome*'. Cardiovascular risk factors occurring together tend to have a multiplicative effect on the overall level of cardiovascular risk. For this reason, it is vital to tackle all cardiovascular risk factors together in diabetes, and not just to focus on glucose levels.

- *Hypertension*. The UKPDS demonstrated that aggressive treatment of hypertension produces a marked reduction in adverse cardiovascular outcomes, both microvascular and macrovascular. A target of 140/85 mmHg is reasonable (Table 19.6). To achieve such a target, the UKPDS found that one-third of patients needed three or more antihypertensive drugs in combination, and two-thirds of treated patients needed two or more.
- *Smoking*: the avoidable risk factor. Never give up efforts to help diabetic patients stop smoking. The opportunity for change may only be grasped if the message is delivered at the right time, which in practice means repeated discussion of the issue.
- *Lipid abnormalities*. Most diabetologists would treat a total cholesterol over 6.5 mmol/L in a young (under 50) diabetic patient with few other risk factors. For diabetics over 50, particularly with clustering of other risk factors, the threshold for treatment would fall to 5.0 mmol/L (Table 19.6).
- *Aspirin* can reduce macrovascular risk, but is associated with a morbidity and mortality from bleeding. The benefits of aspirin outweigh the bleeding risk when the risk of a cardiovascular endpoint is > 30% in the next 10 years. This risk is reached in patients aged under 45 with three strong additional cardiovascular risk factors, aged 45–54 with three additional risk factors, aged 54–65 with two additional risk factors or aged over 65 with just one additional risk factor.
- *ACE inhibitors*. A large randomized international study (HOPE study) has shown that treating people with diabetes and at least one other major cardiovascular risk factor with the ACE-inhibitor ramipril produced a 25–35% lowering of the risk of heart attack, stroke, overt nephropathy or cardiovascular death over a 4.5-year period. If this finding is replicated in other studies, the use of ACE inhibitors in such patients will become general.

Microvascular complications

In contrast to macrovascular disease, which is prevalent in the West as a whole, microvascular disease is specific to diabetes. Small blood vessels throughout the body are affected but the disease process is of particular danger in three sites:

- retina
- renal glomerulus
- nerve sheaths.

Diabetic retinopathy, nephropathy and neuropathy tend to manifest 10–20 years after diagnosis in young patients. They present earlier in older patients, probably because these have had unrecognized diabetes for months or even years prior to diagnosis. Genetic factors appear to contribute to the susceptibility to microvascular disease. Diabetic siblings of diabetic patients with renal and eye disease have a three- to fivefold increased risk of the same complication in both type 1 and type 2 patients. There are racial differences in the overall prevalence of nephropathy. In the USA prevalence is thus: Pima American Indians > Hispanic/Mexican > US black > US white patients. A search for the genes responsible is under way; areas on chromosomes 3 and 7 are implicated by genome scanning.

Diabetic eye disease

Diabetes can affect the eyes in a number of ways. The most common and characteristic form of involvement is *diabetic retinopathy*. About one in three young people in this patient population is likely to develop visual problems, and in the UK 5% have in the past become blind after 30 years of diabetes. Indeed, diabetes has been the most common cause of blindness in the population as a whole up to the age of 65 years, but its contribution is falling.

Other forms of eye disease may also occur:

- *The lens* may be affected by reversible osmotic changes in patients with acute hyperglycaemia, causing blurred vision, or by cataracts.
- *New vessel formation* in the iris (rubeosis iridis) may develop as a late complication of diabetic retinopathy and can cause glaucoma.
- *External ocular palsies*, especially of the sixth nerve, can occur (a mononeuritis).

The natural history of retinopathy (Fig. 19.13)

Diabetes causes increased thickness of the capillary basement membrane and increased permeability of the retinal capillaries. Aneurysmal dilatation may occur in some vessels, while others become occluded. These changes are first detectable by fluorescein angiography: a fluorescent dye is injected into an arm vein and photographed in transit through the retinal vessels. This technique is not necessary to screen effectively for retinal disease. After 20 years of type 1 diabetes, almost all patients have some retinopathy, and 60% progress to sight-threatening proliferative retinopathy (Fig. 19.14). Without treatment, 50% of proliferative patients become blind within 5 years.

Background retinopathy (Fig. 19.13b,c)

The first abnormality visible through the ophthalmoscope is the appearance of dot 'haemorrhages', which are actually due to capillary microaneurysms. Leakage of blood into the deeper layers of the retina produces the characteristic 'blot' haemorrhage, while exudation of

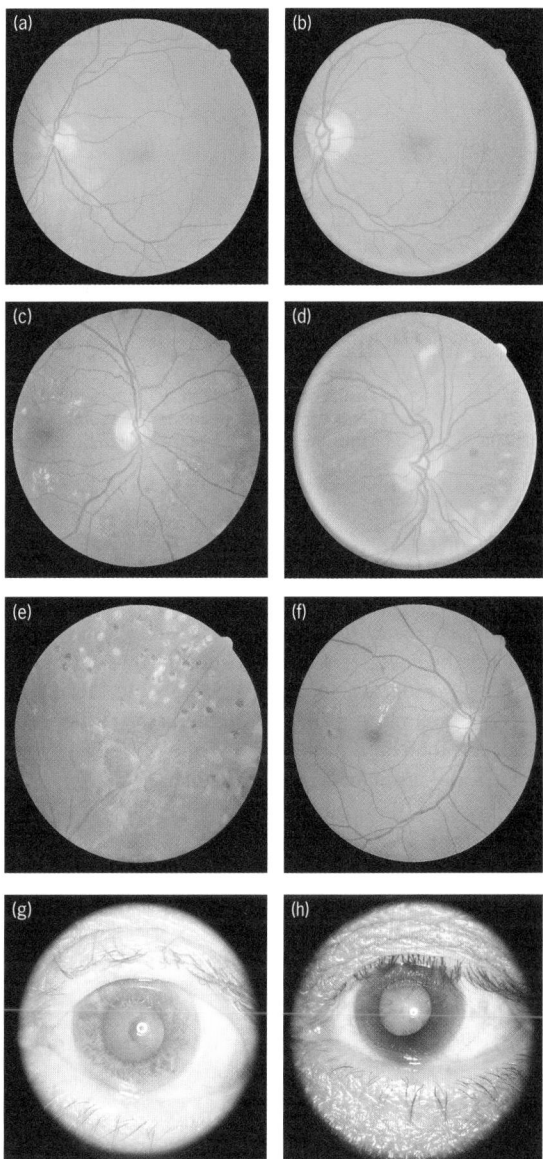

Fig. 19.13 Features of diabetic eye disease. (a) The normal macula (centre) and optic disc. **(b)** Dot and blot haemorrhages (early background retinopathy). **(c)** Hard exudates are present in addition in background retinopathy. **(d)** Multiple cotton-wool spots indicate pre-proliferative retinopathy requiring routine ophthalmic referral. **(e)** Multiple frond-like new vessels, the hallmark of proliferative retinopathy. White fibrous tissue is forming near the new vessels, a feature of advanced retinopathy (this eye also illustrates multiple xenon arc laser burns superiorly). **(f)** Exudates appearing within a disc-width of the macula are a feature of an exudative maculopathy. **(g)** Central and **(h)** cortical cataracts can be seen against the red reflex with the ophthalmoscope.

fluid rich in lipids and protein give rise to hard exudates. These have a bright yellowish white colour and are often irregular in outline with a sharply defined margin. These changes rarely develop in young patients with a duration of diabetes under 10 years, but by 20 years virtually all eyes will manifest at least the

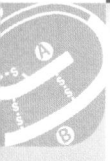

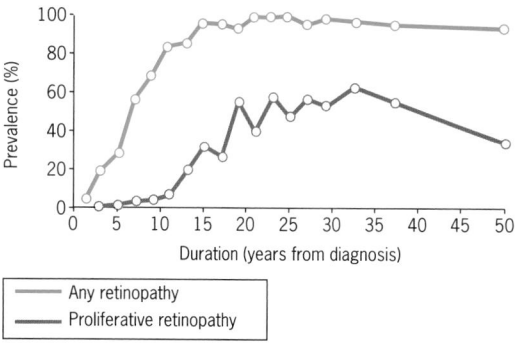

Fig. 19.14 **Prevalence of retinopathy in relation to duration of the disease in patients with insulin-dependent diabetes mellitus diagnosed under the age of 33 years.** Almost all eventually develop background change and 60% progress to proliferative retinopathy. From *Ophthalmology* (1984) **102**: 520.

occasional microaneurysm on careful ophthalmoscopy. In contrast, retinopathy may be present at diagnosis or shortly thereafter in older patients. Background retinopathy does not in itself constitute a threat to vision but may progress to two other distinct forms of retinopathy: maculopathy or proliferative retinopathy. Both are the consequence of damage to retinal blood vessels and resultant retinal ischaemia.

Diabetic maculopathy

This may lead to blindness in the absence of proliferation and particularly affects the older patient with type 2 diabetes. Macular oedema is the first feature of maculopathy and may in itself result in permanent macular damage if not treated early. The first, and only, sign of this is deteriorating visual acuity and this early condition cannot be diagnosed with standard ophthalmoscopy. This is why it is essential to screen patients with diabetes regularly for changes in visual acuity. In most cases, however, maculopathy does not generate sufficient oedema to cause early loss of acuity. The process may then be detected in its later stages as encroachment of hard exudates and haemorrhages on the macular area. These changes are easily visible on ophthalmoscopy, but only through fully dilated pupils.

Pre-proliferative retinopathy

Progressive retinal ischaemia will, in some patients, cause background retinopathy to progress to pre-proliferative, sight-threatening retinopathy. The earliest sign is the appearance of 'cotton-wool spots', representing oedema resulting from retinal infarcts (Fig. 19.13d). They may also occur in severe hypertensive retinopathy. The term 'soft exudate' is often used synonymously but is best avoided. Cotton-wool spots are greyish white, have indistinct margins and a dull matt surface, unlike the glossy appearance of hard exudates. Other features of pre-proliferative retinopathy are described in Table 19.9.

Proliferative retinopathy

Hypoxia is thought to be the signal for formation of new vessels. These lie superficially or grow forward into the vitreous, resembling fronds of seaweed. They branch repeatedly, are fragile, bleed easily (because they lack the normal supportive tissue) and may give rise to a fibrous-tissue reaction (Fig. 19.13e). With advanced retinopathy, haemorrhages can be preretinal or into the vitreous. A vitreous haemorrhage presents as a loss of vision in one eye, sometimes noticed on waking, or as a floating shadow affecting the field of vision. Ophthalmoscopy gives the appearance of a featureless, grey haze. Partial recovery of vision is the rule, as the blood is reabsorbed, but repeated bleeds may occur.

Loss of vision may also result from fibrous proliferation associated with new vessel formation. This may give rise to traction bands that contract with the course of time, producing retinal detachment.

Table 19.9
Pathological changes in the peripheral retina (excluding the macula) in diabetic retinopathy: the action needed

	Fundoscopy/photography findings	Action needed
Background retinopathy	Microaneurysms (dot haemorrhages) Blot haemorrhages Hard exudates	Annual screening only
Pre-proliferative retinopathy	Cotton wool spots Venous beading Venous loops Intraretinal microvascular abnormalities	Non-urgent referral to an ophthalmologist
Proliferative retinopathy	New blood vessel formation Preretinal (subhyaloid) haemorrhage Vitreous haemorrhage	Urgent referral to an ophthalmologist
Advanced retinopathy	Retinal fibrosis Traction retinal detachment	Urgent referral to an ophthalmologist – but much vision already lost

Cataracts

Senile cataracts develop some 10–15 years earlier in diabetic patients than in the remainder of the population. The risk of cataracts was lower in the UKPDS intensively controlled group.

Juvenile or 'snowflake' cataracts are much less common. These are diffuse, rapidly progressive cataracts associated with very poorly controlled diabetes. They should be distinguished from temporary lens changes that occasionally appear during hyperosmolar states and resolve when the hyperglycaemia is brought under control.

Examination

Careful systematic examination of the eye is essential. Visual acuity and eye movements are tested, and 15–30 minutes before the eye is examined the pupils are dilated with a mydriatic such as tropicamide 0.5%. Dilating drugs should not be used, however, in patients with a history of glaucoma, except with the advice of an ophthalmologist. The ophthalmologic examination begins at arm's length. At this distance, cataracts are silhouetted against the red reflex of the retina. The ophthalmoscope is advanced until the retina is in focus. The examination begins at the optic disc, moves through each quadrant in turn, and ends with the macula (since this is least comfortable for the patient). The ophthalmoscope is then adjusted to the +10 dioptre lens for examination of the cornea, anterior chamber and lens. The location of abnormalities should always be sketched in the notes for future reference.

Management of diabetic eye disease (Table 19.9)

The DCCT and UKPDS show that the risk of developing diabetic eye disease can be reduced by striving for aggressive metabolic control of the diabetes. There is no specific medical treatment for background retinopathy. Smoking and hypertension worsen the rate of progression and need treatment. Development or progression of retinopathy may be accelerated by rapid improvement in glycaemic control, pregnancy and in those with nephropathy, and these groups need frequent monitoring. All patients with retinopathy should be examined regularly by a diabetologist or ophthalmologist. Early referral to an ophthalmologist is essential in the following circumstances:

- deteriorating visual acuity
- hard exudates encroaching on the macula
- pre-proliferative changes (cotton-wool spots or venous beading)
- new vessel formation.

The ophthalmologist may perform fluorescein angiography to define the extent of the problem. Maculopathy and proliferative retinopathy are often treatable by retinal laser photocoagulation; in the latter condition early effective therapy reduces the risk of visual loss by about 50%. The value of photocoagulation is particularly marked in those with disc (as against peripheral) new vessels. In one trial only 15% of treated, as against 50% of untreated, eyes with disc new vessels progressed to legal blindness. Treatment in this case is by panretinal photocoagulation. Surgery can be performed to try to salvage some vision after vitreous haemorrhage and to treat traction retinal detachment in advanced retinopathy.

The diabetic kidney

The kidney may be damaged by diabetes in three main ways:

- glomerular damage
- ischaemia resulting from hypertrophy of afferent and efferent arterioles
- ascending infection.

Diabetic nephropathy

Epidemiology

Clinical nephropathy secondary to glomerular disease usually manifests 15–25 years after diagnosis and affects 25–35% of patients diagnosed under the age of 30 years. It is the leading cause of premature death in young diabetic patients. Older patients also develop nephropathy, but the proportion affected is smaller. Some centres have reported a falling incidence rate of diabetic nephropathy in type 1 diabetes. This may reflect good-quality local care for diabetes rather than a change in the natural history of the disease itself. As people with type 2 diabetes develop diabetes progressively younger, a rising incidence rate is seen.

Pathophysiology

The earliest functional abnormality in the diabetic kidney is renal hypertrophy associated with a raised glomerular filtration rate. This appears soon after diagnosis and is related to poor glycaemic control. As the kidney becomes damaged by diabetes, the afferent arteriole (leading to the glomerulus) becomes vasodilated to a greater extent than the efferent glomerular arteriole. This increases the intraglomerular filtration pressure, further damaging the glomerular capillaries. This increased intraglomerular pressure also leads to increased shearing forces locally which are thought to contribute to mesangial cell hypertrophy and increased secretion of extracellular mesangial matrix material. The process eventually leads to glomerular sclerosis. The initial structural lesion in the glomerulus is thickening of the basement membrane. Associated changes may result in disruption of the protein cross-linkages that make the membrane an effective filter. In consequence, there is a progressive leak of large molecules (particularly protein) into the urine.

Albuminuria

The earliest evidence of this is 'microalbuminuria' – amounts of urinary albumin so small as to be undetectable by dipsticks (see p. 595). Microalbuminuria may be tested for by radioimmunoassay or by using special dipsticks. It is a predictive marker of progression to nephropathy in type 1 diabetes, and of increased cardiovascular risk in type 2 diabetes. Microalbuminuria may, after some years, progress to intermittent albuminuria followed by persistent proteinuria. Light-microscopic changes of glomerulosclerosis become manifest; both diffuse and nodular glomerulosclerosis can occur. The latter is sometimes known as the *Kimmelstiel–Wilson lesion*. At the later stage of glomerular sclerosis, the glomerulus is replaced by hyaline material.

At the stage of persistent proteinuria, the plasma creatinine is normal but the average patient is only some 5–10 years from end-stage renal failure. The proteinuria may become so heavy as to induce a transient nephrotic syndrome, with peripheral oedema and hypoalbuminaemia.

Patients with nephropathy typically show a normochromic normocytic anaemia and a raised erythrocyte sedimentation rate (ESR). Hypertension is a common development and may itself damage the kidney still further. A rise in plasma creatinine is a late feature that progresses inevitably to renal failure, although the rate of progression may vary widely between individuals.

The natural history of this process is shown in Figure 19.15.

Ischaemic lesions

Arteriolar lesions, with hypertrophy and hyalinization of the vessels, can occur in patients with diabetes. The appearances are similar to those of hypertensive disease and lead to ischaemic damage to the kidneys.

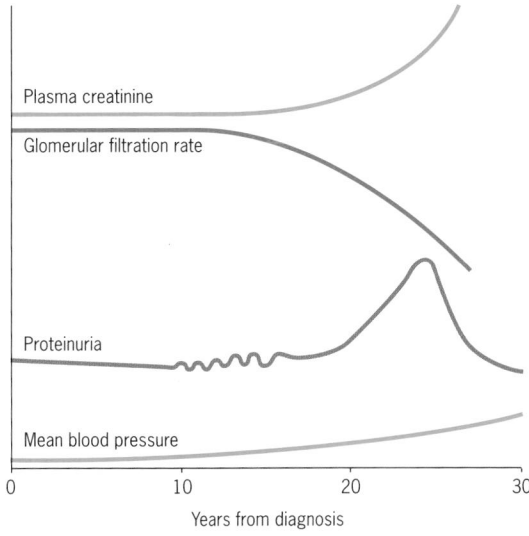

Fig. 19.15 **Schematic representation of the natural history of nephropathy.** The typical onset is 15 years after diagnosis. Intermittent proteinuria leads to persistent proteinuria. In time, the plasma creatinine rises as the glomerular filtration rate falls.

Infective lesions

Urinary tract infections are relatively more common in women with diabetes, but this does not apply to men. Ascending infection may occur because of bladder stasis resulting from autonomic neuropathy, and infections more easily become established in damaged renal tissue. Autopsy material frequently reveals interstitial changes suggestive of infection, but ischaemia may produce similar changes and the true frequency of pyelonephritis in diabetes is uncertain. Untreated infections in diabetics can result in renal papillary necrosis, in which renal papillae are shed in the urine, but this complication is rare.

Diagnosis and management

The urine of all diabetic patients should be checked regularly for the presence of protein. Many centres also screen younger patients for microalbuminuria since there is evidence that meticulous glycaemic control or early antihypertensive treatment at this stage may delay the onset of frank proteinuria. Once proteinuria is present, other possible causes for this should be considered (see below), but once these are excluded, a presumptive diagnosis of diabetic nephropathy can be made. For practical purposes this implies inevitable progression to end-stage renal failure, although the time course can be markedly slowed by early aggressive antihypertensive therapy. Clinical suspicion of a non-diabetic cause of nephropathy may be provoked by an atypical history, the absence of diabetic retinopathy (usually but not invariably present with diabetic nephropathy) and the presence of red-cell casts in the urine. Renal biopsy should be considered in such cases, but in practice is rarely necessary or helpful. The risk of intravenous urography is increased in diabetes, especially if patients are allowed to become dehydrated prior to the procedure, and a renal ultrasound is preferable but not so informative. A 24-hour urine collection is performed to quantify protein loss and to measure creatinine clearance, and regular measurement is made of the plasma creatinine level.

Investigations to detect other treatable causes of nephropathy include urine microscopy and culture, serum protein electrophoresis, serum calcium, serum urate, ESR and antinuclear factor.

Management

The management of diabetic nephropathy is similar to that of other causes of renal failure, with the following provisos:

- Aggressive treatment of blood pressure with a target below 135/85 mmHg has been shown to slow the rate of deterioration of renal failure considerably. Angiotensin-converting enzyme inhibitors or an angiotensin receptor II antagonist are the drugs of choice (see p. 825). These drugs should also be used in normotensive patients with persistent microalbuminuria.

- Oral hypoglycaemic agents partially excreted via the kidney (e.g. chlorpropamide) must be avoided.
- Insulin sensitivity increases and drastic reductions in dosage may be needed.
- Associated diabetic retinopathy tends to progress rapidly, and frequent ophthalmic supervision is essential.

Management of end-stage disease is made more difficult by the fact that patients often have other complications of diabetes such as blindness, autonomic neuropathy or peripheral vascular disease. Vascular shunts tend to calcify rapidly and hence chronic ambulatory peritoneal dialysis may be preferable to haemodialysis. The failure rate of renal transplants is somewhat higher than in non-diabetic patients. A segmental pancreatic graft is sometimes performed at the same time as a renal graft. Although pancreatic transplants have a limited viability, owing to progressive fibrosis within the graft, they may give the patient a year or so of freedom from insulin injections.

Diabetic neuropathy

Diabetes can damage peripheral nervous tissue in a number of ways. The vascular hypothesis postulates occlusion of the vasa nervorum as the prime cause. This seems likely in isolated mononeuropathies, but the diffuse symmetrical nature of the common forms of neuropathy implies a metabolic cause. Since hyperglycaemia leads to increased formation of sorbitol and fructose in Schwann cells, accumulation of these sugars may disrupt function and structure.

The earliest functional change in diabetic nerves is delayed nerve conduction velocity; the earliest histological change is segmental demyelination, caused by damage to Schwann cells. In the early stages axons are preserved, implying prospects of recovery, but at a later stage irreversible axonal degeneration develops.

The following varieties of neuropathy occur (Fig. 19.16):

- symmetrical mainly sensory polyneuropathy (distal)
- acute painful neuropathy
- mononeuropathy and mononeuritis multiplex
  (a) cranial nerve lesions
  (b) isolated peripheral nerve lesions
- diabetic amyotrophy
- autonomic neuropathy.

Symmetrical mainly sensory polyneuropathy

This is often unrecognized by the patient in its early stages. Early clinical signs are loss of vibration sense, pain sensation (deep before superficial) and temperature sensation in the feet. At later stages patients may complain of a feeling of 'walking on cotton wool' and can lose their balance when washing the face or walking in the dark owing to impaired proprioception. Involvement of the hands is much less common and results in a 'stocking and glove' sensory loss. Complications include unrecognized trauma, beginning as blistering due to an ill-fitting shoe or a hot-water bottle, and leading to ulceration.

Sequelae of neuropathy. Involvement of motor nerves to the small muscles of the feet gives rise to interosseous wasting. Unbalanced traction by the long flexor muscles leads to a characteristic shape of the foot, with a high arch and clawing of the toes, which in turn leads to abnormal distribution of pressure on walking, resulting in callus formation under the first metatarsal head or on the tips of the toes and perforating neuropathic

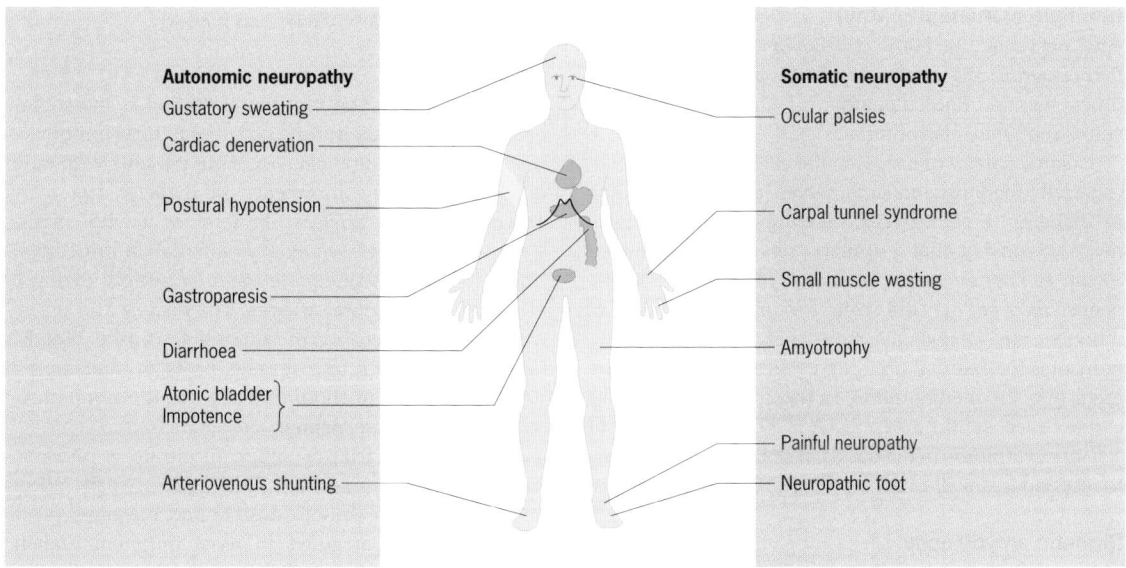

Autonomic neuropathy
Gustatory sweating
Cardiac denervation
Postural hypotension
Gastroparesis
Diarrhoea
Atonic bladder
Impotence
Arteriovenous shunting

Somatic neuropathy
Ocular palsies
Carpal tunnel syndrome
Small muscle wasting
Amyotrophy
Painful neuropathy
Neuropathic foot

Fig. 19.16 **The neuropathic man.**

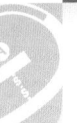
ulceration. Neuropathic arthropathy (Charcot's joints) may sometimes develop in the ankle. The hands show small-muscle wasting as well as sensory changes, but these signs and symptoms must be differentiated from those of the carpal tunnel syndrome, which occurs with increased frequency in diabetes and may be amenable to surgery.

Acute painful neuropathy

A diffuse, painful neuropathy is less common. The patient describes burning or crawling pains in the feet, shins and anterior thighs. These symptoms are typically worse at night, and pressure from bedclothes may be intolerable. It may present at diagnosis or develop after sudden improvement in glycaemic control (e.g. when insulin is started). It usually remits spontaneously after 3–12 months if good control is maintained. A more chronic form, developing later in the course of the disease, is sometimes resistant to almost all forms of therapy. Neurological assessment is difficult because of the hyperaesthesia experienced by the patient, but muscle wasting is not a feature and objective signs can be minimal.

Management is firstly to explore for non-diabetic causes such as a non-metastatic effect of malignancy, vitamin B_{12} deficiency, alcoholic neuropathy, HIV-related neuropathy and drug-related neuropathy (e.g. isoniazid, nitrofurantoin). Explanation and reassurance about the high likelihood of remission within months may be all that is needed. Tricyclic antidepressants, gabapentin, mexiletine and carbamazepine all reduce the perception of neuritic pain somewhat, but usually not as much as patients hope for. Topical capsaicin-containing creams help some patients. A few report that acupuncture has helped.

Mononeuritis and mononeuritis multiplex (multiple mononeuropathy)

Any nerve in the body can be involved in diabetic mononeuritis; the onset is typically abrupt and sometimes painful. Radiculopathy (i.e. involvement of a spinal root) may also occur.

Isolated palsies of nerves to the external eye muscles, especially the third and sixth nerves, are more common in diabetes. A characteristic feature of diabetic third nerve lesions is that pupillary reflexes are retained owing to sparing of pupillomotor fibres. Full spontaneous recovery is the rule for most episodes of mononeuritis. Lesions are more likely to occur at common sites for external pressure palsies or nerve entrapment (e.g. the median nerve in the carpal tunnel). The carpal tunnel syndrome (p. 1213) is a common cause for sensory symptoms in the hands in diabetes, but appears to respond less well to decompression.

Diabetic amyotrophy

This condition is usually seen in older men with diabetes. Presentation is with painful wasting, usually asymmetrical, of the quadriceps muscles. The wasting may be very marked and knee reflexes are diminished or absent. The affected area is often extremely tender. Extensor plantar responses sometimes develop and CSF protein content is elevated. Diabetic amyotrophy is usually associated with periods of poor glycaemic control and may be present at diagnosis. It often resolves in time with careful control of the blood glucose.

Autonomic neuropathy

Asymptomatic autonomic disturbances can be demonstrated on laboratory testing in many patients, but symptomatic autonomic neuropathy is rare. It affects both the sympathetic and parasympathetic nervous systems and can be disabling.

The cardiovascular system

Vagal neuropathy results in tachycardia at rest and loss of sinus arrhythmia. At a later stage, the heart may become denervated (resembling a transplanted heart). Cardiovascular reflexes such as the Valsalva manoeuvre are impaired. Postural hypotension occurs owing to loss of sympathetic tone to peripheral arterioles. A warm foot with a bounding pulse is sometimes seen in a polyneuropathy as a result of peripheral vasodilatation.

Gastrointestinal tract

Vagal damage can lead to gastroparesis, often asymptomatic, but rarely leading to intractable vomiting. Diarrhoea often occurs at night accompanied by urgency and incontinence. Diarrhoea and steatorrhoea may occur owing to small bowel bacterial overgrowth; treatment is with antibiotics such as tetracycline.

Bladder involvement

Loss of tone, incomplete emptying, and stasis (predisposing to infection) can occur, and may ultimately result in an atonic, painless, distended bladder.

Impotence

This is common. The first manifestation is incomplete erection which may in time progress to total impotence; retrograde ejaculation also occurs in patients with autonomic neuropathy. Impotence in diabetes has many causes including anxiety, depression, alcohol excess, drugs, primary or secondary gonadal failure, hypothyroidism, and inadequate vascular supply owing to atheroma in pudendal arteries. The history and examination should focus on these possible causes. Blood is taken for LH, FSH, testosterone, prolactin and thyroid function. Treatment should ideally include sympathetic counselling of both partners.

A therapeutic trial of sildenafil citrate, a phosphodiesterase type-5 inhibitor, which enhances the effects of nitric oxide on smooth muscle and increases penile blood flow, is warranted in most impotent diabetic patients who do not suffer from angina or previous myocardial infarction (contraindications). If sildenafil succeeds, it is worth trying without it after a few months of success, since sometimes potency will continue unaided after confidence is restored. Sixty per cent of diabetic patients can be expected to benefit from this therapy.

There are alternatives for patients who fail to improve with sildenafil, who dislike the side-effects (headache and a green tinge to vision the next day) or those in whom it is contraindicated. Alprostadil (prostaglandin E1 preparation) may be given after suitable training as a small pellet inserted with a device into the urethra (125 μg initially with a maximum of 1 mg). It has a lower success rate than intracavernosal injection treatment, but is less invasive. If the partner is pregnant, barrier contraception must be used to keep prostaglandin away from the fetus.

Patients can be trained by a clinician or impotence nurse specialist in the intracavernosal injection of alprostadil to cause erection. Papaverine (smooth muscle relaxant) and phentolamine and moxisylyte (thymoxamine) (α-adrenoceptor blockers) are sometimes also used. Small doses are given initially, increasing if no effect occurs until an adequate period of erection occurs after injection and sexual stimulation. Intracavernosal injections will fail if the blood supply to the penis is sufficiently low. Side-effects include local reactions (e.g. discomfort, haematoma, fibrosis) and priapism. Patients should be given contact details for urgent treatment should erection last for more than 3 hours. Treatment of priapism should be given well before 6 hours have elapsed. It consists of inserting a 19 gauge butterfly needle into the cavernous tissue and aspirating blood with a 50 mL syringe until detumescence has occurred, if necessary repeating on the other side. If this fails, cautious intracavernosal injection of an α-adrenoceptor agonist such as phenylephrine, metaraminol or epinephrine (adrenaline) may be undertaken with monitoring of pulse and blood pressure. Vacuum devices provide a non-pharmaceutical aid for impotence. A Perspex tube with a seal in the base is placed over the penis and a vacuum pump draws blood into the organ. Tumescence is maintained by slipping a tight rubber band over the base of the penis (and then removing the Perspex tube) until intercourse is complete. Many patients having found a means for restoring potency rarely use it, but feel comforted in having a solution available 'should they need it'.

The diabetic foot

Ten to fifteen per cent of diabetic patients develop foot ulcers at some stage in their lives. Diabetic foot problems are responsible for nearly 50% of all diabetes-related hospital admissions. Fifty per cent of all lower limb amputations are performed on people with diabetes. Many such amputations could be delayed or prevented by more effective patient education and medical supervision. Ischaemia, infection and neuropathy combine to produce tissue necrosis. Although all these factors may coexist, the ischaemic and the neuropathic foot (Table 19.10) can be distinguished.

Management

Many diabetic foot problems are avoidable, so patients need to learn the principles of foot care (Table 19.11). Older patients should visit a chiropodist regularly and should not cut their own toe-nails. Once tissue damage has occurred in the form of ulceration or gangrene, the aim is preservation of viable tissue. The four main threats to the skin and subcutaneous tissues are infection, ischaemia, abnormal pressure and contamination of the wound environment.

- *Infection.* This can take hold rapidly in a diabetic foot. Early antibiotic treatment is essential, with antibiotic therapy adjusted in the light of culture results. The organisms grown from the skin surface may not be the organism causing deeper infection. Collections of pus are drained and excision of infected bone is needed if osteomyelitis develops and does not respond to appropriate antibiotic therapy. Regular X-rays of the foot are needed to check on progress.
- *Ischaemia.* The blood flow to the feet is assessed clinically or with the Doppler ultrasound stethoscope. Femoral arteriography may indicate localized areas of occlusion amenable to bypass surgery or angioplasty. Relatively few patients fall into this category, and the risks (deterioration leading to amputation) and benefits of surgical intervention need careful consideration.

Table 19.10

Distinguishing features between ischaemia and neuropathy in the diabetic foot

	Ischaemia	Neuropathy
Symptoms	Claudication	Usually painless
	Rest pain	Sometimes painful neuropathy
Inspection	Dependent rubor	High arch
	Trophic changes	Clawing of toes
		No trophic changes
Palpation	Cold	Warm
	Pulseless	Bounding pulses
Ulceration	Painful	Painless
	Heels and toes	Plantar

Table 19.11

Principles of diabetic foot care

Inspect feet daily
Seek early advice for any damage
Check shoes inside and out for sharp bodies/areas before wearing
Use lace-up shoes with plenty of room for the toes
Keep feet away from sources of heat (hot sand, hot-water bottles, radiators, fires)
Check the bath temperature before stepping in

- *Abnormal pressure.* An ulcerated site must be kept non-weight-bearing. Resting the affected leg may need to be supplemented with special deep shoes and insoles to move pressure away from critical sites, or by removable or non-removable casts of the leg. After healing, special shoes and insoles are likely to continue to be needed to protect the feet and prevent abnormal pressure repeating damage to a healed area. In neuropathic feet particularly, sharp surgical debridement by a chiropodist is necessary to prevent callus distorting the local wound architecture and causing damage through abnormal pressure on normal skin nearby.
- *Wound environment.* Dressings are used to absorb or remove exudate, maintain moisture, and protect the wound from contaminating agents, and should be easily removable. Expensive new dressings containing growth factors and other biologically active agents may have a role to play in future, but their place is still being assessed.

Foot problems are the major cause of hospital bed occupancy by diabetic patients. Good liaison between physician, chiropodist and surgeon is essential if this period in hospital is to be used efficiently. When irreversible arterial insufficiency is present, it is often quicker and kinder to opt for an early major amputation rather than subject the patient to a debilitating sequence of conservative procedures.

Infections

There is no evidence that diabetic patients with good glycaemic control are more prone to infection than normal subjects. However, poorly controlled diabetes entails increased susceptibility to the following infections:

- *Skin*
  - (a) staphylococcal infections (boils, abscesses, carbuncles)
  - (b) mucocutaneous candidiasis
- *Gastrointestinal tract*
  - (a) chronic periodontitis
  - (b) rectal and ischiorectal abscess formation (when control very poor)
- *Urinary tract*
  - (a) urinary tract infections (in women)
  - (b) pyelonephritis
  - (c) perinephric abscess
- *Lungs*
  - (a) staphylococcal and pneumococcal pneumonia
  - (b) Gram-negative bacterial pneumonia
  - (c) tuberculosis

One reason why poor control lends to infection is that chemotaxis and phagocytosis by polymorphonuclear leucocytes is impaired because at high blood glucose concentrations neutrophil superoxide generation is impaired.

Conversely, infections may lead to loss of glycaemic control, and are a common cause of ketoacidosis.

Insulin-treated patients need to increase their dose by up to 25% in the face of infection, and non-insulin-treated patients may need insulin cover while the infection lasts. Patients should be told never to omit their insulin dose, even if they are nauseated and unable to eat; instead they should test their blood glucose frequently and seek urgent medical advice.

Skin and joints (see also p. 1301)

Joint contractures in the hands are a common consequence of childhood diabetes. The sign may be demonstrated by asking the patient to join the hands as if in prayer; the metacarpophalangeal and interphalangeal joints cannot be apposed. Thickened, waxy skin can be noted on the backs of the fingers. These features may be due to glycosylation of collagen and are not progressive. The condition is sometimes referred to as diabetic cheiroarthropathy.

Osteopenia in the extremities is also described in type 1 diabetes but rarely leads to clinical consequences.

FURTHER READING

Atkinson MA, Eisenbarth GS (2001) Type I diabetes: new perspectives on disease pathogenesis and treatment. *Lancet* **358**: 221–229.

Bain SC, Chowdhury TA (2000) Genetics of diabetic nephropathy and microalbuminuria. *Journal of the Royal Society of Medicine* **93**: 62–66.

Cooper M (1998) Pathogenesis, prevention and treatment of diabetic nephropathy. *Lancet* **352**: 213–219.

Diabetes and the heart (1997) *Lancet* **350** (Suppl 1): 1–32.

Diabetes Control and Complications Trial Research Group (1993) The effect of intensive treatment of diabetes on the development and progression of long-term complications in insulin-dependent diabetes mellitus. *New England Journal of Medicine* **329**: 977–986.

Edmonds ME (1999) Progress in care of the diabetic foot. *Lancet* **354**: 270–272.

Ferris FL, Davis MD, Aiello LM (1999) Treatment of diabetic retinopathy. *New England Journal of Medicine* **341**: 667–678.

Haffner SM (2000) Coronary heart disease in patients with diabetes. *New England Journal of Medicine* **342**: 1040–1042.

HOPE Study Organisation (2000) *Lancet* **355**: 253–259.

Hostetter TH (2001) Prevention of end-stage renal disease in type 2 diabetes. *New England Journal of Medicine* **345**: 910–912.

Ward JD (1996) Diabetic neuropathy in type 2 diabetes. *Diabetologia* **39**: 1676–1678.

Notes on special situations in diabetes

Surgery

Smooth control of diabetes minimizes the risk of infection and balances the catabolic response to anaesthesia and surgery. The procedure for insulin-treated patients is simple:

- Long-acting and/or intermediate insulin should be stopped the day before surgery, with soluble insulin substituted.
- Whenever possible, diabetic patients should be first on the morning theatre list.
- An infusion of glucose, insulin and potassium is given during surgery. The insulin can be mixed into the glucose solution or administered separately by syringe pump. A standard combination is 16 U of soluble insulin with 10 mmol of KCl in 500 mL of 10% glucose, infused at 100 mL/h.
- Postoperatively, the infusion is maintained until the patient is able to eat. Other fluids needed in the perioperative period must be given through a separate intravenous line and must not interrupt the glucose/insulin/potassium infusion. Glucose levels are checked every 2–4 hours and potassium levels are monitored. The amount of insulin and potassium in each infusion bag is adjusted either upwards or downwards according to the results of regular monitoring of the blood glucose and serum potassium concentrations.

The same approach is used in the emergency situation, with the exception that a separate variable-rate insulin infusion may be needed to bring blood glucose under control before surgery.

Non-insulin-treated patients should stop medication 2 days before the operation. Patients with mild hyperglycaemia (fasting blood glucose below 8 mmol/L) can be treated as non-diabetic. Those with higher levels are treated with soluble insulin prior to surgery, and with glucose, insulin and potassium during and after the procedure, as for insulin-treated patients.

Pregnancy and diabetes

Meticulous metabolic control of the diabetes and careful medical and obstetric management is required.

Metabolic control of diabetes in pregnancy

The patient should perform daily home blood glucose profiles, recording blood tests before and 2 hours after meals. The renal threshold falls in pregnancy, and urine tests are therefore of little or no value. Insulin requirements rise progressively, and intensified insulin regimens are generally used. The aim is to maintain blood glucose and fructosamine (or HbA_{1c}) levels as close to the normal range as can be tolerated.

General management

The patient is seen at intervals of 2 weeks or less at a clinic managed jointly by physician and obstetrician. Circumstances permitting, the aim should be outpatient management with a spontaneous vaginal delivery at term. Retinopathy and nephropathy may deteriorate during pregnancy. Expert fundoscopy and urine testing for protein should be undertaken at booking, at 28 weeks and before delivery.

Obstetric problems associated with diabetes

Poorly controlled diabetes is associated with stillbirth, mechanical problems in the birth canal owing to fetal macrosomia, hydramnios and pre-eclampsia. Ketoacidosis in pregnancy carries a 50% fetal mortality, but maternal hypoglycaemia is relatively well tolerated.

Neonatal problems

Maternal diabetes, especially when poorly controlled, is associated with fetal macrosomia. The infant of a diabetic mother is more susceptible to hyaline membrane disease than non-diabetic infants of similar maturity. In addition, neonatal hypoglycaemia may occur. The mechanism is as follows: maternal glucose crosses the placenta, but insulin does not; the fetal islets hypersecrete to combat maternal hyperglycaemia, and a rebound to hypoglycaemic levels occurs when the umbilical cord is severed.

These complications are due to hyperglycaemia in the third trimester. Poor glycaemic control around the time of conception carries an increased risk of major congenital malformations. When a pregnancy is planned, optimal metabolic control should be sought before conception.

Gestational diabetes

This term refers to glucose intolerance that develops in the course of pregnancy and usually remits following delivery. The condition is typically asymptomatic. Women who have a previous history of gestational diabetes, older or overweight women, those with a history of large for gestational age babies and women from certain ethnic groups are at particular risk, but many cases occur in women who are not in any of these categories. For this reason some advocate screening of all pregnant women on the basis of random plasma glucose testing in each trimester and by oral glucose tolerance testing if the glucose concentration is, for example, 7 mmol/L or more. There is no consensus concerning the level of blood glucose which is harmful for the baby, and therefore no consensus concerning cut-off levels for screening and intervention. Since the renal threshold for glucose falls during normal pregnancy and glucose tolerance deteriorates, the condition may easily be misdiagnosed.

Treatment is with diet in the first instance, but most patients require insulin cover during the pregnancy. Insulin does not cross the placenta. Many oral agents cross the placenta and are thus avoided because of the potential risk to the fetus. There is some evidence that glibenclamide may be safe in this situation (p. 1079).

Gestational diabetes has been associated with all the obstetric and neonatal problems described above for pre-existing diabetes, except that there is no increase in the rate of congenital abnormalities. It is likely to recur in subsequent pregnancies. Gestational diabetes is often the harbinger of type 2 diabetes in later life.

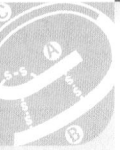

Not all diabetes presenting in pregnancy is gestational. True type 1 diabetes may develop, and swift diagnosis is essential to prevent the development of ketoacidosis. Hospital admission is required if the patient is symptomatic, or has ketonuria or a markedly elevated blood glucose level.

Brittle diabetes

There is no precise definition for this term, which is used to describe patients with recurrent ketoacidosis and/or recurrent hypoglycaemic coma. Of these, the largest group is made up of those who experience recurrent severe hypoglycaemia.

Recurrent severe hypoglycaemia

This affects 1–3% of insulin-dependent patients. Most are adults who have had diabetes for more than 10 years. By this stage endogenous insulin secretion is negligible in the great majority of patients. Pancreatic alpha-cells are still present in undiminished numbers, but the glucagon response to hypoglycaemia is virtually absent. Long-term patients are thus subject to fluctuating hyperinsulinaemia owing to erratic absorption of insulin from injection sites, and lack a major component of the hormonal defence against hypoglycaemia. In this situation epinephrine (adrenaline) secretion becomes vital, but this too may become impaired in the course of diabetes. Loss of epinephrine (adrenaline) secretion has been attributed to autonomic neuropathy, but this is unlikely to be the sole cause; central adaptation to recurrent hypoglycaemia may also be a factor.

The following factors may also predispose to recurrent hypoglycaemia:

- *Overtreatment with insulin.* Frequent biochemical hypoglycaemia lowers the glucose level at which symptoms develop. Symptoms often reappear when overall glucose control is relaxed.
- *An unrecognized low renal threshold for glucose.* Attempts to render the urine sugar-free will inevitably produce hypoglycaemia.
- *Excessive insulin doses.* A common error is to increase the dose when a patient needs more frequent injections to overcome a problem of timing.
- *Endocrine causes.* These include pituitary insufficiency, adrenal insufficiency and premenstrual insulin sensitivity.
- *Alimentary causes.* These include exocrine pancreatic failure and diabetic gastroparesis.
- *Renal failure.* The kidneys are important sites for the clearance of insulin, which tends to accumulate if renal function is lost.
- *Patient causes.* Patients may be unintelligent, uncooperative or may manipulate their therapy.

Recurrent ketoacidosis

This usually occurs in adolescents or young adults, particularly girls. Metabolic decompensation may develop very rapidly. A combination of chaotic food intake and insulin omission, whether consciously or unconsciously, is now regarded as the primary cause of this problem. It almost always occurs in the context of considerable psychosocial problems, particularly eating disorders. This area needs careful and sympathetic exploration in any patient with recurrent ketoacidosis. It is perhaps not surprising that in an illness where much of one's life is spent thinking of and controlling food intake, 30% of women with diabetes have had some features of an eating disorder at some time. Other causes include:

- *Iatrogenic.* Inappropriate insulin combinations may be a cause of swinging glycaemic control. For example, a once-daily regimen may cause hypoglycaemia during the afternoon or evening and pre-breakfast hyperglycaemia due to insulin deficiency.
- *Intercurrent illness.* Unsuspected infections, including urinary tract infections and tuberculosis, may be present. Thyrotoxicosis can also manifest as unstable glycaemic control.

FURTHER READING

Kjos SL, Buchanan TA (1999) Gestational diabetes mellitus. *New England Journal of Medicine* **341**: 1749–1756.
Steel JM, Johnstone FD (1996) Guidelines for the management of insulin-dependent diabetes mellitus in pregnancy. *Drugs* **52**(1): 60–70.
Tattersall RB (1997) Brittle diabetes revisited. *Diabetic Medicine* **14**(2): 99–110.

Hypoglycaemia in the non-diabetic

Hypoglycaemia develops when hepatic glucose output falls below the rate of glucose uptake by peripheral tissues. Hepatic glucose output may be reduced by:

- the inhibition of hepatic glycogenolysis and gluconeogenesis by insulin
- depletion of hepatic glycogen reserves by malnutrition, fasting, exercise or advanced liver disease
- impaired gluconeogenesis (e.g. following alcohol ingestion).

In the first of these categories, insulin levels are raised, the liver contains adequate glycogen stores, and the hypoglycaemia can be reversed by injection of glucagon. In the other two situations, insulin levels are low and glucagon is ineffective. Peripheral glucose uptake is accelerated by high insulin levels and by exercise, but these conditions are normally balanced by increased glucose output.

The most common symptoms and signs of hypoglycaemia are neurological. The brain consumes about

50% of the total glucose produced by the liver. This high energy requirement is needed to generate ATP used to maintain the potential difference across axonal membranes.

Insulin or sulphonylurea therapy for diabetes accounts for the vast majority of cases of severe hypoglycaemia encountered in an accident and emergency department.

Insulinomas

Insulinomas are pancreatic islet cell tumours that secrete insulin. Most are sporadic but some patients have multiple tumours arising from neural crest tissue (multiple endocrine neoplasia). Some 95% of these tumours are benign. The classic presentation is with fasting hypoglycaemia, but early symptoms may also develop in the late morning or afternoon. Recurrent hypoglycaemia is often present for months or years before the diagnosis is made, and the symptoms may be atypical or even bizarre; the presenting features in one series are given in Table 19.12. Common misdiagnoses include psychiatric disorders, particularly pseudodementia in elderly people, epilepsy and cerebrovascular disease. Whipple's triad remains the basis of clinical diagnosis. This is satisfied when:

- symptoms are associated with fasting or exercise
- hypoglycaemia is confirmed during these episodes
- glucose relieves the symptoms.

A fourth criterion – demonstration of inappropriately high insulin levels during hypoglycaemia – may usefully be added to these.

The diagnosis is confirmed by the demonstration of hypoglycaemia in association with inappropriate and excessive insulin secretion. Hypoglycaemia is demonstrated by:

- Measurement of *overnight fasting* (16 hours) glucose and insulin levels on three occasions. About 90% of patients with insulinomas will have low glucose and non-suppressed (normal or elevated) insulin levels.
- A prolonged 72-hour *supervised fast* if overnight testing is inconclusive and symptoms persist.

Autonomous insulin secretion is demonstrated by lack of the normal feedback suppression during hypoglycaemia. This may be shown by measuring insulin, C-peptide or proinsulin during a spontaneous episode of hypoglycaemia.

Table 19.12
Presenting features of insulinoma

Diplopia
Sweating, palpitations, weakness
Confusion or abnormal behaviour
Loss of consciousness
Grand mal seizures

Treatment of insulinoma

The most effective therapy is surgical excision of the tumour, but insulinomas are often very small and difficult to localize. Many techniques can be used to attempt to localize insulinomas. Sensitivity and specificity vary between centres and between operators. These include highly selective angiography, contrast-enhanced high-resolution CT scanning, scanning with radio-labelled somatostatin (some insulinomas express somatostatin receptors), and endoscopic and intraoperative ultrasound scanning. Venous sampling for the detection of 'hot spots' of high insulin concentration in the various intra-abdominal veins is still used occasionally.

Medical treatment with diazoxide is useful when the insulinoma is malignant, in patients in whom a tumour cannot be located, and in elderly patients with mild symptoms. Symptoms may also remit on treatment with a somatostatin analogue (octreotide or lanreotide).

Hypoglycaemia with other tumours

Hypoglycaemia may develop in the course of advanced neoplasia and cachexia, and has been described in association with many tumour types. Certain massive tumours, especially sarcomas, may produce hypoglycaemia owing to the secretion of insulin-like growth factor-1. True ectopic insulin secretion is extremely rare.

Postprandial hypoglycaemia

If frequent venous blood glucose samples are taken following a prolonged glucose tolerance test, about one in four subjects will have at least one value below 3 mmol/L. The arteriovenous glucose difference is quite marked during this phase, so that very few are truly hypoglycaemic in terms of arterial (or capillary) blood glucose content. Failure to appreciate this simple fact led some authorities to believe that postprandial (or reactive) hypoglycaemia was a potential 'organic' explanation for a variety of complaints that might otherwise have been considered psychosomatic. An epidemic of false 'hypoglycaemia' followed, particularly in the USA. Later work showed a poor correlation between symptoms and biochemical hypoglycaemia. Even so, a number of otherwise normal people occasionally become pale, weak and sweaty at times when meals are due, and report benefit from advice to take regular snacks between meals.

True postprandial hypoglycaemia may develop in the presence of alcohol, which 'primes' the cells to produce an exaggerated insulin response to carbohydrate. The person who substitutes alcoholic beverages for lunch is particularly at risk. Postprandial hypoglycaemia sometimes occurs after gastric surgery, owing to rapid gastric emptying and mismatching of nutrient absorption and insulin secretion. This is referred to as 'dumping' but it is now rarely encountered (see p. 276).

Hepatic and renal causes of hypoglycaemia

The liver can maintain a normal glucose output despite extensive damage, and hepatic hypoglycaemia is uncommon. It is particularly a problem with fulminant hepatic failure.

The kidney has a subsidiary role in glucose production (via gluconeogenesis in the renal cortex), and hypoglycaemia is sometimes a problem in terminal renal failure.

Hereditary fructose intolerance occurs in 1 in 20 000 live births and can cause hypoglycaemia (see p. 1115).

Endocrine causes of hypoglycaemia

Endocrine disorders resulting in deficiencies of hormones antagonistic to insulin are rare but well-recognized causes of hypoglycaemia. These include hypopituitarism, isolated adrenocorticotrophic hormone (ACTH) deficiency, and Addison's disease.

Drug-induced hypoglycaemia

Many drugs have been reported to produce isolated cases of hypoglycaemia, but usually only when other predisposing factors are present:

- Sulphonylureas may be used in the treatment of diabetes or may be taken by non-diabetics in suicide attempts.
- Quinine may produce severe hypoglycaemia in the course of treatment for falciparum malaria.
- Salicylates may cause hypoglycaemia following accidental ingestion by children, but this complication is very rare in adults.
- Propranolol has been reported to induce hypoglycaemia in the presence of strenuous exercise or starvation.
- Pentamidine may cause hypoglycaemia when used in the treatment of resistant pneumocystis pneumonia in people with AIDS.

Alcohol-induced hypoglycaemia

Alcohol inhibits gluconeogenesis. Alcohol-induced hypoglycaemia was first described in poorly nourished chronic alcoholics but may also present in binge drinkers and in children who have taken relatively small amounts of alcohol, since they have a diminished hepatic glycogen reserve. The clinical presentation is with coma and hypothermia.

Factitious hypoglycaemia

This is a relatively common variant of self-induced disease and is much more common than an insulinoma. Hypoglycaemia is produced by surreptitious self-administration of insulin or sulphonylureas. Many patients in this category have been extensively investigated for an insulinoma. Measurement of C-peptide levels during hypoglycaemia should identify patients who are injecting insulin; sulphonylurea abuse can be detected by chromatography of plasma or urine.

FURTHER READING

Markes V, Teale JD (1996) Investigation of hypoglycaemia. *Clinical Endocrinology* **44**: 133–136.

Disorders of lipid metabolism

Lipid physiology

Lipids are insoluble in water, and are transported in the bloodstream as macromolecular complexes. In these complexes, lipids (principally triglyceride, cholesterol and cholesterol esters) are surrounded by a stabilizing coat of phospholipid. Proteins (called apoproteins) embedded into the surface of these 'lipoprotein' particles exert a stabilizing function and allow the particles to be recognized by receptors in the liver and the peripheral tissues. The structure of a chylomicron (one type of lipoprotein particle) is illustrated in Figure 19.17.

Five principal types of lipoprotein particles are found in the blood (Fig. 19.18). They are structurally different and can be separated in the laboratory by their density and electrophoretic mobility. The larger particles give postprandial plasma its cloudy appearance. More than half of all patients aged under 60 with angiographically confirmed coronary artery disease have a lipoprotein disorder.

The genes for all the major apoproteins and that for the low-density lipoprotein (LDL) receptor have been isolated, sequenced and their chromosomal sites mapped. Production of abnormal apoproteins is known to produce, or predispose to, several types of lipid disorder, and it is likely that others will be discovered.

Chylomicrons (Fig. 19.18)

Chylomicrons are synthesized in the small intestine postprandially, passing initially into the intestinal lymphatic drainage, then along the thoracic duct into the bloodstream. They contain triglyceride and a small amount of cholesterol and its ester, and provide the main mechanism for transporting the digestion products

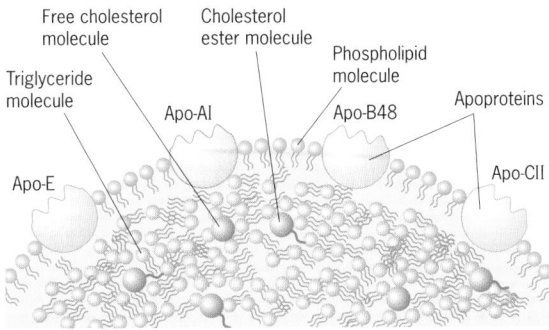

Fig. 19.17 Schematic diagram of a chylomicron particle (75–1200 nm) showing apoproteins lying in the surface membrane.

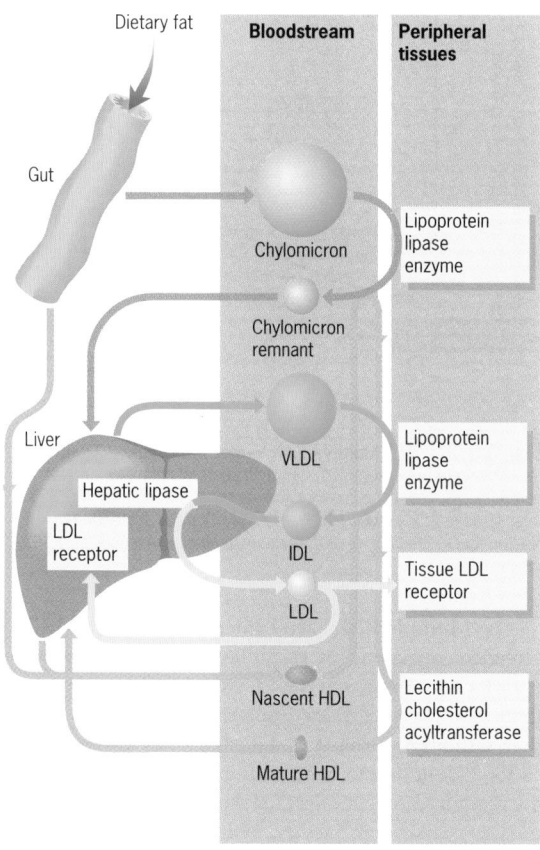

Fig. 19.18 Schematic representation of the sites of origin, interaction between, and fate of, the major lipoprotein particles.

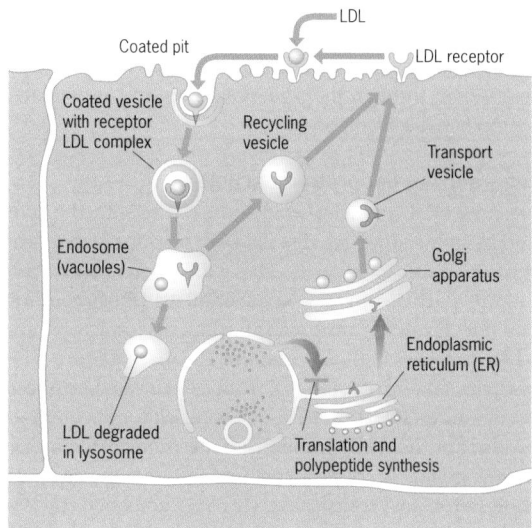

Fig. 19.19 **Receptor-mediated endocytosis.** LDL receptors are formed in the endoplasmic reticulum and transported via the Golgi apparatus to the surface of a hepatocyte. LDLs bind to these receptors, are internalized and taken up by the endosome. The receptor is recycled back to the surface, while the LDL is broken down by the lysosomes, freeing cholesterol needed for membrane synthesis.

of dietary fat to the liver and peripheral tissues. Each newly formed chylomicron contains several different apoproteins (B-48, A-I, A-II), and acquires apoproteins C-II and E by transfer from high-density lipoprotein (HDL) particles in the bloodstream. Apoprotein C-II binds to specific receptors in adipose tissue and skeletal muscle and the liver and allows the endothelial enzyme, lipoprotein lipase, to remove most of the triglyceride from the particle. The remaining chylomicron remnant particle, which contains the bulk of the original cholesterol, is taken up by the liver by mechanisms which are not fully understood, possibly mediated by apoprotein E.

Very-low-density lipoprotein (VLDL) particles
(Fig. 19.18)

These are synthesized continuously in the liver and contain most of the body's endogenously synthesized triglyceride and a smaller quantity of cholesterol. They are the body's main source of energy during prolonged fasting. Apoprotein B-100 is an essential component of VLDL. Apoproteins C-II and E are incorporated later into VLDL by transfer from HDL particles. As they pass round the circulation, VLDL particles bind through apoprotein C-II allowing triglyceride to be progressively

removed by lipoprotein lipase in the capillary endothelium. This leaves a particle, now depleted of triglyceride and apoprotein C-II, called an intermediate-density lipoprotein (IDL) particle.

Intermediate-density lipoprotein particles
(Fig. 19.18)

These have apoprotein B-100 and apoprotein E molecules on the particle surface. Most IDL particles bind to liver LDL receptors through the apoprotein E molecule and are then catabolized. Some IDL particles have further triglyceride removed (by the enzyme hepatic lipase), producing LDL particles.

Low-density lipoprotein particles (Fig. 19.18)

LDL particles are the main carrier of cholesterol, and deliver it both to the liver and to peripheral cells. The surface of the LDL particle contains a single apoprotein B-100, and also apoprotein E. The apoprotein B-100 is the principal ligand for the LDL clearance receptor. This receptor lies within coated pits on the surface of the hepatocyte. Once bound to the receptor, the coated pit invaginates and fuses with liposomes which destroy the LDL particle (Fig. 19.19). The number of hepatic LDL clearance receptors regulates the circulating LDL concentration, which is also influenced by controlling the activity of the rate-limiting enzyme in the cholesterol synthetic pathway, hydroxymethylglutaryl coenzyme A (HMG-CoA) reductase.

LDL particles can deposit lipid into the walls of the peripheral vasculature. Not all the cholesterol synthesized by the liver is packaged immediately into lipoprotein particles. Some is oxidized into bile salts. Both bile salts and cholesterol are excreted in the bile: both are then reabsorbed through the terminal ileum and recirculated (enterohepatic circulation).

High-density lipoprotein particles (Fig. 19.18)

Nascent HDL particles are produced in both the liver and intestine. They are disc shaped, seemingly inert and contain apoprotein A-I. They are transmuted into mature particles by the acquisition of phospholipids, and the E and C apoproteins from chylomicrons and VLDL particles in the circulation. The more mature HDL particles take up cholesterol from cells in the peripheral tissues aided by cholesterol-efflux regulatory protein – a product of the ATP-binding cassette transporter 1 gene (*ABC1* gene). As it is taken up, the enzyme lecithin-cholesterol acyl-transferase (LCAT), activated by the apoprotein A on the particle's surface, esterifies the sequestered cholesterol. The HDL particle transports cholesterol away from the periphery and may transfer it indirectly to other particles such as VLDL in the circulation or deliver its cholesterol directly to the liver (reverse cholesterol transport) and steroid-synthetic tissues (ovaries, testes, adrenal cortex).

This direct delivery takes place through scavenger-receptor B1. In experimental animals the absence of scavenger-receptor B1 dramatically accelerates the development of atheroma, and genetically programmed overproduction suppresses atheroma formation.

Measurement

When a laboratory measures fasting serum lipids, the majority of the total cholesterol concentration consists of LDL particles with a 20–30% contribution from HDL particles. The triglyceride concentration largely reflects the circulating number of VLDL particles, since chylomicrons are not normally present in the fasted state. If the patient is not fasted, the total triglyceride concentration will be raised owing to the additional presence of triglyceride-rich chylomicrons.

Epidemiology and lipids

LDL and total cholesterol

Population studies have repeatedly demonstrated a strong association between both total and LDL cholesterol concentration and coronary heart risk. There is a strong link between mean fat consumption, mean serum cholesterol concentration and the prevalence of coronary heart disease between countries. The exception is France where the cardiovascular risk is only moderate – perhaps owing to high alcohol consumption. Studies of migrants, particularly of Japanese men migrating to Hawaii, have shown that as diet changes, and cholesterol concentrations rise, so does the cardiovascular risk. Such studies show the importance of the environment rather than the genetic make-up of a population.

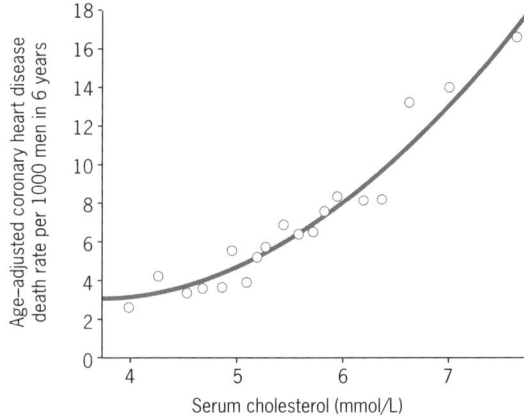

Fig. 19.20 The Multiple Risk Factor Intervention Trial: relationship between levels of serum cholesterol and risks of fatal coronary artery disease in a longitudinal study of more than 361 000 men screened for entry into the trial. From Stamler J, Wentworth D, Neaton JD (1986) *Journal of the American Medical Association* **256**: 2823.

The Multiple Risk Factor Intervention Trial (MRFIT) screened one-third of a million American men for various cardiovascular risk factors and then followed them for 6 years. Data from this study have shown that although cardiovascular risk rises progressively as total cholesterol concentration increases (Fig. 19.20), the risk increase is modest for individuals with no other cardiovascular risk factors. With each additional risk factor the effect produced by the same difference in cholesterol concentration becomes greatly magnified. The Framingham Study has reproduced these findings in a separate population.

HDL cholesterol

Epidemiological studies have shown that higher HDL concentrations protect against cardiovascular disease. HDL also has effects on the function of platelets and of the haemostatic cascade. These properties may favourably influence thrombogenesis.

VLDL particles (triglycerides)

There is a relatively weak independent link between raised concentrations of (triglyceride-rich) VLDL particles and cardiovascular risk. Very raised triglyceride concentrations (> 6 mmol/L) cause a greatly increased risk of acute pancreatitis and retinal vein thrombosis. Hypertriglyceridaemia tends to occur in association with a reduced HDL concentration. Much of the cardiovascular risk associated with 'hypertriglyceridaemia' turns out on multivariate analysis to be due to the associated low HDL levels and not to the hypertriglyceridaemia itself.

Chylomicrons

Excess chylomicrons do not confer an excess cardiovascular risk, but raise the total plasma triglyceride concentration.

Hyperlipidaemia

Hyperlipidaemia results from genetic predisposition interacting with an individual's diet.

Secondary hyperlipidaemia

If a lipid disorder has been detected it is vital to carry out a clinical history, examination and simple special investigations to detect causes of secondary hyperlipidaemia (Table 19.13), which may need treatment in their own right. Hypothyroidism, diabetes, renal disease and abnormal liver function can all raise plasma lipid levels, and can be excluded by measuring thyroid-stimulating hormone, fasting blood glucose concentration, urea and electrolyte concentrations, and liver biochemistry.

Classification, clinical features and investigation of primary hyperlipidaemias

As the genetic basis of lipid disorders becomes clearer, the genetic classification of Goldstein and colleagues is proving of greater clinical relevance than the Fredrickson (WHO) classification (based on the pattern of lipoproteins found in plasma). The lack of direct correspondence between these two systems of classification can be confusing. For clarity we have used the functional/genetic classification and not the Fredrickson classification. This has the advantage that the genetic disorders may be grouped by the results of simple lipid biochemistry into causes of:

- disorders of VLDL and chylomicrons – hypertriglyceridaemia alone
- disorders of LDL – hypercholesterolaemia alone
- disorders of HDL
- combined hyperlipidaemia.

Disorders of VLDL and chylomicrons – hypertriglyceridaemia alone

The majority of cases appear to be due to multiple genes acting together to produce a modest excess of circulating concentration of VLDL particles, such cases being termed polygenic hypertriglyceridaemia.

In a proportion of cases there will be a family history of a lipid disorder or its effects (e.g. pancreatitis). Such cases are often classified as familial hypertriglyceridaemia. The defect underlying the vast majority of such cases is not understood. The main clinical feature is a history of attacks of pancreatitis or retinal vein thrombosis in some individuals.

Lipoprotein lipase deficiency and apoprotein C-II deficiency

These are rare diseases which produce greatly elevated triglyceride concentrations owing to the persistence of chylomicrons (and not VLDL particles) in the circulation. The chylomicrons persist because the triglyceride within cannot be metabolized if the enzyme lipoprotein lipase is defective, or because the triglycerides cannot gain access to the normal enzyme owing to deficiency of the apoprotein C-II on their surface. Patients present in childhood with eruptive xanthomas, lipaemia retinalis and retinal vein thrombosis, pancreatitis and hepatosplenomegaly. If not identified in childhood it can present in adults with gross hypertriglyceridaemia resistant to simple measures. The presence of chylomicrons floating like cream on top of fasting plasma suggests this diagnosis. It is confirmed by plasma electrophoresis or ultracentrifugation. An abnormality of apoprotein C can be deduced if the hypertriglyceridaemia improves temporarily after infusing fresh frozen plasma, and lipoprotein lipase deficiency is likely if it does not.

Disorders of LDL – hypercholesterolaemia alone

Heterozygous familial hypercholesterolaemia is an autosomal dominant monogenic disorder present in 1 in 500 of the normal population. The average primary care physician would therefore be expected to have four such patients on his or her list, but because of clustering within families the prevalence is lower in some lists and much higher in others. There is an increased prevalence in some racial groups (e.g. French Canadians, Finns, South Africans). Surprisingly, most individuals with this disorder remain undetected. Patients may have no physical signs, in which case the diagnosis is made on the presence of very high plasma cholesterol concentrations which are unresponsive to dietary modification and are associated with a typical family history of early cardiovascular disease. Diagnosis can more easily be made if typical clinical features are present. These include xanthomatous thickening of the Achilles tendons and xanthomas over the extensor tendons of the fingers. Xanthelasma may be present, but is not diagnostic of familial hypercholesterolaemia.

The genetic defect of this disorder is the underproduction or malproduction of the LDL cholesterol receptor in the liver (Table 19.14). Over 150 different

Table 19.13
Causes of secondary hyperlipidaemia

Hypothyroidism
Diabetes mellitus (when poorly controlled)
Obesity
Renal impairment
Nephrotic syndrome
Dysglobulinaemia
Hepatic dysfunction
Drugs:
    Oral contraceptives in susceptible individuals
    Retinoids, thiazide diuretics, corticosteroids, opDDD (used in the treatment of Cushing's syndrome)

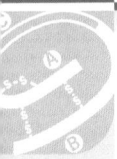
Table 19.14
The genetic defects underlying the common lipoprotein disorders

Disorder	Affected gene	Chromosome	Frequency
Common disorders			
Heterozygous familial hypercholesterolaemia	LDL receptor	19	1:500
Familial defective apoprotein B	Apo B-100	2	1:700
Hypobetalipoproteinaemia	Apo B-100	2	1:1000
Familial combined hyperlipidaemia	As yet unknown	As yet unknown	1:200
Familial hypertriglyceridaemia	As yet unknown	As yet unknown	1:500
Some rarer disorders			
Homozygous familial hypercholesterolaemia	LDL receptor	19	1:1 000 000
Lipoprotein lipase deficiency	As yet unknown	As yet unknown	1:1 000 000 (homozygous)
Apoprotein C-II deficiency	Apo C-II	19	40 cases

mutations in the LDL receptor have been described to date. Fifty per cent of men with the disease will die by the age of 60, most from coronary artery disease, if untreated.

Homozygous familial hypercholesterolaemia is very rare indeed. Affected children have no LDL receptors in the liver. They have a hugely elevated LDL cholesterol concentration, and massive deposition of lipid in arterial walls, the aorta and the skin. The natural history is for death from ischaemic heart disease in late childhood or adolescence. Repeated plasmapheresis has been used to remove LDL cholesterol with some success in these patients. Liver transplantation offers the possibility of cure, but the numbers of patients having undergone this procedure is small. The possibility of gene therapy offers a glimmer of hope on the horizon for affected individuals.

Mutations in the apoprotein B-100 gene cause another relatively common single gene disorder. Since LDL particles bind to their clearance receptor in the liver through apoprotein B-100, this defect also results in high LDL concentrations in the blood, and a clinical picture which closely resembles classical heterozygous familial hypercholesterolaemia. The two disorders can be distinguished clearly only by genetic tests. The approach to treatment is the same.

Polygenic hypercholesterolaemia is a term used to lump together patients with raised serum cholesterol concentrations, but without one of the monogenic disorders above. They exist in the right-hand tail of the normal distribution of cholesterol concentration. The precise nature of the polygenic variation in plasma cholesterol concentration remains unknown. Variations in the apoprotein E gene (chromosome 19) appear to contribute towards the problem in some individuals in this heterogeneous group.

Disorders of HDL – normal total cholesterol and triglycerides

Tangier disease

Tangier disease is an autosomal recessive disorder characterized by a low HDL cholesterol concentration. Cholesterol accumulates in reticuloendothelial tissue and arteries causing enlarged orange-coloured tonsils

and hepatosplenomegaly. Cardiovascular disease, corneal opacities and a polyneuropathy also occur. This has recently been discovered to be due to a mutation in the ATP-binding cassette transporter 1 gene (*ABC1* gene – see HDL physiology above) which normally promotes cholesterol uptake from cells by HDL particles.

Other mutations in this gene have been found in a few families with autosomal dominant HDL deficiency. It is as yet unknown whether abnormalities of this gene contribute to the low HDL cholesterol concentrations commonly seen in cardiovascular disease patients.

Combined hyperlipidaemia (hypercholesterolaemia and hypertriglyceridaemia)

The most common patient group is a polygenic combined hyperlipidaemia. Patients have an increased cardiovascular risk due to both high LDL concentrations and suppression of HDL by the hypertriglyceridaemia.

Familial combined hyperlipidaemia

This is relatively common, affecting 1 in 200 of the general population. The genetic basis for the disorder has not yet been characterized. It is diagnosed by finding raised cholesterol and triglyceride concentrations in association with a typical family history. There are no typical physical signs.

Remnant hyperlipidaemia

This is a rare (1 in 5000) cause of combined hyperlipidaemia. It is due to accumulation of LDL remnant particles and is associated with an extremely high risk of cardiovascular disease. It may be suspected in a patient with raised total cholesterol and triglyceride concentrations by finding xanthomas in the palmar creases (diagnostic) and the presence of tuberous xanthomas typically over the knees and elbows (Fig. 19.21). Remnant hyperlipidaemia is almost always due to the inheritance of a variant of the apoprotein E allele (apoprotein E2) together with an aggravating factor such as another primary hyperlipidaemia. When suspected clinically the diagnosis can be confirmed using ultracentrifugation of plasma, or phenotyping apoprotein E.

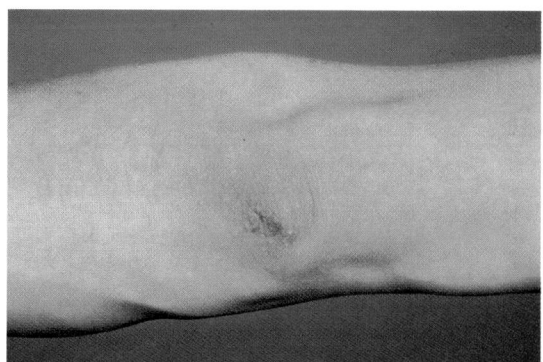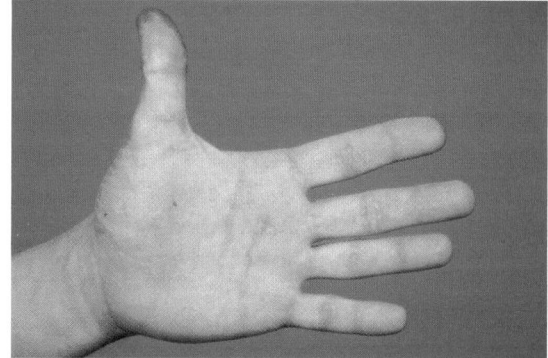

Fig. 19.21 Tuberous xanthomata behind the elbow and lipid deposits in the hand creases in a patient with remnant hyperlipidaemia.

Therapies available to treat hyperlipidaemia

The lipid-lowering diet

Studies have shown that dietitians helping patients to adjust their own diet to meet the nutritional targets set out below produce a better lipid-lowering effect than does the issuing of standard diet sheets and advice from a doctor. The main elements of a lipid-lowering diet are set out below.

Reduce the total fat intake

Dairy products and meat are the principal sources of saturated fat in the diet. Intake of these products should therefore be reduced, and fish and poultry should be substituted. Visible fat and skin should be removed before cooking and preparing meat dishes. Meat products including sausages and reconstituted meats (such as 'luncheon meat') should be avoided since the concentration of fat is unknown and often high. Baking and grilling of meats reduces the fat content and is preferred to frying. Low-fat or cottage cheese and skimmed or semi-skimmed milk should be substituted for the standard full-fat varieties. Pastries and cakes contain large quantities of fat and should be avoided. The overall aim should be to decrease fat intake such that it is providing approximately 30% of the total energy intake in the diet. Further reduction in fat intake is unacceptable to many patients.

Substitution with monounsaturates and polyunsaturates

Monounsaturated oils, particularly olive oil, and polyunsaturated oils such as sunflower, safflower, corn and soya oil, should be used in cooking instead of saturated fat-rich alternatives.

Reduce the dietary cholesterol intake

Liver, offal and fish roes should be avoided. Although eggs and prawns are rich in cholesterol their total contribution to the body's cholesterol pool is small and they can still be part of a balanced lipid-lowering diet.

Increase the intake of fibre (non-starch polysaccharides, NSPs)

Food high in soluble fibre, such as pulses, legumes, root vegetables, leafy vegetables, and unprocessed cereals, help reduce circulating lipid concentrations. These should be substituted in the diet in the place of higher-fat alternatives.

Reduce alcohol consumption

Excess alcohol is an important cause of secondary hyperlipidaemia, and may worsen primary lipid disorders.

Achieve an ideal bodyweight

Treatment of obesity is particularly important in the management of hyperlipidaemia, both because it will exacerbate the lipid disorder itself, and because obesity is an independent cardiovascular risk factor.

Consider foods containing stanol esters

Plant stanols reduce the absorption of cholesterol from the intestine by competing for space in the micelles that deliver lipid to the mucosal cells of the gut. They are largely unabsorbed and excreted in the stool. Increasing the amount of plant stanol in the diet 10-fold by using a margarine (e.g. Benecol) containing added stanol esters lowers LDL cholesterol by approximately 0.35–0.5 mmol/L. A reduction in the risk of heart disease of about 25% would be expected if this reduction in LDL cholesterol was applied to a population.

Fibrates (Table 19.15)

Fibrates raise HDL concentrations (beneficial) and reduce LDL cholesterol concentrations by 10–15% and are useful in patients with modest hypercholesterolaemia. Gemfibrozil has been demonstrated to reduce the incidence of cardiovascular events in a carefully performed large randomized double-blind placebo-controlled primary prevention trial (the Helsinki Heart Study) of patients with moderate hypercholesterolaemia. No similar trials have been carried out to assess the benefit of the other fibrates. Clofibrate is rarely used and is associated with an increased incidence of gallstones.

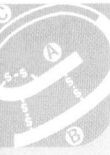
Table 19.15
Drugs used in the management of hyperlipidaemia

Drug	Mechanism of action	Contraindications and adverse reaction	Expected lipid-lowering effect	Long-term safety
Fibric acid derivatives e.g. Gemfibrozil Bezafibrate Fenofibrate Ciprofibrate	Complex and not fully understood 1. Limit substrate availability for hepatic triglyceride synthesis 2. Modulate LDL/ligand interaction 3. Promote action of lipoprotein lipase 4. Stimulate reverse transport of cholesterol	*Contraindications* Severe hepatic or renal impairment, gall bladder disease, pregnancy *Adverse effects* Reversible myositis, nausea, predispose to gallstones, non-specific malaise, impotence	Reduction of LDL cholesterol by 10–15% and triglycerides by 25–35% HDL cholesterol concentrations increase by 0–15% (newer agents often have greater beneficial effect on HDL)	No knowledge of effect on developing fetus Avoid in women of childbearing age Medium-term safety appears good but there is little really long-term experience
Cholesterol-binding resins e.g. Cholestyramine Colestipol	Anion exchange resins Bind bile acids in the gut, preventing enterohepatic circulation This promotes liver to convert cholesterol to bile acids Also stimulates formation of hepatic LDL receptors which take up more cholesterol from the circulation	*Adverse effects* Gastrointestinal adverse effects predominate: nausea, flatulence, abdominal bloating, alteration in bowel habit Palatability is a problem for some *Counselling* Other drugs bind to resins and should be taken 1 h before or 4 h afterwards	8–15% reduction in LDL Little or no effect on HDL cholesterol 5–15% rise in triglyceride concentration	Not systemically absorbed Safety profile is good and theoretically resins are of low risk in women of childbearing age Fat-soluble vitamin supplements may be required in children, pregnancy and breast-feeding
HMG-CoA reductase inhibitors ('statins') e.g. Simvastatin Pravastatin Atorvastatin Fluvastatin	Inhibit the rate-limiting step in cholesterol synthesis	*Contraindications* Active liver disease, pregnancy, lactation *Adverse effects* Derangement of liver function tests (recommended to measure liver function before and periodically during treatment) Myositis. Interferes with ciclosporin elimination and raises its blood concentration	30–40% reduction in LDL cholesterol Moderate reduction in triglycerides or moderate elevation of HDL cholesterol	Undetermined
Nicotinic acid and derivatives e.g. Nicotinic acid Acipimox	Unclear Probably inhibit lipid synthesis in the liver by reducing free fatty acid concentrations owing to an inhibitory effect on lipolysis in fat tissue	*Contraindications* Pregnancy, breast-feeding *Adverse effects* Value limited by frequent side-effects: headache, flushing, dizziness, nausea, malaise, itching, abnormal liver function Glucose intolerance, hyperuricaemia, activation of peptic ulcers, hyperpigmentation may occur	Reduce LDL and triglycerides by 5–10% Modest HDL increase	Medium-term safety known but marred by the adverse effects listed
ω-3 marine triglycerides	Reduce hepatic VLDL secretion	Occasional nausea and belching	Reduce triglycerides in severe hypertriglyceridaemia No favourable change in other lipids, and may aggravate hypercholesterolaemia in a few patients	No long-term experience

Bile acid binding resins (Table 19.15)

These produce an 8–15% reduction in LDL cholesterol concentration. Colestyramine has been shown to reduce the incidence of cardiovascular events in hypercholesterolaemic patients in a carefully performed randomized double-blind placebo-controlled primary prevention trial (the Lipid Research Clinics Trial). The safety profile of these drugs is good and their long-term safety is established. They are particularly useful when a lipid-lowering agent needs to be given to women of childbearing age (they are not absorbed from the gut). They have a synergistic effect when given with an HMG-CoA reductase inhibitor. This combination can reduce LDL cholesterol concentrations by 50–60%.

HMG-CoA reductase inhibitors (statins)
(Table 19.15)

These reduce LDL cholesterol concentrations by 30–40%. Two large secondary prevention trials – the Scandinavian Simvastatin Survival Study (4S) and the Cholesterol and Rare Events (CARE) trial – and one large primary prevention study, the West of Scotland Coronary Prevention Study (WOSCOPS) have demonstrated clearly the benefits of two drugs, simvastatin and pravastatin, in reducing both mortality and cardiovascular morbidity in hypercholesterolaemic patients, whether they are well or already have had a heart attack or angina (Fig. 19.22). The CARE trial went further in showing that cholesterol-lowering therapy using pravastatin reduced the risk of another heart attack in patients with cholesterol concentrations in the upper half of the normal range (4.0–6.0 mmol/L).

Should all post-infarct patients and hypercholesterolaemic patients be on a lipid-lowering drug? The greater an individual's overall cardiovascular risk, the more the cost/benefit ratio leans towards benefit (see p. 770).

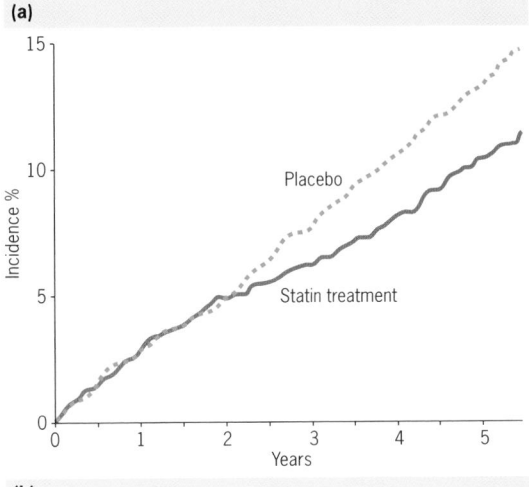

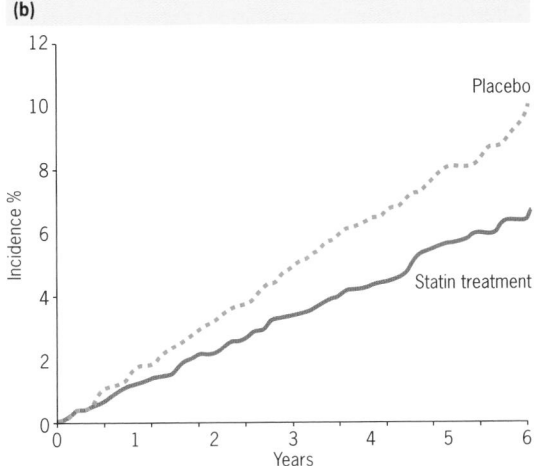

Fig. 19.22 Fatal coronary heart disease and non-fatal myocardial infarction according to treatment group in two trials: **(a)** WOSCOPS (6595 men studied) and **(b)** CARE (4159 studied, predominantly men).

Management of specific hyperlipidaemias

Screening

Most patients with hyperlipidaemia are asymptomatic and have no clinical signs. Many are discovered during the screening of high-risk individuals. Whose lipids should be measured?

There are great doubts as to whether blanket screening of plasma lipids is warranted. Selective screening of people at high risk of cardiovascular disease should be undertaken, to include those with:

- a family history of coronary heart disease (especially below 50 years of age)
- a family history of lipid disorders
- the presence of a xanthoma
- the presence of xanthelasma or corneal arcus before the age of 40 years
- obesity
- diabetes mellitus
- hypertension
- acute pancreatitis
- those undergoing renal replacement therapy.

Where one family member is known to have a monogenic disorder such as familial hypercholesterolaemia (1 in 500 of the population), siblings and children must have their plasma lipid concentrations measured. It is also worth screening the prospective partners of any patients with this heterozygous monogenic lipid disorder because of the small risk of producing children homozygous for the condition.

Acute severe illnesses such as myocardial infarction can derange plasma lipid concentrations for up to 3 months. Plasma lipid concentrations should be measured either within 48 hours of an acute myocardial infarction (before derangement has had time to occur) or 3 months later.

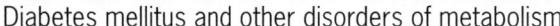
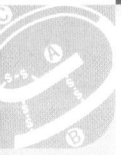

Serum cholesterol concentration does not change significantly after a meal and as a screening test a random blood sample is sufficient. If the total cholesterol concentration is raised, HDL cholesterol, triglyceride, and LDL cholesterol concentrations should be quantitated on a fasting sample. If a test for hypertriglyceridaemia is needed, a fasting blood sample is mandatory.

Hypertriglyceridaemia

A serum triglyceride concentration below 2.0 mmol/L is normal. In the range 2.0–6.0 mmol/L no specific intervention will be needed unless there are coincident cardiovascular risk factors, and in particular a strong family history of early cardiovascular death. In general, patients should be advised that they have a minor lipid problem, offered advice on weight reduction if obese, and advice on correcting other cardiovascular risk factors.

If the triglyceride concentration is above 6.0 mmol/L there is a risk of pancreatitis and retinal vein thrombosis. Patients should be advised to reduce their weight if overweight and start a formal lipid-lowering diet (see below). A proportion of individuals with hypertriglyceridaemia have livers which respond to even moderate degrees of alcohol intake by allowing accumulation or excess production of VLDL particles. If hypertriglyceridaemia persists, lipid measurements should be repeated before and after a 6-week interval of complete abstinence from alcohol. If a considerable improvement results, lifelong abstinence may prove necessary. Other drugs, including thiazides, oestrogens and glucocorticoids, can have a similar effect to alcohol in susceptible patients.

If the triglyceride concentration remains elevated above 6.0 mmol/L, despite the above measures, drug therapy is warranted. A fibric acid derivative is the agent of first choice. Nicotinic acid may be used in addition but its side-effects are often a problem. Fish oil capsules which contain ω-3 long-chain fatty acids are also effective in lowering triglyceride concentrations.

The severe hypertriglyceridaemia associated with the rare disorders of lipoprotein lipase deficiency and apoprotein C-II deficiency may require restriction of dietary fat to 10–20% of total energy intake and the use of special preparations of medium-chain triglycerides in cooking in place of oil or fat. Medium-chain triglycerides are not absorbed via chylomicrons (see p. 286).

Hypercholesterolaemia (without hypertriglyceridaemia)

Management of hypercholesterolaemia can be divided into primary prevention (end-organ damage has not yet occurred) and secondary prevention (end-organ damage – heart attacks and strokes – has already occurred). In both groups other treatable cardiovascular risk factors, including smoking, hypertension and excess weight, should also be addressed in tandem with treatment of hyperlipidaemia. The most important fact to be borne in mind is that cardiovascular risk factors (i.e. the above together with a family history of premature cardiovascular disease and gender) tend to cluster together in individuals and their effects on overall risk are multiplicative rather than additive. The level at which to intervene pharmacologically depends on an assessment of overall cardiovascular risk and of the likely benefits of risk reduction. Table 19.16 can be used as a guide to levels where treatment can be considered in the light of clinical circumstances.

Primary prevention for hypercholesterolaemic patients

Prescribe a lipid-lowering diet. Perimenopausal women should be offered female hormone replacement therapy (HRT) as the risk of cardiovascular disease rises sharply after the menopause and HRT reduces this risk even in normocholesterolaemic women. A small number of women respond adversely to exogenous oestrogens, with a rise in lipids; measurement of fasting lipid levels is therefore necessary shortly after starting treatment.

A guide to level of serum cholesterol at which drug treatment can reasonably be started is shown in Table 19.16.

An array of risk prediction tables are now available to allow quantification of the risk of a patient having a cardiovascular event within the next 10 years. Some advocate the use of these risk tables as a guide to treatment – for example if the 10-year risk reaches the 15% or

Table 19.16
Concentrations of cholesterol at which to consider drug treatment in the general population following failure of diet alone

Clinical context	Total cholesterol (mmol/L)	LDL cholesterol (mmol/L)	HDL cholesterol (mmol/L)
Secondary prevention (known coronary artery disease)	> 5.0	> 3.0	> 1.0
Primary prevention Genetic lipid problem, or two of smoking, diabetes, hypertension	> 6.5	> 3.8	No study data
Asymptomatic men (positive family history)	> 6.5	> 3.8	No study data
Asymptomatic men (no family history)	> 7.8	> 4.5	No study data

the 30% level. We side with those who have reservations over their use. Such risk analyses are a useful approach in helping to decide whether to use treatments such as aspirin. Aspirin probably has no effect until the day an atherosclerotic plaque ruptures, when it may then prevent thrombosis leading to a heart attack or stroke. Furthermore it has a significant associated morbidity and mortality (from bleeding). At a 10-year cardiovascular risk level of 15% the benefit/risk ratio for aspirin becomes favourable. At the 30% level the benefits are clear.

In contrast the use of lipid-lowering agents, if initially tolerated, has a low associated morbidity and mortality. These agents probably reduce the rate of atheroma accumulation over a period of decades. When a patient is young the chance that atheroma will be bad enough to cause a heart attack or stroke within the next 10 years will be small, even if atheroma is accumulating at a swift rate. The level of cardiovascular risk will only rise to the 15% or 30% level when the patient gets older. Yet it seems bizarre not to treat the gradual accumulation of atheroma when the patient is young with a low 10-year risk, and then to start treatment when age causes the 10-year risk levels to rise to a particular threshold, if all other factors are the same. In choosing whether or not to prescribe we prefer to consider 'will he/she live long enough to collect some pension and see his/her grandchildren?' rather than 'will he/she have a heart attack or stroke within the next 10 years?'. The answers to these two questions are very different.

Individuals with familial hypercholesterolaemia often require treatment with both diet and more than one cholesterol-lowering drug. Concurrent therapy with HMG-CoA reductase inhibitors and fibrates is usually avoided, in view of their overlapping side-effects, but in very severe cases such mixed therapy has been undertaken under very close supervision.

Secondary prevention
Studies have shown a clear reduction in mortality, and hypercholesterolaemic patients should be started on a statin at lower serum cholesterol levels than for primary prevention (Table 19.16). Patients with normal total cholesterol levels but low HDL levels (and often raised triglycerides) have been shown to have a reduced cardiovascular risk on treatment with the fibrate gemfibrozil.

Combined hyperlipidaemia (hypercholesterolaemia and hypertriglyceridaemia)
Treatment is the same for all varieties of combined hyperlipidaemia. For any given cholesterol concentration the hypertriglyceridaemia found in the combined hyperlipidaemias increases the cardiovascular risk considerably. Treatment is aimed at reducing serum cholesterol below 6.5 mmol/L and triglycerides below 2.0 mmol/L.

Therapy is with diet in the first instance and with drugs if an adequate response has not occurred. Fibric acid derivatives are the treatment of choice since these reduce both cholesterol and triglyceride concentrations, and also have the benefit of raising cardioprotective HDL concentrations. The combination of a fibric acid derivative and bile acid binding resin is of considerable use when a fibrate alone produces an insufficient reduction in LDL cholesterol. Nicotinic acid can be used in addition, although its unwanted effects render it a third-line agent.

Other lipid disorders

Hypolipidaemia
Low lipid levels can be found in severe protein–energy malnutrition. They are also seen occasionally with severe malabsorption and in intestinal lymphangiectasia.

Hypobetalipoproteinaemia (Table 19.14) is a benign familial condition which is being increasingly recognized. The cholesterol levels are in the range 1–3.5 mmol/L.

Abetalipoproteinaemia
This is described on page 298.

FURTHER READING

Anonymous (1996) Management of hyperlipidaemia. *Drug and Therapeutics Bulletin* **34**(12): 89–93.

Dammerman M, Breslow JL (1995) Genetic basis of lipoprotein disorders. *Circulation* **91**: 505–512.

Farmer JA, Gotto AM (1996) Choosing the right lipid-regulating agent: a guide to selection. *Drugs* **52**: 649–661.

Garber AM, Browner WS, Hulley SB (1996) Cholesterol screening in asymptomatic adults – revisited. *Annals of Internal Medicine* **124**: 518–531.

Grundy SM (1997) Cholesterol and coronary heart disease: the 21st century. *Archives of Internal Medicine* **157**: 1177–1184.

Knopp RH (1999) Drug treatment of lipid disorders. *New England Journal of Medicine* **341**: 498–511.

Law M (2000) Plant sterol and stanol margarines and health. *British Medical Journal* **320**: 861–864.

Owen JS (1999) Role of ABC1 gene in cholesterol efflux and atheroprotection. *Lancet* **354**: 1402–1403.

Sacks FM, Pfeffer MA et al. (1996) The effect of pravastatin on coronary events after myocardial infarction in patients with average cholesterol levels. *New England Journal of Medicine* **335**: 1001–1009.

Scandinavian Simvastatin Survival Study Group (1994) Randomised trial of cholesterol lowering in 4444 patients with coronary heart disease. *Lancet* **334**: 1383–1389.

Shepherd J, Cobbe SM et al. (1995) Prevention of coronary heart disease with pravastatin in men with hypercholesterolaemia. *New England Journal of Medicine* **333**: 1301–1307.

Thompson GR (1997) What targets should lipid-modulating therapy achieve to optimize the prevention of coronary heart disease? *Atherosclerosis* **131**: 1–5.

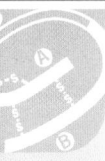

Inborn errors of carbohydrate metabolism

Glycogen storage disease

All mammalian cells can manufacture glycogen, but the main sites of its production are the liver and muscle. Glycogen is a high-molecular-weight glucose polymer. In glycogen storage disease there is either an abnormality in the molecular structure or an increase in glycogen concentration owing to a specific enzyme defect. Almost all these conditions are autosomal recessive in inheritance and present in infancy, except for McArdle's disease, which presents in adults.

Table 19.17 shows the classification and clinical features of some of these diseases.

Galactosaemia

Galactose is normally converted to glucose. However, a deficiency of the enzyme galactose-1-phosphate uridyl-transferase or, less commonly, uridine diphosphate galactase-4-epimerase results in accumulation of galactose-1-phosphate in the blood. The transferase deficiency, inherited as an autosomal recessive, is due in 70% of patients to a mutation Q188R in which arginine is substituted for glutamine. Galactose ingestion (i.e. milk) leads to inanition, failure to thrive, vomiting, liver disease, cataracts and developmental delay. A lactose-free diet stops the acute toxicity but poor growth and problems with speech and mental development still occur with the transferase deficiency.

Prenatal diagnosis and diagnosis of the carrier state are possible by measurement of the level of galactose-1-phosphate in the blood.

Galactokinase deficiency also results in galactosaemia and early cataract formation.

Defects of fructose metabolism

Absorbed fructose is chiefly metabolized in the liver to lactic acid or glucose. Three defects of metabolism in the liver and intestine occur; all are inherited as autosomal recessive traits:

- *Fructosuria* is due to fructokinase deficiency. It is a benign asymptomatic condition.

Table 19.17
Some glycogen storage diseases

Type	Affected tissue	Enzyme defect	Clinical features	Tissue needed for diagnosis*	Outcome
Liver glycogenoses					
I (Von Gierke)	Liver, intestine, kidney	Glucose-6-phosphatase	Hepatomegaly, hypoglycaemia, stunted growth, obesity, hypotonia	Liver	If patients survive initial hypoglycaemia, prognosis is good; hyperuricaemia is a late complication
III (Forbes)	Liver, muscle (abnormal glycogen structure)	Glycogen debranching enzyme	Like type I	Leucocytes, liver, muscle	Good prognosis but progressive neuropathy and cardiomyopathy
IV (Anderson)	Liver (abnormal glycogen structure)	Branching enzyme	Failure to thrive, hepatomegaly, cirrhosis and its complications	Leucocytes, liver, muscle	Death in first 5 years
VI (Hers)	Liver	Liver phosphorylase or phosphorylase kinase	Hepatomegaly with hypoglycaemia in childhood	Liver	Good
Muscle glycogenoses					
II (Pompé)	Liver, muscle, heart	Lysosomal acid α-glucosidase	Heart failure, cardiomyopathy	Fibroblasts, muscles	Death in first 6 months; juvenile and adult variants seen
V (McArdle)	Muscle only	Phosphorylase	Muscle cramps and myoglobinuria after exercise (in adults)	Muscle	Normal life-span; exercise must be avoided
VII (Tarui)	Muscle	Phosphofructokinase	Like type V	Muscle	Like type V

*Tissue obtained is used for the biochemical assay of the enzyme

- *Hereditary fructose intolerance* is due to fructose-1-phosphate aldolase deficiency. Fructose-1-phosphate accumulates after fructose ingestion, inhibiting both glycogenolysis and gluconeogenesis, resulting in symptoms of severe hypoglycaemia. Hepatomegaly and renal tubular defects occur but are reversible on a fructose- and sucrose-free diet. Intelligence is normal and there is an absence of dental caries.
- *Hereditary fructose-1,6-diphosphatase deficiency* leads to a failure of gluconeogenesis. Infants present with hypoglycaemia, ketosis and lactic acidosis. Dietary control can lead to normal growth.

Pentosuria

Pentosuria is due to reduced activity of NADP-linked sylitol dehydrogenase. It has no clinical significance.

Inborn errors of amino acid metabolism

Inborn errors of amino acid metabolism are chiefly inherited as autosomal recessive conditions. The major ones are shown in Table 19.18.

Table 19.18
The major inborn errors of amino acid metabolism

Disease	Enzyme defect	Incidence	Biochemical and clinical features	Treatment	Prognosis
Albinism	Tyrosinase	1 in 13 000	Amelanosis: whitish hair, pink-white skin, grey-blue eyes Nystagmus, photophobia, strabismus	Symptomatic	Good
Alkaptonuria	Homogentisic acid oxidase	1 in 100 000	Homogentisic acid polymerizes to produce a black-brown product that is deposited in cartilage and other tissue (ochronosis)	None	Good
Homocystinuria Type I	Cystathionine synthetase		Homocystine is excreted in urine	–	–
			Mental handicap	–	–
			Marfan-like syndrome	–	–
			Thrombotic episodes	–	–
Type II	Methylene tetrahydrofolate reductase		Survivors have mental retardation	–	Mainly die as neonates
Phenylketonuria	Phenylalanine hydroxylase	1 in 20 000	Brain damage with mental retardation and epilepsy Phenylpyruvate and its derivatives excreted in urine	Diet low in phenylalanine in first few months of life prevents damage	Good but some intellectual impairment
Histidinaemia	Histidase	Very rare	Mental retardation	–	–
'Maple syrup' disease	Branched-chain ketoacid dehydrogenase	Very rare	Failure to thrive Fits, neonatal acidosis and severe cerebral degeneration Valine, isoleucine and their derivatives are excreted in urine A milder form is seen	–	Early death
Oxalosis (hyperoxaluria)	Alanine: glyoxylate aminotransferase	Very rare	Nephrocalcinosis, renal stones, renal failure due to deposition of calcium oxalate Prenatal and early diagnosis now possible	–	Liver transplantation ? Gene therapy

There are many other enzyme defects producing, for example, alaninaemia, ammonaemia, argininaemia, citrullinaemia, isovaleric acidaemia, lysinaemia, ornithinaemia or tyrosinaemia

Amino acid transport defects

Amino acids are filtered by the glomerulus, but 95% of the filtered load is reabsorbed in the proximal convoluted tubule by an active transport mechanism. Aminoaciduria results from:

- abnormally high plasma amino acid levels (e.g. phenylketonuria)
- any inherited disorder that damages the tubules secondarily (e.g. galactosaemia)
- tubular reabsorptive defects, either generalized (e.g. Fanconi syndrome) or specific (e.g. cystinuria).

Amino acid transport defects can be congenital or acquired.

Generalized aminoacidurias

Fanconi syndrome

This occurs in a juvenile form (De Toni–Fanconi–Debré syndrome); in adult life it is often acquired through, for example, heavy metal poisoning, drugs or some renal diseases. There is defective tubular reabsorption of:

- most amino acids
- glucose
- urate
- phosphate, resulting in hypophosphataemic rickets
- bicarbonate, with failure to transport hydrogen ions, causing a renal tubular acidosis that then produces a hyperchloraemic acidosis.

Other abnormalities include:

- potassium depletion, primary or secondary to the acidosis
- polyuria
- increased excretion of immunoglobulins and other low-molecular-weight proteins.

Various combinations of the above abnormalities have been described.

The juvenile form begins at the age of 6–9 months, with failure to thrive, vomiting and thirst. The clinical features are as a result of fluid and electrolyte loss and the characteristic vitamin D-resistant rickets.

In the adult, the disease is similar to the juvenile form, but osteomalacia is a major feature.

Treatment of the bone disease is with large doses of vitamin D (e.g. 1–2 mg of 1α-hydroxycholecalciferol with regular blood calcium monitoring). Fluid and electrolyte loss need to be corrected.

Lowe's syndrome (oculocerebrorenal dystrophy)

In this syndrome there is generalized aminoaciduria combined with mental retardation, hypotonia, congenital cataracts and an abnormal skull shape.

Specific aminoacidurias

Cystinuria

There is a defective tubular reabsorption and jejunal absorption of cystine and the dibasic amino acids, lysine, ornithine and arginine. Inheritance is either completely or incompletely recessive, so that heterozygotes who have increased excretion of lysine and cystine only can occur. Cystine absorption from the jejunum is impaired but, nevertheless, cystine in peptide form can be absorbed. Cystinuria leads to urinary stones and is responsible for approximately 1–2% of all urinary calculi. The disease often starts in childhood, although most cases present in adult life.

Treatment is with a high fluid intake in order to keep the urinary cystine concentration low. Patients are encouraged to drink up to 3 L over 24 hours and to drink even at night. Penicillamine should be used for patients who cannot keep the cystine concentration of their urine low.

The condition cystinosis (see p. 1117) must not be confused with cystinuria.

Hartnup's disease

There is defective tubular reabsorption and jejunal absorption of most neutral amino acids but not their peptides. The resulting tryptophan malabsorption produces nicotinamide deficiency (see p. 236). Patients can be asymptomatic, but others develop evidence of pellagra, with cerebellar ataxia, psychiatric disorders and skin lesions. Treatment is with nicotinamide which often brings about considerable improvement.

Tryptophan malabsorption syndrome (blue diaper syndrome)

This is due to an isolated transport defect for tryptophan: the tryptophan excreted oxidizes to a blue colour on the baby's diaper.

Familial iminoglycinuria

This occurs when there is defective tubular reabsorption of glycine, proline and hydroxyproline. It seems to have few clinical effects.

Methionine malabsorption syndrome

This is due to failure to absorb and excrete methionine, and results in diarrhoea, vomiting and mental retardation. Patients characteristically have an oast-house smell.

Lysosomal storage diseases

Lysosomal storage diseases are due to inborn errors of metabolism which are mainly inherited in an autosomal recessive manner.

Glucosylceramide lipidoses: Gaucher's disease

This is the most prevalent lysosomal storage disease and is due to a deficiency in glucocerebrosidase, a specialized lysosomal acid β-glucosidase. This results in accumulation of glucosylceramide in the lysosomes of the reticuloendothelial system, particularly the liver, bone marrow and spleen. Several mutations have been characterized in the glucocerebrosidase gene, the most common being a single base change causing the substitution of arginine for serine; this is seen in 70% of Jewish patients. The typical Gaucher cell, a glucocerebroside-containing reticuloendothelial histiocyte, is found in the bone marrow.

There are three clinical types, the most common presenting in adult life with an insidious onset of hepatosplenomegaly. There is a high incidence in Ashkenazi Jews (1 in 3000 births), and patients have a characteristic pigmentation on exposed parts, particularly the forehead and hands. The clinical spectrum is variable, with patients developing anaemia, evidence of hypersplenism and pathological fractures that are due to bone involvement. Nevertheless, many have a normal life-span.

Acute Gaucher's disease presents in infancy or childhood with rapid onset of hepatosplenomegaly, with neurological involvement owing to the presence of Gaucher cells in the brain. The outlook is poor.

Some patients with non-neuropathic Gaucher's disease show considerable improvement with infusion of alglucerase (mannose-terminated placental or human recombinant glucocerebrosidase).

Sphingomyelin cholesterol lipidoses: Niemann–Pick disease

The disease is due to a deficiency of lysosomal sphingomyelinase which results in the accumulation of sphingomyelin cholesterol and glycosphingolipids in the reticuloendothelial macrophages of many organs, particularly the liver, spleen, bone marrow and lymph nodes. The disease usually presents within the first 6 months of life with mental retardation and hepatosplenomegaly. Typical foam cells are found in the marrow, lymph nodes, liver and spleen.

The mucopolysaccharidoses (MPSs)

These are a group of disorders caused by the deficiency of lysosomal enzymes required for the catabolism of glycosaminoglycans (mucopolysaccharides).

The catabolism of dermatan sulphate, heparan sulphate, keratin sulphate or chondroitin sulphate may be affected either singularly or together.

Accumulation of glycosaminoglycans in the lysosomes of various tissues results in the disease. Ten forms of MPS have been described; all are chronic but progressive and a wide spectrum of clinical severity can be seen within a single enzyme defect. The MPS types show many clinical features though in variable amounts, with dysostosis, abnormal facies, poor vision and hearing and joint dysmobility (either stiff or hypermobile) being frequently seen. Mental retardation is present in, for example, Hurler (MPS IH) and San Filippo A (MPS IIIA) types, but normal intelligence and life-span are seen in Scheie (MPS IS). α-L-Iduronidase infusion reduces lysosomal storage, resulting in clinical improvement.

The GM2 gangliosidoses

In these conditions there is accumulation of GM2 gangliosides in the central nervous system and peripheral nerves. It is particularly common (1 in 2000) in Ashkenazi Jews. *Tay-Sachs disease* is the severest form where there is a progressive degeneration of all cerebral function, with fits, epilepsy, dementia and blindness, and death usually occurs before 2 years of age. The macula has a characteristic cherry spot appearance.

Fabry's disease

This X-linked recessive condition is due to a deficiency of the lysosomal hydrolase α-galactosidase causing an accumulation of glycosphingolipids with terminal α-galactosyl moieties in the lysosomes of various tissues including the liver, kidney, blood vessels and the ganglion cells of the nervous system. The patients present with peripheral nerve involvement, but eventually most patients develop renal problems in adult life.

Diagnosis

Many of the sphingolipidoses can be diagnosed by demonstrating the enzyme deficiency in the appropriate tissue.

Prenatal diagnosis is possible in a number of the conditions by obtaining specimens of amniotic cells. Carrier states can also be identified, so that sensible genetic counselling can be given.

FURTHER READING

Cox TM (2001) Gaucher's disease. *Quarterly Journal of Medicine* **94**: 399–402.

Cystinosis

Cystine accumulates within the lysosomes of most tissues, but particularly the kidneys. This is due to a defect of cystine transport across the lysosomal membrane. There are two cystinosis phenotypes, nephropathic and non-nephropathic.

The common nephropathic form presents in the first year of life with failure to thrive. This results from the renal tubular Fanconi syndrome caused by cystine deposits in the kidney. Renal damage progresses and visual impairment occurs as the result of cystine

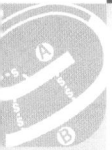
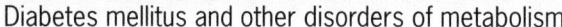

deposits in the retina and cornea. Renal transplantation relieves the kidney problems, but cystine accumulation continues to occur.

The nephropathic form can present in older children and in adults, when the condition tends to be less aggressive.

The non-nephropathic form presents in children with visual impairment. The kidneys seem not to be affected.

Amyloidosis

Amyloidosis is a disorder of protein metabolism in which there is an extracellular deposition of pathologic insoluble fibrillar proteins in organs and tissues. Characteristically, the amyloid protein consists of β-pleated sheets that are responsible for its insolubility and resistance to proteolysis.

Amyloidosis can be acquired or inherited. Classification is based on the nature of the precursor plasma proteins that form the fibrillar deposits. The process for the production of these fibrils appears to be multifactorial and differs amongst the various types of amyloid.

AL amyloidosis

This is a plasma cell dyscrasia, related to multiple myeloma, in which clonal plasma cells in the bone marrow produce immunoglobulins that are amyloidogenic. This may be the outcome of destabilization of light chains owing to substitution of particular amino acids into the light chain variable region. There is a clonal dominance of amyloid light (AL) chains – either the dominant κ or λ isotype – which are excreted in the urine (Bence Jones proteins). This type of amyloid is often associated with lymphoproliferative disorders, such as myeloma, Waldenström's macroglobulinaemia or non-Hodgkin's lymphoma.

Familial amyloidoses

These are autosomally dominant transmitted diseases where the mutant protein forms amyloid fibrils, starting usually in middle age. The most common form is due to a mutant – transthyretin – which is a tetrameric protein with four identical subunits. It is a transport protein for thyroxine and retinol-binding protein and mainly synthesized in the liver. Over 50 amino acid substitutions have been described; for example, a common substitution is that of methionine for valine at position 30 (Met 30) in all racial groups, and alanine for threonine (Ala 60) in the English and Irish. These substitutions destabilize the protein, which precipitates following stimulation, and can cause disorders such as familial amyloidotic polyneuropathy (FAP) or cardiomyopathy. Major foci of FAP occur in Portugal, Japan and Sweden.

Other less common variants include mutations of apoprotein A-I, gelsolin, fibrinogen Aα and lysozyme.

Reactive systemic (secondary) amyloidoses

These are due to amyloid formed from serum amyloid A (SAA) which is an acute phase protein. It is, therefore, related to chronic inflammatory disorders and chronic infection.

Clinical features

Immunoglobulin light chain-associated (AL) (primary) amyloidosis

The clinical features are related to the organs involved. These include the kidneys (presenting with proteinuria and the nephrotic syndrome) and the heart (presenting with heart failure). Autonomic and sensory neuropathies are relatively common, and carpal tunnel syndrome with weakness and paraesthesia of the hands may be an early feature. Sensory neuropathy is common. There is an absence of central nervous system involvement.

On examination, hepatomegaly and rarely splenomegaly, cardiomyopathy, polyneuropathy and bruising may be seen. Macroglossia occurs in about 20% of cases.

Familial transthyretin-associated (ATTR) amyloidosis

In this condition peripheral sensorimotor and autonomic neuropathy is more common, with symptoms of autonomic dysfunction, diarrhoea and weight loss. Renal disease is less prevalent than with AL amyloidosis. Macroglossia does not occur. Cardiac problems are usually those of conduction. There may be a family history of unidentified neurological disease.

Other hereditary systemic amyloidoses include other familial amyloid polyneuropathies (e.g. Portuguese, Icelandic, Dutch). There is a familial Creutzfeldt–Jakob disease. In familial Mediterranean fever, renal amyloidosis is a common serious complication.

AA (reactive or secondary) amyloidosis

This depends on the nature of the disorder. Chronic inflammatory disorders include rheumatoid arthritis, inflammatory bowel disease, and untreated familial Mediterranean fever. In developing countries it is still associated with infectious diseases such as tuberculosis, bronchiectasis and osteomyelitis. AA amyloidosis often presents with renal disease, with hepatomegaly and splenomegaly. Macroglossia is not a feature and cardiac involvement is rare.

Cerebral amyloidosis, Alzheimer's disease and transmissible spongiform encephalopathy

The brain is a common site of amyloid deposition, although it is not directly affected in any form of acquired systemic amyloidosis. Intracerebral and cerebrovascular amyloid deposits are seen in Alzheimer's disease. Most cases are sporadic, but hereditary forms caused by mutations have been reported. In hereditary spongiform encephalopathies several amyloid plaques have been seen.

Amyloid deposits are frequently found in the elderly, particularly cerebral deposits of A4 protein. This is also seen in Down's syndrome. Apoprotein E (involved in LDL transport, see p. 1105) interacts directly with β-A4 protein in senile plaques and neurofibrillary tangles in the brain. The gene for apoprotein E is on chromosome 19 and may be an important susceptibility factor in the aetiology of Alzheimer's disease.

Local amyloidosis

Deposits of amyloid fibrils of various types can be localized to various organs or tissues (e.g. skin, heart and brain) and amyloid syndrome due to β_2-microglobulin deposition as amyloid fibrils is seen in patients on long-term haemodialysis (see p. 655).

Diagnosis

This is based on clinical suspicion and, if possible, on tissue histology. Amyloid in tissues appears as an amorphous, homogeneous substance that stains pink with haematoxylin and eosin and stains red with Congo red. It also has a green fluorescence in polarized light. Tissue can be obtained from the rectum or gum. The bone marrow may show plasma cells in primary amyloidosis or a lymphoproliferative disorder. A paraproteinaemia and proteinuria with light chains in the urine may be seen in AL amyloidosis. In secondary or reactive amyloidosis there will be an underlying disorder. Scintigraphy using ^{123}I-labelled serum amyloid P component is useful for the assessment of AL, ATTR and AA amyloidosis, but it is not widely available.

Treatment

This is symptomatic or the treatment of the associated disorder. The nephrotic syndrome and congestive cardiac failure require the relevant therapies. Treatment of any inflammatory source or infection should be instituted. Colchicine may help familial Mediterranean fever. Chemotherapy is showing some efficacy in AL amyloidosis. In ATTR amyloidosis where transthyretin is predominantly synthesized in the liver, liver transplantation (when there would be a disappearance of the mutant protein from the blood) is now considered as the definitive therapy.

FURTHER READING

Falk RH, Comenzo RL, Skinner M (1997) The systemic amyloidoses. *New England Journal of Medicine* **337**: 898–909.

The porphyrias

This heterogeneous group of rare inborn errors of metabolism is caused by abnormalities of enzymes involved in the biosynthesis of haem, resulting in overproduction of the intermediate compounds called 'porphyrins' (Fig. 19.23). The porphyrias show extreme genetic heterogeneity. For example, in acute intermittent porphyria more than 90 mutations have been identified in the porphobilinogen deaminase gene. One mutation has a high prevalence in patients in northern Sweden, suggesting a common ancestor.

Structurally, porphyrins consist of four pyrrole rings. These pyrrole rings are formed from the precursors glycine and succinyl-CoA, which are converted to δ-amino-laevulinic acid (δ-ALA) in a reaction catalysed by the enzyme δ-ALA synthetase. Two molecules of δ-ALA condense to form a pyrrole ring.

Porphyrins can be divided into uroporphyrins, coproporphyrins or protoporphyrins depending on the structure of the side-chain. They are termed type I if the structure is symmetrical and type III if it is asymmetrical. Both uroporphyrins and coproporphyrins can be excreted in the urine.

The sequence of enzymatic changes in the production of haem is shown in Figure 19.23. The chief rate-limiting step is the enzyme δ-ALA synthetase, as an increase in this enzyme results in an overproduction of porphyrins. Haem provides a negative-feedback mechanism on this enzyme.

In porphyria the excess production of porphyrins occurs either in the liver (hepatic porphyria) or in the bone marrow (erythropoietic porphyria), but porphyrias can also be classified in terms of clinical presentation as *acute* or *non-acute*. Acute porphyrias usually produce neuropsychiatric problems and are associated with excess production and urinary excretion of δ-ALA and porphobilinogen; these metabolites are not increased in non-acute porphyrias. The second control mechanism is therefore porphobilinogen deaminase (see Fig. 19.23); this is depressed or normal in the acute porphyrias and raised in non-acute cases.

A classification of porphyrias is given in Table 19.19.

Acute intermittent porphyria

This is an autosomal dominant disorder. Presentation is in early adult life, usually around the age of 30 years, and women are affected more than men. It may be precipitated by alcohol and drugs such as barbiturates and oral contraceptives, but a wide range of lipid-soluble drugs have also been incriminated. The abnormality lies at the level of porphobilinogen deaminase in the haem biosynthetic pathway (see Fig. 19.23).

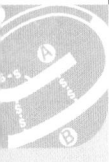
Glycine + succinyl CoA

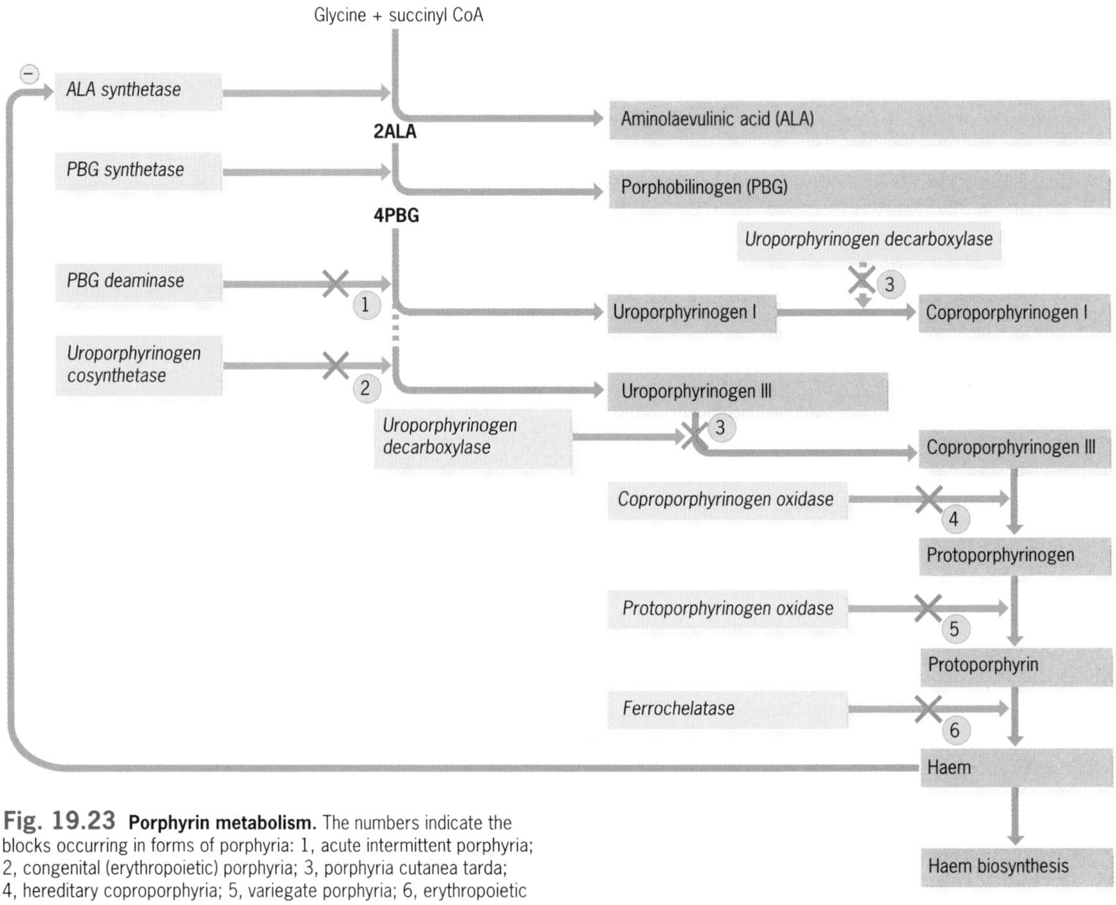

ALA synthetase → Aminolaevulinic acid (ALA)

2ALA

PBG synthetase → Porphobilinogen (PBG)

4PBG

Uroporphyrinogen decarboxylase

PBG deaminase ✕ 1 → Uroporphyrinogen I ✕ 3 → Coproporphyrinogen I

Uroporphyrinogen cosynthetase ✕ 2 → Uroporphyrinogen III

Uroporphyrinogen decarboxylase ✕ 3 → Coproporphyrinogen III

Coproporphyrinogen oxidase ✕ 4 → Protoporphyrinogen

Protoporphyrinogen oxidase ✕ 5 → Protoporphyrin

Ferrochelatase ✕ 6 → Haem

Haem biosynthesis

Fig. 19.23 Porphyrin metabolism. The numbers indicate the blocks occurring in forms of porphyria: 1, acute intermittent porphyria; 2, congenital (erythropoietic) porphyria; 3, porphyria cutanea tarda; 4, hereditary coproporphyria; 5, variegate porphyria; 6, erythropoietic protoporphyria.

Table 19.19
The classification of porphyrias

	Hepatic	Erythropoietic
Acute	Acute intermittent porphyria Variegate porphyria Hereditary coproporphyria	
Non-acute	Porphyria cutanea tarda	Congenital porphyria Erythropoietic protoporphyria

Diagnosis

Presentation is with:

- abdominal pain, vomiting and constipation (90%)
- polyneuropathy (motor, but occasionally sensory) (70%)
- hypertension and tachycardia (70%)
- psychiatric disorders (such as depression, anxiety and frank psychosis) (50%).

The diagnosis should be considered whenever there is a combination of these cardinal features or a family history of porphyria.

The urine turns red-brown or red on standing. A classic bedside test for excess porphobilinogen may be performed by adding one volume of urine to one volume of Ehrlich's aldehyde, which produces a pink colour. If excess porphobilinogen is present, the pink colour persists when two volumes of chloroform are added. A negative test does not exclude an attack. A positive test should be confirmed by a specific assay.

Other investigations

- **Blood count**. This is usually normal, with occasional neutrophil leucocytosis.
- **Liver biochemical tests.** There is elevated bilirubin and amino transferase.
- **Serum urea** is often raised.
- **Faecal and urinary porphyrins** confirm the type of porphyria.

Screening

Family members should be screened to detect latent cases. Urinalysis is not adequate but measurement of erythrocyte porphobilinogen deaminase and ALA synthetase is extremely sensitive.

Management

Management of the acute episodes is largely supportive. A high carbohydrate intake is maintained (this has an indirect effect on porphyrin overproduction), and a narcotic is given for pain. Intravenous haem arginate (human hemin) infusion is of benefit in reducing the duration of attacks.

Management in the remission period is by avoidance of possible precipitating factors, particularly drugs and alcohol.

Other acute porphyrias

Variegate porphyria

This combines many of the features of acute intermittent porphyria with those of a cutaneous porphyria. A bullous eruption develops on exposure to sunlight owing to the activation of porphyrins deposited in the skin. There is an increased production of protoporphyrinogens owing to an abnormality of protoporphyrinogen oxidase in the haem biosynthetic pathway (see Fig. 19.23).

Fluorescence emission spectroscopy of plasma differentiates this from other acute and cutaneous porphyrias.

Hereditary coproporphyria

This is extremely rare and broadly similar in presentation to variegate porphyria. The distinction is based on biochemical analysis.

Porphyria cutanea tarda (cutaneous hepatic porphyria) (see also p. 1301)

This condition, which has a genetic predisposition, presents with a bullous eruption on exposure to sunlight; the eruption heals with scarring. Alcohol is the most common aetiological agent but HCV, iron overload or HIV can also precipitate the disease. There is an abnormality in hepatic uroporphyrinogen decarboxylase. Evidence of biochemical or clinical liver disease may also be present. Polychlorinated hydrocarbons have been implicated and porphyria cutanea tarda has been seen in association with benign or malignant tumours of the liver.

The diagnosis depends on demonstration of increased levels of urinary uroporphyrin. Histology of the skin shows subepidermal blisters with perivascular deposition of periodic acid–Schiff-staining material. The serum iron and transferrin saturation are often raised. Liver biopsy shows mild iron overload as well as features of alcoholic liver disease.

Remission can be induced by venesection; this should be repeated if the urinary uroporphyrin rises in the remission phase. Chloroquine may also have a useful role in promoting urinary excretion of uroporphyrins.

Erythropoietic porphyrias

Congenital porphyria

This is extremely rare and is transmitted as an autosomal recessive trait. Its victims show extreme sensitivity to sunlight and develop disfiguring scars. Dystrophy of the nails, blindness due to lenticular scarring, and brownish discoloration of the teeth also occur.

Erythropoietic protoporphyria

This is more common than congenital porphyria and is inherited as an autosomal dominant trait. It presents with irritation and a burning pain in the skin on exposure to sunlight. Hepatic involvement may also occur. Diagnosis is made by fluorescence of the peripheral red blood cells and by increased protoporphyrin in the red cells and stools. Oral β-carotene provides effective protection against solar sensitivity, but the reason for this is not known.

FURTHER READING

Elder GH, Hift RJ, Meissner PN (1997) The acute porphyrias. *Lancet* **349**: 1613–1617.

CHAPTER BIBLIOGRAPHY

Scriver CR, Beaudet AL, Sly WS, Valle D (2000) *The Metabolic Basis of Inherited Disease*, 8th edn. New York: McGraw-Hill.

Neurological disease

Epidemiology

Clinical neurology is a diverse and complex subject. The wide range of conditions seen in the UK is summarized in Table 20.1.

Table 20.1
Incidence rates for commoner neurological conditions/100 000/year in the UK

Headaches (GP consultations)	2200
Cerebrovascular events	205
Shingles (herpes zoster)	140
Diabetic neuropathy	54
Compressive neuropathies	49
Epilepsy	46
Parkinson's disease	19
Post-herpetic neuralgia	11
Primary CNS tumour	10
Essential tremor	8
Trigeminal neuralgia	8
Meningitis	7
Multiple sclerosis	7
Severe brain injury	7
Subarachnoid haemorrhage	6
Subdural haematoma	6
Metastatic CNS tumour	4
Presenile dementia	4
Cerebral palsy	3
Guillain–Barré syndrome	3
Myasthenia gravis	3
Transient global amnesia	3
Motor neurone disease	2

History, symptoms and signs

The *methods* of recording the history and basic examination are outside the scope of this chapter. Notes should read chronologically and portray the story given by the patient, or relative. Pattern recognition – interpretation of history, symptoms and examination – is very reliable. Practical experience is vital. There are three critical questions:

- What is/are the site(s) of the lesion(s)?
- What is the likely pathology?
- Does a recognizable disease fit this pattern?

This is the essence of clinical diagnosis. The aim in this section is to mention several common problems and to relate these to core neuroanatomy.

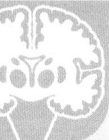

Headaches

Headache is an almost universal experience, and one of the most common symptoms in general and neurological practice. It varies from an infrequent and trivial nuisance to a symptom of serious disease.

Mechanism

Pain receptors are located at the base of the brain in arteries and veins and throughout the meninges, extracranial vessels, muscles of the scalp, neck and face, paranasal sinuses, eyes and teeth. Curiously, brain itself is almost devoid of pain receptors.

Head pain is mediated by mechanical receptors (e.g. stretching of meninges) and chemical receptors (e.g. 5-hydroxytryptamine and histamine stimulation). Nerve impulses travel centrally via the fifth and ninth cranial nerves and via upper cervical sensory roots.

The majority of headaches are benign, but the diagnostic issue – and usual source of concern – is that some are caused by serious disease. The following are some useful clinical pointers.

Chronic (benign) and recurrent headaches

Almost all recurring headaches lasting hours or days – band-like, generalized head pains, with a history going back for several years or months – are vaguely ascribed to muscle tension, and/or migraine (see p. 1206). Depression often accompanies them.

In localized pain of short duration, lasting some minutes or hours, sinusitis, glaucoma and migrainous neuralgia (p. 1203) should also be considered. Malignant hypertension, with arterial damage and brain swelling, occasionally causes headache (see p. 821). Headaches are not caused by high blood pressure alone.

Eyestrain from underlying refractive error is not itself a cause of headache, though new prescription lenses sometimes provoke pain.

Pressure headaches

Intracranial mass lesions displace and stretch the meninges and basal vessels. Pain is provoked when these structures are shifted either by a mass itself or by changes in cerebrospinal fluid (CSF) pressure, e.g. coughing. Cerebral oedema around brain tumours causes further shift. These 'pressure headaches' typically become worse on lying down.

Any headache, however mild, that is present on waking and made worse by coughing, straining or sneezing may well be due to a mass lesion. Vomiting often accompanies pressure headaches. Such headaches are caused early, over weeks, by posterior fossa masses (and see hydrocephalus, p. 1201), but over a longer timescale – months or even years – by hemisphere tumours.

A rare cause of prostrating headache with lower limb weakness is an intraventricular tumour causing intermittent hydrocephalus.

Headache of subacute onset

The onset and progression of a headache over days or weeks with or without the features of a pressure headache should always raise the suspicion of an intracranial mass lesion or serious intracranial disease. Encephalitis (see p. 1194), viral meningitis (p. 1192) and chronic meningitis (p. 1194) should also be considered.

Headaches with scalp tenderness

Patches of exquisite tenderness overlying superficial scalp arteries are caused by giant cell arteritis (see p. 1203), which develops almost exclusively in patients aged over 50 years.

Headache following head injury

Subdural haematoma (see p. 1172) must be considered. However, the vast majority of post-trauma headaches lasting days, weeks or months are not associated with any serious intracranial pathology.

A single episode of severe headache

This common emergency is caused by one of the following:

- subarachnoid haemorrhage
- migraine, or other benign headaches
- meningitis (occasionally).

Particular attention should be paid to the suddenness of onset (suggestive of a subarachnoid haemorrhage), neck stiffness and vomiting (any meningeal irritation), or rash and fever (bacterial meningitis).

Difficulty walking and falls

A change in gait is a common presenting complaint in neurology; the main causes are given in Table 20.2. Arthritis and muscle pain also alter gait, making it stiff and slow (antalgia). Falls, especially in the elderly, are a common and important cause of morbidity. The pattern of abnormal gait is valuable diagnostically.

Spasticity

Spasticity (see p. 1144), particularly in extensor muscles, with or without pyramidal weakness, causes stiffness and jerkiness of walking. The toes of shoes catch level ground, and become scuffed. The pace shortens but a

---

Table 20.2
Common neurological patterns of difficulty walking

Spasticity/hemiparesis
Parkinson's disease
Cerebellar ataxia
Sensory loss (joint position/loss)
Distal weakness
Proximal weakness
Apraxia of gait

narrow base is maintained. Clonus may be noticed as involuntary extensor rhythmic jerking of the legs.

When the problem is predominantly unilateral and weakness is marked (in a hemiparesis), the weaker leg drags stiffly and is circumducted.

Parkinson's disease (see p. 1182)

There is muscular rigidity throughout leg extensors and flexors. While power is preserved, the gait slows. The pace shortens to a shuffle; the base remains narrow. Falls occur. A stoop becomes apparent and arm swinging is diminished. The gait becomes festinant (hurried) in small rapid steps. There is particular difficulty initiating movement and turning quickly. Retropulsion describes small backwards steps, taken involuntarily when a patient is stopped or is halted.

Cerebellar ataxia (see also p. 1147)

In disease of the lateral cerebellar lobes the stance becomes broad-based, unstable and tremulous. Ataxia describes this state of imperfect control. The gait tends to veer towards the side of the more affected cerebellar lobe.

In disease confined to the cerebellar vermis, a midline structure, the trunk becomes unsteady without limb ataxia. There is a tendency to fall backwards or sideways – truncal ataxia.

Sensory ataxia

Peripheral sensory lesions (e.g. polyneuropathy, p. 1214) cause ataxia when there is loss of perception of joint position – proprioception. Broad-based, high-stepping, or stamping gait develops. This ataxia is made worse by removal of additional sensory input, such as in darkness. First described in the sensory ataxia of tabes dorsalis (p. 1196), this is the basis of the positive Romberg's test. Ask the patient to close the eyes while standing: observe whether or not they become unstable (and prevent falling).

Lower limb weakness

When weakness is distal, the leg has to be lifted over obstacles. When ankle dorsiflexors are weak, such as in a common peroneal nerve palsy (see p. 1213), the foot, having been lifted, returns to the ground with a visible and audible slap.

Weakness of proximal lower limb muscles (e.g. in polymyositis or muscular dystrophy) leads to difficulty in rising from sitting or squatting. Once upright, the patient walks with a waddling gait, the pelvis being ill-supported by each lower limb as it carries the full weight of the body.

Apraxia of gait

With frontal lobe disease (e.g. tumour, hydrocephalus, infarction), there is disorganization of walking as an acquired skill. Leg movement is normal when sitting or lying but initiation and organization of walking fail. This is apraxia of gait – a failure of the skilled movement of walking. Shuffling small steps (marche à petits pas), difficulty initiating walking (gait ignition failure) and undue hesitancy may predominate. Urinary incontinence and dementia are often present.

Falls

Falls, especially in the elderly, are a major cause of morbidity and a reason for hospital admission, for example following hip or upper limb fracture. Often no precise cause can be found. A multifactorial approach is essential and includes reviewing risk factors such as rugs, stairs, footwear and additional aids at home.

Dizziness, vertigo, blackouts and 'collapse'

Dizziness covers many complaints, from a vague feeling of unsteadiness to severe, acute vertigo. It is frequently used to describe light-headedness felt in anxiety and panic attacks, during palpitations, and in syncope or chronic ill-health. Therefore, the real nature of this symptom must be determined.

Vertigo – an illusion of movement – is a more definite symptom. It is usually a sensation of rotation, or tipping in which the patient feels that the surroundings are spinning or moving. It is distinctly unpleasant and often accompanied by nausea or vomiting. For causes of vertigo, see page 1139.

Blackout, like dizziness, is a descriptive term implying either altered consciousness, visual disturbance or falling. Epilepsy, syncope, hypoglycaemia, anaemia must be considered. However, commonly no sinister cause is found. A careful history, particularly from an eye-witness, is essential.

Collapse is a vague term but often used. It is not a diagnosis and medically, its use should be avoided.

FURTHER READING

Lance JW, Goadsby PJ (1998) *Mechanism and Management of Headache*. Oxford: Butterworth-Heinemann.
van Weel C, Vermuelen H, van den Bosch W (1995) Falls: a community perspective. *Lancet* **345**: 1549–1551.

Neurological examination

A short five-part examination is shown in Practical box 20.1, and a full ten-part examination in Practical box 20.2.

Formulation

The relevant findings are drawn together in a brief written diagnostic summary. This will form the basis for investigations, transfer of information, and management.

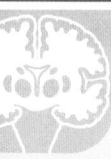

Practical box 20.1

Five-part short neurological examination

1 Look at the patient
General demeanour
Speech
Gait
Arm swinging

2 Examine the head
Fundi
Pupils
Eye movements
Facial movements
Tongue

3 Examine the upper limbs
Posture of outstretched arms
Wasting, fasciculation
Power, tone
Coordination
Reflexes

4 Examine the lower limbs
Power (hip flexion, ankle dorsiflexion)
Tone
Reflexes
Plantar responses

5 Assess sensation
Ask the patient

Table 20.3
Six grades of muscle power

Grade	Definition
5	Normal power
4	Active movement against gravity and resistance
3	Active movement against gravity
2	Active movement with gravity eliminated
1	Flicker of contraction
0	No contraction

Practical box 20.2

Ten-part neurological examination

1 State of consciousness, arousal, appearance (e.g. coma)

2 Mental state, attitude, insight (see Box 21.5, p. 1230)

3 Cognitive function
Orientation in time and place, recall of recent and distant events (memory, level of intellect, language and speech/cerebral dominance, other disorders of skilled function, e.g. apraxia)

4 Gait and Romberg's test

5 Skull shape – circumference, bruits

6 Neck – stiffness, palpation and auscultation of carotid arteries

7 Cranial nerves (see Table 20.5)

8 Motor system
Upper limbs:
Wasting and fasciculation
Posture of arms: drift, rebound, tremor
Tone: spasticity or extrapyramidal rigidity
Power: 0–5 scale (Table 20.3)
Tendon reflexes: + or ++ normal; +++ increased: 0 absent with reinforcement

Thorax and abdomen:
Respiration
Thoracic and abdominal muscles
Abdominal reflexes
Cremasteric reflexes

Lower limbs:
Wasting and fasciculation
Tone, power and tendon reflexes
Plantar responses

9 Coordination and fine movements

10 Sensory system
First, ask whether feeling in the limbs, face and trunk is entirely normal

Posterior columns:
Vibration (using a 128 Hz tuning fork)
Joint position
Light touch
2-point discrimination (normal: 0.5 cm fingertips, 2 cm soles)

Spinothalamic tracts:
Pain: use a split orange-stick or a sterile pin
Temperature: hot or cold tubes

If sensation is abnormal, chart areas involved

Functional neuroanatomy: an introduction

The neurone and synapse (Fig. 20.1)

The neurone is the functional unit of the nervous system. Its cell body and axon terminate in a synapse. The specificity, size and type of each group of neurones vary greatly. One α-motor neurone within the anterior horn of the thoracic spinal cord has an axonal length over 1 metre and innervates between several hundred and 2000 muscle fibres – to form a motor unit. By contrast, some spinal or intracerebral internuncial neurones have axons under 100 μm long and terminate solely on one neuronal cell body.

Neurotransmitters

Synaptic transmission is mediated by neurotransmitters released by action potentials passing down an axon. Neurotransmitters then react with postsynaptic receptors and are removed by transporter proteins. The neurotransmitter–receptor reaction increases ionic permeability and propagates a further action potential. This combination of axonal electrical activity and synaptic chemical release is the basis of all neurological function.

Neurotransmitters include acetylcholine, norepinephrine, (noradrenaline), epinephrine (adrenaline), 5-hydroxytryptamine, gamma-aminobutyric acid (GABA), opioid peptides, prostaglandins, histamine, dopamine, glutamate, nitric oxide, neuromelanin and vasoactive intestinal peptide (VIP). Of these, glutamate is believed to be the principal excitatory neurotransmitter.

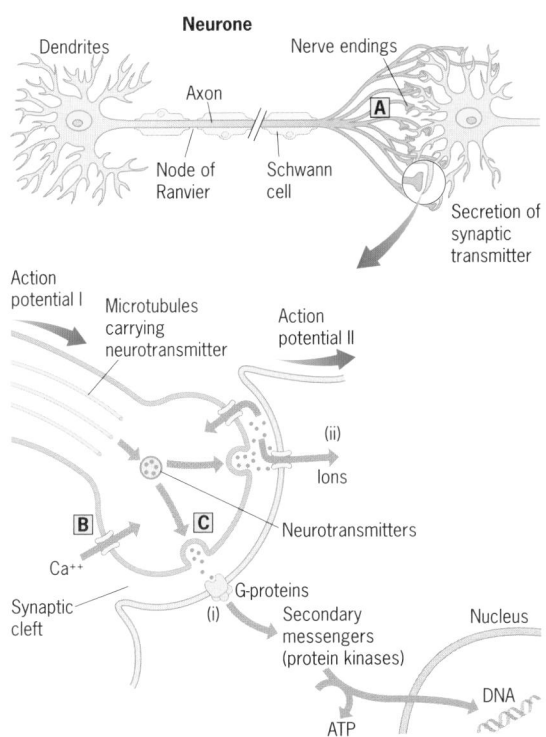

Fig. 20.1 The functional unit: neurone and neurotransmitters.
The action potential (i.e. nerve impulse) travels down the axon.
Microtubules carry the neurotransmitters to the nerve endings **(A)**.
Action potential I depolarizes the synaptic membrane, opening the
voltage-gated calcium channels **(B)**. The influx of calcium causes the
vesicles to fuse with the membrane **(C)**, allowing the neurotransmitter
to (i) bind to the receptor and activate the secondary messenger, which
then modulates gene transcription (see Ch. 3), and also to (ii) open
ligand-gated channels. This allows ions to enter, depolarizes the
membrane and initiates action potential II.

The role of neurotransmitters and transporters in
pathogenesis continues to be evaluated, but it is thought
that a wide variety of acute and chronic neurological
disease may be mediated, at least in part, by a final common pathway of neuronal injury involving excessive
stimulation of glutamate receptors.

Clinical features of focal brain lesions: general mechanisms

Whilst it is unusual to have to recall detailed neuroanatomy, it is necessary to understand how the nervous
system works and how each part is integrated. We need
to be able to recognize, from symptoms and signs, the
site in the nervous system which is malfunctioning; for
example, the left frontal lobe, an internal capsule, or a
seventh cranial (facial) nerve.

Focal lesions of the cerebral cortex, and throughout
the nervous system, cause symptoms and signs by two
processes:

- Suppression of function or *destruction* of neurones and
  surrounding structures (Fig. 20.2). This is the most
  common process – part of the system fails to work.

Site of lesion	Disorder	L	R
Frontal, either	Intellectual impairment Personality change Urinary incontinence Monoparesis or hemiparesis		
Frontal, left	Broca's aphasia		
Temporo-parietal, left	Acalculia Alexia Agraphia Wernicke's aphasia Right–left disorientation Homonymous field defect		
Temporal, right	Confusional states Failure to recognize faces Homonymous field defect		
Parietal, either	Contralateral sensory loss or neglect Agraphaesthesia Homonymous field defect		
Parietal, right	Dressing apraxia Failure to recognize faces		
Parietal, left	Limb apraxia		
Occipital/ occipitoparietal	Visual field defects Visuospatial defects Disturbances of visual recognition		

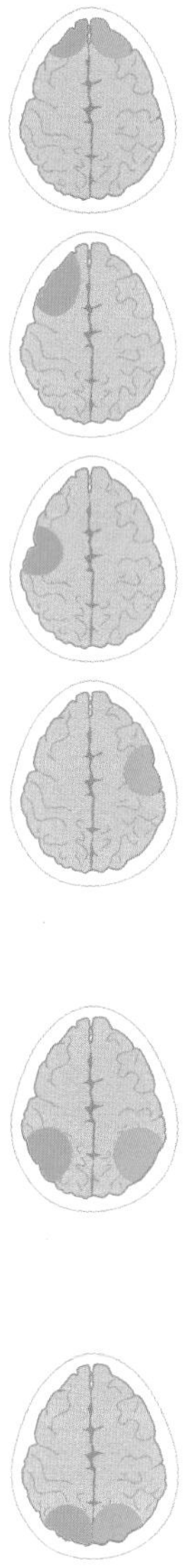

Fig. 20.2 Principal features of destructive cortical lesions
(right-handed individual).

- Synchronous discharge of neurones by *irritative*
  lesions (Fig. 20.3), e.g. brain lesions above the
  tentorium cause epilepsy, either partial or
  generalized.

Localization within the cerebral cortex

This subject causes considerable, and unnecessary difficulty. Work on neuronal networks, functional imaging
and plasticity within the brain has tended to question
traditional views relating to highly specific localization of
function. However, in practical neurology at the bedside,

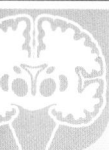

Site of lesion	Effects	L	R
Frontal	Partial seizures – focal motor seizures of contralateral limbs Conjugate deviation of head and eyes away from the lesion		
Temporal	Formed visual hallucinations Complex partial seizures Memory disturbances (e.g. déjà vu)		
Parietal	Partial seizures – focal sensory seizures of contralateral limbs		
Parieto-occipital	Crude visual hallucinations (e.g. shapes in one part of the field)		
Occipital	Visual disturbances (e.g. flashes)		

Fig. 20.3 Effects of an irritative cortical lesion.

it is necessary to understand the main functional roles of the cerebral cortex. The following paragraphs summarize areas of clinical importance.

The dominant hemisphere (usually left)

The concept of cerebral dominance arose with the simple observation that right-handed stroke patients with acquired language disorders had destructive lesions within the left hemisphere. Almost all right-handed and 70% of left-handed people have language function in the left hemisphere.

Destructive lesions within the left fronto-temporo-parietal region cause various disorders of human communication:

- spoken language – *aphasia*, also called *dysphasia*
- writing – *agraphia*
- reading – *acquired alexia*.

Developmental dyslexia describes delayed and disorganized reading and writing ability in children with normal intelligence.

Aphasia

Aphasia is the loss of or defective language because of damage to the speech centres within the left hemisphere.

Some varieties of aphasia

Numerous varieties of aphasia have been described. A brief review follows.

Broca's aphasia (expressive aphasia, anterior aphasia)

A lesion in the left frontal lobe causes reduced fluency of speech with comprehension relatively preserved. The patient makes great efforts to initiate speech. Language is reduced to a few disjointed words and there is failure to construct sentences. Patients who recover from this form of aphasia say that they knew what they wanted to say, but could not get the words out.

Wernicke's aphasia (receptive aphasia, posterior aphasia)

Left temporo-parietal damage leaves language that is fluent but the words themselves are incorrect. This varies from insertion of a few incorrect or nonexistent words into fluent speech to a profuse outpouring of jargon (that is, rubbish with wholly nonexistent words). Severe jargon aphasia may be so bizarre as to be confused with psychotic behaviour.

Patients who have recovered from Wernicke's aphasia say that when aphasic they found speech, both their own and others' like a wholly unintelligible foreign language. They could neither stop themselves nor understand themselves or those around them.

Nominal aphasia (anomic aphasia or amnestic aphasia)

This describes difficulty naming familiar objects. Naming difficulty is an early sign in all types of aphasia. A left posterior temporal/inferior parietal lesion causes a severe, isolated form.

Global aphasia (central aphasia)

This is the combination of the expressive disturbance characteristic of Broca's aphasia and the loss of comprehension of Wernicke's. The patient can neither speak nor understand language. It is due to widespread damage to the areas concerned with speech and is the most common form of aphasia after a severe left hemisphere infarct. Writing and reading are also affected.

Dysarthria

Dysarthria simply means disordered articulation – slurred speech. Language is intact, cf. aphasia. Paralysis, slowing or incoordination of the muscles of articulation or local discomfort causes various different patterns of dysarthria. Examples are the gravelly speech of upper motor neurone lesions of the lower cranial nerves, the ataxic speech of cerebellar lesions, the monotone of Parkinson's disease and speech that fatigues and dies away in myasthenia. Many aphasic patients are also somewhat dysarthric.

The non-dominant hemisphere

Disorders in right-handed patients with right hemisphere lesions are often difficult to recognize. They comprise abnormalities of perception of internal and

Table 20.4
Causes of the amnestic syndrome

Alcohol (Wernicke–Korsakoff syndrome)
Head injury (severe)
Anoxia
Posterior cerebral artery occlusion (bilateral)
Herpes simplex encephalitis
Chronic sedative and solvent abuse
Bilateral invasive tumours
Arsenic poisoning
Following hypoglycaemia

external space. Examples are losing the way in familiar surroundings, failing to put on clothing correctly (*dressing apraxia*), or failure to draw simple shapes – *constructional apraxia*.

Memory and its disorders (see also p. 1265)
Disorders of memory follow damage to the medial surfaces of both temporal lobes and their brainstem connections – the hippocampi, fornices and mammillary bodies. Bilateral lesions are necessary to cause *amnesia*. It is characteristic of all organic disorders of memory that more recent events are recalled poorly, in contrast to the relative preservation of distant memories.

Memory loss (*the amnestic syndrome*) is part of dementia (p. 1266) but also occurs as an isolated entity (Table 20.4).

FURTHER READING

Hoffman B, Lefkowitz R, Taylor P (1996)
Neurotransmission: the autonomic and somatic nervous systems. In: *Goodman and Gilman's The Pharmacological Basis of Therapeutics*, 9th edn. New York: McGraw-Hill.
Masson J, Sagné C, Hamon M, El Mestikawy S (1999)
Neurotransmitter transporters in the central nervous system. *Pharmacological Reviews* **51**: 439–464.

Essential elements of neuroanatomy
For clinical purposes, and particularly in general medical practice, the extreme complexity of neuroanatomy must be reduced to its core elements. The following sections cover:

- cranial nerves
- three systems of motor control:
  (a) corticospinal or pyramidal system
  (b) extrapyramidal system
  (c) cerebellum
- the motor unit
- the reflex arc
- sensory pathways and pain
- control of the bladder and sexual function.

Cranial nerves (see Table 20.5)

I: Olfactory nerve

This sensory nerve arises from olfactory (smell) receptors in the nasal mucosa. Branches pierce the cribriform plate and synapse in the olfactory bulb. The olfactory tract then passes to the olfactory cortex in the anteromedial surface of the temporal lobe.

Anosmia (loss of sense of smell) is caused by head injury and tumours of the olfactory groove (e.g. meningioma, frontal glioma). It is often lost, occasionally permanently, after upper respiratory viral infections and diminished when the nose is blocked.

II: Optic nerve and visual system

The visual pathway is shown in Figure 20.4. The photic energy of light, its amount regulated by the pupillary aperture (see p. 1132), is converted to nerve action potentials by retinal rod, cone and ganglion cells. The lens, under control of the ciliary muscle (see p. 1132), causes the image on the retina to be inverted (1). An object in the lower part of the visual field is projected to the upper retina and one in the temporal field to the nasal retina. Each optic nerve (2), sheathed in pia–arachnoid meninges, carries axons from retinal ganglion cells to the lateral geniculate bodies.

At the optic chiasm (3), fibres travelling in the nasal portions of the optic nerves cross, join uncrossed temporal fibres of each optic nerve and form each optic tract. The fibres synapse at the lateral geniculate body (4). One optic tract thus carries fibres from the temporal ipsilateral retina and the nasal contralateral retina. Some

Table 20.5
Cranial nerves

No.	Name	Main clinical action
I	Olfactory	Smell
II	Optic	Vision, fields, afferent light reflex
III	Oculomotor	Eyelid elevation, eye elevation, ADduction, depression in ABduction, efferent (pupil)
IV	Trochlear	Eye intorsion, depression in ADduction
V	Trigeminal	Facial and corneal sensation, muscles of mastication
VI	Abducens	Eye ABduction
VII	Facial	Facial movement, taste fibres
VIII	Vestibular	Balance
	Cochlear	Hearing
IX	Glossopharyngeal	Sensation – soft palate, taste fibres
X	Vagus	Cough, palatal and vocal cord movements
XI	Accessory	Head turning, shoulder shrugging
XII	Hypoglossal	Tongue movement

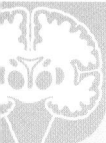

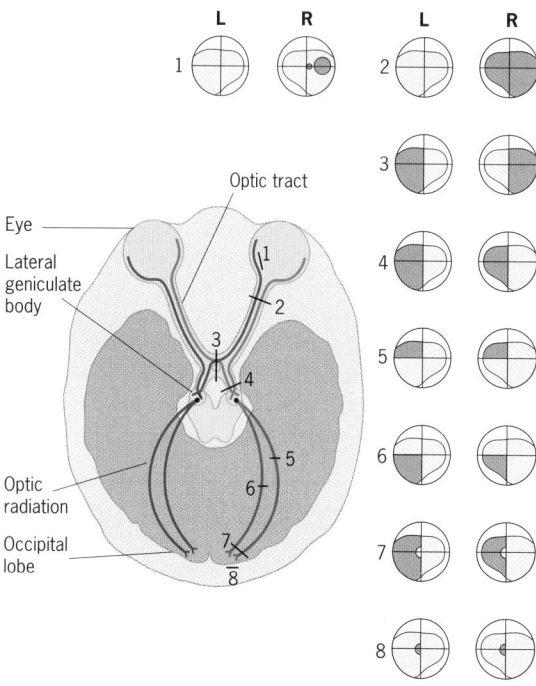

Fig. 20.4 The visual pathway.
1, Paracentral scotoma–retinal lesion.
2, Mononuclear field loss–optic nerve lesion.
3, Bitemporal hemianopia–chiasmal lesion.
4, Homonymous hemianopia–optic tract lesion.
5, Homonymous quadrantanopia–temporal lesion.
6, Homonymous quadrantanopia–parietal lesion.
7, Homonymous hemianopia–occipital cortex or optic radiation.
8, Homonymous hemianopia–occipital pole lesion.
Dark blue = lesion; pale blue = normal field.

optic tract fibres reaching the lateral geniculate bodies pass to the brainstem (see p. 1132) to control refraction (lens) and pupillary aperture.

From the lateral geniculate body, fibres pass in the optic radiation through the parietal and temporal lobes (5 and 6) to reach the visual, or calcarine, cortex of the occipital lobe (7 and 8). The upper retinae (lower visual fields) project in the optic radiation through the parietal lobes to the upper part of the visual cortex, and the lower retinae (upper fields) through the temporal lobes, beneath the parietal, to the lower visual cortex. Impulses reach the cortex in strictly maintained vertical topographical order (i.e. upper field to lower retina, tract, radiation and cortex, and vice versa, lower to upper). Within the visual cortex itself there are synaptic connections between groups of cells which detect lines, orientation, shapes, movement, colour, and depth. These are processed by the neighbouring visual association areas.

Visual field defects caused by lesions of each optic tract, radiation and cortex are called 'homonymous' to indicate the different (i.e. bilateral) origins of each unilateral pathway. (A homonym is the same word used to denote different things.)

Field defects are *hemi*anopic when half the field is affected by a lesion of the optic tract, radiation or cortex (e.g. left homonymous hemianopia), and *quadrant*anopic when a quadrant is affected. Congruous denotes symmetry and incongruous lack of it. Bitemporal defects (damage to crossing nasal fibres) are caused by lesions of the optic chiasm (e.g. pituitary tumour).

Visual acuity

This is recorded with a Snellen chart and/or Near Vision Reading Types and corrected for refractive errors with lenses or a pinhole. The normal acuity is 6/6 to 6/9 in each eye; if less, an explanation is necessary.

Visual loss is due to:

- Ocular causes, e.g. glaucoma, macular degeneration, cataract, retinal detachment, diabetic vascular disease, trachoma, leprosy, vitamin A deficiency, trauma, onchocerciasis (river blindness). All are of major international health and economic importance.
- Lesions of the visual neural pathway (e.g. optic nerve lesions, chiasmal compression, tract, radiation or cortical lesions).

Visual field defects

These are checked by confrontation with white- and red-headed pins and, if abnormal or in doubt, recorded in detail with a Goldmann (or similar) screen. Examples of field defects at different sites are shown in Figure 20.4.

Retinal and local eye lesions (site 1)

Lesions of the retina produce either scotomata (small areas of visual loss) or peripheral visual loss (tunnel vision). Common causes are diabetic retinal vascular disease, glaucoma and retinitis pigmentosa. Local lesions of the eye (e.g. cataract) can also cause visual loss.

Optic nerve lesions (site 2)

Unilateral visual loss, commencing as a central or para-central (off-centre) scotoma, is the hallmark of an optic nerve lesion. A total optic nerve lesion causes unilateral blindness with loss of pupillary light reflex (direct and consensual) when the blind eye is illuminated (see afferent pupillary defect, p. 1132). For causes of optic nerve lesions, see Table 20.6.

The principal pathological appearances of the visible part of the nerve (optic disc) seen on fundoscopy are:

- disc swelling and hyperaemia (papilloedema)
- pallor (optic atrophy).

Papilloedema and optic neuritis

Papilloedema simply means swelling of the papilla – the optic disc. There are many causes (Table 20.7). In all forms of disc oedema there is axonal swelling within the optic nerve, blockage of axonal transport with capillary and venous congestion. Optic neuritis is swelling of the disc and inflammation within the nerve.

Table 20.6
Principal causes of an optic nerve lesion

Optic and retrobulbar neuritis
Optic nerve compression (e.g. tumour or aneurysm)
Toxic optic neuropathy
   (e.g. tobacco, ethambutol, methyl alcohol, quinine)
Syphilis
Ischaemic optic neuropathy (e.g. giant cell arteritis)
Hereditary optic neuropathies
Severe anaemia
Vitamin B_{12} deficiency
Trauma
Infective (spread of paranasal sinus infection or orbital cellulitis)
Papilloedema and its causes (see Table 20.7)
Bone disease affecting optic canal (e.g. Paget's)

Table 20.7
Causes of optic disc swelling (papilloedema)

Raised intracranial pressure	**Venous occlusion**
Brain tumour, abscess, haematoma, intracranial haemorrhage and SAH, idiopathic intracranial hypertension, hydrocephalus, encephalitis	Cavernous sinus thrombosis Central retinal vein thrombosis/occlusion Orbital mass lesions
	Retinal vascular disease
Optic nerve disease	Malignant hypertension
Optic neuritis (e.g. multiple sclerosis)	Vasculitis (e.g. SLE)
Hereditary optic neuropathy	**Metabolic causes**
Ischaemic optic neuropathy (e.g. giant cell arteritis)	Hypercapnia, chronic hypoxia, hypocalcaemia
Toxic optic neuropathy (e.g. methanol ingestion)	**Disc infiltration**
Hypervitaminosis A	Leukaemia, sarcoidosis, optic nerve glioma

SAH, subarachnoid haemorrhage: SLE, systemic lupus erythematosus

The earliest ophthalmoscopic signs of disc swelling are pinkness of the disc followed by blurring and heaping up of its margins, the nasal first. There is loss within the disc of the normal, visible, spontaneous pulsation of the retinal veins. The physiological cup becomes obliterated, the disc engorged and its vessels dilated. Small haemorrhages often surround the disc.

Various conditions simulate true disc oedema. Marked hypermetropic (long-sighted) refractive errors make the disc appear pink, distant and ill-defined. Opaque (myelinated) nerve fibres at the disc margin and hyaline bodies (drusen) can be mistaken for disc swelling.

Disc infiltration also causes first a prominent, then a swollen disc with raised margins (e.g. in leukaemia).

When there is doubt about disc oedema, fluorescein angiography is diagnostic. Fluorescein is injected intravenously: when there is oedema, retinal leakage is seen and photographed.

Early papilloedema from causes other than optic neuritis (see below) often produces few visual symptoms – the underlying disease is the source of the patient's complaints. However, as disc oedema progresses, enlargement of the blind spot and blurring of vision develop. The disc becomes engorged, reducing its arterial blood flow and, then as papilloedema worsens, infarction of the nerve occurs. This causes sudden severe and permanent visual loss.

Optic neuritis

The most common cause of inflammation of the optic nerve is demyelination (e.g. multiple sclerosis). Disc swelling due to optic neuritis is distinguished from other causes of disc oedema by early and severe visual loss.

Retrobulbar neuritis implies that the inflammatory process is within the optic nerve but behind the bulb (i.e. the eye), so that no abnormality is seen at the disc itself in spite of visual impairment.

Leber's hereditary optic neuropathy (LHON)

LHON is a common cause of isolated blindness in otherwise healthy young men. Unilateral or bilateral optic nerve neuropathy develops over the course of days or weeks. There is sometimes disc swelling and telangiectasia around the disc in the acute phase, followed by optic atrophy. Severe bilateral visual loss is usual by the age of 40. Maternal inheritance and genetic analysis have pointed to pathogenic mitochondrial DNA mutations as the cause, many with a mutation at G11778A. Exceptional cases occur in women.

Optic atrophy

Optic atrophy means disc pallor, from loss of axons, glial proliferation and decreased vascularity that follows many pathological processes, e.g. infarction of the nerve from thromboembolism or following papilloedema, inflammation (demyelinating optic neuritis in MS, syphilis, LHON), optic nerve compression, previous trauma, toxic and metabolic causes (vitamin B_{12} deficiency, quinine and methyl alcohol ingestion). Optic atrophy is described as consecutive or secondary when it follows papilloedema of any cause. The degree of visual loss depends upon underlying pathology.

Optic chiasm (site 3)

Bitemporal hemianopic field are the typical defects when a mass compresses the chiasm. Common causes are:

- pituitary neoplasm (p. 1009)
- meningioma
- craniopharyngioma
- secondary neoplasm.

In any case of bilateral visual loss, chiasmal compression must be considered.

Optic tract and optic radiation (sites 4, 5 and 6)

Optic tract lesions (which are rare) cause field defects which are homonymous, hemianopic and often incomplete and incongruous. Optic radiation lesions cause homonymous quadrantanopic defects. Temporal lobe lesions (e.g. tumour or infarction) cause upper quadrantic defects, and parietal lobe, lower.

Occipital cortex (sites 7 and 8)

Homonymous hemianopic defects are produced by unilateral posterior cerebral artery infarction. The macular region of the cortex (at the occipital pole) is spared because it has a separate blood supply from the middle cerebral artery: infarction of one occipital pole alone causes a small, congruous, scotomatous, homonymous hemianopia (8).

Widespread bilateral occipital lobe damage by tumour, trauma or infarction causes cortical blindness (Anton's syndrome). The patient cannot see but characteristically lacks insight into the degree of visual loss and may even deny it. The pupillary responses are normal (see also p. 1167).

Pupils

Sympathetic impulses dilate the pupils. Fibres in the nasociliary nerve pass to the *dilator pupillae* muscle. These arise from the superior cervical ganglion at C2. Sympathetic *pre*ganglionic fibres to the eye (and face) originate in the hypothalamus, pass uncrossed through the midbrain and lateral medulla, and emerge finally from the spinal cord at T1 (close to the lung apex) and form the superior cervical ganglion at C2. *Post*ganglionic fibres leave the ganglion to form a plexus around the carotid bifurcation. Fibres pass to the pupil in the nasociliary nerve from the part of this plexus surrounding the internal carotid artery. Those fibres to the face (sweating and piloerection) arise from the part of the plexus surrounding the external carotid artery. This arrangement has some clinical relevance in Horner's syndrome (p. 1133).

Parasympathetic impulses cause pupillary constriction. Fibres in the short ciliary nerves arise from the ciliary ganglion and pass to the *sphincter pupillae* causing constriction. Parasympathetic pathways and the light reflex mechanism are shown in Figure 20.5.

The light reflex

Afferent fibres (1) in each optic nerve (some crossing in the chiasm) pass to both lateral geniculate bodies (2) and relay to the Edinger–Westphal nuclei (4) via the pretectal nucleus (3).

Efferent (parasympathetic) fibres from each Edinger–Westphal nucleus pass via the third nerve to the ciliary ganglion (5) and thence to the pupil (6).

Light constricts the pupil being illuminated (direct reflex) and, by the consensual reflex, the contralateral pupil.

The convergence reflex

Fixation on a near object requires convergence of the ocular axes and is accompanied by pupillary constriction. Afferent fibres in each optic nerve, which pass through both lateral geniculate bodies, also relay to the convergence centre. This centre receives 1a spindle afferent fibres from the extraocular muscles – principally medial recti – which are innervated by the third nerve.

The efferent route is from the convergence centre to the Edinger–Westphal nucleus, ciliary ganglion and pupils. Voluntary or reflex fixation on a near object is thus accompanied by appropriate convergence and pupillary constriction.

A darkened room makes all pupillary abnormalities easier to see.

Clinical abnormalities of the pupils

Pupillary abnormalities in coma are discussed on page 1161, and in brainstem lesions on page 955.

Physiological changes and old age

A slight difference between the size of each pupil is common (physiological anisocoria) at any age. The pupil tends to become small (3–3.5 mm) and irregular in old age (senile miosis); anisocoria is more pronounced. The convergence reflex becomes sluggish with ageing and a bright light becomes necessary to demonstrate constriction.

Afferent pupillary defect. A blind left eye, for example from previous *complete* section of its optic nerve, has a pupil larger than the right. The features of a left afferent pupillary defect are:

- the left pupil is unreactive to light (i.e. the direct reflex is absent)
- the consensual reflex (constriction of the right pupil when light is shone into the left) is also absent.

Conversely, the left pupil constricts when light is shone in the intact right eye, i.e. the consensual reflex of the right eye is intact.

Relative afferent pupillary defect (RAPD). When there has been *incomplete* damage to one afferent pupillary pathway (i.e. of one optic nerve relative to the other), the difference between the pupillary reaction, and the relative impairment on one side is called a *relative* afferent pupillary defect (RAPD). The sign can provide evidence of an optic nerve lesion, when, for example, retrobulbar neuritis occurred many years previously and there has been apparent complete clinical recovery of vision (p. 1190).

After previous left retrobulbar neuritis:

- Light shone in the left eye causes both left and right pupils to constrict.
- When light is shone into the intact right eye, both pupils again constrict (i.e. right direct and consensual reflexes are intact).
- When the light source is then swung back to the left eye, its pupil dilates, relative to its previous state.

The finding of a left RAPD by the *swinging light test*, showing that the consensual reflex is stronger than the

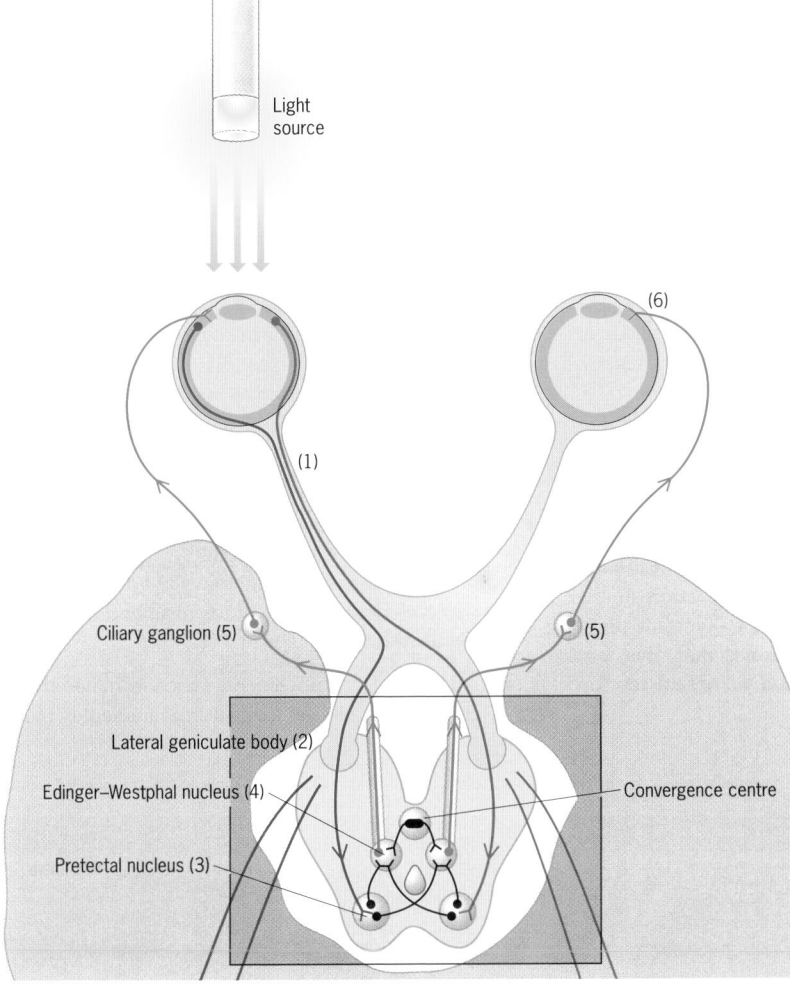

Light
source

(6)

Ciliary ganglion (5)

(5)

Lateral geniculate body (2)

Edinger–Westphal nucleus (4)

Convergence centre

Pretectal nucleus (3)

(1)

Fig. 20.5 Pupillary light reflex.
Afferent pathway.
(1) A retinal image generates action
potentials in the optic nerve.
(2) These travel via axons, some of
which decussate at the chiasm and
pass through the lateral geniculate
bodies.
(3) Synapse at each pretectal nucleus.

Efferent pathway.
(4) Action potentials then pass to each
Edinger–Westphal nucleus of III.
(5) Then, via the ciliary ganglion.
(6) Leading to constriction of pupil.

direct, indicates residual damage in the afferent pupillary fibres of the left optic nerve.

Horner's syndrome

This collection of signs – of unilateral pupillary constriction with slight relative ptosis and enophthalmos – indicates a lesion of the sympathetic pathway on the same side. The conjunctival vessels are slightly injected. Causes of Horner's syndrome are given in Table 20.8. There is loss of sweating of the same side of the face or body; the extent depending upon the level of the lesion:

- Central lesions affect sweating over the entire half of the head, arm and upper trunk.
- Neck lesions proximal to the superior cervical ganglion cause diminished facial sweating.
- Lesions distal to the superior cervical ganglion do not affect sweating at all.

Table 20.8
Causes of Horner's syndrome

Hemisphere and brainstem	Sympathetic chain in neck
Massive cerebral infarction	Following thryoid/laryngeal
Pontine glioma	surgery
Lateral medullary syndrome	Carotid artery occlusion
'Coning' of the temporal lobe	and dissection
	Neoplastic infiltration
Cervical cord	Cervical sympathectomy
Syringomyelia	
Cord tumours	**Miscellaneous**
	Congenital
	Migrainous neuralgia
T1 root	(usually transient)
Bronchial neoplasm (apical)	Isolated and of unknown
Apical tuberculosis	cause
Cervical rib	
Brachial plexus trauma	

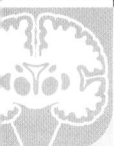

Pharmacological tests help to indicate the level of the lesion. For example, a lesion distal to the superior cervical ganglion causes denervation hypersensitivity of the pupil, which dilates when 1:1000 adrenaline (epinephrine) is instilled. This dose has little effect on the normal pupil or a Horner's pupil from a proximal lesion. In clinical practice the test is of limited value.

Argyll Robertson pupil

This small, irregular (3 mm or less) pupil is fixed to light but constricts on convergence. The lesion is in the brainstem in neural tissue surrounding the aqueduct of Sylvius.

The Argyll Robertson pupil is (almost) diagnostic of neurosyphilis. Similar changes are occasionally seen in diabetes mellitus.

Myotonic pupil (Holmes–Adie pupil)

This is a dilated pupil seen most commonly in young women. It is usually unilateral, and the pupil is often irregular. There is no reaction (or a very slow reaction) to bright light and also incomplete constriction to convergence. The condition is due to denervation in the ciliary ganglion, of unknown cause. The myotonic pupil is of no more pathological significance than this, but is often associated with diminished or absent tendon reflexes.

III, IV, VI: Oculomotor, trochlear and abducens nerves

Mechanisms controlling eye movement are:

- central upper motor neurone mechanisms that drive the normal yoked parallel eye movements (conjugate gaze)
- individual movements generated by each oculomotor, abducens and trochlear nerve.

Conjugate gaze

Fast voluntary and reflex eye movements originate in each frontal lobe. Fibres pass in the anterior limb of the internal capsule and cross in the pons to end in the centre for lateral gaze (paramedian pontine reticular formation – PPRF, Fig. 20.6a), close to each sixth nerve nucleus. The PPRF also receives fibres from:

- the ipsilateral occipital cortex – a pathway concerned with tracking objects
- both vestibular nuclei – pathways linking eye movements with position of the head and neck (doll's head reflexes, p. 955).

Conjugate lateral eye movements are coordinated by the PPRF through the medial longitudinal fasciculus (MLF,

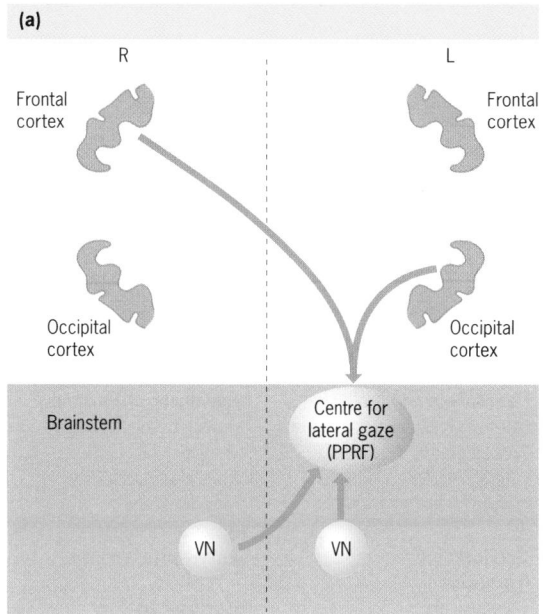

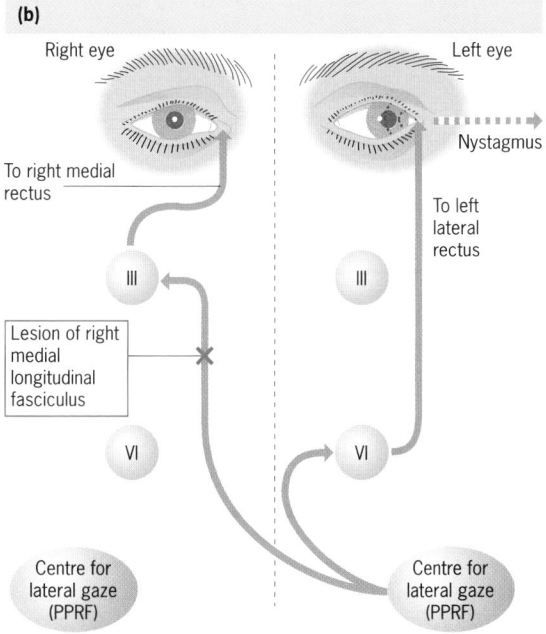

Fig. 20.6 **(a) Principal input to PPRF.** Impulses from the right frontal cortex, the left occipital cortex and both vestibular nuclei (VN) drive the left centre for lateral gaze, or paramedian pontine reticular formation (PPRF).
(b) Principal output from PPRF. Impulses from the PPRF pass via the ipsilateral VIth nerve nucleus to the lateral rectus muscle (ABduction) and via the medial longitudinal fasciculus to the IIIrd nerve nucleus and thus to the opposite medial rectus muscle (ADduction). **X** shows lesion with failure of ADduction of right eye and nystagmus of ABducting left eye.

Fig. 20.6b). Fibres from the PPRF pass both to the ipsilateral sixth nerve nucleus and, having crossed the midline, the opposite third nerve nucleus via the MLF. Each sixth nerve nucleus (supplying lateral rectus) and the opposite third nerve nucleus (supplying medial rectus and others) are thus linked by the MLF, driving the eyes laterally with parallel axes and with the same velocity.

Abnormalities of conjugate lateral gaze

A *destructive lesion* of one side of the brain allows lateral gaze to be driven by the intact opposite pathway. For example, a destructive left frontal lobe lesion (e.g. an infarct) leads to failure of conjugate lateral gaze to the right. In an acute lesion the eyes are often deviated past the midline to the side of the lesion, here to the left, and therefore look towards the normal limbs, as there is usually a contralateral (i.e. right) hemiparesis.

An *irritative left frontal lobe lesion* (e.g. an epileptic focus), stimulates the opposite, right, PPRF and drives lateral gaze away from the side of the lesion (i.e. to the right) during an attack.

In the brainstem itself a unilateral destructive lesion involving the PPRF leads to failure of conjugate lateral gaze towards that side. There is usually a contralateral hemiparesis and lateral gaze is deviated towards the side of the paralysed limbs.

Internuclear ophthalmoplegia

This is due to damage to one MLF. Internuclear ophthalmoplegia (INO) is one of the more common complex brainstem oculomotor signs and is seen frequently in multiple sclerosis.

When present bilaterally, INO is almost pathognomonic of this disease. Unilateral lesions are also caused by small brainstem infarcts. In a right INO there is a lesion of the right MLF (Fig. 20.6b). On attempted left lateral gaze the right eye fails to ADduct. The left eye develops coarse nystagmus in ABduction.

The side of the lesion is on the side of impaired adduction, not on the side of the (obvious, unilateral) nystagmus.

Doll's head reflexes and skew deviation

These are of some diagnostic value in coma (see p. 1162).

Abnormalities of vertical gaze

A failure of up-gaze is caused by upper brainstem lesions, such as a supratentorial mass pressing from above, or a tumour of the brainstem (e.g. a pinealoma). When the pupillary convergence reflex fails as well, this combination is called Parinaud's syndrome.

Defective up-gaze also occurs in certain degenerative disorders (e.g. progressive supranuclear palsy). Some impairment of up-gaze develops as part of normal ageing.

Weakness of extraocular muscles (diplopia)

Diplopia (double vision) indicates weakness of one or more extraocular muscles. The causes are:

- lesions of the third, fourth and/or sixth cranial nerves or nuclei
- disorders of the neuromuscular junction (e.g. myasthenia gravis)
- disease of, or injury to the ocular muscles
- orbital lesions.

Squint (strabismus)

This describes the appearance of the eyes when the visual axes fail to meet at the fixation point, and is either convergent or divergent.

Paralytic squint. Paralytic or incomitant squint occurs when there is an acquired defect of movement of an eye – the usual situation in neurological disease. There is a squint (and hence diplopia) maximal in the direction of action of the weak muscle/s.

Non-paralytic squint. Non-paralytic or concomitant squint describes a squint beginning in childhood in which the angle between the visual axes does not vary when the eyes are moved – the squint remains the same in all directions of gaze. Diplopia is almost never a symptom. The deviating eye (the one that does not fixate) usually has defective vision; this is called *amblyopia ex anopsia*.

Non-paralytic squint may be latent (i.e. only visible at certain times), such as when the patient is tired.

The cover test. The cover test is used principally to assess non-paralytic squint and to recognize latent squint. The patient is asked to fix on a light. A pinpoint reflection is seen in the exact centre of each pupil if there is no squint. The eye that is fixing the light centrally is covered quickly. If a squint has been present the other (uncovered) eye moves to take up central fixation. The test is repeated with the opposite eye. The dominant, fixing eye will not move when the other, squinting, amblyopic eye is covered or uncovered.

Oculomotor (third) nerve

The nucleus of the third nerve lies ventral to the aqueduct in the midbrain. Efferent fibres to four external ocular muscles (superior, inferior and medial recti, and inferior oblique), levator palpebrae superioris and sphincter pupillae (parasympathetic) enter the orbit through the superior orbital fissure.

The common causes of an oculomotor nerve lesion are given in Table 20.9. Signs of a complete third nerve palsy are:

- unilateral complete ptosis
- the eye facing down and out
- a fixed and dilated pupil.

Sparing of the pupil means that parasympathetic fibres which run in a discrete bundle on the superior surface of the nerve remain undamaged, and so the pupil is of

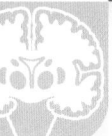

Table 20.9
Common causes of an oculomotor nerve lesion

Aneurysym of the posterior communicating artery
'Coning' of the temporal lobe
Infarction of IIIrd nerve
    In diabetes mellitus
    atheroma
Midbrain infarction
Midbrain tumour

normal size and reacts normally. In diabetes, infarction of the third nerve usually spares the pupil.

In a third nerve palsy the eye can still ABduct (sixth nerve) and rotate inwards or intort (fourth nerve). Preservation of intortion (inward rotation) means that the fourth (trochlear) nerve is intact. In a patient with a right third nerve palsy, when the attempt is made to converge and look downwards, the conjunctival vessels of the right eye are seen to twist clockwise, indicating that the eye is intorting and the fourth nerve is intact (see below).

Trochlear (fourth) nerve

This supplies the superior oblique muscle. An isolated fourth nerve lesion is a rarity. The head is tilted away from the side of the lesion. The patient complains of diplopia when attempting to look down and away from the side affected.

Abducens (sixth) nerve

The abducens nerve supplies the lateral rectus muscle which causes the eye to ABduct.

In a sixth nerve lesion there is a convergent squint with diplopia maximal on looking to the side of the lesion. The eye cannot be ABducted beyond the midline.

There are many causes of a sixth nerve lesion, as the nerve has a long intracranial course. The nerve can be involved within the brainstem (e.g. MS or pontine glioma). In raised intracranial pressure it is compressed against the tip of the petrous temporal bone. The nerve sheath may be infiltrated by tumours, particularly naso-pharyngeal carcinoma. An isolated sixth nerve palsy due to infarction occurs in diabetes mellitus. A sixth nerve lesion is a common sequel of head trauma.

Complete external ophthalmoplegia

Complete external ophthalmoplegia describes the immobile eye when III, IV and VI nerves are paralysed by lesions at the orbital apex (e.g. a metastasis) or within the cavernous sinus (e.g. sinus thrombosis).

V: Trigeminal nerve

This nerve is large, mainly sensory but with some motor fibres.

Sensory fibres (Fig. 20.7; and see Figs 20.11 and 20.12) from the three divisions – ophthalmic (V_1), maxillary (V_2)

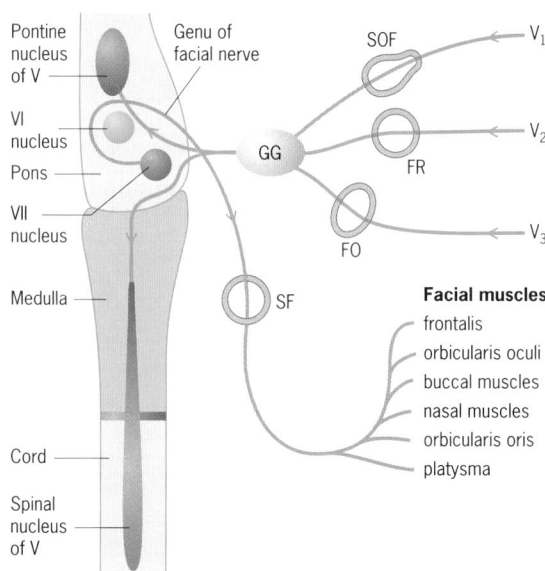

Fig. 20.7 Sensory input of trigeminal nerve (red) and motor output of facial nerve (blue). SOF, superior orbital fissure; FO, foramen ovale; FR, foramen rotundum; GG, Gasserian ganglion; SF, stylomastoid foramen.

and mandibular (V_3) – pass to the trigeminal (Gasserian) ganglion at the apex of the petrous temporal bone, within the cavernous sinus. From here central fibres enter the brainstem. Ascending fibres transmitting the sensation of light touch enter the V nucleus in the pons. Descending fibres carry pain and temperature sensation form the spinal tract of the fifth nerve and end in the spinal V nucleus in the medulla; this extends into the upper cervical cord.

Motor fibres arise in the upper pons and join the mandibular branch to supply the muscles of mastication.

Signs of a V nerve lesion

A complete fifth nerve lesion causes unilateral sensory loss on the face, tongue and buccal mucosa. When motor fibres are damaged the jaw deviates to the side of the lesion as the mouth is opened.

Diminution of the corneal reflex is an early, and sometimes isolated sign of a fifth nerve lesion.

Central (brainstem) lesions of the lower trigeminal nuclei (e.g. in syringobulbia, p. 1206) produce a characteristic circumoral sensory loss.

When the spinal tract (or spinal nucleus) alone is involved, the sensory loss is restricted to pain and temperature sensation, i.e. dissociated (p. 1151).

Causes

Within the *brainstem*, lesions involve the fifth nuclei and central connections, e.g.:

- brainstem glioma
- multiple sclerosis

- infarction
- syringobulbia.

At the *cerebellopontine angle*, the nerve is compressed by:

- acoustic neuroma
- meningioma
- secondary neoplasm.

As these lesions enlarge, the neighbouring seventh and eighth nerves become involved, producing facial weakness and deafness.

At *the apex of the petrous temporal bone*, spreading infection from the middle ear, or a secondary tumour, damages the nerve. The combination of a V nerve lesion with pain and a sixth nerve lesion is called Gradenigo's syndrome.

Within the *cavernous sinus*, the trigeminal (Gasserian) ganglion is compressed by:

- aneurysm of the internal carotid artery
- lateral extension of a pituitary neoplasm
- thrombosis of the cavernous sinus
- secondary neoplasm.

The trigeminal ganglion becomes infected in ophthalmic herpes zoster (p. 1195), the most common lesion of the ganglion itself. Trigeminal postherpetic neuralgia commonly occurs, often affecting the first (ophthalmic) division (p. 1195).

Peripheral branches of the trigeminal nerve are affected by neoplastic infiltration of the skull base.

Trigeminal neuralgia

Trigeminal neuralgia (*tic douloureux*) is a condition of unknown cause, seen most commonly in old age. It is almost always unilateral.

Symptoms

Severe paroxysms of knife-like or electric shock-like pain, lasting seconds, occur in the distribution of the fifth nerve. The pain tends to commence in the mandibular division (V_3) and spreads upwards to the maxillary (V_2) and to the ophthalmic division (V_1). Spasms occur many times a day.

Each paroxysm is stereotyped, brought on by stimulation of a specific and often tiny trigger zone in the face. Washing, shaving, a cold wind or eating are examples of the trivial stimuli that provoke the intense pain. The face may be screwed up in agony (hence the term *tic* – an involuntary movement).

The pain characteristically does not occur at night. Spontaneous remissions last for months or years before recurrence, which is almost inevitable.

Signs

There are no signs of trigeminal nerve dysfunction. The corneal reflex is preserved. Features in the history alone make the diagnosis.

Treatment

The anticonvulsant carbamazepine 600–1200 mg daily reduces the severity of attacks in the majority of patients. Phenytoin, gabapentin and clonazepam are also used, but are less effective.

If drug therapy fails, surgical procedures (radiofrequency extirpation of the ganglion, neurovascular decompression or sectioning of the sensory root) are useful in difficult cases. Alcohol injection into the trigeminal ganglion or peripheral fifth nerve branches can also be carried out.

Secondary trigeminal neuralgia

Trigeminal neuralgia occurs in MS (p. 1190), with tumours of the fifth nerve (e.g. neuroma) and with lesions of the cerebellopontine angle (see below). There are usually physical signs – initially a depressed corneal reflex, progressing to trigeminal sensory loss.

Idiopathic trigeminal neuropathy

A chronic and isolated fifth nerve lesion sometimes develops without apparent cause. When sensory loss is severe, trophic changes (facial scarring and corneal ulceration) develop.

VII: Facial nerve

The facial nerve is largely motor in function, supplying muscles of facial expression. The nerve carries sensory taste fibres from the anterior two-thirds of the tongue via the *chorda tympani*. It also supplies motor fibres to the stapedius muscle. The facial nerve (Fig. 20.7) arises from the seventh nerve nucleus in the pons and leaves the skull through the stylomastoid foramen. Part of each facial nucleus supplying the upper face (principally frontalis muscle) receives supranuclear fibres from each hemisphere. Therefore in a unilateral upper motor neurone lesion of the facial nerve the upper part of the face is usually not affected.

Unilateral facial weakness

Lower motor neurone (LMN) lesions. A unilateral LMN lesion causes weakness of all the muscles of facial expression on the same side. The face, especially the angle of the mouth, falls, and dribbling occurs from the corner of the mouth. There is weakness of frowning (frontalis) and of eye closure since the upper facial muscles are weak. Corneal exposure and ulceration occurs if the eye does not close during sleep. The platysma muscle is also weak.

Upper motor neurone (UMN) lesions. UMN lesions cause weakness of the lower part only of the face on the side opposite the lesion. Frontalis is spared. Thus the normal furrowing of the brow is preserved, and eye

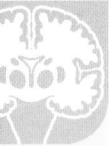

closure and blinking are not affected. The earliest sign is simply slowing of one side of the face, for example on baring the teeth. In UMN lesions, too, there is sometimes relative preservation of spontaneous emotional movement (e.g. smiling) compared with voluntary movement.

Causes of facial weakness

A common cause of facial weakness is a supranuclear (UMN) lesion (e.g. cerebral infarction), leading to UMN facial weakness and hemiparesis.

Lesions at four lower levels are recognized by the association of LMN facial weakness with other signs.

Pons. Here the sixth (abducens) nerve nucleus is encircled by seventh nerve fibres (Fig. 20.7). The sixth nucleus is thus often involved in pontine lesions of the seventh, causing a convergent squint (lateral rectus palsy) with unilateral facial weakness.

When the neighbouring PPRF and corticospinal tract are involved, there is the triple combination of:

- LMN facial weakness
- failure of conjugate lateral gaze (towards the lesion)
- contralateral hemiparesis.

Causes include pontine tumours (e.g. glioma), demyelination and vascular lesions.

The facial nucleus itself is affected unilaterally or bilaterally in poliomyelitis (see p. 52) and in motor neurone disease (p. 1208) – the latter usually bilaterally.

Cerebellopontine angle (CPA). The fifth, sixth and eighth nerves are affected with the seventh where they are clustered together in the CPA. Causes are acoustic neuroma, meningioma and secondary neoplasm.

Petrous temporal bone. The geniculate ganglion (sensory for taste) lies at the *genu* (knee) of the facial nerve (Fig. 20.7). Fibres join the facial nerve in the *chorda tympani* and carry taste from the anterior two-thirds of the tongue. The (motor) nerve to stapedius muscle leaves the facial nerve distal to the *genu*. Facial nerve lesions within the petrous temporal bone cause the combination of:

- loss of taste on the anterior two-thirds of the tongue
- hyperacusis (unpleasantly loud noise distortion) caused by paralysis of stapedius.

Causes include:

- Bell's palsy
- trauma
- middle ear infection
- herpes zoster (Ramsay Hunt syndrome, p. 1138)
- tumours (e.g. glomus tumour).

Skull base, parotid gland and in the face itself. Swelling of the facial nerve within the stylomastoid foramen develops in Bell's palsy (see below). The nerve can be damaged by skull base tumours and in Paget's disease of bone. Branches of the facial nerve that pierce the parotid to supply muscles of facial expression are damaged here by parotid gland tumours, mumps (p. 59), sarcoidosis (p. 897) and trauma. Each nerve is also affected in polyneuritis (e.g. Guillain–Barré syndrome, p. 1214), usually simultaneously.

Weakness of the facial muscles themselves is also seen in primary muscle disease and neuromuscular junction disorders. Weakness is usually symmetrical. Causes include:

- dystrophia myotonica (p. 1224)
- facioscapulohumeral dystrophy (p. 1223)
- myasthenia gravis (p. 1222).

Bell's palsy

This common, acute, isolated facial nerve palsy is probably due to a viral (often herpes simplex) infection that causes swelling of the nerve within the petrous temporal bone and as it traverses the stylomastoid foramen in the skull base.

The patient notices marked unilateral facial weakness, sometimes with loss of taste on the anterior two-thirds of the tongue. Pain behind the ear is common at onset. Diagnosis is made on clinical grounds. No other cranial nerves are involved.

Management and course

Spontaneous improvement of Bell's palsy usually begins during the second week. Thereafter, recovery continues but this may take 12 months to become complete. Occasionally (fewer than 10%) patients are left with a severe, unsightly, residual weakness.

Electrophysiological tests (EMG, p. 1156) are of some help in predicting outcome but rarely used in practice. After the third week, absence of an evoked potential from facial muscles (the nerve is stimulated over the parotid) indicates that recovery is unlikely.

Steroids (e.g. prednisolone 60 mg daily, reducing to nil over 10 days) reduce the proportion of patients left with a severe deficit, provided they are given early. Aciclovir is of unproven value but sometimes given.

Suturing of the upper to lower lid (tarsorrhaphy) is essential to prevent prolonged corneal exposure if the eye cannot be closed. Adhesive tape to hold the eye closed is an invaluable temporary protective measure.

If there is severe late residual paralysis, cosmetic surgery is sometimes helpful.

Bell's palsy occasionally recurs and is very rarely bilateral.

Ramsay Hunt syndrome

This is herpes zoster (shingles) of the geniculate ganglion. There is a facial palsy (identical in appearance to Bell's palsy) with herpetic vesicles in the external auditory meatus (because this receives a sensory twig from the facial nerve) and sometimes on the soft palate. Deafness, or a fifth nerve lesion may occur. Complete recovery is less likely than in Bell's palsy. Treatment for shingles should be given (aciclovir, p. 1277).

Hemifacial spasm

This is an irregular, painless clonic spasm of the facial muscles, usually occurring in middle or old age, and more commonly in women. It varies in severity from a mild inconvenience to a severe and disfiguring condition when it affects all the facial musculature of one side.

The causes are:

- idiopathic
- pressure from vessels in the cerebellopontine angle
- following Bell's palsy
- acoustic neuroma
- Paget's disease in the skull base.

There are clonic spasms of the facial muscles on one side. A mild LMN facial weakness is common.

Management

Mild cases require no treatment. In severe cases, various decompressive procedures on the facial nerve in the cerebellopontine angle are sometimes helpful. Local injection of botulinum toxin into facial muscles reduces the spasm for some months, and can be repeated. Drugs are of no value.

Myokymia

Facial myokymia describes a rare, continuous, fine, sinuous or wave-like movement of the lower face that is seen in brainstem lesions (e.g. multiple sclerosis, brainstem glioma).

The term myokymia is also used to describe the innocent twitching around the eye that commonly occurs in fatigue.

VIII: Vestibulocochlear nerve

This nerve has two parts – cochlear and vestibular.

Cochlear nerve

Auditory fibres from the spiral organ of Corti within the cochlea pass to the cochlear nuclei in the pons. Fibres from these nuclei cross the midline and pass upwards through the medial lemnisci to the medial geniculate bodies and thence to the temporal gyri.

The *symptoms* of a cochlear nerve lesion are deafness and tinnitus. The deafness is called 'sensorineural' (or perceptive) deafness. Clinical detection is by tuning fork (256 Hz, not 128 Hz) tests, principally Rinne's test, which distinguishes conductive from sensorineural deafness:

- The contralateral ear is masked (with the examiner's forefinger).

- The vibrating tuning fork is placed adjacent to the external auditory meatus.
- In sensorineural deafness, perception improves when the base of the vibrating tuning fork is placed on the mastoid process: sound is conducted directly to the ossicles through bone.

Investigations of cochlear lesions

- Pure tone audiometry.
- Measurement of auditory evoked potentials. These record from scalp electrodes the response from a repetitive click auditory stimulus. The level of the lesion may be detected by abnormalities in the response.

Causes of sensorineural deafness are shown in Table 20.10.

Vestibular nerve

Nerve impulses generated by movement of the sensory epithelia of the three semicircular canals, saccule and utricle pass to vestibular nuclei in the pons. The vestibular nuclei are also connected to the cerebellum, nuclei of the ocular muscles, PPRF, extrapyramidal system, reticular formation, temporal lobes and spinal cord.

The maintenance of balance and posture also depends upon the interaction of proprioceptive (joint position sense) impulses passing between the neck, spinal muscles and limbs and the vestibular system.

The *main symptom* of a vestibular lesion is vertigo and loss of balance. Vomiting frequently accompanies acute vertigo of any cause. Nystagmus is the principal physical sign.

Vertigo

Vertigo, the definite illusion of movement of the subject or surroundings, indicates a disturbance of vestibular, eighth nerve, brainstem or, very rarely, cortical function. The principal causes are given in Table 20.11.

Deafness and tinnitus accompanying vertigo indicate that its origin is from the ear or eighth cranial nerve.

Table 20.10
Causes of sensorineural deafness

End organ	Advancing age
	Occupational acoustic trauma
	Ménière's disease
	Drugs (e.g. gentamicin, neomycin)
Eighth nerve lesions	Acoustic neuroma
	Cranial trauma
	Inflammatory lesions:
	Tuberculous meningitis
	Sarcoidosis
	Neurosyphilis
	Carcinomatous meningitis
Brainstem lesions (rare)	Multiple sclerosis
	Infarction

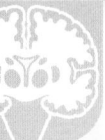
Table 20.11
Principal causes of vertigo

Ménière's disease
Drugs (e.g. gentamicin, anticonvulsant intoxication)
Toxins (e.g. ethyl alcohol)
'Vestibular neuronitis'
Multiple sclerosis
Migraine
Acute cerebellar lesions
Cerebellopontine angle lesions (e.g. acoustic neuroma)
Partial seizures (temporal lobe focus)
Brainstem ischaemia or infarction
Benign paroxysmal positional vertigo

Nystagmus

Nystagmus is a rhythmic oscillation of the eyes. It is a sign of disease of either the ocular or vestibular system and its connections. Nystagmus is classified on its appearance as either *jerk* or *pendular*. For true nystagmus to be present it must be demonstrable within binocular gaze and be sustained.

Jerk nystagmus

Jerk nystagmus (the usual nystagmus of neurological disease) has a fast and a slow component. It is seen in vestibular end-organ, eighth nerve, brainstem, cerebellar and (very rarely) cortical lesions. The direction of nystagmus is decided by the fast component, which can be thought of as a reflex attempt to correct the slower, primary movement.

Considerable difficulties exist when attempts are made to use the direction alone of jerk nystagmus as a localizing sign, although nystagmus is both a common and valuable indication of abnormality within the vestibular system as a whole. The following are useful diagnostic starting points:

- **Horizontal jerk or rotary jerk nystagmus** may be either of peripheral origin (middle ear) or central origin (eighth nerve, brainstem, cerebellum and their connections). In peripheral lesions, nystagmus is usually acute and transient (minutes or hours) and associated with severe prostrating vertigo; in central lesions it is long-lasting (weeks, months or more). Vertigo caused by central lesions tends to wane after days or weeks, the nystagmus outlasting it.
- **Vertical jerk nystagmus.** This is caused only by central lesions.
- **Down-beat jerk nystagmus.** This rarity is caused by lesions around the foramen magnum (e.g. meningioma, cerebellar ectopia).

Pendular nystagmus

Pendular describes movements to and fro that are similar in both velocity and amplitude. Pendular nystagmus

is almost always binocular, horizontal and present in all directions of gaze. Its causes are almost invariably ocular, when there is poor visual fixation (e.g. long-standing, severe visual impairment) or as a congenital lesion, when it is sometimes associated with head-nodding. Exceptionally, it occurs in brainstem disease: a fine pendular, jelly-like nystagmus is a sign of a multiple sclerosis (MS) brainstem plaque, or brainstem glioma.

Investigation of vestibular lesions

Magnetic resonance provides the best structural images of this region.

Caloric tests are used to assess function of the labyrinth. These record the duration of evoked nystagmus when first ice-cold, then warm, water is run into the external meatus. In the normal caloric test:

- ice-cold water in the left ear causes nystagmus with the fast movement to the right
- warm water in the left ear causes nystagmus with the fast movement to the left.

The right ear gives opposite responses. Decreased or absent nystagmus indicates ipsilateral labyrinth, eighth nerve or brainstem involvement. The technique is also used in the diagnosis of brainstem death (p. 955). There are, however, difficulties relating minor abnormalities in caloric tests to clinical symptoms of dizziness.

Vestibular and auditory lesions – central, VIIIth nerve and end organ

Drugs (e.g. anticonvulsant toxicity), alcohol and brainstem vascular disease are common central causes of vertigo. It may also be possible to recognize lesions from clinical features at six distinct levels.

Cerebral cortex. Vertigo is occasionally part of the aura of a partial (temporal lobe) seizure. Vertigo is also a psychological and perceptual sensation when experiencing unaccustomed heights, or in panic attacks. Deafness is very rare in acquired cortical disease; bilateral lesions are necessary.

Pons and brainstem. Vertigo is also common when lesions involve the vestibular nuclei and their connections (demyelination, vascular, tumour, syrinx). A sixth or seventh nerve lesion, internuclear ophthalmoplegia, lower cranial nerve lesions or contralateral hemiparesis will help localization. Nystagmus is frequently present, while deafness is rare. Transient vertigo occurs in basilar migraine (p. 1202), in syncope, and occasionally in hypoglycaemic attacks; its site of origin is often difficult to ascertain.

Cerebellum. Nystagmus, towards the side of a cerebellar mass (e.g. tumour, haemorrhage or infarct) develops. Limb ataxia is usually present. Bilateral cerebellar, or cerebellar connexion disease (e.g. olivo-ponto-cerebellar degeneration) causes bilateral nystagmus. Deafness does not occur.

Cerebellopontine angle. Sensorineural deafness and vertigo occur. Sixth, seventh and fifth nerve lesions develop, followed by cerebellar signs (ipsilateral) and later pyramidal signs (contralateral). Nystagmus is often present. Causes include acoustic neuroma (p. 1199), meningioma and secondary neoplasm, carcinomatous meningitis and inflammatory lesions (Table 20.11).

Petrous temporal bone. Facial weakness (seventh nerve) often accompanies the eighth nerve lesion. Causes include trauma, middle ear infection, secondary neoplasm and Paget's disease of bone (see also Gradenigo's syndrome, p. 1137).

End organs (cochlear and semicircular canals). Causes include:

- Ménière's disease
- drugs (e.g. gentamicin)
- noise (acoustic trauma, p. 997)
- middle ear infection
- mumps
- 'vestibular neuronitis'
- benign paroxysmal positional vertigo
- advancing age
- intrauterine rubella
- congenital syphilis.

Ménière's disease

This condition is characterized by recurrent attacks of the three symptoms – vertigo, tinnitus and deafness. It is associated with a dilatation of the endolymph system of unknown cause.

Symptoms

Sudden, unprovoked attacks of vertigo with vomiting and loss of balance last from minutes to hours. Tinnitus and deafness accompany an attack but may be overshadowed by the degree of vertigo. Attacks are recurrent over months or years. Ultimately deafness develops and vertigo ceases.

Signs

Nystagmus often accompanies an attack. Sensorineural deafness is present.

Management

Medical treatment consists of rest and vestibular sedatives (e.g. cinnarizine, betahistine, prochlorperazine), but is unsatisfactory. Each attack is, however, self-limiting.

Recurrent severe attacks may require surgery, such as surgical endolymph drainage, ultrasound destruction of the labyrinth or vestibular nerve section.

'Vestibular neuronitis'

This common but poorly understood syndrome describes an acute attack of isolated severe vertigo with nystagmus, often with vomiting, but without loss of hearing. It is believed to follow or accompany viral infections that affect the labyrinth or vestibular nerve.

The disturbance lasts for several days or weeks but is self-limiting and rarely recurs. Treatment is with vestibular sedatives. The condition is sometimes followed by benign positional vertigo. Very similar symptoms can be caused by demyelination or vascular lesions within the brainstem, but usually other abnormalities are almost invariably apparent (see above).

Benign paroxysmal positional vertigo (BPPV)

Positional vertigo is vertigo precipitated by head movements, usually into a particular position. It may occur when turning in bed or on sitting up. The onset is typically sudden and distressing. Vertigo is transient, lasting seconds or minutes. The phenomenon fatigues (becomes less severe on repeated movement).

Vertigo can be produced by moving the patient's head suddenly (Hallpike's test). There is a latent interval of a few seconds, followed by nystagmus, which fatigues on repeating the test several times, though repetition is unpleasant for the patient.

Whilst no serious underlying cause is found for BPPV, it is a distressing syndrome that sometimes follows vestibular neuronitis (see above), head injury or ear infection. It usually lasts for some months. There are no sequelae, although it sometimes recurs.

Positional nystagmus (and vertigo) that is immediately apparent on movement (i.e. there is no latent interval) and that persists (it does not fatigue) is occasionally seen with cerebellar mass lesions.

Vertigo is treated symptomatically with vestibular sedative drugs. The evidence base for these compounds is limited. Vestibular exercises (Cawthorne Cooksey exercises) are also recommended. In these, the head and neck are rotated to provoke, and hence fatigue, the unpleasant illusion of movement.

Lower cranial nerves IX, X, XI, XII

The glossopharyngeal (IX), vagus (X) and accessory (XI) nerves arise in the medulla and leave the skull base together through the jugular foramen. The hypoglossal (XII) also arises in the medulla but leaves the skull through the anterior condylar foramen. All four lower cranial nerves lie close together, just outside the skull, and are related to the carotid artery and ascending sympathetic innervation to the eye.

Glossopharyngeal (IX)

This mixed nerve is largely sensory. Sensory fibres supply all sensation to the tonsillar fossa and pharynx (the afferent pathway of the gag reflex), and taste to the posterior third of the tongue.

Motor fibres supply the stylopharyngeus muscle, autonomic fibres supply the parotid gland, and a sensory branch supplies the carotid sinus.

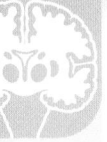
Vagus (X)

This mixed nerve, largely motor, supplies the striated muscle of the pharynx (efferent pathway of the gag reflex), larynx (including the vocal cords via the recurrent laryngeal nerves) and upper oesophagus. There are sensory fibres from the larynx. Parasympathetic fibres supply the heart and abdominal viscera.

Accessory (XI)

This motor nerve supplies the trapezius stomamastoid muscles.

Hypoglossal (XII)

This motor nerve supplies the tongue.

Ninth and tenth nerve lesions

Isolated nerve lesions are most unusual, since disease at the jugular foramen affects both nerves and sometimes the accessory nerve.

A unilateral ninth nerve lesion causes diminished sensation on the same side of the pharynx. A tenth nerve palsy produces ipsilateral failure of voluntary and reflex elevation of the soft palate, which is drawn over to the opposite side.

Bilateral combined lesions of the ninth and tenth nerves cause visible weakness of elevation of the palate, depression of palatal sensation and loss of the gag reflex. The vagal recurrent laryngeal branches are involved. The cough is depressed and the vocal cords paralysed. The patient complains of difficulty in swallowing, hoarseness, nasal regurgitation and choking (particularly with fluids) – a dangerous situation. *Bulbar palsy* is a general term describing palatal, pharyngeal and tongue weakness of LMN type (p. 1142).

Ninth and tenth nerve lesions often accompany eleventh and twelfth nerve lesions. Causes are given in Table 20.12.

Table 20.12

Principal causes of ninth, tenth, eleventh and twelfth nerve lesions

Within the brainstem
Infarction
Syringobulbia
Motor neurone disease (motor fibres)
Poliomyelitis (motor fibres)

At the skull base (jugular and anterior condylar foramina)
Carcinoma of nasopharynx
Glomus tumour
Neurofibroma
Jugular venous thrombosis (XIIth is spared)
Trauma

Within the neck and nasopharynx
Carcinoma of nasopharynx
Metastases
Polyneuropathy
Trauma

Recurrent laryngeal nerve lesions. Paralysis of this branch of each vagus causes hoarseness (dysphonia) and failure of the forceful, explosive part of voluntary and reflex coughing. There is no visible weakness of the palate but vocal cord paralysis is seen endoscopically. Bilateral acute lesions (e.g. postoperatively) are a serious emergency and cause respiratory obstruction.

The left recurrent laryngeal nerve (which loops beneath the aorta) is more commonly damaged than the right.

Causes of recurrent laryngeal nerve lesions include:

- mediastinal primary tumours (e.g. thymoma)
- secondary spread from carcinoma of the bronchus
- aneurysm of the aorta
- trauma or surgery to the neck
- glossopharyngeal neuralgia (rare).

Glossopharyngeal neuralgia. This describes intensely painful, paroxysmal neuralgic spasms of the pharynx triggered repeatedly by swallowing. There are no physical signs. Treatment of this rare condition is with carbamazepine (see trigeminal neuralgia, p. 1137) or section of the nerve in the pharynx.

Table 20.12 shows the principal causes of lesions.

Eleventh nerve lesions

A lesion of the eleventh nerve causes weakness of sternomastoid (rotation of the head and neck to the opposite side) and trapezius (shoulder shrugging). Section of the nerve is followed by persistent neuralgic neck pain and is often accompanied by other lower cranial nerve lesions (see Table 20.12).

Twelfth nerve lesions

LMN lesions of the twelfth nerve lead to unilateral tongue weakness, wasting and fasciculation. When protruded the tongue deviates towards the weaker side. For the principal causes, see Table 20.12.

Bilateral supranuclear (UMN) twelfth nerve lesions (see below) produce slow, limited tongue movements; the tongue is stiff and cannot be protruded far. Fasciculation is absent.

Brain stem lesions

Bulbar palsy

Bulbar palsy describes weakness of LMN type of muscles whose cranial nerve nuclei lie in the medulla (the 'bulb'). Paralysis of bulbar muscles is caused by disease of lower cranial nerve nuclei (e.g. motor neurone disease), lesions of ninth to twelfth cranial nerves (Table 20.12), malfunction of their neuromuscular junctions (e.g. myasthenia gravis, botulism), or disease of muscles themselves (e.g. muscular dystrophies).

Pseudobulbar palsy

This describes bilateral supranuclear (UMN) lesions of lower cranial nerves producing weakness and poverty of movement of the tongue and pharyngeal muscles. (This resembles, superficially a bulbar palsy, hence the term *pseudo*bulbar.) The findings in pseudobulbar palsy are a stiff, slow, spastic tongue (that is not wasted), dysarthria with a stiff, slow, spastic voice sounding dry and gravelly, and dysphagia. The gag and palatal reflexes are preserved. The jaw jerk is exaggerated. Emotional lability (inappropriate laughing or crying) often accompanies pseudobulbar palsy. The principal causes are:

- motor neurone disease, in which there are often both upper UMN and LMN lesions (i.e. elements of both pseudobulbar *and* bulbar palsy)
- multiple sclerosis, mainly as a late event
- cerebrovascular disease, typically in multi-infarct dementia
- following severe head injury.

Great difficulty swallowing, dysarthria and a slow tongue also develop in late stages of Parkinson's disease. This is distinct from both pseudobulbar and bulbar palsy.

Motor control systems

There are three systems:

- The *corticospinal* (or pyramidal) system originates in the cerebral cortex and delivers information to the anterior horn cells of the spinal cord. This system enables purposive, skilled, strong and organized movement to take place. Defective function within the pathway is recognized by a distinct pattern of loss of skilled voluntary movement, spasticity and reflex change. This is seen, for example, in a hemiparesis or hemiplegia.
- The *extrapyramidal* system facilitates fast, fluid movements that the corticospinal system has generated. Defective function is recognized usually by slowness (bradykinesia), stiffness (rigidity) and/or disorders of movement (rest tremor, chorea and other dyskinesias). Frequently, one sign (e.g. stiffness, tremor or chorea) will predominate, depending upon the site and nature of the pathology. Mixtures of these features, and the lack of clear pathological anatomy makes classification of movement disorders difficult.
- The *cerebellum* and its connections have a role in coordinating the smooth movement initiated by the corticospinal system, and in the regulation of balance. Cerebellar disease leads to unsteadiness and jerkiness of movement (ataxia), with characteristic physical signs of past pointing, action tremor and incoordination, or ataxia of gait and/or the trunk.

Each of the three motor control systems also relies upon connections with the other two, and with sensory input, from proprioception (joint position), reticular formation, vestibular system and from special senses.

Corticospinal or pyramidal system

The corticospinal tracts originate in neurones of the fifth layer of the cortex and terminate at the motor nuclei of the cranial nerves and anterior horn cells of the spinal cord. The nerve fibre pathways of particular importance (Fig. 20.8) in clinical diagnosis congregate in the internal

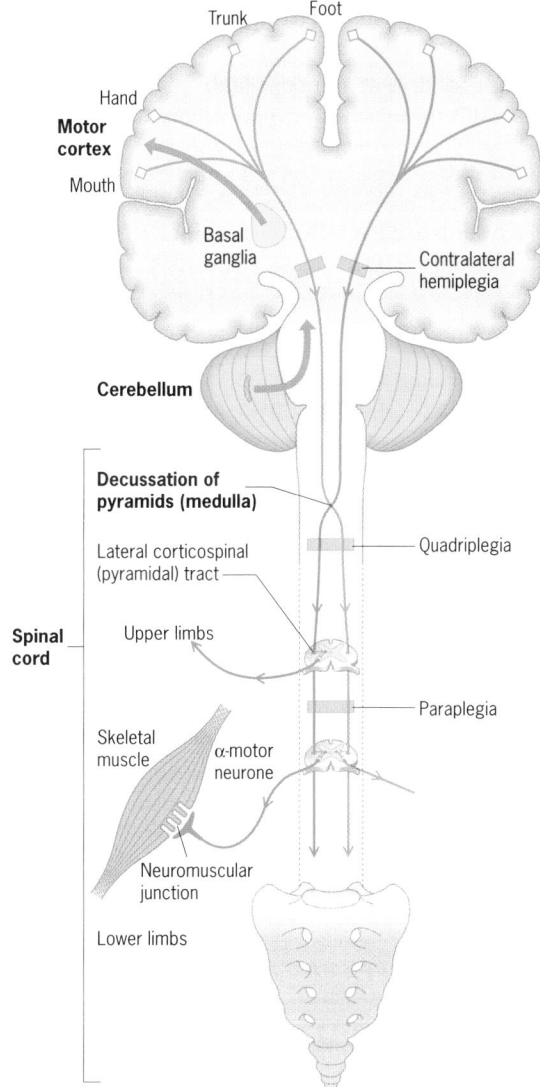

Fig. 20.8 The motor system. Lesions are shown on the *right* hand side of the figure.

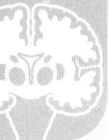

capsule and cross in the medulla (decussation of the pyramids), passing to the contralateral halves of the spinal cord as the crossed lateral corticospinal tracts. This is the *pyramidal system*, disease of which causes upper motor neurone (UMN) lesions. *Pyramidal* is simply a descriptive term that draws together the anatomy and physical signs of lesions of this pathway. It is used here interchangeably with the term UMN.

A small proportion of the corticospinal outflow remains uncrossed (the anterior corticospinal tracts), but this is not of relevance in clinical practice.

Clinical characteristics of pyramidal lesions (see Table 20.13)

The signs of an early pyramidal lesion may be minimal. Weakness, spasticity or changes in superficial reflexes may predominate and the absence of one group of signs does not exclude a UMN lesion.

Pyramidal drift of an upper limb

Normally, the outstretched upper limbs are held symmetrically, even when the eyes are closed. With a pyramidal (UMN) lesion, when both upper limbs are held outstretched, palms uppermost, the affected limb drifts downwards and medially. The forearm tends to pronate and the fingers flex slightly. This upper limb sign is often first to occur, sometimes before weakness or reflex changes become obvious.

Weakness and loss of skilled movement

A unilateral pyramidal (UMN) lesion above the decussation in the medulla (e.g. an infarct in the internal capsule) causes weakness of the opposite limbs, i.e. a contralateral hemiparesis. When acute and complete, this weakness will be immediate and dense – a stroke from an internal capsule infarct causing a hemiplegia (see below). In slowly progressive lesions (e.g. a cortical glioma) a characteristic pattern of increasing weakness emerges in the hemiparetic limbs. In the upper limb flexors remain stronger than extensors, while in the lower limb extensors remain stronger than flexors. In the upper arm the weaker movements are thus shoulder

abduction and elbow extension; in the forearm and hand, wrist and finger extensors and abductors are weaker than their antagonists.

In the lower limb weaker movements are hip flexion and abduction, knee flexion, and ankle dorsiflexion and eversion. In addition to weakness, there is loss of skilled movement. For example, fine finger and toe control diminishes. Muscle wasting (except from disuse) is not a feature of pyramidal lesions. Muscles remain normally excitable electrically.

When the UMN lesion is below the decussation of the pyramids, i.e. in the cervical spinal cord, the hemiparesis is on the same side as the lesion. This situation is unusual.

Increase in tone (spasticity)

An acute lesion of one pyramidal tract (e.g. the internal capsule stroke mentioned above) causes initially flaccid paralysis, and loss of tendon reflexes. Increase in tone follows within several days owing to loss of the inhibitory effect of the corticospinal pathway and an increase in spinal reflex activity. This increase in tone affects all muscle groups on the side affected but is detectable most easily in stronger muscles. The tone itself is characterized by changing resistance to passive movement; the change is sudden – the clasp-knife effect. The tendon reflexes in the affected limbs become exaggerated and clonus is often evident.

Changes in superficial reflexes

The normal flexor plantar response becomes extensor (a positive Babinski). In a severe lesion (e.g. the internal capsule infarct) this extensor response can be elicited from a wide area of the affected limb. As recovery progresses, the area that is receptive diminishes until only the posterior third of the lateral aspect of the sole is receptive. The stimulus should be unpleasant (an orange-stick is the correct instrument). An extensor plantar is certain when the dorsiflexion of the great toe is accompanied by fanning (abduction) of the other toes. The abdominal (and cremasteric reflexes) are abolished on the affected side.

Clinical patterns of UMN disorders

There are two main patterns of UMN (pyramidal) lesions: hemiparesis and paraparesis.

Hemiparesis means a degree of weakness of the limbs of one side; it is usually (but not always, see above) caused by a lesion within the brain. *Paraparesis* means a degree of weakness of *both* lower limbs and is characteristically diagnostic of a spinal cord lesion, though bilateral brain lesions occasionally can also cause a similar picture.

Hemi*plegia* and para*plegia* strictly indicate *total* paralysis, but are often used loosely to describe severe weakness.

Table 20.13
Evidence of an upper motor neurone lesion

Drift of upper limb
Weakness with a characteristic distribution
Increase in tone of spastic type
Exaggerated tendon reflexes
An extensor plantar response
Loss of fine finger/toe movements
Loss of abdominal reflexes
No muscle wasting
Normal electrical excitability of muscle

Hemiparesis

The level within the corticospinal tract is recognized by various accompanying features.

Motor cortex. Weakness and/or loss of skilled movement localized to one contralateral limb (an arm or a leg – monoplegia) or part of a limb (e.g. a weak hand) is characteristic of an isolated lesion of the motor cortex (e.g. a secondary neoplasm). There may also be a defect in higher cortical function (e.g. aphasia when the speech area is affected). Focal epilepsy may occur.

Internal capsule. Since all corticospinal fibres become tightly packed as they reach the internal capsule, occupying about 1 cm², a small lesion causes a large deficit. For example, an infarct of a small branch of the middle cerebral artery (p. 1166) causes a sudden, dense, contralateral hemiplegia that includes the face.

Pons. A pontine lesion (e.g. a plaque of multiple sclerosis) is rarely confined only to the corticospinal tract. As adjacent structures such as the sixth and seventh nuclei, MLF and PPRF (p. 1134), are involved, there are other localizing signs – VI and VII nerve palsies, internuclear ophthalmoplegia (INO) or a lateral gaze palsy, with contralateral hemiparesis.

Spinal cord. An isolated lesion of a single lateral corticospinal tract within the spinal cord (e.g. in the cervical region) causes an ipsilateral UMN lesion, the level indicated by a reflex level (e.g. absent biceps C5/6 jerk), the presence of a Brown–Séquard syndrome and muscle wasting at the level of the lesion (p. 1151).

Paraparesis (Table 20.14)

Paraparesis indicates bilateral damage to the corticospinal tracts. Spinal cord compression (p. 1206) or other cord disease is the usual cause, but cerebral lesions occasionally can produce paraparesis. Paraparesis, including here tetraparesis or quadriparesis (interchangeable terms), is a feature of many neurological conditions, recognizable by additional clinical features, making this differential diagnosis one of pivotal importance in neurology.

Extrapyramidal system

The extrapyramidal system is a general term without an absolute definition for the motor structures of the basal ganglia. These consist of the corpus striatum (i.e. caudate nucleus + globus pallidus + putamen), subthalamic nucleus, substantia nigra and parts of the thalamus. In basal ganglia/extrapyramidal disorders, either or both of two features become apparent in the limbs and axial muscles:

- reduction in speed, known as bradykinesia (slow movement) or akinesia (no movement), with muscle rigidity

Table 20.14
Causes of a spastic paraparesis

Spinal lesions
Spinal cord compression (see Table 20.49)
Multiple sclerosis
Myelitis (e.g. varicella zoster virus)
Motor neurone disease
Subacute combined degeneration of the cord
Syringomyelia
Syphilis
Familial or sporadic paraparesis
Vascular disease of the cord
Non-metastatic manifestation of malignancy
Tropical spastic paraparesis (HTLV-1)
HIV-associated myelopathy

Cerebral lesions*
Parasagittal cortical lesions:
   Meningioma
   Venous sinus thrombosis
Hydrocephalus
Multiple cerebral infarction

---

* All are rare causes of a paraparesis
HTLV-1, human T-cell leukaemia virus

- involuntary movements (e.g. tremor, chorea, hemiballismus, athetosis, dystonia).

Extrapyramidal disorders are classified broadly on clinical grounds into akinetic–rigid syndromes (p. 1182) in which poverty of movement predominates, and dyskinesias, in which there are a variety of excessive involuntary movements (p. 1186).

The most common serious extrapyramidal disorder is Parkinson's disease.

Essential anatomy

The corpus striatum lies close to the substantia nigra, thalami and subthalamic nuclei. There are interconnections between these structures, cerebral cortex, cerebellum and reticular formation, cranial nerve nuclei (particularly vestibular) and spinal cord (Fig. 20.9).

Function and dysfunction

The overall function of this complex system is modulation of cortical motor activity by a series of servo loops, between cortex and basal ganglia. Figure 20.9 is a simplified outline of the anatomy.

It is now clear that in many involuntary movement disorders there are substantial and specific changes in neurotransmitters (Table 20.15) rather than anatomical lesions discernable on imaging or at autopsy. The probable neurotransmitters in extrapyramidal pathways are outlined in Figure 20.9; changes in Parkinson's disease, chorea and hemiballismus are discussed below. The complexity of the situation is evident.

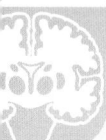

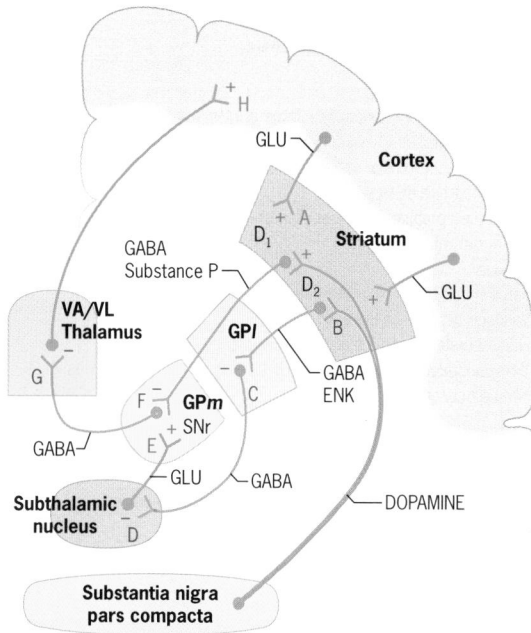

Fig. 20.9 Extrapyramidal system: scheme of connections and neurotransmitters. GLU, glutamate; ENK, enkephalin; GABA, gamma-aminobutyric acid; VA, ventral anterior; VL, ventrolateral; GP*l*, lateral globus pallidus; GP*m*, medial globus pallidus; SN*r*, substantia nigra pars reticulata.

A proposed model of principal basal ganglia pathways

1. Direct pathway from striatum to medial globus pallidus (GP*m*) and substantia nigra pars reticulata (SN*r*). Inhibitory synapse F, GABA and substance P.
2. Indirect pathway from striatum to globus pallidus; via lateral globus pallidus (GP*l*; inhibitory synapse C, GABA, enkephalin) and subthalamic nucleus inhibitory synapse D, GABA). Terminates in GP*m*–SN*r* (in excitatory synapse E, glutamate).
3. Direct pathways, both inhibitory and excitatory from substantia nigra pars compacta (SN*c*) to striatum. Synapse A, dopamine, D_1, excitatory; and synapse B, D_2, inhibitory.
4. GP*m* and SN*r* to thalamus. Synapse G, GABA.
5. Thalamus to cortex. Excitatory, synapse H.
6. Cortex to striatum. Excitatory, glutamate.

The model helps explain how basal ganglia disease can either reduce excitatory thalamo-cortical activity at synapse H, i.e. movement – causing bradykinesia, or increase it, causing hyperkinesia.

Parkinson's disease. This condition is characterized by slowness, stiffness and rest tremor (p. 1182). Degeneration in SN*c* causes loss of dopamine activity in the striatum. Dopamine is excitatory for synapse A and inhibitory for synapse B. Through the direct pathway

Table 20.15

Changes in the major neurotransmitter profile in Parkinson's and Huntington's diseases

Condition	Site	Neurotransmitter
Parkinson's disease	Putamen	Dopamine ↓ 90% Norepinephrine (noradrenaline) ↓ 60% 5-HT ↓ 60%
	Substantia nigra	Dopamine ↓ 90% GAD + GABA ↓↓
	Cerebral cortex	GAD + GABA ↓↓
Huntington's disease	Corpus striatum	Acetylcholine ↓↓ GABA ↓↓ Dopamine: normal GAD + GABA ↓↓

GABA, γ-amino butyric acid; GAD, glutamic acid decarboxylase, the enzyme responsible for synthesizing GABA; 5-HT, 5-hydroxytryptamine

there is reduced activity at synapse F, leading to increased inhibitory output (G) and decreased cortical activity (H).

Also in Parkinson's disease, in the indirect pathway dopamine deficiency results in disinhibition of neurones synapsing at C. This leads to reduced activity at D, and to increased activity of neurones in the subthalamic nucleus. There is excess stimulation at synapse E, enhancing further inhibitory output of GP*m*–SN*r*.

The net effect via both pathways is to inhibit the ventral anterior (VA) and ventrolateral (VL) nuclei of the thalamus at synapse G. Cortical (motor) activity at H is thus reduced.

Levodopa used in the treatment of Parkinson's disease (p. 1184) induces its unwanted dyskinesias by increasing dopamine activity at synapses A and B, reversing the sequences in both direct and indirect pathways.

Huntington's disease. This is an inherited dementia (p. 1186) with progressive jerky movements (chorea). Chorea may result from damage to neurones (GABA, enkephalin) in the indirect pathway from striatum to GP*l*, reducing activity at synapse C. In turn, there is increased inhibition of subthalamic neurones at D, reduced stimulation at E and decreased inhibition of VA/VL at G. Cortical activity at H increases.

Hemiballismus. This describes wild, flinging limb movements usually caused by a small infarct in the subthalamic nucleus. This reduces excitatory activity at synapse E, resulting in a reduction of inhibition at G with increased activity of thalamo-cortical neurones and increased activity at H.

Cerebellum

The third system of motor control is involved with coordination, rather than speed. Ataxia, i.e. unsteadiness, is characteristic when it malfunctions.

The cerebellum receives afferent fibres from:

- proprioceptive organs in joints and muscles
- vestibular nuclei
- basal ganglia
- the corticospinal system
- olivary nuclei.

Efferent fibres pass from the cerebellum to:

- each red nucleus
- vestibular nuclei
- basal ganglia
- corticospinal system.

Each lateral cerebellar lobe coordinates movement of the ipsilateral limb. The vermis (a midline structure) is concerned with maintenance of axial (midline) posture and balance.

Cerebellar lesions

Expanding mass lesions within the cerebellum obstruct the aqueduct to cause hydrocephalus, with severe pressure headaches, vomiting and papilloedema. Coning of the cerebellar tonsils (p. 1200) through the foramen magnum and respiratory arrest occur, often within hours. Rarely tonic seizures (sudden attacks of stiffness) of the limbs occur in cerebellar lesions.

Lateral cerebellar lobes

A lesion within one cerebellar lobe (e.g. a tumour or infarction) causes disruption of the normal sequence of movements (dyssynergia) on the same side. Ataxia and other signs develop.

Unlike in Parkinson's disease, the neurotransmitter changes in cerebellar disease are poorly understood.

Posture and gait. The outstretched arm is held still in the early stages of a cerebellar lesion, cf. the drift of a pyramidal lesion, but there is rebound upward overshoot when the limb is pressed downwards and released by the examiner. Gait becomes ataxic with a broad base; the patient falters towards the side of the lesion.

Tremor and ataxia. Movement is imprecise in direction, in force and in distance (dysmetria). Rapid alternating movements (tapping, clapping or rotary hand movements) are clumsy and disorganized (dysdiadochokinesis). Intention tremor (action tremor, with past-pointing) is seen when finger–nose–finger and heel–shin tests are performed. The speed of movement is preserved, cf. extrapyramidal disease.

Nystagmus. Coarse horizontal nystagmus (p. 1140) develops with lateral cerebellar lobe lesions. Its direction is towards the lesion.

Dysarthria. A halting, jerking dysarthria results – the scanning speech of cerebellar lesions (usually bilateral).

Other signs. Titubation – rhythmic tremor of the head in either to and fro (yes–yes) movements or rotary (no–no) movements – also occurs, mainly when cerebellar connections are involved (e.g. in essential tremor and MS, pp. 1186 and 1189). Hypotonia (floppy limbs)

Table 20.16
Principal causes of cerebellar syndromes

Tumours	Haemangioblastoma
	Medulloblastoma
	Secondary neoplasm
	Compression by acoustic neuroma
Vascular lesions	Haemorrhage
	Infarction
	Arteriovenous malformation
Infection	Abscess
	HIV
	Kuru
Developmental	Arnold-Chiari malformation
	Basilar invagination
	Cerebral palsy
Toxic and metabolic	Anticonvulsant drugs
	Chronic alcohol abuse
	Following carbon monoxide poisoning
	Lead poisoning
	Solvent abuse
Inherited	Friedreich's ataxia
	Ataxia telangiectasia
	Essential tremor
Miscellaneous	Multiple sclerosis
	Hydrocephalus
	Postinfective cerebellar syndrome of childhood
	Hypothyroidism
	Non-metastatic manifestation of malignancy
	Cerebral oedema of chronic hypoxia

and depression of reflexes are also sometimes seen with cerebellar disease, but are usually of little value as localizing signs. Pendular (i.e. slow) reflexes also occur.

Midline cerebellar lesions

Midline cerebellar vermis lesions have a dramatic effect on the equilibrium of the trunk and axial musculature. This is truncal ataxia – difficulty standing and sitting unsupported, with a rolling, broad, ataxic gait. Lesions of the flocculonodular region of the cerebellum cause vertigo, vomiting and ataxia of gait if they extend to the roof of the fourth ventricle.

Table 20.16 summarizes the main causes of cerebellar disease.

Tremor

Tremor means a regular and sinusoidal oscillation of part of the body. Different varieties are outlined below. Pathological anatomy and neurotransmitter changes remain largely unknown.

Postural tremor

Everyone has a physiological tremor (often barely perceptible) of the outstretched hands at 8–12 Hz. This is increased with anxiety, hyperthyroidism and certain drugs (sympathomimetics, sodium valproate, lithium)

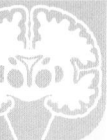
or in mercury poisoning. A coarse, postural tremor is seen in chronic alcohol abusers and in benign essential tremor (usually at 5–8 Hz). Postural tremor does not worsen on movement, though it may become more obvious.

Intention tremor

Tremor exacerbated by action, with past-pointing and accompanying slowness and incoordination of rapid alternating movement (dysdiadochokinesis), occurs in cerebellar lobe disease and with lesions of cerebellar connections. Titubation (head tremor) and nystagmus may be present.

Rest tremor

This occurs typically in Parkinson's disease. Tremor is noticeably at its worst at rest, usually between 4 and 7 Hz and is sometimes described as pill-rolling – between the thumb and index finger.

Other tremors

Coarse tremor is seen following lesions of the red nucleus (e.g. infarction, demyelination) and rarely with frontal lobe lesions.

FURTHER READING

Elble R (2000) Origins of tremor. *Lancet* **355**: 1113–1114.

Lower motor neurone (LMN) lesions

The LMN is the motor pathway from the anterior horn cell (or cranial nerve nucleus) via a peripheral nerve to the motor endplate.

The motor unit consists of a single anterior horn cell, the single fast-conducting motor nerve fibre that leaves the spinal cord via the anterior root, and the group of muscle fibres (100–2000) being supplied via the mixed peripheral nerve. Anterior horn cell activity is modulated by impulses from:

- the corticospinal tracts
- the extrapyramidal system
- the cerebellum
- afferent fibres from posterior roots.

Signs of lower motor neurone lesion

These are seen in the voluntary muscles which depend upon their nerve supply, not only to produce movement but also for metabolic integrity. Signs follow rapidly if the LMN is interrupted at any point in its course (Table 20.17). Muscle wasting appears within 3 weeks of the development of an LMN lesion. Fasciculation (visible muscle twitching) occurs and is due to contractions of denervated single motor units. Fibrillation potentials are seen when denervated muscle is sampled electrically (p. 1156).

Table 20.17
Signs of a lower motor neurone lesion

Weakness
Wasting
Hypotonia
Reflex loss
Fasciculation
Contractures of muscle   } long term effects
'Trophic' changes in skin and nails }

NB: Fibrillation potentials can be detected electromyographically, see page 1156.

Causes

Examples of LMN lesions at various levels are:

- cranial nerve nuclei and anterior horn cell – Bell's palsy, motor neurone disease, poliomyelitis
- spinal root – cervical and lumbar disc protrusion, neuralgic amyotrophy (see p. 1218)
- peripheral (or cranial) nerve – nerve trauma or entrapment (see p. 1212), mononeuritis multiplex (p. 1213).

Spinal reflex arc

The components of the spinal reflex arc are illustrated in Figure 20.10. The stretch reflex is the physiological basis for all tendon reflexes. For example, in the knee jerk a

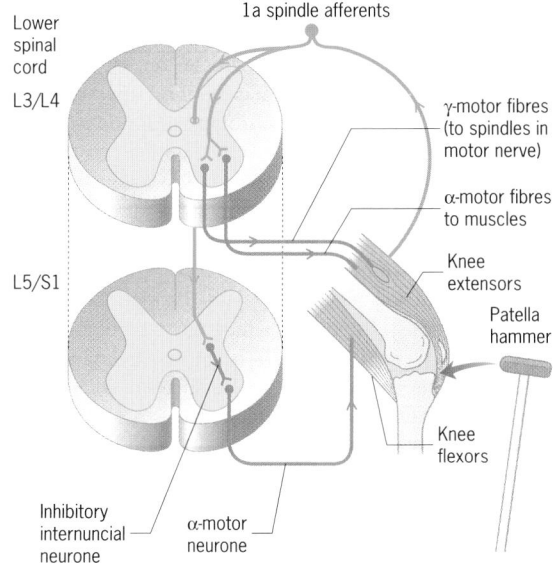

Fig. 20.10 **The knee jerk: a spinal reflex arc.** Sudden stretching of a tendon generates sensory action potentials in 1a muscle spindle afferents. These synapse with γ motor fibres (to spindles) and α motor fibres. Motor action potentials generated cause muscle contraction. There is also inhibition of knee flexion.

Table 20.18
Spinal levels of tendon reflexes

Spinal level	Reflex
C5–6	Supinator
C5–6	Biceps
C7	Triceps
L3–4	Knee
S1	Ankle

tap on the patellar tendon activates stretch receptors in the quadriceps. Impulses in first-order sensory neurones pass directly to LMNs (L3 and L4) that contract quadriceps.

Loss of a tendon reflex is caused by a lesion anywhere along the spinal reflex path. The reflex lost indicates the level of the lesion (Table 20.18).

Reinforcement
Distraction of the patient's attention, clenching the teeth or pulling of the interlocked fingers enhances reflex activity. Such reinforcement manoeuvres should be carried out before a reflex is recorded as absent.

Sensory pathways and pain

Peripheral nerves and spinal roots
Peripheral nerves carry all modalities of sensation from either free or specialized nerve endings to the dorsal root ganglia and thus to the cord. The sensory distribution of spinal roots (dermatomes) is shown in Figure 20.11.

Spinal cord (Fig. 20.12)
Posterior columns
Axons in the posterior columns whose cell bodies are in the ipsilateral gracile and cuneate nuclei in the medulla carry the sensory modalities of vibration sense, joint position (proprioception), light touch and two-point discrimination. Axons from second-order neurones then cross the midline in the brainstem to form the medial lemniscus and pass to the thalamus.

Spinothalamic tracts
Axons carrying pain and temperature sensation synapse in the dorsal horn of the cord, cross the cord and pass as the spinothalamic tracts to the thalamus and reticular formation.

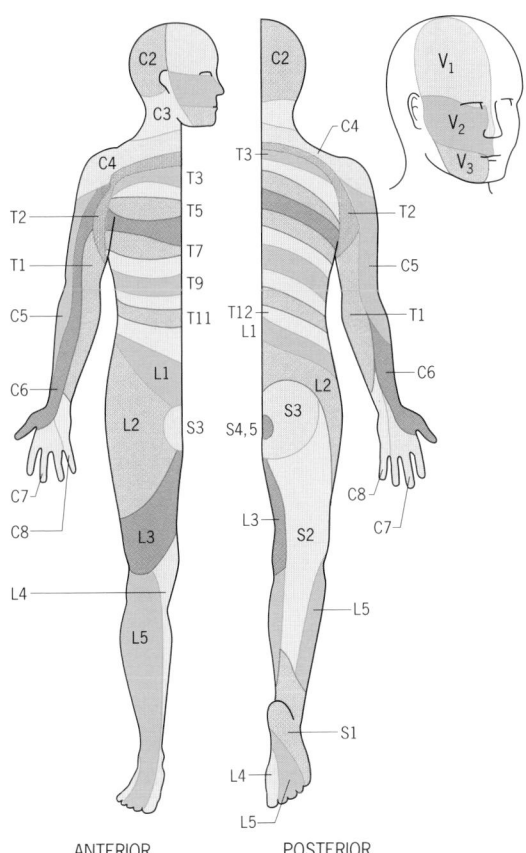

Fig. 20.11 Dermatomes of spinal roots and ophthalmic (V_1), maxillary (V_2) and mandibular (V_3) divisions of the trigeminal nerve.

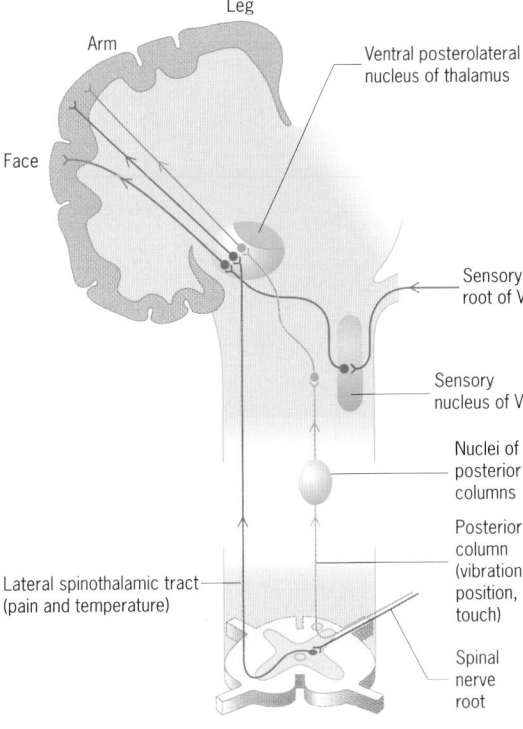

Fig. 20.12 Principal sensory pathways. Posterior columns remain uncrossed until the medulla. The spinothalamic tracts cross close to their entry into the spinal cord.

1149

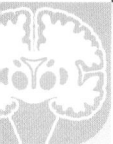

Sensory cortex

The projection of fibres from the thalamus to the sensory cortex of the parietal region is shown in Figure 20.12. Connections also exist between the thalamus and the motor cortex.

Lesions of the sensory pathways

(Fig. 20.13)

Paraesthesiae, numbness and pain are the principal symptoms of sensory lesions. The quality and distribution of symptoms usually suggest the site of pathology.

Peripheral nerve lesions

Symptoms are felt in the distribution of the affected peripheral nerve (p. 1212).

Section of a sensory nerve is followed by complete sensory loss. Nerve entrapment (p. 1212) causes numbness, pain and tingling. Tapping the site of compression sometimes causes a sharp, electric-shock-like pain in the distribution of the nerve, such as at the wrist in the carpal tunnel syndrome (Tinel's sign).

Neuralgia

Neuralgia refers to local pain of great severity in the distribution of a damaged nerve. Examples are:

- trigeminal neuralgia (p. 1137)
- postherpetic neuralgia (p. 1195)
- complex regional pain syndrome type 2 (causalgia) – a chronic burning pain that occasionally follows nerve section. It is seen sometimes after amputation.

Spinal root lesions

Root pain

The pain of root compression is felt in the myotome supplied by that root, and there is also a tingling discomfort in the dermatome. The pain is made worse by manoeuvres that either stretch the nerve root (e.g. the limitation

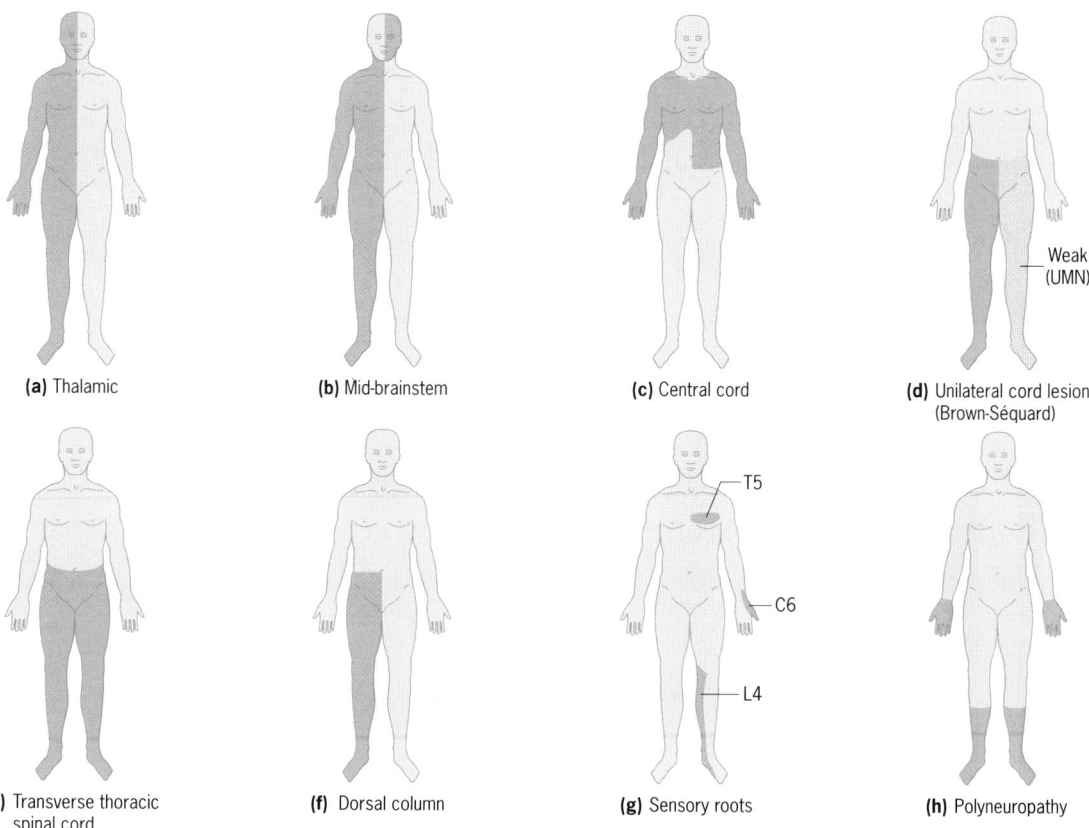

(a) Thalamic   **(b)** Mid-brainstem   **(c)** Central cord   **(d)** Unilateral cord lesion (Brown-Séquard)   Weak (UMN)

(e) Transverse thoracic spinal cord   **(f)** Dorsal column   **(g)** Sensory roots   T5, C6, L4   **(h)** Polyneuropathy

Fig. 20.13 Principal patterns of loss of sensation. (a) Thalamic lesion: sensory loss throughout opposite side. **(b)** Brainstem lesion (rare): contralateral sensory loss below face and ipsilateral loss on face. **(c)** Central cord lesion, e.g. syrinx: 'suspended' areas of loss, often asymmetrical and 'dissociated', i.e. pain and temperature loss but light touch remaining intact. **(d)** 'Hemisection' of cord or unilateral cord lesion = Brown–Séquard syndrome: contralateral spinothalamic (pain and temperature) loss with ipsilateral weakness and dorsal column loss below lesion. UMN, upper motor neurone. **(e)** Transverse cord lesion: loss of all modalities below lesion. **(f)** Isolated dorsal column lesion, e.g. demyelination: loss of proprioception, vibration and light touch. **(g)** Individual sensory root lesions, e.g. C6 (cervical root compression), T5 (shingles), L4 (lumbar root compression). **(h)** Polyneuropathy: distal sensory loss.

of straight leg raising in lumbar disc prolapse) or increase the pressure in the spinal subarachnoid space (coughing and straining).

Cervical and lumbar disc protrusions (p. 1218) are common causes of root lesions.

Dorsal spinal root lesions

Section of a dorsal root causes loss of all modalities of sensation in the appropriate dermatome (Fig. 20.11). However, the overlap with adjacent dermatomes may make it difficult to detect anaesthesia if a single root is destroyed.

Lightning pains. Tabes dorsalis (now a rarity in the UK) is a form of neurosyphilis that causes low-grade inflammation of the dorsal roots and root entry zone of the spinal cord. Irregular, sharp, momentary stabbing pains (like lightning) involve one or two spots, typically in a calf, thigh or ankle.

Spinal cord lesions

Posterior column lesions

These cause:

- tingling
- electric-shock-like sensations
- clumsiness
- numbness
- band-like sensations.

These symptoms are lateralized but often felt vaguely without a clear sensory level. On examination, position sense, vibration sense, light touch and two-point discrimination are lost below the level of the lesion. Loss of position sense produces the stamping gait of sensory ataxia (p. 1125).

Lhermitte's phenomenon

An electric-shock-like sensation radiates down the trunk and limbs when the neck is flexed. This indicates a cervical cord lesion. Lhermitte's sign is common in acute exacerbations of MS (p. 1189). It also occurs in cervical spondylotic myelopathy (p. 1218), subacute combined degeneration of the cord (p. 1216), radiation myelopathy (p. 1207), and occasionally in cord compression.

Spinothalamic tract lesions

Pure spinothalamic lesions cause isolated contralateral loss of pain and temperature sensation below the level of the lesion. This is called dissociated sensory loss – pain and temperature are dissociated from light touch, which remains preserved. This is seen typically in syringomyelia where a cavity occupies the central spinal cord.

The spinal level is modified by the lamination of fibres within the spinothalamic tracts. Fibres from the lower spinal roots lie superficially and are therefore damaged first by compressive lesions from outside the cord. As an external compressive lesion (e.g. a midthoracic extradural meningioma; Fig. 20.14) enlarges, the spinal sensory level ascends as deeper fibres become involved. Conversely, a

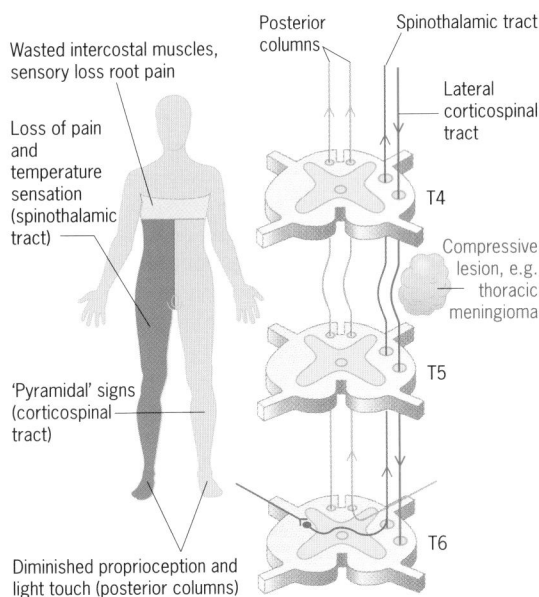

Fig. 20.14 **Clinical features of spinal cord compression.**

central lesion of the cord (e.g. a syrinx, p. 1206) affects the deeper fibres first.

Spinothalamic tract lesions cause loss of pain perception (resulting in painless burns and minor injuries) and loss of temperature sensation (inability to distinguish hot from cold). Perforating ulcers and neuropathic joints (Charcot joints) develop.

Spinal cord compression (Fig. 20.14)

This important syndrome causes a progressive spastic paraparesis (or tetraparesis/quadriparesis) with sensory loss below the level of the lesion. Sphincter disturbance is common.

Root pain is frequent but not invariable. It is felt characteristically at the site of compression. With a lesion of the thoracic cord (e.g. an extradural meningioma), pain radiates in a band around the chest and is made worse by coughing, straining and jarring, as the meningeal sheaths of nerve roots are stretched.

Involvement of one spinothalamic tract (contralateral loss of pain and temperature) together with one corticospinal tract (ipsilateral pyramidal signs) is known as the Brown–Séquard syndrome of hemisection of the cord. The patient complains of numbness on one side and weakness on the other. Paraparesis and spinal cord disease are discussed further on page 1205.

Pontine lesions

Since lesions in the pons (e.g. an MS plaque) lie above the decussation of the posterior columns, and the medial lemniscus and spinothalamic tracts are close together, there is loss of all forms of sensation on the side opposite the lesion. The III, IV, V, VI and VII cranial nerve nuclei are often also involved (Fig. 20.12) and allow recognition of the level.

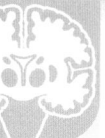

Thalamic lesions

Thalamic pain, also called the thalamic syndrome, is usually caused by a small thalamic infarct. The stroke patient develops a hemiparesis and sensory loss. The weakness recovers partially or completely but there remains a constant very severe deep-seated burning pain in the paretic limbs. Movement does not change the pain, which continues night and day. Extreme anguish is usual and the secondary depression may lead to suicide. Thalamic lesions may also produce loss of all modalities of sensation on the opposite side of the body; this is an unusual clinical picture.

Parietal cortex lesions

Sensory loss, neglect of one side, apraxia (p. 1125) and subtle disorders of sensation occur. Pain is not a feature of destructive cortical lesions. Irritative phenomena (e.g. partial sensory seizures from a glioma) arising in the parietal cortex cause tingling sensations in a limb, or elsewhere.

FURTHER READING

Donaghy M (1997) *Neurology – Oxford Core Texts*. Oxford: Oxford University Press.

Pain

Pain is an unpleasant and unique physical and psychological experience. Acute pain serves a biological purpose (e.g. withdrawal of a limb) and causes sympathetic hyperactivity. It is typically self-limiting, when healing is complete. Chronic pain (e.g. causalgia, p. 1150) lasts many months, far longer than the time required for healing.

Essential physiology of pain

Pain perception is mediated by free nerve endings, the terminations of finely myelinated A-delta and of non-myelinated C fibres. Chemicals released locally as a result of injury either produce pain by direct stimulation or by sensitizing the nerve endings. A-delta fibres give rise to perception of sharp, immediate pain which is followed by slower-onset, duller, more diffuse and prolonged pain mediated by slower-conducting C fibres.

Sensory impulses enter the cord via dorsal spinal roots. Within it, impulses ascend either in each dorsal (posterior) column or in each spinothalamic tract. The cells of the grey matter in the spinal cord are arranged in laminae labelled I to X from dorsal to ventral. A fibres terminate in laminae I and V and excite second-order neurones which send fibres to the contralateral side via the anterior commissure and up the anterolateral column in the direct spinothalamic tract. C fibres mostly terminate in the substantia gelatinosa (laminae II and III). A series of short fibres give rise to long axons which pass through the anterior commissure to the contralateral side and up the spino-reticulo-thalamic tract.

The spinothalamic tracts carry impulses which localize pain. Thalamic pathways to and from the cortex mediate emotional components.

Sympathetic activity increases pain – for example, increasing blood flow in a painful limb.

The gate theory of pain

Gate theory proposes that the entry of afferent impulses is monitored by the cells of the substantia gelatinosa (see above), which acts as a regulator determining whether or not sufficient activity penetrates to fire secondary neurones in the dorsal horn. Each gate is influenced by descending activity from the brain. This can override spinal cord regulatory mechanisms and alter how far the gate is open.

Endogenous opiates

The endorphin family of peptides have opioid activity and probably account for the very real effects of placebo, stress reducers and acupuncture analgesia. They are neurotransmitters acting at inhibitory synapses via δ, κ and μ receptors.

Management of chronic pain (see also p. 530)

Chronic pain is gravely disabling and distressing, and taxing to treat. Multidisciplinary pain-relief clinics are helpful in providing specific and supportive therapy. Pain control should, however, be part of all doctors' skills.

A management plan for intractable pain, when it is often difficult to find the precise cause, has seven components.

Diagnostic

Rigorous attention must be paid to the question of diagnosis, reviewing the history (first hand), the investigations, and radiology. A specific surgical approach may then become apparent (e.g. pain in undiagnosed spinal stenosis, trigeminal neuralgia, glossopharyngeal neuralgia, or discovery of syringomyelia in intractable upper limb pain).

Psychological

Chronic pain influences quality of life and lifestyle. Clinical depression (p. 1235) is almost universally associated with chronic pain even when the underlying pathology is benign. Perhaps paradoxically a relative minority of patients suffering pain from secondary cancer are clinically depressed despite the gravity of their disease. Antidepressant drugs and modification of lifestyle are of help in improving the quality of life. Perseverance and compliance with therapy is an invariable issue.

Analgesics (see p. 508)

Co-analgesics

Co-analgesics are drugs that have a primary use in conditions other than pain but are also effective, either alone or when added to conventional analgesics. Examples are non-steroidal anti-inflammatory drugs used in bone pain or tricyclic antidepressants and anticonvulsants used in deafferentation pain (p. 509). Calcium-channel blockers (nifedipine) improve sympathetically mediated pain, as occurs in, for example, Raynaud's disease. Muscle relaxants, antibiotics and steroids by injection each relieve pain when used in appropriate situations (e.g. severe spasticity, infection, and inflammatory arthropathy, respectively).

Stimulation
Acupuncture, ice, heat, ultrasound, massage, transcutaneous electrical nerve stimulation (TENS) and spinal cord stimulation all achieve analgesia by a gating effect on large myelinated nerve fibres.

Nerve blocks
Pain pathways can be blocked either temporarily by local anaesthetic or permanently with phenol, or with radiofrequency lesions. Examples are:

- somatic blocks
  (a) peripheral nerve and plexus injections
  (b) epidural and spinal analgesia
- sympathetic blocks
  (a) sympathetic ganglia and nerve ending injections
  (b) central epidural and spinal sympathetic blockade.

Neurosurgery
Highly specialized and sometimes controversial techniques have a place alongside pharmacological remedies. Examples are dorsal rhizotomy, sympathectomy, cordotomy and neurostimulation.

FURTHER READING

Wall PD, Melzack R (1999) *Textbook of Pain*. 4th edn. Edinburgh: Churchill Livingstone.
Lancet (1999) Pain Series. **353**: May–June.

Control of the bladder and sexual function

Changes in the pattern of micturition and the failure of normal sexual activity are diagnostic symptoms in sacral, spinal cord and cortical disease.

Essential anatomy and function
The three efferent LMN pathways to the bladder are shown in Table 20.19.

Afferent fibres (T12–S4) record changes in pressure within the bladder and tactile sensation in the genitalia. When the bladder is distended, continence is maintained

Table 20.19
The three efferent pathways to the bladder and genitalia

Nerve supply	Function
Sympathetic T12–L2	Bladder wall relaxation Internal sphincter contraction Orgasm, ejaculation
Parasympathetic S2–4	Bladder wall contraction Internal sphincter relaxation Penis and clitoris erection/engorgement
Pudendal nerves (Somatic)	External sphincter (skeletal muscle)

by reflex suppression of the parasympathetic outflow, and reciprocal activation of the sympathetic, both being subject to cortical (voluntary) control. Voiding takes place by parasympathetic activation of the detrusor muscle, and relaxation of the internal sphincter.

Cortical awareness of bladder fullness is located in the post-central gyrus, parasagittally, while initiation of micturition is in the pre-central gyrus. Voluntary control of micturition is located in the frontal cortex, parasagittally.

Disorders of micturition: incontinence
Three neurological patterns of bladder dysfunction cause urinary incontinence. These may be hard to separate clinically.

Cortical.
- Frontal lesions cause socially inappropriate micturition.
- Pre-central lesions cause difficulty initiating micturition.
- Post-central lesions cause loss of sense of bladder fullness.

Spinal cord. Bilateral UMN lesions (pyramidal tracts) cause frequency of micturition and incontinence. The bladder is small and unusually sensitive to small changes in intravesical pressure (hypertonic bladder). Frontal lobe lesions also sometimes cause a hypertonic bladder. **Lower motor neurone.** Sacral lesions (conus medullaris, sacral roots and pelvic nerve lesions, which need to be bilateral) cause a flaccid, atonic bladder, which overflows without warning.

Impotence
Failure of penile erection often has a mixed aetiology rather than being due solely to either an organic or psychological cause. The emotional aspects of impotence are discussed no further here, but are of great importance. Depression is a common cause, and a common effect. Endocrine aspects of impotence are discussed on page 1021. Erectile dysfunction is treated with sildenafil by mouth.

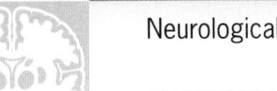

FURTHER READING

Fowler CJ (ed) (1999) *Neurology of Bladder, Bowel and Sexual Dysfunction.* Boston: Butterworth Heinemann.
Sildenafil for erectile dysfunction (1998) *Drugs & Therapeutics Bulletin* **36**: 81–83.

Neurological investigations

These consist largely of imaging preceded by routine investigations (Table 20.20).

Neuroradiology

Skull and spinal X-rays

These are useful for:

- fractures of the skull vault or base
- skull lesions (e.g. metastases, osteomyelitis, Paget's disease, abnormal skull foramina, fibrous dysplasia)
- enlargement or destruction of the pituitary fossa – intrasellar tumour, raised intracranial pressure
- intracranial calcification – tuberculoma, oligodendroglioma, wall of an aneurysm, cysticercosis.

Spinal X-rays show fractures, congenital bone lesions (e.g. cysts), destructive lesions (infection, metastasis) or degeneration change – spondylosis.

Imaging of the brain and spinal cord

The availability of techniques varies widely both between and within different countries. Brain CT is now widely available world-wide. MRI of both brain and spinal cord is rapidly becoming a standard test, superseding both brain CT, and traditional contrast and CT myelography.

Computed tomography: CT (Fig. 20.15)

A collimated X-ray beam moves synchronously with its detectors across a slice of brain between 2 mm and 13 mm thick. The transmitted X-irradiation from an element, or pixel, of that slice (< 1 mm^2) is computer-processed and a value (Hounsfield number) assigned to its density (air = -1000 units; water = 0; bone = $+1000$ units).

The difference in X-ray attenuation (density) between bone, brain and CSF makes it possible to distinguish among normal and infarcted tissue, tumour, extravasated blood, or oedema.

Enhancement with intravenous contrast media helps delineate areas of increased blood supply and oedema.

CT imaging of the spinal cord (CT myelography) and the cerebral ventricles (ventriculography) is occasionally performed with isohexal as contrast.

CT is safe apart from occasional systemic reactions to contrast; the irradiation involved is small.

Value of CT

CT scanning demonstrates:

- cerebral tumours
- intracerebral haemorrhage and infarction
- subdural and extradural haematoma
- free blood in the subarachnoid space (subarachnoid haemorrhage, see p. 1172)
- lateral shift of midline structures and displacement/enlargement of the ventricular system
- cerebral atrophy
- spinal trauma (with CT myelography).

CT imaging, within its limitations, shows that the brain is anatomically normal, which provides reassurance.

Limitations of CT

- Lesions under 1 cm diameter may be missed.
- Lesions with attenuation close to that of bone may be missed if near the skull.
- Lesions with attenuation similar to that of brain are poorly imaged (e.g. MS plaques, isodense subdural haematoma).
- CT images sometimes miss lesions within the posterior fossa.
- The spinal cord is not imaged directly by CT (contrast is necessary).
- Results are poor when patients cannot cooperate – a general anaesthetic is occasionally required.

Magnetic resonance imaging: MRI (Fig. 20.15)

The hydrogen nucleus is a proton whose electrical charge creates a local electrical field. These protons are aligned by a sudden strong magnetic impulse. Protons

Table 20.20
Value of routine investigations in neurology

Test	Yield	Condition
Urinalysis	Glycosuria	Polyneuropathy
	Ketones	Coma
	Bence Jones protein	Cord compression
Blood picture	↑ MCV	B$_{12}$ deficiency
	↑ ESR	Giant cell arteritis
Blood glucose	Hypoglycaemia	Coma
	Hyperglycaemia	Coma
Serum electrolytes	Hyponatraemia	Coma
	Hypokalaemia	Weakness
Serum calcium	Hypocalcaemia	Tetany, spasms
Serum creatine phosphokinase	Raised	Muscle disease
Chest X-ray	Lytic bone or mass lesion	Bronchial cancer, thymoma

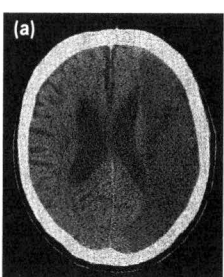

(a) CT: Massive middle cerebral artery infarct.

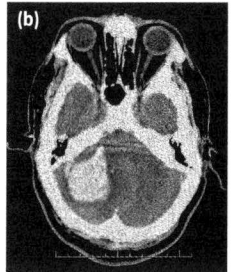

(b) CT: Cerebellar haemorrhage.

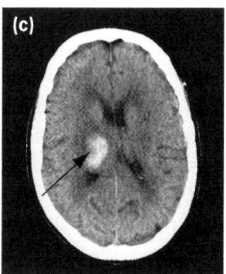

(c) CT: Thalamic haemorrhage.

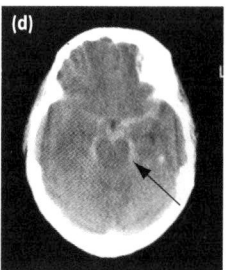

(d) CT: Subarachnoid haemorrhage.

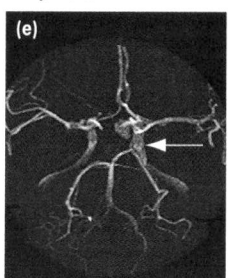

(e) MRA: Posterior communicating artery aneurysm.

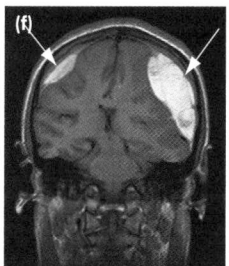

(f) MR (T1): Bilateral subdural haematomas.

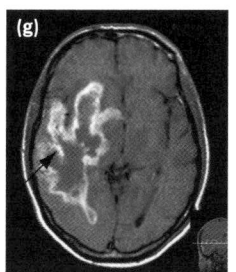

(g) MR (T1): Glioblastoma multiforme.

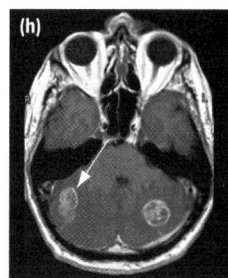

(h) MR (T1): Bilateral cerebellar metastases.

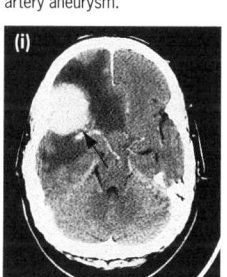

(i) CT: Right frontal meningioma.

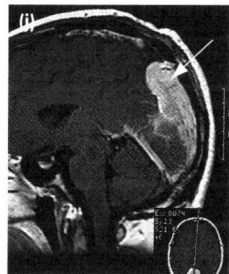

(j) MR (T1): Falx (occipital) meningioma.

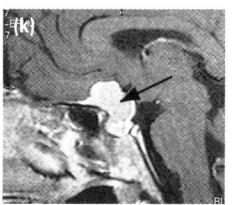

(k) MR (T1): Suprasellar meningioma.

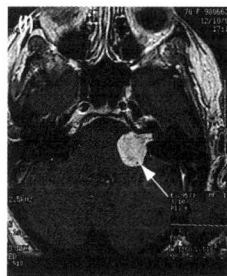

(l) MR (T1): Acoustic neuroma (Schwannoma) in internal auditory meatus.

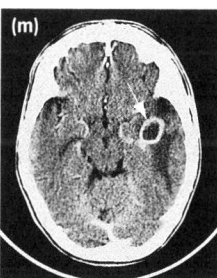

(m) MR: Pyogenic brain abscess.

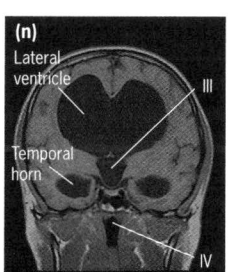

(n) MR (T1): Communicating hydrocephalus.

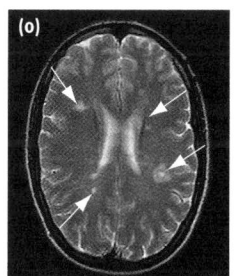

(o) MR (T2): Multiple sclerosis.

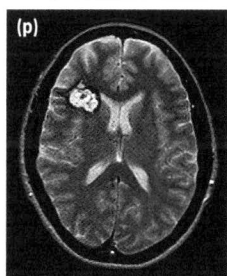

(p) MR (T2): Symptomless cavernous haemangioma.

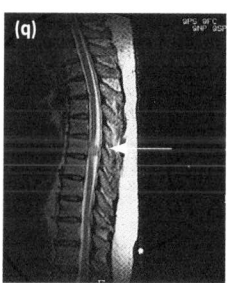

(q) MR (T2): Thoracic meningioma (cord compression).

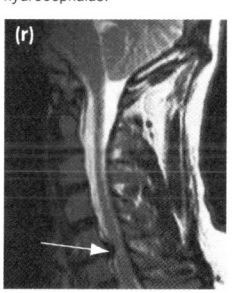

(r) MR (T2): C5/6 disc.

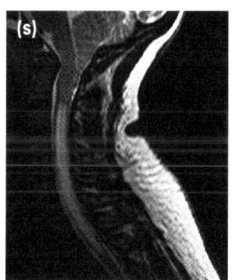

(s) MR: Cervical syrinx (cavity).

Fig. 20.15 Examples of CT and MRI imaging.

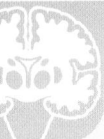

are then imaged with radiofrequency waves at right angles to their alignment. The protons resonate and spin, then revert to their normal alignment. As they do so, images are made at different phases of relaxation, known as T1, T2 and other sequences. These sequences are then recorded. From the timings of these sequences, referred to as different weightings, the recorded images are compared with each other. Gadolinium is used as an intravenous contrast medium.

Value of MRI

There are principal advantages of MRI over CT:

- MR distinguishes between brain white and grey matter.
- Spinal cord and nerve roots are imaged directly.
- Pituitary imaging.
- Resolution of MRI is greater than CT (lesions around 0.5 cm are seen).
- No radiation is involved.
- Magnetic resonance angiography (MRA) images blood vessels without the need for contrast.

Brain tumours, infarction and haemorrhage or haematoma, plaques of MS, the posterior fossa and foramen magnum region are demonstrated well on MRI. In the spinal cord, MRI shows intrinsic and extrinsic tumours, syringomyelia, cord compression and vascular malformations.

Limitations of MRI

Limitations of MRI are principally time and cost. Imaging a single region takes about 30 minutes. As with CT, patients do need to cooperate: claustrophobia is an issue within the confined space of an MR tube. A general anaesthetic may be necessary. Patients with pacemakers or with metallic bodies in the brain cannot be imaged.

Doppler studies

B-mode ultrasound is valuable in the detection of stenosis of the carotid arteries.

Digital cerebral and spinal angiography, and myelography

In many centres where MRI is available, these techniques are now greatly restricted in their application. Contrast is injected intra-arterially or intravenously to demonstrate the arterial and venous systems. *Digital subtraction angiography* (DSA), using computerized subtraction has almost entirely replaced traditional percutaneous angiography. No anaesthetic is usually necessary. However, arterial studies still carry a small mortality and risk of stroke (less than 1%). Carotid and vertebral arteriography images aneurysms, arteriovenous malformations and venous occlusion. Films of the aortic arch and the carotid and vertebral arteries demonstrate occlusion, stenoses and atheromatous plaques. Spinal angiography images arteriovenous malformations of the cord.

Myelography is almost obsolete, having been replaced by MRI. Water-soluble radiopaque dye is injected via the lumbar (or rarely cervical) subarachnoid space and imaged by conventional X-rays or CT. This aids diagnosis of cord tumours and other causes of cord compression. Radiculography is this examination confined to the lumbosacral region to image nerve roots.

Isotope bone scanning

The radioisotope [⁹⁹ᵐTc]-pertechnetate is injected intravenously. This is of value in detection of vertebral and skull lesions (e.g. metastases). Isotope brain scanning for intracranial lesions has been entirely superseded by CT and MRI.

Positron emission tomography (PET) and single proton emission computed tomography (SPECT)

These research tools map brain function in specific areas by tracking uptake and metabolism of radioisotopes. There are difficulties using these tests in clinical practice: the range of normality is poorly defined.

Electroencephalography (EEG)

The electroencephalogram (Fig. 20.16) is recorded from scalp electrodes on 16 channels simultaneously for 10–30 minutes. The main value of the EEG is in diagnosing epilepsy and diffuse brain diseases. Videotelemetry combines continuous EEG and video recording, and is valuable in the specialist assessment of difficult cases of episodes of disturbed consciousness.

Epilepsy

Spikes, or spike-and-wave abnormalities, are the hallmarks of epilepsy, but it should be emphasized that patients with epilepsy often have a normal EEG between seizures (p. 1176).

Diffuse brain disorders

Recognizable patterns of slow-wave EEG abnormalities appear in encephalitis, prion (Creutzfeldt–Jakob) disease and metabolic states (e.g. hypoglycaemia and hepatic coma).

Brain death

The EEG is isoelectric (i.e. flat). EEG is no longer necessary to confirm brain death (p. 955).

Electromyography and nerve conduction studies

Electromyography

A concentric needle electrode is inserted into voluntary muscle. The amplified recording is viewed on an oscilloscope and heard through a speaker. Three main features can be demonstrated:

- a normal interference pattern
- denervation and reinnervation
- myopathic, myotonic or myasthenic changes (p. 1222).

(a) 500 µV gain level   **(b)** 100 µV gain level

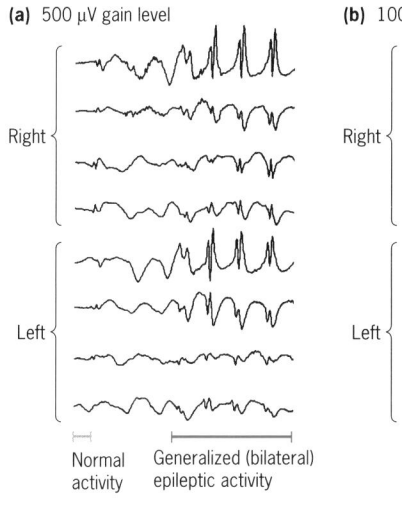
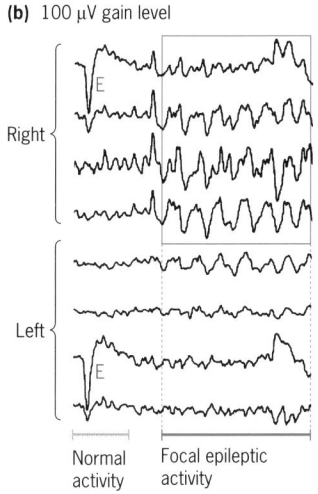

Right

Left

E

Right

Left

E

Normal   Generalized (bilateral)
activity   epileptic activity

Normal   Focal epileptic
activity   activity

Fig. 20.16 Examples of EEG traces.
(a) Normal activity followed by generalized epileptic spikes in all leads. **(b)** Normal activity followed by focal spikes in right leads. E, eye-movement artefact.

Peripheral nerve conduction

Four measurements are of principal value in the diagnosis of neuropathies and nerve entrapment:

- mean nerve (motor and sensory) conduction velocity (Fig. 20.17)
- distal motor latency
- sensory action potentials
- muscle action potentials.

Cerebral-evoked potentials

Visual-evoked potentials record the time for a visual stimulus to reach the occipital cortex. Their value is chiefly in documenting previous retrobulbar neuritis (p. 1190), which leaves a permanent delay in latency despite recovery of vision.

Similar techniques are used for auditory and somatosensory potentials (from the ear or a limb). These are also used during neurosurgery to monitor brain and spinal cord function.

Examination of the cerebrospinal fluid (CSF)

(Table 20.21 and Practical box 20.3)
The indications for lumbar puncture are:

- diagnosis of meningitis and encephalitis
- intrathecal injection of contrast media and drugs
- diagnosis of subarachnoid haemorrhage (sometimes)
- measurement of CSF pressure, e.g. idiopathic intracranial hypertension (p. 1201)
- removal of CSF therapeutically, e.g. idiopathic intracranial hypertension
- diagnosis of miscellaneous conditions, e.g. MS, neurosyphilis, sarcoidosis, Behçet's disease, neoplastic involvement, certain polyneuropathies.

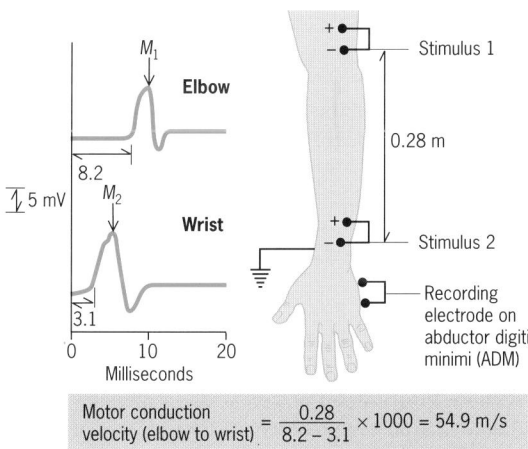

M_1

Elbow

8.2

5 mV M_2

Wrist

3.1

0   10   20
Milliseconds

+
− Stimulus 1

0.28 m

+
− Stimulus 2

Recording electrode on abductor digiti minimi (ADM)

| Motor conduction velocity (elbow to wrist) | $= \dfrac{0.28}{8.2 - 3.1} \times 1000 = 54.9 \text{ m/s}$ |

Fig. 20.17 Measurement of mean (motor) conduction velocity (MCV) in the ulnar nerve. A recording electrode on the abductor digiti minimi records the muscle action potential (*M*) from the ulnar nerve at the elbow (stimulus 1) and at the wrist (stimulus 2). From these values the motor conduction velocity can be calculated:

M_1 = muscle action potential (MAP) from stimulus 1
M_2 = MAP from stimulus 2
T_1 = time from elbow to recording electrode
T_2 = time from wrist to recording electrode

$$\text{MCV} = \frac{\text{distance in metres}}{T_1 - T_2} \times 1000 = \text{metres per second.}$$

Table 20.21
The normal CSF

Appearance	Crystal clear, colourless
Pressure	60–150 mm of H_2O with patient recumbent
Cell count	$< 5/mm^3$
	No polymorphs
	Mononuclear cells only
Protein	0.2–0.4 g/L
Glucose	$^2/_3$ to $^1/_2$ of blood glucose
IgG	< 15% of total CSF protein
Oligoclonal bands	Absent

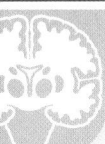

Practical box 20.3

Lumbar puncture

Lumbar puncture should *not* be performed in the presence of raised intracranial pressure or when an intracranial mass lesion is a possibility.

Technique

- The patient is placed on the edge of the bed in the left lateral position with the knees and chin as close together as possible. The procedure should be explained carefully to the patient, and consent obtained.
- The third and fourth lumbar spines are marked. The fourth lumbar spine usually lies on a line joining the iliac crests.
- Using sterile precautions, 2% lidocaine (lignocaine) is injected into the dermis by raising a bleb in either the third or fourth lumbar interspace.
- The special lumbar puncture needle is pushed through the skin in the midline. It is pressed steadily forwards and slightly towards the head, with the head and spine bolstered horizontally with pillows.
- When the needle is felt to penetrate the dura mater, the stylet is withdrawn and a few drops of CSF are allowed to escape.
- The CSF pressure can now be measured by connecting a manometer to the needle. The patient's head must be on the same level as the sacrum. Normal CSF pressure is 60–150 mmH$_2$O. It rises and falls with respiration and the heart beat, and rises on coughing.
- Specimens of CSF are collected in three sterilized test-tubes and sent to the laboratory. An additional sample in which the sugar level can be measured, together with a simultaneous blood sample for blood sugar measurement, should be taken when relevant (e.g. in meningitis).

- Record the naked-eye appearance of the CSF: clear, cloudy, yellow (xanthochromic), red.
- Patients are usually asked to lie flat after the procedure to avoid a subsequent headache, but this manouevre is probably of little value.
- Analgesics may be required for post-LP headaches.

Contraindications for lumbar puncture

- Suspicion of a mass lesion in the brain or spinal cord. Caudal herniation of the cerebellar tonsils ('coning') may occur if an intracranial mass is present and the pressure below is reduced by removal of CSF. In suspected meningococcal infection, it is usual to avoid LP because of the risk of 'coning' (see p. 1200).
- Any cause of raised intracranial pressure.
- Local infection near the site of puncture.
- Congenital lesions in the lumbosacral region (e.g. meningomyelocele).
- Platelet count below 40 × 10^9/L and other clotting abnormalities, including anticoagulant drugs.
- Unconscious patients and those with papilloedema must have a CT scan before lumbar puncture.

Notes

- These contraindications are relative. There are circumstances when lumbar puncture is carried out in spite of them.
- The composition of the normal CSF is shown in Table 20.21.

Meticulous attention should focus on microbiological studies in suspected central nervous system infection. Close liaison between clinician and microbiologist is essential. Specific techniques (e.g. polymerase chain reaction to identify meningococci or other bacteria) are sometimes invaluable. Repeated diagnostic CSF examination is often necessary in chronic infections, such as tuberculosis.

Biopsy

Interpretation of brain, muscle and nerve histology requires a specialist neuropathology service.

Brain

Brain biopsy (e.g. of a non-dominant frontal lobe) is sometimes used to diagnose inflammatory and degenerative brain diseases. CT- and MR-guided stereotactic biopsy of intracranial mass lesions are now standard procedures.

Muscle

Biopsy, with light microscopy, electron microscopy and biochemical analysis where appropriate, elucidates diagnosis of inflammatory, metabolic and dystrophic disorders of muscle (p. 1223).

Peripheral nerve

Biopsy, usually of one sural nerve, at the ankle, aids diagnosis in certain polyneuropathies (e.g. due to vasculitides).

Psychometric assessment

Psychometric testing is valuable for measuring cognitive function. Preservation of verbal IQ (a measure of past attainments) in the presence of deterioration of performance IQ (a measure of present abilities) is an important indicator of physical impairment of cognitive function, for example following brain injury or in dementia. Low subtest scores (e.g. for block design, various aspects of memory, visual, speech and constructional skills) indicate impaired function of specific regions of the brain.

The main limitation of these techniques is that depression and lack of attention reduces scores. Also, opinions sometimes vary greatly between clinical psychologists about interpretation of agreed numerical values of tests, particularly after brain injury – a matter which limits the clinical value of the tests themselves.

Specialized tests in specific diseases

Certain tests are employed in the diagnosis of individual (and often rare) neurological diseases. Examples are:

- antiphospholipid antibody and detailed clotting studies in stroke (p. 466)
- antibody to acetylcholine receptor protein in myasthenia gravis (p. 1222)
- serum copper and caeruloplasmin in Wilson's disease (p. 377)
- blood lactate studies (failure to rise on exercise) in McArdle's syndrome
- serum phytanic acid (elevated) in Refsum's disease
- serum long-chain fatty acid (present) in adrenoleucodystrophy
- genetic studies – e.g. Huntington's disease, hereditary sensorimotor neuropathies (p. 1216).

Unconsciousness and coma

The central ascending reticular formation (or reticular activating substance), extending from the lower brainstem to the thalamus, influences the state of arousal. Our state of consciousness is the product of complex interactions between parts of the reticular formation itself, cortex and brainstem, and all sensory stimuli reaching them.

Disturbed consciousness: definitions

Each term simply describes a recognizable state, either normal or pathological.

- **Consciousness** means a state of wakefulness with awareness of self and surroundings.
- **Clouding of consciousness** means reduced wakefulness and/or self-awareness, sometimes with confusion; the term is used more in psychiatry than clinical neurology.
- **Confusion** is the state of altered consciousness in which the subject is bewildered and misinterprets his or her surroundings.
- **Sleep** is the state of *normal* mental and physical inactivity from which the subject can be roused.
- **Stupor** is an *abnormal*, sleepy state from which the subject can be aroused by stimuli, applied vigorously or repeatedly. The term is also used to describe various psychiatric states, e.g. catatonic and depressive stupor (p. 1261).
- **Delirium** is a state of high arousal (seen typically in *delirium tremens*, p. 1257) in which there is confusion and often visual hallucination.
- **Coma** is a state of unrousable unresponsiveness. The Glasgow Coma Scale for grading coma, particularly in head injury, is shown in Table 20.22.

Mechanisms of coma

Altered consciousness is produced by three mechanisms affecting brainstem, reticular formation and cerebral cortex.

Table 20.22
Glasgow Coma Scale

	Score		Score
Eye opening (E)		**Verbal response (V)**	
Spontaneous	4	Orientated	5
To speech	3	Confused conversation	4
To pain	2	Inappropriate words	3
No response	1	Incomprehensible sounds	2
		No response	1
Motor response (M)			
Obeys	6		
Localizes	5		
Withdraws	4		
Flexion	3		
Extension	2		
No response	1		

Glasgow Coma Scale = $E + M + V$
(GCS minimum = 3: maximum = 15)

- *Diffuse brain dysfunction.* Generalized severe metabolic or toxic disorders (e.g. alcohol abuse, sedative drugs, uraemia and septicaemia) depress/inhibit overall brain function.
- *Direct effect within the brainstem.* A lesion within the brainstem itself damages/inhibits the reticular activating system.
- *Pressure effect on the brainstem.* A mass lesion within the cerebral hemisphere or cerebellum compresses the brainstem, inhibiting the ascending reticular activating system.

A single focal hemisphere (or cerebellar) lesion does not produce coma unless it compresses or damages the brainstem. Oedema frequently surrounds a mass lesion, contributing to its effects.

Other states of unresponsiveness must be distinguished from coma; this sometimes causes difficulty. The features of these are shown in Table 20.23 and illustrated in Figure 20.18.

Persistent vegetative state and locked-in syndrome

- *The persistent vegetative state* (PVS) is a sequel of, for example, widespread cortical damage after head injury. It implies loss of sentient behaviour. The patient perceives little or nothing but lies apparently awake, breathing spontaneously. The brainstem is normal.
- *The locked-in syndrome* is a state of unresponsiveness due to massive brainstem damage below the level of the third nerve nuclei. The patient has a functioning cerebral cortex and is thus unlike a PVS patient, fully aware but cannot move or communicate except by vertical eye movement.
- *Brainstem death* is discussed on page 955.

Distinction between these states is essential before major issues regarding prognosis, quality of life, and cessation of supportive care can be addressed.

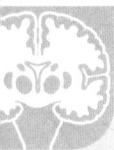

Table 20.23
Differentiation of forms of unresponsiveness

Condition	Vegetative state	Locked-in syndrome	Coma	Brainstem death
Self-awareness	Absent	Present	Absent	Absent
Cyclical eye opening	Present	Present	Absent	Absent
Glasgow Coma Scale	E4, M1–4, V1	E4, M1, V1	E1–2, M1–4, V1–2	E1, M1–2, V1
Motor function	No purposeful movement	Eye movement preserved in the vertical plane and able to blink volitionally	No purposeful movement	None or only reflex spinal movement
Pain perception	No/little	Yes	No/little	No
Respiration function	Normal	Normal	Depressed or varied	Absent
EEG activity	Delta theta; or slow alpha	Usually normal	Delta or theta, sometimes silent	Electrocerebral silence or theta
Cerebral metabolism	Reduced by 50% or more	Minimally or moderately reduced	Reduced by 50% or more	Greatly reduced or absent
Prognosis	Depends on cause and length	Depends on cause; recovery unlikely	Recovery, vegetative state, or death within 2–4 weeks	No recovery

Modified from Working Group of Royal College of Physicians (1996) The permanent vegetative state. *Journal of the Royal College of Physicians of London* **30**: 119–121.

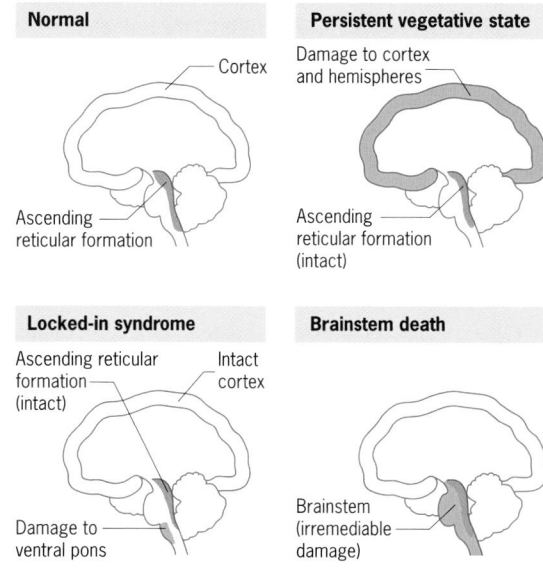

Fig. 20.18 Basic anatomy of altered consciousness.
Adapted from Bates D Coma and brain stem death *Medicine* 2000;
28:7: 65–70 with kind permission of the Medicine Publishing Company.

Unresponsiveness of psychological origin is also a cause of apparent coma. In this vestibulo-ocular reflexes remain intact (p. 000).

Causes

The principal causes of coma and stupor are shown in Table 20.24. A common cause of coma in the UK is self-poisoning. World-wide, in malarial zones, or in travellers from them, cerebral malaria is a frequent cause.

Table 20.24

Examples of mechanisms of principal causes of coma

Diffuse brain dysfunction

Drug overdose, alcohol abuse
CO poisoning, anaesthetic gases
Hypoglycaemia, hyperglycaemia
Hypoxic/ischaemic brain injury
Hypertensive encephalopathy (p. 1167)
Severe uraemia (p. 647)
Hepatocellular failure (p. 372)
Respiratory failure with CO_2 retention (p. 865)
Hypercalcaemia, hypocalcaemia
Hypoadrenalism, hypopituitarism and hypothyroidism (Ch. 18)
Hyponatraemia, hypernatraemia
Metabolic acidosis
Hypothermia, hyperpyrexia
Trauma (following closed head injury)
Epilepsy (following a generalized seizure)
Encephalitis, cerebral malaria, septicaemia
Subarachnoid haemorrhage
Metabolic rarities (e.g. porphyria)
Cerebral oedema from chronic hypoxia (p. 945)

Direct effect within brainstem

Brainstem haemorrhage or infarction
Brainstem neoplasm (e.g. glioma)
Brainstem demyelination
Wernicke-Korsakoff syndrome
Trauma

Pressure effect on brainstem

Hemisphere tumour, infarction, abscess, haematoma, encephalitis or trauma
Cerebellar mass lesions

The unconscious patient

Immediate assessment

Actions which take seconds are essential (see Table 20.25).

A history should be gleaned from relatives, friends, paramedics or police. Many people with diabetes mellitus, epilepsy or hypoadrenalism, or who take corticosteroids, carry identification.

Further examination

- The depth of coma should be assessed and recorded (Table 20.22).
- A full general and neurological examination should be carried out.

General examination

Many clues to the cause of coma become evident.

Temperature

Body temperature is raised in infection and hyperpyrexia, and subnormal in hypothermia. Measure it!

Skin

Look for cyanosis, jaundice, purpura, rashes, pigmentation, injection marks, and trauma.

Skin texture and hydration

The skin is coarse and dry in hypothyroidism.

Breath

Sniff the breath for ketones, alcohol, hepatic and uraemic fetor.

Respiration

Depressed but regular respiration occurs in many states of stupor and light coma. As any coma deepens, or in normal deep sleep, there are pauses in regular respiration. Some patterns of abnormal respiration are of diagnostic importance:

- *Cheyne–Stokes respiration* (periodic respiration) is alternating hyperpnoea and apnoea. In primary neurological disease this points to bilateral cerebral dysfunction, usually deep in the hemispheres or in the upper brainstem, and is a sign of incipient coning. This respiratory pattern also occurs in metabolic comas, if there is CO_2 retention from pulmonary disease, with chronic hypoxia at high altitude above 3500 m and in normal people during sleep.
- *Kussmaul (acidotic) respiration* is deep, sighing hyperventilation seen principally in diabetic ketoacidosis and uraemia.
- *Central neurogenic (pontine) hyperventilation* describes sustained, rapid, deep breathing seen with pontine lesions. It may be episodic, i.e. switch abruptly on and off.

Table 20.25
The unconscious patient: immediate actions

Examine	Findings	Potential action
Airway	Clear?	Maintain; intubate?
Pulse	Absent?	Cardiopulmonary resuscitation
Pupils	Fixed, dilated?	
Head	Trauma	Observe and investigate
Spinal	Trauma	Immobilize

- *Ataxic respiration* is shallow, halting, irregular respiration that occurs when the medullary respiratory centre is damaged. It frequently precedes death.
- *Vomiting, hiccup and excessive yawning* often indicate a lower brainstem lesion in a stuporose patient.

Neurological examination in coma

Head, neck and spine

Note trauma, skull burr-holes, cranial bruits, neck stiffness.

Pupils

Record size and reaction to light. The following patterns are seen:

- *Dilatation of one pupil*, which becomes fixed to light, indicates herniation of the uncus of the temporal lobe (coning) which compresses the third nerve. This is a neurosurgical emergency (possibly subdural/extradural haematoma).
- *Horner's syndrome* (ipsilateral pupillary constriction and ptosis, p. 1133) occurs with lesions of the hypothalamus and also, rarely, in coning.
- *Bilateral mid-point reactive pupils* (i.e. normal pupils) are characteristic in metabolic comas and following most CNS-depressant drugs except opiates.
- *Bilateral light-fixed, dilated pupils* are a cardinal sign of brainstem death. They also occur in deep coma of any cause, but particularly in coma due to barbiturate intoxication or hypothermia.
- *Bilateral pinpoint*, light-fixed pupils occur with pontine lesions (e.g. a pontine haemorrhage) that interrupt sympathetic pathways, and with opiate drugs.
- *Bilateral mid-position light-fixed or slightly dilated light-fixed pupils* (4–6 mm), which are sometimes irregular, are seen when brainstem damage interrupts the light reflex.

Mydriatic drugs administered in coma can confuse diagnosis. Other pupillary changes due to drugs are mentioned on page 975. Previous pupillary surgery can also sometimes cause diagnostic difficulty.

Fundi

Look for papilloedema and retinal haemorrhage.

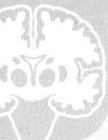

Ocular movements

The ocular axes are usually slightly divergent in coma. Slow, roving, side-to-side eye movements are seen in light coma.

Vestibulo-ocular reflexes. Passive head turning produces conjugate ocular deviation away from the direction of induced head rotation (doll's head reflex). This reflex is lost in very deep coma and is absent in brainstem lesions, and thus in brainstem death. Its practical value in coma is somewhat limited.

Calorics. Slow tonic ocular deviation towards the irrigated ear is seen when ice-cold water is run into the external auditory meatus; this is the caloric or vestibulo-ocular reflex and indicates an intact brainstem. In coma, this test is used mainly in the diagnosis of brainstem death (p. 954).

Abnormalities of conjugate gaze (see also p. 1135).

- *Sustained conjugate lateral deviation* occurs towards the side of a destructive frontal lesion (the eyes look towards the normal limbs). Rarely, an irritative lesion in one frontal region (e.g. an epileptic focus from a glioma) drives the eyes away from the affected side, so conjugate deviation is away from the side of the lesion. In a pontine, brainstem lesion, when one paramedian pontine reticular formulation (PPRF) itself is damaged (p. 1135), sustained conjugate lateral deviation occurs away from the side of the lesion, towards the paralysed limbs, because the opposite PPRF is active.
- *Skew deviation* (one eye deviated up and the other down) indicates a brainstem or cerebellar lesion.
- *Ocular bobbing* describes sudden, brisk, downward-diving eye movements seen in pontine (or cerebellar) haemorrhage.

Other spontaneous eye movements (other than roving eye movements) are distinctly unusual in coma of any cause.

Lateralizing signs. Coma makes it difficult to recognize focal neurological signs. The following are helpful and indicate the side of a lesion:

- *Response to visual threat* in a stuporose patient. Asymmetry suggests hemianopia.
- *Facial appearance.* Drooping of one side, unilateral dribbling, or blowing in and out of the paralysed cheek.
- *Tone.* Unilateral flaccidity or spasticity may be the only sign of hemiparesis.
- *Asymmetrical response to painful stimuli.*
- *Asymmetry of plantar responses.* Both are often extensor in deep coma of any cause.
- *Asymmetry of tendon reflexes.*
- *Asymmetry of decerebrate and decorticate posturing.*

Investigations

In many instances the explanation for coma becomes evident (e.g. head injury, cerebral haemorrhage, self-poisoning). If the cause remains unclear, further investigations are needed.

Blood and urine

- *Drugs screen* (e.g. salicylates, diazepam, narcotics, amfetamines)
- *Routine biochemistry* (urea, electrolytes, glucose, calcium, liver biochemistry)
- *Metabolic and endocrine studies* (TSH, serum cortisol)
- *Blood cultures*
- *Rarities*, such as cerebral malaria (thick blood film) or porphyria, are often forgotten.

Imaging

CT or MR brain imaging may indicate an otherwise unsuspected mass lesion or intracranial haemorrhage.

CSF examination

Lumbar puncture should be performed in coma only after careful risk assessment. It is usually contraindicated when an intracranial mass lesion is a possibility. CT is necessary to exclude this. CSF examination is likely to alter therapy only if undiagnosed meningoencephalitis or other identifiable infection is present.

Electrophysiological tests

EEG is of some value in the diagnosis of metabolic coma, and encephalitis.

Management

Comatose or stuporose patients – be they in ITU, on a general ward, on a trolley in A&E, at home or at the roadside – need immediate careful nursing, meticulous attention to the airway, and frequent monitoring of vital functions.

Longer-term requirements are:

- skin care – turning, removal of jewellery, avoidance of pressure sores and pressure palsies
- oral hygiene – mouth washes, suction
- eye care – taping of lids, prevention of corneal damage, irrigation
- fluids – intragastric or i.v. fluids
- calories – liquid diet through a fine intragastric tube, 1255 kJ (3000 kcal) daily
- sphincters – catheterization only when essential (Paul's tubing if possible); avoid constipation (evacuate rectum).

FURTHER READING

Posner MJ (1994) Attention: the mechanisms of consciousness. *Proceedings of the National Academy of Sciences USA* **91**: 7398–7403.

The permanent vegetative state (1996) Review. *Journal of the Royal College of Physicians* **30**: 119–121.

Cerebrovascular disease and stroke

Stroke is the third most common cause of death in developed countries. The age-adjusted annual death rate from strokes is 116 per 100 000 population in the USA and some 200 per 100 000 in the UK, some 12% of all deaths; it is higher in black African populations than in Caucasian. Stroke is uncommon below the age of 40 years and is more common in males. The death rate following a stroke is around 25%. Hypertension is the most important treatable risk factor. Stroke is decreasing in the 40–60 age range as hypertension is treated; however, in the elderly, it remains a major cause of morbidity and mortality.

Cerebrovascular disease comprises:

- thromboembolic infarction (80%)
- cerebral and cerebellar haemorrhage (10%)
- subarachnoid haemorrhage (about 5%)
- dissection of carotid and vertebral vessels (<3%)
- cortical venous and dural venous sinus thrombosis (<1%)
- subdural and extradural haemorrhage/haematoma.

The latter are usually regarded as surgical issues but can cause diagnostic difficulty.

Definitions

These, though valuable clinically, are arbitrary:

- **Stroke.** To the general public, stroke means a weakness, either permanent or transient on one side, often with loss of speech. It is *defined* as a focal neurological deficit due to a vascular lesion lasting longer than 24 hours. Onset is usually rapid. Hemiplegia following middle cerebral arterial thromboembolism is the typical example.
- **Completed stroke** means the deficit has become maximal, usually within 6 hours.
- **Stroke-in-evolution** describes progression during the first 24 hours.
- **Minor stroke.** Patients recover without significant deficit, usually within a week.
- **Transient ischaemic attack** (TIA). This means a focal deficit, such as a weak limb, aphasia or loss of vision, lasting from a few seconds to 24 hours. There is complete clinical recovery. The attack is usually of sudden onset. TIAs have a tendency to recur, and to herald thromboembolic stroke.

The vague term 'cerebrovascular accident' should be avoided.

Pathophysiology

Different pathological processes may cause similar clinical events in cerebrovascular disease.

Completed stroke

One of four mechanisms is the usual cause:

- arterial embolism from a distant site and subsequent brain infarction
- atheromatous carotid or vertebral artery occlusion and subsequent brain infarction
- atheromatous arterial thrombosis within a cerebral vessel and subsequent brain infarction
- haemorrhage into the brain.

Less commonly, other processes cause stroke, or a similar clinical event:

- venous infarction
- carotid or vertebral artery dissection
- air embolism (and see diving, p. 995) and fat embolism
- multiple sclerosis – a plaque of demyelination
- mass effects of expanding lesions (e.g. brain tumour, abscess, subdural haematoma)
- arteritis, e.g. neurosyphilis, systemic lupus erythematosus.

Transient ischaemic attack (TIA) (p. 1165)

TIAs are *usually* the result of the passage of microemboli, but as in stroke different mechanisms produce similar clinical events. For example, TIAs may be caused by a fall in cerebral perfusion (e.g. because of a cardiac dysrhythmia, postural hypotension or decreased flow through atheromatous carotid and vertebral arteries); infarction is then usually averted by autoregulation (p. 1165). Small areas of brain infarction following thrombosis or haemorrhage may occasionally cause a clinical TIA. Rarely, brain tumours and subdural haematomas cause episodes indistinguishable from thromboembolic TIAs. The clinical TIA is thus not an entirely reliable indicator of the cause.

The principal sources of emboli to the brain are thrombi and atheromatous plaques within the great vessels, the carotid and vertebral systems, or in the heart. Cardiac thrombi (mural and valvular) follow atrial fibrillation, itself often secondary to valvular disease, or myocardial infarction.

Thromboembolism from sources outside the brain generates 70% of all strokes and 80% of TIAs.

Risk factors and primary prevention

There are extreme difficulties of data collection and methodology in apportioning risk factors in stroke. The principal accepted risk factors and the effect of altering them are drawn together in Table 20.26.

In *primary* prevention, the following general measures reduce stroke incidence:

- treatment of hypertension (of vital importance)
- cessation of smoking
- active lifestyle
- moderate alcohol consumption

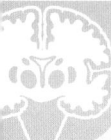

Table 20.26
Reducing stroke risk

Risk factor or intervention	Reduction in stroke risk		
	Cerebral infarction	Cerebral haemorrhage	Subarachnoid haemorrhage
Hypertension: treat	++	++	Possible
Smoking: cessation	++	+	Probable
Lifestyle: more active	+	0	0
Alcohol intake: moderate	+	0	0
Myocardial infarction: statin therapy	+	0	0
Raised haematocrit: reduce	+	0	0
Atrial fibrillation: anticoagulation	+	(Possibly increased risk)	0
Sleep apnoea: treat	0	0	0
Obesity: weight reduction	Probable	Probable	0
Diabetes: good control	Probable	0	0
Postmenopause: HRT	0	0	0

++, major correlation with reduced risk; +, moderate correlation with reduced risk

- reduction of LDL-cholesterol with statins (p. 1111)
- anticoagulation in atrial fibrillation.

Other factors are shown in Table 20.26. Low-dose aspirin in symptomless populations has been advocated but there are still insufficient data. Postmenopausal HRT has so far shown no benefit.

Cerebral and cerebellar haemorrhage
Here particular risk factors are hypertension, anticoagulant and antiplatelet drugs, bleeding disorders, preexisting cerebral aneurysm.

Rarer risk factors and other causes of stroke
- Thrombocythaemia and thrombophilia (protein C deficiency, factor V Leiden) are weakly associated with arterial stroke but predispose to cerebral venous thrombosis.
- Anticardiolipin antibodies causing acquired abnormalities of thrombolysis are associated with arterial thrombotic stroke in younger patients.
- Endocarditis (p. 793) – a thromboembolic stroke may be the presenting feature.
- Low-dose oestrogen-containing oral contraceptives do not increase the risk of stroke significantly in healthy women but probably do so when there are other risk factors, e.g. untreated hypertension or smoking.
- Migraine is a rare cause of cerebral infarction (p. 1202).
- Vasculitis (SLE, polyarteritis nodosa, giant cell arteritis, granulomatous CNS angiitis) are rare causes of stroke.
- Amyloidosis can present as recurrent cerebral haemorrhage (p. 1118).
- Hyperhomocysteinaemia predisposes to thrombotic stroke.

CADASIL (cerebral dominant arteriopathy with subcortical infarcts and leucoencephalopathy) is a rare inherited cause of stroke and vascular dementia. There is a defect in the *NOTCH3* gene on chromosome 19. Characteristic damage to small brain arterioles follows and multiple infarcts are seen on imaging. Familial migraine and depression commencing in youth are associated with CADASIL; typically these progress, with TIA and stroke in the third and fourth decades to dementia and death in the sixth.

Vascular anatomy (Figs 20.19–20.21)
Knowledge of normal arterial anatomy and likely sites of atheromatous plaques and stenoses helps understanding of the main syndromes.

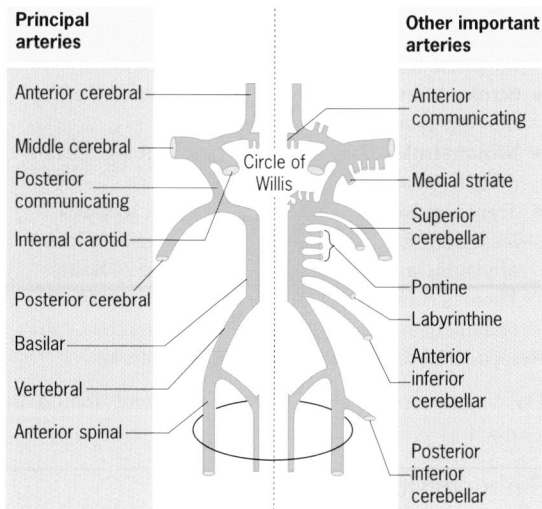

Fig. 20.19 Diagram of arteries supplying the brain.

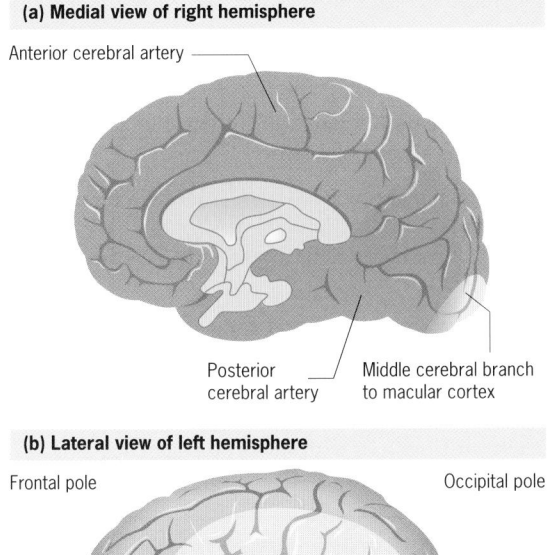

(a) Medial view of right hemisphere

Anterior cerebral artery

Posterior cerebral artery

Middle cerebral branch to macular cortex

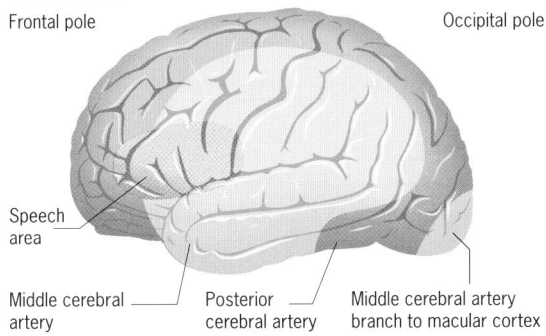

(b) Lateral view of left hemisphere

Frontal pole

Occipital pole

Speech area

Middle cerebral artery

Posterior cerebral artery

Middle cerebral artery branch to macular cortex

Fig. 20.20 Distribution of the three major cerebral arteries.

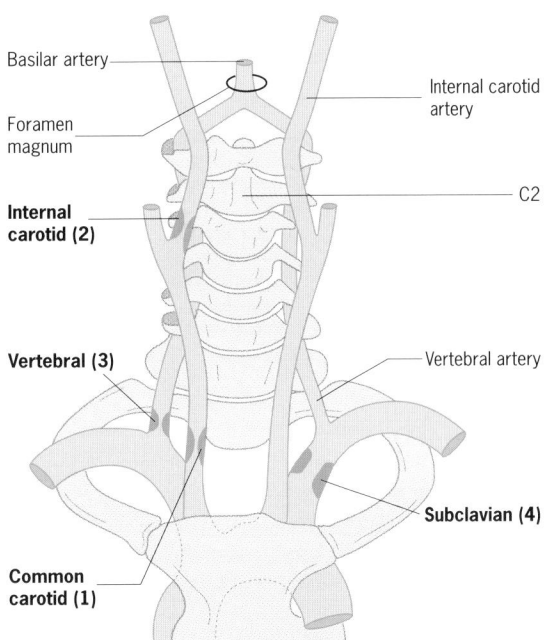

Basilar artery

Foramen magnum

Internal carotid (2)

Vertebral (3)

Common carotid (1)

Internal carotid artery

C2

Vertebral artery

Subclavian (4)

Fig. 20.21 Principal sites of atheromatous stenoses in **extracerebral arteries:** common carotid; internal carotid; vertebral; subclavian.

The circle of Willis is supplied by the two internal carotid arteries and by the basilar artery. The distribution of the anterior, middle and posterior cerebral arteries that supply the cerebrum is shown in Figure 20.20.

Stenoses and plaques proximal to the circle of Willis are common at five sites (positions 1–4 are shown in Fig. 20.21):

- origins of common carotid arteries **(1)**
- origins of internal carotid arteries **(2)**
- carotid artery syphon – within the cavernous sinus
- origins of vertebral arteries **(3)**
- subclavian vessels **(4)**.

Autoregulation

The smooth muscle of small intracerebral arteries responds directly to changes in pressure gradient across the vessel wall. In the normal situation, constant cerebral blood flow (CBF) is maintained by mean arterial blood pressures between 60 and 120 mmHg (i.e. CBF is independent of perfusion pressure).

In disease states, CBF autoregulation may fail. Contributory causes are:

- severe hypotension with systolic BP <75 mmHg
- severe hypertension with systolic BP >180 mmHg

- increase in blood viscosity – polycythaemia
- raised intracranial pressure
- increase in arterial P_{CO_2} and/or fall in arterial P_{O_2}.

Transient ischaemic attacks

Symptoms

TIAs cause sudden loss of function, usually within seconds, and last for minutes or hours (but by definition <24 hours). The site of damage is often suggested by the type of attack.

Features

The clinical features of the principal forms of TIA are given in Table 20.27. Hemiparesis and aphasia are the most common but two other events will be mentioned briefly here.

Amaurosis fugax

This is a sudden transient loss of vision in one eye. When due to the passage of emboli through the retinal arteries, arterial obstruction is sometimes visible through an ophthalmoscope during an attack. A TIA causing an episode of amaurosis fugax is often the first clinical evidence of internal carotid artery stenosis, which may herald a hemiparesis. Amaurosis fugax also occurs as a benign event in migraine.

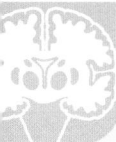

Table 20.27
Features of transient ischaemic attacks

Anterior circulation	Posterior circulation
Carotid system	**Vertebrobasilar system**
Amaurosis fugax	Diplopia, vertigo, vomiting
Aphasia	Choking and dysarthria
Hemiparesis	Ataxia
Hemisensory loss	Hemisensory loss
Hemianopic visual loss	Hemianopic visual loss
	Transient global amnesia
	Tetraparesis
	Loss of consciousness (rare)

Transient global amnesia

Episodes of amnesia lasting for several hours, occurring principally in people over 65, and followed by complete recovery are presumed to be caused by posterior circulation ischaemia. The exact pathology of this striking but unusual event is unknown. Episodes rarely recur.

Clinical findings in TIA

The diagnosis of TIA is often based solely upon its description; it is unusual to witness an attack oneself. Consciousness is usually preserved in TIA.

There may be clinical evidence of a source of embolus, such as:

- carotid arterial bruit (stenosis)
- atrial fibrillation or other dysrhythmia
- valvular heart disease or endocarditis
- recent myocardial infarction
- difference between right and left brachial BP (subclavian stenosis).

An underlying condition may be evident:

- atheroma
- hypertension
- postural hypotension
- bradycardia or low cardiac output
- diabetes mellitus
- rarely, arteritis, polycythaemia
- antiphospholipid syndrome (p. 560).

Differential diagnosis

TIAs must be distinguished, usually on clinical grounds, from other transient episodes (p. 1180). Occasionally, events identical to TIAs are produced by mass lesions of the brain.

Focal epilepsy is distinguished by accompanying irritative phenomena (e.g. limb jerking) and characteristically progression over minutes. In a TIA, deficit is usually apparent immediately. However, involuntary limb movements do occur occasionally in TIAs.

The focal prodrome of migraine, sometimes causes diagnostic confusion. Headache, common but not invariable in migraine, is rare in TIA. Migrainous visual disturbances are not seen in TIA.

Prognosis

Prospective studies have shown that five years after a single thromboembolic TIA:

- 30% of patients will have had a stroke, a third in the first year
- 15% of patients will have suffered a myocardial infarct.

TIA in the anterior cerebral circulation carries a more serious prognosis than one in the posterior circulation.

TIA: investigations and management

These are discussed with stroke on page 1169.

Typical stroke syndromes

Cerebral infarction

Major thromboembolic cerebral infarction usually causes an obvious stroke. Some small infarcts may cause TIAs, while others are silent. The clinical picture is thus very variable and depends on the infarct site and extent. Clinical diagnosis of the precise vascular territory is often inaccurate. Nevertheless, the general site of damage may be deduced from the physical signs (e.g. cortex, internal capsule, brainstem).

Clinical features

The most common stroke is caused by infarction in the internal capsule following thromboembolism in a middle cerebral artery branch. A similar picture is caused by internal carotid occlusion (Fig. 20.21). Limb weakness on the opposite side to the infarct develops over seconds, minutes or hours (occasionally longer). There is a contralateral hemiplegia or hemiparesis. Aphasia is usual when the dominant hemisphere is affected. One side of the face is weak. Weak limbs are at first flaccid and areflexic. Headache is unusual. Consciousness is usually preserved. Exceptionally, an epileptic seizure occurs at the onset of a stroke.

After a variable interval, usually several days, the reflexes return, becoming exaggerated. An extensor plantar response appears. Weakness is maximal at first; recovery gradually over days, weeks or many months can occur.

Brain infarction following carotid or vertebral artery dissection

This accounts for less than one-fifth of strokes below age 40 and is sometimes a sequel of head or neck trauma. Stroke or TIAs occur, often with neck pain at the site of dissection, with migraine-like symptoms.

Brainstem infarction

Infarction in the brainstem causes complex patterns of dysfunction depending on the site of the lesion and its relationship to the cranial nerve nuclei, long tracts and brainstem connections (Table 20.28).

- *The lateral medullary syndrome*, also called posterior inferior cerebellar artery (PICA) thrombosis, or Wallenberg's syndrome, is the most widely recognized syndrome of brainstem infarction. This is caused by PICA or vertebral artery thromboembolism (Fig. 20.22 and Table 20.29).
- *Coma* follows damage to the brainstem reticular activating system.
- *The locked-in syndrome* is caused by upper brainstem infarction (p. 1159).
- *Pseudobulbar palsy* (p. 1143) is caused by lower brainstem infarction.

Other patterns of infarction

Lacunar infarction

Lacunes are small (<1.5 cm³) areas of infarction seen on MRI or at autopsy. Hypertension is commonly present. Minor strokes (e.g. pure motor stroke, pure sensory stroke, sudden unilateral ataxia and sudden dysarthria with a clumsy hand) are syndromes caused typically by single lacunar infarcts. Lacunar infarction is often symptomless.

Hypertensive encephalopathy (see also p. 000)

This describes various neurological sequelae of malignant hypertension with occlusion of small arteries. Severe headaches, TIA, stroke, and rarely subarachnoid haemorrhage occur. Papilloedema may develop, either as part of an ischaemic optic neuropathy or following brain swelling due to multiple acute infarcts.

Multi-infarct dementia (vascular dementia)
(see also p. 1265)

Multiple lacunes or larger infarcts cause the picture of generalized intellectual loss that is seen in patients with advanced cerebrovascular disease. The condition tends to occur with a stepwise progression over months or years with each subsequent infarct. There is dementia, pseudobulbar palsy and a shuffling gait with small steps – the *marche à petits pas*, sometimes called atherosclerotic parkinsonism. There may be confusion clinically with idiopathic Parkinson's disease. *Binswanger's disease* is an imaging term describing low-attenuation areas in cerebral white matter on CT, with dementia, TIAs and stroke episodes in hypertensive patients.

Infarction in the visual cortex

Posterior cerebral artery infarction or infarction of the middle cerebral artery macular branch causes combinations of hemianopic visual loss and cortical blindness (Anton's syndrome, Fig. 20.20).

Weber's syndrome

This is ipsilateral third nerve paralysis with a contralateral hemiplegia due to a lesion in one half of the midbrain. Paralysis of upward gaze is usually present.

Table 20.28
Features of brainstem infarction

Clinical feature	Structure involved
Hemiparesis or tetraparesis	Corticospinal tracts
Sensory loss	Medial lemniscus and spinothalamic tracts
Diplopia	Oculomotor system
Facial numbness	Fifth nerve nuclei
Facial weakness (lower motor neurone)	Seventh nerve nucleus
Nystagmus, vertigo	Vestibular connections
Dysphagia, dysarthria	Ninth and tenth nerve nuclei
Dysarthria, ataxia, hiccups, vomiting	Brainstem and cerebellar connections
Horner's syndrome	Sympathetic fibres
Altered consciousness	Reticular formation

Table 20.29
Clinical signs in the lateral medullary syndrome

Ipsilateral	Contralateral
Facial numbness (Vth)	Spinothalamic sensory loss
Diplopia (VIth)	Hemiparesis (mild, unusual)
Nystagmus	
Ataxia (cerebellar)	
Horner's syndrome	
Ninth and tenth nerve lesions	

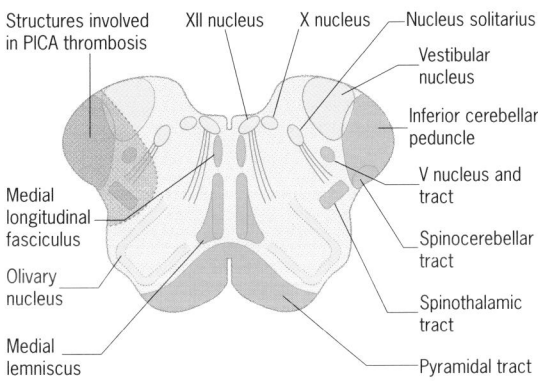

Fig. 20.22 **Cross-section of medulla showing posterior inferior cerebellar artery (PICA) thrombosis (left side).**

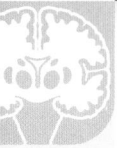

Watershed (or borderzone) cerebral infarction

This describes the multiple cortical infarcts that follow prolonged periods of very low perfusion (e.g. from hypotension after massive myocardial infarction or following cardiac bypass surgery). Borderzones between areas supplied by the anterior, middle and posterior cerebral arteries are damaged. Cortical visual loss, memory loss and intellectual impairment are typical. In severe cases a persistent vegetative state develops (p. 1159).

Management of cerebral infarction

Examination of the airway and of swallowing is essential. The possible sources of embolus should be sought (e.g. carotid bruit, atrial fibrillation, valve lesion, evidence of endocarditis, previous emboli or TIA) and hypertension and postural hypotension assessed. The brachial blood pressure should be measured in each arm; a difference of more than 20 mmHg is suggestive of subclavian artery stenosis. The neurological deficit should be carefully documented.

Stroke: immediate care and thrombolysis

(Box 20.1)

There is broad agreement that dedicated stroke units with multidisciplinary, organized team care deliver a higher standard of care to patients than a general ward,

reducing mortality and long-term disability. National (and international) guidelines have contributed to stroke management by demonstrating the evidence base for this and establishing clear protocols.

After any stroke, immediate, continued and meticulous attention to the airway and to swallowing is essential. The initial decision to admit a stroke patient to hospital depends upon the clinical state and facilities available. Table 20.30 outlines the current guidelines for thrombolysis. Aspirin 300 mg daily should be given as soon as a diagnosis of ischaemic stroke or thromboembolic TIA is confirmed, reducing to 75 mg after several days.

Box 20.1

Stroke: immediate management issues

1. **Admit to multidisciplinary hospital stroke unit if possible.**

2. **General medical measures**
   Care of the unconscious patient (p. 1161)
   Oxygen by mask
   Assessment of swallowing
   Check BP and look for source of emboli.

3. **Is thrombolysis to be considered?**
   If so (see text and Table 20.30) immediate brain imaging is essential.

4. **Brain imaging**
   CT scans will usually be the only emergency imaging available. This will indicate whether there has been brain infarction, haemorrhage or other pathology.

5. **Cerebral infarction**
   If CT shows infarction, give aspirin (300 mg/day initially) antiplatelet therapy if no contraindications, consider alteplase thrombolysis, which must be started within 3 hours of stroke; informed consent is essential.

6. **Cerebral haemorrhage**
   If CT shows haemorrhage, do not give any therapy that may interfere with clotting.
   Neurosurgery may be required.

Table 20.30
Thrombolysis in acute ischaemic stroke

Eligibility

Age ≥18 years
Clinical diagnosis of acute ischaemic stroke
Assessed by experienced team
Measurable neurological deficit
Timing of symptom onset well established
CT or MRI and blood test results available
CT or MRI consistent with diagnosis
Treatment could begin within 180 minutes of symptom onset

Exclusion criteria

Symptoms minor or improving rapidly
Haemorrhage on pretreatment CT or MRI
Suspected subarachnoid haemorrhage
Active bleeding from any site
Gastrointestinal or urinary tract haemorrhage in last 21 days
Platelet count $< 100 \times 10^9$/litre
Recent treatment with heparin and activated partial thromboplastin time above normal
Recent treatment with warfarin and INR elevated
Major surgery or trauma in last 14 days
Recent post-myocardial infarction pericarditis
Neurosurgery, serious head trauma or stroke in last 3 months
History of intracranial haemorrhage (any time)
Known arteriovenous malformation or aneurysm
Recent arterial puncture at non-compressible site
Recent lumbar puncture
Blood pressure consistently >185 systolic or >110 diastolic
Abnormal blood glucose (< 3 mmol/litre or > 20 mmol/litre)
Suspected or known pregnancy
Active pancreatitis
Epileptic seizure at stroke onset

Dose of intravenous tissue plasminogen activator
Total dose 0.9 mg/kg (maximum 90 mg)
10% of total dose as initial intravenous bolus over 1 minute
Remainder infused intravenously over 60 minutes

Source: National Institute of Neurological Disorders and Stroke protocol; from *Medicine* (2000) **28**(7): 62

Management of the unconscious patient is described on page 1161.

Investigations

The purpose of investigations in both stroke and TIA is:

- to confirm clinical diagnosis
- to distinguish between haemorrhage and thromboembolic infarction
- to look for underlying causes of disease and to direct therapy, either medical or surgical.

Routine preliminary investigations in thromboembolic stroke and TIA with their potential yields are listed in Box 20.2. Blood cultures should be taken if there is any possibility of endocarditis. Autoantibody studies, e.g. antinuclear factor (ANF), double-stranded DNA (dsDNA), should be performed in young patients to exclude diseases such as systemic lupus erythematosus (SLE). Detailed clotting studies (anticardiolipin antibodies, protein C, antithrombin, factor V Leiden polymorphism) are indicated in those under 60 with an unexplained TIA or stroke, or with suspected venous thrombosis.

Imaging of TIA and stroke patients

CT and MRI. CT imaging will usually demonstrate the site of a lesion and distinguish immediately between haemorrhage (p. 1171) and infarction; this should be carried out in the majority of cases. Over 90% of all infarcts are detectable at 1 week. MRI is more sensitive in detecting infarction than CT. Imaging will also show unexpected mass lesions, such as subdural haematoma, tumour or abscess.

Carotid Doppler and duplex scanning. Ultrasound studies are of value in screening for arterial stenosis and occlusion: in skilled hands they demonstrate accurately the degree of internal carotid artery stenosis.

Vascular imaging. Magnetic resonance angiography or digital subtraction angiography is valuable in anterior circulation TIAs to confirm surgically accessible arterial stenoses, mainly internal carotid artery stenosis. Most normotensive patients with TIA or stroke in the anterior circulation – who recover well – should have vascular imaging if ultrasound suggests carotid stenosis. Even in more elderly patients, the results of endarterectomy are excellent if cases are selected carefully and internal carotid stenosis is greater than 70%. Vertebral and arch angiography are now rarely performed following posterior circulation TIAs and strokes unless there is a clinical suggestion of subclavian artery disease.

Lumbar puncture. This is indicated only in unusual circumstances, such as when blood syphilitic serology is positive.

Long-term management
Medical therapy

All risk factors (Table 20.26) should be identified and, if possible, treated. For primary prevention, see page 1154.

Antihypertensive therapy

Control of high blood pressure is the single most important factor in primary stroke prevention. The transient hypertension often seen after acute stroke usually does not require treatment with hypotensive drugs provided the diastolic pressure does not remain consistently higher than 100 mmHg. If hypertension is sustained it needs treatment (p. 823), but the pressure must be lowered slowly to avoid a sudden fall in cerebral perfusion pressure.

Antiplatelet therapy (also p. 466)

Long-term soluble aspirin (75 mg daily) reduces substantially the incidence of further infarction after thromboembolic TIA or stroke. Aspirin inhibits cyclo-oxygenase, which converts arachidonic acid to prostaglandins and thromboxanes. The predominant therapeutic effect is to reduce platelet aggregation. Clopidogrel, dipyridamole and ticlopidine are also used (p. 467). The combination of aspirin 75 mg daily and dipyridamole 200 mg twice daily is probably the best combination long term for reduction of further thromboembolic stroke or TIA.

Anticoagulants

Heparin and warfarin should be given when there is atrial fibrillation, other paroxysmal dysrhythmias or when there are certain cardiac valve lesions (uninfected)

Box 20.2

Stroke: further investigation

Further investigation

- Routine bloods (for polycythaemia, infection, vasculitis, thrombophilia, syphilitic serology, clotting studies, autoantibodies, lipids)
- Chest X-ray
- ECG
- Carotid Dopplers
- Angiography

Further management

- Appropriate drugs for hypertension, heart disease, diabetes, other medical conditions
- Other antiplatelet agents, e.g. dipyridamole
- Question of endarterectomy
- Question of anticoagulation – Table 20.31
- Speech therapy, dysphagia care, physiotherapy, occupational therapy
- Specific neurological issues, e.g. epilepsy, pain, incontinence
- Preparations for future care

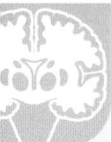
or cardiomyopathies. Brain haemorrhage must be excluded by CT/MRI. All patients on anticoagulants must be aware of the small risks of cerebral (and other) haemorrhage. The drugs are potentially dangerous in the 2 weeks following cerebral infarction because of the risk of provoking cerebral haemorrhage. There are wide differences in clinical practice here. Table 20.31 outlines the issues in secondary stroke prevention.

Other measures
Polycythaemia and clotting abnormalities should be treated if found (p. 466).

Surgical approaches
Internal carotid endarterectomy
This operation is considered in TIA or stroke patients shown to have internal carotid artery stenosis that narrows the arterial lumen by more than 70%. In these patients, successful surgery reduces the risk of further TIA/stroke by approximately 75%. The operation has a mortality around 3%, and a similar risk of stroke. Percutaneous transluminal angioplasty (stenting) is an alternative procedure to direct surgery in specialized units. Endarterectomy is not usually recommended when internal carotid artery stenosis is less than 70%, or an incidental finding in a symptomless patient. Other vascular operations have been popular but none are now commonly performed.

Strokes in the elderly
The yield of investigation in stroke falls with age, and there is a tendency to avoid devoting resources to the rehabilitation of the elderly stroke patient. Age itself is no barrier to recovery and this group of patients probably benefit most from high standards of care. It is particularly important in elderly patients to consider their frequent social isolation, possible pre-existing cognitive impairment, their nutrition, skin and sphincter care, and, repeatedly, reassess the ability to swallow safely. Carotid endarterectomy in patients over 75 years carries little more risk than in younger age groups.

Rehabilitation: physiotherapy and speech therapy
Skilled physiotherapy has particular value in the first few weeks after stroke. It relieves spasticity, prevents contractures and teaches patients to use walking aids. The benefit of physiotherapy for the longer-term outcome is still inadequately researched. Baclofen (a GABA agonist) is sometimes helpful in the management of severe spasticity following stroke.

In aphasia, the trained speech therapist has a vital understanding of the patient's problems and frustration. It is, however, possible that spontaneous return of speech is hastened as much by normal conversation with a relative as by a therapist. If the patient cannot swallow safely without the risk of aspiration, either nasogastric feeding or percutaneous gastrostomy will be needed. Video-fluoroscopy is helpful here.

Both physiotherapy and speech therapy have an undoubted psychological role. Stroke is frequently a devastating event and, particularly when it occurs during working life, radically alters the patient's remaining years. Many become unemployable and lose independence. The financial consequences are usually great. Loss of self-esteem makes secondary depression common.

Following early recovery from stroke, aids and modifications may be necessary at home. For example: stair rails, portable lavatories, bath rails, hoists, sliding boards, wheelchairs, tripods, altering doorways and sleeping arrangements, stair lifts and kitchen modifications.

Table 20.31
Stroke prevention: indications for considering anticoagulants

Indication	Comment
Valvular heart disease	Heparin/warfarin is of clear benefit in chronic rheumatic heart disease, particularly mitral stenosis

Recent MI
    Intracardiac thrombus
    Atrial fibrillation
	Heparin/warfarin should be given if there is evidence of intracardiac thrombus. Anticoagulants long term reduce stroke incidence in atrial fibrillation

Acute internal carotid artery thrombus Acute basilar artery thrombus Internal carotid artery dissection Extracranial vertebral artery dissection	Anticoagulants are reserved for imaging-confirmed cases of arterial thrombosis or dissection. They have not been shown to be beneficial in stroke prevention after thromboembolism from carotid or vertebrobasilar sources
Prothrombic states, e.g. protein C deficiency	Consider anticoagulation in consultation with a haematologist
Recurrent TIAs or stroke on full antiplatelet therapy	If no remediable cause, a trial of anticoagulants may be justified
Cerebral venous thrombosis including sinus thrombosis	Benefits of anticoagulation outweigh risks of haemorrhage

Modified from Brown M (2000) *Medicine* **28**(7): 64

Liaison between a hospital-based neurology community care team, locally based therapists and primary care physician is valuable.

Prognosis

Twenty-five per cent of patients die within 2 years of a stroke. Around 30% of this group die in the first month. This early mortality is lower for thromboembolic infarction (death in under a quarter) than for intracerebral haemorrhage (death in around three-quarters). A poor outcome is likely when there is coma, a defect in conjugate gaze and severe hemiplegia. Many of the complications that lead to early death in stroke, particularly in the elderly, are preventable – for example, aspiration. Coordinated care in a stroke unit reduces these risks.

Recurrent strokes are, however, common (10% in the first year) and many patients die subsequently from myocardial infarction. Of initial stroke survivors, some 30–40% remain alive after 3 years.

Gradual improvement usually follows stroke, although the late residual deficit may be severe. Of those who survive, about one-third return to independent mobility and one-third have serious disability requiring permanent institutional care.

The outlook for recovery of language is variable. If, in general, the patient is intelligible at 3 weeks, the prognosis for fluent speech is good. Many stroke patients are, however, left with word-finding difficulties.

Intracranial haemorrhage

This comprises:

- intracerebral and cerebellar haemorrhage
- subarachnoid haemorrhage
- subdural and extradural haemorrhage/haematoma.

Intracerebral haemorrhage
Aetiology

Intracerebral haemorrhage causes around 10% of strokes. Rupture of microaneurysms (Charcot–Bouchard aneurysms, 0.8–1.0 mm diameter) and degeneration of walls of small deep penetrating arteries are the principal pathology. In this setting haemorrhage is usually massive, often fatal and occurs in chronic hypertension and at well-defined sites – basal ganglia, pons, cerebellum and subcortical white matter.

In normotensive patients, particularly over 60 years *lobar* intracerebral haemorrhage occurs – in the frontal, temporal, parietal or occipital cortex. Cerebral amyloid angiopathy is the underlying cause in some of these cases; the tendency to rebleed may be associated with particular apolipoprotein E genotypes.

Recognition

At the bedside, there is no entirely reliable way of distinguishing between intracerebral haemorrhage and thromboembolic infarction. Both produce stroke.

Intracerebral haemorrhage, however, tends to be dramatic with severe headache. It is more likely to lead to coma than thromboembolic stroke.

Intracerebral haemorrhage is seen on CT imaging almost immediately (cf. infarction, p. 1169) as intracerebral, intraventricular, or subarachnoid blood.

Management

The principles of management for haemorrhagic stroke are those for cerebral infarction. The immediate prognosis is less good. Urgent neurosurgical clot evacuation is considered when an intracerebral haematoma expands, causing deepening coma and coning (occasionally in lobar haemorrhage but particularly in cerebellar haemorrhage, see below). The outlook in this situation is usually poor. Antiplatelet drugs and, of course, anticoagulants are contraindicated. Control of hypertension is vital.

Cerebellar haemorrhage

There is headache and rapid reduction of consciousness with signs of brainstem origin (e.g. nystagmus, ocular palsies). The gaze deviates to the side of the haemorrhage. Skew deviation (p. 1147) may be present. There are unilateral or bilateral cerebellar signs, if the patient is awake. Cerebellar haemorrhage can cause acute hydrocephalus. Emergency surgical evacuation of the clot is usually necessary.

Subarachnoid haemorrhage

Subarachnoid haemorrhage (SAH) describes spontaneous rather than traumatic arterial bleeding into the subarachnoid space, and is usually clearly recognizable clinically by its dramatic onset. SAH accounts for some 5% of strokes and has an annual incidence of 6 per 100 000.

Causes

The causes of SAH are shown in Table 20.32. It is unusual to find any contributing disease.

Table 20.32
Underlying causes of subarachnoid haemorrhage

Saccular ('berry') aneurysms	70%
Arteriovenous malformation (AVM)	10%
No lesion found	20%

Rare associations
Bleeding disorders
Mycotic aneurysms (endocarditis)
Acute bacterial meningitis
Brain tumours (e.g. metastatic melanoma)
Arteritis (e.g. systemic lupus erythematosus)
Spinal AVM (spinal haemorrhage only)
Coarctation of the aorta
Marfan's syndrome, Ehlers–Danlos syndrome
Polycystic kidneys

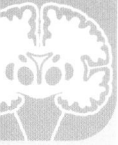

Saccular (berry) aneurysms (Fig. 20.15, p. 1155)

Saccular aneurysms develop during life on the circle of Willis and adjacent arteries. Common sites are at the following arterial junctions:

- between the posterior communicating artery and the internal carotid artery – posterior communicating artery aneurysm
- between the anterior communicating artery and anterior cerebral artery – anterior communicating artery aneurysm
- at a bifurcation or at the trifurcation of the middle cerebral artery – middle cerebral artery aneurysm.

Other aneurysm sites are on the basilar, posterior inferior cerebellar, intracavernous internal carotid and ophthalmic arteries. Saccular aneurysms are an incidental finding in 1% of autopsies and can be multiple.

Aneurysms cause symptoms either by spontaneous rupture, when there is usually no preceding history, or by direct pressure on surrounding structures; for example, an enlarging unruptured posterior communicating artery aneurysm is the commonest cause of a painful third nerve palsy (p. 1136).

Arteriovenous malformation (AVM)

This is a collection of arteries and veins of developmental origin, usually within the hemisphere. An AVM may also cause epilepsy, often focal. Once an AVM has ruptured the tendency is to rebleed at a rate of 10% per year.

Cavernous haemangiomas ('cavernomas') are common (<0.5% of population) and consist of collections of capillary vessels; they are frequently symptomless. Cavernomas sometimes have a genetic basis, with linkage to two loci on chromosome 7q. Rarely cavernomas cause seizures or bleed; exceptionally they are a cause of sudden death from massive haemorrhage. Surgery for cavernomas is rarely appropriate.

Clinical features of SAH

The onset of SAH of any cause is a sudden devastating headache, often occipital. This is usually followed by vomiting and often by loss of consciousness. The patient remains comatose or drowsy for several hours to several days. Less severe headaches cause diagnostic difficulties (p. 1124), but SAH is a possible diagnosis in any sudden headache.

On examination, following major SAH there is neck stiffness and a positive Kernig's sign. Papilloedema is sometimes present and accompanied by retinal haemorrhages and subhyaloid haemorrhage (massive retinal haemorrhage tracking beneath the hyaloid membrane). Minor bleeds cause few physical signs, but almost invariably cause headache.

Investigations

CT imaging is the initial investigation of choice. Subarachnoid or intraventricular blood is usually seen. Lumbar puncture is not necessary if SAH is confirmed by CT, but should be considered if doubt remains. The CSF becomes yellow (xanthochromic) several hours after SAH.

MR angiography is usually performed in all potentially fit for surgery, i.e. generally in those who are below 65 years and not in coma, to establish the cause and site of the bleeding.

Differential diagnosis

SAH must be differentiated from severe migraine. This is sometimes difficult. *Thunderclap headache* is a term used variously to describe either the onset of SAH, or a sudden headache, without obvious migrainous features for which no cause is ever found. The onset of acute bacterial meningitis occasionally causes a very abrupt headache, when a meningeal microabscess ruptures. Subarachnoid bleeding also occasionally occurs at the onset of acute bacterial meningitis.

Complications

Blood in the subarachnoid space can lead to obstruction of CSF flow and hydrocephalus. This can be asymptomatic but is a cause of deteriorating conscious level the days or weeks after SAH. Diagnosis is by CT. Shunting may be required.

Severe arterial spasm (visible on cerebral angiography and a cause of coma or stroke) sometimes complicates SAH. It is a poor prognostic sign.

Management

All surviving SAH cases should be discussed urgently with a specialist centre for a decision about angiography and possible surgery. Nearly half the cases of SAH are either dead or moribund before they reach hospital. Of the remainder, a further 10–20% die in the early weeks in hospital from rebleeding. Delay in diagnosis of minor SAH without coma (or mistaking the sudden headache for migraine) contributes to this mortality.

Patients who remain comatose or with persistent severe deficits have a poor prognosis. In others, where angiography demonstrates aneurysm, a direct neurosurgical approach to clip the neck of the aneurysm is carried out. In selected cases the results of surgery are excellent. Invasive radiological techniques, such as inserting a fine wire coil into an aneurysm are also used. Direct surgery, microembolism and focal radiotherapy ('gamma knife') are used in AVM.

The immediate treatment of patients with SAH is bed rest and supportive measures. Hypertension should be controlled. Dexametasone is often prescribed, to reduce cerebral oedema; it also is believed to stabilize the blood–brain barrier. Nimodipine, a calcium-channel blocking agent, has been shown to reduce mortality.

Subdural and extradural haemorrhage and haematoma

These cause death after head injury unless treated promptly.

Subdural haematoma (SDH) (Fig. 20.15, p. 1155)

SDH means accumulation of blood in the subdural space following rupture of a vein. It is almost always due to head injury, which may be trivial. The interval between injury and symptoms may be days, weeks or months. Chronic, and unsuspected SDH is common in the elderly and in patients with alcohol abuse.

Headache, drowsiness and confusion are common; the symptoms are indolent and often fluctuate. Focal deficits such as hemiparesis or sensory loss develop. Epilepsy occasionally occurs. Stupor and coma gradually ensue.

Extradural haemorrhage

This follows a linear skull vault fracture tearing a branch of the middle meningeal artery. Blood accumulates rapidly over minutes or hours in the extradural space. The most characteristic picture is of a head injury with a brief duration of unconsciousness followed by a lucid interval of recovery. The patient then develops a progressive hemiparesis and stupor, and rapid transtentorial coning, with first an ipsilateral dilated pupil, followed by bilateral fixed dilated pupils, tetraplegia and respiratory arrest. An acute *sub*dural haemorrhage presents in a similar way.

Management

Suspected extradural or subdural haemorrhage needs immediate imaging.

Extradural bleeding requires urgent neurosurgery. If performed early, the outlook is excellent. When far from specialist neurosurgical help (e.g. in wartime or at sea), surgical drainage through a skull burr-hole has been lifesaving when an extradural has been diagnosed on clinical grounds alone.

Subdural bleeding tends to cease spontaneously, and allows more conservative management, sometimes without surgery. Even large subdural collections resolve. Progress can be assessed with serial imaging. Close liaison with a neurosurgeon is essential.

Cortical venous thrombosis and dural venous sinus thrombosis

Intracranial venous thromboses are unusual complications of skull and paranasal (air) sinus infection, dehydration or severe intercurrent illness. When they arise apparently *de novo*, there is an association with pregnancy and hormonal contraceptive agents, the antiphospholipid syndrome (p. 560) and other thrombophilic states.

Cortical venous thrombosis

The venous infarct caused by the thrombosis leads to headache, focal signs (e.g. hemiparesis) and/or epilepsy. There is often a fever.

Dural venous sinus thromboses

Cavernous sinus thrombosis causes ocular pain, fever, proptosis and chemosis. An external and internal ophthalmoplegia with papilloedema develop.

Sagittal and lateral sinus thrombosis cause raised intracranial pressure with headache, fever, papilloedema and often epilepsy.

Management

MRI, MRA and the venous phase of angiography show occluded sinus or veins. Treatment is with antibiotics, anticonvulsants and anticoagulants.

FURTHER READING

Alberts M (1999) Diagnosis and treatment of ischemic stroke. *American Journal of Medicine* **106**: 211–221.

Bath PMW, Lees KR (2000) ABC of arterial and venous disease: acute stroke. *British Medical Journal* **320**: 920–923.

Bath PMW, Lees KR, Naylor AR (2000) ABC of arterial and venous disease: secondary prevention of TIA and stroke. *British Medical Journal* **320**: 991–995.

Brown MM (2000) Stroke. *British Medical Bulletin* **56**

Rudd AG, Wade D, Irwin P (2000) The national clinical guidelines for stroke. *Journal of the Royal College of Physicians of London* **34**: 131–133.

Sacco R (2000) Lobar intracerebral haemorrhage. *New England Journal of Medicine* **342**: 276–279.

Van Gijn J (2000) Cerebral venous thrombosis. *Journal of the Royal Society of Medicine* **93**: 230–233.

Epilepsy and causes of loss of consciousness

Epilepsy

A seizure is a convulsion or transient abnormal event resulting from a paroxysmal discharge of cerebral neurones. Epilepsy is the continuing tendency to have such seizures, even if a long interval separates attacks. A generalized convulsion (i.e. a grand mal fit) is the most common recognized event. Epilepsy is common. Over 2% of the population have two or more seizures during their lives and in 0.5% epilepsy is an active problem. In a typical UK general practice the incidence is 46/100 000/year; approximately 65 people suffer their first seizure each day. Often no clear cause is found for seizures with onset in adult life: sometimes (though unusually) epilepsy is caused by a brain tumour or follows a stroke. Around 250 000 people take anticonvulsant drugs, the mainstay of treatment. Neurosurgery (temporal lobectomy) is also valuable in selected cases.

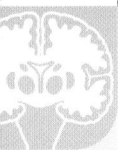

Mechanisms

Spread of electrical activity between cortical neurones is normally restricted. Synchronous discharge of neurones in normal brain takes place in restricted groups whose limited discharges are responsible for the normal EEG rhythms. During a seizure, large groups of neurones are activated repetitively and hypersynchronously. There is failure of inhibitory synaptic contact between neurones. This causes EEG high-voltage spike-and-wave activity, the electrophysiological hallmark of epilepsy.

A partial seizure is epileptic activity confined to one area of cortex with a recognizable clinical pattern (Fig. 20.23). This activity either remains *focal* or spreads to generate epileptic activity in both hemispheres – and thus a *generalized* seizure. This spread is called *secondary* generalization of the partial seizure. The focal onset of a seizure may not be clinically evident; this means that an *apparent* tonic–clonic seizure may be either a generalized major convulsion or a tonic–clonic seizure which began as a partial seizure but without clinical evidence of its focal origin.

An area of brain is or becomes epileptogenic either because neurones have a predisposition to be hyperexcitable, for example following abnormal migration patterns *in utero*, or because they acquire this tendency. Trauma or brain neoplasms are examples of acquired conditions that alter the seizure threshold of neurones.

Seizure threshold

Each individual has a threshold for seizure activity. Experimentally some chemicals (e.g. pentylenetetrazol, a toxic gas) induce seizures in all subjects. Individuals who are more likely to have seizures in response to various stimuli, for example flashing lights, are said to have low seizure thresholds. This is a concept, not a measurement.

Classification

There are various classifications of epilepsy: these confuse the issue. Seizures are classified here by clinical pattern (Table 20.33).

- *Generalized* implies abnormal electrical activity that is bilateral in the brain with bilateral motor manifestations. Consciousness is impaired.
- *A partial seizure* describes a localized seizure without loss of awareness.
  - simple – without loss of consciousness
  - complex – with loss of awareness
- *Unclassifiable seizure*.

Generalized seizure types

Tonic–clonic seizures (grand mal seizures, generalized major convulsions)

Following a vague warning, the tonic phase commences. The body becomes rigid, for up to a minute. The patient utters a cry and falls, sometimes suffering serious injury. The tongue is usually bitten. There may be incontinence of urine or faeces.

The clonic phase then begins, a generalized convulsion, with frothing at the mouth and rhythmic jerking of muscles. This lasts from a few seconds to several minutes. Seizures are usually self-limiting, followed by drowsiness, confusion or coma for several hours.

Table 20.33
The commoner types of epilepsy
Abridged from International League against Epilepsy

1. Generalized seizure types
  A Absence seizures
    (a) Typical absences with 3 Hz spike-and-wave discharge (*petit mal*)
    (b) Atypical absences with other EEG changes
  B Myoclonic seizures
  C Tonic–clonic seizures (*grand mal*, major convulsion)
  D Tonic seizures
  E Akinetic seizures

2. Partial seizure types
These start by activation of a group of neurones in one part of one hemisphere. They are also called 'focal seizures'

  A Simple partial seizures (no impairment of consciousness) (e.g. Jacksonian seizures)
  B Complex partial seizures (impairment of consciousness)
  C Partial seizures evolving to tonic–clonic seizures
  D Apparent generalized tonic–clonic seizures, with EEG but not clinical evidence of focal onset

3. Unclassifiable seizures
Seizures which do not fit in one of the above categories

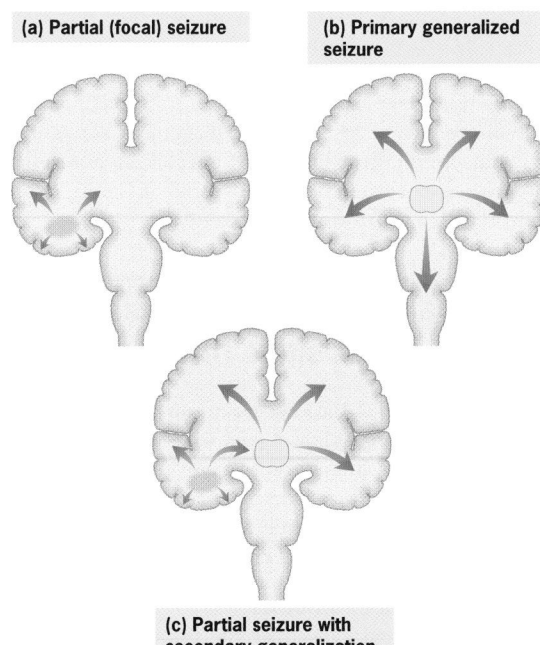

Fig. 20.23 Seizure types. (a) Partial (focal) seizure. **(b)** Primary generalized seizure. **(c)** Partial seizure with secondary generalization.

(a) Partial (focal) seizure

(b) Primary generalized seizure

(c) Partial seizure with secondary generalization

Typical absences (petit mal)

This generalized epilepsy almost invariably begins in childhood. Each attack is accompanied by 3 Hz spike-and-wave EEG activity (Fig. 20.16, p. 1157). Activity ceases, the patient stares and pales slightly for a few seconds. The eyelids twitch; a few muscle jerks may occur. After an attack, normal activity is resumed. Typical absence attacks are never due to acquired lesions such as tumours. They are a developmental abnormality of neuronal control. Children with typical absence attacks tend to develop generalized tonic–clonic seizures in adult life (known as *primary generalized epilepsy*). *Petit mal* describes only these 3 Hz absence seizures. Clinically similar absence attacks are also caused by partial seizures of temporal lobe origin, a source of some confusion.

Other generalized seizure types

Myoclonic seizures describe isolated muscle jerking. *Tonic* seizures describe intense stiffening of the body not followed by convulsive jerking. *Atonic* seizures cause sudden loss of tone, with falling and loss of consciousness.

Partial seizure types

Partial seizures (focal seizures)

A partial or focal seizure (simple or complex, see above) implies that an area of brain (e.g. a temporal lobe) has generated abnormal electrical activity that may spread. The seizure frequently has clinical features that provide evidence of its site.

An *aura* describes effects of initial focal electrical events, such as an unusual smell, tingling in a limb or a strange inner feeling often recognized by the patient as a warning of an impending seizure.

Jacksonian, or focal motor seizures

These simple partial seizures originate in the motor cortex. Jerking movements typically begin at the angle of the mouth or in the thumb and index finger, spreading to involve the limbs on the side opposite the epileptic focus. The clinical evidence of this spread of activity is called the *march* of the seizure. With a frontal lesion, conjugate gaze (p. 1135) deviates away from the irritative epileptic focus. This is called an adversive seizure. Weakness of the convulsing limbs for several hours sometimes follows a seizure – a *Todd's paralysis*.

Temporal lobe seizures

These partial seizures, either simple or complex, describe feelings of unreality (*jamais vu*) or undue familiarity (*déjà vu*) with the surroundings. Absence attacks, vertigo, visual hallucinations (i.e. visions or faces) are other examples of temporal lobe seizures.

Many other types of partial seizure occur, such as autonomic disturbances with piloerection, flushing, and overbreathing, strange smells (frontal cortex), sensory disturbances (parietal cortex), crude visual shapes (occipital cortex), or strange sounds (auditory cortex).

Table 20.34
Aetiological and precipitating factors in epilepsy

Genetic predisposition
Developmental, e.g. hamartomas, neuronal migration abnormalities
Trauma and surgery
Pyrexia
Intracranial mass lesions
Vascular, e.g. cerebral infarction, arteriovenous malformation
Drugs and drug withdrawal
Encephalitis and inflammatory conditions
Metabolic abnormalities, e.g. porphyria, hypocalcaemia
Neural degenerative disorders
Provoked seizures, e.g. photosensitivity, sleep deprivation

Aetiology and precipitants (Table 20.34)

A definite cause for epilepsy is found in under a third of cases in UK community surveys: cerebrovascular disease accounts for some 15%, cerebral tumours for 6%, alcohol-related seizures for 6% and post-traumatic epilepsy 2%. Rarer causes are hippocampal sclerosis (resection may be possible), malformations of cortical development, vascular malformations, hamartomas, low-grade gliomas; epilepsy in these cases is often refractory to drug therapy.

Genetic predisposition and developmental anomalies

The genetics of epilepsies is exceedingly complex. Over 200 genetic disorders list epilepsy among their features, but account for less than 1% of patients with seizures. This gives rises to complex syndromic classifications. Overall about 30% of patients with epilepsy have a history of seizures in first-degree relatives. Usually the mode of inheritance is uncertain; a low seizure threshold appears to run in some families. Generalized typical absence seizures (*petit mal*, 3Hz spike-and-wave) or primary generalized epilepsy are often inherited as an autosomal dominant trait with variable penetrance. Primary epilepsies are due to complex developmental abnormalities of neuronal control; there are abnormalities in synaptic connections, and anomalies in neurotransmitter distribution and release. Neuronal migration defects in utero, dysplastic areas of cerebral cortex and hamartomas contribute to the cause of seizures that develop in infancy and in adult life.

Trauma, hypoxia and surgery

Perinatal trauma (cerebral contusion and haemorrhage) and fetal anoxia are common causes of childhood seizures. Hypoxic damage to the hippocampi (mesial temporal sclerosis) is another childhood cause of epilepsy.

Brain injury is sometimes followed by epilepsy within the first week (early epilepsy) or many months or years later (late epilepsy). To cause epilepsy, the injury must (usually) be sufficient to cause coma. Early epilepsy, a depressed skull fracture, penetrating brain

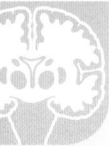

injury, cerebral contusion, dural tear or intracranial haematoma increases the incidence of late post-traumatic epilepsy.

Seizures follow some 10% of neurosurgical operations on the cerebral hemispheres.

Pyrexia

Convulsions sometimes occur when children under 5 years have high fevers (febrile convulsions). In the majority there is no tendency for seizures to recur and (largely for social reasons) these are not usually classed as epilepsy.

Brain tumours (and abscesses)

Mass lesions in the cortex cause epilepsy – either partial or secondary generalized seizures. If epilepsy develops in adult life, the chance of finding an unsuspected tumour is around 3%.

Hydrocephalus (p. 1201) also lowers seizure threshold.

Vascular

Seizures sometimes follow cerebral infarction, especially in elderly people. This is the principal reason for a peak in the incidence of epilepsy late in life. A brain arteriovenous malformation may present with seizures.

Alcohol, drugs and drug withdrawal

Chronic alcohol abuse is a common cause of seizures. These occur either while drinking heavily or during periods of withdrawal. Alcohol-induced hypoglycaemia also provokes attacks (p. 1104).

Phenothiazines, monoamine oxidase inhibitors, tricyclic antidepressants, amfetamines, lidocaine (lignocaine), propofol and nalidixic acid sometimes provoke fits, either in overdose or at therapeutic doses in individuals with a low seizure threshold.

Withdrawal of anticonvulsant drugs (especially phenobarbital) and benzodiazepine withdrawal may provoke seizures.

Encephalitis and inflammatory conditions

Seizures are frequently the presenting feature of encephalitis, cerebral abscess, cortical venous thrombosis, and neurosyphilis. They also occur in chronic meningitis (e.g. tuberculosis) and may rarely be the first sign of bacterial meningitis.

Metabolic abnormalities

Seizures are seen with the following:

- hypocalcaemia
- hypoglycaemia
- hyponatraemia
- acute hypoxia
- porphyria
- uraemia
- hepatocellular failure
- mitochondrial disease.

Degenerative brain disorders

Seizures can occur in Alzheimer's disease and in many rarer degenerative diseases. Epilepsy is three times commoner in multiple sclerosis patients than in the general population.

Provoked seizures (e.g. photosensitivity)

Seizures are occasionally precipitated by flashing lights or a flickering television screen. This photosensitivity can be recorded on occipital EEG electrodes. Rarely other stimuli (e.g. music) provoke attacks.

Sleep deprivation

A convulsion sometimes follows missing a night's sleep in a susceptible person.

Diagnosis and investigations

The history from a witness is crucial. The onset, setting, and stages of attacks are of importance. Neurological examination may be normal or point to a clinical diagnosis (e.g. hemiparesis and papilloedema in a hemisphere tumour). General medical screening, including serum calcium and an ECG should be carried out. The differential diagnosis is from other attacks of disturbed consciousness (p. 1180).

Electroencephalography

The EEG remains a useful test, despite limitations. It should be performed after a first fit.

- *During a seizure* the EEG is almost invariably abnormal, because spikes reach the brain surface.
- *EEG evidence of seizure activity* is shown typically by focal cortical spikes (e.g. over a temporal lobe) or by generalized spike-and-wave activity. Epileptic activity is continuous in *status epilepticus*.
- *3 Hz spike-and-wave activity* occurs specifically in *petit mal* (Fig. 20.16, p. 1157). This is always present during an attack and is frequently seen in between attacks.
- *A normal EEG between attacks* (interictal) does not in any way exclude epilepsy. Many people with epilepsy have normal interictal EEGs.
- *An abnormal interictal EEG* does not prove that one particular attack was epileptic and should not be used to make a diagnosis.
- *EEG videotelemetry* is used to study attacks of uncertain nature (e.g. non-epileptic attack disorder, p. 1156).

CT and/or MR imaging

The trend is towards sophisticated imaging of all new cases of epilepsy when resources permit. In practice, CT is a reasonable screening test in most adults to diagnose unsuspected mass lesions. MR is used for detailed study, particularly in the selection of cases for epilepsy surgery.

Treatment

Emergency measures

When faced with a seizure it is best simply to ensure that the patient comes to as little harm as possible, and that the airway is maintained both during a prolonged seizure and in postictal coma. Wooden mouth gags, tongue forceps and physical restraint cause injury.

Most seizures last only minutes and end spontaneously. A prolonged seizure – longer than 3 minutes – or repeated seizures outside hospital are best treated with rectal diazepam (10 mg), or intravenous diazepam. If there is any suspicion of hypoglycaemia, take blood for glucose and give i.v. glucose. *Serial* epilepsy describes repeated seizures with brief periods of recovery. These may lead to *status epilepticus*. Sudden death in a seizure is unusual but does occur.

Status epilepticus

This medical emergency means continuous seizures without recovery of consciousness. It should be assumed if prolonged serial seizures (two or more) occur with incomplete recovery of consciousness. Status has a mortality of 10–15% from cardiorespiratory failure. Over 50% of cases occur without a previous history of epilepsy. However, about a quarter of patients with apparent refractory status have *pseudostatus* (non-epileptic attack disorder): the iatrogenic morbidity of inappropriate treatment in these patients is significant.

Management. See Practical box 20.4.

Focal status also occurs. In *absence* status, for example, status is non-convulsive – the patient is in a continuous, distant, stuporose state. *Epilepsia partialis continua* is continuous seizure activity in one part of the body, such as a finger or a limb, without loss of consciousness. This is often due to a cortical neoplasm or, in the elderly, a cortical infarct.

Anticonvulsant drugs

Drugs are indicated when there is a firm clinical diagnosis of recurrent seizures, or a substantial risk of recurrence. Anticonvulsant use carries the stigma of epilepsy. Acceptance by patients is essential, and their understanding of potential unwanted effects. For both partial and generalized seizures, prescribe monotherapy with an established anticonvulsant of proven efficacy (Table 20.35). The dose is increased until seizure control is achieved or tolerance exceeded. If control is not achieved a second drug is added. Many new anticonvulsants have been marketed in the 1990s (Table 20.36). Unfortunately there remain different views about the most appropriate drugs for each variety of seizure.

Drug levels. Serum levels of most anticonvulsants can be monitored. With phenytoin the therapeutic level is well-defined and this should be usually be monitored every few months (Table 20.37). Therapeutic serum levels of other anticonvulsants are less useful. Routine

---

✚ Practical box 20.4

Management of status epilepticus

Several treatment schedules exist. Issues of prime importance are the speed with which convulsive activity is treated, the accuracy of diagnosis and need for continued monitoring and cardiorespiratory support – this must be available. An ITU is essential for optimum management.

- At home, give immediate diazepam 10–20 mg i.v. at 5 mg/min and repeat once. If immediate i.v. access is impossible, give rectal diazepam, or rectal paraldehyde.
- Arrange immediate admission to hospital.
- Administer oxygen, monitor ECG, BP, routine bloods (include alcohol, calcium, magnesium, drug screen, anticonvulsant levels). Exclude hypoglycaemia: treat if present.
- Give thiamine i.v. (250 mg) if nutrition poor or alcohol abuse suspected. (In the UK parenteral vitamin B and C, one pair of high-potency i.v. ampoules over 10 minutes.)
- *Anticonvulsants:*
  1. Give lorazepam i.v. 4 mg at 2 mg/min. Respiratory depression, hypotension and cardiac dysrhythmias may occur. (Lorazepam 4 mg vial)
  2. Reinstate previous anticonvulsant drugs. Establish whether the patient has had adequate phenytoin recently. Measure levels as an emergency if service available.
  3. If seizures continue, consider i.v. phenytoin or fosphenytoin (if patient is not already loaded with these drugs).

- Phenytoin: give 15 mg/kg i.v. diluted to 10 mg/mL in normal saline into a large vein at less than 50 mg/min. (Phenytoin sodium 250 mg 5 mL ampoule)
- Fosphenytoin: this is a pro-drug of phenytoin and can be given faster than phenytoin. Doses are expressed in phenytoin equivalents (PE): fosphenytoin 1.5 mg = 1 mg phenytoin.
- Give 15 mg/kg (PE) fosphenytoin (15 mg × 1.5 = 22.5 mg) diluted to 10 mg/mL in normal saline at 50–100 mg (PE)/min. (Fosphenytoin sodium 750 mg 10 mL ampoule)
  4. If status continues, give phenobarbital 10 mg/kg diluted 1 in 10 in water for injection at < 100 mg/min. (Phenobarbital 200 mg/mL 1 mL vial in propylene glycol 90% with water for injection 10%). Intravenous clonazepam, paraldehyde and clomethiazole are also used.
  5. If, despite these measures, status persists > 90 minutes, use thiopentone or propofol anaesthesia with assisted ventilation.

- EEG monitoring is valuable if there is doubt about the nature of status.
- CT scanning may reveal an underlying cause for status.
- Remember: 25% of apparent status turns out to be *pseudostatus*.
- Remember: potential unwanted effects of the drugs (e.g. hypotension, cardiac arrest) and the need for continuous cardiorespiratory monitoring.

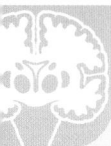

Table 20.35
Principal antiepileptic drugs and common seizure types

Drug	Partial	2° generalized	Tonic–clonic	3 Hz absence	Myoclonic
Carbamazepine	+	+	+	−	−
Ethosuximide	0	0	0	+	0
Phenobarbital	+	+	+	0	+ (?)
Phenytoin	+	+	+	−	−
Primidone	+	+	+	0	?
Valproate	+	+	+	+	+

+, efficacy proven/probable; 0, ineffective; − *worsens* seizures; ?, unknown
After Brodie MJ *Lancet* 2000 **356**: 324

Table 20.36
Newer antiepileptic drugs and common seizure types

Drug	Partial	2° generalized	Tonic–clonic	3 Hz absence	Myoclonic
Felbamate	+	+	?+	?+	?
Gabapentin	+	+	?+	0	?−
Lamotrigine	+	+	+	?	+
Levetiracetam	+	+	+	0	0
Oxcarbazepine	+	+	+	+	+
Tiagabine	+	+	?	?	?
Topiramate	+	+	+	?	+
Vigabatrin	+	+	?+	−	−

+, efficacy proven/probable; 0, ineffective; −, *worsens* seizures; ?, unknown

Table 20.37
Doses and therapeutic levels of antiepileptic drugs

	Usual adult daily dose (mg)	Therapeutic range (μmol/L)
Phenytoin	300–500	40–80
Carbamazepine	400–1000	20–50
Valproate	800–2000	200–700

Table 20.38
Some idiosyncratic unwanted effects of anticonvulsant drugs

Drug	Non-dose-related side-effects
Phenytoin	Rashes Blood dyscrasias Lymphadenopathy Systemic lupus erythematosus Toxic epidermal necrolysis
Carbamazepine	Rashes Blood dyscrasias, particularly severe leucopenia Toxic epidermal necrolysis
Sodium valproate	Anorexia Hair loss Liver damage
Lamotrigine	Toxic epidermal necrolysis
Vigabatrin	Retinal damage (visual field constriction) Psychological change

estimations are not usually performed, unless compliance or toxicity are issues.

Unwanted effects of drugs. Intoxication with all anticonvulsants causes ataxia, nystagmus and dysarthria. Chronic phenytoin causes gum hypertrophy, hypertrichosis, osteomalacia, folate deficiency, polyneuropathy and encephalopathy. A wide range of potential unwanted effects are known. See Table 20.38 for some serious idiosyncratic (i.e. non-dose-related) side-effects. The majority of severe skin reactions (e.g. toxic epidermal neurolysis) following phenytoin, carbamazepine, valproate and phenobarbital occur within the first 8 weeks of treatment.

Three drugs now rarely commenced outside a specialist centre are phenobarbital and its derivative primidone (drowsiness, cognitive impairment) – though phenobarbital still has a place in status – and vigabatrin (visual fields defects).

Refractory epilepsy

Despite medical therapy seizures persist in some 20% of cases of apparent primary generalized epilepsy and up to 35% of cases of partial epilepsy. Rigorous attention to diagnosis, to drug compliance, to trials of different drugs and consideration of surgical approaches to treatment can help reduce this burden.

Epilepsy in the elderly

Some 25% of new cases of epilepsy develop over the age of 65. Many patients have cerebrovascular disease, neurodegenerative conditions or brain tumours. The onset of seizures commonly leads to loss of independence and to physical injuries and their complications (e.g. subdural haematomas). With adequate anticonvulsants, control of seizures can be achieved in some 70% of this vulnerable population.

Women, epilepsy and anticonvulsants

Fertility. There is some reduction of fertility in epileptic populations. This is multifactorial. One-third of women with epilepsy have some ovarian abnormality – irregular menstrual cycles, anovulatory cycles and polycystic ovaries. These are probably more frequent in patients taking sodium valproate.

Birth defects. The overall risk of birth defects in babies of mothers who take one anticonvulsant is around 7%, higher than the 3% in the general population. Counselling before conception is essential. Some women choose to stop anticonvulsants before becoming pregnant. If drugs are continued, monotherapy with a first-line drug is preferable with folic acid (5 mg/day) supplement. Vitamin K 20 mg orally should also be taken daily during the week before delivery to prevent neonatal haemorrhage (caused by inhibition of vitamin K transplacental transport).

Contraception. Anticonvulsants that induce enzymes (e.g. carbamazepine, phenytoin and phenobarbital) reduce the efficacy of oral contraceptives; valproate does not. A combined contraceptive pill containing at least 50 mg of oestrogen should be used, or an IUCD or barrier methods of contraception.

Breast-feeding. Mothers taking the established drugs (Table 20.35) need not in general be discouraged from breast-feeding – though individual drug manufacturers are often hesitant about giving absolute assurance that there is no identifiable risk to the baby.

Drug withdrawal

Epilepsy, when controlled, may remain in remission. Drug withdrawal is sometimes possible, and this question is often raised. Successful withdrawal is only achieved in less than 50%. Recurrence of seizures can cause considerable difficulty when a driving licence has been regained. (Remember, this is either on or off drugs.) The UK Driving Licensing Authority (DVLA Swansea) recommend that patients do not drive while anticonvulsants are reduced and for 6 months after stopping them. Careful discussion and full explanation is necessary. Withdrawal should not usually be considered until all fits have been absent for at least 2–3 years.

Neurosurgical treatment

Several surgical approaches are used in epilepsy. The most important is amputation of the non-dominant anterior temporal lobe in a patient with uncontrolled seizures and hippocampal sclerosis defined by imaging and confirmed by EEG. In these highly selected cases (under 1% of all patients with epilepsy) in a specialist centre this surgical treatment is highly effective with cure rates (complete seizure cessation) over 50%. Section of the corpus callosum and hemispherectomy are also used. Vagus nerve stimulation is also under study as a treatment; its mechanism is unclear.

Social consequences

The great majority of patients with epilepsy are managed by a general practitioner or as a hospital outpatient, and suffer infrequent seizures. In a very small minority who have exceedingly frequent seizures, treatment in hospital or even residential care is necessary.

There remains, however, a considerable stigma attached to the word epilepsy, an important fact to be considered when the nature of attacks is uncertain. Employers are reluctant to accept people with epilepsy.

Both adults and children with epilepsy should be encouraged to lead lives as unrestricted as reasonably possible, though with simple, sensible provisos such as avoiding swimming alone and dangerous sports such as rock-climbing or solo canoeing. Domestic issues are also important, such as leaving unlocked the bathroom or lavatory door. Support groups and information services are of value to patients and their families.

Driving and epilepsy

It is illegal to drive a motor vehicle if any form of seizure or any episode of unexplained loss of consciousness has occurred during the previous year. There is some variation between different countries. In the UK those who have suffered from epilepsy cannot legally hold a Group 1 driving licence (for a car or motorcycle) unless they satisfy the following legal criteria, whether on or off treatment. The regulations state:

- A person who has suffered an epileptic attack whilst awake must refrain from driving for 1 year from the date of the attack before a driving licence may be issued.
- A person who has suffered a single epileptic attack whilst asleep must also refrain from driving for 1 year from the date of that attack, unless they have had attacks exclusively whilst asleep over a period of 3 years and no awake attacks, i.e. attacks occurring exclusively in sleep must be shown to have occurred over a 3-year period.
- In any event, the driving of a vehicle by such a person should not be likely to cause danger to the public.

For UK Group 2 drivers (vocational and for truck drivers) regulations are stricter. Persons with previous seizures must meet *all* these three criteria:

- They must have been free of attacks for at least 10 years.

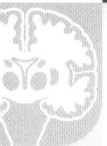
- They must not have taken anticonvulsants during this 10 years.
- They do not have any continuing liability to seizures.

Stringent regulations also exist for potential aircraft pilots, sea captains, divers and other similar activities. The correct diagnosis of an attack at any age is therefore of major social and legal importance. It is an essential medical requirement to inform patients of the law. In the UK the patient should then write to the licensing authorities.

FURTHER READING

At a Glance Guide to the Current Medical Standards of Fitness to Drive (2000) Swansea: Drivers Medical Unit, DVLA

Brodie MJ, French JA (2000) Management of epilepsy in adolescents and adults. *Lancet* **356**: 323–329.

Crawford P et al. (1999) Best practice guidelines for the management of women with epilepsy. *Seizure* **8**: 201–217.

Duncan JA, Shorvon SD, Fish DR (1995) *Clinical Epilepsy.* Edinburgh, Churchill Livingstone.

Engel J, Pedley T (1998) *Epilepsy. A Comprehensive Textbook.* Vols 1–3. Philadelphia: Lippincott-Raven.

Kwan P, Brodie MJ (2000) Early identification of refractory epilepsy. *New England Journal of Medicine* **342**: 314–319.

Stephen LJ, Brodie MJ (2000) Epilepsy in elderly people. *Lancet* **355**: 1441–1446.

Treitman DM et al. (1998) A comparison of four treatments for generalised convulsive status epilepticus. *New England Journal of Medicine* **339**: 792–798.

UK PATIENT SUPPORT GROUP

National Society for Epilepsy, Chesham Lane, Chalfont St Peter, Bucks SL9 0RJ.
www.epilepsyuse.org.uk

Other attacks of disturbed consciousness; falls (Table 20.39)

Episodes of transient disturbance of consciousness and falls are common clinical problems. It is usually possible to distinguish between a fit (i.e. a seizure), a faint (i.e. syncope), and other types of attack from the history and an eye-witness account. The term 'collapse' is non-diagnostic and to be avoided. Falls must be distinguished from episodes of disturbed consciousness. The precise cause of falls in the elderly, with their important sequelae such as a femoral fracture, often remains ill-defined. Falls without loss of awareness are common in Parkinson's disease.

Syncope; vasovagal attacks; drop attacks

(see also p. 708)

Sudden reflex bradycardia with vasodilatation both peripheral and splanchnic leads to loss of consciousness

Table 20.39
Causes of attacks of disturbed consciousness and falling

Epilepsy
Syncope (situational or vasovagal)
    Simple faints
    Cough
    Effort
    Micturition
    Carotid sinus
    Autonomic failure
    Basilar migraine
Cardiac dysrhythmias
Drop attacks
Hydrocephalus
Transient ischaemic attacks
Panic attacks
Non-epileptic attacks (pseudoseizures)
Hyperventilation
Night terrors   } in children
Breath-holding   }
Hypoglycaemia
Hypocalcaemia
Vertigo
Choking
Drug reactions
Carcinoid syndrome
Phaeochromocytoma

– a fainting attack. This is simple syncope (also known as neurocardiogenic syncope), a common response to prolonged standing, fear, venesection or pain. Syncope almost never occurs in the recumbent posture. The subject falls to the ground and is unconscious for less than 2 minutes. Recovery is rapid. Jerking movements can occur. Incontinence of urine is exceptional.

This is the simple faint that over half the population experience at some time, particularly in childhood, in youth or in pregnancy. Syncope occurs with severe anaemia at any age.

Syncope occurs after micturition in men, particularly at night, and in either sex when the venous return to the heart is obstructed by breath-holding and severe coughing.

Postural hypotension causes syncope in patients with impaired autonomic reflexes (e.g. in the elderly), in autonomic neuropathy, or with older ganglion-blocking drugs used in hypertension, with phenothiazines, levodopa or tricyclic antidepressants.

Transient cerebral ischaemia in the posterior cerebral circulation also leads to episodic loss of consciousness. Patients sometimes faint during a severe 'basilar' migraine.

The rare syndrome of carotid sinus syncope is due to excessive sensitivity of the sinus to external pressure. This tends to occur in elderly patients who lose consciousness after touching the neck.

Cardiac arrhythmias (cardiac syncope, Stokes–Adams attacks; p. 738) cause recurrent episodes of loss of onsciousness, particularly in the elderly. There is sometimes a preceding warning of palpitation (either fast or slow). Loss of consciousness is sudden and accompanied by pallor. Exceptionally, there are convulsive movements – anoxic convulsions. Flushing may be seen on recovery. The usual cardiac arrhythmias causing episodic   loss of consciousness are paroxysmal bradycardias (e.g. complete heart block) or ventricular dysrhythmias. Supraventricular tachycardias rarely cause syncope.

Effort syncope (syncope on exertion) is of cardiac origin and occurs in aortic stenosis and hypertrophic cardiomyopathy (p. 812).

Drop attacks are instant unexpected episodes of lower limb weakness with falling, largely in women over 60 years. They are believed to be due to sudden change in lower limb tone, presumably of brainstem origin. Awareness is preserved. They used to be regarded as forms of TIA, from which they are distinct, as other vascular events do not follow them. Sudden attacks of leg weakness also occur in hydrocephalus.

Syncope: investigation and management

Syncope and related conditions where cerebral blood flow falls can usually be distinguished from epilepsy on the clinical history alone. A witness account is extremely valuable: persistent jerking movements, incontinence and post-episode confusion with amnesia are very suggestive of a fit, and rare with a faint. Cardiac monitoring is used to detect dysrhythmia. Tilt testing (p. 722) is sometimes useful in the diagnosis of neurocardiogenic syncope.

The immediate management of syncope, or impending syncope, is to lay the patient down, to lift the legs and to record the pulse. In rare circumstances where cerebral blood flow cannot be restored (e.g. propped upright in a dentist's chair), syncope can be followed by cerebral infarction.

Other conditions

Panic attacks; hyperventilation; non-epileptic attacks (pseudoseizures).

Panic attacks are usually associated with an autonomic disturbance, such as tachycardia, sweating and piloerection. Consciousness is usually preserved and the attacks often recognized by the patient. Hyperventilation is common both during a panic attack and as a cause of panic (see Box 21.11).

Overbreathing causes alkalosis that leads to lightheadedness, sometimes with circumoral and peripheral tingling and tetany, e.g. carpopedal spasm (p. 1063). Occasionally there is loss of consciousness.

Non-epileptic attacks (pseudoseizures) regularly cause difficulty. Attacks often resemble grand mal fits. Usually there are bizarre limb movements, but on occasion there is extreme difficulty in separating these attacks from epilepsy. EEG videotelemetry is valuable. Apparent status epilepticus can be produced by non-epileptic

attacks. The prolactin level is of some diagnostic value: it rises during a true grand mal seizure but not during a pseudoseizure (or a partial seizure).

Hypoglycaemia (see also p. 1102). Hypoglycaemia causes attacks in which the patient either feels unwell or loses consciousness, sometimes with a convulsion. There is often some warning, with hunger, shaking and sweating. Prompt recovery occurs with intravenous (or oral) glucose. Prolonged hypoglycaemia causes widespread cerebral damage. Hypoglycaemic attacks unrelated to diabetes are rare (but see p. 1102). Malaise after fasting or in the early morning does not indicate organic disease.

Hypocalcaemia (see also p. 1062). A grand mal fit may accompany hypocalcaemia, as the seizure threshold is lowered.

Vertigo. Acute vertigo can be severe enough to cause prostration: consciousness is sometimes lost for a few seconds.

Choking. Choking causes sudden loss of speech, with intense coughing and laryngeal spasm, followed by hypoxia, when laryngeal obstruction is partial. When a large food bolus completely blocks the larynx, the person becomes blue and silent. Death occurs if this obstruction is not relieved promptly by the Heimlich manoeuvre (p. 861). Gravity – holding the person upside down – is also useful.

Drug reactions. Acute dystonic reactions (oculogyric crises, p. 1186) are sometimes mistaken for epilepsy. Consciousness is preserved.

Carcinoid syndrome and phaeochromocytoma (pp. 299 and 1066). Flushing and palpitation is sometimes mistaken for anxiety, or a partial seizure.

Sleep and its disturbances

(see also p. 1240)

Sleep is required on a regular basis as it preserves recent memory, refreshing both cognitive and emotional equilibrium, and avoids neurotransmitter depletion. Poorly understood neurotransmitter pathways – including those involving hypothalamic hypocretin (orexin) neuropeptides – between cortex and reticular formation are involved in production and maintenance of sleep.

In insomnia, sleep is fitful (p. 1240). Less time than usual is spent in REM sleep. In old age, sleep requirement falls to as little as 4 hours a night. In practice, insomnia itself is rarely a feature of serious organic neurological disease.

Narcolepsy and cataplexy

Narcoleptic attacks are periods of irresistible sleep, i.e. excessive daytime drowsiness, in inappropriate circumstances. Episodes tend to occur when there is little distraction, after meals, while travelling in a vehicle,

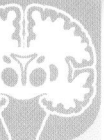
though sometimes without obvious cause. Genetically, narcolepsy is strongly associated with HLA-DR2 and HLA-DQBl*0602 antigens. There are suggestions that narcolepsy patients positive for these antigens have sub-normal hypocretin 1 levels in CSF.

Cataplexy is sudden loss of lower limb tone – falling with preservation of consciousness. Attacks are often set off by sudden surprise or emotion.

The two conditions sometimes coexist and are accompanied by vivid hypnagogic hallucinations (i.e. on falling asleep), hypnopompic hallucinations (i.e. on waking), with sleep paralysis – a frightening inability to move whilst drowsy. The EEG remains normal during and between attacks.

Treatment

Methylphenidate, dexamfetamine, modafinil, or small doses of tricyclic antidepressants, particularly clomi-pramine, are used, rarely with great success. Siberian ginseng (*Elenthrococcus serticosus*) and St John's Wort (*Hypericum perforatum*) are also used.

Sleep apnoea (see p. 869)

Insomnia (see p. 1240)

FURTHER READING

George CFP, Singh S (2000) Hypocretin (orexin) pathway in sleep. *Lancet* **355**: 6–7.
Schneerson J (2000) *Handbook of Sleep Medicine*. Oxford: Blackwell.

Movement disorders

Disorders of movement form a substantial part of neurodegenerative diseases. They divide broadly into akinetic–rigid syndromes, where there is loss of movement with increase in tone (also called parkinsonism), and dyskinesias, where there are added uncontrollable movements. Precise anatomical and neurotransmitter profile changes are often hard to define. Both parkinsonism and dyskinesia may coexist in some conditions, leading to various confusing classifications. Table 20.40 outlines the principal clinical varieties: idiopathic Parkinson's disease (an akinetic–rigid syndrome) and essential tremor (a dyskinesia) are much the commonest movement disorders.

Table 20.40
A classification of movement disorders

Akinetic-rigid syndromes
Idiopathic Parkinson's disease
Drug-induced parkinsonism (e.g. phenothiazines)
MPTP-induced parkinsonism
Postencephalitic parkinsonism
Parkinsonism-plus
Childhood akinetic–rigid syndrome

Dyskinesias
Essential tremor
Chorea
Hemiballismus
Myoclonus
Tic or 'habit spasms'
Torsion dystonias

MPTP, 1-methyl-4-phenyl-1,2,3,6-tetrahydropyridine

FURTHER READING

Martin JB (1999) Molecular basis of the neurodegenerative disorders. *New England Journal of Medicine* **340**: 1970–1980.

Akinetic–rigid syndromes

Idiopathic Parkinson's disease

In 1817, James Parkinson, a physician in Hoxton, London, published *The Shaking Palsy*, the monograph describing a condition that is common and world-wide, with prevalence of 150/100 000 increasing sharply in those over 70 years. The disease is clinically and pathologically distinct from other parkinsonian syndromes.

There are few real clues as to the cause of the common and apparently sporadic idiopathic Parkinson's disease (PD). The relatively uniform world-wide prevalence would suggest that an environmental agent is not responsible. Some factors possibly involved are the following.

Nicotine. Several epidemiological studies suggest the curious and unexplained fact that the disease is less prevalent in tobacco smokers than in lifelong abstainers.

MPTP. Minute doses of the pyridine compound, methylphenyltetrahydropyridine (MPTP) cause a severe parkinsonian syndrome. The significance between this and idiopathic Parkinson's disease remains unclear. Suggestions that environmental MPTP-like herbicides are implicated remain entirely unsubstantiated.

Encephalitis lethargica. Some survivors of the presumed viral *encephalitis lethargica*, developed severe parkinsonism. However, it is not thought that idiopathic Parkinson's disease is related to an infective agent.

Genetic factors. Whilst not usually familial, there is clustering of early-onset Parkinson's disease in some families. Mutations of the alpha-synuclein gene and ubiquitin carboxyl-terminal hydrolase L1 (*UCHL1*), on chromosomes 2p13 and 4p14-16.3 respectively, account for occasional cases. Mutations in the parkin gene on chromosome 6 have been found in families with autosomal recessive cases of PD and some young apparently sporadic cases. Parkin mutations probably account for most PD cases with onset below the age of 40. Mutant parkin proteins are unable to interact and ubiquinate forms of α-synuclein allow it to accumulate (see below). The role of this mechanism in the large majority of older, sporadic cases is unclear.

Pathology

In the *pars compacta* of the *substantia nigra* progressive cell degeneration and neuronal eosinophilic inclusion bodies (Lewy bodies) are seen. These contain protein filaments of ubiquitin and alpha-synuclein. Degeneration also occurs in other basal ganglia nuclei. Biochemically there is loss of dopamine (and melanin) in the striatum that correlates well with the areas of cell loss and also with the degree of akinesia.

Clinical symptoms

The combination of tremor, rigidity and akinesia develops slowly, over months or several years, together with changes in posture. The most common initial symptoms are tremor and slowness. Patients complain that limbs and joints feel stiff and ache and that fine movements are difficult. Slowness causes characteristic symptoms of difficulty in rising from a chair or getting into or out of bed. Writing becomes small (micrographia) and spidery, with a tendency to tail off at the end of a line. Other evidence often comes from relatives who have noted slowness and an impassive facial expression. The disease is almost always more prominent on one side.

Clinical signs

Diagnosis is usually immediate from the overall appearance.

Tremor

This is a characteristic 4–7 Hz rest tremor usually decreased by action and increased by emotion with pill-rolling movements between thumb and forefinger.

Rigidity

Stiffness develops that can be felt throughout the range of limb movement and is equal in opposing muscle groups – in sharp contrast to the selective increase in tone found in spasticity. This 'lead pipe' rigidity is usually more marked on one side and is also present in the neck and axial muscles.

Rigidity is usually more easily felt when a joint is moved slowly and gently. When one arm is being examined, its tone increases when the opposite arm is moved actively. When stiffness is combined with tremor, smooth 'lead-pipe' rigidity is broken up into a jerky resistance to passive movement, a phenomenon known as cogwheeling, or cogging.

Akinesia

Poverty and slowing of movement (bradykinesia) is an additional handicap, distinct from rigidity. There is difficulty initiating movement. Rapid fine finger movements, such as piano-playing, become indistinct, slow and tremulous. The facial immobility gives a mask-like semblance of depression. The frequency of spontaneous blinking is reduced, producing a serpentine stare.

Postural changes

A stoop is characteristic. Gait becomes, hurrying (festinant) and shuffling with poor arm swinging. The posture is sometimes called 'simian' to describe the ape-like forward flexion, immobility and lack of facial expression. Balance is impaired, but despite this the gait retains a narrow base. Falls are common as the usual corrective righting reflexes fail, the sufferer toppling like a falling tree.

Speech

Pronunciation is initially a monotone but progresses to characteristic tremulous slurring dysarthria, the result of combined akinesia, tremor and rigidity. Speech may eventually be lost completely (anarthria). Dribbling and dysphagia develop.

Gastrointestinal and other symptoms

These include heartburn, dysphagia, constipation and weight loss. Urinary difficulties are common, especially in men. The skin is greasy and sweating is excessive.

Natural history and other features

Parkinson's disease worsens over some years, beginning as a mild inconvenience but slowly progressing. Remissions are unknown except for rare and remarkable short-lived periods of release. These tend to occur at times of great emotion, fear or excitement, when the sufferer is released for seconds or minutes and able to move quickly.

While bradykinesia and tremor worsen, power remains normal until immobility makes its assessment difficult. Patients often complain bitterly of limb and joint discomfort. There is no sensory loss. The reflexes are brisk; their asymmetry follows the increase in tone. The plantar responses remain flexor. Cognitive function is preserved, at least early in the condition. Dementia often develops in the late stages. Anxiety and depression are common.

The rate of progression is very variable, with a benign form running over several decades. Usually the course is over 10–15 years, with death resulting from bronchopneumonia.

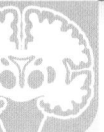

Differential diagnosis

There is no laboratory test for Parkinson's disease. Diagnosis consists of recognizing the clinical pattern. Conventional imaging (MR) is unhelpful. PET scanning is used in research. Idiopathic Parkinson's disease must be distinguished from other akinetic–rigid syndromes.

Certain diffuse or multifocal brain diseases cause some features of parkinsonism, i.e. the slowing, rigidity and tremor seen in idiopathic Parkinson's disease. Examples are Alzheimer's disease, multi-infarct dementia, sequelae of repeated head injury (e.g. in boxers, p. 1205), and the late effects of severe hypoxia or carbon monoxide poisoning. Slowing also occurs in hypothyroidism, and in depression.

Treatment

While no drugs alter the course of Parkinson's disease, levodopa and/or dopaminergic agonists produce striking initial symptomatic improvement. These drugs should be avoided until they are clinically necessary because of delayed unwanted effects (see below). Catechol-O-methyl transferase inhibitors are also used as supplementary therapy. Older treatments such as the antimuscarin trihexyphenidyl (benzhexol) did little for symptoms and frequently caused mental confusion; they are of some help in severe tremor. Selegeline, a monoamine oxidase B inhibitor, may delay the need for levodopa therapy by some months. Antioxidants are also used with this aim, but their value is unproven. A scheme for the mechanism of action of drugs in Parkinson's disease is shown in Figure 20.24.

Levodopa

Levodopa is combined with an aromatic amino acid decarboxylase inhibitor – benserazide (co-beneldopa, as Madopar) or carbidopa (co-careldopa, as Sinemet). The decarboxylase inhibitor reduces peripheral side-effects, principally nausea, of levodopa and its metabolites. Levodopa treatment is commenced (co-beneldopa 62.5 mg or co-careldopa 110 mg, one tablet three times daily) and gradually increased.

The great majority of patients with idiopathic Parkinson's disease (but not other parkinsonian syndromes) improve initially with levodopa. The response in severe, previously untreated Parkinson's disease is sometimes dramatic.

Unwanted effects of levodopa therapy

Nausea and vomiting are the most common immediate symptoms of a levodopa dose being too large. Confusion, formed visual pseudo-hallucinations and chorea also occur with excessive single doses. There are difficult issues with long-term levodopa. After several years the drug gradually becomes ineffective, even with increasing doses. As treatment continues, episodes of immobility develop (freezing). Falls are common. Fluctuation in response to levodopa also appears, its effect apparently

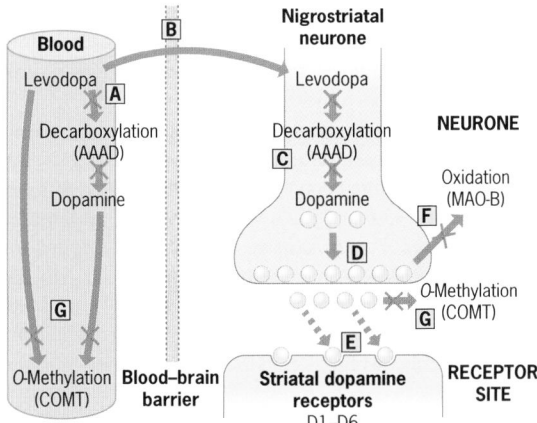

Fig. 20.24 **Drugs in Parkinson's disease: a nigrostriatal neurone and striatal dopamine receptors.** Levodopa crosses the blood–brain barrier, enters a neurone and is converted to dopamine.

A. Carbidopa and benserazide reduce peripheral conversion of levodopa to dopamine by AAAD, thus reducing side-effects of excess circulating dopamine.
B. Dietary amino acids from a high-protein meal may inhibit active transport into brain by competing with levodopa.
C. Levodopa is converted (AAAD) to dopamine in nigrostriatal neurones.
D. At the nerve terminal, amantadine enhances dopamine release.
E. Dopamine agonist drugs react with dopamine receptors.
F. Selegeline, the MAO-B inhibitor, blocks dopamine breakdown.
G. Entacapone, a COMT inhibitor, prolongs dopamine activity by blocking breakdown.

AAAD, aromatic amino acid decarboxylase; COMT, catechol-O-methyl transferase.

turning on and off, causing freezing alternating with dopa-induced dyskinesias, chorea and dystonic movements. Levodopa's duration of action shrinks, with dyskinesia becoming prominent several hours after the dose (end-of-dose dyskinesia). The patient begins to suffer not only from Parkinson's disease but also from a chronic levodopa-induced syndrome.

Levodopa therapy does not alter the natural progression of Parkinson's disease. After 5 years' treatment, around half of Parkinson's patients suffer from minor or major unwanted effects of therapy. The more distressing problems are difficult and often largely insoluble. Approaches to treatment of these complications include:

- Shortening the interval between levodopa doses and increasing each dose.
- Selegiline, a type B monoamine oxidase inhibitor, inhibits catabolism of dopamine in the brain. This sometimes smoothes out the response to levodopa. (Selegeline alone may also delay the need for levodopa therapy by some months.)
- Dopaminergic agonists (see below) are added, or replace levodopa.
- Entacapone, a catechol-O-methyl transferase inhibitor, is used.
- Drug holidays – periods of drug withdrawal – are occasionally helpful. They require close supervision since severe relapse may follow levodopa withdrawal.

Dopamine receptor agonists

Bromocriptine, lisuride, pergolide, cabergoline, prami-pexole and ropinirole are oral directly acting dopamine receptor agonists, acting principally on D_1 and D_2 receptors, and also on receptors D_{3-5}. These are used as an alternative or an addition to levodopa therapy.

Apomorphine, a potent D_1 and D_2 agonist given by subcutaneous metered infusion is an effective method of smoothing out fluctuations in response to levodopa. Skilled nursing is required to train patients and relatives to set up the infusion pump. Vomiting is a common unwanted effect. Haemolytic anaemia is an unusual side-effect of apomorphine.

Dopamine receptor agonists are in general less effective than levodopa in treating symptoms in Parkinson's disease, but are associated with fewer late unwanted dyskinetic effects.

There is much variation in clinical practice between different regimens of levodopa and dopamine receptor agonists, either singly or in combination. Some neurologists tend to use the receptor agonists as a primary treatment, before levodopa. There is an increasing trend towards delaying the start of drug treatment until this is clinically essential, using a directly acting agonist in PD as initial below the age of 70, and levodopa for older cases.

COMT inhibition

Levodopa undergoes *O*-methylation by catechol-*O*-methyl transferase. Entacapone inhibits this reaction; the drug is marketed to reduce end-of-dose fluctuations in response to levodopa.

Other agents

Antioxidant compounds such as vitamins C and E possibly acting as neuroprotective agents are sometimes prescribed. Their role is uncertain. Amantadine, originally marketed as an antiviral drug occasionally has a modest effect. Anticholinergics, e.g. trihexyphenidyl (benzhexol) are also used.

Stereotactic neurosurgery

Small stereotactic lesions, usually unilateral placed in the ventrolateral nucleus of the thalamus (thalamotomy) or in the globus pallidus (pallidotomy), were used widely before levodopa. When successful, surgery still provides effective, if temporary improvement in severe tremor and dyskinesia with minor relief of bradykinesia. Thalamic stimulation is also used.

Tissue transplantation

Transplantation of fetal or autologous dopamine-containing adrenal medulla and glial cell-line neurotrophic releasing factor (GDNF) into the cerebral ventricles or basal ganglia, though technically feasible, has not produced any major clinical improvement in the majority of patients with Parkinson's disease. This was despite early promise and compelling laboratory studies in rats with MPTP-induced parkinsonism.

The surgical treatments above are restricted to specialist centres – it seems unlikely that they will ever have a major role in a common world-wide disease.

Physiotherapy and physical aids

Skilled and determined physiotherapy can improve gait and help overcome particular problems. Practical guidance is of value:

- clothing – avoid zips, fiddly buttons and lace-up shoes
- cutlery – use built-up handles
- chairs – high upright rather than deep, low chairs
- rails – near lavatory and bath
- shoes – should be easy to put on and have smooth soles
- flooring – vinyl is often safer than carpet.

Walking aids are often a hindrance in the early stages, but later a frame or a tripod may be helpful. All attempts must be made to prevent falls, the effects of which may be catastrophic.

Psychiatric aspects

Depression is common in Parkinson's disease as symptoms worsen. SSRIs are the drugs of choice. Tricyclic antidepressants (e.g. amitriptyline) have extrapyramidal side-effects. Type A monoamine oxidase inhibitors (e.g. phenelzine) are absolutely contraindicated with levodopa.

All antiparkinsonian drugs can cause nocturnal visual hallucinations, which may exacerbate any underlying cognitive impairment.

Other akinetic–rigid syndromes

Drug-induced parkinsonism

Reserpine and methyldopa (drugs once used to treat hypertension), phenothiazines and butyrophenones induce a parkinsonian syndrome, with slowness and rigidity but usually little tremor. Tricyclic antidepressants also cause some slowing. These unwanted effects tend not to progress. Symptoms respond poorly, if at all, to levodopa and usually disappear when the drug causing them is stopped.

Neuroleptics and movement disorders

Neuroleptic drugs (i.e. phenothiazines and butyrophenones) also produce movement disorder.

- **Akathisia.** This is a restless, repetitive and irresistible need to move.
- **Acute dystonic reactions.** These sometimes follow, dramatically and unpredictably, single doses of neuroleptics, and related drugs widely used as

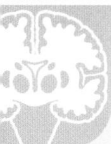

antiemetics and vestibular sedatives (such as prochlorperazine and metoclopramide). Spasmodic torticollis, trismus and oculogyric crises (i.e. episodes of sustained upward gaze) occur. These acute dystonias respond promptly to i.v. anticholinergics such as benztropine (1–2 mg) or procyclidine 5–10 mg. Both the offending drug, and all drugs from the same group, should be avoided subsequently.

- **Chronic tardive dyskinesias**. These are mouthing and lip-smacking grimaces of the face and neck. These disabling disorders tend to occur several years after commencing neuroleptic therapy and may be made temporarily worse when the dose of the drug is reduced. Resolution seldom occurs even when the drug is stopped.

Post-encephalitic parkinsonism and MPTP
(see p. 1182)

Parkinsonism-plus

This describes rare disorders in which there is parkinsonism with additional features and pathology. *Progressive supranuclear palsy* (Steele–Richardson–Olzewski syndrome) is the most common parkinson-plus disorder, and consists of parkinsonism, axial rigidity, falls, dementia, and inability to move the eyes vertically or laterally. Other examples are multiple system atrophies, such as olivo-ponto-cerebellar degeneration and primary autonomic failure (Shy–Drager syndrome).

These conditions tend to be progressive, unresponsive to levodopa and cause death within a decade.

Akinetic–rigid syndromes in children

A group of extremely rare disorders cause akinetic–rigid syndromes primarily under 20 years of age.

Wilson's disease

This rare and treatable disorder of copper metabolism is inherited as an autosomal recessive. There is deposition of copper in the brain, particularly in the basal ganglia, in the cornea and in the liver (p. 376), where it causes cirrhosis. All young patients either with an akinetic–rigid syndrome or with cirrhosis should be screened for Wilson's disease as neurological damage is irreversible unless early treatment is instituted. This akinetic–rigid syndrome and/or dyskinesias is followed by progressive intellectual impairment. Diagnosis and treatment with the chelating agent penicillamine is discussed on page 377.

Athetoid cerebral palsy

Writhing limb movements, sometimes with dystonia, occur in cerebral palsy following kernicterus. Dystonia tends to progress. This is now rare following prophylactic eradication of rhesus haemolytic disease with anti-D immunoglobulin.

Dyskinesias

Benign essential tremor

This common condition, often inherited as an autosomal dominant trait, causes 5–8 Hz tremor, usually worst in the upper limbs. The head is often tremulous (titubation) and also the trunk. Pathologically there is patchy neuronal loss in the cerebellum and its connections. Tremor is seen when the hands adopt a posture, such as holding a glass or a spoon. Essential tremor may be seen at any age but occurs most frequently in the elderly. It is slowly progressive but rarely produces a severe disability. Writing is shaky and untidy but micrographia is absent. Anxiety exacerbates the tremor, sometimes dramatically. In essential tremor, shaking occasionally occurs at rest, as in Parkinson's disease, or on action, as in cerebellar disease.

Treatment is often unnecessary, and unsatisfactory. Many patients are reassured to find they do not have Parkinson's disease, with which essential tremor is often confused.

Small amounts of alcohol, β-adrenergic blockers (propranolol) and the anticonvulsant primidone may help the tremor: sympathomimetics (e.g. salbutamol) make it worse. The antidepressant mirtazapine is being assessed for efficacy in treatment of tremor. Stereotactic thalamotomy and thalamaic stimulation are helpful in very severe essential tremor.

Chorea

Chorea describes jerky, quasi-purposive and sometimes explosive fidgety movements, flitting around the body. Causes of chorea are listed in Table 20.41.

Huntington's disease

Relentlessly progressive chorea and dementia, usually in middle life but sometimes in childhood, are hallmarks of this inherited disease. Prevalence world-wide

Table 20.41
Causes of chorea

Huntington's disease
Sydenham's chorea
Benign hereditary chorea
Abetalipoproteinaemia (see p. 298) with chorea
Chorea associated with:
    Drugs – phenytoin, levodopa, alcohol
    Thyrotoxicosis, pregnancy and oral contraceptive pill
    Systemic lupus erythematosus
    Polycythaemia vera
    Encephalitis lethargica
    Stroke (basal ganglia)
    Rarities (tumour, trauma, subdural haematoma, following carbon monoxide poisoning, paroxysmal choreoathetosis, Wilson's disease, dentato-rubro-pallido-luysian atrophy)

is about 5 in 100 000. Inheritance is as an autosomal dominant trait with full penetrance; children of an affected parent have a 50% chance of developing Huntington's disease. Previous family history is often concealed, either by design or default. A mutation has been identified in the distal short arm of chromosome 4 (4p16.3) with a variable expansion of a CAG-repeat sequence located in exon 1 of a large gene containing 67 exons. This results in translation of an extended gluta-mine sequence in *huntingtin*, the protein product of the gene. Huntingtin is expressed throughout the body. Its function is unclear. The majority of adult Huntington cases have CAG expansions of 40–55 repeats, while expansions of greater than 70 repeats are associated with onset of the disease in childhood.

Pathology

Cerebral atrophy progresses, with marked loss of small neurones in the caudate nucleus and putamen. Changes in neurotransmitters occur:

- *reduction* in enzymes synthesizing acetylcholine (choline acetyl transferase) and GABA in the striatum
- *increased* transglutaminase (which catalyses aggregates of *huntingtin*) in cortex, cerebellum and corpus striatum
- *depletion* of GABA, angiotensin-converting enzyme and met-enkephalin in substantia nigra
- *high* somatostatin levels in the corpus striatum.

These changes may be secondary to cell damage. In contrast to Parkinson's disease, dopamine and tyrosine hydroxylase activity remain normal.

Management and course

Other causes of chorea should be considered and investi-gated. Imaging in Huntington's, if it is possible with the chorea, shows caudate nucleus atrophy. There is steady progression, of both dementia and chorea. No treatment arrests the disease, although phenothiazines (e.g. sulpiride) may reduce chorea, by causing drug-induced parkinsonism. Tetrabenazine helps to control movements. Death usually occurs some 10–20 years from the onset.

Mutation analysis, which is accurate and specific, is available for presymptomatic testing of family mem-bers. This raises ethical problems: centres performing these tests have a common nationally agreed protocol for counselling.

Sydenham's chorea (St Vitus's dance)

This is a postinfective chorea occurring largely in chil-dren and young adults. Streptococcal infection is one cause: under half the cases follow within 3 months of rheumatic fever (p. 79). It may recur, or appear, in adult life during pregnancy as chorea gravidarum or in those taking hormonal contraceptives. In each case there is a diffuse mild encephalitis.

The onset of chorea is usually gradual over a few weeks. Irritability, emotional lability, and inattentiveness herald fidgety movements, sometimes predominantly unilateral. A minority of patients become confused. Although rheumatic heart disease is sometimes found, the patient is usually afebrile and lacks other features of rheumatic fever (p. 79). Antistreptolysin-O (ASO) titre and ESR are often normal. Patients may require sedation but recovery occurs spontaneously within weeks or months. Phenoxymethylpenicillin should continue to the age of 20 to prevent rheumatic heart disease.

Hemiballismus (see p. 1146 and Fig. 20.9)

Hemiballismus (also called hemiballism) describes vio-lent swinging movements of one side caused usually by infarction or haemorrhage in the contralateral sub-thalamic nucleus.

Myoclonus

Myoclonus is sudden, involuntary jerking of a single muscle or a group of muscles. It occurs in a wide range of disorders and is sometimes provoked by sudden stimuli such as loud noise.

Benign essential myoclonus

Nocturnal myoclonus – sudden jerking of the body or a limb on falling asleep – is extremely common and not pathological.

Paramyoclonus multiplex describes widespread, ran-dom muscle jerking usually occurring in adolescence. Fits do not occur.

Myoclonus in epilepsy

Muscle jerking occurs in many different forms of epilepsy.

Progressive myoclonic epilepsies

These rare conditions include familial and metabolic disorders where myoclonus accompanies progressive encephalopathy. *Lafora body disease* is an example, a syndrome of myoclonus, epilepsy and dementia, with mucopolysaccharide inclusion bodies in neurones, liver cells and intestinal mucosa.

Static myoclonic encephalopathy

Non-progressive myoclonus sometimes develops fol-lowing recovery from severe cerebral anoxia.

Tics

Repetitive twitching movements of the face, neck or hand are part of our normal motor gestures. Patients or their relatives seek advice when movements become fre-quent or irritating. Simple transient tics (e.g. sniffing or a particular facial grimace) are common in childhood, but may persist into adult life. The borderland between normal and pathological is vague.

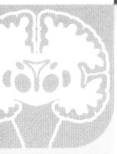

Gilles de la Tourette syndrome

This describes multiple tics (of motor and vocal types) along with behavioural disorders including attention-deficit-hyperactivity disorder (ADHD) and obsessive-compulsive disorder (OCD). It can be accompanied by explosive barking and grunting of sexual obscenities and gestures. The condition develops in childhood or adolescence, more commonly in males, and is lifelong. It is an inherited organic basal ganglia disorder due to a developmental disorder of synaptic neurotransmission. Treatment with haloperidol is sometimes helpful.

Torsion dystonias

Dystonia means movement caused by prolonged muscular contraction – part of the body is thrown into spasm. A brief explanatory classification of these unusual basal ganglia conditions is given in Table 20.42. Their cause is largely unknown.

Primary torsion dystonia (dystonia musculorum deformans)

Dystonia affecting gait and posture commences in childhood and progresses, spreading to all parts of the body over one to four decades. Cognitive function is not impaired. Spontaneous remissions very occasionally occur. This rare disease is usually inherited as an autosomal dominant. A PTD gene has been located on chromosome 9 (9q34); this is a deletion of three base pairs encoding an ATP-binding protein torsin A.

Dopamine-responsive dystonia (DRD)

This lower limb dystonia is almost completely abolished by small doses of levodopa. Typically it causes dystonic difficulty in walking in childhood. The usual form is autosomal dominant DRD with a point mutation of the GTP cyclohydrolase 1 gene on chromosome 14q22.3.

Spasmodic torticollis

Dystonic spasms gradually develop around the neck, usually in the third to fifth decade. These cause the head to turn (torticollis) or to be drawn backwards (retrocollis) or forwards (antecollis). Minor dystonic movements often also affect the trunk and limbs. A curious feature in some patients is a single trigger area, often on the jaw. A gentle touch with a fingertip at this specific site relieves the spasm temporarily. Torticollis may remit but often persists indefinitely.

Writer's cramp

This is a specific inability to perform a previously highly developed skilled movement, especially writing, owing to a curious dystonic posturing. It occurs particularly in those who spend many hours each day writing, and is thus seen less frequently now than in former years. Other skilled functions of the hand are normal and there are no other neurological signs. Prolonged rest sometimes seems to help the condition. It can, however, become a major disability.

Blepharospasm and oromandibular dystonia

These consist of spasms of forced blinking or involuntary movement of the mouth and tongue (e.g. lip-smacking and protrusion of the tongue and jaw). Speech may be affected.

Treatment

All dystonic movement disorders are particularly difficult to help. Butyrophenones (e.g. haloperidol and sulpiride) and anticholinergics (e.g. trihexyphenidyl (benzhexol)) are sometimes helpful. Botulinum toxin carefully sited by injection can help, temporarily, blepharospasm, torticollis and writer's cramp. Neurosurgical treatment, principally stereotactic thalamotomy for torticollis, or neurostimulation brings some temporary alleviation in selected cases.

Table 20.42
A classification of dystonias

Generalized dystonia
Primary torsion dystonia (PTD)
Dopamine-responsive dystonia (DRD)
Drug-induced dystonia (e.g. metoclopramide)
Symptomatic dystonia (e.g. after encephalitis lethargica or in Wilson's disease)
Paroxysmal dystonia (very rare, familial, with marked fluctuation)

Focal dystonia
Spasmodic torticollis
Writer's cramp
Oromandibular dystonia
Blepharospasm
Hemiplegic dystonia (e.g. following stroke)

FURTHER READING

Brooks DJ (2000) Dopamine agonists: their role in the treatment of Parkinson's disease. *Journal of Neurology Neurosurgery and Psychiatry* **68**: 685–690.

Deuschl G (2000) New treatment options for tremor. *New England Journal of Medicine* **342**: 505–507.

Hallett M (1999) One man's poison – clinical applications of botulinum toxin. *New England Journal of Medicine* **341**: 119–120.

Jankovic J (2001) Tourette's syndrome. *New England Journal of Medicine* **345**: 1184–1190.

Lücking C et al. (2000) Association between early-onset PD and mutations in the parkin gene. *New England Journal of Medicine* **342**: 1560-1567.

Marsden CD, Fahn S (eds) (1994) *Movement Disorders*. Oxford: Butterworth-Heinemann.

Schapira AVH (1999) Science, medicine and the future: Parkinson's disease. *British Medical Journal* **318**: 311–314.

Multiple sclerosis (MS)

Prevalence

MS is a common disease of unknown cause in which there are multiple plaques of demyelination within the brain and spinal cord. These are disseminated in time and place, hence the old name disseminated sclerosis. There is genetic predisposition, an acquired defect in the oligodendroglial cells that produce myelin and a demyelinating inflammatory response mediated by CD4 T cells directed against unknown antigens. The most common age of onset is between 20 and 45 years. It is more common in women. In the UK, over 50 000 people are disabled by MS.

The disease occurs world-wide, but prevalence varies widely, being directly proportional to distance from the equator. At latitudes of 50–65 degrees north, roughly from southern England to Iceland, prevalence is 60–100 per 100 000 people; at latitudes less than 30 degrees north prevalence is less than 10 per 100 000; and at the equator it is a rarity. In the southern hemisphere the trend is similar, with progressive increase in prevalence away from the equator.

Aetiology

The precise cause of the disease is unknown.

Familial incidence, HLA linkage and migration

First-degree relatives of a patient have an increased chance of developing MS, although there is no clear-cut pattern of inheritance. There is a concordance rate of 31% amongst monozygotic twins.

In Caucasians in northern Europe and the USA, there is a positive association between MS and antigens HLA-A3, B7, D2 and DR2. Immigrants from low to high prevalence zones (e.g. from near the equator to northern Europe) acquire the prevalence of the country of their destination, provided they arrive before the age of 10.

Infection

Although efforts to transmit MS experimentally have been uniformly unsuccessful, an abnormal immune response in many MS patients produces increased titres of serum and CSF antibodies to many common viruses, particularly measles. No definite links exist between MS and any known infection. Some epidemic transmissible zoonoses, such as scrapie, the demyelinating disease in sheep, have some similarities to MS. Human T-cell leukaemia virus 1 (HTLV-1) in humans causes tropical spastic paraparesis (p. 1145); this seems to have no relevance to MS.

Diet

It has been suggested that MS is related to consumption of large quantities of animal fats. Surveys in Norway have shown that MS is distinctly uncommon in coastal

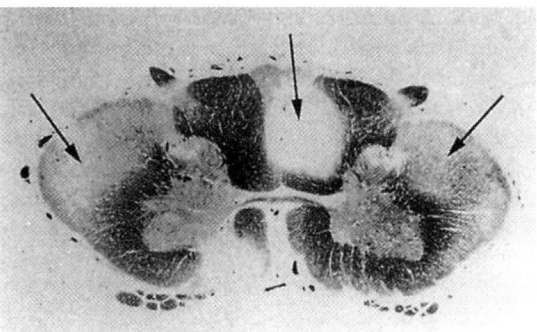

Fig. 20.25 **Multiple sclerosis.** Cross-section of the spinal cord showing demyelination (arrows) in the posterior column and lateral corticospinal tracts. Courtesy of Professor WI Macdonald.

fishing communities compared with agricultural areas. The role of diet is particularly difficult to evaluate.

Pathology (Fig. 20.25)

The essential features are plaques of demyelination, initially 2–10 mm in size. These lesions are perivenular and have a predilection for distinct sites within the brain and spinal cord:

- optic nerves
- periventricular region
- brainstem and its cerebellar connections
- cervical spinal cord – corticospinal tracts and posterior columns.

Acute relapses are caused by focal inflammatory demyelination. Inflammation causes local production of nitric oxide by macrophages, which damages central nerve fibres. Remission occurs when the inflammation decreases. Demyelination also occurs and helps recovery. When damage is severe, secondary permanent axonal destruction follows. In the cord, plaques rarely destroy large groups of neighbouring anterior horn cells – so that focal muscle wasting is unusual. Demyelination in MS never occurs in myelin sheaths of peripheral nerves.

Clinical features

No single group of signs or symptoms is entirely diagnostic of MS. Despite this, the disease is often recognizable on clinical grounds. There are two principal patterns:

- relapsing and remitting MS
- primary progressive MS (c. 20% of cases).

Relapsing and remitting disease may develop into a progressive form (secondary progressive MS). The clinical defects are largely due to nerve conduction blocks, directly from demyelination and indirectly from inflammation.

Occasionally (< 10%) the condition runs a fulminating course over some months (fulminant MS).

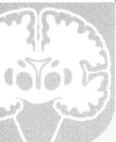

Three characteristic and common presentations of relapsing and remitting MS are described below.

Optic neuropathy (ON)

Symptoms

Blurring of vision in one eye develops over hours or days, varying between a sensation of looking through frosted glass to severe unilateral visual loss, but rarely complete blindness. Mild ocular pain is usual. Recovery occurs, typically within 1 or 2 months. Bilateral ON occasionally occurs.

Signs

The optic disc appearance depends upon the site of the plaque within the optic nerve. When the lesion is in the nerve head there is disc swelling (optic neuritis, p. 1131). If the lesion is several millimetres behind the disc there are often no ophthalmoscopic features – 'the doctor sees nothing and the patient sees nothing'. This is retrobulbar neuritis.

Worsening of vision in ON during a fever, in hot weather or after exercise is known as Uthoff's phenomenon – central conduction is slowed by an increase in local body temperature.

Disc swelling from optic neuritis causes early visual acuity loss, thus distinguishing it from disc swelling from raised intracranial pressure – the latter causes late and sudden visual loss.

A relative afferent pupillary defect (p. 1132) is often recognizable from the early stages. This usually persists after recovery.

Late sequelae of optic neuropathy

There are usually no residual symptoms, but small scotomata and defects in colour vision can be found. Following optic neuropathy, disc pallor appears (optic atrophy), first on the temporal side. Visual evoked responses (VER) remain abnormal (see below).

Brainstem demyelination

An acute episode affecting the brainstem causes various combinations of diplopia, vertigo, facial numbness and/or weakness or dysphagia. Pyramidal signs in the limbs occur when the corticospinal tracts are involved. A typical picture is sudden diplopia and vertigo with nystagmus, but without tinnitus or deafness. This lasts for some weeks before recovery. Diplopia in MS is the result of many different lesions – a sixth nerve lesion and internuclear ophthalmoplegia (INO) are two examples.

Spinal cord lesion

Spastic paraparesis developing over days or weeks (p. 1145) is the typical result of a plaque of demyelination in the cervical or thoracic cord. There is difficulty in walking and sensory disturbance. Lhermitte's sign may be present (p. 1151). Urinary symptoms are common.

Unusual presentations

Epilepsy and trigeminal neuralgia (p. 1137) occur more commonly in MS patients than in the general population. Tonic spasms or brief spasms of a limb are other unusual presentations. Organic psychosis is occasionally seen in early MS.

End-stage multiple sclerosis

In the later stages, MS causes severe disability with a combination of spastic tetraparesis, ataxia, optic atrophy, nystagmus, brainstem signs (e.g. bilateral INO), pseudobulbar palsy, and incontinence of urine. Dementia is common. Death follows from uraemia and/or bronchopneumonia.

Differential diagnosis

Few other neurological diseases of young people follow a similar relapsing and remitting course. Thromboembolism causes events with more sudden onset. Other degenerative conditions, such as Friedreich's ataxia, are gradually progressive, without remissions. Following an isolated neurological event it is often impossible to be sure, even with MR imaging, whether or not a lesion is due to MS. The pattern of subsequent lesions leads to the clinical diagnosis. Remissions may last for several or more years; their length is unpredictable and the mechanism of relapse and remission unclear.

Individual plaques (e.g. in optic nerve, brainstem or cord) must be distinguished from mass, vascular or other inflammatory lesions. Of the latter, CNS sarcoidosis, SLE and Behçet's syndrome may mimic relapsing MS. Adrenoleucodystrophy (a disorder of saturated fatty acid deposition in lipid-containing tissues) can cause a progressive paraparesis identical to chronic progressive MS.

Investigations

MRI of brain and spinal cord is the first-line investigation where available. Multiple plaques are visible, principally in the periventricular region (Fig. 20.15o, p. 1155), brainstem, and cervical cord. Lesions are rarely visible on CT. Peripheral blood and urine tests are unhelpful.

With diagnostic MR images and a compatible clinical picture, CSF examination is often unnecessary but would show, in 80% of cases, oligoclonal IgG bands indicating immunoglobulin production within the CNS in response to an unknown antigen, and a raised mononuclear cell count of 5–60 cells/mm^3.

Electrophysiological tests

Delay in visual-evoked responses (VER) follows optic neuropathy. As some ON attacks are subclinical, a delayed VER can provide evidence of a previous optic nerve lesion. This provides valuable evidence of a second CNS lesion in, for example, an undiagnosed and apparently solitary spinal cord lesion.

Brainstem and somatosensory evoked potentials become delayed when these pathways have been damaged. Peripheral nerve studies are normal and EEG unhelpful.

Management and prognosis

Once diagnosed, practical decisions need to be taken about employment, home and plans for the future in the face of a potentially disabling disease. There is no curative treatment.

There is no method of predicting the course of MS. There is wide variation in severity. Many patients continue to live self-sufficient, productive lives while others become gravely disabled.

Straightforward advice, tempered with reassurance of the benign course of many cases of MS is important. The MS Society, a national UK charity, and others have helpful literature.

Therapy

Many forms of MS treatment have been marketed, among them cryotherapy, pyrotherapy, radiotherapy, various vaccines, purified TB protein derivative (PPD), transfer factor, electrical stimulation, gluten-free diets, sunflower seed oil, arsenicals and hyperbaric oxygen. None has been shown to improve outcome.

- Short courses of corticosteroids, such as i.v. methylprednisolone for several days, are used widely in relapses and do sometimes reduce their severity. They do not influence long-term outcome.
- Beta-interferon (both interferon beta 1b and 1a) by self-administered injection is available in relapsing and remitting disease. This reduces the relapse rate by a third and prevents an increase in lesions seen on MRI over time. Long-term outcome seems unaltered. Unwanted effects are 'flu-like symptoms and irritation at the injection site. Cost–benefit analyses are serious issues with beta-interferon: the drug is expensive.
- Immunosuppressants (azathioprine, cyclophosphamide) are also used, but there is little consensus about their role.
- Other new therapies, such as glatiramer acetate reduce the frequency of relapses but are less effective in slowing the progression of disability.

The rehabilitative approach in MS

There is much to be done for a patient with any chronic disabling disease. Practical advice at work, on walking aids, wheelchairs, car conversions, alterations to houses and gardens is needed, from professionals with experience of rehabilitation. Wide-ranging support – for fear, reactive depression and sexual difficulties – is also helpful. Multidisciplinary team liaison between patient, carers, medical practitioners, and therapists is essential.

Treatment of intercurrent infections is necessary. Urinary infection frequently exacerbates the symptoms.

Urinary incontinence may be helped by oxybutinin and/or intermittent self-catheterization.

Physiotherapy is of particular value in reducing the pain and discomfort of spasticity, particularly flexor spasms of the lower limbs. Muscle relaxants (e.g. baclofen, benzodiazepines and dantrolene) are also sometimes helpful. Injected botulinum toxin is sometimes used for severe spasticity. Prevention of pressure sores is vital. 4-Amidopyridine is sometimes used on a trial basis to improve strength, and amantadine for general fatigue.

FURTHER READING

Confaureux C et al. (2000) Relapses and progression of disability in multiple sclerosis. *New England Journal of Medicine* **343**: 1430–1438.

Goodkin DE (1999) Interferon *beta* therapy for multiple sclerosis. *Lancet* **352**: 1486–1490.

Kraft GH (1999) Rehabilitation still the only way to improve function in MS. *Lancet* **354**: 2016–2017.

Lublin FD, Reingold SC (1996) Defining the clinical course of MS: results of an international survey. *Neurology* **46**: 907–911.

Noseworthy JH et al. (2000) Multiple sclerosis. *New England Journal of Medicine* **343**: 938–952.

Paty DW, Arnold DL (2002) The lesions of multiple sclerosis. *New England Journal of Medicine* **346**: 199–200.

UK NATIONAL CHARITY

The MS Society www.mssociety.org.uk

CNS infection and inflammation

Meningitis

The word 'meningitis' usually describes inflammation owing to infective agents (Table 20.43). Microorganisms reach the meninges either by direct extension from the ears, nasopharynx, cranial injury or congenital meningeal defect, or by bloodstream spread. Immunocompromised patients (e.g. HIV, cytotoxic drugs) are at increased risk of meningeal infection by unusual organisms. Non-infectious causes of inflammation include malignant cells, drugs and blood following subarachnoid haemorrhage.

Pathology

In acute bacterial meningitis, the pia–arachnoid is congested with polymorphs. A layer of pus forms that may organize to form adhesions, causing cranial nerve palsies and hydrocephalus.

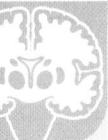

Table 20.43
Infective causes of meningitis in the UK

Bacteria
*Neisseria meningitidis**
*Streptococcus pneumoniae**
Staphylococcus aureus
Streptococcus Group B
Listeria monocytogenes
Gram-negative bacilli
Mycobacterium tuberculosis
Treponema pallidum

Viruses
Enteroviruses
    Echo
    Coxsackie
Mumps
Herpes simplex
HIV
Epstein–Barr virus

Fungi
Cryptococcus neoformans
Candida
(*Coccidioides immitis, Histoplasma capsulatum, Blastomyces
    dermatitidis* in USA)

* These organisms account for 70% of acute bacterial meningitis outside
the neonatal period. A wide variety of infective agents are responsible for
the remaining 30% of cases. *Haemophilus influenzae b* has been
eliminated as a cause in the UK by immunization

Table 20.44
Clinical clues in meningitis

Clinical feature	Probable cause
Petechial rash	Meningococcal infection
Skull fracture Ear disease Congenital CNS lesion }	Pneumococcal infection
Immunocompromised patients	HIV opportunistic infection
Rash or pleurodynia	Enterovirus infection
International travel	Poliomyelitis Malaria
Occupational history (working with drains, canals, polluted river water, recreational swimming): prostration, myalgia, conjunctivitis and jaundice	Leptospirosis

In chronic infection (e.g. TB), the brain is covered in a viscous greyish green exudate with numerous meningeal tubercles. Adhesions are invariable. Cerebral oedema is common in any bacterial meningitis.

In viral meningitis there is a predominantly lymphocytic inflammatory CSF reaction without pus formation, polymorphs or adhesions; there is little or no cerebral oedema unless encephalitis develops.

Clinical features
The meningitic syndrome

This is a simple clinical triad: headache, neck stiffness and fever. Photophobia and vomiting are often present. In acute bacterial infection there is usually intense malaise, fever, rigors, severe headache, photophobia and vomiting. This develops within hours or minutes. The patient is irritable and often prefers to lie still. Neck stiffness and a positive Kernig's sign usually appear within hours.

In less severe cases (e.g. many *viral* meningitides) there are less prominent meningitic signs, but fatal *bacterial* infection may also be indolent, with a deceptively mild onset – *apparently mild* clinical pictures are diagnostically unreliable. Misinterpretation has led to many fatalities.

In uncomplicated meningitis, consciousness remains intact, although the patient with a high fever may be delirious. Progressive drowsiness, lateralizing signs and cranial nerve lesions indicate complications such as venous sinus thrombosis (p. 1173), severe cerebral oedema, hydrocephalus, or an alternative diagnosis such as cerebral abscess (p. 1198) or encephalitis (p. 1194). Papilloedema may develop.

Specific varieties of meningitis
Clinical clues point to the diagnosis (Table 20.44).

Acute bacterial meningitis
The onset is typically sudden, with rigors and a high fever. Meningococcal meningitis is often heralded by a petechial or other rash, sometimes sparse (see Emergency box 20.1). The meningitis may be part of a generalized meningococcal septicaemia (p. 78). Acute septicaemic shock may develop in any bacterial meningitis.

Viral meningitis
This is almost always a benign, self-limiting condition lasting 4–10 days. Headache may follow for some months but there are no serious sequelae.

Chronic meningitis (see below)
Differential diagnosis
It may be difficult to distinguish between the sudden headache of subarachnoid haemorrhage, migraine and acute meningitis. Meningitis should be considered seriously in anyone with a sudden headache, and anyone with headache and fever. Neck stiffness should be assessed carefully – it may not be obvious. Chronic meningitis sometimes resembles an intracranial mass lesion, with headache, epilepsy and focal signs. Cerebral malaria often mimics bacterial meningitis.

Management
Recognition and immediate treatment of acute bacterial meningitis is vital. In this acute illness, minutes save

lives. The condition is lethal, and even with optimal care mortality is around 15%.

When meningococcal meningitis is diagnosed clinically by the petechial rash, immediate parenteral antibiotic treatment should be given before any investigations (see Emergency box 20.1). Lumbar puncture is usually contraindicated if the clinical diagnosis is meningococcal disease, because coning of the cerebellar tonsils may follow – the organism is found by blood culture. If a presumptive diagnosis of the organism can be made (e.g. pneumococcus is likely when there is sinus infection or skull fracture), treatment should also be started immediately. A scheme for immediate antibiotic treatment in acute bacterial meningitis is given in Table 20.45.

Thereafter, if there is any suspicion of an intracranial mass lesion, an immediate CT scan should be carried out. Lumbar puncture should follow if deemed safe. Typical CSF changes are shown in Table 20.46. CSF pressure is characteristically elevated.

Blood should be taken for cultures and glucose level as well as for routine tests. Chest and skull films should be taken if appropriate.

CSF stains demonstrate organisms (e.g. Gram-positive intracellular diplococci – pneumococcus; Gram-negative cocci – meningococcus). Ziehl–Nielsen stain demonstrates acid-fast bacilli (tuberculosis), though organisms are rarely numerous. Indian ink stains fungi.

It cannot be emphasized enough that meticulous attention should focus on microbiological studies in suspected CNS infection. Close liaison between clinician and microbiologist is essential. Specific techniques (e.g. polymerase chain reaction to identify meningococci and other bacteria) are sometimes invaluable. Syphilitic serology should always be carried out.

The clinical picture and CSF examination should thus determine a presumptive cause of acute meningitis within several hours. Typically treatment must begin before an absolute diagnosis (of the actual organism) is achieved.

If bacterial meningitis is diagnosed, discussion with the microbiologist should extend to the choice of antibiotics, drug resistance, recent infections in the locality, and questions of barrier nursing and prophylaxis.

In bacterial meningitis in children, dexamethasone is also given as this reduces the frequency of complications, particularly deafness.

Intrathecal antibiotics are no longer given in meningitis.

Local infection (e.g. an infected paranasal sinus) should be treated, surgically if necessary. Surgical repair of depressed skull fracture or meningeal tear may be required.

Prophylaxis

Meningococcal infection condition should be notified to local public health authorities, and advice sought

Emergency box 20.1

Meningococcal meningitis and meningococcaemia: emergency treatment

Suspicion of meningococcal infection is a medical emergency requiring treatment *immediately* medical contact takes place. In meningococcal meningitis, fever, headache and neck stiffness are accompanied or heralded by a petechial, or non-specific blotchy red rash. However, all these features may not be present – and meningococcal infection may sometimes begin as an apparently intercurrent, non-serious viral infection.

The *immediate* management of suspected meningococcal infection is benzylpenicillin 1200 mg (adult dose) either by slow i.v. injection or intramuscularly, prior to investigations. Cefotaxime 1 g i.v. is an alternative in cases of penicillin allergy. In this condition, minutes count and any delay is unacceptable.

On arrival in hospital, routine tests including blood cultures should be carried out *immediately*, and a close lookout kept for the emergence of septicaemic shock. For further management and prophylaxis, see text.

Table 20.45
Antibiotics and acute bacterial meningitis

Organism	Antibiotic	Alternative (e.g. allergy)
Unknown pyogenic	Cefotaxime	Benzylpenicillin and chloramphenicol
Meningococcus	Benzylpenicillin	Cefotaxime
Pneumococcus	Cefotaxime	Penicillin
Haemophilus	Cefotaxime	Chloramphenicol

Table 20.46
Typical CSF changes in meningitis

	Normal	Viral	Pyogenic	Tuberculosis
Appearance	Crystal-clear	Clear/turbid	Turbid/purulent	Turbid/viscous
Mononuclear cells	< 5 mm^3	10–100 mm^3	< 50 mm^3	100–300 mm^3
Polymorph cells	Nil	Nil*	200–300/mm^3	0–200/mm^3
Protein	0.2–0.4 g/L	0.4–0.8 g/L	0.5–2.0 g/L	0.5–3.0 g/L
Glucose	$^2/_3 > ^1/_2$ blood glucose	$> ^1/_2$ blood glucose	$< ^1/_2$ blood glucose	$< ^1/_2$ blood glucose

* Some polymorph cells may be seen in the early stages of viral meningitis and encephalitis

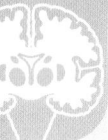
about immunization and prophylaxis of contacts with rifampicin. *MenC*, a meningococcal C conjugate vaccine is available and is part of routine childhood UK immunization. Reported cases have reduced. This vaccine should be given to case contacts. A combined A and C meningococcal vaccine is sometimes used for travel purposes. There is no vaccine for Group B.

Recurrent pneumococcal meningitis, e.g. after a CSF leak following skull fracture, can be prevented by a polyvalent vaccine.

Hib, the *Haemophilus influenzae* vaccine is given routinely in childhood in the UK: this has virtually eliminated a previously common cause of childhood meningitis.

Chronic meningitis

Tuberculous meningitis (TBM) and cryptococcal meningitis commence typically with vague headache, lassitude, anorexia and vomiting. Acute meningitis can occur but is unusual; meningitic signs usually take some weeks to develop. Drowsiness, focal signs (e.g. diplopia, papilloedema, hemiparesis) and seizures are common. Syphilis, sarcoidosis and Behçet's syndrome also cause chronic meningitis. In some chronic cases a cause is never found.

Management of TBM

This is a common and serious disease world-wide. Brain imaging may show meningeal enhancement, hydrocephalus and tuberculomas (p. 1198); it may, however, remain normal. Typical CSF changes are seen in Table 20.46. In many cases organisms – which are sparse – will not be seen on Ziehl–Nielson staining. Repeated diagnostic CSF examination is often necessary.

In TBM it will be some weeks before CSF cultures are confirmatory: treatment with antituberculous drugs (p. 895) – rifampicin, isoniazid and pyrazinamide – must commence on a presumptive basis and continue for at least 9 months. Relapses and complications (e.g. seizures, hydrocephalus) are common in TBM. The mortality remains over 60% even with early treatment.

Malignant meningitis

Malignant cells can cause a subacute or chronic non-infective meningitic process. A meningitic syndrome, cranial nerve palsies, paraparesis and root lesions are seen, often in confusing and fluctuating patterns. The CSF cell count is raised, with high protein and low glucose. Treatment with intrathecal cytotoxic agents is rarely helpful.

Cells in a sterile CSF

Diagnostic difficulties arise when there is a raised CSF cell count but no evident infecting organism. The usual situation is a mixture of lymphocytes and polymorphs, i.e. a CSF pleocytosis. Table 20.47 outlines conditions where this occurs.

Table 20.47
Causes of sterile CSF (pleocytosis)

Partially treated bacterial meningitis	Cerebral venous thrombosis
Viral meningitis	Cerebral infarction
Tuberculosis or fungal infection	Following subarachnoid haemorrhage
Neoplastic meningitis	Encephalitis, including HIV
Parameningeal foci (e.g. paranasal sinus)	Rare causes (e.g. cerebral malaria, sarcoidosis, Behçet's syndrome,
Syphilis	Lyme disease, endocarditis,
Intracranial abscess	cerebral vasculitis/angiitis)

FURTHER READING

Buttery JP, Moxon ER (2000) Designing meningitis vaccines. *Journal of the Royal College of Physicians of London* **34**: 1263–1268.

Department of Health (1999) Replacement Chapter 23 in 'Immunisation Against Infectious Disease. 1996'. [PL CMO (99) 4, PL CNO (99) 8, PL CPHO (99) 3].

Morley SL, Levin M (1998) Bacterial meningitis. *Prescribers' Journal* **38**: 129–141.

INFORMATION FOR PATIENTS

Knowing about meningitis and septicaemia (a leaflet for parents). Department of Health, PO Box 410, Wetherby LS23 7LN.

UK NATIONAL CHARITY

www.meningitis-trust.org.uk

Encephalitis

Encephalitis is inflammation of brain parenchyma, usually viral. Brain inflammation also develops secondarily in bacterial and fungal meningitis.

Acute viral encephalitis

The usual organisms cultured from adult UK cases are herpes simplex, ECHO, Coxsackie, mumps and Epstein–Barr viruses. Adenovirus, varicella zoster, influenza, measles and other viruses are rarer; in many cases a viral aetiology is presumed but not confirmed.

Epidemic and endemic viral encephalitides occur world-wide, for example:

- Japanese encephalitis in South East Asia
- Ross River fever in Australia
- California encephalitis in the USA
- Ömsk haemorrhagic fever in Russia
- Tick-borne flavivirus encephalitis in Sweden and Central Europe
- West Nile encephalitis in Egypt and Sudan.

Epidemic viral encephalitides with new or unusual organisms are common. For example, encephalitis caused by Nipah-virus, hitherto not known to cause disease in man, occurred in 1998 in abattoir workers in Malaysia; in New York in 1999 West Nile virus caused an encephalitis epidemic. Rabies (p. 60) is a variety of sporadic viral encephalitis.

Clinical features
Many encephalitides are mild and self-limiting. In a minority, more serious illness develops with high fever, headache, mood change and drowsiness over several hours to several days. Focal signs, seizures and coma ensue. Death, or severe lasting brain injury follows. Herpes simplex virus (HSV-1) accounts for many of these severe infections in Britain. Mortality remains around 20%. In South East Asia, Japanese arbovirus encephalitis is more usual, causing a serious illness with higher mortality than herpes simplex.

Differential diagnosis
This includes:

- bacterial meningitis with cerebral oedema
- cerebral venous thrombosis
- cerebral abscess
- acute disseminated encephalomyelitis (see below)
- cerebral malaria
- toxic confusional states
- septicaemia, febrile illness.

Investigations
CT and MR imaging show diffuse areas of oedema, often in the temporal lobes. EEG shows characteristic slow wave changes; this is useful in doubtful cases. A normal EEG is exceptional in encephalitis. CSF shows a raised cell count. Specific viral blood and CSF serology is helpful. Brain biopsy is seldom performed.

Treatment
Suspected herpes simplex encephalitis is treated immediately with intravenous aciclovir, the active form of which inhibits DNA synthesis. Phosphorylation of aciclovir is dependent upon viral thymidine kinase; the drug is thus specific for herpesvirus infections. A poor outlook usually follows coma whether or not aciclovir has been given. Supportive measures are required for comatose patients; seizures are treated with anticonvulsants.

Prophylactic immunization against Japanese encephalitis is sometimes advised for travellers to endemic areas in South East Asia.

FURTHER READING

Editorial (2000) Exotic diseases close to home. *Lancet* **354**: 1221.

Whitley RJ, Gnann JW (2002) Viral encephalitis. *Lancet* **359**: 507–514.

Acute disseminated encephalomyelitis (ADEM)
ADEM follows many common viral infections (e.g. measles, varicella zoster, mumps and rubella) and rarely immunization against rabies, influenza or pertussis. The clinical syndrome is often similar to acute viral encephalitis, with added focal brainstem and/or spinal cord lesions due to demyelination (MS, p. 1189). Viral particles are not present in the multiple foci seen on T2-weighted MR images. Prognosis is variable. Mild cases recover completely, but after severe coma mortality is around 25%. Survivors often have permanent brain damage. Treatment is supportive with steroids and anticonvulsants.

Myelitis

Myelitis means spinal cord inflammation causing paraparesis or tetraparesis. This occurs with varicella zoster or postinfective encephalomyelitis (ADEM). Poliomyelitis is a specific spinal cord anterior horn cell enterovirus infection (p. 51). Transverse myelitis is mentioned on page 1207.

Herpes zoster (shingles)

This is a recrudescence of varicella zoster virus infection within dorsal root ganglia, the original infection having been acquired in an attack of chickenpox many years previously. Chickenpox and shingles viruses are identical.

Clinical features
The rashes of shingles are described on page 1277.

In the cranial nerves, herpes zoster has a predilection for the fifth and seventh nerves. Ophthalmic herpes is infection of the first division of the fifth nerve and may lead to corneal scarring and secondary panophthalmitis. Geniculate herpes (the geniculate ganglion of the VIIth nerve) is also called Ramsay Hunt syndrome (p. 1138). Local complications of shingles are secondary bacterial infection, very rarely purpura and necrosis in the affected segment (*purpura fulminans*), generalized herpes zoster, and postherpetic neuralgia. Myelitis, meningo-encephalitis and motor radiculopathy (usually lumbar or brachial) also follow varicella zoster. Treatment with aciclovir is described above.

Postherpetic neuralgia
Postherpetic neuralgia is pain in the zone of previous shingles; this occurs in some 10% of patients (often elderly). Burning, continuous pain responds poorly to all analgesics. Depression is almost universal. Treatment is unsatisfactory but there is a trend towards gradual

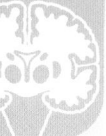

recovery over 2 years. Amitryptyline is commonly used and recently methylprednisolone intrathecally has been shown sometimes to be beneficial.

Neurosyphilis

Syphilis is described on page 125. Tertiary neurosyphilis described below is now rare. A variety of syndromes occur, sometimes in mixed forms.

Asymptomatic neurosyphilis

This describes positive CSF serology without signs.

Meningovascular syphilis

This causes:

- subacute meningitis with cranial nerve palsies and papilloedema
- a gumma – a chronic expanding intracranial mass
- paraparesis caused by a spinal meningovasculitis.

Tabes dorsalis

Demyelination in the dorsal roots causes a complex deafferentation syndrome. The elements of tabes are:

- lightning pains (p. 1151)
- ataxia, stamping gait, reflex and sensory loss, muscle wasting
- neuropathic joints (Charcot joints)
- Argyll Robertson pupils (p. 1134)
- ptosis and optic atrophy.

General paralysis of the insane (GPI)

The grandiose title describes madness and weakness. GPI dementia is, however, often similar to that of Alzheimer's disease (p. 1264). Progressive cognitive decline, seizures, brisk reflexes, extensor plantar reflexes and tremor develop. Death follows within 3 years. Argyll Robertson pupils are usual.

Other forms of neurosyphilis

In *congenital* neurosyphilis (acquired in utero), features of both tabes dorsalis and GPI develop in childhood – taboparesis.

In *secondary* syphilis, a self-limiting meningeal reaction occurs. This is either symptomless or may cause subacute meningitis.

Treatment

Benzylpenicillin 1 g daily by injection for 10 days in primary infection eliminates the risk of future tertiary syphilis. Established neurological disease can be arrested but not usually reversed. Parenteral penicillin is given for 2–3 weeks. Allergic reactions (Jarisch–Herxheimer reactions) may occur; high-dose steroid cover is usually given (of no proven benefit) with penicillin to reduce severity.

HIV and neurology (p. 136)

HIV-infected individuals frequently present with or develop a wide variety of neurological conditions that require speedy and expert treatment. In addition, these patients have a high rate of cerebrovascular disease.

Brain and meningeal disease

Meningitis

Acute aseptic meningitis is a primary HIV infection. Spontaneous recovery is usual.

Chronic meningitis occurs with fungal infections (e.g. *Cryptococcus neoformans* or *Aspergillus*), tuberculosis, *Listeria, Escherichia coli* or other organisms. Aggressive treatment is essential.

Diffuse encephalopathies

AIDS-dementia complex (ADC). This diffuse, progressive, usually fatal HIV-related dementia, is sometimes associated with a cerebellar syndrome.

Encephalitis and brain abscess. Toxoplasma, cytomegalovirus, herpes simplex, and other organisms cause a severe and often fatal encephalitis, commonly with multiple brain abscesses.

CNS lymphoma. This is a progressive disease with a poor prognosis (p. 144).

Progressive multifocal leucoencephalopathy. PML is due to papovavirus (p. 50).

Spinal cord disease

Paraparesis occurs in HIV in several clinical settings:

- acute transverse myelitis – a primary HIV myelitis with spontaneous recovery
- myelopathy due to infection, e.g. herpes simplex, zoster or cytomegalovirus
- CNS lymphoma (causing cord compression or malignant meningitis).

Peripheral nerve disease

Neuropathies (particularly sensory) occur:

- mononeuropathy (e.g. a common peroneal nerve lesion)
- mononeuritis multiplex (p. 1213)
- polyneuropathy (p. 1217).

An autonomic neuropathy also occurs (p. 136)

Management of HIV

This is discussed on page 146. The incidence of many of the above conditions is reduced because of the use of HAART.

FURTHER READING

Guiloff R (1999) Infections in the immunocompromised and post transplant patient. I & II. *CPD Bulletin Neurology* **1**: 3–7, 46–50.

Other infections

Many other infections involve the central nervous system and are discussed in Chapter 2, e.g. rabies, tetanus, botulism, Lyme disease, leprosy and poliomyelitis.

Creutzfeldt–Jakob disease (CJD) (p. 63)

Sporadic, iatrogenic and familial forms. This rare slowly progressive dementia develops usually after 50 years of age and is recognized pathologically by spongiform changes in the brain. CJD, a prion (proteinaceous infectious particle) disease, occurs world-wide and is transmitted by an agent resistant to many sterilization processes. Prion protein (PrP) diseases are associated with accumulation of a disease-related isoform, PrP^{Sc}, derived from its normal cellular precursor, PrP^{C}. Sporadic CJD cases are usually single. Transmission from surgical specimens, autopsy transplant material (e.g. corneal grafts), and human growth hormone has also occurred (iatrogenic CJD). Iatrogenic CJD has a long incubation period, up to 5 years. Death is invariable within 6 months of clinical onset in both iatrogenic and sporadic forms. No treatment alters the course. There is a rare familial form of CJD. CJD pathology is very similar to bovine spongiform encephalopathy (BSE, 'mad cow disease'), recognized first in Britain in the early 1980s.

Incidence. Sporadic CJD occurs world-wide with an annual incidence <1 per million; some 30–55 cases occur annually in the UK. The numbers have not been rising. The incidence of iatrogenic CJD is lower, between 0 and 6 UK cases annually. Familial CJD cases, 0–4 annually in Britain, are associated with mutations of the prion protein (PrP) gene. An even rarer form, the Gerstmann–Straüssler–Scheinker syndrome, is an inherited autosomal recessive condition, typified by chronic progressive ataxia and terminal dementia, with duration 2–10 years.

Variant CJD (vCJD) was noted in Britain in 1995 and numbers of infected cases are rising. vCJD cases are younger than sporadic cases with a mean age of 29 years. Early symptoms are neuropsychiatric, followed by ataxia, and dementia with myoclonus or chorea. vCJD has a longer course than the sporadic form – up to several years. vCJD and BSE are caused by the same prion strain, giving rise to speculation that transmission from animal to human food chain has occurred, with infection from BSE-infected cattle to humans (p. 63). A common source of infection for both man and cattle is an alternative explanation.

Kuru

This dementia and cerebellar ataxia, another prion disease, is described on page 63. Spongiform change occurs in the brain, very similar to CJD.

Miscellaneous inflammatory conditions

Subacute sclerosing panencephalitis (SSPE)

Persistence of measles antigen in the CNS is believed to cause this rare late sequel of measles. Progressive mental deterioration, fits, myoclonus and pyramidal signs develop, usually in a child. Diagnosis is confirmed by high measles antibody titre in blood and CSF. Measles immunization protects against SSPE, which is now almost unknown in the UK.

Progressive rubella encephalitis

Some 10 years after primary rubella infection, this syndrome, rarer than SSPE, causes progressive mental impairment, fits, optic atrophy, cerebellar and pyramidal signs. Antibody to rubella viral antigen is produced locally within the CNS. This condition has not been seen following rubella immunization.

Reye's syndrome (see also p. 385)

This severe encephalitic illness of children is accompanied by fatty infiltration of liver, with hypoglycaemia.

Mollaret's meningitis

This describes recurrent self-limiting episodes of aseptic meningitis (i.e. where no bacterial cause is found) over many years. A recurrent viral infection is postulated.

Vogt–Koyanagi–Harada syndrome

This obscure recurrent inflammation of cells of neural crest origin causes uveitis, meningoencephalitis, vitiligo, deafness and alopecia.

Toxic leukoencephalopathy

This disorder is due to exposure to a wide variety of agents, such as drugs (illicit and therapeutic, e.g. chemotherapy), cranial irradiation and environmental toxins. Damage to the cerebral white matter is seen on MRI. Clinical features vary from forgetfulness and dementia to confusional state.

Myalgic encephalomyelitis (ME, epidemic neuromyasthenia, chronic fatigue syndrome)

(see p. 1234)

Neurosarcoidosis

Sarcoid CNS lesions with or without systemic sarcoidosis, cause chronic meningoencephalitis, spinal cord disease, cranial nerve palsies, particularly bilateral seventh nerve lesions, polyneuropathy, and myopathy (p. 897).

Behçet's syndrome (see also p. 568)

Behçet's three principal features are recurrent oral and/or genital ulceration, inflammatory ocular disease

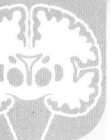

and neurological syndromes. Brainstem and cord lesions, aseptic meningitis (meningitis with cells in CSF but no infective agent), encephalitis and cerebral venous thrombosis occur in less than a third of cases.

Granulomatous (or isolated, primary cerebral) angiitis

In this rare condition there is necrotizing inflammation of segments of brain and leptomeningeal vessels. Stroke-like episodes, seizures and confusional states develop. There is some response to steroid and immunosuppressive therapy.

Brain and spinal abscesses

Brain abscess (see Fig. 20.15m, p. 1155)

This focal bacterial infection behaves as an expanding mass (p. 1200). Typical bacteria are *Streptococcus milleri*, *Bacteroides* species and staphylococci. Mixed infections are common. Multiple abscesses develop, particularly in HIV-positive patients. Fungi also cause brain abscesses. A parameningeal infective focus (e.g. ear, nose, paranasal sinus, skull fracture) or a distant source of infection (e.g. lung, heart, abdomen) may be present. Frequently, however, no cause is found. An abscess is 10 times rarer than a brain tumour in the UK.

Clinical features

Headache, focal signs (e.g. hemiparesis, aphasia, hemianopia), epilepsy and raised intracranial pressure develop. Fever, leucocytosis and raised ESR are usual though not invariable. Abscesses may also be indolent, developing over weeks, particularly in the cerebral hemispheres. Cerebellar abscesses tend to develop rapidly over days or hours, producing hydrocephalus.

Management

Urgent imaging is essential. The search for a local focus of infection should include a detailed examination of the skull, ears and paranasal sinuses; distant foci, such as the heart and abdomen should be considered. Lumbar puncture without prior imaging is contraindicated in suspected brain abscess, and rarely gives diagnostically useful information if an abscess is present.

Treatment demands liaison between neurosurgeon and microbiologist. Surgical decompression may be necessary if parenteral antibiotics are unsuccessful. Despite treatment, mortality remains high at around 25%. Epilepsy is common in survivors.

Brain tuberculoma

Tubercle bacilli cause chronic caseating intracranial granulomas – tuberculomas. These are the most common intracranial masses in countries such as India where TB is common. Brain tuberculomas either present as mass lesions de novo or develop during tuberculous

meningitis. They can also be symptomless, appearing on imaging as areas of intracranial calcification. Spinal cord tuberculomas also occur.

Subdural empyema and intracranial epidural abscess

Intracranial subdural empyema is a collection of subdural pus, usually secondary to local skull or middle ear infection. The features are similar to those of a cerebral abscess. Imaging is diagnostic.

In intracranial epidural abscess, a thin layer of pus tracks along the epidural space causing sequential cranial nerve lesions, typically without evidence of raised pressure. There is usually evidence of local infection, e.g. the middle ear. CT imaging is sometimes normal, as the layer of pus is thin (1–3 mm). MRI is the test of choice. Drainage is required, with appropriate antibiotics.

Spinal epidural abscess

Staphylococcus aureus is the usual organism, reaching the spine via the bloodstream, possibly from a boil. Fever and usually back pain are followed by paraparesis and/or root lesions. Emergency imaging and antibiotics are essential. Surgical decompression is often necessary.

FURTHER READING

Chief Medical Officer (November 1998) Update 20 *New variant Creutzfeldt–Jakob disease*. London: Department of Health.
Collinge J (1999) Variant Creutzfeldt–Jakob disease. *Lancet* **354**: 317–323.
Filley CM, Kleinschmidt-DeMasters BK (2001) Toxic leukoencephalopathy. *New England Journal of Medicine* **345**: 425–432.
Johnson TJ, Gibbs CJ (1998) Creutzfeldt–Jakob disease and related transmissible spongiform encephalopathies. *New England Journal of Medicine* **339**: 1994–2004.
Scully RE et al. (2000) Granulomatous angiitis. *Case Records of the Massachusetts General Hospital* **342**: 957–965.

Brain tumours

Primary intracranial tumours account for some 10% of neoplasms. The most common tumours are outlined in Table 20.48. See also Figure 20.15 (p. 1155). In general medical practice in the UK, metastases are the most common intracranial tumours. Symptomless meningiomas are commonly found on imaging or at autopsy.

Gliomas

These malignant intrinsic tumours originate in neuroglia, usually within the cerebral hemispheres. Their cause is unknown. Glioma is occasionally associated

Table 20.48
Relative frequency of common intracranial tumours on the basis of clinical presentation

Tumour	Approximate relative frequency
Metastases	50%
Bronchus	
Breast	
Stomach	
Prostate	
Thyroid	
Kidney	
Primary malignant (glioma)	35%
Astrocytoma	
Oligodendroglioma	
Benign	15%
Meningioma	
Neurofibroma	

with neurofibromatosis. Primary intracranial malignant tumours tend to spread by direct extension; they virtually never metastasize outside the CNS.

Astrocytomas
These gliomas arise from astrocytes. They are classified histologically into grades I–IV. Grade I astrocytomas grow slowly over many years, while grade IV tumours cause death within several months. *Cystic* astrocytomas of childhood are relatively benign, and usually cerebellar.

Oligodendrogliomas
These arise from oligodendrocytes. They grow slowly, usually over several decades. Calcification is common.

Meningiomas (Fig. 20.15i, j, k, p. 1155)
These benign tumours arise from the arachnoid membrane and may grow to a large size, usually over years. When close to the skull they erode bone. They often occur along the intracranial venous sinuses, which they may invade. They are rare below the tentorium. Sites of predilection are the parasagittal region, sphenoidal ridge, subfrontal region and skull base.

Neurofibromas (Schwannomas)
These solid benign tumours arise from Schwann cells and occur principally in the cerebellopontine angle, where they arise from the eighth nerve sheath (acoustic neuroma) (p. 1141).

Other neoplasms
Other less common neoplasms include:

- cerebellar haemangioblastoma
- ependymoma of the fourth ventricle
- colloid cyst of the third ventricle
- pinealoma

- chordoma of the skull base
- glomus tumour – of the jugular bulb
- medulloblastoma – a cerebellar childhood tumour
- craniopharyngioma (p. 1010)
- cerebral lymphoma.

Pituitary tumours
These are discussed on page 1009.

Clinical features
Mass lesions within the brain produce symptoms and signs by three mechanisms:

- by direct mass effect on structures that are either destroyed or suffer impairment of function
- by secondary effects of raised intracranial pressure and shift of intracranial contents (e.g. papilloedema, vomiting, headache)
- by provoking either generalized or partial seizures.

Although neoplasms, either secondary or primary, are the most common mass lesions in the UK, cerebral abscess, tuberculoma, subdural and intracranial haematoma can also produce symptoms and signs that are clinically indistinguishable.

Direct effects of mass lesions
The hallmark of a direct effect of a mass is local progressive deterioration of function. Tumours can occur anywhere within the brain. Three examples are given:

- *A left frontal meningioma* caused a frontal lobe syndrome over several years – a vague disturbance of personality, apathy and impairment of intellect. Expressive aphasia was followed by a progressive right hemiparesis as the corticospinal pathways became involved. As the mass enlarged further, pressure headaches and papilloedema developed.
- *A right parietal lobe glioma* caused a left homonymous field defect (optic radiation). Cortical sensory loss in the left limbs and left hemiparesis followed over 3 months. Partial seizures (episodes of tingling of the left limbs) developed.
- *A left eighth nerve sheath neurofibroma* (an acoustic neuroma or Schwannoma) growing in the cerebellopontine angle over 3 years caused progressive perceptive deafness (VIII), vertigo (VIII), numbness of the left side of the face (V) and facial weakness (VII), followed by cerebellar ataxia on the same side. Papilloedema is a late sequel.

With a hemisphere tumour, epilepsy and the direct effects commonly bring the patient to seek medical attention initially. The rate of tumour progression varies greatly, from a few days or weeks in a highly malignant glioma, to several years in the case of a slowly enlarging mass, such as a meningioma. Cerebral oedema surrounds mass lesions: it is difficult on clinical grounds to distinguish its effect from that of the mass itself.

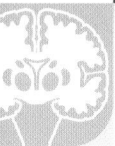

Raised pressure and shift of intracranial contents

Raised intracranial pressure causing headache, vomiting and papilloedema is an important, though relatively unusual, presentation of a mass. These symptoms usually imply hydrocephalus – obstruction to CSF pathways. Typically this is produced early by posterior fossa masses (which obstruct the aqueduct and fourth ventricle) but later with lesions above the tentorium. Shift of the intracranial contents produces symptoms and signs that coexist with the direct effects of an expanding mass:

- *Distortion of the upper brainstem,* as midline structures are displaced either caudally or laterally by a hemisphere mass (Fig. 20.15, p. 1155). This causes impairment of consciousness.
- *Compression of the medulla,* by herniation of the cerebellar tonsils caudally through the foramen magnum – an example of coning – causes impairment of consciousness, respiratory depression, bradycardia, decerebrate posturing and death.
- *False localizing signs* – false only because they do not point directly to the site of the mass.

Three examples of false localizing signs are:

- *A sixth nerve lesion,* first on the side of a mass and later bilaterally. This is caused as the nerve is compressed during its long intracranial course.
- *A third nerve lesion* develops as the temporal lobe uncus herniates caudally, compressing the third nerve against the petroclinoid ligament. The first sign is ipsilateral pupil dilatation as parasympathetic fibres are compressed.
- *Hemiparesis on the same side as a hemisphere tumour* (i.e. the side you would not expect) is produced by compression of the contralateral cerebral peduncle within the brainstem on the free edge of the tentorium.

These false localizing signs, though unusual, are of importance because they indicate that shift of brain has occurred.

Seizures

Partial seizures, simple or complex, that may evolve to generalized tonic–clonic seizures, are characteristic features of many hemisphere masses, whether malignant or benign. Their features are of localizing value (p. 1175).

Investigations

CT and MR imaging

Imaging, usually with contrast, is mandatory when a tumour is suspected. There are, however, limitations to imaging, i.e. cerebral abscess, cerebral infarction as well as benign and malignant tumours have characteristic, but not entirely diagnostic, appearances.

Technetium brain scan

This is of value in diagnosis of destructive skull vault or skull base lesions.

EEG

The EEG is rarely of help in diagnosis. One exception is in cerebral abscess, where characteristic marked focal slow waves are seen.

Skull films (p. 1154)

Skull vault lesions may be seen (e.g. metastases). In pituitary lesions, changes in the dorsum sellae and clinoid processes develop. In hemisphere tumours, plain films have no value.

Routine tests

Since metastases are common, routine tests such as a chest X-ray should be performed.

More specialized neuroradiology

Angiography and volumetric MRI are occasionally used to define blood supply or changing size.

Lumbar puncture

Lumbar puncture is initially contraindicated when the differential diagnosis includes any mass. Examination of CSF rarely yields diagnostically useful information in this situation. The procedure may be followed by immediate herniation of the cerebellar tonsils and should be carried out only after imaging, and after careful consideration.

Biopsy and tumour removal

Stereotactic biopsy via a skull burr-hole is usually carried out to diagnose histologically a suspected hemisphere malignancy. Open exploration at craniotomy is usually carried out when a symptomatic meningioma is found.

Management

Cerebral oedema surrounding a tumour is rapidly reduced by corticosteroids; intravenous or oral dexamethasone is given. Intravenous mannitol, an osmotic diuretic, is also used to reduce oedema. Epilepsy is treated with anticonvulsants.

Whilst complete surgical removal of a brain tumour is an objective, it is not always possible, nor is surgery always necessary. Follow-up with serial imaging is sometimes preferable initially. At surgical exploration, some benign tumours can be entirely removed (e.g. acoustic neuromas, some parasagittal meningiomas). With a brain malignancy it is rarely possible to remove an infiltrating mass. Biopsy and debulking are achieved.

Within the posterior fossa, tumour removal is often necessary because of raised pressure and the danger of coning. Overall mortality for posterior fossa exploration remains around 10%.

Radiotherapy is usually given to gliomas and metastases. An isolated posterior fossa metastasis can sometimes be excised successfully. Chemotherapy has little real value in the majority of primary or secondary brain tumours; vincristine and procarbazine are used. Temozolomide has an active metabolite which interrupts DNA replication by methylation of the 06 position of guanine. Trials suggest a marginal benefit only. Most malignant brain tumours continue to have a poor prognosis despite advances in imaging, surgery, chemotherapy and radiotherapy – less than 50% survival for high-grade gliomas at 2 years. Difficult issues surround the management of these patients.

Idiopathic intracranial hypertension (benign intracranial hypertension)

This syndrome, once called *pseudotumor cerebri*, is included under brain tumours because marked papilloedema develops. There is neither a mass nor an increase in ventricular size. The condition occurs mainly in obese young women with vague menstrual irregularities. Headaches and visual blurring (caused by severe papilloedema) are common. A sixth nerve palsy may be present, as a false localizing sign. The CSF pressure is elevated with normal constituents. Imaging is normal. Steroid therapy is sometimes thought to be a cause and many other drugs have occasionally been implicated. Other causes of papilloedema should be excluded. Sagittal sinus thrombosis sometimes causes a similar picture.

The condition is benign only in that it is not fatal. Infarction of the optic nerve occurs, with consequent visual loss when papilloedema is severe and long-standing. Thiazide diuretics and acetazolamide appear to reduce the intracranial pressure in this condition. Weight reduction is important. Surgical decompression or shunting is sometimes necessary.

FURTHER READING

Batchelor T (2000) Temozolomide for malignant brain tumours. *Lancet* **355**: 1115–1116.

Davies E, Clarke C, Hopkins A (1996) Malignant cerebral glioma. *British Medical Journal* **313**: 1507–1512.

De Angelis LM (2001) Brain tumors. *New England Journal of Medicine* **343**: 114–123.

Pitts LH, Jackler RK (1998) Treatment of acoustic neuromas. *New England Journal of Medicine* **339**: 1471–1473.

Hydrocephalus

Hydrocephalus means an excessive volume of CSF within the cranium. In practice the term hydrocephalus describes different syndromes in which there is, or has been, obstruction to CSF outflow with consequent high pressure and dilatation of the cerebral ventricles. Also, exceptionally an increase in CSF production occurs.

Infantile hydrocephalus

Head enlargement in infancy occurs in 1 in 2000 live births. There are several causes:

- *Arnold–Chiari malformation.* There is elongation of the medulla. Abnormal cerebellar tonsils descend into the cervical canal. Associated spina bifida is common. Syringomyelia may develop (p. 1206).
- *Dandy–Walker syndrome.* There is cerebellar hypoplasia and obstruction to fourth ventricle outflow foramina.
- *Stenosis of the aqueduct of Sylvius* (Fig. 20.15, p. 1155). This is either congenital or acquired following neonatal meningitis or haemorrhage.

No evident cause may be found.

Hydrocephalus in adult life

Hydrocephalus can be an unsuspected symptomless finding on imaging, or infantile hydrocephalus can become apparent in adult life. Combinations of headache, cognitive impairment, vomiting, papilloedema, ataxia and bilateral pyramidal signs occur. Hydrocephalus may develop in other circumstances:

- *Posterior fossa and brainstem tumours* obstruct the aqueduct or fourth ventricular outflow.
- *Following subarachnoid haemorrhage, head injury or meningitis* (particularly tuberculous),
- *A third ventricle colloid cyst* causes lateral ventricle enlargement, headache and papilloedema. These rare intraventricular tumours also sometimes produce intermittent hydrocephalus, recurrent prostrating headaches with episodes of lower limb weakness.
- *Choroid plexus papilloma* (extremely rare) secretes CSF.

Treatment

Ventriculo-atrial or ventriculo-peritoneal shunting becomes necessary when progressive hydrocephalus causes symptoms. Neurosurgical removal of tumours should be carried out where appropriate, sometimes urgently.

Normal pressure hydrocephalus

This rare syndrome describes enlarged cerebral ventricles without cortical atrophy, with dementia, urinary incontinence and gait apraxia, usually in the elderly. CSF constituents and pressure are characteristically normal. Ventriculo-peritoneal shunting occasionally helps.

Headache, migraine and facial pain

'Tension' headache

The vast majority of chronic and recurrent headaches are believed to be due to neurovascular irritation and tension within scalp muscles. Despite universal occurrence,

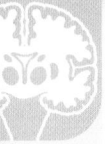

precise mechanisms of common headache remain obscure. What is certain is that most headaches are benign. Tight band sensations, pressure behind the eyes, throbbing and bursting sensations are common.

There may be obvious precipitating factors such as worry, noise, concentrated visual effort or fumes. Depression is also a frequent underlying cause. Tension headaches are often attributed to cervical spondylosis, refractive errors or high blood pressure; evidence for these associations is poor. Headaches also follow even minor head injuries. There are no abnormal physical signs other than tenderness and tension in the nuchal and scalp muscles.

Management
This involves:

- firm reassurance
- avoiding causes
- analgesics – limited amounts
- physical treatments – massage, icepacks, relaxation
- antidepressants – when indicated
- drugs for migraine (see below).

Imaging is often needed for reassurance.

Migraine
Migraine is recurrent headache associated with visual and gastrointestinal disturbance. The borderline between migraine and tension headaches is vague. Over 10% of any sampled population have had these symptoms.

Mechanisms
Precise mechanisms of migraine are unknown. Genetic factors probably play a role; a rare form of familial migraine is associated with a mutation in the alpha-1 subunit of the P/Q-type voltage-gated calcium channel on chromosome 19.

The headache of migraine, often throbbing, is due to vasodilatation or oedema of blood vessels, with stimulation of nerve endings near affected extracranial and meningeal arteries. Release of vasoactive substances such as nitric oxide is thought to have a role. Serum 5-hydroxytryptamine rises at the onset of prodromal symptoms and falls during the headache. Magnesium deficiency, neural excitation by glutamate and aspartate, changes in the hypothalamic–pituitary axis and in endogenous opioids have all been suggested.

Cerebral features, such as tingling limbs, aphasia and weakness, are caused by focal depression of cortical function.

Definite precipitating factors are unusual. Some patients complain of symptoms at times of relaxation (weekend migraine). Others find that chocolate (high in phenylethylamine) and cheese (high in tyramine) precipitate attacks. Migraine is common around puberty, at the menopause and premenstrually, and sometimes increases in severity or frequency with hormonal contraceptives, in pregnancy and with the onset of hypertension. There is no reason to suppose that the development of migraine is suggestive of any major intracranial lesion. However, since migraine is so common, an intracranial mass and migraine sometimes occur together by coincidence. Rarely, migraine follows a head injury; this can be minor.

Clinical patterns
Migraine attacks vary from intermittent headaches indistinguishable from tension headaches to discrete episodes that mimic thromboembolic cerebral ischaemia. Distinction between variants is somewhat artificial. Migraine can be separated into phases:

- well-being before an attack (occasional)
- prodromal symptoms
- headache, nausea, vomiting.

Migraine with aura (classical migraine)
Prodromal symptoms are usually visual and related to depression of visual cortical function or retinal function. There are unilateral patchy scotomata (when the retina is affected) or cortical hemianopic symptoms. Teichopsia (flashes) and fortification spectra (jagged lines resembling battlements) are common. Transient aphasia sometimes occurs, together with tingling, numbness or vague weakness of one side. The patient feels nauseated. The prodrome lasts from 15 minutes to an hour or more. Headache then follows. This is occasionally hemicranial (i.e. splitting the head) but often begins locally and becomes generalized. Nausea increases and vomiting follows. The patient is irritable and prefers a darkened room. Superficial temporal arteries are engorged and pulsating. After several hours the attack ceases, sometimes with a diuresis. Deep sleep often ensues.

Migraine without aura (common migraine)
This is the usual variety. Prodromal visual symptoms are vague. There is recurrent headache accompanied by nausea and malaise.

Basilar migraine
Prodromal symptoms include circumoral tingling, tongue numbness, vertigo, diplopia, transient visual disturbance, blindness, syncope, dysarthria and ataxia. These occur either alone or progress to a migrainous headache.

Hemiparetic migraine
This rarity is classical migraine with hemiparetic features. Recovery occurs within 24 hours. Exceptionally, cerebral infarction and hemiplegia occurs.

Ophthalmoplegic migraine
This is a third nerve, or exceptionally a sixth nerve palsy with a migraine. This is rare and difficult to distinguish

from other causes of a third nerve palsy (p. 1135) without investigation.

Facioplegic migraine

This rarity is unilateral facial weakness during a migraine.

Differential diagnosis

The onset of sudden headache may be similar to meningitis or SAH.

Hemiplegic, visual and hemisensory symptoms must be distinguished from thromboembolic TIAs (p. 1166). In TIAs maximum deficit is present immediately and headache is unusual.

Unilateral tingling or numbness should be distinguished from sensory epilepsy (partial seizures). In epilepsy distinct march (progression) of symptoms is usual.

Management

General measures include:

- reassurance and relief of anxiety
- avoidance of dietary factors – rarely helpful.

Patients taking hormonal contraceptives may benefit from a brand change, or trying without. Severe hemiplegic symptoms are an indication for stopping hormonal contraceptives.

During an attack. Paracetamol or other simple analgesics should be given, with an antiemetic such as metoclopramide if necessary. Repeated use of analgesics leads to further headaches. Triptans (5-HT$_1$ agonists) are also helpful. In some 30% of cases where there is recurrent severe migraine, sumatriptan, zolmitriptan, naratriptan and rizatriptan are of value either by prompt self-administered subcutaneous injection, or orally by wafer or inhaler. Ergotamine tartrate (1–2 mg orally or rectally, 360 mg by inhaler or 0.25–0.5 mg by injection) is also sometimes helpful if given early. Ergotamine and triptans should be avoided when there is vascular disease.

Prophylaxis. It is difficult to discern placebo effects of prophylactic drugs in migraine. When drugs are necessary, the following are helpful:

- pizotifen (an antihistamine and a 5-HT antagonist) 0.5 mg at night for several days, increasing to 1.5 mg at night – common side-effects are slight weight gain and drowsiness
- propranolol 10 mg three times daily, increasing to 40–80 mg three times daily
- methysergide (a 5-HT antagonist) 2–6 mg daily – an occasional side-effect is periaortitis (p. 634) which precludes use for longer than 6 months.
- amitriptyline: 10–30 mg at night is sometimes helpful.

Sodium valproate, verapamil, nifedipine and naproxen are also used.

Facial pain

The face is richly supplied with pain-sensitive structures – the teeth, gums, sinuses, temporomandibular joints, jaw and eyes. Disease of these causes facial pain. Facial pain is also caused by specific neurological conditions.

Trigeminal neuralgia (p. 1137), trigeminal nerve lesions (p. 1136) and postherpetic neuralgia (p. 1195) are described elsewhere.

Cluster headache (migrainous neuralgia)

This condition, distinct from migraine despite its name, describes recurrent bouts of excruciating unilateral pain that wake the patient. Attacks cluster around one eye. It affects adults, commencing in the third and fourth decades and is more common in men. Alcohol sometimes provokes an attack, and also experimentally, nitroglycerin. There are suggestions that there is a change in grey matter density on functional imaging in the posterior hypothalamus. The pain rises to a crescendo over half an hour and lasts for several hours. Vomiting occurs. One cheek and nostril feel congested. Transient ipsilateral Horner's syndrome is common.

Despite very severe pain there are no serious sequelae. Attacks recur at intervals over several years but tend to disappear after 55. Analgesics are unhelpful. Triptans may abort an attack. Prophylactic migraine drugs are of little value. Lithium carbonate (400–1200 mg daily) sometimes has a dramatic effect in preventing attacks: the drug level should be monitored. Inhalation of oxygen sometimes helps stop an attack.

Paroxysmal hemicrania

Episodic paroxysmal hemicrania is a rare condition describing unilateral sudden, brief (< 20 minutes) pains with characteristics of cluster headaches. The pains may occur many times each day. Typically they respond to indometacin.

Atypical facial pain

Facial pain for which no cause can be found is seen in the elderly, mainly in women. It is believed to be a somatic equivalent of depression. Tricyclic antidepressants are sometimes helpful.

Other causes of facial pain

Facial pain occurs in variants of migraine and in giant cell arteritis (see below).

Giant cell arteritis (GCA, cranial arteritis, temporal arteritis) (see also p. 566)

This condition is a granulomatous arteritis of unknown aetiology occurring chiefly over the age of 60. It affects extradural arteries. Other forms of arteritis, such as SLE and microscopic polyangiitis, can occasionally present with similar features. GCA is closely related to polymyalgia rheumatica and can coexist.

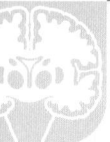

Neurological disease

Clinical features

Headache

Headache is almost invariable in GCA. Pain is felt over inflamed superficial, temporal or occipital arteries. Touching the skin over the inflamed vessel (e.g. combing hair) causes pain. Arterial pulsation is soon lost and the artery becomes hard, tortuous and thickened. The skin over the vessels may become red. Rarely, gangrenous patches appear in the scalp.

Facial pain

Pain in the face, jaw and mouth is caused by inflammation of facial, maxillary and lingual branches of the external carotid artery in GCA. Pain is characteristically worse on eating (jaw claudication). Opening the mouth and protruding the tongue becomes difficult. A painful, ischaemic tongue occurs rarely.

Visual problems

Visual loss owing to arterial inflammation and occlusion occurs in 25% of cases of untreated GCA. Posterior ciliary artery occlusion causes anterior ischaemic optic neuropathy in three-quarters of these cases. Other mechanisms are central retinal artery occlusion, cilioretinal artery occlusion and posterior ischaemic optic neuropathy. There is sudden uniocular visual loss, either partial or complete, and usually painless. Amaurosis fugax (p. 1165) may precede permanent blindness.

When the posterior ciliary vessels are affected, ischaemic optic neuropathy causes the disc to become swollen and pale; retinal branch vessels usually remain normal. When the central retinal artery is occluded, there is sudden permanent unilateral blindness, disc pallor and visible retinal ischaemia. Bilateral blindness may develop.

Rare complications

Brainstem ischaemia, cortical blindness, ischaemic neuropathy of peripheral or cranial nerves, and involvement of the aorta, coronary, renal and mesenteric arteries are sometimes seen.

Investigations

The ESR is greatly elevated, 60–100 mm/hour being common. Exceptionally the ESR remains normal. CRP and plasma α_2-globulins are raised and albumin occasionally reduced. Normochromic normocytic anaemia develops.

The diagnosis should be established immediately by superficial temporal artery biopsy because of the risk of blindness. A segment 1 cm (or longer) should be excised because characteristic arterial granulomatous inflammation (lymphocytes, plasma cells, multinucleate giant cells, internal elastic lamina destruction) is patchy.

Treatment

Immediate high doses of steroids (prednisolone, initially 60–100 mg daily) should be started in a patient with typical features, even before biopsy. The dose is reduced as the ESR falls. A frequent feature of treated GCA is that headache subsides within hours of the first large steroid dose. Opinions differ about the need for long-term steroids. Since the risk of visual loss persists over many years, neurologists and ophthalmologists treating these patients tend to recommend long-term treatment. Rheumatologists seeing polymyalgia rheumatica cases tend to stop steroids after a year or more depending on the ESR or CRP.

FURTHER READING

Bateman N (2000) Triptans and migraine. *Lancet* **355**: 860–861.
Goadsby PJ et al. (2002) Migraine – current understanding and treatment. *New England Journal of Medicine* **346**: 257–270.
Hayreh SS (2000) Steroid therapy for visual loss in patients with GCA. *Lancet* **355**: 1572–1573.
Lance J, Goadsby P (1998) *Mechanism and Management of Headache*. Oxford: Butterworth Heinemann.
May A, Bahra A, Büchel C, Frackowiak R, Goadsby P (1998) Hypothalamic activation in cluster headache attacks. *Lancet* **352**: 275–278.

Traumatic brain injury

In most western countries head injury accounts for about 250 hospital admissions per 100 000 population annually. Traumatic brain injury (TBI) is the preferred term. For each 100 000 people, 10 die annually; 10–15 are transferred to a neurosurgical unit – the majority of these require rehabilitation for a prolonged period of 1–9 months. The *prevalence* of survivors with a major persisting handicap is around 100 per 100 000. Road traffic accidents and alcohol abuse are the principal aetiological factors in this major cause of morbidity and mortality. The following paragraphs mention issues that indicate the severity of TBI.

Skull fractures

Linear skull fracture of the vault or base is one indication of the severity of a blow, but is itself not necessarily associated with any neurological sequelae. Healing takes place and surgery is rarely needed. *Depressed* skull fracture is followed by a high incidence of post-traumatic epilepsy. Surgical elevation and debridement are usually necessary.

Principal local complications of skull fracture are:

- *meningeal artery rupture* – causing extradural haematoma (p. 1173)
- *dural vein tears* – causing subdural haematoma (p. 1173) or CSF rhinorrhoea/otorrhoea with the risk of meningitis.

Mechanisms of brain damage

Older classifications attempted to separate *concussion* (transient coma for hours followed by apparent complete clinical recovery) from brain *contusion* (prolonged coma, with brain damage and focal signs). Pathological support for this division is poor. Mechanisms of TBI are complex and interrelated:

- axonal and neuronal damage – shearing and rotational stresses on decelerating brain, often at sites distant from impact (*contracoup* effect)
- axonal and neuronal damage from direct trauma
- brain oedema
- raised intracranial pressure
- brain hypoxia
- brain ischaemia.

Clinical course

In a mild TBI a patient is first stunned or dazed for a few seconds or minutes. Loss of consciousness is transient and following this the patient is alert, and there is little or no post-traumatic amnesia. The duration of unconsciousness and particularly of post-traumatic amnesia (PTA) helps grade severity. PTA over 24 hours indicates severe TBI. The Glasgow Coma Scale (GCS, p. 1159) is used to record the degree of coma and TBI; this has prognostic value. A GCS below 5/15 at 24 hours implies severe injury; 50% of such patients die or remain in a persistent vegetative state (p. 1159). Prolonged coma of up to several weeks is, however, occasionally followed by good recovery.

Recovery may take many weeks or months. During the first few weeks, patients are often intermittently restless and/or lethargic and have focal neurological deficits, such as hemiparesis or aphasia. Gradually they become more aware, but despite being awake, may remain in post-traumatic amnesia, being unable to lay down any memory of current events. This sometimes lasts several weeks, and may not be obvious clinically. PTA is the best predictor of outcome. PTA lasting 2 weeks predicts that persistent organic cognitive deficit is almost inevitable, although return to unsupported paid work is possible.

Late sequelae

Sequelae of TBI are major causes of morbidity and have important social and medicolegal consequences. They include:

- *Incomplete and prolonged recovery* – e.g. cognitive impairment, hemiparesis.
- *Post-traumatic epilepsy* (p. 1175).
- *Chronic traumatic encephalopathy* – this follows repeated (and often minor) injuries. This 'punch drunk' syndrome is cognitive impairment with extrapyramidal and pyramidal signs. It is seen principally in professional boxers.
- *The post-traumatic* (*post-concussional*) *syndrome.* This describes the vague complaints of headache, dizziness and malaise that follow even minor head injuries. Litigation is frequently an issue. Depression is prominent. Symptoms may be prolonged.

- *Benign paroxysmal positional vertigo* (BPPV, p. 1141).
- *Chronic subdural haematoma* (p. 1173).
- *Hydrocephalus* (p. 1201).

Immediate management

Attention to the airway is vital. If there is coma, depressed fracture or suspicion of an intracranial haematoma, discussion with a neurosurgical unit is essential. Indications for brain imaging (mainly CT) following head injuries vary between different countries – from imaging of all minor head injuries in some US centres to more considered and stringent criteria elsewhere.

In many severe TBI cases, assisted ventilation will be needed. Intracranial pressure monitoring is valuable. Care of the unconscious patient is described on page 1162. Prophylactic anticonvulsant treatment has been shown to be of no value in prevention of late post-traumatic epilepsy.

Rehabilitation

TBI cases require skilled, prolonged and energetic support. Survivors with severe physical and cognitive deficits require rehabilitation in a specialized unit. Rehabilitation includes intensive physiotherapy and care from a multidisciplinary team with both physical and psychological skills. Many survivors are left with cognitive problems – amnesia, neglect, disordered attention and motivation, and behavioural/emotional problems – temper dyscontrol, depression and grief reactions. Long-term attention for both patients and families is necessary.

FURTHER READING

Annegers JF, Hauser AW, Coan SP, Rocca WA (1998) A population based study of seizures after traumatic brain injuries. *New England Journal of Medicine* **338**: 20–24.

Chadwick D (2000) Seizures and epilepsy after TBI. *Lancet* **355**: 334–335.

Editorial (1997) Best practice in traumatic brain injury. *Lancet* **349**: 1041–1042.

Greenwood RJ (ed) (2000) *Neurological Rehabilitation*, 2nd edn. Edinburgh: Churchill Livingstone.

Haydel MJ et al. (2000) Indications for CT in patients with minor head injury. *New England Journal of Medicine* **343**: 100–105.

Shajar J (2000) Traumatic brain injury. *Lancet* **356**: 923–929.

Diseases of the spinal cord

The cord extends from C1 (i.e. its junction with the medulla) to the vertebral body of L1 where it is called the conus medullaris. Blood supply is from the anterior spinal artery and a plexus on the posterior cord. This network is supplied by vertebral arteries, thyrocervical trunk and several branches from lumbar and intercostal vessels.

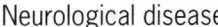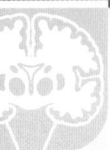

Spinal cord compression

(Table 20.49)

Principal features of chronic and subacute cord compression are of radicular pain at the level of compression, spastic paraparesis or tetraparesis, and sensory loss below the compression.

For example, in compression at T6 a band of pain radiates around the thorax; it is characteristically worse on coughing or straining. Spastic paraparesis develops over months, days or hours, depending upon underlying pathology. Numbness commencing in the feet rises to the level of compression. This is called the sensory level. Retention of urine and constipation develop.

Cord compression is a medical emergency. It is sometimes difficult to distinguish chronic progressive cord compression from other (medical) causes of worsening paraparesis and tetraparesis on clinical grounds alone: the principal reason for this is that pain at a sensory level can be absent, even when severe cord compression is present.

Spinal cord neoplasms (Table 20.50)

Extramedullary tumours, both extradural and intradural, cause cord compression gradually over weeks to months, with root pain and a sensory level (p. 1151).

Intramedullary tumours (e.g. glioma) typically have a very slowly progressive course over many years. Sensory disturbances similar to syringomyelia may appear (p. 1207).

Disc and vertebral lesions

Central cervical disc protrusion and thoracic disc protrusion causing cord compression are considered on page 1219.

Spinal epidural abscess

This is described on page 1192.

Epidural haemorrhage and haematoma

These are rare sequelae of anticoagulant therapy, bleeding disorders and trauma. A rapidly progressive cord lesion develops.

Tuberculosis

Spinal tuberculosis is the commonest cause of cord compression in countries where tuberculosis is common. There is destruction of vertebral bodies and disc spaces, with spread of infection along the extradural space. Cord compression and paraparesis follow, progressing to complete paralysis – Pott's paraplegia.

Management

Early recognition of cord compression is vital. Plain spinal films show degenerative bone disease and destruction of vertebrae by infection or neoplasm.

Table 20.49
Causes of spinal cord compression

Spinal cord neoplasms (see Table 20.50)	Epidural haemorrhage
Disc and vertebral lesions	Rarities
Chronic degenerative	Paget's disease, scoliosis and vertebral anomalies
Trauma	Epithelial, endothelial and parasitic cysts
Inflammatory	Aneurysmal bone cyst
Epidural abscess	Vertebral angioma
Tuberculosis	Haematomyelia, arachnoiditis
Granuloma	Osteoporosis with fracture
Vertebral neoplasms	Arteriovenous malformation
Metastases	
Myeloma	

Table 20.50
Principal spinal cord neoplasms

Extradural	Extramedullary
Metastases	Meningioma
Bronchus	Neurofibroma
Breast	Ependymoma
Prostate	
Lymphoma	**Intramedullary**
Thyroid	Glioma
Melanoma	Ependymoma
	Haemangioblastoma
	Lipoma
	Arteriovenous malformation
	Teratoma

Routine tests (e.g. chest X-ray) may indicate a primary neoplasm or infection. MR identifies most lesions and, where it is available, has entirely replaced contrast myelography. Surgical exploration is frequently necessary. If decompression is not performed sufficiently promptly, irreversible cord damage may follow. Results are excellent if benign tumours are removed early.

Other causes of paraparesis

Paraparesis (and tetraparesis) is a feature of many neurological conditions recognizable by their clinical patterns, making clinical differential diagnosis of fundamental importance in practice. These diseases are shown in Table 20.14 (p. 1145); most are mentioned elsewhere in this chapter.

Syringomyelia and syringobulbia

The syrinx, a fluid-filled cavity within the cervical or thoracic spinal cord is the essential feature. Syringobulbia means a cavity in the brainstem.

Aetiology and mechanism

Classical syringomyelia is associated with the Arnold–Chiari malformation (see p. 1210). Bony anomalies at the foramen magnum, spina bifida (p. 1210), arachnoiditis, hydrocephalus (p. 1201) and intrinsic cord tumours (e.g. glioma and ependymoma) are sometimes also followed by syrinx formation, and its subsequent enlargement. It is believed that with an anatomical abnormality at the foramen magnum, normal pulsatile CSF pressure waves are transmitted to the soft fragile tissues of the cervical cord and brainstem, causing secondary cavity formation. The syrinx is in continuity with the central canal of the cord. Cord trauma can be followed by cavity formation that can progress.

Pathological anatomy

The expanding cavity gradually destroys spinothalamic neurones, anterior horn cells, lateral corticospinal tracts, and trigeminal nuclei, sympathetic trunk, ninth, tenth, eleventh and twelfth nerve nuclei and the vestibular system if disease extends into the medulla.

Clinical features

Patients with classical syringomyelia associated with the Arnold–Chiari malformation usually develop symptoms at the age of 20–30. Upper limb pain exacerbated by exertion or coughing is typical. Spinothalamic sensory loss (pain and temperature) leads to painless upper limb burns, and trophic changes. Difficulty in walking with paraparesis develops. The following are typical signs of a cervical syrinx (Fig. 20.15 (s), p. 1155):

- *Areas of 'dissociated' sensory loss*, i.e. spinothalamic loss without loss of light touch. Bizarre patterns are seen.
- *Loss of upper limb reflexes.*
- *Muscle wasting* in the hand and forearm.
- *Spastic paraparesis* – initially mild and symptomless.
- *Neuropathic joints*, trophic skin changes (scars, nail dystrophy) and ulcers.
- *Brainstem signs* – as the syrinx extends into the brainstem (syringobulbia), there is tongue atrophy and fasciculation, bulbar palsy, nystagmus, Horner's syndrome, hearing loss and impairment of facial sensation.

Course, investigation and management

Syringomyelia is gradually progressive over several decades. Sudden deterioration sometimes follows minor trauma, or apparently spontaneously. MR imaging demonstrates the cavity and herniation of the cerebellar tonsils.

There is no curative treatment. Surgical decompression of the foramen magnum sometimes slows deterioration.

Metabolic and toxic cord disease

Vitamin B₁₂ deficiency (p. 418)

Subacute combined degeneration of the cord resulting from vitamin B_{12} deficiency is the most common example of metabolic disease causing spinal cord damage. Cord lesions probably due to multiple B-vitamin deficiencies are also seen in severe malnutrition.

Lathyrism

This curiosity is an endemic spastic paraparesis of central India caused by the toxin beta-(N)-oxalylamino-L-alanine. It occurs when excessive quantities of a drought-resistant pulse, *Lathyrus sativa*, are consumed.

Konzo; tropical ataxic neuropathy

In West Africa and the West Indies inadequate preparation of *cassava* root allows ingestion of cyanogenic glycosides. A subacute spastic paraparesis follows; this is called *konzo*. Tropical ataxic neuropathy consists of sensory ataxia, loss of reflexes, deafness and optic atrophy. This is believed to be the result of chronic low-level exposure to these glycosides.

Acute transverse myelopathy (transverse myelitis)

This term is used to describe acute inflammation of the cord and paraplegia or paraparesis occurring with viral infections, MS, mixed connective tissue disease and other inflammatory and vascular disorders – for example HIV, syphilis, radiation myelopathy, or anterior spinal artery occlusion. MRI or myelography is usually required to exclude cord compression.

Anterior spinal artery occlusion

Cord infarction, causing an acute paraplegia or tetraplegia, or paresis occurs in many thrombotic or embolic vascular diseases – for example, endocarditis, severe hypotension, atheroma, diabetes mellitus, polycythaemia, syphilis and polyarteritis. Infarction sometimes occurs during surgery to the posterior mediastinum, or follows aortic dissection and trauma. It occasionally occurs as an isolated event.

Radiation myelopathy

A mild paraparesis and sensory loss sometimes develops within several weeks to a year after radiotherapy. Particular care is taken to shield the cord during radiotherapy.

Management of paraplegia

General considerations

The general health and morale should be considered carefully and regularly. Any intercurrent infection is potentially dangerous and should be recognized and treated early. Chronic renal failure is a common cause of death. The paraplegic patient needs skilled and prolonged nursing care. Particular problems are discussed below.

Bladder

Catheterization is usually necessary initially. Many patients manage to self-catheterize, or reflex bladder emptying develops, initiated by abdominal pressure. Frèe urinary drainage is essential to avoid stasis – subsequent infection and calculi.

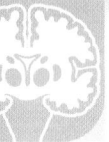
Bowel

Constipation and faecal impaction must be avoided. Manual evacuation is necessary following acute paraplegia, but reflex rectal emptying later develops.

Skin care

The risk of pressure sores is great. Meticulous attention must be paid to cleanliness and to turning the patient every 2 hours. The sacrum, iliac crests, greater trochanters, heels and malleoli should be inspected frequently. Ripple mattresses and water beds are useful. If pressure sores develop, plastic surgical repair should be considered. Pressure palsies (e.g. of ulnar nerves) must be avoided.

Lower limbs

Passive physiotherapy helps to prevent contractures in paralysed limbs. Severe spasticity, with flexor or extensor spasms, may be helped by baclofen, diazepam or dantrolene sodium.

Rehabilitation

Many patients with traumatic paraplegia or tetraplegia return to full or partial self-sufficiency and a wheelchair existence. Specialist advice from a skilled rehabilitation unit is necessary. Lightweight, specially adapted wheelchairs are available. 'Paraplegics' have demanding practical, psychological and social needs but with guidance and help can often return to an active role in society.

Degenerative neuronal diseases

Degenerative underlines our incomplete understanding of these progressive nervous system diseases. The molecular and genetic basis of these conditions is the subject of intense study.

Motor neurone disease (MND)

In this common disease there is progressive degeneration of lower and upper *motor* neurones (LMNs, UMNs) in the spinal cord, in somatic cranial nerve motor nuclei and within the cortex. Most MND is sporadic and of entirely unknown cause. It is thought that relentless degeneration of motor nerve cells is programmed genetically. Abnormal mRNA splicing of the excitatory amino-acid transporter *EAAT2* gene, a major glial transporter, was once thought to be specific for MND but is sometimes found in normal people. Oxidative neuronal damage, aggregation of abnormal neuronal proteins, glutamate mishandling and abnormalities of neurofilament-mediated axonal transport are believed to be involved.

There is a familial form of MND in which there are mutations in the gene (on chromosome 21q) encoding the free radical scavenging enzyme copper/zinc superoxide dismutase (SOD-1).

Incidence of the sporadic form is around 2/100 000/ year, with a slight male predominance and onset in middle life.

Clinical features

The sensory system is not involved. In the common, sporadic form of MND, four broad patterns are seen:

- progressive muscular atrophy
- amyotrophic lateral sclerosis (ALS)
- progressive bulbar and pseudobulbar palsy
- primary lateral sclerosis (rare).

Although useful as a means of recognizing the disease, these are not distinct aetiological or pathological variants; they usually merge as the condition worsens. Other classifications are also used.

Progressive muscular atrophy

Wasting beginning often in the small muscles of one hand spreads inexorably throughout the arm. Although it may begin unilaterally, wasting soon follows on the opposite side. Fasciculation is common. It is due to spontaneous firing of abnormally large motor units formed by branching fibres of surviving axons that are striving to innervate muscle fibres that have lost their nerve supply. Cramps may occur but pain does not.

The physical signs are of wasting and weakness, with fasciculation that is often widespread. Tendon reflexes are lost when the reflex arc is interrupted by anterior horn cell loss, but are preserved or exaggerated when there is loss of corticospinal motor neurones.

Amyotrophic lateral sclerosis (ALS)

Lateral sclerosis means disease of the lateral corticospinal tracts (i.e. one cause of spastic paraparesis). Amyotrophy means simply muscle atrophy – unusual in most other forms of spastic tetraparesis or paraparesis. The clinical picture is a progressive spastic tetraparesis or paraparesis with added lower motor neurone signs and fasciculation. ALS is the term usually given to motor neurone disease in the USA.

Progressive bulbar and pseudobulbar palsy

Here the brunt falls initially upon the lower cranial nerve nuclei and their supranuclear connections. Dysarthria, dysphagia, nasal regurgitation of fluids and choking are common symptoms. For reasons unknown, this form of MND is more common in women than in men. Characteristic features are of a bulbar and pseudobulbar palsy, (p. 1142), with mixed UMN and LMN signs in the lower cranial nerves – for example, a wasted fibrillating tongue with a spastic weak palate. Eye movements remain unaffected in all forms of MND. There are no cerebellar or extrapyramidal signs. Awareness is preserved and dementia unusual. Sphincter disturbance occurs late, if at all.

Primary lateral sclerosis

This describes a rare form of MND in which features are confined to upper motor neurones. There is a progressive tetraparesis with terminal pseudobulbar palsy.

Diagnosis

There are no specific tests; diagnosis is clinical – and usually MND is an easily identifiable condition. Exclusion of other conditions is necessary in atypical cases by neurophysiological studies (EMG and nerve conduction). Cervical radiculopathy and myelopathy and the rare (almost extinct) syphilitic cervical pachymeningitis can cause diagnostic difficulty. Motor neuropathies and spinal muscular atrophies sometimes resemble the progressive muscular atrophy form of MND – their course is more prolonged. Kennedy's syndrome, an X-linked bulbar and spinal muscular atrophy sometimes causes confusion; UMN signs are not seen in this condition.

Bulbar myasthenia gravis (p. 1222) may sometimes appear similar in the early stages.

Multifocal motor neuropathy (p. 1213) causes distal weakness with LMN signs; antibodies to GM_1 ganglioside are present and conduction block seen on electrophysiological studies.

Denervation, a feature in all forms of MND except primary lateral sclerosis is confirmed by electromyography. This characteristically shows chronic partial denervation with preserved motor conduction velocity. CSF constituents are usually normal; CSF protein may be slightly raised.

Course and management

Remission is unknown. The disease progresses, spreading gradually, and causes death, often from bronchopneumonia. Survival for more than 3 years is unusual, although there are rare MND variants in which patients survive for a decade or longer.

No treatment has been shown to influence outcome, although riluzole, a sodium-channel blocker that inhibits glutamate release has been shown to slow progression slightly, particularly in patients with disease of bulbar onset. Contentious issues surround the cost-effectiveness of this expensive drug. Ventilatory support and feeding via gastrostomy helps prolong survival for some months. Giving accurate advice to patients with MND is particularly difficult.

Spinal muscular atrophies

These rare genetically determined disorders of the motor neurone give rise to slowly progressive, usually symmetrical, muscle wasting and weakness. An acute infantile type (Werdnig–Hoffmann disease), a chronic childhood type (Kugelberg–Welander disease) and adult forms are recognized. Clinically these conditions may be confused with muscular dystrophies (p. 1223), hereditary neuropathies or MND.

FURTHER READING

Martin JB (1999) Molecular basis of the neurodegenerative disorders. *New England Journal of Medicine* **340**: 1970–1980.

Mitsumoto H (2000) Disorders of upper and lower motor neurones. In: Bradley W, Daroff RB, Fenichel GM, Marsden CD (eds) *Neurology in Clinical Practice*. Boston: Butterworth Heinemann.

Parton MJ, Lyall R, Leigh PN (1999) Motor neurone disease and its management. *Journal of the Royal College of Physicians of London* **33**: 212–218.

Shaw P (1999) Motor neurone disease. *British Medical Journal* **318**: 1118–1121

Dementia

This diffuse deterioration in brain neuronal function is produced by different pathological processes. The most common is Alzheimer's disease. Dementia is discussed on page 1264.

Congenital and inherited diseases

Cerebral palsy

This describes disorders apparent at birth or in childhood due to neonatal brain damage. Deficits are non-progressive. Mental retardation, varying from severe intellectual impairment to mild learning disorders, is common in all forms of cerebral palsy, but severe physical disability is not necessarily associated with cognitive defect.

The precise cause of damage in an individual child may be difficult to determine. The following are responsible:

- hypoxia in utero and/or during parturition
- neonatal cerebral haemorrhage and/or infarction
- trauma, neonatal or during parturition
- prolonged seizures – *status epilepticus* or hypoglycaemia
- kernicterus.

Clinical features

Failure to achieve normal milestones is often the earliest feature. More specific motor syndromes become apparent later in childhood or, rarely, in adult life.

Spastic diplegia

This is spasticity (predominantly of lower limbs) with scissoring of gait.

Athetoid cerebral palsy

This is described on page 1186.

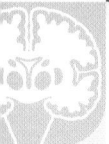

Infantile hemiparesis

Hemiparesis may be noted at birth or later. Limb hemiatrophy with contralateral hemisphere atrophy is usual. Seizures are common.

Congenital ataxia

This is incoordination and hypotonia of limbs and trunk.

Dysraphism

Failure of normal fusion of the fetal neural tube leads to a group of congenital anomalies. Folate deficiency during pregnancy is a contributory factor and supplements are always given (p. 238).

Anencephaly

This is absence of brain and skull and is incompatible with life.

Meningoencephalocele

Brain and meninges extrude through a midline skull defect – protrusion can be minor or massive.

Spina bifida

There is failure of lumbosacral neural tube fusion. Several varieties occur.

Spina bifida occulta

This is failure of vertebral arch fusion alone. Clinical abnormalities are rare. X-rays show the bony anomaly (3% of population). A dimple or a tuft of hair may overlie the anomaly, which is commonly lumbar.

Meningomyelocele and myelocele with spina bifida

Meningomyelocele consists of elements of spinal cord and lumbosacral roots contained within a meningeal sac. This herniates through a vertebral defect. In severe cases both lower limbs and sphincters are paralysed. The lumbosacral defect is visible at birth. Meningocele is a meningeal defect alone.

Basilar impression of skull (platybasia)

This is usually a congenital anomaly. There is invagination of the foramen magnum and skull base upwards. Lower cranial nerves, medulla, upper cervical cord and roots are affected. The *Arnold–Chiari malformation* is often present in which aberrant cerebellar tissue extends through the foramen magnum. Basilar invagination also develops in Paget's disease and rarely in osteomalacia (p. 584). Clinical features are spastic tetraparesis with cerebellar and lower brainstem signs.

Neuroectodermal syndromes

These are disorders in which tissue derived from ectoderm forms tumours and hamartomas, with lesions in the skin, eye and nervous system.

Neurofibromatosis (von Recklinghausen's disease)

This is characterized by multiple skin neurofibromas and pigmentation. The neurofibromas arise from the neurilemmal sheath. One new case occurs in every 3000 live births. The mode of inheritance is autosomal dominant.

Clinical features (see also p. 1300)

Clinically neurofibromatosis is divided into type 1 (peripheral >70%) and type 2 (central). The abnormal gene for NF1 is on chromosome 17 (q11.2) and for NF2 on chromosome 22 (q12.2). The main application for these genetic markers is potential antenatal diagnosis and counselling. A wide variety of abnormalities occur.

Peripheral (NF1)

Skin neurofibromas present as subcutaneous, soft, sometimes pedunculated, tumours (p. 1300). They increase in numbers throughout life.

Multiple café-au-lait patches – pale brown macules 1–20 cm diameter – develop. Isolated patches are common in the normal population; more than five patches is suggestive of neurofibromatosis.

Central (NF2)

Many neural tumours occur:

- eighth-nerve sheath neurofibroma (acoustic neuroma, often bilateral)
- spinal cord and other nerve root neurofibroma
- meningioma
- glioma (including optic nerve glioma)
- plexiform neuroma (massive cutaneous overgrowth)
- cutaneous neurofibroma – these are few.

Rarely, the benign tumours undergo sarcomatous change.

Associated abnormalities

- Scoliosis
- Orbital haemangioma
- Local gigantism of a limb
- Phaeochromocytoma and ganglioneuroma
- Renal artery stenosis
- Pulmonary fibrosis
- Obstructive cardiomyopathy
- Fibrous dysplasia of bone.

Treatment

Surgery may be necessary for cosmetic reasons. Tumours causing pressure within the nervous system require excision, if feasible.

Tuberous sclerosis (epiloia)

This rare autosomal dominant condition comprises adenoma sebaceum, epilepsy and mental retardation (often severe).

Adenoma sebaceum

Reddish nodules (angiofibromas) develop on the cheeks in childhood.

Other lesions

These include shagreen patches, amelanotic naevi, retinal phakomas (glial masses), renal tumours, glial overgrowth in brain and gliomas. Cardiac rhabdomyomas, hamartomas of lung and kidney, and polycystic kidneys also occur.

Sturge–Weber syndrome (encephalofacial angiomatosis)

There is an extensive port-wine naevus on one side of the face (usually in the distribution of a division of the fifth nerve) and a leptomeningeal angioma. Epilepsy is common. Familial occurrence is exceptional.

von Hippel–Lindau syndrome (retinocerebellar angiomatosis)

This is dominantly inherited. Retinal and cerebellar haemangioblastomas develop or, less commonly, haemangioblastomas of the cord and cerebrum. Renal, adrenal and pancreatic tumours (and haemangioblastomas) may also be found. Polycythaemia sometimes occurs.

Numerous other disorders can be classified here – for example, ataxia telangiectasia (p. 1211) and Osler–Weber–Rendu syndrome (p. 458).

Spinocerebellar degenerations

The classification of this large group of rare inherited disorders is complex. Three conditions will be mentioned here.

Friedreich's ataxia

This is an autosomal recessive progressive degeneration of dorsal root ganglia, spinocerebellar tracts, corticospinal tracts and cerebellar Purkinje cells. Most patients are homozygous for the GAA triplet expansion in the Friedreich's ataxia gene. This gene, mapped to chromosome 9q13, encodes a mitochondrial protein (fraxatin) of unknown function. Impaired mitochondrial ATP is likely to be involved. The expression of fraxatin is decreased in Friedreich's patients. Progressive difficulty walking occurs around the age of 12 years. Death is usual before 40. However, with the identification of the gene, patients have been diagnosed in middle age. Clinical findings:

- ataxia of gait and trunk
- nystagmus (25%)
- dysarthria
- absent lower limb joint position and vibration sense
- absent lower limb reflexes
- optic atrophy (30%)
- pes cavus
- cardiomyopathy.

Hereditary spastic paraparesis

Isolated progressive paraparesis runs in some families. Inheritance is variable. Additional features including cerebellar signs, pes cavus, wasted hands and optic atrophy are sometimes seen. The conditions are usually mild and progress slowly over many years.

Ataxia telangiectasia (see also p. 213)

This rare, autosomal recessive condition is a progressive ataxic syndrome in childhood and early adult life. There is striking telangiectasia of the conjunctiva, nose, ears and skin creases. There are also defects in cell-mediated immunity and antibody production. A defect in DNA repair has been demonstrated. Death is usual by the third decade, either from infection or from lymphoreticular malignancy.

FURTHER READING

Wood N, Harding A (2000) Cerebellar and spinocerebellar disorders. In: Bradley W, Daroff RB, Fenichel GM, Marsden CD (eds) *Neurology in Clinical Practice*. Boston: Butterworth Heinemann.

Peripheral nerve disease

The various nerve fibre types are shown in Table 20.51. All are myelinated except C fibres that carry impulses from pain receptors.

Table 20.51
Fibre types in peripheral nerves

Type	Fibre diameter (mm)	Conduction velocity (m/s)	Function
Aα	10–18	90	Primary spindle afferents α-motor neurones
Aγ	4–8	30	γ-afferents; motor to muscle spindles
Aδ	2–6	30	Fast pain afferents
C	1–2	<1	Slow pain and temperature afferents Autonomic postganglionic

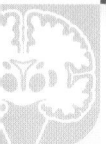

Mechanisms of damage to peripheral nerves

Peripheral nerve consists of two principal cellular structures – the axon, with its anterior horn cell, and the myelin sheath, produced by Schwann cells between each node of Ranvier. Blood supply is via *vasa nervorum*. Six principal mechanisms, some coexisting, cause nerve malfunction.

Demyelination

When the Schwann cell is damaged, the myelin sheath is disrupted. This causes marked slowing of conduction. This occurs in Guillain–Barré syndrome, in post-diphtheritic neuropathy and in hereditary sensorimotor neuropathies.

Axonal degeneration

The primary lesion affects the axon, which dies back from the periphery. Conduction velocity tends to remain normal (cf. demyelination) because axonal continuity is maintained in surviving fibres. Axonal degeneration occurs typically in toxic neuropathies.

Wallerian degeneration

This describes changes following nerve section. Both axon and distal myelin sheath degenerate over several weeks.

Compression

Focal demyelination at the point of compression develops with myelin sheath disruption. This occurs typically in entrapment neuropathies such as the carpal tunnel syndrome.901

Infarction

Microinfarction of *vasa nervorum* occurs in arteritis, e.g. polyarteritis nodosa, Churg–Strauss syndrome (p. 901), and in diabetes mellitus. Wallerian degeneration occurs distal to the ischaemic area.

Infiltration

Peripheral nerves are infiltrated by inflammatory cells in sarcoidosis or leprosy, or by malignant cells.

Nerve regeneration

Regeneration occurs either by remyelination, when recovering Schwann cells spin new myelin sheaths around the axon, or by axonal growth down the nerve sheath and axonal sprouting from the stump. Axonal growth takes place at a rate of up to 1 mm daily.

Definitions (Fig. 20.26)

- **Neuropathy** means a pathological process affecting a peripheral nerve or nerves.
- **Mononeuropathy** is a process affecting a single nerve.
- **Mononeuritis multiplex** (multiple mononeuropathy, or multifocal neuropathy) affects several or multiple nerves.

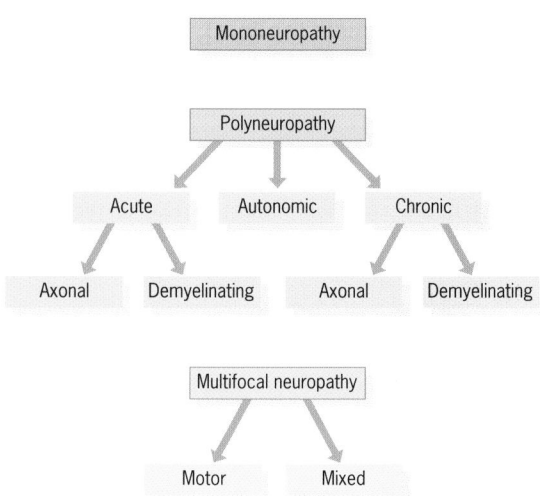

Fig. 20.26 Classification of neuropathies. Modified from Winer JB, Neuropathies *Medicine* 2000; **28:8**: 112–117 with kind permission of the Medicine Publishing Company.

- **Polyneuropathy** is a diffuse, symmetrical disease, usually extending proximally – acute, subacute or chronic. Its course is progressive, relapsing or towards recovery. Polyneuropathies may be acute or chronic, progressive or relapsing, motor, sensory, sensorimotor (i.e. mixed) or autonomic. They are classified broadly into demyelinating and axonal types, depending upon which principal pathological process predominates. It is often impossible to separate the two clinically. Many different classifications exist and many systemic diseases cause neuropathies; this causes some confusion.
- **Radiculopathy** means disease affecting nerve roots.

Diagnosis is made by clinical pattern, electrical tests, nerve biopsy (usually sural or radial) and the identification of systemic or genetic disease.

Mononeuropathies

Peripheral nerve compression or entrapment (Table 20.52)

Nerve damage by compression is either acute (e.g. due to a tourniquet or other sustained pressure) or chronic, such as in entrapment neuropathy. In both, demyelination predominates, but some distal axonal degeneration occurs. Acute compression usually affects nerves exposed anatomically, e.g. common peroneal nerve at fibula head. Entrapment develops in relatively tight anatomical passages, e.g. the carpal tunnel.

These conditions are diagnosed largely by clinical features. Diagnosis is confirmed by nerve conduction studies and electromyography. The most common are mentioned below. All are more common in people with diabetes. In countries where leprosy is prevalent

Table 20.52
Nerve compression and entrapment

Nerve	Site of entrapment or compression
Median	Carpal tunnel
Ulnar	Cubital tunnel
Radial	Spiral groove of humerus
Posterior interosseous	Supinator muscle
Lateral cutaneous of thigh ('meralgia paraesthetica')	Inguinal ligament
Common peroneal	Neck of fibula
Posterior tibial	Flexor retinaculum (tarsal tunnel)

an apparently isolated nerve lesion can be caused by this disease.

Carpal tunnel syndrome (p. 522)

This is the common condition of median nerve compression at the wrist. Many cases are idiopathic, but this entrapment neuropathy is sometimes seen in:

- hypothyroidism
- diabetes mellitus
- pregnancy and obesity
- rheumatoid arthritis
- acromegaly.

There is nocturnal tingling and pain in the hand (and sometimes forearm) followed by weakness of thenar muscles. Wasting of abductor pollicis brevis develops, with sensory loss in the palm and radial three-and-a-half fingers. Tinel's sign may be positive, i.e. tapping the nerve in the carpal tunnel reproduces tingling and pain.

Treatment with a splint at night or a local steroid injection in the wrist gives temporary relief. When the condition occurs in pregnancy, owing to fluid retention, it is often self-limiting. Surgical decompression of the carpel tunnel is a simple and definitive treatment.

Ulnar nerve compression

The nerve is compressed in the cubital tunnel (at the elbow). This follows ulnar fractures or prolonged/recurrent pressure.

Wasting of ulnar innervated muscles develops (hypothenar muscles and interossei) with sensory loss in the ulnar one-and-a-half fingers. Decompression and transposition of the nerve at the elbow may be necessary.

The deep, solely motor, branch of the ulnar nerve may be damaged in the palm by recurrent pressure from tools, e.g. a screwdriver, crutches or cycle handlebars.

Radial nerve compression

The radial nerve is compressed acutely against the humerus, e.g. when the arm is draped over a hard chair for several hours (Saturday night palsy). Wrist drop and weakness of brachioradialis and finger extension follow. Recovery is usual though not invariable within 1–3 months.

Meralgia paraesthetica

Entrapment of the lateral cutaneous nerve of the thigh beneath the inguinal ligament causes burning, tingling and numbness on the anterolateral aspect of the thigh. Many patients are obese; weight reduction helps relieve symptoms. Division of the inguinal ligament is not usually effective.

Common peroneal nerve palsy

When the common peroneal (lateral popliteal) nerve is compressed against the head of the fibula following prolonged squatting, wearing a plaster cast, prolonged bed rest or coma, there is foot drop and weakness of ankle eversion. Frequently no such cause is found. A patch of numbness on the anterolateral border of the shin or dorsum of the foot develops. Recovery is usual, though not invariable within several months.

Multifocal neuropathy (mononeuritis multiplex, multiple mononeuropathy)

This occurs in:

- diabetes mellitus
- leprosy (commonest cause world-wide)
- vasculitis
- sarcoidosis
- amyloidosis
- malignancy
- neurofibromatosis
- HIV infection
- Guillain–Barré syndrome (typically polyneuropathy, p. 1214)
- idiopathic multifocal motor neuropathy.

Diagnosis is largely clinical, supported by electrical studies. Several nerves become affected sequentially or simultaneously, e.g. ulnar, median, radial and lateral popliteal nerves. When multifocal neuropathy is symmetrical, there may be difficulty distinguishing it clinically from polyneuropathy. Treatment is usually that of the underlying disease.

Idiopathic multifocal motor neuropathy

A distal motor neuropathy (often asymmetrical and predominantly in the hands) of unknown cause develops gradually over months with profuse fasciculation – hence the confusion with motor neurone disease (p. 1208). Conduction block and denervation are seen electrically. Antibodies to the ganglioside GM_1 are found in over 50% of cases – a non-specific finding for they are also seen in other neuropathies, e.g. Guillain–Barré syndrome.

Treatment with i.v. immunoglobulin or cyclophosphamide may slow the condition.

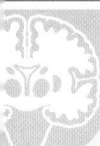

Polyneuropathies

Many toxins and disease processes cause polyneuropathy (see below), though the aetiology often remains obscure even after detailed study. The most common presentation is an acute, chronic or subacute sensorimotor neuropathy. A classification is given in Table 20.53.

Guillain-Barré syndrome (GBS)
Clinical features

This is the most common acute polyneuropathy (3/100 000/year); it is usually demyelinating (occasionally axonal) and probably has an autoallergic basis. GBS is a monophasic illness – it does not recur. It is also known as acute inflammatory or postinfective neuropathy, and acute inflammatory demyelinating polyradiculoneuropathy. It has become clear that the clinical spectrum of demyelinating GBS extends to an acute motor axonal neuropathy, and the Miller–Fisher syndrome – a rare proximal form that affects ocular muscles and causes ataxia.

Paralysis follows 1–3 weeks after an infection that is often trivial, and often unidentified. *Campylobacter jejuni* and cytomegalovirus infections are well-recognized causes of severe GBS. The infecting organisms induce humoral responses against peripheral nerves. 'Molecular mimicry', the sharing of homologous epitopes between microorganism liposaccharides and ganglioside components of nerves (e.g. GM_1), is a potential mechanism for these cross-reactions.

The patient complains of weakness of distal limb muscles and/or distal numbness. This ascends, progressing over several to 21 days. In mild cases there is little disability before spontaneous recovery begins, but in some 20% respiratory and facial muscles become weak. The patient may become completely paralysed. Weakness, areflexia and sensory loss progress, ascending from fingers and toes. Autonomic features (see below) are sometimes seen.

Diagnosis

This is established on clinical grounds and confirmed by nerve conduction studies; these show slowing of conduction in the common demyelinating form, prolonged distal motor latency and/or conduction block. CSF protein is typically raised to 1–3 g/L. The cell count and sugar level remain normal.

Differential diagnosis includes other paralytic illnesses such as poliomyelitis, botulism, cord compression or primary muscle disease.

Course and management

Paralysis may progress rapidly (hours/days) to require ventilatory support. It is essential that ventilation is monitored (vital capacity, blood gases) repeatedly to recognize emerging respiratory muscle weakness.

Table 20.53
Varieties of polyneuropathy

Guillain–Barré syndrome (acute postinfective polyneuropathy)
Chronic inflammatory demyelinating polyneuropathy
Diphtheritic polyneuropathy
Idiopathic sensorimotor neuropathy
Toxic, metabolic and vitamin deficiency neuropathies (Table 20.54)
Hereditary sensorimotor neuropathies e.g. Charcot–Marie Tooth
Other polyneuropathies
   Neuropathy in cancer
   Neuropathies in systemic diseases
   Autonomic neuropathy
   HIV-associated neuropathy
   Critical illness neuropathy

Subcutaneous heparin should be given to reduce the risk of venous thrombosis.

High-dosage intravenous γ-globulin reduces the duration and severity of paralysis. There is some anxiety about using this pooled blood product. Patients should be screened for IgA deficiency before γ-globulin is given – severe allergic reactions due to IgG antibodies may occur when IgA congenital deficiency is present. Plasmapheresis is also of proven benefit in shortening disability. Corticosteroids were used for many years but have been shown to be of no value. Recovery begins (whether or not treatment is given) between several days and 3 weeks from the outset. Prolonged ventilation may be necessary. Improvement towards independent mobility is gradual over many months; it may be incomplete.

Chronic inflammatory demyelinating polyneuropathy (CIDP)

This polyneuropathy recognized in the 1980s, develops over weeks or months, usually with a relapsing and remitting course over years. CSF protein is raised and usually segmental demyelination is seen in peripheral nerves, with Schwann cells arranged in lamellae – hence a descriptive pathological term – onion bulb. CIDP responds to steroids and to i.v. γ-globulin, which is used in exacerbations. In some cases plaques resembling MS lesions are seen on MRI in brain and spinal cord.

Outlook is variable, but with therapy many CIDP cases run a benign course over many years. Recovery occasionally occurs. There are several CIDP varieties – the usual demyelinating form, an axonal form, and multifocal neuropathy.

Diphtheritic neuropathy (p. 68)

Palatal weakness followed by pupillary paralysis and a sensorimotor neuropathy occur several weeks after faucial infection.

Idiopathic chronic sensorimotor neuropathy

The patient complains of progressive symmetrical numbness and tingling in hands and feet, spreading proximally in glove and stocking distribution. There is distal weakness which also ascends. Rarely cranial nerves are affected. Tendon reflexes become absent. Symptoms may progress over many months, remain static or occasionally remit. Autonomic features are sometimes seen.

Nerve conduction and electromyography show either axonal degeneration or demyelination, or features of both these processes. Peripheral nerve biopsy is helpful in classifying some of these cases, in particular diagnosing chronic inflammatory demyelinating polyneuropathy (see above) and unsuspected vasculitis.

Cranial polyneuropathy

This describes simultaneous or sequential cranial nerve lesions, which occur in malignant infiltration, particularly with lymphomas, and in sarcoidosis.

Toxic, metabolic and vitamin-deficiency neuropathies

The most common are shown in Table 20.54. All are due to impairment of normal axonal and/or myelin metabolism.

Metabolic neuropathies

Diabetes mellitus

Several varieties of neuropathy occur in diabetes:

- symmetrical sensory polyneuropathy
- acute painful neuropathy
- mononeuropathy and multiple mononeuropathy:
  – cranial nerve lesions
  – isolated peripheral nerve lesions (e.g. median)
- diabetic amyotrophy
- autonomic neuropathy.

These are discussed in more detail on page 1097.

Uraemia

Progressive sensorimotor neuropathy develops in chronic uraemia. The response to dialysis is variable but the neuropathy usually improves after renal transplantation.

Thyroid disease

A mild chronic sensorimotor neuropathy is sometimes seen in both hyperthyroidism and hypothyroidism (pp. 1040 and 1037). Myopathy also occurs in hyperthyroidism (p. 1041).

Porphyria

In acute intermittent porphyria (p. 1119) there are episodes of a severe, mainly proximal, neuropathy, sometimes associated with abdominal pain, confusion and later coma. Alcohol and barbiturates may precipitate attacks.

Amyloidosis

See page 1118. Either a polyneuropathy or a multifocal neuropathy develops.

Refsum's disease

This is a rare condition inherited as an autosomal recessive trait. There is a sensorimotor polyneuropathy with ataxia, retinal damage and deafness. It is due to a defect in phytanic acid metabolism.

Toxic neuropathies

Alcohol

Polyneuropathy, mainly in the lower limbs, occurs with chronic excess alcohol. Calf pain is common. Thiamine is the treatment, but the response is variable, even with complete abstention. A recurrence or progression of the neuropathy occurs if even small amounts of alcohol are consumed.

Drugs and industrial toxins

Many drugs and a wide variety of industrial toxins cause polyneuropathy. The more important drugs are shown in Table 20.55.

Table 20.54
Toxic, metabolic and vitamin-deficiency neuropathies

Metabolic	Toxic
Diabetes mellitus	Drugs (Table 20.55)
Uraemia	Alcohol
Hepatic disease	Industrial toxins, e.g. lead
Thyroid disease	
Porphyria	**Vitamin deficiency**
Amyloid disease	B_1 (thiamin)
Malignancy	B_6 (pyridoxine)
Refsum's disease	Nicotinic acid
	B_{12}

Table 20.55
Drug-related neuropathies

Drug	Neuropathy	Mode/site of action
Phenytoin Chloramphenicol Procarbazine Metronidazole	Sensory	Axon
Isoniazid	Sensory	Pyridoxine metabolism
Dapsone Gold Amphotericin	Motor	Axon
Nitrofurantoin Vincristine Chlorambucil Disulfiram Cisplatin	Sensorimotor	Axon
Perhexiline (not available in UK)	Sensorimotor	Myelin

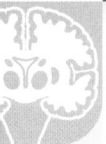
Industrial toxins

A wide variety of toxins have been shown to cause neuropathies:

- Lead poisoning – motor neuropathy
- Acrylamide (plastics industry), trichlorethylene, hexane and other fat-soluble hydrocarbons (e.g. glue-sniffing, p. 1259) – progressive sensorimotor polyneuropathy.
- Arsenic and thallium – polyneuropathy, initially sensory.

Vitamin-deficiency neuropathies

Vitamin deficiencies cause nervous system diseases that are largely preventable and potentially reversible if treated early – and inexorably progressive if not. Deficiency states occur in malnutrition, when they are commonly multiple.

Thiamin (vitamin B₁)

Dietary deficiency causes *beriberi* (p. 235). Principal features are polyneuropathy and cardiac failure. Thiamin deficiency also leads to an amnestic syndrome (Wernicke–Korsakoff psychosis, p. 236 and below); alcohol abuse is the commonest cause in western countries and rarely anorexia nervosa. Other neurological consequences of alcohol are summarized in Table 20.56.

Wernicke–Korsakoff syndrome. This thiamine-responsive *encephalopathy* is due to ischaemic damage in the brainstem and its connections. It consists of:

- *Eye signs* – nystagmus, bilateral lateral rectus palsies, conjugate gaze palsies, fixed pupils and, rarely, papilloedema
- *Ataxia* – broad-based gait, cerebellar signs and vestibular paralysis (absent calorics)
- *Cognitive change* – amnestic syndrome (confabulation), restlessness, stupor, coma
- *Hypothermia and hypotension* – due to hypothalamic involvement; rare.

Wernicke–Korsakoff syndrome is underdiagnosed. Erythrocyte transketolase activity is reduced but the test is of limited practical value because it is rarely available. Thiamine should be given parenterally if the diagnosis is in question. The drug is harmless. Untreated Wernicke–Korsakoff syndrome commonly leads to a severe irreversible amnestic state (Table 20.4, p. 1129) and residual brainstem signs.

Pyridoxine (vitamin B₆)

Deficiency causes a mainly sensory neuropathy. In practical terms this is seen as limb numbness developing during anti-TB therapy in slow isoniazid-acetylators (p. 967). Prophylactic pyridoxine 10 mg daily is given with isoniazid.

Vitamin B₁₂ (cobalamin)

Deficiency causes disease of the brain, spinal cord and peripheral nerves.

Subacute combined degeneration of the cord (SACD). Combined spinal cord and peripheral nerve damage is a sequel of Addisonian pernicious anaemia and rarely other causes of vitamin B₁₂ deficiency (p. 418).

The patient complains initially of numbness and tingling of fingers and toes. There is combined distal sensory loss, particularly posterior column, absent ankle jerks (neuropathy), with cord disease – exaggerated knee jerks, extensor plantar responses. Optic atrophy and retinal haemorrhage may occur. In later stages sphincter disturbance, severe generalized weakness and dementia develop. Exceptionally dementia develops in the early stages. Without treatment SACD is fatal within 5 years.

Macrocytosis with megaloblastic changes in bone marrow are usual but not invariable in SACD. Parenteral B₁₂ reverses peripheral nerve damage but has little effect in the spinal cord and brain.

Hereditary sensorimotor neuropathies (HMNS)

These form large and complex groups, phenotypically similar but genetically heterogeneous.

Charcot–Marie–Tooth disease

Charcot–Marie–Tooth (CMT) disease also called peroneal muscular atrophy describes a common clinical phenotype – of distal limb wasting and weakness that slowly progresses over many years, mostly in the legs, with variable loss of sensation and reflexes. In advanced disease, distal wasting is so marked that the legs are said to resemble inverted champagne bottles. Mild cases have pes cavus and clawing of the toes that can pass unnoticed. Many genetic variants of the CMT phenotype are recognized:

- HMSN Ia (CMT 1A) – the commonest, autosomal dominant (AD) demyelinating neuropathy caused by duplication (or point mutation) of a 1.5 megabase

---

Table 20.56
Neurological effects of ethyl alcohol

Acute intoxication	Epilepsy (3–10%)
Disturbance of balance, gait and speech	Acute intoxication
	Alcohol withdrawal
Coma	Hypoglycaemia
Head injury and its sequelae	Cerebellar degeneration
	Cerebral infarction
Alcohol withdrawal	Cerebral atrophy
'Morning shakes'	Dementia
Tremor of arms and legs	Central pontine myelinolysis
Delirium tremens	Marchiafava–Bignami syndrome
Thiamin deficiency	(a rare degeneration of the
Polyneuropathy	corpus callosum)
Wernicke–Korsakoff syndrome	

portion p11.2 of chromosome 17 encompassing the peripheral myelin protein 22 gene (*PMP22*)

- HMSN Ib (CMT 1B) – the second commonest, an AD demyelinating neuropathy due to mutations in the myelin protein zero (*P0*) gene on chromosome 1
- HMSN II (CMT 2) – an axonal neuropathy (rare) also caused by *P0* gene mutations
- distal spinal muscular atrophy – this is a rare cause of the clinical CMT phenotype
- optic atrophy, deafness, retinitis pigmentosa and spastic paraparesis are sometimes seen in other HMSN variants
- a sex-linked form is due to an abnormality in the connexin gene (p. 178).

HMSN III

This rare demyelinating sensory neuropathy of childhood (Déjérine–Sottas disease) leads to severe incapacity during adolescence. CSF protein is greatly elevated to 10 g/L or more, and nerve roots become greatly hypertrophied. Point mutations either of *PMP22* gene, or of *P0*, generate this phenotype.

Other polyneuropathies
Neuropathy in cancer

Polyneuropathy is seen as a non-metastatic manifestation of malignancy, sometimes with anti-Hu antibodies. Polyneuropathy occurs in myeloma and other dysproteinaemic states, probably owing to impaired perfusion of nerve trunks or to demyelination associated with allergic reactions within peripheral nerves. Individual nerves are sometimes infiltrated with metastatic malignant cells.

Neuropathies in systemic diseases

Vasculitic neuropathy occurs in SLE (see p. 559), polyarteritis nodosa (p. 567), Churg–Strauss syndrome (p. 910), rheumatoid disease (p. 543), sarcoidosis and giant cell arteritis (p. 566). Both multifocal neuropathy and symmetrical sensorimotor polyneuropathy develop.

POEMS syndrome. This rare condition consists of chronic inflammatory demyelinating **P**olyneuropathy, **O**rganomegaly (hepatomegaly 50%), **E**ndocrinopathy (gynaecomastia and atrophic testes), an **M** protein band on electrophoresis with less than 5% of plasma cells in bone marrow, and **S**kin hyperpigmentation.

Autonomic neuropathy

Autonomic neuropathy causes postural hypotension, urinary retention, impotence, diarrhoea (or occasionally constipation), diminished sweating, impaired pupillary responses and cardiac arrhythmias. This develops in diabetes mellitus, in amyloidosis and may complicate Guillain–Barré syndrome. Many varieties of neuropathy cause autonomic failure to a mild, and often subclinical, degree. Occasionally, when there is damage to small myelinated and non-myelinated B and C fibres, clinical features of the autonomic neuropathy predominate, e.g. in diabetes.

HIV-associated polyneuropathies

A wide variety of neuropathies occur in HIV patients. Inflammatory demyelinating neuropathies indistinguishable from Guillain–Barré and CIDP are seen early in HIV infection, particularly during seroconversion. The most common neuropathy is a chronic distal, symmetrical painful neuropathy.

Rarely, a severe lumbosacral polyradiculoneuropathy develops, with a profound lower limb flaccid paralysis, areflexia and sphincter dysfunction. Multifocal neuropathy is also seen (p. 1213).

All HIV-associated neuropathies respond poorly to retroviral therapy.

Critical illness polyneuropathy (p. 950)

Some 50% of critically ill ITU patients with multiple organ failure and sepsis develop electrical features of an axonal polyneuropathy. The severe inflammatory response following infection or trauma appears to initiate events that lead to impaired neural microcirculation. Clinically, distal weakness and depressed reflexes are seen during recovery from the critical illness, less commonly than electrical changes might suggest. Resolution is usual.

Plexus and nerve root lesions

The common conditions that cause these lesions are summarized in Table 20.57.

Thoracic outlet syndrome

A fibrous band or cervical rib extending from the tip of the transverse process of C7 to the first rib stretches across the lower brachial plexus roots (C8 and T1). There is forearm pain (ulnar border), T1 sensory loss and thenar muscle wasting, principally abductor pollicis

Table 20.57
Principal causes of plexus and nerve root lesions

Plexus
Trauma
Malignant infiltration
Cervical rib (thoracic outlet syndrome)
Neuralgic amyotrophy

Nerve root
Trauma
Herpes zoster
Meningeal inflammation (e.g. syphilis, arachnoiditis)
Tumours (neurofibroma, metastases)
Cervical and lumbar spondylosis

brevis. Horner's syndrome may develop. The rib or band can be excised.

In some patients the rib or band causes subclavian artery or venous occlusion. Neurological and vascular problems rarely occur together. Thoracic outlet syndrome is also used, rather vaguely, to describe various painful upper limb symptoms.

Neuralgic amyotrophy

This is a clinically distinct condition with severe pain in the muscles of one shoulder followed by wasting, usually of infraspinatus, supraspinatus, deltoid and serratus anterior muscles. The demyelinating brachial plexopathy develops over several days. The cause is unknown; since the condition sometimes follows viral infection or immunization, an allergic basis is postulated.

Recovery of wasted muscles occurs over some months.

Malignant infiltration

Metastatic disease of nerve roots of the brachial or lumbosacral plexus causes a painful radiculopathy. A common example is an apical bronchial neoplasm (Pancoast's tumour) that causes a T1 lesion and involves the sympathetic outflow. There is wasting of small muscles of the hand, pain, T1 sensory loss and ipsilateral Horner's syndrome. This also occurs in apical tuberculosis.

Cervical and lumbar spondylosis

Spondylosis (Tables 10.3 and 10.6) describes degenerative changes within vertebrae and intervertebral discs that occur during ageing or secondarily to trauma or rheumatoid disease. Several, often related, factors produce the signs and symptoms, including:

- osteophytes – local bony overgrowth (spurs or bars)
- congenital narrowing of the spinal canal
- intervertebral disc degeneration with posterior or lateral disc protrusion
- ischaemic changes in the cord and nerve roots.

Changes on plain X-rays are common in the mid and lower cervical and lower lumbar region in the normal population and correlate poorly with symptoms and signs. Narrowing of disc spaces, osteophytes, narrowing of exit foramina, and narrowing of the spinal canal are seen. Unsuspected malignancy or osteomyelitis may also be shown.

In these common clinical syndromes MRI is the investigation of choice.

Lateral cervical disc protrusion (Fig. 20.27)

The patient complains of pain in the arm. A C7 protrusion is the most common lesion. There is root pain, which radiates into the C7 myotome (triceps, deep to scapular and extensor aspect of forearm), with a sensory disturbance, tingling, and numbness in the C7 dermatome.

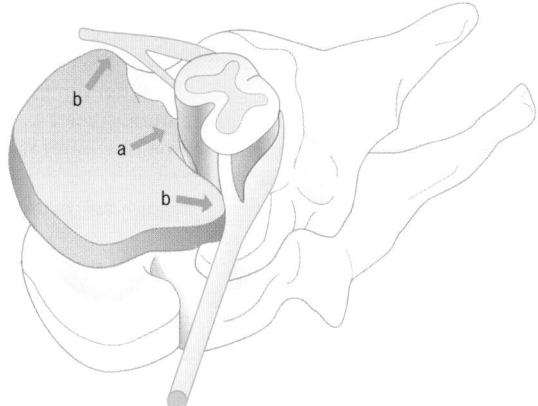

Fig. 20.27 Central and lateral disc protrusions. (a) Central disc protrusion compressing spinal cord. **(b)** Lateral disc protrusion compressing nerve roots.

In a C7 root lesion there is:

- weakness/wasting – triceps, wrist and finger extensors
- loss of the triceps jerk (C7 reflex arc)
- C7 dermatome sensory loss.

Although the initial pain is often very severe, most cases recover with rest and analgesics. It is usual to immobilize the neck. Where recovery is delayed, disc protrusion with root compression is seen on MRI or myelography and surgical root decompression usually performed.

Lateral lumbar disc protrusion

The L5 and S1 roots are commonly compressed by lateral prolapse of the L4–L5 and L5–S1 discs, respectively. There is low back pain and sciatica (pain radiating down the buttock and lower limb). The onset is typically acute. It sometimes follows lifting a heavy weight, bending or minor injury. When the pain follows such an event, it is tempting to ascribe the condition entirely to it. However, lateral lumbar disc protrusion is commonly apparently spontaneous, and lifting or injury are usually only precipitating events in an established and inevitable process.

Straight-leg raising is limited. There is loss of reflexes (e.g. ankle jerk in a complete S1 root lesion) and weakness of plantar flexion (S1). Sensory loss is found in the affected dermatome.

Most cases of sciatica resolve with rest and analgesics. In the minority, MRI is necessary and laminectomy is indicated when a substantial disc lesion is shown.

Acute low back pain

Acute low back pain is an extremely common problem. Most cases are of disc origin (discogenic) or the pain arises from the facet joints. It is unusual that it causes clinically significant nerve root compression. Bed rest for back pain, and rest on hard boards, has long been advocated. However, recent studies suggest that patients should be recommended to be as active as possible and to seek manipulative treatment.

Central disc protrusion (p. 1151)

Central cervical disc protrusion (cervical myelopathy). Posterior disc protrusion (Fig. 20.15r), common at C4–C5, C5–C6 and C6–C7 levels, causes spinal cord compression. Congenital spinal canal narrowing, osteophytic bars and ischaemia are contributory factors. The patient complains of difficulty in walking. Frequently there are no neck symptoms. Spastic paraparesis (or tetraparesis) is found, with variable sensory loss. A reflex level in the upper limbs and evidence of lateral disc protrusion may coexist. MRI or myelography is necessary to demonstrate the level and extent of cord compression. Neck manipulation should be avoided, and a collar fitted.

Cervical laminectomy or anterior fusion of the vertebral bodies with removal of the disc may be necessary when cord compression is severe or progressive. The results of surgery are variable. Simple functional tests are valuable in assessing patients before and after surgery. Complete recovery of the pyramidal signs is unusual, although progression may be halted.

Central thoracic disc protrusion

Central protrusion of a thoracic disc is a rare cause of paraparesis.

Central lumbosacral disc protrusion

A central disc protrusion causes a *cauda equina* syndrome with back pain, bilateral weakness of the lower limbs, sacral numbness, retention of urine, impotence and areflexia. Many nerve roots are involved. The onset is either acute (a cause of an acute flaccid paraparesis) or chronic, when intermittent claudication occurs. A *cauda equina* syndrome should be suspected immediately if a patient with back pain develops retention of urine or sacral numbness. Urgent imaging and surgical decompression is indicated for this emergency. Neoplasms in the lumbosacral region cause a similar picture.

Spinal stenosis

Narrowing of the spinal canal is developmental and frequently symptomless. Congenital narrowing of the cervical canal predisposes the cervical cord to damage from minor disc protrusion. In the lumbar region, further narrowing of the canal by a disc protrusion is a cause of root pain, or buttock and lower limb claudication. As the patient walks, nerve roots become hyperaemic and swell. This causes buttock and lower limb pain with numbness. Surgical decompression is required.

FURTHER READING

Hahn A (1998) Guillain–Barré syndrome. *Lancet* **352**: 635–641.
Royal College of General Practitioners (1996) *The Management of Acute Low Back Pain.* London: RCGP.
Singh A, Crockard HA (1999) Quantitative assessment of cervical spondylotic myelopathy by a simple walking test. *Lancet* **354**: 370–373.

Non-metastatic manifestations of malignancy

Many neurological syndromes may accompany malignancy in the absence of metastases. Clinical pictures include:

- sensorimotor neuropathy (p. 1214)
- mononeuritis multiplex (p. 1213)
- cranial polyneuropathy (p. 1215)
- Lambert–Eaton myasthenic–myopathic syndrome (LEMS, p. 1223)
- motor neurone disease variants (p. 1208)
- spastic paraparesis (p. 1206)
- cerebellar syndrome (p. 1147)
- dementia and encephalopathy (p. 1264)
- progressive multifocal leucoencephalopathy (p. 50).

Mechanisms remain obscure. The clinical importance is that the neurological syndrome sometimes precedes clinical signs of the neoplasm – often a small-cell bronchial carcinoma or lymphoma.

Diseases of voluntary muscle

Definitions

- **Myopathy** describes diseases of voluntary muscle generally.
- **Myositis** indicates inflammation.
- **Muscular dystrophy** describes inherited disorders with progressive weakness.
- **Myasthenia** means fatiguable (worse on exercise) weakness.
- **Myotonia** is sustained contraction/slow relaxation seen in myotonias.
- **Channelopathy** describes disorders of ion channels within muscle cells.

Weakness is the predominant feature of primary muscle disease. Its distribution and pattern is of diagnostic importance. For classification, see Table 20.58. Only the more common conditions are mentioned below.

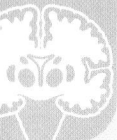

Table 20.58
Classification of muscle disease

Acquired myopathies	Genetically determined myopathies
Inflammatory myopathy	**Muscular dystrophies**
Polymyositis	Duchenne muscular dystrophy
Alone	Facioscapulohumeral dystrophy
With skin lesions	Limb girdle dystrophy
(dermatomyositis)	
With collagen disease	**Myotonias**
With malignancy	Dystrophia myotonica
Viral, bacterial and parasitic	Myotonia congenita
infection	
Sarcoidosis	**Channelopathies**
	(periodic paralyses)
Metabolic and endocrine	Hypokalaemic periodic paralysis
myopathy	Hyperkalaemic periodic paralysis
Corticosteroids/Cushing's	Normokalaemic periodic paralysis
syndrome	
Thyroid disease	**Specific metabolic**
Calcium metabolism disorders	**myopathies** (e.g.)
Hypokalaemia	Myophosphorylase deficiency
Ethanol	Other defects of glycogen
Drugs	and fatty acid metabolism
	Mitochondrial disease
Myasthenic disorders	(ragged red muscle fibres)
Myasthenia gravis	Malignant hyperpyrexia
Lambert–Eaton	
myasthenic–myopathic	
syndrome (LEMS)	

Pathophysiology

Muscle fibres are affected by:

- acute inflammation and fibre necrosis (e.g. polymyositis, infection)
- chronic degeneration (e.g. Duchenne muscular dystrophy)
- infiltration by inflammatory tissue (e.g. sarcoidosis)
- fibre hypertrophy and regeneration
- ion-channel, immunological and mitochondrial disorders.

Examples of the latter are:

- In *myasthenia gravis*, antibodies to postsynaptic membrane acetylcholine receptor protein cause blocking of neuromuscular transmission.
- In *Lambert–Eaton myasthenic–myopathic syndrome* (LEMS), antibodies to muscle calcium-channel components are found.
- In *myotonias*, defective chloride ion membrane conductance is associated with delayed muscle relaxation.
- In *McArdle's syndrome*, myophosphorylase deficiency produces weakness after exercise.
- In *mitochondrial disease*, various ATP enzyme defects cause weakness.

Investigations

Diagnosis is made by the recognition of a clinical pattern in many muscle diseases. The distribution of weakness, wasting or hypertrophy, and muscle consistency (e.g. induration) should be noted.

Serum muscle enzymes

Serum creatine phosphokinase (and aldolase) is greatly elevated in many dystrophies (e.g. Duchenne muscular dystrophy) and in inflammatory disorders of muscle, particularly polymyositis. These enzymes are normal in myasthenia gravis and LEMS, and usually remain normal in myotonias and chronic partial denervation.

Neurogenetic tests

Genetic probes in propositus and family members are helpful in the diagnosis of muscular dystrophies.

Electromyography

When a muscle is weak the normal interference pattern is reduced. Changes in interference pattern indicate:

- *Myopathy.* Short-duration spiky polyphasic muscle action potentials are seen. Spontaneous fibrillation is occasionally recorded.
- *Denervation.* Fibrillation potentials of about 1 ms in duration and 50–200 mV in amplitude are seen.
- *Myotonic discharges.* A characteristic high-frequency whine is heard on the loudspeaker.
- *Decrement and increment.* In myasthenia gravis, a characteristic decrement in evoked muscle action potential follows motor nerve stimulation. The reverse is seen (i.e. an increment in repetitive response) in the rare LEMS, p. 1223.

Muscle biopsy

Histology of muscle fibre types (type 1, slow; type 2, fast), denervation, inflammation, dystrophic changes and muscle histochemistry are performed. Electron microscopy is sometimes necessary. In chronic partial denervation, fibre type grouping (i.e. groups of atrophic fibres of the same fibre type) is seen. Hypertrophic fibres also occur. In acute denervation, small angulated fibres are seen scattered randomly between normal fibres. In dystrophies and myositis, the muscle fibres are diffusely abnormal, the nuclei become central, and invasion by inflammatory cells and/or necrosis occurs. Considerable experience is required to assess these changes accurately.

Imaging

MR images show characteristic changes within muscles in some cases of myositis.

Inflammatory myopathies

Polymyositis

This group of disorders is characterized by non-suppurative skeletal muscle inflammation. Muscles are weak and usually painful. In many cases there are skin changes (dermatomyositis, p. 1298) or other connective tissue diseases (p. 557).

Clinical features

Isolated polymyositis is a rare disease, most common in the fourth and fifth decades. Proximal weakness causes difficulty in rising from a chair, climbing stairs or lifting. Weakness is typically proximal. Weak muscles ache and are sometimes tender and indurated. The course is variable, from a mild condition to a severe progressive disability. If the disease progresses, widespread weakness and wasting develop, with dysphagia, respiratory muscle weakness and cardiac involvement.

Investigations

Preliminary investigations show a raised ESR and a mild normochromic normocytic anaemia. ANF is sometimes positive. The serum creatine phosphokinase is usually greatly elevated. EMG shows myopathic changes. Occasionally fibrillation potentials occur and cause diagnostic difficulty. Muscle biopsy shows inflammatory changes with mononuclear cell infiltration.

Differential diagnosis

Muscular dystrophies rarely progress as rapidly as polymyositis and there is no muscle pain. Pseudo-hypertrophy, which occurs in some dystrophies, does not occur in polymyositis. There is no family history. Motor neurone disease is always eventually accompanied by upper motor neurone signs, and prominent fasciculation is common.

Treatment

Corticosteroids with azathioprine or cyclophosphamide reduce symptoms in about 75% of cases. Only rarely does polymyositis cause death.

Viral, bacterial and parasitic myositis

Muscle tissue is involved in many infections; see Table 20.59.

Table 20.59
Muscle involvement in infections

Myalgia	Influenza viruses
Bornholm's disease	Coxsackie B5
Acute polymyositis, with myoglobinuria	Coxsackie B6, ECHO 9
Acute suppurative (tropical) myositis	*Staphylococcus* spp.
Gas gangrene (clostridial myositis)	*Clostridium perfringens*
Necrotizing myositis	*Streptococcus* spp.
Tuberculous myositis (rare)	*Mycobacterium tuberculosis*
Trichinosis	*Trichinella spiralis*
Cysticercosis	*Taenia solium* (larval form)
Hydatid disease	*Echinococcus granulosus*
Toxoplasma myositis	*Toxoplasma gondii*
Sarcosporidiosis	*Sarcocystis lindemanni*
Chagas' disease	*Trypanosoma cruzi*
Actinomycosis	*Actinomyces* spp.

Myopathy in sarcoidosis and rheumatoid disease

In sarcoidosis, a subacute myopathy sometimes occurs, either with limb muscle swelling and induration, or with wasting. This is usually during pulmonary sarcoidosis, but occasionally it is isolated. Sarcoid nodules in muscle are seen on biopsy. Treatment is with steroids.

In rheumatoid disease, a rare localized nodular myositis causes painful swelling of limb, trunk and facial muscles.

Metabolic and endocrine myopathies

Corticosteroids and Cushing's syndrome

Proximal weakness occurs with prolonged high-dose steroid therapy, particularly with *9-alpha*-fluorinated steroids such as dexamethasone and triamcinolone and in Cushing's syndrome (p. 1052). Selective type-2 fibre atrophy is seen on biopsy.

Thyroid disease (see also p. 1035)

Several myopathies occur. Thyrotoxicosis is sometimes accompanied by severe proximal myopathy. There is also an association between thyrotoxicosis and myasthenia gravis, and between thyrotoxicosis and hypokalaemic periodic paralysis (p. 1224). Both associations are seen more frequently in South East Asia. In ophthalmic Graves' disease, there is swelling and lymphocytic infiltration of extraocular muscles (p. 1044).

Hypothyroidism is sometimes associated with muscle pain and stiffness, resembling myotonia. A proximal myopathy also occurs.

Disorders of calcium metabolism

Proximal myopathy develops in hypocalcaemia and rickets and osteomalacia of any cause (p. 584).

Hypokalaemia

Acute hypokalaemia (e.g. in diuretic therapy) causes a severe flaccid paralysis that is reversed by potassium, given slowly (p. 684). Chronic hypokalaemia (also commonly caused by diuretics) gives rise to a mild, mainly proximal, weakness. See also periodic paralysis (p. 1224).

Alcohol

Severe myopathy with muscle pain, necrosis and myoglobinuria occurs in acute alcoholic excess. A similar syndrome occurs in diamorphine and amfetamine addicts. A subacute proximal myopathy occurs with chronic alcohol abuse.

Drugs

Drug-induced muscle disorders have been described. These include proximal myopathy (steroids), muscle weakness (lithium), myositis-like syndrome (fibrates), rhabdomyolysis (a fibrate combined with a statin), and

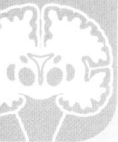
malignant hyperpyrexia (p. 1224). All are rare, and most respond to drug withdrawal.

The neuromuscular junction

Myasthenia gravis

This acquired condition is characterized by weakness and fatiguability of proximal limb, ocular and bulbar muscles. The heart is not affected. The prevalence is about 4 in 100 000. It is twice as common in women as in men, with a peak age incidence around 30.

The cause is unknown. IgG antibodies to acetylcholine receptor protein are found. Immune complexes (IgG and complement) are deposited at the postsynaptic membranes, causing interference with and later destruction of the acetylcholine receptor.

Thymic hyperplasia is found in 70% of myasthenic patients below the age of 40 years. In 10% of patients a thymic tumour is found, the incidence increasing with age; antibodies to striated muscle can be demonstrated in these patients. Young patients without a thymoma have an increased association with HLA-B8, and DR3.

There is an association between myasthenia gravis and thyroid disease, rheumatoid disease, pernicious anaemia and SLE. Transient myasthenia gravis is sometimes caused by D-penicillamine treatment in rheumatoid disease.

Clinical features

Fatiguability is seen in many muscles. Proximal limb muscles, extraocular muscles, and muscles of mastication, speech and facial expression are those commonly affected in the early stages. Respiratory difficulties may occur.

Complex extraocular palsies, ptosis and fluctuating proximal weakness are found. The reflexes are initially preserved but may be fatiguable, i.e. disappear. Muscle wasting is sometimes seen after many years.

Investigations

The clinical picture of fluctuating weakness is often diagnostic. Early symptoms of weakness and fatigue are frequently dismissed by attending doctors.

Serum acetylcholine receptor antibodies

These disease-specific IgG antibodies are present in 90% of cases of generalized myasthenia gravis. The antibodies are found in no other condition. In pure ocular myasthenia they are detectable in 50% of cases.

Nerve stimulation

There is a characteristic decrement in the evoked muscle action potential following continued stimulation of the motor nerve.

Tensilon (edrophonium) test

The anticholinesterase edrophonium (10 mg) is injected i.v. as a bolus after a 1–2 mg test dose. Improvement in weakness occurs within seconds and lasts for 2–3 minutes when the test is positive. To be certain, it is wise to have an observer present and to perform a control test using an injection of saline. Occasionally edrophonium causes bronchial constriction and syncope, and testing must not be carried out without facilities for resuscitation.

Other tests

Preliminary tests may show a thymoma on chest X-ray that can be confirmed by mediastinal imaging or with CT or MR imaging. Routine peripheral blood studies are normal – the ESR is not raised, and CPK normal. Autoantibodies to striated muscle, intrinsic factor or thyroid may be found. Rheumatoid factor and antinuclear antibody tests may be positive. Muscle biopsy is usually not performed but ultrastructural abnormalities can be seen.

Course and management

Myasthenia gravis fluctuates in severity; most cases have a protracted, lifelong course. Respiratory impairment, dysphagia and nasal regurgitation occur; emergency assisted ventilation may be required in myasthenic crises. Simple monitoring tests, such as the duration the arm can be held outstretched, and the vital capacity, are useful.

Exacerbations are usually unpredictable and unprovoked but may be brought on by infections, by aminoglycosides or other drugs. Enemas (magnesium sulphate) may provoke severe weakness.

Treatment

Oral anticholinesterases

Pyridostigmine (60 mg tablet) is the drug most widely used. Its duration of action is 3–4 hours. The dose (usually 4–16 tablets daily) is determined by the patient's response. Pyridostigmine prolongs acetylcholine action by inhibiting cholinesterase. Overdose of anticholinesterase causes severe weakness (a cholinergic crisis). Colic and diarrhoea may occur with anticholinesterases. Oral atropine 0.5 mg with each dose helps to reduce this. Anticholinesterases help weakness but do not alter the natural history of myasthenia.

Thymectomy

Thymectomy improves prognosis, particularly in women below 40 years with positive receptor antibodies and a history of myasthenia of less than 10 years. Some 60% of non-thymoma cases improve; the precise reason is unclear. If a thymoma is present, surgery is necessary to remove a potentially malignant tumour; it is less usual for myasthenia to improve.

Immunosuppressant drugs

Corticosteroids are often used. There is improvement in 70% of cases, although this may be preceded by an initial relapse. Azathioprine is often used in addition.

Plasmapheresis and immunoglobulin therapy

During exacerbations these interventions are of value.

Lambert–Eaton myasthenic–myopathic syndrome (LEMS)

This rare non-metastatic manifestation of small-cell carcinoma of the bronchus is due to defective acetylcholine release at the neuromuscular junction. Proximal muscle weakness, sometimes involving the ocular and bulbar muscles is found, with absent reflexes. Weakness tends to improve after a few minutes' muscular contraction, and absent reflexes return, (cf. myasthenia). Diagnosis is confirmed by EMG and repetitive stimulation of a motor nerve. Antibodies to P/Q-type voltage-gated calcium channels are found in most cases (90%). 3,4-diaminopyridine is used in treatment, with variable effect.

Other rare myasthenic syndromes exist, for example congenital myasthenia.

Muscular dystrophies

These progressive genetically determined disorders of skeletal and sometimes cardiac muscle have a complex clinical and neurogenetic classification.

Duchenne muscular dystrophy (DMD)

This is inherited as an X-linked recessive disorder, though one-third of cases are spontaneous mutants. DMD occurs in 1 in 3000 male infants. The DMD locus has been localized to the Xp21 region of the X chromosome; there is absence of the gene product – the protein *dystrophin*, which is a rod-shaped cytoskeletal muscle protein. DMD is usually obvious by the fourth year, and often causes death by 20.

Dystrophin is essential for cell membrane stability, and deficiency leads to reduction in three glycoproteins (now called α-, β- and γ-sarcoglycan) which link dystrophin to laminin within the cell membrane.

Becker's muscular dystrophy is a disabling condition but milder than Duchenne; it develops in young adults. It is also due to a mutation and abnormalities in dystrophin.

Clinical features

The boy with DMD is noticed to have difficulty in running and in rising to an erect position from the floor, when he has to use the hands to climb up his legs (Gowers' sign). There is initially a proximal limb weakness with pseudohypertrophy of the calves. The myocardium is affected. The boy becomes severely disabled by the age of 10.

Investigations

Diagnosis is often made on clinical grounds alone. Creatine phosphokinase is grossly elevated (100–200 times normal). Muscle biopsy shows characteristic variation in fibre size, fibre necrosis, regeneration and replacement by fat, and on immunochemical staining an absence of dystrophin. EMG shows a myopathic pattern.

Table 20.60
Limb-girdle and facioscapulohumeral dystrophies

	Limb-girdle	Facioscapulohumeral
Inheritance	Autosomal recessive	Autosomal dominant
Onset	10–20 years	10–40 years
Muscles affected	Shoulder and pelvic girdle	Face, shoulder and pelvis
Progress	Severe disability within 20–25 years	Normal life expectancy slow progression
Pseudo-hypertrophy	Rare	Very rare

Management

There is no curative treatment. Passive physiotherapy helps to prevent contractures in the later stages of the disease. Portable respiratory support gives a substantially improved life expectancy.

Carrier detection. A female with an affected brother has a 50% chance of carrying the gene. In carrier females, 70% have a raised creatine phosphokinase level and the remainder usually have electromyographic abnormalities or changes on biopsy. Accurate carrier and prenatal diagnosis can be made using cDNA probes that are co-inherited with the DMD locus.

Genetic advice and counselling about possible termination of pregnancy should be given. Determination of fetal sex by amniocentesis and selective abortion of a male fetus is sometimes carried out. Many proven carrier females choose not to have offspring.

Limb girdle and facioscapulohumeral dystrophy

These less severe but disabling dystrophies are summarized in Table 20.60. There are many other varieties of muscular dystrophy. Most are associated with a sarcoglycan deficiency. Genes for various limb girdle muscular dystrophies (LGMD) have been located; some of the proteins for which they code, e.g. calpain, are known. Type 1 LGMD is a rare autosomal dominant condition. Type 2 LGMD includes all recessive varieties, further subdivided, e.g. LGMD2A (calpain III deficiency), LGMD2C (γ-sarcoglycan deficiency).

FURTHER READING

Emery AEH (2002) The muscular dystrophies. *Lancet* **359**: 687–695.

Myotonias

These are characterized by continued, involuntary, muscle contraction after cessation of voluntary effort. The EMG is characteristic (p. 1156). Patients with myotonia tolerate general anaesthetics poorly. The two most common myotonias are mentioned below. Since there is

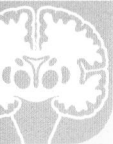

defective skeletal muscle cell chloride ion membrane conductance, myotonias are also classified as channelopathies (see below).

Dystrophia myotonica

This autosomal dominant condition is a genetic disorder with triple repeat mutations (p. 179). It causes progressive distal muscle weakness, with ptosis, weakness and thinning of the face and sternomastoids. Myotonia is usually present. The muscle disease is part of a larger syndrome comprising:

- cataracts
- frontal baldness
- intellectual impairment (mild)
- cardiomyopathy and conduction defects
- small pituitary fossa and hypogonadism
- glucose intolerance
- low serum IgG.

This gradually progressive disease usually becomes evident between 20 and 50 years. There is correlation between disease severity, age at onset and approximate size of triple repeat mutations. Phenytoin or procainamide sometimes helps the myotonia slightly.

Myotonia congenita (Thomsen's disease)

An isolated autosomal dominant myotonia, usually mild, becomes evident in childhood. The myotonia, which persists, is accentuated by rest and by cold. Diffuse muscle hypertrophy occurs – the patient appears to have well-developed muscles.

Channelopathies

A wide variety of conditions are now included within this group – see also myotonias (above) and Lambert–Eaton myasthenic-myopathic syndrome (p. 1223).

Hypokalaemic periodic paralysis

This channelopathy is characterized by generalized weakness, including the speech and bulbar muscles, that often starts after a heavy carbohydrate meal or after a period of rest after exertion. Attacks last for several hours. It is often first noted in the teenage years and tends to remit after the age of 35 years. The serum potassium is usually below 3.0 mmol/L in an attack. The weakness responds to the administration of potassium chloride. It is usually an autosomal dominant trait caused by mutations in a muscle voltage-gated calcium channel (CACLN1A3).

Similar weakness also occurs in hypokalaemia due to diuretics, and occurs with thyrotoxicosis.

Hyperkalaemic periodic paralysis

This condition, also autosomal dominant, is characterized by attacks of weakness sometimes precipitated by exercise. Attacks start in childhood and tend to remit after the age of 20 years. Attacks last from 30 minutes to 2 hours. Myotonia may occur. Serum potassium is raised. An attack can be terminated by giving intravenous calcium gluconate or chloride. There are point mutations in a muscle voltage-gated sodium channel (SCN4A).

A very rare normokalaemic, sodium-responsive periodic paralysis also occurs.

FURTHER READING

Benatar MG (1999) Calcium channelopathies. *Quarterly Journal of Medicine* **92**: 133–141.

Metabolic myopathies

This is a large complex group of rare, genetically determined muscle diseases. Three will be mentioned here.

Myophosphorylase deficiency (McArdle's syndrome)

This is an autosomal recessive disorder in which lack of skeletal muscle myophosphorylase causes easy fatiguability and severe cramp on exercise, with myoglobinuria. Venous lactate during ischaemic exercise does not increase; this is the basis of a test for McArdle's syndrome.

Malignant hyperpyrexia

Widespread skeletal muscle rigidity and hyperpyrexia developing as a sequel to general anaesthesia or neuroleptic drugs (e.g. haloperidol) is due to a genetic defect in the sarcoplasmic reticulum calcium-release channel. Sudden death during or after anaesthesia may occur in this rare condition, sometimes inherited as an autosomal dominant trait. Dantrolene is useful in controlling rigidity.

Mitochondrial diseases (p. 173)

These comprise a complex group of disorders involving muscle, peripheral nerves and CNS. They are characterized by morphological and biochemical abnormalities in mitochondria, with several unusual genetic characteristics, for example the maternal inheritance of mitochondrial DNA. The disease spectrum is large, ranging from optic atrophy (see Leber's hereditary optic neuropathy, p. 1131) to myopathies, neuropathies and encephalopathy. MELAS (mitochondrial encephalomyopathy, lactic acidosis, stroke-like episodes) is one well-recognized form. Chronic progressive ophthalmoplegia (CPEO) is another, and MERRF describes the occurrence of myoclonic epilepsy and 'ragged red' muscle fibres on biopsy. Further developments in this complex field continue.

FURTHER READING

Leonard JV, Shapira AHV (2000) Mitochondrial respiratory chain disorders I and II. *Lancet* **355**: 299–304, 389–394.

Psychological medicine

Introduction

Psychiatry is the branch of medicine that is concerned with the study and treatment of disorders of mental function. Psychological medicine, or liaison psychiatry, is the discipline within psychiatry that is concerned with psychiatric and psychological disorders in patients who have physical complaints or conditions. This chapter primarily will concern itself with this particular branch of psychiatry.

Many doctors believe that psychiatric disorders imply that the cause or even the disorder itself is psychological. 'All your tests are negative so it must be "all in your mind".' But absence of evidence is not the same as evidence of absence. The last 10 years has seen an explosion of research which has consistently shown that the brain is functionally or anatomically abnormal in most if not all psychiatric disorders. This evidence is breaking down long-held beliefs that diseases are either physical or psychological. We now know that doctors must consider both physical and psychological factors, and their interactions, in order to understand and thus help their patients. This philosophical change of approach rejects the Cartesian dualistic approach of the mind/body *medical model* and replaces it with the more holistic *biopsychosocial model*.

Epidemiology (Box 21.1)

The prevalence of psychiatric disorders in the community in the UK is about 20%, mainly composed of depressive and anxiety disorders and substance misuse (mainly alcohol). The prevalence is about twice as high

---

Box 21.1

The approximate prevalence of psychiatric disorders in different populations

	% (approx.)
Community	20%
Neuroses	16%
Psychoses	0.5%
Alcohol misuse	5%
Drug misuse	2% (an underestimate)
(total in community 20% due to comorbidity)	
Primary care	25%
General hospital outpatients	30%
General hospital inpatients	40%

in patients attending the general hospital, with the highest rates in the accident and emergency department and medical wards. The higher rates in the general hospital are due to several factors, such as admission for deliberate self-harm, a psychiatric disorder or treatment causing physical harm (e.g. alcohol-induced hepatitis or lithium-related renal failure), and physical presentations of psychiatric disorders (such as weight loss due to anorexia nervosa).

Culture and ethnicity

Culture and ethnicity can alter either the presentation or the prevalence of psychiatric ill-health. Biological factors in mental illness are usually similar across cultural boundaries whereas psychological and social factors will vary. For example, the prevalence and presentation of schizophrenia vary little between countries, suggesting that biological factors are operating independently of cultural factors. In contrast, conditions in which social factors play more of a role vary between cultures, so that anorexia nervosa is found more often in developed cultures. Culture can also influence the presentation of illnesses, such that physical symptoms are more common presentations of depressive illness in Asia than in Europe.

The psychiatric history

The purpose of the history is to help to make a diagnosis, determine possible aetiology and estimate prognosis. Data may be taken from several sources, including interviewing the patient, a friend or relative (usually with the patient's permission), or their general practitioner. The patient interview enables a doctor to establish a relationship with the patient and is the primary way to make a psychiatric diagnosis. Box 21.2 gives essential guidance on how to safely conduct such an interview. At the same time it is worth remembering that it is very unlikely that a patient will physically harm a healthcare professional. When interviewing a patient for the first time follow the guidance outlined in Chapter 1 (see p. 11).

The history consists of:

- *Reason for referral* – a brief statement of why and how the patient came to the attention of the doctor.
- *Complaints* – as reported by the patient.
- *Present illness* – a detailed account of the illness from the earliest time at which a change was noted until the patient came to the attention of the doctor.
- *Past psychiatric history* – previous episodes of psychiatric illness and their treatments, including responses and adverse reactions. Always ask after previous episodes of self-harm.
- *Past medical history* – this should include emotional reactions to illness and procedures.

> ### Box 21.2
>
> **The essentials of a safe psychiatric interview**
>
> - **Beforehand:** Ask someone senior who knows the patient whether it is safe to interview the patient alone.
> - **Access to others:** If in doubt, interview in the view or hearing of others, or accompanied by another member of staff.
> - **Setting:** If safe; in a quiet room alone for confidentiality, not by the bed.
> - **Seating:** Place yourself between the door and the patient.
> - **Alarm:** If available, find out where the alarm is and how to use it.

- *Family history* – focusing on the way the parents or carers cared (physically and emotionally) for the patient, and the occurrence of both mental and physical illnesses in first-degree relatives.
- *Personal (biographical) history* – a short biography that covers childhood difficulties including both abuse and neglect, educational problems (e.g. bullying and truanting), qualifications (to judge premorbid intelligence), job problems, sexual relationships, children, present housing, financial situation, bereavements and life stresses. Ways of asking awkward questions might include:
  - 'Do you feel able to tell me what memory most upsets you/makes you angry?'
  - 'Are you able to say what you have done in the past that you most regret?'
  - 'How well do you get on with your partner? Are you happy in every way? Are there any problems in your sexual life that you think I should know about?'
- A *reproductive history* in women should include menstrual problems, pregnancies, terminations, miscarriages, contraception and the menopause, if relevant.
- *Personality* – this helps to determine prognosis and response to treatment. The doctor should find out how other people would describe the patient. Is the patient generally a worrier, shy, introverted, dependent on others, passive, aggressive, irritable, over-emotional, prone to moodiness, conscientious, or perfectionist? These are all personality traits that predict a poorer outcome in both medical and psychiatric disorders.
- *Drug history* – both prescribed and over-the-counter medication, the use (units per week) and abuse of alcohol, tobacco, caffeine, and illicit drugs.
- *Forensic history* – you should carefully explain that you need to ask about this since ill-health can sometimes lead to problems with the law.
  - 'Have you ever had any legal problems or contact with the police or courts?'

Particularly note any violent or sexual offences. This is part of a *risk assessment* and is necessary in order to assess potential risks to those close to the patient as well as staff. Ask the patient what is the worst harm they have ever inflicted on someone else, which will give an indication of the potential for violence.

- A *systematic review* of physical symptoms is particularly necessary in patients complaining of physical symptoms.

The mental state examination (MSE)

The history will already have assessed several aspects of the MSE, but the interviewer will need to expand several areas as well as test specific areas, such as cognition.

Appearance and general behaviour

State and colour of clothes, facial appearance, eye contact, posture and movement provide information about a patient's affect. Patients with *psychomotor retardation* due to a depressive illness sit with shoulders hunched, immobile, tearful, with a downcast gaze. Depressed individuals tend to wear clothes with dark colours. Agitation (seen with depressive illness) and anxiety causes an easy startle response, sweating, tremor, restlessness, fidgeting, visual scanning (for danger) and even pacing up and down. Patients with mania are often physically overactive and disinhibited, wearing colourful clothes. Someone who is actively hallucinating will seem distracted and suddenly stop talking or listening and stare intently at a particular place in the room.

Mood and affect

The patient has an *emotion or feeling*, tells the doctor their *mood* and the doctor observes their *affect*. In psychiatric disorders, mood may be altered in three ways:

A persistent change in mood

- *Depression* is a lowering of mood, such as feeling sad, tearful, melancholic or low in spirits. Some patients report *anhedonia*, which is a lack of positive pleasure or loss of interest. Depression is the cardinal feature of depressive illness. Sometimes the word 'depression' is used as shorthand to describe a depressive illness. *Diurnal variation* in mood, feeling worse on waking, suggests a more severe illness, whereas a *reactive mood*, in which the patient can sometimes respond positively, indicates less severity.
- *Anxiety* is a feeling of constant, inappropriate or excessive worry, fear, apprehension, tension or inner restlessness, seen in anxiety and depressive disorders and drug withdrawal.

- *Elation* is a feeling of high spirits, exuberant happiness, vitality and even ecstasy, seen in mania and acute drug intoxication.
- *Irritability* can be either expressed (as in a temper or impatience) or an internal feeling of exasperation or anger, seen in both mania and depressive illness, especially in men.
- *Blunting* of affect is a total absence of emotion, seen most commonly in chronic schizophrenia.

Fluctuating or labile mood

This occurs when different emotions rapidly follow one another, so that a patient is crying one moment and laughing the next. This can occur in mixed affective states (see p. 1241). Alternatively the patient is easily and excessively emotional over banal events or news, but the emotion is transient. This is seen in both a pseudobulbar palsy, commonly following a cerebrovascular accident (see p. 1143), and with mild depressive illnesses.

Inconsistent or incongruous mood

This occurs when emotional expression fails to match thoughts and actions. For example, a patient may laugh when describing the death of a close relative. This can occur in schizophrenia. Such incongruity needs to be distinguished from the embarrassed laughter that indicates that someone is ill at ease when talking about a distressing subject.

Speech

Disorders of thinking are usually recognized from the patient's speech.

Disorders of the stream of thought

These are abnormalities in the amount and speed of the thoughts experienced.

Pressure of speech occurs in mania and can be recognized by loudness, rapidity, and difficulty in interrupting speech.

Poverty of speech is the opposite experience, when there appears to be an absence of any thought and patients report their minds to be empty. It occurs in depressive illness.

Thought block occurs in schizophrenia. There is an abrupt and complete interruption of the stream of thought, so the mind goes blank. Patients may interpret the experience in an unusual way (e.g. thought withdrawal; see below).

Disorders of the form of thought

Flight of ideas. The patient's thoughts rapidly jump from one topic to another, such that one train of thought is not completed before another appears. It is often produced by clang associations (the use of two or more words with a similar sound: 'sun, son, song'), punning, rhyming, and responding to distracting cues in the immediate surroundings. Flight of ideas is characteristic of mania and often accompanies pressure of speech.

Perseveration is the persistent and inappropriate repetition of the same thoughts or actions. It occurs in frontal lobe disorders.

Loosening of associations is manifested by a loss of the normal structure of thinking. The most striking impression is a lack of clarity so that it is impossible to understand what is being said. There are several forms. Knight's move or derailment denotes an illogical transition from one topic to another, in the absence of flight of ideas. When this abnormality is extreme and disrupts the grammatical structure of speech, it is termed 'word salad'.

Thought broadcast is when the patient experiences their thoughts as being understood by others without talking, as though their thoughts are literally being broadcast to all around them.

Thought insertion occurs when a patient's thought is perceived as being planted in their mind by someone else.

Thought withdrawal occurs when a patient experiences their thoughts being taken away from them, without their control.

The latter three types of thought disorders are all *first rank symptoms*, which Schneider suggested were pathognomonic of schizophrenia (see p. 1261).

Thought content

Thought content refers to the worries and preoccupations manifested by the patient and elicited at interview. Abnormal beliefs and experiences are, of course, part of the thought content, but are regarded as sufficient to be discussed separately (see below).

- An *obsessional rumination* is a recurrent, persistent thought, impulse, image or musical theme that enters the mind despite the individual's effort to resist it. The individual recognizes that the obsessional thought is their own, but it is usually unpleasant and often 'out of character', such as the thought that the patient has accidentally killed someone while driving their car. Common obsessions concern dirt, contamination and orderliness.
- A *compulsion* is a repetitive and seemingly purposeful action performed in a stereotyped way, referred to as a *compulsive ritual*. Compulsions are accompanied by a subjective sense that they must be carried out (or the patient will be overwhelmed by either anxiety or a superstitious belief that something bad will occur) and by an urge to resist. Compulsive rituals are used to counteract ruminations, so patients repetitively wash their hands to diminish the fear of contamination with dirt.

Insight and illness beliefs

Insight is the degree to which a person recognizes that he or she is unwell, and is minimal in patients with a psychosis. Illness beliefs are the patient's own explanations of their ill-health, including diagnosis and causes. These beliefs should be elicited because they can help to determine prognosis and compliance with treatment, with any disease.

Abnormal beliefs

The main form of abnormal belief is the *delusion* (Box 21.3). Delusions can be primary or secondary.

- Primary delusions are rare and appear suddenly and with full conviction but without any preceding mental events. For example, a patient on being offered a glass of wine suddenly believes that this indicates that he is Jesus Christ.
- Secondary delusions are derived from a preceding morbid experience, such as a depressed mood or an auditory hallucination.

Delusions are also classified according to their content, and include persecutory delusions, delusions of reference, guilt, worthlessness, nihilism, religious delusions, and delusions of grandeur, jealousy or control. These are further defined when discussed in relation to specific conditions.

Feelings, thoughts or actions may also be interpreted by the patient as being under the control of some external power. Such *passivity* experiences are first rank symptoms and are regarded as diagnostic of schizophrenia (see p. 1261). Patients may develop secondary delusions that explain this alien control as a result of witchcraft, hypnosis, radio waves or television – so-called delusions of passivity.

Delusions should be distinguished from *overvalued ideas* – deeply held personal convictions that are understandable when the individual's background is known.

Ideas of reference that fall short of delusions are held by people who are particularly self-conscious. Such individuals cannot help feeling that people take particular notice of them in public places, laugh at them or pass comment about them. Such a feeling is not delusional in

---

Box 21.3

Delusion

Delusion is defined as an abnormal belief that is:

- held with absolute conviction
- not amenable to reason or modifiable by experience
- not shared by those of a common cultural or social background
- experienced as a self-evident truth of great personal significance
- usually false

that individuals who experience it realize that it originates within themselves and that they are no more noticeable than anyone else, but nevertheless cannot dismiss the feeling.

Abnormal perceptions

- *Illusions* are misperceptions of external stimuli and are most likely to occur when the general level of sensory stimulation is reduced.
- *Hallucinations* are defined in Box 21.4. Healthy people occasionally experience hallucinations, such as in normal grief, or during the transition between sleeping and waking (hypnagogic and hypnapompic). Hallucinations can be elementary (e.g. bangs, whistles) or complex (e.g. faces, voices, music), and may affect any of the perceptions: auditory, visual, tactile, gustatory, olfactory or of deep sensation.
- *Pseudohallucinations* are usually auditory, and are either true externally sited hallucinations, but with insight into their imaginary nature, or are sited within internal space (e.g. 'I heard a voice in my head speak to me.'). They can occur in mood disorders and do not indicate a psychosis.
- *Depersonalization* is a change in self-awareness such that the person feels unreal or detached from their body. The individual is aware, however, of the subjective nature of this alteration.
- *Derealization* is the unpleasant feeling that the external environment has become unreal and/or remote; patients may describe themselves as though they are in a dream-like state. Both this and depersonalization can occur in healthy people when they are tired, after sensory deprivation and when using hallucinogenic drugs. They also occur in anxiety disorders, schizophrenia and temporal lobe epilepsy.
- *Déjà vu* is a sudden familiarity with a situation or event as having been encountered before when it is in fact novel.
- *Jamais vu* is the reverse experience when there is failure to recognize a situation or event that has been encountered before. Déjà vu experiences occur in healthy people as well as in extreme anxiety states.

Box 21.4

Hallucination

An hallucination is defined as a perception in the absence of a stimulus. It is:

- a false perception and not a distortion
- perceived as inhabiting objective space
- perceived as having qualities of normal perception
- perceived alongside normal perceptions
- independent of the individual's will.

Both types of experience can occur in temporal lobe epilepsy (see p. 1175).

- Increased sensitivity of perceptions, such as *photosensitivity* and *phonosensitivity*, occurs in anxiety disorders (e.g. increased sensitivity to the neon strip-lights and noise in a supermarket in agoraphobia) as well as neurological disorders such as migraine.

Cognitive state

Examination of the cognitive state is necessary to diagnose organic brain disorders, such as delirium and dementia. Poor concentration, confusion and memory problems are the most common subjective complaints. Clinical testing is a screening of cognitive functions, which may suggest the need for more formal psychometry. A premorbid estimate of intelligence can be made from asking the patient the final year level of education and the highest qualifications or skills achieved.

Testing can be divided into tests of diffuse and focal brain functions.

Diffuse functions

Orientation in time, place and person. *Consciousness* can be defined as the awareness of the self and the environment. *Clouding of consciousness* is more accurately a fluctuating level of awareness and is commonly seen in delirium.

Attention is tested by saying the months or days backwards.

Verbal memory. Ask the patient to repeat a name and address with 10 or so items, noting how many times it takes to recall it 100% accurately (normal is 1 or 2) (*immediate recall* or *registration*).

Ask the patient to try to remember it and then ask it of them again after 5 minutes (0 or 1 error is normal) (*short-term memory*).

Long-term memory. Ask the patient if they can recall the news of that morning or recently. If they are not interested in the news, find out their interests and ask relevant questions (about their football team or favourite soap opera). *Amnesia* is literally an absence of memory and *dysmnesia* indicates a dysfunctioning memory.

Focal functions

Frontal, temporal and parietal function tests are covered on page 1128. *Frontal lobe skills* are difficult to test at the bedside. Note any *disinhibited behaviour* not explained by another psychiatric illness, such as mania. *Sequential tasks* are tested by asking the patient to alternate making a fist with one hand at the same time as a flat hand with the other. Ask the patient to tap a table once if you tap twice and vice versa. Note any *motor perseveration* whereby the patient cannot change the movement once established. Observe for *verbal perseveration*, in which the patient repeats the same answer as given previously for a different question. *Abstract thinking* is measured by asking the meaning of common proverbs, a literal meaning suggesting frontal lobe dysfunction, assuming reasonable premorbid intelligence.

Mini-mental state examination

Box 21.5 gives the 'mini-mental state' examination of cognitive function. This is a 5-minute bedside test that is useful as a screen and in assessing the degree of cognitive dysfunction in patients with diffuse brain disorders. It correlates well with more time-consuming Intelligence Quotient (IQ) tests, but it will not as easily pick up cognitive problems caused by focal brain lesions. A score of 23 or less will pick up about 90% of patients with cognitive impairments, with about 10% false positives.

Defence mechanisms

Although not strictly part of the mental state examination it is useful to be able to identify psychological defences in ourselves and our patients. Defence mechanisms are mental processes that are usually unconscious. The defence mechanisms described below are among the most commonly used and are useful in understanding many aspects of behaviour.

- *Denial* is similar to repression and occurs when patients behave as though unaware of something that they might be expected to know. One example would be a patient who, despite being told that a close relative has died, continues to behave as though the relative were still alive.
- *Displacement* involves the transferring of emotion from a situation or object with which it is properly associated to another that gives less distress.
- *Identification* refers to the unconscious process of taking on some of the characteristics or behaviours of another person, often to reduce the pain of separation or loss.
- *Projection* involves the attribution to another person of thoughts or feelings that are in fact one's own.
- *Regression* is the adoption of primitive patterns of behaviour appropriate to an earlier stage of development. It can be seen in ill people who become child-like and highly dependent.
- *Repression* is the exclusion from awareness of memories, emotions and/or impulses that would cause anxiety or distress if allowed to enter consciousness.
- *Sublimation* refers to the unconscious diversion of unacceptable behaviours into acceptable ones.

The relevant physical examination

This should be guided by the history and mental state examination. Particular attention should usually be paid to the neurological and endocrinological examinations when organic brain syndromes and affective illnesses are suspected.

Box 21.5

The mini-mental state examination

Orientation
Score one point for each correct answer:
What is the: time, date, day, month, year?   Maximum: 5 points

What is the name of: this ward, hospital, district, town, country?   5 points

Registration
Name three objects only once. Score up to a maximum of 3 points for each correct repetition.   3 points

Repeat the objects until the patient can repeat them accurately (in order to test recall later).

Attention and calculation
Ask the patient to subtract 7 from 100 and then 7 from the result four more times.
Score 1 point for each correct subtraction.   5 points

Recall
Ask the patient to repeat the names of the three objects learnt in the registration test.   3 points

Language
Score 1 point for each of two simple objects named (e.g. pen and a watch).   2 points

Score 1 point for an accurate repetition of the phrase: 'No ifs, ands or buts'.   1 point

Give a 3-stage command, scoring 1 point for each part correctly carried out; e.g. 'With the index finger of your right hand touch your nose and then your left ear'.   3 points

Write 'Close your eyes' on a blank piece of paper and ask the patient to follow the written command. Score 1 point if the patient closes the eyes.   1 point

Ask the patient to write a sentence. Score 1 point if the sentence is sensible and contains a noun and a verb.   1 point

Draw a pair of intersecting pentagons with each side approximately 1 inch long. Score 1 point if it is correctly copied.   1 point

TOTAL MAXIMUM SCORE   30 POINTS

From: Folstein MF, Folstein SE, McHough PR (1975) 'Mini-mental state': a practical method for grading the cognitive state of patients for the clinician. *Journal of Psychiatric Research* **12**: 189–198

Summary or formulation

When the full history and mental state have been assessed, the doctor should make a concise assessment of the case, which is termed a *formulation*. In addition to summarizing the essential features of the history and examination, the formulation includes a differential diagnosis, a discussion of possible causal factors, and an outline of further investigations or interviews needed. It concludes with a concise plan of treatment and a statement of the likely prognosis.

Classification of psychiatric disorders

The classification of psychiatric disorders into categories is mainly based on symptoms, since there are currently few diagnostic tests for psychiatric disorders. The fourth edition of the *Diagnostic and Statistical Manual of the American Psychiatric Association* (DSM-IV) provides descriptions of diagnostic categories in order to enable clinicians and investigators to diagnose, communicate about, study and treat people with various mental disorders. This scheme has five axes:

I   Psychiatric disorders
II Personality disorders, learning difficulty
III General medical conditions
IV Psychosocial and environmental problems
V   Overall level of functioning

Psychiatric classifications have traditionally divided up disorders into neuroses and psychoses.

Neuroses are illnesses in which symptoms vary only in severity from normal experiences. *Psychoses* are illnesses in which symptoms are qualitatively different from normal experience, with little insight into their nature.

There are several problems with a neurotic–psychotic dichotomy. Firstly, neuroses may be as severe in their effects on the patient and their family as psychoses. Secondly, neuroses may cause symptoms that fulfil the definition of psychotic symptoms. For instance, someone with anorexia nervosa may be convinced that they are fat when they are thin, and this belief would meet all the criteria for a delusional belief. Yet we would traditionally classify the illness as a neurosis.

Another classification system – the *International Classification of Mental and Behavioural Disorders* (ICD-10) has been published by the World Health Organization. This system has largely abandoned the traditional division between neurosis and psychosis, although the terms are still used. The disorders are now arranged in groups according to major common themes (e.g. mood disorders, schizophrenia and other delusional disorders). A classification of psychiatric disorders derived from ICD-10 is shown in Table 21.1, and this is the classification mainly used in this chapter.

FURTHER READING

American Psychiatric Association (1994) *Diagnostic and Statistical Manual of Mental Disorders (DSM–IV).* Washington, DC: APA.
World Health Organization (1992) *The ICD-10 Classification of Mental and Behavioural Disorders: Clinical Descriptions and Diagnostic Guidelines.* Geneva: World Health Organization.

Table 21.1
International classification of psychiatric disorders (ICD-10)

Organic disorders
Mental and behavioural disorders due to psychoactive substance use
Schizophrenia and delusional disorders
Mood (affective) disorders
Neurotic, stress-related and somatoform disorders
Behavioural syndromes
Disorders of adult personality and behaviour
Mental retardation

World Health Organization (1992) *The ICD-10 Classification of Mental and Behavioural Disorders.* Geneva: World Health Organization

Causes of a psychiatric disorder

A psychiatric disorder may result from several causes. It is most helpful to divide causes into the three 'P's: predisposing, precipitating and perpetuating factors.

- *Predisposing factors* often stem from early life and include genetic, pregnancy and delivery, previous traumas and personality factors.
- *Precipitating (triggering) factors* may be physical, psychological or social in nature. Whether they produce a disorder depends on their nature, severity and the presence of predisposing factors. For instance a death of a close rather than distant family member is more likely to precipitate a depressive illness or pathological grief reaction in someone who has not come to terms with a previous bereavement.
- *Perpetuating (maintaining) factors* prolong the course of a disorder after it has occurred. Again they may be physical, psychological and/or social and several are often active and interacting at the same time. For example, high levels of criticism at home combined with taking cannabis, as relief from the criticism, may help to maintain schizophrenia.

Psychiatric aspects of physical disease

Patients with physical illnesses are more likely to suffer from psychiatric disorders than those who are well. The most common psychiatric disorders in physically ill patients are mood or adjustment disorders and acute organic brain disorders (delirium). The relationship between psychological and physical symptoms may be understood in one of three ways:

- Psychological distress and disorders can precipitate physical diseases (e.g. anorexia nervosa causing cardiac arrhythmias, due to hypokalaemia).
- Physical diseases and their treatments can cause psychological symptoms or ill-health (Table 21.2).

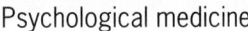 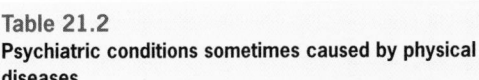

Table 21.2
Psychiatric conditions sometimes caused by physical diseases

Psychiatric disorder/symptom	Physical disease
Depressive illness	Hypothyroidism
	Cushing's syndrome
	Steroid treatment
	Brain tumour
Anxiety disorder	Thyrotoxicosis
	Hypoglycaemia (transient)
	Phaeochromocytoma
	Complex partial seizures (transient)
	Alcohol withdrawal
Irritability	Post-concussion syndrome
	Frontal lobe syndrome
	Hypoglycaemia (transient)
Memory problem	Brain tumour
	Hypothyroidism
Altered behaviour	Acute drug intoxication
	Postictal state
	Acute delirium
	Dementia
	Brain tumour

Table 21.3
Factors increasing the risk of psychiatric disorders in the general hospital

Patient factors	Physical conditions
Previous psychiatric history	Chronic ill-health
Current social or interpersonal stresses	Chronic pain
Homeless	Life-threatening illness
Recent alcohol misuse	Recent bad prognostic news
	Disabling condition
	Brain disease
	Recent live birth, still-birth or miscarriage
	Functional (psychosomatic) illness

Setting	Treatment
A&E department	Certain drugs (e.g. dopamine agonists)
Neurology, oncology and endocrinology wards	Second postoperative day
Intensive care unit	Surgery affecting body image (e.g. emergency stomata)
Renal dialysis unit	

- Physical and psychological symptoms and disorders may be independently co-morbid, particularly in the elderly.

Common psychiatric disorders in the general hospital

Delirium is the commonest psychosis seen in the general hospital, with dementia being the commonest chronic organic brain disorder seen. Mood disorders, particularly depressive illness, are common in patients with chronic painful conditions (severe arthritis), disabling illnesses (after a stroke), and after being given a life-threatening diagnosis, such as cancer. Other factors also increase the risk of a psychiatric disorder in someone with a physical disease (Table 21.3).

Differences in treatment

Although the basic tenets are the same as in treating psychiatric illnesses in the physically healthy, there are some differences:

- *Uncertainty* regarding the physical diagnosis or prognosis, with its attendant tendency to imagine the worst, is often a triggering or maintaining factor, particularly in an adjustment or mood disorder. Good two-way communication between doctor and patient, with time taken to listen to the patient's concerns, is often the most effective 'antidepressant' available.
- A careful history may reveal the role of a *physical disease or treatment* exacerbating the psychiatric condition, which should then be addressed (see Table 21.2). For example, the dopamine agonist bromocriptine can precipitate a psychosis.

- When prescribing psychotropic drugs, the dose should be reduced in disorders affecting *pharmacokinetics*, e.g. fluoxetine in renal or hepatic failure.
- It is more necessary to check for *drug interactions*, e.g. lithium and non-steroidal anti-inflammatories; lithium and thiazide diuretics. Drug interactions are most likely to occur when a patient is acutely admitted to hospital, already taking psychotropics.
- Sometimes a physical treatment may be planned that may exacerbate the psychiatric condition. An example would be high-dose steroids as part of the next cycle of chemotherapy in a patient with leukaemia and depressive illness. Careful thought should be given to the particular priority for the patient at that moment. It is often useful to discuss the clinical dilemma with a psychiatrist.
- Always consider the risk of *suicide* in an inpatient with a mood disorder and take steps to reduce that risk; for example, moving the patient to a room on the ground floor and/or having a registered mental nurse attend the patient while at risk.

Severe behavioural disturbance

Patients with aggressive or violent behaviour cause understandable apprehension in all staff, and are most commonly seen in the accident and emergency department. Information from anyone accompanying the patient, including police or carers, can help considerably. Box 21.6 gives the main causes of disturbed behaviour.

Management of the severely disturbed patient

The primary aims of management are control of dangerous behaviour and establishment of a provisional diagnosis. Three specific strategies may be necessary when dealing with the violent patient:

- reassurance and explanation
- physical restraint
- medication.

The majority of disturbed patients are themselves frightened, as well as frightening, and may feel threatened by those around them, misinterpreting the actions of others. Staff should always explain the situation and their intentions. This simple strategy may calm a patient sufficiently to be interviewed and allow an appropriate examination.

If the behaviour remains severely disturbed, it may be necessary to restrain patients from harming themselves or others. If planned, this should be done with sufficient numbers of trained staff; at least one person per limb and another two in charge or delivering medication. Once brought under physical control, the patient should be held in the prone position, in order to protect the airway and allow access for intramuscular medication.

In these circumstances it is usually necessary to administer medication while the patient is restrained and they should not be released until they are visibly calmed. Management depends on the provisional diagnosis. 'Rapid tranquillization' should be employed when the patient has a psychosis, so long as the Mental Health Act has been used (see p. 1269) or the situation is so dangerous that the doctor is acting under 'common law'. Moderate doses of a neuroleptic or benzodiazepine should be given at regular, comparatively short intervals (30–60 minutes) intramuscularly, if oral administration is not possible. In most situations a single dose of medication should be enough to allow more definitive management to take place. Both neuroleptic drugs and benzodiazepines may be used as tranquillizers. Used in combination they have a synergistic action and it has been shown to reduce the total amount of neuroleptic required to treat acute psychosis. A simple regimen of an intramuscular butyrophenone (see p. 1262) may be used in most situations. Haloperidol (5–10 mg) may be used in patients under 60 years old. This dose should be reduced in the elderly and those with known cardiac or hepatic disease. The patient should be observed for up to 1 hour before a further dose is administered. In the case of continuing disturbance, it may be preferable to administer an adjunctive intramuscular benzodiazepine (lorazepam 2 mg) rather than a further dose of neuroleptic. Breathing, pulse rate and blood pressure should be monitored for hypotension, arrhythmias and respiratory difficulty.

The sick role and illness behaviour

The *sick role* describes behaviour usually adopted by ill people. Such people are not expected to fulfil their normal social obligations. They are treated with sympathy by others and are only obliged to see their doctor and take medical advice or treatments.

Illness behaviour is the way in which given symptoms may be differentially perceived, evaluated and acted (or not acted) upon by different kinds of persons. We all have illness behaviour when we choose what to do about a symptom. Going to see a doctor is generally more likely with more severe and more numerous symptoms and greater distress. It is also more likely in introspective individuals who focus on their health.

Abnormal illness behaviour occurs when there is a discrepancy between the objective somatic pathology present and the patient's response to it, in spite of adequate medical investigation and explanation.

Functional or psychosomatic disorders: medically unexplained symptoms

'Functional' disorders are illnesses in which there is no obvious pathology or anatomical change in an organ (thus in contrast to 'organic') and there is a presumed dysfunction in an organ or system. The word *psychosomatic* has had several meanings, including psychogenic, 'all in the mind', imaginary and malingering. The modern meaning is that psychosomatic disorders are syndromes of unknown aetiology in which both physical and psychological factors are likely to be causative. The psychiatric classification of these disorders would be *somatoform disorders*, but they do not fit easily within either medical or psychiatric classification systems, since they occupy the hinterland between them. Medically unexplained symptoms and syndromes are important because they are so common in both the general hospital and primary care. Over half the outpatients in gastroenterology and neurology clinics have medically unexplained symptoms. Because orthodox medicine has not been particularly effective in treating or understanding these disorders, many patients perceive their doctors as unsympathetic and seek out complementary treatments of uncertain efficacy. Examples of functional disorders are shown in Table 21.4.

Table 21.4
Functional or psychosomatic syndromes (medically unexplained symptoms)

'Tension' headaches	Chronic or post-viral fatigue
Atypical facial pain	syndrome
Atypical chest pain	Multiple chemical sensitivity
Fibromyalgia (chronic	Premenstrual syndrome
widespread pain)	Irritable or functional bowel
Other chronic pain	syndrome
syndromes	Irritable bladder syndrome

Table 21.5
Aetiological factors commonly seen in functional disorders

Predisposing:
Perfectionist, obsessional and introspective personality traits
Childhood traumas (physical and sexual abuse)
Similar illnesses in first-degree relatives

Precipitating (triggering):
Infections
    Chronic fatigue syndrome (CFS)
    Irritable bowel syndrome (IBS)
Psychologically traumatic events (especially accidents)
Physical injuries ('fibromyalgia' and other chronic pain syndromes)
Life events that precipitate changed behaviours (e.g. going off sick)
Incidents where the patient believes others are responsible

Perpetuating (maintaining):
Inactivity with consequent physiological adaptation (CFS and 'fibromyalgia')
Avoidant behaviours – multiple chemical sensitivities (MCS), CFS
Maladaptive illness beliefs (that maintain maladaptive behaviours) (CFS)
Excessive dietary restrictions ('food allergies')
Stimulant drugs
Sleep disturbance
Mood disorders
Somatization disorder
Unresolved anger or guilt
Unresolved compensation

Because epidemiological studies suggest that having one of these syndromes significantly increases the risk of having another, some doctors believe that these syndromes represent different manifestations in time of *'one functional syndrome'*, which is indicative of a *somatization* process. Functional disorders also have a significant association with psychiatric disorders, especially depressive and panic disorders as well as phobias. Against this view is the evidence that the majority of primary care patients with most of these disorders do not have either a psychiatric disorder or other functional disorders. It also seems that it requires a major stress or a psychiatric disorder in order for such sufferers to attend their doctor for help, which might explain why doctors are so impressed with the associations with stress and psychiatric disorders. Doctors have historically tended to diagnose 'stress' or 'psychosomatic disorders' in patients with symptoms that they cannot explain. History is full of such disorders being reclassified as research clarifies the pathology. A recent example is writer's cramp (p. 1188) which most neurologists now agree is a dystonia rather than a neurosis.

Chronic fatigue syndrome (CFS)
There has probably been more controversy over the existence and aetiology of CFS than any other functional syndrome in recent years. This is reflected in its uncertain classification as *neurasthenia* in the psychiatric classification and *myalgic encephalomyelitis* (ME) under neurological disorders. There is now good evidence for this syndrome, although the diagnosis is made clinically and by exclusion of other fatiguing disorders. Its prevalence is 0.5% in the UK, although abnormal fatigue as a symptom occurs in 10–20%. It occurs most commonly in women between the ages of 20 and 40 years old. The cardinal symptom is chronic fatigue made worse by minimal exertion. The fatigue is usually physical and mental, with associated poor concentration, impaired registration of memory, irritability, alteration in sleep pattern (either insomnia or hypersomnia), and muscular pain. The name myalgic encephalomyelitis (ME) is decreasingly used within medicine because it implies a pathology for which there is no evidence.

Aetiology
Functional disorders often have aetiological factors in common with each other (see Table 21.5), as well as more specific aetiologies. For instance, CFS can be triggered by certain infections, such as infectious mononucleosis and viral hepatitis. About 10% of patients with infectious mononucleosis have CFS 6 months after the infectious onset, yet there is no evidence of persistent infection in these patients. Those fatigue states which clearly do follow on a viral infection can be classified as *post-viral fatigue states*. Other aetiological factors include physical inactivity and sleep difficulties. Immune and endocrine abnormalities noted in CFS may be secondary to the inactivity or sleep disturbance commonly seen in patients. Mood disorders are present in a large minority of patients, and can cause problems in diagnosis because of the large overlap in symptoms. These mood disorders may be secondary, independent (co-morbid), or primary with a misdiagnosis of CFS. The role of stress is uncertain, with some indication that the influence of stress is mediated through consequent psychiatric disorders exacerbating fatigue, rather than any direct effect.

Management
The general principles of the management of functional disorders are given in Box 21.7. Specific management of CFS should include a mutually agreed and supervised programme of gradually increasing activity. However, few patients regard themselves as cured after treatment.

It is sometimes difficult to persuade a patient to accept what are inappropriately perceived as 'psychological therapies' for such a physically manifested condition. Antidepressants do not work in the absence of a mood disorder or insomnia.

Prognosis

This is poor without treatment, with less than 10% of hospital attenders recovered after a year. Outcomes are worse with increasing age, co-morbid mood disorders, and the conviction that the illness is entirely physical.

Fibromyalgia (chronic widespread pain: CWP)

This controversial condition of unknown aetiology overlaps with chronic fatigue syndrome, with both conditions causing fatigue and sleep disturbance (see p. 1234). Diffuse muscle and joint pains are more constant and severe in CWP, although the 'tender points', previously considered to be pathognomonic, are now known to be ubiquitous, associated with psychological distress, and of no diagnostic importance (p. 530). CWP occurs most commonly in women aged 40–65 years old, with a prevalence in the community of between 1 and 11%. There are associations with depressive and anxiety disorders, other functional disorders, physical deconditioning and a possibly characteristic sleep disturbance (see Table 21.5).

Management

Apart from the general principles in Box 21.7, management also consists of symptomatic analgesia, reversing the sleep disturbance, and a physically orientated rehabilitation programme. A recent meta-analysis suggests

---

> ### Box 21.7
>
> #### Management of functional disorders
>
> The first principle is the identification and treatment of maintaining factors (e.g. dysfunctional beliefs and behaviours, mood and sleep disorders).
>
> - Communication
>   Explanation of ill-health, including diagnosis and causes
>   Education about management (including self-help leaflets)
> - Stopping drugs (e.g. caffeine causing insomnia, analgesics causing dependence)
> - Rehabilitative therapies
>   Cognitive behaviour therapy (to challenge unhelpful beliefs and change coping strategies)
>   Supervised and graded exercise therapy (to reduce inactivity and improve fitness)
> - Pharmacotherapies
>   Specific antidepressants for mood disorders, analgesia and sleep disturbance
>   Symptomatic medicines (e.g. appropriate analgesia, taken only when necessary)

---

that tricyclic antidepressants that inhibit reuptake of both serotonin and norepinephrine (noradrenaline) (e.g. amitriptyline, dosulepin (dothiepin)) have the greatest effect on sleep, fatigue and pain. The doses used were too low for antidepressant efficacy and the drugs may work through their hypnotic and analgesic effects.

Other chronic pain syndromes

A chronic pain syndrome is a condition of chronic disabling pain for which no medical cause can be found. The psychiatric classification would be a persistent *somatoform pain disorder*, but this is unsatisfactory since the criteria include the stipulation that emotional factors must be the main cause, and it is clinically difficult to be that certain. The main sites of chronic pain syndromes are the head, face, neck, lower back, abdomen, genitalia and all over (CWP: fibromyalgia). 'Functional' low back pain is the commonest 'physical' reason for being off sick long-term in the UK (p. 522). Quite often a minor abnormality will be found on investigation (such as mild cervical spondylosis on the neck X-ray), but this will not be severe enough to explain the severity of the pain and resultant disability. These pains are often unremitting and respond poorly to analgesics. Sleep disturbance is almost universal and co-morbid psychiatric disorders are found in a large minority.

Aetiology

The perception of pain involves sensory (nociceptive), emotional and cognitive processing in the brain. Functional brain scans suggest that the brain may respond abnormally to pain in these conditions. This could be related to conditioned behavioural and physiological responses to the initial acute pain. The brain may then adapt to the prolonged stimulus of the pain by changing its central processing. The prefrontal cortex, thalamus and cingulate gyrus seem to be particularly affected and some of these areas are involved in the emotional appreciation of pain in general. Thus it is possible to start to understand how beliefs, emotions and behaviours might influence the perception of chronic pain (see Table 21.5).

Management

Management involves the same principles as used in other functional syndromes (Box 21.7). Since analgesics are rarely effective, and can cause long-term harm, patients should be encouraged to gradually reduce their use. It is often helpful to involve the patient's immediate family or partner, to ensure that the partner is also supported and not unconsciously discouraging progress.

Specific drug treatments are few. Nerve blocks are not usually effective. Anticonvulsants such as carbamazepine and gabapentin may be given a therapeutic trial if the pain is thought to be neuropathic (see p. 530). The antidepressant *dosulepin (dothiepin)* is an effective

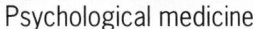

treatment in half of patients with atypical facial pain, and this effect seems to be independent of dosulepin's effect on mood. Another tricyclic antidepressant, *amitriptyline*, is more effective than a selective serotonin reuptake inhibitor (SSRI) in tension headaches, which might be related to its independent analgesic effect. Amitriptyline has the added bonus of increasing slow wave sleep, which may be why it is more effective than NSAIDs in chronic widespread pain. Tricyclic antidepressants that affect both serotonin and norepinephrine (noradrenaline) reuptake (e.g. p. 1245) seem to be more effective than more selective norepinephrine reuptake inhibitors, e.g. in neuropathic pain. There is some preliminary evidence that tricyclics are superior to SSRIs in chronic pain syndromes.

Irritable bowel syndrome

This is one of the commonest functional syndromes, affecting some 10–30% of the population in the UK. The clinical features and management of the syndrome and the related *non-ulcer dyspepsia* are described in more detail on page 324. Although the majority of sufferers with the irritable bowel syndrome (IBS) do not have a psychiatric disorder, depressive illness should be excluded in patients with constipation and a poor appetite. Anxiety disorders should be excluded in patients with nausea and diarrhoea. Persistent abdominal pain or a feeling of emptiness may occasionally be the presenting symptom of a severe depressive illness, particularly in the elderly, with a *nihilistic delusion* that the body is empty or dead inside (see p. 1242).

Management

This is dealt with in more detail on page 327 and in Box 21.7. Seeing a physician who provides specific education that particularly addresses individual illness beliefs and concerns can provide lasting benefit. Psychological therapies that help the more severely affected include biofeedback, hypnotherapy, cognitive behaviour therapy and brief interpersonal psychotherapy. If indicated, the choice of antidepressant should be determined by the effects of these drugs on bowel transit times, with tricyclic antidepressants normally slowing and selective serotonin reuptake inhibitors (SSRIs) (p. 1244) normally speeding up transit times.

Multiple chemical sensitivity, candida hypersensitivity, and food allergies

Some complementary health practitioners, doctors, and patients themselves make diagnoses of multiple chemical sensitivities (MCS) (e.g. to foods, smoking, perfumes, petrol), candida hypersensitivity, and allergies (to food, tap-water, and even electricity). Symptoms and syndromes attributed to these putative disorders are numerous and variable and include all the functional disorders, *mood disorders*, and *arthritis*. Scientific support for the existence of these disorders has been hard to acquire, particularly when double-blind methodologies have been used.

Type 1 hypersensitivities to foods such as nuts certainly exist, although they are fortunately uncommon (approximately 3 per 1000) (see p. 213). Direct specific food intolerances also occur (e.g. chocolate with migraine, caffeine with IBS).

Candidiasis can occur in the gastrointestinal tract in immunocompromised individuals, such as those with AIDS. Vaginal candidiasis can occur after antibiotic treatment in otherwise healthy women. A double-blind and controlled study of nystatin in women, diagnosed as having candidiasis hypersensitivity syndrome, showed that vaginal candida was the only symptom relieved more by nystatin than placebo. There is little evidence of candida having a systemic role in other symptoms. In spite of this evidence, the patient is often convinced of the legitimacy and usefulness of these diagnoses and their treatments.

Aetiology

Surveys of patients diagnosed with MCS or food allergies have shown high rates of current and previous psychiatric disorders (especially mood and anxiety disorders) (see Table 21.5). Eating disorders (p. 1266) should be excluded in patients with food intolerances. Some patients, taking very low carbohydrate diets as putative treatments, may develop reactive hypoglycaemia after a high carbohydrate meal, which they then interpret as a food allergy. A recent study showed how classical conditioning can produce intolerances to foods and smells in healthy people, which may be a causative mechanism in some patients with intolerance. This study supports the existence of these intolerance conditions, but suggests they may be conditioned responses with attendant physiological consequences. This might explain why double-blinding abolishes the reaction to the stimulus.

Management

The general principles in Box 21.7 apply. If one assumes a phobic or conditioned response is responsible, graded exposure (systematic desensitization) to the conditioned stimulus may be worthwhile. Preliminary studies do suggest that this approach may successfully treat such intolerances, in the context of cognitive behaviour therapy.

Premenstrual syndrome

The premenstrual syndrome (PMS) consists of both physical and psychological symptoms that regularly occur during the premenstrual phase and substantially diminish or disappear soon after the period starts. Physical symptoms include headache, fatigue, breast tenderness, abdominal distension and fluid retention. Psychological symptoms can include irritability, emotional lability or low mood, and tension. Recent research supports the existence of a *late luteal dysphoric syndrome*, with mood symptoms predominating. Women who generally suffer from mood disorders may be more prone to experience this syndrome. The prevalence of PMS does not vary between cultures and is reported by the majority of women at some time in their lives. Severely disabling PMS occurs in about 3% of women. The cause of the premenstrual syndrome remain unclear, although exacerbating factors include some of those outlined in Table 21.5. Recent research suggests that abnormalities of reproductive hormone receptors may play a role.

Management

The general principles in Box 21.7 apply. Treatments with vitamin B$_6$ (p. 237), diuretics, progesterone, oral contraceptives, oil of evening primrose and oestrogen implants or patches (balanced by cyclical norethisterone) remain empirical. Psychotherapies aimed at enhancing the patient's coping skills can reduce disability. Two trials suggest that graded exercise therapy improves symptoms. Several studies have now demonstrated that SSRIs (p. 1244) are effective treatments for the premenstrual dysphoric syndrome.

The menopause

The clinical features and management of the menopause are described on page 1017. A recent prospective study has shown that there is no increased incidence of depressive disorders at this time. Such a significant bodily change, sometimes occurring at the same time as children leaving home, is naturally accompanied by an emotional adjustment that does not normally amount to a pathological state.

FURTHER READING

Lishman WA (1998) *Organic Psychiatry: The Psychological Consequences of Cerebral Disorder.* Oxford: Blackwell Science.
Royal College of Physicians and Royal College of Psychiatrists (1995) *The Psychological Care of Medical Patients: Recognition of Need and Service Provision.* London: Royal College of Physicians.
Whiting G et al. (2001) Interventions for the treatment and management of Chronic Fatigue Syndrome. *Journal of the American Medical Association.* **286**: 1360–1368.
Wessely S, Nimnuan C, Sharpe M (1999) Functional somatic syndrome: one or many? *Lancet* **354**: 936–939.

Somatoform disorders

As explained in the section on functional disorders (p. 1233), the classification of somatoform disorders is unsatisfactory because of the uncertain nature and aetiology of these disorders. However, there are certain disorders, beyond those described in 'functional disorders', that present frequently and coherently enough to be usefully recognized.

Somatization disorder

One in ten patients presenting with a functional disorder will fulfil the criteria of a chronic somatization disorder, sometimes known as *Briquet's syndrome*. The condition is composed of multiple, recurrent, medically unexplained physical symptoms, usually starting early in adult life. Exhaustion, dizzy spells, headaches, hypersensitivity to light and noise, paraesthesiae, abdominal neck and back pain, nausea, sexual symptoms, and abnormal skin sensations are among the most common complaints, but symptoms may be referred to almost any part or bodily system. The usually female patient has often had multiple medical opinions and repeated negative investigations. Medical reassurance that the symptoms do not have a demonstrable physical cause fails to reassure the patient, who will continue to 'doctor-shop'. The patient is usually reluctant to accept a psychological and/or social explanation for the symptoms even when such a link seems obvious. Abnormal illness behaviour is evident and patients can be attention-seeking and dependent on doctors. Yet they can complain about the medical care and attention they have previously received.

The aetiology is unknown, but both mood and personality disorders are often also present. It is often associated with dependence upon or misuse of prescribed medication, usually sedatives and analgesics. There is often a history of significant childhood traumas, or chronic ill-health in the child or parent, which may play an aetiological role (see Table 21.5). The condition is probably the somatic presentation of psychological distress, although iatrogenic damage (from postoperative and prescribed-drug-related problems) soon complicates the clinical picture. The course of the disorder is chronic and disabling, with long-standing family, marital and/or occupational problems.

Hypochondriasis

The conspicuous feature is a preoccupation with an assumed serious disease and its consequences. Patients commonly believe that they suffer from cancer or AIDS, or some other serious condition. Characteristically, such patients repeatedly request laboratory and other investigations to either prove they are ill or reassure themselves that they are well. Such reassurance rarely lasts long before another cycle of worry and requests begins. The symptom of hypochondriasis may occur secondary to or associated with a variety of psychiatric disorders, particularly depressive and anxiety disorders. Occasionally the hypochondriasis is delusional, secondary to schizophrenia or a depressive psychosis. Hypochondriasis may coexist with physical disease but the diagnostic point is that the patient's concern is disproportionate and unjustified.

Management of somatoform disorders

The principles outlined in Box 21.7 also apply to these disorders. Patients most appreciate discussion and explanation of their symptoms. Further management consists of ceasing reassurance that no serious disease has been uncovered, since this simply reinforces dependence on the doctor. The doctor should sensitively explore possible psychological and social difficulties, if possible by demonstrating links between symptoms and stresses. Useful questions to ask include:

'When were you last completely well and happy?'

Such a patient may have trouble remembering such a time, which helps to support the diagnosis, and leads to a discussion as to why they have never been well or happy.

'What can't you do now because you are unwell?'
'What changes has your ill-health caused in your close relationships?'

These questions usually give information that can be used to formulate an agreed plan of management. Repeated laboratory investigations should be discouraged. It is vital that all members of staff and close family members adopt the same approach to the patient's problems. Such patients often consciously or unconsciously split both medical staff and family members into 'good' and 'bad' (or caring and uncaring) people, as a way of projecting their distress. Since these disorders have a poor prognosis, the aim is to minimize disability. A contract of mutually agreed care involving the appropriate professionals (general practitioner, and a choice of psychotherapist, health psychologist, complementary health professional, physician or psychiatrist), with agreed frequency of visits and a review date, can be helpful in managing the condition.

Cognitive behaviour therapy has now been shown to provide effective rehabilitation in significant numbers of patients suffering from a somatoform disorder.

Dissociative (conversion) disorders

Until recently these disorders were known as 'hysteria'; but because the word hysteria is sometimes used pejoratively to describe extravagant behaviour, the term is now inappropriate.

A *dissociative disorder* is a condition in which there is a profound loss of awareness or cognitive ability with no medical explanation. The term dissociative indicates the disintegration of different mental activities, and covers such phenomena as amnesia, fugues, and pseudoseizures (non-epileptic fits).

The term *conversion* was introduced by Freud to explain how an unresolved conflict could be converted into usually symbolic physical symptoms as a defence against it. Such symptoms commonly include paralysis, abnormal movements, sensory loss, aphonia, disorders of gait, and pseudocyesis (false pregnancy). The lifetime prevalence has been estimated at 3–6 per 1000 in women, with a lower prevalence in men. Most cases begin before the age of 35 years. Dissociation is unusual in the elderly.

Clinical features

The various symptoms are usually divided into dissociative and conversion categories (Table 21.6). Dissociative disorders have the following four characteristics that are necessary in order to make the diagnosis:

- They occur in the absence of physical pathology that would explain the symptoms.
- They are produced unconsciously.
- The illness is always triggered by an unresolved conflict or life event.
- Symptoms are not caused by overactivity of the sympathetic nervous system.

Other characteristics include:

- Symptoms and signs often reflect a patient's ideas about illness.
- Patients may take up the symptoms of a relative/friend who has been ill.
- There is usually abnormal illness behaviour, with obvious exaggeration of disability.
- *Primary gain* is the immediate relief from the emotional conflict.
- *Secondary gain* refers to the social advantage gained by the patient by being ill and disabled (sympathy of family and friends, being off work, disability pension).
- There may be a curious lack of concern about the symptoms or disability ('belle indifference').
- Physical disease is not uncommonly present (e.g. pseudoseizures in someone with epilepsy).

Dissociative *amnesia* commences suddenly. Patients are unable to recall long periods of their lives and may even deny any knowledge of their previous life or personal identity. In a dissociative *fugue*, patients not only lose their memory but wander away from their usual surroundings, and, when found, deny all memory of their whereabouts during this wandering. The differential diagnosis of a fugue state includes postictal automatism, depressive illness and alcohol abuse.

Table 21.6
Common dissociative/conversion symptoms

Mental	Physical
Amnesia	Paralysis
Fugue	Disorders of gait
Pseudodementia	Tremor
Multiple personality	Aphonia
Psychosis	Mutism
	Sensory symptoms
	Globus hystericus
	Hysterical fits
	Blindness

Dissociative *pseudodementia* involves memory loss and behaviour that initially suggest severe and generalized dementia. A differential diagnosis is depressive pseudodementia (see p. 1242).

Multiple personality disorder is rare, but dramatic, and may be no more than the consequence of suggestion on the part of a psychotherapist. There are rapid alterations between two or more 'personalities' in the same person, each of which is repressed and dissociated from the other 'personalities'. A differential diagnosis is rapid cycling *manic depressive disorder* which would explain sudden apparent changes in personality.

Epidemic or *'mass hysteria'* usually occurs in institutions for girls or young women, in which the combined effects of suggestion and shared anxiety produce outbreaks of sickness or disturbed behaviour, often following sudden illnesses in leaders of the group at a time of threatened or actual social change.

Differential diagnosis

Dissociation is usually a stable and reliable diagnosis over time, although high rates of co-morbid mood and personality disorders are found in chronic sufferers. Particular care should be taken to make the diagnosis on positive grounds, and not simply on the basis of an absence of a medical diagnosis. Care should also be taken to exclude or treat co-morbid psychiatric disorders.

Aetiology

Recent preliminary research with functional brain scans suggests that dissociation involves different areas of the brain from simulation, supporting the unconscious mechanisms first suggested by Charcot (see Fig. 21.1). This research would suggest that there is a disinhibition of voluntary will at an unconscious level, so that the patient can no longer *will* the function to happen.

The psychoanalytical theory of dissociation is that it is the result of emotionally charged memories that are repressed into the unconscious at some point in the past. Symptoms are explained as the combined effects of repression and the symbolic conversion of this emotional energy into physical symptoms. This hypothesis is difficult to test, although there is some evidence that patients with dissociative disorders are more likely to have suffered childhood abuse, particularly when the abuse was both sexual and physical and started early in childhood. Caution should be taken with any such history obtained by therapies that 'recover' childhood memories that were previously completely unknown to the patient.

Patients with dissociative disorders by definition adopt both the sick role and abnormal illness behaviour, with consequent secondary gains that help to maintain the illness.

Management

The treatment of dissociation is similar to the treatment of somatoform disorders in general, outlined above and

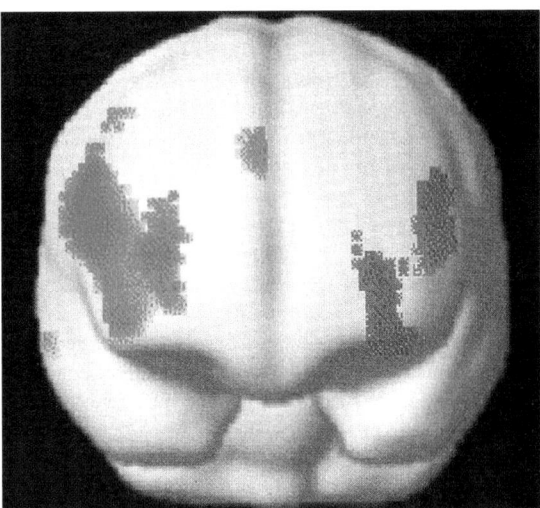

Fig. 21.1 **Statistical parametric maps superimposed on an MRI scan of the anterior surface of the brain, orientated as though looking at a person head on.** Red region shows hypofunction of patients with conversion motor symptoms. Green region shows hypofunction of healthy controls feigning the same motor abnormality. Reproduced from Spence SA, Crimlisk HL, Cope H, Ron MA, Grasby PM (2000) Discrete neurophysiological correlates in prefrontal cortex during hysterical and feigned disorders of movement. *Lancet* **355**:1243–1244, © The Lancet Ltd. 2000, with permission.

in Box 21.7. The first task is to engage the patient and their family with a model of the illness that makes sense to them, is acceptable, and leads to the appropriate management. An invented example of a suitable explanation is given below:

You told me about the tremendous shock you felt when your mother suddenly died. This was particularly the case since you hadn't spoken to her for so long beforehand, after that big disagreement with her over your wedding to John. You weren't able to say good-bye before she died. Your brain was overloaded with grief, guilt and anger all at once. I wonder whether that is why you aren't able to speak now. I wonder whether it's difficult to think of anything to say that would make things right, particularly since you can't speak with your mother now.

Such an explanation would be modified by mutual discussion until an agreed understanding was achieved, which would serve as a working model for the illness. Provision of a rehabilitation programme that addresses both the physical and psychological needs and problems of the patient would then be planned. A graded and mutually agreed plan of a return to normal function can usually be led by the appropriate therapist (e.g. speech therapist for dysphonia, physiotherapist for paralysis). At the same time a psychotherapeutic assessment should be made in order to determine the appropriate form of psychotherapy. For instance, couple therapy will address a significant relationship difficulty; individual psychotherapy could ease an unresolved conflict from childhood.

Abreaction brought about by *hypnosis* or by intravenous injections of small amounts of midazolam may produce a dramatic, if short-lived, recovery. In the abreactive state, the patient is encouraged to relive the stressful events that provoked the disorder and to express the accompanying emotions; i.e. to abreact. Such an approach has been useful in the treatment of acute dissociative states in wartime, but appears to be of much less value in civilian life. It should only be contemplated in the presence of an anaesthetist with suitable resuscitation equipment to hand.

Hypnotherapy is psychotherapy while the patient is in an hypnotic trance, the idea being that therapy is more possible because the patient is relaxed and not using repression. This may allow the therapist access to the previously unconscious emotional conflicts or memories. There are no published trials of this technique in dissociation, which Freud gave up as unsuccessful in order to found psychoanalysis, but some hypnotherapists claim good results. Care should be taken to avoid a catastrophic emotional reaction when the patient is suddenly faced with the previously repressed memories.

Prognosis

Most cases of recent onset recover quickly with treatment, which is why a positive diagnosis should be made early, rather than sending the patient on to the next medical specialist. Those cases that last longer than a year are likely to persist, with entrenched abnormal illness behaviour patterns that are hard to shift.

FURTHER READING

Crimlisk HL, Bhatia K, Cope H, David A, Marsden CD, Ron MA (1998) Slater revisited: 6 year follow up study of patients with medically unexplained symptoms. *British Medical Journal* **316**: 582–586.

Mersky H (1995) *The Analysis of Hysteria*, 2nd edn. Gaskell: London.

Sleep difficulties (p. 1181)

Sleep is divided into *rapid eye movement* (*REM*) and *non-REM* sleep. As drowsiness begins, the alpha rhythm on an EEG disappears and is replaced by deepening slow wave activity (non-REM). After 60–90 minutes, this slow wave pattern is replaced by low amplitude waves on which are superimposed rapid eye movements lasting a few minutes. This cycle is repeated during the duration of sleep, with the REM periods becoming longer. REM sleep is accompanied by dreaming and physiological arousal. Slow wave sleep is associated with release of anabolic hormones and cytokines, with an increased cellular mitotic rate. It helps to maintain host defences, metabolism and repair of cells. For this reason slow wave sleep is increased in those conditions where growth or conservation is required (e.g. adolescence, pregnancy, thyrotoxicosis).

Insomnia is difficulty in sleeping; a third of adults complain of insomnia and in a third of these it can be severe.

Primary sleep disorders include sleep apnoea (p. 869), narcolepsy (see p. 1181), the *restless legs syndrome* (*Ekbom's*) (see p. 648) and its related *periodic leg movement disorder*, in which the legs (and sometimes the arms) jerk while asleep.

Delayed sleep phase syndrome occurs when the circadian pattern of sleep is delayed so that the patient sleeps from the early hours until mid-day or later. *Night terrors*, *sleep-walking* and *sleep-talking* are non-REM phenomena, most commonly found in children, which can recur in adults when under stress or suffering from a mood disorder.

Psychophysiological insomnia commonly occurs with functional, mood and substance misuse disorders, and when under stress (see Box 21.8). It can often be triggered by one of these factors, but then become a habit on its own, driven by anticipation of insomnia and day-time naps. Insomnia causes day-time sleepiness and fatigue, with consequences such as road traffic accidents. Assessment should pay particular attention to mood, life difficulties, and drug intake (especially alcohol, nicotine and caffeine). *Initial insomnia* (trouble getting off to sleep) is common in mania, anxiety, depressive disorders and substance misuse. *Middle insomnia* (waking up in the middle of the night) occurs with medical conditions, such as sleep apnoea and prostatism. *Late insomnia* (early morning waking) is caused by depressive illness and malnutrition (anorexia nervosa).

Habitual alcohol consumption should be carefully estimated since even a small excess can be a potent cause of insomnia, as well as recent withdrawal. *Caffeine* is perhaps the most commonly taken drug in the UK,

---

Box 21.8

Common causes of insomnia

Psychiatric disorders
Mood disorders (mania, depressive and anxiety disorders)
Delirium and dementia

Drug use or misuse
Addictive drug withdrawal (alcohol, benzodiazepines)
Stimulant drugs (caffeine, amfetamines)
Prescribed drugs (steroids, dopamine agonists)

Physical conditions
Pain (classically with carpal tunnel syndrome)
Nocturia (e.g. from prostatism)
Malnutrition

Primary sleep disorders
Sleep apnoea
Restless legs syndrome

and its effects are easily underestimated. Six cups (not mugs) of real coffee a day are likely to cause insomnia in the average healthy adult. Caffeine is not only found in tea and coffee, but is also found in chocolate, cola drinks and some analgesics. Prescription drugs that can either disturb sleep or cause vivid dreams include most appetite suppressants, glucocorticoids, dopamine agonists, lipid-soluble beta-blockers (e.g. propranolol) and certain psychotropic drugs (especially when first prescribed; e.g. fluoxetine, reboxetine, risperidone).

Hypersomnia is not uncommon in adolescents with depressive illness, occurs in narcolepsy, and may temporarily follow infections such as infectious mononucleosis.

Management of insomnia

This is particularly determined by diagnosis. Where none is immediately apparent, it is worth educating the patient about sleep hygiene. Simple measures such as decreasing alcohol intake, having supper earlier, exercising daily, having a bath prior to going to bed and establishing a routine of going to bed at the same time should be tried. Relaxation techniques and cognitive behaviour therapy have a role in those with intractable insomnia. Short half-life benzodiazepines can be useful for acute insomnia, but should not be used for more than 2 weeks continuously to avoid dependence. Recently introduced non-benzodiazepine hypnotics (zopiclone, zolpidem) are said not to cause dependence and tolerance, but act on the same receptors, and should still be used with caution beyond 2 weeks. Certain antihistamines (e.g. promethazine) and antidepressants (e.g. amitriptyline, trimipramine, trazodone) are not addictive and can be used as hypnotics in low dose, with the added advantage of improving slow wave sleep. The commonest side-effects are morning sedation and weight gain.

FURTHER READING

Shapiro CM (ed.) (1993) *ABC of Sleep Disorders.* London: BMJ.

Mood (affective) disorders

Classification

The central and common feature of these disorders is an abnormality of mood. Mood is best considered in terms of a continuum ranging from severe depression at one extreme to severe mania at the other, with the normal, stable mood at the centre (Fig. 21.2). Mood disorders are divided into bipolar and unipolar affective disorders. In bipolar affective disorder (otherwise known as manic-depressive disorder) patients suffer bouts of both depression and mania. In unipolar affective disorder patients suffer from depressive mood swings alone, although they are commonly recurrent. Although mania

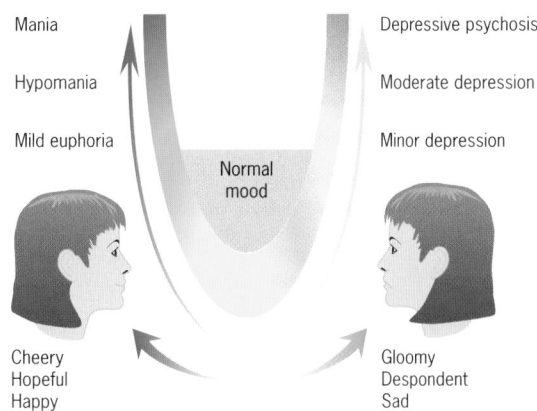

Fig. 21.2 Continuum of normal and abnormal mood.

can rarely occur by itself without depressive mood swings (thus being classified as unipolar) it is far more commonly found in association with depressive swings, even if sometimes it takes several years for the first depressive illness to appear. Hypomania is mild mania. Dysthymia is a chronic low-grade depressive illness.

Depressive disorders

Depressive disorders or 'episodes' are primarily classified as bipolar or unipolar and secondarily as mild, moderate or severe, with or without somatic symptoms. Severe depressive episodes are divided according to the presence or absence of psychotic symptoms. About 10% of patients with depressive illness are eventually found to have bipolar illnesses.

Clinical features of depressive disorder

Whereas everyone will at some time or other feel cheesed off, fed up or down in the dumps, it is when such symptoms become qualitatively different, pervasive, or interfere with normal functioning that a depressive illness has occurred. Depressive disorder, clinical or 'major' depression is characterized by disturbances of mood, speech, energy and ideas (Table 21.7). Patients often describe their symptoms in physical terms. Marked fatigue and headache are the two most common physical symptoms in depressive illness and may be the first symptoms to appear. Patients describe the world as looking grey, themselves as lacking a zest for living and devoid of pleasure and interest in life (anhedonia). Anxiety and panic attacks are common; secondary obsessional and phobic symptoms may emerge. Symptoms should last for at least 2 weeks and should cause significant incapacity (e.g. trouble working or relating to others) to be considered an illness.

In the more severe forms, diurnal variation in mood can occur, feeling worse in the morning after waking in the early hours with apprehension. Suicidal ideas are

Table 21.7
Clinical features of depression

Characteristic	Clinical appearance
Mood	Depressed, miserable or irritable
Talk	Impoverished, slow, monotonous
Energy	Reduced, lethargic
Ideas	Feelings of futility, guilt, self-reproach, unworthiness, hypochondriacal preoccupations, worrying, suicidal thoughts, delusions of guilt, nihilism and persecution
Cognition	Impaired learning, pseudodementia in elderly patients
Physical	Early waking, poor appetite and weight loss, constipation, loss of libido, impotence, fatigue, bodily aches and pains
Behaviour	Retardation or agitation, poverty of movement and expression
Hallucinations	Auditory – often hostile, critical

more frequent, intrusive and prolonged. Delusions of guilt, persecution and bodily disease are not uncommon, along with second person auditory hallucinations insulting the patient or suggesting suicide. In severe depressive illness, particular in the elderly, concentration and memory can be so badly affected that the patient appears to have dementia (pseudodementia). Delusions of poverty and non-existence (nihilism) occur particularly in this age group. Suicide is a real risk, with the lifetime risk being approximately 5% in primary care patients, but 15% in those with depressive illness severe enough to warrant admission to hospital.

Epidemiology

About a third of the population will feel unhappy at any one time, but this is not the same as depressive illness. The point prevalence of depressive illness is 5% in the community, with a further 3% having dysthymia (see below). It is more common in women, but there is no increase with age, and no difference by ethnic group or socio-economic class (apart from an inverse relationship only with dysthymia). Married and never married people have similar prevalence rates, with separated and divorced people having two to three times the prevalence. Some studies have suggested that depressive illness is becoming more common.

Depressive illnesses are more common in the presence of:

- physical diseases, particularly if chronic, stigmatizing or painful
- excessive and chronic alcohol use (probably the most depressing drug humans use)
- social stresses, particularly loss events, such as separation, redundancy and bereavement
- interpersonal difficulties with those close to the patient, especially when socially humiliated
- lack of social support, with no confiding relationship.

Depressed patients with another physical disorder view themselves as more sick and visit their doctors almost four times as often as the non-depressed physically ill, stay in hospital longer, comply less with medical advice and medication, and undergo more medical and surgical procedures. Depressive illness may be associated with increased mortality (excluding suicide) in patients with physical illness, such as myocardial infarct.

Dysthymia

Dysthymia is a more mild depressive illness that lasts intermittently for 2 years or more and is characterized by tiredness and low mood, lack of pleasure, low self-esteem, and a feeling of discouragement. The mood relapses and remits, with several weeks of feeling well, soon followed by longer periods of being unwell. It can be punctuated by depressive episodes of more severity; so-called 'double depression'.

Seasonal affective disorder

Seasonal affective disorder is characterized by recurrent episodes of depressive illness occurring during the winter months in the northern hemisphere. Symptoms are similar to those found with *atypical depressive illness*, in that patients complain of hypersomnia, increased appetite (with carbohydrate craving) and weight gain, with profound fatigue. Such patients have a higher prevalence of bipolar affective disorder, and some doctors are uncertain whether the condition is different from normal depressive illness, with the accentuation of mood that naturally occurs by season. However, there is evidence that seasonal depressive illness can be successfully treated with bright light therapy given in the early morning, which causes a phase advance in the circadian rhythm of melatonin. In contrast, the same treatment given in the early evening, with consequent phase delay of melatonin secretion, is less antidepressant. Selective serotonin reuptake inhibitors (SSRIs) are alternative treatments.

Differential diagnosis

The differential diagnoses of depressive illness are shown in Table 21.8. Other psychiatric disorders are the most common misdiagnoses. 90% of patients presenting with a depressive illness, while misusing alcohol, will no longer be depressed 2 weeks after their last drink.

Pathological (abnormal) and normal grief are described on page 1253. Pathological grief is closely associated with depressive illness.

Investigations

A corroborative history can be valuable in helping to exclude differential diagnoses such as alcohol misuse and elucidating maintaining factors such as the relationship with a partner. Physical investigations should be guided by the history and examination. They will often include measurement of free T_4 and TSH (particularly in

Table 21.8
Common differential diagnoses of depressive illness

Other psychiatric disorders
Alcohol misuse
Amfetamine (and derivatives) misuse and withdrawal
Borderline personality disorder
Dementia
Delirium
Schizophrenia
Normal and pathological grief

Organic (secondary) affective illness
Physical causes which are both necessary and sufficient as a cause
    Cushing's syndrome
    Thyroid disease (although sometimes depression persists after
      treatment)
    Hyperparathyroidism
    Corticosteroid treatment
    Brain tumour (rarely without other neurological signs)

women), calcium, sodium, potassium, mean corpuscular volume, gamma glutamyl transpeptidase, haemoglobin, white cell count, ESR or plasma viscosity. Less commonly a chest X-ray, antinuclear antibody, morning and evening cortisols, electroencephalogram or a brain scan are indicated.

The aetiology of unipolar depressive disorders
The aetiology of unipolar depressive disorders is multifactorial and a mixture of genetic and environmental factors.

Genetic
Unipolar depression is probably polygenic, but no linkage has been firmly identified. The risk of unipolar depression in a first-degree relative of a patient is approximately three times the risk of the non-affected. The concordance of unipolar depression in monozygotic twins is between 30 and 60%, the concordance increasing with more recurrent illnesses. The issue is complicated by the genetic influence on sleep habits, 'neurotic' personality, and even life events, which are all involved in the genesis of depressive illness.

Biochemical
The monoamine theory of depressive illness is supported by the efficacy of monoamine reuptake inhibitors and the depressive effect of dietary tryptophan depletion. Neuroendocrine tests also suggest that the serotonin neurotransmitter system is downregulated. 5-HT_{1a} and 5-HT_2 receptor subtypes are thought most likely to be involved. Receptor-labelled functional brain scans suggest that dopamine underactivity is related to psychomotor retardation.

Hormonal
Cushing's syndrome is the most potent cause of 'organic' depressive illness, with 50–80% of patients with Cushing's suffering from a depressive illness. Corticosteroid treatment causes significant mood disturbance. Nearly half of patients with 'functional' depressive illness have raised cortisol levels, and this is associated with adrenal gland enlargement. Hypercortisolaemia can cause hippocampal damage, which has been found in chronic severe depressive illness. All these data suggest that cortisol may play a role in causing depressive illness.

In contrast *atypical depressive illness*, with prominent hypersomnia and weight gain, is associated with a downregulated hypothalamic–pituitary–adrenal axis, supporting the heterogeneity of depressive disorders.

Sleep
A reduced time between onset of sleep and REM sleep (shortened REM latency) and reduced slow wave sleep both occur in depressive illness. We now know that these abnormalities are persistent in some patients when they are not depressed. Families with several sufferers of depressive illness can share these traits, suggesting that sleep patterns may be inherited and predispose to depression.

Psychological
Poor parenting and physical or sexual abuse in childhood all predispose adults to depressive illness, but the effect is non-specific. Both 'neurotic' (emotional) and perfectionist personality traits are risks for depressive illness, and these may be determined as much by genetic factors as early environment.

Social
Thirty per cent of women will develop a depressive illness after a severe life event or difficulty, such as a divorce, and this is compounded by low self-esteem and a lack of a confiding relationship. Unemployment is a significant risk factor in men.

An integrated model of aetiology
Stress is more likely to trigger depressive illness in a person predisposed by lack of social support and/or certain personality traits. Stress in turn triggers various brain changes in both stress hormones (such as the release of corticotropin-releasing hormone) and neurotransmitters (e.g. serotonin) that are both known to be altered in depressive illness. We can thus start to glimpse the model of an integrated biopsychosocial model of depressive illness. This model challenges dualistic ideas that depressive illnesses are either psychological or physical; depressive illnesses involve both the mind and the body, which are themselves indivisible.

Puerperal affective disorders
Affective illnesses and distress are common in women soon after they have given birth. Such disturbances are usually divided into maternity blues, postpartum

(puerperal) psychosis and postnatal depressive illness. '*Maternity blues*' describe the brief episodes of emotional lability, irritability and tearfulness that occur in about 50% of women 2–3 days postpartum, which resolve spontaneously in a few days.

Postpartum psychosis occurs once in every 500–1000 births. Over 80% of cases are affective in type and the onset is usually within the first 2 weeks following delivery. In addition to the classical features of an affective psychosis, disorientation and confusion are often noted. Severely depressed patients may have delusional ideas that the child is deformed, evil or otherwise affected in some way, and such false ideas may lead to either attempts to kill the child or suicide. The response to speedy treatment is generally good. The recurrence rate for a psychosis in a subsequent puerperium is 20–30%.

Non-psychotic *postnatal depressive disorders* occur during the first postpartum year in 10% of mothers, especially in the first 3 months. Risk factors are first pregnancy, poor relationship with the partner, ambivalence about the pregnancy, and emotional personality traits. Depressive illness after childbirth is clinically similar to other depressive illnesses, but lack of emotional bonding with the baby is common.

Treatment of depressive illness
The patient needs to know the diagnosis to provide understanding and rationalization of the overwhelming distress inherent in depressive illness. Knowing that self-loathing, guilt and suicidal thoughts are caused by the illness can be 'antidepressant' on its own. The further treatment of depressive disorders involves physical, psychological and social interventions (Box 21.9). Patients who are actively suicidal, severely depressed or with psychotic symptoms should be admitted (necessary for perhaps 1 in 1000 patients with clinical depression in primary care). This provides the patient a break from self-care, and allows support, listening, observation, prevention of suicide, and close monitoring of treatments. Avoid the pitfall of not treating a depressive illness just because it seems an 'understandable' reaction to serious illness or difficult circumstances. This is particularly likely to happen if the patient is elderly, severely or even terminally ill.

Drugs used in the treatment of clinical depression
Recreational drugs such as alcohol should be stopped. Prescribed medicines suspected of exacerbating depression, such as corticosteroids, should be gradually stopped or reduced to a safe minimum.

The first course of antidepressant drugs is effective in relieving clinical depression in 60–70% of patients, if given in adequate doses for a sufficient time to the correctly diagnosed patient. Such treatment is more successful when accompanied by sufficient patient education and regular follow-up, particularly in the first

---

Box 21.9

Management of depressive illness

Physical
Stop depressing drugs (alcohol, steroids)
Regular exercise (good for mild to moderate depression)
Antidepressants (choice determined by side-effects, co-morbid illnesses and interactions)
Adjunctive drugs (e.g lithium; if no response to two different antidepressants)
Electroconvulsive therapy (ECT) (if life-threatening or non-responsive)

Psychological
Education and regular follow-up by same professional
Cognitive behaviour therapy (CBT) (most effective psychotherapy in clinical depression)
Other indicated psychotherapies (couple, family, interpersonal therapies)

Social
Financial: eligible benefits, debt counselling
Employment: acquire or change the job or career
Housing: adequate, secure tenancy, safe, social neighbours
Young children: child-care support

Treatments combined
The most effective treatment is a mixture of CBT and an antidepressant

---

6 weeks of treatment. Dysthymia responds less well to antidepressants than does a depressive episode.

The commonest two pharmacological types of antidepressants are tricyclic antidepressants (TCAs) and selective serotonin reuptake inhibitors (SSRIs). All antidepressants have similar efficacy and speed of onset. Choice depends on their side-effects, which can be used to positive effect (sedating drugs given at night to enhance sleep), and their safety. Patients should be warned about side-effects and that it will take 2 or more weeks before a positive benefit is apparent. Drugs should normally be started at a low dose and increased, depending on side-effects and efficacy. A course of antidepressants should be given until 4 months after recovery to prevent relapse. The two greatest problems with these drugs are persuading the patient to take them and compliance, since 80% of the UK public wrongly believe that they are addictive.

Psychotic depression needs either electroconvulsive therapy or a combination of an antidepressant and an antipsychotic drug.

Selective serotonin reuptake inhibitors (SSRIs)
SSRIs selectively inhibit the reuptake of the monoamine serotonin (5-HT) within the synapse, and are thus termed 'selective serotonin reuptake inhibitors' or SSRIs. Citalopram, fluvoxamine, fluoxetine, paroxetine and sertraline have the advantage of causing less serious or disabling side-effects than tricyclics. For instance, SSRIs

do not cause significant weight gain. Because of their long half-lives they can also be given just once a day, normally in the morning after breakfast. For these reasons patients comply more with treatment and therefore SSRIs are now first-line treatments for depressive disorders. Normal doses are between 20 and 60 mg, with sertraline and fluvoxamine needing higher doses. The most common side-effects resemble a 'hangover' and include nausea, vomiting, headache, diarrhoea and dry mouth. Insomnia and paradoxical agitation can occur when first starting the drugs. One in five patients also has sexual side-effects, such as impotence and loss of libido. Those SSRIs with a short half-life (e.g. paroxetine) can cause a *serotonin syndrome* if they are suddenly stopped. This unpleasant *discontinuity syndrome* is characterized by shivering, anxiety, incoordination, restlessness, myoclonus, hyperreflexia, and diarrhoea. Patients should be warned not to leave out a dose and to gradually reduce SSRIs when stopping them.

Tricyclic antidepressants (TCAs)

Dosulepin (dothiepin), imipramine and amitriptyline are the three most commonly used in the UK, but many related compounds have been introduced, some having fewer autonomic and cardiotoxic effects (e.g. trazodone, lofepramine). These drugs potentiate the action of the monoamines, norepinephrine (noradrenaline) and serotonin, by inhibiting their reuptake into nerve terminals (Fig. 21.3(c)). Other tricyclics in common use include nortriptyline, doxepin and clomipramine. Depending on the particular drug, normal doses are between 75 and 150 mg. Having been available for more than 40 years, there is more evidence of the effectiveness of TCAs in depressive illness than for any other group of antidepressants. They are the drugs most commonly used in severe depressive illness.

TCAs have a number of side-effects (Table 21.9). In long-term treatment or prophylaxis, weight gain is most troublesome. Because of their toxicity in overdose, it is wisest NOT to prescribe them to potentially suicidal outpatients, without careful monitoring or giving the drugs to a reliable family member to look after.

SNaRIs, NaSSAs and NaRIs: the new antidepressants

The latest generation of antidepressants block a number of different neurotransmitter receptors both at the synapse and elsewhere. Their different receptor profiles cause different side-effects.

Venlafaxine is a potent *blocker* of both *serotonin* and *noradrenaline (norepinephrine) reuptake (SNaRI)*. It has negligible affinity for other neurotransmitter receptor sites and so produces less sedation and fewer anticholinergic effects. It can be given in slow-release form with the advantage of once-daily dosage. Nausea is the commonest side-effect and high doses can occasionally cause hypertension. It does not cause weight gain.

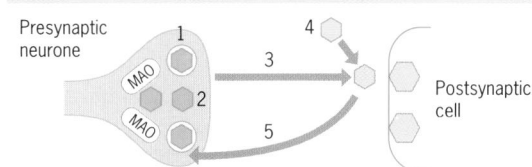

(a) Normal synapse

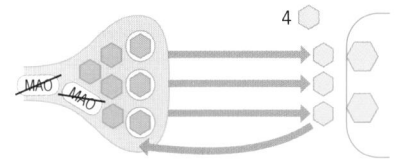

(b) Monoamine oxidase inhibition

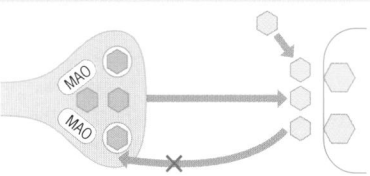

(c) Monoamine reuptake inhibition

Fig. 21.3 **Mechanism by which monoamine oxidase inhibitors and monoamine reuptake inhibitors influence indirectly and directly acting sympathomimetic amines.** 1. Granular store of catecholamine; 2. free cytoplasmic catecholamine; 3. catecholamine released into synaptic cleft by nerve impulse or indirectly acting amine such as ephedrine or tyramine; 4. exogenously administered, directly acting amine such as norepinephrine (noradrenaline); 5. reuptake of catecholamine into the neurone, terminating its action. **(a)** Normal synapse; **(b)** monoamine oxidase inhibition e.g. phenelzine leads to increased catecholamine release by nerve impulse and potentiation of the effect, or sympathomimetic amine; **(c)** monoamine reuptake inhibition, e.g. tricyclics, leads to increased effects of transmitter or administered amine.

Table 21.9
Side-effects of tricyclic antidepressants

Anticholinergic effects	Convulsant activity
Dry mouth	Lowered seizure threshold
Constipation	
Tremor	**Other effects**
Blurred vision	Weight gain
Urinary retention	Sedation
	Mania (rarely)
Cardiovascular	
QT prolongation	
Arrhythmias	
Postural hypotension	

Nefazodone is a potent 5-HT$_2$ receptor antagonist, with weak SNaRI activity. It is more sedating than venlafaxine, also causes nausea, but has few anticholinergic effects and does not cause weight gain. Sexual dysfunction is rare.

Mirtazapine is a 5-HT$_2$ and 5-HT$_3$ receptor antagonist and a potent α$_2$-adrenergic blocker. The consequent effect is to *increase* both *noradrenaline (norepinephrine)* and *selective serotonin transmission*: an *NaSSA*. It can be given at night to aid sleep and rarely causes sexual side-effects. Mirtazapine can be sedating in low dose and can cause weight gain.

Reboxetine is a *selective noradrenaline (norepinephrine) reuptake inhibitor (NaRI)*. It is not sedating and may help reduced motivation and energy. Weight gain is not reported. Dry mouth, insomnia, constipation, urinary hesitancy and tachycardia are reported side-effects.

Monoamine oxidase inhibitors (MAOIs)

These act by irreversibly inhibiting the intracellular enzymes monoamine oxidase A and B, leading to an increase of norepinephrine (noradrenaline), dopamine and 5-hydroxytryptamine in the brain (see Fig. 21.3(b)). Because of their side-effects and restrictions while taking them, they are rarely used by non-psychiatrists. Psychiatrists use them as a second-line treatment of depressive illnesses, particularly with atypical presentations (p. 1243). The most widely used is phenelzine, which is given in doses of 30–60 mg daily. Side-effects include increased appetite, weight gain, sexual dysfunction and insomnia. MAOIs also produce a severe and dangerous hypertensive reaction with foods containing tyramine or dopamine and therefore a restricted diet is prescribed. Tyramine is present in cheese, pickled herrings, yeast extracts, certain red wines, and any food, such as game, that has undergone partial decomposition. Dopamine is present in broad beans. MAOIs interact with drugs such as pethidine and can also occasionally cause liver damage. MAOIs should not normally be given within 2 weeks of a serotonin reuptake inhibitor, depending on half-lives.

Reversible inhibitors of monoamine A (RIMAs)

Reversible inhibitors of monoamine oxidase A (RIMAs) are now available. An example is moclobemide; usual dose 300 mg daily. These drugs appear to have fewer side-effects (insomnia and headache, but some sexual problems) and constitute a low risk in overdose. Patients prescribed such antidepressants should be told that they can eat a normal diet, but should be careful to avoid excessive amounts of food rich in tyramine (see above).

Antidepressant use in general medicine

In patients with cardiac disease, SSRIs, lofepramine and trazodone are preferred over more quinidine-like compounds. MAOIs, mirtazapine and nefazodone do not affect epileptic thresholds. SSRIs are metabolized by the cytochrome p450 system, unlike venlafaxine, mirtazapine and reboxetine, which therefore have fewer drug interactions. Care should be taken not to prescribe antidepressants while a patient is taking the herbal antidepressant St John's wort, which interacts with serotonergic drugs in particular. Doses of antidepressants should initially be halved in the elderly and in patients with renal or hepatic failure.

Antidepressants should be avoided if possible in pregnancy and breast-feeding. If other treatments are ineffective, the risks of drug therapy should be balanced against no treatment, which can affect fetal progress and the future mother–child bonding. Tricyclic antidepressants are generally believed to be safe in pregnancy, with no statistical increase in congenital malformations in fetuses exposed to them. However, occasionally their anticholinergic side-effects produce jitteriness, sucking problems and hyperexcitability in the new-born. Postpartum plasma levels of babies breast-fed by treated mothers are negligible. SSRIs do not seem to be teratogenic but manufacturers advise against their use in pregnancy, until more data are available. MAOIs should be avoided during pregnancy because of the possibility of a hypertensive reaction in the mother.

Electroconvulsive therapy (ECT)

Although the use of ECT is declining in the UK, it is still the treatment of choice in severe life-threatening depressive illness, particularly when psychotic symptoms are present. It is sometimes essential treatment when the patient is dangerously suicidal or refusing to eat and drink. The treatment involves the passage of an electric current across two electrodes applied to the anterior temporal areas of the scalp, in order to induce an epileptic fit. The fit is the essential part of the treatment. Before the treatment is given, the patient is given a general anaesthetic and receives a muscle relaxant to prevent injury during the fit. Treatments are normally given twice a week for 3–6 weeks.

ECT is a controversial treatment, yet it is remarkably safe and free of serious side-effects. Postictal confusion and headache are not uncommon, but transient. Short-term retrograde amnesia and a temporary defect in new learning can occur during the weeks of treatment, but these are short-lived effects.

Uncommonly used treatments

Transcranial magnetic stimulation (TMS) is an experimental treatment, with promising preliminary results. Psychosurgery is very occasionally considered in patients with severe intractable depressive illness, when all other treatments have failed (see p. 1255). A third improve remarkably, while a further third improve somewhat.

Psychological treatments

Cognitive behaviour therapy (CBT)

Aaron Beck developed CBT in the 1960s to reverse the negative cognitive triad with which patients regarded themselves, their situation and their futures. It involves the identification of the automatic dysfunctional thinking that maintains the negative perceptions that feed depression. They commonly include catastrophizing (e.g. making a 'mountain out of a mole-hill'), overgeneralizing (e.g. 'I failed an exam; therefore I am a failure as a person.'), categorical ('black or white') thinking (e.g. 'My work is either perfect or abysmal.'). CBT then involves identifying the links between these thoughts, consequent behaviour, and feeling low, and then testing their logic. This is done by considering the evidence either in the therapy sessions (e.g. Q: 'Did you pass the other exams you took?' A: 'Yes; I guess I did.') or by behavioural 'experiments' (e.g. showing the 'abysmal' work to a colleague and asking their opinion).

There is good evidence that CBT is as effective as antidepressant drugs for mild and moderate depressive illness. CBT is also effective in preventing a relapse of clinical depression. CBT is an effective treatment not only for depressive illness, but also for anxiety disorders and functional disorders (see pp. 1252 and 1234). It has even been shown to help reduce the severity of delusions in schizophrenia.

Interpersonal psychotherapy

American work shows that this psychotherapy is probably as effective as antidepressants in mild and moderate clinical depression. The therapist focuses on a patient's interpersonal relationships involved in or affected by their illness (especially relationship changes or deficiencies), using problem-solving techniques to help the patient to find solutions.

Other psychotherapies

Couple therapy is particularly effective when a patient with clinical depression is in a relationship with problems (practical, emotional or sexual). Both the patient and partner attend therapy. *Family therapy* is effective not only in a family with problems, but also as a way of helping the family to help the patient get better. It may involve understanding one family member's 'depression' as a systemic 'solution' for a wider problem within the family.

Social treatments

Many patients with clinical depression have associated social problems (see Box 21.9). Assistance with social problems can make a significant contribution to clinical recovery. Other social interventions include the provision of group support, social clubs, occupational therapy and referral to a social worker. Educational programmes, self-help groups, and informed and supportive family members can help improve outcome.

Prognosis

The majority of patients have recovered by 6 months in primary care and 12 months in secondary care. About a quarter of patients attending hospital with depressive illnesses will have a recurrence within a year, and three quarters will have a relapse within 10 years. Patients with recurrent depressive illnesses should be offered prevention. This may involve CBT that concentrates on relapse prevention, other forms of psychotherapy, or

antidepressant medication. Full-dose antidepressants are the most effective prophylaxis in recurrent depressive disorders.

FURTHER READING

Kent JM (2000) SNaRIs, NaSSAs, and NaRIs: new agents for the treatment of depression. *Lancet* **355**: 911–918.
Lader M, Cowan P (2001) Depression. *British Medical Bulletin* **57**.
Müller-Oerlinghausen B et al. (2002) Bipolar disorder. *Lancet* **359**: 241–247.
Whooley MA, Simon GE (2000). Managing depression in medical outpatients. *New England Journal of Medicine* **343**: 1942–1950.

Mania and hypomania

The clinical features of mania reflect a marked elevation of mood, characterized by euphoria, overactivity and disinhibition (Table 21.10). Hypomania is the mild form of mania. Hypomania lasts a shorter time and is less severe, with no psychotic features and less disability. Hypomania can be distinguished from normal happiness by its persistence, non-reactivity (not provoked by good news and not affected by bad news) and social disability. Mania almost always occurs as part of a bipolar affective disorder. The social disability of mania can be severe, with disinhibited behaviour leading to significant debts (from overspending and over-generosity), lost relationships (from promiscuity), social ostracism and lost employment (from reckless or disinhibited behaviour).

Some patients have a *rapid cycling* illness, with frequent swings from one mood state to another. A *mixed affective state* occurs when features of mania and depressive illness are seen in the same episode. *Cyclothymia* is a personality trait with spontaneous swings in mood not sufficiently severe or persistent enough to warrant another diagnosis.

Table 21.10
Clinical features of mania

Characteristic	Clinical appearance
Mood	Elevated or irritable
Talk	Fast, pressurized, flight of ideas
Energy	Excessive
Ideas	Grandiose, self-confident, delusions of wealth, power, influence or of religious significance, sometimes persecutory
Cognition	Disturbance of registration of memories
Physical	Insomnia, mild to moderate weight loss, increased libido
Behaviour	Disinhibition, increased sexual activity, excessive drinking or spending
Hallucinations	Fleeting auditory or, more rarely, visual

Differential diagnosis

Acute intoxication with recreational drugs, such as amfetamines, its derivatives (MDMA: Ecstasy), and cocaine can mimic mania. Long-term use of cannabis can also induce an illness with manic features. In one study a quarter of patients with Cushing's syndrome had a secondary manic illness during their illness. Similarly corticosteroids can induce mania less commonly than depressive illness. Dopamine agonists (e.g. bromocriptine) are also known to sometimes induce secondary mania. The excited phase of catatonic schizophrenia can sometimes be mistaken for mania.

Epidemiology

The lifetime prevalence of bipolar affective disorder is 1% across the world. Unlike unipolar depressive illness, it is equally common in men and women, supporting its different aetiology. There is no variation by socioeconomic class or race. The mean age of onset is 21; earlier than unipolar depression. The higher prevalence found in divorced people is probably a consequence of the condition.

Aetiology

Genetic

There is strong evidence for the genetic aetiology in this disorder. There is a 60–80% concordance rate in monozygotic twins, compared to 15% in dizygotic twins, suggesting a high rate of heritability. Adoption studies show similar rates, so this high rate is probably genetic and not due to the family environment. Linkage studies have so far proved disappointing, suggesting there is no single gene with a large effect. Instead it is likely that the condition will prove to be caused by several genes acting together.

Biochemical

It is difficult to carry out research on patients with acute mania, so studies are few. Brain monoamines seem to be increased in mania. Patients with mania tend not to suppress their cortisol levels with dexamethasone, suggesting a similar pattern of non-suppression as seen in severe depressive illness.

Psychological

The effect of life events is much weaker in bipolar compared to unipolar illnesses, with most effect apparent at first onset. Similarly, personality does not seem to be a major influence, in contrast to unipolar depression, although there is some evidence of a link with creativity and divergent thinking that is an advantage in the right occupation.

Treatment of mania

Acute mania

Acute mania is treated with lithium and/or antipsychotic (neuroleptic) drugs. Lithium is the treatment of choice for acute mania in the absence of severe hyperactivity. The advantage of lithium is the lack of motor side-effects seen with neuroleptics (bipolar patients are particularly prone to tardive dyskinesia). The main disadvantage is slow speed of response (normally 2 weeks). The dose of lithium depends on whether citrate or carbonate is used.

Haloperidol and the more sedating chlorpromazine are commonly used neuroleptics, either orally or intramuscularly. Doses are similar to those used in schizophrenia. The behavioural excitement and overactivity are usually reduced within days, but elation, grandiosity and associated delusions often take longer to respond. Severe mania is best treated with a combination of lithium and a neuroleptic, allowing the neuroleptic to be withdrawn after the first 2 or 3 weeks. First attacks of mania usually require treatment for up to 3 months. The anticonvulsants carbamazepine and sodium valproate are also helpful in hypomania or in rapidly cycling illnesses (see below).

Prevention

Since bipolar illnesses tend to be relapsing and remitting, prevention of relapse is the major therapeutic challenge in the management of bipolar affective disorder. A patient who has experienced more than two episodes of affective disorder within a 5-year period is likely to benefit from preventative treatments.

Lithium

Lithium (carbonate or citrate) is the main agent used for prophylaxis in patients with repeated episodes of bipolar illness. It is rapidly absorbed into the gastrointestinal tract and more than 95% is excreted by the kidneys; small amounts are found in the saliva, sweat and breast milk. Renal clearance of lithium correlates with renal creatinine clearance. Lithium is a mood-stabilizing drug that prevents mania more than depression. It reduces the frequency and severity of relapses by half and reduces the likelihood of suicide. Its mode of action is unknown, but lithium is known to act on the serotoninergic system. Poor responses to lithium are associated with a negative family history, an unstable premorbid personality, and a rapid cycling illness.

Patients should be screened for thyroid (free T_4, TSH and thyroid autoantibodies) and renal disease (urea and creatinine concentrations, 24-hour urinary volume) before starting on lithium. Lithium interferes with thyroid function and can produce frank hypothyroidism. The presence of thyroid autoantibodies increases the risk, so it is worthwhile measuring these before treatment. Long-term treatment with lithium causes two renal problems; nephrogenic diabetes insipidus (DI) and reduced creatinine clearance (see p. 590). The therapeutic range for prophylaxis is 0.5–1.0 mmol/L. Lithium levels should be checked every 3 months, along with regular thyroid (free T_4 and TSH) and renal function tests. The best screen for DI is to ask the patient about polyuria and polydipsia. Tests should include serum urea and creatinine, and 24-hour urinary volume if DI is suspected. A creatinine clearance should be carried out if glomerular disease is suspected. Patients should carry a lithium card with them at all times.

Other side-effects of lithium include:

- nausea and diarrhoea
- a fine tremor (15%)
- polyuria and polydipsia (see above)
- weight gain, mainly through increased appetite.

Lithium toxicity begins to occur when the serum concentration exceeds 1.5 mmol/L. Symptoms include drowsiness, nausea, vomiting, blurred vision, a coarse tremor, ataxia and dysarthria. Toxicity is more likely when the patient is dehydrated or with a drug interaction increasing concentrations. Such symptoms progress to delirium and convulsions, and coma and death can occur. As a rule, lithium is not advised during pregnancy, particularly in the first trimester, because of an increased risk of fetal malformation (Ebstein's anomaly). Between 25% and 30% of women with a history of bipolar disorder relapse within 2 weeks of delivery. Restarting lithium within 24 hours of delivery (if the mother is prepared to forgo breast-feeding) markedly reduces the risk of relapse.

Anticonvulsant, mood-stabilizing drugs

Carbamazepine and *sodium valproate* are used both in prophylaxis and treatment of manic states. Some patients who do not respond to lithium may respond to these anticonvulsants or a combination of both. Patients with rapid cycling illnesses show a better response to anticonvulsants than to lithium. For antimanic treatment, dosage in the initial stage of treatment will be 200 mg twice daily of carbamazepine, increasing to a normal dose of 800 to 1000 mg. It may be given as a slow-release formulation. Sodium valproate is given at slightly higher doses of 600 mg initially, increased to a normal dose of 1–2 grams per day. Both carbamazepine and valproate can be teratogenic (neural tube defects) and should be avoided in pregnancy. Other side-effects of these drugs are given on page 1178.

Prognosis

The average duration of a manic episode is 2 months, with 95% making a full recovery in time. Recurrence is the rule in bipolar disorders, with up to 90% relapsing within 10 years.

FURTHER READING

Daly I (1997) Mania. *Lancet* **349**: 1157–1160.

Suicide and attempted suicide (deliberate self-harm) (see also p. 973)

Suicide accounts for 2% of male and 1% of female deaths in England and Wales each year, equivalent to a rate of 8 per 100 000. The rate increases with age, peaking for women in their sixties and for men in their seventies. Suicide is the second most common cause of mortality in 15- to 34-year-olds, and rates in young men are increasing alarmingly. In contrast, suicide rates have declined markedly in older men and in women of all ages. Approximately 15% of people who have suffered a severe depressive disorder (requiring admission) will eventually commit suicide. Suicide rates in schizophrenia sufferers are likewise high, being 20–50 times the rate in the general population; 20–40% of people with schizophrenia make suicide attempts, and 9–13% are successful. A Finnish study suggests that the suicide rate is higher in women who have sustained a miscarriage or undergone an induced abortion, whereas it is significantly reduced in women who are pregnant. The highest rates of suicide have been reported in Hungary (40 per 100 000), while the lowest are those of Spain (3.9 per 100 000) and Greece (2.8 per 100 000), but such variations may reflect differences in reporting, which may be related to religion, as much as genuine differences. Factors that increase the risk of suicide are indicated in Table 21.11.

A distinction must be drawn between those who attempt suicide – deliberate self-harm (DSH) – and those who succeed (suicides). In this regard the following points should be considered:

- The majority of cases of DSH occur in people under 35 years of age.
- The majority of suicides occur in people over 60 years of age.
- Suicides are more common in men, while DSH is more common in women.

Table 21.11
Factors that increase the risk of suicide

Male sex
Older age
Living alone
Immigrant status
Recent bereavement, separation or divorce
Recent loss of a job or retirement
Living in a socially disorganized area
Family history of affective disorder, suicide or alcohol abuse
Previous history of affective disorder, alcohol or drug abuse
Previous suicide attempt
Addiction to alcohol or drugs
Severe depression or early dementia
Incapacitating painful physical illness

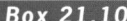

Guidelines for the assessment of patients who harm themselves

Questions to ask: be concerned if positive answer
- Was there a clear precipitant/cause for the attempt?
- Was the act premeditated or impulsive?
- Did the patient leave a suicide note?
- Had the patient taken pains not to be discovered?
- Did the patient make the attempt in strange surroundings (i.e. away from home)?
- Would the patient do it again?

Other relevant factors
- Has the precipitant or crisis resolved?
- Is there continuing suicidal intent?
- Does the patient have any psychiatric symptoms?
- What is the patient's social support system?
- Has the patient inflicted self-harm before?
- Has anyone in the family ever taken their life?
- Does the patient have a physical illness?

Indications for referral to a psychiatrist
Absolute indications include:
- Clinical depression
- Psychotic illness of any kind
- Clearly preplanned suicidal attempts which were not intended to be discovered
- Persistent suicidal intent (the more detailed the plans, the more serious the risk)
- A violent method used.

Other common indications include:
- Alcohol and drug abuse
- Patients over 45 years, especially if male, and young adolescents
- Those with a family history of suicide in first-degree relatives
- Those with serious (especially incurable) physical disease
- Those living alone or otherwise unsupported
- Those in whom there is a major unresolved crisis
- Persistent suicide attempts
- Any patients who give you cause for concern.

- Suicides are more common in older men, but rates in young men are rising fast throughout the UK and Western Europe.
- Suicides in women are slowly falling in the UK.
- Approximately 90% of cases of DSH involve self-poisoning.
- A formal psychiatric disorder is common retrospectively in suicide, but unusual in DSH.

There is, however, an overlap between DSH and suicide. Between 1% and 2% of people who attempt suicide will kill themselves in the year following DSH. In the UK, over 100 000 suicide attempts are made each year, and the overwhelming majority of these are seen and treated within accident and emergency departments.

The guidelines given in Box 21.10 for the assessment of such patients will help ensure that the risk factors relating to suicide are covered. Indications for referral to a psychiatrist before discharge from hospital are also given.

In general, it is worth trying to interview a family member or close friend and check these points with them. Requests for immediate represcription on discharge should be denied, except in cases of essential medication (e.g. for epilepsy). In such cases, however, only 3 days' supply of medication should be given, and the patient should be requested to report to their general practitioner or to their psychiatric outpatient clinic for further supplies. Occasionally involuntary admission under the Mental Health Act (1983) will be required (p. 1269).

FURTHER READING

Henry JA (1996) Suicide risk and antidepressant treatment. *Journal of Psychopharmacology* **19**: 39–40.

The anxiety disorders

These are conditions in which anxiety dominates the clinical symptoms. They are classified according to whether the anxiety is persistent (general anxiety) or episodic, with the episodic conditions classified according to whether the episodes are regularly triggered by the same cue (phobia) or not (panic disorder). The differential diagnoses of anxiety disorders are given in Table 21.12.

General anxiety disorder

This occurs in 4% of the population and is more common in women. Symptoms are persistent and often chronic. General anxiety disorder (GAD) and its related panic disorder are differential diagnoses for medically unexplained symptoms, owing to the many physical symptoms that are caused by these conditions.

Clinical features
The physical and psychological symptoms are outlined in Table 21.13. The patient looks worried, has a tense posture, restless behaviour, a pale and sweaty skin. The

Table 21.12
Anxiety disorders – the differential diagnosis

Psychiatric disorder	Physical disorder
Depressive illness	Hyperthyroidism
Obsessive compulsive disorder	Hypoglycaemia
Presenile dementia	Phaeochromocytoma
Alcohol dependence	
Drug dependence	
Benzodiazepine withdrawal	

Table 21.13
Physical and psychological symptoms of anxiety

Physical symptoms	
Gastrointestinal	*Nervous system*
Dry mouth	Fatigue
Difficulty in swallowing	Blurred vision
Epigastric discomfort	Dizziness
Aerophagy	Headache
'Diarrhoea' (usually frequency)	Sleep disturbance
Respiratory	**Psychological symptoms**
Feeling of chest constriction	Apprehension and fear
Difficulty in inhaling	Irritability
Overbreathing	Difficulty in concentrating
	Distractability
Cardiovascular	Restlessness
Palpitations	Sensitivity to noise
Awareness of missed beats	Depersonalization
Feeling of pain over heart	Derealization
Genitourinary	
Increased frequency	
Failure of erection	
Lack of libido	

Box 21.11

The hyperventilation syndrome

Features

Panic attacks – fear, terror and impending doom – accompanied by some or all of the following:

- dyspnoea (trouble getting a good breath in)
- palpitations
- chest pain or discomfort
- choking sensation
- dizziness
- paraesthesiae
- sweating
- carpopedal spasms.

Cause

Overbreathing leading to a decrease in $P_a\text{co}_2$ and an increase in arterial pH.

Diagnosis

- A provocation test – voluntary overbreathing for 2–3 minutes – provokes similar symptoms; rebreathing from a large paper bag relieves them.
- Blood gases

Management

- Explanation and reassurance is given.
- The patient is trained in relaxation techniques and slow breathing.
- The patient is asked to breathe into a closed paper bag.

patient takes time to go to sleep, and when asleep wakes intermittently with worry dreams. Associated conditions include the hyperventilation syndrome, which is even more common in panic disorder (Box 21.11). The patient will sigh deeply, particularly when talking about the stresses in their life.

Mixed anxiety and depressive disorder

This disorder is probably the commonest mood disorder in primary care, in which there are equal elements of both anxiety and depression, showing how closely associated these two abnormal mood states are.

Panic disorder

Panic disorder is diagnosed when the patient has repeated sudden attacks of overwhelming anxiety, accompanied by severe physical symptoms, usually related to both hyperventilation (Box 21.11) and sympathetic nervous system activity. The prevalence is 1%. Patients with panic disorder often have catastrophic illness beliefs during the panic attack, such as convictions that they are about to die from a stroke or heart attack, or that they suffer from multiple sclerosis (MS). The fear of a stroke is related to dizziness and headache. Fear of a heart attack accompanies chest pain (atypical chest pain), and the fear of MS follows paraesthesiae.

Aetiology

General anxiety and panic disorder occurs four or more times as commonly in first-degree relatives of affected patients, suggesting a genetic influence. Sympathetic nervous system overactivity, increased muscle tension and hyperventilation are the common pathophysiological mechanisms. Psychodynamic theory suggests that

anxiety is the emotional response to the threat of a loss, whereas depression is the response to the loss itself. There is some evidence that being bullied, with the explicit threats involved, leads to anxiety disorders in young people.

Phobic (anxiety) disorders

Phobias are common conditions in which intense fear is triggered by a single stimulus, or set of stimuli, that are predictable and normally cause no particular concern to others (e.g. agoraphobia, claustrophobia, social phobia). This leads to avoidance of the stimulus (see Box 21.12). The patient knows that the fear is irrational, but cannot control it. The prevalence of all phobias is 8%, with many patients having more than one. Many phobias of 'medical' stimuli exist (e.g. of doctors, dentists, hospitals, vomit, blood and injections) which affect the patient's ability to receive adequate healthcare.

Box 21.12

Phobias

A phobia is an abnormal fear and avoidance of an everyday object or situation.
Phobias are common (8% prevalence), disabling, and treatable with behaviour therapy.

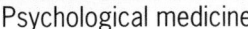

Aetiology

Phobias may be caused by classical conditioning, in which a response (fear and avoidance) becomes conditioned to a previously benign stimulus (a lift) often after an initiating shock (being stuck in a lift). In children, phobias can arise through imagined threats (e.g. stories of ghosts told in the playground). Women have twice the prevalence of most phobias than men. Phobias aggregate in families, but genetic factors are probably weak.

Agoraphobia

Translated as 'fear of the market place', this common phobia (4% prevalence) presents as a fear of being away from home, with avoidance of travelling, walking down a road, and shops being common presentations. This can be a very disabling condition, since the patient can be too unwell to ever leave home, particularly by themselves. It is often associated with *claustrophobia*, a fear of enclosed spaces.

Social phobia

This is the fear and avoidance of social situations: crowds, strangers, parties and meetings. Public speaking would be the sufferer's worst nightmare. It is suffered by 2% of the population.

Simple phobias

The commonest is the phobia of spiders (arachnophobia), particularly in women. The prevalence of simple phobias is 7% in the general population. Other common phobias include insects, moths, bats, dogs, snakes, heights, thunderstorms and the dark. Children are particularly phobic about the dark, ghosts and burglars, but the large majority grow out of these fears.

Treatment of anxiety disorders

Psychological treatments

For many people with brief episodes of an anxiety disorder, a discussion with a doctor concerning the nature of anxiety is usually sufficient.

- *Relaxation* techniques can be effective in mild/moderate anxiety. This can be achieved in many ways, including complementary techniques such as meditation and yoga. Conventional relaxation training involves slow breathing, muscle relaxation, and mental imagery.
- *Anxiety management training* involves two stages. In the first stage, verbal cues and mental imagery are used to arouse anxiety. In the second stage, the patient is trained to reduce this anxiety by relaxation, distraction and reassuring self-statements.
- *Biofeedback* is useful for showing patients that they are not relaxed, even when they fail to recognize it, having become so used to anxiety. Biofeedback involves feeding back to the patient a physiological measure that is abnormal in anxiety. These measures may include electrical resistance of the skin of the palm, heart rate, muscle electromyography, or breathing pattern.
- *Behaviour therapies* are treatments derived from experimental psychology that are intended to change behaviour and thus symptoms. The most common and successful behaviour therapy (with 80% success in some phobias) is *graded exposure*, otherwise known as *systematic desensitization*. This is the treatment of choice for a phobia. Firstly, the patient rates the phobia into a hierarchy or 'ladder' of worsening fears (e.g. in agoraphobia: walking to the front door with a coat on; walking out into the garden; walking to the end of the road). Secondly, the patient practises exposure to the least fearful stimulus until no fear is felt. The patient then moves 'up the ladder' of fears until they are cured.
- *Cognitive behaviour therapy* (CBT) (see p. 1246) is the treatment of choice for panic disorder and general anxiety disorder because the therapist and patient need to identify the mental cues (thoughts and memories) that may subtly provoke exacerbations of anxiety or panic attacks. CBT also allows identification and alteration of the patient's 'schema', or way of looking at themselves and their situation, that feeds anxiety.

Drug treatments

Drugs used in the treatment of anxiety can be divided into two groups: those that act primarily on the central nervous system, and those that block peripheral autonomic receptors.

- *Benzodiazepines* are centrally acting anxiolytic drugs. They bind to specific receptors that stimulate release of the inhibitory transmitter γ-aminobutyric acid (GABA). Diazepam (5 mg twice daily, up to 10 mg three times daily in severe cases) and chlordiazepoxide have relatively long half-lives (20–40 hours) and are used as anti-anxiety drugs in the short term. Side-effects include sedation and memory problems and patients should be advised not to drive while on treatment. They can cause dependence and tolerance within 4–6 weeks, particularly in dependent personalities. The withdrawal syndrome (Table 21.14) can occur after just 3 weeks of continuous use and is particularly severe when high doses have been given for a longer time. Thus, if a benzodiazepine drug is prescribed for anxiety, it should be given in as low a dose and for not more than 2 weeks continuously. A withdrawal programme from chronic use includes changing the drug to the long-acting diazepam, followed by a very gradual reduction in dosage.
- *Buspirone* (5–10 mg three times daily) is a 5-HT$_{1A}$ partial agonist that is anxiolytic after 2 weeks of treatment. It is not yet established as a treatment in the UK. It does not seem to help panic disorder.

Table 21.14
Withdrawal syndrome with benzodiazepines

Insomnia
Anxiety
Tremulousness
Muscle twitchings
Perceptual distortions
Hypersensitivities (light, sound, touch)
Convulsions

- Most SSRIs (e.g. paroxetine, sertraline, citalopram), venlafaxine, MAOIs (phenelzine) and moclobemide (a RIMA) are useful symptomatic treatments for general anxiety and panic disorders, as well as some phobias (social phobia). Imipramine is an established symptomatic treatment for panic disorder, and other tricyclics such as amitriptyline and clomipramine are probably equally effective. Treatment response is often delayed several weeks; a trial of treatment should last 3 months.
- Many of the symptoms of anxiety are due to an increased or sustained release of epinephrine (adrenaline) and norepinephrine (noradrenaline) from the adrenal medulla and sympathetic nerves. Thus, *beta-blockers* such as propranolol (20–40 mg two or three times daily) are effective in reducing peripheral symptoms such as palpitations, tremor and tachycardia, but do not help central symptoms such as anxiety.

Acute stress reactions and adjustment disorders

Acute stress reaction

This occurs in individuals without any other psychiatric disorder, in response to exceptional physical and/or psychological stress. While severe, such a reaction usually subsides within hours or days. The stress may be an overwhelming traumatic experience (e.g. accident, battle, physical assault, rape) or a sudden change in the social circumstances of the individual, such as a bereavement. Individual vulnerability and coping capacity play a role in the occurrence and severity of an acute stress reaction, as evidenced by the fact that not all people exposed to exceptional stress develop symptoms. Symptoms usually include an initial state of feeling 'dazed' or numb, with inability to comprehend the situation. This state may be followed either by further withdrawal from the situation or by anxiety and overactivity. Autonomic signs of arousal, including tachycardia, sweating and hyperventilation, are commonly present. The symptoms usually appear within minutes of the stressor and disappear within 2–3 days.

Adjustment disorder

This disorder can follow an acute stress reaction and is common in the general hospital. This is a more prolonged (up to 6 months) emotional reaction to bad news or a significant life event, with low mood joining the initial shock and consequent anxiety, but not of sufficient severity to fulfil a diagnosis of a mood or anxiety disorder. Supportive counselling is usually a successful treatment, allowing facilitation of unexpressed feelings, elucidation of unspoken fears, and education about the likely future.

Pathological (abnormal) grief

This is a particular kind of adjustment disorder. It can be characterized as excessive and/or prolonged grief, or even absent grieving with abnormal denial of the bereavement. Usually the relative will be stuck in grief, with insomnia and repeated dreams of the dead person, anger at doctors or even the patient for dying, consequent guilt in equal measure, and an inability to 'say good-bye' to the loved person by dealing with their effects. *Guided mourning* uses cognitive and behavioural techniques to allow the relative to stop grieving and move on in life.

Normal grief immediately follows bereavement, is expressed openly, and allows a person to go through the social ceremonies and personal processes of bereavement. The three stages are firstly shock and disbelief, secondly the emotional phase (anger, guilt and sadness) and thirdly acceptance and resolution. This normal process of adjustment may take up to a year, with movement between all three stages occurring in a sometimes haphazard fashion.

Post-traumatic stress disorder (PTSD)

This arises as a delayed and/or protracted response to a stressful event or situation of an exceptionally threatening nature, likely to cause pervasive distress in almost anyone. Causes include natural or human disasters, war, serious accidents, witnessing the violent death of others, being the victim of sexual abuse, rape, torture, terrorism or hostage-taking. Predisposing factors such as personality, previously unresolved traumas, or a history of psychiatric illness may prolong the course of the syndrome. These factors are neither necessary nor sufficient to explain its occurrence, which is most related to the intensity of the trauma, the proximity of the patient to the traumatic event, and how prolonged or repeated it was. Recent functional brain scan research suggests a possible neurophysiological relationship with OCD (p. 1255).

Clinical features

The typical symptoms of PTSD include:

- *'flashbacks'* – repeated vivid reliving of the trauma in the form of intrusive memories, often triggered by a reminder of the trauma
- *insomnia*, usually accompanied by nightmares, the nocturnal equivalent of flashbacks

- *emotional blunting*, emptiness or 'numbness', alternating with …
- *intense anxiety* at exposure to events that resemble an aspect of the traumatic event, including anniversaries of the trauma
- *avoidance* of activities and situations reminiscent of the trauma
- *emotional detachment* from other people
- *hypervigilance* with autonomic hyperarousal and an enhanced startle reaction.

This clinical picture represents the severe end of a spectrum of emotional reactions to trauma, which might alternatively take the form of an adjustment or mood disorder. The course is often fluctuating but recovery can be expected in two-thirds of cases at the end of the first year. Complications include depressive illness and alcohol misuse. In a small proportion of cases the condition may show a chronic course over many years and a transition to an enduring personality change.

Treatment and prevention

Compulsory *psychological debriefing* immediately after a trauma does not prevent PTSD and may be harmful. Behaviourally based therapies should be offered for those with symptoms. It can be normalizing to have therapy in groups with other patients who have suffered similar trauma. A recently introduced therapy is *eye movement desensitization and reprocessing* (EMDR). Further work is necessary before we can be sure of its place in management. SSRIs, venlafaxine and nefazodone have a place in the management of chronic PTSD, but drop-out from pharmacotherapy is common.

The adult consequences of childhood sexual and physical abuse

Estimates of the prevalence of childhood sexual abuse (CSA) vary depending on definition but there is reasonable evidence that 20% of women and 10% of men suffered significant, coercive and inappropriate sexual activity in childhood. The abuser is usually a member of the family or known to the child and preadolescent girls are at greatest risk. The likelihood of long-term consequences are determined by:

- an earlier age of onset
- the severity of the abuse
- the repeated nature and duration of the period of abuse
- the association with physical abuse.

Consequent adult psychiatric disorders include depressive illness, substance misuse, eating disorders, borderline personality disorder and deliberate self-harm. Other negative outcomes include a decline in socio-economic status, sexual problems, prostitution, and difficulties in trusting those closest to the patient.

Psychodynamic psychotherapy

Psychodynamic psychotherapy is derived from psychoanalysis and is based on a number of key analytical concepts. These include Freud's ideas about psychosexual development, defence mechanisms, free association as the method of recall, and the therapeutic techniques of interpretation, including that of transference, defences and dreams. Such therapy usually involves once-weekly 50-minute sessions, the length of treatment varying between 3 months and 2 years. The long-term aim of such therapy is twofold: symptom relief and personality change. Psychodynamic psychotherapy is classically indicated in the treatment of unresolved conflicts in early life, as might be found in non-psychotic and personality disorders, but to date there is a lack of convincing evidence concerning its superiority over other forms of treatment.

FURTHER READING

Shapiro F (1995) *Eye Movement Desensitisation and Reprocessing*. New York: Guildford Press.
Yehudi R (2002) Post-traumatic stress disorder. *New England Journal of Medicine* **346**: 108–114.

Obsessive–compulsive disorder

Obsessive–compulsive disorder (OCD) is characterized by obsessional ruminations and compulsive rituals. It is particularly associated with and/or secondary to both depressive illness and *Gilles de la Tourette syndrome* (p. 1188). The prevalence is up to 2% in the general population and there is an equal distribution by gender.

Clinical features

The obsessions and compulsions are so persistent and intrusive that they greatly impede a patient's functioning and cause considerable distress. There is a constant need to check that things have been done correctly, and no amount of reassurance can remove the small amount of doubt that persists. Some rituals are derived from superstitions, such as actions repeated a required number of times, with the need to start again if interrupted. When severe and primary, OCD can last for many years and is resistant to treatment. However, obsessional symptoms commonly occur in other disorders, most notably general anxiety disorder, depressive illness and schizophrenia, and disappear with the resolution of the primary disorder.

Minor degrees of obsessional symptoms and compulsive rituals or superstitions are common in people who are not ill or in need of treatment, particularly in times of stress. The mildest grade is that of obsessional personality traits such as over-conscientiousness, tidiness, punctuality and other attitudes and behaviours indicating a strong tendency towards conformity and

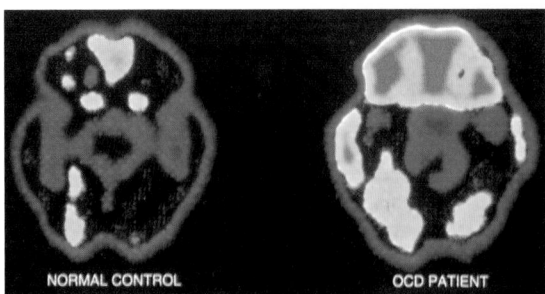

Fig. 21.4 PET images of (left) a normal patient and (right) an obsessive-compulsive disorder (OCD) patient. The right image shows the hyperactivity of the orbitofrontal cortex which is a consistent finding in this condition. Baxter R et al. *Archives of General Psychiatry* **44**: 211, with permission.

inflexibility. Such individuals are *perfectionists* who are intolerant of shortcomings in themselves and others, and take pride in their high standards. When such traits are so marked that they dominate other aspects of the personality, in the absence of clear-cut OCD, the diagnosis is obsessional (anankastic) personality (see p. 1269).

Aetiology
Genetic
OCD is found in 5–7% of the first-degree relatives but few studies have been published.

Basal ganglia dysfunction
OCD is associated with a number of neurological disorders involving dysfunction of the striatum, including Parkinson's disease, Sydenham's and Huntington's chorea. OCD can follow head trauma. Neuroimaging suggests that abnormalities exist in the frontal lobe and basal ganglia (Fig. 21.4). Hyperactivity of the orbitofrontal cortex has been a consistent finding in brain imaging research on OCD patients. The PET images shown here are from the initial report of this finding by a research group at the University of California at Los Angeles. More recent work suggests the caudate nucleus is smaller than in healthy controls.

Serotonin
Serotonin function is probably abnormal in patients with OCD. Serotonin reuptake inhibitors are effective drugs. Postsynaptic serotonin receptor hypersensitivity may follow chronically low levels of synaptic serotonin.

Conditioning
This suggests that compulsive rituals are classically conditioned avoidance responses, which therefore lend themselves to treatment with graded exposure therapy.

Treatment
Psychological treatments
A behaviour therapy that is particularly effective for rituals is *response prevention*. Patients are instructed not to carry out their rituals. There is an initial rise in distress but with persistence both the rituals and the distress diminish. Patients are encouraged to practise response prevention, while returning to situations that normally make them worse.

Modelling involves the therapist demonstrating to the patient what is required and encouraging the patient to follow this example. In the case of hand-washing rituals, this might involve holding an allegedly contaminated object and carrying out other activities without washing, the patient being encouraged to follow suit.

Thought stopping can reduce obsessional ruminations. The patient is taught to arrest the obsessional thought by arranging a sudden intrusion (e.g. snapping an elastic band, clicking the fingers).

Cognitive behaviour therapy allows these techniques as behavioural experiments along with the identification and challenging of the illness-maintaining schema.

Physical treatment
Anxiolytic drugs provide short-term symptomatic relief for overwhelming anxiety on a short-term basis.

Serotonin reuptake inhibitors are the mainstay of drug treatment. Their efficacy is independent of their antidepressant action. Clomipramine is the tricyclic most commonly used in the UK. Specific side-effects include significant tremor and postural hypotension.

Selective serotonin reuptake inhibitors (SSRIs) have been shown to be effective in reducing OCD symptoms, but the doses required are usually some 50–100% higher than those effective in depression. Three months' treatment with high doses may be necessary for a positive response. Positive correlations between reduced severity of OCD and decreased orbitofrontal and caudate metabolism following behavioural and SSRI treatments have been demonstrated in a number of studies.

Psychosurgery
Psychosurgery is very occasionally recommended in cases of chronic and severe OCD that has not responded to other treatments. The development of stereotactic techniques has led to the replacement of the earlier, crude leucotomies with more precise surgical interventions such as subcaudate tractotomy and cingulotomy, with small yttrium radioactive implants, which induce lesions in the cingulate area or the ventromedial quadrant of the frontal lobe. Psychosurgery is now performed only in a few specialist centres in the UK, and formal and detailed consent requirements are laid down in the appropriate mental health act.

Prognosis
Two-thirds of cases improve within a year. The remainder run a fluctuating or persistent course. The prognosis is worse when the personality is anankastic and the OCD is primary and severe.

Alcohol misuse and dependence

A wide range of physical, social and psychiatric problems are associated with excessive drinking. *Alcohol misuse* occurs when a patient is drinking in a way that regularly causes problems to the patient or others.

- The *problem drinker* is one who causes or experiences physical, psychological and/or social harm as a consequence of drinking alcohol. Many problem drinkers, while heavy drinkers, are not physically addicted to alcohol.
- *Heavy drinkers* are those who drink significantly more in terms of quantity and/or frequency than the is safe to do so long-term.
- *Binge drinkers* are those who drink excessively in short bouts, usually 24–48 hours long, separated by often quite lengthy periods of abstinence. Their overall monthly or weekly alcohol intake may be relatively modest.
- *Alcohol dependence* is defined by a physical dependence on or addiction to alcohol. The term *'alcoholism'* is a confusing one with off-putting connotations of vagrancy, 'meths' drinking and social disintegration. It has been replaced by the term *'alcohol dependence syndrome'*.

Epidemiology of alcohol misuse

A survey of drinking in England and Wales found that 15% of men admitted drinking more than 35 units per week and 4% of women drank more than 25 units per week. In the survey, 4% of men and 2% of women reported alcohol withdrawal symptoms.

Approximately one in five male admissions to acute medical wards are directly or indirectly due to alcohol. Between 33% and 40% of accident and emergency attenders have blood alcohol concentrations above the present UK legal limit for driving. People with serious drinking problems have a two to three times increased risk of dying compared to members of the general population of the same age and sex.

Table 21.15 provides an approximate estimate of what can be expected in an average individual in the way of behavioural impairment resulting from a particular blood alcohol level. The usual drink (1 unit of alcohol: $\frac{1}{2}$ pint of ordinary beer, a pub measure of wine) contains about 8 g of absolute alcohol and raises the blood alcohol concentration by about 15–20 mg/dL, the amount that is metabolized in 1 hour.

Detection

Alcohol misuse should be suspected in any patient presenting with one or more physical problems commonly associated with excessive drinking (see p. 250). Alcohol misuse may also be associated with a number of psychiatric symptoms/disorders and social problems (Table 21.16).

Table 21.15
Approximate correlation between blood alcohol level and behavioural/motor impairment

Rising blood alcohol (mg/dL)	Expected effect
20–99	Impaired coordination, euphoria
100–199	Ataxia, poor judgement, labile mood
200–299	Marked ataxia and slurred speech; poor judgement, labile mood, nausea and vomiting
300–399	Stage 1 anaesthesia, memory lapse, labile mood
400+	Respiratory failure, coma, death

Table 21.16
Common alcohol-related psychological and social problems

Psychological	Social
Depression	Marital and sexual difficulties
Anxiety and phobias	Family problems
Memory disturbances	Child abuse
Personality disturbances	Employment problems
Delirium tremens	Financial difficulties
Attempted suicide	Accidents at home, on the roads, at work
Pathological jealousy	Delinquency and crime
	Homelessness

Guidelines

The patient's frequency of drinking and quantity drunk during a typical week should be established. Alcohol consumption can be assessed on the basis of units of alcohol.

- Drinking up to 21 units of alcohol a week for men and 14 units for women carries no long-term health risk.
- There is unlikely to be any long-term health damage with 21–35 units (men) and 14–25 units (women), provided the drinking is spread throughout the week.
- Beyond 36 units a week in men and 24 units a week in women, damage to health becomes increasingly likely.
- Drinking above 50 units a week in men (35 units in women) is a definitive health hazard.

Diagnostic markers of alcohol misuse

Laboratory parameters indicating alcohol misuse are often called markers of recent alcohol misuse. Elevated γ-glutamyl transpeptidase (γ-GT) and mean corpuscular volume (MCV) may indicate alcohol excess in the last few weeks. Blood or breath alcohol are useful tests in anyone suspected of very recent drinking.

Alcohol dependence syndrome

DSM-IV describes dependence as 'a pattern of repeated self-administration that usually results in tolerance,

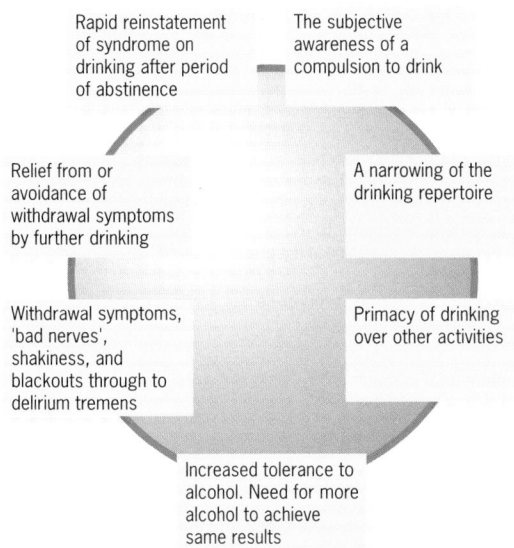

Fig. 21.5 Elements of the alcohol-dependence syndrome.

Table 21.18
Diagnostic criteria for alcohol withdrawal syndrome

Any three of the following:
Tremor of outstretched hands, tongue or eyelids
Sweating
Nausea, retching or vomiting
Tachycardia or hypertension
Anxiety
Psychomotor agitation
Headache
Insomnia
Malaise or weakness
Transient visual, tactile or auditory hallucinations or illusions
Grand mal convulsions

withdrawal and compulsive drug-taking behaviour', the essential element of which is the continued use of the substance despite significant substance-related problems. Figure 21.5 outlines the main characteristics of the syndrome but these do not necessarily present in any particular order. Symptoms of alcohol dependence in a typical order of occurrence are shown in Table 21.17. Diagnostic criteria for alcohol withdrawal syndrome are shown in Table 21.18.

The course of the alcohol dependence syndrome

About 25% of all cases of alcohol misuse will lead to chronic alcohol dependence. This most commonly ends in social incapacity, death or abstinence. Alcohol dependence syndrome usually develops after 10 years of heavy drinking (3–4 years in women). In some individuals who use alcohol to alter consciousness, obliterate conscience and defy social canons, dependence and apparent loss of control may appear in only a few months or years.

Table 21.17
Symptoms of alcohol dependence

Unable to keep a drink limit	Trembling after drinking the
Difficulty in avoiding getting drunk	day before
Spending a considerable	Morning retching and vomiting
time drinking	Sweating excessively at night
Missing meals	Withdrawal fits
Memory lapses, blackouts	Morning drinking
Restless without drink	Increased tolerance
Organizing day around drink	Hallucinations, frank delirium
	tremens

Delirium tremens (DTs)

Delirium tremens is the most serious withdrawal state and occurs 1–3 days after alcohol cessation, so is commonly seen a day or two after admission to hospital. Patients are disorientated, agitated, and have a marked tremor and visual hallucinations (e.g. insects or small animals coming menacingly towards them). Signs include sweating, tachycardia, tachypnoea and pyrexia. Complications include dehydration, infection, hepatic disease or the Wernicke–Korsakoff syndrome (p. 1216).

Causes of alcohol dependence

Genetic factors. Sons of alcohol-dependent people who are adopted by other families are four times more likely to develop drinking problems than are the adopted sons of non-alcohol misusers. Genetic markers include dopamine-2 receptor allele A1, alcohol dehydrogenase subtypes and monoamine oxidase B activity, but they are not specific.

Environmental factors. A Boston follow-up study showed that one in ten boys who grew up in a household where neither parent misused alcohol subsequently became alcohol dependent, compared with one in four of those reared by alcohol-misusing fathers and one in three of those reared by alcohol-misusing mothers.

Biochemical factors. Several factors have been suggested, including abnormalities in alcohol dehydrogenase, neurotransmitter substances and brain amino acids, such as GABA. There is no conclusive evidence that these or other biochemical factors play a causal role.

Psychiatric illness. This is an uncommon cause of addictive drinking but it is a treatable one. Some depressed patients drink excessively in the hope of raising their mood. Patients with anxiety states or phobias are also at risk.

Excess consumption in society. The prevalence of alcohol dependence and problems correlates with the general level (per capita consumption) of alcohol use in a society. This, in turn, is determined by factors that may control overall consumption – including price, licensing laws, the number and nature of sales outlets, and the customs of society concerning the use and misuse of alcohol.

Treatment

Psychological treatment of problem drinking

Successful identification at an early stage can be a helpful intervention in its own right. It should lead to:

- the provision of information concerning safe drinking levels
- a recommendation to cut down where indicated
- simple support and advice concerning associated problems.

Successful alcohol counselling involves *motivational enhancement* (*motivational therapy*), feedback, education about adverse effects of alcohol, and agreeing drinking goals. A motivational approach is based on five stages of change: precontemplation, contemplation, determination, action and maintenance. The therapist uses motivational interviewing and reflective listening to allow the patient to persuade himself along the five stages to change.

This technique, cognitive behaviour therapy and 12-step facilitation (as used by Alcoholics Anonymous (AA)) have all been shown to reduce harmful drinking. With addictive drinking, self-help group therapy, which involves the long-term support by fellow members of the group (e.g. AA), is helpful in maintaining abstinence. Family and marital therapy involving both the alcohol misuser and spouse may also be helpful.

Drug treatments of problem drinking

Alcohol withdrawal and DTs

Addicted drinkers often experience considerable difficulty when they attempt to reduce or stop their drinking. Withdrawal symptoms are a particular problem and delirium tremens needs urgent treatment (Box 21.13). In the absence of DTs, alcohol withdrawal can be treated on an outpatient basis, using one of the fixed schedules in Box 21.13, so long as the patient attends daily for medication and monitoring, and has good social support. Outpatient schedules are sometimes given over 5 days. Long-term treatment with benzodiazepines should not be prescribed in those patients who continue to misuse alcohol. Many alcohol misusers add dependence on diazepam or chlormethiazole to their problems.

Drugs for prevention of alcohol dependence

Naltrexone, the opioid antagonist (50 mg per day), reduces the risk of relapse into heavy drinking and the frequency of drinking. *Acamprosate* (1–2 g per day) is a drug that affects several receptors including those for GABA, norepinephrine (noradrenaline) and serotonin. There is good evidence that it reduces drinking frequency. Neither drug seems particularly helpful in maintaining abstinence. Both drug effects are enhanced by combining them with counselling.

> ### Box 21.13
>
> ### Management of delirium tremens (DTs)
>
> **General measures**
> Admit the patient to a medical bed.
> Correct electrolyte abnormalities and dehydration.
> Treat any co-morbid disorder (e.g. infection).
> Give oral thiamine (200 mg daily) in the absence of Wernicke–Korsakoff (W–K) syndrome.
> Give parenteral thiamine in the presence of a W–K encephalopathy.
> Give prophylactic phenytoin or carbamazepine, if previous history of withdrawal fits.
>
> **Specific drug treatment**
> One of the following orally:
> - Diazepam 10–20 mg
> - Chlordiazepoxide 30–60 mg
> - Lorazepam 2–4 mg
>
> *Repeat 1 hour after last dose depending on response.*
>
> *Fixed-schedule regimens:*
> - Diazepam 10 mg every 6 hours for 4 doses, then 5 mg 6-hourly for 8 doses
> - Chlordiazepoxide 30 mg every 6 hours for 4 doses, then 15 mg 6-hourly for 8 doses
> - Lorazepam 2 mg every 6 hours for 4 doses, then 1 mg 6-hourly for 8 doses
>
> *Provide additional benzodiazepine when symptoms and signs are not controlled.*

Drugs such as *disulfiram* react with alcohol to cause unpleasant acetaldehyde intoxication and histamine release. A daily maintenance dose means that the patient must wait until the disulfiram is eliminated from the body before drinking safely. There is mixed evidence of efficacy.

One trial has suggested that fluoxetine is helpful in the treatment of patients who have both a depressive illness and alcohol dependence.

Outcome

Research suggests that 30–50% of alcohol-dependent drinkers are abstinent or drinking very much less up to 2 years following traditional intervention. It is too early to be certain of the long-term outcome of patients treated with the latest psychological therapies and pharmacotherapies.

FURTHER READING

Fiellin DA, Reid MC, O'Connor PG (2000) New therapies for alcohol problems: application to primary care. *American Journal of Medicine* **108**: 227–237.

Mayo-Smith MF (1997) Pharmacological management of alcohol withdrawal: a meta-analysis and evidence-based practice guideline. *Journal of the American Medical Association* **278**: 144–151.

Drug misuse and dependence

In addition to alcohol and nicotine, there are a number of psychotropic substances that are taken for their effects on mood and other mental functions (Table 21.19).

Causes of drug misuse

There is no single cause of drug misuse and/or dependence. Three factors appear commonly, in a similar way to alcohol problems:

- the availability of drugs
- a vulnerable personality
- social pressures, particularly from peers.

Once regular drug-taking is established, pharmacological factors are particularly important in determining dependence.

Solvents

One per cent of adolescents in the UK sniff solvents for their intoxicating effects. Tolerance develops over weeks or months. Intoxication is characterized by euphoria, excitement, a floating sensation, dizziness, slurred speech and ataxia. Acute intoxication can cause amnesia and visual hallucinations. About 300 teenagers die each year from asphyxiation or acute poisoning.

Amfetamines and related substances

These have temporary stimulant and euphoriant effects that are followed by fatigue and depression, with the latter sometimes prolonged for weeks. Psychological rather than true physical dependence is the rule with 'Speed'. In addition to a manic-like presentation, amfetamines can produce a paranoid psychosis indistinguishable from acute paranoid schizophrenia.

Ecstasy

'Ecstasy' is the street name for 3,4-methylenedioxymethamfetamine (MDMA), a psychoactive phenylisopropylamine, synthesized as an amfetamine derivative. It is a psychodelic drug which is often used as a 'dance' drug at 'raves'. It has a brief duration of action (4–6 hours). There is evidence that repeated use of MDMA can cause permanent neurotransmitter changes in the brain. Deaths have been reported from malignant hyperpyrexia and dehydration. Acute renal and liver failure can occur.

Cocaine

Cocaine is a central nervous system stimulant (with similar effects to amfetamines) derived from *Erythroxylon coca* trees grown in the Andes. In purified form it may be taken by mouth, sniffed or injected. If cocaine hydrochloride is converted to its base ('crack') it can be smoked. This causes an intense stimulating effect and 'free-basing' is common. Compulsive use and dependence occur more

Table 21.19
Commonly used drugs of misuse and dependence

Stimulants	Narcotics
Methylphenidate	Morphine
Phenmetrazine	Heroin
Phencyclidine ('angel dust')	Codeine
Cocaine	Pethidine
Amfetamine derivates	Methadone
Ecstasy (MDMA)	

Hallucinogens	Tranquillizers
Cannabis preparations	Barbiturates
Solvents	Benzodiazepines
LSD	
Mescaline	

LSD, lysergic acid diethylamide

frequently among users who are free-basing. Dependent users take large doses and alternate between the withdrawal phenomena of depression, tremor and muscle pains, and the hyperarousal produced by increasing doses. Prolonged use of high doses produces irritability, restlessness, paranoid ideation and occasionally convulsions. Persistent sniffing of the drug can cause perforation of the nasal septum. Overdoses cause death through myocardial infarction, hyperthermia and arrhythmias (p. 981).

Hallucinogenic drugs

Hallucinogenic drugs, such as lysergic acid diethylamide (LSD) and mescaline, produce distortions and intensifications of sensory perceptions, as well as frank hallucinations in acute intoxication. Psychosis is a long-term complication.

Cannabis

Cannabis is a drug widely used in some subcultures. It is derived from the plant *Cannabis sativa*. It can cause tolerance and dependence. The drug, when smoked, seems to exaggerate the pre-existing mood, be it depression, euphoria or anxiety. It may have specific analgesic properties. An amotivational syndrome has been reported with chronic daily use. There is disagreement over whether it can produce a psychosis (see below).

Tranquillizers

Drugs causing dependence include barbiturates and benzodiazepines. Benzodiazepine dependence is common and may be iatrogenic, when the drugs are prescribed and not discontinued. Discontinuing treatment with benzodiazepines may cause withdrawal symptoms (see Table 21.14). For this reason, withdrawal should be supervised and gradual.

Opiates

Physical dependence occurs with morphine, heroin and codeine as well as with synthetic and semisynthetic

Table 21.20
Opiate withdrawal syndrome

Yawning Rhinorrhoea Lacrimation Pupillary dilatation Sweating Piloerection Restlessness	12–16 hours after last dose of opiate
Muscular twitches Aches and pains Abdominal cramps Vomiting Diarrhoea Hypertension Insomnia Anorexia Agitation Profuse sweating Weight loss	24–72 hours after last dose of opiate

Table 21.21
Length of time urine toxicology screens are likely to remain positive after abstinence

Substance	Usual time positive
Amfetamines	48 hours
Barbiturates	
Short-acting	24 hours
Long-acting	7+ days
Benzodiazepines	3+ days
Cannabinols	5+ days
Cocaine	3+ days
Codeine	48 hours
Morphine	48 hours

opiates such as methadone and pethidine. These substances display cross-tolerance – the withdrawal effects of one are reduced by administration of one of the others. The psychological effect of such substances is of a calm, slightly euphoric mood associated with freedom from physical discomfort and a flattening of emotional response. This is believed to be due to the attachment of morphine and its analogues to receptor sites in the CNS normally occupied by endorphins. Tolerance to this group of drugs is rapidly developed and marked, but is rapidly lost following abstinence. The opiate withdrawal syndrome consists of a constellation of signs and symptoms (Table 21.20) that reaches peak intensity on the second or third day after the last dose of the opiate. These rapidly subside over the next 7 days. Withdrawal is dangerous in patients with heart disease or other chronic debilitating conditions.

Opiate addicts have a relatively high mortality rate, owing to both the ease of accidental overdose and the blood-borne infections associated with shared needles. Heart disease (including infective endocarditis), tuberculosis and AIDS are common causes of death, while tetanus, malaria and the complications of hepatitis B and C are also common.

Treatment of chronic misuse

Blood and urine screening for drugs are required in circumstances where drug misuse is suspected (Table 21.21). When a patient with an opiate addiction is admitted to hospital for another health problem, advice should be sought from a psychiatrist or the patient's drug clinic regarding management of their addiction while an inpatient.

The treatment of chronic dependence is directed towards helping the patient to live without drugs. Patients need help and advice in order to avoid a withdrawal syndrome. Alternatively, patients can be helped to minimize harm to themselves and others. Some patients with opiate addiction who cannot manage such a regimen may be maintained on oral methadone. In the UK, only specially licensed doctors may legally prescribe heroin and cocaine to an addict for maintenance treatment of addiction. An overdose should be treated immediately with the opioid antagonist naloxone.

Drug psychoses

Drug-induced psychoses have been reported with amfetamine and its derivatives, cocaine, and hallucinogens. It can occur acutely after drug use, but is more usually associated with chronic misuse. Psychoses are characterized by vivid hallucinations (usually auditory, but often in more than one sensory modality), misidentifications, delusions and/or ideas of reference (often of a persecutory nature), psychomotor disturbances (excitement or stupor) and an abnormal affect. ICD-10 requires that the condition occurs within 2 weeks and usually within 48 hours of drug use and that it should persist for more than 48 hours but not more than 6 months.

While cannabis use can result in acute anxiety, depression or hallucinations, it is uncertain whether cannabis can produce a more persistent psychosis. Manic-like psychoses occurring after long-term cannabis use have been described, but seem more likely to be related to the toxic effects of heavy ingestion, being quickly resolved. However, a large Swedish prospective study found a significant risk of schizophrenia occurring in soldiers smoking cannabis years earlier. Present evidence suggests that cannabis increases the risk of developing schizophrenia in individuals so predisposed, and can aggravate the psychosis once it is established.

FURTHER READING

Chick J, Cantwell R (1994) *Seminars in Alcohol and Drug Misuse*. London: Gaskell.

Johns A (2001) Psychiatric effects of cannabis. *British Journal of Psychiatry* **178**: 116–122.

Williams H, Salter M, Ghodse AH (1996) Management of substance misusers on the general hospital ward. *British Journal of Clinical Practice* **50**: 94–98.

Schizophrenia

The group of illnesses conventionally referred to as 'schizophrenia' is diverse in nature and covers a broad range of perceptual, cognitive and behavioural disturbances. The point prevalence of the condition is 0.5% throughout the world, with equal gender distribution. A physician primarily needs to know how to recognize schizophrenia, what problems it might present with in the general hospital, and how it is treated.

Causes

No one cause has been identified to date. Schizophrenia is likely to be a disease of neural disconnection caused by an interaction of genetic and multiple environmental factors that affect brain development. The genetic aetiology is likely to be polygenic and non-mendelian. Brain scans and histology often show ventricular enlargement and disorganized cytoarchitecture in the hippocampus, supporting the neurodevelopmental theory of aetiology. Dopamine receptors are upregulated in the mesolimbic system, but the serotonin system may also be involved.

Clinical features

The illness can begin at any age but is rare before puberty. The peak age of onset is in the early twenties. The symptoms that have been considered as diagnostic of the condition have been termed *first rank symptoms* and were described by the German psychiatrist Kurt Schneider. They consist of:

- auditory hallucinations in the third person, and/or voices commenting on their behaviour
- thought withdrawal, insertion and broadcast
- primary delusion
- delusional perception
- somatic passivity and feelings – patients believe that thoughts, feelings or acts are controlled by others.

The more of these symptoms a patient has the more likely the diagnosis is schizophrenia. Other symptoms of acute schizophrenia include behavioural disturbances, other hallucinations, secondary (usually persecutory) delusions and blunting of mood. Schizophrenia is sometimes divided into 'positive' (type 1) and 'negative' (type 2) types:

- Positive schizophrenia is characterized by acute onset, prominent delusions and hallucinations, normal brain structure and function, a biochemical disorder involving dopaminergic transmission, good response to neuroleptics, and better outcome.
- Negative schizophrenia is characterized by a slow, insidious onset, a relative absence of acute symptoms, the presence of apathy, social withdrawal, lack of motivation, underlying brain structure abnormalities, and poor neuroleptic response.

Chronic schizophrenia

This is characterized by long duration and 'negative' symptoms of underactivity, lack of drive, social withdrawal and emotional emptiness.

Differential diagnosis

Schizophrenia should be distinguished from:

- organic mental disorders (e.g. partial complex epilepsy)
- mood (affective) disorders (e.g. mania)
- drug psychoses (e.g. amfetamine psychosis)
- personality disorders (schizotypal).

In older patients, any acute or chronic brain syndrome can present in a schizophrenia-like manner. A helpful diagnostic point is that clouding of consciousness and disturbances of memory do not occur in schizophrenia, and visual hallucinations are unusual.

A *schizoaffective psychosis* describes a clinical presentation in which clear-cut affective and schizophrenic symptoms coexist in the same episode.

Prognosis

The prognosis of schizophrenia is variable. A review of treatment studies suggests that 15–25% of schizophrenics recover completely, about 70% will have relapses and may develop mild to moderate negative symptoms, while about 10% will become seriously disabled.

Treatment

The best results are obtained by combining drug and social treatments.

Antipsychotic (neuroleptic) drugs

These act by blocking the D_1 and D_2 groups of dopamine receptors. Such drugs are most effective against acute, positive symptoms and are least effective in the management of chronic, negative symptoms. Complete control of positive symptoms can take up to 3 months and premature discontinuation of treatment can result in relapse.

As antipsychotic drugs block both D_1 and D_2 dopamine receptors, they usually produce extrapyramidal side-effects. This limits their use in maintenance therapy of many patients. They also block adrenergic and cholinergic receptors and thereby cause a number of unwanted effects (Table 21.22). An infrequent but potentially dangerous unwanted effect is the neuroleptic malignant syndrome (Box 21.14).

Pregnancy. Data on the potential teratogenicity of antipsychotic (neuroleptic) medications are still limited. The disadvantages of not treating during pregnancy have to be balanced against possible developmental risks to the fetus. The butyrophenones (e.g. haloperidol) are probably safer than the phenothiazines. Subsequent management decisions on dosage will depend primarily on the ability to avoid side-effects,

Table 21.22
Unwanted effects of neuroleptic drugs

Common effects	Rare effects
Motor	*Hypersensitivity*
Acute dystonia	Cholestatic jaundice
Parkinsonism	Leucopenia
Akathisia	Skin reactions
Tardive dyskinesia	
	Others
Autonomic	Precipitation of glaucoma
Hypotension	Galactorrhoea
Failure of ejaculation	Amenorrhoea
	Cardiac arrhythmias
Anticholinergic	Seizures
Dry mouth	
Urinary retention	
Constipation	
Blurred vision	
Metabolic	
Weight gain	

since the antiparkinsonian agents are still believed to be teratogenic and should be avoided.

Phenothiazines
Phenothiazines are the group of neuroleptics used most extensively. Chlorpromazine (100–1000 mg daily) is the drug of choice when a more sedating drug is required. Trifluoperazine is used when sedation is undesirable. Fluphenazine decanoate is used as a long-term prophylactic to prevent relapse, as a depot injection (25–100 mg i.m. every 1–4 weeks).

Butyrophenones
The butyrophenones (e.g. haloperidol 2–30 mg daily) are also powerful antipsychotics, used in the treatment of acute schizophrenia and mania. They are highly likely to cause a dystonia and/or extrapyramidal side-effects, but are much less sedating than the phenothiazines. A third of patients with acute schizophrenia will have a good response to haloperidol and a further third will make a partial response.

Atypical antipsychotics
These drugs are 'atypical' in that they block D_2 receptors less than D_1 and thus cause less extrapyramidal side-effects and less tardive dyskinesia.

    Clozapine. Clozapine is used in patients with intractable schizophrenia who have failed to respond to at least two conventional antipsychotic drugs. This drug is a dibenzodiazepine with a relative high affinity for D_1 compared with D_2 dopamine receptors, muscarinic and α-adrenergic receptors. It also blocks 5-HT$_2$ and 5-HT$_1$ receptors. Functional brain scans have shown that clozapine selectively blocks limbic dopamine receptors more than striatal ones, which is probably why it causes considerably fewer extrapyramidal side-effects.

Box 21.14

Neuroleptic malignant syndrome

Neuroleptic malignant syndrome occurs in 0.2% of patients on neuroleptic drugs, particularly potent dopaminergic antagonists such as haloperidol.

Symptoms appear a few days to a few weeks after initiation of therapy and consist of:
- hyperthermia
- muscle rigidity
- autonomic instability (tachycardia, labile BP, pallor)
- fluctuating level of consciousness.

Investigations show:
- ↑ creatine phosphokinase
- ↑ WBC
- abnormal liver biochemistry.

Treatment:
- stop drug
- *Specific*
  bromocriptine – to enhance dopaminergic activity
  dantrolene – to reduce muscle tone
- *Non-specific*
  general management including temperature reduction.

NB. No treatment has proven benefit

Clozapine has been shown to exercise a dramatic therapeutic effect on both intractable positive and negative symptoms. However, clozapine is expensive and produces severe agranulocytosis in 1–2% of patients. Therefore it can only be prescribed to registered patients by doctors and pharmacists registered with the Clozaril patient-monitoring service. The starting dose is 25 mg per day with a maintenance dose of 150–300 mg daily. White cell counts should be monitored weekly for 18 weeks and then 2-weekly for the length of treatment. In addition to its antipsychotic actions, clozapine may also help reduce aggressive and hostile behaviour and the risk of suicide. It can cause considerable weight gain and sialorrhoea. There are some reports of an increased incidence of diabetes mellitus.

    Risperidone is a benzisoxazole derivative with combined dopamine D_2-receptor and 5-HT$_2$-receptor blocking properties. Dosage ranges from 6–10 mg per day. The drug is not markedly sedative and the overall incidence and severity of extrapyramidal side-effects is lower than with more conventional antipsychotics.

    Olanzapine has affinity for 5-HT$_2$, D_1, D_2 and muscarinic receptor sites. Clinical studies indicate it to have a lower incidence of extrapyramidal side-effects. The apparent better compliance with the drug may be related to its lower side-effect profile and its once-daily dosage of 5–10 mg. Weight gain is a problem with long-term treatment.

    Neither risperidone nor olanzapine seem as specific a treatment for intractable chronic schizophrenia as clozapine.

Psychological treatment

This consists of reassurance, support and a good doctor–patient relationship. Psychotherapy of an intensive or exploratory kind is contraindicated. In contrast, recent research shows that cognitive behaviour therapy can help reduce the intensity of delusions.

Social treatment

Social treatment involves attention being paid to the patient's environment and social functioning. Family education can help relatives and partners to provide the optimum amount of emotional and social stimulation, so that not too much emotion is expressed (a risk for relapse). Sheltered employment is usually necessary for the majority of sufferers if they are to work.

Medical presentations related to treatment

The motor side-effects of neuroleptics are the commonest reason for a patient with schizophrenia to present to a physician, followed by deliberate self-harm. *Acute dystonia* normally arises in patients newly started on neuroleptics, causing a *torticollis*. Extrapyramidal side-effects are common and present in the same way as Parkinson's disease. *Akathisia* is a motor restlessness, most commonly affecting the legs. It is similar to the restless legs syndrome (p. 648), but apparent during the day.

Amenorrhoea and galactorrhoea can be caused by dopamine antagonists. Postural hypotension can affect the elderly and neuroleptics can be the cause of delirium in the elderly, if their anticholinergic effects are prominent. The medical emergency of the neuroleptic malignant syndrome is featured in Box 21.14.

FURTHER READING

McGrath J, Emmerson WB (1999) Fortnightly review: treatment of schizophrenia. *British Medical Journal* **319**: 1045–1048.

McGufffin P, Neilson M (1999) Science, medicine, and the future: behaviour and genes. *British Medical Journal* **319**: 37–40.

Organic mental disorders

Organic brain disorders result from structural pathology, as in dementia, or from disturbed central nervous system (CNS) function, as in fever-induced delirium. They do not include mental and behavioural disorders due to alcohol and misuse of drugs, which are classified separately.

Delirium

Delirium, also termed *toxic confusional state* and *acute organic reaction*, is an acute or subacute brain failure in which impairment of attention is accompanied by abnormalities of perception and mood. It is the most common psychosis seen in the general hospital. Ten to twenty per cent of surgical and medical inpatients have delirium during their admission. The degree of impairment classically fluctuates, so that there are intermittent lucid periods. Confusion is usually worse at night, with consequent sleep reversal, so that the patient is asleep in the day and awake all night. During the acute phase, thought and speech are incoherent, memory is impaired and misperceptions occur. Episodic visual hallucinations (or illusions) and persecutory delusions may occur. As a consequence, the patient may be frightened, suspicious, restless and uncooperative.

A developing, deteriorating or damaged brain predisposes a patient to develop delirium (Table 21.23).

A large number of diseases may cause delirium, particularly in elderly patients. Some causes of delirium are listed in Table 21.24. Delirium tremens should be considered in the differential (p. 1257) as well as Lewy body dementia (p. 1265).

Table 21.23
Predisposing factors in delirium

Extremes of age (developing or deteriorating brain)
Damaged brain
    Any dementia (most common predisposition)
    Previous head injury
    Alcoholic brain damage
    Previous stroke
Dislocation to an unfamiliar environment (e.g. hospital admission)
Sleep deprivation
Sensory extremes (overload or deprivation)
Immobilization

Table 21.24
Some common causes of delirium

Systemic infection
Any infection, particularly
  with high fever (e.g. malaria,
  septicaemia)
	Intracranial causes
	Trauma
	Tumour
	Abscess
	Subarachnoid haemorrhage

Metabolic disturbance Hepatic failure Renal failure Disorders of electrolyte balance Hypoxia	Epilepsy

Vitamin deficiency
Thiamin
  (Wernicke–Korsakoff syndrome,
  beriberi)
Nicotinic acid (pellagra)
Vitamin B_{12}
	Drug intoxication
	Anticonvulsants
	Anticholinergics
	Anxiolytic/hypnotics
	Tricyclic antidepressants
	Dopamine agonists
	Digoxin

Endocrine disease Hypothyroidism Cushing's syndrome	**Drug/alcohol withdrawal** **Postoperative states**

Investigation and treatment

Investigation and treatment of the underlying physical disease should be undertaken (Table 21.24). The patient should be carefully nursed and rehydrated in a quiet single room with a window that does not allow exits. If a high fever is present, the temperature should be reduced. All current drug therapy should be reviewed and, where possible, stopped. Psychoactive drugs should be avoided if possible (because of their own risk of exacerbating delirium). In severe delirium, haloperidol is probably an effective choice, the daily dose usually ranging between 1.5 mg (in the elderly) to 30 mg per day. If necessary, the first dose can be administered intramuscularly. Olanzapine has recently been shown to be an effective alternative.

Prognosis of delirium

Delirium usually clears within a week or two, but brain recovery usually lags behind the recovery of the causative physical illness. The prognosis depends not only on the successful treatment of the causative disease, but also on the underlying state of the brain. Twenty-five per cent of the elderly with delirium will have an underlying dementia; 15% of patients do not survive their underlying illness; 40% are in institutional care at 6 months.

Dementia

Dementia is an acquired global impairment of intellect, memory and personality, but without impairment of consciousness. There is often an associated deterioration in emotional control, social behaviour and motivation. Dementia is used both to refer to the primary dementing illness, such as Alzheimer's disease, as well as the process itself, which may be secondary to some other disease (e.g. hypothyroidism). *Presenile dementia* is the term used for patients under 65 years of age and senile dementia for older patients. However, there is no clinical difference.

Dementia affects about 10% of those aged over 65 years and 20% of those over 80 years of age. The causes of dementia are shown in Table 21.25. The majority of cases are due to Alzheimer's disease (AD).

Differential diagnosis

This includes a depressive disorder with *pseudodementia*, in which many of the features of an early dementia, especially memory impairment, slowed thinking, and lack of spontaneity are apparent. Patients with pseudodementia often have a previous history of depression or a family history of mood disorder. Successful treatment of the mood disorder results in restoration of intellectual function. Delirium and mild or moderate learning difficulties are also differential diagnoses.

Alzheimer's disease

This is a primary degenerative brain disease of unknown aetiology that is insidious in onset, followed by gradual deterioration and death in about 10 years.

Table 21.25
Causes of dementia

Degenerative	**Traumatic**
Alzheimer's disease	Post-head injury
Lewy body dementia	Punch drunk syndrome
Frontotemporal dementia	(boxers)
Huntington's disease	
Parkinson's disease	**Intracranial space-occupying**
Normal pressure	**lesions**
hydrocephalus	Subdural haematoma
	Tumours
Vascular	
Cerebrovascular disease	**Anoxic**
Cranial arteritis	Cardiac arrest
	Respiratory failure
Metabolic	Carbon monoxide poisoning
Uraemia	
Liver failure	**Infections**
Remote effects of carcinoma	Encephalitis of any cause
	Creutzfeldt–Jakob disease
Toxic	HIV infection
Alcohol	Syphilis
Occupational exposure	
(e.g. chemicals)	**Endocrine**
Heavy metals (e.g. lead)	Hypothyroidism
	Hypocalcaemia
Vitamin deficiency	
B_{12}	
Thiamin	

The onset can be in middle adult life or even earlier, but the incidence is higher in later life. Patients particularly at risk of developing Alzheimer's disease are those who have a family history, who have sustained a head injury, or have Down's syndrome.

Clinical features of Alzheimer's disease

The cardinal clinical deficits include:

- impaired ability to learn new information or to recall previously learned information
- a decline in language function and, in particular, increased difficulty with names and understanding what is being said (nominal and comprehensive dysphasia)
- dyspraxia – an impaired ability to carry out motor activities, despite intact motor function
- agnosia – the failure to recognize or identify objects despite intact sensory function
- impairment of executive functioning – planning, organizing, sequencing, abstracting.

Behavioural changes are common, including wandering, agitation and aggression. Persecutory delusions occur in up to 50% of patients. Depressive symptoms are also common, but severe depression is not usual, related to the lack of insight.

Pathophysiology of Alzheimer's disease

Neuropathological changes include neuronal reduction, neurofibrillary tangles, senile neurotic plaques and a variable amyloid angiopathy. These changes are particularly seen in the hippocampus, substantia innominata, locus ceruleus and the temicroparietal and frontal cortices. Neurofibrillary tangles are found within the cell body and are made up of paired helical filaments containing the microtubular associated protein, tau. Ubiquitin is found in association with the neurofibrillary tangles. Senile plaques, consisting of a central core of amyloid, develop progressively. Aggregation of amyloid appears to be a central event. Cerebral amyloid plaques are extracellular deposits of amyloid β-protein (Aβ). Recent studies have shown that the enzyme β-seretase (as well as δ-seretase) produces Aβ.

Neurochemical changes occur, including a marked reduction in the enzyme choline acetyltransferase, in acetylcholine itself, and in other neurotransmitters and neuromodulators.

Aetiology

Linkage studies in presenile AD have identified gene loci on chromosomes 1, 14 and 21, with the 14q chromosome link being considered as responsible for 50% of presenile cases. The gene for the precursor protein of amyloid is localized close to the defect on chromosome 21.

A gene locus on chromosome 19q is linked to late-onset AD. A candidate gene in this region encodes the apolipoprotein E. The apolipoprotein E gene is present in the general population in three alleles, ε2, ε3 and ε4. Genetic linkage studies have shown that the ε4 allele is a major risk factor for Alzheimer's disease in all ethnic groups studied and all age groups, but especially the younger. The ε2 allele is under-represented in AD. It has been suggested that the accumulation of β amyloid protein is more extensive in subjects with the ε4 allele than in those without it, whereas the presence of allele ε2 may be associated with less amyloid protein. The great majority of cases of AD are sporadic and of late onset.

Increased free radical formation and impaired antioxidant defences may play a role in the neurodegenerative process. There is a 25–35% reduction in the free radical defence enzyme superoxide dismutase in the frontal cortex and hippocampus. Antioxidant therapy is suggested for treatment (see below).

Vascular dementia (multi-infarct dementia)

This is the second most common cause of dementia and is distinguished from Alzheimer's disease by its history of onset, clinical features and subsequent course. There is usually a history of transient ischaemic attacks with brief impairment of consciousness, fleeting pareses or visual loss. The dementia may follow a succession of acute cerebrovascular events or, less commonly, a single major stroke. Vessel occlusion is the most common cause of vascular dementia, and this may produce a variety of cognitive deficits depending on the site of the ischaemic damage. Multi-infarct dementia results from involvement of several vessels supplying the cerebral

cortex and subcortical structures and is typically associated with signs of cortical dysfunction.

Dementia with Lewy bodies (DLB)

This is probably the most common neurodegenerative disorder after Alzheimer's and multi-infarct dementia, accounting for between 15 and 35% of all dementias. Lewy bodies are neuronal inclusion bodies, which seem to be markers for neuronal loss. They are also found in Parkinson's disease. The clinical presentation is similar to delirium, with fluctuating episodes of confusion, attention problems, and especially visual hallucinations. If prescribed, neuroleptics of all sorts are especially likely to cause an extrapyramidal syndrome and increase mortality. Patients commonly fall down.

Other dementias

Dementia can be due to several disorders including Creutzfeldt–Jakob disease (original and new variant), Huntington's disease, Parkinson's disease and HIV infection (AIDS dementia).

In *frontotemporal dementia* (Pick's disease), a progressive dementia occurs, commencing in middle life and characterized by slowly progressing changes of social, behavioural and personality deterioration. This is followed by impairment of intellect, memory and language. The prevalence is 2–3% of all dementias. The characteristic neuropathological change is that of selective atrophy of the frontal and temporal lobes with silver-staining cytoplasmic inclusion bodies (Pick's bodies). There are no senile plaques or neurofibrillary tangles in excess of that seen in normal ageing, and this distinguishes Pick's disease from Alzheimer's.

Diagnosis of dementia

Dementia is diagnosed clinically by the history and examination, especially cognitive testing (see p. 1229), but it can be confirmed by psychometric testing (e.g. the Wechsler scale). The history must also be taken from someone who has known the patient for a long time. Secondary causes (Table 21.25) are infrequent (10%), but must be excluded as some causes are potentially reversible. Investigations should include blood tests and radiology (Box 21.15).

Management of dementia

The introduction of acetylcholine esterase inhibitors has for the first time suggested a treatment, based on a pathological finding commonly seen in AD. Examples of these drugs include tacrine, donepezil and rivastigmine. Preliminary studies have shown that these drugs delay and sometimes reverse intellectual decline in those patients who can tolerate the side-effects. Patients who respond to the drug usually improve to the level of function present 6–12 months previously. Tacrine therapy requires that a patient has a well-established diagnosis of AD, normal liver biochemistry and a caregiver

---

Box 21.15

Diagnosis of dementia

Blood tests	**Radiology**
Full blood count	Chest X-ray
ESR or C-reactive protein	CT or MRI scan to
Urea and electrolytes	confirm the presence
Blood glucose	of cortical atrophy
Liver biochemistry	and to exclude other
Serum calcium	lesions, such as a
Vitamin B_{12}, folate	brain tumour
TSH, T_4, T_3	EEG (occasionally)
Syphilis serology	
HIV antibodies (after counselling)	

---

willing to give the drug four times daily and to ensure that liver biochemistry is tested as required. Donepezil is the first drug to be licensed in the UK for the treatment of AD. Its benefits appear modest, but it is easily administered and its side-effect profile is favourable.

HRT in postmenopausal women and NSAIDs have shown protective effects against developing AD.

Organic amnestic (dysmnesic) syndrome

This is characterized by a marked impairment of memory occurring in clear consciousness and not as part of a delirium or dementia. Long-term memory is less affected than short-term memory. Often the patient is blandly unconcerned and commonly confabulates. One of the most common causes is severe thiamin deficiency secondary to chronic alcohol misuse (Korsakoff's syndrome), but other less common causes are shown in Table 20.4.

FURTHER READING

Cummings JL (1995) Dementia: the failing brain. *Lancet* **345**: 1481–1484.

Donaldson C, Tarrier N, Burns A (1997) The impact of the symptoms of dementia on caregivers. *British Journal of Psychiatry* **170**: 62–66.

Drachman DA, Leber P (1997) Editorial: Treatment of Alzheimer's disease. *New England Journal of Medicine* **336**: 1245–1249.

McKeith IG, O'Brien JT, Ballard C (1999) Diagnosing dementia with Lewy bodies. *Lancet* **354**: 1227–1228.

Eating disorders

Obesity

This is the commonest eating disorder (see p. 241), which has become epidemic in some developed countries. It is usually caused by a combination of constitutional and social factors, but binge eating disorder and psychological determinants of 'comfort eating' should be excluded.

Anorexia nervosa

The main clinical criteria for diagnosis are:

- a bodyweight more than 15% below the standard weight, or a body mass index (BMI) below 17.5 (ICD-10)
- weight loss is self-induced by avoidance of fattening foods, vomiting, purging, exercise, or appetite suppressants
- a distortion of body image so that the patient regards herself as fat when she is thin
- a morbid fear of fatness
- amenorrhoea in women.

Clinical features include:

- onset usually in adolescence
- a previous history of chubbiness or fatness
- the patient generally eats little
- amenorrhoea – an early symptom; in 20% it precedes weight loss
- binge eating
- usually a marked lack of sexual interest
- lanugo hair.

The physical consequences of anorexia include sensitivity to cold, constipation, hypotension and bradycardia. In most cases, amenorrhoea is secondary to the weight loss. Vomiting and abuse of purgatives may lead to hypokalaemia and alkalosis.

Prevalence

Case register data suggest a rate of 1–10 per 100 000 females aged between 15 and 34 years. Surveys have suggested a prevalence rate of 1–2% among schoolgirls and university students. However, many more young women have amenorrhoea accompanied by less weight loss than the 15% required for the diagnosis. The condition is much less common among men (ratio of 1 : 10). The onset in women is usually at between 16 and 17 years of age and it seldom occurs after the age of 30 years.

Aetiology
Biological factors

Genetic. Six to ten per cent of siblings of affected women suffer from anorexia nervosa. There is an increased concordance amongst monozygotic twins, suggesting a genetic predisposition.

Hormonal. The reductions in sex hormones and the hypothalamic–pituitary–adrenal axis are secondary to malnutrition and usually reversed by refeeding.

Psychological factors

Individual. Anorexia nervosa has often been seen as an escape from the emotional problems of adolescence and a regression into childhood. Patients will often have had dietary problems in early life. Perfectionism and low self-esteem are common antecedents. Recent studies suggest that survivors of childhood sexual abuse are at risk of developing an eating disorder, usually anorexia nervosa, in adolescence.

Family. Families of such patients are allegedly characterized by overprotection, inflexibility and lack of conflict resolution. Anorexia is alleged to prevent dissension in families. However, a recent case control study suggested that there is no more evidence of these factors in families of anorexia nervosa than in control families with a child with an established physical disease.

Social and cultural factors

There is a higher prevalence in higher social classes, and a high rate in certain occupational groups (e.g. ballet dancers and nurses) and in societies where cultural value is placed on thinness.

Prognosis

The condition runs a fluctuating course, with exacerbations and partial remissions. Long-term follow-up suggests that about two-thirds of patients maintain normal weight and that the remaining one-third are split between those who are moderately underweight and those who are seriously underweight. Indicators of a poor outcome include:

- a long initial illness
- severe weight loss
- older age at onset
- bulimia (see below), vomiting or purging
- personality difficulties
- difficulties in relationships.

Suicide has been reported in 2–5% of patients with chronic anorexia nervosa. The mortality rate per year is 0.5% from all causes. More than one-third have recurrent affective illness, and various family, genetic and endocrine studies have found associations between eating disorders and depression. Fifty per cent of patients make a full recovery, 30% a partial recovery and 20% none.

Treatment

Treatment can be conducted on an outpatient basis unless the weight loss is severe and accompanied by marked physical symptoms, dizziness and weakness and/or electrolyte and vitamin disturbances. Hospital admission may then be unavoidable and may need to be on a medical ward initially. Rarely the patient's weight loss may be so severe as to be life-threatening. If the patient cannot be persuaded to enter hospital, compulsory admission may have to be used. Inpatient treatment goals include:

- establishing a good relationship with the patient
- restoring the weight to a level between the ideal bodyweight and the patient's ideal weight

- the provision of a balanced diet, building up to 12.6 MJ (3000 calories) in three to four meals per day
- the elimination of purgative and/or laxative use and vomiting.

Outpatient treatment can be conducted on cognitive behavioural or dynamic psychotherapeutic lines or on a combination of both. Setting up a therapeutic alliance is vital. Individual psychotherapy is better than family therapy if the patient has left home, and vice versa. Motivational enhancement techniques are being used with some success.

Drug treatment has met with limited success, except to symptomatically treat insomnia and depressive illness.

Bulimia nervosa

This refers to episodes of uncontrolled excessive eating, which are also termed 'binges'. There is a preoccupation with food and a habitual adoption of certain behaviours that can be understood as the patient's attempts to avoid the fattening effects of periodic binges. These behaviours include:

- self-induced vomiting
- laxative abuse
- misuse of drugs – diuretics, thyroid extract or anorectics.

Additional clinical features include:

- physical complications of vomiting:
  (a) cardiac arrhythmias
  (b) renal impairment – consequences of low K^+
  (c) muscular paralysis
  (d) tetany – from hypokalaemic alkalosis
  (e) swollen salivary glands – from vomiting
  (f) eroded dental enamel
- associated psychiatric disorders:
  (a) depressive illness
  (b) alcohol misuse
- fluctuations in bodyweight
- menstrual function – periods irregular but amenorrhoea rare
- personality – perfectionism and low self-esteem present premorbidly.

The prevalence of bulimia in community studies is high; it affects between 5% and 30% of girls attending high schools, colleges or universities in the USA. Bulimia is sometimes associated with anorexia nervosa. A premorbid history of dieting is common. The prognosis for bulimia nervosa is better than for anorexia nervosa.

Binge eating disorder

This is bulimia without the vomiting and other weight-reducing strategies.

Treatment

Cognitive behaviour therapy has been shown to be more effective than both interpersonal psychotherapy and drug treatments. SSRIs (fluoxetine) are also an effective treatment, even in the absence of a depressive illness.

FURTHER READING

Becker AE, Grinspoon SK, Klibanski A, Herzog DB (1999) Current concepts: eating disorders. *New England Journal of Medicine* **340**: 1092–1098.

Connan F, Treasure J (2000) Working with adults with anorexia nervosa in an out-patient setting *Advances in Psychiatric Treatment* **6**: 135–144.

Sexual disorders

Sexual disorders can be divided into sexual dysfunctions, deviations, and gender role disorders (Table 21.26).

Sexual dysfunction

Sexual dysfunction in men refers to repeated inability to achieve normal sexual intercourse, whereas in women it refers to a repeatedly unsatisfactory quality of sexual satisfaction. Problems of sexual dysfunction can usefully be classified into those affecting sexual desire, arousal and orgasm. Among men presenting for treatment of sexual dysfunction, impotence is the most frequent complaint. The prevalence of premature ejaculation is low, while ejaculatory failure is rare.

Sexual drive is affected by constitutional factors, ignorance of sexual technique, anxiety about sexual performance, medical and psychiatric conditions and certain drugs (Tables 21.27 and 21.28).

The treatment of sexual dysfunction involves careful assessment, the participation (where appropriate) of the patient's partner, and specific therapeutic techniques, including relaxation, behavioural therapy (Masters and Johnson) and psychotherapy. The introduction of sildenafil has introduced an effective therapy for male impotence (see p. 1021).

Sexual deviation

Nowadays, sexual deviations are more likely to be regarded as unusual forms of behaviour than as illnesses. Doctors are only likely to be involved when the behaviour involves breaking the law (e.g. paedophilia or bestiality) and when there is a question of an associated mental or physical disorder. Homosexuality was formerly classified as an illness but it is now an accepted alternative sexual lifestyle. Men are more likely to have sexual deviations than women.

Gender role disorders

Transsexualism involves a disturbance in gender identity in which the patient is convinced that their body is the wrong gender. A person's gender identity refers to the individual's sense of masculinity or femininity as distinct from sex. It is thought to arise from a biological component (prenatal endocrine influences), psychological imprinting and social conditioning. Disturbances in

---

Table 21.27
Medical conditions affecting sexual performance

Endocrine	**Neurological**
Diabetes mellitus	Neuropathy
Hyperthyroidism	Spinal cord lesions
Hypothyroidism	
	Musculoskeletal
Cardiovascular	Arthritis
Angina pectoris	
Previous myocardial infarction	**Respiratory**
Disorders of peripheral circulation	Asthma
	COPD
Hepatic	
Cirrhosis, particularly alcohol-related	**Psychiatric**
	Depressive illness
Renal	Substance misuse
Renal failure	

Table 21.26
Classification of sexual disorders

Sexual dysfunction	Sexual deviations	Disorders of the gender role
Affecting sexual desire Low libido	**Variations of the sexual 'object'** Fetishism Transvestism	Transsexualism
Impaired sexual arousal Erectile impotence Failure of arousal in women	Paedophilia Bestiality Necrophilia	
Affecting orgasm Premature ejaculation Retarded ejaculation Orgasmic dysfunction in women	**Variations of the sexual act** Exhibitionism Voyeurism Sadism Masochism Frotteurism	

Table 21.28
Drugs affecting sexual arousal

Male arousal	Female arousal
Alcohol	Alcohol
Benzodiazepines	CNS depressants
Neuroleptics	Antidepressants (SSRIs)
Cimetidine	Oral combined contraceptives
Opiate analgesics	Methyldopa
Methyldopa	Clonidine
Clonidine	
Spironolactone	
Antihistamines	
Metoclopramide	
Diuretics	
Beta-blockers	
Cannabis	

Alcohol increases the desire but diminishes the performance

these three areas have variously been blamed for the cause of transsexualism.

For males, treatment includes oestrogen administration and, if surgery is to be recommended, a period of living as a woman as a trial beforehand. In the case of female transsexuals, treatment involves surgery and the use of methyltestosterone.

FURTHER READING

Halaris A (ed.) (1997) Sexual dysfunction. In: *Baillière's Clinical Psychiatry: International Practice and Research*, Vol 3. London: Baillière Tindall.
Watson JP, Davies T (1997) ABC of mental health: psychosexual problems. *British Medical Journal* **315**: 239–242.

Personality disorders

These disorders comprise deeply ingrained and enduring patterns of behaviour which manifest themselves as inflexible responses to a broad range of personal and social situations. Personality disorders are developmental conditions that appear in childhood or adolescence and continue into adult life. They are not secondary to another psychiatric disorder or brain disease, although they may precede or coexist with other disorders. In contrast, personality change is acquired, usually in adult life, following severe or prolonged stress, extreme environmental deprivation, serious psychiatric disorder or brain injury or disease.

Personality disorders are usually subdivided according to clusters of traits that correspond to the most frequent or obvious behavioural manifestations. The main categories of personality disorder are described below.

Borderline (emotionally unstable). Such people act impulsively and develop intense, but short-lived, emotional attachments to others. They describe chronic internal emptiness with frequent self-harm, self-abuse (eating disorders, substance misuse) and they may develop transient psychotic features of uncertain significance. There is often a strong family history of mood disorders.

Paranoid. A paranoid personality is characterized by extreme sensitiveness, suspiciousness, litigiousness, a tendency to excessive self-importance, and a preoccupation with unsubstantiated conspiratorial explanations of events.

Schizoid. A schizoid personality is characterized by emotional coldness and detachment, a limited capacity to express emotions, indifference to praise or criticism, an almost invariable preference for solitary activities, lack of close friendships, and a marked insensitivity to prevailing social norms and conventions.

Antisocial. An antisocial personality is characterized by a callous unconcern for the feelings of others, an incapacity to maintain enduring relationships, a very low tolerance of frustration, an incapacity to experience guilt and to profit from experience, and a marked proneness to rationalize and blame others.

Histrionic. A histrionic personality is characterized by self-dramatization, theatricality, suggestibility, shallow and labile emotions, a continual seeking for excitement and appreciation by others, and an inappropriate seductiveness in appearance or behaviour.

Anankastic (obsessive–compulsive). Such a personality is characterized by feelings of excessive doubt and caution, preoccupation with details, rules, lists, order, perfectionism, excessive conscientiousness, scrupulousness, excessive pedantry, rigidity and stubbornness, and intrusion of unwelcome thoughts or impulses.

Dependent. People with dependent personality encourage others to make their personal decisions, subordinate their needs to others on whom they are dependent, are unwilling to make demands on others, feel unable to care for themselves, are preoccupied with fears of being abandoned. Such patients have a limited capacity to make everyday decisions without an excessive amount of advice and reassurance from others.

Many individuals with disturbed personalities do not fit neatly into such categories, but manifest a mixture of features.

Psychiatry and the law

The law in most developed countries provides for the compulsory admission and/or treatment of mentally disordered persons for their own protection and/or the protection of others and for mitigation in the case of mentally disordered individuals who commit a criminal offence (see also p. 6). In England and Wales the Act of Parliament that is crucially involved is the Mental Health Act 1983, although a new Act is about to go

Table 21.29

Commonly used sections of the Mental Health Act 1983

Section	Duration	Signatures required	Purpose
2	28 days	Two doctors (one approved) plus nearest relative or social worker	Assessment and treatment
3	6 months	Two doctors (one approved) plus nearest relative or social worker	Treatment
4	72 hours	One doctor plus relative or social worker	Emergency admission
5(2)	72 hours	Doctor in charge of patient's care	Emergency detention of a patient already in hospital
5(4)	6 hours	Nurse (RMN)	Emergency detention of a patient already in hospital
136	72 hours	Police officer	Psychiatric assessment of those in public places thought by police to be mentally ill and in need of a place of safety

through parliament. The Mental Health (Scotland) Act 1984 and the Mental Health (Northern Ireland) Order 1986 contain clauses broadly similar to those in England and Wales.

Apart from one provision of the National Assistance Act 1948, the Mental Health Act 1983 is the only method whereby individuals can legally be deprived of their liberty without having committed a crime or being suspected of committing a crime. It is, therefore, necessary that doctors understand the seriousness of their responsibility and the details of the legislation.

There are three conditions that need to be met before an appropriate compulsory section form is signed. The patient must be:

- suffering from a defined mental disorder
- at risk to his/her and/or other people's health or safety
- unwilling to accept hospitalization voluntarily.

The reasons why there is no alternative approach to the treatment suggested for the patient should be outlined. Sexual deviance or alcohol/drug dependence are not defined mental disorders, but otherwise the definition of mental disorder is broad. Any registered medical practitioner may sign a medical recommendation under the Act, but the added signature of a specialist psychiatrist is needed for compulsory orders lasting for more than 72 hours. Unless the patient is already in hospital, the nearest relative or an approved mental health social worker is also required to sign the application form. Relevant sections of the Act are detailed in Table 21.29.

Physicians are likely to be involved in sections 5(2) and 2. It should be remembered that a section does not give a doctor the right to treat a physical disease, although it could be argued that a section would apply if the physical disease was causing the mental disorder (e.g. delirium). This has never been legally tested.

Although much of the process of detention against one's will is formalized, there is no liability for a doctor who acts in good faith with a patient's best interests at heart. Clearly written medical notes, accepted forms of treatment and common sense remain the basis of good practice.

FURTHER READING

Duggan C (ed.) (1997) Assessing risk in the mentally disordered. *British Journal of Psychiatry* **170** (Suppl 32).

CHAPTER BIBLIOGRAPHY

Davies T, Craig TKJ (1998) *ABC of Mental Health.* London: BMJ Books.

Goldberg D (ed.) (1997) *Maudsley Handbook of Practical Psychiatry*, 3rd edn. Oxford: Oxford University Press.

Gelder M, Gath D, Mayou R, Cowen P (1996) *Oxford Textbook of Psychiatry*, 3rd edn. Oxford: Oxford University Press.

Johnstone EC, Freeman CPL, Zealley AK (1998) *Companion to Psychiatric Studies*, 6th edn. Edinburgh: Churchill Livingstone.

Shorter E (1998) *A History of Psychiatry*. Chichester: John Wiley.

Stahl SM (2000) *Essential Psychopharmacology*, 2nd edn. Cambridge: Cambrige University Press

Skin disease 22

Introduction

Skin diseases are common throughout the world. In developing countries, infectious diseases such as tuberculosis, leprosy and onchocerciasis are common, whereas in developed countries, inflammatory disorders such as eczema and acne are common. Skin disorders can be inherited, e.g. Ehlers–Danlos syndrome, a part of normal development, e.g. acne vulgaris, or may present as part of a systemic disorder, e.g. systemic lupus erythematosus (SLE).

Approximately 25% of the UK population will develop a skin problem and, although self-medication is common, skin disease still accounts for 10% of the workload of family doctors. The common reasons for this are itching or pain, which can interfere with people's ability to function normally or to sleep; rashes which cause anxiety, depression and lack of self-confidence and can lead to social isolation if obviously visible; and an inability to work, because certain dermatoses (such as allergic hand eczema in a builder or hairdresser) can interfere with or even prevent working.

Rarely skin disease can be fatal. Examples are malignant melanoma, toxic epidermal necrolysis and pemphigus.

Structure and function of the skin

The skin consists of four distinct layers: the epidermis, the basement membrane zone, the dermis and the subcutaneous layer (Fig. 22.1). The functions are summarized in Box 22.1.

Box 22.1

Functions of the skin

- Physical barrier against friction and shearing forces
- Protection against infection, chemicals, ultraviolet irradiation, particles
- Prevention of excessive water loss or absorption
- Ultraviolet-induced synthesis of vitamin D
- Temperature regulation
- Sensation (pain, touch and temperature)
- Antigen presentation/immunological reactions/wound healing

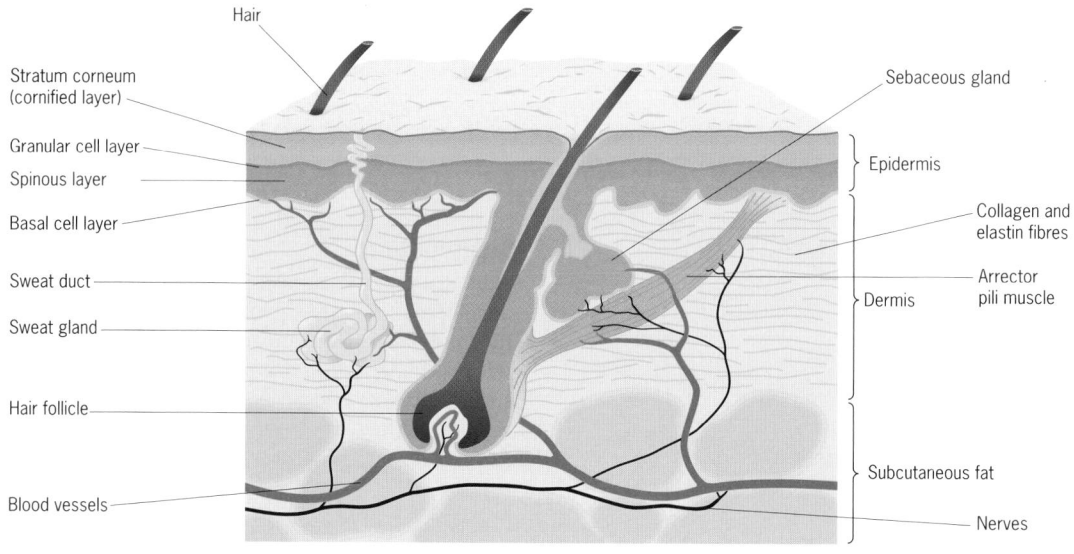

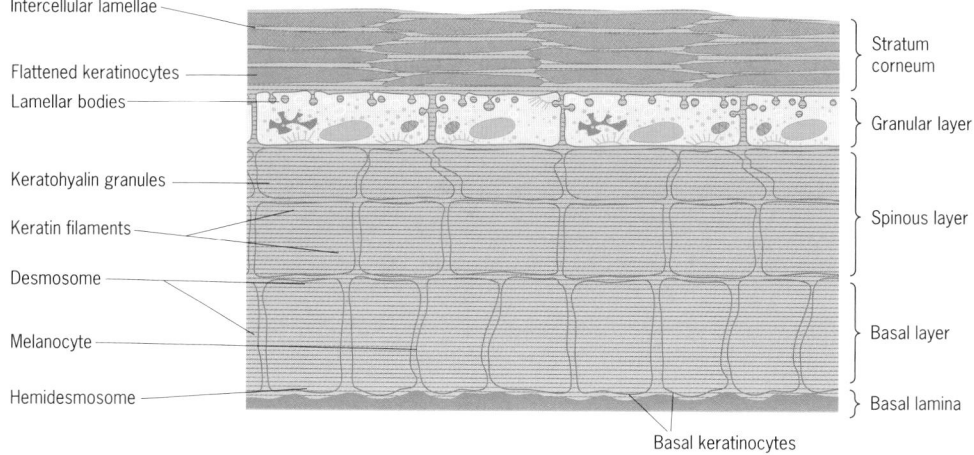

Fig. 22.1 The structure of the skin.

The epidermis

The epidermis is a stratified epithelium of ectodermal origin that arises from dividing basal keratinocytes. The downward projections of the epidermis into the dermis are called the 'rete ridges'. The lower epidermal cells (basal layer) produce a variety of keratin filaments and desmosomal proteins (e.g. desmoglein and desmoplakin), which make up the 'cytoskeleton'. This confers strength to the epidermis and prevents it shedding off. Higher up in the granular layer, complex lipids are secreted by the keratinocytes and these form into intercellular lipid bilayers which act as a semipermeable skin barrier. The upper cells (stratum corneum) lose their nuclei and become surrounded by a tough impermeable 'envelope' of various proteins (loricrin, involucrin, filaggrin and keratin). Changes in lipid metabolism and protein expression in the outer layers allow normal shedding of keratinocytes.

Keratinocytes can secrete a variety of cytokines (e.g. interleukins, interferon, tumour necrosis factor alpha) in response to tissue injury or in certain skin diseases. They therefore play a role in immune function, cutaneous inflammation and tissue repair.

Other cells in the epidermis

Melanocytes are found in the basal layer and secrete the pigment melanin, which protects against UV irradiation. Racial differences are due to variation in melanin production, not melanocyte numbers.

Merkel cells are also found in the basal layer and originate either from neural crest or epidermal keratinocytes. They are numerous on finger tips and in the oral cavity and play a role in sensation.

Langerhans' cells are dendritic cells found in the suprabasal layer. They derive from the bone marrow and as they express the cytokine CCR6, they are guided to normal skin, which contains a CCR6 agonist called macrophage inflammatory protein 3α. Langerhans' cells endocytose extracellular antigens and also act as antigen-presenting cells.

Basement membrane zone (see Fig. 22.26)

The basement membrane zone is a complex proteinaceous structure consisting of type IV and VII collagen, hemidesmosomal proteins, integrins and laminin. Inherited or autoimmune-induced deficiencies of these proteins can cause skin fragility and a variety of blistering diseases (see p. 1302).

The dermis

The dermis is of mesodermal origin and contains blood and lymphatic vessels, nerves, muscle, appendages (e.g. sweat glands, sebaceous glands and hair follicles) and a variety of immune cells such as mast cells and lymphocytes. It is a matrix of collagen and elastin in a ground substance.

The sweat glands

Eccrine sweat glands are found throughout the skin except the mucosal surfaces.

Apocrine sweat glands are found in the axillae, anogenital area and scalp and do not function until puberty.

The sweat glands and vasculature are involved in temperature control.

The sebaceous glands

These are inactive until puberty. They are responsible for secreting sebum or grease onto the skin surface (via the hair follicle) and are found in high number on the face and scalp.

Nerves

The skin is richly innervated. These fibres allow sensation of touch, pain, itch, vibration and change in temperature.

Hair

Hairs arise from a downgrowth of epidermal keratinocytes into the dermis. The hair shaft has an inner and outer root sheath, a cortex and sometimes a medulla. The lower portion of the hair follicle consists of an expanded bulb (which also contains melanocytes) surrounding a richly innervated and vascularized dermal papilla. The hair regrows from the bulb after shedding.

There are three types of hair:

- *terminal* – medullated coarse hair, e.g. scalp, beard, pubic
- *vellus* – non-medullated fine downy hairs seen on the face of women and in prepubertal children
- *lanugo* – non-medullated soft hair on newborns (most marked in premature babies) and occasionally in people with anorexia nervosa.

All hair follicles follow a growth cycle: anagen (growth phase), catagen (involution phase), telogen (shedding phase). At any one time, most hairs (> 90%) will be in the anagen phase, which is typically 3–5 years for scalp hair.

Grey hair is due to decreased tyrosinase activity in the hair bulb melanocytes. White hair is due to total loss of these melanocytes.

Nails

Nails are tough plates of hardened keratin which arise from the nail matrix (just visible as the moon-shaped lunula) under the nail fold. It takes 6 months for a finger-nail to grow out fully and 1 year for a toe-nail.

The subcutaneous layer

The subcutaneous layer consists predominantly of adipose tissue as well as blood vessels and nerves. This layer provides insulation and acts as a lipid store.

Approach to the patient

The *history* should aim to elicit the following points:

- time course of rash
- distribution of lesions
- symptoms (e.g. itch or pain)
- family history (especially of atopy and psoriasis)
- drug/allergy history
- past medical history
- provocating factors (e.g. sunlight or diet)
- previous skin treatments.

Examination entails looking at *and* feeling a rash (for terminology, see Table 22.1). It should include an assessment of nails, hair, and mucosal surfaces, even if these are recorded as unaffected. The following terms are used to describe distribution: flexural, extensor, acral (hands and feet), symmetrical, localized, widespread, facial, unilateral, linear, centripetal (trunk more than limbs), annular and reticulate (lacy network or mesh like).

Investigation. With regard to investigation, clinical acumen remains the most useful tool in dermatology but a variety of tests are useful in confirming a diagnosis (Table 22.2).

FURTHER READING

Montagna W, Kligman AM, Carlisle KS (1992) *Atlas of Normal Human Skin*. New York: Springer Verlag.
Paus R, Cotsarelis G (1999) The biology of hair follicles. *New England Journal of Medicine* **341**: 491–497.
Rees J (1999) Understanding barrier function of the skin. *Lancet* **354**: 1491–1492.
Robert C, Kupper TS (1999) Inflammatory skin diseases, T cells, and immune surveillance. *New England Journal of Medicine* **341**: 1817–1828.

Table 22.1
Morphological description of skin lesions

Atrophy	Thinning of the skin
Bulla	A large fluid-filled blister
Crusted	Dried serum or exudate on the skin
Ecchymosis	Large confluent area of purpura ('bruise')
Erosion	Denuded area of skin (partial epidermal loss)
Excoriation	Scratch mark
Fissure	Deep linear crack or crevice (often in thickened skin)
Lichenified	Thickened epidermis with prominent normal skin markings
Macule	Flat, circumscribed non-palpable lesion
Nodule	Large papule (> 0.5 cm)
Papule	Small palpable, circumscribed lesion (< 0.5 cm)
Petechia	Pinpoint-sized macule of blood in the skin
Plaque	Large flat-topped, elevated, palpable lesion
Purpura	Larger macule or papule of blood in the skin which does not blanch on pressure
Pustule	Yellowish white pus-filled lesion
Scaly	Visible flaking and shedding of surface skin
Telangiectasia	Abnormal visible dilatation of blood vessels
Ulcer	Deeper denuded area of skin (full epidermal and dermal loss)
Vesicle	A small fluid-filled blister
Weal	Itchy raised 'nettle rash'-like swelling due to dermal oedema

Table 22.2
Investigations used in skin disorders

Test	Use	Clinical example
Skin swabs	Bacterial culture	Impetigo
Blister fluid	Electron-microscopy and viral culture	Herpes simplex
Skin scrapes	Fungal culture Microscopy	Tinea pedis Scabies
Nail sampling	Fungal culture	Onychomycosis
Wood's light	Fungal fluorescence	Scalp ringworm Erythrasma
Blood tests	Serology Autoantibodies	Streptococcal cellulitis Discoid lupus erythematosus
	HLA typing DNA analysis	Dermatitis herpetiformis Epidermolysis bullosa
Skin biopsy	Histology Immunohistochemistry Immunofluorescence Culture	General diagnosis Cutaneous lymphoma Immunobullous disease Mycobacteria/fungi
Patch tests	Allergic contact eczema	Hand eczema
Urine	Dipstick	Diabetes mellitus

Infections

Bacterial infections

The skin's normal bacterial flora prevents colonization by pathogenic organisms. A break in epidermal integrity by trauma, leg ulcers, fungal infections (e.g. athlete's foot) or abnormal scaling of the skin (e.g. in eczema) can allow infection. If reinfection occurs, this may be due to asymptomatic nasal carriage of bacteria or the presence of other infected close contacts.

Impetigo
Impetigo is a highly infectious skin disease most common in children (Fig. 22.2). It presents as weeping, exudative areas with a typical honey-coloured crust on the surface. It is spread by direct contact. The term 'scrum pox' is impetigo spread between rugby players. Occasionally this infection can cause blistering ('bullous impetigo') due to bacterial toxins. *Staphylococcus aureus* is implicated in over 90% of cases but rarely group A *Streptococcus* can be responsible. Therefore skin swabs should always be taken.

Treatment
Localized disease is treated with topical fusidic acid (three times daily) and the antiseptic povidone iodine for 1 week. Extensive disease is treated with oral antibiotics for 7–10 days (flucloxacillin 500 mg four times daily for *Staphylococcus*; penicillin V 500 mg four times daily for *Streptococcus*). Other close contacts should be examined and children should avoid school for 1 week after starting therapy. If impetigo appears resistant to treatment or recurrent, take nasal swabs and check other family members. Nasal mupirocin (three times daily for 1 week) is useful to eradicate nasal carriage. Its use in hospitals should be avoided if possible.

Cellulitis
This presents as a hot, sometimes tender area of confluent erythema of the skin owing to infection of the

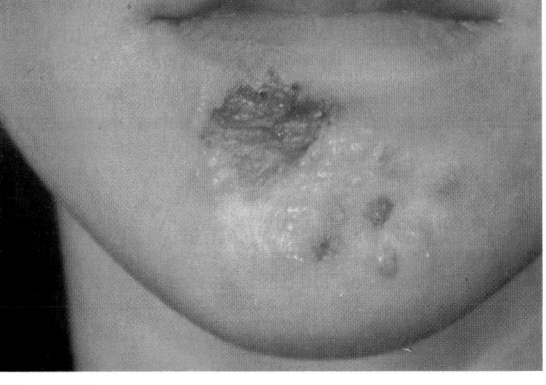

Fig. 22.2 Impetigo – crusted blistering lesions on the chin.

deep subcutaneous layer. It often affects the lower leg, causing an upwards-spreading, hot erythema. It may also be seen affecting one side of the face. Patients are often unwell with a high temperature. It is usually caused by a streptococcus. There may be an obvious portal of entry for infection, such as a recent abrasion or a venous leg ulcer. The web spaces of the toes should be examined for evidence of fungal infection. Skin swabs are usually unhelpful. Confirmation of infection is best done serologically by streptococcal titres.

Erysipelas is the term used for a more superficial infection of the dermis and upper subcutaneous layer that presents clinically with a well-defined edge. However, both erysipelas and cellulitis overlap, so it is often impossible to make a meaningful distinction.

Treatment

Penicillin V or erythromycin (both 500 mg four times daily) is given. If the disease is advanced, treatment may need to be given intravenously for 3–5 days followed by 1–2 weeks of oral therapy. Any identifiable underlying cause should be treated. If cellulitis is recurrent, low-dose antibiotic prophylaxis (e.g. penicillin V 500 mg twice daily) should be given.

Ecthyma

Ecthyma is also an infection due to *Streptococcus* sp. or *Staphylococcus aureus* or occasionally both. It presents as chronic well-demarcated, deeply ulcerative lesions sometimes with an exudative crust. It is commoner in developing countries, being associated with poor nutrition and hygiene. It is rare in the UK but is seen more commonly in intravenous drug abusers and people with HIV.

Treatment is with penicillin V and flucloxacillin (both 500 mg four times daily) for 10–14 days.

Erythrasma

Erythrasma is caused by *Corynebacterium minutissimum*. It usually presents as an orange-brown flexural rash, and is often seen in the axillae or toe web spaces (Fig. 22.3). It is frequently misdiagnosed as a fungal infection. The

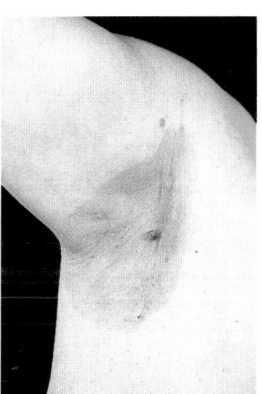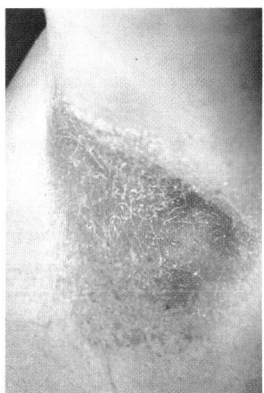

Fig. 22.3 Erythrasma of the axilla, showing pink fluorescence under Wood's light.

rash shows a dramatic coral pink fluorescence under Wood's (ultraviolet) light.

Treatment is with topical fusiden acid three times daily for 7 days, or with oral erythromycin 500 mg four times daily for 7–10 days.

Folliculitis

Folliculitis is an inflammation of the hair follicle. It presents as itchy or tender papules and pustules. *Staphylococcus aureus* is frequently implicated. It is commoner in humid climates and when occlusive clothes are worn. A variant occurs in the beard area (called 'sycosis barbae') which is commoner in black Africans. This is probably caused by the ability of shaved hair to grow back into the skin, especially if the hair is naturally curly. Extensive, itchy folliculitis of the upper trunk and limbs should alert one to the possibility of underlying HIV infection.

Treatment is with topical antiseptics, topical antibiotics (e.g. fusidic acid) or oral antibiotics (e.g. flucloxacillin 500 mg or erythromycin 500 mg both four times daily for 2–4 weeks).

Boils (furuncles)

Boils are a rather more deep-seated infection of the skin, often caused by *Staphylococcus*. They can cause painful red swellings. They are commoner in teenagers and often recurrent. Recurrent boils may rarely occur in diabetes mellitus or in immunosuppression. Large boils are sometimes called 'carbuncles'.

Treatment is with oral antibiotics (e.g. erythromycin 500 mg four times daily for 10–14 days) and occasionally incision and drainage. Antiseptics such as povidone iodine, chlorhexidine (as soap) and a bath oil (e.g. Oilatum plus™) can be useful in prophylaxis.

Hidradenitis suppurativa

This is a rare condition characterized by a painful, discharging, chronic inflammation of the skin at sites rich in apocrine glands (axillae, groins, natal cleft). The cause is unknown but it is commoner in females, and within some families it appears to be inherited in an autosomal dominant fashion. Clinically it presents after puberty with papules, nodules and abscesses which often progress to cysts and sinus formation. With time, scarring may arise. The condition follows a chronic relapsing/remitting course.

Treatment is very difficult but antibiotics, oral retinoids and co-cyprindiol ('2 mg cyproterone acetate + 35 μg ethinylestradiol' in females only) have been tried. They should be used as for acne vulgaris (p. 1292). Severe recalcitrant cases have been treated occasionally with surgery and skin grafting.

Pitted keratolysis

This is a superficial infection of the horny layer of the skin caused by a *Corynebacterium*. It frequently involves

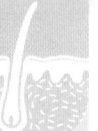

the sole of the forefoot and appears as numerous small punched-out circular lesions of a rather macerated skin (e.g. as seen after prolonged immersion). There may be an associated hyperhidrosis of the feet and a prominent odour.

Treatment. Topical antibiotics (e.g. fusidic acid or clindamycin, applied thrice daily for 2–4 weeks) and topical anti-sweating lotions are effective therapies.

Erysipeloid

This is a very rare infection due to *Erysipelothrix insidiosa*. It is seen in people who handle raw meat (especially pork) and fish. The organism gains entry through breaks in the skin. It presents as a spreading well-demarcated purplish red lesion, usually on the fingers, hands or forearms. There are no systemic symptoms.

Treatment is with penicillin V or oxytetracycline (both 500 mg four times daily for 7–10 days).

Mycobacterial infections

Leprosy (Hansen's disease) (p. 82)

Leprosy usually involves the skin, and the clinical features depend on the body's immune response to the organism *Mycobacterium leprae*.

Indeterminate leprosy is the commonest clinical type, especially in children. This presents as hypopigmented or erythematous circular macules with occasional mild anaesthesia and scaling. This may resolve spontaneously or progress to one of the other types. Biopsy reveals a perineural granulomatous infiltrate and scant acid-fast bacilli.

Tuberculoid leprosy presents with a few hypopigmented or erythematous plaques with an active erythematous, raised rim. Lesions are usually markedly anaesthetic, dry and hairless, reflecting the nerve damage. Nerves may be enlarged and palpable. Biopsy shows a granulomatous infiltrate centred on nerves, but no organisms.

Lepromatous leprosy presents with multiple inflammatory papules, plaques and nodules. Loss of the eyebrows ('madarosis') and nasal stuffiness is common. Skin thickening and severe disfigurement may follow. Anaesthesia is much less prominent. Biopsy shows numerous acid-fast bacilli.

Diagnosis and treatment are discussed on page 84.

Skin manifestations of tuberculosis

Tuberculosis can occasionally cause skin manifestations:

- *Lupus vulgaris* usually arises as a post-primary infection. It usually presents on the head or neck with red-brown nodules which look like apple jelly when pressed with a glass slide. They heal with scarring, and new lesions slowly spread out to form a chronic solitary erythematous plaque. Chronic lesions are at high risk of developing squamous cell carcinoma.

- *Tuberculosis verrucosa cutis* arises in people who are partially immune to tuberculosis but who suffer a further direct inoculation in the skin. It presents as warty lesions on a 'cold' erythematous base.

- *Scrofuloderma* arises when an infected lymph node spreads to the skin causing ulceration, scarring and discharge.

- *The tuberculides* are a group of rashes caused by an immune manifestation of tuberculosis rather than direct infection. Erythema nodosum is the commonest and is discussed on page 1297. Erythema induratum ('Bazin's disease') produces similar deep red nodules but these are usually found on the calves rather than the shins and they often ulcerate.

Atypical mycobacteria

Atypical (non-tuberculous) mycobacteria can occasionally infect the skin. *Mycobacterium marinum* is found in fish tanks and occasionally swimming pools. It can gain access via a break in the skin and then causes deep granulomatous nodules, often in a linear fashion.

Viral infections

Viral exanthem

This is probably the commonest type of virally induced rash. It presents clinically as a widespread non-specific erythematous maculopapular rash, often in the prodromal phase of illness. It probably arises because of circulating immune complexes of antibody and viral antigen localizing to dermal blood vessels. The rash can be caused by many different viruses (e.g. echovirus, parvovirus, human herpes virus-6, Epstein–Barr virus; see p. 49) and so is rarely diagnostic. The rash will resolve spontaneously in 7–10 days.

Slapped cheek syndrome (erythema infectiosum, fifth disease)

This affects children and is caused by parvovirus B19 (see p. 51). It is a mild viral illness which is followed by an intense erythema on the cheeks ('slapped cheeks') and a reticulate erythema on the proximal limbs.

Herpes simplex virus (see also p. 46)

Herpes simplex virus (HSV) occurs as two genomic subtypes. HSV type 1 is spread by direct contact and droplet infection. Most people are affected in early childhood but the infection is usually subclinical. Occasionally it can cause a self-limiting pyrexial primary illness with either clusters of painful blisters on the face or a painful gingivostomatitis. Once infected, cell-mediated immunity develops. In some individuals this response is poor and they may get recurrent attacks of HSV, often manifest as cold sores. Immunosuppression can also cause a recrudescence of HSV. HSV can also autoinoculate into sites of trauma and present as painful blisters/pustules. For example they may be seen on the fingers of healthcare workers ('herpetic whitlow').

HSV type 2 infections occur mainly after puberty and usually affect the genital area. Infections are often symptomatic and transmitted sexually. However, HSV type 1 can also be found in the genital area because of orogenital contact.

Other rare complications of HSV infection include corneal ulceration, eczema herpeticum (p. 1283), chronic perianal ulceration in AIDS patients and erythema multiforme (p. 1297).

Treatment

Oral aciclovir (200 mg five times daily for 5 days) is used for primary HSV and painful genital HSV. Recurrent cold sores are treated with antiviral agents, e.g. aciclovir or famciclovir cream (see Table 2.14) but this must be used early to be effective in shortening an attack. Intravenous aciclovir must be used in immunosuppressed patients.

Varicella zoster virus

Varicella zoster virus (VZV) causes the common childhood infection called chickenpox. It is discussed on page 48. It also causes herpes zoster.

Herpes zoster (shingles)

'Shingles' results from a reactivation of the VZV. It may be preceded by a prodromal phase of tingling or pain which is then followed by a painful and tender blistering eruption in a dermatomal distribution (Fig. 22.4 and Fig. 2.17, p. 48). The blisters occur in crops, may become pustular and then crust over. The rash lasts 2–4 weeks and is usually more severe in the elderly. Occasionally more than one dermatome is involved.

Complications of shingles include severe, persistent pain (post-herpetic neuralgia), ocular disease (if ophthalmic nerve involved) and rarely motor neuropathy.

Treatment

Herpes zoster requires adequate analgesia and antibiotics (if secondary bacterial infection is present). Oral aciclovir 800 mg, five times daily for 7 days helps shorten the attack if given early in the illness. Valaciclovir 1 g or famciclovir 500 mg three times daily for 7 days can also be used. High-dose intravenous aciclovir is needed for immunosuppressed patients. It is unclear how useful aciclovir therapy is in preventing prolonged postherpetic neuralgia.

Human papilloma virus

Human papilloma virus (HPV) is responsible for the common cutaneous infection of 'viral warts'. There are more than 70 subtypes as detected by DNA hybridization. All can cause overgrowth of differentiated squamous epithelium.

Common warts are papular lesions with a coarse roughened surface, often seen on the hands and feet, but also on other sites. Small black dots (bleeding points) are often seen within the lesion (Fig. 22.5). Children and adolescents are usually affected. Spread is by direct contact and is also associated with trauma.

Plantar warts (verrucae) is the term used for lesions on the soles of the feet. They often appear flat ('inward growing') although they have the same papillomatous surface change and black dots are often revealed if the skin is pared down (unlike callosities). Warts may be painful or tender if they are over pressure points or around nail folds.

Filiform warts occur on the face, at the nasal vestibule or around the mouth. They are elongated with a horny cap.

Plane warts are much less common and are caused by certain HPV subtypes. They are clinically different and appear as very small, flesh-coloured or pigmented, flat-topped lesions (best seen with side-on lighting) with little in the way of surface change and no black dots within them. They are usually multiple and are frequently found on the face or the backs of the hands.

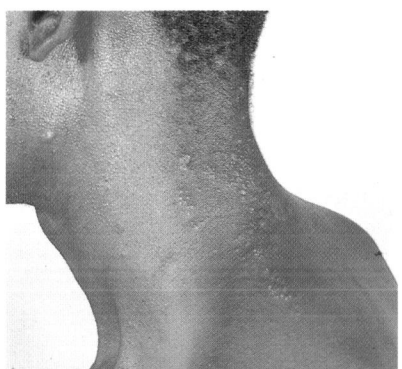

Fig. 22.4 **Herpes zoster in an African** (courtesy of Dr P Matondo, Lusaka, Zambia).

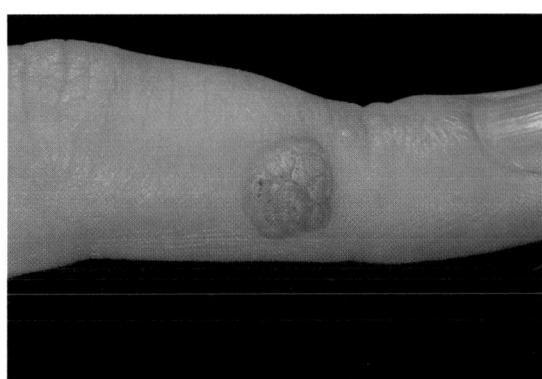

Fig. 22.5 Viral wart.

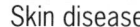

Anogenital warts are usually seen in adults and are normally transmitted by sexual contact. They are rare in childhood and, whilst child sex abuse should always be considered, it should be remembered they may well have been transmitted through non-sexual contact. HPV subtypes 16 and 18 are potentially oncogenic and are associated with cervical and anal carcinomas.

Treatment

Common warts on the skin are surprisingly difficult to treat effectively but they almost always resolve spontaneously after months to years (with no scarring), presumably because of cell-mediated immune recognition. When they do resolve, they tend to do so rapidly within a few days.

Regular use of a topical keratolytic agent (e.g. 2–10% salicylic acid) over many months with weekly paring of the lesion helps speed up resolution in some patients and remains the mainstay of treatment. A course of cryotherapy (freezing) can also help. Cautery, surgery, carbon dioxide laser, alpha-interferon injection and bleomycin injection have all been used with variable success. These treatments may be very painful and can cause permanent scarring.

Genital warts (see p. 129) are usually treated with either cryotherapy, trichloracetic acid, 5% imiquimod cream or topical podophyllin. Patients with genital warts (and their sexual partners) must be screened for other sexually transmitted diseases.

Molluscum contagiosum ('water blisters')

Molluscum contagiosum is a common cutaneous infection of childhood caused by a pox virus. Clinically, lesions are multiple small (1–3 mm) translucent papules which often appear to look like fluid-filled vesicles but are in fact solid. Individual lesions may have a central depression called a punctum. They exhibit the Köbner phenomenon (p. 1288). They can occur at any body site including the genitalia. Transmission is by direct contact. Occasionally lesions may be up to 1 cm in diameter ('giant molluscum'). They are said to be more extensive in children with atopic eczema, which may just reflect that scratching aids their spread.

They usually continue to occur in crops over 6–12 months and rarely require treatment as they spontaneously resolve. Any form of localized trauma, including scratching, helps speed up resolution and cryotherapy may be considered in an older child. Molluscum in an adult, especially if giant, should raise the underlying possibility of immunosuppression, especially HIV infection.

Orf

Orf is a disease of sheep (and occasionally goats) due to a pox virus infection. It causes a vesicular and pustular rash around the mouths of young lambs. People who come into contact with the affected fluid may develop lesions on the hands. Clinically they appear as 1–2 cm reddish papules with a surrounding erythema which usually become pustular. The lesion(s) resolves spontaneously after 4–6 weeks and immunity lasts lifelong. Occasionally orf is complicated by erythema multiforme (p. 1297).

Fungal infections

Fungi are primitive, saprophytic organisms found throughout our environment. Fungal skin disease (mycosis) has a high prevalence in humans, with 'thrush' and 'athlete's foot' being two of the commonest examples. In the immunosuppressed, mycoses can be widespread and life-threatening. There are three groups of pathogenic fungi that commonly affect the outer layer of skin or keratinizing epithelium: dermatophytes, *Candida albicans* and pityrosporum.

Dermatophyte infection

By definition, dermatophytes cause a 'ringworm' type of rash. The three main genera responsible are *Trichophyton*, *Microsporum* and *Epidermophyton*. These organisms are identified by microscopy and culture of skin, hair or nail samples. The clinical appearance of mycoses depends in part on the organism involved, the site affected and the host reaction. All are spread by direct contact from other humans or from infected animals. The use of communal showers and swimming baths and the sharing of towels or sportswear aids indirect fomite transmission.

Tinea corporis

Ringworm of the body usually presents with slightly itchy, asymmetrical, scaly patches which show central clearing and an advancing, scaly, raised edge. Occasionally vesicles or pustules may be seen in the edge. Central clearing is not a universal feature and it is recommended that all asymmetrical scaly lesions should be scraped for fungus. Ringworm of the face (tinea faciei) often arises after the use of topical steroids. It tends to be more erythematous and less scaly than trunk lesions and it may become itchy after sun exposure.

Tinea cruris

Ringworm of the groin is extremely common worldwide. Early on, the lesions appear as well-demarcated red plaques with an arc-like border extending down the upper thigh (Fig. 22.6). Central clearing may appear and a few pustules or vesicles may be seen if inflammation is intense. Satellite lesions, suggestive of *Candida*, are not present.

Tinea pedis

Athlete's foot may be confined to the toe clefts, where the skin looks white, macerated and fissured. It may also be more diffuse, usually causing a diffuse scaly

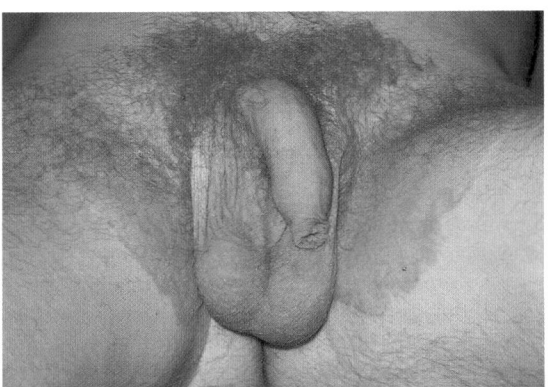

Fig. 22.6 **Tinea cruris** – ringworm of the groin.

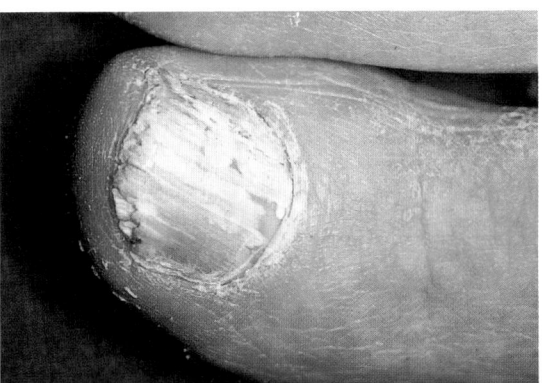

Fig. 22.7 **Dermatophyte infection of the nail showing a white crumbling dystrophy.**

erythema of the soles spreading on to the sides of the foot. Annular lesions rarely occur and can lead to misdiagnosis. There may be an associated hyperhidrosis and fungal involvement of one or more toe-nails. In severe infection, a strong inflammatory reaction can occur causing pustules or blistering and this often leads to a misdiagnosis of pompholyx-type eczema.

Tinea manuum

Ringworm of the hands also presents with a diffuse erythematous scaling of the palms with variable skin peeling and skin thickening. Annular lesions are rare at this site.

Tinea capitis

Scalp ringworm infections are continuing to increase in developed countries although the rate of increase is beginning to slow. Fungus may confine itself to within the hair shaft (endothrix) or spread out over the hair surface (ectothrix). The latter can cause fluorescence under a Wood's lamp (ultraviolet light). Scalp ringworm is spread by close contact (especially in schools and households) and may also be spread indirectly by hairdressers. The number of new cases has risen enormously in the large cities in developed countries. Increase in travel and immigration has allowed the spread of different pathogenic fungi (e.g. *Trichophyton tonsurans* from Central America, *Trichophyton violaceum* from India and Pakistan) into new countries where overcrowding and poor social conditions have allowed spread. The majority of UK cases are currently due to *T. tonsurans* (which does not show fluorescence).

Tinea capitis is much commoner in children, especially those of black African origin whose scalp and hair seems more susceptible to fungal invasion. The clinical appearance of scalp ringworm is highly variable, making underdiagnosis a very real problem. At mildest, there may be some diffuse scaling with no hair loss – similar to dandruff. The more typical appearance is of circular scaly patches in the scalp with associated alopecia and broken hairs. As the host's immune response increases,

a few pustules may appear and an exudate may be present. At worst, a full-blown 'kerion' develops; a boggy swollen mass with copious quantities of discharging pus and exudate accompanied by severe alopecia. This is still poorly recognized and inappropriately treated with antibiotics and attempted surgical drainage.

Extensive infection is occasionally accompanied by a widespread papulopustular rash on the trunk. This is a so-called 'Id reaction' and probably relates to the host immune response to the fungus. It seems commoner in black African children. It resolves when the fungal infection is treated.

Tinea unguium

Ringworm of the nails is increasingly common with age and frequently ignored as it is often asymptomatic. Clinically this presents as asymmetrical whitening (or yellowish black discoloration) of one or more nails, which usually starts at the distal or lateral edge before spreading throughout the nail (Fig. 22.7). The nail plate appears thickened. Crumbly white material appears under the nail plate and this is the best specimen to obtain for mycology sampling. The nail plate may become destroyed with advanced disease.

'Tinea incognito'

This is the term used to describe a fungal skin infection that has been modified by therapy with a topical steroid. The clinical appearance is variable but may show a non-specific erythema with little in the way of scaling or a few reddish nodules. The history of the rash improving with treatment (owing to the suppression of inflammation) but worsening and spreading every time it is stopped is typical. Skin scrapings for mycology or even a biopsy should confirm the diagnosis.

Treatment

Localized ringworm of the body or flexures is treated with topical antifungal creams (clotrimazole, miconazole, terbinafine or amorolofine applied three times daily for

1–2 weeks). More widespread infection, including tinea pedis, tinea manuum and tinea capitis, requires oral antifungal therapy. Itraconazole (100 mg daily) and terbinafine (250 mg daily) are the most effective drugs used for periods of 1–2 months, but are not currently licensed for use in children. High-dose griseofulvin is still used in children for scalp ringworm (15–20 mg/kg/day for 8 weeks).

Tinea unguium of the toe-nails is the most resistant to treatment. Itraconazole (100 mg daily, or 200 mg twice daily for 1 week per month 'pulsed therapy') or terbinafine (250 mg daily) given for 3 months will cure up to about 80% of cases.

Candida albicans (see also p. 94)

Candida albicans is a yeast that is sometimes found as part of the body's flora, especially in the gastrointestinal tract. It acts as an opportunist, taking hold in the skin when there is a suitable warm moist environment such as in nappy rash (p. 1317) or intertrigo in obese individuals (Fig. 22.8).

The flexural areas affected are red with a rather ragged peeling edge that may contain a few small pustules. Small circular areas of erythema or small papules and pustules may be seen in front of the advancing edge (satellite lesions). *Candida* may also affect the moist interdigital clefts of the toes and mimic tinea pedis. In people who have their hands immersed frequently in water (e.g. cleaners, nurses) *Candida* may cause infection in the macerated skin of the finger web spaces or the damaged skin around the nail folds ('chronic paronychia'). Nail infection may mimic tinea unguium. It can infect mucosal surfaces of the mouth or genital tract. This tends to occur in patients taking broad-spectrum antibiotics (owing to suppression of protective bacterial flora) or in immunosuppressed patients. Clinically superficial white or creamy pseudomembranous plaques appear, which can be scraped off leaving raw areas underneath.

Treatment

Treatment is aimed at removing any underlying predisposing factor and applying topical antifungal creams, e.g. clotrimazole or miconazole (or the equivalent as mouth lozenges/pessaries). *Candida* nail infections require systemic antifungal therapy with an imidazole such as itraconazole (100 mg daily for 3 months). Recurrent candidiasis is relatively common, especially in women. Diabetes mellitus should always be excluded. Repeated topical treatment or an oral imidazole may be needed.

Pityrosporum

This yeast occurs as part of the normal flora of human skin. Colonization is prominent in the scalp, flexures and upper trunk. There are two morphological variants called *Pityrosporum ovale* and *Pityrosporum orbiculare* and the mycelial form of this yeast is called *Malassezia furfur*. *Pityrosporum* can overgrow in some individuals and has been implicated in three dermatoses:

- pityriasis versicolor
- seborrhoeic dermatitis (p. 1285)
- pityrosporum folliculitis.

Pityriasis versicolor

This is a relatively common condition of young adults caused by infection with *Pityrosporum*. In Caucasians it presents most commonly on the trunk with reddish brown scaly macules which are asymptomatic. In black-skinned individuals (or in whites who are sun-tanned) it more commonly presents as macular areas of hypopigmentation. Inappropriate use of topical steroids tends to spread the rash.

Diagnosis can be confirmed by skin scrapings or Wood's light examination (yellow fluorescence).

Treatment is with selenium sulphide shampoo (apply to body and remove after 30 minutes and repeat daily for 1 week) or a topical imidazole cream (twice daily for 10 days). Oral itraconazole (100 mg twice daily for 1 week) can be used for resistant cases. The pigmentation takes months to recover, even after successful treatment. The condition may recur but can be retreated.

Pityrosporum folliculitis

This is common in young adult males and characterized by small itchy papules and pustules on the upper back which are centred on hair follicles. It is commoner in people with Down's syndrome. It responds well to ketoconazole shampoo or a topical imidazole cream (twice daily for 2 weeks).

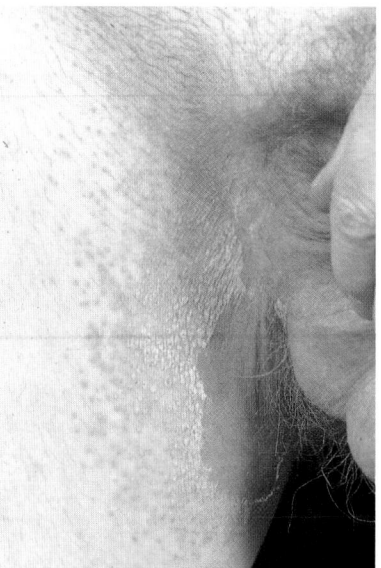

Fig. 22.8 Intertrigo with satellite lesions typical of candidiasis.

Infestations

Scabies

Scabies is an intensely itchy rash caused by the mite *Sarcoptes scabiei*. It can affect all races and people of any social class. It is most common in children and young adults but can affect any age group. There are 300 million cases of scabies in the world each year. It is commoner in poorer countries with social overcrowding.

Scabies is spread by prolonged close contact such as within households or institutions, and by sexual contact. It presents clinically with itchy red papules (or occasionally vesicles and pustules) which can occur anywhere in the skin but rarely on the face, except in neonates. The distribution of lesions is often suggestive of the diagnosis (Fig. 22.9). Sites of predilection are between the web spaces of the fingers and toes, on the palms and soles, around the wrists and axillae, on the male genitalia, and around the nipples and umbilicus.

The pathognomonic sign is of linear or curved skin burrows but these are not always present. The pruritus is normally worse at night. Excoriations and secondary bacterial infection may complicate the rash. Scabies can be confirmed by taking skin scrapings of a lesion and examining a potassium hydroxide preparation for the mite and/or its eggs by microscopy.

Treatment

This involves application of a topical scabicide (e.g. malathion or 5% permethrin). For the treatment to be successful, the following factors should be noted:

- All the skin below the neck should be treated, including the genitalia, palms and soles, and under the nails. Treat the head and neck regions in infants (up to age 2 years).
- All close contacts should be treated at the same time even if asymptomatic.
- Reapply scabicide to the hands if they are washed during the treatment period.
- Patients should be warned that the pruritus may persist for up to 4 weeks after successful treatment. Adjunct treatment with crotamiton cream, an emollient or a mild topical steroid is helpful.
- A patient information leaflet about therapy helps improve compliance.

Benzyl benzoate is still used occasionally but it can be very irritant. Lindane is a cheap therapy which is still used in many countries but there are concerns about resistance to this drug and possible neurotoxic side-effects.

Crusted scabies (Norwegian scabies)

Crusted scabies is a clinical variant that occurs in immunosuppressed individuals where huge numbers of

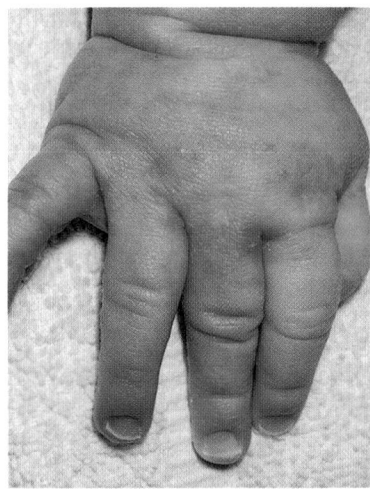

Fig. 22.9 **Scabies** – itchy papules and pustules centred on the web spaces of the hand.

mites are carried in the skin. The patient is extremely infectious after relatively minimal contact, which is unfortunate as the diagnosis is often delayed. Clinically this presents as hyperkeratotic crusted lesions, especially on the hands and feet. Itch is often absent or minimal. Lesions may progress such that the patient has a widespread erythema with irregular crusted plaques. It can therefore mimic infected eczema or psoriasis.

Treatment is with careful barrier nursing, repeated applications of a scabicide and in resistant cases, oral ivermectin (100–200 µg/kg – two doses 1 week apart) may be given but this is an unlicensed use.

Lice infection

Lice are blood-sucking ectoparasites that can affect humans in three ways.

Head lice (pediculosis capitis)

Head lice is a common infection world-wide, affecting predominantly children and being commoner in females. Spread is by direct contact and encouraged by overcrowding. It usually presents with itch or scalp excoriations. Occasionally, erythematous papules on the neck may be seen.

Diagnosis can be confirmed by the presence of eggs ('nits') seen tightly bound to the hair shaft. Adult lice may be seen rarely in heavy infection. School nurses and parents are usually adept at this.

Treatment varies in different areas depending on local policy and resistance patterns. Malathion, phenothrin and permethrin applications are the most commonly used but resistance to all these agents is common. Treatment is usually repeated after 7 days and metal nit combs may help remove the eggs. Some areas in the UK have given up with specific anti-lice treatments but have a policy of treating schools and family members with

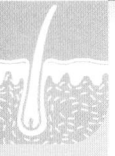

regular nit-combing, shampooing and conditioning of the hair. However, a recent study showed that chemical therapies are more effective than physical treatments, but more studies are needed.

Body lice (pediculosis corporis)

Body lice is a disease of poverty and neglect. It is rarely seen in developed countries except in homeless individuals and vagrants. It is spread by direct contact or sharing infested clothing. The lice and eggs are rarely seen on the patient but are commonly found on the clothing. It presents with itch, excoriations and sometimes post-inflammatory hyperpigmentation of the skin.

Treatment consists of malathion or permethrin for the patient and high-temperature washing and drying of clothing.

Pubic lice (crabs, phthiriasis pubis)

Pubic lice are transmitted by direct contact, usually sexual. It presents with itching, especially at night. Lice can be seen near the base of the hair, with eggs somewhat further up the shaft. Occasionally eyebrows, eyelashes and the beard area are affected.

Treatment is as for head lice but all sexual contacts should be treated and other sexually transmitted diseases should be screened for. Pubic lice of the eyelashes is treated with white soft paraffin thrice daily for 1–2 weeks.

Arthropod-borne diseases ('insect bites' or papular urticaria)

These depend on contact with an animal (e.g. dog, cat, bird) that is infected with fleas ('*Ctenocephalides*'). The animal itself may be itchy with scaly and thickened skin. These fleas can also live in soft furnishings (e.g. carpets and beds) even after the animal has been removed. Bites present as itchy urticated lesions which are often grouped in clusters. The legs are most commonly affected. It is not unusual for an individual to react badly to bites when other family members seem unaffected. Anti-flea treatment of the animal and furnishings is required.

FURTHER READING

Chew AL, Bashir SJ, Maibach HI (2000) Treatment of head lice. *Lancet* **356**: 523–524.

Chosidow O (2000) Scabies and pediculosis. *Lancet* **355**: 819–826.

Mandell GL, Douglas RG Jr, Bennett JE (eds) (1995) *Principles and Practice of Infectious Diseases,* 4th edn. New York: Churchill Livingstone.

Manders SM (1998) Toxin-mediated streptococcal and staphylococcal disease. *Journal of the American Academy of Dermatology* **39**: 383–398.

Papulo-squamous/inflammatory rashes

Eczema

The term 'eczema' derives from the Greek word for 'boiling', which reflects that the skin can become so acutely inflamed that fluid weeps out or vesicles appear. It is synonymous with the term dermatitis and the two words are interchangeable. In the developed world, eczema accounts for a large proportion of skin disease, in both hospital and community-based populations. It is estimated that 10% of people have some form of eczema at any one time, and up to 40% of the population will have an episode of eczema during their lifetime.

All eczemas (see Table 22.3) have some features in common and there is a spectrum of clinical presentation from acute through to chronic. Vesicles or bullae may appear in the acute stage if inflammation is intense. In subacute eczema the skin can be erythematous, dry and flaky, oedematous, and crusted (especially if secondarily infected). Chronic persistent eczema is characterized by thickened or lichenified skin. Eczema is nearly always itchy. Histologically 'eczematous change' refers to a collection of fluid in the epidermis between the keratinocytes ('spongiosis') and an upper dermal perivascular infiltrate of lymphohistiocytic cells. In more chronic disease there is marked thickening of the epidermis ('acanthosis').

Atopic eczema

This type of eczema (often called 'endogenous eczema') occurs in individuals who are 'atopic' (p. 874). It is common, occurring in up to 5% of the UK population. It is commoner in early life, occurring at some stage during childhood in up to 10–15% of all children.

Aetiology

The exact pathophysiology is not fully understood but there is a selective activation of Th2-type CD4 lymphocytes in the skin, which drives the inflammatory process. There is undoubtedly a strong hereditary component but the condition appears to be both polygenic and influenced by environmental factors. A positive

Table 22.3
Classification of eczema

Endogenous	Exogenous
Atopic eczema	Contact eczema – irritant
Discoid eczema	Contact eczema – allergic
Hand eczema	Photosensitive eczema
Seborrhoeic eczema	
Venous ('gravitational') eczema	
Asteatotic eczema	

family history of atopic disease, e.g. asthma, is often present: there is a 90% concordance in monozygotic twins but only 20% in dizygotic twins. Genetic studies in atopy have so far shown linkage to three different loci. Linkage has been demonstrated between atopy and the β-subunit of the high-affinity IgE receptor (on chromosome 11q13) but this site does not demonstrate linkage with familial atopic eczema. Polymorphisms in the mast cell chymase gene have also been associated with atopic eczema – thus genetic heterogeneity is likely. It may be that certain genes are more important in developing eczema rather than asthma, and other genes may be important in determining severity of the disorder or age of onset. If one parent has atopic disease, the risk for a child of developing eczema is about 20–30%. If both parents have atopic eczema, the risk is greater than 50%.

Exacerbating factors

Strong detergents, chemicals and even woollen clothes can be irritant and exacerbate eczema. Infection, either in the skin or systemically, can also lead to a deterioration, possibly by a superantigen effect. Teething is another factor in young children. Severe anxiety or stress appears to exacerbate eczema in some individuals. Cat and dog fur can certainly make eczema worse, possibly by both allergic and irritant mechanisms. The role of house dust mite and diet is less clear cut. There is some evidence that food allergens may play a role in triggering atopic eczema and that dairy products may be important in exacerbating eczema in a few selected infants under 12 months of age.

Clinical features

Atopic eczema can present as a number of distinct morphological variants. The commonest presentation is of itchy erythematous scaly patches, especially in the flexures such as in front of the elbows and ankles, behind the knees (Fig. 22.10) and around the neck. In infants, eczema often starts on the face before spreading to the body. Very acute lesions may weep or exude and can show small vesicles. Scratching can produce

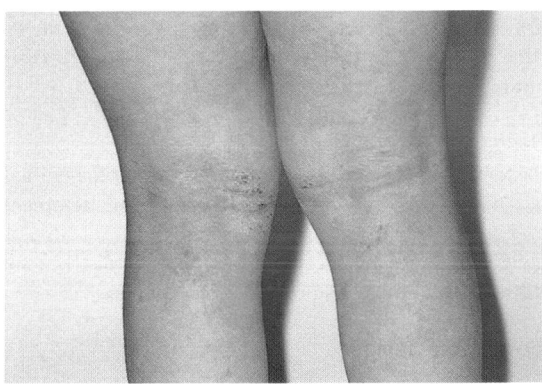

Fig. 22.10 Atopic eczema behind the knees.

excoriations, and repeated rubbing produces skin thickening (lichenification) with exaggerated skin markings.

In patients with pigmented skin, eczema often shows a reverse pattern of extensor involvement. Also, the eczema may be papular or follicular in nature and lichenification is common. A final problem in pigmented skin is of post-inflammatory hyper- or hypopigmentation which is often very slow to fade after control of the eczema.

Associated features

Involvement of the nail bed may produce pitting and ridging of the nails. In some atopic individuals the skin of the upper arms and thighs may feel roughened because of follicular hyperkeratosis ('keratosis pilaris'). The palms may show very prominent skin creases ('hyperlinear palms'). There may be an associated dry 'fish-like' scaling of the skin, which is non-inflammatory and often prominent on the lower legs ('ichthyosis vulgaris').

Complications

Broken skin commonly becomes secondarily infected by bacteria. This is usually due to *Staphylococcus aureus* although streptococci can colonize eczema, especially in macerated flexural areas such as the neck and groin. Clinically this infection may appear as crusted, weeping impetigo-like lesions. Occasionally *Pseudomonas* can be grown from skin swabs but this rarely causes a clinical problem. Cutaneous viral infections (e.g. viral warts and molluscum) are often widespread in atopic eczema and are probably spread by scratching. HSV can cause a widespread eruption called eczema herpeticum (Kaposi's varicelliform eruption). This can occasionally be a very severe infection and has rarely caused death. This appears as multiple small blisters or punched-out crusted lesions associated with malaise and pyrexia, and needs rapid treatment with oral aciclovir. Intravenous aciclovir may be needed if the infection is severe. Ocular complications of atopic eczema include conjunctival irritation and less commonly keratoconjunctivitis and cataract. Retarded growth may be seen in children with chronic severe eczema; it is due to the disease itself and not the use of topical steroids.

Investigations

The diagnosis of atopic eczema is normally clinical. Atopy is characterized by high serum IgE levels or high specific IgE levels to certain ingested or inhaled antigens. The latter can be tested by radio-immunoabsorbent assay (RAST tests) of blood, or indirectly by skin prick testing (p. 854). A peripheral blood eosinophilia may also be seen.

Prognosis

The majority of children with early-onset atopic eczema will spontaneously improve and 'clear' before the

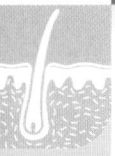
teenage years, 50% being clear by the age of 6. A few will get a recurrence as adults, even if just as hand eczema. However, if the onset of eczema is late in childhood or in adulthood, the disorder follows a more chronic remitting/relapsing course.

Treatment (Box 22.2)

General measures

These include avoiding known irritants (especially soaps or furry animals), wearing cotton clothes, and not getting too hot. Manipulating the diet (e.g. a dairy-free diet) is rarely beneficial except in a few children, especially those under 12 months of age. Any change in diet should be done under supervision, especially with growing children who may need supplements such as calcium.

Topical therapies

Topical therapies (p. 1310) are sufficient to control atopic eczema in most people, and the following 'triple' combination often helps:

- topical steroid twice daily when needed
- emollient frequently (see Table 22.17)
- bath oil and soap substitute (e.g. aqueous cream).

Written information or a practical demonstration of how to apply these treatments improves compliance.

Use of topical steroids. Unjustified fear about the dangers of topical steroids has often led to undertreatment of eczema. Providing appropriate-strength steroid preparations are used for the right body site, these compounds can be used quite safely on a long-term *intermittent* basis. Topical steroids can be divided into four groups depending on their potency (Table 22.4).

The following guidelines should be followed to allow their safe use in common chronic inflammatory skin conditions.

- The face should be treated with mild steroids.
- In adults, the body should be treated with either mild, moderately potent or diluted potent steroids.
- In young children, the body should be treated with mild and moderately potent steroids.
- Potent steroids may be used for short courses (7–10 days).
- Treatment of the palms and soles (but not the dorsal surfaces) may require potent or very potent steroids as the skin is much thicker.
- Regular use of emollients may lessen the need for steroid use.
- Only use steroids on inflamed skin. Do not use as an emollient.
- 'Apply sparingly' means use sufficient to leave a glistening surface to the skin after application.
- Use weaker steroid preparations in flexures (e.g. the groin, and under breasts) as apposition of the skin at these sites tends to occlude the treatment and increase absorption.

Box 22.2

Management of atopic eczema

- Education and explanation
- Avoidance of irritants/allergens
- Emollients
- Bath oils/soap substitutes
- Topical steroids
- Adjunct therapies:
  sedating antihistamines
  occlusive bandaging
  oral antibiotics
- Phototherapy/systemic therapy (for severe cases)

Table 22.4
Classification of topical steroids by potency

Very potent	0.05% clobetasol proprionate 0.3% diflucortolone valerate
Potent	0.1% betamethasone valerate 0.025% fluocinolone acetonide
Diluted potent	0.025% betamethasone valerate 0.00625% fluocinolone acetonide
Moderately potent	0.05% clobetasone butyrate 0.05% alclometasone diproprionate
Mild	2.5% hydrocortisone 1% hydrocortisone

Antibiotics

These are needed for bacterial infection and are usually given orally for 7–10 days. Flucloxacillin (500 mg four times daily) is effective against *Staphylococcus*, and penicillin V (500 mg four times daily) acts against *Streptococcus*. Erythromycin (500 mg four times daily) is useful if there is allergy to penicillin. Topical antiseptics may be useful in cases of recurrent infection but they can be irritant. They are usually added to the bath water rather than directly onto the skin. Combination topical steroid/antibiotic creams can also be used for short periods.

Sedating antihistamines

These, e.g. oral hydroxyzine 25 mg, are useful at night-time. They help by their sedative properties, not by their antihistamine activity.

Bandaging

Paste bandaging can be useful for resistant or lichenified eczema of the limbs. It helps absorption of treatment and acts as a barrier to prevent scratching. Wet tubular gauze bandages are useful for inpatient therapy but are difficult and time-consuming to use at home.

Second-line agents

These may be considered in severe non-responsive cases, especially if the eczema is significantly interfering with an individual's life (e.g. growth, sleeping, school-work or job). Ultraviolet phototherapy (see p. 1294), prednisolone (doses up to 30 mg daily), ciclosporin (3–5 mg/kg daily) and azathioprine (1–2 mg/kg daily) (p. 1303) can all be effective treatments. However, they all have side-effects and the risk/benefit ratio must be openly discussed with the patient before they are used.

Use of ciclosporin. Ciclosporin is a selective immuno-suppressant that inhibits interleukin-2 production by T lymphocytes. A large number of other drugs interact with ciclosporin (e.g. erythromycin, NSAIDs) and should be avoided. Renal damage and hypertension are the two most serious side-effects, so blood pressure and serum creatinine should be measured every 6 weeks. Creatinine clearance should be measured yearly in people on long-term therapy. Renal damage becomes increasingly common with time and tends to be dose-dependent. Hypertrichosis, paraesthesia and nausea are less serious side-effects. Pregnancy should be avoided.

Discoid eczema (nummular eczema)

Discoid eczema is a morphological variant of eczema, characterized by well-demarcated scaly patches especially on the limbs, and this can be confused sometimes with psoriasis. It is commoner in adults and can occur in both atopic and non-atopic individuals. It tends to follow an acute/subacute course rather than a chronic pattern. There is often an infective component (*Staphylococcus aureus*).

Hand eczema

Eczema may be confined to the hands (and feet). It can present with:

- itchy vesicles or blisters of the palm and along the sides of the fingers (also called 'pompholyx') (Fig. 22.11)
- a diffuse erythematous scaling and hyperkeratosis of the palms
- a scaling and peeling most marked at the finger tips.

Hand eczema is not unusual in atopics but more frequently occurs in non-atopic individuals and a cause is not always found. A history of contact with irritants (e.g. detergents, chemicals) and an occupational history should be sought, especially in finger-tip eczema. Patch testing for specific allergic or contact eczema should always be considered, as up to 10% of individuals with hand eczema will show a positive test. Finally, look for evidence of fungal infection, as this can occasionally induce a secondary pompholyx of the hands or feet (a so-called 'Id reaction').

Seborrhoeic eczema
Aetiology

Overgrowth of *Pityrosporum ovale* (also called *Malassezia furfur* in its hyphal form) together with a strong cutaneous immune response to this yeast produces the characteristic inflammation and scaling of seborrhoeic eczema. The condition is more common in parkinsonism as well as in HIV disease.

Clinical features

Seborrhoeic eczema affects body sites rich in sebaceous glands, although these do not appear to play a role in its cause. Three age groups are affected:

- *In childhood* it is common and presents in the first few months of life as 'cradle cap' in most babies. This may in part be due to the effect of maternal androgens on infant sebaceous glands. Yellowish, greasy, thick crusts are seen on the scalp. A more widespread erythematous, scaly rash can be seen over the trunk, especially affecting the nappy area. Unlike with atopic eczema, the child is normally unbothered, as there is little associated pruritus. The rash normally improves spontaneously after a few weeks.
- *In young adults* (especially males) it occurs in 1–3% of the population. The rash is more persistent and presents as an erythematous scaling along the sides of the nose (Fig. 22.12), in the eyebrows, around the eyes and extending into the scalp (which shows marked dandruff). It may affect the skin over the

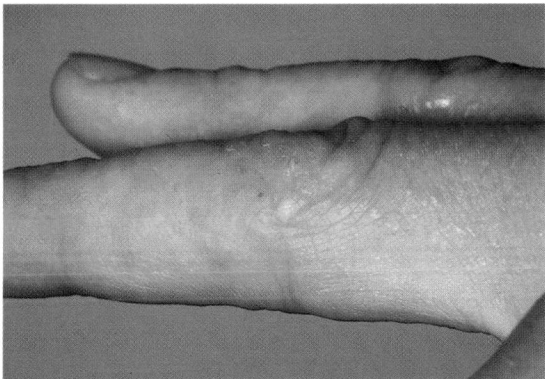

Fig. 22.11 **Pompholyx eczema** (courtesy of Dr A Bewley, London).

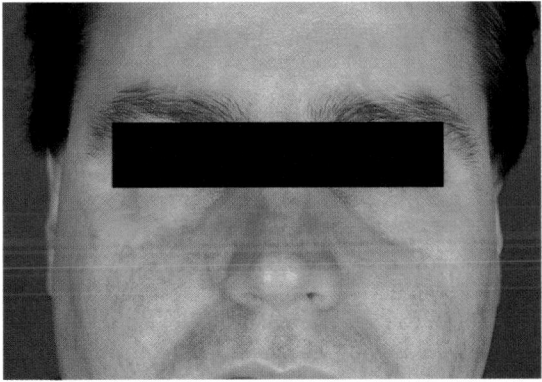

Fig. 22.12 Seborrhoeic eczema affecting the sides of the nose.

sternum and of the glans penis. A blepharitis may also be present.

- *In elderly people* seborrhoeic eczema can be more severe and progress to involve large areas of the body and even cause erythroderma.

Treatment

This is suppressive rather than curative. A combination of a mild steroid ointment (e.g. 1% hydrocortisone applied twice daily) and a topical antifungal cream (e.g. miconazole cream applied twice daily) will help to control the eruption. Two per cent sulphur or 2% salicylic acid can be added to help control resistant cases. Ketoconazole shampoo and arachis oil are useful for the scalp. Emollients and a soap substitute are useful adjuncts.

Venous eczema (varicose eczema, gravitational eczema)

This type of eczema occurs on the lower legs because of chronic venous hypertension (usually of more than 2 years' duration) (see p. 1308). The exact cause remains unknown but it has been suggested that venous hypertension causes endothelial hyperplasia and extravasation of red and white blood cells, which in turn causes inflammation, purpura and pigmentation.

Clinical features

Venous eczema tends to occur in older people, especially women. It usually appears on the lower legs around the ankles. There may be a past history of venous thrombosis or previous surgery for varicose veins. Brownish pigmentation (haemosiderin) may be seen in the skin and a venous leg ulcer or varicose veins may be present.

Superimposed contact eczema is common in venous eczema patients, especially when there have been chronic venous leg ulcers. This is usually due to an allergic reaction to topical therapies or skin dressings. Patch testing should always be done in treatment-resistant cases.

Treatment

This should include emollients and a moderately potent topical steroid but the most important part of therapy is the use of support stockings or compression bandages, which together with leg elevation help reverse the underlying venous hypertension (p. 1309).

Asteatotic eczema (winter eczema, eczema craquelé, senile eczema)

This is a dry plate-like cracking of the skin with a red, eczematous component which occurs in elderly people. It occurs predominantly on the lower legs and the backs of the hands, especially in winter. The exact cause is unknown but the repeated use of soaps in the elderly is undoubtedly a factor as well as the loss of the stratum corneum lipids with age. Rarely, asteatotic eczema can be the presenting sign of hypothyroidism or can follow the commencement of diuretic therapy.

Treatment

Avoiding soaps, and the regular use of emollients and bath oils should be encouraged. Humidifying centrally heated rooms may help. If the skin is very inflamed, a mild topical steroid can be used.

Contact and irritant eczema

Eczema can be caused by a variety of environmental agents (exogenous eczema). One may suspect this if the eczema is in an unusual or localized distribution (Fig. 22.13), especially if there is no personal or family history of atopic disease. A history of an exacerbation of eczema at the workplace is also suggestive. This can happen by two mechanisms: direct irritation or an allergic reaction (type IV delayed hypersensitivity). A detailed history of occupation, hobbies, cosmetic products, clothing and contact with chemicals is necessary.

Irritant eczema can occur in any individual. It often occurs on the hands after repeated exposures to irritants such as detergents, soaps or bleach. It is therefore common in housewives, cleaners, hairdressers, mechanics and nurses.

Contact eczema occurs after repeated exposure to a chemical substance but only in those people who are susceptible to develop an allergic reaction. It is common, occurring in up to 4% of some populations. Many substances can cause this type of reaction but the commoner culprits are nickel (in costume jewellery and buckles), chromate (in cement), latex (in surgical gloves), perfume (in cosmetics and air fresheners), and plants (such as primula or compositae). A good history is necessary and if suspicious, patch testing should be arranged to prove any allergy.

Treatment

This is as for atopic eczema, as well as strict avoidance of any causative agent. This may also involve the wearing of protective clothing such as gloves, or in extreme cases (such as with chromate sensitivity in builders) even changing occupation or hobbies.

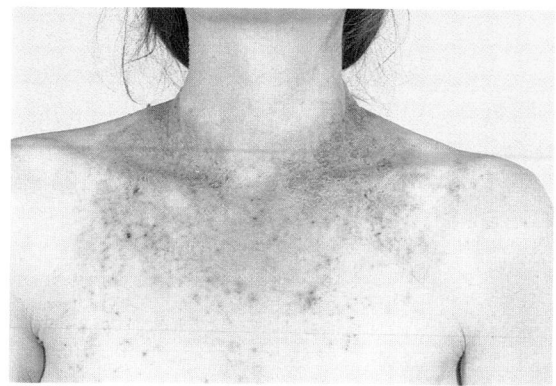

Fig. 22.13 Contact eczema secondary to perfume allergy.

Photosensitive eczema

This is discussed on page 000.

Nodular prurigo/lichen simplex (neurodermatitis)

These two terms are applied to a pattern of cutaneous response to scratching or rubbing in the absence of an underlying dermatosis. It is more common in Asians and also in black African and Oriental patients.

Lichen simplex appears as thickened, scaly and hyper-pigmented areas of lichenification (Fig. 22.14). It starts with intense itching that becomes tender with increased rubbing or scratching. It is rare before adolescence and is commoner in females. Common sites are the nape of the neck, the lateral calves, the upper thighs, the upper back and the scrotum or vulva but any accessible site can be affected.

Nodular prurigo is a different pattern of cutaneous response to scratching, rubbing or picking. It is a chronic unremitting condition which is often resistant to treatment. Individual, itchy papules and domed nodules appear especially on the upper trunk and the extensor surfaces of the limbs. They show significant surface damage from scratching.

These two conditions overlap, with some patients showing mixed features. Atopic individuals seem predisposed to develop these conditions (in the absence of obviously active eczema). However, they can occur in non-atopics. Emotional stress appears to be a contributory factor in many of these patients.

The diagnosis is made by exclusion of other pathologies and may require a skin biopsy. General medical causes of pruritus should be excluded (p. 1299). In the elderly, nodular prurigo may be an early sign of bullous pemphigoid, before the more typical blistering phase has appeared.

Treatment

This is often difficult as symptoms can be intractable. Very potent topical steroids (e.g. 0.05% clobetasol propionate) with occlusive tar bandaging may sometimes help. Intralesional steroids can also be useful but there is a risk of atrophy. For resistant cases (especially of prurigo lesions), phototherapy (p. 1294) and even ciclosporin (3–5 mg/kg/day) can be considered but the risk/benefit ratio must be discussed with the patient as these therapies are potentially toxic.

Psoriasis

Psoriasis is a common papulo-squamous disorder affecting 2% of the population and is characterized by well-demarcated, red scaly plaques. The skin becomes inflamed and hyperproliferates to about 10 times the normal rate. It affects males and females equally and can affect all races. The age of onset occurs in two peaks. Early onset (age 16–22) is commoner and is often associated with a positive family history. Late-onset disease peaks at age 55–60 years.

Aetiology

The condition appears to be polygenic but is also dependent on certain environmental triggers. Twin studies show 73% concordance in monozygotic twins compared with 20% in dizygotic pairs. Three genetic regions (on chromosome 6p21, 17q and 4q) have been shown to be involved in psoriasis but it is likely that more genetic loci are involved. Infection (group A *Streptococcus*), drugs (e.g. lithium), ultraviolet light, alcohol abuse and possibly stress may be important triggers or exacerbating factors in certain individuals. The exact aetiology is unknown but psoriasis may be a T-lymphocyte driven disorder with a possible altered response from the keratinocyte (Box 22.3). Interferon, interleukins (IL-1, -2, -8), and growth factors (TGF-α and TNF-α) are raised and adhesion molecules upregulated. Immune complexes to epidermal antigens are seen in the psoriatic lesions.

Box 22.3

Evidence that psoriasis is a T-lymphocyte driven disorder

- Group A streptococcal sore throats can set off guttate psoriasis, possibly by immune cross-reactivity or by a superantigen mechanism.
- There is an association between psoriasis and HLA-cw6.
- One of the earliest histological changes in a new psoriatic lesion is the infiltration of T lymphocytes.
- Certain immunosuppressive therapies (e.g. ciclosporin, tacrolimus and anti-CD4 monoclonal antibody) are useful in treating psoriasis.
- Selective expansion of T-cell clones occurs and proliferating T cells associate with antigen-presenting cells in psoriatic lesions.
- The immune dysfunction seen in patients with AIDS may be associated with a deterioration of their psoriasis.

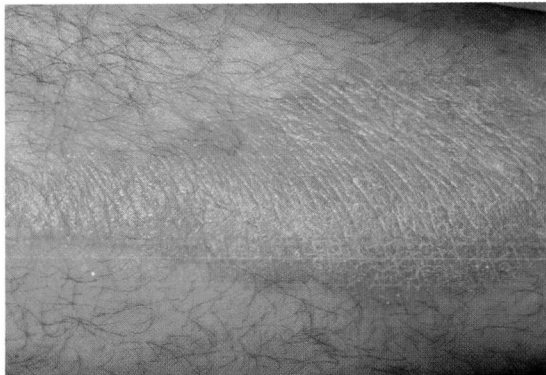

Fig. 22.14 Lichen simplex from chronic rubbing.

Pathology

Skin biopsy shows acanthosis and parakeratosis, reflecting the increase in skin turnover. The granular layer is often absent. Polymorphonuclear abscesses may be seen in the upper epidermis. The epidermal rete ridges appear elongated and clubbed as they fold down into the dermis. Dermal changes include capillary dilatation surrounded by a mixed neutrophilic and lymphohistiocytic perivascular infiltrate.

Clinical features

Psoriasis can present in different clinical patterns but they may overlap between the different forms. Certain drugs can make psoriasis worse – notably lithium, antimalarials and rarely beta-blockers.

Chronic plaque psoriasis

This is the 'common' type of psoriasis. It is characterized by pinkish red scaly plaques, especially on extensor surfaces such as knees (Fig. 22.15a) and elbows. The lower back, ears and scalp are also commonly involved. New plaques of psoriasis may occur at sites of skin trauma – the so-called Köbner phenomenon. The lesions can become itchy or sore.

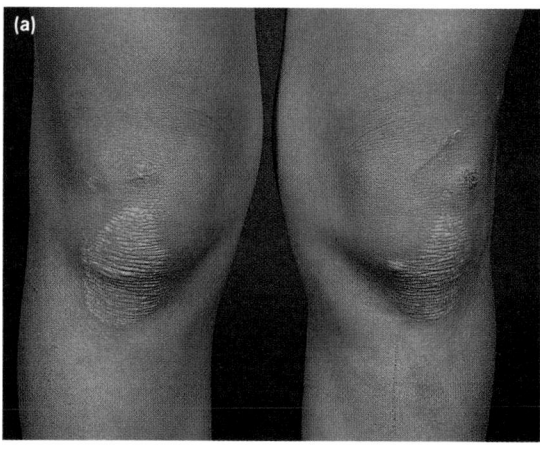

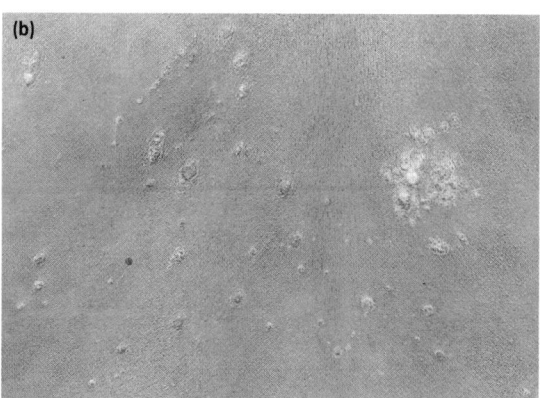

Fig. 22.15 **(a) Psoriasis of the knees. (b) Guttate psoriasis in an African** (courtesy of Dr P Matondo, Lusaka, Zambia).

Flexural psoriasis

This tends to occur in later life. It is characterized by well-demarcated, red glazed plaques confined to flexures such as the groin, natal cleft and sub-mammary area. As these sites are apposed there is rarely any scaling. In the absence of psoriasis elsewhere the rash is often misdiagnosed as candida intertrigo but the latter will normally show satellite lesions.

Guttate psoriasis

'Raindrop-like' psoriasis is a variant most commonly seen in children and young adults (Fig. 22.15b). An explosive eruption of very small circular or oval plaques appears over the trunk about 2 weeks after a streptococcal sore throat. It usually resolves spontaneously over 1–2 months even without treatment (see below).

Erythrodermic and pustular psoriasis

These are the most severe types of psoriasis reflecting a widespread intense inflammation of the skin. They can occur together ('Von Zumbusch' psoriasis) and may be associated with malaise, pyrexia and circulatory disturbance. This form can be life-threatening. The pustules are not infected but are sterile collections of inflammatory cells. There is also a more localized variant of pustular psoriasis that confines itself to the hands and feet (palmo-plantar psoriasis) but is not associated with severe systemic symptoms. This latter type is more common in heavy cigarette smokers.

Associated features

Nails. Up to 50% of individuals with psoriasis develop nail changes (Fig. 22.16) and, rarely, these can precede the onset of skin disease. There are five types of nail change: (a) pitting of the nail plate; (b) distal separation of the nail plate (onycholysis); (c) yellow-brown discoloration; (d) subungual hyperkeratosis; (e) rarely, a damaged nail matrix and lost nail plate. Treatment of nail dystrophy is very difficult.

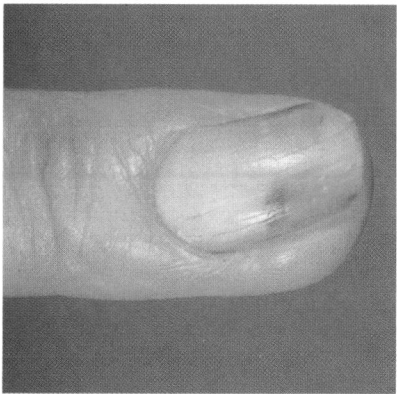

Fig. 22.16 **Psoriasis on the nail** – yellowish brown discoloration and distal nail plate separation (onycholysis) due to psoriasis.

Arthritis. Up to 5% of individuals develop psoriatic arthritis and most of these will have nail changes (p. 1288). Five patterns are recognized: (a) distal interphalangeal arthritis; (b) peripheral mono- or oligoarthritis; (c) symmetrical 'rheumatoid arthritis pattern' but seronegative; (d) spondylitis or sacro-iliitis (especially if HLA-B27 positive); and (e) rarely, arthritis mutilans causing destruction and resorption of bone leading to telescoping of affected digits (p. 549).

Prognosis

Most individuals who develop chronic plaque psoriasis will have the condition lifelong. It fluctuates in severity and there are no available tests to predict outcome. Guttate psoriasis resolves spontaneously and in up to a third of individuals does not recur. However, two-thirds will go on to get recurrent guttate attacks or will progress to chronic plaque psoriasis.

Treatment

This is concerned with control rather than cure. It should be tailored to the patient's wishes and not just to the doctor's assessment of disease severity.

Most patients with *chronic plaque psoriasis* can be improved with topical therapies.

Emollients should always be used to hydrate the skin. Mild to moderate topical steroids, calcipotriol (a synthetic vitamin D_3 analogue), 0.05% tazarotene (a retinoid) and purified coal tar are the most popular specific therapies. Salicylic acid can be a useful adjunct. All should be applied once to twice daily to palpable lesions. Once lesions have flattened, therapy can be discontinued. Dithranol can also be helpful but it causes staining of the skin and clothing and it may prove difficult to use at home on a regular basis. It is normally applied for 20–60 minutes and then washed off. It must be applied carefully to the lesions as it causes irritation to normal skin. Dithranol is more likely to induce remission than other topical therapies. Tazarotene (a retinoid) has recently been used topically for mild to moderate plaque psoriasis affecting up to 10% of the skin.

Topical therapies are sometimes used in combination with UVB or PUVA. The 'Goeckerman regime' consists of tar and UVB; the 'Ingram's regime' consists of dithranol and UVB.

Guttate psoriasis is usually treated with topical therapies and/or UVB phototherapy.

Flexural psoriasis is usually treated with mild steroid and/or tar topical creams. Calcipotriol and tazarotene tend to cause irritation in the flexures.

Palmo-plantar psoriasis is treated with very potent topical steroids, coal tar paste or local hand and foot PUVA.

Psoriasis unresponsive to topical therapies requires the use of phototherapy (UVB and PUVA) or systemic therapy (such as methotrexate, acitretin, ciclosporin or hydroxycarbamide (hydroxyurea)).

Management of *erythrodermic psoriasis* also requires systemic therapy (but not phototherapy) as well as general supportive measures (p. 1296).

All systemic treatments must be monitored for toxicity.

Use of methotrexate. Methotrexate is normally given once weekly. Some patients experience severe nausea on the day they take it. Pregnancy should be avoided. Some patients are allergic to methotrexate and develop a pyrexia and mouth ulceration. Regular blood tests need to be done to monitor for bone marrow suppression and liver damage. Alcohol must be avoided as this increases the risk of hepatotoxicity. NSAIDs should also be avoided. Long-term users will need a liver biopsy every 2–3 years to monitor for hepatic damage.

Urticaria

Urticaria (hives, 'nettle rash') is a common skin condition characterized by the acute development of itchy weals or swellings in the skin because of leaky dermal vessels (Fig. 22.17). Urticaria is described as 'acute' if it lasts less than 6 weeks and 'chronic' if it persists beyond this.

Aetiology

The final event in pathogenesis involves degranulation of cutaneous mast cells, which releases a number of inflammatory mediators (including histamine) which in turn make the dermal capillaries leaky. In most cases the underlying cause is unknown. Occasionally urticaria is secondary to viral or parasitic infection, drug reactions (e.g. aspirin or penicillin allergy), food allergy (e.g. to strawberries, food colourings or seafood), or rarely systemic lupus erythematosus. There is evidence for an autoimmune aetiology in some of the 'idiopathic' cases, as certain individuals develop autoantibodies against the high-affinity IgE receptor alpha subunit of the mast cell. Urticaria is commoner in atopic individuals and usually presents in children and young adults.

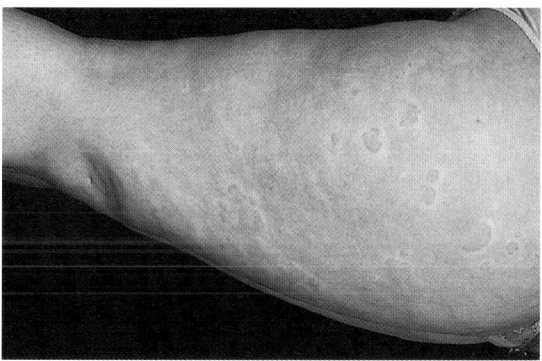

Fig. 22.17 Urticaria.

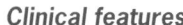

Clinical features

The history is of cutaneous swellings or weals developing acutely over a few minutes. They can occur anywhere on the skin and last between minutes and hours before resolving spontaneously. Lesions are intensely itchy and show no surface change or scaling. Lesions are normally erythematous but if very acutely swollen, they may appear flesh-coloured or whitish and people often mistake them for blisters. Severe urticaria with subcutaneous involvement can present as soft tissue swelling (angio-oedema) especially around the eyes, the lips and the hands. This can be very alarming to the patient. It can also be dangerous if mucosal areas such as the mouth and larynx are involved but fortunately this is very rare.

Physical urticarias

Occasionally urticaria can be caused by physical stimuli such as cold (cold urticaria), deep pressure (delayed pressure urticaria), stress or heat (cholinergic urticaria), sunlight (solar urticaria, p. 1294), water (aquagenic urticaria) or chemicals such as latex (contact urticaria).

Cholinergic urticaria is one of the commonest physical urticarias and has rather different clinical lesions from the other forms. Small itchy papules rather than weals appear on the upper trunk and arms after exercise or anxiety.

Pressure can cause two types of urticaria. More superficial pressure can cause *dermographism*, which is relatively common. This presents as urticated weals occurring a few minutes after application of light pressure. Even scratching or rubbing will bring up linear weals in dermographic individuals. *Delayed pressure urticaria* is rare and occurs as deep swellings some hours after pressure is removed (e.g. on the soles of the feet or under a tight belt).

Investigations

A careful history is necessary for the diagnosis. Routine investigation is probably not justified unless the history suggests one of the underlying causes listed above. The physical urticarias should be reproducible by applying the relevant stimulus.

Treatment

Any identifiable underlying cause should be treated appropriately. Patients should avoid salicylates and opiates as they can degranulate mast cells. Oral antihistamines (H_1 blockers) are the most important part of treating the idiopathic cases. Therapy should be started with regular use of a non-sedating antihistamine (e.g. cetirizine 10 mg daily or loratadine 10 mg daily). If control proves difficult, addition of a sedating antihistamine or an H_2 blocker may be helpful. Dietary manipulation (e.g. additive and colouring free diets) may help a small proportion of patients with chronic urticaria but it is generally unrewarding. Angio-oedema of the mouth and throat may require urgent treatment with intravenous steroids and subcutaneous epinephrine (see Emergency box 16.1).

Prognosis

Most cases of 'idiopathic' urticaria last a few weeks to months before disappearing spontaneously. The majority of these will be controlled with an antihistamine. A small percentage of people go on to develop chronic urticaria, which can last for several months or years. The physical urticarias (especially cholinergic urticaria) are more persistent, often lasting for years, and they are often resistant to therapy.

Urticarial vasculitis

This is a variant of urticaria and should be suspected if individual urticarial lesions last longer than 24 hours and leave bruising behind after resolution. The diagnosis is confirmed by skin biopsy. A full vasculitis screen should be carried out for an underlying cause (p. 565).

Treatment is with oral dapsone (50–100 mg daily) or immunosuppressants.

Hereditary angio-oedema

This is an extremely rare autosomal dominant condition due to an inherited deficiency of C1 esterase inhibitor, a component of the complement system. The defect is due to either reduced function or reduced absolute levels. Serum C2 and C4 levels are normally low but C1 and C3 are normal. Rarely this condition is acquired and associated with lymphoma or SLE. These types show low C1 esterase inhibitor levels but also low C1 levels.

Clinical features

It presents with attacks of non-itchy cutaneous angio-oedema (but no urticaria) which may last up to 72 hours. It may also present with recurrent abdominal pain (due to intestinal oedema) and there may be a family history of sudden death (due to laryngeal involvement). A non-specific erythematous rash may precede an attack of angio-oedema but urticaria is not a feature.

Treatment

In the acute setting, treatment is with C1 esterase inhibitor concentrates and fresh frozen plasma. Epinephrine (adrenaline) and steroids are often ineffective. Maintenance treatment with the anabolic steroid stanozolol (or danazol) stimulates an increase in hepatic synthesis of C1 esterase inhibitor but this should not be used in children. Family members should be screened.

Pityriasis rosea

Pityriasis rosea is a self-limiting rash seen in adolescents and young adults. The cause is unknown but it is thought to be a viral or post-viral rash. There is an increased incidence in spring and autumn and outbreaks may occur in institutions.

Clinical features

The rash consists of circular or oval pink macules with a collarette of scale and is more prominent on the trunk than the limbs. The long axis of the oval lesions tends to run along dermatomal lines giving a 'Christmas tree' pattern on the back. The rash may be preceded by a large solitary patch with peripheral scaling ('herald patch') and this is most commonly found on the trunk. The rash is usually asymptomatic and spontaneously resolves over 4–8 weeks.

Treatment

Treatment is not normally required but 1% menthol in aqueous cream may help relieve any itch. In persistent cases UVB may be helpful.

Lichen planus

Lichen planus is a pruritic inflammatory dermatosis that is commonly associated with mucosal involvement and rarely with nail dystrophy and scarring alopecia.

The cause is unknown but it has been postulated that a T-cell driven immune mechanism is involved. This stems from the fact that an almost identical rash can be caused by certain drugs (e.g. gold, levamisole, penicillamine or antimalarials) or by graft-versus-host disease.

Pathology

A mixed lymphohistiocytic infiltrate is seen at the dermoepidermal junction, which becomes ragged and saw-toothed. The basal layer shows liquefactive degeneration with the production of colloid bodies in the upper dermis. There may be acanthosis and a hyperkeratosis of the epidermis.

Clinical features

The rash is characterized by small, purple flat-topped, polygonal papules that are intensely pruritic (Fig. 22.18). It is common on the flexors of the wrists and the lower legs but can occur anywhere. There may be a fine lacy white pattern on the surface of lesions (Wickham's striae). Lesions may fuse into plaques, especially on the lower legs and in black Africans. Hyperpigmentation is common after resolution of lesions, especially in patients with pigmented skin. Atrophic, hypertrophic and annular variants can occur. Lichen planus lesions often localize to scratch marks. If lesions occur in the scalp, they may cause a scarring alopecia.

Mucosal involvement is common. The mouth is the most commonly affected but the anogenital region, and rarely the oesophagus, can be involved. It can present as lacy white streaks, white plaques or as ulceration. The

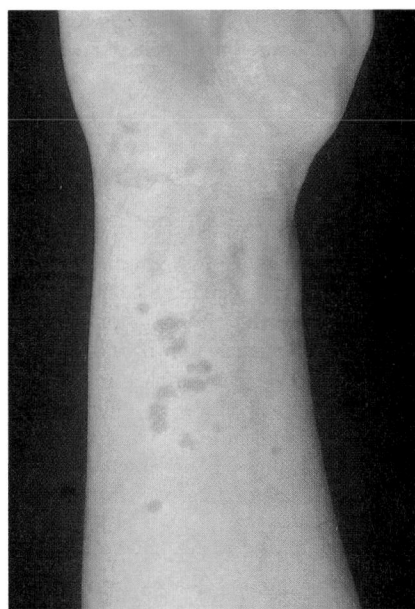

Fig. 22.18 Lichen planus.

prominent mucosal symptom is of pain rather than itch. Nails may be dystrophic and can be lost altogether (with scarring and 'wing' formation) in severe disease.

Prognosis

The condition often clears by 18 months but can recur at intervals. The hypertrophic and atrophic variants, and mucosal disease are more persistent, lasting years. Ulcerative mucosal disease is premalignant.

Treatment

This requires the use of potent topical steroids (0.05% clobetasol proprionate) and occasionally oral prednisolone (30 mg daily for 2–4 weeks). Occlusion of topical treatments can be helpful. Resistant cases may respond to PUVA, oral retinoids (0.5 mg/kg/day) or azathioprine (1–2 mg/kg/day).

Granuloma annulare

Granuloma annulare is a dermatosis predominantly of children and young adults. It is characterized by clusters of small dermal papules (with no surface change) that often form into rings or part of a ring. They are common on the dorsal surface of the hands and feet. They are flesh coloured or slightly erythematous and are usually asymptomatic. As they heal the centre becomes dusky and altered in texture. A deep form, which is tender, exists in children. Diffuse granuloma annulare may be associated with diabetes mellitus. The pathology shows a granulomatous dermal infiltrate with foci of degeneration of collagen (necrobiosis). Spontaneous resolution often occurs but cryotherapy or triamcinolone injection may help localized disease.

Lichen sclerosus et atrophicus

Lichen sclerosus et atrophicus is an inflammatory dermatosis that occurs in all age groups and particularly affects the anogenital region. It is more common in females. It presents with atrophic ivory-white macules with a well-defined edge on the vulva, glans penis, foreskin or perianal skin. Telangiectasia may be seen over the surface. Occasionally lesions involve the shaft of the penis and the urethral meatus. Lesions are often itchy but may be sore at times. Long-standing vulval lesions may be associated with fissuring and a marked loss of architecture, especially of the clitoral hood and the labium minora, which may become fused. Early lesions in young girls may present as haemorrhagic blisters and these are occasionally mistaken as signs of sexual abuse. Involvement of the foreskin can cause phimosis, and urethral disease may interfere with micturition. Perianal lesions may fissure and cause constipation.

Rarely lichen sclerosus can affect non-genital skin, but this is most common in females and clinically it may show rather more hyperkeratosis and follicular plugging than is seen in the anogenital region.

If the clinical picture is unclear, diagnosis may require biopsy to exclude genital lichen planus and extramammary Paget's disease. Vulval scarring can also occur with cicatricial pemphigoid (p. 1303), so occasionally immunofluorescence studies may be needed.

Treatment with very potent topical steroids helps control the symptoms. Hydroxychloroquine (200 mg twice daily) helps resistant cases. The condition may burn itself out after many years, especially in children. There is a risk of developing squamous cell carcinoma in long-standing lesions.

FURTHER READING

Charman C (1999) Clinical evidence – atopic eczema. *British Medical Journal* **318**: 1600–1604.

Coleman R et al. (1997) Genetic studies of atopy and atopic dermatitis. *British Journal of Dermatology* **136**: 1–5.

Granstein RD (2001) New treatments for psoriasis. *New England Journal of Medicine* **345**: 284–287.

Kaplan AL (2002) Chronic urticaria and angiooedema. *New England Journal of Medicine* **346**: 175–179.

Mitchell T, Paige D, Spowart K (1998) *Eczema and Your Child – A Parent's Guide*. UK: Class Publishing.

Reynolds NJ (1997) Recent advances in atopic dermatitis. *Journal of the Royal College of Physicians of London* **31**: 241–245.

Williams EH (2000) *Atopic Dermatitis*. Cambridge: Cambridge University Press.

Facial rashes

Facial rashes often cause diagnostic confusion but a close examination of the clinical signs should help differentiate the underlying cause (Table 22.5). All facial rashes, by virtue of their visibility, can cause significant distress to the patient and this should never be underestimated.

Acne vulgaris

Acne is a common facial rash occurring in adolescence and rarely in early and mid-adult life. The cause is multifactorial but the blockage of pilosebaceous units with surrounding inflammation is the main pathological process and this can occur because of a number of different factors (Fig. 22.19a).

Clinical features

Acne presents in areas rich in sebaceous glands such as the face, back and sternal area. The three cardinal features are:

- open comedones (blackheads) or closed comedones (whiteheads)
- inflammatory papules
- pustules (Fig. 20.19b).

The skin may be very greasy (seborrhoea). Rupture of the inflamed lesions may lead to deep-seated dermal inflammation and nodulocystic lesions, which are more likely to cause facial scarring. A premenstrual exacerbation of acne is sometimes noticed. There is a tendency for spontaneous improvement over a number of years but acne can persist unabated into adult life.

A number of clinical variants exist:

- *Infantile acne.* Facial acne is occasionally seen in infants and is sometimes cystic. It is thought to be due to the influence of maternal androgens and resolves spontaneously.
- *Steroid acne.* Acne may occur secondary to corticosteroid therapy or Cushing's syndrome. Comedones and cysts are rare in this variant but involvement of the back and shoulders (rather than the face) is common. Clinically the rash often appears as a pustular folliculitis.
- *Oil acne.* This is an industrial disease seen in workers who have prolonged contact with oils

Table 22.5
Causes of facial rashes

Acne vulgaris	Perioral dermatitis
Rosacea	Photosensitivity
Seborrhoeic eczema	Sarcoidosis
Atopic eczema	Chronic discoid lupus erythematosus
Contact eczema	Systemic lupus erythematosus
Dermatomyositis	Subacute lupus erythematosus

(a)

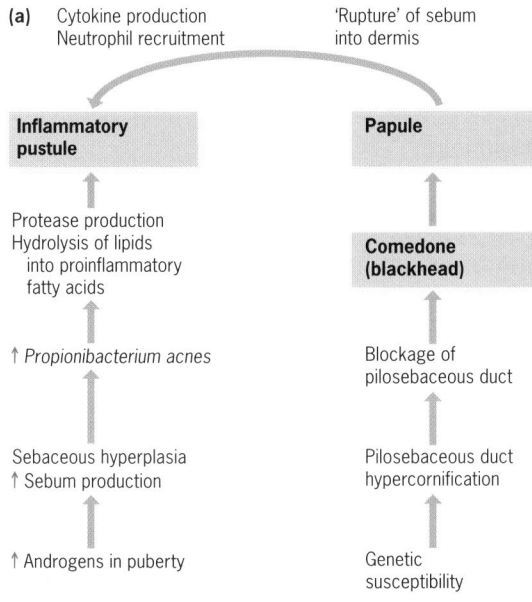

Cytokine production
Neutrophil recruitment

'Rupture' of sebum
into dermis

| Inflammatory pustule |

↑ Protease production
Hydrolysis of lipids
into proinflammatory
fatty acids

↑ *Propionibacterium acnes*

Sebaceous hyperplasia
↑ Sebum production

↑ Androgens in puberty

| Papule |

| Comedone (blackhead) |

Blockage of
pilosebaceous duct

Pilosebaceous duct
hypercornification

Genetic
susceptibility

(b)

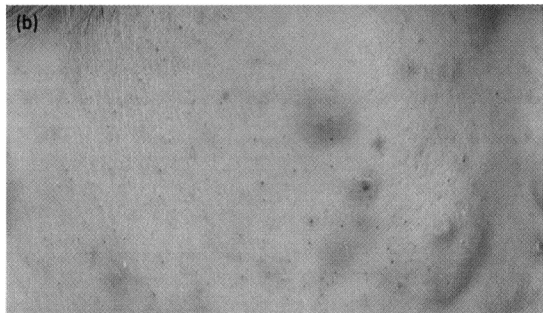

Fig. 22.19 (a) **Pathophysiology of acne vulgaris.** (b) **Acne vulgaris.**

or other hydrocarbons and is common on the legs and other exposure sites.

- *Acne fulminans.* This is a rare variant seen most commonly in young male adolescents. Severe necrotic and crusted acne lesions appear, associated with malaise, pyrexia, arthralgia and bone pain (due to sterile bone cysts). It requires urgent treatment with oral prednisolone (30–40 mg daily) and analgesics followed by a course of oral isotretinoin (see below).
- *'Follicular occlusion triad'.* This is a rare disorder most commonly seen in black Africans. It is characterized by the presence of severe nodulocystic acne, dissecting cellulitis of the scalp (p. 1316) and hidradenitis suppurativa (p. 1275). It has been suggested that this is caused by a problem of follicular occlusion rather than having an infective aetiology.

Treatment

Treatment is aimed at decreasing sebum production, decreasing bacteria, normalizing duct keratinization or decreasing inflammation.

Regular washing with acne soaps to remove excess grease should be encouraged as normal soaps can be comedogenic. 'Picking' should be discouraged.

First-line therapy

Mild acne can respond to a variety of topical agents such as antibiotics (tetracycline, clindamycin), keratolytics (benzoyl peroxide), topical retinoids (tretinoin) or retinoid-like agents (adapalene). If these fail, second-line agents should be added.

Second-line therapy

- *Low-dose oral antibiotic therapy* often helps but must be given for at least 3–4 months. Oxytetracycline 500 mg twice daily is often used first. Minocycline 100 mg daily, erythromycin 500 mg twice daily or trimethoprim 100 mg twice daily are alternatives.
- An extra treatment 'cyproterone acetate 2 mg/ ethinylestradiol 35 μg' (co-cyprindiol) can be considered in females if there is no contraindication to oral contraception. This acts as a normal combined contraceptive but has antiandrogen activity. It may take 6–8 months to have its maximum effect.
- *UVB phototherapy* can be helpful but is rarely used since the development of retinoid drugs.

Third-line therapy

Third-line treatment with a retinoid drug (isotretinoin) should be given if:

- the above measures fail
- there is nodulocystic acne with scarring
- there is severe psychological disturbance.

Use of retinoids (isotretinoin or acitretin). Retinoids are synthetic vitamin A analogues that affect cell growth and differentiation. They are very teratogenic.

Isotretinoin is a 'hospital-only drug' in most countries because of its teratogenicity and is restricted to the use of dermatologists. A pregnancy test is advisable prior to its use in fertile women. It is given as a 4-month course at a dose of 0.5–1 mg/kg/day. Over 90% of individuals will respond to this therapy and 65% of people will obtain a long-term 'cure'.

Patients must avoid pregnancy during therapy and for 1 month after stopping isotretinoin (but for 2 years after stopping acitretin as it is very lipophilic). Both drugs cause drying of the skin, especially of the lips. Hair thinning and exercise-induced myalgia are not uncommon. Blood count, liver biochemistry and fasting lipids need to be monitored during therapy. Retinoids may also cause depression.

Rosacea

Rosacea (Fig. 22.20) is a common inflammatory rash predominantly affecting the face. The onset is usually in middle age and it is commoner in women. It often causes significant psychological distress.

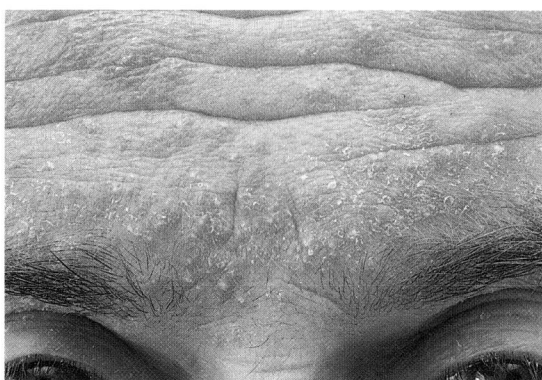

Fig. 22.20 Rosacea. Papules and pustules on a background erythema. There are no comedones.

The cause is unknown. Theories have suggested an underlying problem in vasomotor stability of blood vessels or a role for the skin mite *Demodex* but there is little evidence to confirm these speculations.

Clinical features

The cardinal features are of facial flushing, inflammatory papules and pustules affecting the nose, forehead and cheeks. The flushing may precede the other signs by some years. There are no comedones. Additional features may include dilated blood vessels (telangiectasia), inflammation of the eyelid margins (blepharitis), keratitis and sebaceous gland hypertrophy especially of the nose. The latter is commoner in men and can cause a disfiguring enlargement of the nose called rhinophyma. The flushing may be exacerbated by alcohol, hot drinks, sunlight and changes in ambient temperature. Prolonged use of topical steroids can exacerbate or trigger the condition. As the disease progresses, the flushing may be replaced by a permanent erythema.

Treatment

This is suppressive rather than curative. Long-term use of topical 0.075% metronidazole may help. Avoid topical steroids. A 3-month course of oral tetracycline (500 mg twice daily) is also helpful. Oral metronidazole (400 mg twice daily) or oral isotretinoin (0.5–1 mg/kg/day) is occasionally given in resistant cases (p. 1293). The papules and pustules tend to respond best to therapy but repeat courses may be necessary. The flushing and erythema are often resistant to treatment; cosmetic camouflage can be helpful. Rhinophyma can be treated with plastic surgery or by carbon dioxide laser.

Perioral dermatitis

Perioral dermatitis is a common rash found around the mouth, especially in young females. The exact cause is unknown but it often has an iatrogenic component as topical steroids often exacerbate the condition in the long term.

Clinical features

It presents with erythema, scaling, papules and occasionally pustules around the mouth. It usually spares a halo of skin immediately adjacent to the lips.

Treatment

Treatment involves stopping topical steroids, although they may have to be withdrawn slowly to prevent too severe a rebound after withdrawal. The mainstay of treatment is with a 3- to 4-month course of low-dose oxytetracycline or erythromycin (both 500 mg twice daily).

FURTHER READING

Leyden JJ (1997) Therapy for acne vulgaris. *New England Journal of Medicine* **336**: 1156–1162.
Munro CS (1997) Acne. *Journal of the Royal College of Physicians* **31**: 360–363.
Webster GF (1999) Acne vulgaris: state of the science. *Archives of Dermatology* **135**: 1101–1102.

Photodermatology

Sunlight – light in the ultraviolet (UV) part of the spectrum – combines short, medium and long wavelengths (UVC, UVB and UVA respectively). Both UVB and UVA can penetrate the atmosphere and reach the skin. This light energy is potentially mutagenic and carcinogenic but it can also suppress cutaneous inflammation. Thus UV irradiation can both *cause* skin disease and be used to *treat* it.

Photosensitive rashes usually appear on sites exposed to the sun's rays, such as the face, the anterior 'V' of the chest, the ears and the backs of the hands. Certain 'protected' areas are characteristically spared, such as under the chin or the upper eyelid and between the finger webs. Porphyria, drug sensitivity and lupus erythematosus should be excluded in all photosensitive patients.

Photosensitive rashes may be divided into photo-exacerbated/provoked rashes and the idiopathic photodermatoses (Table 22.6). The former are discussed on pages 558 (SLE), 236 (pellagra) and 1121 (porphyria).

Phototherapy and photoprotection
Phototherapy

UVB and UVA are both used in the treatment of inflammatory dermatoses. They have a suppressive effect on cutaneous inflammation and there is increasing evidence that they can suppress systemic immunoreactivity to some degree. However, both types can cause skin ageing and predispose to skin malignancy if excessive doses are used. This is more of a problem in white-skinned individuals. Unaffected regions of skin or high-risk areas like the scrotum can be screened during phototherapy.

Table 22.6
Differential diagnosis of photosensitive rashes

Photoexacerbated/provoked rashes

Systemic disease	SLE, CDLE, SCLE (p. 1299)
Metabolic disease	Porphyrias (pp. 1121 and 1301), pellagra (p. 236)
Drugs	Thiazides, phenothiazines, tetracyclines, amiodarone
Plant phototoxins	Phytophotodermatitis (photosensitivity induced by contact of the skin with certain plants, e.g. celery, hogweed, rue)
Skin disease	Rosacea Rarely atopic eczema, psoriasis, lichen planus (these normally improve in sunlight)

Idiopathic photodermatoses
Polymorphic light eruption
Chronic actinic dermatitis
Solar urticaria

CDLE, chronic discoid lupus erythematosus
SCLE, subacute cutaneous lupus erythematosus

UVB is more likely to burn but it is less carcinogenic than UVA. It is used in the treatment of eczema and psoriasis (especially in children) and is usually given three times per week for 6–10 weeks. Eye protection needs to be worn during therapy.

Narrow-band UVB (311 nanometer) is superseding broad-band UVB because it is much more effective in the treatment of eczema and psoriasis. Animal and in vitro studies show it to be less carcinogenic than PUVA but long-term data in humans are not yet available.

UVA is relatively ineffective on its own so is used in conjunction with a photosensitizer ('psoralen'); hence the term 'PUVA'. The psoralen can be given by mouth or applied to the skin in bath water. PUVA is given twice per week and eye protection must been worn *for the whole of the treatment day* as the psoralen sensitizes the retina. It is more effective than UVB but is limited by its carcinogenic potential. A maximum dose is given over a lifetime depending on skin type (1000 joules or 200 sessions approximately). It is used for many conditions including psoriasis, eczema, cutaneous T-cell lymphoma, some photosensitive dermatoses and vitiligo.

Sunbeds are used for tanning and consist of predominantly UVA light; they are therefore rarely effective in treating skin disease. If used frequently there may be an increased risk of skin cancer.

Photoprotection
There are two broad classes of sunblock cream: they either absorb UV light (e.g. aminobenzoic acid or methoxycinnamate) or reflect it (e.g. titanium dioxide). Most modern creams protect against UVA and UVB to varying degrees. UVB protection is graded by the 'sun protection factor' (SPF): an SPF of 15 implies you can spend 15 times as long in the sun before burning,

providing it is applied correctly. SPFs above 15 confer little extra protection. There is no standardized way of assessing efficiency against UVA. Some sunscreens (especially aminobenzoates) may rarely cause photosensitization. This can be proven by photopatch testing.

Idiopathic photodermatoses

Polymorphic light eruption (PLE)
This is the most common photosensitive eruption in temperate regions, affecting up to 10–20% of the population. It is most common in young women. In many it is mild and often goes undiagnosed. An itchy rash appears some hours after sun exposure, which is strictly confined to the exposed sites. Lesions may be papules, vesicles or plaques. They can last for several hours or several days. The condition starts in spring and often improves during the summer because of skin 'hardening'.

Treatment
Avoidance of sunlight and the use of sunblocks are helpful in mild cases. Topical steroids help treat an attack. In those individuals who only get PLE after very intense sun exposure (e.g. on sunny holidays) a short course of oral prednisolone (30 mg daily for 7–10 days) will often prevent or treat an attack. For resistant cases, 'desensitization' with low-dose PUVA (or narrow-band UVB) in the springtime may be required but patients will need to 'top up' their sun exposure from natural sunlight during the summer to keep their skin desensitized.

Chronic actinic dermatitis (photosensitive eczema, actinic reticuloid)
This is a relatively rare type of eczema, occurring in a photosensitive distribution over the face, neck and hands. It typically affects middle-aged or elderly males. There may be a pre-existing eczema, so the subsequent development of photosensitivity is often missed. This is further confounded by the fact that the eczema usually will spread to affect skin not exposed to sunlight, and the patient can become erythrodermic. The skin has typical features of eczema but there is often marked skin thickening. Histology is often atypical and can look almost lymphoma like. The diagnosis can be confirmed by specialist monochromator light-testing. The most severe cases can even be exacerbated by artificial lighting, as these patients can become exquisitely photosensitive.

Treatment
This consists of strict avoidance of sunlight, including the use of high-factor sunblocks and screening of house and car windows. Topical steroids and emollients are useful in milder cases. Oral prednisolone may be needed and azathioprine (1–2 mg/kg daily) should be considered for long-term suppression. Low-dose PUVA under steroid cover may help with 'desensitization'.

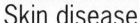
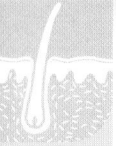
Solar urticaria

This is very rare. Itchy urticarial lesions occur within minutes of sun exposure and characteristically settle within 1–2 hours. Sun avoidance, sunblocks, H_1 antihistamines and low-dose PUVA are all used in treatment.

FURTHER READING

Hawk JLM (ed.) (1999) *Photodermatology*. London: Arnold.

Erythroderma

Erythroderma, meaning 'red skin', refers to the clinical state of inflammation or redness of all (or nearly all) of the skin. It is sometimes called *exfoliative dermatitis*, but dermatitis is not always present. It is commoner in males and later in life. Patients often complain of their skin feeling 'tight' as well as itchy. Long-standing erythroderma is often associated with hair loss, ectropion of the eyelids and even nail shedding. Systemic symptoms are common, such as malaise, pyrexia, widespread lymphadenopathy and possible serious circulatory disturbance. Erythroderma can occasionally lead to death, so it should be regarded as a medical 'emergency'.

Aetiology

There are a number of underlying causes (Table 22.7) and a careful history should be sought, paying particular attention to previous skin disease and any drug history. Examination should specifically look for pustules and nail changes suggestive of psoriasis. A skin biopsy may further help to elucidate the cause, especially of cutaneous lymphoma. Techniques such as T-cell receptor gene rearrangement studies (looking for evidence of clonal T-cell expansion in the skin and blood) are also useful in the diagnosis of lymphoma.

A number of cases defy an exact diagnosis. Lymph node biopsy should be considered in lymphoma. In non-malignant disease lymph nodes normally show non-specific, reactive (dermatopathic) changes.

Complications

The skin is one of the largest organs of the body; perhaps it is no surprise that inflammation of the whole organ can cause metabolic and haemodynamic problems. Examples are:

- high-output cardiac failure from increased blood flow
- hypothermia from heat loss
- fluid loss by transpiration
- hypoalbuminaemia
- increased basal metabolic rate
- 'capillary leak syndrome'.

Capillary leak syndrome is the most severe complication and has been responsible for a fatal outcome in some cases of psoriasis, although this is extremely rare. It is thought that the inflamed skin releases large quantities of cytokines that cause a generalized vascular leakage. This can cause cutaneous oedema but more worryingly can cause leaky vessels in the lungs, resulting in acute lung injury (p. 951).

Treatment

Treatment of erythroderma is best initiated in hospital. Patients must be kept very warm (with space blankets and heaters) and put on fluid-balance charts. Their vital signs should be monitored regularly. Changes in electrolytes, albumin and circulatory status should be corrected. Swabs should be taken to detect any secondary skin infection.

The skin condition is treated with bed rest and either a bland emollient or a mild topical steroid. All unessential drugs should be stopped. Where known, the underlying cause should be treated appropriately. The blanket use of systemic steroid therapy for erythroderma remains controversial in view of possible side-effects.

Advanced capillary leak syndrome will often require specialized haemodynamic management in an intensive care unit.

FURTHER READING

Champion RH, Burton JL, Ebling FJG (eds) (1998) *Textbook of Dermatology*, 6th edn. Oxford: Blackwell Scientific Publications.

Table 22.7
Causes of erythroderma

Common
Atopic eczema
Psoriasis
Drugs (e.g. sulphonamides, gold, sulphonylureas, penicillin, allopurinol, captopril)
Chronic actinic dermatitis/seborrhoeic dermatitis
Idiopathic

Rare
Cutaneous T-cell lymphoma (Sézary syndrome) (p. 1307)
Malignancy (especially leukaemias)
Pemphigus foliaceous
Pityriasis rubra pilaris (a hereditary disorder of keratinization)
HIV infection
Toxic shock syndrome (p. 66)

Cutaneous signs of systemic disease

Some dermatoses are associated with a variety of underlying systemic diseases. Furthermore, some medical conditions may present with cutaneous features.

Erythema nodosum

Erythema nodosum has a number of underlying causes (Table 22.8). It presents as painful or tender dusky blue-red nodules, commonly over the shins or lower limbs, which fade over 2–3 weeks leaving a bruised appearance (see Fig. 22.38). It is most common in young adults, especially females. It may be associated with arthralgia, malaise and fever. Inflammation occurs in the dermis and the subcutaneous layer (panniculitis).

Treatment

Symptoms should be treated with non-steroidal anti-inflammatory drugs (avoid in pregnancy), light compression bandaging and bed rest, as the condition resolves spontaneously. The underlying cause should be treated appropriately. In very persistent cases, dapsone (100 mg daily), colchicine (500 mg twice daily) or prednisolone (up to 30 mg daily) can be useful.

Erythema multiforme

Erythema multiforme (EM) is a hypersensitivity rash of acute onset frequently caused by infection or drugs. A cell-mediated cutaneous lymphocytotoxic response is present. Clinically the lesions can be erythematous, polycyclic, annular or show concentric rings called 'target lesions' (Fig. 22.21). Frank blistering is not uncommon. The rash tends to be symmetrical and commonly affects the limbs, especially the hands and feet, where palms and soles may be involved. Occasionally there is severe mucosal involvement leading to necrotic ulcers of the mouth and genitalia, and a conjunctivitis ('EM major' – previously called Stevens–Johnson syndrome – see Box 22.4). The term 'EM minor' may be used for cases without mucosal involvement.

Erythema multiforme usually resolves in 2–4 weeks. The cause is not found in 50% of cases but the following should be considered:

- herpes simplex virus (the most common identifiable cause)
- other viral infections (e.g. EBV, orf disease)
- drugs (e.g. sulphonamides, anticonvulsants)

Table 22.8
Causes of erythema nodosum

Streptococcal infection*
Drugs* (e.g. sulphonamides, oral contraceptive, aspirin, NSAIDs)
Sarcoidosis*
Idiopathic*
Yersinia infection
Fungal infection (histoplasmosis, blastomycosis)
Tuberculosis
Leprosy
Inflammatory bowel disease
Chlamydia infection

* Common causes in the UK

- mycoplasma infection
- connective tissue disease (e.g. SLE, polyarteritis nodosa)
- HIV infection
- Wegener's granulomatosis
- carcinoma, lymphoma.

Rarely, recurrent erythema multiforme can occur and this is triggered by herpes simplex infection in at least 80% of cases.

Treatment

This is symptomatic and involves treating the underlying cause. Some advocate the use of oral steroids in severe disease but this remains controversial.

Recurrent erythema multiforme can be treated with prophylactic oral aciclovir (200 mg twice daily) even if no cause has been found, as 80% appear to be driven by herpes simplex virus. In resistant cases, azathioprine (1–2 mg/kg daily) is used.

Pyoderma gangrenosum

Pyoderma gangrenosum is a condition of unknown aetiology that presents with erythematous nodules or pustules which frequently ulcerate (Fig. 22.22). The ulcers can be large and grow at an alarming speed. The ulcer has a typical bluish black ('gangrenous') undermined edge and a purulent surface ('pyoderma'). There may be an associated pyrexia and malaise. Biopsy through the ulcer edge shows an intense neutrophilic infiltrate and occasionally a vasculitis, but the diagnosis

> **Box 22.4**
>
> ### Stevens–Johnson syndrome
>
> This term is now used for a mild form of toxic epidermal necrolysis (p. 1314) which shares similar mucosal lesions to 'erythema multiforme major' but does not show typical cutaneous target lesions. Both Stevens–Johnson syndrome and toxic epidermal necrolysis are more likely to be drug induced.

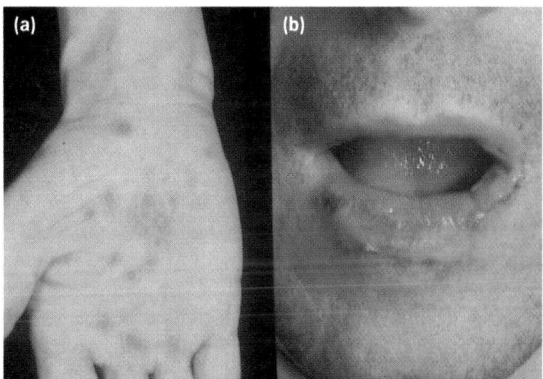

Fig. 22.21 Erythema multiforme major – target lesions of (**a**) the palm and (**b**) with mucosal involvement around the mouth.

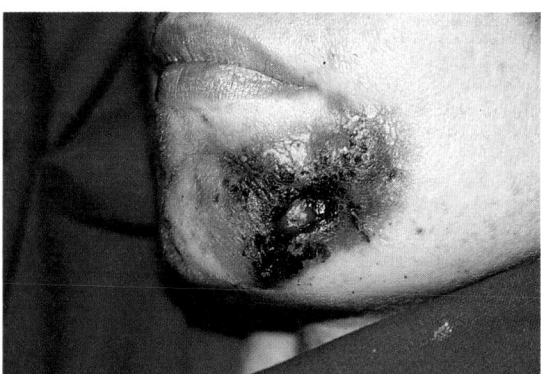

Fig. 22.22 Pyoderma gangrenosum.

depends mostly on the clinical appearance. The main causes are:

- inflammatory bowel disease
- rheumatoid arthritis
- myeloma, monoclonal gammopathy, leukaemia, lymphoma
- liver disease (primary biliary cirrhosis)
- idiopathic (>20% in some series).

Treatment

This is with very potent topical steroids and/or high-dose oral steroids to prevent rapidly progressive ulceration. Oral dapsone and minocycline may help. Other immunosuppressants, such as ciclosporin, are useful in resistant cases. The underlying cause should be treated appropriately.

Acanthosis nigricans

Acanthosis nigricans presents as thickened, hyperpigmented skin predominantly of the flexures (Fig. 22.23). It can appear warty or velvety when advanced. In early life it is seen in obese individuals who have very high levels of insulin owing to insulin resistance. In older people it normally reflects an underlying malignancy (especially gastrointestinal tumours). Rarely it is associated with hyperandrogenism in females.

Treatment

Topical or oral retinoids (0.5 mg/kg/day) may help (p. 1293). Any underlying malignancy should be treated appropriately.

Dermatomyositis (see also p. 563)

The rash is distinctive. Facial erythema and a magenta-coloured rash around the eyes with associated oedema are often present. Bluish red nodules or plaques may be present over the knuckles and extensor surfaces. The nail folds are frequently ragged with dilated capillaries. The diagnosis is made from the clinical appearance, muscle biopsy, EMG and a raised serum creatine phosphokinase. Skin biopsy is not diagnostic.

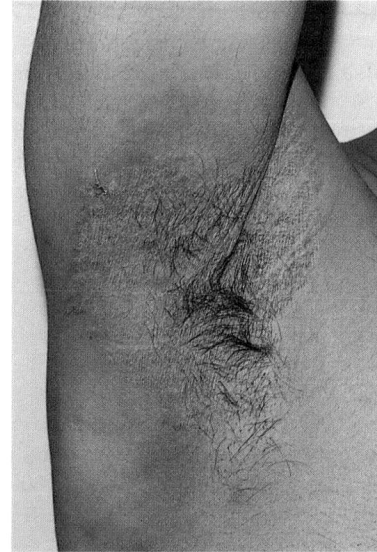

Fig. 22.23 Acanthosis nigricans.

There is a childhood form which usually occurs before the age of 10 and which eventually resolves. This type is often associated with calcinosis in the skin and can cause significant long-term functional problems with weak muscles and contractures. Life-threatening bowel infarction can also occur in the childhood form. The adult form usually occurs after the age of 40. Some cases are associated with an underlying malignancy, whereas others appear to reflect a 'connective tissue disease'. This latter group may overlap with scleroderma and lupus erythematosus.

Treatment

Skin disease may respond to hydroxychloroquine (200 mg twice daily) as well as immunosuppressants, e.g. azathioprine (p. 564).

Scleroderma (see also p. 561)

The term scleroderma refers to a thickening or hardening of the skin owing to abnormal dermal collagen. It is not a diagnostic entity in itself. Systemic sclerosis and morphoea both show sclerodermatous changes but are separate conditions.

Systemic sclerosis (often called scleroderma) has cutaneous and systemic features and is discussed fully on page 561.

Morphoea is confined to the skin and usually presents in children or young adults. It is commoner in females and the cause is unknown. Lesions are usually on the trunk and appear as bluish red plaques which progress to induration and then central white atrophy. A linear variant exists in childhood which is more severe as it can cause atrophy of underlying deep tissues and thus can cause unequal limb growth or scarring alopecia.

Rarely, sclerodermatous skin changes may be seen in chronic Lyme disease (acrodermatitis chronica atrophicans), chronic graft-versus-host disease, polyvinyl chloride disease, eosinophilic myalgia syndrome (due to tryptophan therapy) and bleomycin therapy.

Lupus erythematosus (LE)

There are three clinical variants to this disease but some patients may show features of more than one type:

- chronic discoid lupus erythematosus (CDLE)
- subacute lupus erythematosus (SCLE)
- systemic lupus erythematosus (SLE).

The aetiology is unknown but is presumably a reflection of some abnormality in immune function, as variable autoantibodies may be found in all types. Very rarely it can be induced by certain drugs such as phenothiazines, hydralazine, methyldopa, isoniazid, tetracycline, mesalazine and penicillin.

Chronic discoid lupus erythematosus (CDLE)

CDLE is the most common type of LE seen by dermatologists and more frequently affects females. Clinically it presents with fixed erythematous, scaly, atrophic plaques with telangiectasia, especially on the face or other sun-exposed sites (Fig. 22.24). Hypopigmentation is common and follicular plugging may be apparent. Scalp involvement may lead to a scarring alopecia. Oral involvement (erythematous patches or ulceration) occurs in 25% of cases.

CDLE may be triggered and exacerbated by UV exposure. A few patients may also suffer with Raynaud's phenomenon or unusual chilblain-like lesions (chilblain lupus). Only 5% of cases will go on to develop SLE but this is more common in children. Serum antinuclear factor (ANF) is positive in 30% of cases.

Skin biopsy shows a dense patchy, dermal lymphohistiocytic infiltrate which often is centred around

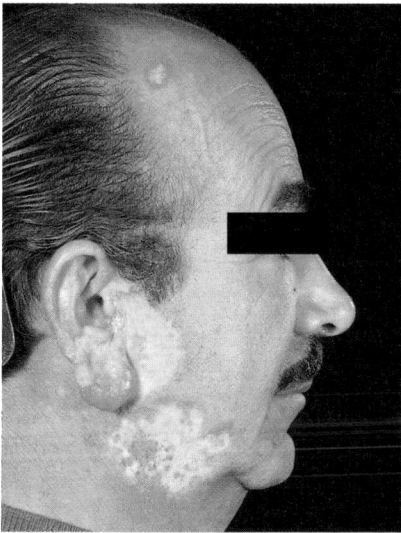

Fig. 22.24 **Chronic discoid lupus erythematosus** showing scaling, atrophy and hypopigmentation.

appendages. Epidermal basal layer damage, follicular plugging and hyperkeratosis may be present. Direct immunofluorescence studies of lesional skin may show the presence of IgM and C3 at the dermoepidermal junction ('lupus band').

Treatment

First-line therapy is with sunscreens and potent topical steroids. Certain oral antimalarials (hydroxychloroquine 100–200 mg twice daily and mepacrine 100 mg daily) can prove very useful and are generally safe for long-term intermittent use. Oral prednisolone is beneficial but its use is limited by its side-effect profile. Azathioprine, retinoids and ciclosporin can be useful in resistant cases.

Prognosis

The disease is usually chronic, although it may fluctuate in severity. CDLE remains confined to the skin in most patients and it will eventually go into remission in up to 50% of cases (after many years).

Subacute lupus erythematosus (SCLE)

SCLE is a rare cutaneous variant of LE. It presents with widespread indurated, sometimes urticated erythematous lesions, often on the upper trunk. The lesions can also be annular. Photosensitivity is often a prominent feature. Complications, such as arthralgia and mouth ulceration, are seen but significant organ involvement is rare. Serum ANF and extractable nuclear antibodies (anti-Ro and anti-La) are usually positive (see p. 516).

Treatment is with oral dapsone, antimalarials or systemic immunosuppression (prednisolone and ciclosporin).

Systemic lupus erythematosus (SLE) (see also p. 557)

The cutaneous involvement of SLE is one of the minor problems of this disease but it is important to recognize as it may be the presenting feature.

Features include macular erythema over the cheeks, nose and forehead ('butterfly rash' – Fig. 22.25). Palmar erythema, dilated nail fold capillaries, splinter haemorrhages and digital infarcts of the finger tips may also be seen but are not always noticed by the patient. Joint swellings, livedo reticularis and purpura are occasionally seen. Rarely SLE can be complicated by an atypical erythema multiforme-like rash ('Rowell's syndrome'). Treatment (p. 560) is usually managed by a rheumatologist.

Pruritus

The mechanisms of pruritus are poorly understood. Evidence suggests that low stimulation of unmyelinated C-fibres in the skin is associated with the sensation of itch (high stimulation produces pain). Histamine, tachykinins (e.g. substance P) and cytokines (e.g. interleukin-2) may also play a role peripherally in the skin. The major nerve pathways for itch and the influence of the central nervous system are not well characterized but opioid

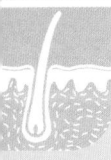

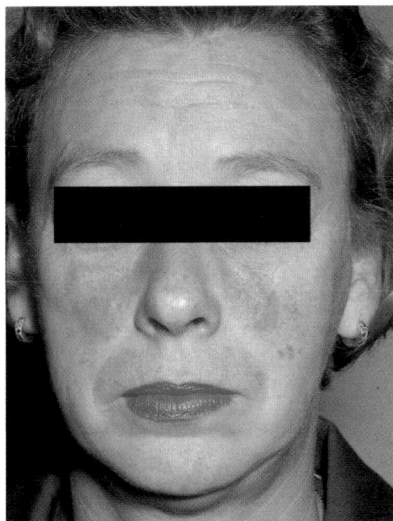

Fig. 22.25 **Systemic lupus erythematosus** – 'butterfly' rash.

μ-receptor-dependent processes can regulate the perception and intensity of itch.

Pruritus (see lichen simplex nodular prurigo/neurodermatitis) in the absence of a demonstrable rash can be caused by a number of different medical problems (Table 22.9).

Asteatotic eczema and cholinergic urticaria are common causes of pruritus where the rash is often missed. The term idiopathic pruritus or 'senile' pruritus probably overlaps with asteatotic eczema and this is common in the elderly.

Treatment involves avoiding soaps, and symptomatic measures (as for asteatotic eczema). Phototherapy may help intractable cases. Oral opiate antagonists, which act centrally, are a new approach for treating pruritus and are currently under assessment. Underlying medical problems should be treated appropriately.

Sarcoidosis (see also p. 897)

Sarcoidosis is a multisystem granulomatous disorder of unknown aetiology. It may present as reddish brown dermal papules and nodules, especially around the eyelid margins and the rim of the nostrils. More polymorphic lesions (papules, nodules and plaques) may appear on the body. It is most common in black Africans where it is often accompanied by hypo- or hyperpigmentation. Rarely it can present with a bluish red infiltrate or swelling, especially of the nose or ears, called lupus pernio. Both these types of lesion can be seen anywhere on the body but are common on the face. Erythema nodosum (p. 1297) of the shins is sometimes seen in acute-onset sarcoidosis. Erythema nodosum is an immunological reaction and not due to sarcoid tissue infiltration. Swollen fingers from a dactylitis may also be present. Whilst sarcoidosis may be confined to the skin, all patients should be investigated for evidence of systemic disease (p. 898).

Table 22.9
Medical conditions associated with pruritus

Iron deficiency anaemia
Internal malignancy (especially lymphoma)
Diabetes mellitus
Chronic renal failure
Chronic liver disease (especially primary biliary cirrhosis and other cholestatic conditions)
Thyroid disease
HIV infection
Polycythaemia vera

Treatment of cutaneous lesions includes very potent topical steroids (0.05% clobetasol proprionate), intra-lesional steroids, oral steroids and occasionally methotrexate or antimalarials.

Neurofibromatosis type 1 (von Recklinghausen's disease) (see also p. 1210)

Type 1 neurofibromatosis is an autosomal dominant condition which often presents in childhood with a variety of cutaneous features. Many cases are new mutations in the *NF1* gene. Early signs include *café au lait* spots (brown macules, greater than 2.5 cm in diameter and more than five lesions) and axillary freckling. Lisch nodules (hyperpigmented iris hamartomas) may be seen in the eyes by slit lamp examination. Later on, fleshy skin tags and deeper soft tumours (neurofibromas) appear and they may progress to completely cover the skin, causing significant cosmetic disability. A number of endocrine disorders may be rarely associated including phaeochromocytoma, acromegaly and Addison's disease.

Tuberous sclerosis (epiloia)

Tuberous sclerosis is also an autosomal dominant condition of variable severity which may not present until later childhood. It is characterized by a variety of hamartomatous growths. The three cardinal features are (a) mental retardation, (b) epilepsy and (c) cutaneous abnormalities – but not all have to be present. The skin signs include:

- adenoma sebaceum (reddish papules/fibromas around the nose)
- periungual fibroma (nodules arising from the nail bed)
- shagreen patches (firm, flesh-coloured plaques on the trunk)
- ash-leaf hypopigmentation (pale macules best seen with UV light)
- forehead plaque (indurated flesh-coloured patch)
- *café au lait* patches
- pitting of dental enamel.

Internal hamartomas can arise in the heart, kidney, retina and CNS. Parents of a suspected case should be carefully examined as they may have a forme fruste of the condition which can manifest just as hypopigmented patches. This would have genetic implications for future offspring.

Diabetes mellitus (see also p. 1100)

Diabetes mellitus can have a number of cutaneous features. Complications of diabetes itself include:

- fungal infection (e.g. candidiasis)
- bacterial infections (e.g. recurrent boils)
- xanthomas
- arterial disease (ulcers, gangrene)
- neuropathic ulcers.

Specific dermatoses of diabetes include:

- necrobiosis lipoidica (a patch of spreading erythema over the shin which becomes yellowish and atrophic in the centre and may ulcerate)
- diffuse granuloma annulare (p. 1291)
- diabetic dermopathy (red-brown flat-topped papules)
- blisters (usually on the feet or hands)
- diabetic stiff skin (tight waxy skin over the fingers with limitation of joint movement owing to thickened collagen – also called cheiroarthropathy).

Chronic liver disease (see also p. 346)

Chronic liver disease may present with jaundice, palmar erythema, spider naevi, white nails, hyperpigmentation and pruritus.

Porphyria cutanea tarda (p. 000) is a rare genetic disorder associated with liver disease usually due to hepatic damage from excessive alcohol consumption or hepatitis C infection. It presents clinically on exposed skin with sun-induced blisters, skin fragility, scarring, milia and hypertrichosis. Treatment of the cutaneous features is with repeated venesection and/or very low-dose chloroquine plus an avoidance of alcohol. There is anecdotal evidence that specific treatment of hepatitis C (p. 1121) will also help the skin, presumably through improving liver function.

Chronic renal failure (see also p. 646)

Chronic renal failure is commonly associated with intractable pruritus. Long-standing renal transplant patients often suffer with recurrent viral warts and squamous cell carcinomas because of the immunosuppression.

Thyroid disease (see also p. 1035)

Hypothyroidism may cause dry firm gelatinous (myxoedematous) skin with diffuse hair thinning and a loss of the outer third of the eyebrows.

Hyperthyroidism may be associated with warm sweaty skin and a diffuse alopecia. Graves' disease is rarely associated with thyroid acropachy ('clubbing' with underlying bone changes) and pretibial myxoedema (a red-brown infiltration of the shins which can become lumpy and tender).

Cushing's syndrome (see also p. 1052)

Cushing's syndrome may cause hirsutism, a moon face, a buffalo hump, stretch marks (striae) and a pustular folliculitis (often called steroid acne) of the skin.

Hyperlipidaemias (see also p. 1107)

Hyperlipidaemias can present with xanthomas, which are abnormal collections of lipid in the skin. All patients with xanthomas should be investigated for hyperlipidaemia, although the most common type called xanthelasma (yellow plaques around the eyes) are usually associated with normal lipids. There are a number of other clinical variants of xanthomas such as (i) tuberous xanthoma (firm orange-yellow nodules and plaques on extensor surfaces), (ii) tendon xanthoma (firm subcutaneous swellings attached to tendons), (iii) plane xanthoma (orange-yellow macules often affecting palmar creases), and (iv) eruptive xanthoma (numerous small yellowish papules commonly on the buttocks).

Cutaneous amyloid

Cutaneous amyloid can be confined to the skin or be part of systemic disease (p. 1118). Macular amyloid is a common purely cutaneous variant seen in Asians. It is characterized by itchy brown rippled macules on the upper back.

Systemic amyloid may be associated with reddish brown papules, nodules or plaques, especially around the eyes, the flexural areas and mucosal surfaces. Distinctive periorbital bruising and macroglossia may also be present.

Systemic malignant disease

Certain rashes may be a non-metastatic manifestation of an underlying malignancy (Table 22.10). Rarely tumours

Table 22.10
Non-metastatic cutaneous manifestations of underlying malignancy

Dermatosis	Tumour
Dermatomyositis	Lung, GI tract, GU tract
Acanthosis nigricans	GI tract, lung, liver
Paget's disease (localized patch of eczema around the nipple)	Ductal breast carcinoma
Erythroderma	Lymphoma/leukaemia
Tylosis (thickened palms/soles)	Oesophageal carcinoma
Ichthyosis (dry flaking of skin)	Lymphoma
Erythema gyratum repens (concentric rings of erythema which change rapidly)	Lung, breast
Necrolytic migratory erythema (burning, geographic and spreading annular areas of erythema)	Glucagonoma

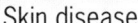

can metastasize to the skin where they normally present as papules or nodules which may proceed to ulceration.

FURTHER READING

Braverman IM (ed.) (1997) *Skin Signs of Systemic Disease*, 3rd edn. Philadelphia: WB Saunders.

Fitzpatrick TB, Eisen AZ, Wolff K, Freedberg IM, Austen KF (eds) (1998) *Dermatology in General Medicine*, 5th edn. New York: McGraw-Hill.

Metze D et al. (1999) Efficacy and safety of naltrexone, an oral opiate receptor antagonist, in the treatment of pruritus in internal and dermatological diseases. *Journal of the American Academy of Dermatology* **41**: 533–539.

Bullous disease

Primary blistering diseases of the skin are rare. A variety of skin proteins are important in holding the skin together. Inherited abnormalities or immune damage of these proteins causes abnormal cell separation, inflammation, fluid accumulation and blistering (Fig. 22.26). The 'level' of blistering determines the clinical picture as well as the prognosis. Therefore skin biopsy for light and electron microscopy together with immunofluorescence (IMF) studies are paramount in diagnosis. However, remember that the commonest causes of skin blistering are chickenpox, herpes, impetigo, pompholyx eczema and insect bite reactions although these are often localized.

Immunobullous disease

Pemphigus vulgaris

Pemphigus vulgaris is a potentially fatal blistering disease occurring in all races but commoner in Ashkenazi Jews and possibly in people from the Indian subcontinent. Onset is usually in middle age and both sexes are affected equally. Prior to the development of oral steroids this condition was frequently fatal. The development of autoantibodies against the desmosomal protein, desmoglein 3, is pathogenic in this disease and they can be measured experimentally as markers of disease activity. Rarely the disease can be drug induced (e.g. penicillamine or ACE inhibitors).

Skin biopsy shows a superficial intraepidermal split just above the basal layer with acantholysis (separation of individual cells). In the rarer variant, pemphigus foliaceous (characterized by anti-desmoglein 1 autoantibodies), the split is higher in the upper epidermis. Both direct IMF of skin (perilesional) and indirect IMF using patients' serum show intercellular staining of IgG within the epidermis.

Clinical features

Mucosal involvement (especially oral ulceration) is common and may be the presenting sign in up to 50% of cases. This may then be followed by the appearance of flaccid blisters, particularly involving the trunk. They tend to be sore rather than itchy. Blistering usually becomes widespread but the blisters rapidly denude; thus pemphigus often presents with erythematous,

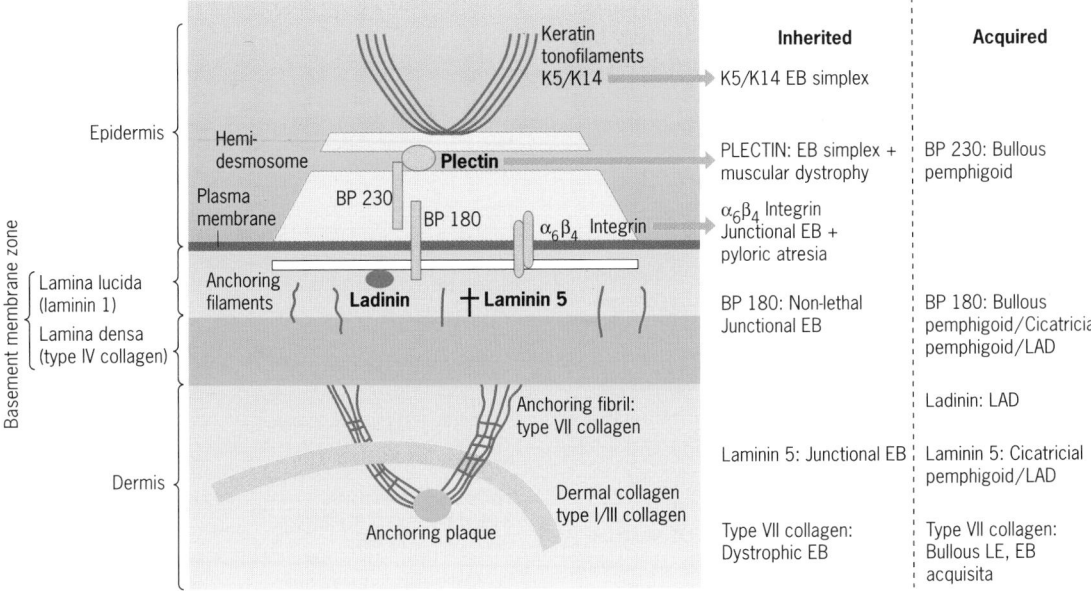

Fig. 22.26 **Section of the basement membrane zone**, showing the structural sites of damage in bullous disorders. LAD, linear IgA disease; EB, epidermolysis bullosa.

weeping erosions. Blisters can be extended with gentle sliding pressure (Nikolsky's sign). Flexural lesions often have a vegetative appearance. In *pemphigus foliaceous* the blisters and erosions often start in a seborrhoeic distribution (scalp, face and upper chest) before becoming more widespread.

Treatment

This is with very high-dose oral prednisolone (60–100 mg daily) or pulsed methylprednisolone and this may need to be lifelong. Therefore other immunosuppressants such as azathioprine (or occasionally cyclophosphamide or ciclosporin) are used as steroid-sparing agents. Intravenous immunoglobulin infusions can be useful in resistant cases.

Whilst treatment is normally effective, perhaps up to 10% of patients may succumb, either because of complications of the disease or more commonly from side-effects of the treatment.

Use of azathioprine. Azathioprine can cause bone marrow suppression and an allergic hepatitis. Therefore blood count and liver biochemical tests should be regularly monitored during therapy (every 6 weeks). Pregnancy should be avoided. Long-term use with other immunosuppressants causes a slightly increased risk of malignancy, especially of the skin.

Bullous pemphigoid

Bullous pemphigoid is more common than pemphigus. It presents in later life (usually over 60 years old) and mucosal involvement is rarer. Autoantibodies against a 230 kDa or 180 kDa hemidesmosomal protein ('bullous pemphigoid antigens 1 and 2') play an aetiological role.

Skin biopsy shows a deeper blister (than in pemphigus) owing to a subepidermal split through the basement membrane. Direct and indirect IMF studies show linear staining of IgG along the basement membrane.

Clinical features

Large tense bullae appear anywhere on the skin (Fig. 22.27) but often involve limbs, hands and feet. They may be centred on an erythematous or urticated background

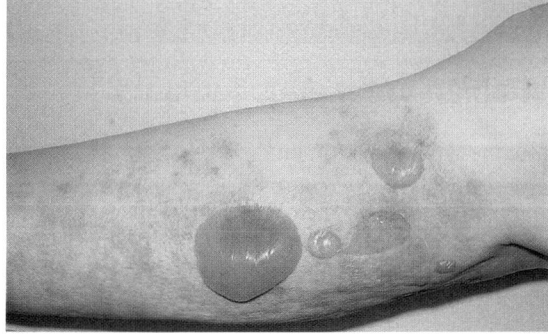

Fig. 22.27 Bullous pemphigoid.

and they can be haemorrhagic. Pemphigoid can be very itchy. Mucosal ulceration is uncommon but a variant of pemphigoid exists which predominantly affects mucosal surfaces with scarring (cicatricial pemphigoid).

Treatment

This is with high-dose oral prednisolone (30–60 mg daily) and steroid-sparing agents such as azathioprine. In general, disease control is easier than with pemphigus. Often, treatment can be withdrawn after 2–3 years. However, pemphigoid treatment often causes side-effects, especially as most patients are elderly. Occasionally localized disease can be controlled with potent topical steroids or oral dapsone.

Dermatitis herpetiformis (see also p. 293)

Dermatitis herpetiformis is a rare blistering disorder associated with gluten-sensitive enteropathy (coeliac disease) and occasionally other organ-specific autoimmune disorders. The HLA associations (B8, DR3, DQ2 in 80–90% of cases) and immunological findings (endomysial, tissue transglutaminase, reticulin and gliadin autoantibodies may be present in serum) are similar to coeliac disease.

Skin biopsy shows a subepidermal blister with neutrophil microabscesses in the dermal papillae. Direct IMF studies of uninvolved skin show IgA in the dermal papillae and patchy granular IgA along the basement membrane. The jejunal mucosa may show partial villous atrophy but the changes tend to be milder than in coeliac disease (p. 293).

Clinical features

Dermatitis herpetiformis is commoner in males and can present at any age but is most likely to appear for the first time in young adult life. It presents with small, intensely itchy blisters of the skin. The lesions have a predilection for the elbows, extensor forearms, scalp and buttocks. The tops of the blisters are usually scratched off; thus crusted erosions are often seen at presentation. Remissions and exacerbations are common.

Treatment

This should always be with a gluten-free diet (GFD). Control of the skin disease can be obtained with oral dapsone (50–200 mg daily) or sulphonamides. If a strict GFD is adhered to, oral medication can often be withdrawn after 2 years. The GFD will need to be lifelong. It protects against the rare complication of small bowel lymphoma.

Use of dapsone. Dapsone frequently causes a mild dose-related haemolytic anaemia (which is usually well tolerated) but the haemolysis can be devastating if there is G6PD deficiency. Liver damage, polyneuropathy and aplastic anaemia can also occur rarely, so regular monitoring of a blood count and liver biochemistry is needed.

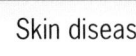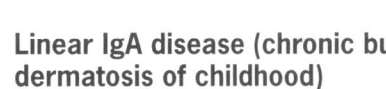

Linear IgA disease (chronic bullous dermatosis of childhood)

Linear IgA disease is a subepidermal blistering disorder of adults and children. Pathogenic autoantibodies can bind to a variety of basement membrane proteins including ladinin, BP 180 antigen and laminin 5. It is the most common immunobullous disease seen in children. Rarely it is drug induced by vancomycin.

Clinical features

Linear IgA disease can present with circular clusters of large blisters, a pemphigoid type of blistering or a dermatitis herpetiformis picture. Mucosal involvement of the mouth, vulva and eyes is not uncommon and can cause scarring. Direct IMF studies of skin show linear IgA deposition along the basement membrane.

Treatment

This is with oral dapsone (50–200 mg daily) or sulphonamides. Occasionally immunosuppression is needed. Many patients show spontaneous resolution after 3–6 years.

Mechanobullous disease (epidermolysis bullosa, 'EB')

These disorders are due to inherited abnormalities in structurally important skin proteins which lead to 'skin fragility'. The resultant blistering tends to arise secondary to trauma and often appears at or shortly after birth. These conditions can be a mild inconvenience, severely disabling or fatal but fortunately are very rare. There are three groups of disorders in which the fundamental gene/protein abnormalities have been characterized. This enables prenatal amniocentesis diagnosis.

Epidermolysis bullosa simplex

This is a group of autosomal dominant genodermatoses characterized by 'superficial' blistering owing to mutations of cytoskeleton proteins within the basal layer of the epidermis, e.g. keratin 5 (chromosome 12q) or keratin 14 (chromosome 17q). Most forms of EB simplex show mild disease with intermittent blistering of the hands and feet, especially in hot weather. The teeth and nails are normal and scarring is absent.

Epidermolysis bullosa dystrophica

This is a group of genodermatoses characterized by 'deeper' blistering associated with scarring and milia formation. The level of split is deep within the basement membrane and is due to a mutation in the *COL-7A1* gene (locus at chromosome 3p21.1) which causes a loss of collagen VII in the anchoring fibrils. Nails, mucosae and even the larynx are often involved. The autosomal dominant variety is milder but the autosomal recessive type produces severe disease with disabling scarring, fusion of digits, joint contractures and dysphagia. Life expectancy is significantly reduced. Repeated scarring can result in the development of multiple squamous cell carcinomas.

Junctional epidermolysis bullosa

This, the most severe form, is characterized by a split in the lamina lucida of the basement membrane and is due to mutations in various proteins, mainly laminin 5 but also $\alpha_6\beta_4$ integrin or the 180 kDa bullous pemphigoid-2 antigen. It presents at birth with widespread blistering and areas of absent skin. Erosions of the central face and hoarseness from laryngeal involvement are common. Nail and teeth abnormalities are also common. Both a lethal and a rarer non-lethal form of junctional EB exist and they show an autosomal recessive inheritance.

Investigation and treatment

Investigation and treatment of EB should be carried out in a specialist centre. Diagnosis at birth on clinical grounds is difficult and should be avoided. Exact diagnosis depends on ultrastructural analysis of induced blisters in the skin and immunohistochemistry. Only then can prognosis and genetic counselling be given accurately to parents. Prenatal diagnosis is available for the more severe forms of EB.

FURTHER READING

Diaz LA, Giudice GJ (2000) End of the century overview of skin blisters. *Archives of Dermatology* **136**: 106–112.
Edelson RL (2000) Pemphigus. Editorial. *New England Journal of Medicine* **343**: 60–61.
Fine JD (1995) Management of acquired bullous skin disease. *New England Journal of Medicine* **333**: 1475–1484.
Nousari HC, Anhalt GJ (1999) Pemphigus and bullous pemphigoid. *Lancet* **354**: 667–672.
Wakelin SH, Black MM (1997) The autoimmune bullous diseases. *Journal of the Royal College of Physicians of London* **31**: 364–368.

Skin tumours

Benign cutaneous tumours

Melanocytic naevi (moles)

Moles are a benign overgrowth of melanocytes that are common in white-skinned people. They appear in childhood and increase in number and size during adolescence and early adult life. They often start as flat brown macules with proliferation of melanocytes at the dermo-epidermal junction (junctional naevi). The melanocytes continue to proliferate and grow down into the dermis (compound naevi), which causes an elevation of the mole above the skin surface. The pigmentation is usually even and the border regular. They eventually mature into a dermal naevus (cellular naevus), often with a loss of pigment.

Blue naevus is an acquired asymptomatic blue-looking mole. It is due to a proliferation of melanocytes deep in the mid-dermis.

Basal cell papilloma (seborrhoeic wart)

This is a common benign overgrowth of the basal cell layer of the epidermis. The lesion can be flesh coloured, brown or even black and often has a greasy appearance. The surface is irregular and warty and the lesions appear very superficial as though stuck on to the skin (Fig. 22.28). Tiny keratin cysts may be seen on the surface. They can be treated with cryotherapy or curettage.

Dermatofibroma (histiocytoma)

Dermatofibromas appear as firm, elevated pigmented nodules which may feel like a button in the skin. A peripheral ring of pigmentation is sometimes seen. They are often found on the leg and are commoner in females. There may be a preceding history of trauma or insect bite. The lesion consists of histiocytes, blood vessels and varying degrees of fibrosis. If symptomatic, excision is required.

Epidermoid cyst (previously 'sebaceous cyst')

Epidermoid cysts present as cystic swellings of the skin with a central punctum. They contain 'cheesy' keratin rather than sebum; thus the old term 'sebaceous cyst' should be avoided. These cysts occasionally rupture causing significant dermal inflammation which is not infected.

Pilar cyst (trichilemmal cyst)

Pilar cysts are smooth cysts without a punctum, usually found on the scalp. They may be multiple and familial.

Keratoacanthoma

Keratoacanthomas are rapidly growing epidermal tumours which develop central necrosis and ulceration (Fig. 22.29). They occur on sun-exposed skin in later life and can grow up to 2–3 cm across. Whilst they may resolve spontaneously over a few months, they are best excised both to exclude a squamous cell carcinoma (which they can mimic) and to improve the cosmetic outcome.

Pyogenic granuloma (granuloma telangiectaticum)

Pyogenic granulomas are a benign overgrowth of blood vessels. They present as rapidly growing pinkish red nodules which are friable and readily bleed. They may follow trauma and are often found on the fingers and lips. They are best excised to exclude an amelanotic malignant melanoma.

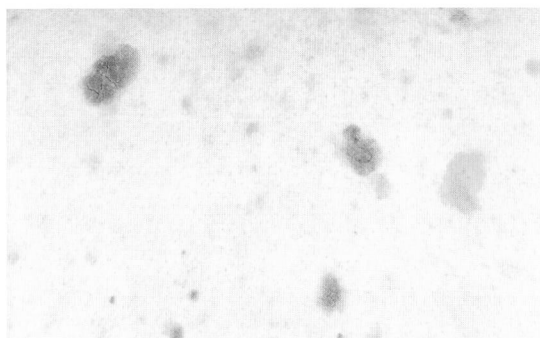

Fig. 22.28 Seborrhoeic wart (basal cell papilloma).

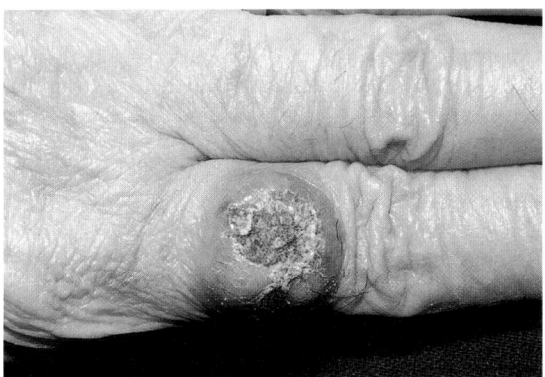

Fig. 22.29 Keratoacanthoma.

Cherry angioma (Campbell de Morgan spots)

They are benign angiokeratomas that appear as tiny pin-point red papules, especially on the trunk, and increase with age. No treatment is required.

Potentially pre-malignant cutaneous tumours

Solar keratoses (actinic keratoses)

These frequently develop later in life in white-skinned people who have had significant sun exposure. They appear on exposed skin as erythematous silver-scaly papules or patches with a conical surface and a red base. The background skin is often inelastic, wrinkled and may show flat brown macules ('liver spots' or solar lentigos) reflecting diffuse solar damage (Fig. 22.30). A small proportion of these keratoses can transform into squamous cell carcinoma but only after many years.

Treatment of lesions is with cryotherapy or topical 5-fluorouracil cream.

Bowen's disease

This is a form of intraepidermal carcinoma-in-situ which rarely can become invasive. It presents on

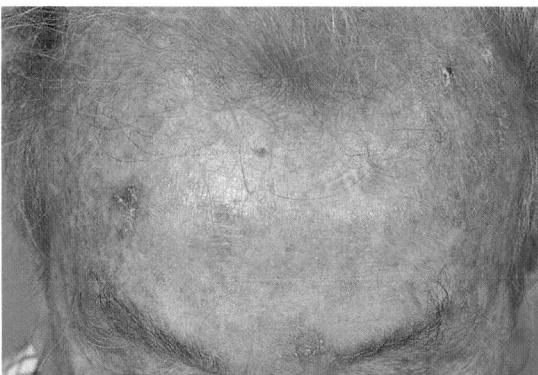

Fig. 22.30 **Solar keratoses with background actinic damage.**

exposed skin as an isolated scaly red patch or plaque looking rather like psoriasis although it has a rather irregular edge. The lesions do not clear but slowly increase in size with time.

Treatment is with topical 5-fluorouracil, cryotherapy or curettage.

Atypical mole syndrome (dysplastic naevus syndrome)

This is often familial. A large number of melanocytic naevi begin to appear in childhood even on unexposed sites. Individual lesions may be large with irregular pigmentation and border, and histologically they may show cytological and architectural atypia but no frank malignant change. Individuals with this condition have an increased risk of developing malignant melanoma. They should have their moles photographed and be regularly reviewed. Suspicious lesions should be excised.

Giant congenital melanocytic naevi

These are very large moles present at birth. They show an increased risk of developing malignant melanoma. Excision should be performed if possible.

Lentigo maligna

This is a slow-growing macular area of pigmentation seen in elderly people, commonly on the face. The border and pigmentation are often irregular. Some people regard this lesion as a melanoma-in-situ. There is an increased risk of developing invasive malignant melanoma. Treatment is by excision.

Malignant cutaneous tumours

Basal cell carcinoma (rodent ulcer)

Basal cell carcinomas are the most common malignant skin tumour and most relate to excessive sun exposure. They are common later in life on exposed sites although rare on the ear. They can present as a slow-growing

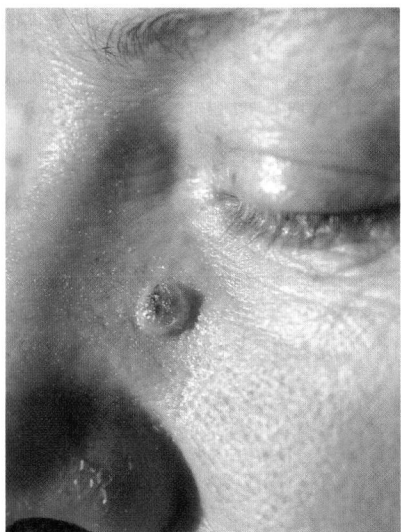

Fig. 22.31 **Ulcerating basal cell carcinoma.**

papule or nodule (or rarely be cystic) which may go on to ulcerate (Fig. 22.31). Telangiectasia over the tumour or a skin-coloured jelly-like 'pearly edge' may be seen. A flat, diffuse superficial form exists and an ill-defined 'morphoeic' variant. Basal cell carcinomas will slowly grow and erode structures if untreated but these tumours almost never metastasize.

Treatment

This is usually with surgical excision although radiotherapy can be useful for large superficial forms. Curettage may occasionally be used in older patients, although not for central facial lesions as they often recur. Very superficial lesions may be treated with cryotherapy but follow-up is advised.

Squamous cell carcinoma

Squamous cell carcinoma is a more aggressive tumour than basal cell carcinoma as it can metastasize if left untreated. Most relate to sun exposure and they can arise in pre-existing solar keratoses or Bowen's disease. They can also arise as a result of chronic inflammation such as in lupus vulgaris. Rarely multiple tumours may arise because of arsenic ingestion in early life. Multiple tumours also occur in people who have had prolonged periods of immunosuppression, such as renal transplant patients where certain human papilloma virus subtypes may be important in malignant transformation.

Clinically the lesions are often keratotic, rather ill-defined nodules which may ulcerate (Fig. 22.32). They can grow very rapidly. Examination of regional lymph nodes is essential. They are most common on sun-exposed sites in later life. One should have a high index of suspicion for ulcerated lesions on the lower lip or ear.

Treatment is with excision or radiotherapy. Curettage should be avoided.

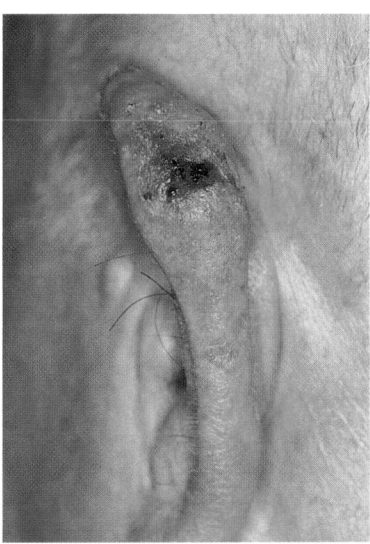

Fig. 22.32 **Squamous cell carcinoma.**

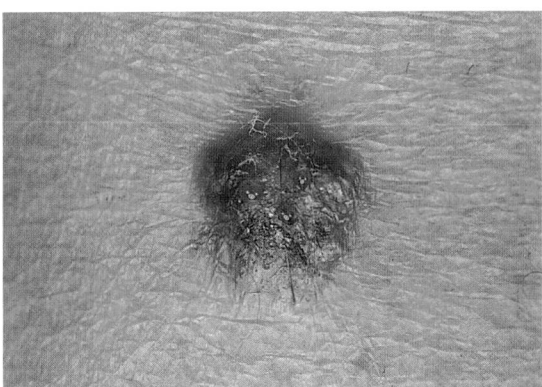

Fig. 22.33 **Nodular malignant melanoma.**

Table 22.11
Clinical criteria for the diagnosis of malignant melanoma

ABCDE criteria (USA)
Asymmetry of mole
Border irregularity
Colour variegation
Diameter > 6 mm
Elevation

The Glasgow 7-point checklist

Major criteria	Change in size
	Change in shape
	Change in colour
Minor criteria	Diameter more than 6 mm
	Inflammation
	Oozing or bleeding
	Mild itch or altered sensation

Malignant melanoma

Malignant melanoma is the most serious form of skin cancer as metastasis can occur early and it causes a number of deaths even in young people. As with other types of skin cancer the incidence is continuing to increase, probably because of excessive exposure to sunlight. The history of childhood sun exposure and intermittent sun exposure appears to be particularly important in the development of malignant melanoma. Other risk factors include atypical mole syndrome, giant congenital melanocytic naevi, lentigo maligna and a positive family history of malignant melanoma. Malignant melanoma is commoner in later life but many young adults are also affected.

Diagnosis of melanoma is not always easy but the clinical signs listed in Table 22.11 help distinguish malignant from benign moles. Examination with epiluminescence microscopy can further help in detecting malignant lesions.

Four clinical types exist:

- *Lentigo maligna melanoma* is where a patch of lentigo maligna develops a papule or nodule signalling invasive tumour.
- *Superficial spreading malignant melanoma* is a large flat irregularly pigmented lesion which grows laterally before vertical invasion develops.
- *Nodular malignant melanoma* (Fig. 22.33) is the most aggressive type. It presents as a rapidly growing pigmented nodule which bleeds or ulcerates. Rarely they are amelanotic (non-pigmented) and can mimic pyogenic granuloma.
- *Acral lentiginous malignant melanoma* arises as pigmented lesions on the palm, sole or under the nail and it usually presents late.

Treatment

This consists of urgent wide excision of the lesion. Histological analysis will determine the depth of invasion ('Clark's level') and the thickness of the tumour ('Breslow thickness'). These two factors help to predict prognosis and 5-year survival rates. Excision and histology interpretation should only be done by experts to ensure optimum treatment and assessment of prognosis. Metastatic disease is best managed by an oncologist and can involve surgery to lymph nodes, radiotherapy, immunotherapy and chemotherapy.

The role of governments and medical personnel in public health education to discourage sunbathing and encourage the use of sunscreens is of the utmost importance in skin cancer prevention.

Cutaneous T-cell lymphoma (mycosis fungoides)

This is a rare type of skin tumour which often follows a relatively benign course. It presents insidiously with scaly patches and plaques which can look eczematous or psoriasiform. Lesions often appear initially on the buttocks. These lesions may come and go or remain persistent over many years. Patients may well die of

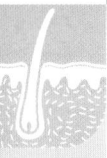

unrelated causes. Skin biopsy confirms the diagnosis showing invasion by atypical lymphocytes. T-cell receptor gene rearrangement studies show that there is often a monoclonal expansion of lymphocytes in the skin.

Occasionally the disease can progress to a cutaneous nodular or tumour stage which may be accompanied by systemic organ involvement. In elderly males the disease may progress rarely to an erythrodermic variant accompanied by lymphadenopathy and peripheral blood involvement ('Sézary syndrome').

All patients should be staged at the time of diagnosis to assess for any systemic involvement.

Treatment

Early cutaneous disease can be left untreated or treated with topical steroids or PUVA. More advanced disease of the skin, or systemic involvement, may require radiotherapy, chemotherapy, immunotherapy or electron beam therapy.

Kaposi's sarcoma

This is a tumour of vascular and lymphatic endothelium that presents as purplish nodules and plaques. There are three types:

- The 'classic 'or 'sporadic' form (as described by Kaposi) occurs in elderly males, especially Jews from eastern Europe. It presents as slow-growing purple tumours in the foot and lower leg which rarely cause any significant problem.
- The 'endemic' form occurs in males from central Africa and shows more widespread cutaneous involvement as well as lymph node (or occasionally systemic) involvement. Oedema is a prominent feature.
- The immunosuppression-related form is more severe and is most common in homosexual patients with HIV (p. 144). Lesions are widespread and often affect the skin, bowel, oral cavity and lungs.

All three types have a strong association with herpes virus type 8 but other factors must be involved as herpes type 8 seroprevalence is up to 10% in the USA and 50% in some African countries. HAART (p. 146) has reduced the incidence of Kaposi's sarcoma.

Treatment

Treatment of advanced Kaposi's sarcoma is with radiotherapy, immunotherapy or chemotherapy.

FURTHER READING

Alam M, Ratner D (2001) Cutaneous squamous cell carcinoma. *New England Journal of Medicine* **344**: 975–983.
Antman K, Chang Y (2000) Kaposi's sarcoma. *New England Journal of Medicine* **342**: 1027–1038.
Gilchrest BA et al. (1999) The pathogenesis of melanoma induced by ultraviolet radiation. *New England Journal of Medicine* **340**: 1341–1348.

Goldberg LH (1996) Basal cell carcinoma. *Lancet* **347**: 663–667.
Hill D (1999) Efficacy of sunscreens in protection against skin cancer. *Lancet* **354**: 699–700.
Kittler H et al. (1999) Morphological changes of pigmented skin lesions: a useful expansion of the ABCD rule for dermatoscopy. *Journal of the American Academy of Dermatology* **40**: 558–562.
Rees J (1997) Skin cancer. *Journal of the Royal College of Physicians of London* **31**: 246–250.

Disorders of blood vessels/ lymphatics

Leg ulcers

Venous ulcers

Leg ulcers are common in Western societies and can have many causes (Table 22.12). Venous ulcers are the most common type in developed countries.

Venous ulcers are the result of sustained venous hypertension in the superficial veins, owing to incompetent valves in the deep or perforating veins or to previous deep vein thrombosis. The increased pressure causes extravasation of fibrinogen through the capillary walls, giving rise to perivascular fibrin deposition, which leads to poor oxygenation of the surrounding skin.

Venous ulcers are common in later life and cause a significant drain on healthcare budgets as they are often chronic and recurrent; they affect 1% of the population over the age of 70 years. They are most commonly found on the lower leg in a triangle above the ankles (Fig. 22.34), and may be associated with:

- venous eczema (p. 1286)
- brown pigmentation from haemosiderin
- varicose veins
- lipodermatosclerosis (the combination of induration, reddish-brown pigmentation and inflammation)
- scarring white atrophy with telangiectasia (atrophie blanche).

Table 22.12
Causes of leg ulceration

- Venous hypertension
- Arterial disease
- Neuropathic (e.g. diabetes, leprosy)
- Neoplastic (e.g. squamous or basal cell carcinoma)
- Vasculitis (e.g. rheumatoid arthritis, SLE, pyoderma gangrenosum)
- Infection (e.g. ecthyma, tuberculosis, deep mycoses, tropical ulcer, syphilis, yaws)
- Haematological (e.g. sickle cell disease, spherocytosis)
- Other (e.g. necrobiosis lipoidica, trauma, artefact)

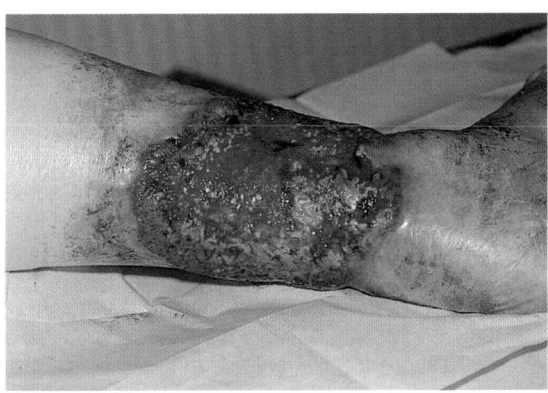

Fig. 22.34 Venous leg ulcer.

Treatment

This is with high-compression bandaging (e.g. Unna boot or four-layer bandaging) and leg elevation to try to decrease the venous hypertension. Doppler studies should always be done before bandaging to exclude arterial disease. This treatment is best delivered in the community by appropriately trained nurses. 'Four-layer bandaging' is increasingly popular as this provides high levels of graduated compression (with pressures decreasing up the leg). The choice of ulcer dressing is less important but one should be chosen to keep the ulcer moist and free of slough and exudate. Up to 80% of ulcers can be healed within 26 weeks. Slower healing rates occur in patients with decreased mobility and if the ulcers are very large, present for longer than 6 months or are bilateral. Diuretics are sometimes helpful to reduce the oedema. Antibiotics are necessary only for overt infection.

Venous leg ulcers can be very painful so adequate analgesia should be given, including opiates if required. Split-thickness skin grafting may be considered in resistant cases. Lifelong support stockings (individually fitted) should be worn after healing.

Underlying venous disease is best investigated with duplex ultrasound or plethysmography. Surgery for purely superficial venous disease can occasionally be useful for ulcer healing but, in general, venous surgery is unhelpful.

Arterial ulcers

Arterial ulcers may present as punched-out, painful ulcers higher up the leg or on the feet. There may be a history of claudication, hypertension, angina or smoking. Clinically the leg may be cold and show pallor. Absent peripheral pulses, arterial bruits and loss of hair may be present. Doppler ultrasound studies will confirm arterial disease and digital subtraction angiography will further delineate the extent and site of the disease.

Treatment depends on keeping the ulcer clean and covered, adequate analgesia and vascular reconstruction if appropriate.

Neuropathic ulcers

Neuropathic ulcers tend to be seen over pressure areas of the feet, such as the metatarsal heads, owing to repeated trauma. These are most commonly seen in diabetics because of peripheral neuropathy. In developing countries leprosy is a common cause.

Treatment depends on keeping the ulcer clean and removing pressure or trauma from the affected area. Diabetics should pay particular attention to foot care and correctly fitting shoes.

Pressure sores (decubitus ulcers, bedsores)

These occur in the elderly, immobile, unconscious or paralysed patients. They are due to skin ischaemia from sustained pressure over a bony prominence, most commonly the heel and sacrum. Normal individuals feel the pain of continued pressure, and even during sleep, movement takes place to change position continually. There are numerous risk factors for development of pressure sores (Table 22.13).

The majority of pressure sores occur in hospital. Seventy per cent appear in the first 2 weeks of hospitalization, and 70% are in orthopaedic patients, especially those on traction. Between 20% and 30% of pressure sores occur in the community.

Eighty per cent of patients with deep ulcers involving the subcutaneous tissue die in the first 4 months.

The early sign of red/blue discoloration of the skin can lead rapidly to ulcers in 1–2 hours. Leaving patients on hard emergency room trolleys, or sitting them in chairs for prolonged periods, must be avoided.

Table 22.13
Risk factors for the development of pressure sores

- Prolonged immobility
  paraplegia
  arthritis
  severe physical disease
  apathy
  operation and postoperative states
  plaster casts
  intensive care

- Decreased sensation
  coma, neurological disease, diabetes mellitus
  drug-induced sleep

- Vascular disease
  atherosclerosis, diabetes mellitus, scleroderma, vasculitis

- Poor nutrition
  anaemia
  hypoalbuminaemia
  vitamin C or zinc deficiency

Management

Prevention

Prevention is better than cure. Specialist 'tissue-viability nurses' help identify at-risk patients and train other medical staff. Several risk-assessment tools have been devised for the immobile patient based on the known risk factors. The 'Norton scale' and Waterlow Pressure Sore Risk Assessment (Box 22.5) are two such validated systems which produce a numerical score, enabling staff to identify those at most risk.

Treatment

- Bed rest with pillows and fleeces to keep pressure off bony areas (e.g. sacrum and heels) and prevent friction.
- Air-filled cushions for patients in wheelchairs.
- Special pressure-relieving mattresses and beds.
- Regular turning, but avoid pressure on hips.
- Ensure adequate nutrition.
- Non-irritant occlusive moist dressings.
- Adequate analgesia (may need opiates).
- Plastic surgery (debridement and grafting).
- Treatment of underlying condition.

Vasculitis (see also p. 564)

Vasculitis is the term applied to an inflammatory disorder of blood vessels which causes endothelial damage. It can be confirmed by skin biopsy. The classification used here (Table 22.14) depends more on the site of the vessel involved than on its size. An alternative classification, depending on size of vessel, is shown in Tables 10.18 and 10.19.

The cutaneous features are of haemorrhagic papules, pustules, nodules or plaques which may erode and ulcerate. These purpuric lesions do not blanche with pressure. Occasionally a fixed livedo reticularis pattern may appear which does not disappear on warming. Pyrexia and arthralgia are common associations even in the absence of significant systemic involvement. Other clinical features depend on the underlying cause.

The most common cutaneous vasculitis is *leucocytoclastic vasculitis*, which usually appears on the lower legs as a symmetrical palpable purpura. It is rarely associated with systemic involvement. This can be caused by drugs or infection but often no cause is found. Whilst it often settles spontaneously, treatment with analgesia,

---

Box 22.5

Pressure sore risk-assessment tools

Norton Scale for Pressure Sores

Physical	Neurology	Activity	Mobility	Incontinence
4 Good	4 Alert	4 Ambulant	4 Full	4 None
3 Fair	3 Apathetic	3 Walks with help	3 Slightly	3 Occasionally
2 Poor	2 Confused	2 Not bound	2 Limited*	2 Usually
1 Very poor	1 Stupor	1 Bedfast	1 Very limited Immobile	1 Double

Norton Scale for Pressure Sores. Low scores carry a high risk

Waterlow Pressure Sore Risk Assessment

Build/weight for height		Visual skin type		Continence		Mobility		Sex Age		Appetite	
Average	0	Healthy	0	Complete	0	Fully mobile	0	Male	1	Average	0
Above average	2	Tissue paper	1	Occasionally	1	Restricted/	1	Female	2	Poor	1
		Dry	1	incontinent		difficult		14–18	1	Anorectic	2
Below average	3	Oedematous	1	Catheter/	2	Restless/	2	50–64	2		
		Clammy	1	incontinent		fidgety		65–75	3		
		Discoloured	2	of faeces		Apathetic	3	75–80	4		
		Broken/spot	3	Doubly incontinent	3	Inert/traction	4	81+	5		

Special risk factors		Assessment value	
1. Poor nutrition; e.g. terminal cachexia	8	At risk	10
2. Sensory deprivation, e.g. diabetes, paraplegia, cerebrovascular accident	6	High risk	15
3. High-dose anti-inflammatory or steroids in use	3	Very high risk	20
4. Smoking 10+ per day	1		
5. Orthopaedic surgery/fracture below waist	3		

Table 22.14
A classification of vasculitis

Necrotizing venulitis
- Septic vasculitis (*Streptococcus*, hepatitis B, dental abscess)
- Allergic 'leucocytoclastic' vasculitis (including Henoch–Schönlein purpura)
- Connective tissue disease (e.g. SLE, rheumatoid arthritis)
- Urticarial vasculitis

Necrotizing arteritis
- Polyarteritis nodosa (classic and microscopic variants)

Granulomatous vasculitis
- Wegener's granulomatosis
- Churg–Strauss disease
- Giant cell arteritis

'Occlusion'
- Cryoglobulinaemia (lymphoma, hepatitis C)
- Dysproteinaemia (Waldenström's macroglobulinaemia)
- Anti-phospholipid syndrome

multiple small vesicles in the skin which weep lymphatic fluid and sometimes blood. They reflect deeper vessel involvement so surgery should be avoided. Cryotherapy or CO_2 laser treatment may help the superficial lesions.

FURTHER READING

Blair SD et al. (1988) Sustained compression and healing of chronic venous leg ulcers. *British Medical Journal* **297**: 1159–1161.
Jeanette CJ, Falk RJ (1997) Small vessel vasculitis. *New England Journal of Medicine* **337**: 1512–1523.
Kani LF et al. (1998) Pressure sores. *Journal of the American Academy of Dermatology* **38:** 517–536.
Nuffield Institute for Health, Leeds; NHS centre for reviews and dissemination, University of York (1995) The prevention and treatment of pressure sores. *Effective Health Care* **2**: 1–16.

support stockings, dapsone or prednisolone may be needed to control the pain and to heal up any ulceration.

Miscellaneous conditions

Klippel–Trenauney–Weber syndrome
Klippel–Trenauney–Weber syndrome refers to a rare condition in which there is an extensive vascular malformation of a limb with both deep and superficial involvement. There is a mixture of capillary and cavernous haemangiomas. There may be an underlying arteriovenous malformation which can cause faster growth of the affected limb. The growth may also be increased by local production of growth factors in the affected limb.

Lymphoedema
Lymphoedema refers to a chronic non-pitting oedema due to lymphatic insufficiency. It is most commonly seen affecting the legs and tends to progress with age. The legs can become enormous and prevent wearing of normal shoes. Chronic disease may cause a secondary 'cobblestone' thickening of the skin. Lymphoedema can be primary (and present early in life) owing to an inherited deficiency of lymphatic vessels (e.g. Milroy's disease) or can be secondary because of obstruction of lymphatic vessels (e.g. filarial infection or malignant disease).

Treatment is with compression stockings and physical massage. If there is recurrent cellulitis, long-term antibiotics are advisable as each episode of cellulitis will further damage the lymph vessels. Surgery should be avoided.

Lymphangioma circumscriptum
Lymphangioma circumscriptum is a rare hamartoma of lymphatic tissue. It usually presents in childhood with

Disorders of collagen and elastic tissue

Ehlers–Danlos syndrome (see also p. 585)
Ehlers–Danlos syndrome can be subdivided into at least 10 variants. They are all inherited disorders causing abnormalities in collagen of the skin, joints and blood vessels. Clinically this causes increased elasticity of the skin, hypermobile joints and fragile blood vessels causing easy bruising. The skin is hyperextensible but recoils normally after stretching. It is easily injured and heals slowly with scarring like tissue paper. Pseudotumours may occur at the sites of scarring (such as elbows and knees), consisting mainly of fat, but calcification can occur.

Pseudoxanthoma elasticum
Pseudoxanthoma elasticum is a rare group of disorders characterized by abnormalities in collagen and elastic tissue affecting the skin, eye and blood vessels. The skin may be loose, lax and wrinkled. It can look yellowish and papular ('plucked chicken skin') and tends to lose its elastic recoil when stretched. Skin changes are best seen in the flexures, especially the sides of the neck. Non-cutaneous features include recurrent gastrointestinal bleeding, early myocardial infarction, claudication and angioid streaks on the retina reflecting disruption of vascular elastic tissue.

Marfan's syndrome (see also p. 803)
Marfan's syndrome is an autosomal dominant disorder of connective tissue affecting 1:5000 of the population world-wide. The basic genetic defect is a mutation in the Marfan syndrome gene (*MFS1*) in the extracellular matrix glycoprotein fibrillin 1 (FBN-1) on chromosome

Skin disease

15q21 but the condition shows both genetic and phenotypic heterogeneity. The syndrome is characterized by tall stature and long thin digits (arachnodactyly). The arm span can exceed the height of the patient and a high arched palate may be present. Lax ligaments results in frequent dislocation of joints. Inguinal and femoral hernias are common. Scoliosis and flat feet may be present. Pulmonary changes include emphysema, diaphragmatic hernia and spontaneous pneumothorax. Degeneration of the media of blood vessels can lead to cardiovascular complications such as aortic and mitral incompetence and aortic aneurysm, and this is a common cause of death in these patients. Eighty per cent of patients will develop aortic complications. Dislocation of the ocular lens is common. Skin changes are usually absent but striae may develop. Patients with homocystinuria (Table 19.18) have similar features.

Management

Diagnosis can be confirmed by studying family linkage to the causative gene (see above) but 25% of patients are affected as a result of a new mutation. These latter patients are severely affected and have a high cardiovascular risk (see p. 803). Patients should be reviewed by an ophthalmologist, an orthopaedic surgeon and a cardiologist to screen for and deal with the above complications. Early treatment of the cardiac complications prolongs survival significantly. Genetic counselling should be offered to families.

Striae

Striae are visible linear scars due to dermal collagen damage and stretching. Histologically a thinned epidermis overlies parallel bundles of fine collagen. They occur commonly over the abdomen and breasts in pregnancy but also occur on the thighs and trunk in rapidly growing adolescents as well as in some obese individuals. They are also seen in Cushing's syndrome and with corticosteroid therapy. Striae are initially reddish blue but fade to white atrophic marks. Puberty-related striae normally disappear completely.

Keloid scars

Keloid scars are characterized by smooth hard nodules (Fig. 22.35) due to excessive collagen production. They may occur spontaneously or follow skin trauma/surgery and they are often itchy. They tend to affect young adults and are much commoner in black Africans. Sites of predilection include the shoulders, upper back and chest, earlobes and the chin. Unlike hypertrophic scars (which fade within 12 months) keloids are persistent and may continue to enlarge.

   Treatment is with triamcinolone injection, compression with silica gels or surgery but the latter must be followed by steroid injection or superficial radiotherapy or it may make the problem worse.

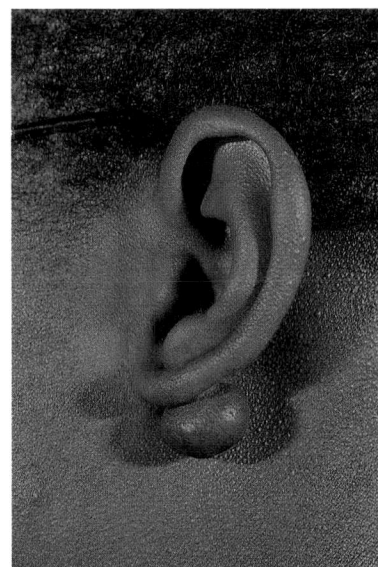

Fig. 22.35 Keloid scar of the lobe of the ear.

FURTHER READING

De Paepe (1999) Dural ectasia and the diagnosis of Marfan's syndrome. *Lancet* **354**: 878–879 (see also p. 910).

Ridley CM, Oriel JD, Robinson AJ (1992) *A Colour Atlas of Diseases of the Vulva*. London: Chapman and Hall.

Royce PM, Steinmann B (eds) (1993) *Connective Tissue and its Heritable Disorders*. New York: Wiley Liss.

Disorders of pigmentation

Hypopigmentation

Vitiligo

Vitiligo is a common disorder of depigmentation which probably has an autoimmune aetiology. Sufferers often have relatives with other organ-specific autoimmune disorders. It presents in childhood or early adult life with well-demarcated macules of complete pigment loss. There is no history of preceding inflammation. Patients are very susceptible to sunburn. Lesions are often symmetrical and frequently involve the face, hands and genitalia (Fig. 22.36). The hair can also depigment. Trauma may induce new lesions. Spontaneous repigmentation can occur and often starts around hair follicles giving a speckled appearance. However, repigmentation is rare if a lesion has persisted for more than 1 year or if the hair is depigmented. The psychological consequences of vitiligo can be devastating especially in Asian or black African people.

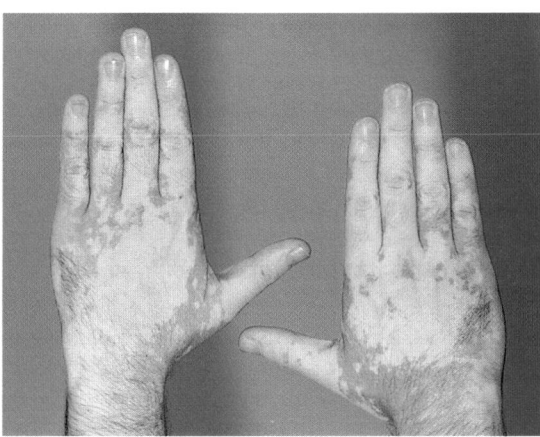

Fig. 22.36 Vitiligo.

Treatment is very unsatisfactory and has no impact on the long-term outcome. Sunblocks should be used to prevent burning. Potent topical steroids or PUVA therapy may help some individuals. If vitiligo is almost universal, depigmentation may be considered as a treatment. Finally, referral to a specialist camouflage clinic can be useful.

Post-inflammatory hypopigmentation

This is one of the most common causes of pale skin. It is much more common in people with pigmented skin. It may be seen as a consequence of eczema, acne or psoriasis and may even be the reason for individuals presenting to a doctor. Providing the skin disease is controlled the pigmentation will recover slowly after many months. Post-inflammatory hyperpigmentation can also occur.

Oculocutaneous albinism

This is a group of rare autosomal recessive disorders affecting the pigmentation of skin, hair and eyes. It can affect all races. Melanocytes are in normal number but have abnormal function. Clinically it presents with universal pale skin, white or yellow hair and a pinkish iris. Photophobia, nystagmus and a squint are also present in most cases.

Treatment involves obsessive protection against sunlight to avoid sunburning and development of skin cancer.

Idiopathic guttate hypomelanosis

This occurs most commonly in black African people and is of unknown aetiology. It presents with small (2–4 mm) asymptomatic porcelain-white macules, often on skin exposed to sunlight. The borders are often sharply defined and angular. There is no effective treatment.

Leprosy (see also p. 82)

Both tuberculoid leprosy and indeterminate leprosy can present with anaesthetic patches of depigmentation and should always be considered in people from endemic regions. Loss of hair and decreased sweating may also be present in the lesions.

Hyperpigmentation

Freckles (ephelides)

These appear in childhood as small brown macules after sun exposure. They fade in the winter months.

Lentigos

These are a more permanent macule of pigmentation similar to freckles but they tend to persist in the winter. Solar lentigos (also called 'liver spots') occur in older people on exposed skin because of actinic damage.

Chloasma

These are brown macules often seen symmetrically over the cheeks and forehead and are most common in women. They can occur spontaneously but are also associated with pregnancy and the oral contraceptive pill.

Metabolic/endocrine effects

A generalized skin darkening can occur with chronic liver disease, especially haemachromatosis. It also is seen sometimes in Cushing's syndrome, Addison's disease (more marked in palmar creases and buccal mucosa) and Nelson's syndrome.

Peutz–Jegher syndrome (p. 299)

This is an autosomal dominant genetic condition. The gene responsible is *LKB1*, a serine-threonine kinase. It presents with brown macules of the lips and perioral region. It is associated with gastrointestinal polyposis which almost never becomes malignant.

Urticaria pigmentosa (cutaneous mastocytosis)

This presents most commonly with multiple pigmented macules in children. These lesions tend to become red, itchy and urticated if they are rubbed (Darier's sign). Occasionally lesions may blister and in the rare congenital, diffuse form of the disease the skin may become thickened and leathery. Skin biopsy shows an excess of mast cells in the skin. Occasionally, systemic symptoms are present such as wheeze, flushing, syncope or diarrhoea, reflecting extensive mast cell degranulation from the skin. Anaphylaxis occurs very rarely and may be precipitated by mast cell degranulators such as aspirin or opiates. The condition spontaneously resolves after some years in children but is persistent in adults.

Rarely there may be infiltration of internal organs with mast cells (*systemic mastocytosis*) especially in adult disease. This can involve any organ but especially the bone (where it can cause severe pain), gastrointestinal tract, liver and spleen. There is a small risk of developing leukaemia if the bone marrow is heavily infiltrated.

FURTHER READING

Levine N (ed.) (1993) *Pigmentation and Pigmentary Disorders.*
  Florida: CRC Press.
Longley J et al. (1995) The mast cell and mast cell disease.
  Journal of the American Academy of Dermatology **32**: 545–561.
Njoo MD et al. (1999) The development of guidelines for
  the treatment of vitiligo. *Archives of Dermatology* **135**:
  1514–1521.

Drug-induced rashes

Drugs can be toxic and teratogenic but they can also cause problems through allergic reactions. This frequently presents in the skin where just about any type of skin rash can arise (Table 22.15), although a widespread symmetrical maculopapular rash is the most common type (Fig. 22.37). 'Fixed drug eruptions' may occur where a rash evolves and resolves at a specific site. The rash is reproduced at exactly the same site after a repeated exposure.

A thorough history is of great value in assessing drug reactions, and a drug cause for any skin condition should always be considered. The use of prick-testing and patch-testing is rarely helpful and not without risk. Drug allergy can only be proven by rechallenging but this is rarely justified as it carries some risks. Rechallenging is occasionally justified for antituberculosis drugs or antiretroviral drugs but this should be

carried out as an inpatient as there is a risk of anaphylaxis. Certain individuals (e.g. those with HIV infections) are more susceptible to drug rashes (Fig. 22.38).

Most rashes will settle spontaneously once the offending agent is removed. The three most serious types of drug rashes are:

- erythroderma (p. 1296)
- toxic epidermal necrolysis
- anticonvulsant hypersensitivity syndrome.

Toxic epidermal necrolysis (TEN) is characterized by a widespread subepidermal blistering and sloughing of most of the skin. The skin may be itchy but typically takes on a burning quality. Fever and mucosal involvement are common. The internal epithelial surfaces (lung, bladder, gastrointestinal tract) are also involved. Multiorgan failure and sepsis often occurs. TEN can be fatal even after drug withdrawal and full intensive care support. Occlusive cutaneous dressings significantly reduce the pain. Ophthalmological assessment and oral hygiene are necessary. Specific medical treatment with

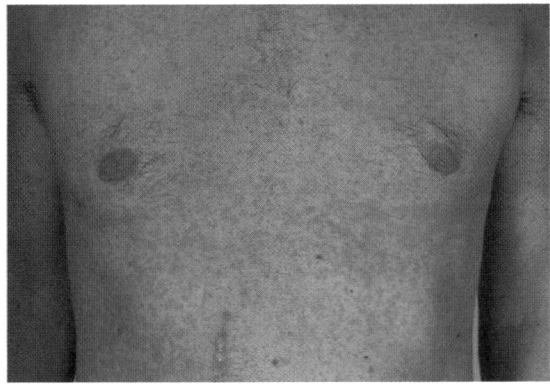

Fig. 22.37 Morbilliform drug rash, due to penicillin allergy.

Table 22.15
Morphological types of drug rashes and some common causes

Maculopapular	Penicillin
Urticaria	Penicillin, aspirin
Vasculitis	Gold, hydralazine
Fixed drug rash	Phenolphthalein in laxatives, tetracyclines, paracetamol
Pigmentation	Minocycline (black), amiodarone (slate grey)
Lupus erythematosus	Penicillamine, isoniazid
Photosensitivity	Thiazides, chlorpromazine, sulphonamide, amiodarone
Pustular	Carbamazepine
Erythema nodosum	Sulphonamides, oral contraceptive
Erythema multiforme	Anticonvulsants
Acneiform	Corticosteroids
Lichenoid	Chloroquine, thiazides, gold, allopurinol
Psoriasiform	Methyldopa, gold, lithium, beta-blockers
Toxic epidermal necrolysis	Penicillin, co-trimoxazole, carbamazepine, NSAIDs
Pemphigus	Penicillamine, ACE inhibitors
Erythroderma	Gold, sulphonylureas, allopurinol

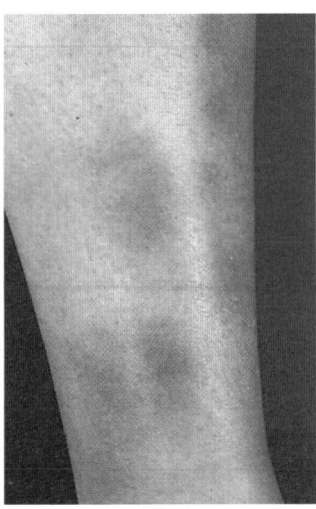

Fig. 22.38 Erythema nodosum in a patient on co-trimoxazole with HIV.

steroids or ciclosporin is controversial and requires further research.

A variant exists called *Stevens–Johnson syndrome* where the damage is restricted to the mucosal surfaces with milder bullous involvement of the skin.

Anticonvulsant hypersensitivity syndrome is characterized by a generalized mucocutaneous rash, fever and lymphadenopathy with variable arthralgia, pharyngitis, periorbital oedema and hepatosplenomegaly. Rarely pustulation of the skin and conjunctivitis are present. The blood may show a peripheral eosinophilia, lymphocytosis with atypical lymphocytes, and raised hepatic enzymes. It can progress to multiorgan failure. This reaction occurs typically 3–4 weeks into therapy. It can occur with any of the aromatic anticonvulsants (carbamazepine, phenytoin, phenobarbital, primidone and clonazepam). As they often cross-react, all these drugs must be avoided in the future. Sodium valproate is a suitable alternative. The potential for cross-reaction with the newer anticonvulsants (vigabatrin and lamotrigine) remains unclear.

FURTHER READING

Becker DS (1998) Toxic epidermal necrolysis. *Lancet* **351**: 1417–1420.
Breathnach SM, Hintner H (1992) *Adverse Drug Reactions and the Skin*. Oxford: Blackwell Scientific Publications.

Disorders of nails

Psoriasis and fungal nail infection are the commonest causes of nail dystrophy and are discussed on pages 1279 and 1288.

- *Nail pitting* can be caused by psoriasis, alopecia areata and atopic eczema. A few pits can be present because of trauma.
- *Onycholysis* (distal nail plate separation) is caused by psoriasis, hyperthyroidism, following trauma and, rarely, a photosensitive reaction to drugs such as tetracyclines.
- *Koilonychia* (thin spoon-shaped nails) can be caused by iron deficiency anaemia or rarely is congenital.
- *Leuconychia* (white nails) is seen in hypoalbuminaemia. A striate congenital leuconychia exists.
- *Beau's lines* (transverse lines) appear as solitary depressions which grow out slowly over many months. They arise because of a severe illness or shock which causes a temporary arrest in nail growth.
- *Yellow-nail syndrome* is a rare disorder of lymphatic drainage. It presents with thickened, slow-growing, yellow nails which may be associated with pleural effusions, bronchiectasis and lymphoedema of the legs.

- *Onychogryphosis* is a gross thickening of the nail which is seen in later life especially in the big toe-nail. There is often a history of preceding trauma. Both psoriasis and fungal infection can also cause nail thickening.
- *Nail–patella syndrome* is an autosomal dominant condition which presents with triangular rather than half-moon shaped lunulae, especially of the thumb and forefingers. The nail plates may be small or dystrophic. The patellae are hypoplastic or absent. Other skeletal anomalies may be present and renal impairment (glomerulonephritis) occurs in up to 30% of individuals.
- *Melanonychia* (longitudinal brown streaks) may be seen as a normal variant in black-skinned patients. In a white patient it may reflect an underlying subungual melanoma, especially if the pigmentation progresses proximally onto the nail fold ('Hutchinson's sign').
- *Clubbing* is discussed on page 845.

FURTHER READING

Baran R, Dawber RPR (eds) (1994) *Diseases of the Nails and their Management*, 2nd edn. Oxford: Blackwell Scientific Publications.

Disorders of hair

Hair loss

Hair loss can be due to a disorder of the hair follicle in which the scalp skin looks normal (non-scarring alopecia) or due to a disorder within the scalp skin that causes permanent loss of the follicle (scarring or cicatricial alopecia). This latter form causes shiny atrophic bald areas in the scalp which are devoid of follicular openings. There are many causes of alopecia to consider (Table 22.16).

Table 22.16
Causes of alopecia

Scarring alopecia	Non-scarring alopecia
Discoid lupus erythematosus	Androgenic alopecia
Kerion (tinea capitis)	Telogen effluvium
Lichen planus	Alopecia areata
Dissecting cellulitis	Trichotillomania (self-induced hair-pulling)
X-irradiation	Tinea capitis
Idiopathic ('pseudopelade')	Traction alopecia
	Metabolic (iron deficiency, hypothyroidism)
	Drug (e.g. heparin, isotretinoin, chemotherapy)

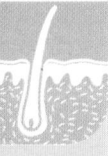

Androgenic alopecia

Androgenic alopecia (male pattern baldness) is the most common type of non-scarring hair loss and depends on genetic factors and an abnormal sensitivity to androgens. It presents in young men with frontal receding followed by thinning of the crown and there is often a positive family history. It also occurs in females but tends to occur at a later age, be milder and show little in the way of frontal recession. If acne and menstrual disturbance are also present one should consider polycystic ovary syndrome and other endocrine disorders of androgens.

Treatment. This may not be required. Topical 5% minoxidil lotion or oral finasteride (1 mg daily) can help arrest progression and may cause a small amount of regrowth, providing it is used early in disease. Finasteride is a selective inhibitor of 5 α-reductase and it can cause side-effects such as loss of libido. It should not be used in females as it can affect the sexual development of a male fetus. However, antiandrogen therapy (e.g. cyproterone acetate or spironolactone) may help some women.

Alopecia areata

Alopecia areata may be regarded as an immune-mediated type of hair loss. It may be associated with other organ-specific autoimmune diseases. It presents in childhood or young adults with patches of baldness. These may regrow to be followed by new patches of hair loss. The presence of broken exclamation mark hairs (narrow at the scalp/wider and more pigmented at the tip) at the edge of a bald area is diagnostic. Regrowth may initially be with white hairs and often occurs slowly over months. Occasionally all the scalp hair is lost (alopecia totalis) and rarely all body hair is lost (alopecia universalis). The nails may be pitted or roughened.

Treatment has no effect on the long-term progression. Potent topical or injected steroids may be of limited use. Topical immunotherapy with diphencyprone or topical 5% minoxidil are occasionally tried but often do not help. Wigs can be provided for severe cases and patient support groups are often beneficial.

Traction alopecia

This refers to the 'mechanical damage' type of hair loss that arises from pulling the hair back into a bun or tight plaiting. It is more common in black Africans.

Telogen effluvium

Telogen effluvium refers to the pattern of diffuse hair loss that occurs some 3 months after pregnancy or a severe illness. It occurs because the 'stress' puts all the hairs into the telogen phase of hair shedding at the same time. The hair fully recovers and the normal staggered hair growth/hair shedding cycle resumes.

Dissecting cellulitis

This is a chronic folliculitis affecting predominantly young black males. It presents with papules and pustules over the occipital region of the scalp with hair loss. If severe, the back of the scalp becomes a boggy swelling (discharging pus) with areas of scarring alopecia. It can be complicated by keloid scar formation ('acne keloidalis nuchae').

Treatment is difficult as antibiotics are rarely useful except in early acute inflammatory episodes. Prolonged courses of isotretinoin can help a few individuals and deep surgical excision with grafting can be used in recalcitrant cases.

Increased hair growth

Hirsutism (p. 1022)

Hirsutism refers to the male pattern of hair growth seen in females. The racial variation in hair growth must be considered. Certain races (e.g. Mediterranean and Asian) have more male pattern hair growth than northern European females. This is not due to excess androgens but may reflect a genetically determined altered sensitivity to them. If virilizing features (deep voice, clitoromegaly, dysmenorrhoea, acne) are present, one should carry out a full endocrine assessment. Hirsutism can cause severe psychological distress to some individuals.

Treatment involves physical methods such as bleaching, waxing, electrolysis and laser therapy. Antiandrogen therapy is occasionally helpful.

Hypertrichosis

Hypertrichosis refers to the state of excessive hair growth at any site and occurs in both sexes. It can be seen in anorexia nervosa, porphyria cutanea tarda and underlying malignancy, and is caused by certain drugs (e.g. ciclosporin, minoxidil).

FURTHER READING

Barth JH (2000) Should men still go bald gracefully? *Lancet* **355:** 161–162.

Dawber R, Van Neste D (1995) *Hair and Scalp Disorders.* London: Martin Dunitz.

Price VH (1999) Treatment of hair loss. *New England Journal of Medicine* **341**: 964–973.

Birth marks/neonatal rashes

Strawberry naevus (cavernous haemangioma)

Strawberry naevus affects up to 1% of infants. It presents at or shortly after birth as a single red lumpy

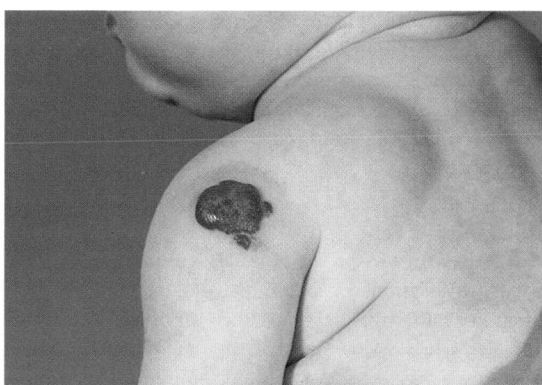

Fig. 22.39 Strawberry naevus.

nodule (Fig. 22.39) that grows rapidly for the first few months. Multiple lesions can be present. They will spontaneously resolve with good cosmesis but this may take up to 7 years for complete resolution. Occasionally plastic surgery is needed after resolution to remove residual slack skin. Reassurance of parents is usually all that is required.

Treatment is indicated if:

- the lesion interferes with feeding or vision
- the lesion ulcerates or bleeds frequently
- the lesion is associated with high-output cardiac failure from shunting of large volumes of blood
- the lesion consumes platelets and/or clotting factors causing potentially life-threatening haemorrhage ('Kasabach–Merritt syndrome').

The latter two complications are very rare and only tend to occur in large lesions with significant deep vessel involvement.

Treatment modalities include intralesional or oral corticosteroids, surgery (for selected lesions), and tunable dye laser (for treating ulceration). Alpha-interferon injections or embolization are only used for life-threatening events.

Port-wine stain (naevus flammeus)

Port-wine stain is also called a capillary haemangioma but strictly speaking it is not a haemangioma but is just an abnormal dilatation of dermal capillaries. It presents at birth as a flat red macular area and is commonly found on the face. It does not improve spontaneously and it may become thickened with time. If the lesion is found in the distribution of the first division of the trigeminal nerve it may be associated with ipsilateral meningeal vascular anomalies which can cause epilepsy and even hemiplegia (Sturge–Weber syndrome). If a port-wine stain involves the skin near the eye, glaucoma is a risk and ophthalmic assessment is mandatory.

Treatment of port-wine stains is ideally carried out with the tunable dye laser.

Milia

'Milk spots' are small follicular epidermal cysts. They are small pinhead white papules commonly found on the face of infants. They resolve spontaneously.

Mongolian blue spot

This appears in infants as a deep blue-grey bruise-like area, usually over the sacrum or back, and is occasionally mistaken as a sign of child abuse. It is due to deep dermal melanocytes. It is very common in Oriental children, less common in black Africans and rare in Caucasians. It has usually disappeared by the age of 7 years.

Toxic erythema of the newborn (erythema neonatorum)

Toxic erythema of the newborn is a term used to describe a common transient blotchy maculopapular rash in newborns. The rash is occasionally pustular but the child is not toxic or unwell. It disappears within a few days, spontaneously.

Nappy rash ('diaper dermatitis')

This is an irritant eczema caused by occlusion of faeces and urine against the skin. It is almost universal in babies. The flexures are usually spared, which is a useful differentiating feature from seborrhoeic and atopic eczema. If satellite lesions are present around the edge, it may indicate a superimposed *Candida* infection.

Treatment involves frequent changing of the nappy and regular application of a barrier cream.

Acrodermatitis enteropathica (p. 239)

This is due to a rare inherited deficiency of zinc absorption. It presents 4–6 weeks after weaning, or earlier in bottle-fed babies. There is an erythematous, sometimes blistering, rash around the perineum, mouth, hands and feet. It may be associated with photophobia, diarrhoea and alopecia.

Treatment is with lifelong oral zinc, which seems to override the poor absorption. The response is rapid.

FURTHER READING

Harper J, Oranje A, Prose N (eds) (2000) *Textbook of Pediatric Dermatology*. Oxford: Blackwell Scientific.
Weinberg S, Prose NS, Kristal L (1998) *Colour Atlas of Pediatric Dermatology*, 3rd edn. New York: McGraw-Hill.

Human immunodeficiency virus and the skin (p. 136)

HIV infection commonly causes significant dermatological problems. A rash may even be the presenting feature of underlying HIV infection. It is estimated that 90% of

HIV-positive patients will suffer with a mucocutaneous disorder during the illness. It is also estimated that up to 30% of people with AIDS will suffer from three different dermatoses. These rashes can often be clinically atypical and difficult to diagnose. One must have a low threshold for skin biopsy and skin culture. On top of this many of the skin problems are resistant to standard treatments. The dermatoses may be arbitrarily divided into six groups; all are seen less frequently since HAART (p. 146).

Cutaneous infection and opportunistic infection

Not surprisingly, infections are increased because of the HIV-induced immune deficiency. Molluscum contagiosum are particularly common, especially on the face. They are often multiple and of a 'giant' size measuring over 1 cm across. Molluscum are rarely seen in adults and they can be the presenting feature of HIV. Other viral infections such as extensive ulcerative herpes or widespread viral warts may be seen. Bacterial infections (e.g. staphylococcal boils) and fungal infections (e.g. ringworm and *Candida*) are also common. Recalcitrant and recurrent oropharyngeal candidiasis is a particular problem.

Opportunistic infections such as cutaneous cytomegalovirus (pustules or necrotic ulcers), sporotrichosis (linear nodules) or cryptococcus (red papules, psoriasiform or molluscum-like lesions) can pose diagnostic difficulties, stressing the need for skin biopsy and culture.

Inflammatory dermatoses

Inflammatory dermatoses show an increased incidence with HIV infection, probably because of an immune dysfunction or imbalance rather than as a consequence of immune suppression. Severe, extensive seborrhoeic eczema is very common and may be a presenting sign of HIV. Other types of eczema, psoriasis, ichthyosis (dry scaly skin), nodular prurigo and pruritus are all common in HIV infection and can be very severe. Granuloma annulare and lichen planus are probably increased in incidence. The treatment of these conditions is difficult as oral immunosuppressive therapies (e.g. prednisolone, ciclosporin) are best avoided. Topical therapies and phototherapy seem relatively safe. Oral retinoids are useful in the management of psoriasis. Highly active antiretroviral therapy (reverse transcriptase inhibitors and protease inhibitors) often helps these conditions, presumably because of a restoration of immune function.

'Autoimmune dermatoses'

Bullous pemphigoid, thrombocytopenic purpura and vitiligo seem to be increased in incidence. The polyclonal stimulation of B lymphocytes by HIV and the resulting abnormal antibody production may be important in their aetiology. Erythroderma is sometimes seen in HIV disease where skin biopsy suggests a 'graft-versus-host disease' mechanism. This presumably reflects a severe underlying immune dysfunction of T lymphocyte control.

Drug rashes

Adverse drug rashes are much commoner in HIV patients. Reactions to co-trimoxazole, dapsone (used in pneumocystis prophylaxis) and antiretroviral drugs appear particularly common. Drug rashes may be severe, resulting in erythroderma or toxic epidermal necrolysis.

Cutaneous tumours

Kaposi's sarcoma (p. 144) may present with purplish nodules and plaques in the skin and on the oral and genital mucosa. It is much commoner in homosexuals with HIV than other groups. Basal and squamous cell carcinomas and benign melanocytic naevi are also increased in incidence, presumably reflecting a loss of immune surveillance.

'Specific' HIV dermatoses

Papular pruritic eruption of HIV ('itchy folliculitis')

Itchy follicular eruptions are common in HIV as CD4 counts decline. The previously described staphylococcal folliculitis, eosinophilic folliculitis, pityrosporum folliculitis, and demodex mite folliculitis are probably all part of a spectrum. The unifying term 'papular pruritic eruption' of HIV is preferable. This presents with intensely itchy papules centred on hair follicles and occurring most commonly over the upper trunk and upper arms. Individual lesions frequently have the top scratched off, leaving a crateriform appearance. The aetiology is unknown but may reflect a hypersensitivity reaction as high IgE and eosinophil counts may be present.

Treatment with oral minocycline, potent topical steroids and emollients may help. Phototherapy or oral isotretinoin are useful in resistant cases.

Oral hairy leucoplakia

This is characterized by white plaques with vertical ridging on the sides of the tongue. Unlike with oral *Candida*, the lesions cannot be peeled off to leave raw areas underneath. It was first recognized in HIV disease but can rarely occur in other forms of immunosuppression. It is thought to be due to co-infection with Epstein–Barr virus.

Treatment with aciclovir, ganciclovir or foscarnet may help.

FURTHER READING

Penneys NS (1995) *Skin Manifestations of AIDS,* 2nd edn. London: Martin Dunitz.

Dermatoses of pregnancy

There are a number of minor skin changes during pregnancy. There is an increase in spider naevi, melanocytic naevi, skin tags and chloasma. The abdomen shows midline pigmentation (linea nigra) and striae (stretch marks). There are four less common skin problems associated with pregnancy.

Polymorphic eruption of pregnancy (PEP)

This rash tends to appear in the last trimester of a first pregnancy in 1 in 160 cases. It is of unknown aetiology and recurs only rarely in subsequent pregnancies. It presents with very itchy urticated papules and plaques and occasionally small vesicles. Lesions usually start on the abdomen and striae but may spread to the upper arms and thighs. The umbilicus may be spared. PEP is commoner in twin pregnancies. The rash is not associated with any maternal or fetal risk. PEP has recently been shown to be associated with low maternal serum cortisol levels.

Treatment is with reassurance, bland emollients and mild topical steroids. The rash disappears after childbirth.

Prurigo of pregnancy

This affects 1 in 300 pregnancies. It usually starts on the abdomen in the third trimester but may persist for some months after delivery. Clustered excoriated papules (prurigo-like lesions) occur on the abdomen and extensor surfaces of the limbs. The cause is unknown but pregnancy-related itch (pruritus gravidarum) may be due to cholestasis (p. 383). Rarely the liver biochemistry is abnormal and urinary HCG levels may be elevated. It can recur in subsequent pregnancies. Some authors believe the condition is associated with an increase in fetal mortality but this remains controversial.

Treatment is with topical steroids and oral antihistamines.

Pruritic folliculitis of pregnancy

This occurs in the second or third trimester of pregnancy and is characterized by an itchy folliculitis which looks similar to steroid-induced 'acne'. It is not associated with any increased maternal or fetal risk.

Treatment with topical benzoyl peroxide and hydrocortisone cream helps to relieve symptoms.

Pemphigoid gestationis (herpes gestationis)

This is the rarest of the pregnancy-related rashes (1 in 60 000). The immune changes of pregnancy appear to set off bullous pemphigoid. It is characterized by an itchy blistering urticated eruption starting on the abdomen but may become widespread. Large bullae may be present. Unlike PEP it can occur early, starting in the second or even first trimester of pregnancy and the umbilicus is often involved. It tends to recur in subsequent pregnancies and at an earlier stage. Diagnosis is confirmed by immunofluorescence of a skin biopsy.

A transient bullous eruption occurs in 5% of infants, presumably owing to transplacental passage of the offending antibody. There is no increase in fetal mortality but there is an increased incidence of prematurity and low birth weight, which is probably due to the autoantibody causing placental insufficiency. Therefore, it seems sensible to keep such pregnancies closely monitored and to advise on hospital rather than home delivery.

Treatment of mild cases may be with potent topical steroids but most cases will require oral corticosteroids. The steroid dose may need to be increased after delivery as there is often a postpartum flare-up of the disease. The rash can be set off again by the oral contraceptive pill and this should be avoided.

FURTHER READING

Bos JD (1999) Reappraisal of dermatoses of pregnancy. *Lancet* **354**: 1140.

Vaughan Jones SA et al. (1999) A prospective study of 200 women with dermatoses of pregnancy correlating clinical findings with hormonal and immunopathological profiles. *British Journal of Dermatology* **141**: 71–81.

Principles of topical therapy

Dermatology is unique in having such direct accessibility to the affected organ. This allows the use of topical treatments, which can avoid certain systemic side-effects.

A topical therapy consists of an *active ingredient*, an appropriate *vehicle* or *base* to deliver this, and often a *preservative* or *stabilizer* to maintain the product's shelf-life. It is important to find a cosmetically acceptable product and to instruct patients about correct usage. Without this, compliance tends to be poor. Perfumed or scented products should be avoided.

Bases and their uses

Creams

These are a semisolid mixture of oil and water held together by an emulsifying agent. They need to have added preservatives such as parabens. They are 'lighter' and rub in more easily than ointments. They have a high cosmetic acceptability and are useful for topical treatments of the face and hands. Aqueous cream is particularly useful as a soap substitute.

Ointments

These are semisolid and contain no water, being based usually on oils or greases such as polyethylene glycol (water soluble) or paraffin (fatty). They feel greasy or sticky to the touch. They are the best treatment for dry, flaky skin disorders as they are good at hydrating the

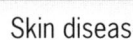

Table 22.17
Emollients commonly used in the UK

Greasy emollients	Lighter creams
Diprobase ointment*	E45 cream*
Oily cream	Diprobase cream*
Unguentum Merck*	Aveeno cream*
50:50 white soft paraffin/liquid paraffin	Aqueous cream

* Trade names

stratum corneum and they deliver an active ingredient (e.g. a steroid) more effectively.

If patients dislike the greasy nature of ointments, a cream is better than no treatment at all, but creams are less effective and do have to be used more frequently. A compromise may be to use a cream on the face and an ointment elsewhere (Table 22.17).

Lotions

These are based on a liquid vehicle such as water or alcohol. They are usually volatile and rapid evaporation promotes a cooling effect on the skin. They are useful for weeping skin conditions and are ideal for use on hairy skin (e.g. the scalp). The cooling effect can be a useful antipruritic. Alcohol-based lotions should be avoided on broken skin as they cause stinging.

Gels

These are semisolid preparations of high molecular weight polymers. They are non-greasy and liquefy on contact with the skin. They are useful for treating hairy skin (e.g. the scalp).

Pastes

Pastes contain a high percentage (> 40%) of powder in an ointment base. They are thick and stiff and difficult to remove from the skin. They are useful when a treatment needs to be applied precisely to a skin lesion without it smearing on to surrounding normal skin. An example would be dithranol in Lassar's paste (used on plaques of psoriasis) as dithranol will burn the surrounding normal skin.

Safety of topical steroids

Providing that preparations of appropriate strength are used for the body site being treated, these compounds can be used safely on a long-term intermittent basis (p. 1284). If

potent steroids are misused they will cause skin atrophy, manifest as striae, wrinkling, fragility and telangiectasia.

Problems with topical therapies

- *Systemic absorption* may occur if large areas of inflamed skin are treated topically, especially if the treatment is occluded with bandages or polyurethane films. Neonates are particularly susceptible to this owing to the relative increase in body surface area to volume.
- *Contact allergy* to topical preparations is not uncommon and may be suspected by unusually resistant disease or by apparent worsening of a condition after application of a substance. It is more common with creams as it is often the result of allergy to the preservative or emulsifying agent. Allergy can also be due to the active ingredient itself (e.g. neomycin or hydrocortisone).
- *Folliculitis* can occur because of blockage of hair follicles. Creams and ointments should be applied to the skin in the same direction as hair growth to try to prevent this blockage. It is a particular problem with the use of ointments in hot weather (especially if under occlusive bandages) and a lighter cream may be more appropriate at this time.

CHAPTER BIBLIOGRAPHY

Champion RH, Burton JL and Ebling FJG (eds) (1998) *Textbook of Dermatology*, 6th edn. Oxford: Blackwell Scientific.
Harper J, Oranje A, Prose N (eds) (2000) *Textbook of Pediatric Dermatology*. Oxford: Blackwell Scientific.
Weedon D (ed) (1997) *Skin Pathology*. Edinburgh: Churchill Livingstone.

UK PATIENT SUPPORT GROUPS

DEBRA (Dystrophic Epidermolysis Bullosa Research Association): DEBRA House, 13 Wellington Business Park, Duke's Ride, Crowthorne, Berkshire RG11 6LS
Hairline International: 1668 High Street, Knowle, West Midlands B93 0LY
National Eczema Society: 163 Eversholt Street, London NW1 1BU
Psoriatic Arthropathy Support Group: D. Chandler, PO Box 111, St Albans, Hertfordshire AL1 3JQ
Psoriasis Association: Milton House, 7 Milton Street, Northampton NN2 7JG
Vitiligo Society: 125 Kennington Road, London SE11 6SF

Index

Page numbers in **bold** refer to major discussions in the text, and usually include aspects such as epidemiology, clinical features, diagnosis, pathology and treatment.

Page numbers in *italics* refer to pages on which tables/information boxes/figures are to be found.

This index is arranged in letter-by-letter order, whereby hyphens and spaces between words are ignored in the alphabetization e.g. (brainstem precedes brain tumours).

vs denotes differential diagnosis

Cross-references in *italics* are either general cross-references, or refer to subentries within the same main entry .

Abbreviations used in subentries include:
AIDS - Acquired Immunodeficiency Syndrome
COPD - Chronic Obstructive Pulmonary Disease
CMV - Cytomegalovirus
HIV - Human immunodeficiency virus
SLE - Systemic lupus erythematosus

Other abbreviations are to be found in the index text

A

A,B,C life support (resuscitation) *730,* *730–731*
ABC transporter superfamily 156
Abdomen
  acute conditions 254, **328–332**
    appendicitis *see* Appendicitis
    gynaecological **330**
    investigations 329–330
    medical causes *329*
    obstruction **331**
    peritonitis *see* Peritonitis
    pseudo-obstruction **331–332**
    referred pain *329*
  clinical examination *see* Abdominal examination
Abdominal actinomycosis 92
Abdominal bruits 256
Abdominal distension
  inspection 255
  myelofibrosis (myelosclerosis) 442
  pain/gas/bloat syndrome 328
Abdominal examination *255,* **255–256**
  acute abdomen **329–330,** 331
  bowel sounds (auscultation) 329
  inspection 255, 329
  ischaemic colitis 314
  palpation 255, *255,* 329
  patient history 328
  percussion 255–256
  see also Abdominal X-ray
Abdominal mass, renal tumours 662
Abdominal pain 254–255
  acute 254, 255
  analgesia 401
  ascites 370
  chronic 254, 255
  colicky 328
  common causes *329*
  constant 328
  epigastric *see* Epigastric pain
  inflammatory 328

left iliac fossa 255
lower abdomen 255
management 328
right hypochondrial 254, 388, 389
specific conditions
  acute abdomen 328, *329*
  acute appendicitis 328
  acute intermittent porphyria 1120
  acute pancreatitis 397
  chronic intestinal ischaemia 297
  chronic pancreatitis 400–401, *401*
  common bile duct stones 390
  Crohn's disease 302
  diabetic ketoacidosis 1089
  α-glucosidase inhibitors adverse effects 1079
  hypercalcaemia 1060
  pain/gas/bloat syndrome 328
  pancreatic carcinoma 402–403
  peritonitis 328
  peritonitis in peritoneal dialysis 654
  porphyrias 1120
  small intestinal disease 289
  ulcerative colitis 305
  Whipple's disease 295
sudden onset 328
upper abdomen 254
Abdominal tuberculosis 333
Abdominal veins, pulmonary emboli 804
Abdominal X-ray 257
  kidneys 596
  specific disorders
    acute abdomen 330
    acute cholecystitis 389
    medullary sponge kidney *627*
    urinary tract infections 618–619
    urinary tract stones *628*
Abducens nerve (VI) **1136**
  lesion 1136
Abetalipoproteinaemia **298,** 1113
  gene defect *178*
ABO blood group **445**
  antibodies 445, *445*
  antigens (A,B,H) 445, *445*

cancer associations 278
genetics 445
incompatibility
  haemolytic disease of newborn and 438–439
  haemolytic transfusion reactions 447–448
  sugar chains 445, *445*
Abortion 432
  acute tubular necrosis association 639
  antiphospholipid syndrome 560
  mifepristone 1027
  septic 639
  see also Prenatal diagnosis
Abreaction, dissociative disorder treatment 1240
Abscess
  amoebic **381,** 891
  anorectal **315**
  Bartholin's 123
  bone in osteomyelitis 557
  brain **1198**
    HIV/AIDS 1196, 1198
  Brodie's 557
  cold 557, 620
  epidural **1198**
  liver **381**
  mycotic 795
  pulmonary 795, 891
    amoebic lung 891
  pyogenic **381**
  spinal cord **1198**
  subphrenic 332
Absorbents, overdose management 977–978
Absorption **284–286**
  colonic 309
  nutrients **285–286**
    carbohydrate 285, *285*
    fats 285–286, *286*
    glucose 285, *285*
    protein 285
    water/electrolytes 286, 309, *309*
  small intestinal, tests 290–291

1321

Index

1327

Index

Index

Index

C

Index

Index

Index

G

Index

Index

Index

Index

J

Index

Index

Index

Index

Index

Index

Index

Index